PRINCIPLES OF
SURGERY

PRINCIPLES OF SURGERY

THIRD EDITION

EDITOR-IN-CHIEF

Seymour I. Schwartz, M.D.
Professor of Surgery
University of Rochester School of Medicine and Dentistry

ASSOCIATE EDITORS

G. Tom Shires, M.D.
Professor and Chairman
Department of Surgery
Cornell University Medical College

Frank C. Spencer, M.D.
Professor and Director
Department of Surgery
New York University School of Medicine

Edward H. Storer, M.D.
Professor of Surgery
Yale University School of Medicine

McGRAW-HILL BOOK COMPANY

New York   St. Louis   San Francisco   Auckland   Bogotá   Düsseldorf
Johannesburg   London   Madrid   Mexico   Montreal   New Delhi
Panama   Paris   São Paulo   Singapore   Sydney   Tokyo   Toronto

NOTICE

Medicine is an ever-changing science. As new research and clinical experience broaden our knowledge, changes in treatment and drug therapy are required. The editors and the publisher of this work have made every effort to ensure that the drug dosage schedules herein are accurate and in accord with the standards accepted at the time of publication. Readers are advised, however, to check the product information sheet included in the package of each drug they plan to administer to be certain that changes have not been made in the recommended dose or in the contraindications for administration. This recommendation is of particular importance in regard to new or infrequently used drugs.

PRINCIPLES OF SURGERY

2 3 4 5 6 7 8 9 0   7 8 3 2 1 0 9

This book was set in Times Roman by York Graphic Services, Inc. The editors were J. Dereck Jeffers, Stuart D. Boynton, and Bob Leap; the designer was Barbara Ellwood; the production supervisor was Robert C. Pedersen. New drawings were done by J & R Services, Inc. The cover was designed by Nicholas Krenitsky.

Library of Congress Cataloging in Publication Data

Main entry under title:

Principles of surgery.

    Bibliography: p.
    Includes index.
    1. Surgery. I. Schwartz, Seymour I.
[DNLM: 1. Surgery. W0100.3 P957]
RD31.P88 1979b   617   78-13763
ISBN 0-07-055735-7

LC CIP DATA (2 vol ed.)

RD31.P88 1979   617   78-6763
ISBN 0-07-055736-5

To students of surgery,
at all levels,
in their quest for knowledge

Contents

List of Contributors

James T. Adams, M.D.
Professor of Surgery, University of Rochester School of Medicine and Dentistry

R. Peter Altman, M.D.
Associate Professor of Surgery, George Washington University; Senior Attending Surgeon, Children's Hospital National Medical Center

Kathryn D. Anderson, M.D.
Assistant Professor of Surgery, George Washington University; Senior Attending Surgeon, Children's Hospital National Medical Center

Richard M. Bergland, M.D.
Associate Professor of Neurosurgery, Harvard; Chief, Division of Neurosurgery, Beth Israel Hospital

George H. Bornside, Ph.D.
Professor of Surgical Research and Microbiology, Louisiana State University School of Medicine

Thomas J. Brobyn, M.D.
Clinical Assistant Professor of Plastic Surgery, Thomas Jefferson University; Associate Chief of Plastic Surgery, Chesnut Hill Hospital

Lester R. Bryant, M.D.
Professor and Chairman, Department of Surgery, East Tennessee State University

Peter C. Canizaro, M.D.
Associate Professor of Surgery, Cornell University Medical College

C. James Carrico, M.D.
Professor of Surgery, University of Washington School of Medicine

Robert A. Chase, M.D.
Professor, Department of Surgery, Stanford University School of Medicine

Isidore Cohn, Jr., M.D.
Professor and Chairman, Department of Surgery,
Louisiana State University School of Medicine

William F. Collins, Jr., M.D.
Professor and Chairman, Section of Neurological
Surgery, Yale University School of Medicine

Robert E. Condon, M.D.
Professor of Surgery, The Medical College of Wisconsin

Lester M. Cramer, M.D.
Clinical Professor of Plastic Surgery, University of
Colorado Medical Center; Chief of Plastic Surgery,
Chesnut Hill Hospital

Joseph N. Cunningham, M.D.
Associate Professor, Department of Surgery, New York
University School of Medicine

P. William Curreri, M.D.
Professor of Surgery and Director, Burn Center, The
New York Hospital—Cornell Medical Center

Louis R. M. Del Guercio, M.D.
Professor and Chairman, Department of Surgery, New
York Medical College

James A. DeWeese, M.D.
Professor of Surgery, University of Rochester School of
Medicine and Dentistry

J. Herbert Dietz, Jr., M.D.
Associate Professor of Rehabilitation (Surgery), Cornell
University Medical College; Chief, Rehabilitation
Service (Surgery), Memorial Sloan-Kettering Cancer
Center

Robert B. Duthie, M.D., M.B.
Nuffield Professor of Orthopedic Surgery, Nuffield
Orthopedic Center, Oxford, England

F. Henry Ellis, Jr., M.D., Ph.D.
Chairman, Department of Thoracic and Cardiovascular Surgery, Lahey Clinic Foundation and New England Deaconess Hospital; Associate Clinical Professor of Surgery, Harvard Medical School

John E. Foker, M.D.
Assistant Professor of Surgery, University of Minnesota

John H. Foster, M.D.
Professor of Surgery, Vanderbilt University School of Medicine

Irwin N. Frank, M.D.
Professor of Surgery, Urology Division, University of Rochester School of Medicine and Dentistry

Donald S. Gann, M.D.
Professor of Surgery, The Johns Hopkins School of Medicine; Director of Emergency Medicine, Johns Hopkins Hospital

Adolph H. Giesecke, Jr., M.D.
Professor and Chairman, Department of Anesthesiology, The University of Texas Southwestern Medical School at Dallas

Stanley M. Goldberg, M.D.
Clinical Professor of Surgery, Director and Head, Division of Colon and Rectal Surgery, Department of Surgery, University of Minnesota Health Sciences Center

Nicholas M. Greene, M.D.
Professor, Department of Anesthesiology, Yale University School of Medicine

Timothy S. Harrison, M.D.
Professor of Surgery and Physiology, The Milton S. Hershey Medical Center, The Pennsylvania State University

Charles M. Haskell, M.D.
Associate Professor of Medicine and Surgery,
Department of Medicine, UCLA School of Medicine,
University of California at Los Angeles

Arthur L. Herbst, M.D.
Professor and Chairman, Department of Obstetrics and
Gynecology, The University of Chicago

Franklin T. Hoaglund, M.D.
Professor and Chairman, Department of Orthopedic
Surgery, University of Vermont College of Medicine

Anthony M. Imparato, M.D.
Professor of Clinical Surgery, New York University
School of Medicine

E. R. Johnson, M.D.
Associate Professor of Physical Medicine and
Rehabilitation, The University of Texas Southwestern
Medical School at Dallas

Robert F. Jones, M.D.
Professor of Surgery, University of Washington School
of Medicine

Ronald C. Jones, M.D.
Professor of Surgery, The University of Texas
Southwestern Medical School at Dallas

Edwin L. Kaplan, M.D.
Professor of Surgery, Pritzker School of Medicine,
University of Chicago

James F. Lee, M.D.
Professor of Anesthesiology, The University of Texas,
Southwestern Medical School at Dallas

Richard R. Lower, M.D.
Professor and Chairman, Division of Thoracic and
Cardiac Surgery, Medical College of Virginia

Robert N. McClelland, M.D.
Professor of Surgery, The University of Texas
Southwestern Medical School at Dallas

Donald F. McDonald, M.D.
Professor, Division of Urology, University of Texas
Medical Branch at Galveston

René B. Menguy, M.D.
Professor of Surgery, University of Rochester School of
Medicine and Dentistry

Calvin Morgan, M.D.
Clinical Assistant Professor of Surgery, East Tennessee
State University

Donald L. Morton, M.D.
Professor of Surgery and Chief, Divisions General
Surgery and Oncology, UCLA School of Medicine,
University of California at Los Angeles

John H. Morton, M.D.
Professor of Surgery, University of Rochester School of
Medicine and Dentistry

John S. Najarian, M.D.
Professor and Chairman, Department of Surgery,
University of Minnesota Health Sciences Center

Santhat Nivatvongs, M.D.
Assistant Professor, Division of Colon and Rectal
Surgery, Department of Surgery, University of
Minnesota Health Sciences Center

W. Spencer Payne, M.D.
Professor of Surgery, Mayo Medical School, Mayo
Graduate School of Medicine, Consultant Section of
Thoracic, Cardiovascular and General Surgery in the
Mayo Clinic and Mayo Foundation

Erle E. Peacock, Jr., M.D.
Professor of Surgery, Plastic Surgery Section, Tulane
University School of Medicine

Malcolm O. Perry, M.D.
Professor of Surgery and Chief, Division of Vascular
Surgery, Cornell University Medical College

Judson G. Randolph, M.D.
Professor of Surgery, George Washington University;
Surgeon-in-Chief, Children's Hospital, National Medical
Center

Benjamin F. Rush, Jr., M.D.
Professor and Chairman, Department of Surgery,
College of Medicine and Dentistry of New Jersey at
Newark

Howard A. Rusk, M.D.
Professor of Rehabilitation Medicine, New York
University School of Medicine

Seymour I. Schwartz, M.D.
Professor of Surgery, University of Rochester School of
Medicine and Dentistry

G. Tom Shires, M.D.
Professor and Chairman, Department of Surgery,
Cornell University Medical College

William Silen, M.D.
Chief of Surgery, Beth Israel Hospital; Professor of
Surgery, Harvard Medical School

Richard L. Simmons, M.D.
Professor of Surgery and Microbiology, Department of
Surgery, University of Minnesota Health Sciences
Center

William H. Snyder, III, M.D.
Associate Professor of Surgery, The University of Texas Southwestern Medical School at Dallas

Frank C. Sparks, M.D.
Professor and Chairman, Department of Surgery, University of Connecticut Health Center, School of Medicine

Dennis D. Spencer, M.D.
Assistant Professor, Section of Neurosurgery, Yale University School of Medicine

Frank C. Spencer, M.D.
Professor and Director, Department of Surgery, New York University School of Medicine

Edward H. Storer, M.D.
Professor of Surgery, Yale University School of Medicine

Erwin R. Thal, M.D.
Associate Professor of Surgery, The University of Texas Southwestern Medical School at Dallas

Donald R. Tredway, M.D., Ph.D.
Associate Professor and Chief, Section of Reproductive Endocrinology, Department of Obstetrics and Gynecology, The University of Chicago

Howard Ulfelder, M.D.
Joe V. Meigs Professor of Gynecology, Harvard Medical School

Joan L. Venes, M.D.
Associate Professor, Section of Neurosurgery, Yale University School of Medicine

Franklin C. Wagner, Jr., M.D.
Associate Professor, Section of Neurosurgery, Yale University School of Medicine

Preface
to the Third Edition

The science of surgery continues to expand and change at a rate which makes only the title of a textbook immutable. The editors remain devoted to the concept of a *modern* source of information and therefore offer this third edition as evidence of their concern. The third edition of *Principles of Surgery* maintains its consistent format, while reflecting the changes which have evolved over the past five years.

There are 15 new authors and approximately 35 percent of the text has been altered. Chapters which were rewritten by new authors include: Endocrine and Metabolic Responses to Injury; Shock; Burns; Chest Wall, Pleura, Lung, and Mediastinum; Peritonitis and Intraabdominal Abscesses, Pituitary and Adrenal; Pediatric Surgery; and Urology. All other chapters have been extensively revised and updated. Each of the chapters in the "Basic Considerations" section have undergone major change—particularly those concerned with oncology and transplantation—reflecting the explosion of knowledge in these areas. The specific organ system chapters have been revised with an emphasis on newly introduced diagnostic techniques and current consensus of opinion regarding management. The References of each chapter have been brought up to date.

The editors wish to thank the readers for their past reception of our efforts, and offer the present work as a statement of our appreciation in the hopes that the third edition serves the same purpose as its two predecessors and is equally well received.

Seymour I. Schwartz

Acknowledgments

The editors appreciate the efforts of all the contributors whose expertise, lucid presentation, and promptness have eased our task. This statement is an expression of particular thanks to Ms. Wendy Husser, Administrative Assistant, who devoted her intellectual energies throughout the entire development of this edition. Finally, once again, the four editors would like to acknowledge the patience, cooperation, and sacrifice on the part of our families, permitting us uncompromised devotion to this project which has now extended over twelve years.

Seymour I. Schwartz

Preface to the First Edition

The raison d'etre for a new textbook in a discipline which has been served by standard works for many years was the Editorial Board's initial conviction that a distinct need for a modern approach in the dissemination of surgical knowledge existed. As incoming chapters were reviewed, both the need and satisfaction became increasingly apparent and, at the completion, we felt a sense of excitement at having the opportunity to contribute to the education of modern and future students concerned with the care of surgical patients.

The recent explosion of factual knowledge has emphasized the need for a presentation which would provide the student an opportunity to assimilate pertinent facts in a logical fashion. This would then permit correlation, synthesis of concepts, and eventual extrapolation to specific situations. The physiologic bases for diseases are therefore emphasized and the manifestations and diagnostic studies are considered as a reflection of pathophysiology. Therapy then becomes logical in this schema and the necessity to regurgitate facts is minimized. In appreciation of the impact which Harrison's *Principles of Internal Medicine* has had, the clinical manifestations of the disease processes are considered in detail for each area. Since the operative procedure represents the one element in the therapeutic armentarium unique to the surgeon, the indications, important technical considerations, and complications receive appropriate emphasis. While we appreciate that a textbook cannot hope to incorporate an atlas of surgical procedures, we have provided the student a single book which will satisfy the sequential demands in the care and considerations of surgical patients.

The ultimate goal of the Editorial Board has been to collate a book which is deserving of the adjective "modern." We have therefore selected as authors dynamic and active contributors to their particular fields. The *au courant* concept is hopefully apparent throughout the entire work and is exemplified by appropriate emphasis on diseases of modern surgical interest, such as trauma, transplantation, and the recently appreciated importance of rehabilitation. Cardiovascular surgery is presented in keeping with the exponential strides recently achieved.

There are two major subdivisions to the text. In the first twelve chapters, subjects that transcend several organ systems are presented. The second portion of the book represents a consideration of specific organ systems and surgical specialties.

Throughout the text, the authors have addressed themselves to a sophisticated audience, regarding the medical student as a graduate student, incorporating material generally sought after by the surgeon in training and presenting information appropriate for the continuing education of the practicing surgeon. The need for a text such as we have envisioned is great and the goal admittedly high. It is our hope that this effort fulfills the expressed demands.

Seymour I. Schwartz

PRINCIPLES OF
SURGERY

Surgically Correctible Hypertension

by John H. Foster

Systemic hypertension and its associated cerebrovascular, renal, and cardiovascular sequelae are among the most common causes of crippling illness and death in the world today. Gordon and Devine estimated in the early 1960s that there were 17 million people with hypertension in the United States; current estimates are that 30 million people have hypertension. Although the vast majority of hypertensive patients have essential hypertension, an increasingly significant percentage, estimated to be between 5 and 10 percent of all hypertensive patients, are being found to have a specific underlying lesion which is surgically correctible.

PHYSIOLOGY AND PATHOPHYSIOLOGY

Blood flows through a series of elastic arterial tubes. The peak pressure within arteries, a reflection of ventricular contraction, is referred to as systolic pressure. Residual resting pressure during ventricular diastole accounts for the diastolic pressure. The accepted upper limit of normal blood pressure in the adult is 140/90 mm Hg. The so-called "normal" varies with age as follows: infants, 70/45 mm Hg, early childhood 85/55 mm Hg, and adolescence 100/75 mm Hg.

The factors influencing arterial blood pressure include (1) viscosity of blood, (2) blood volume, (3) cardiac output, (4) elasticity of arterial wall, and (5) peripheral resistance.

An increase in viscosity results in an increase in resistance to blood flow and may give rise to hypertension, as in polycythemia. An increase in the amount of blood or fluid circulating in the vascular system may also result in hypertension, just as a reduction in the blood volume is manifest by hypotension. The cardiac output, which refers to the volume of blood pumped into the vascular system per unit of time, is an important determinant. An increase in output, as in thyrotoxicosis, may cause hypertension, whereas the decrease which accompanies myocardial disease and cardiomyopathies is attended by hypotension. The arterial wall normally relaxes in systole and contracts in diastole; loss of this function, as in rigid arteriosclerotic vessels, results in increased systolic and decreased diastolic pressure. Perhaps the most important determinant in the development of systemic hypertension is the peripheral resistance within the arteriolar segments of the vascular system. Small changes in arterial caliber result in marked changes in resistance and pressure, chiefly the diastolic pressure.

Although each of these factors may influence the blood pressure, the effect depends largely on the modifying influence of the autonomic nervous system and on renal and hormonal contributions. Reflex arcs within the nervous system control the vasomotor tone, cardiac rate, and cardiac output. Proprioceptors or baroreceptors in the aortic wall and carotid sinus participate in the reflex arcs and play an important role in the regulation of blood pressure.

In most cases of hypertension, little is known about the factors which alter the arteriolar tone and caliber. Age, race, and environment are significant but ill-defined factors in essential hypertension. A more precise role has been determined for certain humoral agents in a small percentage of patients. Excessive production of catecholamines such as epinephrine and norepinephrine by the adrenal medulla in cases of pheochromocytoma has been shown to increase small-vessel tone and consequently increase peripheral resistance. Adrenal cortical hormones have also been implicated in clinical hypertension. Aldosterone, the sodium-retaining hormone of the cortex, has been shown to potentiate the rise in blood pressure caused by pressor agents. Excessive secretion of aldosterone is accompanied by retention of sodium and water, with consequent expansion of the blood volume and resultant hypertension. Although sodium seems to have an unquestioned role in human hypertension, the mechanism or locus of its effect is unclear. The volume-expansion effects of sodium are the most obvious. In addition, an increased sodium content of the vascular wall appears to make the blood vessels more responsive to vasoconstrictor agents. Production or accentuation of experimental hypertension by salt feeding is well documented and carries over into the clinical management of hypertensive patients, where salt restriction is commonly advised. However, the relation between aldosterone and hypertension does not seem to be limited to salt retention and volume expansion. In many cases of malignant hypertension of renovascular origin there is an associated hyperplasia of the cortex and increase in aldosterone secretion, and in such cases the urinary excretion of sodium may be high and the blood volume normal.

The role of other adrenocortical hormones in human hypertension is even more obscure. Hypertension is a manifestation of Cushing's syndrome which is associated with excessive production of cortisol. The effects of this hormone on hypertension have not been defined. In Cushing's syndrome, an increase in aldosterone is inconstant, and hyperresponsiveness of blood vessels to pressor amines, which has been related to an increase in glucocorticoids, has not been observed. Androgenic adrenal tumors are also occasionally associated with hypertension, but the mechanism is obscure.

Humoral mechanisms are also involved in the role of the kidney in the production of hypertension, an area of intense interest and controversy for over half a century. In response to the compromising of the arterial blood supply, the kidney releases renin, which by interaction with a serum globulin produces angiotensin I. A plasma enzyme acts to convert angiotensin I to angiotensin II, which is a powerful vasoconstrictor. Angiotensin also stimulates aldosterone production, which, with its resultant sodium and water retention and expansion of blood volume, plays an important role in the production of hypertension. More obscure renal mechanisms which may play a role in the formation of systemic hypertension include the production of antirenins and vasoexciter material (VEM), which may potentiate arteriolar response to epinephrine, and the excretion or metabolism of circulatory pressor substances.

CLINICAL MANIFESTATIONS

The signs and symptoms of hypertension are rarely to be attributed to the elevated blood pressure per se but rather to the effects of the elevated pressure on a given organ system. Early in the course of hypertension there are usually no signs or symptoms. Headache, weakness, palpitation, and dizziness are among the early symptoms. Epistaxis occurs more frequently in older patients with established hypertension. A history of flushing, sweating, paroxysmal headaches, and episodic hypertension suggests pheochromocytoma. The combination of paresthesia, muscular weakness, transient paralysis, polyuria, and polydipsia is associated with aldosteronism. Urinary tract infection may suggest renal parenchymal disease, and the presence of peripheral vascular disease intensifies suspicion of renal vascular hypertension.

The duration of hypertension and the presence or ab-

sence of visual disturbances, angina, stroke, and myocardial infarction should all be documented, since these provide an index of the severity of hypertension and have prognostic implications.

On physical examination, the finding of a persistently elevated diastolic pressure establishes the diagnosis of systemic hypertension. Vascular changes in the optic fundi, graded on the Keith-Wagener-Barker scale from 0 to 4 for increasing severity, are indicative of general systemic changes and of the degree of hypertension. With all types of hypertension, signs of specific organ involvement may be apparent. These include congestive failure, renal failure, hypertensive encephalopathy, and manifestations of cerebrovascular accident. Certain causes of surgically correctible hypertension are associated with specific findings. Coarctation of the aorta is suggested by decreased femoral pulses and decreased blood pressures in the leg. A loud systolic bruit may be heard over the precordium and posterior chest wall. After the first decade of life, patients have well-developed shoulders and arms, and enlarged collateral arteries are palpable in the musculature of the thorax posteriorly. The finding most suggestive of renovascular hypertension is the presence of a bruit in the upper abdomen. This is most frequently encountered in young females with fibromuscular hyperplasia of the renal artery. Evidence of arteriosclerotic disease of the aorta or of the iliac, femoral, or carotid arteries in hypertensive patients increases the likelihood of similar lesions in the renal arteries.

Cushing's syndrome is associated with the physical findings of central obesity, "buffalo hump," moon face, abdominal striae, ecchymoses, hirsutism, and evidence of osteoporosis. Pheochromocytoma is characterized by sweating, blanching or flushing, syncope, tachycardia, or angina associated with extreme fluctuations in blood pressure. These paroxysms may be induced by painful stimulus, exercise, or palpation of the tumor. The physical manifestations of primary aldosteronism are nonspecific except for those associated with advanced hypokalemic alkalosis, in which a positive Chvostek's sign may be present and carpal spasm may occur when the blood pressure cuff is inflated. Muscle weakness or paralysis also may be noted.

LABORATORY STUDIES

The chest x-ray and electrocardiogram serve as indices for the extent of cardiomegaly and left ventricular hypertrophy. The x-ray may provide the diagnosis in cases of coarctation of the aorta, in which rib notching and the silhouette of a coarcted segment of aorta may be seen. In hyperaldosteronism, the electrocardiogram demonstrates the typical findings of hypokalemia.

Abnormalities demonstrated in routine urine examination such as bacterial growth and proteinuria, accompanied by an elevation of the blood urea nitrogen (BUN) and impaired creatinine clearance, suggest bilateral parenchymal disease. However, these findings do not rule out the possibility of renovascular hypertension. If the urine culture shows bacterial growth, split renal function studies should be delayed until the infection is brought under control.

In pheochromocytoma, a 24-hour urinary output of catecholamines in excess of 200 μg/day and an excretion of the catecholamine metabolite VMA (3-methoxy-4-hydroxymandelic acid) in excess of 7 mg/day are key diagnostic findings. However, certain drugs and foods give false-positive results. The fasting blood sugar level and basal metabolic rate are often elevated. In Cushing's syndrome, the critical determination is an elevated 24-hour urinary output of 17-hydroxysteroids in relation to the daily excretion of creatinine; the fasting blood sugar and glucose tolerance tests often show a diabetic-type response.

In primary aldosteronism, serum electrolyte determinations reveal the potassium to be less than 3 mEq/L and the carbon dioxide more than 30 mEq/L, while the sodium is normal or only slightly increased. The daily urinary potassium excretion exceeds 40 mEq/L, while sodium excretion is normal. The urinary specific gravity is low and there is an alkaline pH. The changes of hypokalemic alkalosis may also occur with secondary aldosteronism related to renovascular hypertension.

CLASSIFICATION

In general, surgically correctible hypertension involves the consideration of diastolic hypertension. Systolic hypertension with normal or decreased diastolic pressure is usually dependent upon cardiac output, and changes in the elasticity of the aortic wall are not commonly associated with pathologic sequelae in the small vessels or target organ systems. Examples of systolic hypertension include arteriovenous fistulas, thyrotoxicosis, and atherosclerosis of the aorta in the elderly patient. Elevation of diastolic pressure is primarily the result of a chronically increased residual resistance in the peripheral vascular bed.

Table 23-1 lists the more important surgically correctible causes of hypertension. Although several entries might be added, those which are included have the greatest practical importance, because of their relative frequency and the lasting benefits which may result from their recognition and treatment. Correction of any of these disease processes may save a patient from a lifetime of antihypertensive drug therapy.

The first three causes listed in the table, i.e., pheochromocytoma, primary aldosteronism, and Cushing's syndrome, are related to abnormalities in the adrenal glands and are discussed in detail in Chap. 37; coarctation of the

Table 23-1. SURGICALLY CORRECTIBLE CAUSES OF HYPERTENSION

Pheochromocytoma
Primary aldosteronism
Cushing's syndrome
Coarctation of the aorta
Renovascular hypertension
Unilateral renal parenchymal disease

Table 23-2. STUDY OF THE HYPERTENSIVE PATIENT FOR EVIDENCE OF A SURGICALLY CORRECTIBLE LESION

History
Physical examination
Roentgenogram of the chest
Electrocardiogram
Laboratory studies:
  Urinalysis, urine culture, and 24-hour urine protein
  Hemogram
  Serum: BUN, creatinine, and cholesterol
  Serum*: CO_2, K, Cl, Na
  Fasting blood sugar and glucose tolerance test
  24-hour urinary excretion of catecholamines†, VMA†, and 17-hydroxy steroids
  24-hour urinary excretion of K and Na
  Creatinine clearance
Special tests:
  Rapid-sequence excretory urogram
  Radioisotope renogram
  Renal arteriography, via aortic injection and selective injection if indicated

If the above studies show or suggest one of the following correctible causes, further procedure is as indicated:

Renal artery stenosis: Split renal function study and renal vein renin assay.
Aldosteronism: Plasma renin activity and aldosterone secretion rates.
Cushing's syndrome: Adrenopituitary function studies.
Pheochromocytoma: Reconfirm results and proceed with operation.
Coarctation of the aorta: Thoracic aortogram.
Unilateral renal parenchymal disease: Split renal function study and renal vein renin assay.

  *Patient should not be receiving diuretic therapy.
  †A number of drugs or foods may cause false-positive results.

aorta is considered in Chap. 18. These causes are briefly summarized in this chapter, with special emphasis on their relation to the diagnostic study of a patient with hypertension.

In September of 1963, at Vanderbilt University Hospital, a careful search was initiated for patients with surgically correctible hypertension. As of July 1, 1972, a total of 1,070 patients with diastolic hypertension had been investigated. In this study, the history, physical examination, and laboratory and special diagnostic studies (Table 23-2) were designed to detect the causes listed in Table 23-1. The results of this study are referred to throughout the chapter. The very low incidence of patients with hypertension secondary to adrenal causes or coarctation of the aorta in this study may be somewhat misleading. In most patients with hypertension secondary to an adrenal pathologic condition the diagnosis of a pheochromocytoma, Cushing's syndrome, or primary aldosteronism is established or strongly suspected before they are referred. Ordinarily such patients are not included in our general study of patients with hypertension; the same is true of most patients with coarctation of the aorta. Therefore the incidence of this condition will be very small, which indeed it is, but not so small as may be indicated.

PHEOCHROMOCYTOMA

Pheochromocytoma is undoubtedly the most dramatic and treacherous of the surgically correctible causes of hypertension. Unfortunately, many reported cases to date have been undiagnosed during the patient's life or have been suspected only at the last minute during a lethal paroxysmal hypertensive crisis and confirmed at autopsy. The incidence of pheochromocytoma even in the hypertensive population is very low. It has been estimated by Barbeau et al. and Kvale et al. that 0.4 to 2 percent of patients with hypertension have a pheochromocytoma. In the 9-year study of 1,070 consecutive hypertensive patients investigated for evidence of a surgically correctible cause, only 3 patients with pheochromocytoma were found at Vanderbilt University Hospital. During that time, approximately 150 patients presented with a clinical picture suggestive of pheochromocytoma which subsequent study failed to confirm.

CLINICAL MANIFESTATIONS AND LABORATORY STUDIES. The clinical manifestations of these neoplasms are related to their secretion of norepinephrine and epinephrine, and the resultant hypertension may be paroxysmal or sustained. It occurs in all age groups, although 80 percent of the reported cases have been in adults. Although pheochromocytoma is rare, the lethal propensities of the tumor in the untreated case and the extremely good result attending well-planned surgical treatment make it important to screen all patients with hypertension for the lesion. From a practical point of view, this can be done by determining the 24-hour urinary excretion of catecholamines (normally less than 100 μg/24 hours) and of the catecholamine metabolite VMA (usually excreted in the urine in excess of 7 mg/24 hours in patients with pheochromocytoma). This latter test is especially useful in patients taking an antihypertensive drug such as alpha-methyldopa, which interferes with the measurement of catecholamine excretion but does not alter the validity of the VMA determination. Other pharmacologic tests useful in the study of patients suspected of having pheochromocytoma are discussed in Chap. 37.

Pheochromocytoma should be strongly suspected in all patients who have hypertensive or hypotensive reactions associated with anesthesia, pregnancy, or antihypertensive drug therapy, and in patients with family histories of pheochromocytoma, von Hippel-Lindau syndrome, von Recklinghausen's disease, or Sipple's syndrome. When performing any diagnostic study which may involve painful stimuli or provoke catecholamine release in a patient suspected of having a pheochromocytoma, adequate means of supporting or lowering the patient's blood pressure should be instantly available. Although aortography may demonstrate the location of a pheochromocytoma, the powerful stimulation attending this procedure can precipitate a paroxysmal crisis, and deaths have resulted. It is for this reason that, in the Vanderbilt University Hospital study protocol for hypertensive patients, the catecholamine and VMA levels are routinely determined before aortography if there is any suggestion of a pheochromocytoma in the history or physical examination. Although we formerly believed that aortography should not be done in the patient with a pheochromocytoma, we now believe that with certain precautions it can be done safely and will provide important localizing information. In general the tumor is very vascular, and an intense tumor stain is demonstrated. Obviously if a palpable adrenal mass is present or is demonstrated on an intravenous pyelogram (IVP), aortography assumes less importance. However, many of the tumors are small, 10 percent occur in extraadrenal locations, and 7 to 11 percent are multiple or bilateral.

TREATMENT. Once the diagnosis of pheochromocytoma has been established, the preoperative preparation becomes very important. The use of alpha- and beta-adrenergic blockage in preparing these patients for operation as well as during and after the operation is presented in Chap. 37. These advances have contributed significantly to the greatly lessened operative mortality noted below. Anesthesia for these operations is critical. There is a paramount need for smooth, nonstressful induction, atraumatic tracheal intubation, and avoidance of anesthetics which stimulate catecholamine release or enhance responsiveness to these amines. The operative approach is shown in Fig. 23-1.

During the last decade, reports by Greer et al., by Hume, and by Scott et al. indicate that better understanding of the pharmacologic problems engendered by pheochromocytoma and adherence to a careful plan of treatment have resulted in a reduction of operative mortality from 25 percent to less than 5 percent. Following removal of the tumor, the majority of patients (70 to 75 percent) become normotensive and remain so. About 25 percent of the patients have persistent mild to moderate hypertension, which is thought to be due to hypertensive vascular changes in the kidney.

PRIMARY ALDOSTERONISM

Primary aldosteronism refers to a syndrome caused by autonomous hypersecretion of aldosterone by hyperplastic

Fig. 23-1. Abdominothoracic approach to the adrenal glands. This approach is preferred in cases of pheochromocytoma and in Cushing's syndrome due to adrenal carcinoma; it allows radical nonmanipulative removal of the adrenal tumor.

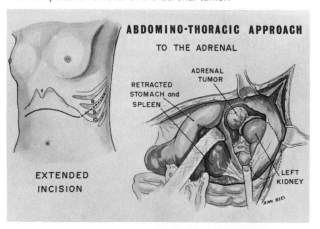

adrenal, or by an adrenal adenoma or (rarely) carcinoma. Aldosterone, a mineral corticoid discovered in 1952, regulates extracellular fluid volume by controlling the excretion and resorption of sodium and water by the kidney. It is the most potent sodium-retaining hormone naturally occurring in man. In 1955, Conn described a syndrome of hypertension, hypokalemia, and alkalosis due to overproduction of aldosterone by an adrenal adenoma. Since that time several hundred cases have been reported.

In the vast majority of reported cases of primary aldosteronism, the cause is an adrenal adenoma. Less frequently, bilateral adrenal hyperplasia with or without nodularity has been reported as causing primary aldosteronism. Adrenal carcinoma is rare as a cause of aldosteronism.

CLINICAL MANIFESTATIONS AND LABORATORY FINDINGS. Conn collected 145 cases and found females predominated 3 to 1. Patients have ranged in age from fifteen to seventy-five years, but most have been in the fourth and fifth decades of life. Hypertension is usually present but is rarely severe. However, it may be associated with headache, cardiomegaly, and retinopathy. In the juvenile cases, severe and even malignant hypertension may occur. Symptoms related to the hypokalemia and alkalosis include muscle weakness, often episodic, which sometimes progresses to paralysis. Paresthesias of the hands and feet are common. Frank tetany may occur, with positive Chvostek's and Trousseau's signs. Polyuria and polydipsia are often prominent. Edema is usually absent.

Laboratory findings include hypokalemia (usually below 3 mEq/L), increased serum bicarbonate, normal or increased serum sodium, and elevated serum pH. Urinary potassium exceeds 40 mEq/24 hours, while urinary sodium is normal. Conn has recently stressed the opinion that hypokalemia may be a late manifestation of the disease and has reported cases of primary aldosteronism with persistent normokalemia. In primary aldosteronism, the plasma renin activity is low and the daily aldosterone secretion rates are high. The reasons for these pathophysiologic changes are discussed in detail in Chap. 37.

Primary aldosteronism is to be suspected in any hypertensive patient with the signs and symptoms listed above, especially the patient with hypertension, lack of edema, low serum potassium level, and increased serum sodium and carbon dioxide. Hypokalemia has proved to be the most valuable simple laboratory test. Plasma renin activity is low, usually 100 m μg/100 ml (nanograms) or less. The definitive diagnosis depends on the finding of a low serum renin with an increased urinary aldosterone excretion. The normal range for the latter study is 3 to 17 μg/24 hours, while in patients with primary aldosteronism the excretion rate may be elevated to levels as high as 160 μg/24 hours.

A number of factors influence the serum potassium, aldosterone, and renin levels, two of the most important being salt restriction and diuretic therapy. Thiazide diuretics cause potassium depletion and hypokalemia. A low-salt diet may prevent the hypokalemia and alkalosis of primary aldosteronism. Finally, a low-salt diet may cause a considerable rise in aldosterone and renin secretion. Patients being screened for evidence of primary aldosteronism should therefore be off diuretic therapy and on a liberal-salt diet (200 mEq sodium for 4 to 5 days) if meaningful serum potassium, aldosterone, and renin levels are to be obtained.

Secondary aldosteronism occurs in renovascular hypertension, congestive heart failure, nephrosis, cirrhosis of the liver, and other edematous states. In all these, the urinary sodium level is low as contrasted to normal or high levels in primary aldosteronism, and plasma renin activity is usually high.

At one point in the initial Vanderbilt University Hospital series of 341 patients with diastolic hypertension, 90 consecutive patients were studied for evidence of primary aldosteronism. After the patients had received a high-salt diet for 4 to 5 days, peripheral venous renin activity and aldosterone secretion rates were determined. Any patient with a suggestive elevation of aldosterone secretion or depression of plasma renin activity was readmitted to the hospital and again studied. Of these 90 patients, none proved to have primary aldosteronism due to an adrenal adenoma; one had a marked decrease in aldosterone secretion following removal of the left adrenal gland and 50 percent of the right adrenal. An initial serum potassium of less than 3.5 mEq/L was encountered in 42 of 341 patients. Many of these patients actually turned out to have a syndrome of hypokalemia, suppressed renin levels even with stimulation, normal aldosterone levels, and hypertension which was controlled by aldactone.

Conn's early estimate that 15 to 20 percent of patients designated as having essential hypertension have primary aldosteronism was excessive. Simpler and better methods of renin and aldosterone assays for widespread use will provide the means of answering many of the troublesome questions about this form of surgically correctible hypertension. Treatment and results are discussed in Chap. 37.

CUSHING'S SYNDROME

In 1932, Harvey Cushing described a syndrome consisting of central obesity ("buffalo hump" and moon face), osteoporosis, amenorrhea, hirsutism, abdominal striae, hypertension, and weakness. Cushing's syndrome is presently defined as a constellation of clinical and metabolic disorders which result from a chronic excess of cortisol (hydrocortisone). The source of the excess cortisol may be an adrenocortical tumor or, more commonly, bilateral adrenocortical hyperplasia under the stimulation of ACTH from the pituitary or a nonendocrine ACTH-secreting tumor of the lung, pancreas, or other organ. Untreated Cushing's syndrome is a highly incapacitating and lethal disorder. With early recognition and treatment a favorable outcome may be expected.

PATHOLOGY. The underlying adrenal pathologic condition in Cushing's syndrome is bilateral adrenocortical hyperplasia in 60 to 70 percent of cases. The remainder have adrenocortical tumors, of which two-thirds are adenomas and one-third carcinomas. The incidence of Cushing's syndrome due to nonendocrine ACTH-secreting tumors (ectopic ACTH syndrome) is unknown, but this type probably accounts for fewer cases than do adrenocortical tumors. In cases due to adrenal hyperplasia under the influence of pituitary ACTH, the pituitary may or may not contain an adenoma.

Normal adults excrete 3 to 12 mg of 17-hydroxycorticosteroids (17-OHCS) in 24 hours, while adults with Cushing's syndrome usually excrete in excess of 12 mg/day. However, it is more accurate to relate the daily urinary output of 17-OHCS to the quantity of creatinine excreted per 24-hour period. In this way variation due to body size and to the collection of less than the 24-hour output can be averted. Normal persons usually excrete 3 to 7 mg of 17-OHCS/Gm of creatinine; with Cushing's syndrome more than 7 mg of 17-OHCS/Gm of creatinine is usually excreted.

CLINICAL MANIFESTATIONS AND LABORATORY FINDINGS. Cushing's syndrome is three times as frequent in females as in males. It is found at all ages but is most common in the third and fourth decades. In children it almost always is due to an adrenocortical tumor, usually a carcinoma. The frequency of the various clinical and metabolic manifestations of the syndrome is shown in Table 23-3.

The florid case of Cushing's syndrome may be recognized by the clinical picture alone. However, many patients present only a few of the classic findings. The basic diagnostic study is the measurement of 24-hour urinary excretion of 17-OHCS. If the 17-OHCS output is abnormally elevated, special adrenopituitary function studies as described by Liddle are performed to confirm the diagnosis and to determine the underlying pathologic condition. These are discussed in detail in Chap. 37.

In the Vanderbilt University Hospital study of 1,070 consecutive hypertensive patients one patient with Cushing's syndrome was encountered. Interestingly enough, the initial determination of 17-OHCS had been in the normal range. Aortography revealed a tumor of the right adrenal gland. Subsequent 17-OHCS determinations and the other tests of adrenopituitary function indicated that the lesion was an adrenal adenoma, and this was confirmed when the tumor was removed.

TREATMENT. Diagnostic precision is important because appropriate therapy depends on recognition of the under-

lying pathologic condition. Before surgical treatment is undertaken, severe metabolic derangements, infections, and complications related to hypertension should be brought under control. The views on treatment expressed here primarily reflect the experience of Liddle's Division of Endocrinology at Vanderbilt University Hospital.

Cushing's Syndrome Due to Adrenal Tumors. The only satisfactory treatment of Cushing's syndrome due to adrenocortical neoplasm is complete surgical removal of the tumor. In cases due to an adenoma, the posterior approach (Fig. 23-2) through the bed of the twelfth rib provides satisfactory exposure. Hayes has advocated bilateral adrenal exploration, because bilateral adenomas are found in about 10 percent of the cases. The most practical approach is perhaps the use of two surgical teams carrying out simultaneous posterior exposure of the two adrenal glands. This approach is less difficult, especially in the obese patient, and is associated with a lower postoperative morbidity than is the transperitoneal approach (Fig. 23-3). Following surgical excision of the adenoma, prompt and permanent regression of the syndrome is to be expected in the overwhelming majority of cases, although the hypertension may take some time to subside completely. An important consequence of "autonomous" production of cortisol by an adrenal tumor is the supression of ACTH production by the pituitary with resultant atrophy of the remaining adrenal tissue. A careful regimen of adrenal substitution therapy (usually hydrocortisone) must be initiated during the operation and continued until it has been demonstrated (by ACTH stimulation tests and 17-OHCS urinary levels) that the remaining adrenal tissue is functionally adequate.

In cases of Cushing's syndrome known or suspected to be due to an adrenocortical carcinoma, a thoracoabdominal incision is preferred so that a radical, nonmanipulative resection can be performed (Fig. 23-1). If preoperative roentgen studies have failed to localize the tumor, the abdominal component of the incision is made first and then extended into the appropriate hemithorax after the tumor has been identified. If the carcinoma can be completely removed, the results are the same as described above for an adenoma; the remarks regarding adrenal substitution therapy also apply. Obviously, if the tumor has metastasized beyond the limits of the resection or if the carcinoma is so extensive as to defy complete excision, the ultimate result is usually poor.

Cushing's Syndrome Due to Ectopic ACTH Syndrome. The only satisfactory treatment of an ACTH-secreting tumor (usually of the lung or the pancreas) is complete surgical removal. This has been accomplished in few cases to date; widespread metastases are usually present by the time the diagnosis is established. Irradiation or chemotherapy has been of little if any benefit in these cases. Bilateral adrenalectomy or therapy with adrenal-inhibiting agents may offer substantial benefit in selected cases, even though it has no influence on the tumor or on ectopic ACTH production.

Cushing's Syndrome Due to Bilateral Adrenocortical Hyperplasia. Treatment is dependent on the severity of the syndrome. If the patient has severe hypertension, osteo-

Table 23-3. FREQUENCY OF THE MANIFESTATIONS OF CUSHING'S SYNDROME
(61 Cases, Vanderbilt University Hospital, 1954–1964)

Manifestation	Frequency, percent
Central obesity	100
Hypertension	83
Impaired glucose tolerance	83
Protein wasting	77
Osteoporosis	70
Hirsutism	70
Weakness	60
Menstrual aberrations	50
Ecchymoses	47
Edema	33
Striae	27

porosis, or psychosis, bilateral total adrenalectomy should be performed. The bilateral posterior approach is preferred for the reasons indicated earlier. Patients so treated usually have complete regression of the syndrome. Lifelong adrenal replacement therapy is required. Mild to moderate hypertension persists in about 10 percent of the cases.

If Cushing's syndrome is only mild to moderate and not associated with the severe manifestations listed above, irradiation of the pituitary with 4,000 to 5,000 r should be the initial treatment. Approximately 30 percent of the patients so treated with irradiation will obtain complete and lasting remission of the syndrome. Patients who fail to respond to this form of therapy should have bilateral adrenalectomy.

Patients with sellar enlargement or neurologic deficits attributable to a pituitary tumor should have the tumor removed. Transsphenoidal hypophysectomy employing magnification technique is being used with increasing frequency and success.

In patients treated by bilateral adrenalectomy as the initial therapy evidence of pituitary tumors may develop subsequently. Thorn has reported the incidence as 15 to 20 percent in his experience; in the Vanderbilt University Hospital experience, as reported by Liddle, it had occurred in three of seven cases. Of 11 patients treated by irradiation and then bilateral adrenalectomy, none had developed evidence of a pituitary tumor; of 18 patients treated with irradiation alone, none had developed evidence of a pituitary tumor. This experience would support the belief that pituitary irradiation lessens the incidence of pituitary tumor in patients who have bilateral adrenalectomy.

Finally, mention must be made of subtotal adrenalectomy in the treatment of Cushing's syndrome with bilateral adrenocortical hyperplasia. Subtotal adrenalectomy refers to complete removal of one adrenal and 80 to 90 percent of the other. This procedure had its origin at the time when adrenal steroid substitution therapy was not available. Persistent severe hypertension has been common in patients with hyperplasia who were treated by subtotal adrenalectomy. As Orth has reported, in our experience every patient treated by subtotal adrenalectomy was a treatment failure.

COARCTATION OF THE AORTA

Coarctation of the aorta is to be suspected in all infants, children, and adults with hypertension. The coarctation can occur anywhere in the aorta from the midpoint of the aortic arch down to the aortic bifurcation; however, 98 percent of coarctations are located in the first part of the descending thoracic aorta. The association of coarctation and systemic hypertension has long been known. It was not until 1945, however, that both Crafoord and Gross performed successful surgical correction of the coarctation and demonstrated that this form of hypertension was surgically correctible.

The mechanism of hypertension in coarctation remains debatable. The explanation that it is caused by mechanical

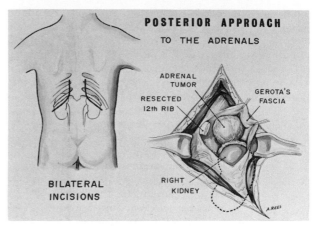

Fig. 23-2. Posterior approach to the adrenal glands. This approach is recommended in cases of Cushing's syndrome due to an adrenal adenoma or bilateral adrenocortical hyperplasia and in primary aldosteronism.

obstruction of the aorta causing increase in resistance to blood flow, with resultant hypertension in the circulation of the arms and head, has never seemed valid, since obstruction of the lower abdominal aorta does not produce hypertension. The experimental studies of Scott and associates have suggested that the coarctation results in reduced renal blood flow and activation of the renal pressor system. Convincing corroborative evidence in patients with coarctation has not yet been presented. Sealy performed angiotensin assays in five patients with coarctation of the aorta and found elevated levels in only two of them.

CLINICAL MANIFESTATIONS AND LABORATORY FINDINGS. The presence of vigorous pulses in the upper extremities and absence or profound decrease in the pulses of the lower extremities provide the basis for prompt recognition of this important cause of hypertension. Decreased blood pressure in the legs, normally 20 to 40 mm Hg higher than in the arms, and a precordial systolic murmur are valuable confirmatory findings. In infants and young children, the blood pressure in the arms may be normal or only mildly elevated. In older children and

Fig. 23-3. Anterior transperitoneal approach to the adrenals for removal of adrenal adenoma or hyperplastic adrenal glands.

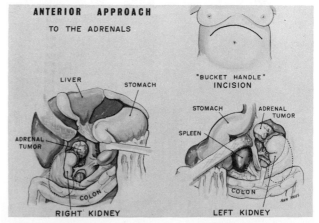

adults, hypertension is the rule. After the first decade of life, the shoulders and arms of a patient with coarctation are often extremely well developed and collateral arterial pulsation can be palpated in the musculature of the posterior thorax. The chest roentgenogram frequently reveals a silhouette of the coarcted segment in the descending thoracic aorta and notching of the ribs due to compensatory changes in the collateral circulation. The electrocardiogram usually shows left axis deviation.

A detailed consideration of coarctation of the aorta is presented in Chap. 18. Suffice it to say that coarctation is an important cause of hypertension which, if not corrected, leads to death in 60 percent of patients before the age of forty years. With surgical treatment, complete remission of the hypertension occurs in 95 percent of patients. In our study of 1,070 hypertensive patients two adults and one teen-ager had coarctation of the thoracic aorta.

RENOVASCULAR HYPERTENSION

Renovascular hypertension may be defined as diastolic hypertension secondary to an occlusive lesion of a main renal artery or segmental renal artery which is sufficiently

Fig. 23-4. Aortogram showing left renal artery stenosis due to atherosclerosis involving orifice and proximal third of the renal artery. Poststenotic dilatation is common with such lesions.

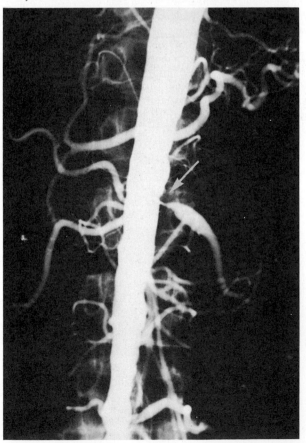

severe to activate the renal pressor mechanism. Interest in renovascular hypertension was initiated by Goldblatt and colleagues in the early 1930s, when they produced persistent hypertension in dogs by constriction of the renal arteries. Thereafter Page, Helmer, and Braun Menendez, with their colleagues, independently described the renin-angiotensin system. For the next two decades attention was focused on the kidney in the etiology of hypertension, although renal artery stenosis was considered to be a relatively uncommon cause of hypertension. Adequate and safe methods of studying renal function and vascular anatomy were not available. Nephrectomy was frequently performed for hypertension with an associated small kidney seen on excretory urography, but remission of the hypertension was observed infrequently. In 1956 Homer Smith reviewed a series of 575 hypertensive patients treated by nephrectomy in which it was observed that only 26 percent were normotensive after 1 year. Smith concluded that nephrectomy should be done only for strict urologic indications and not with any hope of relieving hypertension. At that time vascular surgery was developing rapidly, and new and improved techniques of aortography were being introduced and used with increasing frequency. Renal artery stenosis was seen frequently, and usually in patients with hypertension. The demonstrations by De-Camp and Birchall, Morris et al., DeBakey et al., Dustan et al., and others that normal blood pressure could be restored in many hypertensive patients with obstructive disease of the renal artery by surgical relief of the stenotic lesion initiated the present interest in renovascular hypertension. Refinements in excretory urography and renal arteriography and the development of split renal function studies, isotope renography, better methods of renin-angiotensin assay, and improved surgical techniques followed. All these advances contributed materially to a better understanding of renovascular hypertension and to a better selection of those hypertensive patients who would benefit from surgical treatment.

PATHOLOGY. Arteriosclerosis has been the underlying cause in 60 to 70 percent of the proved cases of renovascular hypertension reported to date. The atherosclerotic lesions usually occur in older patients and more frequently in the male. There is usually an atheromatous plaque situated in the orifice or proximal third of the renal artery (Fig. 23-4). However, the presence of an arteriosclerotic plaque in a renal artery does not necessarily indicate a causal relationship to associated hypertension. Autopsy and arteriographic studies by Eyler et al., Holley et al., and Foster et al. show that over 50 percent of patients after fifty years of age have some degree of arteriosclerotic renal artery stenosis whether they are hypertensive or normotensive. Associated arteriosclerotic disease of other vascular systems is commonly encountered. Bilateral renal artery lesions are present in roughly one-third of patients with renovascular hypertension due to arteriosclerosis (Fig. 23-5). Complete occlusion of a renal artery, with filling of the distal segment of the artery via collaterals, is not uncommon in patients over fifty-five years of age (Fig. 23-6).

Fibromuscular hyperplasia or dysplasia of the renal

artery has been the underlying cause in 20 to 25 percent of the reported cases of renovascular hypertension. Significant series of cases have been reported by Wylie et al., by Hunt et al., by Ernst et al., and by Fry et al. It has usually been observed in young patients, especially women in the twenty-five to forty-five age range. The lesion is characterized by a thickening of the media with a myxomatous-appearing fibrous tissue, which separates and distorts the muscle fibers, and by degenerative and disruptive changes in elastic tissue and smooth muscle. These changes result in lesions of the arterial wall which have been termed *microaneurysms*. Dissecting aneurysms and hematomas have also been observed. The striking feature of fibromuscular hyperplasia is the corrugation of the internal surface of the renal artery caused by alternating zones of hyperplasia and disruption of the media and elastic tissue in the wall of the artery. This corrugation gives the "string of beads" effect seen on renal arteriography (Figs. 23-7 and 23-8).

Earlier it was thought the lesions were unilateral in the majority of cases. However, it has now become apparent that the vast majority are bilateral lesions. The reason for this turnabout is found in the improvements in renal arteriography during the past few years. Selective oblique arteriograms in several projections are demonstrating lesions which previously were undetected. This holds true for both atherosclerotic and fibrodysplastic lesions but most commonly for the latter. Hunt et al. believe that virtually 100 percent of the fibromuscular lesions are bilateral, and our recent experience tends to support this concept. An aortogram in the anteroposterior projection will not suffice to demonstrate many renal artery lesions. The reason for this is shown schematically in Fig. 23-9. The origin of the renal artery may be masked by the aorta in such a projection, and the distal renal artery courses in almost an antero-

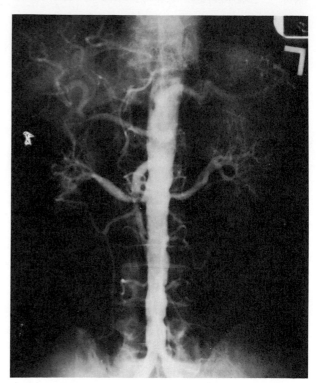

Fig. 23-5. Aortogram showing bilateral renal artery stenosis due to atherosclerosis. About one-third of patients with renovascular hypertension due to atherosclerosis have bilateral lesions.

posterior direction. The lesion is usually located in the middle and distal thirds of the artery, frequently extending into the segmental branches. With multiple renal arteries to one kidney, more than one of the arteries may show fibromuscular hyperplasia. On serial arteriograms over a period of several years, the lesions have been seen to become progressively more severe in some patients.

A variant of fibromuscular hyperplasia called *subadventitial fibroplasia* by McCormack et al. consists of a dense collar of collagen located in the periphery of the media, which is often thinned and disorganized by the fibrous tissue (Fig. 23-10). These lesions also have been most commonly found in females in the twenty-to-forty age

Fig. 23-6. *A.* Aortogram showing complete atherosclerotic occlusion of the left renal artery in a fifty-three-year-old man. Arrow indicates proximal portion of left renal artery which is still patent. *B.* Later film in aortographic series showing filling of the distal portion of the left renal artery via collaterals. Arrow indicates patent distal left renal artery. Lesion is amenable to correction by either bypass grafting or thromboendarterectomy with a patch graft.

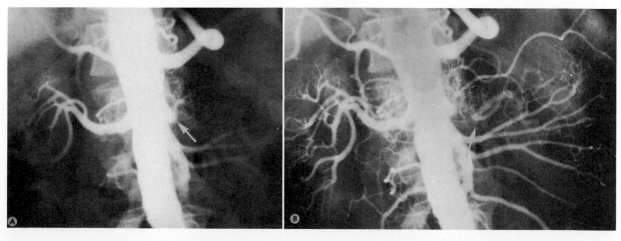

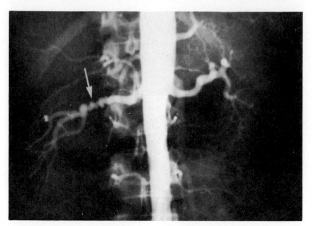

Fig. 23-7. Aortogram showing fibromuscular hyperplasia of the right renal artery with typical "string of beads" effect. Lesions often extend out to or even involve branch arteries. Selective left renal arteriography in this patient showed some lesions which had not been demonstrated by the aortogram.

range. A third variant is the occlusive lesion caused by an intimal fibrous proliferation producing either a discrete short area of stenosis or a long tubular stenosis; this has been called *single mural hyperplasia* (Fig. 23-11). It has been most commonly encountered in the very young patient, less than twenty years of age and as young as four months. Children with unilateral stenosis have been observed by Foster et al. to develop contralateral stenosis in subsequent years.

Harrison and McCormack, and Sheps et al. (1972), have devised a classification of the various fibromuscular lesions which allows recognition on radiograph and has some prognostic implications. These writers feel they can recognize whether the lesion will progress in severity.

The pathogenesis of the fibromuscular dysplasia group of lesions is not known. The lesion does occasionally occur in other arterial systems. Whether it is congenital or acquired is uncertain, and there may be more than one underlying cause. Suggested etiologic factors have been

summarized by Hunt et al.; they include congenital anomaly, intrinsic defects in the elastic tissue, Erdheims' medial necrosis, healed arteritis, and abnormal stretching of arteries, especially in pregnancy.

Less common lesions causing renovascular hypertension are renal artery aneurysm, dissecting aneurysm of the renal artery, embolism with segmental infarction, primary thrombosis, and compression of the artery by a fibrous or muscular band (right crus of diaphragm) or a mass. In the author's experience, segmental infarction, presumably due either to an embolus or a segmental artery thrombosis, has been the third most common cause of proved renovascular hypertension.

PATHOPHYSIOLOGY. Reduction or dampening of the arterial pulse pressure in the renal artery beyond the obstruction is thought to be the stimulus which initiates the renal pressor mechanism. The manner in which this is brought about is not entirely understood. Both Crocker et al. and Tobian have shown that patients with renovascular hypertension frequently have hyperplasia and increased cellularity of the juxtaglomerular apparatus (JGA). The JGA surrounds the afferent arteriole of the cortical nephron and is thought to be the source of renin production. These observations have led to the hypothesis that the JGA contains a volume- or pressure-sensing mechanism which responds to reduced pulse pressure by liberating renin. Renin, a proteolytic enzyme, acts on the substrate angiotensinogen, a globulin produced by the liver and found in the α 2-globulin fraction of plasma, to produce a decapeptide which is designated *angiotensin I*. A plasmolytic converting enzyme splits off the last two amino acids from the apparently inert angiotensin I to produce an octapeptide called *angiotensin II*, which is the active pressor agent. Angiotensin II is an extremely powerful vasoconstrictive substance. On a weight basis, it is approximately ten times as potent a pressor agent as norepinephrine. The biologic properties of angiotensin II have been studied extensively, and it appears well established as the active vasoconstrictive factor in renovascular hypertension. Angiotensin II has other effects which are important in producing hyper-

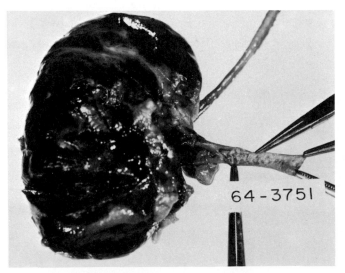

Fig. 23-8. Resected right kidney with renal artery opened longitudinally to show fibrous septa forming corrugated internal surface.

tension. It potentiates the circulatory responses to norepinephrine, and it also stimulates secretion of aldosterone by the adrenal cortex. This latter effect may result in potassium depletion, sodium and water retention, and all the other features of aldosteronism in patients with renovascular hypertension. Recent studies by Louis and his associates have cast some doubt about the role the renin-angiotension system plays in the etiology of experimental renovascular hypertension.

CLINICAL MANIFESTATIONS. The incidence of renovascular hypertension in patients with diastolic hypertension is not known. In a study searching for patients with renovascular hypertension at Vanderbilt University Hospital during the years 1963 to 1972, the incidence was 16 percent. However, this cannot be considered a study of diastolic hypertension in unselected subjects, because of the bias introduced by the physician's referral of a patient to the study. At present it is estimated that 5 percent of patients with diastolic hypertension have renovascular hypertension.

There are no unique features in history, physical examination, or routine laboratory determinations which will differentiate renovascular hypertension from essential hypertension, although a number have been suggested. Most of the classic concepts about essential hypertension are based on patients in whom other causes of hypertension were not excluded. Table 23-4 shows a comparison of the clinical findings in a group of 57 patients with proved renovascular hypertension and a group of 260 patients with essential hypertension. These data still pertain to our larger experience with 1,070 hypertensive patients. Every one of these patients had a complete evaluation, including rapid-

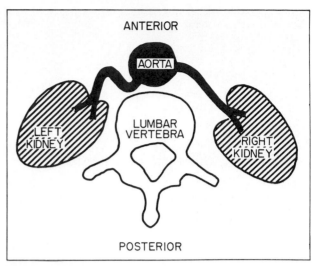

Fig. 23-9. Diagram showing the course of the renal arteries. Lesions in the renal arteries may be masked in the anteroposterior projection. Oblique selective arteriograms are required to demonstrate these lesions.

sequence excretory urography, isotope renography, and renal arteriography. If a renal artery stenosis was found, split renal function study was performed, and in the later period of the study renal vein renin was assayed. The diagnosis of renovascular hypertension was based strictly on a favorable response to surgical treatment, the most critical of diagnostic criteria. In those cases designated as essential hypertension, all tests were normal. Patients with hypertension due to adrenal causes or renal parenchymal disease were eliminated. The reason for the disparate figures under the various clinical observations is that for some patients the pertinent information was not known.

Classic teaching has been that a family history of hypertension suggests essential hypertension, but renovascular hypertension was just as frequently associated with this

Fig. 23-10. *A.* Selective right renal arteriogram of patient with subadventitial fibroplasia; lesion is more disorganized and does not have the regularity of the "strings of beads" effect seen in Fig. 23-7. *B.* Photomicrograph of renal artery with subadventitial fibroplasia. In the upper and lower corners at the right the dense collar of collagen is seen in the peripheral media. Disorganization of the media and intima is also seen.

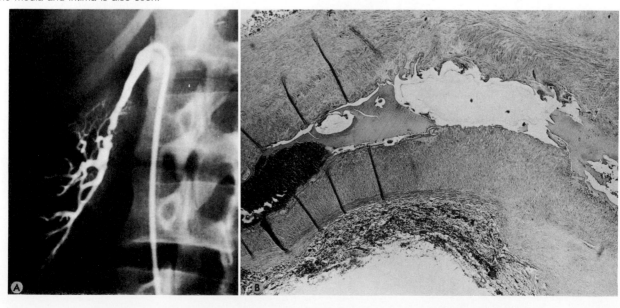

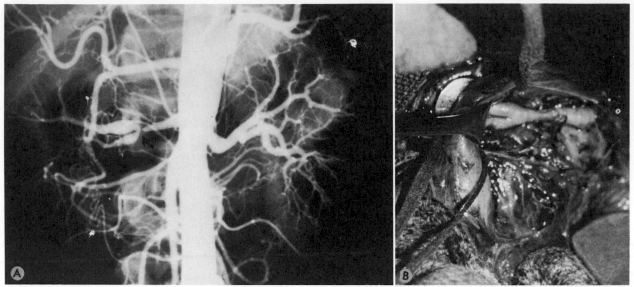

Fig. 23-11. *A.* Aortogram showing single mural hyperplasia of the right renal artery, in an eighteen-year-old girl. *B.* Photograph of the stenosis seen at operation. The vena cava has been retracted to the patient's right to expose the renal artery and the area of stenosis.

observation. A history of recent acceleration of hypertension, recent onset of hypertension, and flank pain or trauma in the hypertensive patient was equally frequent in the two groups. The mean duration of hypertension was but slightly longer in the patient with essential hypertension. Only the finding of an upper abdominal bruit on physical examination provided any differentiation between the two groups, since it was four times more frequent in the renovascular hypertension group. The eye ground changes on fundoscopic examination provided information as to the severity of the hypertension but not as to the origin.

It is commonly stated that hypertension in the young patient is more likely to have a renovascular cause. Figure 23-12 compares patients with renovascular hypertension and those with essential hypertension by decade of life. Again patients with renal parenchymal disease were eliminated, and the diagnoses of essential hypertension and renovascular hypertension were on the same basis as for Table 23-4. The highest incidence of renovascular hypertension was in the first decade of life, the next highest incidence was in the sixty- to sixty-nine-year age group, and surprisingly few instances were found in patients ten to nineteen years of age. It can only be concluded that renovascular hypertension occurs at all ages. Certainly the very young patient with severe hypertension is a

Table 23-4. CLINICAL FINDINGS IN RENOVASCULAR HYPERTENSION AND ESSENTIAL HYPERTENSION
(Vanderbilt University Hospital, 1963–1966)

	Renovascular hypertension		Essential hypertension	
	Number	Percent	Number	Percent
Family history of hypertension	26/51	51	130/245	53
Recent acceleration of hypertension.	7/48	15	31/225	14
Recent onset of hypertension (6 months). . . .	10/50	20	40/230	17
Hypertension associated with history of				
flank pain, hematuria, or renal trauma . . .	4/57	7	18/260	7
Upper abdominal bruit	22/57	40	24/260	9
Duration of hypertension, years:				
Range	0–23		0–28	
Mean	5.4		6.2	

prime suspect, but so is the older hypertensive patient.

LABORATORY FINDINGS. Routine laboratory determinations provide little help in the detection of renovascular hypertension. Only an occasional patient will have secondary aldosteronism with hypokalemic alkalosis. Tarazi et al. have noted an increased incidence of elevated hematocrit level in patients with hypertension secondary to renal artery stenosis, but this was found in only a small percentage (less than 20 percent) of the patients. The urinalysis, phenolsulfonphthalein excretion, and hemogram or serum electrolyte determinations provide few clues as to the cause of the hypertension. Azotemia occurs with equal frequency in renovascular and essential hypertension. The changes of left ventricular hypertrophy found on the chest x-ray or electrocardiogram are helpful in gauging the severity of the hypertension but not in determining the underlying cause.

SELECTION OF PATIENTS FOR INTENSIVE DIAGNOSTIC STUDY. As the foregoing discussion of the clinical characteristics of renovascular hypertension indicates and as will be seen in the discussion of some of the special screening tests, there is no simple way to predict which patient will be found to have renovascular hypertension. This has led to the author's principle that *any patient with significant diastolic hypertension in whom surgical correction would be recommended if a significant lesion were found should have intensive diagnostic study.* This approach eliminates the mildly hypertensive patient and the patient who is an unacceptable operative risk.

SPECIAL DIAGNOSTIC STUDIES. Rapid-Sequence Excretory Urography. This is a simple variation of the standard intravenous pyelogram described by Maxwell et al. The patient, having been dehydrated, receives a rapid intravenous injection of contrast medium, and roentgenograms are made at 1, 2, 3, 4, 5, 10, 15, and 30 minutes. Contrast medium should appear in the calyceal system of the normal kidney on the 2-minute film. Findings suggestive of renovascular hypertension include (1) unilateral delay in appearance of contrast medium, strongly suggesting renal artery stenosis (Fig. 23-13); (2) decrease in renal length greater than 1.5 cm as compared with the contralateral kidney (Fig. 23-14); (3) unilateral decreased concentration or density of the medium on the early films; (4) ureteral notching due to collateral arterial supply; and (5) unilateral hyperconcentration of the medium on the late films (Fig. 23-15), which is explained by the fact that the kidney with a significant renal artery stenosis displays increased tubular resorption of water and sodium, while the contrast medium is a fixed solute and is not resorbed, thus appearing in hyperconcentration on the late films. (This effect may be accentuated by hydrating the patient or even giving an intravenous infusion of a saline solution of urea, so-called "washout" intravenous pyelography.) This phenomenon is the basis of the split renal function tests described below. A further finding on the urogram, defects in the renal silhouette, may indicate segmental infarction (Fig. 23-16).

The urogram also provides important information re-

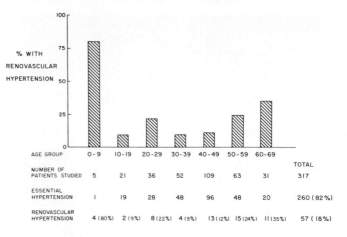

AGE GROUP	0-9	10-19	20-29	30-39	40-49	50-59	60-69	TOTAL
NUMBER OF PATIENTS STUDIED	5	21	36	52	109	63	31	317
ESSENTIAL HYPERTENSION	1	19	28	48	96	48	20	260 (82%)
RENOVASCULAR HYPERTENSION	4 (80%)	2 (9%)	8 (22%)	4 (9%)	13 (12%)	15 (24%)	11 (35%)	57 (18%)

INCIDENCE OF RENOVASCULAR HYPERTENSION AND ESSENTIAL HYPERTENSION BY DECADE OF LIFE
VANDERBILT UNIVERSITY SERIES 1963-1966

Fig. 23-12. Incidence of renovascular hypertension and essential hypertension in 317 hypertensive patients.

garding renal parenchymal disease, e.g., pyelonephritis and hydronephrosis. However, in the recent analysis by Foster et al. of 122 patients with proved renovascular hypertension, the urogram was judged to be normal in 31 percent of the patients. If, as some have advocated, the urogram had been used to determine whether to proceed with further studies (i.e., arteriography), we would have missed almost one-third of the patients with renovascular hypertension. The fact that one-half the false-negative results occurred in patients with bilateral lesions is of interest but does not alter the fact that they would have been missed. A urogram that is abnormal preoperatively but normal postoperatively is very reassuring. On many occasions we have seen a kidney increase in length by 1.5 to 2.0 cm

Fig. 23-13. Two-minute film from a rapid-sequence excretory urogram. Contrast medium is present in the calyceal system on the right; none is seen on the left. This is strongly suggestive of a left renal artery stenosis.

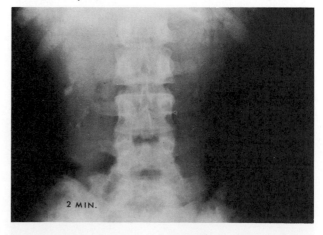

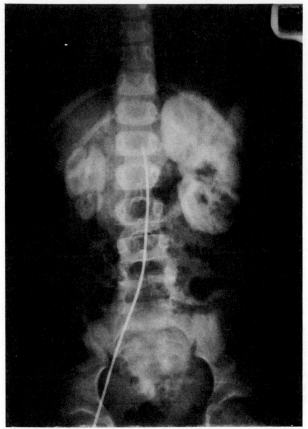

Fig. 23-14. Nephrographic phase of aortogram showing difference in renal size which suggests renal artery stenosis.

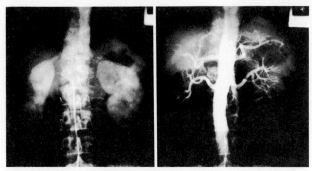

Fig. 23-16. Nephrographic phase of an aortogram showing defect in midportion of the right kidney. This was detected on the excretory urogram. Aortogram shows branch artery to midportion of right kidney completely occluded. Heminephrectomy resulted in remission of hypertension.

by the seventh day following successful operative treatment.

Isotope Renography. The ^{131}I orthoiodohippurate renogram has been widely used in screening hypertensive patients for renovascular hypertension. Tracer doses of the

Fig. 23-15. Late film in excretory urogram showing hyperconcentration of contrast medium in the right renal pelvis, a sign indicative of right renal artery stenosis.

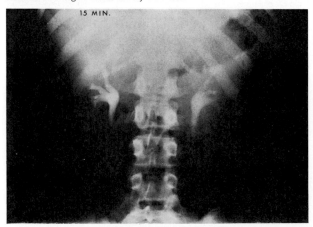

isotope are injected intravenously, and external scintillation counters, placed posteriorly over each kidney, simultaneously record timed uptake and excretion curves. Features characteristic of renal artery stenosis are reduced total height of curve, delayed time to maximal height, and delayed excretion. These abnormalities reflect the degree of reduced renal tubular function and the reduced volume of urine excreted by the ischemic kidney. The test is not specific and must be interpreted with the aid of the excretory urogram. Obstructive uropathy simulates renal ischemia. Pyelonephritis and other parenchymal renal diseases are also responsible for false-positive interpretations in perhaps 20 percent of patients with renovascular hypertension. As with excretory urography, the renogram compares one kidney with the other; hence bilateral renal artery stenosis may not be detected. We have not found the renogram to be particularly helpful in the diagnosis of renovascular hypertension. A triple isotope renogram study is currently being evaluated in the study of patients with hypertension.

Renal Arteriography. If one accepts stenosis of a main or segmental renal artery as part of the definition of renovascular hypertension, renal arteriography becomes the best screening test for renovascular hypertension. Hesitancy to apply arteriography in all patients with diastolic hypertension is related to the fact that the procedure involves a small but definite risk, is expensive, and ordinarily requires that the patient be hospitalized.

A number of methods of obtaining contrast angiographic demonstration of the renal arteries are available. The most widely accepted method is the percutaneous retrograde catheter technique via a femoral artery. Under fluoroscopic control the catheter tip is located in the aorta at the level of the L_1–L_2 interspace; a pressure injector is used to inject the contrast medium, and a rapid film changer is used to obtain serial films. The films will show the aorta, the main renal arteries, the segmental branch arteries, and the entire kidney in the nephrographic phase.

In recent years oblique aortograms and selective renal arteriography, with the catheter tip placed in the renal artery, have been used to obtain additional information. With a catheter selectively placed in a renal artery one

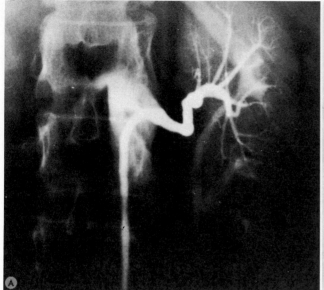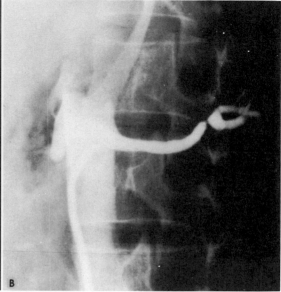

Fig. 23-17. *A.* Left selective renal arteriogram in straight antero-posterior projection; renal artery stenosis is not seen. *B.* Repeat arteriogram with same patient in oblique position shows severe stenosis of distal left renal artery and distal renal artery segment suitable for implantation of an aorticorenal bypass graft utilizing a segment of saphenous vein.

can rotate the patient in various oblique views to demonstrate a severe stenosis which may have appeared to be of questionable significance on straight posteroanterior projection (Fig 23-17). Similarly, in some patients with extensive fibromuscular hyperplasia which on the aortic-injection arteriogram did not appear amenable to surgical correction, a selective arteriogram may show a distal seg-

ment of the renal artery suitable for placement of a bypass graft (Fig. 23-18). Figure 23-9 shows why oblique arteriograms are required in these patients.

In patients with severe arteriosclerotic occlusive disease of the aortoiliac-femoral system it may not be possible or advisable to insert the catheter via a femoral artery. In this situation translumbar aortography or a catheter inserted via an axillary artery may be used to demonstrate the renal arteries.

In the Vanderbilt University Hospital study of 1,070 consecutive hypertensive patients, 1,423 renal arteriograms have been made in the course of initial and follow-up studies. There have been 10 serious complications (0.7 percent): three massive hematomas, one false aneurysm of the femoral artery, thrombosis of the femoral artery in six patients, and one death following aortic surgery for postaortogram thrombosis of the aorta in a patient with severe atherosclerotic occlusive disease.

Fig. 23-18. *A.* Aortogram showing fibromuscular hyperplasia which appears to extend into branch arteries and precludes satisfactory corrective surgery. *B.* Oblique left renal arteriogram in same patient showing distal segment suitable for implantation of a bypass graft (see Fig. 23-23).

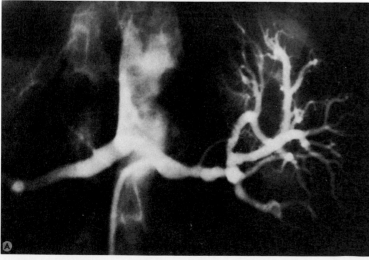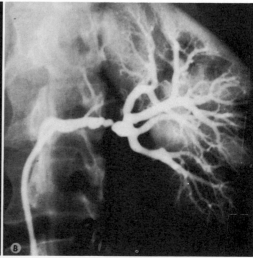

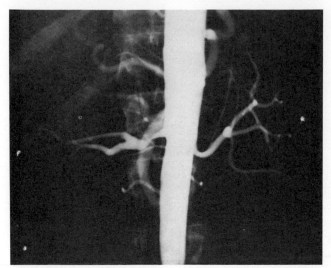

Fig. 23-19. Aortogram showing stenosis of proximal right renal artery due to extrinsic compression of the artery. At operation the right crus of the diaphragm was found to be compressing the artery in this forty-two-year-old man.

Arteriosclerosis is the most common cause of renal artery stenosis, and the lesions are bilateral in about one-third of the cases (Fig. 23-4 and 23-5). The process usually involves the origin and the proximal third of the renal artery; poststenotic dilatation is common with severe lesions. Complete occlusion is not uncommon in patients over fifty years of age; in this circumstance the distal renal artery is usually seen to opacify on the later films via collateral arterial supply (Fig. 23-6).

Fibromuscular hyperplasia is the second most commonly encountered stenosis of the renal artery. The lesion usually involves the middle and distal thirds of the renal artery, and frequently the segmental branch arteries are involved. In women in the twenty-five to forty-five age range the lesion is that of multiple mural hyperplasia with

Fig. 23-20. Incidence of renal artery stenosis, demonstrated by arteriography, in 317 hypertensive patients.

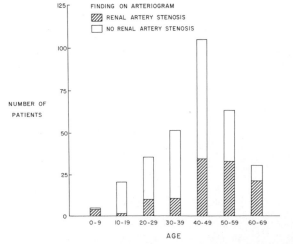

INCIDENCE OF ANGIOGRAPHIC RENAL ARTERY STENOSIS BY DECADE OF LIFE

the "string of beads" appearance (Fig. 23-7). In patients under twenty years of age and in the male in general a single mural hyperplasia (intimal hyperplasia) is more common (Fig. 23-11).

Less common lesions causing renal artery occlusion are aneurysm, embolism or thrombosis, and compression by a fibrous or muscular band or mass (Fig. 23-19).

Figure 23-20 shows the frequency of arteriographic demonstration of a renal artery stenosis in 317 hypertensive patients. Stenosis in patients under thirty years of age was almost exclusively due to fibromuscular dysplasia; arteriosclerosis was the predominant lesion in patients over fifty years of age. Between ages thirty and fifty the incidence of arteriosclerosis and fibromuscular dyplasia was about equal. Table 23-5 shows the arteriographic findings in the larger series of 1,070 patients.

A renal artery stenosis found on arteriogram in hypertensive patients does not establish a causal relationship. Two-thirds of patients over sixty years of age had a stenosis, but Fig. 23-12 shows that only half the stenoses were of proved functional significance. At present there are three ways of determining whether a stenosis is functionally significant: renal biopsy and histologic study of the juxtaglomerular apparatus, reninangiotensin assay, and split renal function study. The first (JGA study) is not very practical, and accumulated experience to date is quite limited. From our experience, if either of the latter two studies are positive, a good blood pressure response following operative treatment can be expected in 90 percent of the patients.

Split Renal Function Studies. In normal persons and persons with essential hypertension the two kidneys seldom vary significantly in their handling of water, sodium, or solutes. In renal artery stenosis a functionally ischemic kidney resorbs sodium and water excessively, while fixed solutes appear in the urine in increased concentration. These characteristics of the ischemic kidney led to the development of a number of tests to determine when a given stenosis is functionally significant. All the tests involve catheterizing the ureters, collecting urine specimens for successive controlled periods of time, and analyzing the urine specimens.

The Howard test was the first such test described. A reduction in urine volume of 50 percent and a reduction in urine sodium concentration of at least 15 percent or an increase of urinary creatinine concentration of at least 15 percent from the involved kidney have functional significance. The Rappaport test is based on sodium/creatinine ratios from each kidney. A tubular rejection fraction ration (TRFR) is obtained by multiplying the sodium/creatinine ratio on the left by that on the right. A ratio of less than 0.6 indicates significant left renal artery stenosis, and a ratio of more than 1.6 implicates the right renal artery. When the values are between 0.6 and 1.6, the test is negative. The Birchall test employs an infusion of hypertonic saline solution (0.25 Gm sodium chloride/100 ml/kg body weight in 45 minutes). Sodium/creatinine urinary concentration ratios from the two kidneys are compared. The larger sodium/creatinine ratio is divided by the smaller one; if the resultant value is 2 or more,

Table 23-5. RESULTS OF EVALUATION OF 1,070 HYPERTENSIVE PATIENTS

	Renal arteriogram	*Renovascular hypertension**
Normal	610 (57%)	—
Renal artery stenosis due to:		
Atherosclerosis	297 (43%)	114
Fibromuscular dysplasia . .	152	51 39% / 16%
Miscellaneous	11	11

*Positive functional tests—split renal function studies or renal venous renin assays.

the test is positive. The smaller ratio indicates the involved kidney. The Stamey test involves osmotic diuresis by means of an intravenous infusion of urea. Para-aminohippurate (PAH), a fixed solute excreted by the kidney but not resorbed by the tubules, is added to the infusion. Functionally significant renal artery stenosis is suggested when the involved kidney shows a 66 percent smaller urine volume and a 100 percent greater PAH concentration than the uninvolved kidney. In the Stamey test one also determines the effective renal plasma flow (ERPF) in each kidney. This is valuable in assessing the function of the contralateral or normal kidney; severely impaired plasma flow usually indicates intrarenal small vessel disease. Table 23-6 shows the results of split renal function studies in patients with functionally significant right renal artery stenosis.

In bilateral renal artery stenosis, the split function studies are frequently difficult to interpret; however, in most cases of bilateral stenosis there is a marked discrepancy in the severity of stenosis on the two sides, and the split function studies demonstrate this functional difference.

The author's experience is limited to the use of the Howard and Stamey tests. The original criteria for the interpretation of these tests were based on a very small number of patients. In the beginning we adhered rigidly to those criteria in selecting patients for operative treatment. However, since 1966 liberalized criteria for a positive test have been used. A recent retrospective study of 41 patients who are unequivocally cured following unilateral renal arterial surgery revealed that the following criteria seem to suffice for a positive test: (1) consistently lateralizing discrepancies in the triplicate samples; (2) Howard test—25 percent reduction in urine volume and 15 percent increase in creatinine from the involved kidney as compared with the contralateral kidney; and (3) Stamey test—25 percent increase in PAH concentration and 25 percent reduction in urine volume in the affected kidney.

Disadvantages of split renal function studies include patient discomfort and occasional complications secondary to the study, e.g., urinary tract infection, ureteral colic, and, rarely, transient ureteral obstruction secondary to edema. A more frequent problem is technical failure to obtain a satisfactory study in about 10 percent of the patients. This occurs most frequently in the male over fifty years of age with prostatic enlargement which interferes with ureteral catheterization.

Renal Venous Renin Assay. If the renin-angiotensin pressor system is the mechanism through which renal artery stenosis causes renovascular hypertension, assay of these substances should afford an accurate way of detecting the disorder. Reports by Fitz, by McPhaul et al., and by Michelakis et al. support this concept. Renin assays, using a radioimmunoassay technique, are now widely available and have proved to be extremely accurate in demonstrating renovascular hypertension. Peripheral venous renin assays are important in detecting primary aldosteronism or other conditions in which renin secretion is severely depressed. However, for the diagnosis of renovascular hypertension, comparative assays of the renin activity in the individual renal veins are usually required. In our initial report, Michelakis et al. stated that the criterion for a positive study was a 1.5 renin ratio when comparing the involved and uninvolved kidneys, and we have continued to use this criterion. Ernst and his associates have indicated that a 1.4 ratio is sufficient, and under certain circumstances (e.g., extensive collateralization) even a smaller ratio is significant.

Disadvantages of the renal vein renin assay are few. Thrombophlebitis subsequent to femoral vein catheterization is occasionally encountered. Catheterization of the renal veins under fluoroscopic control is simple and almost always feasible.

Table 23-6. RESULTS OF SPLIT RENAL FUNCTION STUDIES IN PATIENTS WITH RIGHT RENAL ARTERY STENOSIS

	Right kidney			*Left kidney*			*Serum*		
	Patient 1	*Patient 2*	*Patient 3*	*Patient 1*	*Patient 2*	*Patient 3*	*Patient 1*	*Patient 2*	*Patient 3*
Volume, ml/min	1.6	1.5	2.4	15.2	18.0	23.2			
Na, mEq/L	35.0	43.0	54.0	70.0	93.0	103.0	140.0		
Creatinine, mg/100 ml .	19.0	18.0	16.0	5.0	3.5	3.5	0.67	0.67	0.67
Creatinine clearance, ml/min	55.0	49.0	70.0	138.0	115.0	148.0			
PAH, mg/100 ml	264.0	240.0	216.0	60.0	52.0	48.0	1.84	1.76	1.76
PAH cleared, mg/min . .	4.224	3.600	5.184	9.120	9.360	11.136			
ERPF, ml/min	281	250.0	360.0	605.0	649.0	772.0			
Osmolality, mOsm/kg . .	488	522	532	275	292	309	290	292	299

Relative Value of Split Renal Function Studies and Renal Venous Renin Assays in Renovascular Hypertension. Now that renin assays are fairly widely available, many physicians are using this test alone to determine when a renal artery stenosis is causing hypertension. As mentioned earlier, in our experience when either or both of the tests are positive, a good blood pressure response will follow operative treatment in 90 percent of the cases. We have persisted in using both tests whenever feasible and recommend operative treatment when either is positive. Retrospective analysis of patients who are unequivocally cured following operative treatment of unilateral lesions reveals that about 10 percent had negative or normal split function studies and the same number had negative or normal renin assays. In each of these patients the other test had been positive. There are a number of variables which influence the results of both tests, and these variables are often difficult to control. We think the two tests complement each other and, in addition, the renal function studies provide valuable information regarding the status of the contralateral, or uninvolved, kidney.

Preoperative Renal Biopsy. Vertes et al. have advocated percutaneous biopsy of the kidney in the assessment of patients with renovascular hypertension. They have correctly noted that there are degrees of intrarenal arterial and arteriolar nephrosis which *may* preclude a beneficial result following corrective surgery. The problem has been to determine when such changes exist. Schacht et al., Baker et al., and Strickler have reported patients with renovascular hypertension and a renal biopsy interpreted as moderate or severe who have been cured or unequivocally improved by corrective surgery. In the future a well-controlled retrospective study of a large group of patients with renovascular hypertension may validate the recommendation of Vertes et al. However, it must also be pointed out that the etiology of hypertension does not follow an "all-or-none" law. Patients with severe renovascular hypertension due to an ischemic kidney may also have an element of hypertension as the result of arteriolar nephrosclerosis. Correction of the renovascular lesion will often change such a patient from the category of malignant hypertension to a mild hypertensive categorized as improved in the results of treatment. This has been observed repeatedly in older patients with complete occlusion of a renal artery.

TREATMENT. Selection of Patients for Surgical Treatment. Patients who have significant diastolic hypertension secondary to a functionally significant rental artery stenosis, as demonstrated by split renal function study or renal vein renin assay, and who present a reasonable surgical risk should have corrective surgical treatment. The consideration of surgical risk is relative. A patient with severe or malignant renovascular hypertension, even though cardiac or central nervous system complications may have already occurred, should have corrective surgical treatment if at all possible because of the extremely poor prognosis if the hypertension is not brought under control. Stamey and others have stated that unless the contralateral, uninvolved kidney has a renal plasma flow of 200 ml/minute or more, as determined by split function study, the patient will not benefit from corrective surgery. As with Vertes' opinion regarding nephrosclerosis, future analysis of differential renal function studies in a large number of patients may provide accurate prognostic information of this sort. The author and others have seen patients with unilateral renovascular hypertension and contralateral renal plasma flow of less than 200 ml/minute who have been benefited by corrective surgery.

Preoperative Preparation. If at all possible the patient should be off antihypertensive medication for 10 days or 2 weeks before operation. These agents alter the vasomotor system so that when a general anesthetic is administered, profound vasomotor collapse may occur. Reserpine and other *Rauwolfia* drugs are notorious for this effect: it takes 10 to 14 days for patients on reserpine or guanethidine to become free of their effects. However, there are patients in whom the hypertension is so severe that antihypertensive medication must be continued up to and even during the surgical procedure. This has been demonstrated particularly in young children with malignant hypertension secondary to renal artery stenosis. In such instances control of the blood pressure with alpha-methyldopa, a relatively short-acting agent which does not deplete the nerve endings of norepinephrine stores, has been well tolerated, and vasomotor instability has not been a problem. In general, if the anesthetist knows that the patient has been receiving drugs, anesthesia can be administered safely.

Renal artery reconstruction or nephrectomy should not be undertaken after split renal function study or renal arteriography until it has been determined that these procedures have not caused any degree of renal injury. This is rarely a problem after arteriography, but after split renal function study some degree of ureteral edema is not infrequent. If one adds the trauma of a period of renal artery occlusion or removal of functioning kidney tissue, a disastrous result may ensue. Therefore a 2- or 3-day period should elapse between split renal function study and the surgical procedure, during which the patient's urine output and BUN levels should be monitored. If there is evidence of renal or ureteral injury, the operative procedure should be postponed until the patient has fully recovered.

A blood volume deficit of 500 to 1,740 ml is encountered in 31 percent of patients with renovascular hypertension. Preoperatively the blood volume should be determined, and appropriate correction of plasma or red blood cell deficits should be made to avoid postoperative hypotension and attendant thrombotic complications. In the occasional patient with secondary aldosteronism, metabolic aberrations must be corrected preoperatively.

Operative Treatment. In the selection of an operative procedure for renovascular hypertension, preservation of renal tissue is a prime consideration. Nephrectomy should be done only as a last resort. Patients with both fibromuscular and atherosclerotic lesions frequently have progression of insignificant lesions or develop new lesions in the contralateral renal artery. The younger the patient, the more important this consideration becomes. At present about the only indication for nephrectomy is a destroyed, virtually nonfunctioning kidney.

Adequate exposure for reconstruction of the renal arteries can be obtained through either a long midline incision from the pubic symphysis to the xiphoid or a supraumbilical transverse incision extending from flank to flank. When a coexisting lesion of the abdominal aorta, an aneurysm, or occlusive disease requires attention, the midline incision provides better exposure for dealing with the iliac arteries. Previously we performed bilateral renal biopsy and measurement of pressure gradients across the stenosis in every case. The value of these observations was quite limited, and now these determinations rarely are made. Any value judgment of bilateral renal biopsies must await the report of the pathologists of The Cooperative Study of Renal Arterial Hypertension. They are analyzing biopsy material from several hundred cases. As regards pressure gradients, as Thomas et al. have pointed out, if there is one present, it means the stenosis is significant, but the absence of a gradient is difficult to interpret.

To expose the left renal artery, the entire small bowel is retracted to the right, and the posterior peritoneum overlying the aorta is incised. With appropriate dissection of the surrounding retroperitonal fatty areolar tissue, the left renal vein crossing the aorta is displaced superiorly and the left renal artery exposed. To expose the right renal artery, the inferior vena cava is mobilized and retracted to the right to expose the origin and first portion of the artery. One or more pairs of lumbar veins may be divided in this dissection. To approach the distal right renal artery, the hepatic flexure of the colon and the second portion of the duodenum are mobilized and retracted to the left, and the dissection is carried down to expose the distal right renal vein and artery. This approach is now used in most cases of right renal artery stenosis. It provides the best exposure for an anastomosis between the graft and the renal artery.

The most applicable and most commonly used operative procedure is either a thromboendarterectomy, with or without a patch graft, or some form of bypass graft from the aorta to the renal artery distal to the stenosis (Fig. 23-21). Other operative procedures include splenorenal anastomosis, implantation of the renal artery into the side of the aorta; resection of the lesion with end-to-end anastomosis of the renal artery; and interposition of a graft into the renal artery (Fig. 23-22).

When thromboendarterectomy is performed, the remaining renal artery is usually an extremely delicate and thin-walled structure. A patch graft of autogenous vein or Dacron is often required to avoid narrowing of the renal artery lumen by the suture line. Sometimes a thromboendarterectomy can be performed transaortically after the aorta has been occluded above the renal artery, thus avoiding direct handling and suturing of the renal artery. Transaortic endarterectomy in patients with orificial atherosclerotic lesions has been strongly advocated by Wylie and Starney and their associates.

From a practical point of view, the bypass procedure is the most widely applicable. In dealing with a small renal artery, as in most cases of fibromuscular hyperplasia, a segment of saphenous vein or autologous hypogastric artery lends itself well to a precise, delicate anastomosis with the renal artery (Fig. 23-23). If the distal renal artery is

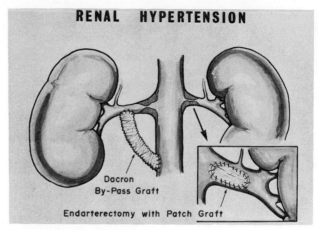

Fig. 23-21. The most commonly employed methods of correcting a renal artery stenosis. Saphenous vein or a Dacron prosthesis may be used for a bypass or patch graft.

large, as is often the case in arteriosclerotic lesions with poststenotic dilatation, a Dacron prosthesis works quite well (Fig. 23-24).

Prior to application of occluding vascular clamps the patient is given 50 mg of heparin intravenously. A mannitol solution is infused intravenously to stimulate osmotic diuresis prior to and during periods of renal artery occlusion. The graft is first anastamosed end to side to the renal artery. This is the more difficult anastomosis and is easier if done first. Occluding vascular clamps are then removed from the renal artery, and a small bulldog clamp is placed across the graft at the anastomotic site. The aortic anastomosis is then done. A recent improvement in technique has been the use of a monofilament polypropylene suture material (Prolene). Previously we had used a braided polyester suture and routinely encountered brisk bleeding from the suture lines requiring administration of 2 or more units of blood and reversal of the heparin with protamine. Since 1971 we have used the polypropylene suture; we have noted minimal anastomotic bleeding, blood transfu-

Fig. 23-22. Various operative procedures available to correct a renal artery stenosis.

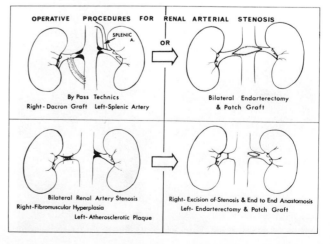

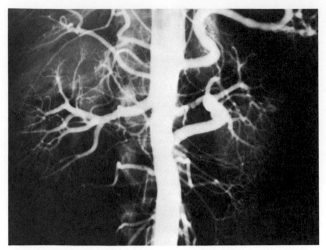

Fig. 23-23. Aortogram showing left aorticorenal bypass graft 1 year after implantation (same patient as Fig. 23-18). The graft is a segment of saphenous vein.

sion rarely has been necessary, and we have not had to give protamine. A review of 38 comparable procedures showed over twice as much blood replacement was required with the braided suture. Examination of the braided suture under the microscope reveals that it is quite porous and has an irregular serrated surface when compared with smooth monofilament material. When the braided suture is pulled through an artery or vein, a sawing effect results which enlarges the hole created by the needle. We believe this is the cause of the greater suture line's bleeding with the braided suture. At any rate the polypropylene suture creates a watertight suture line. It has virtually no drag as it is pulled through the vessel wall. One must take care to avoid a purse-string effect with this suture. For this

Fig. 23-24. Aortogram showing bilateral aorticorenal bypass grafts of crimped Dacron. This aortogram was obtained 4 years after the operation (preoperative aortogram is shown in Fig. 23-5).

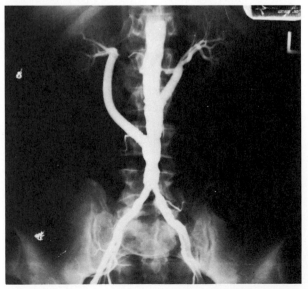

reason the suture line is interrupted in four places, and the arteriotomy is held open widely with traction sutures during the anastomosis.

In constructing an aorticorenal bypass great care must be taken in orienting the course of the graft so as to avoid kinking or twisting. Wylie et al. and Fry and his associates prefer an end-to-end anastomosis between the renal artery and the graft. This technique avoids angulation at the renal artery anastomosis which sometimes causes kinking. If a kink is encountered, the anastomosis must be redone. The best course for the graft from the renal artery to the aorta varies from patient to patient. On the left side the graft usually seems to course better behind the left renal vein. On the right side a retrocaval course usually works best.

If the aortic bifurcation has been resected, because of occlusive disease or aneurysm, and there is a coexisting significant renal artery stenosis, a side-arm bypass graft can be attached in the aortic prosthesis before the graft is interposed between the aorta and iliac arteries and subsequently anastomosed to the renal artery.

Renal transplantation experience has shown that if the vasculature of the donor kidney is washed out and the kidney cooled, tubular necrosis and renal dysfunction are minimized. This technique is now being employed in renal artery reconstructions. When the renal artery is opened, a cannula is inserted and the kidney perfused with 500 ml of a saline solution which has been cooled to 1 to 2°C. The perfusate is collected from the renal vein to prevent its entrance into the systemic circulation. Thereafter the arterial reconstruction is done. This technique produces a core kidney temperature of 16°C. The results with this technique are only preliminary, but they appear to show better tubular function in the early postoperative period, and no complications have attended the procedure. Prior to adoption of this technique, the triple isotope renogram done on the first postoperative day would show normal renal artery blood flow but poor tubular function. With this technique, tubular function appears to be normal or near normal on the first postoperative day. Again, these are preliminary results.

Another perplexing problem has been the patient with renovascular hypertension secondary to stenoses and/or aneurysm in the distal renal artery with extension into the branch renal arteries, usually fibromuscular lesions. A distal renal arterial segment suitable for conventional bypass is not present. In the past for many such patients nephrectomy was performed. However, the propensity for the development of bilateral severe lesions in these patients has dampened any enthusiasm for nephrectomy. In patients with stenoses involving the segmental branch arteries, Fry and his associates adopted a technique of using olive-tipped dilators to dilate these lesions and have presented interesting follow-up arteriographic data supporting the merits of the procedure.

Renal transplantation experience has led to an alternative technique that appears to be applicable in these patients: ex vivo reconstruction of the renal artery. Ota et al., Lim et al., and Belzer as well as others have reported use of this technique. The exact details of the operative procedure have varied from group to group, and the technique is still in the developmental stage. We have employed the procedure in five renal arterial reconstructions, anatomically successful in each instance. The renal artery and vein are divided close to the aorta and vena cava. The kidney is then rotated out on the abdominal wall onto a small operating platform. The ureter has been mobilized to allow this maneuver but has not been divided. The renal vasculature is flushed with 500 ml of a cold (1 to 2°C) saline solution. The artery is then attached to the Belzer apparatus and perfused with an acellular, oxygenated solution. Gravity is used to return the venous effluent to the Belzer pump. Using magnification and 7-0 arterial sutures, the multiple segmental renal artery lesions are repaired. In the case of terminal renal artery aneurysm the branch arteries are implanted into a saphenous vein graft. The artery or vein graft is then implanted into the common iliac artery and the renal vein into the distal vena cava. Ureteral collaterals, in cases of severe stenosis, can lead to significant renal blood flow which appears in the venous effluent. This can be avoided by application of atraumatic Potts ties to the ureteral artery. It is too early to judge this technique, but it appears to be an exciting development in renal artery surgery.

The problem of what to do in case of a severe functionally significant stenosis in one renal artery and a moderate nonsignificant stenosis in the other has not yet been answered objectively. In the opinion of some, performing a bypass on the side with the moderate stenosis adds little time or risk to the operative procedure, may be beneficial in avoiding future problems, and will improve renal blood flow. The evidence supporting this concept at the present time is tenuous.

Postoperative Care. Following renal artery reconstruction the patient is maintained on nasogastric suction and intravenous fluids for 3 to 5 days. Central venous pressure is monitored in the early postoperative period in older patients and in any patient with an impaired myocardial reserve. Most patients have some degree of diuresis following successful repair. In an occasional patient the diuresis may be massive, and severe electrolyte aberrations may ensue if the losses are not replaced. Urine output is monitored hourly via an indwelling catheter, and daily urinary output of sodium, potassium, and chlorides is determined, as are the serum levels of these electrolytes. Significant losses are replaced quantitatively. The patient is weighed daily to gauge fluid balance and to avoid overloading. It is difficult to overemphasize the importance of this simple observation. These patients often have an impaired myocardial reserve, and a fluid overload can result in congestive heart failure, pulmonary edema, and accelerated hypertension.

The blood volume should be determined early in the postoperative period, and the hematocrit should be monitored for several days. Postoperative hypotension and oliguria are usually related to an inadequate blood volume, due either to failure to expand a contracted blood volume preoperatively or to failure to replace operative blood losses.

Severe hypertension in the postoperative period is not an uncommon problem. There are a number of underlying causes: *Hypothermia* with peripheral vasoconstriction is managed by warming the patient and administering Thorazine. *Fluid overload* with increased central venous pressure and weight gain is managed with fluid restriction and judicious diuretic therapy. Finally, a number of patients will have *severe blood pressure elevations* that cannot be explained and must be treated with antihypertensive drugs; alpha-methyldopa is administered intravenously (500 mg every 4 to 6 hours) for several days. If hypertension becomes more severe than it was preoperatively, thrombosis of the reconstruction is to be strongly suspected. An excretory urogram or renogram is helpful in determining whether the kidney is functioning properly; if it is not, renal arteriography should be performed. Thrombosis of a renal artery reconstruction can result in malignant hypertension in a matter of a few days, as reported by Miller and Foster. Revision of the reconstruction or nephrectomy is usually required.

Some degree of transient azotemia is usually observed in patients who have undergone bilateral renal artery operations and in many patients who have had unilateral operation. This is probably due to renal tubular damage secondary to intraoperative renal artery occlusion which has been previously noted, and we are now reluctant to do bilateral simultaneous renal artery reconstructions. The degree of renal injury is usually minor, and with adequate hydration the BUN usually returns to normal by the time the patient is ready for discharge, ordinarily the eighth to tenth postoperative day. Renal failure secondary to tubular necrosis occasionally occurs after surgical treatment of renovascular hypertension. Other postoperative complications that have been recorded are those which might be expected in any seriously ill patient with hypertensive cardiovascular disease: myocardial infarction, congestive heart failure, cerebrovascular accident. Avoidance of hypotension or severe hypertension is the only means of preventing these complications.

RESULTS OF SURGICAL TREATMENT. The bulk of experience with operative treatment of renovascular hypertension has accumulated in the last decade. It is not surprising that there has been considerable variation in classifying the response to surgical treatment. Definition of the term "cure" presents the least problem: adults with documented diastolic hypertension who 3 or more months after surgical treatment have a diastolic blood pressure of less than 90 mm Hg are considered to be cured. It is more difficult to define a cure in children, especially children less than ten years of age.

The blood pressure response in the first 7 to 14 days after operative treatment is not a reliable index to the true response. The combination of the operation and strict bed rest may result in normal blood pressure levels which return to hypertensive levels when the patient resumes normal activity. On the other hand, some patients may remain hypertensive in the early postoperative period and become normotensive several weeks or months later. The greatest problem in defining response to treatment is in patients who are improved by operation but who continue to have a diastolic blood pressure above 90 mm Hg. These patients are largely the elderly, with atherosclerosis, who

Table 23-7. RESULTS OF OPERATIVE TREATMENT
OF RENOVASCULAR HYPERTENSION

Report	Period	Year of report	No. of patients	Cure, percent	Cure and improved, percent	Operative mortality, percent
Michigan	60–61	1962	43	40	82	4.0
Cleveland Clinic	57–61	1963	76	62	78	10.0
UCLA.	59-64	1964	67	37	82	4.0
Baylor	56–64	1966	432	41	81	7.0
Vanderbilt	62–65	1966	35	46	77	6.0
Mayo Clinic*	58–65	1967	100	55	84	0.0
UCSF	52–66	1967	122	37	65	8.0
Virginia	61–67	1968	53	28	75	3.6
Columbia	64–69	1970	40	53	76	2.5
Mayo Clinic†	64–70	1970	46	46	66	6.0
Cooperative Study . . .	61–69	In press	502	47	61	6.8
Vanderbilt‡	62–72	1973	122	70	90	5.4
UCSF§	52–62	1969	41	22	56	15.0
UCSF§	63–68	1969	42	26	74	2.4
Michigan*	61–70	1972	66	62	94	0.0

*None of these patients had simultaneous treatment of extrarenal atherosclerotic vascular lesions.
†All patients had aortic occlusive disease or aneurysm in addition to renal artery stenosis and operative treatment of both.
‡All patients had positive split renal function studies and/or renal venous renin assays.
§Atherosclerotic lesions only.

in addition to a renovascular cause for their hypertension have an underlying essential hypertension or arteriolar nephrosclerosis. "Improvement" has generally been defined as a persistent (i.e., at least 3 months) 20 mm Hg reduction in diastolic pressure. In the future, more rigid criteria for defining improvement should be forthcoming from such groups as The Cooperative Study of Renal Arterial Hypertension, which involves 13 institutions under U.S. Public Health Service sponsorship. The number of patients classified as failures or unimproved after surgical treatment will obviously be influenced by definition of the "improved" category; however, overt failures are quite obvious.

The time lapse between a successful operation for renovascular hypertension and a salutary blood pressure response has been variable. In most patients (perhaps 75 percent) the blood pressure recorded 1 month after operation accurately reflects the ultimate result; but some patients have required 3 months or more to become normotensive. The reasons for this are poorly understood.

Table 23-7 presents a composite view of the response to operative treatment of renovascular hypertension in a number of centers. Methods of selection of patients for operative treatment were varied, as were the criteria used to classify the operative result. The two reports with a 0 percent operative mortality omitted patients with simultaneous treatment of extrarenal atherosclerotic vascular lesions. A similar adjustment of our 1972 series would decrease the number of patients to 106 and the operative mortality to less than 3 percent. The Vanderbilt University Hospital series shows that more than 90 percent of the patients have a good result following operative treatment if the preoperative functional studies were positive. Figure

23-25 shows our yearly incidence of renal artery operations for renovascular hypertension since 1962.

Interest in renovascular hypertension varies widely from one center to another in the United States. In a few institutions the condition is being recognized frequently; however, in most centers it is identified only occasionally or is virtually unknown. There are several reasons for this difference: (1) A prime reason is that in the late 1950s and early 1960s many patients with hypertension and an associated renal artery stenosis had operative treatment but were not benefited. They did not have functional evidence of renovascular hypertension. This experience dampened or extinguished interest in renovascular hypertension. (2) There is widespread belief that renovascular hypertension is a rare condition. Our experience indicates that about 5 percent of patients with diastolic hypertension have renovascular hypertension. By conservative estimate there are at least 30 million patients with hypertension in the United States, or 1.5 million patients with renovascular hypertension. The condition can hardly be considered rare. (3) A multidisciplinary team approach to the study of the patient with hypertension is necessary if patients with renovascular hypertension are to be recognized. The internist is the key physician; if the experience of the 1950s and early 1960s has left him with little interest in renovascular hypertension (Item 1, above) or if he believes renovascular hypertension is rare (Item 2), he will probably treat his hypertensive patients with drugs and not try to find an underlying cause for the high blood pressure. Our group had a slow start, but the medical community has gradually adopted the philosphy of complete study of the patient with hypertension. While we have detailed data on 1,070 hypertensive patients, it is probable that an equal number of hypertensive patients have been evaluated according to the same protocol in our community. This explains the high frequency (16 percent) of renovascular hypertension in the 1,070 patients—many of the patients have been referred after a positive pyelogram or arteriogram.

In the past 15 years there have been tremendous advances in the drug therapy of hypertension. Freis and his associates have presented convincing evidence of the efficacy of antihypertensive drug treatment of hypertension and prevention of the complications attending hypertension. However, drug therapy has many untoward side effects. Most notable is postural hypotension. In many hypertensive patients effective control of the blood pressure is limited to the time spent in the upright position; hypertension during the hours spent in the supine position must be accepted. Control of the supine blood pressure may result in intolerable hypotension in the upright position.

Shapiro and his associates and others have stated that patients with renovascular hypertension who are over fifty years of age should not have operative treatment. From their experience it was felt that the risk is too great and the chance of a good result is too small. They advised drug therapy in this age group. Fifty-two of our patients were over fifty years of age, and 80 percent of them were either cured or improved following operative treatment. The operative mortality (10 percent) was higher in these older patients, but this was primarily because of patients who had simultaneous operative treatment of extrarenal vascular lesions such as an aortic aneurysm or occlusive disease.

A comparative study of drug treatment and operative treatment of renovascular hypertension has not yet been reported. Our group is presently doing such a prospective randomized study, but it is too early to report any results.

Figure 23-25 shows the number of patients a year since 1960 who have had renal artery operations. An analysis of the results of surgical treatment related to the type of renal artery lesion shows that patients with fibromuscular hyperplasia are cured more often (73 percent) than patients with an arteriosclerotic plaque (53 percent), although the improved group of patients contains a higher percentage of patients with arteriosclerosis. If the results of treatment are related to the type of surgical procedure, renal artery reconstruction has resulted in cure in 76 percent, while cure has been effected in 52 percent of nephrectomized patients. However, the nephrectomy series contains a larger proportion of the improved patients.

The severity of arteriolar nephrosclerosis, as determined by study of bilateral renal biopsies, has not correlated well with the response to operative treatment. There is a higher incidence of severe arteriolar nephrosclerosis in the unimproved group and of benign arteriolar nephrosclerosis in the cured group, but there are numbers of patients with severe changes who have been cured and of unimproved patients with benign changes.

Renovascular hypertension due to unilateral stenosis can so severely damage the contralateral kidney that it becomes the more powerful renin-secreting kidney. In this

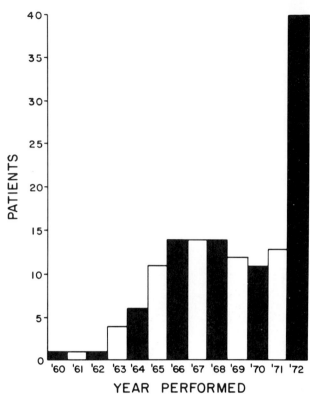

Fig. 23-25. Number of patients undergoing operative treatment for renovascular hypertension each year since 1960 at Vanderbilt University Hospital.

condition, the kidney with the renal artery stenosis is protected from the ravages of severe hypertension. Floyer demonstrated this experimentally in the 1950s, and there have been occasional reports providing human confirmation since that time (Thal et al., Marable et al., Morris et al., and others). We have encountered this situation in two patients, one of whom was reported by McAllister et al. Relief of the hypertension requires unilateral arterial reconstruction and contralateral removal of the kidney which has been destroyed by the hypertension (Fig. 23-26). An interesting observation has emerged from the treatment of these patients and of patients with a solitary kidney with renal artery stenosis—their blood pressure returns to normal immediately following successful operative treatment. This is in contradistinction to many patients with renovascular hypertension due to unilateral stenosis in whom it may require days, weeks, or even months before the blood pressure becomes normal. In these patients, as Alpert et al. have shown, it seems likely that the contralateral kidney has been damaged by hypertension. The ultimate result then depends on whether the damage is reversible; if reversible, considerable time may be required.

The reported incidence of thrombosis or stenosis of a renal artery reconstruction has ranged from 15 to 35 percent. In our experience and in that of Ernst et al. and Fry

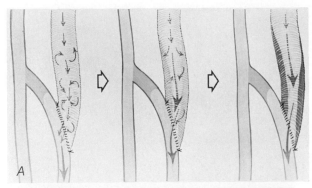

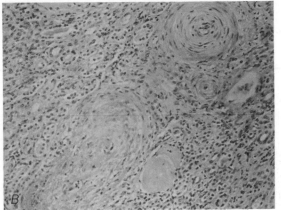

Fig. 23-26. *A.* Dacron graft bypass to right renal artery. *B.* Photomicrograph showing destroyed left kidney which was removed. Arteriolar changes including fibrinoid necrosis are apparent.

et al., thrombosis usually occurs in the first few postoperative days and is due to technical errors in performing the reconstruction. With experience and improved operative technique it has been possible to reduce the frequency of this complication to less than 5 percent. Immediate post-repair arteriograms and flowmeter studies should help reduce this problem further.

Serious postoperative complications have occurred frequently in these patients. Many have compromised cardiac function, and congestive failure and pulmonary edema are common problems unless fluid balance is carefully managed. Table 23-8 lists the complications in 122 patients.

There have been few reported follow-up arteriographic

Table 23-8. POSTOPERATIVE COMPLICATIONS
OF OPERATIVE TREATMENT OF
RENOVASCULAR HYPERTENSION

Complication	No. of Patients
Congestive heart failure	4
Acute tubular necrosis	4
Intestinal obstruction	2
Aortic suture line disruption	1
Basilar artery thrombosis	1
Hemolytic crisis	1
Bracheal plexus stretch injury	1
Renal arteriovenous fistula	1
Abdominal angina	1

data on aorticorenal bypass. Exceptions are the reports of Kaufman et al. and of Ernst et al. Ernst and Fry and their associates have shown that the saphenous vein, used to construct an aorticorenal bypass, almost routinely undergoes uniform dilatation, sometimes progressing to aneurysmal proportions. We have noted these same changes, and vein graft aneurysm has occurred in 2 of 68 patients 4 to 6 years following implantation (Fig. 23-27). Arteriographic follow-up studies of aorticorenal bypass utilizing hypogastric artery are needed.

UNILATERAL RENAL PARENCHYMAL DISEASE

There is an ill-defined group of patients with hypertension who have a small atrophic kidney on one side, a normal or hypertrophic contralateral kidney, and no evidence of main or segmental renal artery stenosis on arteriography. The underlying etiologic factors have usually been unilateral pyelonephritis, congenital hypoplasia, radiation fibrosis, or posttraumatic fibrosis. The problem has been to determine when an atrophic kidney is responsible for the hypertension. For 20 years after Goldblatt's original studies, nephrectomy was frequently performed on the basis of hypertension and an associated small kidney. Although these patients were operated on because it was thought they might have a "Goldblatt kidney," remission in the hypertension was observed infrequently. Smith's review in 1956 of 575 patients indicated that only 26 percent were benefited.

A recent 5-year experience with hypertensive patients, involving careful study in search of an underlying cause, indicates that perhaps 5 percent have a small kidney on one side and no evidence of main or segmental renal artery stenosis on arteriography. The involved kidney may be anywhere from 3 to 7 cm shorter than its mate, and the renal cortex of the involved kidney is proportionately thinned. The uninvolved kidney may be normal in length or hypertrophic (less than 13.5 to 14 cm long). Renal artery stenosis can cause these same changes in kidney length. However, in unilateral parenchymal disease the main renal artery and its segmental branches are uniformly small throughout, without evidence of stenosis or occlusion. In unilateral pyelonephritis, calyceal clubbing is usually seen on the pyelogram. There are often areas in the parenchyma which suggest focal atrophy, and there is distortion of the small intrarenal arterial branches. In so-called "congenital hypoplasia" all the structures are small and may be diminutive but have no distortion or other abnormality.

Recent reports by McDonald, by Hickler, et al., and by Crocker et al. indicate that nephrectomy in patients with unilateral renal parenchymal disease has been accompanied by cure or improvement of their hypertension only if there was evidence of an ischemic pattern on split renal function study. The author's experience indicates that an increase in the renal vein renin from the involved side is equally valid. In the case of a totally nonfunctioning kidney, renal vein renin assays may be the only means of

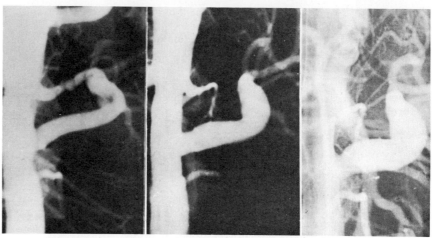

Fig. 23-27. Arteriograms showing a saphenous vein aorticorenal artery bypass 1, 3, and 5 years after implantation. Aneurysmal dilatation is apparent at 5 years.

determining functional significance as regards the hypertension. Hypertension due to unilateral renal parenchymal disease is of unknown pathogenesis but is generally considered to result from activation of the renal pressor mechanism by intrarenal small artery disease.

SURGICAL TREATMENT OF ESSENTIAL HYPERTENSION

During the era 1940 through 1959, before effective antihypertensive drug therapy was available, thoracolumbar sympathectomy or splanchnicectomy was used frequently in the treatment of patients with severe diastolic hypertension. During the latter part of this period, bilateral total or subtotal adrenalectomy alone or in conjunction with thoracolumbar sympathectomy was advocated for control of severe hypertension. The effectiveness of these forms of treatment depends on interrupting the increased peripheral resistance so commonly present in most forms of diastolic hypertension. Beneficial and at times long-lasting results were obtained with these forms of treatment, as documented in reports by Grimson, Smithwick, Zintel, and Jeffers et al. During the following decade these forms of surgical treatment were largely abandoned, being replaced by the use of the potent antihypertensive drugs currently available.

Recently, baropacing of the carotid sinus nerve as a means of decreasing peripheral resistance and thereby lowering the blood pressure has been the subject of experimental and clinical studies reported by Schwartz and Griffith and by Bilgutay and Lillehei. The carotid sinus nerve, a branch of the glossopharyngeal nerve, is the afferent nerve of the carotid baroreceptor reflex and transmits to the medullary vasomotor centers action potentials which originate in the carotid sinus. Under normal conditions, an increase in the intraluminal pressure of the carotid baroreceptor reflexly lowers blood pressure, induces bradycardia, decreases cardiac output, and diminishes venous return. When pressure is lowered in the baroreceptor, the reverse occurs. Chronic neurogenic vasoconstriction is thought to occur when the baroreceptor mechanism loses its efficiency or is "reset" at elevated blood pressure levels. This resetting has been attributed to the development of refractoriness or elevation of the thresholds of the baroreceptors in chronic hypertensive states. McCubbin et al. hypothesized that either the vasomotor centers are altered by hypertension and unable to appreciate afferent stimuli from the baroreceptor organs or there is an adaptation within the baroreceptor, so that an insufficient number of impulses results from the hypertension stimulus. Using electroneurography, they demonstrated that the baroreceptors continued to function in hypertension but that the threshold stimulus required to trigger the receptor was significantly raised. These observations led to Warner's use of electrical stimulation of the carotid sinus nerve to lower systemic blood pressure in the dog. Subsequently, Griffith and Schwartz reported reversal of renal hypertension in dogs by electrical stimulation of the carotid sinus nerve, an observation confirmed by Bilgutay and Lillehei. Chronic electrical stimulation of the carotid sinus nerve as a method of treating hypertension has been applied clinically. The stimulator, or baropacer, was implanted in the neck and connected to the carotid sinus nerve; unilateral stimulation was initially employed, and more recently bilateral stimulation has been used. Schwartz and Griffith have reported encouraging results with treatment of 11 hypertensive patients, and Bilgutay and Lillehei have had favorable experiences with 2 patients.

At present, stimulation of the carotid sinus nerve in the treatment of hypertension must be considered an experimental approach. Two major unresolved questions are whether chronic stimulation will result in fibrosis and destruction of the nerve and whether the baroreceptor system will eventually reset itself so that hypertension will recur. Experience with baropacing continues to accumulate slowly. In addition to controlling hypertension, it has been reported to be useful in management of angina pectoris and paroxysmal supraventricular tachycardia. Recent reports have been summarized by Brest. More study of this method of treatment is needed. It may eventually prove to be a valuable addition to the treatment of hypertension.

Bilateral nephrectomy and renal transplantation for patients with severe essential hypertension and end-stage renal disease are discussed in Chap. 10.

References

Pheochromocytoma

Scott, H. W., Jr., Riddell, D. H., and Brockman, S. K.: Surgical Management of Pheochromocytoma, *Surg Gynecol Obstet,* **120:**707, 1965.

Van Way, C. W., III, Michelakis, A. M., Alper, B. J., Hutcheson, J. K., Rhamy, R. K., and Scott, H. W., Jr.: Renal Vein Renin Studies in a Patient with Renal Hilar Pheochromocytoma and Renal Artery Stenosis, *Ann Surg,* **172:**212, 1970.

Primary Aldosteronism

Conn, J. W.: Primary Aldosteronism: A New Clinical Syndrome, *J Lab Clin Med,* **45:**3, 1955.

———, Cohen, E. L., and Rovner, D. R.: Suppression of Plasma Renin Activity in Primary Aldosteronism, *JAMA,* **190:**125, 1964.

———, ———, ———, and Nesbit, R. M.: Special Communication: Normokalemic Primary Aldosteronism, *JAMA,* **193:**100, 1965.

———, Knoph, R. F., and Nesbit, R. M.: Primary Aldosteronism: Present Evaluation of Its Clinical Characteristics and the Results of Surgery, in E. E. Baulieu and P. Robel, *"Aldosterone,"* Blackwell Scientific Publications, Ltd., Oxford, 1964.

Egdahl, R. H., Kahn, P. C., and Melby, J. C.: Unilateral Adrenalectomy for Aldosteronomas Localized Preoperatively by Differential Adrenal Vein Catheterization, *Surgery,* **64:**117, 1968.

Fishman, L. M., Kuchel, O., Liddle, G. W., Michelakis, A. M., Gordon, R. D., and Chick, W. T.: Incidence of Primary Aldosteronism in Uncomplicated "Essential" Hypertension, *JAMA,* **205:**497, 1968.

Grim, C. E., McBryde, A. C., Glenn, J. F., and Gunnels, J. C., Jr.: Childhood Primary Aldosteronism with Bilateral Adrenocortical Hyperplasia: Plasma Renin Activity As an Aid to Diagnosis, *Pediatrics,* **71:**377, 1967.

Melby, J. C., Spark, R. F., Dale, S. L., Egdahl, R. H., and Kahn, P. C.: Diagnosis and Localization of Aldosterone-Producing Adenomas by Adrenal-Vein Catheterization, *N Engl J Med,* **277:**1050, 1967.

Silen, W., Biglieri, E. G., Slaton, P., and Galante, M.: Management of Primary Aldosteronism, *Ann Surg,* **164:**600, 1966.

Cushing's Syndrome

Cushing, H.: The Basophil Adenomas of the Pituitary Gland and Their Clinical Manifestations, *Bull Johns Hopkins Hosp,* **50:**137, 1932.

Hayes, M.: Operative Treatment of Adrenal Cortical Hyperfunctionary Disease, *Ann Surg,* **154:**33, 1961.

Liddle, G. W.: Tests of Pituitary-Adrenal Suppressibility in the Diagnosis of Cushing's Syndrome, *J Clin Endocrinol Metab,* **20:**1939, 1960.

———: "Cushing's Syndrome: The Adrenal Cortex," Little, Brown and Company, Boston, 1967.

Orth, D. N., and Liddle, G. W.: Results of Treatment in 108 Patients with Cushing's Syndrome, *N Engl J Med,* **285:**243, 1971.

Scott, H. W., Jr.: "Tumors of the Endocrine Glands: Tumors of the Adrenal Cortex and Cushing's Syndrome," Seventh National Cancer Conference Proceedings, p. 513, 1973.

Coarctation of the Aorta

Beattie, E. J., Jr., Cooke, F. N., Paul, J. S., and Orbison, J. A.: Coarctation of Aorta at Level of Diaphragm Treated Successfully with Preserved Human Blood Vessel Graft, *J Thorac Surg,* **21:**506, 1951.

Bjork, V. O., and Intonti, F.: Coarctation of Abdominal Aorta with Right Renal Artery Stenosis, *Ann Surg,* **160:**54, 1964.

Crafoord, C., and Nylin, G.: Congenital Coarctation of the Aorta and Its Surgical Treatment, *J Thorac Cardiovasc Surg,* **14:**347, 1945.

Glenn, F., Keefer, E. B. C., Speer, D. S., and Dotter, C. T.: Coarctation of the Lower Thoracic and Abdominal Aorta Immediately Proximal to the Celiac Axis, *Surg Gynec Obstet,* **94:**561, 1952.

Gross, R. E., and Hufnagel, C. A.: Coarctation of the Aorta: Experimental Studies Regarding Its Surgical Correction, *N Engl J Med,* **233:**287, 1945.

Morris, G. C., Jr., DeBakey, M. E., Cooley, D. A., and Crawford, E. S.: Subisthmic Aortic Stenosis and Occlusive Disease, *Arch Surg,* **80:**87, 1960.

Robicsek, F., Sanger, P. W., and Daugherty, H. K.: Coarctation of the Abdominal Aorta Diagnosed by Aortography: Report of Three Cases, *Ann Surg,* **162:**227, 1965.

Renovascular Hypertension

Belzer, F. O., Salvatierra, O., Palubinskas, A., and Stoney, R. J.: Ex Vivo Renal Artery Reconstruction, *Ann Surg,* **182:**456, 1975.

Dean, R. H., and Foster, J. H.: Criteria for the Diagnosis of Renovascular Hypertension, *Surgery,* **74:**926, 1973.

DeBakey, M. E., Morris, G. C., Jr., Morgen, R. O., Crawford, E. S., and Cooley, D. A.: Lesions of the Renal Artery: Surgical Technic and Results, *Am J Surg,* **107:**84, 1964.

DeCamp, P. T., and Birchall, R.: Recognition and Treatment of Renal Artery Stenosis Associated with Hypertension, *Surgery,* **43:**134, 1958.

Dustan, H. P., Page, I. H., and Poutasse, E. F.: Renal Hypertension, *N Engl J Med,* **261:**647, 1959.

———, ———, ———, and Wilson, L.: An Evaluation of Treatment of Hypertension Associated with Occlusive Renal Arterial Disease, *Circulation,* **27:**1018, 1963.

Ernst, C. B., Bookstein, J. J., Montie, J., Baumgartel, E., Hoobler, S. W., and Fry, W. J.: Renal Vein Renin Ratios and Collateral Vessels in Renovascular Hypertension, *Arch Surg,* **104:**496, 1972.

———, Marshall, F. F., Stanley, J. C., and Fry, W. J.: Autogenous Saphenous Vein for Aortorenal Bypass: A Ten Year Experience, *Arch Surg,* **105:**855, 1972.

Foster, J. H.: Surgically Correctible Hypertension, in S. Schwartz (ed.), "Principles of Surgery," 2d ed., p. 939, McGraw Hill Book Company, 1974.

———, Dean, R. H., Pinkerton, J. A., and Rhamy, R. K.: Ten

Years Experience with the Surgical Management of Renovascular Hypertension, *Ann Surg,* 1973.

————, Klatte, E. C., and Burko, H. C.: Arteriographic Pitfalls in the Diagnosis of Renovascular Hypertension, *Arch Surg,* **99:**792, 1969.

————, Oates, J. A., Rhamy, R. K., Klatte, E. C., Burko, H. C., and Michelakis, A. M.: Hypertension and Fibromuscular Dysplasia of the Renal Arteries, *Surgery,* **65:**157, 1969.

————, ————, ————, Pettinger, W. A., Burko, H. C., Younger, R. K., and Scott, H. W., Jr.: Detection and Treatment of Patients with Renovascular Hypertension, *Surgery,* **60:**240, 1966.

————, Pettinger, W. A., Oates, J. A., Rhamy, R. K., Klatte, E. C., Burko, H. C., Bolasny, B. L., Gordon, R., Puyau, F. A., and Younger, R. K.: Malignant Hypertension Secondary to Renal Artery Stenosis in Children, *Ann Surg,* **164:**700, 1966.

————, Rhamy, R. K., Oates, J. A., Klatte, E. C., Burko, H. C., and Michelakis, A. M.: Renovascular Hypertension Secondary to Atherosclerosis, *Am J Med,* **46:**741, 1969.

Fry, W. J., Brink, B. E., and Thompson, N. W.: New Techniques in the Treatment of Extensive Fibromuscular Disease Involving the Renal Arteries, *Surgery,* **68:**959, 1970.

————, Ernst, C. B., Stanley, J. C., and Brink, B.: Renovascular Hypertension in the Pediatric Patient, *Arch Surg,* **107:**692, 1973.

Goldblatt, H., Lynch, J., Hanzal, R. F., and Summerville, W. W.: Studies on Experimental Hypertension, *J Exp Med,* **59:**347, 1934.

Holley, K. W., Hunt, J. C., Brown, A. L., Kincaid, O. W., and Sheps, S. G.: Renal Artery Stenosis: A Clinical-Pathologic Study in Normotensive and Hypertensive Patients, *Am J Med,* **37:**14, 1964.

Howard, J. E., and Connor, T. B.: Use of Differential Renal Function Studies in the Diagnosis of Renovascular Hypertension, *Am J Surg,* **107:**58, 1964.

Hunt, J. C., Harrison, E. G., Jr., Kincaid, O. W., Bernatz, P. E., and Davis, G. D.: Idiopathic Fibrous and Fibromuscular Stenoses of the Renal Arteries Associated with Hypertension, *Proc Staff Meetings Mayo Clin,* **37:**181, 1962.

Leadbetter, W. F., and Burkland, C. E.: Hypertension in Unilateral Renal Disease, *J Urol,* **39:**611, 1938.

Michelakis, A. M., Foster, J. H., Liddle, G. W., Rhamy, R. K., and Kuchel, O.: Measurement of Renin in Both Renal Veins and Its Use in Diagnosis of Renovascular Hypertension, *Arch Intern Med,* **120:**444, 1967.

Morris, G. C., Jr., DeBakey, M. E., Crawford, E. S., Cooley, D. A., and Zanger, L. C. C.: Late Results of Surgical Treatment for Renovascular Hypertension, *Surg Gynecol Obstet,* **122:**1255, 1966.

Ota, K., Mori, S., Awane, Y., and Ueno, A.: Ex Situ Repair of Renal Artery for Renovascular Hypertension, *Arch Surg,* **94:**370, 1967.

Page, I. H., and Corcoran, A. C.: Hypertension: Review of Humoral Pathogenesis and Clinical Treatment, *Adv Intern Med,* **1:**183, 1942.

Shapiro, A. P., Perez-Stable, E., Scheib, E. T., Bron, K., Montsos, S. E., Bert, G., and Misage, J. R.: Renal Artery Stenosis and Hypertension. Observations on the Current Status of Therapy from a Study of 115 Patients, *Am J Med,* **47:**175, 1969.

Sheps, S. G., Hunt, J. C., and Bernatz, P. E.: Diagnosis of Hypertension Associated with Renal Artery Disease, *Manit Med Rev,* **45:**558, 1965.

Stamey, T. A.: Renovascular Hypertension—1965, *Am J Med,* **38:**829, 1965.

————, Nudelmon, I. J., Good, P. H., Schwentker, F. N., and Hendricks, F.: Functional Characteristics of Renovascular Hypertension, *Medicine (Baltimore),* **40:**347, 1961.

Stanley, J. C., Ernst, C. B., and Fry, W. J.: Fate of 100 Aortorenal Vein Grafts: Characteristics of Late Graft Expansion, Aneurysmic Dilatation and Stenosis, *Surgery,* **74:**931, 1973.

Vaughan, E. D., Jr., Buhler, F. R., Laragh, J. H., Sealey, J. E., Baer, L., and Bard, R. H.: Renovascular Hypertension: Renin Measurements to Indicate Hypersecretion and Contralateral Suppression, Estimate Renal Plasma Flow and Score for Surgical Curability, *Am J Med,* **55:**402, 1973.

Vertes, V., Grauel, J. A., and Stoney, R. J.: Autogenous Tissue Revascularization Technics in Surgery for Renovascular Hypertension, *Ann Surg,* **170:**416, 1969.

Vermeulen, F., Stas, F., Delegher, C., Buyssens, N., et al.: Surgical Correction of Renovascular Hypertension in Children, *J Cardiovasc Surg (Torino),* **16:**21, 1975.

Wylie, E. J., Perloff, D., and Stoney, R. J.: Autogenous Tissue Revascularization Techniques in Surgery for Renovascular Hypertension, *Ann Surg,* **170:**416, 1969.

————, Perloff, D., and Wellington, J. S.: Fibromuscular Hyperplasia of the Renal Arteries, *Ann Surg,* **156:**592, 1962.

Unilateral Renal Parenchymal Disease

McDonald, D. F.: Renal Hypertension without Main Arterial Stenosis: Function Tests Predict Cure., *JAMA,* **203:**130, 1968.

Vaughan, E. D., Jr., Buhler, F. R., Laragh, J. H., Sealey, J. E., Gavras, H., and Baer, L.: Hypertension and Unilateral Parenchymal Renal Disease: Evidence for Abnormal Vasoconstriction-Volume Interaction, *JAMA,* **223:**1177, 1975.

Essential Hypertension

Bilgutay, A. M., and Lillehei, C. W.: Treatment of Hypertension with an Implantable Electronic Device, *JAMA,* **191:**649, 1965.

Brest, A. N.: Carotid Sinus Nerve Stimulation, *Am J Cardiol,* **26:**328, 1970.

Gordon, T., and Devine, B.: "Hypertension and Hypertensive Heart Disease in Adults, United States—1960–62: Vital and Health Statistics Data from the National Health Survey," U.S. Department of Health, Education, and Welfare, National Center for Health Statistics ser. II, no. 13.

Griffith, L. S. C., and Schwartz, S. I.: Reversal of Renal Hypertension by Electrical Stimulation of the Carotid Sinus Nerve, *Surgery,* **56:**232, 1964.

Grimson, K. S.: Total Thoracic and Partial to Total Lumbar Sympathectomy and Celiac Ganglionectomy in the Treatment of Hypertension, *Ann Surg,* **114:**753, 1941.

Jeffers, W. A., Sellers, A. M., Wolferth, C. C., Ross, A. M., and Blakemore, W. S.: Results of Sympathectomy and Adrenalectomy, *Am J Surg,* **107:**211, 1964.

McCubbin, J. W., Green, J. H., and Page, I. H.: Baroreceptor Function in Chronic Renal Hypertension, *Circ Res,* **4:**205, 1956.

Schwartz, S. I., and Griffith, L. S. C.: "Reduction of Hypertension by Electrical Stimulation of the Carotid Sinus Nerve, Baroreceptors and Hypertension," Pergamon Press, New York, 1967.

———, ———, Neistadt, A., and Hagfors, N.: Chronic Carotid Sinus Nerve Stimulation in the Treatment of Essential Hypertension, *Am J Surg,* **114:**5, 1967.

Smithwick, R. H.: Practical Treatment for Hypertension, Splanch-nicectomy, Adrenalectomy, and Nephrectomy, *Postgrad Med,* **34:**32, 1963.

Warner, H. R.: The Frequency-dependent Nature of Blood Pressure Regulation by the Carotid Sinus Studied with an Electric Analog, *Circ Res,* **6:**35, 1958.

Zintel, H. A.: Adrenalectomy versus Sympathectomy: Results of Surgery, in J. H. Moyer (ed.), "Hypertension," p. 695, W. B. Saunders Company, Philadelphia, 1959.

Chapter 24

Manifestations of Gastrointestinal Disease

by **Seymour I. Schwartz** and **Edward H. Storer**

Symptoms represent subjective manifestations of disturbance in function and are not specific for a disease but rather for a pathophysiologic state. In the gastrointestinal tract, the following changes in physiologic function may be implicated: altered secretion, altered motility, inadequate digestion, inadequate absorption, obstruction. The resultant symptoms of gastrointestinal disease include abdominal pain, dysphagia, anorexia, nausea and vomiting, bloating or distension, constipation, and diarrhea.

Signs of gastrointestinal disease are objective demonstrations of a pathologic process. These include tenderness, abdominal wall rigidity, palpable masses, altered bowel sounds, evidence of gastrointestinal bleeding, poor nutrition, jaundice, and stigmata of hepatic dysfunction.

PAIN

Pain (from the Latin *poena,* penalty, punishment, torment) is the predominant sensory experience by which man judges the existence of disease within himself. Like all subjective experiences, pain cannot be satisfactorily defined but is known to us by experience and described by illustration.

Most diseases of the abdominal viscera are associated with pain at some time during their course. Indeed, the correct diagnosis of acute abdominal disorders (the "acute abdomen") usually amounts to the correct identification of the cause of the abdominal pain.

There have been two opposing theories of the nature of pain. Proponents of the *intensity theory* held that pain is the consequence of excessive stimulation of any nerve endings, be they touch, temperature, sight, smell, or taste. Sensations of every order which in moderate degree are rather pleasant become unpleasant when their intensity grows too strong. In this intensity scheme, any nervous pathways are considered potential pain pathways and conduct the impulse patterns that are associated with the perceptions of pain. Integration at the thalamocortical level provides the possibility for impulses received from the same peripheral apparatus to be perceived as pain.

Although there is not yet unequivocal proof that each peripheral nerve fiber is devoted to but one type of sensory modality—pain, touch, cold, or warmth—most physiologists now subscribe to the *specificity theory,* which holds that pain is a separate sensory modality with its own specific neural apparatus. In 1965 Melzak and Wall proposed the *gate-control theory.* They indicated that the specificity theory was strongly supported but disagreed with the proposal that sensation is achieved by a fixed direct-line communication from skin to brain. Their contribution was the suggestion that the amount and quality of perceived pain are determined by many physiological and psychological variables. Modulation of nociceptive impulses occurs at the dorsal horn and at various levels of the ascending afferent systems. Appropriate stimuli initiate impulses in skin, muscle, or viscera. These sensory impulses are transmitted to the posterior horn of the spinal cord in the primary sensory neuron which has its cell body in the dorsal root ganglion. The secondary sensory neuron in the posterior horn transmits the impulses in the contralateral spinothalamic tract to the posterolateral nucleus of the thalamus. The tertiary sensory neuron transmits the impulses from the thalamus to the postcentral gyrus of the cerebral cortex (Fig. 24-1).

Three kinds of pain are recognized and designated: superficial, or cutaneous pain; deep pain from muscles, tendons, joints, and fascia; and visceral pain. The first two may be combined as somatic pain. Knowledge of visceral pain has lagged, in part because of the difficulty of the laboratory investigation of pain, but also because of some early theories which, by the strength of tradition and prestige, delayed progress.

PAIN PATHWAYS. Until well into the twentieth century,

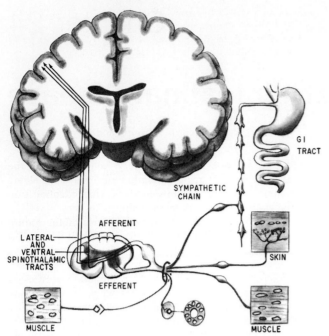

Fig. 24-1. Schematic representation of pathways involved in abdominal pain.

the viscera were thought to be completely insensitive. The first important observer of visceral sensation was William Harvey in the seventeenth century. When the young son of Count Montgomery sustained a chest wound which on healing left the heart exposed, Harvey observed that touching the heart caused not the slightest sensation. After the discovery of local anesthesia, Lennander found that human abdominal viscera are insensitive to cutting, crushing, and even burning. He categorically stated in 1901 that the viscera are wholly insensitive and that only traction or irritation of the parietal peritoneum could cause abdominal pain. The record was set straight in 1911 by Hurst, who demonstrated that distension of any hollow viscus is painful. Ryle amplified this by emphasizing that contraction of smooth muscle of hollow viscera is an adequate physiologic stimulus.

The current and preferable terminology uses the term *visceral afferents* to denote all afferent fibers from the viscera including those which give rise to visceral reflexes as well as those which subserve pain. The terms *autonomic, sympathetic,* and *parasympathetic* are reserved for the visceral *efferent* fibers.

Pain impulses from the abdominal cavity reach the central nervous system by three routes: from the viscera via visceral afferents that travel with (1) the sympathetic and (2) the parasympathetic nerves, and from the parietal peritoneum, body wall, diaphragm, and root of mesenteries via somatic afferents that travel in (3) the segmental spinal nerves or phrenic nerves. Primary sensory neurons for pain, both visceral and somatic, are mostly small (1 to 2 μ), unmyelinated fibers but with some small (3 to 4 μ), myelinated fibers (Gasser classes C and A delta, or groups IV and III in Lloyd's terminology).

The route of a typical afferent from an abdominal viscus is as follows: the axons of nerve endings in the wall of the viscus follow the artery to the aorta and then through the collateral sympathetic ganglion without synapsing. They then enter the splanchnic nerve, traverse the paravertebral sympathetic ganglion, again without synapsing, and join the spinal nerve via the white ramus communicans. The cell body of this primary visceral afferent neuron is located in the spinal ganglion from which central processes are sent to the dorsal horn of the spinal cord via the dorsal root.

The central processes of the primary sensory neuron synapse with at least three distinct spinal tracts: (1) secondary pain neurons whose axons ascend for two or three segments and then cross in the anterior commissure to the anterolateral spinothalamic tract, (2) secondary sensory neurons whose processes ascend the posterior columns, and (3) many small neurons in the substantia gelatinosa which contribute to the tract of Lissauer. As the secondary sensory neurons ascend, collaterals are given off to the reticular substance forming the core of the brainstem, and to the hypothalamus. The role of these extraspinothalamic pathways is uncertain—they may be alternative pain pathways, may inhibit central pain responses, or may be involved in the affective aspects of pain. Sensory tracts synapse in the thalamus with tertiary neurons that project to the cortex. The cortical areas involved with pain are not completely known. Stimulation of various areas of the postcentral gyrus in conscious man produces contralateral paresthesias of small areas of the body, but even total hemispherectomy does not consistently abolish pain, though localization is defective. The functions of the thalamus in man, in contrast to animals, are largely expressed through the cortex. But one function that may have been retained in the evolutionary process is the expression of the affective aspects of sensation. Affectivity—pleasantness and unpleasantness—is considered a primitive function which has remained at the thalamic level despite development of the cerebral cortex.

Though the thalamus and frontal cortex are the principal areas of the brain involved with pain, they cannot be considered as *the* brain centers, since the hypothalamus, the limbic system, the brainstem reticular formation, and the parietal cortex are also involved in pain perception.

Abdominal Pain

Three distinct types of pain are involved in the general symptom complex of abdominal pain: visceral pain, (deep) somatic pain, and referred pain.

VISCERAL PAIN. True visceral pain, or splanchnic pain, arises in abdominal organs invested with visceral peritoneum via impulses conducted to the spinal cord over visceral afferent nerve fibers. As noted above, the viscera are normally insensitive to stimuli that produce pain when applied to the skin. But there is no reason for the viscera to react to these stimuli to which they are not normally exposed, and thus sensitivity has not evolved. Adequate stimuli for visceral pain are those arising from their own environment—pathologic conditions of the viscera. Stimuli that produce pain include increased tension in the wall of hollow viscera from either distension or spastic contraction, stretching of the capsules of solid viscera, ischemia, and certain chemicals. The threshold for pain is lowered by inflammation and by ischemia, so that normal muscular contractions that would ordinarily not be felt may produce pain.

The role of chemical substances in visceral pain is not clear at this time. Experimentally, pain can be produced by the intraarterial injection of acid, alkaline, or hypertonic solutions: lactate, potassium ions, or bradykinin. Potassium which is released from cells by injury or ischemia has long been known as a pain-producing agent, and it has been suggested that the release of intracellular potassium ions may be the actual physiologic stimulus for pain. Lim would classify some pain receptors as chemoceptors and attributes the pain of ischemia to increasing concentrations of hydrogen ions and the pain of inflammation to the accrual of algesic bradykinin peptides.

Visceral pain tends to be rather diffuse and poorly localized, has a high threshold, and exhibits an exceedingly slow rate of adaptation. The high threshold and poor localization are probably in part attributable to the relatively sparse distribution of sensory endings in the viscera. The pain is felt by the patient to be "deep" in those cutaneous areas or zones which correspond roughly to the segmental distribution of somatic sensory fibers which take origin from the same segments of the cord as the visceral afferent fibers from the viscus in question.

With severe visceral or deep somatic pain, concomitant responses, presumably due to autonomic reflexes, may be prominent. These include sweating; nausea, sometimes with vomiting; tachycardia or bradycardia; fall in blood pressure; cutaneous hyperalgesia, hyperesthesia, or tenderness; and involuntary spastic contractions of abdominal wall musculature. The muscular rigidity accompanying severe pain is most marked when the body wall is involved by the pain-inciting lesion, e.g., the boardlike rigidity associated with perforated peptic ulcer. The distribution is regional rather than segmental and thus involves sustained reflexes in several segmental nerves. Maintained muscular rigidity may of itself become painful, so that on occasion the deep muscular tenderness outlasts and outweighs the original visceral pain.

SOMATIC PAIN. Pain arising in the abdominal wall, particularly the parietal peritoneum, root of the mesenteries, and respiratory diaphragm, is mediated by somatic afferents in segmental spinal nerves. Pain from parietal structures is for the most part sharper and brighter than visceral pain; it is well localized close to the site of stimulation; and when the source is on one side of the midline, the pain is also lateralized. Acute appendicitis is a common visceral disease that well illustrates typical visceral and somatic abdominal pain. The visceral pain of early appendicitis is perceived diffusely and dully in the periumbilical and lower epigastric regions, and there is little or no rigidity of the abdominal musculature. Later, when parietal peritoneum becomes involved in the inflammatory process, the somatic component of pain is more severe and sharply localized in the right lower quadrant. There is also cutaneous hyperesthesia, tenderness, and muscular rigidity in the right lower quadrant.

REFERRED PAIN. Visceral disease may give rise to pain localized to more superficial areas of the body, often at a considerable distance from the diseased viscus. The reference is usually dermatomic, but on occasion pain may be referred to the scar of a previous surgical operation, trauma, or localized pathologic process. This is called *habit reference* and implies that pain perception is influenced by the individual's prior pain experience.

There are two major hypotheses of the dermatomic reference of visceral pain: *convergence-facilitation* and *convergence-projection*. MacKenzie believed that visceral afferents have no direct connection to the spinothalamic tracts but can only set up an irritable focus in the spinal segment at which they enter the cord. According to his hypothesis, afferent impulses from surface areas which are arriving in insufficient numbers to be felt as pain by themselves are facilitated by the visceral impulses with the production of cutaneous pain and hyperalgesia. There is little evidence to support this hypothesis of referred pain; in general, neurophysiologists have found that one afferent volley tends to block another. As a matter of fact, in the gate-control hypothesis of Melzack and Wall, input of impulses into the substantia gelatinosa from surface afferents, along with corticospinal impulses, serves to inhibit the transmission of pain, not to facilitate it.

More consonant with current evidence is the convergence-projection hypothesis. Since the pain fibers in the posterior roots greatly outnumber the fibers in the spinothalamic tracts, several pain fibers must converge on one tract fiber. This same convergence may occur at thalmic or cortical levels as well. When afferents from the skin and viscera converge on the same neuron at some point in the pain pathway, the resulting impulses, on projection to the brain, are interpreted as coming from the skin, an interpretation learned from previous experiences in which the same tract fiber was stimulated by cutaneous afferents.

INTRACTABLE PAIN

Fortunately, most abdominal pain is caused by pathologic processes that are amenable to medical or surgical treatment. The control of pain associated with diseases that cannot be satisfactorily treated is one of the most challenging and often frustrating problems the clinician has to face. Examples are unresectable carcinoma of the pancreas and chronic pancreatitis.

Opiate analgesics if given in sufficient dosage can usually control abdominal pain, but at the risk of addiction and negating the patient's ability to function as an effective person. This is probably the best therapy, however, for a patient with incurable disease and a life expectancy of a few weeks or months. It should not be used in patients with severe pain from nonmalignant causes with an unpredictable life expectancy.

Neurosurgical intervention on the pain pathways, though disappointing at times, is the treatment of choice for intractable pain in properly selected patients. Narcotic addiction prior to surgery usually compromises the result, as an addicted patient continues to be addicted even though his pain is relieved by the procedure.

Splanchnicectomy and celiac ganglionectomy can effectively control abdominal pain if somatically innervated structures are not involved in the pain-producing process. When both visceral and somatic pain fibers are involved, posterior rhizotomy or tract interruption is indicated. The spinothalamic tracts are usually interrupted, either by surgical incision or injection of sclerosing chemicals, in the spinal cord a few segments above the segments where the noxious impulses are entering. The interruption has also been done at medullary or mesencephalic levels. After anterolateral chordotomy, pain and temperature sensation are lost, while proprioception and touch are virtually unimpaired. Paresthesias often replace pain in the anesthetic areas, and in a significant number of patients, after about 1 year, the paresthesias become disagreeable and painful. For this reason, root or tract interruption is most useful in patients with intractable pain and a life expectancy of a year or so.

For patients with pain arising from areas too great to be controlled by peripheral interventions, prefrontal lobotomy may be considered. Such lesions do not abolish pain but diminish the reaction to pain. The price paid for such relief, however, includes inability to experience pleasure, as well; i.e., there is a flattening of all affect and the development of a more or less apathetic state.

It is obvious from the above that there is a need for a means to relieve intractable pain which would be non-addicting, would not affect the patient's personality or mind, and would not destroy normal neural tissue. Recent developments in clinical research offer some hope. Shealy et al. have devised and successfully tested a dorsal column stimulator which is now commercially available. In theory, impulses arising from electrostimulation of descending dorsal column fibers are used to inhibit, in accordance with the gate-control theory, prolonged small-fiber afterdischarge which is uniquely related to pain. Electrodes are implanted four to eight segments above the pain input. The external transmitter is controlled by the patient. There is a buzzing or tingling sensation below the site of the stimulator, but pain is usually controlled without significant alteration of normal sensory function. Transcutaneous electrical stimulation has been used effectively to control postoperative pain. Whether this technique can be extended over prolonged periods remains to be evaluated.

ETIOLOGY. Abdominal pain may be caused by a great variety of gastrointestinal and intraperitoneal diseases, and, because of overlapping nerve distribution, the pain may be secondary to extraperitoneal disorders. Pain of intraabdominal origin (Table 24-1) may emanate from the peritoneum, hollow intestinal viscera, solid viscera, mesentery, or pelvic organs, and may be caused by inflammation, mechanical processes such as obstruction or acute distension, and vascular disturbances.

The extraperitoneal causes of abdominal pain are outlined in Table 24-2. Most of the intrathoracic diseases which cause abdominal pain are confused with upper abdominal disorders, since their segmental distribution is similar. The intraspinal diseases have pain patterns which

Table 24-1. GASTROINTESTINAL AND INTRAPERITONEAL CAUSES OF ABDOMINAL PAIN

I. Inflammation
  A. Peritoneum
    1. Chemical and nonbacterial peritonitis—perforated peptic ulcer, gallbladder, ruptured ovarian cyst, mittelschmerz
    2. Bacterial peritonitis
      a. Primary peritonitis—pneumococcal, streptococcal, tuberculous
      b. Perforated hollow viscus—stomach, intestine, biliary tract
  B. Hollow intestinal organs
    1. Appendicitis
    2. Cholecystitis
    3. Peptic ulceration
    4. Gastroenteritis
    5. Regional enteritis
    6. Meckel's diverticulitis
    7. Colitis—ulcerative, bacterial, amebic
    8. Diverticulitis
  C. Solid viscera
    1. Pancreatitis
    2. Hepatitis
    3. Hepatic abscess
    4. Splenic abscess
  D. Mesentery
    1. Lymphadenitis
  E. Pelvic organs
    1. Pelvic inflammatory disease
    2. Tuboovarian abscess
    3. Endometritis
II. Mechanical (obstruction, acute distension)
  A. Hollow intestinal organs
    1. Intestinal obstruction—adhesions, hernia, tumor, volvulus, intussusception
    2. Biliary obstruction—calculi, tumor, choledochal cyst, hematobilia
  B. Solid viscera
    1. Acute splenomegaly
    2. Acute hepatomegaly—cardiac failure, Budd-Chiari syndrome
  C. Mesentery
    1. Omental torsion
  D. Pelvic organs
    1. Ovarian cyst
    2. Torsion or degeneration of fibroid
    3. Ectopic pregnancy
III. Vascular
  A. Intraperitoneal bleeding
    1. Ruptured liver
    2. Ruptured spleen
    3. Ruptured mesentery
    4. Ruptured ectopic pregnancy
    5. Ruptured aortic, splenic, or hepatic aneurysm
  B. Ischemia
    1. Mesenteric thrombosis
    2. Hepatic infarction—toxemia, purpura
    3. Splenic infarction
    4. Omental ischemia
IV. Miscellaneous
  A. Endometriosis

are similar to the referred pain from abdominal pathologic conditions, but they are usually not accompanied by tenderness or muscular rigidity. Inflammation of peripheral nerves, as in the case of herpes zoster, may be accompanied

Table 24-2. EXTRAPERITONEAL CAUSES
OF ABDOMINAL PAIN

Cardiopulmonary	*Vascular*
Pneumonia	Dissection, rupture, or ex-
Empyema	pansion of aortic aneurysm
Myocardial ischemia	Periarteritis
Active rheumatic heart	*Metabolic*
disease	Uremia
Blood	Diabetic acidosis
Leukemia	Porphyria
Sickle cell crisis	Addisonian crisis
Neurogenic	*Toxins*
Spinal cord tumors	Bacterial (tetanus)
Osteomyelitis of spine	Insect bites
Tabes dorsalis	Venoms
Herpes zoster	Drugs
Abdominal epilepsy	Lead poisoning
Genitourinary	*Abdominal wall*
Nephritis	Intramuscular hematoma
Pyelitis	*Psychogenic*
Perinephric abscesses	
Ureteral obstruction (calculi,	
tumors)	
Prostatitis	
Seminal vesiculitis	
Epidydimitis	

by tenderness and pain before the lesion becomes apparent. The pain usually has a distribution similar to myocardial infarction of biliary tract disease.

CLINICAL EVALUATION. Since pain is the subjective reaction to a stimulus which initiates transmission along nerve pathways to cortical centers, the patient's response is dependent upon both physical and psychologic factors. Physical requirements for response to pain include the patient's consciousness to permit perception, and integrity of the entire avenue along which impulses are transmitted to the brain. With repeated stimulation, the cortical threshold becomes lowered, and resistance is reduced along nerve pathways, which results in hypersensitivity and "facilitated pain." Hyperthyroidism, hyperadrenalism, and the menopausal syndrome are all associated with increased response to pain, while hypothyroidism is usually accompanied by an increased pain threshold. Sensitivity alters with age, increasing from infancy to adult life and then gradually diminishing in the elderly patient. The asthenic habitus is generally characterized by increased sensitivity, and the Anglo-Saxon and Nordic types are generally less sensitive and responsive to pain than Latins and Jews.

The physical responses to painful stimuli are also variable. While superficial pain is frequently associated with diffuse sympathetic nervous system stimulation and outpouring of epinephrine as part of a defense reaction, severe deep pain is more often accompanied by bradycardia, hypotension, nausea and vomiting, sweating, and, at times, syncope. Continued pain may cause a decrease in renal blood flow, renal clearance, and oliguria. Cardiac arrythmias may also occur, and, in the extreme case, neurogenic shock may result.

History. In elicting a description of pain, the character, severity, location, timing, and factors which either augment or reduce the pain should all be defined. Certain pathologic states are associated with characteristic pain patterns.

Colic—biliary, ureteral, or intestinal—is intermittent, frequently occurring in waves, and is described as cramping, or the patient may use the very term "colicky." Pain of a penetrating ulcer is "burning," while pain accompanying expansion of an abdominal aneurysm is "boring and pounding." Tabes is manifested by "stabbing" pain, and the pain accompanying pleuritis or perforation of a viscus has also been described as "knifelike."

The severity of the pain is an expression of the intensity of stimuli plus the patient's physical and emotional response. Colicky pain related to acute distension of the biliary tract, intestine, or ureters and pain of neurologic origin such as herpes and tabes all have an extremely high intensity. Pain evoked by inflammatory stimuli is less marked. In patients with peritonitis, the degree of pain and muscular rigidity generally parallel each other. Severe pain may be manifested by physical responses, to which previous reference has been made.

In general, abdominal pains which persist for 6 hours are caused by conditions of surgical significance. However, it is rare for any pain to be absolutely constant. The pain resulting from distension of hollow viscera is generally intermittent, while the pain of peritonitis is most frequently continuous. Pain which awakens the patient from sleep is usually characteristic of organic disease. Ulcer pain frequently occurs at night or prior to a meal, whereas gallbladder pain may be stimulated by eating. Peptic ulcer pain also has a seasonal variation, occurring more frequently in the spring and fall. In addition to the effect of digestion of food on the pain, the effects of position, motion, and respiration have diagnostic importance.

The location of pain should include a description of original situation, any shifting, and radiation. The initial location may better define the visceral involvement, since once peritonitis occurs, pain becomes diffuse. Because of variation in location of the organs and the pathologic processes plus the vagueness of visceral pain, it is difficult to totally exclude diseases on the basic of location, but certain relationships generally pertain (Fig. 24-2). Visceral intestinal pain is usually experienced in the midportion of the abdomen. Duodenal pain is felt in the epigastrium, while the pain of the remainder of the small intestine is characteristically referred to the region of the umbilicus. Pain originating in the large bowel is less well localized and frequently experienced in the hypogastrium. Sigmoid dilatation may result in suprapublic or presacral pain.

The patient's age represents a factor which focuses attention on certain processes. Acute colicky pain in a child under two is suggestive of intussusception, whereas peptic ulcer is extremely uncommon in the young age group. Appendicitis is most frequently a disease of the young adolescent, cholecystitis is more commonly seen in the middle-age group, while diverticulitis rarely occurs before the age of thirty-five.

Vomiting is indicative of severe irritation of the peritoneum, stretching of the mesentery, obstruction, or absorbed toxins. The exact timing of vomiting in relation to the onset of pain is pertinent. Pain almost always precedes vomiting by several hours in patients with appendicitis. Vomiting may also occur early in relation to the onset of

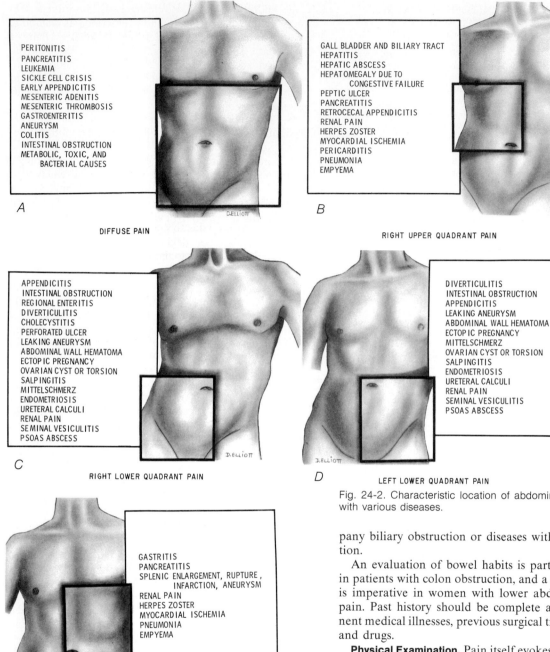

A

PERITONITIS
PANCREATITIS
LEUKEMIA
SICKLE CELL CRISIS
EARLY APPENDICITIS
MESENTERIC ADENITIS
MESENTERIC THROMBOSIS
GASTROENTERITIS
ANEURYSM
COLITIS
INTESTINAL OBSTRUCTION
METABOLIC, TOXIC, AND
     BACTERIAL CAUSES

DIFFUSE PAIN

B

GALL BLADDER AND BILIARY TRACT
HEPATITIS
HEPATIC ABSCESS
HEPATOMEGALY DUE TO
     CONGESTIVE FAILURE
PEPTIC ULCER
PANCREATITIS
RETROCECAL APPENDICITIS
RENAL PAIN
HERPES ZOSTER
MYOCARDIAL ISCHEMIA
PERICARDITIS
PNEUMONIA
EMPYEMA

RIGHT UPPER QUADRANT PAIN

C

APPENDICITIS
INTESTINAL OBSTRUCTION
REGIONAL ENTERITIS
DIVERTICULITIS
CHOLECYSTITIS
PERFORATED ULCER
LEAKING ANEURYSM
ABDOMINAL WALL HEMATOMA
ECTOPIC PREGNANCY
OVARIAN CYST OR TORSION
SALPINGITIS
MITTELSCHMERZ
ENDOMETRIOSIS
URETERAL CALCULI
RENAL PAIN
SEMINAL VESICULITIS
PSOAS ABSCESS

RIGHT LOWER QUADRANT PAIN

D

DIVERTICULITIS
INTESTINAL OBSTRUCTION
APPENDICITIS
LEAKING ANEURYSM
ABDOMINAL WALL HEMATOMA
ECTOPIC PREGNANCY
MITTELSCHMERZ
OVARIAN CYST OR TORSION
SALPINGITIS
ENDOMETRIOSIS
URETERAL CALCULI
RENAL PAIN
SEMINAL VESICULITIS
PSOAS ABSCESS

LEFT LOWER QUADRANT PAIN

Fig. 24-2. Characteristic location of abdominal pain associated with various diseases.

E

GASTRITIS
PANCREATITIS
SPLENIC ENLARGEMENT, RUPTURE,
     INFARCTION, ANEURYSM
RENAL PAIN
HERPES ZOSTER
MYOCARDIAL ISCHEMIA
PNEUMONIA
EMPYEMA

LEFT UPPER QUADRANT PAIN

pain in patients with peritonitis and biliary or ureteral colic. With intestinal obstruction, the interval between the onset of pain and vomiting provides some indication of the level of obstruction. Frequent vomiting is indicative of intestinal obstruction, while a clear emesis may accom-

pany biliary obstruction or diseases with pyloric obstruction.

An evaluation of bowel habits is particularly pertinent in patients with colon obstruction, and a menstrual history is imperative in women with lower abdominal or pelvic pain. Past history should be complete and include pertinent medical illnesses, previous surgical treatment, trauma, and drugs.

Physical Examination. Pain itself evokes physical changes which may be manifested on examination. Hyperalgesia may occur at the site of the original stimulus or in the area of referred pain. Muscle contraction may be a consequence of deep pain, or the muscle spasm itself may be responsible for pain. The autonomic responses to pain include pallor, sweating, nausea, vomiting, bradycardia, hypotension, and syncope. Regard for the patient's general appearance includes his attitude in bed, tissue turgor, respiratory rate, and temperature. Restricted motion in bed suggests peritonitis, whereas writhing is more frequently an accompaniment of biliary or ureteral colic.

The abdomen should be examined in a routine manner

with inspection, auscultation, percussion, and palpation performed sequentially. On inspection, restricted motion of the abdominal wall during respiration suggests diffuse peritonitis. Maintenance of the hip in a position of flexion is suggestive of a psoas abscess, appendicitis, or a pelvic abscess. Auscultation for bowel sounds may reveal the borborygmi associated with mechanical intestinal obstruction, while an absence of bowel sounds is suggestive of diffuse peritonitis. Percussion is performed for the detection of free peritoneal fluid, distension, and the absence of liver dullness associated with a perforated viscus. Palpation should always begin away from the area of pain and include all possible sites for hernia. Superficial palpation may demonstrate hyperesthesia to pinprick or pinching in a segmental area of referred pain. Deep palpation may detect a mass. Muscle rigidity is a relative term, and its evaluation is dependent on the patient's cooperation. Pelvic and rectal examination are integral procedures for the evaluation of the acute surgical abdomen, as is a thorough examination of the chest for cardiac and pulmonary disease.

Laboratory Procedures. The hemogram with specific interest in the white blood cell count to define the presence of an inflammatory process and a hematocrit reading to determine if there is hemoconcentration or anemia should be routine. Urinalysis is directed toward evaluating diabetes, porphyria, the presence of infection, or red cells associated with calculi. An elevated serum amylase level is most frequently associated with acute pancreatitis but does occur with a variety of other intraabdominal processes including perforated viscera, cholecystitis, choledocholithiasis, and intraabdominal bleeding. A sickle cell preparation may be called for in Negroes. Emergency roentgenographic studies include supine films and upright or lateral decubitus films to determine the presence of air within the intestinal lumen or free within the peritoneal cavity. A chest x-ray is particularly applicable in patients over forty with upper abdominal pain, as is an electrocardiogram to rule out mycrocardial ischemia, which may mimic cholecystitis. The determination of the presence of free blood or significant amounts of peritoneal fluid may be accomplished by paracentesis with microscopic examination of the specimen or, in the case of lower abdominal or pelvic pain, culdocentesis and culdoscopy. It is to be emphasized that laparotomy may consitute an important tool in the diagnosis of acute abdominal pain.

DYSPHAGIA

Dysphagia refers to a difficulty in swallowing and is related to either a functional alteration in the mechanism of deglutition or physical encroachment upon the lumen of the esophagus. The term *odynophagia* is used when swallowing is painful.

ACT OF SWALLOWING. This is classically divided into three stages. In the first stage the bolus of food or liquid is voluntarily moved into the pharynx by contraction of the mylohyoid muscle. In the second stage, the material is transported through the pharynx by waves of contractions which are involuntary, or reflex. This reflex is initiated by a stimulus from the base of the tongue, soft palate, uvula, and posterior pharyngeal wall and travels up the glossopharyngeal nerve, the second division of the trigeminal nerve, and the superior laryngeal nerve. The impulses terminate in the medulla and initiate a series of efferent stimuli which coordinate contraction of the pharyngeal constrictors. Elevation of the soft palate closes off the nasopharynx, and contraction of the suprahyoid muscles elevates the larynx and brings it forward, thus closing the entrance into the larynx and trachea. Respiration is inhibited, and the respiratory tract is completely sealed off by approximation of the vocal cords and posterior displacement of the epiglottis. The terminal phase of the second stage is relaxation of the cricopharyngeus muscles, which permits the bolus to enter the upper esophagus.

The third stage of deglutition transports the bolus through the esophagus into the stomach. Waves of positive pressure sweep down the body of the esophagus in an orderly fashion, and the wave of pressure may reach an intensity of 50 to 100 cm of water. This wave is effected by a reflex arc, the afferent impulses of which are carried through the glossopharyngeal nerve and the efferent impulses transported by the vagi. Auerbach's plexuses within the wall of the esophagus are also involved. When distension by a solid bolus of food occurs, secondary peristaltic contractions result in that segment. Nonperistaltic tertiary esophageal contractions are seen in the lower esophagus of normal people after the age of forty. They are important considerations in the differential diagnosis of esophageal varices.

Transport of the bolus through the esophagus is dependent upon the pressure gradient produced by the primary peristaltic contraction plus, in the case of liquids, the effect of gravity. The final phase of deglutition is the propulsion of the bolus from the esophagus into the stomach. This is dependent upon relaxation of the inferior esophageal sphincter, which reacts reflexly and autonomously in response to pressure or peristalsis in the lower esophagus.

ETIOLOGY. Dysphagia may be due to oropharyngeal or esophageal causes. The former includes disorders of the mouth, upper respiratory tract, and pharynx. Any painful lesion of the mouth or tongue including pharyngitis, retropharyngeal abscess, or oral carcinoma may be implicated. Acute thyroiditis is usually accompanied by pharyngeal dysphagia. Neuromuscular disturbances which may affect deglutition include poliomyelitis, syringomyelia, glossopharyngeal neuritis, and myasthenia. Alteration of the muscle itself, as is seen in amyloidosis and scleroderma, also results in dysphagia, which may be either oropharyngeal or esophageal in location.

Esophageal dysphagia is related to a great variety of causes, which are listed in Table 24-3. The level at which the patient localizes a sticking sensation usually corresponds well to the level of the responsible lesion. Dysphagia may be caused by disturbance in esophageal motility with either hypomotility or hypermotility implicated (see Chap. 25). The passage of fluid through the esophagus

Table 24-3. CAUSES OF ESOPHAGEAL DYSPHAGIA

Cause	Predominant sex	Age incidence		Salient historical and related characteristics
		10–45	45 and over	
Carcinoma	Male	Rare	Common	Duration of symptoms less than 2 years; painful swallowing occurs early, dysphagia later.
Peptic esophagitis	Male	Common	Common	Heartburn for years, often preceding dysphagia; odynophagia later.
Achalasia	Male-female	Common	Common	Liquids, especially cold, cause dysphagia early; regurgitation easy; odynophagia mild and late.
Contractile ring	Male	Rare	Common	Brief, intermittent attacks of dysphagia with no interval symptoms.
Diffuse spasm	Male	Rare	Rare	Affects elderly persons; multiple ringlike contractions along esophageal tube.
Zenker's diverticulum	Male	Rare	Rare	Sticking feeling in neck, gurgling on swallowing; occasional regurgitation of decayed food.
Scleroderma	Female	Common	Rare	Skin changes; Raynaud's phenomenon.
Paraesophageal hiatal hernia . . .	Female	Rare	Rare	Attacks of substernal pressure, pain, dysphagia, and belching during meals.
Extrinsic masses		Common	Rare	Symptoms of primary disorder.

SOURCE: After Ingelfinger, *Med Sci,* Apr. 10, 1960, pp. 451–470.

may also be impaired by encroachment upon the lumen. In the proximal esophagus, Zenker's pharyngoesophageal diverticulum, obstructing bands, and hypertrophic spurs of the anterior cervical vertebrae may be implicated. Dysphagia in the region of the cervical esophagus may also be due to esophageal carcinoma, cervical lymphadenopathy, stenosis secondary to ingestion of a caustic substance, or pressure from an enlarged thyroid. In the middle third of the esophagus carcinoma, stenosis, esophagitis, and traction diverticulum all may be causes. In addition, a wide variety of mediastinal inflammatory malignant lesions may encroach upon the lumen. Vascular lesions such as enlargement of the left atrium, aneurysm in the arch of the aorta, and anomalous right subclavian artery are rare causes of dysphagia in this region. In the lower third of the esophagus, primary carcinoma and carcinoma of the stomach with craniad extension represent common causes, particularly in the older age group. Other lower esophageal causes of dysphagia include reflux esophagitis, achalasia, contractile rings, and epiphrenic diverticula.

Dysphagia is a relatively common manifestation of emotional diseases. Inability to swallow accompanies anxiety states, conversion hysteria, and anorexia nervosa.

CLINICAL EVALUATION. History should include a precise description of the symptom with particular reference to the duration, location, and timing in relation to ingestion of food. True dysphagia occurs within 15 minutes of swallowing. The patient can usually pinpoint the site of obstruction. The determination of the amount of weight loss and the presence of associated vomiting are important. Physical examination is directed toward the detection of cervical nodes suggesting mediastinal or esophageal lesions, enlargement of the esophagus, and stigmata of scleroderma. Barium study of the esophagus is frequently diagnostic, and the use of cineroentgenography and/or

manometric motility studies are particularly applicable in determining disorders of motility. In the case of intrinsic esophageal lesions, the ultimate diagnostic study is esophagoscopy with biopsy.

ANOREXIA

Anorexia is the absence of the desire to eat and can be related to a variety of organic and psychologic disturbances. Since appetite is essentially a central phenomenon, anorexia is dependent upon central effects producing a loss of appetite. Animal experiments have demonstrated a feeding center in the lateral hypothalmus and a satiety center in the medial hypothalmus. In most instances, gastric hypofunction, with mucosal pallor and decrease in gastric motility and secretion, has been associated with anorexia, but the stomach itself plays a minor role. Anorexia may also occur when both the secretory and motor activity of the stomach and gastrointestinal tract are increased. Visceral stimuli are generally carried to the midbrain via the vagus, pelvic, and sympathetic nerves, but combined sympathetic and parasympathetic denervation may not alter appetite or preclude the possibility of anorexia. The absence of precise pathophysiologic explanation and the protean disorders associated with the symptom of anorexia make it of little diagnostic significance. Among the organic diseases associated with anorexia are inflammatory processes within the intestinal tract; carcinoma of the stomach, pancreas, and liver; hepatitis and alcoholism; advanced renal disease with uremia; congestive heart failure; and certain endocrine disorders such as panhypopituitarism, adrenal cortical insufficiency, and hyperparathyroidism. Many, if not most, drugs can cause anorexia; there is no medication which consistently increases appetite.

NAUSEA AND VOMITING

Nausea and vomiting may occur separately but are closely allied. Nausea usually refers to the feeling of an imminent desire to vomit. Vomiting may be defined as the forceful expulsion of gastrointestinal contents through the mouth. In most instances, nausea precedes vomiting.

In spite of the frequency and great clinical importance of vomiting, the nervous mechanism of the act and the physical and chemical stimuli are not well understood. Most physiologists have agreed to the existence of a vomiting center and to its location in the reticular core of the medulla oblongata. There are actually two medullary centers concerned with emesis: (1) a sensory "chemoreceptive trigger zone" and (2) an integrated center which is concerned directly with the production of vomiting. The former is implicated in the drug-induced emesis and also in the vomiting associated with uremia, infections, and radiation sickness.

Afferent pathways to the vomiting center emanate from almost all sites in the body. Impulses from the gastrointestinal system pass through the emetic center by way of afferent fibers in both the vagal and sympathetic nerves. Although neither vagotomy nor sympathectomy alone abolishes the vomiting of peritonitis, the vagus is considered the more important afferent pathway from this stimulus. The vomiting induced by intestinal distension is dependent upon afferent impulses transmitted in the sympathetic nerves as evidenced by the fact that denervation of the mesenteric pedicle prevents vomiting associated with distension of that segment. Distension of the gallbladder and extrahepatic biliary tract also causes vomiting which may be obviated by a combination of vagotomy and splanchnicectomy. Pyloric pouch distension vomiting is abolished by vagotomy alone. However, it is known that vomiting may be a consequence of surgical vagotomy and that the higher the vagotomy, the more frequent the incidence of vomiting. In this circumstance, the vomiting is related to esophageal stasis with regurgitation of esophageal content into the pharynx and subsequent pharyngeal irritation.

The act of vomiting is primarily a motor function involving the respiratory and somatic muscular systems in addition to the gastrointestinal tract. Vomiting occurs in the normal fashion following total denervation of the intestine. The efferent neuropathways involve the phrenic nerves to the diaphragm, spinal nerves to the abdominal and intercostal muscles, and efferent visceral fibers along the vagus and sympathetic nerves to the intestine and muscles of the pharynx and larynx. The act of vomiting depends upon the coordinated closure of the glottis, contraction and fixation of the diaphragm in the inspiratory position, closure of the pylorus, and relaxation of the rest of the stomach including the cardia. Relaxation of the upper half of the stomach and the esophageal cardia is followed by peristaltic contractions passing from the midstomach to the incisura angularis. Contraction at the incisura persists and prevents the contents of the stomach from passing into the gastric antrum. This is followed by forceful contraction of the abdominal, diaphragmatic, and intercostal muscles, which transmit a pressure to the stomach and cause regurgitation. Reverse peristalsis in the stomach plays no major role in the mechanism of vomiting. Reverse peristalsis of the small intestine frequently occurs and results in the passage of intestinal contents into the stomach and the presence of bile in the vomitus after repeated retching. However, this type of intestinal activity has been shown to occur normally in the duodenum and does not contribute to the act of vomiting. Vomiting is frequently associated with autonomic activity including pallor, sweating, increased salivation, and cardiovascular changes including irregularity, ectopic beats, heart block, and, rarely, arrest.

All organic diseases of the alimentary tract and its appendages as well as diseases of almost every organ of the body have been associated with vomiting. Derangements of the autonomic nervous system, psychogenic disturbances, and the ingestion of noxious materials may also cause vomiting. A broad spectrum of drugs are considered as emetic agents. These include morphine, cardiac glycosides, quinine and quinidine, veratrine alkaloids, pilocarpine, Pituitrin, Pitocin, acetylcholine, ergot alkalis, atropine, tartar emetic, ipecac, zinc sulfate, and bacterial endotoxins. With each of these causes of vomiting any combination of three major factors may be involved: impulses arising from the gastrointestinal tract, central or cerebral impulses, and chemical materials transported in the blood.

The vomiting associated with shock and severe pain may be related to a reduced blood supply in the cerebral medullary centers or vasoconstriction in the splanchnic areas. Reduction of oxygen supply to the vomiting center has been implicated in the vomiting associated with anemia, vascular occlusion, and increased intracranial pressure. Migraine may also induce vomiting by an effective increase in intracranial pressure with interference of blood supply to the cerebromedullary center. Emetic drugs act in one of two ways, either directly on the cerebrum, hypothalamus, or brainstem or by their irritative effect on the gastric and intestinal mucosa. These two factors may also be involved in vomiting induced by spoiled or contaminated food and the vomiting following the ingestion of alcohol. The vomiting associated with diabetic acidosis, uremia, and Addisonian crisis has been related to changes in electrolytes and, more specifically, acidosis and hyperkalemia affecting the emesis center. An augmented irritability of the emesis center is postulated as playing a significant role in the vomiting of thyrotoxicosis.

The gastrointestinal pathophysiologic processes which lead to vomiting are many and varied. Obstruction to passage of food at any level will eventually be accompanied by vomiting. The higher the obstruction, the more rapid the onset of vomiting. The rapidity is also related to the acuteness of onset, since a gradual obstruction is attended by compensation with stretching of muscle fibers and hypertrophy. Inflammatory diseases and malignant tumors of the stomach are frequent causes of vomiting and are usually preceded by anorexia and nausea. In the child under three months of age, vomiting of clear, non-bile-stained materials is highly suggestive of hypertrophic pyloric stenosis. Acute inflammatory diseases of the intestine and pelvic organs are associated with nausea and vomiting through visceral reflexes; the more common disorders include appendictis, cholecystitis, hepatitis, pancreatitis, and salpingitis.

The pattern of vomiting is of clinical significance. Vomiting without antecedent nausea suggests a central nervous system lesion with increased intracranial pressure, such as hemorrhage or brain tumor. In these cases vomiting is usually sudden in onset and often projectile. Projectile vomiting is also characteristic of hypertrophic pyloric stenosis. Emesis which follows and relieves epigastric pain is usually associated with intragastric lesions or pyloric spasm. Vomiting which immediately follows eating is noted with toxic causes, such as uremia and hyperemesis gravidarum, gastritis, high intestinal obstruction, and gastric neoplasms. Vomiting of large amounts of digested food at 12- to 48-hour intervals is suggestive of chronic pyloric obstruction. Vomiting of feculent material is associated with gastrocolic fistula. Continued retching and vomiting, especially in alcoholics, may lacerate the gastroesophageal mucosa and result in the Mallory-Weiss syndrome with severe bleeding and, at times, exsanguination. An extension of this process is the spontaneous rupture of the esophagus which occurs more frequently in vomiting by the patient with a full stomach.

CONSEQUENCES OF VOMITING. Depending upon the intensity and duration, vomiting may produce hypovolemia, hypokalemia, alteration in the acid-base balance, and the consequences of starvation. Vomitus, without admixture of ingested food, is isoosmotic with the extracellular fluid. However, the electrolyte composition is extremely variable and dependent upon the extent of hydrogen ion excretion.

When hydrogen ion is excreted into the gastric juice, there is a shift of bicarbonate ion into the plasma, and, to maintain electric neutrality of the blood, chloride is excreted into the gastric juice. Concentration of bicarbonate in the plasma is augmented by the loss of chloride and excessive sodium in the vomitus. In general, an inverse relation exists between the concentration of hydrogen ion and sodium ion in the vomitus. Even in the achlorhydric state, when vomiting results in a depletion of sodium chloride and potassium chloride, chloride is excreted in excess of the physiologic proportions of that existent in plasma, i.e., 145 mEq of sodium and 100 mEq of chloride. As the plasma bicarbonate rises, the body compensates by increasing renal excretion of bicarbonate and reducing the rate and depth of respiration to decrease the respiratory loss of $HHCO_3$ to maintain the acid/base ratio. These compensatory features may maintain the normal blood pH, while the urine is alkaline because of excretion of bicarbonate. Determination of plasma electrolytes is only partly informative, since it is dependent upon the relative loss of electrolytes and water and also upon the solutions ingested.

With continued vomiting, the plasma and extracellular potassium concentration becomes reduced as a result of the increased quantities of potassium excreted in the urine in exchange for sodium, which in turn is related to the lack of availability of hydrogen ions depleted by loss in the vomitus. Adrenal cortical stimulation intensifies the potassium loss and potentiates the absorption of bicarbonate by the renal tubular cell. The extracellular and subsequently intracellular potassium concentrations become reduced, sodium cations shift into the cell, and, in order to conserve sodium, an acid urine is formed in the face of generalized alkalosis. This intensifies the alkalosis and sets up a vicious cycle which includes shift of more potassium out of the cell in exchange for sodium.

The fluid loss results in reduction in the circulating blood volume, and in time the consequences of starvation such as cellular breakdown of protein and increased renal load of nitrogenous waste products cause a rise in the BUN (blood urea nitrogen) level. Fat stores are utilized. Ketone bodies are formed, and since they require sodium for excretion, this further depletes the body stores of sodium.

Therapy should be instituted early, correcting relatively minor defects, since advanced deficiencies are critical and difficult to reverse. Drugs used to treat vomiting include anticholinergics, antihistamines, phenothiazine derivatives, and orthopramides.

CONSTIPATION AND DIARRHEA

Alteration in bowel habits may be related to the type of food ingested, psychologic disorders, or lesions in the gastrointestinal tract.

INTESTINAL TRANSIT. The rate of gastric emptying varies with the amount and quality of food and the emotional state of the individual. Generally, the healthy stomach is emptied within 3 to 4 hours, and passage through the duodenum and jejunum is rapid. Digested food usually begins to traverse the ileocolic sphincter in 2 to 3 hours and completes its passage into the cecum in 9 hours. Some delay occurs almost constantly in the distal ileum, where "segmentation" of a radiopaque bolus can be noted. The contents of the small intestine travel at an average rate of 1 in./minute, or 22 ft in 4 hours.

The chyme which enters the cecum is semiliquid in consistency. Most of the absorption of water which occurs in the large intestine takes place in the cecum and ascending colon. The intensity and frequency of muscular contractions increase from the duodenum to the rectum. Mass peristalsis carries the bolus from the hepatic flexure onward. These waves occur at varying times but are known to be frequent after meals, the so-called "gastrocolic reflex." Although some food products are evacuated within 24 hours of ingestion, the major portion requires several days for disposition.

Normally, the fecal bolus does not pass beyond the sigmoid into the rectum until defecation is about to occur. The passage into the rectum is brought about by powerful peristaltic waves with concomitant relaxation of the smooth musculature at the rectosigmoid junction. Distension of the rectum initiates afferent nervous impulses conducted via hypogastric and pelvic nerves to the sacral cord, whence efferent impulses are discharged. The process of defecation may be entirely involuntary but is usually assisted by voluntary contractions of the muscles of the abdomen and diaphragm and voluntary relaxation of the external anal sphincter. The intraluminal pressure is increased, forcing the stool through the relaxed internal sphincter and the voluntarily relaxed external sphincter. The entire colon, distal to the splenic flexure, is usually emptied at one time.

Four types of wave action have been noted in the colon: Type 1 waves are small and of short duration, lasting 5 seconds, and are not propulsive in character. These are not observed roentgenographically and are only noted in a pressure-measuring system. Type 2 waves are characterized by an increase in pressure, and the duration varies between 12 and 120 seconds. They constitute the principal activity in the descending and pelvic segments of the colon. They may or may not be propulsive. Type 3 waves are of low intensity, affecting 10 cm of water pressure and last 1 to 4 minutes. They may play a role in absorption by increasing the luminal pressure. Type 4 waves are strong, propulsive contractions with pressures up to 100 cm of water and effect a mass movement of the fecal bolus. They are commonly noted in patients with ulcerative colitis.

Although intestinal motility continues after transection of the nerves, under normal conditions the vagi, splanchnics, and pelvic nerves do play a significant role. Parasympathetic efferent supply to the small intestine and proximal colon courses over the vagi, while the remainder of the colon innervation is carried over the lower sacral segment via the pelvic nerves. Splanchnic nerves supply sympathetic innervation. The intrinsic myenteric reflexes are the prime movers, but motility is augmented by parasympathetic stimulation, while sympathetic stimulation results in inhibition of tone. Sympathetic stimulation explains the reflex ileus which is known to accompany retroperitoneal trauma or dissection.

The external anal sphincter, a voluntary muscle, receives nerve fibers from the gray matter of the conus terminalis, where the reflex is located. Transection of the cord in this region does not affect reflex contraction. However, if the lower segment of the cord is destroyed, the external sphincter becomes relaxed and no longer contracts. If the afferent nerves are destroyed, the fecal bolus may accumulate without sensation. It has been suggested that the medullary center may be implicated in the act of defecation, since a central nervous system influence is capable of causing either diarrhea or constipation.

In addition to neurogenic factors, chemicals also influence defecation. Acetylcoholine-like drugs increase the tone and activity of the intestine. Pilocarpine causes smooth muscle contraction, while neostigmine and Mecholyl inhibit the destruction of cholinesterase and produce intestinal activity. Serotonin also alters intestinal motility with resultant increased activity. Guanethidine causes increased motility by its inhibitory effect on the sympathetic nerves, and reserpine acts by its effect on serotonin release. Vasopressin is strongly motor to the entire intestine. Potassium is implicated in intestinal motility, since the function of the muscle cell is dependent upon its potassium level. Drugs may also delay the passage of intestinal contents. Morphine and codeine decrease the propulsive motility by resulting in a marked increase in tone. Atropine decreases motility by paralyzing the parasympathetic nerve endings.

Constipation

Constipation may be defined as an abnormal retention of fecal matter or undue delay in discharge when compared with the patient's usual bowel habits. However, the term is used in a variety of ways. It may refer to the fact that the stool occurs with relative infrequency, that the stool is insufficient in quantity, or that it is abnormally hard and dry.

ETIOLOGY. Constipation may be due to psychologic factors, dietary constituents, laxatives and drugs, neurogenic causes, decreased skeletal muscular power, and mechanical factors which are either intrinsic or extrinsic to the gastrointestinal tract.

Psychogenic constipation may be related to improper training, and the symptom frequently dates from early childhood. The end result may be a functional megacolon, which is considered to be more common than Hirschsprung's disease. *Dietary factors* include a lack of bulky foods and the use of laxatives which lead to overstimulation of the bowel with eventual fatigue. Drugs with constipating effects have already been referred to in the section on Intestinal Transit.

Decreased muscular power in the skeletal muscles of the diaphragm, abdominal wall, and pelvic floor may all cause constipation. Weakness of the diaphragm may be associated with a variety of chronic pulmonary diseases, while weakness of the abdominal wall may occur in pregnancy, in the presence of large, rapidly expanding intraabdominal masses, and in patients with marked ascites. Weakness of the pelvic floor is usually a consequence of pregnancy. The role of *atony of the intestinal muscle* is difficult to evaluate and may be of minimal importance. Hypokalemia results in ileus based on this cause. Collagen and endocrine disorders are thought to be associated with intestinal atony. *Neurogenic causes* include tabes dorsalis, multiple sclerosis, spinal cord tumors, and trauma. These lesions may result in deficient reflex activity or may directly destroy or depress the autonomic innervation of the intestine. In Hirschsprung's disease the neurologic deficit in the myenteric and submucosal plexuses interrupts the peristaltic action to that segment. *Factors which are intrinsic to the gastrointestinal tract* and contribute to the symptom of constipation include tumors, fecal impactions, intussusception, and volvulus. The mechanical factor is also implicated at the anal sphincter, when spasm and the voluntary avoidance of defecation because of pain occur in patients with hemorrhoids, fissures, or proctitis. *Extrinsic causes* consist of large intraabdominal masses such as ovarian cysts, fibroids, pregnancy, and obstructing adhesions.

ASSOCIATED SYMPTOMS AND EFFECTS. Obstipation, which is defined as the absence of passage of both flatus and feces, is suggestive of mechanical obstruction. Reflex symptoms accompanying constipation include back and hip pain, headache, and, occasionally, tachycardia. So-called "intestinal toxemia" in patients with chronic constipation remains unproved but probably occurs. Fecal accumulations within the rectum may reach large size and contribute to the formation of anal lesions such as hemorrhoids, fissures, and ulcers. Constipation also has a significant role in the development of colonic diverticula and sigmoid volvulus.

CLINICAL EVALUATION. The history should include complete elaboration of bowel habits and also the patient's dietary intake. Direct questioning concerning the color, consistency, and caliber of the stool, the presence of melena or unaltered blood, mucus, or undigested fats or foods, and the occurrence of tenesmus is indicated. Although abdominal examination may reveal a mass, the rectal is usually the most rewarding aspect of the physical examination. Proctosigmoidoscopy may define the presence of inflammation, tumors, or the melanosis coli of patients who take laxatives chronically. Roentgenographic examination with a barium enema is indicated in all patients with prolonged constipation.

Diarrhea

Diarrhea refers to an excessively rapid evacuation of excessively fluid stool. It may be acute, in which instance it is usually related to dietary, toxic, or infectious causes. When diarrhea is chronic or recurrent, it is more likely a manifestation of gastrointestinal disease.

ETIOLOGY. Even when discussion is limited to chronic diarrhea, classification is at best imperfect.

Functional enterocolonic disease represents the most common cause of chronic diarrhea, which is a relatively frequent manifestaton of emotional disorder. The mechanism has not been defined, and the spectrum of emotions which are associated with diarrhea is great. Emotional problems are major factors in the development of mucous colitis and may play a contributory role in ulcerative colitis.

Organic colonic disease is a frequent cause of diarrhea. Included in this group is ulcerative colitis and granulomatous colitis, diverticulitis, obstructive lesions such as malignancy or fecal impaction, and polyposis. Rarer causes are lymphogranuloma venereum, endometriosis of the colon, and colitis secondary to ingestion of toxic drugs such as the heavy metals. Orally ingested arsenic, mercury, and alcohol in high concentration induce hyperemia and edema of both the small intestine and colon. Villous adenoma is frequently associated with diarrhea because of the large quantity of fluid and mucus excreted by the tumor itself. Diarrhea, paradoxically, may be the presenting manifestation in patients with obstruction, particularly fecal impaction.

Small intestinal causes of diarrhea include regional ileitis, tuberculous enteritis, and a great variety of diseases associated with a defect in absorption. The absorption defect may be primary in such syndromes as sprue or may be secondary to intestinal tumors such as carcinoid, intestinal lipodystrophy, or the Zollinger-Ellison syndrome. Reduction of absorption may also be due to mechanical causes such as extensive enterectomy, fistulas, or enterocolostomy bypassing a significant proportion of the bowel. Malabsorption and diarrhea are also a consequence of the blind loop syndrome.

Gastric factors have been implicated as causes of diarrhea. Diarrhea may be an accompaniment of either hypochlorhydria, such as is seen in achylia gastrica or with gastric neoplasms, and also with the hyperchlorhydria of patients with the Zollinger-Ellison syndrome. Diarrhea is often a major symptom following surgical treatment for peptic ulceration. It is one of the manifestations of the dumping syndrome following gastrectomy, the afferent loop syndrome, gastrojejunal colic fistula, or the inadvertent performance of a gastroileostomy rather than a gastrojejunostomy. Diarrhea is also seen following vagotomy and drainage procedures because of changes in the innervation of the small intestine.

Disorders of the *solid viscera of the gastrointestinal system,* particularly the pancreas and hepatobiliary organs, are also causes of diarrhea. A deficiency of pancreatic juice, such as occurs with chronic pancreatitis and obstructive malignancy, is associated with diarrhea. As has already been mentioned, diarrhea is one of the major manifestations of the non-insulin-secreting islet cell tumor of Zollinger-Ellison. Diarrhea may be a symptom of obstruction of the extrahepatic biliary tract but is more frequently noted with extrahepatic biliary fistulas. It is a major manifestation of the syndrome of watery diarrhea, hypokalemia, and achlorhydria ascribed to secretion of vasoactive intestinal peptide.

Enteric infections and parasitic infestations are characteristically manifested by diarrhea. Included in this group are infections with the viruses, *Salmonella* and *Shigella* and some coliform organisms, and the ominous staphylococcal enterocolitis. The last occurs after antibiotics have eliminated the usual intestinal flora. Amebiasis and leishmaniasis are commonly accompanied by diarrhea, as are the infestations with helminths such as *Ascaris,* liver flukes, schistosomes, and *Trichinella.*

Metabolic disorders may also cause diarrhea. Thyrotoxicosis, with its excitation of the nervous system, results in a marked autonomic hyperactivity and is frequently associated with diarrhea. Parathyroid deficiency with its accompanying hypocalcemia increases neuromuscular excitability and results in a hyperirritable bowel. Medullary carcinoma of the thyroid is frequently associated with diarrhea related to increased secretion of calcitonin. Hypermotility is also noted in uremia. The pathophysiology explaining the diarrhea which is associated with diabetes has not been defined. In these patients, diarrhea has a tendency to occur at night, and antibiotic therapy has induced remission. Patients with Addisonian crisis may also have diarrhea.

A variety of *central nervous system stimulations* result in increased peristaltic contractions in both the small intestine and colon. Diarrhea is seen in patients with tabes dorsalis and intracranial space-occupying lesions and tumors.

Drugs act in different ways to produce diarrhea. Most cathartics result in loose stools because of their muscosal irritating effect or by a hygroscopic effect. Certain drugs administered parenterally cause intestinal hypermotility by their action on the autonomic nervous system. Acetylcholine, neostigmine, and Urecholine are all intestinal stimulants. Intravenously administered serotonin stimulates intestinal peristalsis, and its precursor, 5-hydroxytryptophan, is thought to be the etiologic factor in the diarrhea associated with the carcinoid syndrome.

CONSEQUENCES OF DIARRHEA. The consequences are dependent upon the intensity and duration of the symptom. Severe or prolonged diarrhea may result in dehydration, electrolyte loss, and acidosis. The fecal sodium and chloride concentrations are usually lower than the plasma levels, whereas the potassium and bicarbonate levels are higher. The villous adenoma excretes a fluid which is particularly high in potassium with concentrations many times that of plasma.

Acidosis may result because of a high bicarbonate content in the stool or may be related to the production of acid due to starvation or to the dehydration compromising renal function. Dehydration and acidosis accelerate the body depletion of potassium by a shift of the cation out of the cell in exchange for sodium and hydrogen ions. These factors coupled with the large amount of potassium lost in the stool because of excretion into the intestine in exchange for sodium absorption from the lower small intestine and colon may result in significant hypokalemia.

Plasma or electrolyte determinations do not represent a guide to the severity of volume loss, since this reflection is dependent upon the relative tonicity of the stool with respect to extracellular fluid and the amount of fluid lost. In the absence of associated bleeding, the hematocrit is the better index of the severity of dehydration.

CLINICAL EVALUATION. History. Direct questioning should elicit the duration of diarrhea, the time of day during which diarrhea occurs, the patient's description of the stool, the presence of accompanying pain or urge to defecate, and the presence of other manifestations of gastrointestinal disease such as anorexia, nausea, and vomiting. A family or community history of similar episodes suggests an infectious basis. Diarrhea which alternates with constipation occurs with colon lesions such as carcinoma, diverticulitis, partial intestinal obstruction, and chronic constipation treated with laxatives. Recurrent episodes of diarrhea are characteristic of ulcerative colitis, psychogenic causes, and amebic colitis. Ulcerative colitis may be associated with red stools, while the patient may recognize infestation by the presence of the offending organism in the stool. Large, pale, bulky stools suggest pancreatic deficiency. Large amounts of mucus in the stool are seen in patients with mucous colitis, ulcerative colitis, carcinoma of the colon, and villous adenoma.

Pain is a frequent factor with ulcerative colitis and diverticulitis, and may be present when diarrhea is due to carcinoma. Tenesmus commonly accompanies ulcerative colitis and carcinoma of the rectum and lymphogranuloma venereum. Anorexia, nausea, and/or vomiting are more characteristic symptoms of intestinal malignancy, ulcerative colitis, and severe bacillary or amebic dysentery.

Physical Examination. *Fever* may be present with a variety of inflammatory processes and occurs more rarely as an accompaniment of neoplastic disease with the exception of lymphoma. Arthritis is particularly common in ulcerative colitis, regional enteritis, and lipodystrophy. This also applies to other hypersensitivity reactions such as iritis and erythema nodosum. A palpable *abdominal mass* should be sought. In the left lower quadrant, this may suggest sigmoid carcinoma or diverticulitis with inflammatory obstruction. Granulomas of regional enteritis, amebic infection, and tuberculosis may all cause palpable masses. *Tenderness* suggests regional enteritis, diverticulitis, or intraabdominal inflammatory processes. *Digital examination* of the rectum may define the presence of lymphogranuloma venereum, carcinoma, granulomas, ulcerative colitis, diffuse polyposis, or a fecal impaction. *Proctosigmoidoscopy* should represent an integral part of the examination of the patient with diarrhea. A friable rectal mucosa may suggest ulcerative colitis or amebiasis. The overwhelming majority of patients with ulcerative colitis have lesions which may be visualized by this technique. Malignant lesions, polyps, and villous adenomas can usually be defined by proctosigmoidoscopy.

Stool. The stool should be evaluated for consistency and the presence of mucus and occult and unaltered blood. Fatty stools suggest pancreatic insufficiency or malabsorption. Carcinoma and diverticulitis may be associated with bloody stools. Microscopic examination for ova and parasites is particularly pertinent to the diagnosis of infestations.

Radiological Studies. Abdominal films may demonstrate intestinal obstruction, a mass, or calculi associated with chronic pancreatitis. Barium enema is an essential part of the examination and is frequently diagnostic for ulcerative colitis, tumors, and diverticulitis. Regurgitation at the terminal ileum may define the presence of regional enteritis or tuberculous enteritis. In rare instances, regurgitation of barium into the jejunum or stomach will demonstrate a fistula. The upper gastrointestinal series is also of importance, particularly in determining the presence of gastrocolic fistula, blind loop syndrome, and iatrogenic gastroileostomy. The barium meal may be utilized as a method of determining intestinal transit time in patients with massive resection. Primary malabsorption syndromes may be associated with a small bowel pattern which is quite characteristic. Pancreatography may be indicated.

Laparotomy. In some cases, laparotomy should be considered a diagnostic procedure. Small bowel biopsy is indicated in the differential diagnosis of malabsorption syndrome, regional enteritis, Whipple's disease, lymphomas, and small intestinal tumors.

INTESTINAL OBSTRUCTION

Intestinal obstruction exists when there is interference with the normal aboral progression of intestinal contents. The term *mechanical intestinal obstruction* is used if an actual physical barrier blocks the intestinal lumen. The term *ileus,* though properly a synonym for intestinal obstruction from whatever cause, by common usage now connotes failure of downward progress of bowel contents because of disordered propulsive motility of the bowel.

Gastric outlet obstruction is discussed in Chap. 26, esophageal obstruction in Chap. 25, and mesenteric vascular obstruction in Chap. 35. Discussion of specific entities causing intestinal obstruction in infancy and childhood will be found in Chap. 39.

ETIOLOGY. The causes of mechanical obstruction may be classified according to the manner in which the obstruction is produced: (1) by obturation of the lumen as in gallstone ileus, (2) by encroachment on the lumen by intrinsic disease of the bowel wall as in regional enteritis or carcinoma, or (3) by lesions extrinsic to bowel such as an adhesive band (Table 24-4).

Classification of intestinal obstruction on clinical and pathologic grounds is also necessary. In *simple mechanical obstruction* the lumen is obstructed, but the blood supply

Table 24-4. MECHANISMS OF INTESTINAL OBSTRUCTIONS

Mechanical obstruction of the lumen
  Obturation of the lumen
    Meconium
    Intussusception
    Gallstones
    Impactions—fecal, barium, bezoar, worms
  Lesions of bowel
    Congenital
      Atresia and stenosis
      Imperforate anus
      Duplications
      Meckel's diverticulum
    Traumatic
    Inflammatory
      Regional enteritis
      Diverticulitis
      Chronic ulcerative colitis
    Neoplastic
    Miscellaneous
      K^+-induced stricture
      Radiation stricture
      Endometriosis
  Lesions extrinsic to bowel
    Adhesive band constriction, or angulation by adhesion
    Hernia and wound dehiscence
    Extrinsic masses
      Annular pancreas
      Anomalous vessels
      Abscesses and hematomas
      Neoplasms
  Volvulus
Inadequate propulsive motility
  Neuromuscular defects
    Megacolon
    Paralytic ileus
      Abdominal causes
        Intestinal distension
        Peritonitis
        Retroperitoneal lesions
      Systemic causes
        Electrolyte imbalance
        Toxemias
    Spastic ileus
  Vascular occlusion
    Arterial
    Venous

is intact. If mesenteric vessels are occluded, then *strangulation obstruction* exists. *Closed-loop obstruction* results when both limbs of the loop are obstructed so that neither aboral progression nor regurgitation is possible. Obstruction is further delineated by classification as partial or complete, acute or chronic, high or low, small intestinal or colonic.

INCIDENCE. Because accurate vital statistics are still not universally available in the United States, the overall incidence of intestinal obstruction and the mortality therefrom can be only roughly estimated. Probably about 20 percent of surgical admissions for acute abdominal conditions are for intestinal obstruction.

Adhesive bands are now the most frequent cause of obstruction for all age groups combined. Strangulated groin hernia, formerly the most common cause, is now in second place, with neoplasm of the bowel in third place. In some recently reported series, neoplasm has taken over second place, with hernia now in third. These three etiologic agents account for more than 80 percent of all intestinal obstruction.

The order of frequency differs for different age groups. Hernia is by far the most common cause of obstruction in childhood. Colorectal carcinoma and diverticulitis coli are prominent etiologic agents in the older age group, and these lesions are becoming more prominent in the overall picture as more of the population is living into the geriatric age where these lesions prevail.

The mortality rate from intestinal obstruction was over 50 percent in the United States in the early part of this century. There has been a gradual reduction, the sharpest fall occurring in the decade after World War II. The mortality rate is now under 10 percent. The factors principally responsible for the reduction are (1) recognition of the role of fluid and electrolyte therapy, (2) gastrointestinal decompression by intubation, and (3) antibiotics. Probably equally responsible is the definitive marked rise in surgical standards that occurred in the United States after World War II.

Though the mortality rate is now but one-fifth of the rate in the early twentieth century, it is still distressingly and needlessly high. This death rate could be appreciably lowered if patients with hernias were urged to have their hernias repaired, since herniorrhaphy can now be done with only about a 0.1 to 0.2 percent mortality even in the presence of other chronic systemic disease. A further lowering of the death rate could be attained if a larger percentage of patients could be operated upon before simple mechanical obstruction has progressed to strangulation obstruction with its greatly increased morbidity and mortality.

PATHOPHYSIOLOGY. Though simple mechanical obstruction, strangulation obstruction, and ileus have much in common, there are important differences in pathophysiology and management. Also, colon obstruction differs in some aspects from small bowel obstruction.

Simple Mechanical Obstruction of the Small Intestine. The principal physiologic derangements of the mechanically obstructed intestine with intact blood supply are accumulation of fluid and gas above the point of obstruction and altered bowel motility, which lead also to systemic derangements. These will be considered separately, although such a division is somewhat artificial.

Fluid and Electrolyte Losses. Death from intestinal obstruction was for many years attributed to "toxins" that were absorbed from the intestine. In 1912 Hartwell and Hoguet were able to prolong the life of dogs with high intestinal obstruction by the daily parenteral administration of physiologic saline solution. Gamble later demonstrated that the "toxic" factor in simple mechanical obstruction was actually the loss of fluid and electrolytes from the body by vomiting and by sequestering in the obstructed bowel.

Accumulation of large quantities of fluid and gas within the lumen of the bowel above an obstruction is striking and progressive. Some have felt that the fluid is principally digestive secretions and that obstruction causes hypersecretion of digestive juices. Others have felt that the principal defect is not hypersecretion of digestive juices but rather the inability of the obstructed bowel to absorb water and electrolytes at the normal rate.

Availability of isotopes since about 1940 to measure movements of water and electrolytes in both directions across the intestinal mucosa has greatly simplified these measurements and has produced much quantitative data. It is now clear that the absorption of ingested fluid and of upper gastrointestinal digestive secretions are but a part of a much larger exchange of fluid between the body and the lumen of the gastrointestinal tract. For example, if a fasting adult ingests 1,000 ml of water, about 50 percent is absorbed in 30 minutes. When barium sulfate is mixed with the water, it can be seen fluoroscopically to be distributed throughout the small intestine within 2 or 3 minutes. If D_2O—heavy water—is placed in the intestine, 50 percent of the D_2O reaches the blood within 3 minutes. Thus during absorption there must be a flux of water from blood to intestinal lumen only slightly slower than the flux from the lumen into the blood. The above example suggests that in 30 minutes about 5,000 ml goes from blood to lumen while 5,500 ml is going from lumen to blood, giving a net absorption of 500 ml.

The movement of a substance across the intestinal mucosa (sorption) is equal to the difference between the unidirectional flux from intestinal lumen to blood (insorption) and the opposite flux from blood to lumen (exsorption).

Accumulation of fluid within the bowel—a negative net flux—will result if the flux from lumen to blood (insorption) is decreased or if the flux from blood to lumen (exsorption) is increased. Currently available evidence from animal experiments is conflicting on which mechanism is responsible for the accumulation of fluid within the lumen in intestinal obstruction—increased secretion or decreased absorption.

Shields studied the movement of water, sodium, and potassium across the ileal mucosa of dogs in which obstruction had been produced by transecting the distal ileum and closing both ends. He found that within 12 hours the ileum above the obstruction ceased to absorb (net) and began to secrete water at a steadily increasing rate. This resulted initially from a decrease in the flux from lumen to blood. The flux from blood to lumen continued at a normal rate initially, but after 48 hours the rate of entry

of water increased rapidly and significantly. The findings for sodium and potassium were parallel. At sacrifice, the obstructed bowel was heavier and shorter than the unobstructed bowel, and histologically the veins in the bowel wall were greatly congested and engorged. The part of the intestine distal to the obstruction did not react in the same way as the part of the intestine above. Although the volume of water absorbed by this segment was reduced to one-third of its original rate after 60 hours of obstruction, at no time did exsorption exceed insorption. And at sacrifice there was no edema or congestion of the bowel wall.

Davenport has reported similar studies in which the fluxes across the mucosa of an obstructed ileal segment were measured by placing a radioactive sodium chloride solution in the lumen. Normal fluxes were found in the direction of blood to lumen, but fluxes from lumen to blood were depressed or abolished. As a result, water, sodium, and chloride (and presumably other ions) moved into the obstructed intestinal segment but not out of it, distending it with fluid having approximately the electrolyte composition of plasma.

Further studies are obviously needed to clarify the pathophysiologic mechanism by which the obstructed bowel becomes progressively distended with fluid.

The bowel immediately above the obstruction is the most affected initially. It becomes distended with fluids and electrolytes, and circulation is impaired. With increasing intraluminal pressure the fluid is dispersed orad until it reaches bowel that is still capable of absorbing. When obstruction has been present for a long time, the proximal portions of the intestine also lose their ability to handle fluid and electrolytes, and the entire bowel proximal to the obstruction becomes distended.

A second route of fluid and electrolyte loss is into the wall of the involved bowel, accounting for the boggy edematous appearance of the bowel often seen at operation. Some of this fluid exudes from the serosal surface of the bowel, resulting in free peritoneal fluid. The extent of fluid and electrolyte loss into the bowel wall and peritoneal cavity depends on the extent of bowel involved in venous congestion and edema, and the length of time before the obstruction is relieved.

The most obvious route of fluid and electrolyte loss is by vomiting—or gastrointestinal tube after treatment is initiated. The aggregate of these losses (1) into the bowel lumen, (2) into the edematous bowel wall, (3) as free peritoneal fluid, plus (4) by vomiting or nasogastric suction rapidly depletes the extracellular fluid space, leading progressively to hemoconcentration, hypovolemia, renal insufficiency, shock, and death unless treatment is prompt and resolute. The blood chemistry values to be expected in intestinal obstruction will be found below under Clinical Manifestations.

Intestinal Gas. Much of the distension of the bowel above a mechanical obstruction can be accounted for by the fluid sequestered within the lumen. Intestinal gas is also responsible for distension.

The approximate composition of small intestine gas (Table 24-5) shows that the basic composition is that of air to which small amounts of gases not found in the atmosphere have been added.

Table 24-5. INTESTINAL GAS

Percent

Nitrogen	70
Oxygen	12
Carbon dioxide	8
Hydrogen sulfide	5
Ammonia and amines	4
Hydrogen	1

Gases are absorbed from the intestine at rates that are directly related to the partial pressure of the particular gas in the intestine, in the plasma, and in the air breathed. Thus with nitrogen there is little diffusion, since the partial pressures of the gas are virtually the same in intestine, plasma, and air. On the other hand carbon dioxide diffuses very rapidly, because the partial pressure of carbon dioxide is high in the intestine, intermediate in plasma, and very low in air. For this reason, though carbon dioxide is produced in large amounts in the intestine, it contributes little to gaseous distension because of its rapid diffusibility.

Maddock et al. studied the accumulation of intestinal gas by serial roentgenography in patients who had been prepared for pyelography. He found that by continuous gastric suction, considerable volumes of air were aspirated from the stomach, and when it was kept empty, no increase in intestinal gas occurred. Patients without gastric suction rapidly accumulated gas on the serial x-rays. Nervous patients undergoing pyelography had three times as much air aspirated from their stomachs as calm patients. It is probable that air swallowing is increased in patients with the abdominal discomfort of intestinal obstruction.

Wangensteen produced simple mechanical obstruction of the lower ileum in dogs and found that an average of 328 ml of gas accumulated. Closed-loop obstructions, precluding swallowed air, contained but 12 ml of gas. To elucidate further the role of swallowed air, the cervical esophagus was divided, the proximal end brought to the skin, the distal end closed, and the ileum then divided. Parenteral fluids and electrolytes were given. The average survival was 35 days, and the amount of gas and fluid found in the intestine at autopsy was not great. The control animals—with obstruction but without esophageal transection—lived about 5 days.

On the basis of these and other studies, it is now felt that intestinal gases are principally derived from swallowed air.

Bowel Motility. With obstruction of the lumen, peristalsis becomes violent in an "attempt" to overcome the obstruction. After a short time, continuous peristalsis above the obstruction gives way to regularly recurring bursts of peristaltic activity interspersed with quiescent periods. The duration of the quiescent period is related to the level of the obstruction in the gastrointestinal tract—it is 3 to 5 minutes with high obstruction, 10 to 15 minutes with lower ileal obstruction. These muscular contractions may be of sufficient violence to traumatize the bowel and contribute to the swelling and edema of the bowel wall. As bowel above the obstruction distends, bowel below the obstruction becomes progressively more quiet. This results from an inhibitory reflex initiated by distension of the bowel above.

Strangulated Obstruction. Occlusion of the blood supply to a segment of bowel in addition to obstruction of the lumen is usually referred to as strangulated obstruction. Interference with the mesenteric blood supply is the most serious complication of intestinal obstruction. This frequently occurs secondary to adhesive band obstruction, hernia, and volvulus.

The accumulation of fluid and gas in obstructed loops and the altered motility seen in simple mechanical obstruction are rapidly overshadowed by the consequences of blockage of venous outflow from the strangulated segment—extravasation of bloody fluid into the bowel and bowel wall.

In addition to the loss of blood and plasma-like fluid, the gangrenous bowel leaks toxic materials (not to be confused with the pre-Gamble "toxins") into the peritoneal cavity. These have been variously identified as exotoxins or endotoxins, or toxic hemin breakdown products.

The pathophysiology of the strangulated loop was pointed out in a series of papers by Murphy, Brooks, et al. in the early part of this century. They showed (1) that the contents of an obstructed bowel are toxic; (2) that bacteria are necessary for the production of this toxin; (3) that neither living tissue nor mucous membrane, nor any of the secretions of the mucous membrane, are necessary for the formation of the toxin; (4) that the toxin does not pass through normal mucosa; (5) that absorption of the toxin is more important than its production, as the toxin is physiologically lost if it exists within a loop and is never absorbed; (6) that circulatory damage aids absorptions; and (7) that symptoms may be correlated with the toxin formed in the obstructed intestine.

Recent work by Barnett et al. has reemphasized the role of bacteria. A standard method of producing strangulation obstruction uniformly killed dogs in 24 to 36 hours. Peritoneal fluid from dogs succumbing to obstruction was lethal when injected intravenously into normal animals. If the strangulated segment was enclosed in a plastic bag so that the exuding fluid was kept separate from the abdominal cavity, survival was extended far past the usual lethal period. Furthermore, if the plastic bag with the accumulated fluid and the strangulated segment of intestine was removed, the dogs survived indefinitely. But if the bag was allowed to spill its contents into the peritoneal cavity, the animals died within 8 to 12 hours. The toxicity could be largely counteracted by instilling antibiotics into the obstructed loop of intestine or the plastic bag. Passage through a Seitz filter also removed the toxicity, indicating that bacteria played a major role in these experiments.

Cohn and Atik were able to lower the mortality rate in dogs with a closed loop of ileum from a control level of 91 to 13 percent by instilling antibiotics into the loop, again pointing to the importance of bacteria in strangulation obstruction.

Closed-Loop Obstruction. When both afferent and efferent limbs of a loop of bowel are obstructed, closed-loop intestinal obstruction exists. This is a clinically dangerous form of obstruction because of the propensity for rapid progression to strangulation of the blood supply before the usual manifestations of intestinal obstruction become obvious. Interference with blood supply may occur either from the same mechanism that produced obstruction of the intestine—twist of the bowel on the mesentery, extrinsic band—or from distension of the obstructed loop. The secretory pressure in the closed loop quite rapidly reaches a level sufficient to interfere with venous return from the loop. Widespread distension of the intestine usually does not occur, and so neither does abdominal distension.

Colon Obstruction. The effects on the patient with colon obstruction are usually less dramatic than the effects of small bowel obstruction. First, colon obstruction, with the exception of volvulus, usually does not strangulate. Second, because the colon is principally a storage organ with relatively minor absorptive and secretory functions, fluid and electrolyte sequestration progresses more slowly. Systemic derangements therefrom are of less magnitude and urgency than in small bowel obstruction.

Progressive distension is the most dangerous aspect of nonstrangulated colon obstruction. If the ileocecal valve is incompetent, then partial decompression of the obstructed colon may occur by reflux into the ileum. But if the ileocecal valve is competent, then the colon becomes essentially a closed loop—closed below by the obstructing lesion and above by the competent valve. If the obstruction is not relieved, distension progressing to rupture of the colon threatens. The cecum is the usual site of rupture, because it is the segment of the colon with the largest diameter. According to the law of Laplace, the pressure required to stretch the walls of a hollow viscus decreases in inverse proportion to the radius of curvature. Applying this law to the colon, given an equal pressure throughout the colon, we find that the greatest distension will occur in the portion of the colon with the largest radius (Fig. 24-3).

CLINICAL MANIFESTATIONS. The initial symptoms of simple mechanical intestinal obstruction are abdominal pain, vomiting, and failure to pass gas or feces by rectum. Abdominal distension is a later symptom.

As the bowel obstructs, severe *cramping pain* is felt synchronously with hyperperistalsis. Initially, the waves of cramps are unremitting, but after a short time attacks of pain alternate with quiescent periods during which the patient may feel quite well. The pain is diffuse, poorly localized, and is felt across the upper abdomen in high obstruction, at the level of the umbilicus in low ileal obstruction, in the lower abdomen in colon obstruction, and in the perineum as well as the abdomen in rectosigmoid obstruction. The period between attacks of pain is short with high intestinal obstruction (4 or 5 minutes) and is longer the lower the obstruction (15 to 20 minutes). When obstruction is not relieved, the characteristic colicky pain may cease (as distension becomes extreme) and be replaced by a steady generalized abdominal discomfort. There is no real pain in adynamic ileus, just a steady generalized abdominal discomfort similar to that seen in neglected simple mechanical obstruction. Steady severe

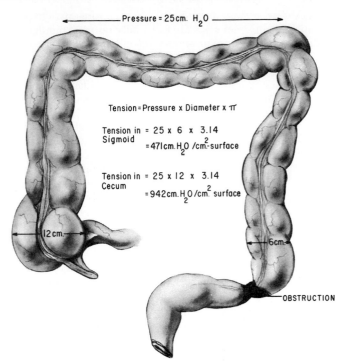

Fig. 24-3. Physics of cecal rupture in colon obstruction.

pain with no quiescent periods is usually indicative of strangulation.

Vomiting, like pain, usually occurs almost immediately after obstruction of the bowel. This early vomiting is "reflex" vomiting and is followed by a variable quiescent period before vomiting resumes. The quiet interval is short in high obstruction but may even be a day or two with low small bowel obstruction. The vomitus frequently becomes thick, dark, and malodorous (i.e., feculent) from stagnation and bacterial action but is not actually regurgitated feces. With high obstruction, vomiting is more frequent and copious and may effectively decompress the obstructed bowel. With low small bowel obstruction, vomiting is less frequent and less productive; little decompression of bowel occurs, because of the excessive length of bowel that the regurgitated material must traverse and because segmentation of the boggy loops prevents regurgitation. Reflex vomiting is unusual in colon obstruction. Thus, vomiting does not occur in most cases until retrograde distension involves the small bowel. When the ileocecal valve is competent, small bowel distension and vomiting may not occur in colonic obstruction.

Failure to pass gas or feces through the rectum is a valuable diagnostic symptom. Gas and feces distal to the obstruction may pass through the rectum after obstruction occurs, however, particularly if the obstruction is high in the jejunum. Cramping pain followed shortly by explosive diarrhea often indicates partial intestinal obstruction.

Abdominal distension is the result of fairly long-standing obstruction. There may be no generalized distension with high small bowel obstruction.

Physical examination of a patient with simple mechanical obstruction within the first 24 hours may yield surprisingly few abnormal findings except during periods of colicky pain. Vital signs are essentially normal, and dehydration and distension are not yet marked. Strangulation obstruction is likely if the patient appears seriously ill during this early period. *Palpation* during colic usually demonstrates muscle guarding; between attacks of pain only slight tenderness remains. A mass or localized area of tenderness usually indicates strangulation. *Auscultation* is of great value: in simple mechanical obstruction the abdomen is quiet except during attacks of colic, at which time the sounds become loud, high-pitched, and metallic and occur in bursts or rushes; in paralytic ileus an occasional isolated bowel sound is heard; gangrenous bowel produces complete silence. By the second or third day of obstruction serious illness is obvious. Dehydration and distension are marked, and vital signs are increasingly abnormal, though frank shock does not occur until very late in simple obstruction.

Laboratory Findings. The loss of large amounts of essentially isotonic extracellular fluid into the intestine is principally responsible for the laboratory findings in simple mechanical obstruction. The body responds to this sudden volume decrease by antidiuresis and renal sodium retention. In the early phases, in which the effects are predominantly those of extracellular fluid loss, the hematocrit rises roughly in proportion to the fluid loss. There is little change in the concentration of sodium, potassium, and chloride in the plasma. Acid-base changes, as manifested by the pH and carbon dioxide, are slight. The markedly reduced urine flow is reflected in a somewhat elevated BUN level. The dehydration and antidiuresis is often so marked that patients may not be able to produce a urine specimen until after intravenous fluid therapy has been started. Urinary specific gravity of 1.025 to 1.030 is the rule; mild proteinuria or acetonuria may also be present.

In the untreated patient, sodium-free water, derived from catabolism of cells and oxidation of fat, tends to restore the acute loss of extracellular fluid volume but at the expense of plasma osmolality. Thus, there is a gradual reduction of the plasma sodium and chloride concentration. Urine volume gradually increases, though not to normal, with excretion of potassium, including the potassium freed by cellular catabolism. The previously noted progressive increase in the hematocrit is halted or actually reversed by the ingress of endogenous water. Acid-base effects are determined by the nature of the fluid lost. Metabolic acidosis due to the combined effects of dehydration, starvation, ketosis, and loss of alkaline secretions is most common. Metabolic alkalosis is infrequent and is principally due to loss of highly acid gastric juice. With great distension of the abdomen, the diaphragm may be sufficiently elevated to embarrass respiration, resulting in carbon dioxide retention and respiratory acidosis.

The white blood cell count is useful in differentiating between different types of obstruction. In general, simple mechanical obstruction calls forth only modest numbers of leukocytes—white blood cell counts often to 15,000 with some shift to the left. White blood cell counts of 15,000 to 25,000/mm³ and marked polymorphonuclear predominance with many immature forms strongly suggest that the

obstruction is strangulated. Very high white cell counts, such as 40,000 to 60,000/mm³, suggest primary mesenteric vascular occlusion.

Serum amylase level elevations may occur in intestinal obstruction and compromise the differential diagnostic value of the test. Amylase gains entry to the blood by regurgitation from the pancreas because of back pressure in the duodenum, or by peritoneal absorption after leakage from dying bowel.

Radiologic Findings. When properly done, this is the most important diagnostic procedure. The films must be of good technical quality—not the type that are made in the emergency room by a substitute technician with a portable x-ray machine.

X-rays should be made as early in the hospitalization as the patient's condition permits—usually within the first hour. Plain films of the abdomen (without contrast medium) in the supine and upright positions, and posteroanterior and lateral views of the chest are obtained. If the patient is too weak to remain in the sitting position for the 15 minutes that is necessary to demonstrate air under the diaphragrm (best seen on the posteroanterior chest film), then a left lateral decubitus film may be substituted.

The diagnostic features that enable one to distinguish in the majority of cases between simple mechanical obstruction, strangulation obstruction, and paralytic ileus are summarized in Table 24-6. Representative films of the three types of obstruction are shown in Fig. 24-4.

Gas-fluid levels are among the important criteria in the x-ray diagnosis of intestinal obstruction. Gas is normally visible in the colon and stomach on plain films of the abdomen in normal adults. Small bowel gas may be visible in infants and occasionally in apparently normal adults. The transit time of swallowed air is normally so rapid that there is an insufficient amount in any one place to show on the x-ray. But if the normal aboral progression of intestinal content is interfered with, then gas collects along with retained fluid and produces gas-fluid levels which are best seen on the upright film of the abdomen. Though gas-fluid levels are highly suggestive of intestinal obstruction (including ileus), they may be seen in other conditions such as extreme aerophagia, gastroenteritis, severe constipation, and sprue.

Additional radiographic studies are sometimes indicated. These are barium enema, intravenous urography, and occasionally administration of contrast medium by mouth or nasogastric tube.

Barium enema is indicated when the clinical picture and plain films suggest colon obstruction, to give information on the type and location of the obstruction. Barium enema is often helpful also when the distribution of gas is not clear on the plain films. Barium enema may be used therapeutically for attempted reduction of nonstrangulated intussusception in children.

The dangers of barium enema in obstruction are the possibility of perforating an inflammatory lesion such as diverticulitis or appendicitis and, secondly, changing a partial colon obstruction to a complete one by forcing barium up past a partially obstructing lesion to form an obstructing concretion of inspissated barium.

Table 24-6. RADIOLOGIC SIGNS IN INTESTINAL OBSTRUCTION

Sign	Simple mechanical obstruction (see Fig. 24-4A)	Strangulation obstruction (see Fig. 24-4B)	Adynamic ileus (see Fig. 24-4C)
Gas in intestine	Large bow-shaped loops in ladder pattern	Little distension, often only single loop	Copious gas diffusely through intestine
Gas in colon	Less than nomal	Less than normal	Increased, scattered through colon
Fluid levels in intestine	Definite	If present, small and localized	Often very large throughout
Tumor.	None	Rounded, smooth, C-shaped margin	None
Peritoneal exudate	None	Present; general haziness may obscure	Present with peritonitis; otherwise absent
Diaphragm	Somewhat elevated; free motion	Diminished motion	Elevated; diminished motion

SOURCE: Adapted from C. E. Welch and J. Frimann-Dahl (see References at end of chapter).

Intravenous urography may be indicated to look for ureteral calculi, which often produce marked paralytic ileus.

The principal indication for administration of contrast medium above an obstruction is to differentiate postoperative ileus from mechanical obstruction. The actual point of obstruction rarely can be demonstrated because of dilution of the contrast medium, but if some medium is seen to go through the gastrointestinal tract, the diagnosis of ileus is strengthened. Some surgeons are loath to give barium above an obstruction and prefer to use a liquid medium such as Hypaque. There is, however, little evidence that small amounts of barium are harmful in small bowel obstruction.

MANAGEMENT. The principles of treatment are fluid and electrolyte therapy, decompression of the bowel, and timed surgical intervention.

Essentially all patients with mechanical intestinal ob-

Fig. 24-4. Plain films of the abdomen in intestinal obstruction. *A.* Simple mechanical obstruction of the small intestine. *B.* Closed-loop obstruction with strangulation. *C.* Postoperative adynamic ileus.

struction except in the immediate postoperative period should be operated upon. The decision to be made is *when* to operate—selection of the optimal time for the individual patient.

Patients with simple mechanical obstruction who can be operated upon within the first 24 hours of the disease do not need extensive preoperative preparation, because water and salt depletion and distension are usually not serious at this stage. After the history and physical examination have established the presumptive diagnosis, laboratory studies should be done, intravenous repletion initiated, decompression started with a nasogastric sump tube in the stomach, and abdominal and chest x-ray films taken on the way to the operating room. This whole process should take less than 2 hours. The mortality rate is less than 1 percent for patients with simple mechanical obstruction who are operated upon within the first 24 hours.

If the obstruction has been present for more than 24 hours when the patient is first seen, depletion and distension may be so severe that if strangulation or closed-loop obstruction seems unlikely, the patient's best interests are served by a period of preparation before the obstruction

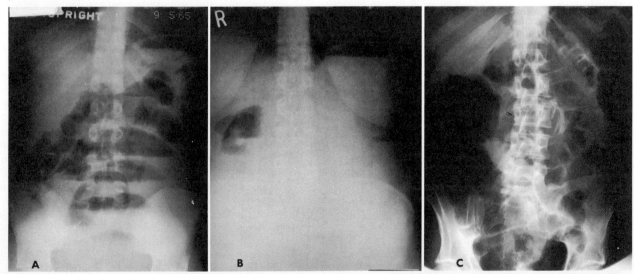

is surgically relieved. In general, the longer the obstruction has existed, the longer it will take to get the patient ready for surgical treatment. Patients with moderate derangements, particularly hypokalemia, usually require 6 to 12 hours; in those with severe problems, 24 to 36 hours may be necessary, mainly because of the hazard of giving intravenous potassium ion faster than it can equilibrate.

With the possible exception of patients with early simple mechanical obstruction, all patients with intestinal obstruction should have a plastic venous catheter threaded into the superior vena cava for frequent measurements of the central venous pressure, as well as for rapid administration of fluid, and an indwelling catheter inserted into the bladder for accurate continual measurement of the urinary output.

The initial hematocrit reading may be used to estimate the extent of extracellular fluid loss, and thus the volume necessary for restoration of this static debt. For example, if the hematocrit has risen to 55 percent, this indicates a loss of approximately 40 percent of the plasma and extracellular fluid volume. In a 70-kg man, this would amount to about 1,100 ml of plasma and 4,000 ml of electrolyte solutions.

Colloid replacement may be either as plasma per se or as human serum albumin, using 1 unit of 12.5 Gm for each 300 ml of plasma required. If acid gastric juice loss is prominent, then normal saline solution is used; otherwise lactated Ringer's solution and 5% dextrose in water in about equal proportions are preferred to replace the lost fluid and to cover maintenance fluid needs. Potassium chloride also will be necessary but should not be given until a good urinary output is established. Antibiotics should also be given in generous dosage and may be added to the intravenous fluids. The choice of antibiotics is a matter of individual preference: the authors currently use a tetracycline and ampicillin.

The rate of fluid administration is best controlled by monitoring the central venous pressure (CVP). Fluids may be given rapidly as long as the CVP remains below 10 to 12 cm of water. The end point of volume replacement is indicated by a sudden rise in the CVP. Other guides are return of skin turgor and the hourly rate of urine production.

The goal in terms of electrolyte concentration and acid-base balance is restoration of these to, or close to, the normal range by the time the volume deficit has been repaired. This is usually possible in patients with reasonably normal renal and pulmonary functions.

When the possibility of strangulation exists, preoperative treatment to fluid-electrolyte normality is not possible or advisable. This is an emergency situation requiring vigorous preparation with blood, plasma, fluids and electrolytes, massive antibiotics, nasogastric suction, and an operation at the earliest possible moment to remove the cause of the strangulation and/or nonviable bowel. Despite application of these principles, the mortality rate in strangulated obstruction is still about 25 percent.

Intubation. Tubes for gastrointestinal aspiration, available in bewildering variety, are basically of but two types: "short" tubes for gastric aspiration and "long" tubes for aspiration of the small intestine. The Levin tube, for nasogastric intubation, is preferred by many surgeons for preoperative gastrointestinal decompression in patients with obstruction. Complete decompression of the gastrointestinal tract is not accomplished, since only the intestinal gas and fluid from the upper intestine that regurgitates into the stomach is removed. The stomach is completely emptied, however, which prevents any possible aspiration during anesthesia, and progression of intestinal distension is halted, since all swallowed air is removed. Nasogastric tubes with a double lumen, one for aspiration plus a small second channel to allow ingress of air into the stomach—the "sump" tube, perform much more efficiently than the old single-lumen tubes.

Long intestinal tubes, of which the Miller-Abbott tubes is the prototype, have a lumen for aspiration plus a mercury-containing balloon or small bag at or near the distal end. When inflated in the intestine, the balloon is carried distad by peristalsis. The purpose of the mercury is to aid in getting the tube through the pylorus. After the tube is passed into the stomach, the patient lies on his right side with feet slightly elevated, so that gravity will help pull the tip of the tube through the pylorus.

In the past, intestinal intubation was advocated for the definitive treatment of simple mechanical intestinal obstruction, and a few surgeons still cling to the belief that a trial of suction therapy is warranted. There is now good evidence that the use of suction as definitive therapy (except as noted below) should be condemned—temporizing may lead to death from strangulation obstruction. For example, Becker analyzed 412 cases of acute intestinal obstruction due to old adhesions and showed that the usual criteria, presence or absence of fever, tachycardia, leukocytosis, a palpable mass, and peritoneal irritation, did not suffice to differentiate simple obstruction from strangulation obstruction. The overall mortality rate in the series was 11.8 percent; in the 52 cases in which tube decompression was abused, the mortality rate was 38.4 percent. Another reason for not using intubation as definitive therapy is an early recurrence rate of over 30 percent. The principal indications now for primary intubation therapy are obstruction in the immediate postoperative period, partial small bowel obstruction, or obstruction due to inflammation which is expected to subside under conservative therapy.

Some surgeons prefer to use a long intestinal tube for preoperative gastrointestinal decompression in patients with obstruction, feeling that decompression of the intestine per se is sufficiently important to warrant the extra time and trouble necessary to pass an intestinal tube as compared to the Levin nasogastric tube. Emptying of the stomach is inadequate with the long tube, however, and a second short tube is required for this purpose.

Operation. Proper timing of the operation for intestinal obstruction is essential. There are four types of obstruction in which the operation should be done as an emergency as soon as possible after admission: strangulation, closed-loop obstruction, colon obstruction, and early simple mechanical obstruction.

The principal hazard to life in strangulation is septic

shock from transperitoneal absorption of toxins spilled from dying bowel. In closed-loop obstruction, which cannot be decompressed by intubation, the hazard is that the loop will strangulate, and it must be treated with the same urgency as strangulation.

In colon obstruction, which also cannot be decompressed by tube, a competent ileocecal valve preventing regurgitation into the ileum converts the colon into a closed loop. Since fluid and electrolyte abnormalities progress slowly in colon obstruction, a brief period of hydration while laboratory studies are being done is all that is necessary before operation. And, as noted above, when patients with simple mechanical obstruction get to the surgeon early in the course of their disease, immediate surgical procedures may be carried out with essentially no mortality. Thus only in *late* simple mechanical obstruction of the small intestine does extensive preparation for operation take priority over immediate operation.

Anesthesia. General anesthesia is safest for the patient and the method of choice from the point of view of both surgeon and anesthesiologist. Endotracheal intubation, at times performed intially under local anesthesia, is particularly indicated to prevent aspiration of regurgitated gastric content. The surgeon should not be tempted to use local anesthesia for abdominal exploration on the assumption that local anesthesia is easier on the poor-risk patient than general anesthesia—it is not! Local anesthesia should be used only when the surgeon knows the cause of the obstruction and plans a limited procedure only, such as cecostomy.

Surgical Procedures. Surgical procedures for the relief of intestinal obstruction may be divided into five categories:

1. Procedures not requiring opening of bowel—lysis of adhesions, manipulation-reduction of intussusception, reduction of incarcerated hernia
2. Enterotomy for removal of obturation obstruction—gallstone, bezoars
3. Resection of the obstructing lesion or strangulated bowel with primary anastomosis
4. Short-circuiting anastomosis around an obstruction
5. Formation of a cutaneous stoma proximal to the obstruction—cecostomy, transverse colostomy (Figs. 24-5 and 24-6).

On opening the peritoneum, the presence or absence of free peritoneal fluid should be noted, as well as the appearance of the fluid. Bloody fluid denotes strangulation, whereas clear straw-colored fluid is found with simple obstruction. The point of obstruction is usually best found by starting in the right lower quadrant. If the cecum is grossly distended, the obstruction is in the colon. If collapsed small bowel is found, then this is followed back to the point of obstruction, thus avoiding evisceration of the proximal distended loops.

The surgeon is sometimes faced with the difficult decision of whether to resect or to replace in the abdomen a loop of intestine of questionable viability. Before release the strangulated loop has a dull purple-red appearance and is devoid of motion. After release there is a dramatic color change to bright red in the obviously viable loop as well as a return of peristalsis. Conversely, in obviously dead bowel there is no color change and no motion after release of the strangulating obstruction. The loop that only partially pinks up and has little or no motion is the problem. It is usually best to wrap the questionable segment in moist laparotomy pads and leave it completely undisturbed for 10 minutes by the clock. If the circulation is obviously better at the end of this time, the loop is replaced in the abdomen. If the viability of the segment is still in doubt, resection should be done. But if a very long segment of bowel is involved, requiring a very extensive resection, then an attempt should be made to restore flow in the larger vessels supplying the segment. Even if this is unsuccessful, one should probably accept the risk of replacing nonviable bowel rather than make an intestinal cripple. The patient is observed very closely; if evidence of progressive toxicity develops, reoperation and resection are done. In any event, reexploration and reevaluation of the status of the bowel about 24 hours later may be advisable.

Decompression of grossly distended intestine during the operative procedure is sometimes necessary, particularly in late simple mechanical obstruction. Operative decompression is still a contentious point. There is no doubt that the operation is facilitated: the site of obstruction is more easily found, the uncontrolled eventration of distended loops through the incision is avoided, the bowel can be returned to the peritoneal cavity without the kinks that may cause segmentation and postoperative obstruction, and closure of the incision is possible without a struggle. Relief of distension also improves the blood supply to the intestine, and peristalsis returns sooner. It is also probable that removal of toxic bowel content is worthwhile. Whereas the normal mucosa is impermeable to these toxins, permeability is affected by impairment of the blood supply, and absorption may occur in compromised bowel.

Operative aspiration can be done in a variety of ways. Multiple needle aspirations are ineffective and definitely increase the morbidity, e.g., a wound infection rate of 20 percent versus a rate of 4 percent in a comparable group of patients without needle aspiration. Decompression with an ordinary suction tip through multiple enterotomies, though effective, is similarly attended by an increased infection rate, plus the risk of small bowel fistula. An effective, safe method of decompression is by passage of a tube from above downward, so that the entire gastrointestinal tract proximal to the obstruction is decompressed. A firm tube with generous lumen (Baker tube) is introduced through a proximal jejunostomy. The tube is advanced by manipulation through the intact bowel until the entire length of involved bowel down to the obstructed segment is pleated on the long tube. The tube is secured in that position for postoperative decompression.

Postoperative Care. The principles of postoperative care are the same as for the preoperative preparation of the patient with obstruction—fluids and electrolytes, antibiotics, and gastrointestinal decompression.

Fluid and electrolyte management is more difficult in the postoperative intestinal obstruction patient than in the usual postoperative abdominal surgical patient because of the large third space of sequestered, isotonic fluid. There is continued loss in the immediate postoperative period

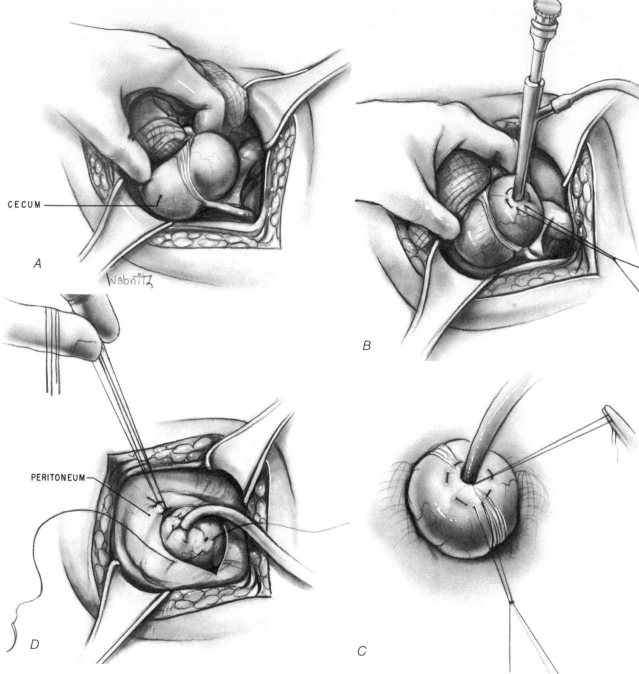

CECUM

A

Wabnitz

B

PERITONEUM

D

C

Fig. 24-5. Tube cecostomy. *A.* A McBurney incision is made in the right lower quadrant, the lateral peritoneal attachment of the cecum is divided, and the cecum is delivered into the wound, using a dry sponge. *B.* The distended cecum is held by the assistant, using gauze sponges, while the surgeon decompresses the cecum with a large trocar connected to suction. If distension is not great, this step may be omitted. *C.* A large rubber tube is then placed in the cecum by enlarging the opening made by the trocar, and the tube is secured in place with two concentric purse-string sutures. *D.* The peritoneum is sutured circumferentially to the cecum. Fascia is approximated; skin and subcutaneous tissues are packed open. The tube is connected to straight drainage.

into the sequestered fluid space. This loss slows in rate, however, and is reversed in direction after a variable period, usually about the third postoperative day. This large autoinfusion, as fluid is picked up by the vascular compartment from the sequestered fluid, must be allowed for in planning the daily ration of intravenous fluid therapy, lest the patient be watered into congestive failure.

Serum sodium and potassium levels must be watched very closely and kept in the normal range. A deficit of

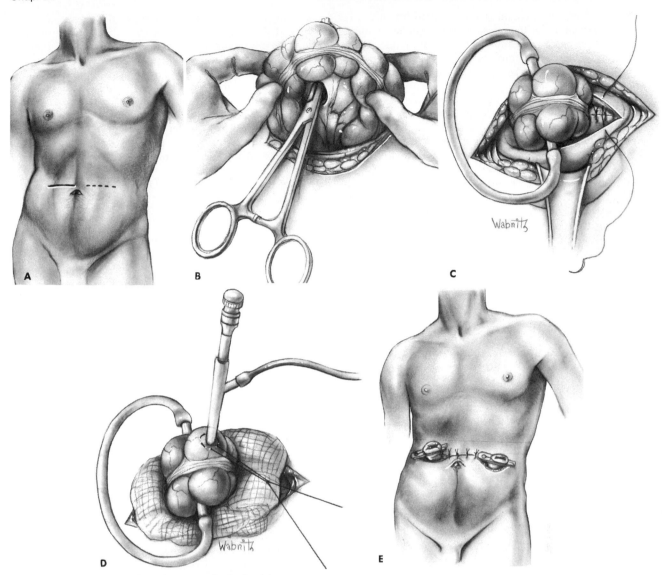

Fig. 24-6. Transverse loop colostomy. *A.* A short transverse incision is made about midway between costal margin and umbilicus. Choice of right or left depends on the type of definitive surgical treatment planned for the future. *B.* After freeing the omentum, an opening is made in an avascular area of the transverse mesocolon close to the bowel. *The middle colic artery must be avoided. C.* A glass rod is inserted through the mesentery and secured in place by rubber tubing. The incision is closed in layers about the colon loop. No sutures are placed in the colon. *D.* If colon distension is extreme, trocar decompression may be done immediately after closing the incision. Otherwise the colostomy is opened with cautery about 24 to 36 hours after operation. *E.* Double-barrel colostomy may be performed initially using deMartel's clamps. A small catheter can be inserted into the proximal limb to achieve immediate decompression.

either or both of these ions is associated with prolonged paralysis of the gastrointestinal tract.

Decompression of the gastrointestinal tract is also harder to handle than in the usual postoperative patient, because restoration of normal propulsive intestinal motility is usually significantly delayed after release of intestinal obstruc-

tion. Whereas bowel function usually resumes on about the third day after abdominal operation, after intestinal obstruction it is often 5 or 6 days before gastrointestinal decompression can be discontinued. After 2 or 3 days of suction drainage it is often advisable to discontinue the suction and vent the intestinal tube to straight drainage only, to minimize fluid and electrolyte losses.

Ileus

Ileus may be divided into three groups: *adynamic, or inhibition, ileus,* in which there is diminished or absent motility because of inhibition of the neuromuscular apparatus; *spastic ileus,* in which the bowel musculature remains tightly contracted without coordinated propulsive motility; and the *ileus of vascular occlusion,* in which the bowel wall is incapable of coordinated motility, because it is dying from ischemia.

Spastic ileus, an uncommon form caused by uncoordinated hyperactivity of the intestine, is seen in heavy-metal poisoning, in prophyria, and sometimes in uremia. Therapy of the intestinal manifestations is usually not indicated—therapy should be aimed at the underlying disorder.

Adynamic ileus of some degree is extremely common, since it occurs after every abdominal operation. The rate of recovery of motor function is different in different segments of the gastrointestinal tract: small bowel motility returns within 24 hours and gastric motility within 48 hours, but colonic inertia persists for 3 to 5 days. Oral intake usually can be resumed on the third or fourth postoperative day. Only when postoperative ileus persists does it become a clinical problem. Common causes of serious degrees of inhibition ileus are many and varied and include intraperitoneal inflammation such as acute appendicitis or acute pancreatitis; retroperitoneal pathologic conditions such as ureteral colic, retroperitoneal hematoma, or fracture of the spine; thoracic lesions such as basal pneumonia or fractured ribs; and systemic causes such as severe toxemia, hyponatremia, or hypokalemia.

Overactivity of the sympathetic system appears to be the common denominator in inhibition ileus associated with many of the lesions listed above; alterations in the composition of the internal environment also playing an important role.

The mechanism by which sympathetic activity brings about inhibition of intestinal motility was studied extensively by Kock, using anesthetized cats. He concluded that centrally induced inhibition of motility is virtually exclusively dependent on the hormonal component of the sympathoadrenal system. Landman and Longmire studied the hormonal influences of peritonitis on paralytic ileus in conscious dogs. Jejunal loops were studied, then subjected to extrinsic denervation by division of the neurovascular pedicle. They found that induction of chemical peritonitis produced atony of the loop with or without innervation and so concluded that inhibition of motility in the denervated loop must be explained on the basis of a blood-borne substance.

CLINICAL MANIFESTATIONS. The primary disease causing the ileus may predominate in the clinical picture, or conversely, in some cases, abdominal findings may so predominate that the primary process is overlooked. In postoperative ileus, the division between physiologic ileus and the undue abnormal prolongation of bowel hypofunction is blurred. Instead of the patient's passing flatus and becoming hungry on about the third day, as expected following abdominal operation, he is noted to be distended and disinterested in food and his surroundings. Examination confirms that there is generalized abdominal distension with tympany and scattered, occasional bowel sounds.

Assistance from the laboratory is needed mainly in evaluating some of the causes of ileus such as acute anemia, sepsis, hyponatremia, hypokalemia, and hypoosmolarity.

As outlined above (Table 24-6 and Fig. 24-4), x-ray can often help in the differential diagnosis between postoperative adynamic ileus and postoperative mechanical obstruction. If the plain films are inconclusive, contrast medium is given by mouth or through a gastrointestinal tube. In inhibition ileus, some medium should reach the cecum in about 4 hours, whereas a stationary column of medium for 3 or 4 hours indicates complete obstruction of the small intestine.

Adynamic ileus characteristically involves both the small and large bowel to a greater or lesser degree. Occasionally, there is marked distension confined largely to the colon without evidence of mechanical obstruction of the bowel itself or interference with its blood supply—pseudoobstruction of the colon or Ogilvie's syndrome. Barium enema is indicated to rule out organic obstruction. Cecal perforation may occur even though mechanical intestinal obstruction is absent.

TREATMENT. The treatment of ileus is essentially the treatment of the primary lesion. Postoperative ileus is caused in the vast majority of patients either by focal inflammation—leaking anastomosis, abscess following contamination—or by gross fluid-electrolyte derangements. When these problems are promptly eradicated, the ileus will take care of itself.

Treatment of the distension is best done by passage of a long tube. Unfortunately it is much more difficult to pass than in mechanical ileus because of the difference in motility of the intestine. If the long tube will not pass the pylorus, then gastric suction should be used and will prevent further distension.

The availability of newer pharmacologic agents that affect gastrointestinal motility has led to renewed interest in this method of treating ileus. In the past, nonoperative techniques were either ineffective or dangerous. Gastrointestinal pacing by means of an electrode in the tip of the nasogastric tube through which physiologic electric currents are delivered appears to be of little value. Similarly, injections of d-pantothenyl alcohol (a component of coenzyme A which is necessary for the production of acetylcholine) have been shown to be ineffective in postoperative ileus.

Vasopressin which causes contraction of smooth muscle, and parasympathomimetic drugs such as neostigmine or Urecholine will often increase intestinal motility but are not safe to use, because perforation of the bowel can result if there is mechanical obstruction. Catchpole and others have shown that if the sympathetics are blocked pharmacologically, then small (and presumably safe) doses of parasympathomimetic drugs will produce effective propulsive gastrointestinal motility.

Rarely, paralytic ileus does not respond to conservative measures—the obstruction does not relent, and operation must be considered. In most such cases, mechanical obstruction will be found. If no mechanical factors are found, a long tube should be manipulated by the surgeon well down into the small bowel. If the ileocecal valve is competent and marked colon distension is present, then cecostomy should be added. The ileus will be made worse by the operation but can now be managed with adequate decompression.

GASTROINTESTINAL BLEEDING: HEMATEMESIS, MELENA, AND RECTAL BLEEDING

Bleeding may be a manifestation of a variety of diseases along the entire length of the gastrointestinal tract from the oropharynx to the anus. Bleeding represents the initial symptom of gastrointestinal disease in more than one-third of these patients, and in 70 percent there is no history of a previous bleeding episode.

DEFINITIONS. *Hematemesis* refers to the vomiting of blood which is either fresh and unaltered or digested by gastric secretion. It is a manifestation of a bleeding site located between the oropharynx and the ligament of Treitz and may be accompanied by simultaneous melena. The character of the specimen depends on the site of bleeding, the rate of hemorrhage, and the rate of gastric emptying. The presence of blood clots reflects massive bleeding, while a coffee-ground vomitus usually indicates a slower rate with retention in the stomach and alteration to form acid hematin.

Melena is usually defined as the passage of a black, tarry stool. Only 50 ml of blood is necessary to produce this sign and, following the cessation of a bleeding of 1,000 ml, the finding may persist for as long as 5 days. A guaiac-positive stool, indicative of occult blood, may persist for 3 weeks following hematemesis or melena. In general, blood from the distal colon is red and not thoroughly mixed with the stool, whereas blood from the upper gastrointestinal tract produces a tarry stool. However, massive bleeding from the upper gastrointestinal tract may be associated with red or currant jelly clots if the bleeding is rapid and the gastrointestinal motility is increased. Red or black stools may also result from the ingestion of food dye substances and iron. The tarry color, which accompanies upper gastrointestinal bleeding, is attributable to the production of acid hematin by action of gastric acid on the hemoglobin or the production of sulfide from heme by the action of hydrogen sulfide on the iron in the heme molecule. Melena without hematemesis generally indicates a lesion distal to the pylorus but has been associated with bleeding varices and gastritis.

CONSEQUENCES OF GASTROINTESTINAL BLEEDING. Hypotension and shock are dependent upon the rate of the bleeding and the patient's response to the blood loss. It is difficult to estimate the amount of blood loss in either the vomitus or stool, because both specimens contain a mixture of multiple components. The hematocrit and hemoglobin levels are unreliable until equilibration occurs, i.e., 6 to 48 hours subsequent to the bleeding, and estimations of blood volume have also proved unreliable, since the error associated with the technique is great and the range of normals for a given physical state is wide. Shortly after bleeding has begun, a vasovagal reaction is associated with bradycardia, whereas with the progression of time the heart rate increases and the cardiac output decreases. The clinical picture of shock may reflect a coronary occlusion or myocardial ischemia precipitated by hemorrhage rather than the consequences of massive blood loss per se. An-

other consequence of hypotension is reduced renal blood flow resulting in either oliguria or anuria.

Azotemia, which is characteristically associated with bleeding esophagogastric varices, also occurs in patients with other types of massive hemorrhage. Blood urea nitrogen levels of 30 mg/100 ml or more occur in two-thirds of patients with bleeding varices, and an elevation of 50 mg/100 ml or more occurs in one-fifth of the cases. Following cessation of the bleeding, normal levels are usually achieved within 3 days. Azotemia usually does not occur with hemorrhage originating in the colon, and since it is dependent upon bacterial action, normal levels may be associated with upper gastrointestinal tract bleeding in patients on antibiotics which sterilize the intestinal flora. The level to which the BUN rises parallels the extent of gastrointestinal bleeding, but it may be potentiated by shock, impairment of renal function, and increased catabolism. In the presence of blood in the intestinal tract renal function can be evaluated by clearance studies.

Upper Gastrointestinal Tract Bleeding

ETIOLOGY. Although a great variety of lesions above the ligament of Treitz have been implicated in the cause of upper gastrointestinal tract hemorrhage, in the vast majority it is due to peptic ulceration, acute mucosal lesions—gastritis and erosions, esophagogastric varices, diaphragmatic hernia, or gastric neoplasms (Table 24-7).

Peptic ulceration represents the most common cause and accounts for one-half to two-thirds of the cases. Hemorrhage from duodenal ulcer occurs four times more frequently than that from gastric ulcer, but since this represents the relative incidence of the two lesions, the two types have an equal tendency to bleed. Massive bleeding occurs in 10 to 15 percent of ulcer patients with hemorrhage and is the first symptom in 16 percent of the patients who bleed. The bleeding is generally caused by the inflammatory process eroding into the regional artery. In the case of duodenal ulcers, the gastroduodenal artery is involved, while the left and right gastric arteries and their branches are most frequently involved with gastric ulcers. Most bleeding ulcers are chronic lesions, and the adjacent arteries suffer from local inflammatory changes. Since hemostasis is dependent on the retraction of the walls of the vessel, persistent bleeding is more likely to occur with chronic lesions and in older patients with atherosclerotic vessels.

Peptic ulceration of the stomal mucosa at the site of a gastroenterostomy is to be considered in any patient who has had previous gastric surgical treatment. It is a more frequent occurrence when less than two-thirds of the stomach has been removed and an accompanying vagotomy has not been performed, especially if there is retained antrum.

The next most common cause of gross upper gastrointestinal tract hemorrhage after peptic ulcer is a diverse group of lesions that can best be collectively termed *acute mucosal lesions* until they are clearly delineated and separated into entities. The reported incidence (Table 24-7)

Table 24-7. ETIOLOGY OF UPPER GASTROINTESTINAL TRACT BLEEDING IN 10,554 CASES

Author	Year	Number of cases	Peptic ulcer percent	Acute mucosal lesions, percent	Esophageal varices, percent	Diaphragmatic hernia, percent	Gastric cancer, percent	Other, percent	Undetermined percent
Jones	1956	1,910	57	29	3	2	2	3	5
Ferguson	1962	1,124	62	4	7	1	4	1	20
Hirschowitz	1963	216	58	22	1	1	1	5	12
Dorsey	1965	405	68	2	2	3	...	5	20
Katz	1970	800	24	33	17	...	...	10	16
Palmer	1970	1,400	45	12	19	8	...	11	7
Schiff	1970	640	53	1	13	2	2	8	21
Halmagyi	1970	199	65	1	7	6	1	15	5
Preston	1970	535	50	2	30	...	...	7	17
Schiller	1970	2,149	45	3	2	...	2	22	26
Foster	1971	296	67	13	9	...	3	4	4
Crook	1972	880	50	19	11	3	2	5	4
Average	...	...	50	13	9	2	2	8	16

ranges from 1 to 33 percent. The true incidence will not be known until endoscopy is universally applied early in the course of upper gastrointestinal tract hemorrhage. Pathologically, these lesions are sometimes single but more often multiple, or the mucosa may be diffusely involved in hemorrhagic necrosis. The process usually does not extend through the muscularis mucosae, and therefore the lesions are technically *erosions,* not true ulcers. In contradistinction to chronic benign ulcers, which are characteristically located in the antrum or on the lesser curvature, the acute erosive lesions are found in the body and fundus of the stomach, sparing the antrum, and on the greater curvature as often as on the lesser.

"Stress ulceration" is a much abused term which if used at all should be confined to the acute gastroduodenal lesions that occur secondary to shock and sepsis following operation, trauma, or burns. McClelland et al. have shown in patients with trauma and hemorrhagic shock that gastric secretion is not increased but that splanchnic blood flow is significantly decreased. They conclude that "ischemic damage to the superficial gastric mucosa may induce stress ulceration." Sepsis also plays a prominent role. Altemeier et al. documented upper gastrointestinal tract bleeding in approximately one-third of surgical patients with septicemia and also implicated the coagulation abnormalities that attend sepsis. Nance et al. found that in germ-free rats subjected to restraint stress there is a marked reduction in the incidence and severity of gastric ulceration as compared to conventional animals and concluded that bacterial factors play a significant role in the pathogenesis of stress ulcers.

Probably closely related to stress erosions is the acute ulceration or erosion of the stomach and duodenum which occurs in burn patients. Such lesions are usually referred to as Curling's ulcers, after the man who described them in 1842. Curling's ulcers occur in about 12 percent of patients hospitalized for burns. The incidence increases with burn size—up to a 40 percent incidence in burns of 70 percent or more of the body surface. Sepsis is an addit-

itive stress. In two-thirds of patients with Curling's ulcer the presenting clinical sign is bleeding, and in 45 percent such bleeding is massive. Though there are many similarities between stress erosions and Curling's ulcers, their distribution is somewhat different: stress erosions are usually multiple and usually in the stomach; Curling's ulcers are about evenly divided between single and multiple, and between stomach and duodenum.

Another eponymic ulcer that is probably closely related to stress erosions is the *Cushing ulcer.* In 1932, Harvey Cushing described a variety of esophagogastroduodenal lesions in nine patients following craniotomy. Since then the belief has persisted that dysfunction in specific areas of the brain leads to gastrointestinal ulceration. In many of these patients, the etiologic factors are probably the same as for patients after any major operation, but there is some evidence that significant gastric hypersecretion may occur after certain intracranial operations or trauma.

Adrenal corticosteroids, given in large doses for prolonged periods, frequently lead to gastroduodenal erosions or ulcers, or to activation of preexisting quiescent peptic ulcers. Patients receiving steroids for rheumatoid arthritis or lupus erythematosus are more prone to this complication than patients with asthma or inflammatory bowel disease. Despite the fact that steroids do not increase the gastric acid output, antacid therapy is often efficacious. The distribution of "steroid ulcers" is much the same as that of postoperative "stress ulcers."

Aspirin and alcohol are the major offenders of a large group of ingested agents that may produce erosive, hemorrhagic gastritis and duodenitis. The incidence with which this lesion is diagnosed is directly related to the degree to which early endoscopic examination is employed. Alcohol is a known gastric secretagogue, but aspirin and similar agents are not; the latter presumably act by increasing back-diffusion of HCl through the gastric mucosa. The hemorrhage is generally mild to moderate but is sometimes massive. Since the gastric mucosa normally renews itself every 48 to 72 hours, the process is self-limited if symptoms can be controlled until mucosal regeneration occurs. Emergency operation for exsanguinating hemorrhage is sometimes necessary.

Esophagogastric varices constitute the most common cause of bleeding in patients with cirrhosis or extrahepatic obstruction of the portal vein. These account for approximately 10 percent of all cases of upper gastrointestinal tract bleeding, but the incidence varies widely, being significantly higher in the hospitals with a large indigent population. Bleeding varices constitute 95 percent of the cases of massive hematemesis in the child, and they are usually associated with extrahepatic obstruction of the portal vein. In cirrhotic patients, varices are the cause of bleeding in 53 percent of the cases, while gastritis is implicated in 22 percent and duodenal and gastric ulcers in 20 percent. Correlation of the lesions and severity of bleeding reveals that in the majority of cases (70 percent) patients with bleeding from varices have severe hemorrhage while 84 percent of patients with bleeding from gastritis demonstrate mild to moderate blood loss. The precipitation of the bleeding episode has been ascribed to two major factors: increased pressure within the varix and ulceration secondary to esophagitis. Although esophagogastric varices are almost always associated with portal hypertension, the diagnosis has been established in occasional patients with normal portal pressures. The veins responsible for the bleeding are usually opened laterally by transmural erosion, and any hemostasis which occurs is dependent upon occlusion of the opening by a thrombus. The bleeding is nearly always associated with hematemesis and is generally very profuse.

Hiatal hernia frequently may be associated with occult bleeding but is usually not a cause of gross upper gastrointestinal tract hemorrhage, accounting for approximately 2 percent of the cases. The bleeding in the sliding hernia is related to reflux peptic esophagitis. Bleeding is more commonly seen with paraesophageal hernias and is thought to be caused by the retention of acid contents within the incarcerated gastric pouch or congestion of the vascular supply of the herniated portion of the stomach.

A variety of miscellaneous lesions account for up to 8 percent of occasional upper gastrointestinal tract bleeding, while in 16 percent the diagnosis is never determined. Neoplasms are uncommonly implicated, and there is evidence that the incidence of carcinoma of the stomach is decreasing in the United States. Bleeding associated with gastric carcinoma is caused by erosion of the tumor into underlying vessels. It is usually mild to moderate, but if a large vessel is involved, massive bleeding can occur. Massive hemorrhage may be the initial symptom in a patient with gastric carcinoma. Other tumors occur less frequently. Leiomyoma and leiomyosarcoma of the stomach or esophagus may be manifested by profuse bleeding, usually in men in the third decade of life. Leukemia with intestinal infiltrates may cause significant gastrointestinal bleeding. Also, polyps, either single, familial, or associated with the Peutz-Jeghers syndrome, are included as neoplastic lesions with a bleeding potential.

Vascular lesions, including angiomas, hereditary hemorrhagic telangiectasia (Rendu-Osler-Weber), and vasculitis,

have all been reported as etiologic factors in upper gastrointestinal tract bleeding. Spontaneous rupture of aortic, hepatic arterial, and splenic arterial aneurysms may produce alarming bleeding. Characteristically, aortic aneurysm is manifested by moderate bleeding which stops for a variable period of time only to recur as massive bleeding.

Inflammation of the mucosa with erosion of small or large vessels may accompany prolapsing gastric mucosa and duodenal diverticula. Prolapsing gastric mucosa, which is usually not considered a common source of bleeding, may be accompanied by moderate blood loss. Similarly, although duodenal diverticula are generally considered to be asymptomatic, massive hemorrhage has accompanied ulceration of this lesion. Hepatic trauma with development of a central or subcapsular hematoma which discharges into the biliary tree is responsible for the development of the syndrome known as hematobilia, which may represent a cause of moderate or massive bleeding. Hematobilia may also occur with cholecystitis, cholelithiasis, and passage of stones. The interval between trauma and the bleeding manifestation is variable. Another traumatic cause of upper gastrointestinal tract bleeding is the Mallory-Weiss syndrome, which consists of linear tears of the esophagogastric junction induced by severe vomiting, usually in alcoholic patients.

DIAGNOSIS. History and Physical Examination. The patient's own account of the amount of bleeding is frequently misleading. Vomiting of large amounts of blood is more suggestive of bleeding ulcer or esophagogastric varices. A history of active ulcer symptoms preceding the hemorrhage with cessation of the pain at the onset of bleeding suggests that the bleeding is originating from the peptic ulcer. However, 20 percent of patients with bleeding have no previous history of ulcer. Although there is an increased incidence of the ulcer diathesis in cirrhotic patients, esophagogastric varices represent the most common cause of bleeding in these patients and account for over 50 percent of the bleeding episodes. Violent retching and vomiting in alcoholics or pregnant women is characteristic of a Mallory-Weiss syndrome. The history should include questions directed toward the recent ingestion of drugs implicated as causes of gastrointestinal bleeding, particularly salicylates, Butazolidin, alcohol, anticoagulants, and steroids. A history regarding the bleeding tendency during childhood, in early adulthood, and in other members of the family focuses on the possibility of hematologic disorders. Previous gastric surgical treatment such as gastroenterostomy or partial gastrectomy directs one's thinking toward the possibility of a marginal ulcer. Heartburn, epigastric substernal pain accentuated by the recumbent position and the ingestion of large meals, suggests the presence of a hiatal hernia. A recent history of upper abdominal or chest trauma is most compatible with a diagnosis of hematobilia, particularly when the bleeding is accompanied by jaundice and intermittent colicky pain.

Examination of the patient with upper gastrointestinal tract bleeding is directed at determining stigmata of the various diseases considered in the etiology. The skin and mucous membranes should be examined for icterus, spider angiomas, liver palms, and decreased hair over the extremity, all suggestive of hepatic disease. The mucous membrane should be investigated for melanin spots of the Peutz-Jeghers syndrome. Hereditary telangiectasia lesions are most common on the lips, tongue, and ears. Lymphadenopathy, particularly in the left supraclavicular region, may suggest a malignant intraabdominal process. Abdominal palpation more commonly reveals tenderness when the bleeding is related to ulcer or gastritis, whereas a palpable liver, particularly when accompanied by splenomegaly and abdominal veins which fill in a centrifugal pattern from the umbilicus, is more indicative of bleeding varices. Examination should always include aspiration via nasogastric tube in order to determine presence of blood at this level and the extent of bleeding at the time of examination.

Special Diagnostic Procedures. The extent of anemia may be assessed by the hematocrit level. It should be appreciated that, with acute blood loss, the initial level may be normal, since the hematocrit reduction does not occur for 4 to 6 hours, during which time equilibration occurs. Repeat hematocrit readings taken at 4- to 6-hour intervals are more meaningful. Leukocytosis, with levels of 25,000, may accompany acute hemorrhage, but more marked increases are suggestive of leukemia. Both the neutrophils and platelets may be reduced in the case of hypersplenism secondary to primary hepatic disease, suggesting bleeding from esophagogastric varices.

Clinical chemistries are directed toward evaluating the extent of bleeding and, particularly, determining the presence of hepatocellular dysfunction. None of the tests define the site of bleeding. A rise in the BUN level parallels the extent of hemorrhage and is related to the absorption of blood products from the gastrointestinal tract, possible associated reduction in renal flow secondary to shock or dehydration, and, at times, the presence of preexisting renal disease. In the presence of marked hepatic dysfunction, the BUN level may not be elevated, since the liver is unable to synthesize urea. In this circumstance, the blood ammonia level is frequently elevated with bleeding varices, since it is related to the extent of portal collateralization and reduced hepatic function. The validity of this test, however, is not uniform. Normal values are present in patients with variceal bleeding. When this test is combined with the BSP (Bromsulphalein test), no diagnostic significance can be attributed if either level is elevated and the other normal. However, when both the blood ammonia and BSP retention levels are elevated, this represents strong evidence of cirrhosis. The BSP retention is particularly applicable to the diagnosis of cirrhosis in patients with massive hemorrhage. Abnormal BSP retention may be related either to liver disease or to shock from hemorrhage regardless of the site. In contrast, a normal value in association with massive bleeding suggests that the liver is not responsible.

Determination of the blood clotting factors is of great importance, particularly in patients bleeding from stress ulceration. Reduced platelet adhesiveness, thrombocytopenia, prolonged prothrombin time, and other clotting defects are common in such patients. The bleeding often stops, obviating emergency operation, following the ad-

ministration of fresh platelet infusions, vitamin K, and fresh frozen plasma.

Rarely, bleeding is so rapid that immediate operation without preoperative diagnostic procedures is necessary to save life. More commonly, transfusions can easily allow time for diagnosis and preparation; further, many patients stop bleeding soon after admission. As the above tests are being done, the patient should be rapidly transfused to circulatory normality, with vital signs, central venous pressure, and urinary output as guides. The stomach should be completely evacuated using iced Ringer's lavage through a nasogastric tube; an Ewald tube may be advisable initially if many large clots are present.

Endoscopy is the first special diagnostic procedure to be considered; it is virtually mandatory if the bleeding is thought to be from esophagogastric varices or from an acute mucosal lesion. Esophagoscopy defines the bleeding point in the case of varices, since liver function tests, manometry, barium x-ray, and isotopic studies merely indicate the presence of portal hypertension or varices but do not determine if these lesions are actually bleeding. The reported esophagscopic accident rate is 0.25 percent, and an experienced endoscopist is required. A 33 percent disagreement rate between two experienced endoscopists evaluating a given group of patients is reported. This is related to the difficulty in differentiating varices and mucosal folds. Gastroduodenoscopy with fiberoptic instruments is particularly valuable in revealing acute gastritis, erosions, and small superficial ulcers that are not demonstrable on upper gastrointestinal tract x-ray.

Radiologic Studies. Selective arteriography of the celiac and superior mesenteric arteries and their branches is a relatively safe and accurate method of identifying active bleeding points in the upper gastrointestinal tract (Fig. 24-7). A skillful experienced radiologist using highly specialized, sophisticated equipment is essential to obtain reliable information. Angiography is usually done after endoscopy if that procedure has not identified the bleeding point. In any event, it must come before the upper gastrointestinal barium x-rays, which will obscure the field. Although bleeding at the rate of 1 to 2 ml/minute can be detected experimentally, bleeding must be at the rate of 3 to 5 ml/minute for accurate clinical angiographic diagnosis. The diagnostic accuracy of angiography in visualizing actively bleeding arterial lesions is about 90 percent; the accuracy in variceal bleeding, using the venous phase of the angiogram, is only about 20 percent.

In addition to diagnosis, selective arterial catheterization can be used for therapy of gastrointestinal bleeding. After the bleeding point is identified, a small therapeutic catheter is guided into the artery supplying the bleeding area, and vasoconstrictive agents, usually vasopressin at the rate of 0.1 to 0.2 units/minute, are infused. In the case of variceal bleeding, the main superior mesentric artery is infused in order to reduce splanchnic blood flow and thus decrease portal vein flow and pressure. In many patients (depending on the nature of the lesion), the bleeding is arrested; in some, bleeding is only partially controlled, and an operation is necessary but can be done under more orderly circumstances. In about 20 percent, vasopressin infusion does not control bleeding. Regional vasoconstrictive therapy should be used only in patients in whom the potential benefit justifies the very considerable risk; Conn et al. have reported a 35 percent complication rate. Also, several comparative studies of systemic intravenous vasopressin versus regional arterial vasopressin have not shown any advantage for the more difficult and dangerous arterial route.

An upper gastrointestinal tract series, the cornerstone of morphologic radiographic diagnosis, should be done next, if endoscopy and arteriography have not revealed the bleeding site. As with endoscopy, the stomach should be evacuated of clots prior to the examination.

In the case of bleeding ulcer, delaying for several days after hemorrhage has ceased does not increase the accuracy of diagnosis. The question of safety in the patient with bleeding has been raised, since the routine gastrointestinal series involves compression which may be attended by increasing hemorrhage. The Hampton technique for demonstration of bleeding ulcers obviates the use of palpation or compression and is attended by a diagnostic accuracy of 86 percent for demonstration of ulcers. The diagnostic accuracy in the case of bleeding varices is approximately 50 percent. Both the Valsalva and Müller maneuvers may occasionally show varices when other methods fail. Roentgenograms have proved of little value in the diagnosis of gastritis with a yield of approximately 25 percent.

Percutaneous splenoportography affords a high yield for the diagnosis of esophageal varices but is rarely performed on an emergency basis. Before carrying out this procedure, a platelet count greater than 50,000 and a prothrombin time greater than 35 percent should be demonstrated.

Splenic pulp manometry has been applied as an emergency test in the differential diagnosis of upper gastrointestinal tract bleeding. A 90 percent accuracy has been reported, but there is a zone of splenic pulp pressures which cannot differentiate variceal bleeding from other causes. In addition, isotopic and splenoportographic studies have demonstrated patients in whom portal hypertension is unaccompanied by the development of a collateral circulation. Finally, the admittedly rare situation of bleeding esophageal varices associated with normal portal pressure would not be diagnosed by this technique.

Balloon tamponade has been used as a diagnostic-therapeutic measure. However, varices are controlled even temporarily in only 65 to 75 percent of patients, and a peptic ulcer may coincidentally stop bleeding after a gastric balloon is inflated.

In some instances, an operation is performed on a patient with massive upper gastrointestinal tract bleeding in whom a diagnosis has not been established preoperatively. Laparotomy is to be considered as an important diagnostic tool. Once the peritoneal cavity has been opened, inspection of the liver may reveal cirrhosis, and distension of the omental vessels may suggest portal hypertension. In most cases, however, a determination of the source of bleeding requires a long gastrotomy which permits visualization of the gastric mucosa and the proximal portions of the duodenum. An attempt should be made to identify duodenal ulcer or a gastric lesion, and if these are not

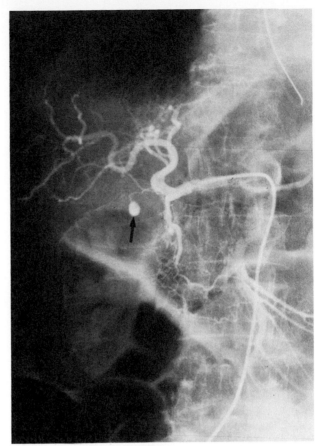

Fig. 24-7. Selective angiography in upper gastrointestinal bleeding. Dye injection into the common hepatic artery has outlined a bleeding duodenal ulcer (arrow). Later films showed a persistent puddling of contrast medium in the duodenum after all intravascular contrast had disappeared.

apparent, traction on the lower end of the nasogastric tube which is brought out through the gastrotomy will often expose the cardiac end of the stomach and distal esophagus to inspection. Intraoperative esophagogastroscopy by the usual route also may be helpful. Occasionally, in the absence of a preopoerative diagnosis, no site of bleeding will be found at operation. In this situation, some surgeons do a vagotomy and drainage procedure; others simply close and hope that if bleeding recurs, the diagnosis can be made at that time and specific therapy instituted. The "blind" gastric resection which was formerly done in this situation has fallen into disfavor.

Lower Gastrointestinal Tract Bleeding

Bleeding distal to the ligament of Treitz is manifested by the passage of tarry stools or unaltered blood (hemochezia) and is characteristically unaccompanied by hematemesis. It is usually moderate or mild but may be massive.

ETIOLOGY. A great variety of lesions extending from the ligament of Treitz to the anus may be implicated as causes of lower gastrointestinal tract bleeding.

Jejunal and Ileal Bleeding. Meckel's diverticulitis, intussusception, and regional enteritis represent the most common causes. Meckel's diverticulitis with associated bleeding occurs most frequently in children, and the bleeding episode is related to gastric mucosa within the diverticulum stimulating ulceration of the adjacent ileum. Ileocecal intussusception is also a lesion of childhood, occurring most commonly before the age of two and attended by a characteristic currant jelly stool. The cause of this mechanical process in childhood is usually undetermined, while ileocecal intussusception in the adult is usually secondary to an intestinal polyp or tumor. Regional enteritis is accompanied by severe melena in approximately 5 percent of the cases, while some rectal bleeding is a common symptom in about 20 percent of the patients with this disease. Although tumors of the small intestine are rare, approximately half are accompanied by bleeding. The neoplasms include leiomyomas, polyps, either single or multiple (familial polyposis), and the polyps of the Peutz-Jegher syndrome. Carcinomas, sarcomas, and leukemias have all been reported to be associated with bleeding, whereas bleeding is an uncommon manifestation of a carcinoid tumor. Hemangiomas, hereditary telangiectasis, microaneurysms of blood vessels within the wall of the intestine, mesenteric thrombosis, drug reactions, and blood dyscrasias all represent rare causes of small intestinal bleeding.

Colonic Bleeding. The common causes include carcinoma, diverticula, colitis, and polyps (Table 24-8). Although carcinoma represents the most common cause of rectal bleeding, the bleeding associated with this lesion is rarely massive. Carcinoma of the right colon, particularly of the cecum, is usually accompanied by melena which may be so subtle that it is not considered until anemia has become established. Diverticulosis presents the most common cause of *massive* rectal bleeding. This is related to erosion of vessels within the neck of the diverticulum. In contrast, the bleeding which accompanies diverticulitis is mild to moderate and is caused by a superficial erosion of smaller vessels on the surface of the mucosa. Although the bleeding which accompanies ulcerative colitis is usually mild to moderate, massive hemorrhage may occur. Polyps

which may be single or multiple and may be located in any segment of the colon represent a relatively frequent source of rectal bleeding. Rarer causes include cecal ulceration, sarcomas, lymphomas, leukemia, hematologic disorders, and impairment of the vascular supply due to mesenteric thrombosis or ischemic colitis, or secondary to aortic resection with interruption of a functionally important inferior mesenteric artery.

Prior to angiography, bleeding lesions of the right colon were thought to be rare, but in the past decade many reports have emphasized that the right colon is a common site of bleeding. Diverticula were thought to be the responsible lesion. Boley and associates have shown that vascular ectasias are probably responsible for much of the right colon bleeding; they suggest that ectasias may be the commonest cause of major lower intestinal bleeding in the elderly. They present evidence that these vascular ectasias: (1) are degenerative lesions of aging and are not congenital or neoplastic; (2) occur in patients over 60 years of age; (3) are not associated with angiomatous lesions of the skin or other viscera; (4) occur in the cecum and proximal ascending colon; (5) are small, usually less than 5 mm in diameter; (6) can be diagnosed only by angiography; and (7) usually cannot be identified by the surgeon at operation or by the pathologist using standard techniques—injecting-clearing techniques must be used.

Rectal and Anal Bleeding. This is usually manifested by unaltered blood on the surface of the stool. The causes include hemorrhoids, and fissures, and proctitis. It is to be emphasized that the presence of hemorrhoids in a patient with rectal bleeding should not preclude investigation of other possible sources, particularly carcinoma.

DIAGNOSIS. A precise description of the bleeding episode and the nature of the stool is indicated. The question of familial polyposis and drug ingestion should be investigated. Physical examination includes a search for skin and mucosal lesions of the hemorrhagic telangiectasis (Rendu-Osler-Weber syndrome) or the Peutz-Jegher syndrome. Abdominal palpation may reveal a mass, tumor, or intussusception, the last frequently accompanied by absence of bowel in the right lower quadrant. Rectal ex-

Table 24-8. INCIDENCE OF RECTAL BLEEDING (1955–1960)

Characteristic lesion	All rectal bleeding, no. of cases	Moderate rectal bleeding, no. of cases	Severe rectal bleeding, no. of cases
Cancer, left colon	75	73	2
Diverticulosis	62	45	17
Ulcerative colitis	39	39	
Polyps	25	23	2
Diverticulitis	16	16	
Cancer, right colon	14	13	1
Miscellaneous	14 (1 each)	12 (1 each)	2 (1 each)
Total	245	221	24

SOURCE: From R. J. Noer et al., Rectal Hemorrhage: Moderate and Severe, *Ann Surg,* 155:794, 1962, and from the Louisville General Hospital and Louisville Veterans Administration Hospital.

amination may be diagnostic for tumor, polyps, or anal lesions. Proctosigmoidoscopy should be done early in the hospital course.

Selective angiography is by far the most accurate method of diagnosis provided there is active bleeding at the rate of at least 2 or 3 ml/minute at the time of the examination. The small intestine and right half of the colon are examined by catheterization of branches of the superior mesenteric artery (Fig. 24-5). Examination of the left colon is sometimes more difficult, since the inferior mesenteric artery may be more difficult to catheterize. As with upper gastrointestinal tract bleeding, regional infusion of vasoconstrictive agents via a catheter in the artery supplying the bleeding site is often an effective method of controlling bleeding.

Barium contrast studies, if needed, should follow angiography so that the contrast material does not obscure the angiographer's field. Barium enema studies, including air contrast, represent a reliable, accurate method of diagnosing colon lesions but yield no information as to whether or not the lesions visualized are responsible for the bleeding. Gastrointestinal series with small bowel follow-through is less productive in the case of lesions of the small intestine. Every effort should be made to demonstrate the bleeding site prior to operation, since diagnosis at the operating table is often not possible.

JAUNDICE

The term *jaundice* is derived from the French word meaning "yellow" and refers to the presence of an excess of bile pigments in the tissues and the serum. It is the presenting sign of a number of hepatic and nonhepatic diseases. The differential diagnosis and management are dependent upon an appreciation of the normal and abnormal variants of bile pigment metabolism. A flow sheet analysis of hyperbilirubinemia is presented in Table 24-9.

NORMAL BILE PIGMENT METABOLISM. The bile pigment bilirubin (Fig. 24-8) is a tetrapyrrole which is formed to the greatest extent from hemoglobin and, to a lesser extent, from myoglobin breakdown and hepatic synthesis itself. When the red blood cell is destroyed by the reticuloendothelial system, either at the end of its natural life span or prematurely, the iron and globin are removed, and the heme ring is opened and transformed into biliverdin, which is green. The latter is reduced to become bilirubin, which is yellow (Fig. 24-9). The bilirubin combines with albumin to form a relatively stable protein-pigment complex and is transported as such to the hepatic parenchymal cell. This complex, which is referred to as *indirect-reacting* bilirubin, since it gives the van den Bergh diazo reaction only after treatment with alcohol and other substances which split the protein bond, is poorly soluble in water and is not excreted in the urine.

In the hepatic parenchymal cell the albumin is removed, and the bilirubin is conjugated with glucuronic acid to form a diglucuronide, which is water-soluble and is excreted into the bile canaliculi. This substance gives an

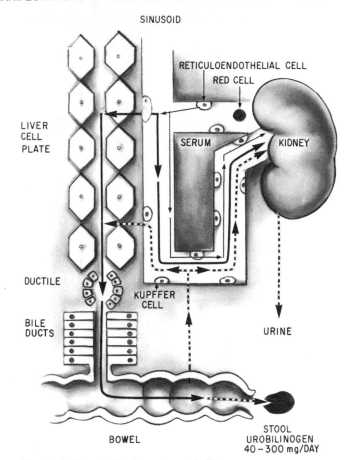

Fig. 24-8. Normal bile pigment metabolism.

Fig. 24-9. Conversion of heme to bilirubin.

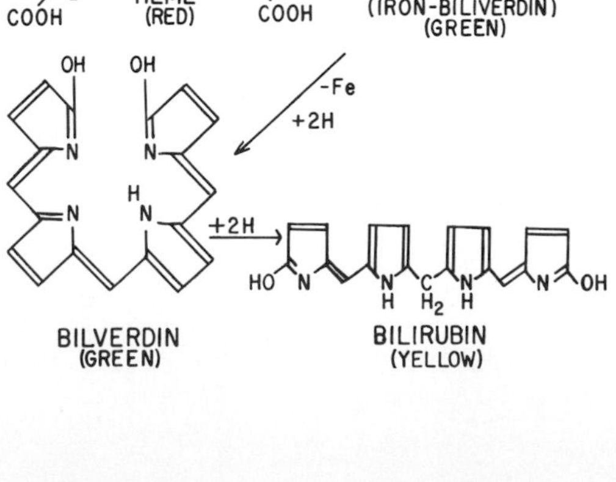

Table 24-9. ANALYSIS OF A CASE OF HYPERBILIRUBINEMIA

Fractionate serum bilirubin and measure urine bilirubin and urobilinogen to determine whether:

I. Unconjugated hyperbilirubinemia
   Determine mechanism on basis of age, clinical features, and laboratory findings:

A. Production of bilirubin beyond excretory capacity. Evidence of:
   1. Hemolysis
      a. Extracorpuscular
         (1) Immune body reactions
             (a) Transfusion reactions
             (b) Erythroblastosis
         (2) Infections and chemicals
         (3) Physical agents
         (4) Secondary hemolysis in pregnancy
      b. Intracorpuscular
         (1) Congenital hemolytic jaundice
         (2) Sickle cell anemia
         (3) Mediterranean anemia
   2. No hemolysis
      a. Pulmonary infarction
      b. Transfusion of aged red blood cells
      c. Hematomas
      d. "Shunt" hyperbilirubinemia

B. Deficient hepatic uptake of bilirubin:
   1. ? Gilbert's disease (normal biopsy, low-grade hyperbilirubinemia)
   2. ? Acquired liver disease

C. Deficient conjugation of bilirubin:
   1. Physiologic jaundice of newborn
   2. Crigler-Najjar syndrome (transferase deficiency)
      a. Inadequate bilirubin glucuronide synthesis
   3. Inhibition of glucuronyl transferase
      a. Large doses of vitamin K analogs in premature infants
      b. Increased level of pregnanediol
      c. Breast milk containing pregnane-3-(a), 20-(β)-diol
      d. Novobiocin
   4. Competitive inhibition
      a. Drugs detoxified as glucuronides

II. Conjugated hyperbilirubinemia
   Determine mechanism on basis of age, clinical features, and laboratory findings:

A. Defect in bilirubin excretion
   Confirm with serum alkaline phosphatase (elevated), cephalin flocculation (normal). In absence of rapid subsidence, exploratory surgery is desirable to differentiate:

1. Extrahepatic biliary obstruction
   Identify by radiologic means and/or direct inspection during surgical intervention.
   a. Calculus
   b. Stricture
   c. Neoplasm

2. Intrahepatic biliary obstruction
   Confirm absence of extrahepatic biliary obstruction with operative or T-tube cholangiography. Identify localization of lesion by surgical biopsy.
   a. Lesion of bile canaliculi
      (1) Drugs
      (2) Viruses
   b. Lesion of bile ductules
      (1) Drugs
      (2) Viruses
   c. Lesion of bile ducts
      (1) Drugs
      (2) Viruses

B. Deficient liver cell secretion of bilirubin
   May need to differentiate from excretory defect by surgical exploration, cholangiography, or biopsy:

1. Persistence of excretory defect in immature liver after development of adequate glucuronide-synthesizing capacity
2. Dubin-Johnson syndrome (biopsy showing characteristic pigment)
3. Rotor syndrome (absence of characteristic pigment)

III. Combined unconjugated and conjugated hyperbilirubinemia
   Determine mechanism on basis of clinical features and laboratory findings:

A. Familial defect or immature liver reflected in partial deficiency of glucuronide formation or excretion

B. Acquired liver cell damage
   Confirm with liver function tests and determine primary abnormality:
1. Deficient hepatic uptake of bilirubin
2. Deficient conjugation of bilirubin
3. Deficient secretion or excretion of conjugated bilirubin

C. Hemolysis with secondary liver damage
   Demonstrate presence of hemolysis:
1. Hepatic damage secondary to shock
2. Hepatic damage secondary to hemolysis

D. Biliary obstruction with secondary liver damage:
1. Bile stasis with secondary injury
2. Ascending cholangitis

SOURCE: Leevy, C. M.: "Evaluation of Liver Function in Clinical Practice," The Lilly Research Laboratories, Indianapolis, Ind., 1965, by permission.

immediate diazo reaction, is therefore termed *direct-reacting*, and is readily passed into the urine. Normally there is less than 1.2 mg of indirect-reacting serum bilirubin and less than 0.3 mg of direct-reacting serum bilirubin per 100 ml of serum.

The conjugated bilirubin, which is excreted via the bile into the intestine, is acted upon by bacteria and undergoes a series of reductive reactions leading to the formation of two groups of compounds, the colorless urobilinogens and the colored urobilin (Fig. 24-10). The normal daily fecal excretion ranges between 40 and 300 mg with an average of 100 to 200 mg. In children values are lower, and in newborn infants, because of the absence of bacterial flora, urobilinogen may be absent. A reduction in enteric bacteria is also responsible for the reduced pigment excretion that accompanies the use of intestinal antibiotics. Some of the urobilinogen is resorbed by way of the portal venous system and returns to the liver, where it is either removed or, to a small extent, excreted in the urine.

ABNORMAL BILE PIGMENT METABOLISM. No classification of jaundice is totally satisfactory. The classification most widely used distinguishes between hemolytic, obstructive, and hepatocellular jaundice. However, it is more reasonable to categorize (1) those disease states in which the bile flow is unimpeded and (2) those types which are associated with an impairment of bile flow (Fig. 24-11).

Normal Bile Excretion. The overproduction of bile pigment from excessive hemolysis creates a situation in which the normal liver is confronted with more pigment than it is able to remove. This occurs in the physiologic jaundice of infancy and all patholigic hemolytic states. However, the reserve capacity of the liver is great, and even when the bilirubin production is increased six times, there is only a 2- to 3-mg rise in the serum bilirubin level per 100 ml. In this situation, the increase in serum bilirubin is in the unconjugated indirect-reacting pigment. No bilirubin appears in the urine, but there is an increase in the fecal and urinary urobilinogen. An excess of bilirubin production also occurs in *shunt hyperbilirubinemia*, in which indirect-reacting bilirubin accumulates in the absence of any reduction in red cell life span.

Constitutional defects of liver function may also cause hyperbilirubinemia without impairment of bile flow. In Gilbert's disease, there is a defect in the bilirubin transport into the liver cell, while in the Crigler-Najjar syndrome the defect is an inability of the liver to conjugate the

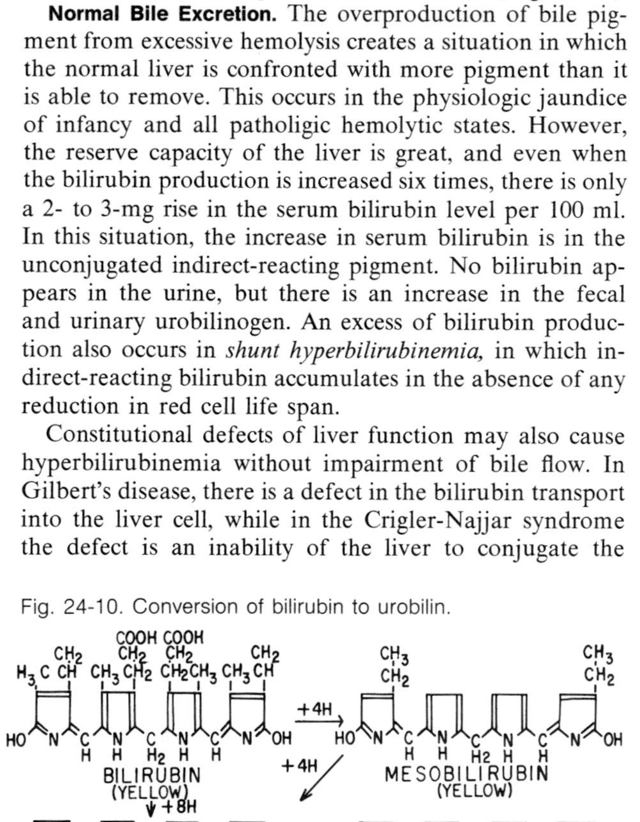

bilirubin with glucuronic acid. In these states, the elevation of bile pigment is in the indirect-reacting fraction. All other hepatic function tests are normal, and no histologic abnormalities are noted. With all the above-mentioned diseases, the bilirubin pigment is attached to the albumin and cannot be excreted by the kidney, thus prompting the term *acholuric jaundice.*

Impaired Bile Excretion. All other lesions are associated with an accumulation of conjugated bilirubin in the blood and impaired excretion. The bilirubin pigment, which is water-soluble, is readily excreted into the urine, which becomes brown. Both the fecal urobilinogen and the urinary urobilinogen are decreased or absent, depending upon the degree of obstruction. Obstructive jaundice may be intrahepatic or extrahepatic.

Intrahepatic Obstructive Jaundice. In the Dubin-Johnson syndrome, which is associated with the appearance of iron-free pigment in the hepatic cells and normal liver function, the hepatic excretion of the conjugated bilirubin is impaired. Intrahepatic cholestasis has also been related to a variety of drugs and hepatocellular diseases. Methyltestosterone and norethandrolone damage the microvilli of the bile canaliculi and may cause jaundice. The phenothiazine drugs, such as chlorpromazine, may evoke a hypersensitivity reaction in a small percentage of patients and result in cholangiolitic hepatitis and intrahepatic cholestasis. A lesion along the excretory path within the liver is believed to cause the obstructive jaundice associated with primary biliary cirrhosis.

The jaundice from hepatocellular degeneration, such as occurs in hepatitis and cirrhosis, is associated with morphologic changes in the parenchymal cells and abnormal liver function tests. With these diseases, a Kupffer cell liver block has been proposed to result in regurgitation of bilirubin from the bile canaliculi into the tissue spaces. This defect, coupled with the reduction in the ability of the liver cell to convert the bilirubin protein to the bilirubin glucuronide, causes a rise in both bilirubin and its conjugates. In contrast to the pure obstructive jaundice, urinary urobilinogen may be increased, since the parenchyma is no longer capable of clearing the serum urobilinogen entering from the intestinal tract. However, the excretion of bile may be so suppressed that virtually no bilirubin reaches the intestine; under these conditions the stools are clay-colored, and the production and resorption of the bilirubin from the intestine is diminished, in which case the urine urobilinogen falls to a low level. In rare instances of intrahepatic bile duct atresia absolute obstruction of the bile conduits within the liver results in jaundice.

Extrahepatic Cholestasis. This is caused by an anatomic obstacle to the flow of bile from the liver to the intestine. The obstacle may be situated anywhere from the junction of the right and left hepatic ducts to the termination of the common bile duct in the duodenum. Atresia, stricture, gallstones, tumors of the bile duct and pancreas, choledochal cysts, and parasites have all been implicated. Obstruction of the extrahepatic ducts results in an increase in the serum bilirubin, particularly the direct-reacting type, the appearance of bile in the urine, and the passage of clay-colored stools. When the total bilirubin level is above

Fig. 24-10. Conversion of bilirubin to urobilin.

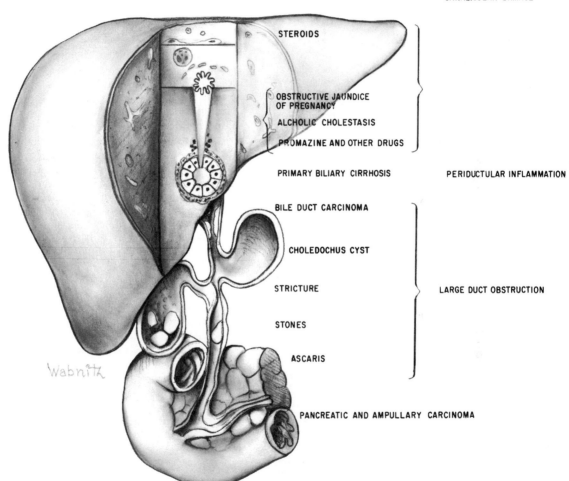

CAUSE OF JAUNDICE

HEMOLYSIS

SHUNT — HYPERBILIRUBINEMIA

GILBERT

NEONATE, CRIGLER - NAJJAR

DUBIN-JOHNSON HYPERBILIRUBINEMIA

STEROIDS

OBSTRUCTIVE JAUNDICE OF PREGNANCY

ALCHOLIC CHOLESTASIS

PROMAZINE AND OTHER DRUGS

PRIMARY BILIARY CIRRHOSIS

BILE DUCT CARCINOMA

CHOLEDOCHUS CYST

STRICTURE

STONES

ASCARIS

PANCREATIC AND AMPULLARY CARCINOMA

POSTULATED DEFECT

EXCESS BILIRUBIN PRODUCTION

BILIRUBIN TRANSPORT

BILIRUBIN CONJUGATION

CONJUGATION TRANSPORT

CANALICULAR DAMAGE

PERIDUCTULAR INFLAMMATION

LARGE DUCT OBSTRUCTION

Fig. 24-11. Abnormal bile pigment metabolism.

3 mg/100 ml, the increases in both the direct- and indirect-reacting fractions parallel one another. With complete and persistent obstruction, the serum bilirubin may plateau, while the fecal and urinary urobilinogen becomes zero. If the obstruction is fluctuating, the levels of these three determinations will change.

EVALUATION AND MANAGEMENT OF THE PATIENT WITH JAUNDICE. For a discussion of neonatal jaundice and biliary atresia see Chap. 31.

Jaundice is apparent when the serum bilirubin level exceeds 2 mg/100 ml. Tissues rich in elastic fibers have a particular affinity for bilirubin, thus accounting for the earlier appearance and greater intensity in the sclerae and in the skin of the face and upper trunk. Jaundice is not a mere reflection of yellow light through the skin from underlying interstitial fluid but rather a deposition in the tissue fibers and cells. Tissues stain more readily with direct bilirubin than with the indirect-reacting fraction. There is a failure to stain in areas of marked edema and vitiligo.

The diagnosis of jaundice attempts to define the precise cause and also is directed toward the division into surgically correctable lesions, on one hand, and other types in which surgical intervention is not indicated.

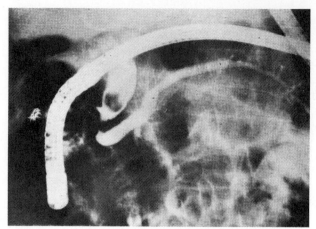

Fig. 24-12. Postcholecystectomy jaundice in a sixty-four-year-old man with recurrent attacks of pancreatitis. Intravenous cholangiogram revealed a dilated common bile duct but no calculus. Note the demonstration by endoscopic retrograde choledochopancreatography of a normal pancreatic duct and dilated common bile duct with a large calculus at its lower end. (*By permission of Surgery, Gynecology & Obstetrics, 138:565, 1974.*)

History. Jaundice secondary to obstruction of the extrahepatic ducts usually starts insidiously and becomes progressively more pronounced. Gastrointestinal disturbances are uncommon, with the exception of those related to biliary calculi. Although, classically, carcinoma of the head of the pancreas is painless, some 20 to 30 percent of these patients do complain of deep epigastric distress or backache. Extrahepatic obstruction associated with ascending cholangitis is accompanied by spiking fevers and abdominal pain. A history of pruritus preceding the onset of jaundice occurs frequently with both extrahepatic biliary obstruction and intrahepatic obstruction secondary to primary cholangiolitis or primary biliary cirrhosis. A detailed family history and history of drug ingestion are imperative before subjecting a patient to surgical treatment, since both constitutional deficiencies and drug-induced jaundice result in a defect in excretion of bile. Loss of appetite, fever, and change of smoking habits are particularly suggestive of hepatitis, and history should be taken of possible contact with persons with known cases and of injections in the previous 6 months. Inquiry into chronic alcohol ingestion is important to rule out jaundice associated with cirrhosis.

Physical Examination. Physical examination also contributes to the diagnosis. Inspection of the skin may reveal a rash, typical of drug reactions, spider angiomas of cirrhosis, or excoriations suggestive of pruritus. Anemia and splenomegaly may be present with hemolytic jaundice. Hepatomegaly and hepatic tenderness are predominant findings with viral hepatitis. A palpable gallbladder in a patient with extrahepatic obstruction occurs more frequently when the obstruction is related to malignancy and less commonly when obstruction is due to biliary calculi. This axiom, known as Courvoisier's law, however, is not universal. Careful search for extrahepatic neoplasm should be made, and the stigmata of portal hypertension including prominent abdominal wall veins and ascites should be investigated.

Laboratory Studies. Hemolytic jaundice is accompanied by anemia and an increased reticulocyte count. Smears for sickle cells, spherocytes, and target cells should be made. The white blood cell count is usually not elevated in viral hepatitis, while it is frequently markedly increased with extrahepatic obstruction and accompanying ascending cholangitis. Stools should be studied for pigment and the presence or absence of guaiac, indicative of bleeding. With carcinoma of the pancreas, approximately one-third of the patients have guaiac-positive stools; this occurs more frequently in patients with obstructive jaundice secondary to carcinoma of the ampulla of Vater.

The so-called "liver function tests" are directed toward assessing the degree of functional impairment of the liver and differentiating between "medical" and "surgical" jaundice. The extreme functional reserve of the liver occasionally produces normal results in the face of significant lesions, and none of the tests provides a pathologic diagnosis. Recently, significant advances in the detection of hepatitis virus have been reported.

Icterus index is a colorimetric evaluation of the serum compared with a chemical standard. It is approximately ten times the value of the serum bilirubin, and jaundice becomes clinically apparent at a level of 16 units. The major application of this procedure is as a rapid screening test to determine whether a more precise measurement of the serum bilirubin is indicated. Serum bilirubin is normally present in concentrations up to 1.5 mg/100 ml and, as previously mentioned, appears both in water-insoluble unconjugated form, which gives the indirect van den Bergh reaction, and the water-soluble conjugated form, which reacts directly. Up to 1.2 mg/100 ml of unconjugated bilirubin is present in the normal serum. Increases in this fraction accompany hemolytic processes such as physiologic jaundice of the newborn, erythroblastosis, and hereditary and acquired hemolytic crises. This fraction is also elevated in the Crigler-Najjar syndrome and in Gilbert's disease. In patients with jaundice secondary to obstruction of the flow of bile or hepatocellular degeneration, the determination of the direct fraction is a more sensitive index of impairment than the total serum bilirubin.

Normally no bilirubin is present in the urine, and bilirubinuria does not accompany hemolytic jaundice or jaundice related to deficiency in the glucuronal transferase system, since the unconjugated fraction, which is increased in these situations, cannot be excreted by the kidney. An elevation in the direct-reacting bilirubin level is associated with bilirubinuria. The production of foam by shaking the urine suggests this elevation. Increased direct-reacting serum bilirubin may not appear in the urine of patients with severe renal failure.

Fecal urobilinogen and to a lesser extent urinary urobilinogen increase with hemolytic jaundice. With obstructive jaundice, the fecal urobilinogen approaches zero, and the urinary urobilinogen follows suit. With hepatocellular jaundice, a mild to moderate decrease in fecal urobilinogen may be associated with an increase in urinary urobilinogen because of a spillover of pigment absorbed from the intestine. A fluctuating fecal or urinary urobilinogen level is suggestive of intermittent hepatic obstruction, most commonly choledocholithiasis.

Enzyme studies are also applicable to the differential diagnosis of jaundice. A markedly elevated serum alkaline phosphatase level is usually associated with obstructive jaundice of either extrahepatic or intrahepatic origin. Elevations in SGOT and SGPT are indicative of hepatocellular disease.

Other laboratory findings, such as a reduction in serum albumin and a reduction in the esterified fraction of the cholesterol, and abnormal turbidity studies are altered with hepatocellular disease. Removal of foreign dye from the liver, either rose bengal or BSP, is dependent upon hepatic blood flow, hepatocellular function, and biliary excretion. The response of prothrombin time to injection of parenteral vitamin K is helpful in establishing a differential diagnosis between hepatocellular and obstructive jaundice. An increase in the prothrombin time within 48 hours of parenteral administration suggests the diagnosis of obstructive jaundice, while a lack of response is more compatible with hepatocellular disease.

Other Diagnostic Procedures. *Radiological Studies.* An x-ray of the abdomen is indicated, since 20 percent of gallstones are radiopaque (see Chap. 31). Oral cholecystography is rarely effective if the serum bilirubin level is above 1.8 mg/100 ml, while intravenous studies are unrewarding if the serum bilirubin level exceeds 3.5 mg/100 ml.

Recent advances which have contributed significantly in the differential diagnosis of jaundice include endoscopic retrograde cholangiopancreatography (ERCP), percutaneous transhepatic cholangiography (PTC) with the skinny Chiba needle, ultrasonography, and computed tomography (CT) scanning. In experienced hands 90 to 95 percent success rates for ERCP (Fig. 24-12) definition of the extrahepatic biliary system have been reported, but in most institutions the yield is less than 65 percent. Cholangitis and pancreatitis are uncommon complications. The technique is uniquely suited to the evaluation of sclerosing cholangitis. In a randomized trial comparing PTC with ERCP for bile duct visualization in deeply jaundiced patients, PTC (see Fig. 31-21) was demonstrated to be the procedure of choice when cholestasis had a surgical cause. PTC was successful in 95 percent of cases with extrahepatic cholestasis and in 25 percent of patients with intrahepatic cholestasis, while ERCP was successful in 62 percent of patients with extrahepatic and 76 percent with intrahepatic cholestasis. In the patient with extrahepatic obstructive jaundice, provision for early operation should be made if bile peritonitis, an uncommon complication, occurs. ERCP is preferred when coagulation defects preclude PTC.

Compound B scanning provides echographic patterns in patients who are deeply jaundiced and whose ducts cannot be visualized with contrast media. Dilated ducts, calculi, and tumors can be defined by serial laminographic scans. (Equipment capable of defining gray scale has increased the sensitivity of this technique.) CT employing the body scanner also will demonstrate dilatation of intrahepatic and/or extrahepatic portions of the biliary tract (Fig. 24-13).

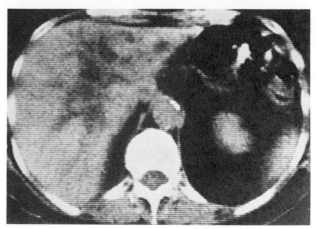

Fig. 24-13. CT scan in a jaundiced woman, showing dilated intrahepatic bile ducts as linear and circular branching structures with an attenuation value approximating water radiating from the porta hepatis. Scans at lower levels showed an enlarged pancreatic head, which proved at operation to contain carcinoma. (*By permission of Radiology, 124:123, 1977.*)

Liver Biopsy. Percutaneous needle biopsy of the liver may, on one hand, prevent procrastination of surgical intervention and progressive parenchymal damage in patients with extrahepatic biliary obstruction; on the other hand, it may preclude laparotomy in patients with severe hepatocellular disease. Patients should be screened for deficiency in the clotting mechanism, and the risk is small. Characteristic lesions of viral hepatitis, cholangiolitic hepatitis, and bile laking suggestive of extrahepatic biliary obstruction can be defined by this technique.

Laparotomy. This is considered an important tool in the diagnostic armamentarium. Laparotomy for obstructive jaundice is never urgent unless there is an acute suppurative cholangitis. Surgical intervention is indicated when other diagnostic procedures have raised a suspicion of extrahepatic obstruction and when the danger of operating on a patient with possible hepatocellular jaundice is considered minimal.

References

Pain

Cope, Z.: "The Early Diagnosis of Acute Abdomen," 14th ed., Oxford University Press, London, 1972.

Lewis, T.: "Pain," The Macmillan Company, New York, 1942.

Lim, R. K. S.: Pain, *Annu Rev Physiol,* **32:**269, 1970.

Long, D. M.: Electrical Stimulation for the Control of Pain, *Arch Surg,* **112:**884, 1977.

Melzack, R., and Wall, P. D.: Pain Mechanisms: A New Theory, *Science,* **150:**971, 1965.

Nathan, P. W.: Pain, *Br Med Bull,* **33:**149, 1977.

Pflug, A. E., and Bonica, J. J.: Physiopathology and Control of Postoperative Pain, *Arch Surg,* **112:**773, 1977.

Ruch, T. C.: Pathophysiology of Pain, in T. C. Ruch and H. D. Patton (eds.), "Physiology and Biophysics," 19th ed., W. B. Saunders Company, Philadelphia, 1965.

Ryle, J. A.: "The Natural History of Disease," 2d ed., Oxford University Press, London, 1948.

Shealy, C. N., Mortimer, J. T., and Hagford, N. R.: Dorsal Column Electroanalgesia, *J Neurosurg,* **32:**560, 1970.

Sweet, W. H.: Pain, in H. W. Magoun (ed.), "Handbook of Physiology" sec. 1, vol. I, "Neurophysiology," American Physiological Society, Washington, 1959.

White, J. C., Smithwick, R. H., and Simeone, F. A.: "The Autonomic Nervous System: Anatomy, Physiology, Surgical Application," 3d ed., The Macmillan Company, New York, 1952.

——— and Sweet, W. H.: "Pain and the Neurosurgeon: A Forty-Year Experience," Charles C Thomas, Publisher, Springfield, Ill., 1969.

Wolff, H., and Wolf, S.: "Pain," 2d ed., Charles C Thomas, Publisher, Springfield, Ill., 1958.

Dysphagia

Davenport, H. W.: "Physiology of the Digestive Tract," 3d ed., Year Book Medical Publishers, Inc., Chicago, 1971.

Glass, G. B. J.: "Introduction to Gastrointestinal Physiology," Prentice-Hall, Inc., Englewood Cliffs, N.J., 1968.

Goyal, R. K., Bauer, J. L., and Spiro, H. M.: The Nature and Location of Lower Esophageal Ring, *N Engl J Med,* **284:**1175, 1971.

Hightower, N. C.: The Physiology of Symptoms: I. Swallowing and Esophageal Motility, *Am J Dig Dis,* **3:**562, 1958.

Ingelfinger, F. J.: Swallowing Disorders in Clinical Practice, *Med Sci,* Apr. 10, 1960, p. 451.

Spiro, H. M.: "Clinical Gastroenterology," The Macmillan Company, New York, 1970.

Anorexia, Nausea, and Vomiting

Borison, H. L., and Wang, S. C.: Physiology and Pharmacology of Vomiting, *Pharmacol Rev,* **5:**193, 1953.

Code, C. F., (sec. ed.): Control of Food and Water Intake, in W. Heidel (ed.), "Handbook of Physiology," sec. 6, vol. I, American Physiological Society, Washington, 1967.

Davenport, H. W.: "Physiology of the Digestive Tract," 3d ed., The Year Book Medical Publishers, Inc., Chicago, 1971.

Drucker, W. R., and Wright, H. K.: Physiology and Pathophysiology of Gastrointestinal Fluids, *Curr Probl Surg,* May, 1964.

Gregory, R. A.: Changes in Intestinal Tone and Motility Associated with Nausea and Vomiting, *J Physiol (Lond),* **105:**58, 1946.

———:The Nervous Pathways of Intestinal Reflexes Associated with Nausea and Vomiting, *J Physiol (Lond),* **106:**95, 1957.

Hawkins, C.: Anorexia and Loss of Weight, *Br Med J,* **2:**1373, 1976.

McGuigan, J. E.: Anorexia, Nausea and Vomiting, in C. M. MacBryde and R. S. Blacklow (eds.), "Signs and Symptoms," 5th ed., J. B. Lippincott Company, Philadelphia, 1970.

Constipation and Diarrhea

Chaudhary, N. A., and Truelove, S. C.: Colonic Motility: A Critical Review of Methods and Results, *Am J Med,* **31:**86, 1961.

Davenport, H. W.: "Physiology of the Digestive Tract," 3d ed., The Year Book Medical Publishers, Inc., Chicago, 1971.

Hurst, A. F.: "Constipation and Allied Intestinal Disorders," 2d ed., Oxford University Press, London, 1921.

Low-Beer, T. S., and Read, A. E.: Diarrhoea: Mechanisms and Treatment, *Gut,* **12:**1021, 1971.

Mellinkoff, S. M. (ed.): "The Differential Diagnosis of Diarrhea," McGraw-Hill Book Company, New York, 1964.

Morrison, A. B., Rawson, A. J., and Fitts, W. T., Jr.: The Syndrome of Refractory Watery Diarrhea and Hypokalemia in Patients with a Noninsulin-secreting Islet Cell Tumor, *Am J Med,* **32:**119, 1962.

Phillips, S. F.: Diarrhea, *Postgrad Med,* **57**(1):65, 1975.

Rabinowitz, R., Farber, M., and Friedman, I. S.: A Depletion Syndrome in Villous Adenoma of the Rectum, *Arch Intern Med,* **109:**265, 1962.

Intestinal Obstruction

Adams, J. T.: Adynamic Ileus of the Colon; an Indication for Cecostomy, *Arch Surg,* **109:**503, 1974.

Baker, J. W., and Ritter, K. J.: Complete Surgical Decompression for Late Obstruction of the Small Intestine, with Reference to a Method, *Ann Surg,* **157:**759, 1963.

Barnett, W. O., Oliver, R. I., and Elliott, R. L.: Elimination of the Lethal Properties of Gangrenous Bowel Segments, *Ann Surg,* **167:**912, 1968.

———, Petro, A. B., and Williamson, J. W.: A Current Appraisal of Problems with Gangrenous Bowel, *Ann Surg,* **183:**653, 1976.

Becker, W. F.: Acute Adhesive Ileus: A Study of 412 Cases with Particular Reference to the Abuse of Tube Decompression in Treatment, *Surg Gynecol Obstet,* **95:**472, 1952.

Berk, J. E., (ed.): "Gastrointestinal Gas," *Ann NY Acad Sci,* **150:**1, 1968.

Billig, D. M., and Jordan, P. H., Jr.: Hemodynamic Abnormalities Secondary to Extracellular Fluid Depletion in Intestinal Obstruction, *Surg Gynecol Obstet,* **128:**1274, 1969.

Boley, S. J., Agrawal, G. P., Warren, A. R., Veith, F. J., Levowitz, B. S., Treiber, W., Dougherty, J., Schwartz, S. S., and Gliedman, M. L.: Pathophysiologic Effects of Bowel Distention on Intestinal Blood Flow, *Am J Surg,* **117:**228, 1969.

Bussemaker, J. B., and Lindeman, J.: Comparison of Methods to Determine Viability of Small Intestine, *Ann Surg,* **176:**97, 1972.

Carmichael, M. J., Weisbrodt, N. W., and Copeland, E. M.: Effect of Abdominal Surgery on Intestinal Myoelectric Activity in the Dog, *Am J Surg,* **133:**34, 1977.

Catchpole, B. N.: Ileus: Use of Sympathetic Blocking Agents in Its Treatment, *Surgery,* **66:**811, 1969.

Clark, D. D., and Hubay, C. A.: Tube Cecostomy: An Evaluation of 161 Cases, *Ann Surg,* **175:**55, 1972.

Cohn, I., Jr., and Atik, M.: Strangulation Obstruction: Closed Loop Studies, *Ann Surg,* **153:**94, 1961.

Davenport, H. W.: "Physiology of the Digestive Tract," 4th ed., The Year Book Medical Publishers, Inc., Chicago, 1977.

Day, E. A., and Marks, C.: Gallstone Ileus, *Am J Surg,* **129:**552, 1975.

Dennis, C.: The Gastrointestinal Sump Tube, *Surgery,* **66:**309, 1969.

Drucker, W. R., and Wright, H. K.: Physiology and Pathophysiology of Gastrointestinal Fluids, *Curr Probl Surg,* May, 1964.

Ellis, H.: Collective Review: The Cause and Prevention of Postoperative Intraperitoneal Adhesions, *Surg Gynecol Obstet,* **133:**497, 1971.

Frimann-Dahl, J.: "Roentgen Examinations in Acute Abdominal Diseases," 3d ed., Charles C Thomas, Publisher, Springfield, Ill., 1974.

Gammill, S. L., and Nice, C. M., Jr.: Air Fluid Levels: Their Occurrence in Normal Patients and Their Role in the Analysis of Ileus, *Surgery,* **71:**771, 1972.

Heimbach, D. M., and Crout, J. R.: Treatment of Paralytic Ileus with Adrenergic Neuronal Blocking Agents, *Surgery,* **69:**582, 1971.

Hubbard, T. B., Jr., Khan, M. Z., Carag, V. R., Albites, V. E., and Hricko, G. M.: The Pathology of Peritoneal Repair: Its Relation to the Formation of Adhesions, *Ann Surg,* **165:**908, 1967.

Kock, N. G.: An Experimental Analysis of Mechanisms Engaged in Reflex Inhibition of Intestinal Motility, *Acta Physiol Scand,* vol. 47 (*Suppl* 164), 1959.

Landman, M. D., and Longmire, W. P., Jr.: Neural and Hormonal Influences of Peritonitis on Paralytic Ileus, *Am Surg,* **33:**756, 1967.

Larsen, E., and Pories, W. J.: Frequency of Wound Complications after Surgery for Small Bowel Obstruction, *Am J Surg,* **122:**384, 1971.

Levitt, M. D., and Bond, J. H., Jr.: Volume, Composition, and Source of Intestinal Gas, *Gastroent,* **59:**921, 1970.

Maddock, W. G., Bell, J. L., and Tremaine, M. J.: Gastrointestinal Gas: Observations on Belching during Anesthesia, Operations and Pyelography; and Rapid Passage of Gas, *Ann Surg,* **130:**512, 1949.

Miller, R. E., and Brahme, F.: Large Amounts of Orally Administered Barium for Obstruction of the Small Intestine, *Surg Gynecol Obstet,* **129:**1185, 1969.

Nachlas, M. M., Younis, M. T., Roda, C. P., and Wityk, J. J.: Gastrointestinal Motility Studies as a Guide to Postoperative Management, *Ann Surg,* **175:**510, 1972.

Nadrowski, L. F.: Pathophysiology and Current Treatment of Intestinal Obstruction, *Rev Surg,* **31:**381, 1974.

Norton, L., Young, D., and Scribner, R.: Management of Pseudo-obstruction of the Colon, *Surg Gynecol Obstet,* **138:**595, 1974.

Öhman, U.: Studies on Small Intestinal Obstruction, I–VI, *Acta Chir Scand,* **141:**413, 417, 536, 545, 763, 771, 1975.

Playforth, R. H., Holloway, J. B., and Griffen, W. O., Jr.: Mechanical Small Bowel Obstruction: A Plea for Earlier Surgical Intervention, *Ann Surg,* **171:**783, 1970.

Price, J. E., Michel, S. L., and Morgenstern, L.: Fruit Pit Obstruction, *Arch Surg,* **111:**773, 1976.

Raf, L.: Causes of Small Intestinal Obstruction, *Acta Chir Scand.,* **135:**67, 1969.

Saegesser, F., and Sandblom, P.: Ischemic Lesions of the Distended Colon: A Complication of Obstructive Colorectal Cancer, *Am J Surg,* **129:**309, 1975.

Schuffler, M. D., Rohrmann, C. A., Jr., and Templeton, F. E.: The Radiologic Manifestations of Idiopathic Intestinal Obstruction, *Am J Roentgenol,* **127:**729, 1976.

Shields, R.: The Absorption and Secretion of Fluid and Electrolytes by the Obstructed Bowel, *Br J Surg,* **52:**774, 1965.

Shin, C-S., Nimmannit, S., Hoff, A., and Enquist, I. F.: Body Fluid Compartments in Patients with Nonstrangulating Obstruction of the Small Intestine, *Surg Gynecol Obstet,* **132:**980, 1971.

Smith, J., Kelly, K. A., and Weinshilboum, R. M.: Pathophysiology of Postoperative Ileus, *Arch Surg,* **112:**203, 1977.

Sufian, S., and Matsumoto, T.: Intestinal Obstruction, *Am J Surg,* **130:**9, 1975.

Sullivan, M. A., Snape, W. J., Jr., Matarazzo, S. A., Petrokubi, R. J., Jeffries, G., and Cohen, S.: Gastrointestinal Myoelectrical Activity in Idiopathic Intestinal Pseudo-obstruction, *N Engl J Med,* **297:**233, 1977.

Sung, D. T. W., and Williams, L. F., Jr.: Intestinal Secretion after Intravenous Fluid Infusion in Small Bowel Obstruction, *Am J Surg,* **121:**91, 1971.

Sykes, P. A., Boulter, K. H., and Schofield, P. F.: The Microflora of the Obstructed Bowel, *Br J Surg,* **63:**721, 1976.

Tibblin, S.: Diagnosis of Intestinal Obstruction with Special Regard to Plain Roentgen Examination of the Abdomen, *Acta Chir Scand,* **135:**249, 1969.

Tinker, M. A., Teicher, I., and Burdman, D.: Cellulose Granulomas and Their Relationship to Intestinal Obstruction, *Am J Surg,* **133:**134, 1977.

Trippestad, A., and Midtvedt, T.: The Role of Hemoglobin for the Lethal Effect of Intestinal Strangulation Fluid, *J Surg Res,* **10:**465, 1970.

Wangensteen, O. H.: "Intestinal Obstruction," 3d ed., Charles C Thomas, Publisher, Springfield, Ill., 1955.

———: Historical Aspects of the Management of Acute Intestinal Obstruction, *Surgery,* **65:**363, 1969.

Weilbaecher, D., Bolin, J. A., Hearn, D., and Ogden, W., II.: Intussusception in Adults, *Am J Surg,* **121:**531, 1971.

Welch, C. E.: "Intestinal Obstruction," The Year Book Medical Publishers, Inc., Chicago, 1958.

Welch, J. P., and Donaldson, G. A.: Management of Severe Obstruction of the Large Bowel Due to Malignant Disease, *Am J Surg,* **127:**492, 1974.

Wojtalik, R. S., Lindenauer, S. M., and Kahn, S. S.: Perforation of the Colon Associated with Adynamic Ileus, *Am J Surg,* **125:**601, 1973.

Wright, H. K., O'Brien, J. J., and Tilson, M. D.: Water Absorption in Experimental Closed Segment Obstruction of the Ileum in Man, *Am J Surg,* **121:**96, 1971.

Yale, C. E.: Ischemic Intestinal Strangulation in Germ-free Rats, *Arch Surg,* **99:**397, 1969.

Gastrointestinal Bleeding

Altemeier, W. A., Fullen, W. D., and McDonough, J. J.: Sepsis and Gastrointestinal Bleeding, *Ann Surg,* **175:**759, 1972.

Athanasoulis, C. A., Baum, S., Rosch, J., Waltman, A. C., Ring, E. J., Smith, J. C., Jr., Sugarbaker, E., and Wood, W.: Mesenteric Arterial Infusions of Vasopressin for Hemorrhage from Colonic Diverticulosis, *Am J Surg,* **129:**212, 1975.

———, ———, Waltman, A. C., Ring, E. J., Imbembo, A., and Vander Salm, T. J.: Control of Acute Gastric Mucosal Hemorrhage: Intra-arterial Infusion of Posterior Pituitary Extract, *N Engl J Med,* **290:**597, 1974.

Bauer, J. J., Kreel, I., and Kark, A. E.: The Use of the Sengstaken-Blakemore Tube for Immediate Control of Bleeding Esophageal Varices, *Ann Surg,* **179:**273, 1974.

Behringer, G. E., and Albright, N. L.: Diverticular Disease of the Colon: A Frequent Cause of Massive Rectal Bleeding, *Am J Surg,* **125:**419, 1973.

Boley, S. J., Sammartano, R., Adams, A., DiBiase, A., Kleinhaus, S., and Sprayregen, S.: On the Nature and Etiology of Vascular Ectasias of the Colon: Degenerative Lesions of Aging, Gastroenterology, 72:650, 1977.

Conn, H. O., Ramsby, G. R., Storer, E. H., Mutshnick, M., Joshi, P. H., Phillips, M. M., Cohen, G. A., Fields, G. N., and Petroski, D.: Intraarterial Vasopressin in the Treatment of Upper Gastrointestinal Hemorrhage: A Prospective, Controlled Clinical Trial, Gastroenterology, 68:211, 1975.

Crook, J. N., Gray, L. W., Jr., Nance, F. C., and Cohn, I., Jr.: Upper Gastrointestinal Bleeding, Ann Surg, 175:771, 1972.

Drapanas, T., Woolverton, W. C., Reeder, J. W., Reed, R. L., and Weichert, R. F.: Experiences with Surgical Management of Acute Gastric Mucosal Hemorrhage: A Unified Concept in the Pathophysiology, Ann Surg, 173:628, 1971.

Dronfield, M. W., McIllmurray, M. B., Ferguson, R., Atkinson, M., and Langman, M. J. S.: A Prospective, Randomized Study of Endoscopy and Radiology in Acute Upper-Gastrointestinal-Bleeding, Lancet, 1:1168, 1977.

Eastwood, G. L.: Does Early Endoscopy Benefit the Patient with Active Upper Gastrointestinal Bleeding? Gastroenterology, 72:737, 1977.

Fischer, R. P., Jelense, S., and Fulton, R. L.: The Maintenance of Gastric Mucosal Barrier during the Early Erosive Gastritis Component of Stress Ulceration, Surgery, 80:40, 1976.

Foster, J. H.: Immediate Results of Emergency Operation for Massive Upper Gastrointestinal Hemorrhage, Am J Surg, 122:387, 1971.

Grace, D. M., Pitt, D. F., and Gold, R. E.: Vascular Embolization and Occlusion by Angiographic Techniques as an Aid or Alternative to Operation, Surg Gynecol Obstet, 143:469, 1976.

Halmagyi, A. F.: A Critical Review of 425 Patients with Gastrointestinal Hemorrhage, Surg Gynecol Obstet, 130:419, 1970.

Hamlyn, A. N., Lunzer, M. R., Morris, J. S., Puritz, H., and Dick, R.: Portal Hypertension with Varices in Unusual Sites, Lancet, 2:1531, 1974.

Harvey, R. F., and Langman, M. J. S.: Late Results of Medical and Surgical Treatment for Bleeding Duodenal Ulcer, Q J Med, 39:539, 1970.

Johnson, W. C., Widrich, W. C., Ansell, J. E., Robbins, A. H., and Nabseth, D. C.: Control of Bleeding Varices by Vasopressin: A Prospective Randomized Study, Ann Surg, 186:369, 1977.

Katon, R. M.: Experimental Control of Gastrointestinal Hemorrhage via the Endoscope: A New Era Dawns, Gastroenterology, 70:272, 1976.

Knauer, C. M.: Mallory-Weiss Syndrome, Gastroenterology, 71:5, 1976.

Langman, M. J. S.: Epidemiological Evidence for the Association of Aspirin and Acute Gastrointestinal Bleeding, Gut, 11:627, 1970.

Le Gall, J. R., Mignon, F. C., Rapin, M., Redjemi, M., Harari, A., Bader, J. P., and Soussy, C. J.: Acute Gastroduodenal Lesions Related to Severe Sepsis, Surg Gynecol Obstet, 142:377, 1976.

McClelland, R. N., Shires, G. T., and Prager, M.: Gastric Secretory and Splanchnic Blood Flow Studies in Man after Severe Trauma and Hemorrhagic Shock, Am J Surg, 121:134, 1971.

Malt, R. A.: Control of Massive Upper Gastrointestinal Hemorrhage, N Engl J Med, 286:1043, 1972.

Matsumoto, T., ed.: "Current Management of Acute Gastrointes-

tinal Hemorrhage," Charles C Thomas, Publisher, Springfield, Ill., 1977.

Menguy, R., and Masters, Y. F.: Gastric Mucosal Energy Metabolism and "Stress Ulceration," Ann Surg, 180:538, 1974.

Meyers, M. A., Alonso, D. R., Gray, G. F., and Baer, J. W.: Pathogenesis of Bleeding Colonic Diverticulosis, Gastroenterology, 71:577, 1976.

Miller, R. D., Robbins, T. O., Tong, M. J., and Barton, S. L.: Coagulation Defects Associated with Massive Blood Transfusions, Ann Surg, 174:794, 1971.

Milliser, R. V., Greenberg, S. R., and Neiman, B. H.: Exsanguinating Stercoral Ulceration, Am J Dig Dis, 15:485, 1970.

Moody, F. G.: Rectal Bleeding, N Engl J Med, 290:839, 1974.

Moss, G.: Cause of Azotemia after Gastrointestinal Hemorrhage: Examining an Old Wives' Tale, Am J Surg, 130:269, 1975.

Nance, F. C., Kaufman, H. J., and Batson, R. C.: The Role of the Microbial Flora in Acute Gastric Stress Ulceration, Surgery, 72:68, 1972.

Netterville, R. E., Hardy, J. D., and Martin, R. S.: Small Bowel Hemorrhage, Ann Surg, 167:949, 1968.

Northfield, T. C., and Smith, T.: Physiologic Significance of Central Venous Pressure in Patients with Hemorrhage, Surg Gynecol Obstet, 135:267, 1972.

Novis, B. H., Duys, P., Barbecat, G. O., Clain, J., Bank, S., and Terblanche, T.: Fibreoptic Endoscopy and the Use of the Sengstaken Tube in Acute Gastrointestinal Hemorrhage in Patients with Portal Hypertension and Varices, Gut, 17:258, 1976.

Nusbaum, M., and Conn, H. O.: Arterial Vasopressin Infusions: Science or Seance?, Gastroenterology, 69:263, 1975.

Parsa, F., Gordon, H. E., and Wilson, S. E.: Bleeding Diverticulosis of the Colon, Dis Colon Rectum, 18:37, 1975.

Pitcher, J. L.: Safety and Effectiveness of the Modified Sengstaken-Blakemore Tube: A Prospective Study, Gastroenterology, 61:291, 1971.

Pruitt, B. A., Foley, F. D., and Moncrief, J. A.: Curling's Ulcer: A Clinical-Pathological Study of 323 Cases, Ann Surg, 172:523, 1970.

Ritchie, W. P., Jr.: Bile Acids, the "Barrier," and Reflux-Related Clinical Disorders of the Gastric Mucosa, Surgery, 82:192, 1977.

Safaie-Shirazi, S., Foster, L. D., and Hardy, B. M.: The Effect of Metiamide, an H_2-Receptor Antagonist, in the Prevention of Experimental Stress Ulcers, Gastroenterology, 71:421, 1976.

Schiff, L.: Hematemesis and Melena, in C. M. MacBryde, (ed.), "Signs and Symptoms," 5th ed., J. B. Lippincott Company, Philadelphia, 1970.

Schiller, K. F. R., Truelove, S. C., and Williams, D. G.: Haematemesis and Melaena, with Special Reference to Factors Influencing the Outcome, Br Med J, 2:7, 1970.

Silen, W.: New Concepts of the Gastric Mucosal Barrier, Am J Surg, 133:8, 1977.

Simonian, S. J., and Curtis, L. E.: Treatment of Hemorrhagic Gastritis by Antacid, Ann Surg, 184:429, 1976.

Sutherland, D., Frech, R. S., Weil, R., Najarian, J. S., and Simmons, R. L.: The Bleeding Cecal Ulcer: Pathogenesis, Angiographic Diagnosis, and Nonoperative Control, Surgery, 71:290, 1972.

Wagner, M., Kiselow, M. C., Keats, W. L., and Jan, M. L.: Varices of the Colon, Arch Surg, 100:718, 1970.

Wilson, W. S., Gadacz, T., Olcott, C., III, and Blaisdell, F. W.: Superficial Gastric Erosions: Response to Surgical Treatment, *Am J Surg,* **126:**133, 1973.

Villar, H. V., Fender, H. R., Watson, L. C., and Thompson, J. C.: Emergency Diagnosis of Upper Gastrointestinal Bleeding by Fiberoptic Endoscopy, *Ann Surg,* **185:**367, 1977.

Yajko, R. D., Norton, L. W., and Eiseman, B.: Current Management of Upper Gastrointestinal Bleeding, *Ann Surg,* **181:**474, 1975.

Jaundice

Blumgart, L. H., Salmon, P. R., and Cotton, P. B.: Endoscopy and Retrograde Choledochopancreatography in Diagnosis of Patient with Jaundice, *Surg Gynecol Obstet,* **138:**565, 1974.

Elias, E., Hamlyn, A. N., Jain, S., Long, R. G., Summerfield, J. A., Dick, R., and Sherlock, S.: A Randomized Trial of Percutaneous Transhepatic Cholangiography with the Chiba Needle versus Endoscopic Retrograde Cholangiography for Bile Duct Visualization in Jaundice, *Gastroenterology,* **71:**439, 1976.

Freimanis, A. T.: Intraabdominal Fluid Collections, in S. Gottlieb and M. Viamonte, Jr. (eds.), "Diagnostic Ultrasound," Chicago, Ill. The American College of Radiology, Committee on New Technology, 1976.

Leevy, C. M.: "Evaluation of Liver Function in Clinical Practice," The Lilly Research Laboratories, Indianapolis, Ind., 1965.

Levitt, R. G., Sagel, S. S., Stanley, R. J., and Jost, R. G.: Accuracy of Computed Tomography of the Liver and Biliary Tract, *Radiology,* **124:**123, 1977.

Popper, H., and Schaffner, F.: "Liver: Structure and Function," McGraw-Hill Book Company, New York, 1957.

Schwartz, S. I.: "Surgical Diseases of the Liver," McGraw-Hill Book Company, New York, 1964.

Thompson, R. P. H.: Recent Advances in Jaundice: Physiology, *Br Med J,* **1:**223, 1970.

Williams, R.: Recent Advances in Jaundice: Medical Aspects of Investigation and Treatment, *Br Med J,* **1:**225, 1970.

Chapter 25

Esophagus and Diaphragmatic Hernias

by W. Spencer Payne and F. Henry Ellis, Jr.

Surgery of the esophagus is primarily a development of the twentieth century, and its major advances have paralleled those of thoracic surgery. Operations on the esophagus were carried out in earlier years, but they were concerned mainly with removal of foreign bodies or with local excision of malignant lesions or diverticula of the cervical esophagus. Transabdominal procedures for the relief of esophageal achalasia were done in the early 1900s, as were staged reconstructive operations for corrosive stricture and malignant lesions; but only later, after the development of techniques permitting intrathoracic operations, was the thoracic portion of this organ approached with confidence. The first successful one-stage transpleural esophagogastrectomy for carcinoma was performed in 1933 by Ohsawa. Marshall was the first to perform this operation successfully in the United States, in 1937. Thereafter, advances in all aspects of thoracic surgery came rapidly, and as a result the esophagus became accessible to the surgeon's knife. The reductions in surgical morbidity and mortality at first were not matched, however, by similar advances in the understanding of the function of the esophagus. Largely as a result of studies of esophageal motility carried out by Ingelfinger and by Code and Schlegel, the surgical approach to esophageal lesions now rests on sounder physiologic grounds.

ANATOMY

The esophagus is a long muscular tube extending downward from the pharynx at the C_6 level and terminating in a region commonly referred to as the "cardia," whose definition is highly variable (Fig. 25-1). In its course between these two points, it occupies in the neck a midline position immediately behind the trachea. In the thorax it inclines posteriorly behind the great vessels, curving slightly to the left to pass behind the left main bronchus, whence it inclines slightly to the right as it continues in the posterior mediastinum. It again deviates to the left behind the pericardial sac, where it runs anterior to the thoracic aorta, crossing it to the left of the midline. It reaches the abdomen through the esophageal hiatus, a noose of diaphragmatic muscle composed chiefly of the right crus of the diaphragm. An esophageal segment of variable length usually occupies an intraabdominal location before joining the stomach at the point referred to as the "cardia." In general, this term applies to a vague region including the lower esophagus, the esophagogastric junction, and the upper portion of the stomach. Identification of the esophagogastric junction by reference to the

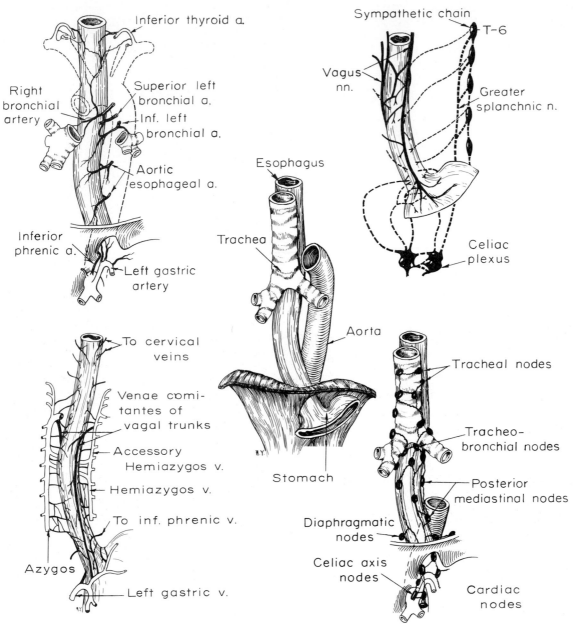

Fig. 25-1. Anatomy of the human esophagus. Upper Left: Arterial supply. Lower left: Venous drainage. Upper right: Innervation. Lower right: Lymphatic system. [*From F. H. Ellis, Jr., The Esophagus, in L. Davis (ed.), "Christopher's Textbook of Surgery," 8th ed., W. B. Saunders Company, Philadelphia, 1964, pp. 591–620.*]

mucosal lining is also difficult. From a practical standpoint, the junction can best be described as that point where the esophageal tube meets the gastric pouch.

There are important supporting structures in the region of the diaphragm and the esophagogastric junction. The anatomy of the diaphragmatic crura varies (Fig. 25-2). The muscle fibers which form the crura arise from the lateral aspects of the second, third, and fourth lumbar vertebrae and pass superiorly and anteriorly past the aorta to form the margins of the esophageal hiatus, inserting into the central tendon of the diaphragm. Many variations may be seen. In the most common, the right crus contributes all the fibers which form the esophageal hiatus and is reinforced by muscle from the left side (Fig. 25-2*A*). The

second most common type is quite similar, but a slip of muscle from the left crus passes behind the esophagus to form part of the right margin of the hiatus (Fig. 25-2*B*). These two variations account for four-fifths of the known variations. The phrenoesophageal membrane or ligament, another important anatomic structure, was described by Laimer in 1883. Composed of mature collagenous fibers, this structure is a continuation of the transversalis fascia of the abdominal parietes and inserts onto the circumference of the lower thoracic esophagus 2 to 3 cm above the true esophagogastric junction. A contribution to this structure is provided by fascia arising from the upper surface of the diaphragm. Further support is provided by the pleura above and the peritoneal reflection below. The fibers themselves fan out and insert into the lower esophagus over a relatively wide zone (Fig. 25-3A).

The blood supply of the esophagus is provided in its cervical portion by the inferior thyroid arteries and in its thoracic portion by the aorta itself and by esophageal branches of the bronchial arteries. Supplemental vessels come from arteries on the abdominal side of the diaphragm as well as branches from intercostal arteries. The venous drainage is more complex. Subepithelial and subvenous channels course longitudinally to empty above into the hypopharyngeal and below into the gastric veins. These channels also penetrate the esophageal muscle, from which they receive branches, and leave the esophagus to form a periesophageal plexus, the longest trunks of which accompany the vagus nerves. Drainage from the cervical portion of the esophagus empties ultimately into the inferior thyroid and vertebral veins, that from the thoracic portion into the azygos and hemiazygos veins, and that from the abdominal portion into the left gastric vein.

The lymphatic vessels run longitudinally in the wall of the esophagus before penetrating the muscle layers to reach regional lymph nodes. Thus malignant lesions of the middle or upper esophagus may metastasize first to the cervical nodes and lesions of the lower esophagus to gastric and celiac nodes. On leaving the esophagus, however, the lymphatic channels go to the nearest group of nodes, which within the thorax are usually identified by their location as tracheal, tracheobronchial, posterior mediastinal, or diaphragmatic nodes.

The esophagus receives both vagal and sympathetic nerves, its upper portion being supplied by the recurrent nerves and branches from the ninth and tenth cranial nerves and the cranial root of the eleventh and by sympathetic nerves. The vagal trunks send branches to the remaining voluntary muscles, and the parasympathetic preganglionic fibers to the smooth muscles. The vagus nerves lie on either side of the esophagus through most of its course, forming a plexus about it. At the hiatus, however, two major trunks emerge, the left one coming to lie anteriorly and the right one posteriorly. The vagal plexuses are joined by mediastinal branches of the thoracic sympathetic chain of the splanchnic nerves. The lower end of the esophagus and the esophagogastric junction zone also receive sympathetic branches from the periarterial plexus along the left gastric and left inferior phrenic arteries.

The esophageal wall is composed of an inner circular layer of muscle and an outer longitudinal layer without a surrounding serosal covering. Striated muscle fibers make a considerable contribution to the outer longitudinal coat in the upper portion of the esophagus, whereas smooth muscle predominates in the lower portion of the esophagus. Measurements of the thickness of the muscle layers of the distal esophageal wall reveal no consistent increase in the segment that corresponds to the physiologic gastro-

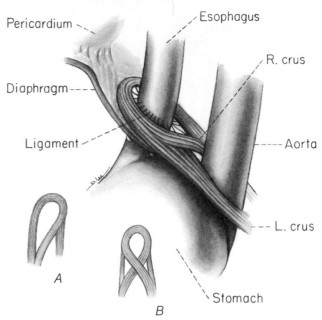

Fig. 25-2. The crura of the diaphragm. *A.* Most common anatomic variation. *B.* Next most common variation.

esophageal sphincter, but an area of thickened muscle known as the gastric sling fibers of Willis can be demonstrated partially encircling the proximal part of the stomach at the esophagogastric junction area (Fig. 25-3B).

There is a prominent submucosa containing mucous

Fig. 25-3. Gross anatomy of region of esophagogastric junction area. *A.* Details of origin and insertion of phrenoesophageal membrane or ligament. *B.* Cross section of distal esophagus and proximal stomach. *C.* Oblique gastric sling fibers.

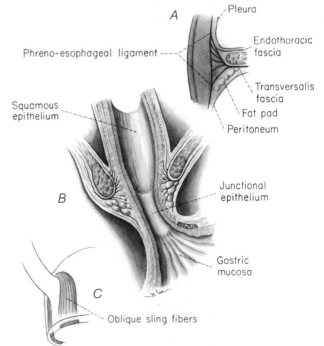

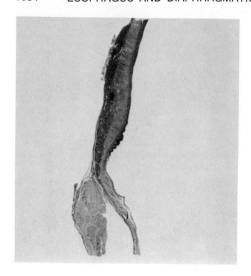 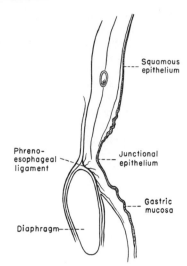

Fig. 25-4. Microscopic anatomy of esophagogastric junction area. Left: Photomicrograph. (Hematoxylin and eosin; ×1.) Right: Schematic representation, showing origin and insertion of phrenoesophageal ligament, diaphragm, and mucosal lining.

glands, blood vessels, Meissner's plexus of nerves, and a rich network of lymphatic vessels. The mucosal lining is characteristically made up of squamous epithelium, although ectopic islands of gastric mucosa have been identified, particularly in the proximal portions of the esophagus. The distal 1 or 2 cm of the esophageal lumen is lined by columnar epithelium, the columnar-squamous junction lying not at the true esophagogastric junction but within the lower esophagus (Figs. 25-3 and 25-4).

PHYSIOLOGY

The esophagus provides a channel by which ingested material is conveyed from the pharynx to the stomach. At

Fig. 25-5. Balloon-covered differential transformer and open-tipped tubes (arrows) used in measurement of esophageal and sphincteric pressures. (From C. F. Code, M. L. Kelley, Jr., J. F. Schlegel, and A. M. Olsen, Detection of Hiatal Hernia during Esophageal Motility Tests, Gastroenterology, 43:521–531, 1962.)

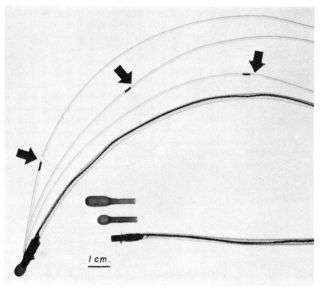

either end of the tube are regulatory mechanisms which assist in this function. Current knowledge of the physiology of the esophagus has been gained by the use of special recording techniques to detect and record intraesophageal pressures. In routine tests, three or four pressure-detecting units (fine water-filled polyethylene tubes attached to strain-gauge manometers) are positioned at various points in the esophagus. Some prefer to use a balloon-covered transducer in addition to tubes with lateral openings at 5-cm intervals (Fig. 25-5). The infusion of saline solution at a constant rate through the open-tipped tubes may provide more accurate pressure recordings. Measurements are made when the esophagus is at rest and after swallowing, the resting pressures being measured while the units are being withdrawn in stepwise fashion from the stomach into the esophagus prior to the recording of deglutition pressures.

At the upper end of the esophagus there is a zone, about 3 cm long, of increased pressure which relaxes promptly with swallowing and contracts thereafter as a wave of high pressure passes through it (Fig. 25-6). Contractions of this sphincter are in peristaltic sequence with those of the pharynx above and the esophagus below, and the primary peristaltic wave of the esophagus is thus initiated. The sphincter relaxes to allow the wave to pass and then closes more tightly. This wave of positive pressure sweeps in an orderly peristaltic fashion down the body of the esophagus, reaching an intensity of 50 to 100 cm H_2O and being somewhat more forceful in the lower esophagus. The resting pressures in the body of the esophagus are normally less than atmospheric pressure, reflecting negative intrathoracic pressure. There is also a zone of increased pressure at the lower end of the esophagus, somewhat longer than that at the upper end (3 to 5 cm long), which can be detected by withdrawing the recording units from the stomach into the esophagus (Fig. 25-7). It is located in the region of the hiatus; in response to a swallowing effort, relaxation of this zone of increased pressure can be identified, along with the immediately following sphincteric contraction in sequence with the peristaltic wave from the esophagus above (Fig. 25-8). This zone is the inferior sphincter of the esophagus.

The details of esophageal innervation remain to be clarified, but esophageal peristalsis seems to be under vagal control, because division of these nerves produces low simultaneous pressures in the body of the esophagus after deglutition. The inferior esophageal sphincter, however, continues to relax with swallowing even after complete denervation, suggesting a certain degree of autonomy.

In spite of the clear demonstration of a physiologic sphincter at the lower end of the esophagus, there remains considerable controversy concerning the exact mechanism by which gastroesophageal reflux is prevented under normal circumstances. Factors that have been suggested as important include the diaphragm, a valve flap mechanism, the gastric sling fibers and the oblique angle of entry, and the mucosal rosette. There is substantial evidence to suggest that the first three are not involved in gastroesophageal competence and that the musculature of the intrinsic sphincter, in combination with prominent folds of epithelial gastric lining at the cardia, comprise the main antireflux mechanisms.

Recent studies by Goyal indicate that the lower esophageal sphincter (LES) is controlled by neural, hormonal, myogenic, and mechanical influences.

In the past some observers believed that the basal sphincter pressure was maintained by continuous vagal tone and that sphincter relaxation was a result of a decrease of tonic vagal activity. However, it is now held that both relaxation and contraction of the LES are due to the vagal transmission of active inhibitory or excitatory impulses but that neither acts as the major determinant of basal LES pressure. The role of sympathetic innervation on the LES is less well understood. Stimulation of alpha-adrenergic receptors causes the LES to contract, and that of beta-adrenergic receptors causes it to relax. It is further hypothesized that sympathetic nerves act to modulate vagal activity on the LES. The fact that complete pharmacologic denervation of the LES does not influence basal sphincter pressure suggests that basal sphincter pressure is not due to tonic autonomic neural activity but that it may be due to tonic myogenic activity of the LES muscle itself.

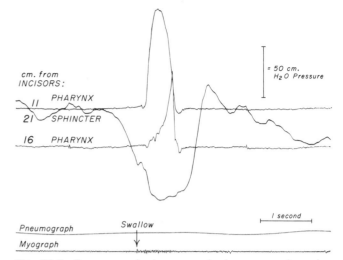

Fig. 25-6. Response of pharynx and pharyngoesophageal sphincter to swallowing and to peristalsis and sphincteric relaxation. (*From C. F. Code and J. F. Schlegel, The Physiologic Basis of Some Motor Disorders of the Oesophagus, in A. N. Smith, "Surgical Physiology of Gastrointestinal Tract," Royal College of Surgeons, Edinburgh, 1963, pp. 1–19.*)

Many hormones have been known to modify basal pressure of the LES. It has been held that circulating gastrin is the major determinant of basal LES pressure and that this effect is modulated by interaction of secretin. However, recent studies do not support these views and suggest that the changes previously observed were obtainable only in response to unphysiologically high levels of these hormones. Other hormones such as prostaglandins, histamine, and serotonin produce less clear or variable effects on LES pressure, depending on experimental conditions.

Thus, at this time it appears that the basal LES pressure is due to background basal tone provided by intrinsic myogenic activity of the sphincter muscle itself and that this tone is modulated by a variety of excitatory and inhibitory neurohormonal influences. The sphincter relaxation is chiefly due to neural activity mediated by inhibitory vagal and extravagal pathways.

Loss of the LES basal tone can occur as a consequence of pregnancy (because of elevated levels of progesterone and estrogens), excessive ingestion of alcohol, smoking, and use of drugs that especially inhibit the LES (atropine, nitrites, beta-adrenergic agents, etc.). The LES basal tone can be enhanced by neutralization of gastric acid and by the administration of drugs such as bethanecol or metoclopramide.

Fig. 25-7. Pressure profiles of normal lower esophageal sphincter, detected by withdrawal of open-tipped tube and small balloon. (*From F. H. Ellis, Jr., The Esophagus, in L. Davis, "Christopher's Textbook of Surgery," 8th ed., W. B. Saunders Company, Philadelphia, 1964, pp. 591–620.*)

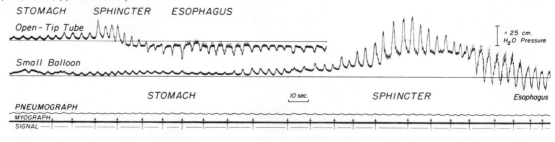

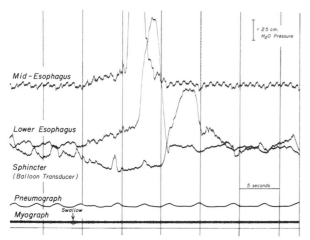

Fig. 25-8. Deglutitive response of inferior esophageal sphincter in healthy subject. Note that relaxation precedes arrival of peristaltic wave in the sphincter. (*From F. H. Ellis, Jr., and W. S. Payne, Motility Disturbances of the Esophagus and Its Inferior Sphincter: Recent Surgical Advances, Adv Surg, 1:179–246, 1965. Copyright 1965 by Year Book Medical Publishers Inc. Used by permission.*)

When the LES is challenged by an increase in intragastric pressure, its resting tone increases. This response is due to a vagus-mediated neural reflex that can be blocked by atropine or vagotomy, as shown by Cohen and Lipshutz. The ability to increase the LES pressure so that it is greater than the rise in intragastric pressure is one of the essential features of the competent LES.

ESOPHAGEAL MOTILITY DISTURBANCES

The development of techniques for physiologic evaluation of esophageal function has permitted the classification of esophageal motility disorders in two main categories: those characterized by hypomotility of the esophagus, such as esophageal achalasia, and those characterized by hyper-

motility, such as diffuse spasm of the esophagus with or without hypertensive gastroesophageal sphincter. Although the causes of these conditions remain in doubt, their clinical and physiologic manifestations are now well known, so surgical treatment can be undertaken on sound grounds in properly selected patients.

Hypomotility

ACHALASIA

Achalasia of the esophagus, or cardiospasm, as it is more commonly but inaccurately known, has been recognized by the medical profession for almost 300 years. As early as 1674, Thomas Willis in his *Pharmaceutice Rationalis* described the symptoms of this condition and advised forceful dilation as treatment. It is a disease characterized by a disturbance of esophageal motility, in which there is absence of peristalsis in the body of the esophagus and failure of the inferior esophageal sphincter to relax in response to swallowing.

The causes of the disease are unknown, although a variety have been suggested, including inherent weakness of the esophagus, spasm of the esophagus, mechanical factors such as external compression or trauma, and congenital factors. Most students of the subject now agree that the disease has a neurogenic basis, and pathologic evidence in support of this theory is provided by demonstration of degeneration or absence of the ganglion cells of Auerbach's plexus in the esophagus of many patients with the disease, a finding first reported by Rake in 1926. Subsequent studies have shown that the changes occur throughout the thoracic esophagus, particularly in the body of the organ, but one-third of the patients are unaffected.

The reason for these nerve cell changes remains obscure; infections due to bacteria or viruses, infestations by para-

Fig. 25-9. Esophageal roentgenograms of achalasia of the esophagus. Left: Mild. Center: Moderate. Right: Severe. (*From A. M. Olsen, S. W. Harrington, H. J. Moersch, and H. A. Andersen, The Treatment of Cardiospasm: Analysis of a Twelve-Year Experience, J Thorac Surg, 22:164–187, 1951.*)

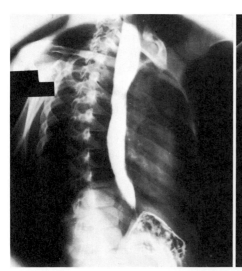
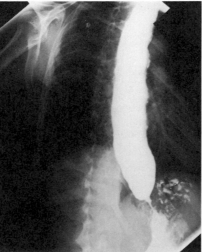
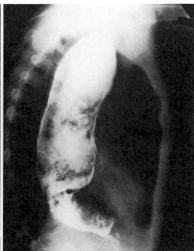

sites, and vitamin deficiencies have all been incriminated. That the primary site of the disorder may be in the extraesophageal nerve supply—either the vagus nerve itself or its central nuclei—has been suggested by pathologic studies of biopsy and autopsy material and by experiments involving the selective destruction of the motor nuclei of the vagus nerve in the medulla of the cat and the dog.

CLINICAL MANIFESTATIONS. Whatever the cause of the disease, its clinical manifestations are now well recognized. It occurs with equal frequency in men and in women, and although it may occur at any age, it is more frequently seen in persons between the ages of thirty and fifty years. The earliest and most constant symptom is obstruction to swallowing, which at first may be intermittent. However, as the condition progresses, difficulty is experienced with all efforts to swallow. As a rule, the patient experiences more difficulty with cold than with warm foods, and solids may at first seem to pass more easily than liquids. Pain is rare and is more likely to occur in the early stages of the disease than later; it becomes less noticeable as the esophagus dilates. Regurgitation of ingested food and liquids is a common symptom and may occur particularly at night when the patient is recumbent, leading to aspiration and the development of pulmonary complications. Carcinoma of the esophagus occurs approximately seven times as often in patients with esophageal achalasia as in the general population.

Roentgenographic studies are helpful in the diagnosis of the disease, because even in the early stages evidence of obstruction at the cardia and slight dilatation of the esophagus may be noted. As the disease progresses, the classic roentgenographic signs develop (Fig. 25-9), the esophagus becoming dilated and its lower portion projecting beaklike into the distal narrowed segment with very little, if any, barium present in the stomach. In some cases, the esophagus may reach huge proportions, so that it may be seen on the ordinary thoracic roentgenogram. Differentiation between early stages of esophageal achalasia and benign stricture or carcinoma of the cardia may be difficult, and esophagoscopy may be required for diagnosis.

PHYSIOLOGIC STUDIES. Confirmation of the clinical diagnosis can be provided by studies of esophageal motility. Such studies demonstrate that the pressure in the body of the esophagus is higher than normal, often being equal to atmospheric pressure, presumably because of esophageal dilatation with retention of food and fluid. In response to a swallowing effort, feeble, simultaneous, repetitive contractions occur throughout the esophagus, but there is no coordinated peristaltic wave (Fig. 25-10). Although relaxation of the upper esophageal sphincter occurs normally, in the majority of cases the lower sphincter fails to relax after swallowing, but the resting pressures within it are usually within normal limits. However, Cohen and Lipshutz carried out manometric studies using perfused polyvinyl catheters and suggested that the lower esophageal sphincter pressure at rest is increased in patients with achalasia to approximately twice that seen in normal subjects. Furthermore, when the sphincter does relax during swallowing, the relaxation is incomplete, and pressures remain higher than gastric pressures. Occasionally contrac-

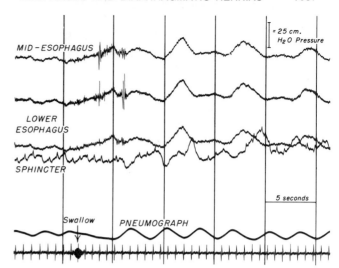

Fig. 25-10. Response to deglutition in achalasia of the esophagus. Feeble simultaneous contractions in response to swallowing occur in the body of the esophagus, with failure of sphincteric relaxation. (*From F. H. Ellis, Jr., and W. S. Payne, Motility Disturbances of the Esophagus and Its Inferior Sphincter: Recent Surgical Advances, Adv Surg, 1:179–246, 1965. Copyright 1965 by Year Book Medical Publishers, Inc. Used by permission.*)

tions of the esophagus and the sphincter may be vigorous, and the term "vigorous achalasia" has been applied to this condition.

TREATMENT. Current knowledge does not permit restoration of the disordered esophageal motility to normal. Effective therapy, therefore, can be directed only to relief of the distal esophageal obstruction. Because diet and drugs are ineffective, this must be accomplished either by forceful dilation of the distal esophagus or by surgical means.

Mechanical, pneumatic, and hydrostatic dilators have been used with success. At the Mayo Clinic, hydrostatic dilation (Fig. 25-11) has been used extensively in the past and has been found to be a useful technique. Sanderson and associates reported good to excellent results in 65 percent of patients observed for an average of $9\frac{1}{2}$ years (Table 25-1). The method is not without risk—an esophageal perforation occurred in about 2 percent of cases.

Limitations of medical therapy, including the use of forceful dilation, have led to surgical efforts to relieve the symptoms of patients with esophageal achalasia. These techniques have included excisional or bypassing procedures and denervation procedures. The latter were ineffective, and the uniform development of severe esophagitis after any procedure which destroys or bypasses the inferior esophageal sphincter has rightly led to their abandonment.

Current surgical therapy stems historically from the double cardiomyotomy first proposed by Heller in 1913. It has been modified by a number of surgeons in subsequent years. The simplest and most effective modification involves an incision through the muscle layers of the distal esophagus, through a thoracic approach. The mucosa is exposed to free completely the narrowed distal esophageal segment of its circular musculature, but the incision is

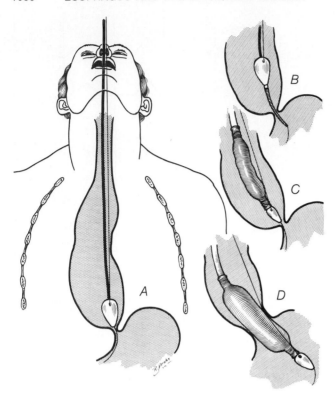

Figure. 25-11. Method of performing hydrostatic dilation. *A.* Passage of #41 F olive-tipped bougie into stomach; *B.* Passage of #50 to 60 F sound guided by flexible wire spiral; *C.* Passage of hydrostatic dilator into esophagogastric junction; *D.* Distension of dilator. (*From A. M. Olsen, S. W. Harrington, H. J. Moersch, and H. A. Andersen, The Treatment of Cardiospasm: Analysis of a Twelve-Year Experience, J Thorac Surg, 22:164–187, 1951.*)

extended onto the stomach only far enough to ensure completeness of this portion of the procedure (Fig. 25-12). Damage to the vagus nerves and the supporting structures about the hiatus is avoided. An operation carried out in the manner described should relieve the distal esophageal obstruction in almost every patient and should rarely lead to esophageal reflux. The addition of such ancillary procedures as gastric drainage operations and vagotomy should not be necessary. Ellis and Olsen reported that 94 percent of 268 patients treated in this fashion were benefited by the operation, and approximately 83 percent had excellent or good results (Table 25-1). More recent reviews of other series confirm our favorable experience with surgical treatment of achalasia.

Because of the superior results obtainable by a properly performed esophagomyotomy, surgery is replacing all other forms of treatment for achalasia. Forceful dilation should be used only for selected patients whose general condition precludes major surgery or for patients who decline to undergo operation. Thus, myotomy should now be offered to all but extremely high-risk patients.

The late results of a properly performed esophagomyotomy are so satisfactory that it is neither advisable nor necessary to consider the performance of ancillary esophageal procedures in all patients at the time of myotomy.

Indeed, Peyton et al. have reported that the performance of an antireflux procedure at operation on all achalasia patients in the absence of a preexistent sliding esophageal hiatal hernia constitutes an overreaction to the 3 percent incidence of incompetence after myotomy alone. Further, the failure rate of antireflux procedures exceeds the failure rate which they are designed to prevent. Fewer than 6 percent of patients have poor results requiring reoperation for any cause. Indeed, the majority of patients requiring reoperation for achalasia require treatment for persistent obstruction at the distal esophagus due to achalasia, not for stricture or esophagitis. In the majority of these patients the previous myotomy is found to have healed and the patients respond rather well to performance of a properly designed procedure with attention to the details outlined.

HYPOTENSIVE LOWER ESOPHAGEAL SPHINCTER

A unified concept of the etiology of gastroesophageal incompetence gained credibility with the objective manometric studies of Cohen and Harris. These investigators were able to differentiate clearly among patients with and without hiatal hernia those with symptoms of reflux and those without, on the basis of level of lower esophageal sphincter pressure. Subsequently, Olsen, Schlegel, and Payne described a group of patients without demonstrable anatomic esophageal hiatal hernia in whom symptomatic reflux was occurring. They were able to differentiate these

Table 25-1. COMPARISON OF TWO METHODS USED IN TREATING ACHALASIA AT THE MAYO CLINIC, 1949 THROUGH 1967

	Hydrostatic dilation (1950 through 1967)	*Esophagomyotomy (1949 through 1966)*
Number of patients	408*	268
Ages, yr	1–85	4–80 (46.5 mean)
Operative mortality, %	0.5†	0.3 (1 of 300)
Follow-up:		
Percent	77	96
Number	313‡	256
Range, yr	1–18	1–17.5
Average, yr	9.5	5.5
Result:		
Excellent, %, (no.)	28 (88)	47 (120)
Good, %, (no.)	65 { 37 (115) } 81 improved	83 { 36 (91) } 94 improved
Fair, %, (no.)	16 (50)	11 (29)
Poor, %, (no.)	19 (58)	6 (16)
Complications:		
Percent	4.6	3.3
Number	19§	11 (11 of 300)¶

*Eighty-two percent (334 patients) dilated once; 16 percent (66 patients) dilated twice; 2 percent (8 patients) dilated three or more times.

†Two patients died from unrelated illness 5 days and 2 weeks, respectively, after dilation.

‡Fifty patients (12 percent) whose initial treatment was dilation subsequently underwent esophagomyotomy because of persistent or recurrent major symptoms.

§Ten patients (2.4 percent) required operation for rupture of distal esophagus; all recovered.

¶Mainly infections; all recovered.

SOURCE: W. S. Payne and F. E. Donoghue, Surgical Treatment of Achalasia, *Mod Treat,* 7:1229–1240, 1970. By permission of Harper & Row, Publishers, Incorporated, New York.

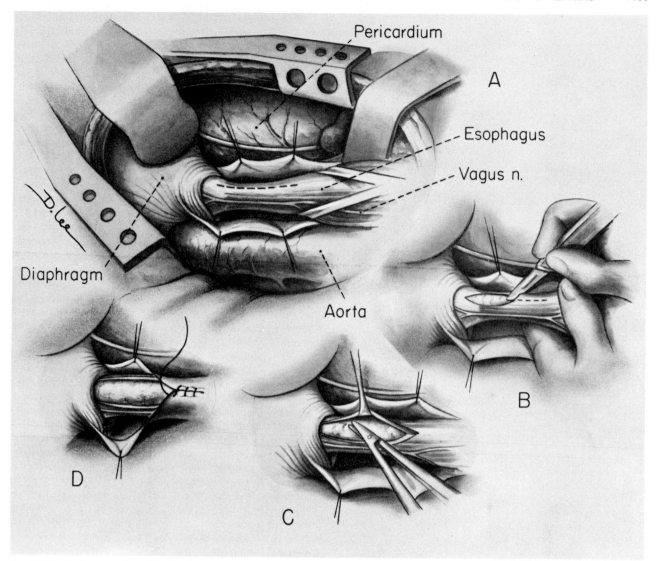

Fig. 25-12. Technique of modified Heller esophagomyotomy for achalasia of the esophagus. *A.* Transthoracic exposure of distal esophagus for esophagomyotomy. The esophagus has been mobilized and elevated from its bed by a Penrose drain. The intended incision is indicated by the dashed line. *B.* Beginning the incision. *C.* Dissection of mucosa from muscularis. *D.* Restoration of esophagogastric junction to intraabdominal position with suture narrowing of esophageal hiatus if necessary. (*From F. H. Ellis, Jr., J. C. Kiser, J. F. Schlegel, R. J. Earlam, J. L. McVey, and A. M. Olsen, Esophagomyotomy for Esophageal Achalasia: Experimental, Clinical, and Manometric Aspects, Ann Surg, 166:640–655, 1967.*)

patients from normal controls on the basis of the level of lower esophageal sphincter pressure. Thus, the concept of a hypotensive lower esophageal sphincter as an isolated clinical entity without hiatal hernia assumed respectability. Such studies have served to emphasize that the restoration of competence is dependent on restoration of sphincter pressure, not on correction of anatomic deformity—a concept that forms the basis of the modern treatment of reflux esophagitis and its complications. As enlightening as this

concept may be, the cause of sphincter failure remains obscure. The treatment of hypotensive lower esophageal sphincter with or without hiatal hernia is discussed further on in detail in the section Complications of Gastroesophageal Reflux.

Though the cause of hypotensive lower esophageal sphincter is unknown in most patients with or without hiatal hernia, it is widely appreciated that certain diseases, such as scleroderma, or certain operations which destroy or bypass the lower esophageal sphincter cause reflux esophagitis and its complications.

Among the postsurgical states that may interfere with the tone and responsiveness of the lower esophageal sphincter are truncal vagotomy, esophagogastrectomy with esophagogastrostomy, and esophagogastric myotomy. Esophagomyotomy may weaken the sphincter but not eliminate it, while esophagogastric myotomy usually totally destroys sphincter tone. Other, largely obsolete procedures that destroy sphincter function include Wendel cardioplasty

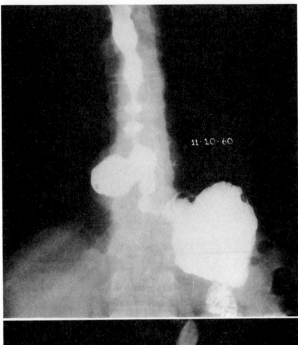

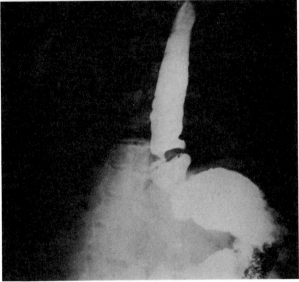

Fig. 25-13. Esophageal roentgenograms of two patients with hypermotility disturbances. Above: Diffuse spasm of esophagus with epiphrenic diverticulum and small hiatal hernia. Below: Hypertensive gastroesophageal sphincter with small hiatal hernia. (*From F. H. Ellis, Jr., and W. S. Payne, Motility Disturbances of the Esophagus and Its Inferior Sphincter: Recent Surgical Advances, Adv Surg, 1:179–246, 1965. Copyright 1965 by Year Book Medical Publishers, Inc. Used by permission.*)

and the Heyrovsky and Gröndahl procedures. Total gastrectomy is usually associated with loss of competence of the lower esophageal sphincter, and special reconstruction of esophagointestinal continuity is required to prevent alkaline biliary reflux. In our experience, reconstruction with a long-limb Roux en Y provides reliable control of this problem. In other situations, though prevention is to be stressed, treatment is usually feasible through performance of one of the antireflux operations.

DIAGNOSTIC STUDIES. Though reflux symptoms are usually clear-cut, further objectivity is achievable through clinical diagnostic testing. Pope has emphasized the value of certain specific objective histologic changes seen in epithelial biopsies in patients with reflux. Such findings are of special diagnostic value in the evaluation of patients with reflux symptoms in whom macroscopic esophagitis is endoscopically absent. Esophageal manometric studies not only define sphincter tone but also identify associated motility disturbances that may require additional management. Introduced by Lind and associates, the abdominal compression test is important in identifying an incompetent sphincter. The procedure consists of raising intragastric pressure by exerting pressure on the abdomen and observing its effect on both the sphincter pressure and the intraluminal esophageal pressure above the sphincter. The normal response is a 1:1 or greater rise of sphincteric pressure in comparison to gastric pressure with no transmission of pressure to the esophagus above the sphincter. In patients with incompetence, there is little or no rise in sphincter pressure with free transmission of intragastric pressure into the esophagus—the so-called common cavity effect. As noted previously, this response is eliminated by vagotomy and use of atropine.

Although many have used radiography, acid perfusion and acid clearing tests, and measurements of pH levels on withdrawal of an electrode from the stomach to the esophagus, it is generally agreed that a far more sensitive test of gastroesophageal reflux is the pH reflux test in which a pH electrode is placed 5 cm above the esophagogastric junction and 0.1 N hydrochloric acid is injected intragastrically. A positive response, indicating free reflux, is a quick drop in pH as recorded on the intraesophageal pH meter. Whereas none of these tests is entirely diagnostic, when taken together they are extremely useful; they provide objective evidence of the existence of reflux. Undoubtedly, they will be used more extensively in the future, not only in the preoperative evaluation of patients with a hypotensive inferior esophageal sphincter but also in the postoperative evaluation of the effectiveness of medical or surgical treatment or both.

Hypermotility

The causes of hypermotility disorders are also unknown, although they too may be related to abnormalities affecting the vagus supply to the organ. Diffuse spasm of the esophagus and hypertensive gastroesophageal sphincter are the conditions under discussion, and there is little evidence that they may be precursors of esophageal achalasia.

CLINICAL MANIFESTATIONS. Differentiation of these conditions from esophageal achalasia can usually be made on clinical grounds. Pain and dysphagia are the predominant symptoms, pain being more pronounced and dysphagia occurring intermittently or not at all. The pain may manifest itself only as a sensation of discomfort under the lower half of the sternum, or it may be severe and colicky, with extension through to the back or into the neck, shoulders, or arms, mimicking cardiac pain. It may be provoked by eating, or it may come on spontaneously, even awakening the patient at night. Patients so afflicted tend to be high-strung and nervous, and the diagnosis of psychoneurosis may be entertained. The symptoms are intermittent and are more likely to be troublesome than incapacitating; even during an attack, the patient seldom appears to be seriously ill.

Abnormalities of the esophageal roentgenogram occur in fewer than half the cases. When present, however, they may be quite striking, ranging from simple narrowing to segmental spasm and finally to extreme changes, including pseudodiverticulosis (Fig. 25-13). A small diaphragmatic hernia is frequently present, and an epiphrenic diverticulum commonly exists. A localized area of obstruction may be detectable in patients with hypertensive gastroesophageal sphincter.

PHYSIOLOGIC STUDIES. Because esophageal roentgenograms may appear normal in patients with these disorders, the diagnosis usually rests on the results of esophageal motility studies. In patients with diffuse spasm, there is a specific abnormal pattern of the deglutitive pressures. A primary peristaltic wave can be recognized over the upper half or two-thirds of the esophagus, but in the lower half or third it is replaced by simultaneous, repetitive, and occasionally prolonged increases in pressure (Fig. 25-14). Evidence of hiatal herniation is common. In most patients, however, there is no evidence of abnormality of the two sphincters unless there is a hypertensive gastroesophageal sphincter, in which case resting pressures in that region are excessive and relaxation may be poor.

TREATMENT. The use of an extended esophagomyotomy for the treatment of patients with "diffuse nodular myomatosis of the esophagus" was suggested in 1950 by Lortat-Jacob. Although physiologic studies were not made in his patients, many probably had forms of esophageal hypermotility disturbances. A similar approach was initiated independently at the Mayo Clinic in 1956 in order to control the severe symptoms of hypermotility disturbance of the esophagus in carefully selected patients.

In many respects, the technique of the operation resembles that used for achalasia of the esophagus. However, the proximal limit of the esophageal muscular incision varies, depending on the preoperative estimate of the extent of the disease as defined by esophageal motility studies. It may occasionally extend as high as the aortic arch (Fig. 25-15). Surgical repair of an associated diaphragmatic hernia is essential. Henderson and associates have stressed the need for an antireflux procedure at operation on all patients with diffuse spasm and extension of the myotomy from the stomach to 10 cm above the aortic end. Flye and Sealy have reported similar good results with long esophagomyotomy, reserving antireflux operations for patients with manifest hernia or incompetence. This treatment is less effective than it is for achalasia; only 78 percent of the patients so treated are benefited. Patients should therefore be selected carefully for this operation, the ideal candidate being an emotionally stable person with serious disability from the disease but without evidence of associated gastrointestinal problems. There should be demonstrable evidence of the severity of the disease in the form of a markedly abnormal esophageal motility pattern, ideally

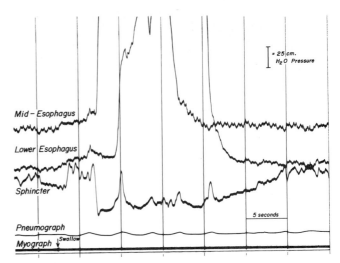

Fig. 25-14. Motility in esophagus and sphincter of patient with diffuse spasm. Note giant repetitive contractions. The sphincter relaxes normally. Peristalsis, although usually absent, is present in this case. (*From F. H. Ellis, Jr., C. F. Code, and A. M. Olsen, Long Esophagomyotomy for Diffuse Spasm of the Esophagus and Hypertensive Gastroesophageal Sphincter, Surgery, 48:155–169, 1960.*)

associated with roentgenographic evidence of esophageal spasm.

DIVERTICULA

Diverticula of the esophagus are among the more common lesions that cause esophageal dysfunction. They may have serious consequences if neglected, but current techniques of management offer a particularly rewarding opportunity for effective surgical treatment.

Typical diverticula of the esophagus are thought to be acquired lesions which result either from the protrusion of mucosa through a defect in the esophageal musculature (pulsion diverticula) or from the traction effect of adjacent inflamed parabronchial lymph nodes (traction diverticula). Such acquired lesions should be clearly differentiated from the rare congenital diverticulum of the esophagus and the occasional duplication, enterogenous cyst, or neoplasm which may have a fistulous communication with the esophageal lumen.

Pharyngoesophageal Diverticulum

The most common diverticulum of the esophagus arises at the pharyngoesophageal junction. Typically, it is located posteriorly in the midline, protruding between the oblique fibers of the inferior pharyngeal constrictor and the transverse fibers of the cricopharyngeus. Although first described in 1769 by the English surgeon Ludlow, Zenker's name has become intimately associated with the condition as the result of his studies on 27 collected cases in 1874.

INCIDENCE, PATHOPHYSIOLOGY, AND ANATOMY. Pharyngoesophageal diverticulum is definitely an acquired abnormality, since it is rarely encountered in patients less

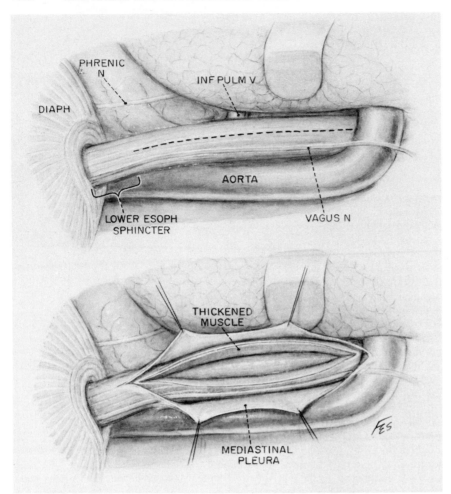

Fig. 25-15. Technique of long esophagomyotomy for diffuse spasm of esophagus. Note that incision extends to the aortic arch and spares the lower esophageal sphincter.

than thirty years old and usually occurs in those more than fifty. Esophageal motility studies have demonstrated premature contraction of the cricopharyngeus muscle in patients with pharyngoesophageal diverticulum. This occurs with sufficient frequency during swallowing that the partial obstructive effects of cricopharyngeal incoordination are implicated in the development of these diverticula. Because of the recurrent pressures involved and the effect of gravity and peristalsis, a globular dependent sac filled with ingested material gradually develops, insinuating itself posteriorly between the esophagus and the cervical vertebrae. In more advanced stages it may descend into the mediastinum.

Since the mouth of the diverticulum is located above the superior esophageal sphincter, there is no barrier to prevent spontaneous pharyngeal reflux and aspiration. Particularly in the sleeping or obtunded patient, this may result in recurrent episodes of airway contamination and aspiration pneumonitis.

CLINICAL MANIFESTATIONS. A sensation of high cervical obstruction to swallowing is the most common symptom. Such patients complain of a noisy, gurgling sound in their throats with drinking and the regurgitation of portions of recent meals into the mouth. Characteristically,

this food is undigested but may have an offensive odor due to decomposition. Frequently such regurgitation is associated with paroxysms of coughing, which may occur either immediately after meals or on reclining and may even awaken the patient from sleep.

The patient with a neglected pharyngoesophageal diverticulum may find eating to be a slow and laborious process, with dysphagia and interruptions by episodes of regurgitation and cough. In the extreme case, fatigue, malnutrition, hoarseness, and suppurative lung disease may further complicate the clinical course. Occasionally, patients with pharyngoesophageal diverticula are unaware of the abnormality until they experience some complication from it.

The diagnosis may be strongly suspected from the patient's history, but it can be firmly established only by roentgenographic examination of the esophagus with contrast medium (Fig. 25-16). Esophagoscopy usually is not necessary.

TREATMENT. In general, any diverticulum arising in the pharyngoesophageal region and producing symptoms warrants treatment. In a given patient, the minimal risks of intervention must be weighed against the severity of symptoms and the risk of present or potential complications arising from the diverticulum.

Currently, most patients with a pharyngoesophageal diverticulum seek medical assistance before severe complications have developed, and little or no preoperative preparation is required. Nonetheless, some effort should be made to ensure that the diverticulum is emptied of all secretions, food, and barium before anesthesia is induced.

If the patient is poorly nourished or dehydrated, appropriate measures should be employed to correct these abnormalities. In such patients it is often possible to give temporary preoperative palliation for dysphagia by performing esophageal dilation.

When aspiration pneumonitis or lung abscess has complicated a diverticulum, attempts should be made to resolve this before proceeding with operation. Occasionally, however, it is necessary to correct the esophageal problem before the pulmonary process will improve.

Although a wide variety of ingenious surgical procedures have been devised and many continue to be used in the treatment of this condition, one-stage diverticulectomy is the method most generally used at the present time. Cricopharyngeal myotomy also is an effective method of treatment. In our experience, dependable results with myotomy are confined to the smaller diverticula, which are less amenable to surgical excision. Therefore, we prefer diverticulectomy for the larger diverticula and myotomy for the smaller diverticula.

Technique of One-Stage Pharyngoesophageal Diverticulectomy. Either regional cervical block or general anesthesia can be used satisfactorily. Local anesthesia has also been particularly effective in elderly, debilitated patients who have complicating cardiovascular or respiratory disease. Because most diverticula tend to extend more to the left in the neck, in 80 percent of Mayo Clinic patients exploration has been from that side. Both the horizontal and the oblique lower cervical incision have been used (Fig. 25-17A). After the incision has been deepened, exposure of the retropharyngeal space and the diverticulum is obtained by retracting the sternocleidomastoid muscle and the carotid sheath and its contents laterally and the thyroid gland and larynx mediad (Fig. 25-17B). The apex of the diverticulum is grasped with an Allis forceps and elevated into the wound. The diverticulum must be thoroughly dissected, so that the neck of the mucosal sac and the surrounding ring of the muscular defect are clearly defined. A curved clamp is placed accurately across the neck of the mucosal sac at right angles to the long axis of the esophagus (Fig. 25-17B). The mucosal diverticular sac is amputated proximal to the clamp and flush with the neck of the sac. Amputation of the sac and suture closure of the esophagus are best accomplished in steps, by placing interrupted fine silk sutures in the mucosa as it is incised (Fig. 25-17B). When the diverticulum is completely excised and the mucosa satisfactorily closed, the muscular and fascial layers of the hypopharynx are closed over the repair in a transverse direction (Fig. 25-17C). A small Penrose rubber drain is placed near the site of repair in the pre-

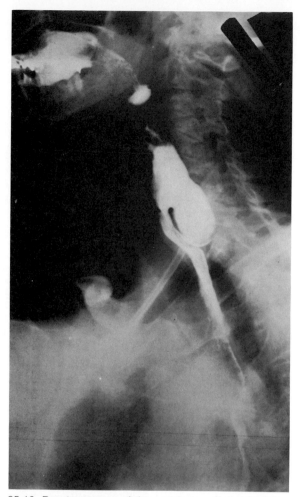

Fig. 25-16. Roentgenogram of the esophagus demonstrating a pharyngoesophageal diverticulum. Note that main lumen is angulated and compressed by this moderate-sized diverticulum. (*From W. S. Payne, and O. T. Clagett, Pharyngeal and Esophageal Diverticula, Curr Probl Surg, April 1965, pp. 1–31. Copyright 1965 by Year Book Medical Publishers, Inc. Used by permission.*)

vertebral space and brought to the outside through the lower end of the incision prior to closure (Fig. 25-17D).

Results of One-Stage Diverticulectomy. During the 28-year period ending December 31, 1971, 828 consecutive patients with pulsion diverticula of the hypopharynx were operated on at the Mayo Clinic by a one-stage procedure. In Clagett and Payne's 1960 review of 478 consecutive one-stage operations performed during the first 14 years of this experience, the surgical mortality was 0.8 percent. Esophagocutaneous fistulas developed postoperatively in 4 of the 478 patients. All fistulas closed spontaneously in 1 to 3 months. There were no instances of serious mediastinal infection. Unilateral paralysis of the vocal cords was noted postoperatively in 11 patients; in only 3 was this paralysis permanent. Symptoms or roentgenologic evidence of recurrence of the diverticulum developed in 6 of 250 patients restudied. All other patients were asymptomatic. In a recent 5- to 14-year follow-up of 164 patients, Welsh and Payne found that 93 percent had good or excel-

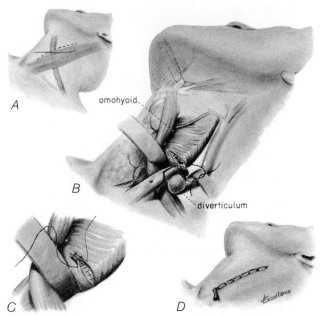

Fig. 25-17. Technique of one-stage pharyngoesophageal diverticulectomy. *A.* Surgical incisions employed when neck is explored from left. Note location of both oblique and horizontal incisions and their relationship to sternocleidomastoid and omohyoid muscles. *B.* Exposure obtained during removal of diverticulum. Note relationship of omohyoid to origin of diverticulum. Curved clamp has been placed across neck of sac, and sac has been amputated and esophageal mucosa closed in steps, with use of "cut-and-sew" technique. *C.* Layer closure of esophagus is completed with approximation of musculofascial tissues. *D.* Single soft-rubber drain is brought from prevertebral space and region of repair to outside through lower end of incision. Platysma and skin are closed in layers. (*From W. S. Payne, and O. T. Clagett, Pharyngeal and Esophageal Diverticula, Curr Probl Surg, April 1965, pp. 1–31. Copyright 1965 by Year Book Medical Publishers, Inc. Used by permission.*)

lent symptomatic results. The late recurrence rate was 3 percent.

Other Techniques. The two-stage diverticulectomy advocated by Lahey and Warren in 1954 is infrequently indicated today except in the late management of a neglected perforated diverticulum. In this procedure the sac is first freed and brought out through the wound. Two weeks later, after the fascial planes have sealed, the sac is removed much as in the one-stage procedure.

Extramucosal cricopharyngeal myotomy is a relatively new procedure in the management of pharyngoesophageal diverticulum. Cross and associates have suggested the use of such a myotomy as an adjunct to one-stage diverticulectomy to prevent recurrence. Belsey uses esophagomyotomy with diverticulopexy. Sutherland has reported the use of cricopharyngeal myotomy as the sole means of treating pharyngoesophageal diverticulum. The technique is certainly an effective means of dealing with smaller diverticula, not only because it reduces the tone of the partially obstructing sphincter, but also because it eliminates the distal support of the diverticular neck and obliterates the

septating spur. Dohlman and Mattsson have accomplished this same reentry effect by an endoscopic diathermic division of the spur formed by the diverticular esophageal wall. The total number of patients treated by cricopharyngeal myotomy, either alone or in conjunction with other techniques, has not been sufficient to permit valid statistical comparisons with diverticulectomy. Nonetheless, myotomy alone appears to be a satisfactory technique for the smaller diverticula. Whether its use in conjunction with diverticulectomy can effect further improvement remains unanswered.

Technique of Cricopharyngeal Myotomy. Surgical exposure is accomplished as described for diverticulectomy (Fig. 25-18).

After the diverticulum is freed to its neck, the transverse fibers of the cricopharyngeal muscle bordering the inferior margin of the neck of the diverticulum are easily identified and incised vertically. The incision is carried down to mucosa and is extended caudad onto the esophagus, the length of the incision averaging about 3 cm. After the myotomy, the esophageal and cricopharyngeal muscles are dissected for half the circumference of the mucosal tube to allow the mucosa to protrude freely through the incision. The cervical wound is then closed, with or without drainage.

Epiphrenic Diverticulum

Probably no other benign condition affecting the esophagus has been so poorly understood for so long as the epiphrenic diverticulum. Unfortunately, lack of basic knowledge concerning pathogenesis has all too often been equated with poor surgical results. Current surgical management permits a safe and often rational approach for most patients with this condition.

INCIDENCE, PATHOPHYSIOLOGY, AND ANATOMY. This diverticulum usually occurs among older persons. As its name implies, the epiphrenic diverticulum usually occurs in the lower thoracic esophagus—typically within 10 cm of the cardia—but may occur at higher levels in the thoracic esophagus. The pathologic anatomy is almost identical with that of pulsion diverticula in the pharyngoesophageal region in that the diverticulum is essentially a herniated sac of mucosa and submucosa protruding through the usual supporting sheath of esophageal musculature. The sac is covered by thin bands of attenuated muscle, which are often not discernible except on microscopic study.

The association of epiphrenic diverticula with motility disturbances and esophageal hiatal hernia was first appreciated by Vinson in 1934. Others since have noted the incidence of associated abnormal esophageal and diaphragmatic conditions to be as high as 75 percent. These and other data suggest that the majority of pulsion diverticula of the lower esophagus develop as the result of abnormal intraesophageal pressures. Allen and Clagett, in a review of 160 patients with epiphrenic diverticulum, found diffuse spasm of the esophagus in 39, esophageal achalasia in 16, esophageal hiatal hernia in 55, and esophagitis and a

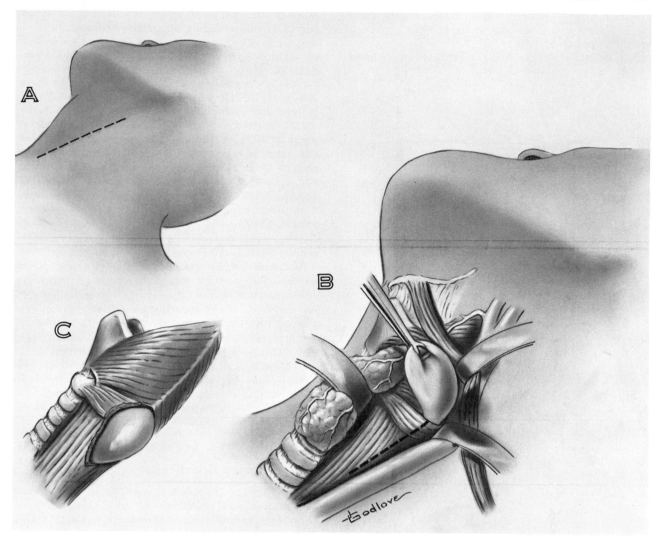

Fig. 25-18. Technique of cricopharyngeal myotomy. *A.* Site of skin incision. *B.* Exposure of diverticulum. Dashed line indicates proposed myotomy site. *C.* Completed operation. (*From F. H. Ellis, Jr., J. F. Schlegel, V. P. Lynch, and W. S. Payne, Cricopharyngeal Myotomy for Pharyngoesophageal Diverticulum, Ann Surg, 170:340–349, 1969.*)

variety of other associated conditions in 18. Only 66 of the 160 patients had no apparent abnormality associated with the epiphrenic diverticulum.

CLINICAL MANIFESTATIONS. Because of the high incidence of abnormal conditions of the esophagus associated with epiphrenic diverticula, it is difficult to be certain which, if any, of a given patient's symptoms are due to the diverticulum. Certainly, as with pharyngoesophageal diverticula, dysphagia and regurgitation are the most frequent complaints, but many patients have no symptoms referable to the esophagus. Habein and associates, in a study of 149 nonsurgical cases, estimated that only 15 to 20 percent of pulsion diverticula in this region produce definite symptoms. As with other diverticula, the regurgitated food is undigested and is recognizable as retention

from a recent meal. The relatively low incidence of tracheobronchial aspiration and suppurative pneumonitis is understandable in view of the distance and the sphincteric and peristaltic barriers between the diverticulum and the pharynx.

The symptoms of epiphrenic diverticulum are less definite than those of pharyngoesophageal diverticulum and may be only suggestive of the diagnosis. Roentgenographic examination of the esophagus with contrast medium is the best means of determining the presence and location of a pulsion diverticulum and the associated conditions (Fig. 25-13, top). Esophagoscopy is not required to establish a diagnosis but should be performed to seek out and define associated esophageal disease. Studies of esophageal motility are essential in current surgical management of epiphrenic diverticulum.

TREATMENT. The management of most epiphrenic diverticula is largely symptomatic. The presence of a defect causing few or no symptoms does not warrant surgical intervention if more serious associated conditions can be excluded. Generally, operation is indicated only when symptoms are progressive and severe or when associated conditions require it.

Surgical Treatment. The chief preoperative consideration

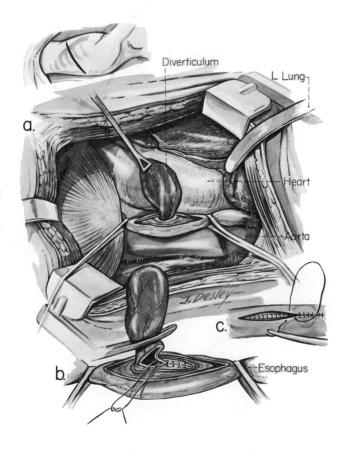

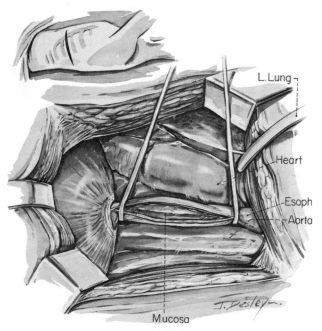

in the treatment of epiphrenic diverticulum is the prevention of aspiration during the induction of anesthesia. In addition to emptying the diverticulum, some consideration should be given to esophageal retention secondary to associated conditions. Occasionally, it is necessary to consider endoscopic evacuation. Often, preoperative esophageal bougienage will effect satisfactory emptying of the esophagus and diverticulum.

Left thoracotomy (Fig. 25-19) should be used almost routinely in the surgical treatment of epiphrenic diverticulum, since this incision provides the necessary exposure for excision of the diverticulum and, more important, is usually required to correct frequently associated esophageal and diaphragmatic conditions. Furthermore, the results of diverticulectomy are more satisfactory if a long, extramucosal esophagomyotomy is routinely performed in all such diverticulectomies along with correction of any other associated defects of the esophagus and diaphragm.

Results of Surgical Treatment. The significance of the present concept of the surgical treatment of pulsion diverticula of the lower esophageal region is clearly apparent on review of the Mayo Clinic experience from 1944 through 1963. Early in this experience, esophagomyotomy was not performed concomitantly with diverticulectomy and correction of associated diaphragmatic hernia. Of 29 patients so treated, 7 had significant postoperative complications (there were 4 recurrent epiphrenic diverticula in this group). Later, esophagomyotomy was performed routinely with diverticulectomy. Of the 11 patients so treated, only 1 had a postoperative complication and none died.

Parabronchial or Midesophageal Diverticulum

Granulomatous infections of mediastinal lymph nodes may cause traction diverticula. Although they occur typically in relation to subcarinal and parabronchial lymph nodes in the middle third of the esophagus, they can occur at any level. Generally these minute triangular esophageal deformities are of little or no clinical significance except as indications of a previous, often healed infection; they produce no esophageal symptoms and require no treat-

Fig. 25-19. Above: Surgical treatment of pulsion diverticulum of lower esophagus. Inset shows placement of left posterolateral thoracotomy incision. *A.* Exposure of diverticulum of esophagus obtained when chest is entered through bed of left eighth rib; note that tapes have been passed around esophagus and esophagus has been rotated to bring diverticulum into view. *B.* Removal of diverticulum and closure of mucosa; note that mucosal sutures are tied with knots within esophageal lumen. *C.* Closure of esophageal musculature over mucosal suture line. Below: Complete long esophagomyotomy, which should be performed concomitantly with diverticulectomy and through the same posterolateral thoracotomy incision. Site of diverticular excision has been rotated back to right and is not visible. A long myotomy incision, extending from cardia to aortic arch, is apparent, with underlying mucosa bulging through incision. If a diaphragmatic hernia is present, it too should be repaired through same incision. (*From W. S. Payne, and O. T. Clagett, Pharyngeal and Esophageal Diverticula, Curr Probl Surg, April 1965, pp. 1–31. Copyright 1965 by Year Book Medical Publishers, Inc. Used by permission.*)

ment. When symptoms are present, they are usually caused by some other, unrelated process.

In the presence of symptoms, the usual studies should be carried out to determine the cause and rule out more serious disease. These include roentgenographic examination, endoscopy, and occasionally motility studies. When active infection is suspected, appropriate skin tests and microbiologic studies are indicated.

Interest in traction diverticula is thus focused chiefly on differentiating them from more serious conditions. Such a diverticulum may, however, be the site of serious, although rare, complications. These include obstruction to swallowing, esophagitis, hemorrhage, perforation with empyema, pericarditis, and tracheobronchial-esophageal fistula. Usually the symptomatic traction diverticulum can be managed by simple excision. Fistulas between the esophagus and lower respiratory tract respond to excision and closure of the communication and interposition of normal tissues to prevent recurrence. Perforation with empyema or pericarditis often requires specific antibiotic

treatment as well as surgical drainage and temporary defunctionalization of the esophagus.

ESOPHAGEAL HIATAL HERNIA

Esophageal hiatal hernias are not only the most common hernias of the diaphragm but also are among the more common abnormalities affecting the upper gastrointestinal tract.

There are basically two main types of esophageal hiatal hernias: the sliding hernia and the paraesophageal hernia. A third type, the short esophagus hiatal hernia, is a complication of gastroesophageal reflux usually associated with a sliding hernia and will be discussed subsequently (Fig. 25-20).

Sliding Hernia

The most common is the sliding hernia, in which there is displacement of the esophagogastric junction and portions of the proximal part of the stomach through the esophageal hiatus into the posterior mediastinum. Although such herniations are known to move in and out of the thorax with changes in intrathoracic and intraabdominal pres-

Fig. 25-20. Two chief varieties of esophageal hiatal hernia. *Left:* Sliding esophageal hiatal hernia. *Right:* Paraesophageal hiatal hernia. (*From J. E. Mobley and N. A. Christensen, Esophageal Hiatal Hernia: Prevalence, Diagnosis and Treatment in an American City of 30,000, Gastroenterology, 30:1, 1956. By permission of Williams & Wilkins Company.*)

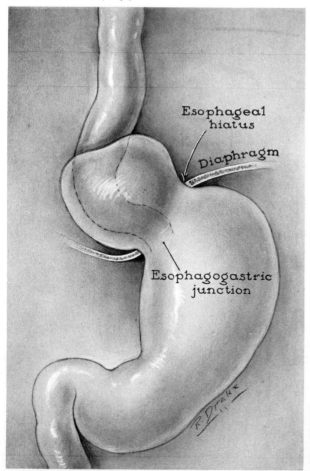
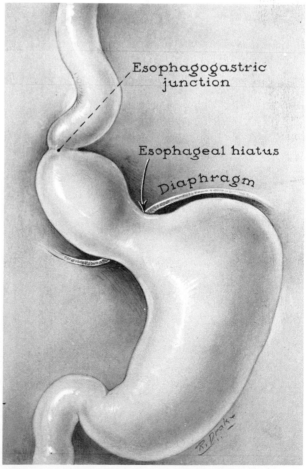

sures, the term *sliding* is applied not because of this behavior but because the hernia has a partial peritoneal sac, the stomach forming the other wall of the hernial sac. In the paraesophageal hiatal hernia, a portion or all of the stomach is displaced into the thorax through the esophageal hiatus alongside the esophagus. The esophagogastric junction is in its normal position while the fundus and successively greater portions of the remainder of the stomach ascend into the thorax.

Gastroesophageal reflux may or may not occur in patients with a sliding esophageal hiatal hernia. In view of the prevalence of the condition (5 per 1,000 population in one series), only a minority ever have significant symptoms of reflux. The presence or absence of reflux in hiatal hernia is directly related to the level of pressure at the inferior sphincter. In fact, Cohen and Harris have suggested that the abnormal anatomy is less important than the abnormal physiology consequent to a hypotensive inferior esophageal sphincter. Reflux is accentuated by certain postural or physiologic changes that are associated with increased intraabdominal or intragastric pressure: stooping, lifting, overeating, or straining.

Fig. 25-21. Belsey Mark IV transthoracic repair of sliding esophageal hiatal hernia. Exposure is gained through a left thoracotomy incision. After complete mobilization of the cardia, the lower 4 cm of esophagus is cleared of connective tissue. *A.* Mattress sutures are placed between gastric fundus and muscular layers of esophagus 1 to 2 cm above and below the esophagogastric junction. *B.* After these mattress sutures are tied, a second row of mattress sutures is placed to imbricate additional fundus onto the lower esophagus. Note that these sutures pass through the hiatus and out through the tendinous portion of the diaphragm. Before these sutures are tied, crural sutures are placed to narrow the esophageal hiatus. *C.* Completed repair after reduction of hernia and tying of sutures to maintain reconstruction. Previously placed crural sutures have been tied behind the esophagus to narrow the hiatus (not shown).

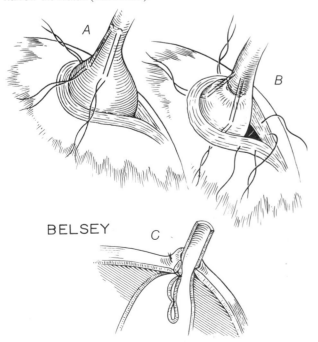

BELSEY

Gastroesophageal reflux in itself would not be deleterious if it were not for the presence of acidic gastric fluid, which in man is secreted continuously. The esophagus appears to be particularly susceptible to the corrosive effects of acidic secretions, as well as to the more alkaline biliary, pancreatic, and intestinal secretions. Fortunately, patients with sliding esophageal hiatal hernias rarely exhibit gastric hypersecretion.

CLINICAL MANIFESTATIONS. Symptoms and complications of gastroesophageal reflux are the major consequences of sliding esophageal hiatal hernia. The majority of these hernias, however, are asymptomatic.

The symptoms of uncomplicated gastroesophageal incompetence are heartburn and regurgitation. The retrosternal or epigastric burning distress is noted particularly after meals; typically, it is accentuated when the patient lies down, stoops, or strains. It is characteristically relieved by sitting and standing or by ingestion of water or antacids. Regurgitation of secretions into the mouth occurs with postural changes and is often described as a hot, bitter, or sour liquid coming into the throat or mouth. Food is regurgitated infrequently, but when it is, it is recent and partially digested and is mixed with gastrointestinal secretions. Dysphagia may occur even in the absence of demonstrable complications such as esophagitis, stricture, or spasm. Other symptoms may be present and may be difficult to differentiate from those due to associated conditions such as coronary artery disease, cholelithiasis, colonic diverticulosis, and duodenal ulcer.

The diagnosis of sliding esophageal hiatal hernia, with or without symptoms, depends almost entirely on demonstrating by roentgenographic examination the protrusion of gastric mucosa through the esophageal hiatus. Although a variety of diagnostic maneuvers have been suggested to aid the roentgenologist, in some patients a sliding hernia, with or without gastroesophageal reflux, may not be apparent unless specifically sought.

Esophagoscopy is indicated in symptomatic patients, particularly those considered for surgical treatment, both to assess esophageal complications and to exclude other, more serious disease. Occasionally studies of esophageal motility are advisable to assist in the diagnosis of sliding hernia, or pH studies may be required for objective evaluation of reflux.

TREATMENT. The treatment of sliding esophageal hiatal hernia with no complications is largely symptomatic. When symptoms are absent or only mild and transient, no therapy is indicated, since the condition is rarely progressive. In other cases the treatment is designed to eliminate gastroesophageal reflux and to minimize its deleterious effects. Such measures as weight reduction, ulcer diet, administration of antacids, elimination of constricting garments, avoidance of stooping, lifting, or straining, and elevation of the head of the bed for sleeping are instituted with these goals in mind. If these medical measures are unavailing or if there are complications, surgical measures may be required for relief of symptoms.

Surgical Treatment. The primary goal of the surgical treatment of sliding esophageal hernia is restoration of gastroesophageal competence. Because restoration of normal anatomy has been found to be an inadequate operation for restoration of normal pressures to the hypotensive sphincter, "antireflux" operations have been devised to accomplish this end more effectively. The operations associated with the names Belsey, Nissen, and Hill are typical of these procedures. All are variations of a basic "wrap-around" procedure, and their success in preventing reflux makes it unnecessary to perform concomitant vagotomy and pyloroplasty unless there is an active duodenal ulcer. The routine use of these additional procedures is discouraged because of their disagreeable side effects.

Belsey's operation (Fig. 25-21) is a transthoracic procedure that creates a segment of intraabdominal esophagus held in place by a buttress of plicated stomach which surrounds approximately 280° of the distal esophagus. Long-term results indicate that the procedure is successful in relieving symptoms in 85 percent of patients and that the recurrence rate varies between 10 and 15 percent, depending on the length of follow-up.

Nissen's fundoplication can be performed either transabdominally or transthoracically (Fig. 25-22). This operation, which totally surrounds the distal esophagus with the adjacent gastric fundus, also produces good clinical results and a low recurrence rate. A worldwide survey of the results of the Nissen operation indicated an overall success rate of 96 percent, failures being usually the result of either recurrent hernia or postoperative reflux. Some dissatisfaction with this procedure has been expressed by Woodward and associates, who found an unacceptably high rate of dysphagia and the so-called gas-bloat syndrome, complications that should be minimal or absent if the procedure is performed in the presence of an indwelling nasogastric tube of ample caliber to prevent excessive narrowing of the distal esophagus. Long-term follow-up, furthermore, showed a regression in the severity of these symptoms when they did occur.

Hill's operation (Fig. 25-23) is basically a posterior gastropexy performed transabdominally, but incorporating plicating sutures to narrow the esophagogastric junction. He reported the cases of 149 patients treated by this technique in an 8-year period, with no deaths and no anatomic recurrences during the follow-up period; 97 percent of the patients were improved.

In addition to these gratifying clinical and roentgenologic results, physiologic studies of postoperative sphincteric function are encouraging. Not only is the amplitude of the lower esophageal sphincteric pressure more than doubled, but also the high-pressure zone is lengthened and the normal neural and hormonal response at the sphincter is restored. Now both experimental and clinical evidence suggest that the 360° wrap afforded by the Nissen fundoplication is the most effective of the three antireflux procedures in restoring lower esophageal sphincter pressure and preventing reflux.

Paraesophageal Hernia

A paraesophageal hiatal hernia is a rare life-threatening entity. Unlike the symptoms of a sliding hernia, which are primarily the result of deranged physiology, the symptoms

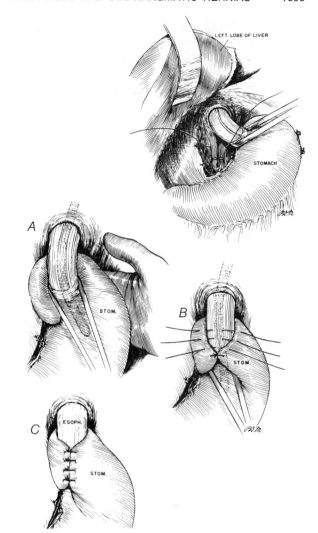

Fig. 25-22. Technique of transabdominal Nissen fundoplication. Above: Abdominal exposure and mobilization of the distal esophagus and upper stomach in preparation for carrying out a fundoplication. *A.* Mobilized fundus is displaced behind the esophagus by the surgeon's right hand. *B.* Placement of sutures so as to encircle the distal esophagus with a generous portion of fundus. Note indwelling #40 F gastric tube. *C.* Completed procedure. (*From F. H. Ellis, Jr., Gastroesophageal Reflux: Indications for Fundoplication, Surg Clin North Am, 51:575–588, 1971.*)

of a paraesophageal hernia result from anatomic defect. Although it may occur in combination with sliding esophageal hernia, in its pure form it is not associated with gastroesophageal reflux. The major complications of paraesophageal hiatal hernia are obstruction and hemorrhage. With these hernias there may be hemorrhage from erosions of the mucosa of the herniated part of the stomach. When a large portion of the stomach or all of it is displaced into the thorax, obstructive symptoms may occur as the result of angulation and compression. Occasionally other viscera, including spleen, colon, and small bowel, may be involved as well as the stomach. Incarceration, hemorrhage, volvulus, and strangulation are major complications of massive

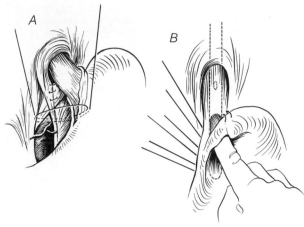

Fig. 25-23. Hill's transabdominal repair of sliding esophageal hiatal hernia. *A*. Reduced esophagogastric junction with crural sutures narrowing the hiatus in place behind esophagus. A single suture is shown incorporating gastrohepatic omentum along lesser curvature of stomach and preaortic fascia. Care is taken in placing sutures to avoid injury to adjacent vagal nerve trunks. Two or three additional sutures are similarly placed on lesser curvature, anchoring stomach posteriorly (posterior gastropexy). *B*. When these sutures are tied, gastric sling fibers should be sufficiently shortened to permit distal phalanx of index finger to invaginate snugly into terminal esophageal lumen alongside Levin tube. Angle of His is further accentuated by placement of sutures between gastric fundus and terminal esophagus. [*From W. S. Payne, and F. H. Ellis, Jr., Diaphragmatic Hernia, in F. H. Ellis, Jr., (ed.), "Lewis-Walters' Practice of Surgery," vol. 5, "Thoracic Surgery," Harper & Row, Publishers, Inc., New York, 1971, chap. 15, pp. 1–59.*]

paraesophageal hernias. Because of the high incidence of serious complications associated with paraesophageal hernia, surgical repair is generally indicated even in the absence of symptoms or complications. The method of repair differs from that described for sliding esophageal hernia. Since the lower esophageal sphincter functions normally, the esophagogastric junctional area is not disturbed. Rather, the herniated fundus is reduced through an abdominal incision, the hernial sac is excised, and the widened hiatus is narrowed by sutures placed in the limbs of the crus anterior to the esophagus as in the technique described by Hill and Tobias (Fig. 25-24). The results of repair of paraesophageal hernias are almost always satisfactory.

COMPLICATIONS OF GASTROESOPHAGEAL REFLUX

Esophagitis

Esophagitis represents a manifestation of the unusual sensitivity of the esophageal mucosa to a variety of agents, particularly strong acids and alkalies, which may be endogenous or exogenous. The most common cause of esophagitis is reflux of acidic gastric juice into the esophagus, a condition resulting from hypotension of the lower

esophageal sphincter (see above). Mucosal inflammation and ulceration occur, and if tissue destruction is severe, a stricture may form during the healing phase. Pathologic study of involved tissues has stressed the superficial nature of the inflammation in most cases, the muscularis propria rarely being involved. Localized marginal esophageal ulceration is common in the presence of a hiatal hernia, whereas extended areas of linear esophagitis are more common in patients with a history of vomiting or duodenal ulcer or both, in surgical patients, and in patients requiring a nasogastric tube.

CLINICAL MANIFESTATIONS. Dysphagia, odynophagia, regurgitation, substernal or epigastric pain, and heartburn are the common symptoms of esophagitis. Dysphagia is more prominent in the later stages of the disease when fibrosis and stricture have occurred. Occasionally, hematemesis or melena may be prominent, although massive gastrointestinal bleeding is rare. Roentgenography is of little value in diagnosing esophagitis but is helpful in excluding a malignant lesion. Since some patients with symptoms of heartburn and regurgitation have normal esophageal mucosa while others have severe esophagitis and even early stricture formation in the absence of typical symptoms, esophagoscopy is required in order to establish a definitive diagnosis.

TREATMENT. Treatment of reflux esophagitis is designed to eliminate gastroesophageal reflux or to minimize its

Fig. 25-24. Technique of surgical repair of paraesophageal hiatal hernia. *A*. Left lobe of liver mobilized and hernia exposed. *B*. Stomach reduced and apex of widened hiatus pulled anteriorly. Sac has been excised. *C*. Hiatus closed anterior to normally placed esophagus with interrupted sutures in crura. [*From F. H. Ellis, Jr., Paraesophageal Hiatus Hernia, in L. M. Nyhus (ed.), "Hernia," 2d ed., J. B. Lippincott Company, Philadelphia, 1977.*]

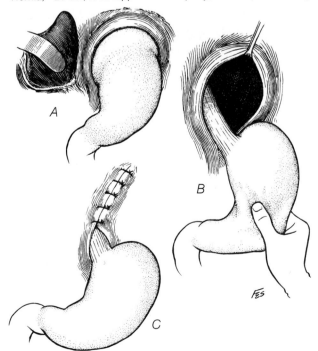

deleterious effects. In the absence of significant complications, a trial of medical treatment is often justified. Weight reduction, ulcer diet, use of antacids, elimination of constricting garments, and elevation of the head of the bed for sleeping all help to minimize reflux and to neutralize gastric acids. If medical measures fail or if there are complications, surgical measures may be required for relief of symptoms. The various operations that will prevent reflux and allow healing of esophagitis have been described previously.

Short Esophagus

If reflux esophagitis is not promptly and effectively managed in its early stages, complications such as fibrosis and scarring with esophageal shortening and, ultimately, stricture may develop.

Congenital shortening of the esophagus rarely if ever occurs, almost all examples of a shortened esophagus being the result of long-standing untreated gastroesophageal reflux, usually in the presence of a sliding esophageal hiatal hernia. Almost always the fibrosis leading to esophageal shortening also results in an esophageal stricture, usually localized to the esophagogastric junction (Fig. 25-25). Medical therapy, unfortunately, is usually ineffective at this stage of the disease, although it should be tried initially. Bougienage sometimes is successful in dilating the stricture and providing an adequate esophageal lumen. If, as often happens, medical treatment is unsuccessful, surgical treatment must be considered, but a complex procedure is frequently required, simple reduction of the hernia alone rarely being successful if there is prominent shortening of the esophagus.

A variety of ingenious operative procedures has been suggested over the years for the management of this severe complication of gastroesophageal reflux, yet agreement is lacking among surgeons as to the best. Though commonly undertaken in the recent past, resection of the stricture is now rarely used. Rather, an esophageal lengthening procedure, the Collis gastroplasty, coupled with an antireflux operation such as the Belsey (Fig. 25-26) or Nissen fundoplication, is preferred. Intraoperative and postoperative dilation of the stricture is performed as indicated until healing occurs. With acid reflux prevented, healing occurs within an adequate time in most cases. In those rare cases in which the stricture is too firm to permit dilation, one of the three procedures illustrated in Fig. 25-27 may be selected.

Lower Esophagus Lined by Columnar Epithelium (Barrett Esophagus)

In 1950, Barrett described a condition in which the lower end of the esophagus is lined by a continuous sheet of gastric epithelium; he postulated that this was of congenital origin. The designation *lower esophagus lined by columnar epithelium* was adopted after Allison and Johnstone demonstrated that the epithelial lining was similar to the columnar epithelium present at the junctional zone and did

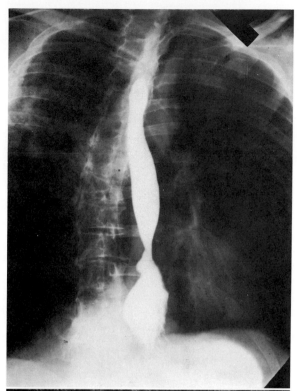

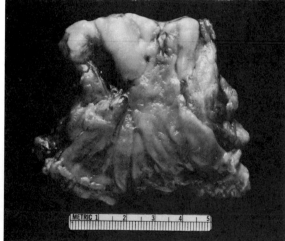

Fig. 25-25. Short-esophagus hiatal hernia with stricture. Above: Esophageal roentgenogram. Below: Resected specimen showing ulceration and stricture.

not contain acid-producing cells. It is now generally agreed that the lesion is acquired rather than congenital in origin, the mucosal changes representing, in patients with esophageal hiatal hernia, a mucosal adaptation to the injurious effects of acidic gastric juice by which the squamous epithelium lining the distal portion of the esophagus is destroyed and replaced with columnar epithelium. It is as yet uncertain whether these epithelial changes are the result of metaplasia or of cephalad growth of functional epithelium from the distal esophagus. This abnormal esophageal lin-

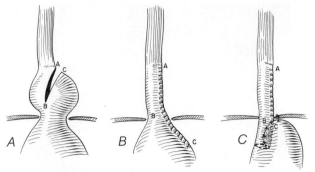

Fig. 25-26. Collis gastroplasty with Belsey hiatal hernia repair for irreversible short esophagus as suggested by Pearson et al. Procedure is effected through a left thoracotomy. *A.* After appropriate mobilization of esophagus and stomach, an incision (A, B, C) in herniated proximal stomach is made parallel with lesser curvature. *B.* Closure of the incision (A, B, C). *C.* Sufficient esophageal length and fundus are acquired to perform a Belsey Mark IV hiatal hernia repair (A, B, C). (*From W. S. Payne and A. M. Olsen, "The Esophagus," Lea & Febiger, Philadelphia. In press.*)

ing may extend to the level of the aortic arch, and ulcer formation may occasionally be demonstrated therein (Barrett's ulcer). A stricture at the columnar-squamous junction is common (Fig. 25-28). The risk of a carcinoma's developing in this abnormal epithelium is high, so that even after treatment the condition of such patients should be closely and carefully followed.

Controversy regarding the nature of this defect is not without therapeutic implications, because if it is an acquired condition secondary to a hiatal hernia, surgical reduction of the hernia should prevent reflux and relieve the symptoms without necessitating removal of the abnormal distal esophagus or of the stricture, which can be successfully dilated once reflux has been eliminated.

CORROSIVE ESOPHAGITIS

The ingestion of strong acid or alkali causes a severe inflammatory reaction of the affected mucosa, known as *corrosive esophagitis.* Lye, a strong cleaning agent containing sodium hydroxide and sodium carbonate, is most commonly responsible for such injuries, although a variety of other fluids, including mineral acids, strong bases, phenol, and organic solvents, can produce similar changes. The nature and concentration of the agent ingested determine the degree and extent of the injury, which may involve limited areas of the esophagus, the entire esophagus, or even the stomach.

PATHOLOGY. The pathologic changes after ingestion of lye have been shown experimentally to consist of edema and congestion of the submucosal layer associated with inflammation and thrombosis of its vessels. Sloughing of the superficial layers occurs, with varying degrees of necrosis of the muscularis, followed by fibrosis and delayed reepithelization. In severe cases the entire mucous membrane of the upper portion of the alimentary tract may slough, with subsequent development of an esophageal stricture.

CLINICAL MANIFESTATIONS. During the acute phase of the reaction, burns of the lips, tongue, mouth, and pharynx are apparent. Pain in the involved region is a common symptom, and there may be associated vomiting. Painful dysphagia is prominent during the acute phase, which lasts from several days to several weeks. As the chronic phase develops, dysphagia may become the predominant symptom as a stricture forms.

Fig. 25-27. Operative procedures for management of short-esophagus diaphragmatic hernia with stricture. Left: Esophagogastrectomy with Roux-en-Y esophagojejunostomy. Center: Esophagogastrectomy with colon interposition and pyloroplasty. Right: Gastric tube of Gavriliu.

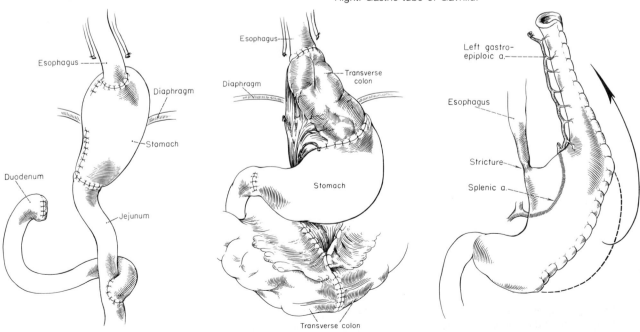

TREATMENT. During the initial period of the injury, appropriate neutralizing agents (such as dilute acidic or alkaline solutions) should be administered to minimize the local effect of the ingested material. Antibiotics are administered to counteract bacterial invasion, and administration of cortisone during the acute phase of the burn has been advocated in order to reduce the incidence and severity of the subsequent stricture formation. Early esophagoscopy is important to determine the extent of the injury and should be repeated every 10 days to 2 weeks to allow proper planning and evaluation of treatment. This can be done safely over a previously swallowed thread, which should be kept in place until the need for dilation has been determined.

Stricture formation is rare if prompt treatment as outlined is initiated. However, should esophagoscopy reveal evidence of stricture formation, dilation of the strictured zone by bougienage over the swallowed thread may be begun within a few weeks of the accident. In some patients, repeated dilation at intervals may be required for prolonged periods, sometimes a year or more. When patients are seen in the chronic phase of the disease and a string has not been ingested previously, it may be necessary to perform gastrostomy for feeding purposes and also for retrograde dilation of the esophageal stricture.

In a small percentage of cases it may become apparent that repeated dilation cannot maintain a satisfactory esophageal lumen. In such cases extensive reconstructive operative procedures are required to establish a satisfactory, functioning esophageal substitute. Many procedures have been devised, including use of skin-lined tubes and segments of intestine or stomach, as reported by Yudin; the Russian surgeons have had extensive experience with these. Total bypass of the strictured esophagus by a segment of right or left colon interposed substernally between the pharynx and stomach is currently preferred. For lesser degrees of stricture, the site of the disease may be approached transthoracically and either resected or bypassed with a segment of jejunum or colon.

ESOPHAGEAL PERFORATION

Irrespective of cause, esophageal perforation or rupture may initiate a virulent periesophageal infection. Prompt recognition and proper treatment may avert death or obviate a prolonged and difficult convalescence. In spite of all efforts, esophageal perforation continues to be associated with high mortality and morbidity.

INCIDENCE. Most esophageal perforations today occur after some form of esophageal instrumentation. The number of such perforations appears to have increased over the past 30 years as a result of the greater use of esophagoscopy, gastroscopy, esophageal dilation, tamponade, and even simple esophageal intubation for diagnosis or treatment.

Of equal interest are those less frequently encountered instances of noninstrumental perforation, which occur as the result of accidental ingestion of foreign bodies or as a consequence of the strain of emesis with or without

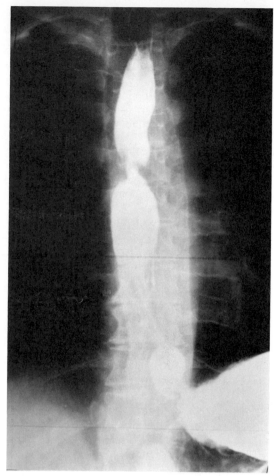

Fig. 25-28. Roentgenogram of esophagus in a patient with Barrett esophagus. Note presence of small diaphragmatic hernia (sliding type) and midesophageal stricture. The tubular structure between stricture and hernia is columnar epithelium-lined esophagus with typical esophageal motility. (*From J. N. Burgess, W. S. Payne, H. A. Andersen, L. H. Weiland, and H. C. Carlson, Barrett Esophagus: The Columnar-Epithelial-Lined Lower Esophagus, Mayo Clin Proc, 46:728–734, 1971.*)

predisposing esophageal disease. A variety of other conditions also have been implicated in the noninstrumental perforation of the esophagus, including "stress" associated with neurologic disease or following operations or burns remote from the esophagus. Infrequently, the esophagus may be perforated as the result of either penetrating or nonpenetrating external trauma.

ETIOLOGY. The wall of the esophagus can be breached in a number of ways by either an instrument or a foreign body: (1) simple penetration of the entire wall of the esophagus, (2) simple splitting or rupture of the esophagus by strain exceeding its circumferential tensile strength, (3) breaking down of the wall of the esophagus by a localized inflammatory process resulting from mucosal tears, (4) perforation through pressure necrosis.

Instrumental and foreign body perforations can occur at any level of the esophagus; however, the sites of normal narrowing are the ones most frequently involved. The narrowest of these is the esophageal introitus and, indeed, accounts for the high incidence of perforations seen in this region. The impingement of the rigid scope on the bodies of hyperextended cervical vertebrae may result in a crushing effect on the mucosa, particularly in the presence of hypertrophic bony spurs.

The second most common site for instrumental and foreign body perforations has been the lower esophagus immediately above the point where the esophagus narrows to pass through the diaphragmatic hiatus. The incidence of perforation at this level is further contributed to by the increased occurrence of disease and the frequent need for endoscopic manipulations in this region. Perforations of the middle third and abdominal part of the esophagus occur infrequently.

The mechanism of postemetic perforation of the lower esophagus has evoked considerable interest. Mackler has shown that the inflation of fresh human cadaver esophagus resulted in simple splitting when the pressure exceeded its circumferential tensile strength. In 95 percent of the 65 specimens studied, such tears occurred in the distal portion of esophagus. Duval, as cited by Kinsella and coworkers,

Fig. 25-29. Lateral roentgenogram of cervical part of spinal column 2 hours after instrumental perforation of the cervical part of the esophagus. Note anterior displacement of trachea by an anterior bulging of the retrovisceral space, emphysema in tissue planes, and hypertrophic bony spurs on lower cervical vertebrae. (*From F. H. Ellis, Jr., and W. S. Payne, Complications of Esophageal and Diaphragmatic Surgery, in C. P. Artz, and J. D. Hardy, "Complications in Surgery and Their Management," 2d ed., W. B. Saunders Company, Philadelphia, 1967.*)

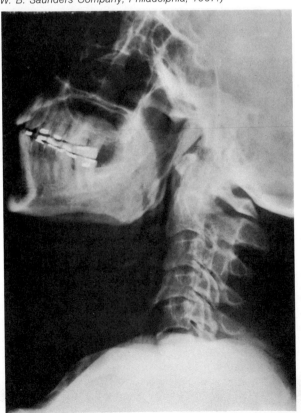

demonstrated that the rapidity of the increase in pressure rather than the amount of pressure per se may be a critical factor in such injuries. The fact that most postemetic perforations occur in adults rather than in children may be explainable by the higher incidence of predisposing factors in adults and especially by the fact that the strength of the esophagus is thirteen times greater in infants (less than one year old) and four times greater in children (less than twelve years old) than it is in adults.

PATHOPHYSIOLOGY. The consequences of esophageal perforation are due to contamination of periesophageal spaces with corrosive digestive fluids, food, and bacteria, which leads to a diffuse cellulitis with localized or extensive suppuration.

Anatomic considerations are important, both in the evolution of signs and symptoms and in treatment. The majority of cervical esophageal perforations are posterior and result in suppuration first in the retrovesical space and then extending along fascial planes into the mediastinum.

Perforations of the anterior wall of the cervical esophagus and those involving the lateral pharyngeal spaces and pyriform fossae enter the pretracheal space. The pretracheal space communicates with the mediastinum via the fascial attachment to the pericardium. The manifestations of perforation depend on the relation of the esophagus to the contiguous spaces. The upper two-thirds of the thoracic esophagus is in close proximity to the right pleural cavity. In its lower third, the esophagus lies adjacent to the left pleural space. In rare cases, the intraabdominal or subphrenic esophagus may be perforated, leading to peritonitis and intraabdominal abscess.

Although the perforation need not be extensive or impressive to produce marked local or systemic reaction, the consequent sequestration of body fluids in the adjacent spaces may add hypovolemia to bacteremic shock. In addition, the accumulation of fluid and leakage of free air from the perforated hollow viscus may significantly interfere with normal cardiorespiratory dynamics.

CLINICAL MANIFESTATIONS. The diagnosis of esophageal perforation depends on an awareness of the circumstances in which it may occur, the patient's symptoms, the presence of physical signs, and the demonstration of the perforation and its secondary manifestations by roentgenography.

Although the symptoms of perforation depend to a large degree on its site and the extent of inflammatory reaction, pain, fever, and dysphagia are the most frequent early complaints. Dyspnea is usually related to pleural space involvement, with or without pneumothorax. Cervical tenderness is an early and constant feature of cervical esophageal perforation. Cervical crepitation may be minimal but is an almost constant finding.

The physical findings with thoracic esophageal perforation are usually limited to the thorax; cervical crepitation may be a feature, but there is usually no cervical tenderness. Auscultation over the heart may elicit signs of mediastinal emphysema (Hamman's sign). Cardiorespiratory embarrassment with shock and cyanosis is more commonly seen early with thoracic and subphrenic esophageal perforations but may not be apparent until a late stage.

Roentgenographic studies are of great assistance in diagnosis. Anterior, posterior, and lateral views of the cervical part of the spinal column often demonstrate pathognomonic signs of cervical perforation (Fig. 25-29). Anterior displacement of the trachea, widening of the retrovisceral space, air in tissue spaces, and occasionally widening of the superior mediastinum are seen. Widening of the superior mediastinum is a common sign in perforation of the cervical or upper thoracic part of the esophagus. Mediastinal emphysema and pleural effusion with or without pneumothorax may be present with thoracic or subphrenic esophageal injuries. Studies with opaque medium are occasionally indicated to localize the site or sites of perforation and to detect associated abnormalities (Fig. 25-30). The medium should be nonirritating and, preferably, absorbable. Endoscopic procedures are rarely indicated in the diagnosis of esophageal perforations except when a foreign body is present.

TREATMENT. While there is wide agreement that most perforations of the esophagus are best treated by immediate surgical exploration, repair if necessary, and drainage, this is neither universally accepted nor always feasible. Parenteral antibiotic therapy plus parenteral fluid and electrolyte correction and support are appropriate measures for all patients with esophageal injury.

Simple surgical exploration and drainage of the retrovisceral space or, on rare occasions, of the pretracheal space is the treatment of choice for cervical esophageal perforations (Fig. 25-31). Suppuration extending as low as the fourth vertebra can be evacuated effectively by this route. The usually encountered early perforation may be small, and the inflammatory reaction may be slight; however, major lacerations occasionally are present and require suture closure, with drainage of considerable retrovisceral and mediastinal collections.

Instrumental and noninstrumental perforations of the thoracic and subphrenic parts of the esophagus are often large and require surgical exploration, repair, and drainage. The upper two-thirds of the esophagus is best approached transpleurally through a right midthoracotomy and the lower third through a lower left thoracotomy. The rare subphrenic lacerations are best explored transabdominally. Gastric decompression, either by nasogastric tube or, rarely, by gastrostomy, is indicated. On occasion, resection of the perforated region and associated esophageal lesion is required.

Late localized cervical and mediastinal abscesses are uncommon complications after adequate early surgical treatment of perforations. When present, they can be drained either by cervical mediastinotomy (Fig. 25-31) or,

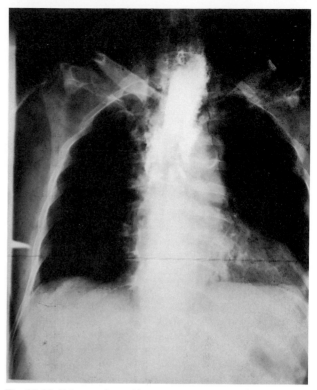

Fig. 25-30. Extravasation of ingested contrast medium into neck and superior mediastinum, pathognomonic of cervical esophageal perforation. Note failure of distal part of esophagus to fill. (*From F. H. Ellis, Jr., and W. S. Payne, Complications of Esophageal and Diaphragmatic Surgery, in C. P. Artz, and J. D. Hardy, "Complications in Surgery and Their Management," 2d ed., W. B. Saunders Company, Philadelphia, 1967.*)

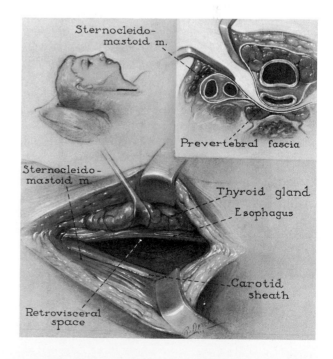

Fig. 25-31. Technique of cervical mediastinotomy. Upper left: Placement of skin incision in lower part of neck. Upper right: Incision is carried deep and mediad, with retraction of sternomastoid muscle and carotid artery laterally and trachea and thyroid mediad. Below: Note accessibility of pretracheal space. Collections as low as fourth thoracic vertebra are adequately drained through such an incision. (*From W. D. Seybold, M. A. Johnson, III, and W. V. Leary, Perforation of the Esophagus: An Analysis of 50 Cases and an Account of Experimental Studies, Surg Clin North Am, August, 1950, pp. 1155–1183.*)

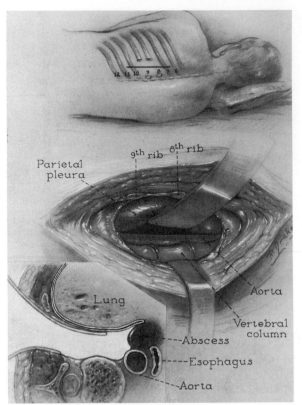

Fig. 25-32. Posteroinferior mediastinotomy. This may be required for extrapleural drainage of a mediastinal abscess. (*From W. D. Seybold, M. A. Johnson, III, and W. V. Leary, Perforation of the Esophagus: An Analysis of 50 Cases and an Account of Experimental Studies, Surg Clin North Am, August, 1950, pp. 1155–1183.*)

if in the lower mediastinum, by posteroinferior mediastinotomy (Fig. 25-32). As a rule, the late development of empyema can be prevented by early and adequate closed intercostal-tube drainage of the pleural space. When empyema occurs, it usually responds to appropriate open or closed drainage; if it does not, thoracotomy may be required for pulmonary decortication.

Esophagopleural or esophagopleural-cutaneous fistulas may occur as a complication of any esophageal perforation. If the esophagus is not obstructed distad and good drainage is provided, such fistulas invariably close with time, provided that no local infection, foreign body invasion, malignant change, or epithelization of the tract is involved. When there is an esophageal fistula, it is best to seek out and treat any factors which may contribute to chronicity. Generally, it is wise to carry out repeated esophageal dilation over a previously swallowed thread during the healing stage of such chronic fistulas, even if no obstruction is demonstrated. With healing, cicatricial narrowing may occur after any perforation.

Tuttle and Barrett stressed the nutritional aspects in cases of esophageal fistula and noted the difficulties attending long-term intravenous maintenance of patients after esophageal perforation. They stressed not only the

desirability but also the feasibility of resuming early oral feeding, even in the presence of a fistula. In a series of late perforations treated by them, the excellent survival rate was attributed to a policy of early intensive effort to confine draining mediastinal abscesses and esophageal fistulas to a small, localized, basal empyema pocket. With this accomplished, a full diet was given by mouth. If the fistula is not too large, most of the food passes to nourish the patient, and adequate drainage provides egress for the remainder.

RESULTS. The results of the surgical treatment of esophageal perforation depend not only on the cause, site, and severity of the reaction but also, to a large extent, on the lapse of time between perforation and treatment and on the type of treatment.

The results of treatment of cervical esophageal perforations, regardless of cause, have been excellent with early cervical exploration and drainage. Even with major injuries with marked contamination and delayed treatment, the results of surgical management have been satisfactory. Although the incidence of complications, secondary procedures, prolonged hospitalization, and late sequelae has been greater in this latter group, the mortality has been negligible.

The results of treatment for perforations involving the thoracic and subphrenic esophagus have been less satisfactory. Delay in diagnosis and treatment beyond 18 hours appears to be a major factor contributing to morbidity and mortality. Recent reports of series of thoracic esophageal perforations mention mortalities in excess of 60 percent with the usual surgical methods in late perforation and between 10 and 30 percent with early treatment.

Not all surgeons agree with the operative management outlined. There are instances of cervical and of thoracic esophageal perforation (usually instrumental) in which it may be possible to use successfully a nonoperative management (parenteral fluids and antibiotics and intercostal tube drainage), because of a late and benign course, or the patient may refuse treatment by other means. Neuhof and Jemerin reported in 1943 that surgical drainage alone resulted in 60 percent survival, whereas conservative nonsurgical management resulted in 16 percent survival. A decade later, Seybold and coworkers and Weisel and Raine reported greatly reduced mortality with early suture closure and drainage of esophageal perforation.

The high mortality associated with late diagnosis and treatment of intrathoracic esophageal perforations has led to the development of a variety of alternative methods of management (Fig. 25-33) which are applicable under a variety of circumstances.

In addition to the multiple procedures illustrated (Fig. 25-33), there is a number of effective technical variants. Thus, in lieu of the gastric patch technique shown, diaphragmatic (Rao et al.), pericardial (Millard), intercostal (Dooling and Zick), and parietal pleural (Grillo and Wilkins) pedicles have been used with success to buttress or augment surgical repair of esophageal perforation. Variations on the esophageal exclusion described by Johnson et al. include the partial exclusion and diversion techniques

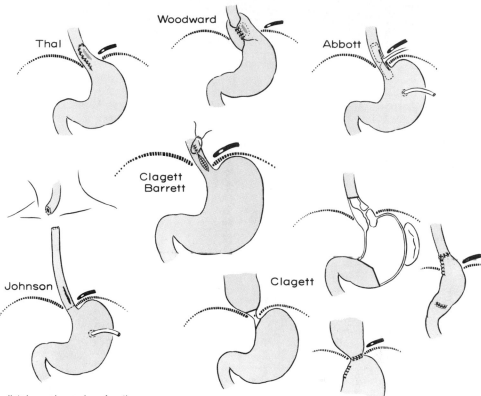

Fig. 25-33. Methods of managing distal esophageal perforations. *Clagett-Barrett:* In absence of delay or severe inflammation, it is usually possible to carry out a primary transthoracic layer closure of a distal esophageal tear with appropriate gastric and pleural space drainage. *Clagett:* In presence of associated cancer or other obstructive esophageal disease, some type of appropriate resection of lesions with esophagogastrostomy may be indicated, as shown by this procedure. *Thal:* Use of gastric fundus as patch for esophageal perforations. *Woodward:* Fundus completely wrapped around esophagus after insertion of fundal patch. *Johnson:* Complete defunctionalization of esophagus for late perforations by creation of proximal cervical esophagostomy, with closure of esophagus above and below. Colon interposition is employed after recovery to reestablish esophagogastric continuity. *Abbott:* Insertion of a Silastic T tube through an esophageal perforation with tube leading from esophagus to outside. With appropriate tube drainage of pleural space, T tube is removed after a few weeks, and resultant fistula closes spontaneously. Gastric decompression is an essential feature in all these repairs, and tube gastrostomy often is preferred. The proper placement of a double-lumen gastrostomy tube with one limb advanced through the pylorus to the jejunum while the other remains in the stomach may permit simultaneous tube feeding and gastric decompression during healing. (*From W. S. Payne and R. H. Larson, Acute Mediastinitis, Surg Clin North Am, 49:999–1009, 1969.*)

reported by Urschel et al. and by Menguy. It is, of course, impossible to prescribe a technique applicable to all thoracic esophageal perforations or even those of a given variety. It is essential, however, to have a clear and concise understanding of the clinical problems and the rational application of multiple available techniques in planning the care of individual patients.

MALIGNANT TUMORS

Both benign and malignant tumors occur in the esophagus, but the vast majority are carcinomas which arise from the epithelial lining of the esophagus and cardia. While these are not the most commonly encountered visceral cancers, they are certainly among the most discouraging from the standpoint of control.

INCIDENCE AND ETIOLOGY. Carcinoma of the esophagus is predominantly a disease of males (male-to-female ratio, 3:1) between the ages of fifty and seventy years. The incidence varies widely throughout the world, being notably high in China, Japan, Scotland, Russia, and the Scandinavian countries. In South Africa incidence is high especially among the native Bantu. Although the basic cause of the disease is unknown, dietary and alcoholic habits, as well as tobacco use, have been implicated. A particularly high incidence has been reported in patients with achalasia and corrosive esophagitis. Joske and Benedict noted an unusually high incidence of cancer of the cervical esophagus in patients with Plummer-Vinson (Paterson-Kelly) syndrome. Other conditions associated with a high incidence of esophageal carcinoma include lye burns, diverticula of the esophagus, the columnar epithelial-lined lower esophagus of Barrett, and the syndrome known as tylosis palmaris et plantaris.

PATHOLOGY. Although almost all malignant tumors arising in the body of the esophagus are squamous cell carcinomas, most of those involving the esophagogastric

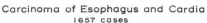

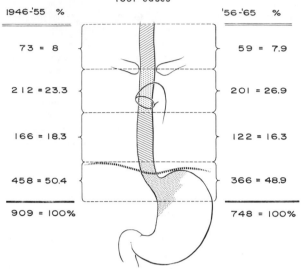

Fig. 25-34. Distribution of 1,657 patients with carcinoma of the esophagus and cardia according to anatomic location. (*From G. H. Gunnlaugsson, A. R. Wychulis, C. Roland, and F. H. Ellis, Jr., Analysis of the Records of 1,657 Patients with Analysis of Carcinoma of the Esophagus and Cardia of the Stomach, Surg Gynecol Obstet, 130:997–1005, 1970. By permission of Surgery, Gynecology & Obstetrics.*)

junction are adenocarcinomas of gastric origin. Figure 25-34 shows the anatomic locations of 1,657 malignant lesions of the esophagus and cardia encountered at the Mayo Clinic from January 1946 through December 1965. It should be noted that almost as many tumors affected the cardia as affected the entire cervical and thoracic segments of the esophagus combined.

The remainder of the malignant tumors of the esophagus are rare sarcomas, mostly leiomyosarcomas. These are predominantly extramucosal, but in contrast to the benign leiomyomas, they tend to ulcerate and calcify. Carcinosarcoma is another uncommon malignant lesion of the esophagus; it is of interest because it appears to be associated with a better prognosis than other malignant neoplasms. Although melanoblasts have never been demonstrated in the human esophagus, there have been reports of primary malignant melanomas of the esophagus.

Some carcinomas develop as bulky, fungating, obstructive growths and others as superficially ulcerated, surface-spreading tumors producing little obstruction. These tumors spread via lymphatic vessels, by direct extension from the esophagus, and by vascular invasion. Tumors of the cervical esophagus disseminate through the lymphatic vessels to cervical nodes, particularly the anterior jugular and supraclavicular nodes. Those arising in the thoracic esophagus spread early to local mediastinal (peritracheal and esophageal) glands as well as supraclavicular and, occasionally, subdiaphragmatic nodes. Those occurring at the cardia may involve local mediastinal as well as subdiaphragmatic nodes. Metastasis through the bloodstream may produce liver, lung, or bone implants. Raven reported

that no lymph node metastases were present in 42 percent of cases in which autopsy was performed, but many of these cases showed extensive local infiltration of vital structures or distant spread which would have precluded complete removal.

CLINICAL MANIFESTATIONS. The earliest and almost constant feature of carcinoma of the esophagus is progressive dysphagia. Initially, it is noted with ingestion of solid foods, but ultimately, the swallowing of even liquids and saliva becomes difficult. Weight loss and weakness are the inevitable consequences of inanition. Aspiration pneumonitis is not infrequent as obstructive symptoms progress. The diagnosis of carcinoma of the esophagus can be made with a high degree of accuracy by the usual roentgenographic examination of the esophagus. This usually demonstrates an irregular, ragged mucosal pattern with annular luminal narrowing. Unlike the more chronic benign obstructive lesions, carcinoma usually is not associated with marked proximal dilatation of the esophagus.

Esophagoscopy should be performed in all patients suspected of having esophageal cancer, irrespective of the interpretation of the roentgenogram, both to establish a tissue diagnosis and to determine accurately the upper limit of the lesion. In lesions involving the upper esophagus, it is usually desirable to perform bronchoscopy to detect malignant involvement of the adjacent tracheobronchial tree. Cytologic study of smears made from suggestive lesions is a valuable diagnostic adjunct. Occasionally, study of esophageal motility may suggest malignant involvement, but this technique is of greater assistance in defining one of the more common motility disturbances as a cause for dysphagia. Occasionally surgical exploration is required to establish the presence or absence of malignant growth when results of diagnostic studies are not definitive.

A report from the Honan Province of China indicates that the application of special screening techniques to a high-risk population permits detection of carcinoma of the esophagus before symptoms develop and at a stage when nearly all cases are resectable, with more than a 70 percent chance of 5-year survival.

TREATMENT. There are only two methods of treatment which offer benefit to patients with carcinoma of the esophagus: surgical resection and irradiation. Neither of these methods is new; hence it is not surprising that there has been no recent notable improvement in survival statistics among patients with this condition.

Squamous cell carcinoma of the esophagus is a radiosensitive and theoretically radiocurable tumor. Unfortunately, although the primary lesion can be controlled, failures result from the presence of tumor outside the irradiated field, and few permanent cures are obtainable. Surgical resection, too, suffers from being a local form of therapy with a high incidence of failure from distant recurrences. Surgical ablation is more effective than radiotherapy in dealing with adenocarcinomas that occur around the distal esophagus and cardia. It is apparent that some form of systemic therapy is desperately needed to deal more effectively with the problem of esophageal malignancy. Combining surgical treatment and radiotherapy has been suggested as a possible means of improving the results of treatment. The main rationale for the use of radiotherapy before operation in a combined program is the local control of microscopic disease, particularly at the margins of the primary tumor and involved nodes. The suggestion also has been made that preoperative radiotherapy might convert a locally unresectable lesion to a resectable one. Unfortunately, existing data comparing different treatment modalities in esophageal carcinoma are far from conclusive. Many studies have been reported, but all of them compare different types of patients or different periods of time. None has been prospective or randomized to eliminate the effects of selection of patients. Thus Pearson's results with radiotherapy alone are far superior to any others yet reported with this method. Yet his report represents selected cases, since about half the patients who entered the study were unable to complete the planned treatment and were excluded from the final results. Furthermore, little emphasis has been placed on the complications of excessive radiotherapy, which, as shown in the series of some investigators, include radiation pneumonitis, myocardial injury, spinal cord injury, tracheoesophageal fistula, hemorrhage, and postradiation strictures.

Palliation in terms of relief of dysphagia is the goal of therapy for most patients; for the few with well-localized lesions there is the possibility of cure. Surgical resection is more effective than radiotherapy in relieving dysphagia (95 percent versus 20 percent) and in increasing mean survival time after treatment (11 months with surgery versus 5 months with radiotherapy).

Proponents of combined therapy cite the improved results in a recent decade compared to that of a previous era when combination therapy was not employed. Interpretation is rendered even more confusing by the fact that in at least one reported series only 25 percent of patients completed the combined protocol.

In a recent decade at the Mayo Clinic, 5-year survival with surgery alone improved 100 percent over that of an earlier period of similar duration simply as the result of increasing operability, higher resectability rates, and lowered hospital mortality.

It is our conclusion that cure is not generally obtainable for the majority of patients with cancer of the esophagus and cardia by currently available means, but that resection provides the most expedient and effective means of restoring function while retaining the possibility of cure. Radiotherapy should be reserved for lesions of the cervical portion of the esophagus that would require laryngectomy for removal. But here, too, the exact site and extent of invasion of the adjacent larynx, trachea, or hypopharynx may dictate palliation by combined or exclusively surgical means. Close collaboration between radiotherapist and esophageal and laryngeal surgeons is desirable. Certain lesions of the thoracic part of the esophagus that appear nonresectable may become resectable with radiotherapy.

In the interest of time, specifically the duration of the patient's disability, staged operations and time-consuming treatments should be minimized or avoided. Selection factors will continue to be used to define those patients who will derive the greatest benefit-to-risk ratio from treatment.

Indications and Preparation for Surgical Treatment. In general, the selection of patients for operation for carcinoma of the esophagus entails careful clinical evaluation to exclude those whose tumor has extended beyond the scope of total surgical excision. Patients with obvious distant metastasis or those showing obvious involvement of vital structures, such as heart, liver, trachea, or aorta, are not generally considered suitable candidates. Survival after incomplete excision under such circumstances usually is not long enough to justify the risk, discomfort, and expense of resective procedures, and other forms of palliation should be considered.

Because of the difficulty in accurately assessing the possibility of total excision of esophageal lesions prior to operation, alternative palliative procedures are not infrequently carried out after the extent of the lesion has been more accurately defined at the time of surgical exploration.

Before undergoing operation for the control of esophageal malignant growths, patients must be in satisfactory condition to tolerate the proposed procedure. Prolonged preoperative preparation usually is not justified, but efforts should be made to restore blood volume, fluid, and electrolyte balance. Swallowing may be temporarily improved by dilation over a thread as a guide. Oral alimentation is doubtless superior to intravenous, but preoperative feeding by gastrostomy or jejunostomy is rarely if ever indicated. It is reasonable to employ parenteral hyperalimentation in the severely nutritionally depleted patient before operation and to continue such nutritional support in the postoperative period until full oral intake is well established. However, operation should not be delayed in some vain hope of restoring body weight in a short time by this or any other means. At best it is aimed at minimizing further negative nitrogen balance in the early postoperative period. Associated pulmonary problems are frequent, particularly emphysema and bronchitis. Occasionally patients with obstructive carcinoma of the esophagus experience aspiration and subsequent suppurative pneumonitis, which should be resolved before definitive surgery.

Technique. The surgical procedure used in the treatment of carcinoma of the esophagus varies with the anatomic location of the tumor.

For carcinomas arising at or near the esophagogastric junction, esophagogastrectomy is usually used. At the Mayo Clinic, a technique similar to that described by Kirklin and Clagett is commonly used. The exposure obtained through a left thoracoabdominal incision (Fig. 25-35) usually permits wide resection of the distal esophagus and proximal part of the stomach, along with spleen, omentum, and regional nodes. When local extension demands it, portions of the pancreas, diaphragm, transverse mesocolon, and colon can be included in the en bloc resection. The point of gastric transection is selected to permit removal of most of the acid-producing portion of the stomach. In creating a tubular gastric remnant of antrum for anastomosis to the esophagus, most of the lesser curvature, along with its lymph node-bearing tissue, is

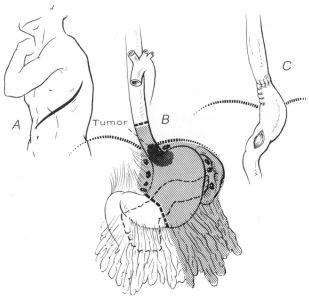

Fig. 25-35. Esophagogastrectomy for lesions of distal esophagus and esophagogastric junction. *A.* Incision. *B.* Shading indicates tissue to be resected. *C.* Completed operation. Note gastric drainage procedure. (*From F. H. Ellis, Jr., Surgical Aspects of Malignant Lesions of the Esophagogastric Junction, in W. H. ReMine, J. T. Priestley, and J. Berkson, "Cancer of the Stomach," W. B. Saunders Company, Philadelphia, 1964, pp. 127–140.*)

excised. Esophagogastrectomy, as described, results in bilateral vagotomy. Gastric retention due to postvagotomy pylorospasm and gastric hypomotility may be minimized by pyloromyotomy or pyloroplasty. The avoidance of gastric retention is particularly desirable in patients in whom

Fig. 25-36. Esophagogastrectomy for lesions of lower and middle thirds of thoracic esophagus. *A.* Incision. Either thoracoabdominal incision or separate thoracic and abdominal incisions may be used. *B.* Shading indicates portion of esophagus to be resected. *C.* Completed operation with high intrathoracic anastomosis. Note gastric drainage procedure. (*From F. H. Ellis, Jr., Treatment of Carcinoma of the Esophagus and Cardia, Proc Staff Meetings Mayo Clin, 35:653–663, 1960.*)

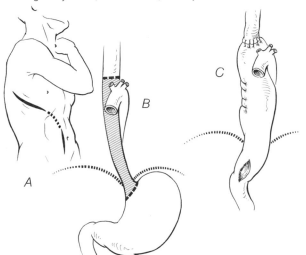

the gastroesophageal sphincter mechanism is resected, because esophageal reflux occurs readily with its destruction. Bombeck and associates have suggested retention of sufficient stomach so that an end-to-side anastomosis between the esophagus and stomach can be effected and a valve-competent plication of stomach about the anastomosis can be developed. Some cardial cancers are found to involve the proximal portion of the stomach extensively, and these are best managed by total gastrectomy. Esophagointestinal continuity under these circumstances must be aimed at preventing reflux of erosive biliary and pancreatic secretions into the esophagus. Payne has found that a long-limb Roux en Y provides the best means of reconstruction to prevent this complication after total gastrectomy.

Although the majority of lesions in the lower half of the esophagus can be managed through a left thoracoabdominal incision, a right thoracotomy is preferred for excision of those lesions arising in the thoracic esophagus at sites above the cardia.

Reconstruction of esophagogastric continuity after resection for thoracic esophageal cancer again depends on the anatomic site of the lesion. For those resections involving the esophagus above the cardia but below the level of the azygos vein, the stomach may be brought into the thorax for anastomosis high in the thorax (Fig. 25-36). For resections for tumors at or above the level of the azygos vein, the colon may be interposed (Figs. 25-37 and 25-38). As with other procedures involving vagal resection, pyloromyotomy or pyloroplasty is a desirable adjunctive procedure.

Colon interposition can be accomplished with either the right or left half of the colon prepared on a pedicle of middle colic vessels. Since there appears to be no disadvantage to using an antiperistaltic segment of large bowel, the left colon is preferred because the length, lumen, and blood supply are more adequate and dependable. Belsey described the use of an isoperistaltic segment of left colon with an inferior mesenteric vascular pedicle.

The use of interposed colon has the advantage of a proximal cervical anastomosis, which, if anastomotic leakage should occur, is less dangerous. Such interposed large bowel may be passed from the abdomen to the neck, either subcutaneously through a presternal tunnel or retrosternally. Occasionally, the interposed colon can be placed in the posterior mediastinal bed of the resected esophagus. In recent years the stomach has gained increasing favor over the colon as the organ to be used to replace resected esophagus or to bypass an unresectable thoracic lesion. Griffen and associates favor a substernal reversed gastric tube of the Gavriliu type. Ong, Akiyama, Le Quesne, and their associates as well as others have favored bringing the gastric fundus to the neck for anastomosis either to the cervical esophagus or, after laryngectomy, to the pharynx. Sufficient length is available to bring the stomach either through the posterior mediastinal esophageal bed or substernally. Advantage over the colon is obvious since only one anastomosis is required.

Alternatives to the use of either colon or stomach after laryngopharyngocervical esophagectomy are locally developed pedicle skin grafts used to restore continuity between the pharynx and the thoracic esophagus. Wooky devised a unilateral, cervically based pedicle graft to create a skin-lined tube to bridge this defect. In more recent years, the medially based deltopectoral skin flap devised by Bakamjian has proved simpler and more reliable (Fig. 25-39).

Results. The results of surgical treatment of carcinoma of the esophagus depend largely on the anatomic site, extent, and type of the tumor. It is apparent from a 1970 review of patients treated at the Mayo Clinic (Table 25-2) that there was a significant increase in resection rates during the period when surgical techniques were being developed and standardized. The 3- and 5-year survival rates after resections for carcinoma at various sites in the esophagus and cardia during that period are shown in Table 25-3. The influence of cell type and of the lymph node metastasis on 5-year survival is clearly apparent on review of follow-up data on patients treated for cancer of the cardia (Table 25-4).

The reader is referred to the earlier section on treatment for a discussion of the results of other methods of definitive treatment.

Palliation. All too often, patients with cancer of the esophagus present with lesions which are not amenable to curative excision. Although malnutrition is related to inanition, patients with cancer of the esophagus cannot be made to live longer by establishing a means of feeding them. Furthermore, it appears that the greatest problem associated with high-grade obstructions of the esophagus is not inanition per se but the inability to cope with the normal salivary secretions, which tend to accumulate in the mouth and to be aspirated if the patient attempts to swallow them. Accordingly, gastrostomy or jejunostomy for feeding are rarely used in the management of these patients. Instead, methods which permit swallowing are preferred. Irradiation or simple bougienage or both may alleviate the esophageal obstruction temporarily in cases of frankly inoperable cancer. For patients found at opera-

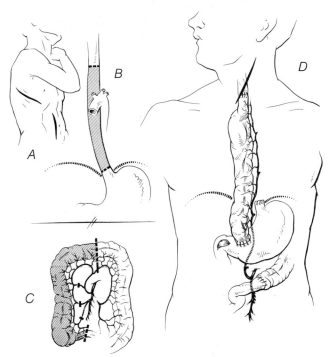

Fig. 25-37. Esophagectomy with interposition of right colon. Procedure may be carried out in one or two stages. *A.* Incision. *B.* Shading indicates portion to be resected. *C.* Mobilization of right colon. *D.* Completed operation. (*From F. H. Ellis, Jr., Treatment of Carcinoma of the Esophagus and Cardia, Proc Staff Meetings Mayo Clin, 35:653–663, 1960.*)

Fig. 25-38. Esophagectomy with interposition of left colon. *A.* Incision. *B.* Shading indicates portion of esophagus to be resected. *C.* Mobilized portion of colon. *D.* Completed operation.

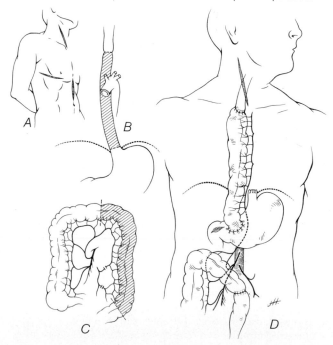

Table 25-2. OPERABILITY AND RESECTABILITY IN 1,657 PATIENTS WITH CARCINOMA OF ESOPHAGUS AND CARDIA

| | Patients | | | |
| | 1946–1955 | | 1956–1965 | |
Operation	No.	Percent	No.	Percent
Resection	245	27	334	45
Exploration	169	19	165	22
None	495	54	249	33
Total	909	100	748	100
Hospital mortality after resection	39	16	39	12

SOURCE: Modified from G. H. Gunnlaugsson, A. R. Wychulis, C. Roland, and F. H. Ellis, Jr., Analysis of the Records of 1,657 Patients with Analysis of Carcinoma of the Esophagus and Cardia of the Stomach, *Surg Gynecol Obstet*, **130:**997–1005, 1970. By permission.

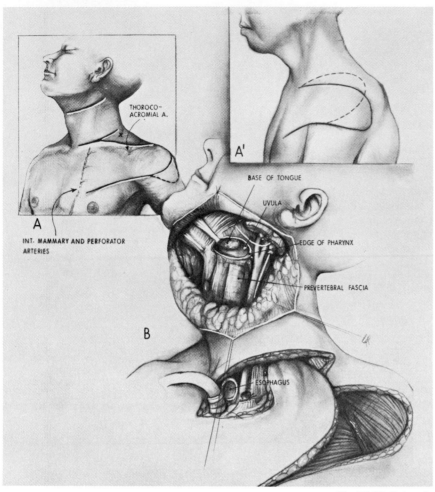

Fig. 25-39. Bakamjian reconstruction of the pharynx and cervical esophagus after laryngectomy and radical neck dissection for pharyngoesophageal malignancy. A medially based deltopectoral skin flap is elevated, rotated, and folded into a tubular conduit between pharynx and esophagus, to which it is anastomosed. At a subsequent stage (not shown) the base of the pedicle is divided and the cervical fistula is closed. (*From J. M. Loré, Jr., "An Atlas of Head and Neck Surgery," vol 1, 2d ed., W. B. Saunders Company, Philadelphia, 1973.*)

tion to have nonexcisable lesions, a plastic tube may be inserted as a palliative measure. Satisfactory palliation occurs in the majority of patients in whom the Celestin tube is employed. Palliative intubation is particularly applicable in patients with obstructive lesions of the lower esophagus. The decision to bypass or exclude a nonresectable thoracic esophageal neoplasm must be decided on an individual basis. Certainly, the experience of Skinner and DeMeester with the Japanese extracorporeal esophagogastric tube suggests that esophageal exclusion can be made more tolerable without resorting to extensive surgical reconstruction. The suggestion of Orringer and Sloan and of Griffen and associates to employ stomach to restore swallowing in all patients with esophageal malignancy, though appealing, has not been widely applied.

BENIGN CYSTS AND TUMORS

Benign cysts and tumors of the esophagus are uncommon but are of clinical concern, not only because they must be differentiated from more serious conditions but also because on occasion they can produce significant clinical symptoms and even threaten life. More than half of

the 246 benign esophageal tumors and cysts seen at the Mayo Clinic before 1973 were surgically or endoscopically removed; the rest were encountered at autopsy (Table 25-5).

Leiomyomas are the most common benign tumors. Those less than 5 cm in diameter are rarely symptomatic. Most leiomyomas occur in the lower half of the esophagus, and the majority of these are extramucosal and can be treated by simple enucleation. Roentgenographic examination often suggests the diagnosis (Fig. 25-40). Those encountered in the region of the esophagogastric junction tend to be large, obstructive lesions and usually require esophagogastrectomy for successful removal.

Cysts are the second most common benign lesions of the esophagus. Most can be removed successfully by enucleation. Complete reduplication is extremely rare.

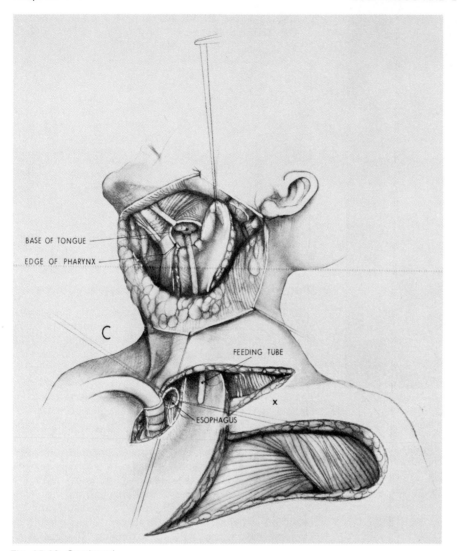

BASE OF TONGUE

EDGE OF PHARYNX

C

FEEDING TUBE

ESOPHAGUS

x

Fig. 25-39. Continued.

Table 25-3. SURVIVAL RATES FOR 3-YEAR AND 5-YEAR PERIODS
AFTER RESECTION FOR CARCINOMA OF THE ESOPHAGUS
AND CARDIA, MAYO CLINIC, 1946–1965

	3-year follow-up				*5-year follow-up*			
	Patients		*Survival*		*Patients*		*Survival*	
Site of resection	*Total*	*Traced*	*No.*	*%*	*Total*	*Traced*	*No.*	*%*
Esophagus:								
Cervical	17	17	3	18	15	15	1	7
Upper thoracic	103	94	17	18	86	82	7	9
Lower thoracic	92	90	30	33	82	79	21	27
Cardia.	367	358	76	21	322	315	40	13
Total	579	559	126	23	505	491	70	14

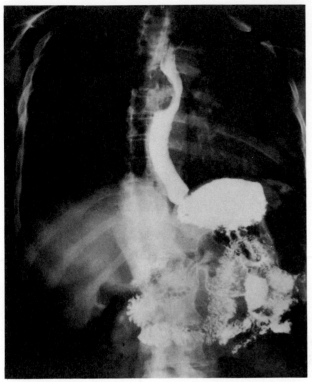

Fig. 25-40. Roentgenogram of esophagus, demonstrating presence of extramucosal filling defect which proved to be a leiomyoma that could be treated by simple enucleation.

A variety of polypoid intraesophageal tumors have been described, including mucosal polyps, chondromas, lipomas, fibrolipomas, and myxofibromas. The smaller lesions can be managed by endoscopic snare; others require esophagotomy for removal.

Table 25-4. 5-YEAR SURVIVAL RATES AFTER RESECTION FOR LESIONS INVOLVING THE ESOPHAGOGASTRIC JUNCTION, MAYO CLINIC, 1946–1963

Pathologic finding	No. of patients	Survival for 5 years or more after hospital dismissal*	
		No.	Percent
Squamous cell epithelium .	24	8	33.3
Negative lymph nodes . .	11	6	54.5
Positive lymph nodes . .	13	2	15.4
Adenocarcinoma.	238	31	13.0
Negative lymph nodes . .	67	18	26.9
Positive lymph nodes . .	171	13	7.6

* Based on traced patients; hospital deaths excluded in calculation of survival rates.
SOURCE: Data compiled from G. H. Gunnlaugsson, A. R. Wychulis, C. Roland, and F. H. Ellis, Jr., Analysis of the Records of 1,657 Patients with Analysis of Carcinoma of the Esophagus and Cardia of the Stomach, *Surg Gynecol Obstet,* **130:**997–1005, 1970.

Table 25-5. 246 BENIGN TUMORS AND CYSTS OF THE ESOPHAGUS SEEN AT THE MAYO CLINIC BEFORE 1973

Type	Total	Type	Total
Leiomyoma	145	Myxofibroma . . .	2
Cyst	55	Fibrolipoma . . .	2
Polyp	12	Neurofibroma . .	2
Papilloma	5	Fibroma	1
Lipoma	5	Lymphangioma .	1
Hemangioma	4	Mucocele	1
Adenoma	3	Duplication	1
Granular cell myoblastoma . .	3	Chondroma	1
Indeterminate	3		

MISCELLANEOUS ESOPHAGEAL LESIONS

Plummer-Vinson (Paterson-Kelly) Syndrome

In 1919, Paterson and Kelly independently described a clinical state with which the names of Plummer and Vinson later became associated in the United States. The typical patient is a middle-aged, edentulous woman with atrophic oral mucosa, spoon-shaped fingers with brittle nails, and a long-standing history of anemia and dysphagia. Because of the common finding of iron-deficiency anemia, the term *sideropenic dysphagia* has been used by some to describe the condition, which is more common in the Scandinavian countries than in the United States. The dysphagia is explained by the endoscopic and roentgenographic demonstration of a fibrous web partially obstructing the esophageal lumen in an eccentric fashion a few millimeters below the cricopharyngeus muscle. A dietary deficiency has been established as the cause, and the condition responds well to iron therapy and forceful dilation of the stricture. In approximately 10 percent of affected persons, a malignant lesion of the oral cavity, hypopharynx, or esophagus develops. The syndrome covers a broad spectrum of clinical entities, and not all patients exhibit hypochromic anemia, nor do they necessarily show evidence of malnutrition. Conversely, not all patients with the other clinical features of the Plummer-Vinson syndrome are found to have esophageal webs. Furthermore, some upper esophageal webs in younger patients who lack the clinical stigmata of the classic syndrome may have a congenital basis.

Lower Esophageal Ring

A ringlike constriction of the lower esophagus has been demonstrated roentgenographically by Schatzki and Gary in patients with hiatal hernia. The majority of patients in whom this abnormality is demonstrated are asymptomatic. However, some complain of dysphagia, and the symptom is directly related to the degree of narrowing produced by the ring. There is controversy as to the exact location of the narrowing, but most investigators believe it to be at the squamocolumnar mucosal junction. This abnormal roentgenographic finding has been related to the presence of a hypertonic inferior esophageal sphincter, an esophageal stricture, or the accordionlike or shortening effect on the esophagus of intrathoracic displacement of the esophagogastric junction in hiatal hernia. That it is truly an organic lesion is now generally accepted, although the cause remains obscure. Incision, resection, or partial excision of the ring should be done at the time of repair of the hiatal hernia in those patients with significant dysphagia not improved by dilation. The pathologic specimens from such procedures show little more than submucosal fibrosis.

Mallory-Weiss Syndrome

In 1929, Mallory and Weiss reported 15 cases of gastrointestinal bleeding after repeated emesis. Linear tears in the mucosa of the esophagogastric junction were demonstrated at postmortem examination in some of these patients. In subsequent years the condition has been noted more commonly and should be considered in the differential diagnosis of patients with unexplained hematemesis. The mechanism of the development of the lacerations is similar to that involved in the development of spontaneous rupture of the esophagus—namely, an explosive vomiting effort against a closed cardia or esophagus. A history of prolonged retching or vomiting, often but not always associated with alcoholism, is characteristic. Early diagnosis can be facilitated by roentgenographic studies to exclude the possibility of other lesions and by endoscopy to identify the site of bleeding. Bleeding may cease with conservative management, but surgical exploration may be required if it persists. The upper end of the stomach should be exposed through a long gastrotomy, and after manual evacuation of clots and the insertion of proper retractors for exposure, the lacerated areas should be repaired with sutures. Prompt arrest of bleeding can be expected with this technique.

Scleroderma and Related Diseases

Sometimes systemic diseases involve the esophagus, and scleroderma is probably the most common disease which gives rise to significant abnormalities of this organ. This disease affects the connective tissues of the body; when the esophagus becomes involved, the characteristic changes are fragmentation and homogenization of the submucosal connective tissue elements. The muscular layers usually are not involved. Motor failure of the esophagus is the characteristic finding on esophageal motility studies, and these findings may often precede the development of significant symptoms. When symptoms develop, dysphagia, regurgitation, and heartburn are common, and because the disease affects the inferior esophageal sphincter, gastroesophageal reflux with esophagitis may occur. At this stage of the disease, an antireflux operation such as the Nissen fundoplication may prove beneficial. As the disease process progresses, fibrosis and shortening of the esophagus ensue, with the development of a hiatal hernia. In advanced cases a stricture may be encountered, requiring forceful dilation for the relief of symptoms. The usual medical measures

to minimize the deleterious effects of gastroesophageal reflux should always be instituted. Resection of the strictured region may occasionally be required when dilation fails to relieve persistent dysphagia.

Dysphagia may occur in most of the so-called collagen diseases, but it is encountered most frequently in dermatomyositis, an incidence of 60 percent being reported by Donoghue and associates. A generalized muscular defect may be demonstrated by esophageal motility studies in patients with this disease. Weakness of the pharyngeal muscles predominates, but the abnormalities in the body of the esophagus resemble those seen in scleroderma. Usually, however, the integrity of the inferior sphincter is maintained. Remission of the disease may occur after administration of corticosteroids.

Neuromuscular Disturbances

Swallowing dysfunction is common in patients with neuromuscular disorders, and the details of these abnormalities can be demonstrated by esophageal motility studies. The most striking abnormalities can be seen in patients with disorders that are primarily myotonic in origin, such as myasthenia gravis and myotonia dystrophica. Rarely do esophageal motility studies give normal results in such patients. In myasthenia gravis, the amplitudes of the peristaltic waves are decreased, and they disappear in the lower esophagus during repetitive swallowing. Motor failure of the esophagus also occurs in myotonia dystrophica, a condition in which both smooth and striated muscles are affected.

A variety of nonspecific abnormalities may be seen in patients with central and peripheral neurologic disorders, usually involving changes in peristalsis. There may be an increase in the number of simultaneous waves, or esophageal spasm may be demonstrated. Some of these changes are seen even in patients with hemiplegia or Parkinson's disease. In amyotrophic lateral sclerosis, the most common finding is the occurrence of feeble peristaltic contractions in place of the vigorous contractions seen normally. Sometimes the contractions are simultaneous and may be repetitive; sphincteric changes are relatively less common. In multiple sclerosis, a variety of abnormalities may be noted, including poor relaxation of the pharyngoesophageal or gastroesophageal sphincter, simultaneous deglutition waves, incoordination of swallowing complexes, and diffuse spasm of the esophagus. Cricopharyngeal dysfunction has been implicated in the genesis of certain cervical dysphagia syndromes seen in a variety of neurologic conditions, especially bulbar poliomyelitis and amyotrophic lateral sclerosis, or after radical oral laryngeal surgery. The exact mechanism of dysphagia awaits clarification, but cricopharyngeal myotomy provides relief in properly selected patients. A similar problem has been described by Henderson and associates in patients with peripheral unilateral recurrent laryngeal nerve paralysis and in patients with gastroesophageal reflux. In classic idiopathic globus sensation, long thought to be a subjective emotional problem, there is demonstrable hypertonicity of the upper esophageal sphincter. The physiologic studies of Winans are particularly pertinent in interpreting reported observations in pharyngoesophageal function.

Acquired Fistulas

Occasionally, a fistulous communication requiring treatment may develop between the esophagus and the lower part of the respiratory tract. Other potential sites of fistulous communication include the aorta, the vena cava, and the heart. The commonest cause of acquired fistula is malignancy and usually represents a preterminal event in the course of incurable carcinoma of the esophagus, the lungs, or the neck structures.

Typically, a fistula between the esophagus and the tracheobronchial tree produces cough on eating or drinking, although it may present more subtly, with pulmonary symptoms alone. The basic principles of surgical treatment include division of the fistulous tract and suture closure of the defect in the esophagus and respiratory tree, with the interposition of viable tissue to prevent recurrence. Additionally, distal esophageal obstruction should be corrected.

The management of congenital tracheoesophageal fistula with and without atresia is discussed in the chapter dealing with pediatric surgery.

OTHER DIAPHRAGMATIC HERNIAS AND CONDITIONS

Although esophageal hiatal hernias are the most common type of diaphragmatic defect, a variety of other congenital and acquired defects and abnormalities may affect this structure and may cause considerable disability or even death unless promptly recognized and appropriately managed.

Posterolateral (Foramen of Bochdalek) Hernias

Congenital hernias through the posterolateral aspect of the diaphragm (pleuroperitoneal canal, or foramen of Bochdalek) are the most common diaphragmatic hernias in infants. This hernia often presents as an acute respiratory emergency at or shortly after birth, depending on the amount of herniated abdominal viscera present in the thorax. Rarely, such defects remain undetected until later childhood.

PATHOLOGY. The normal diaphragm results from the fusion of several anlagen, which completes the separation of the thoracic and abdominal cavities. Essentially, this type of hernia is thought to develop as the result of a failure, on either side, of complete fusion of the pleuroperitoneal folds during the first trimester of gestation. Normally the posterior portion of this embryonic membrane is the last to close; it is known as the *pleuroperitoneal canal,* or *foramen of Bochdalek.*

Initially the pleuroperitoneal folds consist of membranous pleura and peritoneum, between which later grow muscle fibers derived from cervical myotomes. Thus it may be postulated that a foramen of Bochdalek hernia may or may not have a hernial sac, depending on whether the failure of fusion occurs during the late or the initial stage of development. Usually, however, the defect results in a primary failure of the membranous anlage, which results in a muscular defect without a sac. The fact that the left diaphragmatic anlage evolves more slowly than the right might account for the higher incidence of left-sided hernias.

The consequences of such a hernia depend on the mass of abdominal viscera that herniates into the thorax. Although severe respiratory insufficiency may be apparent at birth, an infant may appear to be normal initially and may not have symptoms until the ingestion of air and food causes distension of the herniated hollow viscera. Labored respiration with associated negative intrathoracic pressures may further increase the mass of herniated abdominal organs in the chest.

Usually, prolonged residence of abdominal viscera in the thorax during embryonic development results in severe hypoplasia of the lung on the affected side. Furthermore, the displacement of abdominal viscera into the thorax may result in an abdominal cavity that is too small to accommodate these normal structures. Finally, not uncommon concomitant abnormalities of gastrointestinal rotation and attachment, which may be associated with peritoneal bands, may affect intestinal patency or predispose to a volvulus.

CLINICAL MANIFESTATIONS. Usually, an infant with foramen of Bochdalek hernia presents in a state of acute respiratory emergency, with cyanosis and greatly increased respiratory rate and effort. The affected hemithorax is usually dull on percussion, and there is evidence of shift of mediastinal structures to the opposite side. The diagnosis is almost always apparent on standard roentgenograms of the thorax, which often clearly demonstrate gas-filled intestines. In rare cases, it is difficult to differentiate this process from various inflammatory conditions of the lung, enterogenous cysts, duplications, pneumothorax, lobar emphysema, or other anomalies. Under such circumstances, it is desirable to have the infant ingest an appropriate nonirritating contrast medium.

TREATMENT. Because of the severe, life-threatening respiratory distress associated with this condition, immediate surgical repair is indicated on an emergency basis. The passage of a small catheter into the stomach for decompression may provide temporary improvement and, more important, may prevent progressive distension. Accidental contamination of the respiratory tract may be minimized by keeping the infant in an upright position. A high-oxygen atmosphere may decrease respiratory distress and cyanosis.

Usually, not enough time has elapsed since birth for development of significant fluid and electrolyte problems, and little preoperative preparation is required except to provide an adequate intravenous route for administration of fluids. Peroral tracheal intubation for assisted ventilation may be necessary in severely ill infants.

Technique. Generally, the abdominal route is preferred

in the management of this type of hernia. It provides easy access to the defect, and viscera are more easily reduced and do not interfere with repair when reduced. Furthermore, this route provides easy access for the assessment of associated gastrointestinal anomalies and satisfies the frequent need for the creation of a ventral hernia (to accommodate the reduced viscera) and for gastrostomy. The reduction of the hernial contents from the thorax is often facilitated by the insertion of a catheter or finger through the diaphragmatic defect from below to allow air to enter the thorax as the viscera are removed.

Although commonly of relatively large size, the defect usually can be closed primarily with interrupted nonabsorbable sutures. Occasionally such defects are so large that complete closure by direct suture is difficult or impossible. Under such circumstances it may be necessary to use a patch of plastic material to fill the defect. Rosenkrantz and Cotton have suggested obliterating large diaphragmatic defects by using a flap of innervated muscle, fascia, and peritoneum from the anterior abdominal wall.

A hernial sac should be carefully sought for and removed if present. Repair of the diaphragmatic defect without excision of the sac may result in the formation of an expanding cystic structure that may be as life-threatening as an unrepaired hernia. If such a cyst should develop, simple aspiration will prevent respiratory embarrassment until excision can be accomplished.

It is often tempting to try forceful reexpansion of the hypoplastic lung on the affected side. Such efforts are not only fruitless but may cause irreparable damage and intractable postoperative pulmonary edema. After the abdominal contents are reduced, it seems preferable to adjust intrapleural pressures on the affected side as the defect is closed. This naturally results in a pneumothorax, which will be resorbed as the hypoplastic lung matures and expands during the ensuing days or even months. Fluids may accumulate in the pleural space and may require aspiration.

The occurrence of severe respiratory distress or recurrence of the hernia in the postoperative period can be minimized by appropriate gastrointestinal decompression, usually by tube gastrostomy. Often it is difficult to replace gas-distended intestines in the abdomen, particularly in infants in whom marked distension of the intestine has been allowed to develop. Under such circumstances, attempts at evacuating the intestinal contents may not be adequate, and it may be necessary to create a ventral hernia to provide space for the viscera and to minimize both tension on the repair and dyspnea. When such a hernia is created, one of the difficult postoperative decisions may be the timing of its repair.

Results. In spite of all efforts, severe respiratory and metabolic acidosis may occur in the postoperative period, requiring assisted ventilation and administration of sodium bicarbonate. In any event, postoperative management should include a moist atmosphere high in oxygen, frequent turning of the patient, and aspiration of secretions. Feeding is started when intestinal activity returns. In infants, although recurrences are rare, mortality has ranged

from 12 to 30 percent. However, Cerilli has noted that when the diagnosis was made at the age of two to thirty days, the mortality rate was about one-third that in the immediate neonatal period.

Foramen of Morgagni Hernias

This type of hernia has been called *anterior diaphragmatic, parasternal,* or *retrosternal* hernia but is best known by the eponym *foramen of Morgagni hernia.* The exact cause is unknown. Although generally thought to be due to a congenital defect in the fusion of sternal and costal elements of the diaphragmatic anlage, it is an uncommon hernia in infants and children; the majority of defects are detected in adults.

CLINICAL MANIFESTATIONS. When these hernias occur in infants and children, the manifestations are cardiorespiratory distress and the usual findings associated with foramen of Bochdalek hernia, but the vast majority of Morgagni hernias are detected incidentally as asymptomatic anterior cardiophrenic masses on routine roentgenographic examination of the thorax of adults. Approximately 20 percent of patients have symptoms referable to the hernia; these are predominantly vague, nonspecific gastrointestinal complaints. Almost all these hernias have a hernial sac. Although most contain herniated omentum or colon, portions of liver, small bowel, and stomach have been encountered.

The diagnosis is often obvious on standard roentgenograms of the thorax: gas and fluid are seen in the herniated large bowel. On lateral or stereoscopic views of the thorax, the anterior cardiophrenic location is apparent. In some patients, examination of the colon and, less frequently, of the upper gastrointestinal tract with appropriate contrast medium will establish the nature of such a defect.

TREATMENT. When a definitive clinical diagnosis can be established, it is usually desirable, even in the absence of severe symptoms, to advise repair as an elective prophylactic procedure unless other conditions preclude operation. Under usual circumstances, the simplest and most direct approach is through an upper transabdominal incision (Fig. 25-41). This permits easy access to either a right- or left-sided hernia or to bilateral hernias. Viscera are easily reduced by traction from below. The peritoneal sac is easily excised and the defect readily closed by this route.

When a definitive preoperative diagnosis cannot be established and more serious disease cannot be excluded, the transthoracic approach is indicated. This approach is more difficult technically but affords a better opportunity to deal with other unsuspected pulmonary, diaphragmatic, or paramediastinal conditions that may occur in this region.

Eventration of the Diaphragm

Unilateral elevation of the diaphragm may be a congenital or an acquired abnormality and may be seen in patients of any age. It may occur as the result of anomalous development of the diaphragm or its innervation or as a

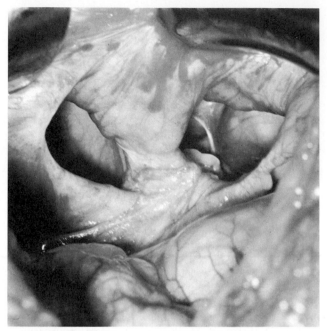

Fig. 25-41. Bilateral foramen of Morgagni hernia as seen at operation from abdominal approach. (*From T. P. Comer, and O. T. Clagett, Surgical Treatment of Hernia of the Foramen of Morgagni, J Thor Surg, 52:461, 1966.*)

result of injury, at birth or later, to the phrenic nerve and diaphragm. This process may affect a portion or all of the hemidiaphragm on one side. It may be impossible to differentiate certain elevations of the diaphragm from congenital hernias, particularly from foramen of Bochdalek hernias. Irrespective of cause, which usually cannot

Fig. 25-42. Diaphragmatic eventration and operative procedures available for its correction. (*From F. H. Ellis, Jr., Eventration: Unilateral Elevation of the Diaphragm, in L. M. Nyhus and H. N. Harkins, "Hernia," J. B. Lippincott Company, Philadelphia, 1964, pp. 554–565.*)

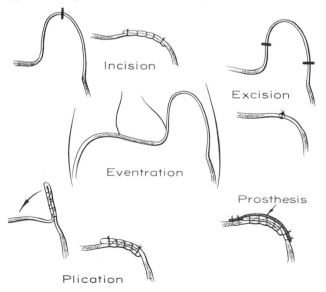

be established with certainty, such abnormalities of the diaphragm are of significance only when they are associated with symptoms or when they cannot be differentiated from more serious conditions.

CLINICAL MANIFESTATIONS. Eventration of the diaphragm causes symptoms as the result of interference with pulmonary ventilation. Typically, symptoms are encountered in infants and in old persons. When seen in the newborn, the symptoms and problems are identical to those of the massive congenital diaphragmatic hernias already described. In the fifth and sixth decades of life, when decreased cardiopulmonary reserve develops in combination with intraabdominal pressure secondary to obesity, digestive and respiratory symptoms related to this abnormality may appear for the first time.

TREATMENT. Prompt emergency treatment is indicated in the newborn infant who is dyspneic and cyanotic. Usually the transabdominal approach is preferred, for the reasons indicated for the repair of foramen of Morgagni hernias. Operation consists of imbrication of the eventrated leaf.

In patients of any age, and particularly in those in whom surgical treatment is contraindicated, if symptoms are not life-threatening, symptomatic palliation is indicated. These measures include restriction of activities, weight reduction, and avoidance of abdominal distension, lifting, or straining.

In older children and adults in whom symptoms are disabling, surgical treatment to restore the diaphragm to its normal position should be considered. Such procedures help to stabilize the mediastinum and permit more normal pulmonary ventilation. The procedure most commonly used is diaphragmatic plication (Fig. 25-42). In adults, the thoracic approach gives better exposure and greater ease of repair than the abdominal approach. When viscera are adherent to the undersurface of the diaphragm, a thoracoabdominal incision may be advantageous.

Rupture of the Diaphragm

Loss of anatomic continuity of the diaphragm may occur under a variety of circumstances and may permit the passage of abdominal contents into the pleural space.

The majority of such ruptures of the diaphragm occur as the result of severe blunt external trauma. Occasionally, some inflammatory process, such as a subphrenic abscess or empyema, will produce a diaphragmatic defect. Penetrating injuries, such as gunshot or stab wounds, are relatively infrequent causes of rupture of the diaphragm. Dehiscence of surgical incisions in the diaphragm may also result in hernia.

CLINICAL MANIFESTATIONS. Irrespective of cause, the majority of ruptures of the diaphragm are on the left, and the symptoms are almost invariably related to the type and amount of herniated abdominal viscera present in the thorax. Clinical manifestations vary from no symptoms to life-endangering problems immediately after injury. Late complications include gastrointestinal hemorrhage and obstructions. With massive herniation, rapidly progressive cardiorespiratory distress poses a life-threatening problem.

Extraneous shadows above the diaphragm, such as a gas-filled or homogeneous area, along with a shift of the mediastinum, are extremely suggestive of a ruptured diaphragm. Occasionally, roentgenographic examination of the gastrointestinal tract is required to establish a diagnosis. With massive herniation of the stomach into the thorax, the passage of a nasogastric tube both confirms the diagnosis and prevents progressive distension.

TREATMENT. Acutely traumatic diaphragmatic hernia is best managed via a transabdominal incision, since associated abdominal visceral injury is common and is best managed via abdominal exposure. Furthermore, acute herniation of abdominal viscera is not associated with adhesions to intrathoracic structures, and reduction is readily effected from below. Late operations are often difficult because of the presence of adhesions, and a transthoracic exploration provides the best exposure for their lysis in preparation for reduction and repair of the hernia. In either early or late intervention, primary suture repair of the diaphragmatic defect is usually possible, but on rare occasions adjacent tissue or even prosthetic material may be required for diaphragmatic closure.

References

General

Code, C. F., Creamer, B., Schlegel, J. F., Olsen, A. M., Donoghue, F. E., and Andersen, H. A.: "An Atlas of Esophageal Motility in Health and Disease," Charles C Thomas, Publisher, Springfield, Ill., 1958.

——— and Schlegel, J. F.: Motor Action of the Esophagus and Its Sphincters, in W. Heidel (ed.), "Handbook of Physiology," sec. 6: "Alimentary Canal," vol. 4, p. 1821, American Physiological Society, Washington, 1968.

Earlam, R.: "Clinical Tests of Oesophageal Function," Grune & Stratton, Inc., New York, 1975.

Ellis, F. H., Jr., and Olsen, A. M.: Achalasia of the Esophagus, *Major Probl Clin Surg,* **9:**1, 1969.

Henderson, R. D.: "Motor Disorders of the Esophagus," Williams & Wilkins Company, Baltimore, 1976.

Ingelfinger, F. J.: Esophageal Motility, *Physiol Rev,* **38:**533, 1958.

Marshall, S. F.: Carcinoma of the Esophagus: Successful Resection of Lower End of Esophagus with Reestablishment of Esophageal Gastric Continuity, *Surg Clin North Am,* **18:**643, 1938.

Ohsawa, T.: Surgery of the Oesophagus, *Arch Jap Chir,* **10:**605, 1933.

Payne, W. S., and Olsen, A. M.: "The Esophagus," Lea & Febiger, Philadelphia, 1974.

Postlethwait, R. W., and Sealy, W. C.: "Surgery of the Esophagus," Charles C Thomas, Publisher, Springfield, Ill., 1961.

Siewert, R., Blum, A. L., and Waldeck, F.: "Funktionsstörungen der Speiseröhre," Springer-Verlag KG, Berlin, 1976.

Skinner, D. B., Belsey, R. H. R., Hendrix, T. R., and Zuidema, G. D.: "Gastroesophageal Reflux and Hiatal Hernia," Little, Brown & Company, Boston, 1972.

Smith, R. A., and Smith, R. E.: "Surgery of the Oesophagus," Butterworth & Co. (Publishers) Ltd., London, 1972.

Vantrappen, G., and Hellemans, J.: "Diseases of the Esophagus," Springer-Verlag New York, Inc., New York, 1974.

Von Hacker, V., and Lotheissen, G.: "Chirurgie der Speiseröhre," vol. 34, Ferdinand Enke, Stuttgart, 1926.

Zaino, C., Jacobson, H. G., Lepow, H., and Ozturk, C. H.: "The Pharyngoesophageal Sphincter," Charles C Thomas, Publisher, Springfield, Ill., 1970.

Anatomy

Butler, H.: The Veins of the Oesophagus, *Thorax,* **6:**276, 1951.

Carey, J. M., and Hollinshead, W. H.: An Anatomic Study of the Esophageal Hiatus, *Surg Gynecol Obstet,* **100:**196, 1955.

Daniels, B. T.: The Phrenoesophageal Membrane, *Am J Surg,* **110:**814, 1965.

Hayward, J.: Phreno-oesophageal Ligament in Hiatal Hernia Repair, *Thorax,* **16:**41, 1961.

Higgs, B., Shorter, R. G., and Ellis, F. H., Jr.: A Study of the Anatomy of the Human Esophagus with Special Reference to the Gastroesophageal Sphincter, *J Surg Res,* **5:**503, 1965.

Laimer, E.: Beitrag zur Anatomie des Oesophagus, *Med Jahrb Wien,* 1883, p. 333.

Listerud, M. B., and Harkins, H. N.: Variations in the Muscular Anatomy of the Esophageal Hiatus: Based on Dissections of Two Hundred and Four Fresh Cadavers, *West J Surg,* **67:**110, 1959.

Swigart, L. L., Siekert, R. G., Hambley, W. C., and Anson, B. J.: The Esophageal Arteries: An Anatomic Study of 150 Specimens, *Surg Gynecol Obstet,* **90:**234, 1950.

Physiology

Botha, G. S. M.: Mucosal Folds at Cardia as a Component of the Gastro-oesophageal Closing Mechanism, *Br J Surg,* **45:**569, 1958.

Braasch, J. W., and Ellis, F. H., Jr.: The Gastroesophageal Sphincter Mechanism: An Experimental Study, *Surgery,* **39:**901, 1956.

Carveth, S. W., Schlegel, J. F., Code, C. F., and Ellis, F. H., Jr.: Esophageal Motility after Vagotomy, Phrenicotomy, Myotomy, and Myomectomy in Dogs, *Surg Gynecol Obstet,* **114:**31, 1962.

Castell, D. O., and Harris, L. D.: Hormonal Control of Gastroesophageal-Sphincter Strength, *N Engl J Med,* **282:**886, 1970.

———, and Levine, S. M.: Lower Esophageal Sphincter Response to Gastric Alkalinization: A New Mechanism for Treatment of Heartburn with Antacids, *Ann Intern Med,* **74:**223, 1971.

Code, C. F., Creamer, B., Schlegel, J. F., Olsen, A. M., Donoghue, F. E., and Andersen, H. A.: "An Atlas of Esophageal Motility in Health and Disease," Charles C Thomas, Publisher, Springfield, Ill., 1958.

———, and Schlegel, J. F.: The Physiologic Basis of Some Motor Disorders of the Oesophagus, in A. N. Smith, "Surgical Physiology of Gastrointestinal Tract," Royal College of Surgeons, Edinburgh, Scotland, 1963.

Cohen, S., and Lipshutz, W.: Anticholinergic Therapy: A Triple Threat to Lower Esophageal Sphincter Competence (Abstract), *Ann Intern Med,* **72:**792, 1970.

——— and ———: Hormonal Regulation of Human Lower Esophageal Sphincter Competence: Interaction of Gastrin and Secretin, *J Clin Invest,* **50:**449, 1971.

Dennish, G. W., and Castell, D. O.: Inhibitory Effect of Smoking on the Lower Esophageal Sphincter, *N Engl J Med,* **284:**1136, 1971.

Dillard, D. H., and Anderson, H. N.: A New Concept of the Mechanism of Sphincteric Failure in Sliding Esophageal Hiatal Hernia, *Surg Gynecol Obstet,* **122**:1030, 1966.

Goyal, R. K.: The Lower Esophageal Sphincter, *Viewpoints Dig Dis,* **8**:1, 1976.

Greenwood, R. K., Schlegel, J. F., Helm, W. J., and Code, C. F.: Pressure and Potential Difference Characteristics of Surgically Created Canine Hiatal Hernia, *Gastroenterology,* **48**:602, 1965.

Gryboski, J. D., Thayer, W. R., Jr., and Spiro, H. M.: Esophageal Motility in Infants and Children, *Pediatrics,* **31**:382, 1963.

Ingelfinger, F. J.: Esophageal Motility, *Physiol Rev,* **38**:533, 1958.

Lind, J. F., Crispin, J. S., and McIvor, D. K.: The Effect of Atropine on the Gastroesophageal Sphincter, *Can J Physiol Pharmacol,* **46**:233, 1968.

Mann, C. V., Ellis, F., H., Jr., Schlegel, J. F., and Code, C. F.: Abdominal Displacement of the Canine Gastroesophageal Sphincter, *Surg Gynecol Obstet,* **118**:1009, 1964.

————, Schlegel, J. F., Ellis, F. H., Jr., and Code, C. F.: Studies of the Isolated Gastroesophageal Sphincter, *Surg Forum,* **13**:248, 1962.

Meiss, J. H., Grindlay, J. H., and Ellis, F. H., Jr.: The Gastroesophageal Sphincter Mechanism: II. Further Experimental Studies in the Dog, *J Thorac Cardiovasc Surg,* **36**:156, 1958.

Vandertoll, D. J., Ellis, F. H., Jr., Schlegel, J. F., and Code, C. F.: An Experimental Study of the Role of Gastric and Esophageal Muscle in Gastroesophageal Competence, *Surg Gynecol Obstet,* **122**:579, 1966.

Esophageal Motility Disturbances

Barker, J. R., and Franklin, R. H.: Heller's Operation for Achalasia of the Cardia: A Study of the Early and Late Results, *Br J Surg,* **58**:466, 1971.

Benz, L. J., Hootkin, L. A., Margulies, S., Donner, M. W., Cauthorne, R. T., and Hendrix, T. R.: A Comparison of Clinical Measurements of Gastroesophageal Reflux, *Gastroenterology,* **62**:1, 1972.

Bombeck, C. T., Helfrich, G. B., and Nyhus, L. M.: Planning Surgery for Reflux Esophagitis and Hiatus Hernia, *Surg Clin North Am,* **50**:29, 1970.

Butin, J. W., Olsen, A. M., Moersch, H. J., and Code, C. F.: A Study of Esophageal Pressures in Normal Persons and Patients with Cardiospasm, *Gastroenterology,* **23**:278, 1953.

Butterfield, D. G., Struthers, J. E., Jr., and Showalter, J. P.: A Test of Gastroesophageal Sphincter Competence: The Common Cavity Test, *Am J Dig Dis,* **17**:415, 1972.

Cassella, R. R., Brown, A. L., Jr., Sayre, G. P., and Ellis, F. H., Jr.: Achalasia of the Esophagus: Pathologic and Etiologic Considerations, *Ann Surg,* **160**:474, 1964.

————, Ellis, F. H., Jr., and Brown, A. L., Jr.: Diffuse Spasm of the Lower Part of the Esophagus: Fine Structure of Esophageal Smooth Muscle and Nerve, *JAMA,* **191**:379, 1965.

Code, C. F., Schlegel, J. F., Kelley, M. L., Jr., Olsen, A. M., and Ellis, F. H., Jr.: Hypertensive Gastroesophageal Sphincter, *Proc Staff Meet Mayo Clin,* **35**:391, 1960.

Cohen, S., and Lipshutz, W.: Lower Esophageal Sphincter Dysfunction in Achalasia, *Gastroenterology,* **61**:814, 1971.

Creamer, B., Donoghue, F. E., and Code, C. F.: Pattern of Esophageal Motility in Diffuse Spasm, *Gastroenterology,* **34**:787, 1958.

Earlam, R. J., Ellis, F. H., Jr., and Nobrega, F. T.: Achalasia of the Esophagus in a Small Urban Community, *Mayo Clin Proc,* **44**:478, 1969.

Effler, D. B., Loop, F. D., Groves, L. K., and Favaloro, R. G.: Primary Surgical Treatment of Esophageal Achalasia, *Surg Gynecol Obstet,* **132**:1057, 1971.

Ellis, F. G.: The Natural History of Achalasia of the Cardia, *Proc R Soc Med,* **53**:663, 1960.

Ellis, F. H., Jr., Code, C. F., and Olsen, A. M.: Long Esophagomyotomy for Diffuse Spasm of the Esophagus and Hypertensive Gastroesophageal Sphincter, *Surgery,* **48**:155, 1960.

————, and Gibb, S. P.: Reoperation after Esophagomyotomy for Achalasia of the Esophagus, *Am J Surg,* **129**:407, 1975.

————, and Olsen, A. M.: Achalasia of the Esophagus, *Major Probl Clin Surg,* **9**:1, 1969.

————, and Payne, W. S.: Motility Disturbances of the Esophagus and Its Inferior Sphincter: Recent Surgical Advances, *Adv Surg,* **1**:179, 1965.

Ferguson, T. B., Woodbury, J. D., Roper, C. L., and Burford, T. H.: Giant Muscular Hypertrophy of the Esophagus, *Ann Thorac Surg,* **8**:209, 1969.

Flye, M. W., and Sealy, W. C.: Diffuse Spasm of the Esophagus, *Ann Thorac Surg,* **19**:677, 1975.

Grimes, O. F., Stephens, H. B., and Margulis, A. R.: Achalasia of the Esophagus, *Am J Surg,* **120**:198, 1970.

Heller, E.: Extramuköse Cardioplastik beim chronischen Cardiospasmus mit Dilatation des Oesophagus, *Mitt Grengeb Med Chir,* **27**:141, 1913.

————, ————, Schlegel, J. F., and Code, C. F.: Surgical Treatment of Esophageal Hypermotility Disturbances, *JAMA,* **188**:862, 1964.

Helsingen, N., Jr.: Oesophagitis following Total Gastrectomy: A Follow-up Study on 9 Patients 5 Years or More after Operation, *Acta Chir Scand,* **118**:190, 1960.

Henderson, R. D., Ho, C. S., and Davidson, J. W.: Primary Disordered Motor Activity of the Esophagus (Diffuse Spasm): Diagnosis and Treatment, *Ann Thorac Surg,* **18**:327, 1974.

————, and Rodney, K.: Tone of the Gastroesophageal Junction: Its Response to Abdominal Compression and to Swallowing, *Can J Surg,* **14**:328, 1971.

Hiebert, C. A.: Primary Incompetence of the Gastric Cardia, *Am J Surg,* **119**:365, 1970.

Higgs, B., Kerr, F. W. L., and Ellis, F. H., Jr.: The Experimental Production of Esophageal Achalasia by Electrolytic Lesions in the Medulla, *J Thorac Cardiovasc Surg,* **50**:613, 1965.

Ismail-Beigi, F., Horton, P. F., and Pope, C. E., II: Histological Consequences of Gastroesophageal Reflux in Man, *Gastroenterology,* **58**:163, 1970.

Jahadi, M. R., and Chandler, J. P.: Detecting Gastroesophageal Reflux by pH Recording and Acid Reflux Test, *Am Surg,* **38**:281, 1972.

Koberle, F.: Megaesophagus, *Gastroenterology,* **34**:460, 1958.

Lind, J. F., Cotton, D. J., Blanchard, R., Crispin, J. S., and Dimopolos, G. E.: Effect of Thoracic Displacement and Vagotomy on the Canine Gastroesophageal Junctional Zone, *Gastroenterology,* **56**:1078, 1969.

————, Warrian, W. G., and Wankling, W. J.: Responses of the Gastroesophageal Junctional Zone to Increases in Abdominal Pressure, *Can J Surg,* **9**:32, 1966.

Lipshutz, W. H., Gaskins, R. D., Lukash, W. M., and Sode, J.:

Pathogenesis of Lower-Esophageal–Sphincter Incompetence, *N Engl J Med,* **289:**182, 1973.

Lortat-Jacob, J.-L.: La Myomatose nodulaire diffuse de l'oesophage, *Acquis Med Recent,* 1950, p. 108.

Maillet, P., Micol, P., Parsal, J. P., Viard, H., and Favre, J.-P.: Les Résultats du traitement chirurgical du méga-oesophage (72 observations), *Ann Chir,* **27:**579, 1973.

Olsen, A. M., and Creamer, B.: Studies of Oesophageal Motility, with Special Reference to the Differential Diagnosis of Diffuse Spasm and Achalasia (Cardiospasm), *Thorax,* **12:**279, 1957.

———, Schlegel, J. F., and Payne, W. S.: The Hypotensive Gastroesophageal Sphincter, *Mayo Clin Proc,* **48:**165, 1973.

Patrick, D. L., Payne, W. S., Olsen, A. M., and Ellis, F. H., Jr.: Reoperation for Achalasia of the Esophagus, *Arch Surg,* **103:**122, 1971.

Peyton, M. D., Greenfield, L. J., and Elkins, R. C.: Combined Myotomy and Hiatal Herniorrhaphy: A New Approach to Achalasia, *Am J Surg,* **128:**786, 1974.

Pope, C. E., II: Pathophysiology and Diagnosis of Reflux Esophagitis, *Gastroenterology,* **70:**445, 1976.

Rapant, V., and Králik, J.: Die Problematik der Therapie der Achalasie der Speiseröhre, *Bruns Beitr Klin Chir,* **218:**12, 1970.

Sanderson, D. R., Ellis, F. H., Jr., Schlegel, J. F., Code, C. F., and Olsen, A. M.: "Syndrome of Vigorous Achalasia: Clinical and Physiologic Considerations," paper presented at meeting of American College of Chest Physicians, Chicago, June 23–27, 1966.

———, ———, and Olsen, A. M.: Achalasia of the Esophagus: Results of Therapy by Dilation, 1950–1967, *Chest,* **58:**116, 1970.

Skinner, D. B., and Booth, D. J.: Assessment of Distal Esophageal Function in Patients with Hiatal Hernia and/or Gastroesophageal Reflux, *Ann Surg,* **172:**627, 1970.

Windsor, C. W. O.: Gastro-oesophageal Reflux after Partial Gastrectomy, *Br Med J,* **2:**1233, 1964.

Diverticula

Allen, T. H., and Clagett, O. T.: Changing Concepts in the Surgical Treatment of Pulsion Diverticula of the Lower Esophagus, *J Thorac Cardiovasc Surg,* **50:**455, 1965.

Belsey, R.: Functional Diseases of the Esophagus, *J Thorac Cardiovasc Surg,* **52:**164, 1966.

Clagett, O. T., and Payne, W. S.: Surgical Treatment of Pulsion Diverticula of the Hypopharynx: One-Stage Resection in 478 Cases, *Dis Chest,* **37:**257, 1960.

Cross, F. S., Johnson, G. F., and Gerein, A. N.: Esophageal Diverticula: Associated Neuromuscular Changes in the Esophagus, *Arch Surg,* **83:**525, 1961.

Dohlman, G., and Mattsson, O.: The Endoscopic Operation for Hypopharyngeal Diverticula: A Roentgencinematographic Study, *Arch Otolaryngol,* **71:**744, 1960.

Ellis, F. H., Jr., Schlegel, J. G., Lynch, V. P., and Payne, W. S.: Cricopharyngeal Myotomy for Pharyngoesophageal Diverticulum, *Ann Surg,* **170:**340, 1969.

Goodman, H. I., and Parnes, I. H.: Epiphrenic Diverticula of the Esophagus, *J Thorac Cardiovasc Surg,* **23:**145, 1952.

Habein, H. C., Jr., Kirklin, J. W., Clagett, O. T., and Moersch, H. J.: Surgical Treatment of Lower Esophageal Pulsion Diverticula, *Arch Surg,* **72:**1018, 1956.

———, Moersch, H. J., and Kirklin, J. W.: Diverticula of the

Lower Part of the Esophagus: A Clinical Study of 149 Nonsurgical Cases, *Arch Intern Med,* **97:**768, 1956.

Lahey, F. H., and Warren, K. W.: Esophageal Diverticula, *Surg Gynecol Obstet,* **98:**1, 1954.

Negus, V. E.: Pharyngeal Diverticula: Observations on Their Evolution and Treatment, *Br J Surg,* **38:**129, 1950.

Putney, F. J., and Clerf, L. H.: Epiphrenic Esophageal Diverticulum, *Ann Otol Rhinol Laryngol,* **62:**803, 1953.

Sutherland, H. D.: Cricopharyngeal Achalasia, *J Thorac Cardiovasc Surg,* **43:**114, 1962.

Vinson, P. P.: Diverticula of the Thoracic Portion of the Esophagus: Report of 42 Cases, *Arch Otolaryngol,* **19:**508, 1934.

Welsh, G. F., and Payne, W. S.: The Present Status of One-Stage Pharyngoesophageal Diverticulectomy, *Surg Clin North Am,* **53:**953, 1973.

Wychulis, A. R., Ellis, F. H., Jr., and Andersen, H. A.: Acquired Nonmalignant Esophagotracheobronchial Fistula: Report of 36 Cases, *JAMA,* **196:**117, 1966.

Esophageal Hiatal Hernia

Allison, P. R.: Reflux Esophagitis, Sliding Hiatal Hernia, and the Anatomy of Repair, *Surg Gynecol Obstet,* **92:**419, 1951.

Battle, W. S., Nyhus, L. M., and Bombeck, C. T.: Nissen Fundoplication and Esophagitis Secondary to Gastroesophageal Reflux, *Arch Surg,* **106:**588, 1973.

Behar, J., Sheahan, D. G., Biancani, P., Spiro, H. M., and Storer, E. H.: Medical and Surgical Management of Reflux Esophagitis: A 38-Month Report on a Prospective Clinical Trial, *N Engl J Med,* **293:**263, 1975.

Belsey, R.: Reconstruction of the Esophagus with Left Colon, *J Thorac Cardiovasc Surg,* **49:**33, 1965.

Bosher, L. H., Jr., Fishman, L., Webb, W. R., and Old, L., Jr.: Strangulated Diaphragmatic Hernia with Gangrene and Perforation of the Stomach, *Dis Chest,* **37:**504, 1960.

Bushkin, F. L., Neustein, C. L., Parker, T. H., and Woodward, E. R.: Nissen Fundoplication for Reflux Peptic Esophagitis, *Ann Surg,* **185:**672, 1977.

Cohen, S., and Harris, L. D.: Does Hiatus Hernia Affect Competence of the Gastroesophageal Sphincter? *N Engl J Med,* **284:**1053, 1971.

Collis, J. L.: An Appraisal of the Methods of Treating Hiatus Hernia and Its Complications, *Ann R Coll Surg Engl,* **46:**338, 1970.

Csendes, A., and Larrain, A.: Effect of Posterior Gastropexy on Gastroesophageal Sphincter Pressure and Symptomatic Reflux in Patients with Hiatal Hernia, *Gastroenterology,* **63:**19, 1972.

Culver, G. J., Pirson, H. S., and Bean, B. C.: Mechanism of Obstruction in Para-esophageal Diaphragmatic Hernias, *JAMA,* **181:**933, 1962.

DeMeester, T. R., Johnson, L. F., and Kent, A. H.: Evaluation of Current Operations for the Prevention of Gastroesophageal Reflux, *Ann Surg,* **180:**511, 1974.

DiMarino, A. J., Rosato, E., Rosato, F., and Cohen, S.: Improvement in Lower Esophageal Sphincter Pressure following Surgery for Complicated Gastroesophageal Reflux, *Ann Surg,* **181:**239, 1975.

Ellis, F. H., Jr., El-Kurd, M. F. A., and Gibb, S. P.: The Effect of Fundoplication on the Lower Esophageal Sphincter, *Surg Gynecol Obstet,* **143:**1, 1976.

Harrington, S. W.: Esophageal Hiatal Diaphragmatic Hernia, *Surg Gynecol Obstet,* **100:**277, 1955.

Hill, L. D.: An Effective Operation for Hiatal Hernia: An Eight Year Appraisal, *Ann Surg,* **166:**681, 1967.

————: Incarcerated Paraesophageal Hernia: A Surgical Emergency, *Am J Surg,* **126:**286, 1973.

————, and Tobias, J. A.: Paraesophageal Hernia, *Arch Surg,* **96:**735, 1968.

Leonardi, H. K., Lee, M. E., El-Kurd, M. F. A., and Ellis, F. H., Jr.: An Experimental Study of the Effectiveness of Various Anti-reflux Operations, *Ann Thorac Surg.* (In press.)

Lipshutz, W. H., Eckert, R. J., Gaskins, R. D., Blanton, D. E., and Lukash, W. M.: Normal Lower-Esophageal-Sphincter Function after Surgical Treatment of Gastroesophageal Reflux, *N Engl J Med,* **291:**1107, 1974.

Mobley, J. E., and Christensen, N. A.: Esophageal Hiatal Hernia: Prevalence, Diagnosis and Treatment in an American City of 30,000, *Gastroenterology,* **30:**1, 1956.

Nissen, R.: Eine einfache Operation zur Beeinflussung der Refluxoesophagitis, *Schweiz Med Wochenschr,* **86:**590, 1956.

Orringer, M. B., Skinner, D. B., and Belsey, R. H. R.: Long-Term Results of the Mark IV Operation for Hiatal Hernia and Analyses of Recurrences and Their Treatment, *J Thorac Cardiovasc Surg,* **63:**25, 1972.

Polk, H. C., Jr.: Fundoplication for Reflux Esophagitis: Misadventures with the Operation of Choice, *Ann Surg,* **183:**645, 1976.

————, and Zeppa, R.: Hiatal Hernia and Esophagitis: A Survey of Indications for Operation and Technic and Results of Fundoplication, *Ann Surg,* **173:**775, 1971.

Pridie, R. B.: Incidence and Coincidence of Hiatus Hernia, *Gut,* **7:**188, 1966.

Rex, J. C., Andersen, H. A., Bartholomew, L. G., and Cain, J. C.: Esophageal Hiatal Hernia: A Ten Year Study of Medically Treated Cases, *JAMA,* **178:**271, 1961.

Woodward, E. R., Thomas, H. F., and McAlhany, J. C.: Comparison of Crural Repair and Nissen Fundoplication in the Treatment of Esophageal Hiatus Hernia with Peptic Esophagitis, *Ann Surg,* **173:**782, 1971.

Complications of Gastroesophageal Reflux

Allison, P. R., and Johnstone, A. S.: The Oesophagus Lined with Gastric Mucous Membrane, *Thorax,* **8:**87, 1953.

Barrett, N. R.: Chronic Peptic Ulcer of the Oesophagus and "Oesophagitis," *Br J Surg,* **38:**175, 1950.

Behar, J., Biancani, P., and Sheahan, D. G.: Evaluation of Esophageal Tests in the Diagnosis of Reflux Esophagitis, *Gastroenterology,* **71:**9, 1976.

Benedict, E. B.: Esophageal Stenosis Caused by Peptic Esophagitis or Ulceration, *Surg Gynecol Obstet,* **122:**613, 1966.

Borrie, J., and Goldwater, L.: Columnar Cell-Lined Esophagus: Assessment of Etiology and Treatment; a 22 Year Experience, *J Thorac Cardiovasc Surg,* **71:**825, 1976.

Bremner, C. G., Lynch, V. P., and Ellis, F. H., Jr.: Barrett's Esophagus: Congenital or Acquired? An Experimental Study of Esophageal Mucosal Regeneration in the Dog, *Surgery,* **68:**209, 1970.

Bugden, W. F., and Delmonico, J. E., Jr.: Lower Esophageal Web, *J Thorac Cardiovasc Surg,* **31:**1, 1956.

Burgess, J. N., Payne, W. S., Andersen, H. A., Weiland, L. H., and Carlson, H. C.: Barrett Esophagus: The Columnar-Epithelial-Lined Lower Esophagus, *Mayo Clin Proc,* **46:**728, 1971.

Collis, J. L.: Gastroplasty, *Thorax,* **16:**197, 1961.

Gavriliu, D.: État actuel du procédé de reconstruction de l'oesophage par tube gastrique (138 malades opérés), *Ann Chir,* **19:**219, 1965.

Hawe, A., Payne, W. S., Weiland, L. H., and Fontana, R. S.: Adenocarcinoma in the Columnar Epithelial Lined Lower (Barrett) Oesophagus, *Thorax,* **28:**511, 1973.

Hill, L. D., Gelfand, M., and Bauermeister, D.: Simplified Management of Reflux Esophagitis with Stricture, *Ann Surg,* **172:**638, 1970.

Moersch, R. N., Ellis, F. H., Jr., and McDonald, J. R.: Pathologic Changes Occurring in Severe Reflux Esophagitis, *Surg Gynecol Obstet,* **108:**476, 1959.

Olsen, A. M., and Harrington, S. W.: Esophageal Hiatal Hernias of the Short Esophagus Type: Etiologic and Therapeutic Considerations, *J Thorac Cardiovasc Surg,* **17:**189, 1948.

Orringer, M. B., and Sloan, H.: Complications and Failings of the Combined Collis-Belsey Operation, *J Thorac Cardiovasc Surg.* (In press.)

Payne, W. S., Andersen, H. A., and Ellis, F. H., Jr.: Reappraisal of Esophagogastrectomy and Antral Excision in the Treatment of Short Esophagus, *Surgery,* **55:**344, 1964.

Pearson, F. G., and Henderson, R. D.: Long-Term Follow-up of Peptic Strictures Managed by Dilatation, Modified Collis Gastroplasty, and Belsey Hiatus Hernia Repair, *Surgery,* **80:**396, 1976.

————, Langer, B., and Henderson, R. D.: Gastroplasty and Belsey Hiatus Hernia Repair: An Operation for the Management of Peptic Stricture with Acquired Short Esophagus, *J Thorac Cardiovasc Surg,* **61:**50, 1971.

Radigan, L. R., Glover, J. L., Shipley, F. E., and Shoemaker, R. E.: Barrett Esophagus, *Arch Surg,* **112:**486, 1977.

Corrosive Esophagitis

Campbell, G. S., Burnett, H. F., Ransom, J. M., and Williams, G. D.: Treatment of Corrosive Burns of the Esophagus, *Arch Surg,* **112:**495, 1977.

Floberg, L. E., and Koch, H.: Effect of Cortisone on Scarification in Corrosive Lesions of Esophagus, *Acta Otolaryngol [Suppl.] (Stockh.),* **109:**33, 1953.

Ogura, J. H., Roper, C. L., and Burford, T. H.: Complete Functional Restitution of the Food Passages in Extensive Stenosing Caustic Burns, *J Thorac Cardiovasc Surg,* **42:**340, 1961.

Viscomi, G. J., Beekhuis, G. J., and Whitten, C. F.: An Evaluation of Early Esophagoscopy and Corticosteroid Therapy in the Management of Corrosive Injury of the Esophagus, *J Pediatr,* **59:**356, 1961.

Yudin, S. S.: The Surgical Construction of 80 Cases of Artificial Esophagus, *Surg Gynecol Obstet,* **78:**561, 1944.

Esophageal Perforation

Abbott, O. A., Mansour, K. A., Logan, W. D., Jr., Hatches, C. R., Jr., and Symbas, P. N.: Atraumatic So-called "Spontaneous" Rupture of the Esophagus: A Review of 47 Personal Cases with Comments on a New Method of Surgical Therapy, *J Thorac Cardiovasc Surg,* **59:**67, 1970.

Barrett, N. R.: Report of a Case of Spontaneous Perforation of the Oesophagus Successfully Treated by Operation, *Br J Surg,* **35:**216, 1947.

Dooling, J. A., and Zick, H. R.: Closure of an Esophagopleural Fistula Using Onlay Intercostal Pedicle Graft, *Ann Thorac Surg,* **3:**553, 1967.

Grillo, H. C., and Wilkins, E. W., Jr.: Esophageal Repair following Late Diagnosis of Intrathoracic Perforation, *Ann Thorac Surg,* **20:**387, 1975.

Johnson, J., Schwegman, C. W., and Kirby, C. K.: Esophageal Exclusion for Persistent Fistula following Spontaneous Rupture of the Esophagus, *J Thorac Cardiovasc Surg,* **32:**827, 1956.

Kinsella, T. J., Morse, R. W., and Hertzog, A. J.: Spontaneous Rupture of Esophagus, *J Thorac Cardiovasc Surg,* **17:**613, 1948.

McBurney, R. P., Kirklin, J. W., Hood, R. T., Jr., and Andersen, H. A.: One-Stage Esophagogastrectomy for Perforated Carcinoma in the Presence of Mediastinitis, *Proc Staff Meet Mayo Clin,* **28:**281, 1953.

Mackler, S. A.: Spontaneous Rupture of the Esophagus: An Experimental and Clinical Study, *Surg Gynecol Obstet,* **95:**345, 1952.

Mengoli, L. R., and Klassen, K. P.: Conservative Management of Esophageal Perforation, *Arch Surg,* **91:**238, 1965.

Menguy, R.: Near-Total Esophageal Exclusion by Cervical Esophagostomy and Tube Gastrostomy in the Management of Massive Esophageal Perforation: Report of a Case, *Ann Surg,* **173:**613, 1971.

Millard, A. H.: "Spontaneous" Perforation of the Oesophagus Treated by Utilization of a Pericardial Flap, *Br J Surg,* **58:**70, 1971.

Neuhof, H., and Jemerin, E. E.: "Acute Infections of the Mediastinum," The Williams & Wilkins Company, Baltimore, 1943.

Payne, W. S., and Larson, R. H.: Acute Mediastinitis, *Surg Clin North Am,* **49:**999, 1969.

Rao, K. V. S., Mir, M., and Cogbill, C. L.: Management of Perforations of the Thoracic Esophagus: A New Technic Utilizing a Pedicle Flap of Diaphragm, *Am J Surg,* **127:**609, 1974.

Seybold, W. D., Johnson, M. A., III, and Leary, W. V.: Perforation of the Esophagus: An Analysis of 50 Cases and an Account of Experimental Studies, *Surg Clin North Am,* **30:**1155, 1950.

Strauch, G. O., and Lynch, R. E.: Subphrenic Extrathoracic Rupture of the Esophagus: First Reported Case, *Ann Surg,* **161:** 213, 1965.

Takaro, T., Walkup, H. E., and Okano, T.: Esophagopleural Fistula as a Complication of Thoracic Surgery, *J Thorac Cardiovasc Surg,* **40:**179, 1960.

Thal, A. P.: A Unified Approach to Surgical Problems of the Esophagogastric Junction, *Ann Surg,* **168:**542, 1968.

Tuttle, W. M., and Barrett, R. J.: Late Esophageal Perforations, *Arch Surg,* **86:**695, 1963.

Urschel, H. C., Razzuk, M. A., Wood, R. E., Galbraith, N. F., and Paulson, D. L.: An Improved Surgical Technique for the Complicated Hiatal Hernia with Gastroesophageal Reflux, *Ann Thorac Surg,* **15:**443, 1973.

Weisel, W., and Raine, F.: Surgical Treatment of Traumatic Esophageal Perforation, *Surg Gynecol Obstet,* **94:**337, 1952.

Worman, L. W., Hurley, J. D., Pemberton, A. H., and Narodick, B. G.: Rupture of the Esophagus from External Blunt Trauma, *Arch Surg,* **85:**333, 1962.

Wychulis, A. R., Fontana, R. S., and Payne, W. S.: Instrumental Perforations of the Esophagus, *Dis Chest,* **55:**184, 1969.

———, ———, and ———: Noninstrumental Perforations of the Esophagus, *Dis Chest,* **55:**190, 1969.

Malignant Tumors

Akakura, I., Nakamura, Y., Kakegawa, T., Nakayama, R., Watanabe, H., and Kakegawa, T.: Surgery of Carcinoma of the Esophagus with Preoperative Radiation, *Chest,* **57:**47, 1970.

Akiyama, H., and Hiyama, M.: A Simple Esophageal Bypass Operation by the High Gastric Division, *Surgery,* **75:**674, 1974.

———, ———, and Miyazono, H.: Total Esophageal Reconstruction after Extraction of the Esophagus, *Ann Surg,* **182:**547, 1975.

———, Sato, Y., and Takahashi, F.: Immediate Pharyngogastrostomy following Total Esophagectomy by Blunt Dissection, *Jap J Surg,* **1:**225, 1971.

Andersen, H. A., McDonald, J. R., and Olsen, A. M.: Cytologic Diagnosis of Carcinoma of the Esophagus and Cardia of the Stomach, *Proc Staff Meet Mayo Clin,* **24:**245, 1949.

Bakamjian, V. Y.: Total Reconstruction of Pharynx with Medially Based Deltopectoral Skin Flap, *NY State J Med,* **68:**2771, 1968.

Bombeck, C. T., Coelho, R. G. P., and Nyhus, L. M.: Prevention of Gastroesophageal Reflux after Resection of the Lower Esophagus, *Surg Gynecol Obstet,* **130:**1035, 1970.

Clifton, E. E., Goodner, J. T., and Bronstein, E.: Preoperative Irradiation for Cancer of the Esophagus, *Cancer,* **13:**37, 1960.

Collis, J. L.: Surgical Treatment of Carcinoma of the Oesophagus and Cardia, *Br J Surg,* **58:**801, 1971.

Department of Surgery, Cancer Institute, Chinese Academy of Medical Sciences: Surgical Treatment of Carcinoma of Esophagus and Gastric Cardia: An Analysis of 1,432 Cases, *Chin Med J [Engl]* n.s., **1:**60, 1975.

Dickson, R. J.: Radiation Therapy in Carcinoma of the Esophagus: A Review, *Am J Med Sci,* **241:**662, 1961.

Duvoisin, G. E., Ellis, F. H., Jr., and Payne, W. S.: The Value of Palliative Prostheses in Malignant Lesions of the Esophagus, *Surg Clin North Am,* **47:**827, 1967.

Ellis, F. H., Jr., and Salzman, F. A.: Carcinoma of the Esophagus: Surgery versus Radiotherapy, *Postgrad Med,* **61:**167, 1977.

Farrell, K. H., Devine, K. D., Harrison, E. G., Jr., and Olsen, A. M.: Granular Cell Myoblastoma of the Esophagus: Incidence and Surgical Treatment, *Ann Otol Rhinol Laryngol,* **82:**784, 1973.

Garfinkle, J. M., and Cahan, W. G.: Primary Melanocarcinoma of the Esophagus, *Cancer,* **5:**921, 1952.

Gavriliu, D.: Aspects of Esophageal Surgery, *Curr Probl Surg,* **12:**36, 1975.

Griffen, W. O., Jr., Daugherty, M. E., McGee, E. M., and Utley, J. R.: Unified Approach to Carcinoma of the Esophagus, *Ann Surg,* **183:**511, 1976.

Gunnlaugsson, G. H., Wychulis, A. R., Roland, C., and Ellis, F. H., Jr.: Analysis of the Records of 1,657 Patients with Analysis of Carcinoma of the Esophagus and Cardia of the Stomach, *Surg Gynecol Obstet,* **130:**997, 1970.

Hawe, A., Payne, W. S., Weiland, L. H., and Fontana, R. S.: Adenocarcinoma in the Columnar Epithelial Lined Lower (Barrett) Oesophagus, *Thorax,* **28:**511, 1973.

Hughes, R. O., and Price, J.: Tylosis and Oesophageal Carcinoma (Letter to the Editor), *Br Med J,* **3:**111, 1971.

Inberg, M. V., Scheinin, T. M., Voutilainen, A., Havia, T., and Nikkanen, T. A. V.: Management of Oesophageal Carcinoma: A Report of 267 Cases, *Scand J Thorac Cardiovasc Surg,* **8:**220, 1974.

Joske, R. A., and Benedict, E. B.: The Role of Benign Esophageal Obstruction in the Development of Carcinoma of the Esophagus, *Gastroenterology,* **36:**749, 1959.

Kirklin, J. W., and Clagett, O. T.: Some Technical Aspects of Esophagogastrectomy for Carcinoma of the Lower Part of the Esophagus and Cardiac End of the Stomach, *Surg Clin North Am,* **31:**959, 1951.

Kiviranta, U. K.: Corrosion Carcinoma of the Esophagus: 381 Cases of Corrosion and Nine Cases of Corrosion Carcinoma, *Acta Otolaryngol (Stockh),* **42:**89, 1952.

Le Quesne, L. P., and Ranger, D.: Pharyngolaryngectomy, with Immediate Pharyngogastric Anastomosis, *Br J Surg,* **53:**105, 1966.

Leverment, J. N., and Milne, D. M.: Oesophagogastrectomy in the Treatment of Malignancy of the Thoracic Oesophagus and Cardia, *Br J Surg,* **61:**683, 1974.

Lewis, I.: The Surgical Treatment of Carcinoma of the Oesophagus: With Special Reference to a New Operation for Growths of the Middle Third, *Br J Surg,* **34:**18, 1946.

McKeown, K. C.: Trends in Oesophageal Resection for Carcinoma: With Special Reference to Total Oesophagectomy, *Ann R Coll Surg Engl,* **51:**213, 1972.

Manning, P. C., Jr., Beahrs, O. H., and Devine, K. D.: Pharyngoesophagoplasty: Interposition of Right Colon; Surgical Treatment of Six Cases of Cancer of the Hypopharynx and Upper Part of the Esophagus, *Arch Surg,* **88:**939, 1964.

Marks, R. D., Jr., Scruggs, H. J., and Wallace, K. M.: Preoperative Radiation Therapy for Carcinoma of the Esophagus, *Cancer,* **38:**84, 1976.

Nakayama, K.: Preoperative Irradiation in the Treatment of Patients with Carcinoma of the Oesophagus and of Some Other Sites, *Clin Radiol,* **15:**232, 1964.

Ong, G. B.: Resection and Reconstruction of the Oesophagus in Oesophageal Cancer, *J Jap Assoc Thorac Surg,* **22:**769, 1974.

Orringer, M. B., and Sloan, H.: Substernal Gastric Bypass of the Excluded Thoracic Esophagus for Palliation of Esophageal Carcinoma, *J Thorac Cardiovasc Surg,* **70:**836, 1975.

Parker, E. F., and Gregorie, H. B.: Carcinoma of the Esophagus: Long-Term Results, *JAMA,* **235:**1018, 1976.

————, ————, Arrants, J. E., and Ravenel, J. M.: Carcinoma of the Esophagus, *Ann Surg,* **171:**746, 1970.

Payne, W. S.: Esophageal Reflux Ulceration: Causes and Surgical Management, *Surg Clin North Am,* **51:**935, 1971.

————, and Bernatz, P. E.: One-Stage Resection and Reconstruction for Carcinoma of the Esophagogastric Junction, in R. L. Varco and J. P. Delaney, "Controversy in Surgery," W. B. Saunders Company, Philadelphia, 1976.

Pearson, J. G.: The Value of Radiotherapy in the Management of Esophageal Cancer, *Am J Roentgenol,* **105:**500, 1969.

People's Republic of China: Surgical Treatment of Cancer of the Esophagus in the County and Commune Hospitals in the Rural Regions (Abstract), *Bull Soc Int Chir,* **34:**281, 1975.

Raven, R. W.: Carcinoma of the Oesophagus: A Clinicopathological Study, *Br J Surg,* **36:**70, 1948.

Skinner, D. B., and DeMeester, T. R.: Permanent Extracorporeal Esophagogastric Tube for Esophageal Replacement, *Ann Thorac Surg,* **22:**107, 1976.

Talbert, J. L., and Cantrell, J. R.: Clinical and Pathologic Characteristics of Carcinosarcoma of the Esophagus, *J Thorac Cardiovasc Surg,* **45:**1, 1963.

Wilson, S. E., Plested, W. G., and Carey, J. S.: Esophagogastrectomy versus Radiation Therapy for Midesophageal Carcinoma, *Ann Thorac Surg,* **10:**195, 1970.

Wooky, H.: Cited by V. Y. Bakamjian, Total Reconstruction of Pharynx with Medially Based Deltopectoral Skin Flap, *NY State J Med,* **68:**2771, 1968.

Wychulis, A. R., Gunnlaugsson, G. H., and Clagett, O. T.: Carcinoma Occurring in Pharyngoesophageal Diverticulum: Report of Three Cases, *Surgery,* **66:**979, 1969.

————, Woolam, G. L., Andersen, H. A., and Ellis, F. H., Jr.: Achalasia and Carcinoma of the Esophagus, *JAMA,* **215:**1638, 1971.

Wynder, E. L., and Bross, I. J.: A Study of Etiological Factors in Cancer of the Esophagus, *Cancer,* **14:**389, 1961.

————, Hultberg, S., Jacobsson, F., and Bross, I. J.: Environmental Factors in Cancer of the Upper Alimentary Tract: A Swedish Study with Special Reference to Plummer-Vinson (Paterson-Kelly) Syndrome, *Cancer,* **10:**470, 1957.

————, and Mabuchi, K.: Etiological and Environmental Factors, *JAMA,* **226:**1546, 1973.

Benign Cysts and Tumors

Johnston, J. B., Clagett, O. T., and McDonald, J. R.: Smooth-Muscle Tumours of the Oesophagus, *Thorax,* **8:**251, 1953.

Moersch, H. J., and Harrington, S. W.: Benign Tumor of the Esophagus, *Ann Otol Rhinol Laryngol,* **53:**800, 1944.

Schmidt, H. W., Clagett, O. T., and Harrison, E. G., Jr.: Benign Tumors and Cysts of the Esophagus, *J Thorac Cardiovasc Surg,* **41:**717, 1961.

Miscellaneous Esophageal Lesions

Adler, R. H.: Congenital Esophageal Webs, *J Thorac Cardiovasc Surg,* **45:**175, 1963.

Creamer, B., Andersen, H. A., and Code, C. F.: Esophageal Motility in Patients with Scleroderma and Related Diseases, *Gastroenterologia,* **86:**763, 1956.

Daly, D. C., Code, C. F., and Andersen, H. A.: Disturbances of Swallowing and Esophageal Motility in Patients with Multiple Sclerosis, *Neurology* (Minneap.), **12:**250, 1962.

Donoghue, F. E., Winkelmann, R. K., and Moersch, H. J.: Esophageal Defects in Dermatomyositis, *Ann Otol Rhinol Laryngol,* **69:**1139, 1960.

Ellis, F. H., Jr.: Upper Esophageal Sphincter in Health and Disease, *Surg Clin North Am,* **51:**553, 1971.

Fisher, R. A., Ellison, G. W., Thayer, W. R., Spiro, H. M., and Glaser, G. H.: Esophageal Motility in Neuromuscular Disorders, *Ann Intern Med,* **63:**229, 1965.

Henderson, R. D., and Pearson, F. G.: Surgical Management of Esophageal Scleroderma, *J Thorac Cardiovasc Surg,* **66:**686, 1973.

———, Boszko, A., and vanNostrand, A. W. P.: Pharyngoesophageal Dysphagia and Recurrent Laryngeal Nerve Palsy, *J Thorac Cardiovasc Surg,* **68:**507, 1974.

———, Woolf, C., and Marryatt, G.: Pharyngoesophageal Dysphagia and Gastroesophageal Reflux, *Laryngoscope,* **86:**1531, 1976.

Kelley, M. L., Jr.: Dysphagia and Motor Failure of the Esophagus in Myotonia Dystrophica, *Neurology (Minneap),* **14:**955, 1964.

Kelly, A. B.: Spasm at the Entrance of the Oesophagus, *J Laryngol Otol,* **34:**285, 1919.

Lam, C. R., Taber, R. E., and Arciniegas, E.: The Nature and Surgical Treatment of Lower Esophageal Ring (Schatzki's Ring), *J Thorac Cardiovasc Surg,* **63:**34, 1972.

Mallory, G. K., and Weiss, S.: Hemorrhages from Lacerations of the Cardiac Orifice of the Stomach Due to Vomiting, *Am J Med Sci,* **178:**506, 1929.

Orringer, M. B., Dabich, L., Zarafonetis, C. J. D., and Sloan, H.: Gastroesophageal Reflux in Esophageal Scleroderma: Diagnosis and Implications, *Ann Thorac Surg,* **22:**120, 1976.

Palmer, E. D.: Disorders of the Cricopharyngeus Muscle: A Review, *Gastroenterology,* **71:**510, 1976.

Paterson, D. R.: A Clinical Type of Dysphagia, *J Laryngol Otol,* **34:**289, 1919.

Payne, W. S., and Olsen, A. M.: "The Esophagus," Lea & Febiger, Philadelphia. (In press.)

Schatzki, R., and Gary, J. E.: Dysphagia Due to a Diaphragm-like Localized Narrowing in the Lower Esophagus ("Lower Esophageal Ring"), *Am J Roentgenol,* **70:**911, 1953.

Smith, A. W. M., Mulder, D. W., and Code, C. F.: Esophageal Motility in Amyotrophic Lateral Sclerosis, *Proc Staff Meet Mayo Clin,* **32:**438, 1957.

Stiennon, O. A.: The Anatomic Basis for the Lower Esophageal Contraction Ring: Plication Theory and Its Applications, *Am J Roentgenol,* **90:**811, 1963.

Treacy, W. L., Baggenstoss, A. H., Slocumb, C. H., and Code, C. F.: Scleroderma of the Esophagus: A Correlation of Histologic and Physiologic Findings, *Ann Intern Med,* **59:**351, 1963.

Watson, W. C., and Sullivan, S. N.: Hypertonicity of the Cricopharyngeal Sphincter: A Cause of Globus Sensation, *Lancet,* **2:**1417, 1974.

Wesselhoeft, C. W., Jr., and Keshishian, J. M.: Acquired Nonmalignant Esophagotracheal and Esophagobronchial Fistulas, *Ann Thorac Surg,* **6:**187, 1968.

Wilkins, E. W., Jr., and Bartlett, M. K.: Surgical Treatment of the Lower Esophageal Ring, *N Engl J Med,* **268:**461, 1963.

Winans, C. S.: The Pharyngoesophageal Closure Mechanism: A Manometric Study, *Gastroenterology,* **63:**768, 1972.

Wychulis, A. R., Ellis, F. H., Jr., and Andersen, H. A.: Acquired Nonmalignant Esophagotracheobronchial Fistula: Report of 36 Cases, *JAMA,* **196:**117, 1966.

Other Diaphragmatic Hernias and Conditions

Beck, W. C., and Motsay, D. S.: Eventration of Diaphragm, *Arch Surg,* **65:**557, 1952.

Bernatz, P. E., Burnside, A. F., Jr., and Clagett, O. T.: Problem of the Ruptured Diaphragm, *JAMA,* **168:**877, 1958.

Butsch, W. L., and Leahy, L. J.: A Technique for the Surgical Treatment of Congenital Eventration of the Diaphragm in Infancy: Report of a Case, *J Thorac Cardiovasc Surg,* **20:**968, 1950.

Cerilli, G. J.: Foramen of Bochdalek Hernia: A Review of the Experience at Children's Hospital of Denver, Colorado, *Ann Surg,* **159:**385, 1964.

Chin, E. F., and Duchesne, E. R.: The Parasternal Defect, *Thorax,* **10:**214, 1955.

Comer, T. P., and Clagett, O. T.: Surgical Treatment of Hernia of the Foramen of Morgagni, *J Thorac Cardiovasc Surg,* **52:**461, 1966.

Effler, D. B.: Allison's Repair of Hiatal Hernia: Late Complication of Diaphragmatic Counterincision and Technique to Avoid It, *J Thorac Cardiovasc Surg,* **49:**669, 1965.

Gross, R. E.: "The Surgery of Infancy and Childhood: Its Principles and Techniques," W. B. Saunders Company, Philadelphia, 1953.

Kenigsberg, K., and Gwinn, J. L.: The Retained Sac in Repair of Posterolateral Diaphragmatic Hernia in the Newborn, *Surgery,* **57:**894, 1965.

Kiesewetter, W. B., Gutierrez, I. Z., and Sieber, W. K.: Diaphragmatic Hernia in Infants under One Year of Age, *Arch Surg,* **83:**561, 1961.

Nylander, P. E. A., and Elfving, G.: Partial Eventration of Diaphragm, *Ann Chir Gynaecol Fenn,* **40:**1, 1951.

Rosenkrantz, J. G., and Cotton, E. K.: Replacement of Left Hemidiaphragm by a Pedicled Abdominal Muscular Flap, *J Thorac Cardiovasc Surg,* **48:**912, 1964.

Snyder, W. H., Jr., and Greaney, E. M., Jr.: Congenital Diaphragmatic Hernia: 77 Consecutive Cases, *Surgery,* **57:**576, 1965.

Chapter 26

Stomach

by **René B. Menguy**

ANATOMY

The J-shaped organ lies between the esophagus and the duodenum, separated from the former by a multicomponent sphincter mechanism and from the latter by the anatomically well-defined pyloric sphincter. The stomach is described as having two borders, or curvatures, known as the lesser and greater curvatures, and two surfaces, anterior and posterior. The two curvatures of the stomach are important surgically, because of their relation to the major vascular and lymphatic arcades of the stomach. The arterial arcade along the lesser curvature is supplied by the left gastric artery, which originates from the celiac axis and divides into the left gastric artery proper, or descending branch, and the ascending esophageal branch, which supplies the cardiac portion of the stomach and the lower esophagus. The left gastric artery connects with the right gastric artery, a branch of the hepatic artery. Along the greater curvature of the stomach lies a vascular arcade formed by the right gastroepiploic artery, a branch of the gastroduodenal artery, sending gastric branches, each of which divides into anterior and posterior rami. At about the midportion of the greater curvature of the stomach, the right gastroepiploic artery connects with the left gastroepiploic artery, which rises from the splenic artery and reaches the greater curvature in the gastrosplenic ligament. The point at which the gastric branches of this vascular arcade change direction corresponds to the midportion of

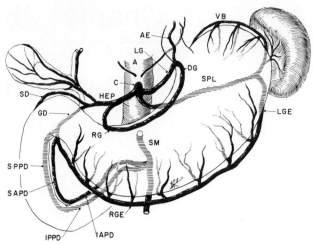

Fig. 26-1. Blood supply of the stomach. C, Celiac artery; LG, left gastric artery; AE, ascending esophageal artery; DG, descending gastric artery; RG, right gastric artery; GD, gastroduodenal artery; RGE, right gastroepiploic artery; LGE, left gastroepiploic artery; SPL, splenic artery; VB, vasa brevia.

the greater curvature. The left gastroepiploic also sends gastric branches to the greater curvature. The arterial arcade along the proximal segment of the greater curvature of the stomach is supplied by vasa brevia, which arise either from the splenic trunk or from the left gastroepiploic artery (Fig. 26-1).

Branches from these two arcades ramify through the entire submucosa, forming a plexus from which branches supply the mucosal membrane of the entire stomach, except for the lesser curvature; this receives its arterial supply directly from branches of the right and left gastric arteries. This anatomic arrangement of the arterial supply to the lesser curvature has been interpreted as rendering the lesser curvature more liable to ischemia. The veins and the lymphatics are distributed along the arterial arcades.

Knowledge of the autonomic nervous supply to the stomach by the vagus nerves is particularly important today because interruption of the parasympathetic supply to the stomach has become an essential part of the surgical treatment of duodenal ulcer. Distribution of vagus nerves

Fig. 26-2. Parasympathetic innervation of the stomach.

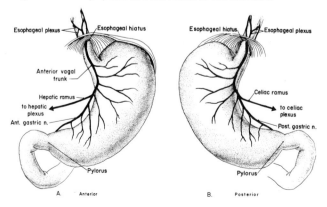

to the stomach is illustrated in Fig. 26-2. The preganglionic fibers in these nerves terminate by synapsing with ganglion cells of Auerbach's plexus located between the longitudinal and circular muscle layers of the stomach. Postganglionic fibers are distributed from these ganglion cells to the submucous (Meissner) network of nerve fibers. These postganglionic fibers are cholinergic. Postganglionic sympathetic fibers from the celiac plexus reach the stomach along the main gastric arteries.

GASTRIC FUNCTION

Three times a day the stomach discharges into the duodenum 500 to 1,000 ml of gastric chyme, a mixture of gastric juice and food subjected to gastric digestion. Actually, the digestive role of the stomach is rather unimportant. When food is chewed carefully, carbohydrates exposed to the action of salivary amylase are hydrolyzed as long as the gastric pH remains elevated, but as gastric pH falls, amylase becomes inactive. The contribution of the stomach to the digestion of dietary protein is minimal; only 10 to 15 percent is reduced to peptones. Although gastric pepsin is a powerful proteolytic enzyme, it can only initiate protein hydrolysis. It also disperses intracellular contents by digesting cell walls. However, denaturation of protein by gastric acid facilitates the action of other proteolytic enzymes of pancreatic and intestinal origin. The contribution of the stomach to lipolysis is negligible. In summary, the stomach decreases the particulate size of foodstuffs, denatures alimentary protein by acidification, and brings ingested materials to levels of temperature and osmolarity which will be tolerated by the mucosa of the proximal small bowel.

Motor Function

The musculature of the stomach differs from that of the remainder of the digestive tract by having three layers instead of two. An outer layer of longitudinal fibers continuous with the longitudinal coat of the esophagus is thickest along the two curvatures. The circular layer is continuous with the circular coat of the esophagus and is thickest over the prepyloric antrum. A deep layer of oblique fibers originates from the left side of the cardia and fans out toward the greater curvature. An important feature of the muscular coat of the stomach is its greater thickness in the prepyloric antrum.

The volume of the stomach fluctuates tremendously. When empty, its volume is 50 ml or less. As food enters its lumen the stomach wall relaxes and allows its volume to increase without a change in intragastric pressure until volumes of greater than 1,500 ml are reached. This ability of the stomach to accommodate a large increase in intraluminal volume without stretching of its walls is known as *receptive relaxation*. At rest, the stomach undergoes transient phases of nonpropulsive motor activity lasting for 5 to 10 minutes, separated by periods of 15 to 20 minutes of quiescence. When food enters the stomach, motor activity gradually increases. The characteristic manifestation of gastric motor activity is a peristaltic wave which originates near the cardia and travels toward the pylorus. At the beginning of a meal these waves are shallow and die out as they reach the antrum. Later, the waves become deeper and sweep over the antrum and pylorus.

The gastric peristaltic wave depends in part upon a reflex arc with afferent signals arising from sensory receptors in the stomach that are stimulated by gastric distension. Ascending fibers of this arc are carried in the vagus nerves, which also carry its efferent branches. During the height of digestion, peristaltic waves occurring at a rhythmic rate of approximately four per minute mix the gastric contents and force chyme into the antrum where gastric digestion occurs. Periodically, a portion of gastric chyme coming from the fundus of the stomach is propelled through the entire length of the antrum, where the greater thickness of the gastric wall increases the propulsive strength of the peristaltic wave. This portion of the stomach has the function of a pump. At rest, the pyloric muscle is relaxed, allowing its borders to be in apposition. Moreover, the absence of a pressure gradient between the stomach and the duodenum prevents the stomach from emptying its contents. As the antral peristaltic wave approaches the pylorus, its strength, as well as its speed, increases so that the antrum contracts almost as a unit; at the same time the pylorus relaxes because of the relaxation that precedes the peristaltic wave. In addition, the gastric peristaltic wave produces a positive pressure gradient from the stomach to the antrum which drives a small fraction of gastric chyme (2 to 6 ml) into the duodenum. At the end of the cycle the peristaltic wave traverses the pylorus, which contracts, and gastric emptying ends for that cycle. The fraction of gastric chyme evacuated into the duodenum is propelled distally by duodenal contractions and is prevented by the closure of the pylorus from refluxing into the stomach.

The entry of gastric chyme into the duodenum initiates "feedback" regulatory mechanisms which alter the rate of gastric emptying. Excessive variations of temperature, of tonicity, or a pH below 3.5 all reduce gastric motility and the rate of gastric emptying. These inhibitory influences are mediated by hormonal substances released from the mucosa of the proximal small intestine under the influence of one of the conditions listed above. These hormones are known as *enterogastrones.* Secretin may be involved in the inhibition of gastric motility occurring when the duodenal pH falls below 3.5 since secretin release from the duodenum is brought about, *inter alia,* by duodenal acidification and since secretin is known to inhibit gastric motility in addition to inhibiting gastrin-stimulated gastric acid secretion. A particularly strong inhibition of gastric motility takes place when the gastric chyme reaching the proximal small intestine has a high fat content. The hormonal substance for the mediation of this gastric inhibition by fat—the first enteric hormone to be called enterogastrone—unlike secretin and cholecystokinin, has not yet been defined as a distinct chemical entity.

Secretory Function

HISTOLOGY. The gastric mucosa is divided into three parts: the *cardiac gland area* forms a 1- to 3-cm-wide strip beginning at the esophagogastric junction; the *fundus or parietal cell area,* primarily responsible for secretion of acid and pepsin, occupies the proximal three-fourths of the gastric mucosa; the *antrum or pyloric gland area* occupies the distal one-fourth of the stomach. The mucosal surface consists of a columnar epithelium. Over the fundus the mucosa is thrown into numerous "rugal" folds which increase its secretory surface. The antral mucosa is almost completely flat. Microscopic examination of the mucosal surface reveals multiple pits or *foveolae* into which open three or four gastric glands. The types of cells lining the gland vary according to the region of the stomach. In the fundus the mucosal surface and the foveolae are lined by *surface mucous cells* containing numerous granules of mucin. At the junction of the body of the gland with the gastric pit, *mucous neck cells* also containing mucin granules are found. The function of these cells will be discussed below. In the upper portion of the gland the predominant cell type is the *parietal cell,* a large pyramidal-shaped cell with the base on the basement membrane of the gland with a centrally placed nucleus and a finely granular, eosinophilic cytoplasm. These cells have the function of producing HCl and, in humans, intrinsic factor. In the

Fig. 26-3. Schematic illustration of a gastric gland. (*From S. Ito et al., J Cell Biol, 16:541, 1963.*)

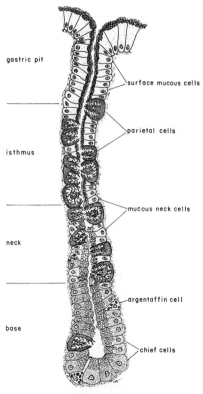

gastric pit

surface mucous cells

parietal cells

isthmus

mucous neck cells

neck

argentaffin cell

base

chief cells

GASTRIC GLAND

deeper portion of the fundic glands the predominant cell type is the *chief cell,* a cuboidal-shaped cell with a basally situated nucleus and a basophilic cytoplasm which is responsible for the elaboration of *pepsinogen.* In addition, true argentaffin and argyrophilic cells, whose functions are not known, are found (Fig. 26-3). The *cardiac glands* are characterized by a shallow foveola and a short length. They are lined mainly by mucous cells. The *pyloric mucosa* is covered by surface mucous cells similar to those lining the remainder of the stomach. The glandular foveolae are deeper than in the fundus and the deeper portions of the glands are coiled. The cells lining the glands are similar to the mucous neck cells in the fundus. The major secretory product of these glands is mucus. Unidentified cells in the pyloric mucosa are responsible for the elaboration of the hormone *gastrin.*

In between the glands and foveolae lies the *lamina propria,* a loose aggregation of connective tissue, lymphocytes, plasma cells, and mast cells containing serotonin and histamine. The mucosa is separated from the submucosa by a thin layer of smooth muscle, the *muscularis mucosae.*

Renewal of the Surface Epithelium. The surface mucous cells lining the lumen undergo continuous renewal due to mitotic activity confined to mucous neck cells situated in the isthmus of the glands. The daughter cells migrate up the walls of the foveolae, reach the surface, and are eventually exfoliated into the lumen. The whole cycle covers approximately 36 hours in the rat, the animal in which this phenomenon, crucial to the health of the mucosa, has been most extensively studied. Although the neck mucous cells differentiate primarily into surface mucous cells, they appear also to contribute to a much slower renewal of chief and parietal cells.

The histology of the superficial duodenal mucosa resembles that of the remainder of the small intestine. The characteristic feature of the mammalian duodenum is the presence in the proximal duodenum of *glands of Brunner.* Situated in the submucosa they empty into the crypts of Lieberkühn via small secretory ducts. Their viscous, mucoid alkaline secretion probably contributes to the protection of the duodenal mucosa against the corrosive action of gastric juice.

METHODS OF STUDYING GASTRIC SECRETION. To study glandular function one must be able to collect the secretory product. For experimental purposes the collection of gastric juice uncontaminated by saliva and food is possible with the gastric pouch preparations devised by Heidenhain and Pavlov, illustrated in Fig. 26-4. A vagally denervated pouch is used to study humoral influences on gastric secretion, since the only systemic connections of the pouch are via its blood supply. A vagally innervated pouch serves to study neural influences on gastric secretion.

Human gastric secretion both in health and disease is measured by placing under radioscopic control the aspirating tip of a tube in the most dependent portion of the stomach. Gastric secretions are withdrawn, preferably by manual suction, for a determined period of time and under various conditions. It is important that the subject be instructed to spit his saliva continuously during the collection.

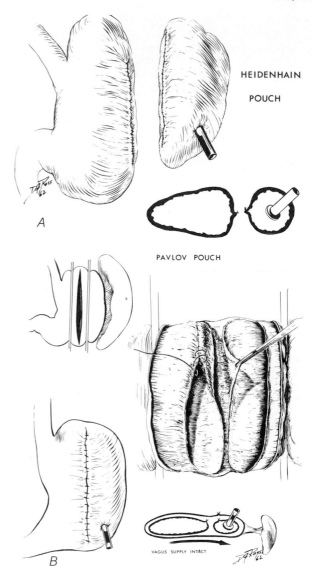

Fig. 26-4. Schematic illustration of (*A*) vagally denervated (Heidenhain) and (*B*) vagally innervated (Pavlov) gastric pouches. [*Reproduced from Ballinger (ed.), "Research Methods in Surgery," Little, Brown and Company, Boston, 1964.*]

COMPOSITION OF GASTRIC JUICE. Gastric secretion is not the simple hydrochloric acid solution often depicted in advertisements for antacids. The components for gastric juice can be divided into two parts: organic and inorganic.

Organic Constituents of Gastric Juice. *Mucus.* Gastric mucus, secreted predominantly by the prepyloric glands but also by the surface epithelial cells lining the stomach, is a heterogeneous mixture of several molecular species. Although their molecular structures are not known, several are glycoproteins of very high molecular weight. These mucoid secretions have characteristic properties of adhesiveness, cohesiveness, and high viscosity, allowing them to form a thin layer adherent to the mucosa. It has been postulated that this layer of mucus limits the access of gastric juice to the underlying epithelium. A corollary of this view is that a deficiency in the quantity of mucus or its quality could lead to peptic ulceration. In addition to these physicochemical properties, the glycoproteins comprising the major portion of gastric mucus are resistant to enzymatic proteolysis, a quality imparted to the molecule of glycoprotein by its carbohydrate prosthetic groups.

Pepsinogen. The important proteolytic enzyme, pepsin, is secreted by the chief cells of the fundus of the stomach in the form of an inactive precursor called *pepsinogen*. The latter is formed by the coupling of the active molecule of pepsin with a peptide called the *pepsin inhibitor*. Below a pH of 5, disassociation of the pepsin inhibitor liberates active pepsin. The activity of pepsin is greatest when the pH of the medium is 2. Above pH levels of 5 peptic activity gradually decreases. Recent studies have shown that human gastric juice contains several types of pepsin with different optimal pH levels.

Pepsinogen is also found in blood and urine. Uropepsinogen undoubtedly comes from the stomach, since it disappears from the urine after a total gastrectomy. Unfortunately, uropepsinogen levels cannot be utilized to measure gastric secretory activity because of a poor correlation between the two.

Intrinsic Factor. Intrinsic factor (IF), discovered by Castle, appears to be a mucoprotein which binds with vitamin B_{12}. The IF-vitamin B_{12} complex renders vitamin B_{12} unavailable to intestinal microorganisms. Dissociation of this complex occurs in the ileum, where vitamin B_{12} is absorbed. The fate of intrinsic factor is unknown. Malabsorption of vitamin B_{12} occurs in patients with pernicious anemia whose stomachs do not elaborate IF, and after total gastrectomy. Vitamin B_{12} deficiency appears only after 3 to 7 years following a total gastrectomy, since the daily needs of vitamin B_{12} are 1 to 2 μg and the normal liver stores approximately 2 mg.

Blood Group Substances. In about 75 percent of the population the stomach secretes into gastric juice the major blood group antigens A, B, and H(O) as well as minor blood group antigens such as the Lewis substances (Le^a and Le^b). Individuals who have the Le^{a+} substance on their red blood cells (about 25 percent of the population are Le^{a+}) in addition to their major blood group antigen do not secrete their major blood group antigens into their gastric juice or saliva, but secrete similar amounts of Lewis^a antigen. For unknown reasons, these individuals, called "nonsecretors," are more liable to duodenal ulceration than "secretors." These blood group antigens found in gastric juice, saliva, and other body fluids are *water-soluble* glycoproteins containing galactose, L-fucose, galactosamine, glucosamine, N-acetylneuraminic acid. The corresponding antigens extractable from red blood cell membranes are alcohol-soluble lipoglycoproteins.

Nonorganic Constituents of Gastric Juice. HCl, secreted by the parietal cells, is the important and characteristic nonorganic constituent of gastric juice. 0.167 N HCl from the parietal cells is admixed with varying amounts of secretions from the other gastric mucosal cells, so that aspirated gastric juice contains Na^+ and K^+, and HCO_3, in addition to HCl. Although the levels of the ions are constantly changing, the average concentrations are Na,

65 mEq; K, 13 mEq; Cl, 100 mEq; and H, 90 mEq. The molar concentration of Cl exceeds that of H^+, because a small amount of "neutral" Cl is secreted as KCl and NaCl. There is a reciprocal relationship between ions, so that as H^+ increases, Na^+ and K^+ decrease. A fundamental consideration in the study of gastric secretory function is the quantification of the concentration of HCl in gastric juice.

Measurement of Gastric Acidity. Juice is collected by one of the methods described above for fixed periods, usually 15 minutes. The H^+ concentration of each sample is estimated by pH measure and by titration to an end point of 7. Results are expressed as mEq HCl/15 minutes [volume of 15-minute sample (liters) $\times$ HCl concentration (mEq/L)].

Mechanism of HCl Secretion. The essential aspects of gastric juice secretion are well established. The parietal cells elaborate hydrogen ion, chloride, water, and intrinsic factor. The chief cells secrete pepsinogen, and chloride may come from other cells as well as from the parietal cells. The principal anion in gastric juice is chloride, and during slow rates of acid secretion, the other cation is sodium. The maximal concentration of acid in the gastric juice is between 140 and 160 mEq/L which represents a concentration gradient over two million times greater than that in the blood bathing the gastric cells. The important questions with respect to the mechanism of HCl secretion are the following: How does the parietal cell establish this concentration gradient? How does the stomach alter it? How does the stomach maintain it?

The actual secretion of hydrogen ion into the canaliculi of the parietal cells against an enormous concentration gradient is dependent upon a "pump" mechanism utilizing energy derived from high-energy substrates. During the secretion it is possible that sodium ion in the glandular tubule is exchanged for hydrogen ion.

It is almost certain that the secretion from a parietal cell always has a "maximal," constant acidity of about 160 to 170 mEq/L. Variations in the concentration of acid in the gastric juice appear due in part to dilution of the parietal cell secretion by alkaline secretions from the other cells. The more important regulatory mechanism may be the variable rate at which hydrogen ion diffuses back from lumen to mucosa. At low rates of acid secretion this back diffusion would be great and would be offset by an enhanced movement of sodium ion from plasma to lumen. The reverse would occur during high rates of secretion.

To explain how the stomach can maintain such an enormous concentration gradient of hydrogen ion between the lumen and the plasma, one must introduce the concept of a gastric mucosal *barrier*.

Gastric Mucosal Barrier. Hydrogen ion in gastric juice is separated from the interior of mucosal cells at two sites, the canaliculi of the parietal cells and the luminal border of the cells lining the glands and the mucosal surface. The two sites form a barrier which gives the stomach its unique property of "holding" a high concentration of HCl in its lumen. To this barrier one must attach a feature of *variable permeability*.

Studies conducted mainly in experimental animals have shown that natural (i.e., normal) differences in mucosal permeability occur from one animal to another and may account in part for individual variations in gastric acidity under standard conditions of gastric stimulation. Intraindividual variations of mucosal permeability to hydrogen ion *under physiologic conditions* remain to be studied. However, the classical studies of Davenport have shown that in contrast to the small permeability of the *normal* gastric mucosa to hydrogen ion, injury of the mucosa with agents such as eugenol, acetic acid, or aspirin in HCl increases its permeability to hydrogen ion enormously. Such an abnormally permeable mucosa can no longer generate or maintain a high concentration of hydrogen ion. It is reasonable to postulate that the stomach's capacity to retain digestive juices within its lumen and away from the mucosal tissues depends upon the integrity of this barrier. In all likelihood this relative impermeability to hydrogen ion results not from a static "barrier" (impervious membrane) but from an ATP(adenosine triphosphate)-dependent, energy-consuming process.

REGULATION OF GASTRIC SECRETION. Stimulation of Gastric Secretion. The mechanisms responsible for a secretory response to a meal have been divided into three phases: the cephalic, gastric, and intestinal phases of gastric secretion. For reasons that will be discussed below, a classification of the stimulatory mechanisms into two phases, vagal-antral and intestinal, is more in agreement with modern physiologic data.

Vagal-Antral Phase. The sight, thought, smell, and taste of food coinciding with the beginning of a meal provoke a strong secretory response. These stimuli are mediated to the stomach by the vagus nerves. This neural influence on gastric secretion is exerted via two mechanisms: a direct stimulating effect on the parietal cells, and an indirect stimulating influence on the parietal cells mediated by the vagally induced release of the hormone *gastrin* by the antrum. Vagal stimulation of gastric secretion can be induced by the administration of insulin (0.2 μg/Kg body weight). The resulting hypoglycemia stimulates vagal centers with a resulting increase in vagal tone. Characteristically, gastric juice secreted in response to vagal stimulation has a high concentration of pepsin.

When the bolus of food enters the stomach, distension of the antrum further enhances the elaboration of the stimulatory hormone *gastrin,* the release of which has already been initiated by vagal stimulation of the antrum.

Gastrin. Although the concept of a humoral phase of gastric secretion originated in 1906 with the work of Edkins, only recently has the concept been fully accepted; that occurred only after Gregory succeeded in extracting pure gastrin from the antral mucosa of man and animals, determined its structure, and synthesized it. Gastrin, the most potent known stimulant of gastric acid secretion, is a heptadecapeptide amide. The principal action of gastrin is a strong stimulation of the secretion of water, electrolytes, and intrinsic factor by the stomach; the secretion of pepsin is stimulated only weakly. Gastrin also stimulates water and electrolyte secretion of the liver, pancreas, and Brunner's glands. It inhibits absorption of water and electrolytes by ileal mucosa. It increases the tone of the lower esopha-

geal sphincter, reduces the tone of the sphincter of Oddi, and increases the motility of the stomach, intestine, and gallbladder. Gastrin also has a potent *trophic* action on the gastric mucosa. These physiologic properties are carried by the C-terminal tetrapeptide amide portion of the molecule (tryp-met-asp-phe-NH$_2$). It is interesting that *cholecystokinin,* a hormone released by the small intestine, has the identical amino acid sequence at its C-terminus. Although these two hormones act on the same targets, the intrinsic activities by which they act on a given site differ. Gastrin is a far more potent stimulus to gastric acid secretion than cholecystokinin. The latter stimulates acid secretion weakly and actually inhibits gastrin-stimulated acid secretion (competitive inhibition). On the other hand, cholecystokinin is a far more potent stimulant of gall bladder motility than gastrin. The structures of gastrins from various mammalian species (man, dog, sheep, hog, cat) are virtually identical. In all species gastrin occurs in two forms: gastrin I, in which a tyrosine residue is nonsulfated, and gastrin II, in which the tyrosine is sulfated. Both forms have the same potency on acid secretion. The gastrin produced by pancreatic islet-cell tumors (Zollinger-Ellison syndrome) and that produced by the human antrum are identical. Both occur as a mixture of gastrins I and II. In the blood gastrin circulates in the form of a larger molecule ("big gastrin") than the 17 amino acid residue polypeptide extractable from the antrum.

Although gastrin is formed in small amounts in the gastric fundus and the proximal small intestine, the principal site of gastrin formation is in the antral mucosa in as-yet-undetermined cells. The release of gastrin into the circulation by the antral mucosa occurs in response to vagal stimulation, to distension of the antrum and to the presence in its lumen of specific secretagogues such as peptone solutions. These factors potentiate each other so that a vagally denervated antrum releases less gastrin in response to a given degree of distension than when its vagal innervation was intact. These stimuli of gastrin release are strengthened when the antral contents are alkaline and are suppressed when the pH in the antrum falls below 2.0.

The release of gastrin from the antral mucosa is blocked by *secretin* and enhanced by *calcium.* In addition, secretin inhibits the action of gastrin on the parietal cell.

In addition to a synergism between vagal innervation of the antrum and gastrin release during mechanical or chemical stimulation of the antrum, gastrin and vagal stimuli act synergistically on the parietal cell. Denervated parietal cells respond less to exogenous gastrin. Therefore, separation of a cephalic, or neural, phase from a gastric, or humoral, phase of gastric secretion is no longer justified.

Synthetic derivatives of gastrin like the pentapeptide (*N-t*-butyloxycarbonyl-B ala-tryp-met-asp-phe-NH$_2$) "pentagastrin" have a potent stimulating effect on gastric secretion and have proved very useful in the experimental and clinical study of gastric acid secretion.

Intestinal Phase. Gastric secretory activity reaches a peak with each meal and then wanes. However, secretion never stops. The stimuli influencing the stomach between meals belong to the intestinal phase of gastric secretion. In an animal with a denervated total gastric pouch and an esophagoduodenal anastomosis, a weak secretory response lasting for 5 or 6 hours occurs several hours after a meal. The stimuli responsible for this phase of gastric secretion are not known. Possibly certain by-products of digestion of dietary substances, such as histamine, formed by the bacterial decarboxylation of histidine, may be involved. An active gastric secretory response follows the direct introduction of peptones or histamine into the small intestine.

Inhibition of Gastric Secretion. Several factors intervene at the end of gastric digestion to inhibit gastric secretory activity. It is convenient to classify these in the same categories considered for the stimulatory factors.

Vagal-Antral Phase. An important mechanism for the decrease in gastric secretion 2 to 3 hours after a meal relates to the decrease in vagal activity. This is an example of inhibition due to removal of a stimulus. The importance of this vagal cutoff can be demonstrated in the experimental animal with a vagally innervated gastric pouch and an esophageal fistula. Sham feeding causes prolonged gastric secretion due to continuous vagal stimulation of the pouch.

Antral distension, an important stimulus to gastrin release from the antrum, subsides with gastric emptying. Moreover, it has been shown that the low pH in the antrum at the end of gastric digestion interrupts gastrin release. This phenomenon of "acid inhibition" is activated when antral contents reach a pH level of 2. In addition, it has been postulated that the acidified antrum releases an inhibitory hormone. However, the existence of this inhibitory chalone remains unproved.

Intestinal Phase. The entry of acid gastric chyme into the duodenum lowers duodenal pH and triggers an important inhibitory mechanism. This phenomenon of duodenal acid inhibition was first demonstrated by Sokolov. Many investigators have confirmed the fact that acidification of the duodenum inhibits both gastric secretion and motility via neural and humoral pathways. Because the hormone secretin inhibits gastrin-stimulated gastric secretion in addition to stimulating pancreatic secretion, it is possible that this hormone, which is released by the acidified duodenum, may mediate duodenal acid inhibition of gastric secretion. In addition to duodenal acid inhibition, the presence of fat in the proximal small intestine decreases gastric secretion and motility. It has been postulated that the mucosa of the duodenum, when in contact with fat, releases a gastric inhibitory chalone known as "enterogastrone."

In addition, extreme variations in tonicity or temperature of chyme entering the duodenum also have a mild inhibitory influence on gastric function.

The cyclic waxing and waning of gastric secretory activity corresponding with meals is due to the smooth interplay of these stimulatory and inhibitory factors. Under certain conditions these physiologic mechanisms become deranged, and altered states of gastric function characteristic of disease occur.

PEPTIC ULCER DISEASE

A peptic ulcer is a mucosal defect located in an area adjacent to or in acid-secreting epithelium. Accordingly, it can be found in the lower esophagus, the body of the stomach, the duodenum, in the jejunum marginal to a surgically constructed gastrojejunostomy and in the ileum at the outlet of a Meckel's diverticulum containing aberrant gastric mucosa. By definition an *ulcer* penetrates beyond the muscularis mucosae whereas an *erosion* is superficial to this layer. Traditionally all "ulcerating" lesions in the gastroduodenal area have been called "peptic ulcers." Recent knowledge has enabled the separation of these lesions into several distinct entities.

1. Duodenal ulcer diathesis
   a. Duodenal ulcer
   b. Ulcer immediately proximal to the pylorus or in the pyloric canal
   c. Combined gastric and duodenal ulcer
2. Gastric ulcer
3. Acute gastric mucosal lesions (erosive gastritis)

At the turn of the century, peptic ulceration became an increasingly important cause of morbidity. Data from the National Center for Health Statistics indicated that the annual prevalence rate for peptic ulcer was 19 per 1,000 adults per year in 1965. This figure was 30 percent greater than the rate for 1959. The total deaths attributed to peptic ulcer were estimated to be 12,500 in 1965.

The incidence of gastroduodenal ulceration and the ratio of duodenal (DU) to gastric ulceration (GU) have changed considerably since the last century when "peptic" ulcers were usually gastric, duodenal ulceration being rarely mentioned by pathologists of the nineteenth century. Acute gastric ulceration in young women was a common clinical problem. At the turn of the century a commonly quoted DU:GU ratio was 1:20. Since then and until the mid-1960s, the incidence of duodenal ulceration has increased, and this, coupled with a decrease in the prevalence of gastric ulceration, has resulted in the generally accepted DU:GU ratio of 10:1. Since the mid-1960s the incidence of duodenal ulceration has, for unknown reasons, decreased by almost 40 percent. This evolution of peptic ulcer disease has not been uniform throughout the world. Certain areas such as Japan and parts of South America remain afflicted with a high incidence of gastric ulceration. Another interesting aspect of the evolution of peptic ulcer disease is the change brought about by violent social upheavals such as the two world wars, during which the incidence of gastric ulceration among the civilian European population on both sides of the conflict increased sharply.

DUODENAL ULCER DIATHESIS

The duodenal ulcer diathesis is characterized by the presence of a chronic ulcer in the duodenal mucosa usually in the base of the bulb on its anterior or posterior wall. Other locations are the superior or the inferior recess of the bulb, the postbulbar mucosa, or rarely, the second portion of the duodenum. As mentioned above, ulcerations located in the pyloric canal or immediately proximal to it belong to the duodenal ulcer diathesis, as do jejunal ulcers appearing at the margin of a gastrojejunostomy after a partial gastrectomy for duodenal ulcer.

Pathogenesis

The best explanation for this condition is that the ulceration results from a relative or absolute excess of acid-peptic gastric secretions. Several arguments support this view.

The average patient with duodenal ulcer has higher rates of gastric acid secretion than an ulcer-free subject of the same age and sex in the general population (Table 26-1).

Conditions producing extremely high rates of gastric acid secretion are associated with a very high incidence of duodenal ulceration.

Continuous stimulation of gastric acid secretion in dogs produces duodenal ulceration.

Constant infusion of acid gastric juice into the duodenum of experimental animals produces duodenal ulceration.

The production of a relative hyperacidity in the gastric outlet zone of dogs by diversion of the alkaline pancreatic secretion to another segment of the gut (Mann-Williamson preparation, Figs. 26-5 and 26-6) results in lesions similar to human duodenal ulcers.

The temporary reduction of gastric acidity by buffers alleviates the symptoms of duodenal ulceration, and healing of the ulcer follows permanent reduction of acidity by surgical means. However, some aspects of the relationship between acid output and duodenal ulceration remain unclear, suggesting

Table 26-1. BASAL AND HISTALOG-STIMULATED GASTRIC SECRETION IN NORMAL SUBJECTS AND IN PATIENTS WITH PEPTIC ULCER OR WITH GASTRIC CANCER

Condition	Basal acid output, mEq/hr	Histalog,* mEq/1 hr post-Histalog
Normal:		
Male	2.44 ± 2.85	11.64 ± 7.62
Female	1.33 ± 2.00	7.53 ± 5.20
Duodenal ulcer:		
Male	5.29 ± 4.63	19.91 ± 9.70
Female	2.87 ± 3.14	13.42 ± 6.87
Gastric ulcer:		
Male	1.45 ± 1.99	9.68 ± 6.97
Female	1.00 ± 1.49	7.95 ± 5.96
Gastric cancer:		
Male	0.45 ± 1.23	3.25 ± 4.79
Female	0.16 ± 0.47	1.46 ± 2.50

*Histalog given in a dose of 0.5 mg/kg of body weight.
SOURCE: Data from Grossman et al., *Gastroenterology,* **45**:14, 1963.

that some factor other than acid-peptic activity may intervene. Although *average* gastric output is higher in patients with duodenal ulcer than in ulcer-free subjects, the values overlap greatly; many patients with an ulcer have normal acid outputs. Even

Fig. 26-5. The similarity between the marginal ulceration that used to occur after a Roux en Y bypass of the duodenum and the ulcer occurring in animals after total diversion of duodenal secretions to the ileum. Both lesions result from hyperacidity of the gastric outlet zone.

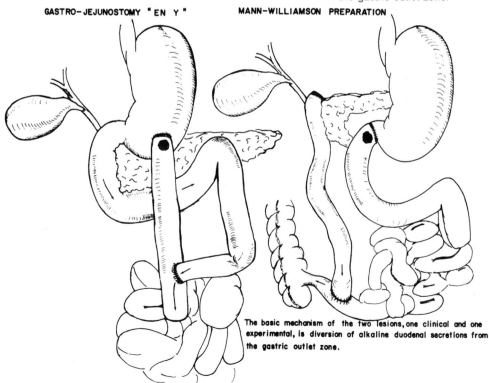

GASTRO-JEJUNOSTOMY "EN Y"   MANN-WILLIAMSON PREPARATION

The basic mechanism of the two lesions, one clinical and one experimental, is diversion of alkaline duodenal secretions from the gastric outlet zone.

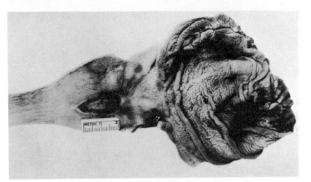

Fig. 26-6. Example of a Mann-Williamson ulcer from Mann's first experiment. (*Courtesy of Dr. Jesse Bollman.*)

more surprising is the absence of duodenal ulceration in some patients with gastric-producing pancreatic islet-cell tumors and enormously elevated levels of acid output.

Unless a serious complication supervenes, most duodenal ulcers heal spontaneously. *Healing is not accompanied by a decrease in gastric acid output.*

ROLE OF PEPSIN. The relation between duodenal ulceration and gastric acidity has evolved because acid output is easily quantified, whereas pepsin output can only be estimated as *peptic activity* in gastric juice. Its role is important since the tissue destruction characteristic of ulcerogenesis requires peptic activity. Yet pepsin cannot be considered separately, any more than can acid be. Human pepsins have acid pH optima. The longer the gastric outlet zone's pH remains within the range where pepsin is active (as when excessive acid output overwhelms the buffering capacity of duodenal secretions), the longer will the duodenal mucosa remain exposed to the proteolytic action of pepsin. Thus gastric acid and pepsins operate in concert, not only in the degradation of dietary protein but also in the mucosal destruction characteristic of ulcerogenesis. As a general rule, the gastric output of peptic activity parallels that of acid.

Because of the importance of the acid-peptic factor many studies of the etiology of duodenal ulceration have been directed at the mechanism of the acid hypersecretion so often present. Several possibilities have been explored.

MECHANISM OF GASTRIC HYPERACIDITY. Excessive Neural Stimulation of Gastric Secretion. It has been suggested that increased vagal impulses of subconscious origin may cause hypersecretion accompanying duodenal ulcer. This theory is based on the well-known fact that vagotomy, when complete, abolishes gastric hypersecretion. This observation, although correct, does not prove the theory, since another influence of the vagus nerves on gastric secretion, in addition to direct and indirect stimulation, is to render the parietal cell more reactive. Therefore, one would expect vagotomy to decrease HCl production regardless of the nature of the abnormal stimulus initially responsible for the hypersecretion.

Excessive Hormonal Stimulation of Gastric Secretion. The recent availability of serum gastrin assay based on radioimmunoassay with antibodies to synthetic human gastrin I has made it possible to estimate serum gastrin levels under various conditions in normal subjects and in patients with duodenal ulceration. McGuigan has found that fasting serum gastrin levels are not higher in patients with duodenal ulceration than in ulcer-free control subjects. However recent studies suggest that serum gastrin levels may reach higher levels than those in normal subjects in response to vagal stimulation. At present the role of gastrin output in the etiology of the common variety of duodenal ulcer (as distinguished from the Zollinger-Ellison syndrome) remains unclear.

Impairment of Physiologic Mechanism Responsible for Gastric Inhibition. This theory has received the least experimental support. Patients with duodenal ulcer appear to have a normal drop in gastric secretion upon acidification of the antrum or the duodenum. However, gastric emptying is more rapid in patients with a duodenal ulcer than in ulcer-free subjects. This, coupled with an augmented acid output, should have an adverse effect on the duodenal mucosa.

Excessive Capacity to Produce Acid. This hypothesis is an attractive one. It has been shown that stomachs of patients with duodenal ulcer contain more parietal cells than those of normal individuals. This in turn causes the greater maximal histamine response often found in patients with duodenal ulcer. Furthermore, the predominance of duodenal ulcer in males may be explained by the fact that, generally men have more parietal cells than women. It would be attractive to view the greater parietal cell mass in patients with duodenal ulcer as a genetically inherited trait, in turn responsible for hypersecretion and duodenal ulcer production. However, it could also represent the result of work hyperplasia in response to an unknown stimulus. The latter explanation appears more valid at present, since recent animal studies have shown that parietal cell hyperplasia accompanies constant gastric stimulation produced by chronic administration of histamine or following construction of an Eck fistula.

Genetic Aspects of Duodenal Ulceration. An excess of peptic ulcer disease exists among siblings of patients with this condition. Moreover, such studies have shown that this predisposition is type-specific; an excess of duodenal ulcer exists among the relatives of patients with a duodenal ulcer and the same is true for gastric ulcer among the relatives of patients with this lesion. In addition, it has been proven by several workers that subjects with blood group O are more prevalent among patients with a duodenal ulcer than in the control population. This relationship is particularly strong for duodenal ulceration complicated by bleeding. Another factor to consider is an individual's "secretor status." Approximately 75 percent of our population secrete into saliva, gastric juice, and urine, water-soluble blood group antigens immunologically identical to the blood group antigens on their red blood cells. They are "secretors." The remainder are all Le^{a+} and instead of their major blood group antigen, they secrete into these body fluids the Lewis antigen. These subjects are "nonsecretors," a state determined by the Le^{a+} phenotype. Nonsecretors are more liable to duodenal ulceration than secretors. It is interesting that the greater risk associated with the nonsecretor status and the risk associated with blood group

O are additive, so that an individual with type O blood who is also a nonsecretor of H(O) antigen in gastric and salivary secretions is almost three times more liable to duodenal ulceration than someone who is A or B and Le^{a-}. There is no explanation for this well-documented phenomenon.

ASSOCIATION OF PEPTIC ULCER WITH OTHER CLINICAL ENTITIES. Extragastric factors appear to influence the stomach in a way not always related to gastric secretion. The greater frequency of duodenal ulcer in association with certain disease entities suggests such relationships.

Pulmonary Disease. Carefully controlled clinical and autopsy studies have shown that in patients with pulmonary emphysema, peptic ulcer is at least three times more common than in the general population. Conversely, emphysema occurs three to four times more often in patients with peptic ulcer than would be expected from the normal incidence of emphysema in the general population. In all the clinical studies of this problem, duodenal ulcer was five times more common than gastric ulcer. The mechanism by which chronic lung disease predisposes to peptic ulceration is not known.

Liver Disease. A relationship between the liver and the stomach was suspected when it was noted that gastric hyperacidity occurred following the construction of an Eck fistula (end-to-side portacaval shunt) in dogs. However, *clinical* data have failed to show a pattern of hyperacidity in patients with Laennec's cirrhosis. In cirrhotics without coexisting duodenal ulcer, gastric hyposecretion and frequent anacidity in response to histamine prevail. In cirrhotics with duodenal ulcer, gastric acidity is higher than in those without an ulcer, but lower than in healthy individuals and much lower than the acidity usually accompanying duodenal ulcer. Gastric acidity is higher in cirrhotics with a portacaval shunt. Moreover, reports of an increased incidence of "peptic ulceration" in patients with cirrhosis have been misleading by their failure to define which type of ulceration is involved. More recent data indicate that cirrhotics are particularly liable to acute erosive gastritis and acute/or chronic gastric ulceration. Duodenal ulceration with its attendant hyperacidity is not appreciably more common in cirrhotics than in the general population.

Exocrine Pancreatic Disease. The evidence for a relationship between the exocrine pancreas and the stomach is based upon the frequency of peptic ulcer, particularly duodenal ulcer, in patients with chronic pancreatitis. Because the earliest manifestation of chronic pancreatitis is a decrease in the concentration of bicarbonate in pancreatic juice, ulceration could be due to a decreased buffering capacity of duodenal secretions. In addition, it has been theorized that patients with chronic pancreatitis may have increased gastric HCl production. This view is founded upon experimental observations of gastric hyperacidity in dogs after ligation of the pancreatic ducts, an experimental situation which simulates human chronic pancreatitis. However, one cannot extrapolate these data to the explanation of the human disease. Patients with chronic pancreatitis do not secrete more acid than healthy subjects.

ENDOCRINE DISORDERS. Zollinger-Ellison Syndrome. In 1955 Zollinger and Ellison described the syndrome now bearing their names. The important aspects of this syndrome are a markedly elevated rate of gastric acid secretion, a very severe duodenal ulcer diathesis, and a non-beta islet-cell tumor of the pancreas. Over half of the tumors are malignant. In 20 percent of cases there is diffuse microadenomatosis of the pancreas, a feature of this condition which prohibits the therapeutic use of tumor excision or partial pancreatectomy. In some instances the islet-cell tumor is found in an extrapancreatic location such as the wall of the first portion of the duodenum. Some cases of this syndrome result from a diffuse hyperplasia of the islets of Langerhans. In some instances the elevated serum gastrin levels may be caused by a hyperplasia of the antral gastrin-producing cells (G cells). It has been definitely proven that the hyperacidity and the ulcer diathesis are due to the release of gastrin by the tumor. Radioimmunoassay with antibodies to synthetic human gastrin I have shown large amounts of gastrin in tumor tissue and the blood of patients with this syndrome. In normal subjects serum gastrin concentrations are usually lower than 200 pg/ml whereas levels higher than 600 pg/ml are found in patients with this syndrome. Strangely, some patients with this syndrome do not develop an ulcer despite enormously elevated rates of acid secretion and instead present with diarrhea, malabsorption, and weight loss. In 20 percent of cases there are other endocrine tumors, often of the parathyroid glands (MEA I).

The ulcer disease associated with this syndrome has characteristic features listed below. It is important that the physician treating a patient with a duodenal ulcer disease recognize these features so that specific diagnostic procedures may be initiated. Although the proportion of duodenal ulcer patients with a Zollinger-Ellison syndrome is well below 1 percent, the consequences of improper treatment are so devastating that early, accurate diagnosis is essential.

1. Although most ulcers associated with this syndrome are in the usual location for duodenal ulcer disease, some may appear in a postbulbar location or even in the jejunum and may be associated with jagged and irregular mucosal folds (Fig. 26-7).
2. The basal acid output is very high, over 20 mEq/hour, and the ratio of the basal acid output to the maximal acid output (obtained with stimulation by Histalog) is usually greater than 60 percent.
3. This syndrome should be suspected when ulcer rapidly and severely recurs after adequate surgical treatment.
4. Severe diarrhea associated with hyperkalemia.
5. Duodenal ulcer in a patient with a functioning endocrine tumor such as a parathyroid adenoma.

The diagnosis may then be confirmed by one or more of the following tests:

Radioimmunoassay of serum gastrin levels. In normal subjects and in patients with the common form of duodenal ulcer, the fasting serum gastrin concentration does not exceed 200 pg/ml. The Zollinger-Ellison syndrome is associated with levels ranging from 200 to 300,000 pg/ml. Although comparable or even higher levels are found in patients with atrophic gastritis, the crucial point is that in this condition the high gastrin levels are associated with a very low gastric acid output: the high gastrin levels result from a lack of inhibition of gastrin release by HCl.

Secretin infusion test. During an intravenous infusion of secretin, both serum gastrin and gastric acid output of normal subjects and of patients with the common form of duodenal ulcer *diminish;* in patients with a Zollinger-Ellison syndrome they *increase* (Fig. 26-8).

Provocative calcium infusion test. In patients with the Zollinger-Ellison syndrome, an intravenous infusion of calcium (5 mg/hour) causes an excessive rise in serum gastrin levels (>500 pg/ml), as well as a greater rise in acid output than in normal subjects or patients with ordinary duodenal ulceration.

Arteriography. Selective celiac and superior mesenteric arteriography are capable of demonstrating a pancreatic lesion in a high percentage of cases of Zollinger-Ellison syndrome caused by a tumor.

Parathyroid Glands. Several clinical studies have demonstrated a slightly higher incidence of duodenal ulcer in patients with primary hyperparathyroidism. It is likely that some of these patients have gastrin-producing pancreatic tumor and Zollinger-Ellison syndrome; in these patients serum gastrin levels are increased by calcium infusions after removal of the parathyroid adenoma. In normal subjects gastric acid secretion is increased by intravenous calcium infusion and, conversely, hypocalcemia is accompanied by a reduction in gastric secretion. These relationships between serum calcium levels and gastric secretion may explain the occasional appearance of a duodenal ulcer in a patient with hypercalcemic hyperparathyroidism and no gastrin-producing pancreatic tumor.

Clinical Manifestations

An active duodenal ulcer reveals its presence by a symptom complex often described as "ulcer pain." The pain of duodenal ulcer is vague and often located in the mid-epigastrium to the right of the midline. The following characteristics should be determined in the evaluation of ulcer distress: the site of the pain, its quality, its radiation, the time of onset in relation to meals, aggravation of pain, relief of pain, and finally the chronology of painful attacks.

The quality of the pain is often the most difficult characteristic to elicit. Classically, it is described as a burning pain. In reality this is rarely accurate. Often, patients complain of a sensation of "pressure," of a "cramp," or of

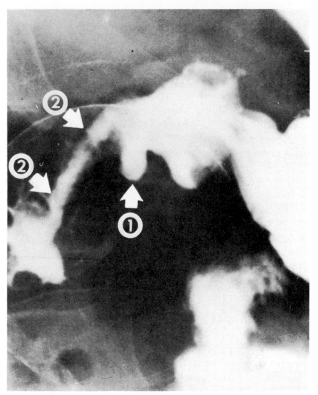

Fig. 26-7. Zollinger-Ellison syndrome. Note large duodenal ulcer crater (1) and irregular appearance of the mucosa of the second portion of the duodenum (2).

"discomfort." Occasionally, a patient describes the sensation of being "hungry." When investigating complaints suggestive of duodenal ulcer, one should open the questioning by asking the patient whether or not discomfort rather than actual pain is experienced. The distinction may seem overly subtle, but to many patients pain is something akin to a toothache. Moreover, the distinction has physiologic relevance, since the painful impulses in visceral disease are carried by the autonomic nervous system and

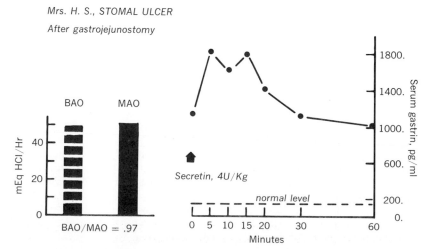

Fig. 26-8. Strongly positive secretin infusion test in a patient with a presumptive diagnosis of Zollinger-Ellison syndrome based upon a high BAO/MAO. Diagnosis was confirmed surgically.

cause different subjective sensations from those mediated by the somatic nervous system.

The epigastric discomfort of duodenal ulcer radiates in a beltlike fashion across the upper abdomen. When the ulcer penetrates posteriorly into the pancreas, the pain radiates to the back at T8 to T10. Occasionally, posterior radiation of pain becomes the dominant symptom, and the author has encountered several patients with duodenal ulcer who were being mistakenly treated for a chronic backache.

Because the epigastric discomfort of active duodenal ulcer is aggravated by fasting, these patients often realize that they must eat frequently. Occasionally, rapid ingestion of excessively cold or excessively warm fluids may aggravate these symptoms. Aspirin is avoided by many patients with duodenal ulcer because of severe symptomatic exacerbation.

Ingestion of anything that dilutes or buffers gastric acid relieves the ulcer pain. Plain water, which dilutes gastric secretions, affords immediate, although very temporary, relief. Milk or antacids which have a buffering capacity give prompt and longer relief.

The symptoms of duodenal ulcer usually occur when the stomach is empty: late in the morning, in midafternoon, and during the middle of the night. This rhythmicity may be lacking in children. A useful symptom in distinguishing a peptic ulcer from psychosomatic gastrointestinal distress is a history of the patient's being awakened by discomfort. This rarely occurs in the absence of organic disease. Night pain reflects the high nocturnal secretion of HCl unbuffered by food.

An important trait of duodenal ulcer is its tendency to chronicity and periodicity. Symptomatic attacks lasting for several weeks are interspersed with months of complete or near-complete absence of symptoms. The relationship of these symptoms to climatic and seasonal variations is well known. In temperate zones, exacerbations and complications occur during fall and spring. This is not true in other parts of the world. This seasonal influence may be related to an increase in volume and acidity of gastric secretion occurring in animals and in man during the autumn and spring. It has also been noticed that exacerbations of the ulcer process are often associated with traumatic emotional experiences. During World War II, admissions for perforated duodenal ulcer in Great Britain increased sharply during heavy air raids.

Diagnosis

RADIOLOGY. Radiologic examination of the duodenum is the most important diagnostic tool available to the clinician. The radiologist looks for two important abnormalities: a crater and duodenal deformity (Figs. 26-9 and 26-10). A crater appears as a barium-filled defect in the duodenal bulb or more frequently as a persistent fleck of barium. The evolutionary pattern of duodenal ulcer is a succession of episodes of ulceration followed by healing; this is what eventually deforms the bulb. At the level of the ulcer a stricture forms, above which the bulb dilates into two or three irregular outpouchings called pseudodiverticula. In

addition, the fibrotic and rigid duodenum fails to fill with barium when pressure is applied to the abdomen. Normally, pressure distends the bulb, because the pyloric sphincter prevents regurgitation of barium into the stomach. A deformed duodenal bulb in a patient with a history suggestive of duodenal ulcer is a reliable radiologic sign and is more often present than a crater.

ENDOSCOPY. With the refinement of fiberoptic instrumentation, this procedure has become a valuable adjunct to radiology. One can evaluate the condition of the esophageal mucosa for the presence of esophagitis, often associated with duodenal ulceration. Superficial gastric lesions such as erosions and antral gastritis may be demonstrated. Duodenal ulcers too shallow to be demonstrated radiologically may be detected, as well as the chronic inflammation of the duodenal mucosa—duodenitis—often found instead of a crater in patients with symptomatic gastric hyperacidity.

GASTRIC ANALYSIS. The value of gastric analysis is often questioned because at least half of the patients with a duodenal ulcer have normal rates of gastric secretion. However, a gastric analysis in patients with a peptic ulcer (including duodenal ulcer and gastric ulcer) may furnish the following information:

Recognition of patients with a duodenal ulcer diathesis due to a functioning endocrine tumor in the pancreas (Zollinger-Ellison syndrome).

Evaluation of the severity of the duodenal ulcer process. Obviously, patients with marked hyperacidity (without pyloric obstruction) have a more severe duodenal ulcer process with a greater expectancy of recurrence after therapy.

Evaluation of the results of therapy. It is useful to compare gastric analysis after surgical treatment for peptic ulcer or after treatment by anticholinergic drugs with control values. Gastric analysis is indispensable for the evaluation of the results of vagotomy.

Differentiation between benign and malignant ulcerations. When an ulcerating gastric lesion is accompanied by high rates of gastric secretion, the lesion may be considered and treated as belonging to a duodenal ulcer diathesis, whether or not a frank duodenal ulcer coexists. This is often true when a gastric ulcer is prepyloric or when a duodenal ulcer has caused pyloric stenosis with gastric stasis and subsequent gastric ulceration. It is very unusual to find gastric adenocarcinoma accompanied by frank hyperacidity.

Augmented Histamine Test. Gastric juice is aspirated in the morning after an overnight fast until the stomach is completely empty. During the test the subject is instructed to spit out his saliva. After removal of residual juice in the stomach, basal secretion is collected for 1 hour. At the end of an hour, Histalog (betazole, 3-β-aminoethylpyrazole dihydrochloride) is injected subcutaneously in a dose of 1.5 mg/kg of body weight. Gastric juice is collected in 15-minute periods for 2 hours after the injection.

Pentagastrin Stimulation Test. Pentagastrin is a synthetic polypeptide containing the five active terminal amino acids of gastrin. An injection of 6 mg/kg of pentagastrin produces a maximal acid output similar to that induced by histamine phosphate or Histalog without side effects. Since it is a more physiologic gastric stimulant, it will probably be used extensively in the future.

Hollander Insulin Test. The Hollander insulin test remains the most reliable method of determining the completeness of vagotomy. The test is based upon the fact that insulin-induced hypoglycemia stimulates gastric secretion only if there are intact vagal pathways to the stomach. The usual indication for the test is an investigation of the reasons for a recurrent ulcer in a patient previously treated by a vagotomy and drainage procedure. The test must be performed in the fasting patient. The stomach is intubated and after its contents have been evacuated, four 15-minute samples of basal secretion are collected. Following this the patient receives 20 units of regular insulin intravenously, and venous blood samples are taken for estimation of blood sugar at the time of the insulin injection and again 30 and 45 minutes later. For 2 hours after the insulin injection, 15-minute aspirates of gastric juice are collected and their volume, pH, and acid concentration are measured. A positive response is indicated by an increase in acid concentration greater than 20 mEq/L over the fasting concentration during the 2 hours following the injection of insulin, provided that the blood sugar falls to at least 35 mg/100 ml. When basal secretions are anacid, an increase in acid concentration greater than 10 mEq/L is considered to represent a positive response.

Management

The treatment of this condition has three aspects: long-term, or supportive, management; the management of an acute exacerbation; and the management of complications.

LONG-TERM MANAGEMENT

Therapy is aimed at decreasing gastric secretion and minimizing its effects on the duodenal mucosa. Many myths are attached to the dietary management of duodenal ulcer. Of these, that of a bland diet is particularly naive. With the exception of alcohol, foods ordinarily consumed by man do not irritate the gastroduodenal mucosa. It is the acid-peptic action of gastric juice that causes the tissue destruction characteristic of a duodenal ulcer. Food buffers gastric juice by accepting hydrogen ion; also, it binds the pepsin in gastric juice to the peptide bonds mobilized by digestion of protein and thus minimizes the ulcerogenic action of gastric juice. Therefore, the important aspect of the dietary management of duodenal ulcer is not what one eats but how one eats. A patient with a duodenal ulcer soon learns that discomfort accompanies an empty stomach. The reason for this must be explained to the patient when he is advised to follow a schedule of frequent feedings: breakfast, snack at midmorning, light lunch, snack at midafternoon, dinner, light snack before retiring. Skim milk rather than cream or half-and-half is taken between meals. Although alcohol in moderation may have beneficial sedative effects, its heavy consumption is harmful, and it should be completely avoided during acute exacerbations. Excessive consumption of fat, which retards gastric emptying and may thus increase gastric acidity by enhancement of the antral phase of gastric secretion, is harmful. Coffee and tea, because of their important secretagogue effects, should be left out.

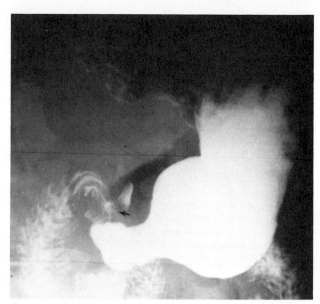

Fig. 26-9. Small ulcer crater (arrow) in the duodenal bulb with minimal deformity of the bulb.

Anticholinergic agents may contribute to the long-term management of duodenal ulcer by decreasing the number of recurrences. Their beneficial effects are, at best, questionable, and because they reduce the tone of the lower esophageal sphincter, they should *never* be used in patients who have associated reflux esophagitis.

Although antacids are often used for the long-term management of duodenal ulcer, they have little value except during exacerbations of the process. The buffering capacity of nonabsorbable antacids is smaller than is usually realized, principally because they are emptied from the stomach rapidly. Absorbable antacids, which are more

Fig. 26-10. Characteristic radiologic findings in duodenal ulcer. Scarring of the bulb resulting in obliteration of the inferior recess of the bulb (1), large crater (2), and narrowing of the lumen at the level of the crater (3).

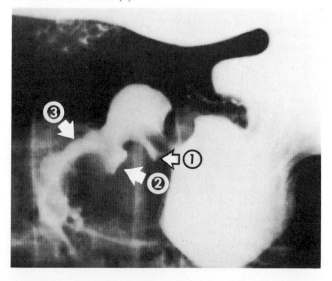

efficient buffers of HCl, may be hazardous when used for longer than a few weeks.

Conventional antihistaminic agents do not inhibit gastric acid secretion. It has been suggested that the action of histamine on secretion is mediated by H_2 receptors structurally different from the H_1 receptors which mediate those histamine effects blocked by conventional antihistaminics. *Metiamide,* a compound which inhibits effects mediated by H_2 but not by H_1 receptors, has been produced by side-chain modifications of histamine. In man, Metiamide inhibits gastric secretory responses to histamine, pentagastrin, insulin, and food. It has been used successfully abroad in the treatment of duodenal ulceration but has since been withdrawn because of its depressing action on the bone marrow. An analog of Metiamide, *Cimetidine,* has identical antisecretory properties but, at least so far, appears free of significant side effects. It has been used with success in Great Britain in the treatment of duodenal ulcer.

It is important that a patient with a duodenal ulcer lead a stereotyped existence, in addition to following the dietary schedule outlined above. Departures from the daily routine of life, whether they be physical or emotional, often precipitate symptomatic relapses. Patients should be warned against excessive smoking, and of course aspirin or aspirin-containing compounds are contraindicated.

MANAGEMENT OF AN ACUTE EXACERBATION

For a mild, symptomatic relapse, a simple intensification of the treatment often suffices. However, a severe relapse requires admission to the hospital for more intensive treatment, which includes (1) complete bed rest, (2) nasogastric suction, (3) antacid therapy, (4) anticholinergics, and (5) sedation.

A remarkable feature of duodenal ulcer is the rapidity with which intractable pain disappears when a patient is hospitalized and isolated from his usual environment. Keeping gastric juices away from the ulcer for 24 to 48 hours by constant suction accelerates healing of an intractable ulcer. After 24 to 48 hours of suction, a gastroduodenal series is obtained to rule out pyloric obstruction. If the stomach empties normally, the patient is given 150 ml of skim milk every 2 hours and 4 Gm of calcium carbonate every alternate 2 hours. The latter is a good buffer of HCl and is safe as long as the patient is free of renal disease and a high urinary output is maintained. Rising serum calcium and BUN (blood urea nitrogen) levels, accompanied by a falling urinary output, require immediate cessation of this antacid therapy and a change to a nonabsorbable antacid. This regimen should be continued for 72 hours or until complete disappearance of epigastric discomfort. It is important to awaken the patient at 3- to 4-hour intervals during the night for administration of milk and antacids. After 3 to 4 days the patient gradually returns to a soft diet with six small and equal feedings.

Anticholinergics are given up to tolerance as indicated by dryness of the mouth. Sedation is obtained with small doses of phenobarbital, which is a very helpful adjunct to the treatment.

At discharge, the patient is instructed to set his alarm for the middle of the night and take some milk and antacid at this time. A month after the onset of the acute exacerbation, the therapeutic regimen can gradually be readjusted to that followed for the long-term management.

INDICATIONS FOR SURGERY

The usual indications for recommending an operation to patients with a duodenal ulcer are intractability, a complication such as uncontrollable bleeding or late-occurring obstruction, and perforation. As a general rule, approximately 20 percent of patients with a duodenal ulcer ultimately require an operation.

INTRACTABILITY. By contrast with massive bleeding, severe pyloric obstruction, and duodenal perforation, which represent incontrovertible indications for surgery, intractability is less readily defined and a less compelling guideline for the clinician. It may be defined as a situation where medical management cannot control the symptoms of the disease. Naturally, the interpretation of intractability as an indication for surgery depends not only on the physician's judgment and the patient's willingness to accept the disability of a chronic disease, but also on the individual patient's circumstances. If the exigencies of an adequate therapeutic regimen—a regular pattern of living and eating, the constant use of antacids, anticholinergic and sedative drugs—are not compatible with the patient's occupation, family status, or finances, surgery might be imposed sooner than the severity of the duodenal ulcer diathesis might otherwise indicate. It is important that the clinician be satisfied that all reasonable avenues of medical management have been properly followed before proceeding with surgery based on the indication of intractability. It is every surgeon's experience that the patients who spontaneously request an operation after an exhaustive trial of medical management, ultimately have the best symptomatic results from surgery.

BLEEDING. Hemorrhage from a duodenal ulcer is responsible for approximately 20 percent of all cases of upper gastrointestinal bleeding. There are two aspects to the management of this complication. First in importance is resuscitation with all the measures used in the treatment of blood loss. In addition the stomach must be decompressed by a large-bore gastric tube such as an Ewald tube and lavaged thoroughly with cold isotonic saline solution to evacuate blood and clots.

After hypovolemic shock, if present, has been controlled, the clinician can proceed with the diagnostic aspect of the management. Patients with bleeding duodenal ulcer often have a previous history of similar episodes. A history of duodenal ulcer distress with its characteristic rhythmicity and periodicity is usually present. Emergency fiberoptic gastroscopy is an important diagnostic maneuver as it helps to exclude bleeding from esophageal or gastric varices in patients with cirrhosis and bleeding from a gastric ulcer or gastric erosions. When a duodenal ulcer is the source of bleeding, the operator may actually see the bleeding lesions, or more often, see blood refluxing into the stomach through the pylorus.

Bleeding from peptic ulcer is often treated by a milk drip. This is superfluous and possibly harmful. The blood already in the stomach is a better buffer than milk. Moreover, distension of the stomach interferes with spontaneous hemostasis which results from contraction of the gastric wall. Usually bleeding subsides with medical measures, and the patient may return to a rigid ulcer regimen for several weeks. Beyond that, the long-term management varies. In a young patient with a short ulcer history, long-term medical management should be continued. However, when the bleeding has been preceded by a long history of ulcer disease or by previous bleeding episodes, an ulcer operation should be considered.

When the ulcer is bleeding actively, the clinician's major concern is to recognize early enough the failure of conservative therapy and recommend an operation. The criterion of massive bleeding is a good guide to follow in determining which cases are surgical. Gastrointestinal bleeding is "massive" when 30 percent of the patient's blood volume must be replaced during 12 hours to maintain stable vital signs. In practice this represents 1,500 to 2,000 ml of blood for an adult of average size. The surgical approach to bleeding peptic ulcer will be described below.

PYLORIC OBSTRUCTION. The management of pyloric obstruction by a chronic duodenal ulcer depends upon the length of the ulcer history. Pyloric obstruction preceded by a short history of peptic ulcer disease usually signifies that the obstruction is due to duodenitis and antral gastritis impairing the propulsive motility of the antrum and active relaxation of the pyloric sphincter. This process is reversible, and normal gastric emptying returns as the inflammatory reaction around the ulcer subsides. Treatment consists of the following:

Nasogastric Suction and Interdiction of Oral Intake. It is important to forbid drinking, which patients often think is permissible because of the relief after gastric decompression.

Fluid and Electrolyte Replacement. Pyloric obstruction often stimulates gastric secretion. Enough fluid and electrolytes may be lost by vomiting to cause *hypochloremic* and *hypokalemic alkalosis*. This metabolic abnormality results from the combined losses of hydrogen, chloride, and potassium ions in gastric juice. The resulting potassium depletion may, in addition, alter renal function so that tubular reabsorption of bicarbonate is increased, thus leading to the characteristic finding of an aciduria associated with the alkalosis. There may also be impairment of the sodium-cation exchange mechanism.

Anticholinergic agents should not be given to patients with pyloric obstruction since they may aggravate the gastric stasis by decreasing gastric motility. When fluoroscopic examination with small amounts of barium shows return of gastric emptying, the patient should resume the rigid ulcer program used for the management of an acute exacerbation. The long-term medical management should be continued. Often after such an episode many years elapse without further symptoms of ulcer.

Pyloric obstruction occurring after a long history of duodenal ulcer distress almost always results from severe cicatricial duodenal deformity, and little can be expected from further conservative management. It is advisable to operate after fluid and electrolyte replacement. Clinging stubbornly to nasogastric suction and fluid and electrolyte

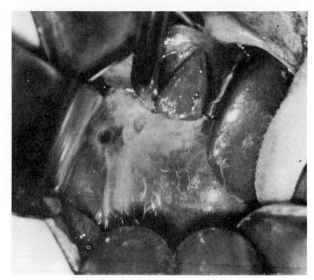

Fig. 26-11. Perforated duodenal ulcer. Note inflammatory exudate around the perforation.

replacement for several weeks in the futile hope of overcoming a cicatricial pyloric stenosis only renders the ultimate and necessary surgical management more difficult. Details of the surgical approach to this problem will be discussed below.

PERFORATION. Free perforation into the peritoneal cavity is the most dramatic and potentially the most lethal complication of duodenal ulcer (Fig. 26-11). Its major symptom is sudden, generalized epigastric pain. The patient can often give the hour and the minute of onset. It is the perforated duodenal ulcer that usually causes the rigid, "boardlike," scaphoid abdomen described as the classic physical finding in acute peritonitis. The large amounts of air in the peritoneal cavity are revealed clinically by an absence of the normal liver dullness. These findings and a history of peptic ulcer disease suffice to make a diagnosis which can be confirmed by a chest x-ray (in preference to an upright view of the abdomen) showing air under one or both sides of the diagram (Fig. 26-12). Occasionally, a perforation is the first manifestation of peptic ulcer disease. The actual perforation is sometimes accompanied by bleeding which, if appreciable, may overshadow the more lethal event. Of crucial importance is the existence of hypovolemic shock. Although the blood pressure may initially be normal, peripheral vasoconstriction, an accelerated pulse, and a decreased urinary output are usually present. The parietal and serosal peritoneum exposed to gastric acid contents undergo a chemical "burn," and changes similar to those of thermal burns occur, i.e., a decrease of plasma volume, a rise in hematocrit, and all the systemic abnormalities characteristic of hypovolemic shock.

The only safe way to treat a perforated duodenal ulcer is by surgical intervention. From time to time it is argued that a patient may be too ill to tolerate an operation. Patients are rarely too ill to tolerate surgical treatment. In this instance the intolerable insult is not the surgical treatment

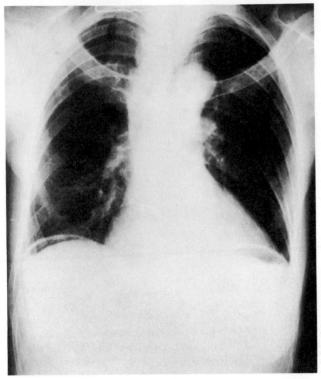

Fig. 26-12. Perforated duodenal ulcer. Note the presence of air under both sides of the diaphragm on this chest film.

but the continued soiling of the peritoneal cavity. Rarely are patients so ill that they fail to improve with preoperative treatment of the hypovolemic shock. These measures are (1) restoration of blood volume by administration of colloid, (2) parenteral fluid and electrolyte therapy, (3) nasogastric suction, and (4) administration of antibiotics.

After these corrective measures the ulcer is sutured or, in selected cases, definitive surgical treatment of the duodenal ulcer diathesis may be carried out. The details of the procedure will be described below.

From time to time, nonoperative treatment of perforated ulcer has been advocated. This consists of nasogastric suction and administration of blood, fluid, and antibiotics. The rationale of this method rests upon the demonstrated ability of perforations to become sealed spontaneously. Unfortunately, this event is unpredictable. If spontaneous closure of small acute ulcers does happen, a chronic indurated ulcer lacks the same potential. Today the risk of a laparotomy is so low that it is safer to operate; operation for a perforated duodenal ulcer is indeed the conservative approach.

The patient's future after closure of a perforated duodenal ulcer depends in part upon the length of the ulcer history prior to the perforation. In young patients with a short ulcer history the perforation is often the first and last manifestation of ulcer disease. However, when a long ulcer history precedes the perforation, over half of the patients continue to suffer. Some patients have another perforation; the author has seen several patients who had

three perforations over a period of several years. Recurrent duodenal ulcer distress after simple closure of a perforation is an indication for operation.

Elective Surgical Treatment of Duodenal Ulceration

HISTORICAL EVOLUTION

Operations on the stomach were first developed for gastric cancer during the latter part of the nineteenth century. *Posterior gastroenterostomy* was devised to overcome gastric outlet obstruction by gastric cancer. The applicability of this operation to the treatment of duodenal ulcer and its complications was then recognized. Since it was known that duodenal ulcer was due in part to the corrosive action of gastric juice on the duodenal mucosa, gastroenterostomy, which diverts secretions from the ulcer bed, appealed to physiology-minded surgeons. Its simplicity, at a time when the mortality and morbidity of intraabdominal operations was high, was also in its favor. This appeal was so great that gastroenterostomy was abandoned in this country only recently and after recognition of postoperative stomal ulceration. This complication was first reported in 1899. By 1930 it was obvious that stomal ulceration complicated 30 percent of posterior gastroenterostomies. As early as 1910, Austrian and German surgeons recognized this and adopted *partial gastrectomy* for duodenal ulcer. Except for a few isolated clinics, it was not until the late 1930s and early 1940s that gastroenterostomy was abandoned in favor of subtotal gastric resection in this country.

The rationale of partial gastrectomy was reduction of gastric acidity by removal of the parietal cell mass. Against this background were many controversial issues on details of technique, such as whether or not resection should encompass the ulcer or whether the reconstruction should be in the form of a gastroduodenostomy or gastrojejunostomy, and in the latter case whether the anastomosis should be antecolic or retrocolic. During the late 1930s, 1940s, and early 1950s, the trend moved toward more radical operations. However, it became evident that although 80 percent gastrectomy effectively cured duodenal ulcer, its sequelae were too frequent and too serious to be discounted. This prompted a search for operations equally effective and less costly in morbidity and mortality. In 1943 the rediscovery of the principle of vagus nerve section by Lester Dragstedt and his associates at the University of Chicago inaugurated a new era in the surgical treatment of ulcer disease. At first the principle of *vagotomy*, as applied by Dragstedt to the treatment of duodenal ulcer, sometimes failed, because the severe gastric stasis due to loss of the coordinated motor function of the pyloric muscle and the antrum produced intolerable side effects; recurrent ulcers, particularly gastric, were common. Addition of a gastric drainage procedure, namely, posterior gastroenterostomy designed to prevent gastric stasis, created an effective operation for duodenal ulcer. Subsequently the principle of vagotomy coupled with a gastric drainage operation—posterior gastroenterostomy, pyloroplasty, or antrectomy—became solidly established. Because of the possibility that some of the undesirable side effects of vagotomy, such as diarrhea, may be due to vagal denervation of the midgut, modifications of vagotomy designed to preserve all but the vagal supply to the stomach and known as *selective vagotomy* have been introduced during the past decade. Although selective vagotomy, which preserves the hepatic and celiac branches, appears to reduce the incidence of diarrhea, it still requires a drainage procedure and thus exposes the patient to the possibility of a postoperative *dumping syndrome*. In 1970, the concept of vagal denervation of the parietal cell area—*highly selective vagotomy, proximal gastric vagotomy*—without a drainage procedure was first tested clinically in Denmark and Great Britain. The early results appear encouraging.

In the ensuing paragraphs some of the advantages and disadvantages of these procedures will be discussed.

GASTROENTEROSTOMY

This operation should never be performed alone for the treatment of duodenal ulcer. Although a gastroenterostomy allows gastric juice to bypass the duodenal lesion, it also allows alkaline pancreatic and biliary secretions to flow into the antrum. Enhancement of antral gastrin mechanism by alkalinization of the antrum was the reason for this operation's frequent failure to cure the duodenal ulcer diathesis. In a dog prepared with a Heidenhain pouch, secretion from the pouch increases appreciably after a gastroenterostomy.

SUBTOTAL GASTRIC RESECTION

This procedure consists of removal of at least the distal 75 percent of the stomach (Fig. 26-13). Alimentary continuity is reestablished by anastomosing the entire section of the gastric pouch (Pólya) or a portion of its section after closure of the lesser curvature (Hofmeister) to the jejunum. The anastomosis may be antecolic or retrocolic. Anastomosis of the gastric remnant to the jejunum by any one of these methods is known as a "Billroth II operation." When the anastomosis joins the gastric remnant to the duodenal stump, the operation is termed "Billroth I." The latter procedure is best applied to the treatment of gastric ulcer and should not be used to treat duodenal ulceration unless supplemented by a vagotomy. The rationale of partial gastrectomy rests upon the assumption that removal of a large portion of the parietal cell mass diminishes gastric secretion. However, the anatomy of the gastric mucosal membrane is such that a 75 to 80 percent gastric resection removes the antrum and only a portion of the parietal cell mass. Moreover, the remaining parietal cells retain their vagal innervation and their responsiveness to other stimuli and therefore a secretory potential capable of causing recurrent ulcers. Recurrent ulceration after a partial gastrectomy for duodenal ulcer appears on the jejunal side of the gastrojejunostomy and is known as a "stomal," or "marginal," ulcer. When a partial gastrectomy alone has been done, the possible causes for the recurrence are (1) inadequate gastric resection; (2) excessively long afferent loop; (3) existence of a remnant of antrum left behind intentionally or inadvertently, resulting in excessive gastric

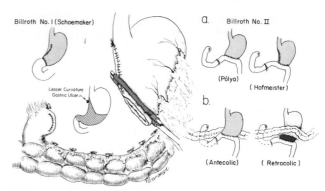

Fig. 26-13. Partial gastrectomy for benign disease. The larger sketch shows the Hofmeister closure of the lesser curvature. This is particularly applicable to the management of high-lying lesser curvature gastric ulcers. Gastrointestinal continuity is reestablished either by a gastroduodenostomy (Billroth I) technique, particularly applicable to gastric ulcer, or by a gastrojejunostomy (Billroth II). The latter may be performed with the full section of the gastric pouch (Pólya) or after resection and closure of the lesser curvature (Hofmeister). The anastomosis may be placed in front of or behind the transverse colon.

stimulation by gastrin released from the antrum bathed by alkaline juices; or (4) presence of a pancreatic islet-cell adenoma of the Zollinger-Ellison variety.

The recurrence rate is particularly high when patients are followed for more than 10 years after the operation. Gastric resection has other drawbacks. Primary is the mortality rate of gastric resection, which ranges from 1.0 percent to as high as 4 or 5 percent. The mortality rate is primarily related to circumferential dissection of the chronically inflamed duodenum, since half of the early postoperative deaths come from nonhealing of the duodenal stump with the formation of a duodenal fistula, with or without generalized peritonitis, or localized subphrenic and subhepatic abscesses.

Without question, a very radical subtotal gastric resection cures the ulcer diathesis. The reductio ad absurdum is the assurance of a zero incidence of recurrent ulcer after a total gastrectomy. However, time has shown that even after lesser resections of the stomach a host of undesirable sequelae related to loss of the reservoir function of the stomach and to impaired digestion and absorption follow in the wake of gastrectomy.

COMPLICATIONS OF PARTIAL GASTRECTOMY. Dumping Syndrome. The salient manifestation of the loss of the reservoir function of the stomach is known as the "dumping syndrome." The latter consists of some of or all the following postcibal symptoms: weakness, sweating, pallor, nausea and/or vomiting, epigastric discomfort, borborygmi, palpitations, dizziness, and diarrhea. These symptoms appear within 10 minutes after a meal and subside after 40 to 60 minutes. They may be accompanied by the following objective findings: tachycardia, tachypnea, elevation in blood pressure, increased small intestinal intraluminal pressure and motility, electrocardiogram changes in the T wave and the S-T segment, decreased plasma volume, decreased plasma potassium and phosphate, increased urinary excretion of uric acid, hyperglycemia, decreased cardiac output, increased digital blood flow, increased renal blood flow, and abnormal intestinal electrical activity. The syndrome is due in part to distension of the jejunum by an outpouring of extracellular fluid into the bowel lumen, which in turn results from the premature entry into the proximal small bowel of hypertonic chyme. Other manifestations, such as apprehension, sweating, and vascular instability, are due to autonomic or adrenomedullary corrective mechanisms. Some patients experience symptoms of hypoglycemia 60 to 90 minutes after a meal, particularly if it is high in carbohydrate content. The exact incidence of the dumping syndrome after gastric resection is unknown. It should be emphasized that some of or all these manifestations follow the administration of a hypertonic meal in virtually every individual who has had a gastric resection. However, only 5 to 10 percent of patients suffer from clinically significant dumping after a gastrectomy. In only 1 or 2 percent of the patients are the symptoms incapacitating. Often dumping is potentiated by the patient's emotional makeup.

Bilious Vomiting. Postoperative bilious vomiting may result from a chronic afferent loop syndrome or from alkaline reflux gastritis.

Chronic afferent loop syndrome is due to a partial obstruction of the afferent loop at, or close to, the stoma. Patients experience dull epigastric discomfort after meals. The distress is completely relieved by the vomiting of large amounts of bilious material which does not contain recently ingested food.

Alkaline reflux gastritis is a postgastrectomy condition due to reflux of bile into the stomach. This causes a chronic gastritis ("peristomal gastritis") which, in turn, leads to *constant* epigastric distress and frequent nausea and vomiting; the vomitus often contains food, since the gastritis impairs gastric emptying. The diagnosis is made by gastroscopy, which shows a fiery red, friable mucosa with superficial erosions. The changes are predominantly in the vicinity of the stoma.

Steatorrhea. Steatorrhea, defined as a fecal excretion greater than 7 percent of ingested fat, occurs more often after a Billroth II type of gastrectomy. The gastrojejunostomy allows gastric chyme to bypass the duodenum and escape the digestive action of pancreatic enzymes and the emulsifying action of bile salts. Undigested food stimulates intestinal motility and is propelled distad before pancreatic secretion and gallbladder emptying can occur. In other words, gastric emptying and pancreatobiliary digestion of dietary fat are out of phase. Steatorrhea occurs in approximately 50 percent of all patients who have had a gastric resection, is rare after gastrojejunostomy or vagotomy alone, but is almost the rule after total gastrectomy. Still another factor in steatorrhea after partial gastrectomy is the so-called "blind loop" syndrome. There may be sufficient stasis in the proximal loop of duodenum to cause bacterial proliferation. Bacterial enzymes are capable of deconjugating bile salts. In turn deconjugated bile salts are irritating to the intestinal mucosa and appear to be responsible for diarrhea. Moreover the altered bile salts are less able to contribute to the formation of lipid micelles essential for normal fat digestion and absorption and thus con-

tribute to the development of steatorrhea. The latter may be corrected by the administration of a broad-spectrum antibiotic.

Anemia. Chronic iron deficiency anemia is another facet of the postgastrectomy state. It occurs in at least 50 percent of patients who have had a partial gastrectomy. Although patients can absorb iron normally after gastrectomy, they cannot increase iron absorption in the face of increased iron losses. About 30 percent of patients have impaired absorption of vitamin B_{12} after a partial gastrectomy, and in about 6 percent megaloblastic anemia develops. The malabsorption usually comes from deficient secretion of intrinsic factor due to loss of gastric tissue and atrophy of the gastric remnant.

Calcium Deficiency. Deficient calcium absorption is another consequence of subtotal gastric resection. Balance studies have shown that as many as 30 percent of patients have an abnormal calcium metabolism 7 to 16 years after gastric resection. In some patients the defect in calcium absorption may lead to osteomalacia.

Small Bowel Obstruction. Small bowel obstruction is an occasional late complication of partial gastrectomy, particularly of the Billroth II variety. A loop of small bowel may herniate through the operative defect in the transverse mesocolon when it has been improperly closed, or a volvulus may form around the gastrojejunostomy.

Gastrocolic Fistula. The stomal ulcer that used to occur so often after gastroenterostomy (done alone without vagotomy) is a particularly virulent type of ulcer diathesis with a great propensity for perforation either into the peritoneal cavity or into the transverse colon, causing a gastrojejunocolic fistula responsible for severe diarrhea, emaciation, and anemia. In the absence of such specific aggravating circumstances as a Zollinger-Ellison syndrome, this particular complication rarely occurs after a gastrojejunostomy constructed in conjunction with an adequate partial gastrectomy. It is not the short-circuiting of gastric contents into the colon that causes the diarrhea, as one would expect, but rather the reflux of feces into the small bowel. The resulting increase in the bacterial population of the proximal gastrointestinal tract probably causes the diarrhea and malabsorption. The latter can be corrected rapidly by a proximal colostomy, which may be necessary to restore proper nutrition before undertaking definitive treatment of the gastrocolic fistula. A gastrocolic fistula is demonstrated much more readily by a barium enema than by an upper gastrointestinal series.

VAGOTOMY

The rationale of vagotomy has been described above. This operation interrupts vagal impulses to the parietal cell gland area and to the antrum. By inhibiting antral motility and rhythmic relaxation of the pyloric sphincter mechanism, it also causes gastric stasis. Many of the patients who had this operation in the 1940s were severely incapacitated by gastric distension, foul eructations, and gastric ulceration. For these reasons vagotomy alone was not a satisfactory operation. By adding an operation which relieves the gastric stasis, all its advantages are conserved without its disadvantages. At present, three types of gastric drainage operations are currently performed: pyloroplasty, gastroenterostomy, and antrectomy, followed by a Billroth I or II type of reconstruction.

The operation of vagotomy and pyloroplasty interrupts neural stimuli to the parietal cells and decreases the responsiveness of the parietal cells to other stimuli. In addition, the antrum is denervated and gastric emptying is enhanced, so that endogenous release of gastrin is depressed. All these factors lower gastric HCl production. Pyloroplasty which defunctionalizes the pyloric sphincter mechanism and corrects a duodenal stricture can be performed according to the Heinecke-Mikulicz, Finney, or Jaboulay techniques (Fig. 26-14). Of these three techniques, the first, in the author's opinion, is the least desirable, since it is more prone to stenosis and dysfunction and is awkward to construct in the face of severe duodenal fibrosis (Fig. 26-15 and Fig. 26-16).

Gastroenterostomy has been proposed by some as the best method of decompressing the stomach in conjunction with a vagotomy. In the author's opinion, gastroenterostomy is less desirable than pyloroplasty, because the normal continuity of the gastroduodenal tract is not respected. The goal of surgery should be restoration, not alteration, of normal physiology. A gastrojejunostomy bypasses the important digestive and absorptive functions of the duodenum. Moreover, this type of anastomosis is subject to mechanical complications leading to gastric outlet obstruction and afferent loop stasis.

Others consider antrectomy the best method of decompressing the stomach with vagotomy, since it removes the source of gastrin. It should be pointed out that if the antrum is preserved, as is the case with a pyloroplasty and vagotomy, it is denervated, and gastrin release is diminished (but not as much as after antrectomy). Therefore, the argument supporting antrectomy is not entirely valid. However, it is true that the lowest rates of recurrence after surgery for duodenal ulcer (1 to 2 percent) have been provided by vagotomy and antrectomy. The "best" recurrence rates observed after vagotomy and simple drainage—pyloroplasty or gastrojejunostomy—have been around 5 percent. However, patients who have had a vagotomy and antrectomy are liable to postgastrectomy symptoms—dumping, etc.—in addition to *postvagotomy episodic diarrhea.*

The operative risk of vagotomy with pyloroplasty or gastroenterostomy is small; in the author's experience the mortality rate is less than 0.5 percent. Many patients experience diarrhea, which usually improves after a few weeks or months but in a few patients (1 to 2%) may persist and may be disabling. The mechanism of the diarrhea is unknown. It is distinguished from the diarrhea associated with the dumping syndrome by its tendency to occur episodically and without relation to meals. In addition it has been suggested that truncal vagotomy predisposes to gallstone formation. This belief is based on the observation that progressive enlargement of the gallbladder is a consequence of complete severance of the vagus nerves and on the impression of some authors that the incidence of cholelithiasis is greater among previously vagotomized pa-

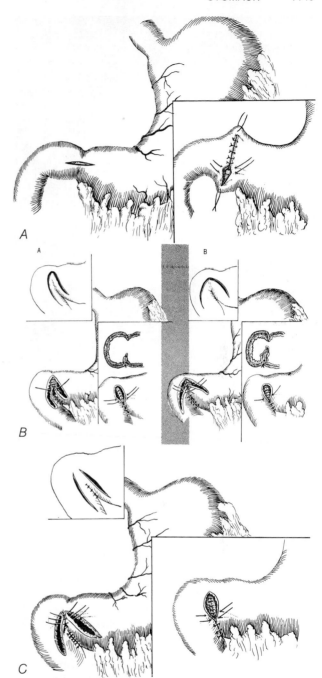

Fig. 26-14. *A.* Heinecke-Mikulicz pyloroplasty: vertical incision 3 cm in length centered on the pyloric ring and closed transversely with one layer of interrupted seromuscular sutures. *B.* Finney pyloroplasty. Insert B demonstrates the correct technique; note the wider septum turned. This leads to malfunction of the pyloroplasty. *C.* Jaboulay pyloroplasty. In reality this is a side-to-side gastroduodenostomy and is an excellent method of drainage when the duodenum is severely scarred.

tients than in the general population. Although the former appears valid, it is also true that in man contraction of the gallbladder is primarily hormone-dependent and that after a vagotomy the gallbladder contracts normally in response

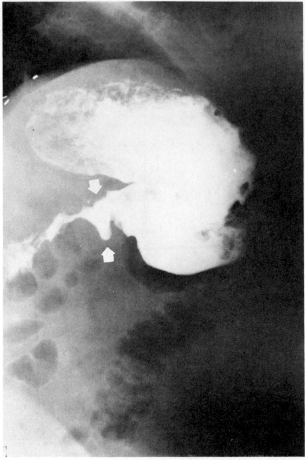

Fig. 26-15. Severe gastric stasis after a vagotomy and a Heineke-Mikulicz pyloroplasty. Note that the stenosis from the patient's duodenal ulcer disease remains *distal* to the pyloroplasty (arrows).

to a test meal. Impressions of an abnormal incidence of cholelithiasis after vagotomy remain unconfirmed. Nevertheless, attempts to prevent postvagotomy diarrhea and biliary dysfunction have led to the introduction of selective vagotomy designed to preserve the celiac branches of the posterior vagus and the hepatic branches of the anterior trunk. Since a selective vagotomy results in complete vagal denervation of the stomach, the procedure requires a supplemental drainage procedure, i.e., pyloroplasty, gastrojejunostomy, or antrectomy with Billroth I or Billroth II reconstruction. Although there appear to be fewer instances of postvagotomy diarrhea after this operation than after truncal vagotomy, the incidence of other sequelae such as dumping and alkaline gastritis is not lessened. The rationale of *highly selective vagotomy* is to interrupt vagal pathways to the fundus and corpus while preserving vagal branches (anterior and posterior nerves of Latarjet) going to the antrum. The vagally innervated antrum maintains a normal pumping function, and, as amply demonstrated by clinical experience, a *drainage procedure is not necessary.* This eliminates the risk of any sequelae associated with a drainage procedure, as well as technical problems related

to invasion of the gastrointestinal lumen: leaking suture line, intraabdominal abscess, and wound infection (Fig. 26-17).

APPLICATION TO DUODENAL ULCERATION. Today fewer and fewer surgeons continue to treat duodenal ulceration with a two-thirds partial gastrectomy. The operations most commonly applied to the treatment of this condition are vagotomy—truncal or selective—*and drainage*—antrectomy, gastroenterostomy, or pyloroplasty. It is a surprising fact that whenever the worth of these various procedures has been subjected to rigorous clinical experimentation, no *significant* differences in results have been found among them. However, some generalizations regarding these procedures can be made. In general the operative mortality is higher for procedures involving resection of the stomach (distal partial gastrectomy or vagotomy and antrectomy) than for vagotomy and simple drainage. Weight loss or inability to maintain a preoperative weight, steatorrhea, and symptoms of "dumping" occur more often after partial gastrectomy and vagotomy with antrectomy than after vagotomy and simple drainage. However, recurrence is least common after vagotomy and antrectomy (approximately 2 percent) and greatest (approximately 7 percent) after vagotomy and simple drainage. The recurrence rate after two-thirds partial gastrectomy lies between these two extremes.

Some argue that the lower mortality of a vagotomy and simple drainage makes the slightly greater recurrence rate acceptable. Others believe that this benefit may be canceled by the mortality and morbidity of additional surgery for recurrent ulceration. Rather than adopting a rigid attitude, an experienced surgeon will select the operation best suited to an individual patient. He may perform a vagotomy and antrectomy in a good-risk patient with a severe ulcer diathesis and reserve vagotomy and simple drainage for cases where the risk of a resection is enhanced by very severe duodenal inflammation or advanced age and associated diseases. At the time of writing, highly selective vagotomy remains under clinical trial. Although the initial results have been almost uniformly good, it is still too early to compare recurrence rates with those of the other established procedures.

Surgical Treatment of Complications of Duodenal Ulceration

BLEEDING

The general management of a patient bleeding from a peptic ulcer has been discussed previously. Details of the surgical management follow.

The failure of medical measures to control the bleeding is the indication of laparotomy. The criterion usually followed is that of massive bleeding, i.e., bleeding which requires replacement of 30 percent of the patient's blood volume over a period of 12 hours to maintain stable vital signs. At the time of laparotomy the duodenum is inspected carefully for signs of scarring and inflammation. If none is found, the stomach is carefully palpated after opening the gastrocolic ligament. If the duodenum is scarred or the serosa of the anterior duodenal wall is stippled and edematous, a vertical incision extending 1 to $\frac{1}{2}$ cm on either side of the pylorus is made. A duodenal ulcer, if present, is usually located in the first portion of the duodenum. An arterial "spurter" may be seen in the base of the ulcer which should be carefully oversewn with two mattress sutures of 2-0 chromic catgut placed on either side of the arterial defect. If possible, one should try to undermine the mucosa so that it can be closed over the ulcer by one or two sutures after suture ligature of the bleeding artery. When suturing a very large ulcer, the author usually places a piece of muscle from the rectus into the base of the ulcer and holds it in place with a mattress suture. The vertical incision over the pylorus is incorporated into a Finney pyloroplasty, and a vagotomy is performed. Whether or not an ulcer is found in the duodenum, a vertical gastrotomy is then made in the midportion of the stomach. One should search for a bleeding gastric ulcer, even though a duodenal ulcer has been found, because of the frequent association of gastric and duodenal ulcer. Frequently hemorrhage from an ulcer ceases with the induction of anesthesia, and the finding of an active crater in the duodenum is not sufficient assurance that it was the source of bleeding. After the gastrotomy incision has been made, retractors are placed in the lumen of the stomach, and the entire mucosal surface is carefully examined. It is often necessary to irrigate the gastric lumen thoroughly to evacuate blood and clots. Some bleeding ulcers are small and easily hidden by a mucosal fold. If the fundic mucosa is not exposed, the greater curvature is mobilized so that by pushing on the anterior or posterior surface of the stomach the fundic mucosa may be turned inside out into the gastrotomy incision. A bleeding gastric ulcer should be oversewn carefully, after a four-quadrant biopsy of the lesion.

The superiority of the concept of vagotomy and simple drainage over partial gastrectomy has been most obvious when applied to the surgical treatment of massively bleeding duodenal ulcer. Under these conditions the operative mortality of gastrectomy approached 20 percent. The current experience is that massively bleeding duodenal ulcer can be managed by vagotomy and pyloroplasty with suture ligation of the ulcer, with a mortality rate close to that expected for elective surgery.

PYLORIC OBSTRUCTION

The proper timing of surgical treatment in the management of pyloric obstruction due to a duodenal ulcer has been discussed above. The obstruction is usually due to a duodenal ulcer, although a gastric ulcer in the pyloric canal ("channel ulcer") or a prepyloric ulcer can cause enough fibrosis of the antrum to obstruct the gastric outlet. The operation should relieve the obstruction and control the duodenal ulcer diathesis, goals which can be achieved by a vagotomy and pyloroplasty. Often the deformity of the duodenum is so severe that a Heineke-Mikulicz pyloroplasty is technically not feasible. Under these conditions, it is usually possible to construct a Finney or a Jaboulay type of pyloroplasty without difficulty. Faced with a severely deformed duodenum, some surgeons prefer a gas-

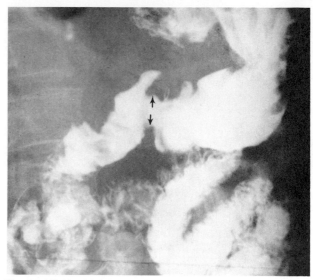

Fig. 26-16. Note by comparison with Fig. 26-15 the excellent gastric drainage obtained with a Jaboulay pyloroplasty. Arrows indicate the margins of the pyloroplasty.

trojejunostomy to a pyloroplasty. Occasionally a patient has such a severe distension of the stomach that the tone of the muscularis of the stomach has been lost. In these patients, the delay in gastric emptying often accompanying vagotomy may be more severe. When such far-advanced gastric distension is encountered, a subtotal gastric resection may be preferable to a vagotomy and drainage procedure.

Fig. 26-17. Diagram of the three types of vagotomy.

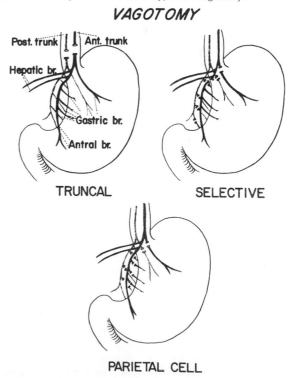

VAGOTOMY

TRUNCAL   SELECTIVE

PARIETAL CELL

PERFORATION

The goal of surgical treatment is to prevent further contamination of the peritoneal cavity. The exploration should be carried out through a short incision either in the upper midline or in the right upper quadrant. Over 75 percent of the perforations occur in the anterior wall of the first portion of the duodenum. Varying amounts of food debris and inflammatory exudate occupy the peritoneal cavity. The perforation should be closed with one or two mattress sutures of 2-0 silk, the ends of which are tied over a fold of omentum to reinforce the closure. After the perforation has been closed, the peritoneal cavity should be cleansed of debris and inflammatory exudate by repeated irrigation of the peritoneal cavity, of the subhepatic and suprahepatic spaces, of the paracolic gutters, and of the pelvic cavity with several gallons of normal saline solution. One can thus prevent localized intraperitoneal abscesses, formerly a frequent complication of perforated duodenal ulcer.

A controversial point is the one of definitive treatment of the duodenal ulcer diathesis at the time of exploration for perforation. This matter should be left to the judgment of the individual surgeon. However, a third of the patients remain symptom-free after the perforation has been closed; for them definitive treatment would not be justified. Experience has shown that the patients whose ulcer symptoms recur after closure of a perforation have long antecedent histories of ulcer. Therefore, in selected patients, i.e., those with long histories of ulcer distress in whom exploration is carried out a short time after the perforation, a vagotomy and pyloroplasty can be done safely. The pyloroplasty incision is carried through the perforation with excision of its margins.

MARGINAL ULCER

A marginal ulcer after partial gastrectomy is notoriously refractory to medical management and usually requires additional surgical procedures. Unless clinical evidence for a Zollinger-Ellison syndrome is present, a vagotomy, transabdominal or transthoracic, is the preferred treatment (Fig. 26-18). When a marginal ulcer occurs in a patient who has had a vagotomy and drainage operation (gastroenterostomy with or without antrectomy), one should first of all determine the completeness of the vagotomy by a Hollander test. Recurrence due to incomplete vagotomy is managed by re-vagotomy and antrectomy. Recurrence despite a complete vagotomy usually results from gastric stasis due to malfunction of the stoma and requires another abdominal exploration, at which time the findings dictate the choice of procedure, i.e., closure of gastrojejunostomy and construction of a pyloroplasty, antrectomy, etc. The possibility of endocrine adenomatosis, however, should always be considered when the clinician is confronted by recurrent ulcer disease. Should the proper diagnostic tests for a Zollinger-Ellison syndrome, including radioimmunoassay of serum gastrin, indicate that a recurrent ulcer is associated with a gastrin-producing pancreatic islet-cell tumor, the only course of management should be complete removal of the target organ: a total gastrectomy. It is futile to attempt to treat what is usually a fulminating ulcer diathesis by lesser resections since even minuscule gastric remnants may under these conditions secrete huge amounts of acid. Equally futile are attempts to reduce serum gastrin levels by searching for and removing these islet-cell tumors, because they are so often multiple and microscopic and/or malignant and have already metastasized. It is particularly important to remove the entire stomach when faced with a Zollinger-Ellison syndrome due to metastatic islet-cell tumor, because it has been shown that these tumors grow very slowly and may actually regress after the stomach has been removed. It is the fulminating ulcer diathesis, not the tumor, which is the lethal factor.

SURGICAL TREATMENT OF SEQUELAE OF ULCER SURGERY

Usually the undesirable side effects of ulcer operations become less noticeable as time goes by. But in a small percentage of patients (<5 percent), crippling symptoms persist. Fortunately, these are often amenable to surgical

Fig. 26-18. *A*. Large marginal ulcer crater 4 years after partial gastrectomy for duodenal ulcer (1). *B*. Seven days posttransthoracic vagotomy; the stoma (2) is now free of ulceration.

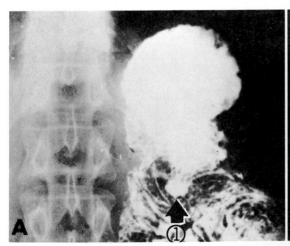
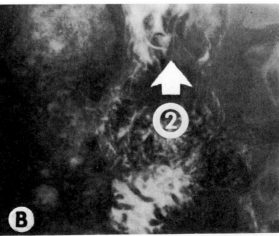

correction. The problems encountered most often are *alkaline reflux gastritis, dumping syndrome,* and *episodic* (postvagotomy) *diarrhea.*

Alkaline reflux gastritis is usually associated with a prior gastrectomy and gastrojejunostomy with or without vagotomy. It is corrected by converting the gastrojejunostomy to a Roux en Y arrangement, which effectively diverts bile-containing duodenal juices from the gastric pouch. If not already done, *vagi must be divided.*

A dumping syndrome which does not respond to conservative measures such as a dry, high-protein, low-carbohydrate diet and which persists for more than 2 years after the initial surgery, may be appreciably improved by interposing a *reversed loop* of jejunum, 6 to 8 cm in length, between the gastric pouch and the duodenum. The symptoms of episodic diarrhea may be corrected in a similar fashion by reversing a short (4 to 6 cm) segment of intestine at a point about 100 cm distal to the gastric outlet.

GASTRIC ULCERATIONS

Chronic Gastric Ulcer

Although the term gastric encompasses the antral, fundic, and cardiac segments of the stomach, it has been shown that most chronic gastric ulcers appear in antral mucosa.

DIFFERENCES BETWEEN DUODENAL AND GASTRIC ULCERATION

As will be pointed out below, some ulcers located in the *stomach* actually behave like *duodenal* ulcers. However, some important features separate duodenal ulceration from high-lying gastric ulcers.

SEX. Although both types of ulcer are more prevalent among men, the ratio of men to women is only 2:1 for gastric ulcer as compared with a ratio of 6 or 7:1 for duodenal ulcer. During the decade 1950–1960 the mortality rate for gastric ulcer among women increased by 26 percent and among men decreased by 20 percent.

AGE. By contrast with duodenal ulcer, a disease of middle-aged men (thirty-five to forty-five), the incidence of gastric ulcer increases steadily with age.

FAMILIAL FACTOR. There is an excess of peptic ulcer among the siblings of patients with peptic ulcer disease. Moreover, such studies have shown that the predisposition to an ulcer is type-specific. An excess of gastric ulcer exists among the relatives of patients with gastric ulcer and the same is true for duodenal ulcer among the relatives of patients with this lesion. In addition, there exists among patients with duodenal ulcer a preponderance of blood group O whereas high-lying gastric ulcers tend to be associated with blood group A.

EPIDEMIOLOGY. In most countries, including the United States, duodenal ulcer prevails over gastric ulcer by a ratio of 6:1 or 7:1. However, in some countries such as Japan, where gastric ulceration causes 90 percent of all peptic ulcer deaths, the reverse is true.

ENVIRONMENT. Duodenal ulcer tends to occur more often in individuals working under conditions of tension in positions of responsibility: skilled workers, foremen, executives, etc. Gastric ulcer, on the other hand, occurs more often in unskilled workers and is two to five times more prevalent in the poorer social classes than in the upper social strata.

GASTRIC SECRETORY ACTIVITY. Patients with a duodenal ulcer have higher average rates of gastric secretion than ulcer-free individuals. On the other hand, patients with gastric ulcer have normal or slightly lower than normal levels of HCl secretion (with exceptions to be discussed below).

RESPONSE TO TREATMENT. Duodenal ulcers usually respond well to medical management, whereas gastric ulcers require an operation more often. However, the recurrence rate after operations for duodenal ulcer is higher than is the case for gastric ulcer.

No longer is it believed that gastric ulcers can become malignant. Benign gastric ulcers remain benign and gastric cancers start de novo.

ETIOLOGY OF CHRONIC GASTRIC ULCERATION

The pathophysiology of chronic gastric ulcer is more complex than that of duodenal ulceration. In recent years several etiological factors have been studied.

CHRONIC GASTRITIS AND REDUCED MUCOSAL RESISTANCE. The presence of atrophic gastritis in the stomachs of patients with gastric ulcer, a phenomenon exhaustively studied by DuPlessis, is an important clue to the cause of chronic gastric ulcer. DuPlessis found atrophic gastritis in 61 of 75 stomachs with a gastric ulcer. The ulcer always appeared in chronically inflamed and atrophic mucosa and gastric ulcers located in the body of the stomach were always associated with gastritis extending into the fundus. It has been proposed that the chronic gastritis which appears to favor the formation of a gastric ulcer is due to the chronic reflux of bile into the stomach. Reflux of bile into the stomach can be demonstrated more often in patients with a chronic gastric ulcer than in patients with duodenal disease. Experimental preparations designed to allow bile to bathe the gastric mucosa continuously result in the development of a chronic gastritis which is strikingly similar to the human disease. The gastric mucosa near the stoma of a gastrojejunostomy always shows changes of chronic gastritis. These observations suggest that the reflux of bile-containing duodenal secretions into the stomach over a long time causes chronic gastritis which in turn lessens the resistance of the gastric mucosa to ulceration. Since chronic gastritis is associated with an atrophy of the acid-secreting apparatus, these changes also explain the reduced output of HCl associated with many (but not all) gastric ulcers.

DRUG-INDUCED CHRONIC GASTRIC ULCERATION. In about 20 percent of patients with gastric ulcer, chronic gastritis is absent and the etiological mechanism described in the previous paragraph is not applicable. Of the other possible etiological factors, drug-induced chronic gastric ulceration has received the most interest in recent years. This interest began when it was noticed that the incidence of chronic gastric ulcer in young women in New South Wales (Australia) began to increase in 1943. In subsequent studies a significant association was found between *gastric ulcers in women* and the chronic use of aspirin-containing preparations. No such association was found for duodenal ulcer in either sex or for gastric ulcer in men. Although aspirin, because of its universal use, is the most important of the "ulcerogenic drugs," this phenomenon was first noticed after the introduction of the adrenocorticosteroids. It is now a generally accepted fact that the therapeutic use of steroids particularly for rheumatoid arthritis may be complicated by the development of a chronic *gastric* ulceration. Phenylbutazone and Indomethacin are also occasionally responsible for causing a gastric ulcer. All the drugs—aspirin, steroids, Phenylbutazone, Indomethacin—known to be capable of producing an ulcer have similar antirheumatic, anti-inflammatory properties. The exact mechanisms by which these drugs cause gastric ulceration is not known. However, studies from the author's laboratory have shown that all of these drugs reduce substantially the ability of the gastric mucosa to secrete mucus, which may favor ulcer formation since the layer of mucus covering the gastric epithelium is believed to play a role in mucosal defense mechanisms against ulceration (Fig. 26-19).

HEREDITARY FACTORS. As previously mentioned there is an inherited predisposition to one type or the other of peptic ulceration. This phenomenon has received considerable support with respect to duodenal ulceration from the well-documented association between blood group O and duodenal ulceration. Unfortunately, a relationship between blood group phenotypes and *gastric* ulceration remained buried by the anatomical classification of peptic ulcers into duodenal and gastric. When Johnson separated gastric ulcers into three categories (lesions in the corpus of the stomach without abnormalities of the duodenum, pylorus, or prepyloric region; gastric ulcers associated with an active duodenal ulcer or with a scarred duodenum; and gastric ulcers situated close to the pylorus), he found a significant excess of blood group A among the patients in the first category. Patients in the other two categories showed the strong association with blood group O characteristic of duodenal ulceration. Although these observations do not provide an explanation for the greater susceptibility to gastric ulceration associated with blood group A (any more than we understand the reason for the association between blood group O and duodenal ulceration) they at least have formed the basis for a more rational classification of gastric ulceration to be discussed below.

GASTRIC ACIDITY. As in the case of duodenal ulceration (DU), a *chronic* gastric ulcer (GU) does not occur in the absence of gastric secretion of HCl and pepsin. However, whereas duodenal ulceration is associated, on the average, with excessive gastric acidity, patients with gastric ulcer (anatomic classification) secrete, on the average, normal amounts of acid (Table 26-1). Nevertheless, a frequently cited theory of gastric ulceration attributes the process to gastric hyperacidity due to gastric stasis. This view is based on the frequency with which a gastric ulcer is associated with an active duodenal ulcer or a scarred duodenum. The incidence of combined GU-DU is approximately 25 percent of all chronic gastric ulcers. Because the duodenal ulcer usually precedes the appearance of the gastric lesion, it has been assumed that the gastric stasis produced by the duodenal ulcer increases antral release of gastrin, and the resulting hyperacidity would lead to the formation of the gastric ulcer.

Actually, much of the confusion surrounding the possible role of an augmented acid-peptic factor in the etiology of chronic gastric ulceration is cleared when one departs from a purely anatomic definition of a gastric ulcer. On the basis of physiologic data one may separate chronic ulcers located in the stomach into two categories. On the one hand, there are lesions located near the pylorus or in the pyloric canal or associated with an active duodenal ulcer. When these lesions are analyzed separately, one finds that they are associated with blood group O and *with rates of gastric secretion greater than those of normal subjects and close to the range commonly found in patients with a duodenal ulcer.* On the other hand, lesions located in the body of the stomach, in addition to being associated with blood group A, as previously mentioned, are characterized by a *reduced* gastric output of acid.

The following classification of chronic gastric ulcer summarizes the foregoing discussion of the etiological aspects of this lesion.

Fig. 26-19. Bars represent volume (in milliliters) of gastric antral mucus secreted during a daily 3-hour collection period. Note the decrease in the rate of secretion under the influence of cortisone. (*Reproduced from Menguy and Masters, Surgery, 54:19, 1963.*)

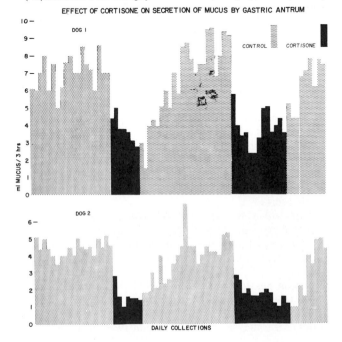

EFFECT OF CORTISONE ON SECRETION OF MUCUS BY GASTRIC ANTRUM

Type	Location	Etiological Relationship
I	High-lying, lesser curvature	Chronic gastritis, blood group A
II	Prepyloric or associated with a duodenal ulcer or scarred duodenum	Hyperacidity
III	Random, may be on greater curvature	Drug-induced: aspirin, steroids, Indomethacin, Phenylbutazone

CLINICAL MANIFESTATIONS

Symptomatic differences between gastric and duodenal ulcer are subtle. As with duodenal ulcer the distress of a gastric lesion occurs when the stomach is empty and is relieved by food and antacids. The astute physician may recognize some differences. The pain is often to the left of the midline. The patient with a gastric ulcer may experience discomfort ("burning," "pressure," "gas") immediately after drinking hot or cold liquids, alcohol or highly spiced foods, raw fruits, and vegetables. Sometimes, and this is characteristic of penetrating gastric ulcers, food does not relieve the distress (as it does with duodenal ulcer), but, on the contrary aggravates it. Sometimes, a gastric ulcer may remain asymptomatic until its presence is manifested by a serious complication such as bleeding or perforation.

The greater seriousness of gastric ulceration by comparison with duodenal ulceration is emphasized by the fact that gastric ulceration, although less common than the duodenal disease, is responsible for at least one-half of all ulcer deaths. Perhaps because patients with a gastric ulcer are older, the consequences of such ulcer-related complications as hemorrhage and perforation are compounded by associated age-related conditions. Moreover, even when the age factor is discounted, the mortality rate of perforated gastric ulcer is greater than that of perforated duodenal ulcer. The gravity of perforated gastric ulcer may result from a higher incidence of intraperitoneal septic complications caused by the heavy bacterial growth to be expected in the hypochlorhydric stomachs of patients with a gastric ulcer.

Another feature of chronic gastric ulceration is the tendency for it to recur after healing. One may expect that in at least 50 percent of cases the lesion will recur during the two years following initial healing of the lesion. This recurrence rate seems to be particularly high for gastric ulcers associated with a duodenal ulcer.

DIAGNOSIS

The roentgenographic demonstration of an ulcerating lesion in the stomach is the most important step in the diagnosis. Once the presence of an ulcerating lesion has been recognized, its benign or malignant nature must be established. It is vital that all of the information that roentgenography, gastroscopy, and cytology can provide be applied to this end.

ROENTGENOGRAPHY. Roentgenographic demonstration of a gastric ulceration is the first and most important step in the diagnosis. After its discovery, the benign or malignant nature of the ulceration must be determined. This diagnosis is based upon certain characteristic roentgenographic features.

The projection of the base of the ulcer with respect to the gastric wall is important. When the base lies in or outside the gastric contour, the ulcer is probably benign. If the base lies inside the gastric contour, and particularly if it is located in a space-occupying gastric mass, it is probably malignant. Rigidity of the gastric wall in the vicinity of the ulceration indicates malignancy. An ulcer

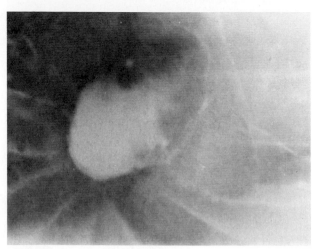

Fig. 26-20. Large benign gastric ulcer crater. Note that gastric mucosal folds radiate toward the ulcer.

with a regular round or oval shape has greater chance of being benign, whereas irregular or asymmetric craters are often malignant. When the mucosal folds in the vicinity of the ulcer radiate toward the ulcer, the latter is probably benign (Fig. 26-20). A gastric ulcer accompanied by a duodenal ulcer or a deformity of the duodenal bulb is probably benign. The size of the ulceration is of diagnostic importance only if it is small. A diameter of less than 1 cm probably indicates a benign lesion.

Without question, the most valuable roentgenologic feature is the relation of the ulceration to the contour of the gastric wall. As can be seen in Fig. 26-21, a benign gastric ulcer crater extends beyond the contour of the wall. The margin surrounding the ulcer is smooth and slightly rolled. The healing ulcer fills with granulation tissue and assumes a pyramidal shape as it gradually becomes smaller and

Fig. 26-21. Benign gastric ulcer. Sequential films at 2-week intervals on the same patient. A. The base of the ulcer extends beyond the contour of the gastric wall. Some edema surrounds the ulcer. B. Good healing of the crater is evidenced by the pyramidal shape it has assumed. Note mucosal folds radiating toward the crater. C. Complete healing with scarring and stellar configuration of mucosal folds.

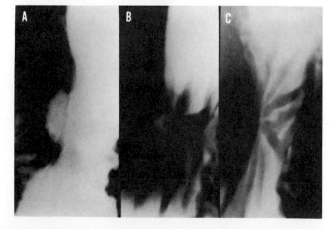

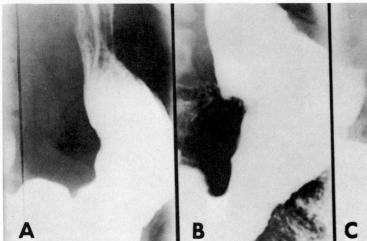
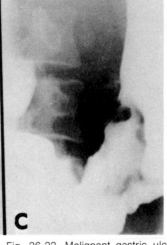

closes. By contrast, Fig. 26-22 illustrates a malignant ulcer which has the appearance of a broad plateau projecting into the lumen of the stomach. Mucosal folds do not reach the mass because of infiltration of the mucosa around the ulcer by carcinomatous tissue. Digestion of the tumor mass by acid-peptic juice results in the formation of a crater in its center.

The accuracy with which a gastric carcinoma may be recognized varies with its location. The diagnosis of fundic

Fig. 26-22. Malignant gastric ulceration. Sequential films in a patient who refused surgical intervention. *A.* and *B.* The ulcer does not extend beyond the contour of the stomach but is contained in a broad plateau projecting into the lumen. Inexorable progression of the lesion is obvious.

Fig. 26-23. Single malignant cell demonstrated upon cytologic study of gastric aspirate from a patient with a small malignant ulceration.

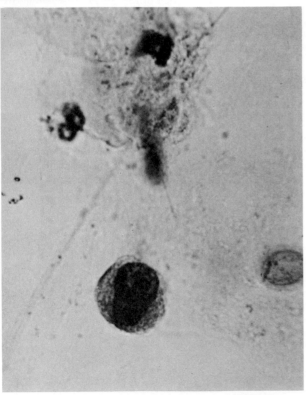

lesions is unreliable because of the difficulty in filling this portion of the stomach with barium. Recognition of lesions in the antrum is more accurate. In general, the accuracy of radiologic interpretation approximates 90 percent.

GASTROSCOPY. Direct visualization of a gastric lesion is a very useful adjunct to the differential diagnosis, particularly since the introduction of the fiberoptic instrumentation which has made the procedure a simple and safe one. The endoscopic diagnosis of an ulcerating lesion is based on the gross features of the lesion: a smooth, regular, round punched-out lesion with a clean white base and radiating folds is likely to be benign, whereas an irregular lesion with a dirty-looking base and heaped-up edges is more likely to be malignant. The value of gastroscopy has been enhanced by the capability, provided by the newer instrumentation, of brushing cytology and biopsy under direct vision. Because of the small amount of material sampled, the latter techniques are associated with false negative results even in the hands of experienced operators.

EXFOLIATIVE CYTOLOGY. The value of cytology in separating benign from malignant gastric ulcerations has been proved only in centers where the procedure has been applied as a research arm of medicine or pathology. The morphologic features of malignant exfoliated cells (Fig. 26-23) include increased nuclear-cytoplasmic ratio, hyperchromasia, irregular clumping of chromatin, increased number and size of nucleoli, and "signet ring" appearance of cells. It must be stressed that the value of the procedure depends upon the experience of the cytologist. A negative cytological study cannot stand alone and can serve only to reinforce an impression of benignancy provided by other methods. A positive result must of course be accepted as a formal indication of malignancy even though false-positive results do occur.

GASTRIC ANALYSIS. Approximately one-half of patients

with a gastric carcinoma are achlorhydric; i.e., the pH of gastric juice remains above 3.5 even during stimulation with secretagogues. However, because the presence of even high concentrations of HCl in gastric juice does not exclude the possibility of a malignant gastric ulcer, gastric analysis has only limited value in the differential diagnosis of gastric ulcerations.

ACCURACY OF DIFFERENTIAL DIAGNOSIS. It is often claimed that the combined use of roentgenography, gastroscopy, biopsy (endoscopic), and cytology provide the clinician with almost 100 percent accuracy in differentiating benign from malignant gastric ulcerations. It should be pointed out that because of the recent decrease in the incidence of gastric cancer only about 8 percent of ulcerating lesions in the stomach are malignant. In other words, if one were to approach all gastric ulcerations as being benign one would be "correct" in at least 90 percent of instances. In the author's opinion the "almost 100 percent accuracy" is due to the smaller number of cancers, some of which are all too obvious. It is with the small number of potentially curable gastric cancers associated with many of the features of a benign ulcer that the diagnostic tools described above may be severely taxed.

In clinical practice one often relies upon the test of healing to make this crucial diagnosis (Fig. 26-21). The test is based on the generally valid assumption that malignant ulcerations rarely show sustained healing. But, in fact, they can heal sufficiently to satisfy radiological criteria of healing. In a recent study of 638 patients with a gastric ulceration, 25 proved to have a cancer. In 4 of the 25 patients with gastric cancer, the initially detected ulceration had appeared benign radiologically and subsequently healed with medical treatment. The correct diagnosis was made only 9 to 19 months later.

MEDICAL TREATMENT OF CHRONIC GASTRIC ULCERATION

If all of the diagnostic procedures described above indicate that the lesion is benign, medical treatment based on the following measures is instituted.

ABSTINENCE FROM SMOKING. This—and bed rest—is the only measure which has been shown to accelerate healing.

ABSOLUTE BED REST. This is an important feature of the treatment and, at least initially, should be in-hospital, the best environment for the intense diagnostic and therapeutic program required for this potentially serious disease.

ANTACID THERAPY. Although gastric acidity is usually lower in patients with a gastric ulcer, it remains true that a peptic ulcer does not occur in the absence of HCl. If the already low levels of gastric acid accompanying gastric ulcer can be lowered even more, the ulcer often heals rapidly. As mentioned previously, effective antacid therapy is provided by absorbable antacids such as calcium carbonate in doses of 4 Gm every 2 hours (after excluding organic renal disease).

DIET. A multiple-feeding program keeps gastric juice buffered by food. There may be merit in avoiding foods with roughage such as raw fruit and vegetables.

AVOIDANCE OF GASTRIC STASIS. Anticholinergics are contraindicated because of their inhibitory action on gastric motility.

NEW MEASURES. Carbenoxolone sodium, a compound synthesized from an essential ingredient of licorice, has recently been found to accelerate the rate of healing of gastric ulcers in ambulatory patients. It has been postulated that this occurs via an enhanced secretion of gastric mucus. The main side effect of carbenoxolone is an aldosterone-like activity which may precipitate congestive heart failure in elderly patients.

INDICATIONS FOR SURGERY

If one excludes from this discussion obviously malignant lesions for which the decision to operate should not be in question, this decision is based upon the behavior of the lesion and its potential for complications, recurrence, or prolonged morbidity. The following features of gastric ulceration should suggest the advisability of an operation.

Gastric ulcers associated with a duodenal ulcer are more liable to recur after healing and deserve an early operation.

Pyloric canal "channel" ulcers are often severely symptomatic and respond poorly to medical treatment.

When there is evidence of deep penetration, the risk of a serious complication such as perforation or hemorrhage is higher and warrants early consideration of surgery.

Very large or so-called "giant" gastric ulcers should be treated surgically. In addition to the hazard of complications, the healing of these lesions often causes sufficient scarring to impair gastric emptying.

Ulcers failing to undergo a 50 percent reduction in size over a 3-week period of medical treatment are best treated surgically.

The recurrence of a gastric ulcer should, in the absence of a contraindication, be considered as an indication for surgery.

And above all, should there be *the slightest doubt* about the benignancy of the lesion, surgical intervention should be advised without undue delay.

Acute Gastric Mucosal Lesions

An *erosion* is a mucosal defect that does not penetrate deeper than the muscularis mucosae. A lesion extending beyond this layer is an *ulcer*. A condition characterized by profuse bleeding from multiple gastric *erosions* was described for the first time in 1898 by Dieulafoy who used the term of "exulceratio simplex" to describe it. Since then such terms as "acute erosive gastritis," "acute hemorrhagic gastritis," "Cushing's ulcer," "Curling's ulcer," and "stress ulcer" have been employed. Because the cause of these acute, superficial mucosal lesions remains poorly defined it seems preferable to refer to them as "acute gastric mucosal (AGM) lesions" which cause "acute gastric mucosal bleeding."

The true incidence of this condition was not appreciated until recently when the introduction of fiberoptic endoscopic instrumentation made it practically feasible to examine the gastric mucosa in most cases of upper gastrointestinal bleeding. As long as emergency radiological examination of the stomach was the mainstay of the workup of the "upper gastrointestinal bleeder," the importance of AGM lesions was not appreciated because erosions, when present, would result in a negative radiological study. The latter would often be interpreted as "bleeding probably due to peptic ulcer." It is now apparent that gastric erosions are responsible for at least 20 percent of all cases of upper gastrointestinal bleeding.

PATHOLOGIC ANATOMY

The main gross feature is the presence of mucosal erosions, usually multiple, ranging in size from barely visible petechiae, to round lesions about 1 cm in diameter (Fig. 26-24). In addition one may find acute penetrating ulcers often with an irregular "geographic" contour particularly when the condition complicates a stressful situation (see below). The lesions may involve any segment of the stomach and particularly after a "stress" may be found in the duodenum. The mucosal erosion is the main microscopic feature of this condition. It is preceded by the development of focal mucosal hemorrhagic and coagulative necrosis. As the foci of necrotic mucosa slough, erosions based on the muscularis mucosae are left. These erosions rapidly heal without scarring. Elsewhere, one finds mucosal and submucosal edema and hemorrhage. Antecedent chronic, atrophic gastritis may be present in some patients, particularly in those where AGM bleeding is not precipitated by one of the usual "causes" of this condition (see below).

ETIOLOGY

The appearance of acute gastric erosions is often preceded by one of the following situations:

Stress: trauma; burns; surgical operations. The complication of any one of these situations by *sepsis* is particularly conducive to the development of AGM lesions.

Alcohol.

Drugs: aspirin, steroids, Indomethacin, Phenylbutazone.

No apparent cause. Patients in whom AGM lesions do not appear to have been precipitated by one of the "causes" listed above often have an underlying chronic, atrophic gastritis which seems to predispose the gastric mucosa to this acute condition.

Although it is not known why stress or drugs should cause mucosal erosions, the following etiological mechanisms have been investigated.

GASTRIC HYPERSECRETION. Because of the role played by an excessive gastric output of acid in some types of ulceration, a similar relationship has been investigated for AGM lesions, but with scant success. Although gastric hyperacidity has been found in patients having undergone neurosurgical operations, operations particularly susceptible to this complication, a consistent pattern of hyperacidity has never been found in burned patients, who are most prone to AGM lesions. Moreover viable microorganisms have been found on the gastric mucosa of burned patients. This finding is not consistent with gastric acidity. Whenever this factor has been studied it has been found that stressful situations suppress rather than stimulate gastric acid secretion. Drug-induced AGM lesions are probably not acid related since these drugs have no important action on gastric secretion, except for the steroids which, when given over many days, increase acid secretion slightly. The development of AGM lesions in patients with atrophic gastritis and pernicious anemia suggests that mucosal erosions may appear in the absence of measurable amounts of gastric acid.

ABNORMAL GASTRIC MUCOSAL BARRIER. Normally the permeability of the gastric mucosal membrane to hydrogen ion is limited. This relative impermeability is responsible for the extremely high gradient in HCl concentration between the lumen of the stomach and the extracellular fluid compartment. Recent studies suggest that experimental conditions simulating those commonly associated with the clinical development of AGM lesions, such as hemorrhagic shock, increase the permeability of the gastric mucosa to hydrogen ion. It has been suggested that hypochlorhydria often found in critically ill patients may be due to this

Fig. 26-24. Gross appearance of gastric mucosal erosions. In this instance, the lesions were caused by aspirin.

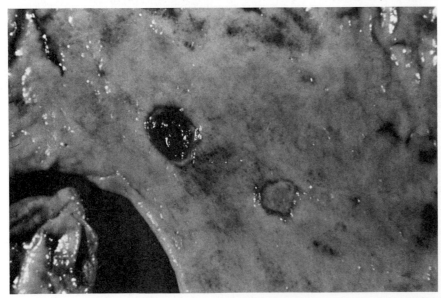

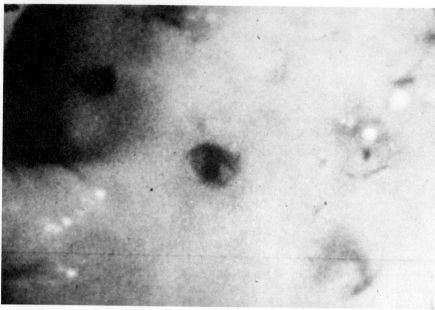

Fig. 26-25. Endoscopic appearance of erosive gastritis.

loss of hydrogen ion by back diffusion rather than from an absolute reduction in gastric acid secretion. With respect to the mechanism of drug-induced erosive gastritis, Davenport found that after canine stomachs had been exposed to aspirin, mucosal damage with fluid and ionic diffusion into the lumen occurred. He postulated that the increased permeability of the mucosa to hydrogen ion leads to gross mucosal injury and bleeding. Other factors which may play a role in the development of mucosal erosions under the influence of stress and "ulcerogenic drugs" are related to the mucous layer lining the mucosa and the rate at which the mucosa is capable of renewing itself. Studies from the author's laboratory have shown that steroids reduce the rate of gastric mucous secretion as well as the rate of epithelial cell turnover in the canine stomach, changes which should affect adversely the ability of the mucosal membrane to maintain its integrity.

CLINICAL MANIFESTATIONS

It may be redundant to point out that the salient clinical feature of AGM lesions or "hemorrhagic gastritis" is bleeding. Some aspects of the bleeding merit discussion. The hemorrhage may be occult and discovered only at autopsy. Signs of hemorrhagic shock may be misinterpreted in a patient already burdened with several potentially lethal problems. One must be alert to this possibility in all severely stressed patients (particularly when sepsis enters the picture). The interval between the stressful incident (trauma, operation) and the appearance of bleeding seems to be approximately 6 days. When AGM lesions complicate a severe illness or multiple injuries, the patient's primary problems may completely overshadow the bleeding. There may be, particularly in burned patients, penetrating acute ulcers. A free perforation may be masked by the symptoms of the primary problems and by the bleeding.

DIAGNOSIS OF AGM LESIONS

The most important diagnostic step is early endoscopy (Fig. 26-25). It is important to realize that the shallow erosions which characterize this condition cannot be demonstrated by conventional barium meal roentgenographic studies; these can only serve to interfere with subsequent endoscopy. Moreover, endoscopy must be performed early, while the hemorrhage is active. If the examination is delayed, these lesions, which heal rapidly, may be completely missed. Selective arteriography is gaining favor as a diagnostic method for this condition. However, it provides less specific information on the source of bleeding, is more hazardous, and, in patients with severely diseased arteries, may be impossible to perform.

MEDICAL TREATMENT OF AGM LESIONS

As with any condition associated with blood loss, adequate replenishment of the blood volume is very critical. It is even more critical in stress-related AGM lesions because hypovolemia and inadequate tissue perfusion pose another burden on a patient already seriously ill. The replacement, although aggressive, must be accurate with due allowance for the patient's cardiac reserve, which in the cirumstances often surrounding AGM lesions may be marginal.

Gastric cooling, which may prevent further mucosal injury by reducing gastric secretion and peptic activity, appears to have some merit in this condition although it has only questionable value in arresting bleeding from gastric or duodenal ulcers. The best way to cool the stomach is to lavage it extensively with iced saline solution via an Ewald tube, a method which also allows one to empty the stomach of blood and thus facilitate endoscopy.

Recently some success in arresting hemorrhage from AGM lesions has been reported with selective catheterization of the celiac axis and infusion of Pitressin or epinephrine into the vascular bed of the stomach.

Surgical Treatment of Chronic Gastric Ulceration

The elective surgical management of a chronic gastric ulcer depends upon the type of gastric ulceration.

If the ulcer belongs to the type and category of high-lying gastric ulcerations associated with chronic gastritis and gastric acid hyposecretion (approximately 75 percent of chronic gastric ulcerations), the best method of treatment is a partial gastrectomy. It is especially important to carry the resection high on the lesser curvature of the stomach to remove all of the antral mucosa. The absence of duodenal scarring not only eliminates the technical problems associated with this operation when it is done for duodenal ulceration, but also allows one to reestablish gastrointestinal continuity by a Billroth I gastroduodenostomy. The limited extent of the resection and the gastroduodenal anastomosis reduce the incidence of the various symptoms associated with the postgastrectomy state. Experience accumulated over the past two decades indicates that the operative mortality of elective gastrectomy for chronic gastric ulceration is 1 percent or lower. The long-term results with respect to ulcer recurrence are excellent and it has been customary to compare the good results after gastrectomy for gastric ulcer with the accepted recurrence rate of about 5 percent after the same but more extensive operation for duodenal ulcer. Recurrence rates ranging from 0 to 1 percent are representative of the results that one has learned to expect after partial gastrectomy for chronic gastric ulcer.

When dealing with a Type II lesion characterized by associated duodenal ulceration or a scarred duodenal bulb and/or by an abnormally high rate of gastric acid secretion or by the location of the lesion in the pyloric canal or immediately proximal to it, the goal of therapy should be reduction of acid secretory activity rather than excision of all of the antral mucosa. Vagotomy and a drainage procedure such as a pyloroplasty, or a distal antrectomy are the procedures of choice. Naturally, a careful four-quadrant biopsy of the lesion should be carried out whenever the ulcer is to be left in situ. It should be mentioned at this juncture that during the early and mid-1960s there was a wave of interest in the application of vagotomy and pyloroplasty (with a four-quadrant biopsy of the ulcer) to *all* cases of gastric ulceration. The results published to date suggest that the recurrence rate is prohibitively high. However, as mentioned above, this approach has a sound rationale when reserved for those gastric ulcers which belong to the duodenal ulcer diathesis.

Chronic gastric ulcers associated with ulcerogenic drugs are often quite large when detected, are liable to severe complications, do not always respond promptly to removal of the responsible agent and in the author's experience are best treated by a partial gastrectomy.

Surgical Treatment of Acute Gastric Mucosal Lesions

As previously indicated, bleeding from multiple, superficial gastric erosions is one of the most common causes of upper gastrointestinal bleeding. Fortunately the hemorrhage ceases spontaneously in the majority of cases. But when surgery becomes necessary, the choice of an appropriate operation may be difficult. For many years the operation most commonly performed for this condition was a partial gastrectomy. An all-too-common sequela was persistent bleeding due to overlooked erosions or new lesions in the remaining gastric mucosa. Because of this problem, Sullivan and Waddel advocated vagotomy and pyloroplasty along with multiple-suture-ligatures of the bleeding lesions through a wide gastrotomy. This approach, initially satisfactory in their hands, has been used widely but with mixed results. As reported by various authors, the rate of rebleeding cases after this operation ranges from 15 to 100 percent. All too often patients with this condition are so desperately ill because of the condition which may have precipitated the erosive gastritis that they cannot tolerate the continued bleeding, much less the reoperation to control it. For this reason the author has suggested that when erosive gastritis requires an operation, it should be tailored to the individual patient. When the patient is desperately ill, usually because of the condition responsible for the erosive gastritis (severe burns, multiple injuries, sepsis), the operation performed should be one which precludes further bleeding, i.e. a near-total gastrectomy. But if the patient's condition is good enough to allow him to tolerate rebleeding (and, possible reoperation) after a more conservative procedure, a vagotomy and hemigastrectomy or vagotomy and pyloroplasty with suture-ligation of all visible bleeding points through a large gastrotomy should be carried out.

It is important to stress that fatalities from this condition often result from the primary precipitating illness and its complications, of which erosive gastritis and massive bleeding may be one of several. The least the surgeon can do is to ensure that bleeding isn't the last straw.

MISCELLANEOUS SURGICAL DISEASES

Acute Gastric Dilatation

This condition may occur after operations on the stomach or the upper abdomen and after certain types of trauma, particularly of the chest. It is especially common in women and children and is more likely to occur in patients who are partially conscious and receiving oxygen through a nasal catheter or artificial respiration without a properly cuffed tracheostomy tube. A particularly lethal combination is the administration of oxygen via a nasal catheter in a patient with an indwelling nasogastric tube. There are occurrences on record (and probably many more not on record) in which the oxygen line was inadvertently connected to the gastric tube, resulting in severe distension and bursting of the stomach. The error is obviously so easy to commit by nonprofessional personnel that one should never give oxygen therapy via a nasal catheter to a patient with a Levin tube in the stomach.

The usual mechanism of acute gastric dilatation is a vicious cycle of gastric distension compounded by the patient's efforts at belching, which result only in swallowing more air, which increases the distension, and so on. As the stomach becomes distended, interstitial fluid seeps into its lumen; in addition, gastric secretion is stimulated by the distension. In this manner, several liters (up to 4 or 5) may accumulate in the stomach. Distension of this degree can lead to death by dehydration and fall in plasma volume, and by interference with cardiac and pulmonary function from compression of the diaphragm. In any patient with the conditions described above, the onset of hiccuping, regurgitation of small amounts of fluid, a rise in pulse rate, and tympany over the epigastrium should lead to the recognition of acute gastric dilatation and indicate the need for immediate insertion of a nasogastric tube. Acute gastric dilatation can be rapidly fatal if not corrected. Death often results from acute pulmonary edema caused by sudden aspiration of gastric contents into the tracheobronchial tree.

Mallory-Weiss Syndrome

The pathologic basis of this syndrome is the development of longitudinal mucosal tears along the gastroesophageal junction. By definition, the tears involve only the mucosa and submucosa. They lie in the region of the cardia. Profuse gastric hemorrhage is the salient clinical manifestation. Most cases of this syndrome have been associated with acute alcoholic debauches, and it has been surmised that the lacerations result from violent retching motions forcing gastric contents against a contracted cardia. The laceration may involve the full thickness of the cardia with or without extension into the esophagus. Spontaneous rupture of the gastroesophageal junction (Boerhave's syndrome) is almost invariably fatal if not recognized and treated promptly. The perforation may cause signs of peritonitis when located below the phrenoesophageal ligament; when involving the esophagus above the latter structure, signs of mediastinitis with severe retrosternal pain, high fever, crunching precordial sounds, and a *characteristic air fluid level in the posterior mediastinum* may occur. Occasionally both the mediastinum and the peritoneal cavity may be involved.

Prolapse of Gastric Mucosa

The major clinical manifestations are delayed gastric emptying and episodes of vomiting, accompanied by epigastric fullness. Roentgenographic studies may show the prolapse of antral folds into the duodenum (Fig. 26-26). It should be pointed out that such a prolapse may be found in otherwise asymptomatic patients. Therefore, one should rule out very carefully the existence of other diseases before attempting specific treatment of a mucosal prolapse. This treatment consists of antrectomy and reconstruction of gastroduodenal continuity by a Billroth I anastomosis.

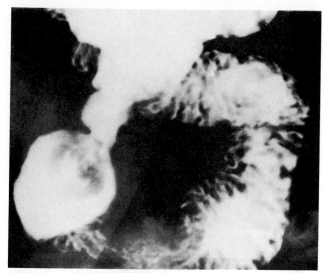

Fig. 26-26. Prolapse of gastric mucosa into the duodenum. Patient also has a small prepyloric gastric ulcer on the lesser curvature.

Gastritis

ATROPHIC GASTRITIS

The diagnosis of atrophic gastritis is usually a clinical one and is based upon demonstrated hypochlorhydria or achlorhydria. At gastroscopy one may see a thinning of the gastric mucosal membrane, through which vessels are visible, and flattening of the rugal folds. A decrease in number of the gastric glands with a chronic inflammatory reaction in the mucosa and intestinalization of the gastric mucosal membrane constitute the histologic picture. In some patients with this condition, circulating antibodies to parietal cells have been demonstrated. Malabsorption of vitamin B_{12} may or may not be present.

CORROSIVE GASTRITIS

Although the ingestion of caustic agents usually causes more damage to the esophagus than to the stomach, occasionally enough material may reach the stomach to cause acute gastritis. In extreme cases of this condition, the injury may involve the full thickness of the gastric wall with resulting perforation. Total gastrectomy becomes necessary as a lifesaving measure. In less severe instances of corrosive gastritis, the caustic material pooling in the more dependent portion of the stomach results in scarring and pyloric obstruction, requiring a gastrojejunostomy to relieve the obstructive process (Fig. 26-27).

EOSINOPHILIC GASTRITIS

This rare condition is characterized by a chronic inflammatory infiltrate in the wall of the stomach and sometimes of the proximal small bowel. The infiltrate is of the granulomatous variety, and eosinophilia may be present. Occasionally the chronic inflammation may cause sufficient scarring and thickening of the gastric wall to mimic the

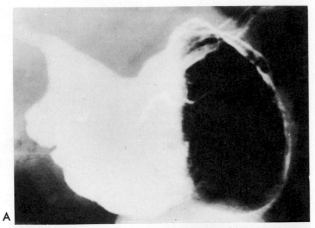

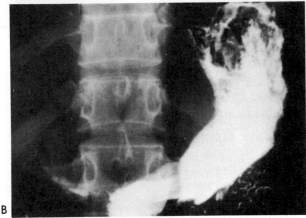

Fig. 26-27. *A.* Corrosive gastritis due to ingestion of concentrated HCl. Healing with severe cicatricial contraction of the antrum. *B.* Obstruction relieved by a gastrojejunostomy.

gross appearance of a gastric carcinoma, particularly of the linitis plastica variety. Gastric ulceration may occur.

HYPERTROPHIC GASTRITIS

This condition was first described by Ménétrier (polyadénomes en nappe). The clinical significance of giant hypertrophic gastritis is poorly understood. It is often a roentgenographic finding of enlarged rugal folds requiring a diagnosis between hypertrophic gastritis and a gastric lymphoma. This diffuse enlargement of the rugal folds is often found in association with polyendocrine adenomatosis in the Zollinger-Ellison syndrome. Under these conditions, the enlarged rugal folds represent a hyperplasia of the gastric mucosal membrane. Hypertrophic gastritis is often associated with an increased permeability of the gastric mucosal barrier to serum proteins and loss of albumin into the lumen.

Gastric Volvulus

The symptomatic triad of gastric volvulus consists of the following: (1) severe nausea with a paradoxical inability to vomit, (2) localized epigastric pain, and (3) impossibility of introducing a stomach tube. These lesions are idiopathic or secondary to such conditions as eventration of the diaphragm and paraesophageal hiatal hernia. Incarceration of the displaced stomach in a paraesophageal hernia sac may cause occult bleeding and anemia or massive bleeding. The treatment requires surgical reduction of the volvulus.

Foreign Bodies

Clinicians are frequently confronted with a patient, often a child, who has inadvertently or intentionally swallowed a foreign body. One should adopt an attitude of watchful expectation unless the object has sharp projections which could injure the mucosal membrane or is obviously too large to pass the pylorus. In patients with a duodenal ulcer, small gastric foreign bodies which might otherwise enter the duodenum are often retained in the stomach and may precipitate pyloric obstruction. When it becomes obvious that the foreign body is not passing through the pylorus or is causing symptoms, it should be removed surgically. Before opening the abdomen, it is worthwhile to pass a flexible gastroscope into the stomach under general anesthesia and attempt removal with the biopsy attachment.

BEZOARS

Bezoars are concretions formed by the swallowing of material retained in the stomach. They may be:

1. Trichobezoars (balls formed from hair eaten by children, usually girls)
2. Phytobezoars (balls formed from vegetable fibers, such as those of persimmons)

Symptomatic bezoars require surgical removal only when they cannot be broken down by the intragastric administration of a preparation of *cellulose.* Because of the reduced gastric acidity and motility produced by a vagotomy for duodenal ulcer, patients who have had this operation seem more prone to developing phytobezoars. They must be cautioned against eating large amounts of highly fibrous fresh fruits.

GASTRIC CANCER

INCIDENCE. For unknown reasons the incidence of gastric cancer has been falling during recent decades. In the United States the age-adjusted mortality rate from gastric cancer fell from 29 per 100,000 in 1930 to 20 per 100,000 in 1945, to 13 per 100,000 in 1955 and to 7 per 100,000 in 1966. During the same time, deaths from all cancers increased from 197,042 in 1948 to 245,070 in 1956. The same phenomenon has been observed in the Netherlands, Norway, and Great Britain. By contrast, gastric cancer has become more prevalent in Japan, Chile, Iceland, Finland, and the Scandinavian countries. In Japan, gastric cancer constitutes slightly more than one-half of all cases of cancer. It is interesting to note that as the decrease in gastric cancer was taking place in the United States, the incidence of colonic cancer increased, so that today the colon is the most common location of cancers of the gut.

ETIOLOGY. The cause of gastric cancer remains unknown. Nevertheless it is associated with several factors which may eventually provide a clue to its etiology.

Environmental Factors. In the United States, as well as in several other countries, the frequency of gastric cancer increases with the distance from the equator. It has already been pointed out that the incidence of gastric cancer is considerably higher in Japan than it is in the United States. However, it is appreciably lower in Japanese immigrants to the United States. The incidence of gastric cancer in Japanese born in the United States is no greater than in Caucasian Americans.

Elsewhere, the incidence of gastric cancer has been found to be higher in the city than in the surrounding rural areas. Moreover, in urban areas, gastric cancer was more prevalent among laborers than among artisans and white collar workers.

Diet. Although a possible correlation between diet and gastric cancer has been studied extensively, consumption of cabbage is the only dietary factor correlating with gastric cancer in the United States. Countries with a high incidence of gastric cancer also have a high consumption of fish. Whether it is the fish itself or whether it is the cooking in superheated oils and fats or smoking that is responsible remains to be proved. Others have incriminated the salty and spicy foods so characteristic of the Japanese diet.

Heredity. The risk of developing a gastric cancer is greater than expected among the male and female relatives of patients with gastric cancer.

The interaction between gastric cancers and ABO blood groups may be a related phenomenon. Many controlled studies have shown an excess of blood group A and a deficiency of blood group O in comparison with control patients from the same population. These studies indicate that blood group A increases the risk of gastric cancer by about 20 percent, a proportional increase which remains the same regardless of the local overall incidence of gastric cancer. There does not appear to be a correlation between ABO blood groups and the site of origin of the tumor in the stomach.

Sex. As with other tumors of the gut, gastric cancer is more prevalent among men than among women. This male predominance appears greater during the fifth, sixth, and seventh decades of life and greater for tumors originating in the fundus than for tumors growing in the antrum.

Atrophic Gastritis and Achlorhydria. Several prospective studies have shown that individuals with atrophic gastritis when followed over many years eventually proved to have an incidence of gastric cancer of about 10 percent. This is in comparison with similar prospective studies of subjects with a normal gastric mucosa in whom no gastric cancers developed during the same period. Studies such as these have shown conclusively that gastritis with *intestinal metaplasia* found in the mucosa around a carcinoma or in areas remote from the tumor represents a premalignant state rather than a secondary reaction induced by the

cancer. The atrophic gastritis accompanying gastric cancer may be of the diffuse, "autoimmune" type associated with pernicious anemia or of the multifocal "simple" variety. Recent studies suggest that the latter is numerically a more important precursor of gastric cancer than the former.

It is well known that achlorhydria exists in approximately one-half of patients with gastric cancer. The atrophic gastritis which almost invariably accompanies a gastric cancer is sufficient to account for this phenomenon.

Relationship between Gastric Ulcer and Gastric Cancer. In the past, one of the most controversial questions concerning gastric carcinoma was its relationship to benign gastric ulcer. For many years it was believed that benign ulcers often underwent malignant degeneration. This view has been discredited; it is now generally agreed that an ulcer either is malignant from the beginning or remains benign. The respective locations of benign gastric ulcers and gastric cancers argue against a common etiology. The majority of benign gastric ulcers occur on the lesser curvature. By contrast, 40 to 71 percent of cancers appear in the antrum. Occasionally, a pathologist discovers neoplastic cells in the margin of what appears to be a benign gastric ulcer. This may result from necrosis of carcinoma or may represent coincidental development of carcinoma in the vicinity of a benign gastric ulcer. At present, the important question raised by the finding of a gastric ulceration is not whether it may become malignant but whether it is, in fact, benign or malignant.

CLINICAL MANIFESTATIONS. The clinical manifestations of gastric carcinoma are so vague and misleading that a tumor may develop and become inoperable while a patient is being followed carefully. The most frequent symptom is weight loss. Lesions in the prepyloric antrum interfere with gastric emptying and cause gastric stasis and vomiting. The vomitus often has a characteristic coffee-ground appearance due to slow bleeding from the tumor. Anorexia, particularly pronounced for meat, postprandial fullness, and indigestion occur in one-fourth of the cases. As an early symptom pain is unreliable but is often present in far-advanced cases and under these conditions represents extragastric invasion by the tumor. The chronic slow bleeding from a fungating tumor often causes an iron deficiency anemia accompanied by weakness, dizziness, and dyspnea upon exertion. Occasionally, the first manifestation of a gastric carcinoma is an acute peritonitis due to a perforation of the malignant ulceration. A mass is present in one-third of the cases and, although an ominous sign, does not always signify inoperability. As a general rule, it can be said that when many of or all these symptoms are present, the chances for operative cure are minimal. Experience indicates that survival after curative operation is longer when the tumor has been asymptomatic.

LABORATORY AND DIAGNOSTIC STUDIES. Discussed previously under the heading Roentgenography in the section on Gastric Ulceration.

PATHOLOGY. Gross Appearance. According to their gross appearance, gastric carcinomas may be classified as follows.

Polypoid or Fungating. The lesion forms a bulky mass

protruding into the gastric lumen. This type is more often located in the cardia or the fundus. Most of these tumors have the histologic appearance of well-differentiated adenocarcinoma.

Ulcerative. Most of these malignant ulcerations are located on the lesser curvature or in the prepyloric antrum, and about half are moderately well-differentiated adenocarcinomas. This is the variety that may be confused clinically with a benign gastric ulcer.

Infiltrating. This type infiltrates the gastric wall diffusely and forms sessile intraluminal masses. The histologic appearance is more often that of a poorly differentiated adenocarcinoma. Linitis plastica, or "leather bottle stomach" (Fig. 26-28), is simply a variant of infiltrating gastric carcinoma. The lesion is characterized by a profound desmoplasia with sections of the gastric wall appearing thickened by a grayish white infiltrate. Histologic sections contain large amounts of fibrous tissue with rare signet ring cells often in "single file." Gland formation is sparse. The infiltrating *"diffuse"* form of gastric adenocarcinoma carries the worst prognosis.

Histology. The histologic classification of gastric carcinoma is based upon the degree of cellular anaplasia. This classification has some prognostic value. For instance, the

Fig. 26-28. Radiologic appearance of a stomach diffusely infiltrated with adenocarcinoma of the linitis plastica variety. This is the typical "leather-bottle stomach."

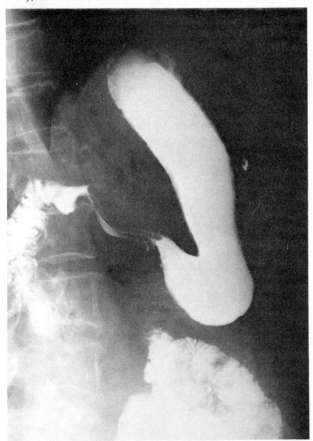

5-year survival after curative operation for low-grade carcinoma without nodes is approximately 50 percent. The 5-year survival rate for highly undifferentiated carcinomas is much lower.

One of the characteristics of gastric carcinoma is a tendency to intramural extension via lymphatic channels. In tumors involving the gastric antrum, submucosal invasion of the duodenum along subserosal lymphatics occurs in 43 percent of the cases. In tumors of the fundus and cardia, spread into the esophagus along submucosal lymphatics is frequent. Therefore, the lines of surgical transection should be placed well beyond the palpable margins of the tumor, since the distance involved by the intramural spread ranges from 3 to 6 cm. It seems to be greater for the esophagus than for the duodenum.

Lymphatic Spread. Invasion of the regional lymphatics in carcinoma of the stomach is often extensive and is present in 50 to 70 percent of the cases in which curative operation is attempted. If one includes cases in which surgical treatment is carried out for palliation, the incidence of lymph node metastasis is as high as 75 percent. Metastases to regional lymphatics from an adenocarcinoma of the stomach characteristically involve four zones of spread, listed below.

Infiltrating adenocarcinoma spreads to these regional lymph nodes more often than the polypoid variety. Recent studies have shown that the zone 2 groups of lymph nodes are involved in 30 percent of the cases of carcinoma involving the distal portion of the stomach. This finding has prompted some workers to include the spleen in the en bloc resection of the stomach and zones of lymphatic spread.

Zone 1 consists of nodes and lymphatic vessels located in the gastrocolic ligament around the right gastroepiploic vessels. Drainage to this group of lymph nodes comes from the pyloric portion of the greater curvature. Lymph flow from this area goes to the pylorus and then to the celiac and aortic nodes.

Zone 2 consists of nodes and lymphatic vessels situated in the gastrocolic and gastrosplenic ligaments around the left gastroepiploic vessels. This group of lymph nodes drains the cardia and fundus of the stomach. From here, lymph reaches the splenic vessels along the upper border of the pancreas and then the preaortic lymph nodes.

Zone 3 is situated around the left gastric artery along the proximal two-thirds of the stomach and drains the proximal portion of the lesser curvature of the stomach. From here, lymph reaches nodes around the celiac axis. Lymph from the nodes located around the cardia may drain into periesophageal nodes.

Zone 4 drains the pylorus and distal portion of the lesser curvature. Lymph from these nodes, situated above the pylorus and first portion of the duodenum, drains into hepatic nodes located around the hepatic artery, and from there to celiac and preaortic nodes.

Extramural Spread. Gastric adenocarcinoma also spreads by direct invasion of surrounding structures. Those most frequently involved are the liver, the pancreas, and the transverse colon. In addition, after the serosa of the stomach has been invaded, cells become seeded directly into the peritoneal cavity and form widespread serosal tumor implants. Implants occur with characteristic frequency in the rectovesical or rectouterine cul de sac (Blumer's shelf) and in the ovary (Krukenberg's tumor).

Staging of Gastric Cancer. The accurate staging of each gastric tumor is essential for prognosis in a given case and for the meaningful evaluation of various therapeutic modalities. A widely adapted staging scheme is the one recently proposed by the American Joint Committee for Cancer Staging and End Results Reporting. This staging system, known as the TNM system, is based upon the degree of penetration of the primary tumor into the wall of the stomach, upon spread to regional lymph nodes, and upon the presence or absence of metastatic tumor in distant organs. The size of the primary lesion, its location in the stomach, and its degree of histologic differentiation all have no weight in this staging scheme and in the ultimate prognosis of an individual lesion.

Three components comprise this TNM system:

1. The status of the primary tumor, designated by the letter "T," expressed by the degree of penetration of the tumor through the gastric wall.
   - T1. Tumor confined to the mucosa.
   - T2. Tumor involving all layers of the gastric wall including the serosa but not extending through the serosa.
   - T3. Tumor extends through the serosa with or without invasion of adjacent structures.
   - T4. Diffuse infiltration of all layers of the gastric wall. The lesion has no demonstrable boundaries (linitis plastica).
   - TX. Degree of involvement of gastric wall not determined.
2. The status of the regional lymph nodes, designated by the letter N.
   - N0. Lymph nodes free of tumor.
   - N1. Metastatic deposits in the perigastric lymph nodes adjacent to the primary tumor.
   - N2. Metastatic deposits in the perigastric lymph nodes remote from the tumor or on both gastric curvatures.
   - NX. Presence or absence of lymph node metastases not determined.
3. The status of distant organs and tissues with respect to metastatic spread, designated by the letter M.
   - M0. No distant metastasis.
   - M1. Distant metastasis demonstrated clinically, radiologically, or surgically in remote tissues or organs and including nodes beyond the regional lymph nodes but excluding direct invasion by the primary tumor.

On the basis of the preceding classification of the extent of the disease in a given case the following scheme of staging is being widely adopted.

Stage I
A. Tumor confined to the mucosa without tumor deposits in the regional lymph nodes or remote tissues. (T1, N0, M0.)
B. Tumor extending to but not through the serosa without tumor deposits in the regional lymph nodes or remote tissues. (T2, N0, M0.)
C. Tumor extending through the serosa with or without invasion of adjacent structures and without tumor deposits in the regional lymph nodes or remote tissues. (T3, N0, M0.)

Stage II
Diffuse involvement of the gastric wall (linitis plastica) without node involvement or distant metastasis. (T4, N0, M0.)

Or, any degree of involvement of the gastric wall with tumor deposits in the regional lymph nodes but without distant metastasis. (T1, N1, M0; T2, N1, M0; T3, N1, M0; T4, N1, M0.)

Stage III
Any degree of involvement of the gastric wall accompanied by metastatic deposits in perigastric lymph nodes remote from the tumor or on both gastric curvatures but without metastasis in remote tissues or organs. (T1, N2, M0; T2, N2, M0; T3, N2, M0; T4, N2, M0.)

Stage IV
Any gastric carcinoma with distant metastasis regardless of the status of the primary tumor or the perigastric lymph nodes.

TREATMENT. At present the only way of curing carcinoma of the stomach is to remove the involved stomach before the advent of metastases or invasion extending beyond the confines of the stomach and the adjacent channels of lymphatic spread. The history of surgical operation for gastric cancer goes back to 1881, when the first successful partial gastrectomy was performed by Billroth. Schlatter, in 1897, performed the first total gastrectomy for gastric cancer. With perfection of surgical techniques and of preoperative and postoperative care, surgical operations for gastric carcinoma became more and more extensive. In the 1940s routine total gastrectomy for gastric carcinoma was employed in several clinics as the method of choice. Because of lymphatic spread to lymph nodes along the superior border of the pancreas and along the celiac axis, several writers have described inclusion of the body and tail of the pancreas, the spleen, the hepatic artery up to the junction of the gastroduodenal artery, the gastrocolic ligament, and the omentum in the block of tissue resected with the stomach. The mortality rate of such extensive procedures has been as high as 50 percent. However, technical improvements have reduced the mortality of extensive operations to below 10 percent. But time has shown that the 5-year survival rate after surgical treatment has not been appreciably increased by extending the scope of the operation. As a result, there has been a return to less extensive procedures, and the approach followed by many surgeons at present is as follows.

For carcinomas involving the distal portion of the stomach, which represents the majority of gastric carcinomas, the operation performed is a radical distal subtotal gastric resection, removing approximately 80 percent of the stomach. The operation is extended distally to include the first portion of the duodenum, so that lymph nodes and lymphatic channels in the pyloric region may be removed. Because of the frequent involvement of nodes in the gastrosplenic ligament, the spleen and the greater omentum are included in the bloc of resected tissue. The left gastric artery is divided at its origin, and the entire gastrohepatic omentum is removed in continuity with the specimen. Gastrointestinal continuity is reestablished by anastomosing the remaining gastric pouch either to the first portion of the duodenum as a Billroth I type of anastomosis or to the jejunum as a Billroth II procedure, which may be antecolic or retrocolic. A total gastrectomy including the omentum, the spleen, the first portion of the duodenum, and possibly the celiac artery if surrounded by involved nodes is reserved for more extensive tumors, particularly of the fundus. *Adjunctive* chemotherapy, preferably with several drugs, should be started as soon as possible after the patient's recovery from surgery. At present, this represents the only hope of improving the survival rate.

It is important that the operating surgeon thoroughly explore the abdomen before attempting to remove the gastric tumor. Hepatic metastases, ascitic fluid in the peritoneal cavity, visible serosal implants, implants in the rectouterine or rectovesical pouch preclude curative surgical operation. To attempt heroic resective surgical treatment under these conditions is simply a refusal to acknowledge that the tumor has extended beyond the limits where resection can be carried out with a reasonable expectation of a cure. Because of the frequency with which one of the reasons mentioned above renders a gastric carcinoma inoperable, palliation is a frequent consideration. The main indications for palliative surgery are pyloric obstruction, bleeding, or impending perforation.

Under these conditions a limited gastric resection, when technically feasible, appears to provide more satisfactory results than a bypass procedure such as a gastroenterostomy. From time to time one may have to consider palliative procedures for problems created by a recurrence following a previous curative resection. A particularly distressing problem is the severe dysphagia caused by massive local recurrence around an esophagojejunostomy after a previous total gastrectomy. This situation cannot

be controlled by a feeding jejunostomy since one of the symptoms is the inability to swallow salivary secretions with consequent aspiration pneumonitis. We have achieved worthwhile palliation under these circumstances by bypassing the obstruction with a long jejunal loop brought up through the left leaf of the diaphragm and anastomosed to the esophagus above and to an unobstructed loop of small bowel below.

PROGNOSIS. Data indicating a slight improvement in the results of surgical treatment of gastric cancer are summarized in Fig. 26-29. It is quite obvious that although the results, expressed as 5-year survival rates of operated patients, may appear encouraging on the surface, they are in actuality quite dismal when one considers the 5-year survival rate of all patients with gastric cancer, which remains around 15 percent. This, of course, is due to the fact that only half of the patients with gastric cancer are operable with the goal of cure. The most significant factor in determining the prognosis of a patient with gastric carcinoma operated on for cure is the presence or absence of lymph node metastases. Only 7 percent of patients with metastases to regional lymph nodes survive for more than 5 years after the operation. By contrast, 35 percent of the patients can be expected to survive after gastrectomy if the regional nodes are uninvolved. More recent figures suggest that the 5-year survival rate in the absence of lymph node involvement in some hands may be as high as 45 percent.

MISCELLANEOUS TUMORS

Malignant Tumors

LEIOMYOSARCOMA

These lesions comprise approximately 1 percent of all gastric malignant tumors. They usually form bulky intraluminal tumors, although they may infiltrate the gastric wall widely or grow extraluminally. A characteristic of intraluminal leiomyosarcomas is necrosis of the core of the tumor with formation of a huge ulceration within the tumor mass. The prognosis for 5-year survival following gastric resection is good (67 percent).

LYMPHOMA

Gastric lymphomas represent approximately 2 percent of gastric malignant tumors. Radiologically, they often present as ill-defined gastric masses, frequently with diffuse thickening of the rugal folds. The treatment of gastric lymphoma consists of a radical subtotal resection followed by postoperative radiation. The 5-year survival rate following this form of therapy is approximately 40 percent.

Benign Tumors

Polypoid adenomas or polyps of the stomach represent the most frequent benign gastric tumors. They are often single but may be multiple, and have demonstrated a propensity for malignant degeneration. There is an in-

Fig. 26-29. Ultimate survival rates for all patients with diagnosed gastric carcinoma. Note that from about 1910 to 1965 the greatest improvements have been in the rates of operability and resectability. (*Reproduced from W. H. ReMine, J. T. Priestley, and J. Berkson, "Cancer of the Stomach," W. B. Saunders Company, Philadelphia, 1964.*)

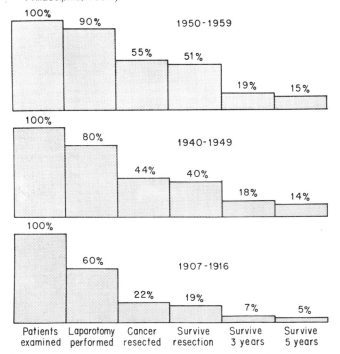

100%	90%	55%	51%	19%	15%
		1950-1959			
100%	80%	44%	40%	18%	14%
		1940-1949			
100%	60%	22%	19%	7%	5%
		1907-1916			
Patients examined	Laparotomy performed	Cancer resected	Survive resection	Survive 3 years	Survive 5 years

creased incidence of carcinoma with polyps above 3 cm. Treatment consists of resection of the polyp with a rim of normal mucosa around it. A partial gastrectomy should be performed for diffuse gastric polyposis. If the latter involves the entire stomach, a total gastrectomy should be considered, because of the malignant potential of these lesions. However, before resecting the stomach, it should be definitely ascertained that one is dealing with gastric polyps and not a giant hypertrophic gastritis. In the latter condition, the giant rugal folds often simulate polyps. Other common benign tumors of the stomach are, in order of decreasing frequency, aberrant pancreatic tumors, leiomyomas, neurogenic tumors, fibromas, and lipomas. The majority of these tumors are asymptomatic and usually are discovered incidentally during an upper gastrointestinal tract series.

References

Anatomy

Bentley, F. H., and Barlow, T. E.: Stomach: Vascular Supply in Relation to Gastric Ulcer, *Surg Prog, 1952,* Butterworth & Co., London, 1953.

Gastric Function

Anderson, S., and Olbe, L.: Gastric Acid Secretory Responses to Gastrin and Histamine in Dogs before and after Vagal Denervation of the Gastric Pouch, *Acta Physiol Scand,* **60:**51, 1964.

Brackney, E. L., Thal, A. P., and Wangensteen, O. H.: Role of duodenum in the control of gastric secretion, *Proc Soc Exp Biol Med,* **88:**302, 1955.

Brunschwig, A., Rasmussen, R. A., Camp, E. J., and Moe, R.: Gastric Secretory Depressant in Gastric Juice, *Surgery,* **12:**887, 1942.

Card, W. I., and Marks, I. N.: The Relationship between the Acid Output of the Stomach following "Maximal" Histamine Stimulation and the Parietal Cell Mass, *Clin Sci,* **19:**147, 1960.

Code, C. F., and Watkinson, G.: Importance of Vagal Innervation in the Regulatory Effect of Acid in the Duodenum on Gastric Secretion of Acid, *J Physiol* (*Lond*), **130:**233, 1955.

Davenport, H. W., Warner, H. A., Code, C. F.: Functional Significance of Gastric Mucosal Barrier to Sodium, *Gastroenterology,* **47:**142, 1964.

Davenport, H. W.: Destruction of the Gastric Mucosal Barrier by Detergents and Urea, *Gastroenterology,* **54:**175, 1968.

Edkins, J. S.: The Chemical Mechanism of Gastric Secretion, *J Physiol* (*Lond*), **34:**133, 1906.

Gibson, R., Hirschowitz, B. I., and Hutchison, G.: Actions of Metiamide, an H_2-Histamine Receptor Antagonist on Gastric H^+ and Pepsin Secretion in Dogs, *Gastroenterology,* **67:**93, 1974.

Gregory, R. A.: The Effect of Portal Venous Occlusion on Gastric Secretion, *J Physiol* (*Lond*), **137:**760, 1957.

—— and Tracy, H. J.: The Constitution and Properties of Two Gastrins Extracted from Hog Antral Mucosa. I. The Isolation of Two Gastrins from Hog Antral Mucosa. II. The Properties of Two Gastrins Isolated from Hog Antral Mucosa. W. H.

Taylor: A Note on the Nature of the Gastrin-like Stimulant Present in Zollinger-Ellison Tumors, *Gut,* **5:**103, 1964.

Isenberg, J. I.: Gastric Secretory Testing, in M. H. Sleisenger and J. S. Fordtran (eds.), "Gastrointestinal Disease," pp. 536–554, W. B. Saunders Company, Philadelphia, 1973.

Lebedinskaja, S. I.: Über die Magensekretion bei Eckschen Fistelhunden, *Z Gesamte Exp Med,* **88:**264, 1933.

Max, M., and Menguy, R.: Influence of Adrenocorticotropin, Cortisone, Aspirin and Phenylbutazone on the Rate of Exfoliation and the Rate of Renewal of Gastric Mucosal Cells, *Gastroenterology,* **58:**329, 1970.

McGuigan, J. E.: Immunochemical Studies With Synthetic Human Gastrin, *Gastroenterology,* **54:**1005, 1968.

McGuigan, J. E., and Trudeau, W. L.: Serum Gastrin Concentrations in Pernicious Anemia, *N Engl J Med,* **282:**358, 1970.

McGuigan, J. E., and Trudeau, W. L.: Studies With Antibodies to Gastrin: Radioimmunoassay in Human Serum and Physiological Studies, *Gastroenterology,* **58:**139, 1970.

Menguy, R.: Studies on the Role of the Pancreatic and Biliary Secretion in the Mechanism of Gastric Inhibition by Fat, *Surgery,* **48:**195, 1960.

——: Effect of Biliary Diversion from the Small Intestine on Gastric Secretory Activity in Dogs, *Gastroenterology,* **41:**568, 1961.

——: Pathogenesis of Mann-Williamson Ulcer. III. Effect of Excluding Pancreatic or Biliary Secretions from the Intestine on Gastric Secretion and Liver Function, *Surgery,* **54:**495, 1963.

—— and Masters, Y. F.: Effect of Cortisone on Mucoprotein Secretion by Gastric Antrum of Dogs: Pathogenesis of Steroid Ulcer, *Surgery,* **54:**19, 1963.

Nyhus, L. M., Chapman, N. D., DeVito, R. V., and Harkins, H. N.: The Control of Gastrin Release: An Experimental Study Illustrating a New Concept, *Gastroenterology,* **39:**582, 1960.

Passaro, E. P., and Grossman, M. I.: Effect of Vagal Innervation on Acid and Pepsin Response to Histamine and Gastrin, *Am J Physiol,* **206:**1068, 1964.

Porter, R. W., Brady, J. V., Conrad, M. A., Mason, J. W., Galambos, R., and Rioch, D. M.: Some Experimental Observations on Gastrointestinal Lesions in Behaviorally Conditioned Monkeys, *Psychosom Med,* **20:**379, 1958.

Shay, H.: Stress and Gastric Secretion, *Gastroenterology,* **26:**316, 1954.

Silen, W., Hein, M. F., and Harper, H. A.: The Influence of the Liver upon Canine Gastric Secretion, *Surgery,* **54:**29, 1963.

——, Skillman, J. J., Hein, M., and Harper, H. A.: The Effect of Biliary Obstruction upon Canine Gastric Secretory Activity, *J Surg Res,* **2:**197, 1962.

Sircus, W.: The Intestinal Phase of Gastric Secretion, *Q J Exp Physiol,* **38:**91, 1953.

Skillman, J. J., Silen, W., Harper, H. A., Neely, J. C., and Simmons, E. L.: Effect of Hepatocellular Injury on Gastric Secretion in Dogs, *Surg Forum,* **12:**276, 1961.

Sokolov, A. P.: Analysis of the Secretory Work of the Stomach in the Dog, thesis, St. Petersburg, 1904.

Stavney, L. S., Kato, T., Savage, L. E., Harkins, H. N., and Nyhus, L. M.: Parietal Cell Reactivity, *Surg Gynecol Obstet,* **118:**1269, 1964.

Trudeau, W. L., McGuigan, J. E.: Relations between Serum

Gastrin Levels and Rates of Gastric Hydrochloric Acid Secretion, *N Engl J Med,* **284:**408, 1971.

Uvnas, B.: The Part Played by the Pyloric Region in the Cephalic Phase of Gastric Secretion, *Acta Physiol Scand,* **4**(Suppl. 13):1942.

Villarreal, R., Ganong, W. F., and Gray, S. J.: Effect of Adrenocorticotrophic Hormone upon the Gastric Secretion of Hydrochloric Acid, Pepsin and Electrolytes in the Dog, *Am J Physiol,* **183:**485, 1955.

Walsh, J. H., and Grossman, M. I.: Gastrin, *N Engl J Med,* **292:**1324, 1975.

Wolf, S., and Wolff, H. G.: "Human Gastric Function," Oxford University Press, London, 1943.

Woodward, E. R., Lyon, E. J., Landor, J., and Dragstedt, L. R.: The Physiology of the Gastric Antrum: Experimental Studies on Isolated Antral Pouches in Dogs, *Gastroenterology,* **27:**766, 1954.

———, Robertson, C., Fried, W., and Schapiro, H.: Further Studies on the Isolated Gastric Antrum, *Gastroenterology,* **32:**868, 1957.

Peptic Ulcer Disease

Brooks, J. R., and Eraklis, A. J.: Factors Affecting the Mortality from Peptic Ulcer, *N Engl J Med,* **271:**803, 1964.

Clarke, J. S., Costarella, R., and Ward, S.: Gastric Secretion in the Fasting State and after Antral Stimulation in Patients with Cirrhosis and Portacaval Shunts, *Surg Forum,* **9:**417, 1958.

———, McKissock, P. K., and Cruze, K.: Studies on the Site of Origin of the Agent Causing Hypersecretion in Dogs with Portacaval Shunt, *Surgery,* **46:**48, 1959.

———, Ozeran, R. S., Hart, J. C., Cruze, K., and Crevling, V.: Peptic Ulcer following Portacaval Shunt, *Ann Surg,* **148:**551, 1958.

Doll, R., and Buch, J.: Hereditary Factors in Peptic Ulcer, *Ann Eugenics,* **15:**135, 1950.

———, Swynnerton, B. F., and Newell, A. C.: Observations on Blood Group Distribution in Peptic Ulcer and Gastric Cancer, *Gut,* **1:**31, 1960.

Dragstedt, L. R.: The Etiology of Gastric and Duodenal Ulcers, *Postgrad Med,* **15:**99, 1954.

DuPlessis, D. J.: Some Aspects of the Pathogenesis and Surgical Management of Peptic Ulcers, *S Afr Med J,* **34:**101, 1960.

Flint, F. J., and Warrack, A. J.: Acute Peptic Ulceration in Emphysema, *Lancet,* **2:**178, 1958.

Grossman, M. I., Kirsner, J. B., and Gillespie, I. E.: Basal and Histalog-stimulated Gastric Secretion in Control Subjects and in Patients with Peptic Ulcer or Gastric Cancer, *Gastroenterology,* **45:**14, 1963.

Kammerer, W. H., Freiberger, R. H., and Rivelis, A. L.: Peptic Ulcer in Rheumatoid Patients on Corticosteroid Therapy: Clinical Experimental and Radiologic Study, *Arthritis Rheum,* **1:**122, 1958.

Katz, D., Douvres, P., Weisberg, H., McKinnon, W., Glass, G. B. Jerzy: Early Diagnosis of Upper Gastrointestinal Hemorrhage, *JAMA,* **188:**405, 1964.

Kern, F., Jr., Clark, G. M., and Lukens, J. G.: Peptic Ulceration Occurring during Therapy for Rheumatoid Arthritis, *Gastroenterology,* **33:**25, 1957.

Lambling, A., Gosset, J., Bertrand, I., and Viau, P.: Le genie evolutif de la maladie ulcereuse avant et pendant la guerre, *Paris Med,* **36:**146, 1946.

Meltzer, L. E., Bockman, A. A., Kanenson, W., and Cohen, A.: Incidence of Peptic Ulcer among Patients on Long term Prednisone Therapy, *Gastroenterology,* **35:**351, 1958.

Menguy, R., and Masters, Y. F.: Effects of Aspirin on Gastric Mucous Secretion, *Surg Gynecol Obstet.,* **120:**92, 1965.

Muir, A., and Cossar, I. A.: Aspirin and Ulcer, *Br Med J,* **2:**7, 1955.

Ostrow, J. D., Timmerman, R. J., and Gray, S. J.: Gastric Secretion in Human Hepatic Cirrhosis, *Gastroenterology,* **38:**303, 1960.

Palmer, E. D.: Cyclic Dynamism in Ulcer Disease, *Surg Gynec Obstet,* **130:**709, 1970.

Spicer, C. C., Stewart, D. N., and Winser, D. M. deR.: Perforated Peptic Ulcer during the Period of Heavy Air Raids, *Lancet,* **1:**14, 1944.

Stolzer, B. L., Barr, J. H., Jr., Eisenbeis, C. H., Jr., Wechsler, R. C. and Margolis, H. M.: Prednisone and Prednisolone Therapy in Rheumatoid Arthritis: Clinical Evaluation with Emphasis on Gastrointestinal Manifestations in 156 Patients Observed for Periods of 4 to 14 months, *JAMA,* **165:**13, 1957.

Trudeau, W. L., and McGuigan, J. E.: Serum Gastrin Levels in Patients with Peptic Ulcer Disease, *Gastroenterology,* **59:**6, 1970.

Welsh, J. D., and Wolf, S.: Geographical and Environmental Aspect of Peptic Ulcer, *Am J Med,* **29:**754, 1960.

Winkelman, E. I., and Summerskill, W. H. G.: Gastric secretion in Relation to Gastrointestinal Bleeding from Salicylate Compounds, *Gastroenterology,* **40:**56, 1961.

Zasly, L., Baum, G. L., and Rumball, J. M.: A Study of Gastric Secretions in Chronic Obstructive Pulmonary Emphysema, *Dis Chest,* **38:**69, 1960.

Zollinger, R. M., Elliott, D. W., Endahl, G. L., Grant, G. N., Goswitz, J. T., and Taft, D. A.: Origin of the Ulcerogenic Hormone in Endocrine Induced Ulcer, *Ann Surg,* **156:**570, 1962.

——— and ———: Primary Peptic Ulcerations of the Jejunum Associated with Islet-cell Tumors of the Pancreas, *Ann Surg,* **142:**709, 1955.

Duodenal Ulcer Diathesis

Amdrup, B. M., and Griffith, C. A.: Selective Vagotomy of the Parietal Cell Mass. I. With preservation of the innervated antrum and pylorus, *Ann Surg,* **170:**207, 1969.

Bruce, J., Card, W. I., Marks, I. N., and Sircus, W.: The Rationale of Selective Surgery in the Treatment of Duodenal Ulcer, *J R Coll Surg Edinb,* **4:**85, 1959.

Burns, G. P., Cheng, F. C. Y., Cox, A. G., Payne, R. A., Spencer, J., and Welbourn, R. B.: Significance of Early and Late Positive Responses to Insulin Hypoglycaemia in Patients with Intact Vagi, *Gut,* **10:**820, 1969.

Cushing, H.: Peptic Ulcers and the Interbrain, *Surg Gynecol Obstet,* **55:**1, 1932.

Davies, R. E., and Longmuir, N. M.: Production of Ulcers in Isolated Frog Gastric Mucosa, *Biochem J,* **42:**621, 1948.

Desbaillets, L., and Menguy, R.: Influence of Corticotrophic Hormone on the Secretion of Gastric Mucus, *Surg Forum,* **17:**291, 1966.

Donegan, W. L., and Spiro, H. M.: Parathyroids and Gastric Secretion, *Gastroenterology,* **38:**750, 1960.

Dragstedt, L. R.: Pathogenesis of Gastroduodenal Ulcer, *Arch Surg,* **44:**438, 1942.

Dragstedt, L. R.: Vagotomy for Gastroduodenal Ulcer, *Ann Surg,* **122:**973, 1945.

———— and Owens, F. M., Jr.: Supradiaphragmatic Section of Vagus Nerves in Treatment of Duodenal Ulcer, *Proc Soc Exp Biol Med,* **53:**152, 1943.

————: The Role of the Nervous System in the Pathogenesis of Duodenal Ulcer, *Surgery,* **34:**902, 1953.

Elliott, D. W., Taft, D. A., Passaro, E., and Zollinger, R. M.: Pancreatic Influences on Gastric Secretion, *Surgery,* **50:**126, 1961.

Ellison, E. H., and Wilson, S. D.: Zollinger-Ellison Syndrome: Re-appraisal and Evaluation of 206 Registered Cases, *Ann Surg,* **160:**512, 1964.

Elman, R., and Hartmann, A. F.: Spontaneous Peptic Ulcers of Duodenum after Continued Loss of Total Pancreatic Juice, *Arch Surg,* **23:**1030, 1931.

Emas, S., and Grossman, M. I.: Effect of Truncal Vagotomy on Acid and Pepsin Responses to Histamine and Gastrin in Dogs, *Am J Physiol,* **212:**1007, 1967.

Evans, D. A. P.: The Fucose and Agglutinogen Contents of Saliva in Subjects with Duodenal Ulcers, *J Lab Clin Med,* **55:**386, 1960.

Evans, R., Zajtchuk, R., and Menguy, R.: Role of Vagotomy and Gastric Drainage in the Surgical Treatment of Duodenal Ulcer: Results of a 10-year Experience at the University of Chicago Hospitals, *Surg Clin North Am,* **47:**141, 1967.

Farris, J. M., and Smith, G. K.: Vagotomy and Pyloroplastry for Bleeding Duodenal Ulcer, *Am J Surg,* **105:**388, 1963.

Fox, P. S., Hofmann, J. W., DeCosse, J. J., and Wilson, S. D.: The Influence of Total Gastrectomy on Survival in Malignant Zollinger-Ellison Tumors, *Ann Surg,* **180:**558, 1974.

Garrido-Klinge, G., and Pena, L.: Gastroduodenal ulcer in High Altitudes (Peruvian Andes), *Gastroenterology,* **37:**390, 1959.

Gillespie, G., Gillespie, I. E., and Kay, A. W.: An Analysis of the Insulin Test after Vagotomy Using Single and Multiple Criteria, *Gut,* **9:**470, 1968.

Goligher, J. C., Pulvertaft, C. N., deDombal, F. T., Clark, C. G., Conyers, J. T., Duthie, H. L., Feather, D. B., Latchmore, A. J. C., Matheson, T. S., Shoesmith, J. H., Smiddy, F. G., and Willson-Pepper, J.: Clinical Comparison of Vagotomy and Pyloroplasty with Other Forms of Elective Surgery for Duodenal Ulcer, *Br Med J,* **2:**787, 1968.

Gregory, R. A., Tracy, H. J., French, J. M., and Sircus, W.: Extraction of a Gastrin-like Substance from a Pancreatic Tumor in a Case of Zollinger-Ellison Syndrome, *Lancet,* **1:**1045, 1960.

Grossman, M. I., Matsumoto, K. K., and Lichter, R. J.: Fecal Blood Loss Produced by Oral and Intravenous Administration of Various Salicylates, *Gastroenterology,* **40:**383, 1961.

Herrington, J. L., Sawyers, J. L., and Scott, H. W., Jr.: A Twenty-five Year Experience with Vagotomy-Antrectomy, *Arch Surg,* **106:**469, 1973.

Hollander, F.: Laboratory Procedures in the Study of Vagotomy, *Gastroenterology,* **11:**419, 1948.

Holle, F., and Andersson, S. (eds.): "Vagotomy: Latest Advances with Special Reference to Gastric and Duodenal Ulcer Disease," Springer-Verlag, New York, 1974.

Johnston, D., and Wilkinson, A. R.: Highly Selective Vagotomy without a Drainage Procedure in the Treatment of Duodenal Ulcer, *Br J Surg,* **57:**289, 1970.

Kramer, P., and Markarian, B.: Gastric Acid Secretion in Chronic Obstructive Pulmonary Emphysema, *Gastroenterology,* **38:**295, 1960.

McGuigan, J. E., and Trudeau, W. L.: Serum Gastrin Levels Before and After Vagotomy and Pyloroplasty or Vagotomy and Antrectomy, *N Engl J Med,* **286:**184, 1972.

Myhill, J., and Piper, D. W.: Antacid Therapy of Peptic Ulcer, *Gut,* **5:**581, 1964.

Oberhelman, H. A., Jr., Nelson, T. S., Johnson, A. N., Jr., and Dragstedt, L. R., II: Ulcerogenic Tumors of the Duodenum, *Ann Surg,* **153:**214, 1961.

Ostrow, J. D., Blanshard, G., and Gray, S. J.: Peptic Ulcer in Primary Hyperparathyroidism, *Am J Med,* **29:**769, 1960.

Rogers, H. M., Keating, F. R., Morlock, C. G., and Braker, N. W.: Primary Hypertrophy and Hyperplasia of the Parathyroid Glands Associated with Duodenal Ulcer, *Arch Intern Med,* **79:**307, 1947.

Roth, J. L. A.: Clinical Evaluation of the Caffeine Gastric Analysis in Duodenal Ulcer Patients, *Gastroenterology,* **19:**199, 1951.

Sawyers, H. L., and Scott, H. W., Jr.: Selective Gastric Vagotomy with Antrectomy or Pyloroplasty, *Ann Surg,* **174:**541, 1971.

Schlaeger, R., LeMay, M., and Wermer, P.: Upper Gastrointestinal Tract Alterations in Adenomatosis of the Endocrine Glands, *Radiology,* **75:**517, 1960.

Spencer, J. A., Morlock, C. G., and Sayre, G. P.: Lesions in the Upper Portion of the G. I. Tract Associated with Intracranial Neoplasms, *Gastroenterology,* **37:**20, 1959.

Tompkins, R. K., Kraft, A. R., Zimmerman, E., Lichtenstein, J. E., and Zollinger, R. M.: Clinical and Biochemical Evidence of Increased Gallstone Formation after Complete Vagotomy, *Surgery,* **71:**196, 1972.

Weinberg, J. A.: Treatment of the Massively Bleeding Duodenal Ulcer by Ligation, Pyloroplasty and Vagotomy, *Am J Surg,* **102:**158, 1961.

Wormsley, K. G., and Grossman, M. I.: Maximal Histalog Test in Control Subjects and Patients with Peptic Ulcer, *Gut,* **6:**427, 1950.

Gastric Ulcerations

Billington, B. P.: Observations from New South Wales on the Changing Incidence of Gastric Ulcer in Australia, *Gut,* **6:**121, 1965.

Black, R. B., Roberts, G., and Rhodes, J.: The Effect of Healing on Bile Reflux in Gastric Ulcer, *Gut,* **12:**552, 1971.

Burge, H.: The Etiology of Lesser-Curve Gastric Ulceration. Its Treatment by Vagotomy and Pyloroplasty, *De Med Tuenda,* **1:**16, 1964.

Chapman, B. L., and Duggan, J. M.: Aspirin and Uncomplicated Peptic Ulcer, *Gut,* **10:**443, 1969.

Davenport, H. W.: Is the Apparent Hyposecretion of Acid by Patients with Gastric Ulcer a Consequence of a Broken Barrier to Diffusion of Hydrogen Ions into the Gastric Mucosa? *Gut,* **6:**513, 1965.

Dragstedt, L. R., Oberhelman, H. A., Jr., Evans, S. O., and Rigler,

S. P.: Antrum Hyperfunction and Gastric Ulcer, *Ann Surg,* **140:**396, 1954.

Duggan, J. M., and Chapman, B. L.: The Incidence of Aspirin Ingestion in Patients with Peptic Ulcer, *Med J Aust,* **7:**797, 1970.

DuPlessis, D. J.: Pathogenesis of Gastric Ulceration, *Lancet,* **1:**974, 1965.

Farris, J. M., and Smith, G. K.: Some Other Operations for Gastric Ulcer, *Surg Clin North Am,* **46:**329, 1966.

Farris, J. M., and Smith, G. K.: Treatment of Gastric Ulcer (in situ) by Vagotomy and Pyloroplasty. A Clinical Study, *Ann Surg,* **158:**461, 1963.

Flint, F. J., and Grech, P.: Pyloric Regurgitation and Gastric Ulcer, *Gut,* **11:**735, 1970.

Gear, M. W. L., Truelove, S. C., and Whitehead, R.: Gastric Ulcer and Gastritis, *Gut,* **12:**639, 1971.

Harvey, H. D.: Twenty-five Years Experience with Elective Gastric Resection for Gastric Ulcer, *Surg Gynecol Obstet,* **113:**191, 1961.

Henley, W. H., and Bowers, R. F.: Observations of Surgical Therapy for Gastric Ulcer, *Arch Surg,* **90:**205, 1965.

Johnson, H. D.: Gastric Ulcer: Classification Blood Group Characteristics, Secretion Patterns and Pathogenesis, *Ann Surg,* **162:**996, 1965.

Kraft, R. O., Myers, J., Overton, S., and Fry, W. J.: Vagotomy and the Gastric Ulcer, *Am J Surg,* **121:**122, 1971.

Lampert, E. G., Waugh, J. M., and Dockerty, M. D.: The Incidence of Malignancy in Gastric Ulcers Believed Preoperatively to Be Benign, *Surg Gynecol Obstet,* **91:**673, 1950.

Larson, N. E., Cain, J. C., and Bartholomew, L. G.: Prognosis of the Medically Treated Small Gastric Ulcer. I. Comparison of Follow Data in Two Series, *N Engl J Med,* **264:**119, 1961.

Lawson, H. H.: Gastritis and Gastric Ulceration, *Br J Surg,* **53:**493, 1966.

Lawson, H. H.: Effect of Duodenal Contents on the Gastric Mucosa Under Experimental Conditions, *Lancet,* **1:**469, 1964.

Levrat, M., Pasquier, J., Martin, F., and Truchot, R.: Les ulceres medicamentaux de la grande courbure, *Arch Mal App Dig Nut,* **54:**305, 1965.

Mauer, E. F.: Toxic Effects of Phenylbutazone (Butazolidin); Review of Literature and Report of Twenty-third Death Following Its Use, *N Engl J Med,* **253:**404, 1955.

Menguy, R., and Max, M.: Influence of Bile on the Canine Gastric-Antral Mucosa, *Am J Surg,* **119:**177, 1970.

Ruding, R.: Gastric Ulcer and Antral Border, *Surgery,* **61:**495, 1967.

Stemmer, E. A., Zahn, R. L., Hom, L. W., and Connolly, J. E.: Vagotomy and Drainage Procedures for Gastric Ulcer, *Arch Surg,* **96:**586, 1968.

Veterans Administration Cooperative Study on Gastric Ulcer, *Gastroenterology,* **61:**567, 1971.

Wanka, J., Jones, L. I., Wood, P. H. N. and Dixon, St. J.: Indomethacin in Rheumatic Diseases: A Controlled Clinical Trial, *Ann Rheum Dis,* **23:**218, 1964.

Weisberg, H., and Glass, G. B.: Coexisting Gastric and Duodenal Ulcers; A Review, *Am J Dig Dis,* **8:**992, 1963.

Woodward, E. R., Eisenberg, M. M., and Dragstedt, L. R.: Recurrence of Gastric Ulcer After Pyloroplasty, *Am J Surg,* **113:**5, 1967.

Zahn, H. L., Stemmer, E. A., Hom, L. W., and Connolly, J. E.: Delayed Recurrence of Gastric Ulcer Following Vagotomy and Drainage Procedures, *Am Surg,* **34:**757, 1968.

Acute Gastric Mucosal Lesions

Bryant, L. R., and Griffen, W. O.: Vagotomy and Pyloroplasty: An Inadequate Operation for Stress Ulcers, *Arch Surg,* **93:**16, 1966.

Davenport, H. W.: Damage to the Gastric Mucosa: Effects of Salicylates and Stimulation, *Gastroenterology,* **49:**189, 1965.

Davenport, H. W.: Gastric Mucosal Injury by Fatty and Acetylsalicylic Acids, *Gastroenterology,* **46:**245, 1964.

Dieulafoy, G.: Exulteratio Simplex: L'Intervention Chirurgicale dans les Hematemèses Foudroyantes Consécutives, *Bull Acad Med,* **39:**49, 1898.

Ferguson, H. L., and Clarke, J. S.: Treatment of Hemorrhage from Erosive Gastritis by Vagotomy and Pyloroplasty, *Am J Surg,* **112:**739, 1966.

Fletcher, D. G., and Harkins, H. N.: Acute Peptic Ulcer as a Complication of Major Surgery, Stress or Trauma, *Surgery,* **36:**212, 1954.

Flowers, R. S., Kyle, K., and Hoerr, S. O.: Postoperative Hemorrhage from Stress Ulceration of the Stomach and Duodenum, *Am J Surg,* **119:**632, 1970.

Gilchrist, R. K., and Chun, N.: Severe Hemorrhage in Presumed Peptic Ulcer: Surgical Treatment in the Absence of Demonstrable Lesion, *Arch Surg,* **69:**366, 1954.

Goodman, A. A., and Frey, C. F.: Massive Upper Gastrointestinal Hemorrhage Following Surgical Operations, *Ann Surg,* **167:**180, 1968.

Harjola, P. A., and Sivula, A.: Gastric Ulcerations Following Experimentally Induced Hypoxia and Hemorrhagic Shock, *Ann Surg,* **163:**21, 1966.

Kirtley, J. A., Scott, H. W., Sawyers, J. L., Graves, H. A., and Lawler, M. R.: The Surgical Management of Stress Ulcers, *Ann Surg,* **169:**801, 1969.

Langman, M. J. S., Hansky, J. H., Drury, R. A. B., and Avery Jones, F.: The Gastric Mucosa in Radiologically Negative Acute Gastrointestinal Bleeding, *Gut,* **5:**550, 1964.

Law, E. J., Day, S. B., and MacMillan, B. G.: Autopsy Findings in the Upper Gastro-Intestinal Tract of 81 Burn Patients, *Arch Surg,* **102:**412, 1971.

Lucas, C. E., Sugawa, C., Riddle, J., Rector, F., Rosenberg, B., and Walt, A. J.: Natural History and Surgical Dilemma of "Stress" Gastric Bleeding, *Arch Surg,* **102:**266, 1971.

Menguy, R., Desbaillets, L., and Masters, Y. F.: Mechanism of Stress Ulcer: Influence of Hypovolemic Shock on Energy Metabolism in the Gastric Mucosa, *Gastroenterology,* **66:**46, 1974.

Menguy, R., Gadacz, T., and Zajtchuk, R.: The Surgical Management of Acute Gastric Mucosal Bleeding, *Arch Surg,* **99:**198, 1969.

Nusbaum, M., Baum, S., and Kuroda, K.: Selective Intra-arterial Infusion of Vasoactive Agents in the Control of Gastrointestinal Bleeding, *Arch Surg,* **97:**1005, 1968.

O'Neill, J. A., Pruitt, B. A., and Moncrief, J. A.: Surgical Treatment of Curling's Ulcer, *Surg Gynecol Obstet,* **126:**40, 1968.

Palmer, E. D.: Hemorrhage from Erosive Gastritis and its Surgical Implications, *Gastroenterology,* **36:**856, 1959.

Skillman, J. J., Bushnell, L. S., Goldman, H., and Silen, W.: Respiratory Failure, Hypotension, Sepsis and Jaundice: A Clinical Syndrome Associated with Lethal Hemorrhage from Acute Stress Ulceration of the Stomach, *Am J Surg,* **117:**523, 1969.

Skillman, J. J., and Silen, W.: Acute Gastroduodenal "Stress" Ulceration: Barrier Disruption of Varied Pathogenesis, *Gastroenterology,* **59:**478, 1970.

Sullivan, R. C., and Waddell, W. R.: Accumulated Experience with Vagotomy and Pyloroplasty for Surgical Control of Hemorrhagic Gastritis, *Am J Surg,* **116:**745, 1968.

Winawer, S. J., Bejar, J., and Zamcheck, N.: Recurrent Massive Hemorrhage in Patients with Achlorhydria and Atrophic Gastritis, *Arch Intern Med,* **120:**327, 1967.

Miscellaneous Surgical Diseases

Booher, R. J., and Grant, R. N.: Eosinophilic Granuloma of the Stomach and Small Intestine, *Surgery,* **30:**388, 1951.

Bruno, M. S., Grier, W. R. N., and Ober, W. B.: Spontaneous Laceration and Rupture of Esophagus and Stomach: Mallory-Weiss Syndrome, Boerhaave Syndrome, and Their Variants, *Arch Intern Med,* **112:**574, 1963.

DeBakey, M., and Ochsner, A.: Bezoars and Concretions, *Surgery,* **4:**934, 1938; **5:**132, 1939.

Dobbins, W. O.: Mallory-Weiss Syndrome: A Commonly Overlooked Cause of Upper Gastrointestinal Bleeding: Report of Three Cases and Review of the Literature, *Gastroenterology,* **44:**689, 1963.

Feldman, M., Morrison, S., and Myers, P.: The Clinical Evaluation of Prolapse of the Gastric Mucosa into the Duodenum, *Gastroenterology,* **22:**80, 1952.

Fieber, S. S.: Hypertrophic Gastritis: Report of 2 Cases and Analysis of 50 Pathologically Verified Cases from the Literature, *Gastroenterology,* **28:**39, 1955.

Mallory, G. K., and Weiss, S.: Hemorrhages from Lacerations of the Cardiac Orifice of the Stomach Due to Vomiting, *Am J Med Sci,* **178:**506, 1929.

Gastric Cancer

Ackerman, N. B.: An Evaluation of Gastric Cytology: Results of a Nationwide Survey, *J Chronic Dis,* **20:**621, 1967.

Aird, I., Bentall, H. H., and Fraser-Roberts, J. A.: A Relationship between Cancer of the Stomach and the ABO Blood Groups, *Br Med J,* **1:**799, 1953.

Berkson, J., Walters, W., Gray, H. K., and Priestley, J. T.: Mortality and Survival in Cancer of the Stomach: A Statistical Summary of the Experience of the Mayo Clinic, *Proc Staff Meetings Mayo Clin,* **27:**137, 1952.

Blendis, L. M., Beilby, J. O. W., Wilson, J. P., Coles, M. J., and Hadley, G. D.: Carcinoma of the Stomach: Evaluation of Individual and Combined Diagnostic Accuracy of Radiology, Cytology and Gastrophotography, *Br Med J,* **1:**656, 1967.

Brown, P. M., Cain, J. C., and Dockerty, M. B.: Clinically "Benign" Gastric Ulcerations Found to Be Malignant at Operation, *Surg Gynecol Obstet,* **112:**82, 1961.

Eisenberg, H., and Shambaugh, E.: Cancer of the Gastrointestinal Tract: Trends in Incidence and Mortality Rates. In: "Proceedings of the Sixth National Cancer Conference," p. 417, J. B. Lippincott Company, Philadelphia, 1968.

Gilbertsen, V. A.: Results of Treatment of Stomach Cancer, An Appraisal of Efforts for More Extensive Surgery and a Report of 1,983 Cases, *Cancer,* **23:**1305, 1969.

Huppler, E. G., Priestley, J. T., Morlock, C. G., and Gage, R. P.: Diagnosis and Results of Treatment in Gastric Polyps, *Surg, Gynecol Obstet,* **110:**390, 1960.

Kennedy, B. J.: TNM Classification for Stomach Cancer, *Cancer,* **26:**971, 1960.

Scott, H. W., Jr., and Longmire, W. P., Jr.: Total Gastrectomy. Report of Sixty-three Cases, *Surgery,* **26:**488, 1949.

"Staging System for Carcinoma of the Stomach, 1971," American Joint Committee for Cancer Staging and End Results Reporting, Chicago, 1971.

Stout, A. P.: Tumors of the Stomach, in "Atlas of Tumor Pathology," sec. VI, fascicle 21, Armed Forces Institute of Pathology, Washington, 1953.

Strode, J. E.: Malignant Lesions of the Stomach in Hawaii: Experiences with 350 Patients, *Surgery,* **49:**573, 1961.

Walker, I. R., Strickland, R. G., Ungar, B., and MacKay, I. R.: Simple Atrophic Gastritis and Gastric Carcinoma, *Gut,* **12:**906, 1971.

Welch, C. E., and Wilkins, E. W., Jr.: Carcinoma of the Stomach, *Ann Surg,* **148:**666, 1958.

Zinninger, M. M.: Extension of Gastric Cancer in the Intramural Lymphatics and its Relation to Gastrectomy, *Am Surg,* **20:**920, 1954.

Chapter 27

Small Intestine

by **Edward H. Storer**

Inflammatory Diseases

Regional Enteritis
Tuberculous Enteritis
Typhoid Enteritis

Neoplasms

Benign Neoplasms
    Peutz-Jeghers Syndrome
Malignant Neoplasms
    Carcinoids

Diverticular Disease

Meckel's Diverticulum
Duodenal Diverticula
Jejunal and Ileal Diverticula

Miscellaneous Problems

Ulcer of the Small Intestine
Ingested Foreign Bodies
Fistula
Pneumatosis Cystoides Intestinalis
Blind Loop Syndrome
Short Bowel Syndrome
Intestinal Bypass
    Morbid Obesity
    Hyperlipidemia

The length of the human small intestine at autopsy, after separation from its mesentery, is 6 to 8 m. In life, however, the intestine is about 3 m long because of a constant base-line state of muscular contraction. Estimates of the absorbing surface vary from 2.2 m² to larger than a tennis court depending on whether the microvilli are included in the estimate. Despite this impressive length and surface area, the small intestine is much less susceptible to primary disease than the stomach or colon—except for its first 3 cm, the duodenal bulb. Disease is as frequent in the first 3 cm as in all of the remaining 300 cm combined.

The small intestine has been relatively inaccessible for nonoperative diagnostic procedures compared to stomach or colon. Recent additions to the diagnostic armamentarium are proving to be of value in selected types of small bowel disease. Mucosal biopsies obtained with the peroral biopsy capsule are often diagnostic in diffuse mucosal diseases. Selective mesenteric angiography is often helpful in cases of discrete lesions that have vascular abnormalities such as neoplasms, vascular malformations, or actively bleeding lesions. Fiberoptic endoscopy of the duodenum and proximal jejunum is now a feasible clinical procedure.

Some diseases affecting the small intestine are discussed in other chapters: intestinal obstruction, Chap. 24; mesenteric vascular disease, Chap. 35; diseases of the intestine in infancy and childhood, Chap. 39; the intestine in trauma, Chap. 6; duodenal and gastrojejunal peptic ulcer, Chap. 26; and carcinoma of the second part of the duodenum, Chap. 32.

INFLAMMATORY DISEASES

Regional Enteritis

This is a chronic, sclerosing granulomatous disease of the gastrointestinal tract of unknown cause. Soon after Crohn's separation, in 1932, of what he initially called "terminal ileitis" from other chronic granulomas of the intestine, it was recognized that the disease, though most common in the terminal ileum, may affect any segment of the small or large bowel, so the term "regional enteritis" is now used in the United States. The eponym "Crohn's disease" is commonly employed elsewhere.

INCIDENCE. Though regional enteritis is the most common surgical disease of the small intestine, it is quite uncommon compared to other gastrointestinal diseases such as peptic ulcer or actue appendicitis. The range of incidence in the United States and Europe was estimated in 1972 to be two to four new cases per year per 100,000 population. Crohn's disease has its highest incidence in the United States, followed by the United Kingdom and Scandinavia. It is infrequent in Central Europe and only occasionally seen in Africa, Asia, and South America. The incidence is about three times higher in Jews than in non-Jews, appreciably higher in whites than in nonwhites, and slightly higher in males. The disease is seen in all age groups but is most frequent in young adults; the average age at onset of symptoms is twenty-seven years.

PATHOLOGY, PATHOGENESIS, AND ETIOLOGY. The usual sequence in discussion of a disease entity is etiology, pathogenesis, pathology. This sequence is here reversed in order to relate pathologic findings, which are well known, to hypotheses concerning pathogenetic and etiologic factors, which are not known.

Intestinal segments involved in chronic regional enteritis present a very characteristic appearance at operation. Diseased segments are beefy, dull purple-red, thickened to two or three times normal diameter, and covered with strands and patches of thick gray-white exudate. Mesenteric fat tends to grow over the serosa so that it nearly encompasses the bowel in areas of maximal involvement. The thickened bowel wall is very firm, rubbery, and virtually incompressible. Involved segments are often adherent to adjacent loops or other viscera, or several loops may be matted together into a bulky conglomerate mass. Internal fistulas are frequently present in such adherent areas. The mesentery of the segment is characteristically greatly thickened, dull, and rubbery, and contains lymph node masses up to 3 or 4 cm in size. The uninvolved proximal bowel is often dilated because of the considerable degree of obstruction present in the diseased segment.

Three striking abnormalities are seen in areas of maximal involvement on opening a resected specimen: tremendous thickening of the bowel wall, the submucosa showing the greatest increase in breadth; marked narrowing of the lumen; and varying degrees of mucosal nodularity, ulceration, and destruction.

Diseased tissues are less strikingly abnormal in the acute phase of regional enteritis. Early changes are principally marked hyperemia, dullness and fine granularity of the serosal surface, edema and soft thickening of the bowel wall, and edema of the corresponding mesentery. Moderately enlarged soft mesenteric lymph nodes are frequently but not invariably present.

The relationship of "acute regional enteritis" to the classical chronic form is unclear. Acute enteritis is usually discovered at laparotomy for suspected appendicitis. Only a minority of these patients progress to chronic regional enteritis; in the majority the process subsides without medical or surgical therapy. Some acute regional enteritides may be attributable to specific agents such as enteroviruses or Yersinia species, and perhaps also to allergic phenomena.

Regional enteritis may involve any segment of the gastrointestinal tract from esophagus to rectum. Isolated involvement of esophagus, stomach, or duodenum are rare, however. Granulomatous disease limited to the colon occurs fairly frequently and is discussed in Chap. 28. There are three principal patterns of involvement of the small intestine that occur in about 95 percent of all patients with this disease. The most frequent site of involvement is the terminal ileum, and in nearly one-half this is the only segment involved. In the classic terminal ileitis pattern there is an abrupt demarcation at the ileocecal valve with minimal or no cecal abnormality. Maximal disease of bowel and mesentery extends proximally for 15 to 25 cm, beyond which the degree of involvement diminishes fairly rapidly to dilated but otherwise normal proximal small bowel and accompanying mesentery. In about one-third of patients both small and large bowel are involved. The disease is often continuous, since terminal ileum is the most frequently involved segment of small bowel, and cecum and right colon the most frequent site of colonic involvement. This is not invariable, however, and areas of disease may be separated by segments of essentially normal bowel—"skip areas." The third pattern, jejunoileitis, extensively involves the distal one-half of the jejunum and proximal one-half of ileum. Infrequently, multiple diseased segments of varying lengths involve the entire length of small bowel.

Microscopic features of regional enteritis are somewhat variable, but histologic features occur with sufficient consistency to create a pattern that, while not specific, is characteristic of the disease. Some understanding of pathogenesis may be gained by observing the progression of changes from early to late phases of regional enteritis.

The most striking finding in the early phase is a marked edema of the entire bowel wall, but especially the submucosa. The edema is accompanied by lymphangiectasis and hyperemia. Mucosa is essentially normal except for an increase in the proportion of goblet cells. A fibrinopurulent exudate is invariably present on the serosal surface. Granulomas are not found in the early phase.

In the intermediate phase, though edema and lymphangiectasis persist, thickening of the bowel wall is more attributable to fibrosis of submucosa and subserosa. Small focal ulcers that rarely penetrate the muscularis mucosa are numerous, and the lamina propria is infiltrated with lymphocytes, plasma cells, and variable numbers of eosinophils. In the submucosa, the extensive fibrosis is fine and fibrillar in character and is accompanied by diffuse infiltration of mononuclear cells and prominent hypertrophy and hyperplasia of lymphoid follicles. The muscularis propria also demonstrates hypertrophy, fibrosis, and cellular infiltrate but to a lesser degree than the submucosa. Granulomas may be present, particularly in the submucosa, subserosa, or regional lymph nodes. They resemble the epithelioid giant cell granulomas of tuberculosis but do not caseate and do not contain tubercle bacilli, and thus are often called "sarcoidlike granulomas."

Coarse dense fibrosis of submucosa and subserosa characterizes the late phase. The degree of fibrosis is disproportionate and suggests that it is not a simple process of repair and replacement of damaged tissue but rather an altered tissue reactivity that is peculiar to the disease process. The mucosa is denuded over wide areas. Where mucosal islands are present, villi are blunted or absent and glands atrophied, producing a picture resembling colonic mucosa. Small mucous glands deep in the mucosa resemble the glands of the pyloric region and are termed "aberrant pyloric glands," or "Brunner's gland metaplasia." Deep ulcers are often present, surrounded by focal areas of suppuration. Progression through the entire bowel wall may occur, producing a fistulous tract. Sarcoidlike granulomas are frequently but by no means invariably present.

The marked lymphangiectasia which is invariably present in regional enteritis has led to speculation that progressive obstructive lymphangitis is the principal primary pathogenetic mechanism, all other changes being secondary. Some have suggested that primary mesenteric adenitis initiates the process. Experimentally, lymphatic obstruction with lymphedema, chronic inflammatory changes, and fibrosis of the submucosa has been produced by feeding finely divided silicates to laboratory animals. Ulcerogranulomatous lesions similar to regional enteritis are not produced, however, nor is foreign material in significant amounts detectable in the diseased tissues of regional enteritis.

Until 1932, regional enteritis was probably most frequently misdiagnosed as hyperplastic tuberculosis. As noted above, the granulomas in regional enteritis do not caseate, and tubercle bacilli cannot be isolated. Antituberculosis chemotherapy has no beneficial effect in patients with regional enteritis.

Similarities between sarcoidosis and Crohn's disease suggest an etiologic relationship. Histologically, both diseases often have noncaseating epithelioid cell granulomas with Langhans' giant cells, both may respond to corticosteroid therapy, and both are associated with some depression of cell-mediated immune reactions. But sarcoid is thought to be a systemic disease with involvement of many sites, principally lungs, lymph nodes, skin, liver, and spleen, whereas, the granulomas of regional enteritis are found only in the gastrointestinal tract, mesenteric nodes, and occasionally the liver. The Kveim test, which is positive in about 80 percent of patients with active sarcoidosis, is nearly always negative in Crohn's disease. (In the early 1970s, there were several reports of positive Kveim tests in about 50 percent of patients with Crohn's disease. These were apparently false positives attributable to defective batches of Kveim antigen.)

Crohn, in his original paper, proposed that terminal ileitis may have a specific infectious causative agent, but despite countless investigations, no infectious agent has yet fulfilled Koch's postulates. Interest was rekindled in 1970 by Mitchell and Rees, who reported sarcoidlike granulomas in the footpads of mice which had been injected months earlier with homogenates of intestine and mesenteric lymph nodes from a patient with Crohn's disease. Some investigators have been unable to repeat this work, but others have confirmed and extended the observations. Granulomas have been induced in rabbit intestine by intraileal injection of tissue from a patient with Crohn's disease. These lesions can be serially passed by intravenous, footpad, or intraileal injection in both mice and rabbits. Tissues from patients without inflammatory bowel disease do not produce granulomas. The pathogenicity of Crohn's tissues is maintained after 220 nm filtration and freezing at $-70°C$, but is removed by autoclaving. This suggests a virus as the transmissible agent but does not rule out L-forms or mycoplasmas. Two groups have subsequently cultured viruses from intestinal tissues of patients with a variety of chronic gastrointestinal disorders including Crohn's disease. It is not clear at this point, however, what role, if any, these viruses play in Crohn's disease. They may be innocent passenger viruses in a diseased bowel.

The possibility that immune mechanisms play a role in the initiation and/or perpetuation of inflammatory bowel disease is also receiving considerable attention. Shorter has proposed that these diseases are the result of a local hypersensitivity reaction. Initial sensitization of the gut-associated lymphoid tissues is thought to occur in the neonatal period when the mucosal barrier is incomplete, permitting penetration of enterobacteria and macromolecules. Reexposure to bacteria and intestinal antigens may occur in later life if the normal mucosal integrity is damaged by gastroenteritis, bacillary dysentery, amebic colitis, ischemic episodes, or even metabolic alterations induced by psychologic stress. This reexposure then causes the local primary cellular, immune-mediated hypersensitivity reaction resulting in inflammatory bowel disease.

Whether or not immune phenomena are involved in the intestinal disease per se, it is entirely possible that some of the extraintestinal manifestations, such as erythema nodosum and peripheral arthritis, are mediated by circulating antigen-antibody complexes originating in the diseased bowel. The systemic manifestations usually improve following resection of the diseased bowel.

From 10 to 15 percent of patients with inflammatory bowel disease have a relative with the disease, which suggests genetic transmission. It now seems clear that these are not classic genetically transmitted disorders but may represent the combined interaction of several genes, the multifactorial type of inheritance, interacting with environmental influences in susceptible individuals.

Many clinicians feel that emotional stress is important in the initiation and perpetuation of inflammatory bowel disease—that these are psychosomatic phenomena. There is no convincing scientific evidence to date to support this. But evaluation of psychological influences is difficult when the patient already has the somatic disease when first seen. Cause and effect are difficult to identify at this point.

Crohn's statement that "the actual etiology is completely unknown" is still essentially true.

CLINICAL MANIFESTATIONS. The symptom pattern depends largely upon the anatomic site of involvement, extent of disease process, and presence or absence of complications. Onset is varied. Some patients present with only a febrile illness without localizing symptoms or signs. Careful questioning will usually elicit a history of abdominal discomfort that increases after eating, mild anorexia, and loose stools.

In about 10 percent of patients, more frequently in the young, the onset is acute and mimics acute appendicitis. There is midabdominal or right lower quadrant pain and tenderness, low-grade fever, leukocytosis, often nausea and vomiting, occasionally diarrhea. The correct diagnosis in acute regional enteritis is usually made only at operation.

In the majority of patients the onset is insidious, the course protracted and slowly progressive. Symptomatic periods are interspersed with symptom-free periods, but the symptomatic periods gradually become more frequent, more severe, and longer-lasting. Pain or discomfort is the most frequent and occasionally the only symptom. It is usually of an intermittent peristaltic type and early in the course is precipitated by dietary indiscretion. This cramping may gradually take on the characteristics of frank partial obstruction with distension and visible bowel loops. A second type of pain is a constant aching or soreness and usually implies advanced disease. Tenderness and a palpable mass nearly always accompany this type of pain.

Diarrhea is the next most frequent symptom and is

present, at least intermittently, in about 85 percent of patients. The frequency of stools is not great compared to ulcerative colitis, numbering two to five daily, and, unlike ulcerative colitis, the stools rarely contain mucus, pus, or blood.

Fever is present in about one-third of these patients; moderate weight loss, loss of strength, and easy fatigability, in over one-half. Frank nutritional disorders and steatorrhea are uncommon prior to surgical treatment. Extraintestinal manifestations, although quite rare, comprise a lengthy list: ankylosing spondylitis, migratory polyarthritis, erythema nodosum, pyoderma gangrenosum, pericholangitis, hepatic fatty infiltration, portal fibrosis, cholelithiasis, uveitis, periureteric fibrosis producing hydronephrosis, pancreatic fibrosis, and secondary amyloidosis.

Presenting symptoms in some patients may be those of a complication of regional enteritis: intestinal obstruction, confined perforation with abscess or internal fistula, free perforation with peritonitis, perianal abscesses or fistulas, or hemorrhage. About 40 cases of adenocarcinoma of the small bowel associated with regional enteritis have been reported. Though the number is small, it is probably significant because carcinoma of the ileum is a rare disease. Immunosuppression from chronic corticosteroid administration may play a role. The prognosis is poor: the 5-year survival rate is less than 10 percent, compared to about 21 percent for carcinoma of the ileum not associated with regional enteritis.

Complete obstruction is uncommon in contrast to partial obstruction. Emergency operation for obstruction per se

Fig. 27-1. Small bowel barium meal radiograph of a patient with regional enterocolitis. Arrows point to a string sign in the terminal ileum.

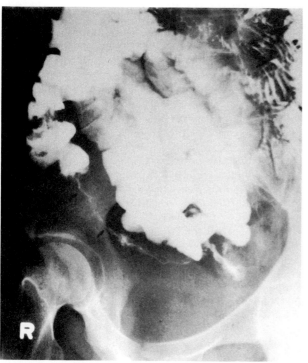

is usually not necessary, since most patients respond rather quickly to nonoperative measures. Elective operative treatment for the high-grade partial obstruction is usually indicated, however, as soon as the patient can be prepared.

Perforation as the result of an ulcer burrowing through the entire thickness of the bowel wall occurs in 15 to 20 percent of patients. Rarely, the perforation is into the free peritoneal cavity; confined perforation is the rule, resulting in abscesses or internal fistulas. Fistulization may be into another loop of intestine, small or large, urinary bladder, or vagina. Enterocutaneous fistulas do not occur in patients not operated upon but are common after operation. Perianal or perirectal abscesses and fistulas are also a common manifestation of regional enteritis with a reported frequency varying from 14 to 50 percent. The pathogenesis of this complication is not understood, since the abscesses or fistulas usually do not communicate with the diseased small bowel.

Frank hemorrhage producing hematochezia or melena is a rare complication of regional enteritis in contrast to ulcerative colitis. Occult bleeding sufficient to produce anemia is common, however.

ROENTGENOGRAPHIC FINDINGS. Barium enema with ileocecal reflux usually suffices to demonstrate involvement of the terminal ileum. Small bowel barium meal study should also be done to identify other possible sites of small bowel involvement.

With severe disease, the wall is thickened and rigid and encroaches on the lumen so that only a thin trickle of barium is seen, producing the string sign of Kantor (Fig. 27-1). Thickening of the wall and mesentery increases the space between the hoselike loops. In areas of lesser involvement, the mucosal pattern is grossly distorted with thick, irregular folds. Fistulas may be seen but are often obscured by overlapping loops.

TREATMENT. There is no curative therapy, either medical or surgical, for regional enteritis. Despite the fact that medical therapy is symptomatic and empiric, this form of therapy is indicated until a serious complication supervenes, because the recurrence rate after operation is so high. Medical therapy is directed at relieving abdominal pain, treating infection, controlling diarrhea, and correcting deficiencies in hemoglobin, protein, electrolytes, and vitamins.

Systemic antibiotics are often of value in the management of suppurative complications but have little or no effect on the primary disease process and should not be given for prolonged periods. Nonabsorbable antibiotics, particularly salicylazosulfapyridine, do sometimes exert a beneficial effect on the symptoms and should be tried. Results of treatment with corticotropin or corticosteroids have been disappointing. There is no clear evidence that they have exerted any favorable influence in mitigating the complications of stenosis, perforation, and fistula formation, and may increase the postoperative morbidity in patients who subsequently must have surgical therapy. Nevertheless some patients do appear to be benefited, so that a course of steroid therapy is probably worthwhile. Improvement of mood and appetite, more than antiinflammatory effect, are the principal benefits.

Despite the paucity of evidence implicating immune mechanisms in regional enteritis, immunosuppressive therapy is currently very popular. Azathiaprine, the antimetabolite used by most, has not caused serious toxicity when used in modest doses. Amelioration of the disease may be attributable to the anti-inflammatory effects of azathiaprine and not to immunosuppression. Hepatotoxicity, bone marrow depression, masking of infectious complications, and in the long run, increased oncogenesis are hazards. The usefulness of immunosuppressive therapy is still uncertain. Controlled studies have not provided clear-cut evidence to support its effectiveness, though some patients improve dramatically. It may be that there is a small subset of Crohn's patients, not yet identified, in whom immunosuppression will be the preferred mode of therapy.

A major advance in the nonoperative therapy of inflammatory bowel disease has been the elemental diet and total parenteral nutrition. The elemental diet provides a high-caloric, high-nitrogen, fat-free, zero-residue substrate which is absorbed in the upper part of the small bowel. This can be given to nearly all patients with Crohn's disease, even during acute exacerbations. Parenteral hyperalimentation, since it is not as safe as the oral elemental diet, should be reserved for patients with active upper intestinal disease or small bowel fistulas. Operation can often be avoided by the use of this nutrition therapy. It is also useful for getting patients in optimal shape for operation.

Failure of medical therapy results from progression of the disease process at the established existing sites of disease. Longitudinal extension along the bowel rarely occurs prior to surgical intervention.

Surgical Therapy. *Indications.* In general, failure of medical therapy to ameliorate the disease and prevent complications is the indication for operative intervention. Surgical treatment is used to correct complications that are themselves producing serious symptoms. The majority of patients with chronic regional enteritis will eventually require operation at least once in the course of their disease. Specific indications, in descending order of frequency, are obstruction; persistent, symptomatic abdominal mass or abscess; fistula, internal and/or external; perirectal fistulas that do not respond to local therapy; and intractability, or continued downhill course despite medical therapy. Uncommon indications are free perforation, hemorrhage, growth retardation in children, and blind loop syndrome. Contraindications for surgical therapy include acute regional enteritis, mucosal or superficial enteritis, and extensive jejunoileitis with involvement of all or a large part of the small bowel.

Procedure. Three surgical approaches are available: simple bypass of the diseased segment, bypass with exclusion, and resection of the diseased segment with primary anastomosis (Fig. 27-2). The choice of procedure depends on the findings at operation and the preference of the surgeon.

Simple bypass is rarely used now for a single short segment of disease because fecal diversion is incomplete, but it is the procedure of choice in extensive disease with several stenotic segments requiring surgical relief. Bypass in the form of a gastrojejunostomy instead of resection is also preferred for obstructive gastroduodenal Crohn's disease.

Bypass with exclusion was popular for a time, because it could be done with a lower mortality-morbidity rate than resection but with about the same recurrence rate as resection. It was also hoped that diversion of the fecal stream would permit healing in the excluded bowel, and that restoration of normal continuity might then be feasible. This has proved to be a forlorn hope most of the time. Disease in the excluded bowel does usually become quiescent but only rarely does the excluded segment "heal" sufficiently to permit restoration of continuity. On the contrary, active disease sometimes continues, with persistence of fistulas, bleeding, and symptoms and signs of continuing inflammation. Bypass with exclusion is now used in elderly, poor-risk patients; in patients who have had several prior resections and can ill afford to lose any more bowel; and in patients in whom resection would necessitate entering an abscess or endangering normal structures. It must be kept in mind that the proximal end of the bypassed segment can be brought out onto the abdominal wall as a mucous fistula, permitting introduction of topical therapy directly to the diseased area. If new, effective topical agents become available, bypass with exclusion will need to be resurrected.

The procedure now preferred by most surgeons is conservative resection of the grossly diseased intestine along with its mesentery. Current evidence indicates that results are not improved by increasing the margins of normal tissue proximal and distal to the diseased intestine. Thus the proximal margin should be through soft, pliable bowel—dilatation does not necessarily indicate disease—and microscopic control of margins with frozen sections is not helpful and is often confusing. The distal line of resection (with disease in the terminal ileum) should be in the ascending colon although the standard right colectomy is technically easier. Nor should any attempt be made to remove all enlarged mesenteric lymph nodes, since this does not change the rate of recurrence and may endanger the blood supply of otherwise normal intestine.

There has been considerable controversy in the past whether to do an appendectomy when enteritis is encountered at laparotomy done for suspected appendicitis because of the very appreciable incidence of postoperative enterocutaneous fistula through the incision. It now seems clear that appendectomy should be done except when the cecum at the base of the appendix is involved in the inflammation. Up to 90 percent of patients with acute regional enteritis do not progress to the chronic form, and it has been shown that postoperative fistulas, when they do occur, usually arise in the diseased ileum and not in the appendiceal stump.

Results. The operative mortality rate is now about 4 percent in most series and is about the same for all three procedures. The morbidity is appreciable and is higher in patients who have been on large doses of steroids for prolonged periods at the time of operation. Principal complications are enterocutaneous fistula, intraperitoneal or wound sepsis, and prolonged postoperative ileus.

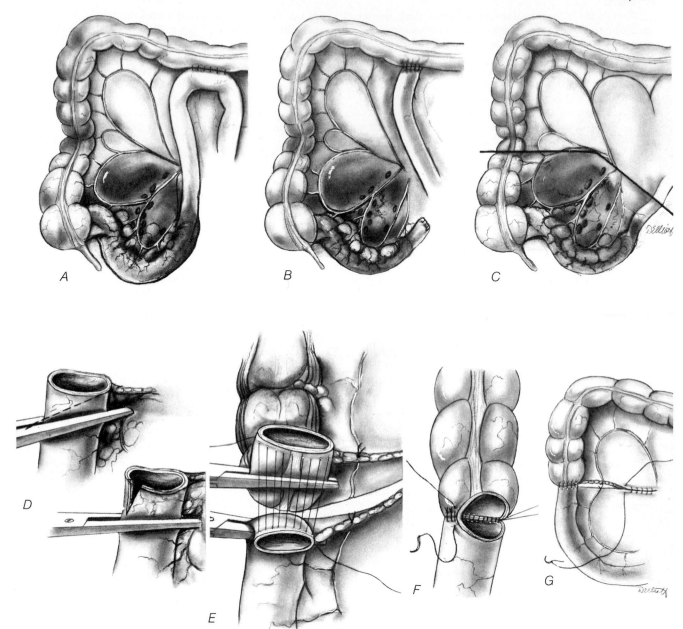

A

B

C

D

E

F

G

The recurrence rate is from 35 to 50 percent overall. It is lower in elderly patients and higher in the young. Recurrences may be more frequent and occur sooner after each successive operation for regional enteritis. These postoperative recurrences characteristically develop in the neoterminal ileum and end abruptly at the colon. The fact that about one-half of surgically treated patients will at some time have a symptomatic or radiographic recurrence of disease does not negate the great benefit to be derived from properly timed surgical therapy. One-half do not have recurrence—they are completely rehabilitated. Many of the patients with recurrence have substituted a disabling life-threatening complication for a relatively mild recurrence that is managed very well by proper medical therapy.

Regional enteritis is not a particularly fatal disease ini-

Fig. 27-2. Operations for regional enteritis. *A.* Simple side-to-side ileocolostomy bypass. *B.* Bypass with exclusion. The ileum is divided proximal to any evidence of disease; the distal end is closed or brought out as a mucous fistula; the proximal end is anastomosed end-to-side into the colon. *C* through *G.* Resection with primary anastomosis. *C.* Extent of bowel and mesentery to be resected. *D.* Insert: Methods of increasing the diameter of end of ileum to be anastomosed. The clamp may be placed obliquely or an incision made on the antimesenteric border. *E.* Placing the posterior outer suture line. The discrepancy in diameter of the bowel ends is eliminated by placing the two end sutures first, then progressively bisecting intervening spaces with successive sutures. *F.* Placing the anterior inner suture line—an infolding, hemostatic running stitch. *G.* The anastomosis completed with interrupted sutures in the outer anterior row. The cut edges of mesenteries of ileum and colon are approximated.

tially or at any one time, but becomes progressively more dangerous as the years go by. In general the death rate of persons with this disease is about twice that for the normal population.

Tuberculous Enteritis

Tuberculosis of the gastrointestinal tract occurs in two forms. Primary infection is usually due to the bovine strain of *Mycobacterium tuberculosis* and results from ingesting infected milk. This is now rare in the United States but is still common in undeveloped countries. Secondary infection, due to the human strain, results from the swallowing of bacilli by patients with active pulmonary tuberculosis. Chemotherapy has markedly decreased the incidence of secondary tuberculous enteritis, so that it now occurs in only about 1 percent of patients with pulmonary tuberculosis.

The ileocecal region is the site of involvement in about 85 percent of patients with tuberculous enteritis, presumably because of the abundance of lymphoid tissue in this area.

Primary tuberculous enteritis often produces minimal symptoms unless dissemination to other organs occurs. Occasionally a hypertrophic reaction produces contracture and stenosis of the lumen of distal ileum, cecum, and ascending colon. Such involvement may produce symptoms, signs, and radiographic findings that are indistinguishable from those of carcinoma of the colon, and surgical exploration with biopsy may be advisable. If the diagnosis is suspected preoperatively, chemotherapy, consisting of isoniazid, 100 mg three times a day, and para-aminosalicylic acid (PAS), 3 Gm three times a day, should be administered for about 2 weeks. Streptomycin, 0.5 Gm, twice daily, is started the day before operation. If tuberculosis is found at operation, all drugs are continued—streptomycin for 1 to 2 weeks, isoniazid and PAS at the same dose for 1 year after the patient has become asymptomatic. Surgical therapy of hypertrophic tuberculous enteritis is usually inadvisable unless high-grade stenosis dictates immediate relief. Right colectomy is applicable if the involved segment is short and clearly defined, otherwise ileocolic bypass is the safer procedure.

Symptoms of the more common ulcerative form of tuberculous enteritis secondary to pulmonary disease are also variable, and the diagnosis may be made only by routine radiographic intestinal examination of patients with pulmonary tuberculosis. When present, symptoms consist of alternating constipation and diarrhea associated with crampy lower abdominal pain. In severe cases, diarrhea is persistent, and anemia and inanition are progressive. The diagnosis can usually be made by barium enema examination. Early in the disease, irritability of the terminal ileum and cecum causes rapid emptying of barium from the affected segment. Later, intestinal contours become spiculated as folds stiffen and thicken. Ulceration may be visible, followed by fibrosis, narrowing, and shortening of the area. Clinical confirmation of a presumptive diagnosis may be obtained by a prompt response to antituberculous chemotherapy. Surgical therapy is contraindicated except for the rare complications of perforation, obstruction, or hemorrhage. Chemotherapy which is prescribed for the pulmonary disease usually brings about healing of the intestinal lesions.

Typhoid Enteritis

This is an acute, systemic infection of several weeks' duration, caused by *Salmonella typhosa* and manifested by fever, headache, prostration, cough, maculopapular rash, abdominal pain, and leukopenia. There is hyperplasia and ulceration of Peyer's patches of the intestine, mesenteric lymphadenopathy, splenomegaly, and parenchymatous changes in the liver. Confirmation of diagnosis is obtained by culturing *S. typhosa* from blood or feces or by finding a high titer of agglutinins against the O and H antigens.

Typhoid fever is still a major disease in areas of the world that have not yet attained high public health standards, but the incidence has progressively declined in the United States since 1900. The death rate, which was formerly about 10 percent, is now about 2 percent, in large part because of the specific antimicrobial chloramphenicol, which was introduced in 1948.

Chloramphenicol is given orally in doses of 50 mg/kg of body weight per day in four divided doses until the temperature is normal, then reduced to 30 mg/kg/day for a total of 2 weeks. Ampicillin is also effective and should be given intravenously or intramuscularly in doses of 1 Gm every 6 hours for 2 weeks. Severely toxic patients who do not respond well within 1 week should also receive prednisone in doses of 15 mg four times a day the first day, 10 mg four times a day the second, and 5 mg four times a day the third day. When given with appropriate antibiotic therapy, prednisone does not increase the risk of complications.

Gross hemorrhage occurs in 10 to 20 percent of hospitalized patients, even while they are on adequate therapy. Transfusion therapy is indicated and usually suffices. Every effort should be made to avoid operation, since the bleeding is often from multiple ulcers and the bowel is exceedingly friable. Rarely, laparotomy must be done for uncontrollable, life-threatening hemorrhage.

Perforation, through ulcerated Peyer's patches, is usually in the terminal ileum, and occurs in about 2 percent of cases. Operative treatment is indicated unless the patient is moribund, since localization or walling-off of the perforation is uncommon. Simple closure of the perforation, along with appropriate toilette of the peritoneal cavity, usually suffices. With multiple perforations, which occur in about one-fourth of patients, resection with primary anastomosis is preferred. The mortality rate of those with free perforation is about 10 percent.

NEOPLASMS

Neoplasms of the small bowel are uncommon. Despite the much greater length and surface area of the small bowel, colonic neoplasms occur forty times as frequently.

Though the numbers are small, the variety is great, since virtually all the cells that histologically make up the small bowel give rise to benign and malignant neoplasms. Benign and malignant lesions are reported to occur with about equal frequency in clinical series, while benign lesions are more frequent in autopsy series. Two interesting clinical syndromes are associated with small bowel neoplasms: the Peutz-Jeghers syndrome and the malignant carcinoid syndrome.

Benign Neoplasms

Histologic types of small bowel benign tumors and their relative incidence are shown in Table 27-1. This information should be considered only as a rough approximation, since it is a compilation from many reports, some clinical, some necropsy, utilizing varied terminology. For example, adenomas are the most frequent tumor in one review but are not even mentioned in another review because of subclassification.

About 15 percent of benign tumors are found in the duodenum; about 25 percent in the jejunum, principally in the upper one-third; and about 60 percent in the ileum, principally the lower one-third. All ages are affected with the peak incidence, in clinical cases, in the fourth decade.

CLINICAL MANIFESTATIONS. An appreciable number of small bowel benign tumors apparently cause no serious symptoms during life and are incidental findings at autopsy. The diagnosis is delayed or missed in many clinical cases because symptoms may be absent or vague and nonspecific until significant complications have developed; physical examination rarely provides any clue unless intestinal obstruction is present; and roentgenographic small bowel studies and selective angiography, the only specific diagnostic aids, may fail to demonstrate an existing tumor even though it is suspected clinically. In only about one-half of small bowel tumors found at operation has the correct diagnosis been made preoperatively.

The two most common clinical manifestations of small bowel tumors are bleeding and obstruction. Rarely, perfo-

ration of the bowel wall occurs, resulting in abscess or internal fistula formation, peritonitis, or pneumatosis cystoides intestinalis. Bleeding occurs in about one-third of patients but is rarely gross hemorrhage. More commonly bleeding is occult and intermittent, producing guaiac-positive stools and iron-deficiency anemia. Leiomyomas and hemangiomas are the lesions that most often cause bleeding. The differential diagnosis of small bowel bleeding should include hereditary hemorrhagic telangiectasia, or Osler-Rendu-Weber syndrome. This is transmitted as a simple dominant trait and is manifested by multiple telangiectases of bowel, skin, and mucous membranes.

Intestinal obstruction may be produced either by encroachment on the lumen by the tumor, in which case obstruction is usually chronic and partial, or by intussusception, with the tumor acting as the intussusceptum. Intussusception in adults differs from that seen in children. An organic cause is demonstrable in about 80 percent of adults; benign neoplasm is the organic cause in nearly one-half. Adults often have "chronic" intussusception with recurrent bouts that resolve by spontaneous reduction.

ROENTGENOGRAPHIC FINDINGS. Small bowel barium meal studies are indicated when clinical findings suggest small bowel neoplasms. Accuracy of diagnosis varies from 50 to 90 percent depending on the nature of the lesion and on the diligence with which the examination is done. Oral barium should not be given to patients with findings of complete or high-grade partial obstruction.

TREATMENT. Surgical removal of benign tumors is nearly always indicated because of the risk of complications if untreated and because the diagnosis of benignity can be made with certainty only by microscopic examination of the resected tumor. Segmental resection with primary anastomosis is usually necessary except in very small lesions. The entire bowel should be searched for other lesions, since they are often multiple.

PEUTZ-JEGHERS SYNDROME

This is an uncommon familial disease manifested by intestinal polyposis and melanin spots of the oral mucosa, lips, palms of the hands, and soles of the feet. Over 300 cases have been reported since Peutz first described the syndrome in 1921 and Jeghers et al. rediscovered it in 1949. Inheritance is as a simple mendelian dominant. Both males and females carry the factor, and there is a high degree of penetrance. A single pleiotropic gene is responsible for both the polyps and melanin spots. Pigmentation without polyposis and polyposis without pigmentation have been reported.

Jejunum and ileum are the most frequently involved portion of the gastrointestinal tract, polyposis being found in essentially all cases reported. Colon and rectum are also involved in about one-third, stomach in about one-fourth. The polyps were initially thought to be adenomas but are now thought by most to be hamartomas and thus without malignant potential (Fig. 27-3). There are several single-case reports of malignant tumors of the gastrointestinal tract in patients with the Peutz-Jeghers syndrome. In a few of these patients, the malignant process appeared to be related to Peutz-Jeghers polyps. It is not yet clear whether

Table 27-1. TYPES AND RELATIVE FREQUENCY OF SMALL BOWEL BENIGN NEOPLASMS

Neoplasms	Percent
Leiomyomas	17
Lipomas	16
Adenomas	14
Polyps	14
Polyposis, Peutz-Jeghers	3
Hemangiomas	10
Fibromas	10
Neurogenic tumors	5
Fibromyomas	5
Myxomas	2
Lymphangiomas	2
Fibroadenomas	1
Others	1

this represents coincidence or a malignant potential in the syndrome.

Recurrent colicky abdominal pain caused by transient intussusception is the most frequent symptom. Abdominal pain with a palpable mass is present in about one-third of patients. Hemorrhage occurs less frequently.

Surgical therapy is required for obstruction or bleeding, but the procedure should be limited to relieving the complication only, i.e., polypectomy or minimal resection. The wide distribution and large number of polyps usually preclude removal of all polyps, lest the patient be left a cripple from the short bowel syndrome.

Malignant Neoplasms

Malignant tumor of the small bowel is relatively infrequent, comprising about 2 percent of gastrointestinal malignant neoplasms. Adenocarcinoma is the most frequent, followed by carcinoid, lymphoma, and sarcoma, principally leiomyosarcoma. Adenocarcinoma occurs with about equal frequency in duodenum, jejunum, and ileum; the others occur predominantly in the ileum.

CLINICAL MANIFESTATIONS. Clinical manifestations fall roughly into three groups: diarrhea with large amounts of mucus, and tenesmus; obstruction with nausea, vomiting, and cramping abdominal pain; and chronic blood loss with anemia, weakness, guaiac-positive stools, and occasionally melena or hematochezia. As with benign neoplasms, symptoms of malignant neoplasms are often present for many months before the diagnosis is made, emphasizing the insidious nature of small bowel lesions.

TREATMENT. The therapy of choice is wide resection including regional lymph nodes. This requires pancreatoduodenectomy in duodenal lesions. If spread of disease precludes curative resection, short-circuiting procedures usually offer worthwhile palliation. The overall resectability rate of small bowel malignant neoplasms is about 40 percent. The 5-year survival of all diagnosed cases is about 20 percent in adenocarcinoma, 35 percent in lymphoma, and 40 percent in leiomyosarcoma. Carcinoids are discussed below. Postoperative irradiation is indicated in the lymphomas but is of no value in the other lesions. Similarly chemotherapy has little to offer except in the lymphomas.

Two variant lymphomas of the small intestine are of special interest. After many years of malabsorption due to celiac sprue, a small percentage of patients develop lymphoma. The cell type is most frequently histiocytic lymphoma (formerly called reticulum cell sarcoma), followed by Hodgkin's sarcoma and mixed-cell lymphoma. The second variant, so-called Mediterranean-type lymphoma, was first found in non-European Jews and Arabs in the Middle Eastern countries; hence the name. Patients with this lymphoma have monoclonal alpha heavy chains of immunoglobulin in the serum and urine, and a high percentage also have a heavy plasma-cell infiltration of the intestinal mucosa and lymph nodes away from the areas of lymphoma. The prognosis in both the celiac-associated and Mediterranean lymphomas is much worse than in the conventional small intestine lymphoma.

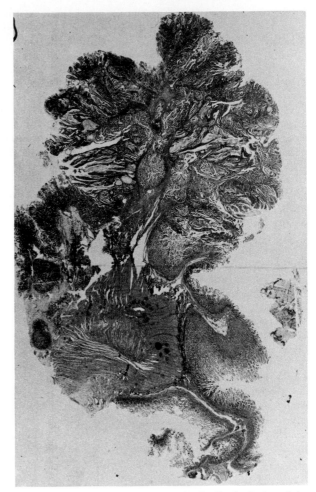

Fig. 27-3. Low-power photomicrograph of a Peutz-Jeghers jejunal polyp. Instead of one predominant cell as seen in most intestinal polyps, these contain all cells of normal intestinal mucosa interspersed within bands of smooth muscle—a hamartoma.

CARCINOIDS

Carcinoids are of particular interest because of their great variability in malignant potential and because of an unusual clinical syndrome associated with them.

The first histologic description of these tumors was published in 1808. Ninety-nine years later the term "carcinoid" was applied to emphasize biologic benignity (erroneously) despite morphologic resemblance to carcinoma. Their true potential for biologic malignancy was first recognized in 1911 but has only recently been generally accepted. Masson identified the cell of origin of carcinoids as the Kultschitzsky cell because of a similar affinity of cytoplasmic granules for silver and named these lesions "argentaffin tumors." Masson also suggested that argentaffin tumors are endocrine in nature. Between 1953 and 1954, three groups independently described the malignant carcinoid syndrome, and shortly thereafter the biochemical abnormalities responsible for the syndrome were elucidated.

Carcinoid tumors can occur anywhere in the gastrointestinal tract that Kultschitzsky cells occur—from gastric cardia to anus. The appendix is most frequently involved (46 percent), followed by ileum (28 percent) and rectum (17 percent). Other locations are shown in Table 27-2. Outside the gastrointestinal tract, carcinoid tumor is found in the bronchus and has been reported in ovarian and sacrococcygeal teratoma.

The malignant potential and the ability to metastasize appear to be related to the site of origin and size of the primary. Only about 3 percent of appendiceal carcinoids metastasize, but about 35 percent of ileal carcinoids do (Table 27-2). Seventy-five percent of gastrointestinal carcinoids are less than 1 cm in diameter, and only 2 percent of this group have metastasized. About 20 percent of the primary tumors are 1 to 2 cm in diameter, and about half of this group have metastasized. Only about 5 percent are over 2 cm in diameter; 80 to 90 percent of these have metastasized. No primary carcinoid of the gastrointestinal tract exceeding 3 cm in diameter has been reported. Carcinoids of the small bowel are multiple in 30 percent of cases, rarely so in the appendix. This tendency to multicentricity exceeds that of any other malignant neoplasm of the gastrointestinal tract. Another unusual and, to date, unexplained feature of carcinoids of the bowel is the frequent coexistence of a second primary malignant neoplasm of a different histologic type. A second primary neoplasm was found in 29 percent of patients in one large series.

Carcinoids present grossly as slightly elevated, smooth, rounded yellow-gray or tan nodules. They are apt to be overlooked by radiologist and surgeon unless carefully searched for because of their small size and submucosal location. The mucosa over carcinoids is usually intact but may ulcerate. Narrowing of the lumen is produced, not by the bulk of the tumor per se, but by a fibrous reaction around the tumor. Also, metastasis to mesentery usually results in kinking and fixation of the bowel both by an extensive desmoplastic reaction and by very large secondary tumor masses—in contrast to the characteristically small primary.

Symptomatology is similar to that seen in other small bowel tumors as outlined above unless the malignant carcinoid syndrome is present. The radiographic picture may resemble regional enteritis if infiltration of the bowel wall and mesentery has caused narrowing and fixation of a loop. Small, noninfiltrating carcinoids are difficult to detect.

TREATMENT. The magnitude of the indicated surgical resection of small bowel carcinoids is determined by the presence or absence of metastases and the size of the primary tumor. If the primary is less than 1 cm in diameter and no extension or metastasis is demonstrable, local excision is adequate therapy. A standard cancer operation is indicated for lesions of less than 1 cm with demonstrable spread of disease, for multiple primaries, and for all primary lesions of the intestine that exceed 1 cm in diameter. Since most of the tumors are in the distal ileum, adequate resection of node-bearing tissue usually requires right colectomy with the accompanying mesentery in addition to distal ileum. Even with widespread metastatic disease that precludes resection for cure, removal of all resectable tumor tissue is usually indicated, since very significant palliation often results. Bypass procedures are used in poor-risk patients with disseminated disease. Streptozotocin and 5-fluorouracil, singly or in combination, are sometimes helpful.

The overall 5-year survival rate following resection of malignant carcinoids of the small bowel is about 50 percent. If a "curative resection" is done, about 70 percent live 5 years. Even with palliative therapy, about 25 percent live 5 years. One patient is reported who lived in comfort for 14 years with known unresectable tumor in mesenteric and aortic nodes, only to die of unrelated disease.

Malignant Carcinoid Syndrome

This syndrome comprises a group of striking and debilitating symptoms, involving six different organ systems, that can be divided into episodic and permanent manifestations (Fig. 27-4). Episodic manifestations include cutaneous flushing, hyperperistalsis and diarrhea, asthma, and hemodynamic alterations that may result in vasomotor collapse. Permanent manifestations are facial hyperemia, peripheral edema, cutaneous lesions of pellagra, and valvular heart disease. The syndrome was initially thought to be due to excessive amounts of circulating serotonin that was being produced by functioning carcinoid tumors. Some recent observations indicate, however, that this simple hypothesis is inadequate and the biochemical aspects of the malignant carcinoid syndrome are much more complex than first thought.

Serotonin, one of the biologically active peptides, was first isolated in 1948, the formula of 5-hydroxytryptamine was applied in 1949, and it was synthesized in 1951. Serotonin secretion by Kulschitzsky cells was demonstrated in 1952, and in 1953 serotonin was extracted from a carcinoid tumor found at autopsy. Shortly thereafter, the clinical

Table 27-2. DISTRIBUTION OF GASTROINTESTINAL CARCINOIDS: INCIDENCE OF METASTASES AND OF CARCINOID SYNDROME

Site	Cases	Average % metastasis	Cases of carcinoid syndrome
Esophagus	1	. . .	0
Stomach	93	23	8
Duodenum	135	20	4
Jejunoileum	1,032	34	91
Meckel's diverticulum	42	19	3
Appendix	1,686	2	6
Colon	91	60	5
Rectum	592	18	1
Ovary	34	6	17
Biliary tract	10	30	0
Pancreas	2	. . .	1
	3,718		136

SOURCE: From Wilson, Cheek, Sherman, and Storer, 1970.

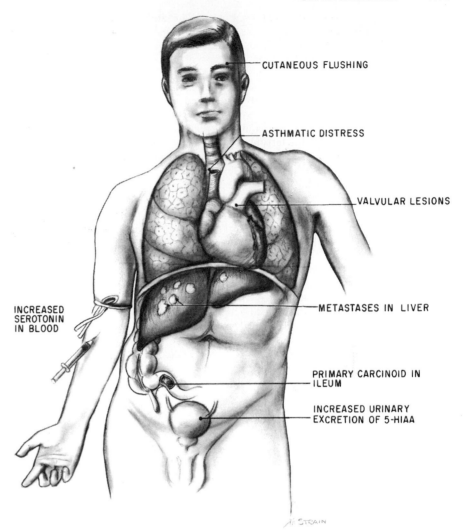

Fig. 27-4. Clinical manifestations of malignant carcinoid syndrome.

syndrome of functioning malignant carcinoids was described and overproduction of serotonin implicated in the pathogenesis of the syndrome.

Serotonin is derived in the body from the essential amino acid tryptophan:

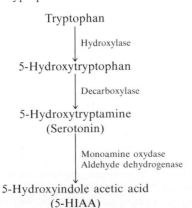

Normally only about 1 percent of dietary tryptophan is metabolized in this manner. Functioning carcinoid tumors may divert as much as 60 percent into the serotonin pathway, leaving less tryptophan available for the formation of other substances such as niacin and body protein, which, along with diarrhea and decreased food intake, contribute to development of pellagra and protein deficiency.

Serotonin is broken down in the liver to 5-HIAA, which is excreted in the urine. This is the basis of a test for the presence of functioning carcinoid tumors: 5-HIAA excretion in normal persons is 2 to 10 mg/day. With functioning tumors the excretion is greatly increased, being 50 to 600 mg/day.

5-HIAA is biologically inactive. Thus carcinoids drained by the portal vein may elaborate tremendous amounts of serotonin without producing the malignant carcinoid syndrome. Release of serotonin into the systemic circulation occurs most frequently with carcinoid metastases in the liver, occasionally with metastases in other sites drained by systemic veins, or from primary carcinoids outside the portal area, such as ovary or bronchus.

Functioning carcinoids may produce, in addition to

serotonin, 5-hydroxytryptophan, kallikrein, histamine, and ACTH. Also, a functioning tumor of the duodenum which morphologically and functionally has features of both foregut carcinoids and islet-cell tumors of the pancreas has been implicated in the Zollinger-Ellison syndrome.

CLINICAL MANIFESTATIONS. Cutaneous phenomena are the most characteristic and frequently recognized manifestations of the malignant carcinoid syndrome. Flushing is the most common early symptom and is present in most but not all patients. It is characteristically episodic and of short duration initially. During the flush, the face, neck, arms, and upper trunk are involved by a dusky red hyperemia, often with a cyanotic hue. This may be accompanied by pruritus, sweating, edema of face and hands, paresthesias, tachycardia, and occasionally vasomotor collapse. Vascular collapse and death occurring during induction of anesthesia have been reported. The flushing episodes usually occur spontaneously but may be precipitated by emotional stress, ingestion of food or alcohol, or defecation. As the syndrome progresses, permanent reddening of the skin occurs and telangiectases appear on the cheeks, nose, and forehead. A permanent cyanotic hue is often seen even in patients without valvular heart disease and with normal arterial oxygen saturation.

Diarrhea is a significant complaint in over 80 percent of patients with the carcinoid syndrome. This is characteristically sudden in onset, watery, not bloody, and more frequent in the morning. Audible borborygmus and cramping abdominal pain frequently accompany the stools. Abdominal symptoms may or may not be related to episodes of flushing. Malabsorption is occasionally seen with severe, long-continued diarrhea.

Peripheral edema is present in about 70 percent of patients and may occur in the absence of valvular heart disease or hypoaluminemia. Periodic increases in venous pressure during flushing and the antidiuretic effect of serotonin may play a role.

Asthmatic attacks, usually concurrent with flushing attacks, have been reported in about 25 percent of patients with the syndrome. Severe bronchoconstriction has occurred during anesthetic induction.

Cardiac involvement is a late development in the syndrome and occurs in about one-half of cases. This peculiar form of valvular disease affects primarily the tricuspid and pulmonic valves; mitral and aortic valve lesions also occur but much less frequently. The valve cusps are progressively thickened, shortened, and narrowed, producing stenosis of the pulmonic valve and usually both stenosis and insufficiency of the tricuspid valve.

The role of serotonin as the sole mediator of all of the varied manifestations has been placed in doubt by some recent observations. Some patients with the carcinoid syndrome have normal levels of 5-HIAA in the urine. Conversely, some patients with grossly elevated levels of serotonin in peripheral blood do not exhibit any of the manifestations of the syndrome. Further, intravenous infusion of pure serotonin does not elicit all the manifestations of the clinical syndrome. Considerable work has been done on the pathogenesis of cutaneous flushing. The levels of circulating serotonin do not correlate with episodes of flushing in patients with the syndrome, and only atypical flushing is produced by infused serotonin. Typical attacks of flushing can usually be induced by intravenous administration of small doses of epinephrine. There is evidence that the flush is not caused by a local response to epinephrine but is mediated through the release of other substances, probably bradykinin. Typical flushing in carcinoid syndrome patients can also be produced by giving synthetic bradykinin. Kallikrein, an enzyme that catalyzes the formation of kinin peptides, as well as kininogen and histamine, has been found in carcinoid tumors. It would appear that carcinoid tumors have multiple endocrine capacities and that several biologically active peptides and amines may be involved. This could account for the variability of clinical syndromes encountered as well as for the discrepancies in the serotonin hypothesis.

DIAGNOSTIC FINDINGS. The syndrome is easily recognized when fully manifest, but a single symptom or sign may be the only clinical evidence of a functioning carcinoid. Knobby hepatomegaly is often present, since the syndrome is nearly always produced by massive liver metastases. Radioisotope scan is useful to document the presence of space-occupying lesions in the liver. Needle biopsy of one of the palpable nodules frequently establishes a histologic diagnosis. Flush induction by intravenous epinephrine is a useful bedside test. The initial dose is 1 μg, with subsequent doses of 2 μg, 5 μg, and 10 μg if necessary. Appearance of a flush, usually associated with hypotension and tachycardia, between 45 and 90 seconds after injection is considered positive. A negative result consists of no reaction or transient facial blanching or transient hypertension.

A 4-hour intravenous infusion of calcium also has been used successfully to provoke attacks in patients suspected of having the carcinoid syndrome.

The most practical laboratory test is the quantitative determination of urinary 5-HIAA. Patients with the syndrome excrete more than 40 mg/day compared to a normal excretion of less than 10 mg/day. A negative test makes the diagnosis of functioning carcinoid unlikely, but there are occasional patients who excrete increased amounts of serotonin instead of 5-HIAA. The qualitative test for urinary 5-HIAA is of some value as a screening procedure, but false positives and false negatives can occur after the ingestion of certain drugs.

TREATMENT. Surgical removal of all neoplastic tissue is rarely possible, except for solitary bronchial or ovarian carcinoids or fortuitously located liver metastases. Exploration is indicated, however, in essentially all patients with malignant carcinoid syndrome. Removal of as much tumor, primary and metastatic, as possible should be attempted even though the line of resection crosses gross tumor. Very remarkable amelioration of symptoms for prolonged periods is the rule rather than the exception when subtotal resection of tumor can be done. Ligation of the hepatic artery in an attempt to deprive the metastases of blood supply has also been reported to be effective.

Drug therapy is of some value for controlling symptoms. The antiserotonin agents methysergide, cyprohepadine, and p-chlorophenylalanine have proved to be helpful in controlling the bowel symptoms, but not flushing, in some patients. Methyldopa is occasionally effective. Empirically, opiates can usually control the diarrhea. Flushing attacks sometimes are ameliorated by the phenothiazines or by α-adrenergic blocking agents such as phentolamine or phenoxybenzamine. Rather marked decreases in carcinoid syndrome symptomatology have been obtained occasionally with corticosteroid therapy. Cancer chemotherapy with the combination of 5-fluorouracil and streptozotocin has yielded some palliation of the syndrome in a small group of patients. Since streptozotocin has little hematologic toxicity, it can be combined with 5-FU at essentially full doses of each agent. Such treatment should be initiated cautiously lest tumor necrosis produce a fatal carcinoid crisis.

DIVERTICULAR DISEASE

Meckel's Diverticulum

The most frequently encountered diverticulum of the small intestine is named for Johann Meckel, who described this structure in 1809. The embryology of Meckel's diverticulum and related anomalies, and diseases of these structures occurring in infancy and childhood, are discussed in Chap. 39.

Meckel's diverticulum is found on the antimesenteric border of the ileum about 2 ft, rarely more than 3 ft, from the ileocecal valve. A persistent band or sinus may connect with the umbilicus. Many of these diverticula are incidental findings at laparotomy or necropsy. Clinically important manifestations are found primarily in childhood, over 60 percent occurring before age ten.

The most common complication of Meckel's diverticulum in the adult, in contrast to the child, is intestinal obstruction. This may result from volvulus or kinking around a band running from the tip of the diverticulum to umbilicus, abdominal wall, or mesentery; or it may be caused by intussusception with the diverticulum as the intussusceptum.

Bleeding is also a common manifestation. This is due to peptic ulceration produced by secretion of acid-pepsin by ectopic gastric mucosa in the diverticulum. Melena is usual, but frank hemorrhage with passage of dark red clots also occurs. Preoperative diagnosis is sometimes possible utilizing abdominal scanning following the administration of radiotechnicium which has an affinity for gastric parietal cells.

Meckel's diverticulitis, clinically indistinguishable from appendicitis, is the third complication in the adult. The incidence of perforation and peritonitis is about 50 percent.

Meckel's diverticulum as a primary lesion should be considered in patients who present with mechanical obstruction of the ileum, with low small bowel hemorrhage, or with signs of inflammation or peritonitis in the midabdomen or lower abdomen. Treatment is prompt surgical intervention with removal of the offending diverticulum by diverticulectomy or resection of the segment of ileum bearing the diverticulum.

Soltero and Bill have challenged the time-honored dictum that incidentally encountered Meckel's diverticula should be removed prophylactically. They estimate that only about 4 percent of diverticula ever become diseased and that thus the morbidity of incidental removal outweighs the potential disease prophylaxis.

Duodenal Diverticula

This is an uncommon lesion, seen in about 1 percent of patients studied by upper gastrointestinal roentgenography. These diverticula, composed only of mucosa and submucosa, are usually single and project mediad from the concavity of duodenum in the region of the head of the pancreas. Nonspecific epigastric symptoms are present in about 10 percent of patients; bleeding and perforation occasionally occur. The morbidity and mortality of these complications is high because of difficulty in diagnosis leading to delay in treatment.

The clinical manifestations of perforated duodenal diverticula are those of other acute gastrointestinal diseases so that the diagnosis is usually made at laparotomy. The inflammatory mass may obstruct the common bile duct and/or the major pancreatic duct producing jaundice and/or pancreatitis. Enteroliths are sometimes found and may be the proximal cause of the inflammation. The perforation is usually walled-off in the retroperitoneal space producing an abscess or phlegmon. Drainage of the collection and gastrojejunostomy is the procedure of choice. Decompression of biliary and pancreatic ducts also may be necessary.

In patients with bleeding or with symptomatic but uncomplicated diverticula, diverticulectomy is indicated. This can usually be done by rolling the duodenum and pancreas forward by the Kocher maneuver. Excision is performed in such a manner as to leave a transverse opening, which is closed with interrupted inverting nonabsorbable sutures. Diverticula imbedded in the pancreas are more safely approached through an anterior duodenotomy. The sac is invaginated and amputated, and the defect closed from within the lumen. Removal of asymptomatic or incidentally encountered diverticula is not advisable.

Jejunal and Ileal Diverticula

Diverticula of the small intestine are distinctly uncommon lesions, being seen in from 0.1 to 0.5 percent of small bowel barium studies. Most are found in the jejunum and are usually multiple. Like duodenal diverticula, these are composed only of mucosa and submucosa. They lie on the mesenteric border, often projecting between the leaves of the mesentery.

Symptoms of partial upper small bowel obstruction may be produced by pressure from a distended or inflamed diverticulum or by adhesions from the diverticulum to surrounding viscera. Acute diverticulitis and hemorrhage from ulceration in a diverticulum have been reported.

Since diverticula are usually limited to the upper small bowel, resection of the segment is usually advisable for obstruction or hemorrhage. Drainage and bypass may be done for diverticulitis with perforation if primary resection appears hazardous. Blind-loop symptoms can usually be controlled with broad-spectrum antibiotics. Asymptomatic diverticula require no treatment.

MISCELLANEOUS PROBLEMS

Ulcer of the Small Intestine

Ulcer of the small intestine of unknown cause has been the subject of sporadic reports since it was first described by Baillie in 1795. A total of 76 cases were reported in the American and European literature between 1936 and 1955. Perforation was the most frequent complication; stenosis occurred in 32 percent.

In 1964, two reports suggested a possible relationship between the administration of thiazide diuretics in combination with enteric-coated potassium chloride and the development of small intestinal ulceration and stenosis. Accordingly a survey of 440 hospitals was made and data obtained on 484 patients with ulcers of the small intestine. Fifty-seven percent of the patients had received diuretics or potassium chloride. The typical ulcerations were reproduced in dogs and monkeys by oral administration of enteric-coated potassium chloride, but not by thiazides. Accordingly, enteric-coated potassium preparations were withdrawn from the United States drug market. A new, slow-release wax matrix formulation of potassium chloride has greatly decreased but has not eliminated gastrointestinal ulceration.

Potassium chloride ulcers are strikingly uniform. There is a circumferential, sharply limited mucosal ulceration overlying a zone of cicatricial narrowing. The width of the ulcerated zone averages 1 cm. Potassium chloride locally in concentrations exceeding 10 percent causes, sequentially, venous spasm and stasis, submucosal edema, segmental hemorrhagic infarction, ulceration, and stenosis.

Symptoms produced by potassium chloride ulcers are most frequently due to stenosis and consist of postprandial cramping abdominal pain, nausea, vomiting, and intermittent fullness. Hemorrhage and perforation are occasionally seen.

Once symptomatic, these lesions nearly always require surgical therapy. Resection of the involved segment with primary anastomosis is the procedure of choice.

Ingested Foreign Bodies

A wide variety of objects, potentially capable of penetrating the wall of the alimentary tract, are swallowed, usually accidentally but sometimes intentionally by the mentally deranged. These include glass and metal fragments, pins, needles, cocktail toothpicks, fish bones, coins, whistles, toys, and broken razor blades.

Treatment is expectant, since the vast majority pass without difficulty. If the object is radiopaque, progress can be followed by serial plain films. Catharsis is contraindicated.

Sharp, pointed objects such as sewing needles, may penetrate the bowel wall. If abdominal pain, tenderness, fever, and/or leukocytosis occur, immediate surgical removal of the offending object is indicated. Abscess or granuloma formation are the usual outcome without surgical therapy.

Fistula

Enterocutaneous fistulas of the mesenteric small intestine are nearly always secondary to operation—less than 2 percent of fistulas result from bowel disease or trauma per se. In some patients there are contributing factors, such as: preoperative radiotherapy, intestinal obstruction, inflammatory bowel disease, mesenteric vascular disease, and intraabdominal sepsis. But in the majority surgical misadventures are the primary cause. These include anastomotic leak, inadvertent injury of bowel or blood supply at operation, laceration of bowel by wire mesh or retention sutures, and retained sponges.

Diagnosis of small bowel fistula is usually not difficult. When the damaged area of the small bowel breaks down and discharges its contents, dissemination may occur widely in the peritoneal cavity producing the picture of generalized peritonitis. More commonly, however, the process is more or less walled-off to the immediate area of the leak, with formation of an abscess. This in turn presents at the operative incision, so that when a few skin sutures are removed to ascertain why the incision is becoming red and tender, contents of the abscess are discharged and the fistula established. Initially the discharge may be purulent or bloody, but this is followed in a day or two by drainage of obvious small bowel contents. If the diagnosis is in doubt, confirmation can be obtained by oral administration of a nonabsorbable marker such as charcoal or Congo red.

Small bowel fistulas are classified according to their location and daily volume flow, since these factors dictate treatment, as well as morbidity and mortality rates. In general, the higher the fistula in the intestine, the more serious the problem. Proximal fistulas have a greater fluid and electrolyte loss, the drainage has a greater digestive capacity, and an important segment is not available for food absorption. It is important therefore, as soon as the patient's condition is stabilized, to identify the site of the fistula, and secondly, to ascertain if there is distal obstruction, since fistulas will not close in the presence of distal obstruction. Upper gastrointestinal series with small bowel follow-through and barium enema studies usually yield this information. Fistulograms may also be helpful not only to delineate the fistula but also to determine the extent of the associated abscess cavity.

Initial priorities in management are concerned with fluid and electrolyte replacement, control of the fistula, and control of sepsis. Fluid losses in high fistulas, particularly if the patient is still febrile and has a persistent ileus with attendant high nasogastric suction losses, may require heroic volumes of replacement fluids. A central venous catheter with around-the-clock therapy is usually in order.

Fistula care consists of cleaning up any residual sepsis, protecting the skin, and measuring the output. Early on, a soft rubber sump works well but should be abandoned as soon as possible in favor of a cement-on collection device lest the bowel opening be kept open by the tube. Occasionally a circular-frame bed can be used allowing gravity drainage when the patient is prone. The skin surrounding the fistula must be protected from excoriation by the digestive enzymes particularly in high jejunal fistulas. This is usually best accomplished by the frequent application of karaya powder. Aluminum paste or zinc oxide are also useful. Control of sepsis requires administration of appropriate antibiotics plus establishment of free drainage of the process at the site of the fistula. Some patients may have additional pockets of suppuration apart from the fistula site. The peritoneum often can handle these, but surgical drainage may also be necessary.

Nutrition rapidly becomes a major consideration in patients with small bowel fistulas. Fortunately two recent developments now allow effective therapy: intravenous hyperalimentation, and elemental oral diets. The oral route is to be preferred whenever possible because of the hazard of prolonged intravenous therapy in the presence of sepsis and antibiotics. If the fistula is in the ileum or lower jejunum, oral elemental diets work well even though the fistula output may be increased. With proximal jejunal fistulas, feeding can often be carried out via a tube which has been threaded past the fistula.

With proper supportive care, and in the absence of distal obstruction, up to 40 percent of small bowel fistulas can be expected to close spontaneously. But if the fistula is not closing satisfactorily in 2 or 3 weeks, then operative intervention likely will be necessary and should not be delayed. Hopefully, by this time the patient's condition is stable; sepsis is under control and he is in anabolic phase as the result of vigorous nutritional therapy.

The preferred procedure is resection of the portion of bowel containing the fistula(s) with primary anastomosis. Distal obstruction, if present, must also be corrected at the same time. Simple closure of the fistulous openings is almost invariably unsuccessful and should not be attempted, but closure may be successful if a loop of uninvolved jejunum is used as a serosal patch to buttress the repair. If resection or serosal patch technique is not possible or is felt to be unduly hazardous, then a staged procedure should be elected. The fistula is not disturbed; afferent and efferent loops are found and divided, and an anastomosis made between proximal and distal ends, thus completely excluding the fistula (Fig. 27-5). The bowel ends on the fistulous segment are oversewn, or brought to the skin as mucous fistulas. The diseased segment is left in place to be removed at a later, safer time. Bypass with proximal exclusion only (Fig. 27-5) is inferior to complete bypass but may be indicated in very poor-risk patients or where the distal bowel cannot be mobilized. Simple side-to-side bypass without exclusion is without merit.

The overall mortality rate in enterocutaneous fistulas of the small bowel is still more than 20 percent. It is higher in jejunal fistulas and significantly lower in ileal fistulas.

Pneumatosis Cystoides Intestinalis

This is an uncommon condition manifested by multiple gas-filled cysts of the gastrointestinal tract. The cysts are either submucosal or subserosal and vary in size from microscopic to several centimeters in diameter. The jejunum is most frequently involved, followed by the ileocecal region and colon. Gas cysts are associated with other lesions of the gastrointestinal tract in about 85 percent of cases. Pneumatosis not associated with other lesions (15 percent) is called "primary."

Grossly the cysts resemble cystic lymphangiomas or hydatid cysts. On section, the involved portion has a honeycomb appearance. The cysts are thin-walled and break easily. Spontaneous rupture gives rise to pneumoperitoneum.

Symptoms are nonspecific and in "secondary" pneumatosis may be those of the associated disease. In primary pneumatosis, symptoms, when present, resemble those of irritable bowel syndrome. Diagnosis is usually made radiographically (Fig. 27-6). No treatment is necessary unless one of the very rare complications supervenes, such as rectal bleeding, cyst-induced volvulus, or tension pneumoperitoneum. Prognosis in most patients is that of the underlying disease. The cysts may disappear spontaneously or may persist for prolonged periods without serious symptoms.

Blind Loop Syndrome

This is a rare clinical syndrome manifested by diarrhea, steatorrhea, anemia, weight loss, abdominal pain, multiple vitamin deficiencies, and neurologic disorders. The underlying cause is not a blind loop per se but stagnation of small intestinal contents by stricture, stenosis, fistulas, blind pouch formation, or diverticula. The bacterial flora are altered in the stagnant area, both in number and in kind. The bacteria successfully compete for vitamin B_{12}, producing a systemic deficiency of B_{12} and megaloblastic anemia. Steatorrhea also occurs; bacteria in the stagnant area deconjugate bile salts, causing disruption of micellar solubilization of fats. There may also be absorptive defects of other macro- and micronutrients. The mechanism of these defects is not clear at this time.

The syndrome can be confirmed by a series of laboratory investigations. First, a Schilling test (cobalt 60—labeled B_{12} absorption) is performed; this should reveal a pernicious anemia type of urinary excretion of vitamin B_{12} (0 to 6 percent, compared with the normal of 7 to 25 percent). The test is then repeated with the addition of intrinsic factor. In true pernicious anemia the excretion should rise to normal; in the blind loop syndrome, the addition of intrinsic factor will not increase the excretion of B_{12}. Next, the patient is given a course of tetracycline for 3 to 5 days, and the Schilling test is repeated. With blind loop syndrome, absorption of cobalt 60—labeled B_{12}—returns to normal; this does not occur in the macrocytic anemia due to steatorrhea. Whereas patients with the blind loop syndrome respond to tetracyclines and parenteral B_{12} therapy,

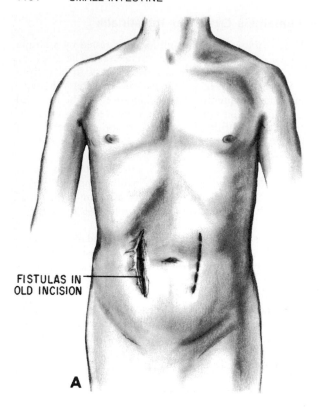

FISTULAS IN
OLD INCISION

A

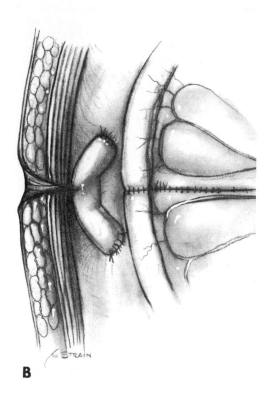

B

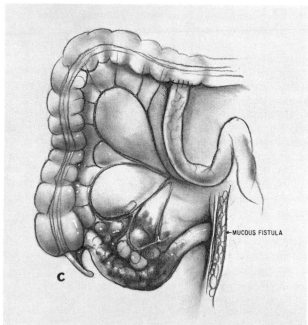

←MUCOUS FISTULA

C

Fig. 27-5. Exclusion of a fistula. *A.* Placement of incision in uninvolved area of abdomen. *B.* Complete exclusion. Intestinal loops leading to and from the fistulous areas are divided and anastomosed end-to-end. The ends of the fistulous loop are oversewn or brought out as mucous fistulas. *C.* Exclusion with bypass. The intestine is divided above the fistula, and continuity is restored by anastomosis of proximal bowel to normal bowel distal to the fistula. Both procedures avoid dissection in inflamed tissue. A second operation to excise the diseased loop is necessary.

surgical correction of the condition producing stagnation and blind loop syndrome effects a permanent cure and therefore is indicated.

Short Bowel Syndrome

Emergency massive resection of small bowel must sometimes be done when extensive frank gangrene precludes revascularization. Mesenteric occlusion, midgut volvulus, and traumatic disruption of the superior mesenteric vessels are the most frequent causes. Short bowel syndrome may also be the end result in patients with severe recurrent regional enteritis in whom several bowel resections have been done.

No nutritional deficits are produced by resection of the entire jejunum. Loss of the entire ileum is compatible with essentially normal nutrition, though B_{12} replacement will always be necessary since the sole site of absorption is the lower ileum and adaptation does not occur. Though there is considerable individual variation, in general, resection of up to 70 percent can be tolerated if the terminal ileum and ileocecal valve can be preserved. If these are resected, nutrition can be severely impaired by a 50 to 60 percent small bowel resection. A few patients with resections of 95 to 100 percent of the small bowel have survived. Until recently it was possible for such patients to live only in the hospital. It is now possible, by use of the Scribner technique of parenteral nutrition with an implanted right atrial catheter, for selected anenteric patients to live outside the hospital.

PATHOGENESIS. Absorption defects in short bowel syndrome may be divided into three categories: vitamin B_{12}, fat, and water and electrolytes.

Fat presents the absorbing mechanism with its greatest problem, since it, of the three major nutrients, is least efficiently absorbed. Fat can be absorbed, however, by both jejunum and ileum. Three reasons for fat malabsorption have been elucidated recently. Gastric hypersecretion of hydrochloric acid is produced by massive intestinal resection. A low pH in the bowel interferes with digestion and shortens the transit time, thus shortening digestion-absorption time. A second factor is interruption of the normal enterohepatic circulation of bile salts. Absorption of bile salts occurs in the ileum. If the ileum is missing or diseased, bile salts are lost instead of recirculating, producing a relative bile-salt deficiency and a defect in the intraluminal phase of fat absorption. The third factor is a corollary of the second. Soaps and fatty acids formed during fat digestion, if not absorbed, are very irritative to the colonic mucosa, further increasing diarrhea and steatorrhea. Castor oil and soapsuds enemas are effective by virtue of this same chemical mechanism.

Fluid and electrolyte depletion are a function of short transit time and watery diarrhea. These are all rapidly absorbed in all segments of the small intestine.

TREATMENT. The key to treatment of the short bowel syndrome is control of diarrhea and steatorrhea. This requires patient trial and error, since what works in one may be of no value in another.

Pullan has divided the course of patients after partial

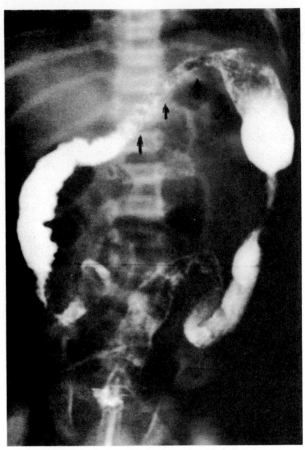

Fig. 27-6. Barium enema radiograph of an infant with pneumatosis cystoides coli. Arrows point to several submucosal gas cysts.

Table 27-3. SUMMARY OF TREATMENT OF THE SHORT GUT SYNDROME

Stage	Signs	Treatment
First Stage	Diarrhea exceeds 7–8 bowel movements per day or more than 2½ liters per day	(a) Only intravenous fluids (b) Control diarrhea (c) Maintain fluid and electrolyte balance
Second Stage	Diarrhea less than 2 liters per day	(a) Continue intravenous fluids to give calories (b) Start hypotonic oral fluids to maintain fluid and electrolyte volume, consider space diets, add carbohydrates and proteins, medium chain triglycerides
Third Stage	Stabilization of diarrhea on fat-free diet	(a) Add fat (b) Adjust weight to gut length (c) Consider adjunctive surgical procedures to control gastric hypersecretion and motility

SOURCE: From H. K. Wright and M. D. Tilson: The Short Gut Syndrome; Pathophysiology and Treatment, *Curr Probl Surg,* June, 1971. Copyright © 1971 by Year Book Medical Publishers. Used by permission.

enterectomy into three stages. Wright and Tilson use these clinical stages as a basis for treatment (Table 27-3).

Drugs to slow intestinal motility, such as Lomotil or codeine, are usually helpful. Oral calcium carbonate decreases diarrhea by neutralizing hydrochloric acid and free fatty acids. Dietary fat is restricted to 30 to 50 Gm daily to minimize steatorrhea. Medium chain triglycerides, which are water-soluble and thus absorbed into the portal vein instead of lacteals, are worthwhile in some patients but poorly tolerated by others. Similarly, oral bile salts to increase fat absorption help some patients but increase diarrhea by their cathartic effect in others. Cholestyramine, an agent that sequesters bile acids, is often useful in patients with resections of less than 100 cm, but is of no value in patients with greater resections. Electrolyte losses, particularly calcium and potassium, must be closely watched and replaced parenterally as needed.

A number of surgical procedures have been tried in an attempt to ameliorate the short bowel syndrome. This includes reversal of a segment of intestine, recirculating loops, artificial sphincters, and vagotomy-pyloroplasty. The usefulness, if any, of the procedures is certainly unclear at this time. It is certain, however, that no accessory procedures should be done at the time of the initial surgery, but should only be considered 6 to 12 months after resection in patients who cannot maintain weight within 30 percent of normal without intravenous supplementation. Vagotomy-pyloroplasty may be required in a few patients for demonstrated gastric hypersecretion that is producing severe steatorrhea out of proportion to the length of bowel resection because of acid inhibition of lipase activity.

The hope of the future is probably allotransplantation of a segment of intestine. The procedure is technically feasible as shown by the studies of Ruiz et al. (in association with Lillehei). Four human allotransplants have been unsuccessful with no patient surviving a month. The major unsolved problem at present is control of the immunologic response. When the entire small bowel is allotransplanted in dogs, the grafted intestine remains viable, but the host is killed by a massive graft-versus-host reaction, presumably because of the massive amount of lymphoid tissue in the intestine. The group of Holmes et al. (in association with Fortner) has suggested that intestinal segments 4 to 5 feet in length should provide adequate function and that rejection may be easier to control.

Fig. 27-7. Bypass operations. *A.* Payne-DeWind operation. The proximal 35 cm of jejunum is anastomosed end-to-side to the ileum 10 cm above the ileocecal valve. *B.* Scott operation. The proximal 30 cm of jejunum is anastomosed end-to-end to the distal 15 cm of ileum. The proximal end of the divided ileum is anastomosed to the transverse colon. *C.* Mason operation. The distal 90 percent of the stomach is surgically excluded; the proximal pouch is anastomosed by a narrow stoma to the jejunum. *D.* Buchwald-Varco operation. The distal one-third of the small intestine is excluded; the proximal intestine is anastomosed end-to-side to the ascending colon.

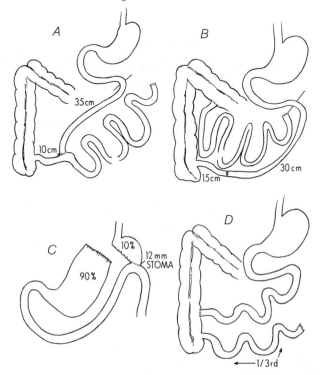

Intestinal Bypass

MORBID OBESITY

A surgically created short-gut malabsorption syndrome has become a rather widely used method of treating massive exogenous obesity that has proved refractory to all other efforts at control. The original operation, anastomosis of the proximal jejunum to the transverse colon, had to be abandoned because of an unacceptable rate of complications. The two most popular operations currently are diagramed in Fig. 27-7*A* and *B.* An alternate method of surgical therapy of obesity is the gastric exclusion operation (Fig. 27-7*C*). This operation limits food intake by reducing the reservoir capacity of the stomach to 10 percent of normal.

Before operative management of obesity is considered, a fully informed patient and his internist must agree that operation is now the logical next step in the management of the patient's problem—that all else has been tried and has failed. In addition to massive obesity per se, other indications for weight-reduction surgery are Pickwickian syndrome, adult-onset diabetes, and essential hypertension. The best results have been in patients between the ages of eighteen and thirty years. Jejunoileal bypass should not be done in growing patients since intellectual, skeletal, and reproductive growth may be adversely affected.

Satisfactory weight loss without serious complications is attained in about 80 percent of patients, with the most overweight patients losing the most weight. Weight loss goes on for 12 to 18 months; the weight then usually plateaus at a level still considerably above the ideal but well below the preoperative weight. Adaptation of the gut, as described above under Short Bowel Syndrome, is the principal reason for the plateau.

The operative mortality rate of jejunoileostomy is 2 to 5 percent. The morbidity, as always in operations on very obese patients, is appreciable and includes atelectasis, pneumonia, wound infection and dehiscence, and thromboembolism. These must be weighed, however, against the risks of untreated massive obesity.

The late mortality rate has been about 10 percent, one-half the deaths being from liver failure. Late complications are many and formidable; they include hepatic steatosis, cirrhosis, and failure; hyperoxaluria and calcium oxalate urinary tract calculi; hyperbilirubinemia and gallstones; electrolyte imbalances including hypocalcemia, hypomagnesemia, and hypokalemia; avitaminoses; psychologic problems and emotional upsets; loss of hair; polyarthropathy; pancreatitis; blind loop syndrome; pneumatosis cystoides intestinalis; colonic pseudoobstruction; intussusception of bypassed jejunum; and bypass enteritis.

Hepatic failure has been the most serious of the late complications of jejunoileal bypass for obesity. Essentially all massively obese patients have slight to moderate hepatic steatosis prior to operation—the steatosis of hyperphagia. The amount of fat in the liver usually increases postoperatively, particularly in those patients who are losing weight rapidly, then decreases as the patient's weight plateaus. Frank cirrhosis has developed in a few patients. The majority of investigators feel that this post-bypass hepatic dysfunction is a form of kwashiorkor, i.e., protein malnutrition in the presence of adequate or high carbohydrate intake. There is also some evidence from the laboratory that overgrowth of bacteria, particularly bacteroides, in the excluded intestine contributes to the hepatic dysfunction. As noted above, the hepatic dysfunction spontaneously ameliorates as the patient's weight stabilizes in most cases, but in a small percentage of patients (the exact number not yet known) a severe liver failure syndrome intervenes which is fatal if not promptly diagnosed and vigorously treated. It is particularly dangerous because the ordinary liver function tests do not herald the incipient crisis. The diagnosis, at present, is made on clinical grounds. The failure is manifested by marked anorexia, nausea, vomiting, and crampy abdominal pain. Fluid retention is manifested by weight gain, peripheral edema, and ascites. The most striking laboratory findings are profound hypoalbuminemia and hypokalemia. Liver function tests, including conjugated bilirubin, become markedly abnormal. The immediate treatment is massive infusions of albumin and potassium plus parenteral alimentation with amino acid solutions containing little or no carbohydrate. Reversal of the shunt after the patient's condition is stabilized is usually advisable unless the hepatic dysfunction can be managed with amino acid supplements.

Most of the weight lost by these morbidly obese persons after a shunt represents lost fat and water. Whether or not significant lean body mass is also lost is not yet settled. Most investigators who have done body composition studies have found that lean body mass is also lost, but some others have found that such loss is insignificant. The reasons for the differences are not apparent at this time. If it is confirmed that lean tissue is lost, then the validity of the procedure will be in question.

In some 10 or 15 percent of patients in whom jejunoileal bypass has been performed it becomes necessary to revise or to reverse the shunt. The principal indications have been hepatic failure, unmanageable electrolyte and metabolic imbalances, persistent uncontrollable diarrhea or associated severe anorectal problems, excessive or excessively rapid weight loss, and inadequate weight loss. It is imperative that the patient be carefully prepared for the reversal operation by vigorous appropriate parenteral therapy. Several weeks in the hospital may be required to attain the optimum state for reoperation.

Griffen and associates have conducted a prospective comparison of gastric and jejunoileal bypass for morbid obesity. In patients examined one year after operation, they found that the jejunoileal bypass resulted in a somewhat greater weight loss—average of 69 kg versus 51 kg, the risk of immediate operative complications was equal, but the gastric bypass led to fewer late complications, less need for rehospitalization, less medication requirement, and no increase in liver disease. If these results hold up with time and are confirmed by others, then gastric bypass should be the preferred operation for treatment of morbid obesity.

HYPERLIPIDEMIA

Surgical bypass of a portion of the small intestine is also a useful method of treating hypercholesterolemia and hypertriglyceridemia. The operation (Fig. 27-7D), designed by Buchwald and Varco, short-circuits the distal 200 cm or one-third the small intestine length, whichever is greater. This operation, though associated with diarrhea at times, does not cause significant weight loss and is not associated with the undesirable side effects of the jejunoileal bypass.

This procedure lowers serum cholesterol level by two mechanisms: by interfering with the absorption of cholesterol by short-circuiting the usual site of absorption, and secondly, by increasing cholesterol and bile acid excretion, which accelerates cholesterol turnover.

Clinical metabolic studies have demonstrated a 60 percent decrease in cholesterol absorption, a 40 percent reduction in serum cholesterol, and more than a 50 percent reduction in plasma triglycerides. About 70 percent of patients with angina have had improvement or total remission of symptoms after this operation. Thus partial ileal bypass appears to be an effective method of lipid reduction. It is obligatory in its actions, safe, and associated with minimal side effects.

References

General

Broido, P. W., Gorbach, S. L., and Nyhus, L. M.: Microflora of the Gastrointestinal Tract and the Surgical Malabsorption Syndromes, *Surg Gynecol Obstet,* **135:**449, 1972.

Christensen, J.: The Controls of Gastrointestinal Movements: Some Old and New Views, *New Engl J Med,* **285:**85, 1971.

Colcock, B. P., and Braasch, J. W.: Surgery of the Small Intestine in the Adult, in "Major Problems in Clinical Surgery," vol. VII, W. B. Saunders Company, Philadelphia, 1968.

Creamer, B. (ed.): "The Small Intestine," Year Book Medical Publishers, Inc., Chicago, 1974.

Gangl, A., and Ockner, R. K.: Intestinal Metabolism of Lipids and Lipoproteins, *Gastroenterology,* **68:**167, 1975.

Grand, R. J., Watkins, J. B., and Torti, F. M.: Development of the Human Gastrointestinal Tract, *Gastroenterology,* **70:**790, 1976.

Kagnoff, M. F.: Induction and Paralysis: A Conceptual Framework from Which to Examine the Intestinal Immune System, *Gastroenterology,* **66:**1240, 1974.

Mallory, A., Kern, F., Jr., Smith, J., and Savage, D.: Patterns of Bile Acids and Microflora in the Human Small Intestine, *Gastroenterology,* **64:**26, 1973.

Pearse, A. G. E., Polak, J. M., and Bloom, S. R.: The Newer Gut Hormones. Cellular Sources, Physiology, Pathology, and Clinical Aspects, *Gastroenterology,* **72:**746, 1977.

Scott, B. B., and Losowsky, M. S.: Peroral Small-Intestine Biopsy: Experience with the Hydraulic Multiple Biopsy Instrument in Routine Clinical Practice, *Gut,* **17:**740, 1976.

Trier, J. S.: Diagnostic Value of Peroral Biopsy of the Proximal Small Intestine, *N Engl J Med,* **285:**1470, 1971.

Inflammatory Diseases

Beeken, W. L., Mitchell, D. N., and Cave, D. R.: Evidence for a Transmissible Agent in Crohn's Disease, in "Clinics in Gastroenterology," vol. 5, p. 289, W. B. Saunders Company, Philadelphia, 1976.

Block, G. E., Enker, W. E., and Kirsner, J. B.: Significance and Treatment of Occult Obstructive Uropathy Complicating Crohn's Disease, *Ann Surg,* **178:**322, 1973.

———, Moossa, A. R., and Simonowitz, D.: The Operative Treatment of Crohn's Disease in Childhood, *Surg Gynecol Obstet,* **144:**713, 1977.

Cave, D. R., Mitchell, D. N., and Brooke, B. N.: Experimental Animal Studies of the Etiology and Pathogenesis of Crohn's Disease, *Gastroenterology,* **69:**618, 1975.

Crohn, B. B., Ginzburg, L., and Oppenheimer, G. D.: Regional Ileitis: Pathological and Clinical Entity, *JAMA,* **99:**1323, 1932.

Das, P., and Shukla, H. S.: Clinical Diagnosis of Abdominal Tuberculosis, *Br J Surg,* **63:**941, 1976.

DeDombal, F. T., Burton, I. L., Clamp, S. E., and Goligher, J. C.: Short-term Course and Prognosis of Crohn's Disease, *Gut,* **15:**435, 1974.

Dunne, W. T., Cooke, W. T., and Allan, R. N.: Enzymatic and Morphometric Evidence for Crohn's Disease as a Diffuse Lesion of the Gastrointestinal Tract, *Gut,* **18:**290, 1977.

Eade, M. N., Cooke, W. T., and Williams, J. A.: Clinical and Hematologic Features of Crohn's Disease, *Surg Gynecol Obstet,* **134:**643, 1972.

Farmer, R. G., Hawk, W. A., and Turnbull, R. B., Jr.: Indications for Surgery in Crohn's Disease: Analysis of 500 Cases, *Gastroenterology,* **71:**245, 1976.

Freeman, J. B., Egan, M. C., and Millis, B. J.: The Elemental Diet, *Surg Gynecol Obstet,* **142:**925, 1976.

Gitnick, G. L., Arthur, M. H., and Shibata, I.: Cultivation of Viral Agents from Crohn's Disease: A New Sensitive System, *Lancet,* **2:**215, 1976.

Glass, R. E., and Baker, W. N. W.: Role of the Granuloma in Recurrent Crohn's Disease, *Gut,* **17:**75, 1976.

Glotzer, D. J., and Silen, W.: Surgical Management of Regional Enteritis, *Gastroenterology,* **61:**751, 1971.

Gump, F. E., Sakellariadis, P., Wolff, M., and Broell, J. R.: Clinical-Pathological Investigation of Regional Enteritis as a Guide to Prognosis, *Ann Surg,* **176:**233, 1972.

Kewenter, J., Hulten, L., and Kock, N. G.: The Relationship and Epidemiology of Acute Terminal Ileitis and Crohn's Disease, *Gut,* **15:**801, 1974.

Kim, J.-P., Oh, S.-K., and Jarrett, F.: Management of Ileal Perforation due to Typhoid Fever, *Ann Surg,* **181:**88, 1975.

Kirsner, J. B.: Genetic Aspects of Inflammatory Bowel Disease, in "Clinics in Gastroenterology," vol. 2, p. 557, W. B. Saunders Company, Philadelphia, 1973.

Klein, M., Binder, H. J., Mitchell, M., Aaronson, R., and Spiro, H.: Treatment of Crohn's Disease with Azathioprine: A Controlled Evaluation, *Gastroenterology,* **66:**916, 1974.

MacPherson, B. R., Albertini, R. J., and Beeken, W. L.: Immunological Studies in Patients with Crohn's Disease, *Gut,* **17:**100, 1976.

Marshak, R. H., and Lindner, A. E.: Roentgen Features in Crohn's Disease, in "Clinics in Gastroenterology," vol. 1, p. 411, W. B. Saunders Company, Philadelphia, 1972.

Menguy, R.: Surgical Management of Free Perforation of the Small Intestine Complicating Regional Enteritis, *Ann Surg,* **175:**178, 1972.

Mitchell, D. N., and Rees, R. J. W.: Agent Transmissible from Crohn's Disease Tissue, *Lancet,* **2:**168, 1970.

Morson, B. C.: Pathology of Crohn's Disease, in "Clinics in Gastroenterology," vol. 1, p. 265, W. B. Saunders Company, Philadelphia, 1972.

Mottet, N. K.: Histopathologic Spectrum of Regional Enteritis and Ulcerative Colitis, in "Major Problems in Pathology," vol. II, W. B. Saunders Company, Philadelphia, 1971.

Nesbit, R. R., Jr., Elbadawi, N. A., Morton, J. H., and Cooper, R. A., Jr.: Carcinoma of the Small Bowel, a Complication of Regional Enteritis, *Cancer,* **37:**2948, 1976.

Nugent, F. W., Richmond, M., and Park, S. K.: Crohn's Disease of the Duodenum, *Gut,* **18:**115, 1977.

Reilly, J., Ryan, J. A., Strole, W., and Fischer, J. E.: Hyperalimentation in Inflammatory Bowel Disease, *Am J Surg,* **131:**192, 1976.

Rocchio, M. A., MoCha, C.-J., Haas, K. F., and Randall, H. T.: Use of Chemically Defined Diets in the Management of Patients with Acute Inflammatory Bowel Disease, *Am J Surg,* **127:**469, 1974.

Sachar, D. B., Taub, R. N., and Janowitz, H. D.: A Transmissible Agent in Crohn's Disease? New Pursuit of an Old Concept, *N Engl J Med,* **293:**354, 1975.

Senewiratne, B., and Senewiratne, K.: Reassessment of the Widal Test in the Diagnosis of Typhoid, *Gastroenterology,* **73:**233, 1977.

Shorter, R. G., Huizenga, K. A., and Spencer, R. J.: A Working Hypothesis for the Etiology and Pathogenesis of Non-specific Inflammatory Bowel Disease, *Am J Dig Dis,* **17:**1024, 1972.

Simonowitz, D., Block, G. E., Riddell, R. H., Kraft, S. C., and Kirsner, J. B.: The Production of an Unusual Tissue Reaction in Rabbit Bowel Injected with Crohn's Disease Homogenates, *Surgery,* **82:**211, 1977.

Smith, L. H., and Hofmann, A. F.: Acquired Hyperoxaluria, Urolithiasis, and Intestinal Disease: A New Digestive Disorder? *Gastroenterology,* **66:**1257, 1974.

Steinberg, D. M., Cooke, W. T., and Williams, J. A.: Abscess and Fistulae in Crohn's Disease, *Gut,* **14:**865, 1973.

Tandon, H. D., and Prakash, A.: Pathology of Intestinal Tuberculosis and Its Distinction from Crohn's Disease, *Gut,* **13:**260, 1972.

Thayer, W. R., Jr.: Are the Inflammatory Bowel Diseases Immune Complex Diseases? *Gastroenterology,* **70:**136, 1976.

Truelove, S. C., and Penn, A. S.: Course and Prognosis of Crohn's Disease, *Gut,* **17:**192, 1976.

Vantrappen, G., Ponette, E., Geboes, K., and Bertrand, P.: Yersinia Enteritis and Enterocolitis: Gastroenterological Aspects, *Gastroenterology,* **72:**220, 1977.

Walker, W. A., and Isselbacher, K. J.: Uptake and Transport of Macromolecules by the Intestine, Possible Role in Clinical Disorders, *Gastroenterology,* **67:**531, 1974.

Weakley, F. L., and Turnbull, F. L.: Recognition of Regional Ileitis in the Operating Room, *Dis Colon Rectum,* **14:**17, 1971.

Whorwell, P. J., and Wright, R.: Immunological Aspects of Inflammatory Bowel Disease, in "Clinics in Gastroenterology," vol. 5, p. 303, W. B. Saunders Company, Philadelphia, 1976.

Neoplasms

Barry, R. E., and Read, A. E.: Coeliac Disease and Malignancy, *Q J Med,* **42:**665, 1973.

Brown, N. K., and Smith, M. P.: Neoplastic Diathesis of Patients with Carcinoid, *Cancer,* **32:**216, 1973.

Bussey, H. J. R.: Gastrointestinal Polyposis, *Gut,* **11:**970, 1970.

Calman, K. C.: Why Are Small Bowel Tumours Rare? An Experimental Model, *Gut,* **15:**552, 1974.

Davis, Z., Moertel, C. G., and McIlrath, D. C.: The Malignant Carcinoid Syndrome, *Surg Gynecol Obstet,* **137:**637, 1973.

Fu, Y.-S., and Perzin, K. H.: Lymphosarcoma of the Small Intestine, *Cancer,* **29:**645, 1972.

Gardner, B., Dollinger, M., Silen, W., Back, N., and O'Reilly, S.: Studies of the Carcinoid Syndrome: Its Relationship to Serotonin, Bradykinin, and Histamine, *Surgery,* **61:**846, 1967.

Jeghers, H., McKusick, V. A., and Katz, K. H.: Generalized Intestinal Polyposis and Melanin Spots on the Oral Mucosa, Lips and Digits, *N Engl J Med,* **241:**993, 1949.

Kaplan, E. L., Jaffe, B. M., and Peskin, G. W.: A New Provocative Test for the Diagnosis of the Carcinoid Syndrome, *Am J Surg,* **123:**173, 1972.

Lewin, K. J., Kahn, L. B., and Novis, B. H.: Primary Intestinal Lymphoma of "Western" and "Mediterranean" Type, Alpha Chain Disease and Massive Plasma Cell Infiltration, *Cancer,* **38:**2511, 1976.

McDermott, W. V., and Hensle, T. W.: Metastatic Carcinoid to the Liver Treated by Hepatic Dearterialization, *Ann Surg,* **180:**305, 1974.

McKittrick, J. E., Lewis, W. M., Doane, W. A., and Gerwig, W. H.: The Peutz-Jeghers Syndrome, *Arch Surg,* **103:**57, 1971.

Masson, P.: Carcinoids (Argentaffin-Cell Tumors) and Nerve Hyperplasia of Appendicular Mucosa, *Am J Pathol,* **4:**181, 1928.

Moertel, C. G.: Clinical Management of Advanced Gastrointestinal Cancer, *Cancer,* **36:**675, 1975.

Postlethwait, R. W.: Gastrointestinal Carcinoid Tumors: A Review, *Postgrad Med,* **40:**445, 1966.

Ranchod, M., and Kempson, R. L.: Smooth Muscle Tumors of the Gastrointestinal Tract and Retroperitoneum, *Cancer,* **39:**257, 1977.

Reid, J. D.: Intestinal Carcinoma in the Peutz-Jeghers Syndrome, *JAMA,* **229:**833, 1974.

Sheahan, D. G., Martin, F., Baginsky, S., Mallory, G. K., and Zamcheck, N.: Multiple Lymphomatous Polyposis of the Gastrointestinal Tract, *Cancer,* **28:**408, 1971.

Teitelbaum, S. L.: The Carcinoid. A Collective Review, *Am J Surg,* **123:**564, 1972.

Wilson, H., Cheek, R. C., Sherman, R. T., and Storer, E. H.: Carcinoid Tumors, in "Current Problems in Surgery," The Year Book Medical Publishers, Inc., Chicago, 1970.

Wilson, J. M., Melvin, D. B., Gray, G. F., and Thorbjarnarson, B.: Primary Malignancies of the Small Bowel: A Report of 96 Cases and Review of the Literature, *Ann Surg,* **180:**175, 1974.

——, ——, ——, and ——: Benign Small Bowel Tumor, *Ann Surg,* **181:**247, 1975.

Diverticular Disease

Altemeier, W. A., Bryant, L. R., and Wulsin, J. H.: The Surgical Significance of Jejunal Diverticulosis, *Arch Surg,* **86:**732, 1963.

Economides, N. G., McBurney, R. P., and Hamilton, F. H., III: Intraluminal Duodenal Diverticulum in the Adult, *Ann Surg,* **185:**147, 1977.

Herrington, J. L., Jr.: Spontaneous Asymptomatic Pneumoperito-

neum: A Complication of Jejunal Diverticulosis, *Am J Surg,* **113:**567, 1967.

Kellum, J. M., Boucher, J. K., and Ballinger, W. F.: Serosal Patch Repair for Benign Duodenocolic Fistula Secondary to Duodenal Diverticulum, *Am J Surg,* **131:**607, 1976.

Kilpatrick, Z. M., and Aseron, C. A.: Radioisotope Detection of Meckel's Diverticulum Causing Acute Rectal Hemorrhage, *N Engl J Med,* **287:**653, 1972.

Localio, S. A., and Stahl, W. M.: Diverticular Disease of the Alimentary Tract. II. The Esophagus, Stomach, Duodenum and Small Intestine, in "Current Problems in Surgery," The Year Book Medical Publishers, Inc., Chicago, 1968.

Roses, D. F., Gouge, T. H., Scher, K. S., and Ranson, J. H. C.: Perforated Diverticula of the Jejunum and Ileum, *Am J Surg,* **132:**649, 1976.

Soltero, M. J., and Bill, A. H.: The Natural History of Meckel's Diverticulum and Its Relation to Incidental Removal, *Am J Surg,* **132:**168, 1976.

Ulcer of the Small Intestine

Guest, J. L.: Nonspecific Ulceration of the Intestine: Collective Review, *Surg Gynecol Obstet,* **117:**409, 1963.

McMahon, F. G., and Akdamar, K.: Gastric Ulceration after "Slow-K," *N Engl J Med,* **295:**733, 1976.

Foreign Bodies

Maleki, M., and Evans, W. E.: Foreign-body Perforation of the Intestinal Tract, *Arch Surg,* **101:**475, 1970.

Fistula

Aguirre, A., Fischer, J. E., and Welch, C. E.: The Role of Surgery and Hyperalimentation in Therapy of Gastrointestinal-Cutaneous Fistulae, *Ann Surg,* **180:**393, 1974.

Gross, E., and Irving, M.: Protection of the Skin around Intestinal Fistula, *Br J Surg,* **64:**258, 1977.

Hill, G. L., Mair, W. S. J., Edwards, J. P., Morgan, D. B., and Goligher, J. C.: Effect of a Chemically Defined Liquid Diet on Composition and Volume of Ileal Fistula Drainage, *Gastroenterology,* **68:**676, 1975.

Jones, S. A., and Steedman, R. A.: Management of Chronic Infected Intestinal Perforations by the Serosal Patch Technic, *Am J Surg,* **117:**731, 1969.

MacFadyen, B. V., Jr., Dudrick, S. J., and Ruberg, R. L.: Management of Gastrointestinal Fistulas with Parenteral Hyperalimentation, *Surgery,* **74:**100, 1973.

MacFarlane, M., and Frawley, J. E.: A Technique for Drainage of Enterocutaneous Fistulas, *Surg Gynecol Obstet,* **141:**263, 1975.

Roback, S. A., and Nicoloff, D. M.: High Output Enterocutaneous Fistulas of the Small Bowel, *Am J Surg,* **123:**317, 1972.

Sheldon, G. F., Gardiner, B. N., Way, L. W., and Dunphy, J. E.: Management of Gastrointestinal Fistulas, *Surg Gynecol Obstet,* **133:**385, 1971.

Pneumatosis Cystoides Intestinalis

Feinberg, S. B., Schwartz, M. Z., Clifford, S., Buchwald, H., and Varco, R. L.: Significance of Pneumatosis Cystoides Intestinalis after Jejunoileal Bypass, *Am J Surg,* **133:**149, 1977.

Reyna, R., Soper, R. T., and Condon, R. E.: Pneumatosis Intestinalis, *Am J Surg,* **125:**667, 1973.

Blind Loop Syndrome

Aabakke, J., and Schjonsby, H.: Value of Urinary Simple Phenol and Indican Determinations in the Diagnosis of the Stagnant Loop Syndrome, *Scand J Gastroentol,* **11:**409, 1976.

Ellis, H., and Smith, A. D. M.: The Blind-loop Syndrome, in "Monographs in the Surgical Sciences," The Williams & Wilkins Company, Baltimore, 1967.

Fromm, D.: Ileal Resection, or Disease, and the Blind Loop Syndrome: Current Concepts of Pathophysiology, *Surgery,* **73:**639, 1973.

Short Bowel Syndrome

Binder, H. J.: Fecal Fatty Acids—Mediators of Diarrhea? *Gastroenterology,* **65:**847, 1973.

Dowling, R. H.: Intestinal Adaptation, *N Engl J Med,* **288:**520, 1973.

Hofmann, A. F.: Bile Acid Malabsorption Caused by Ileal Resection, *Arch Intern Med,* **130:**597, 1972.

Mackby, M. J.: The Short Bowel Revisited, *Surgery,* **79:**1, 1976.

Riella, M. C., and Scribner, B. A.: Five Years' Experience with a Right Atrial Catheter for Prolonged Parenteral Nutrition at Home, *Surg Gynecol Obstet,* **143:**205, 1976.

Weser, E.: The Management of Patients after Small Bowel Resection, *Gastroenterology,* **71:**146, 1976.

Winchester, D. P., and Dorsey, J. M.: Intestinal Segments and Pouches in Gastrointestinal Surgery, *Surg Gynecol Obstet,* **132:**131, 1971.

Wright, H. K., and Tilson, M. D.: The Short Gut Syndrome. Pathophysiology and Treatment, in "Current Problems in Surgery," The Year Book Medical Publishers, Inc., Chicago, 1971.

Intestinal Bypass

Brown, R. G., O'Leary, J. P., and Woodward, E. R.: Hepatic Effects of Jejunoileal Bypass for Morbid Obesity, *Am J Surg,* **127:**53, 1974.

Buchwald, H., Moore, R. B., and Varco, R. L.: Ten Years Clinical Experience with Partial Ileal Bypass in Management of the Hyperlipidemias, *Ann Surg,* **180:**384, 1974.

Cegielski, M. M., Organ, C. H., Jr., and Saporta, J. A.: Revision of Intestinal Bypass Procedures, *Surg Gynecol Obstet,* **142:**829, 1976.

DeWind, L. T., and Payne, J. H.: Intestinal Bypass Surgery for Morbid Obesity, *JAMA,* **236:**2298, 1976.

Dudrick, S. J., Daly, J. M., Castro, G., and Akhtar, M.: Gastrointestinal Adaptation following Small Bowel Bypass for Obesity, *Ann Surg,* **185:**642, 1977.

Griffen, W. O., Jr., Young, V. L., and Stevenson, C. C.: A Prospective Comparison of Gastric and Jejuno-ileal Bypass for Morbid Obesity, *Ann Surg,* **186:**500, 1977.

Holmes, J. T., Yeh, S. D. J., Winawer, S. J., Kawano, N., and Fortner, J. G.: Absorption Studies in Canine Jejunal Allografts, *Ann Surg,* **174:**101, 1971.

Mason, E. E., Printen, K. J., Hartford, C. E., and Boyd, W. C.: Optimizing Results of Gastric Bypass, *Ann Surg,* **182:**405, 1975.

Malt, R. A., and Guggenheim, F. G.: Surgery for Obesity, *N Engl J Med,* **295:**43, 1976.

Moxley, R. T., III, Pozefsky, T., and Lockwood, D. H.: Protein Nutrition and Liver Disease after Jejunoileal Bypass for Morbid Obesity, *N Engl J Med,* **290:**921, 1974.

Ruiz, J. O., Uchida, H., Schultz, L. S., and Lillehei, R. C.: Problems in Absorption and Immunosuppression after Entire Intestinal Allotransplantation, *Am J Surg,* **123:**297, 1972.

Scott, H. W., Jr.: Metabolic Surgery for Hyperlipidemia and Atherosclerosis, *Am J Surg,* **123:**3, 1972.

———, Dean, R., Shull, H. J., Abram, H. S., Webb, W., Younger, R. K., and Brill, A. B.: New Considerations in Use of Jejuno-ileal Bypass in Patients with Morbid Obesity, *Ann Surg,* **177:**723, 1973.

Spanier, A. H., Kurta, R. S., Shibata, H. R., MacLean, L. D., and Shizgal, H. M.: Alterations in Body Composition following Intestinal Bypass for Morbid Obesity, *Surgery,* **80:**171, 1976.

Toledo-Pereyra, L. H., Simmons, R. L., and Najarian, J. S.: Prolonged Survival of Canine Orthotopic Small Intestinal Allografts Preserved for 24 Hours by Hypothermic Bloodless Perfusion, *Surgery,* **75:**368, 1974.

Chapter 28

Colon, Rectum, and Anus

by **Edward H. Storer, Stanley M. Goldberg, and Santhat Nivatvongs**

The principal functions of the colon are water absorption and storage of feces. The cecum receives about 500 ml of chyme from the ileum daily. This is dehydrated in the right half of the colon to about 150 ml—the daily volume of feces. Thus only about 5 percent of water absorption in the intestinal tract occurs in the colon. The left colon functions principally as a storage organ. Voluntary control of defecation is regulated by rectum and anus. Their principal function in our society is to allow defecation only at socially convenient times. The colon, rectum, and anus therefore play a relatively unimportant role in the bodily economy; completely normal biologic existence is possible following total proctocolectomy. They are indispensable, however, for a comfortable life in society without the constant risk of embarrassment.

Though the colon, rectum, and anus are relatively unimportant biologically, they are one of the most important organ systems clinically because of the high incidence and variety of diseases associated with these organs. About 10 million persons now living in the United States have diverticulosis coli; about 20 million harbor *Endamoeba histolytica* in their colons. Primary chronic ulcerative colitis is fortunately uncommon, for it is one of the most miserable chronic diseases known to mankind. A diagnosis of carcinoma of the colon or rectum was made for the first time in 101,000 Americans in 1977. This is the most common internal cancer in the United States and causes 51,300 deaths annually—about 13 percent of all cancer deaths. Some 11 million Americans have colonic polyps, which are thought to be premalignant lesions. The number of persons with hemorrhoids and anorectal fissures and fistulas cannot even be estimated—there are countless millions.

INFLAMMATORY DISEASES

Ulcerative Colitis

Idiopathic nonspecific ulcerative colitis is an uncommon inflammatory disease involving primarily mucosa and submucosa of the colon. Both acute and chronic forms are seen. Though colitis (segmental colitis, right-sided colitis, Crohn's disease of the colon) was recognized as an entity distinct from ulcerative colitis in 1932, the distinction has gradually gained acceptance only since about 1959. Thus reports prior to 1959 are of limited value. Strenuous efforts were aimed for a time at clear separation of the two forms of idiopathic colitis, but there is now a growing tendency to emphasize their similarities and to refer to them together as "inflammatory bowel disease."

INCIDENCE. Most information on incidence and prevalence of ulcerative colitis has been derived from hospital admission records. This data may be misleading, because patients with chronic ulcerative colitis tend to gravitate to large teaching centers and because the composition of the population from which the patients were drawn is not known. Ulcerative colitis has been studied recently in four populations of known composition in Baltimore, Maryland, in Rochester, Minnesota, in Oxford, England, and in Norway. The average annual incidence rate (the number of patients affected by the disease for the first time in a given year divided by the number of people at risk in that year) for idiopathic ulcerative colitis in white adults was 4.6 per 100,000 in Baltimore, 3.4 in Rochester, 6.5 in Oxford, and 2.1 in Norway.

The incidence of ulcerative colitis in Jews is about three times the rate in non-Jews; females are affected more than males by a ratio of about 5:4. Blacks probably have a significantly lower incidence than whites, but valid large-scale studies are not available. The disease affects all age groups, with the highest incidence in the third and fourth decades. In the United States, ulcerative colitis is seen more frequently in the North and East—more frequently than can be accounted for by differences in Jewish and black populations.

The familial incidence of ulcerative colitis is higher than would be expected from chance alone, but the rate is not striking and may be due to environmental factors, not heredity. In a study of 2,000 patients with ulcerative colitis, 26 had positive family histories; in another study of 1,084 patients, 66 reported colitis in other family members.

ETIOLOGY. Ulcerative colitis is still idiopathic despite many years of study and voluminous publications by persons of diverse interests and backgrounds. Clinical investigation is difficult, because the course of the disease is unpredictable and characterized by spontaneous and unexplained remissions.

Laboratory investigation of ulcerative colitis is handicapped because there is still no disease of other animals,

either spontaneous or experimentally induced, that closely resembles the human disease. A form of colitis occurs infrequently in boxer dogs that has some of the characteristics of ulcerative colitis but also some of the characteristics of Crohn's colitis and of Whipple's disease. The cause of canine colitis is unknown, and the condition cannot be induced at will. Ulcerative colitis-like lesions of the cecum and colon have been induced in small laboratory animals by the feeding of carrageenan, a hydrocolloid extracted from seaweed, and by the feeding of two pepsin inhibitors, sodium lignosulfonate and sulfated amylopectin. This is a convenient laboratory model but unfortunately appears to have little or no relationship to the human disease. Carrageenan is widely used as a food additive and as a medicine; the pepsin inhibitors are commercially available for the treatment of peptic ulcer.

The similarity of the clinical picture in idiopathic ulcerative colitis to that of the specific dysenteries has led to attempts to implicate specific microorganisms. There are a few documented cases of chronic ulcerative colitis following proved *Shigella* or amebic dysentery, but such cases are the exception and not the rule. Specific therapy directed against *Shigella* or *E. histolytica* rarely exerts any beneficial effect on the course of the ulcerative colitis. Furthermore, the incidence of ulcerative colitis is low where these specific dysentery infections are endemic. Other organisms that have been proposed as specific etiologic agents include an enteric diplostreptococcus and *Bacterium necrophorum*. New evidence for a transmissible infectious factor has been presented by Cave and associates, who injected filtered homogenates of ulcerative colitis tissues into rabbits and produced histologic changes in the rabbit colon that resemble those in the human disease. These data suggest a virus but do not rule out L forms or mycoplasmas.

The generally favorable influence of adrenal corticosteroids on the course of chronic ulcerative colitis has led to a revival of the thesis that allergy or hypersensitivity plays a role in the genesis of the disease. Occasional patients have a remarkable remission of symptoms following omission of milk and milk products from their diets. Antibodies to cow's milk proteins can be demonstrated in some patients with ulcerative colitis, and it has been suggested that this may be attributable to early weaning with ingestion of cow's milk formula before fourteen days of age. This exposes the infant to foreign proteins at a time of immunologic tolerance and permissive absorption of whole proteins. But circulating antibodies to cow's milk protein can be found in control patients with the same frequency as in patients with ulcerative colitis. Furthermore, circulating antibodies to milk proteins are not correlated with the presence or absence of clinical intolerance to milk. The occasional intolerance to milk may be related to a secondary deficiency in intestinal lactase rather than to a specific allergy.

Shorter and associates have proposed that the inflammatory bowel diseases are produced by local hypersensitivity reactions. Initial sensitization of the gut-associated lymphoid tissues is thought to occur in the neonatal period before the mucosal barrier is complete, permitting penetration of enterobacteria and macromolecules. Reexposure to bacteria and intestinal antigens may occur in later life if the mucosal integrity is damaged by infection, ischemia, or even metabolic alterations induced by emotional stress. Antigen reexposure then causes the local primary cellular immune-mediated hypersensitivity reaction, with the production of inflammatory bowel disease.

Hemorrhagic colitis somewhat resembling the human disease has been produced in several different laboratory animals by the administration of anticolonic antisera. These experimental immune lesions of the colon do not completely reproduce human ulcerative colitis, and their occurrence does not necessarily imply any connection with the natural genesis of human ulcerative colitis. They demonstrate only that the colon can generate autoimmune reactions. Immunosuppressive drugs, particularly azathioprine, might be expected to exert a beneficial effect if ulcerative colitis is truly an autoimmune disease. The results to date are inconclusive: some but not all patients are improved, and the benefit is slower and less marked than with corticosteroids.

Studies indicate that sensitized lymphocytes play an important role in autoimmunity in ulcerative colitis and suggest that a more fruitful approach would be via the cellular factors of hypersensitivity rather than circulating antibodies. It has been clearly demonstrated that circulating lymphocytes, but not sera, from patients with ulcerative colitis are cytotoxic for human fetal or adult colon epithelial cells. Lymphocytes from normal controls are not cytotoxic.

Mast cells, in the connective tissue of the colon, have been shown to contain histamine, serotonin, heparin, chymase, tryptase, and other biologically active substances. Sommers has proposed that mucosal hyperemia and persistent edema in ulcerative colitis are attributable to local excesses of histamine released by an increased colonic population of mast cells and that release of stored serotonin by mast cells is an exacerbating factor. This hypothesis has not yet received experimental confirmation; indeed one study reported normal levels of histamine in the blood, urine, and colonic mucosa of patients with ulcerative colitis.

The left colon has been shown in the laboratory to respond to parasympathomimetic drugs, to serotonin, and to emotional tension by sustained high-tension contractions that shorten and narrow the organ. Extravasation of blood is the first change one might expect in a mucosa rendered turgid because of impedance of venous outflow by sustained muscle contraction.

Numerous attempts to implicate mental disorders in the etiology of ulcerative colitis have produced no convincing evidence. Patients with psychoses or depressive reactions are not prone to develop ulcerative colitis, nor has functional bowel distress been observed to lead to ulcerative colitis. Whereas it is certainly true that ulcerative colitis patients manifest abnormalities of the psyche, such abnormalities may well be the effect, not the cause, of the disease—a somatopsychic rather than a psychosomatic disorder. Esler and Goulston have assessed the levels of anxiety and neuroticism in patients with ulcerative colitis and in general medical patients; there was no significant difference in these dimensions of personality. Mendeloff and associates compared life stresses in patients with ulcerative colitis and control subjects drawn from the same population group. They concluded that "this and other studies fail to support the thesis that ulcerative colitis is a paradigm of psychosomatic illness."

Despite these observations, many clinicians still have the impression that emotional stress, particularly if the patient's reaction is one of hopelessness and helplessness, often seems to trigger exacerbations of chronic ulcerative colitis, and in a small but definite percentage emotional stress appears to precipitate the disease. Conversely, emotional stress, hopelessness, and helplessness are virtually ubiquitous in our society, and yet ulcerative colitis remains an uncommon disease.

The search for a single cause of ulcerative colitis may be unrealistic. The colon can respond to injury (in the broad sense) in a limited number of ways. Several etiologic factors may have in common the initial injury to colonic mucosa in biologically predisposed individuals. Perpetuation of the process could well be due to a different mechanism(s).

PATHOLOGY. The rectum is the most frequently involved portion of the bowel in idiopathic ulcerative colitis. It is the earliest site of involvement in patients in whom the disease spreads proximally and in some is the only site of involvement. In more than half, the entire colon is diseased. With less than total involvement, disease is always in continuity—there are no skip areas, in contrast to Crohn's colitis—and the lesion is usually in the left colon, rarely the right colon alone. The terminal ileum is involved for a short distance in continuity with cecal involvement in up to 10 percent—so-called "backwash ileitis." Involvement is segmental in more than 50 percent in Crohn's colitis and affects the proximal colon more frequently than the distal. A comparison of the two forms of colitis will be found in Table 28-1.

Grossly, the serosal surface is probably essentially normal early in the disease, since ulcerative colitis initially involves the mucosa and submucosa. In advanced cases, as seen at operation or at necropsy, the bowel is greatly shortened, the sigmoid redundancy is lost, and the right and left colon segments occupy a more medial position than normal. The mesentery is contracted, edematous, and somewhat thickened, but this is much less marked than with Crohn's colitis, and large lymph node masses are conspicuously absent in ulcerative colitis. The serosal surface of the bowel is dull and grayish but with little or no exudate unless perforation has occurred. The wall is moderately thickened and firm. Contained perforations on the mesenteric margin are frequent, with abscess formation. Abscesses are also frequently encountered at the sites of stricture formation. Fistulas, except perianal, are rare in ulcerative colitis compared to Crohn's colitis. With fulminating acute colitis, the entire bowel wall is hemorrhagic and very friable, with numerous areas of necrosis.

The mucosal surface in advanced chronic ulcerative

Table 28-1. DIFFERENTIATION OF ULCERATIVE COLITIS FROM CROHN'S DISEASE OF THE COLON

Features	*Ulcerative colitis*	*Crohn's disease*
Pathology	Essentially mucosal	Transmural
Rectal involvement and distribution of the disease	Rectal involvement almost invariable (95%); spread is in continuity to the rest of the colon	Rectum frequently (50%) spared; distribution often segmental
Cobblestoning of mucosa	Unusual	Common
Extensive small bowel involvement	Never	May occur
Anorectal complications (e.g., perineal fistulas, rectovaginal fistulas, anal fissures)	Uncommon	Common
Abdominal wall or inter-fistulas	Never	Frequent
Granulomatous foci	Absent	Present in two-thirds
Lymph nodes	Reactive hyperplasia	Often granulomatous foci
Ulceration	Diffuse distribution	Longitudinal or serpiginous ulcers with normal mucosa in between
Benign colonic or rectal strictures	Rare (about 10%)	Common
Bleeding	Very common	Less common
Inflammatory abdominal mass	Never	Sometimes
Sigmoidoscopy	Diffuse involvement	Submucosal edema with heaping up of the mucosa to give a cobblestone appearance; discrete ulcerations with normal intervening mucosa

SOURCE: L. Wise, G. Efron, D. G. Glotzer, and R. B. Turnbull, Jr.: Symposium: Ulcerative Colitis and Crohn's Disease, *Contemp Surg,* **2**:95, 1973.

colitis is even more strikingly abnormal than the serosa. Bloody pus covers the ragged, moth-eaten-appearing surface. Irregular, shallow, linear, often anastomosing ulcers interspersed with islands of swollen mucosa—"pseudo polyps"—account for the characteristic appearance.

Biopsies of the rectal mucosa afford the opportunity to observe the disease histologically in all stages. The earliest lesion develops in the bases of the crypts of Lieberkühn, where neutrophils can be seen passing between the lining cells to accumulate inside the crypt lumen or lamina propria. The accumulation of neutrophils, plus eosinophils, red blood cells, and serum, forms the microscopic "crypt abscess" which is a characteristic feature of the disease. These may rupture through the mucosal surface, forming a microulcer, or into the submucosa. Whereas crypt abscesses may be seen in other inflammatory diseases of the bowel, they are always present in ulcerative colitis and in much greater numbers. With progression, numerous crypts are involved, and large areas of their walls break down, liberating exudate into the submucosa and producing widespread ulceration. As the disease becomes chronic, lymphocytes, plasma cells, and macrophages infiltrate the mucosa and submucosa. Eosinophils and increased numbers of mast cells also may be present. In advanced cases, all layers of the bowel wall are involved in acute and chronic inflammation and in fibrosis. The mucosa is absent over wide areas and replaced by granulation tissue. Pseudopolyps between the denuded areas consist of inflamed edematous mucosa or vegetative proliferations of granulation tissue.

CLINICAL MANIFESTATIONS. Idiopathic ulcerative colitis may be divided into three forms according to the clinical course: acute, fulminant; chronic, continuous; and chronic-relapsing-remitting.

The disease has an abrupt onset in about one-third of patients but fortunately runs a fulminant course in less than 10 percent. Rarely fulminant colitis is superimposed as an exacerbation upon the chronic form. Unrelenting diarrhea, preceded by severe lower abdominal cramps, continues day and night. Incontinence is frequent; tenesmus and urgency are marked. Stools are small in amount but may number 30 to 40 per day and consist of bloody mucus, pus, and watery fecal material. Systemic toxicity is striking, with fever spiking to 39 or 40°C. The malignant diarrhea rapidly produces extreme dehydration, hypokalemia, anemia, hypoproteinemia, and marked weight loss with gaunt facies and sunken eyeballs. Heroic nonoperative therapy brings the process under control in some patients, but many require urgent operative therapy because of failure to respond or for a complication—hemorrhage, colonic perforation, or toxic megacolon. The mortality rate in fulminant colitis is still about 20 percent.

The relapsing-remitting form is much more common and is seen in over two-thirds of all patients with chronic ulcerative colitis. The course is variable and characterized by almost unpredictable exacerbations and remissions. Recurrences are often associated with emotional stress, physical fatigue, respiratory infections and other acute illnesses, dietary indiscretions, use of antibiotics and cathartics, and, in women, menses and pregnancy. Bloody diarrhea is the predominant symptom. The onset is acute in some, but more commonly the diarrhea has gradually become worse for a considerable period, recurring periodically, with essentially normal bowel habits during remissions. Lower abdominal cramping is nearly always present in the earlier phases, but when the bowel becomes scarred, thickened, and shortened, cramping is less marked. Cramping is followed shortly by urgency and tenesmus, and the painful passage of a small watery stool consisting of an admixture of stool, mucus, blood, and pus. In later stages, cramping may not be present to warn of impending defecation, which then occurs unexpectedly, accounting for some of the anxiety and insecurity that colitis patients often exhibit. Anorexia is marked during relapses. This, combined with the considerable continuing caloric loss by diarrhea, causes rapid and appreciable weight loss and malnutrition.

COMPLICATIONS. Complications of chronic ulcerative colitis are numerous and varied, and are frequently of sufficient gravity of themselves to require definitive surgical therapy of the primary colonic disease. Systemic complications include electrolyte deficiencies, microcytic anemia, hypoproteinemia, avitaminoses, amyloidosis, osteoporosis, amenorrhea, retarded sexual development, and retarded growth. Serious complications in other organs or systems include arthritis, ankylosing spondylitis, and sacroileitis; conjunctivitis, iritis, and episcleritis; gallstones, fatty liver, hepatitis, pericholangitis, cirrhosis, and carcinoma of the bile ducts; erythema nodosum, pyoderma gangrenosum, aphthous stomatitis, and clubbing of the fingers; pyelonephritis and urolithiasis; interstitial pancreatitis; peripheral neuropathy and vascular thromboses. Colonic complications include gross hemorrhage; stricture formation with partial obstruction; perforation, either free, producing peritonitis, or confined, with abscess or fistula formation; perianal and perirectal abscesses and fistulas; malabsorption; carcinoma of the colon; and toxic megacolon.

Toxic Megacolon. Toxic megacolon is a dreaded complication of ulcerative colitis that fortunately occurs in only 2 to 5 percent of patients with the disease. It is a manifestation of fulminant colitis and usually occurs with the initial acute episode, less frequently during a relapse of the remitting type, rarely in the chronic, continuous form of ulcerative colitis.

The cause of toxic dilatation is not known. The loss of tone, contractility, and propulsive motility have been attributed by some to necrotizing inflammation of the smooth muscle of the bowel and by others to damage of the myenteric plexus. Barium enema during a period of severe diarrhea is almost surely a precipitating factor. Other factors that may play a role include hypokalemia, hypomagnesemia, hypoproteinemia, opiates, and anticholinergics. Corticosteroids apparently do not play an etiologic role but may mask symptoms, particularly those of perforation of the megacolon.

The diagnosis should be immediately suspected in any patient with active colitis who has a sharp decrease in the number of daily stools without a corresponding amelioration in general status. Bloody rectal discharges may continue but with little gas or feces. The patient is obviously severely toxic, febrile, apathetic, and obtunded. Abdominal distension is progressive, and bowel sounds are hypoactive or absent. Plain abdominal roentgenograms show marked gaseous distension, particularly of the transverse colon.

Since toxic megacolon is a reversible process, a trial of intensive nonoperative therapy is indicated, with the patient watched very closely for actual or impending perforation. Therapy consists of intestinal decompression, antibiotics, correction of electrolyte deficits, discontinuance of opiates and anticholinergics, blood and albumin transfusions, and intravenous alimentation. If the patient has been receiving steroids, these are continued; if not, it is not clear whether initiation of steroid therapy is helpful or harmful.

Efficacy of therapy is measured by frequent plain films of the abdomen to evaluate the diameter of the dilated colon and watch for free air or intraabdominal collections, resumption of bowel function, fever, leukocytosis, and frequent physical examination of the abdomen. If the patient improves or at least the rapid downhill course is arrested, then medical therapy is continued. Operative intervention is indicated for perforation, deterioration in clinical status, or failure to improve after several days of intensive therapy. Most surgeons have preferred total or subtotal colectomy and ileostomy. The mortality rate has been at least 20 percent and much higher in some series, but recent studies indicate that much lower mortality rates are attainable if the patients are operated upon early in the course before colonic perforation and progressive metabolic deterioration have occurred. Turnbull and associates prefer the operation of ileostomy-colostomy, particularly if sealed-off perforations are suspected at laparotomy. They have reported a series of 42 patients so treated with only one death. If the patient with toxic megacolon has been treated medically or by Turnbull's procedure, definitive total colectomy–permanent ileostomy should be carried out electively as soon as the patient's condition warrants.

Carcinoma of the Colon. Carcinoma of the colon is a late complication of chronic ulcerative colitis, particularly of the smoldering, chronic, continuous form of the disease. Reported frequency of cancer in ulcerative colitis ranges from 0.7 to 17 percent but is usually about 3 percent. The most reliable current estimate would indicate that cancer in patients with chronic ulcerative colitis is about ten times as common as in the general population.

Factors affecting the frequency of cancer in colitis include extent of colonic involvement, duration of disease, and age at onset. In patients with total colitis cancer develops much more frequently than in those with left-sided colitis or ulcerative proctitis. Duration of the disease is also important, since most studies indicate that the risk of cancer is very low in the first 10 years of colitis but then rises to a risk of about 4 percent per year. Age at onset of colitis is the third factor; the incidence of cancer in colitis beginning before the age of twenty-five years is twice as great as in those with symptoms beginning after age twenty-five. The average age at the time of diagnosis of cancer in patients with ulcerative colitis is about thirty-seven years; in patients with idiopathic colon cancer, sixty-five years.

Carcinomas arising in ulcerative colitis are distributed more evenly throughout the colon as compared with the usual high incidence in the sigmoid and rectum. The growths are often multiple and commonly flat and infiltrating, and there is a high incidence of poorly differentiated and mucus-secreting types. These carry a poor prognosis. Neoplasia occurs in abnormal regenerated mucosa—the malignant potential of pseudopolyps is universally regarded as almost nil.

The most frequent symptoms of neoplasm simulate those of an exacerbation of ulcerative colitis—diarrhea, abdominal pain, rectal bleeding, and weight loss. Symptoms different from colitis—abdominal pain unrelated to defecation, and constipation—are unfortunately usually associated with far advanced cancer.

The prognosis for cancer arising in ulcerative colitis is much worse than for idiopathic colon cancer, probably because of the more frequent occurrence of more malignant histologic varieties and because of difficulty in diagnosis. The overall 5-year survival in idiopathic cancer is about 40 percent; for colitic cancer, it is less than 20 percent.

Diagnosis continues to be difficult and uncertain before the carcinoma is quite extensive. Morson proposed that certain premalignant histologic changes in rectal biopsies herald the development of carcinoma elsewhere in the ulcerative colitis colon—but this has not yet proved to be reliable. Nor is the carcinoembryonic antigen test reliable; the test is sometimes positive in patients with ulcerative colitis alone without carcinoma and sometimes negative in patients with early carcinomas. Fibercolonoscopy is emerging as an accurate diagnostic modality and will probably become the preferred method. Visual identification of carcinoma in a universally diseased mucosa is difficult, but most lesions can be detected by biopsy permitting histologic verification. Barium enema roentgenography is still the standard diagnostic tool but is considerably less accurate in diagnosing carcinoma in the presence of ulcerative colitis than in the otherwise normal colon.

The specter of carcinoma must influence the management of patients with chronic ulcerative colitis of many years' duration. The diagnosis of cancer in the ulcerative colitis colon is difficult, and the required studies are not without hazard. At present, any patient who has had active universal colitis for 10 years should be strongly urged to have a total colectomy–permanent ileostomy.

DIAGNOSIS. The diagnosis of nonspecific ulcerative colitis is one of exclusion of the specific causes of diarrhea and ulcerative colitis. Diseases to be evaluated by appropriate bacteriologic, serologic, chemical, radiologic, and sigmoidoscopic techniques include amebiasis, bacillary dysentery, intestinal tuberculosis, diverticulitis, lymphogranuloma venereum, carcinoma coli, malignant carcinoid syndrome, celiac disease, nontropical sprue, malabsorption syndrome, and ischemic colitis.

Sigmoidoscopy and colonoscopy, including biopsy, are the most reliable procedures for establishing the diagnosis of nonspecific ulcerative colitis. The endoscopic appearance of the rectal mucosa, while characteristic, is not pathognomonic for nonspecific ulcerative colitis. For this reason, bacteriologic and histologic examination of biopsy material is essential. Hyperemia, edema, and small, scattered, pinpoint ulcerations are seen in the early stages. The mucosa is friable and bleeds easily when touched. Later, the pinpoint ulcerations enlarge and coalesce to form larger ulcers which are usually covered with bloody pus. After several exacerbations and healing, the mucosa develops a finely granular appearance. Healing is also evidenced by submucosal scarring with small, irregular pearly plaques visible through the mucosa. With advanced disease, gross areas of ulceration are surrounded by irregular pseudopolypoid islands of abnormal mucosa. Additional findings include stricture formation, carcinoma, perianal abscesses and fistulas, and stenosis and fissures, and thrombosed hemorrhoids.

Barium enema is also helpful but should be given with caution, if at all, during acute exacerbations of the disease. Extensive preparation is unnecessary; a single low-pressure saline enema usually suffices; oral laxatives should not be given. Early in the disease, barium enema examination may be within normal limits, or irritability may be noted. With established disease there is some loss of haustration; fine ulcerations and alterations of the reticular mucosal pattern are seen on the postevacuation films. When the ulcers become larger and more numerous, the colon appears characteristically stippled and serrated. With moderately advanced disease, pseudopolyposis shows as multiple lucencies in the barium column—the "cobblestone" picture. In far advanced disease the lumen is narrowed, the bowel is rigid and shortened, haustra are absent, and the mucosal pattern is completely disorganized—the hose-like colon (Fig. 28-1).

TREATMENT. The primary treatment of nonspecific ulcerative colitis is medical. Since the specific cause of the disease is not known, there is no specific treatment. The components of therapy are antidiarrheal agents, antimicrobials, corticosteroids, diet, vitamin and mineral supplements, and general support.

Antidiarrheal agents are of some value in most patients but should be used with caution, since they may be implicated in the genesis of toxic megacolon. Most frequently used are diphenoxylate hydrochloride with atropine (Lomotil), codeine, paregoric, and calcium carbonate powders. Kaolin and pectin are of little value.

Salicylazosulfapyridine (Azulfidine), an oral nonabsorbable sulfonamide, is the antimicrobial of choice and should be tried in all patients on nonoperative therapy. It is not clear whether the benefit is derived from the antimicrobial action of the sulfa portion or the anti-inflammatory action of the salicylic acid component. Antibiotics are of no value in uncomplicated ulcerative colitis and should be used only for purulent complications such as abscesses or impending perforation.

Corticosteroid therapy of ulcerative colitis is controversial. There is no doubt that many patients are significantly benefited. This has been shown by serial rectal biopsies to be truly organic and not merely due to the sense of well-being, increased appetite, and reduction of fever which occur as a by-product of steroid therapy. On the other hand, some patients are not helped; morbidity is significantly higher in patients who subsequently require operative therapy; symptoms of perforation and peritonitis may be masked; and Cushing's syndrome is produced by prolonged therapy. In seriously ill patients, steroid therapy should be initiated with intravenous ACTH, 40 I.U. every 12 hours, or continuous intravenous prednisolone, 100 mg/day. If remission is achieved, oral prednisolone can be used after a few days. If there is no significant improvement in 7 to 10 days, colectomy must be seriously considered, since it is unlikely that nonoperative therapy will be successful.

Maintenance steroid therapy is with oral prednisone, starting at 60 mg daily in divided doses and tapering as rapidly as possible to 15 mg or less. The principal role of maintenance therapy is the control of symptoms; maintenance steroids do not abort exacerbations. Therefore every effort should be made to wean the patient completely. If a daily maintenance level of more than 15 mg prednisone is required to control symptoms for any length of time, then operative therapy should be advised. Retention enemas containing water-soluble corticosteroids are often beneficial in patients with disease limited to the rectum or left colon.

Rigid dietary restrictions have not been shown to be worthwhile. Every effort should be made to offer these patients a balanced diet of foods that appeal to them—served expeditiously and not allowed to stand on a cart until both hot foods and cold foods have reached room temperature. A milk-free diet should be tried, to observe possible benefit.

Vitamins A, C, and D and calcium are usually necessary. With very active disease and inadequate alimentation parenteral B complex should be given daily. Supplemental iron is given for iron-deficiency anemia. Potassium supplements are used during steroid therapy.

Supportive therapy consists of physical and emotional rest. Formal psychiatric therapy is rarely indicated and is sometimes harmful. The indicated psychotherapy should be given by a trusted sympathetic physician with a sincere interest in all the patient's problems.

Immunosuppressive therapy, based on the hypothesis that ulcerative colitis is an autoimmune disease, has had very limited success. Further trials, under rigidly controlled conditions, are indicated, but immunosuppressive therapy certainly cannot be recommended for general use at this time. These drugs may interfere with normal immunologic homeostasis, enhance oncogenic viruses, and repress im-

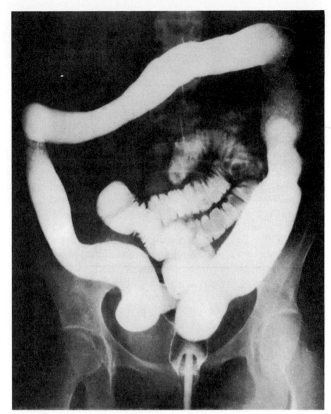

Fig. 28-1. Barium radiograph of chronic idiopathic ulcerative colitis. Note shortening of colon, absence of haustrations, destruction of mucosal pattern. Ileum is not affected.

munologic mechanisms for the surveillance and rejection of malignant cells. Thus there may be an added neoplastic risk in patients with ulcerative colitis who are already more vulnerable to colonic carcinoma.

Operative Therapy. Seventy-five to eighty percent of patients with idiopathic ulcerative colitis are more or less satisfactorily managed medically. Surgical therapy cures the disease, but because proper surgical therapy necessitates a permanent ileostomy, physicians and patients are understandably reluctant to agree to definitive surgical therapy until absolutely necessary.

Indications for emergency surgical intervention include uncontrollable hemorrhage, complete intestinal obstruction, free perforation with peritonitis, and toxic megacolon. Elective indications include partial intestinal obstruction; confined perforation with abscess formation; failure of medical management to control the disease; carcinoma; developmental retardation, either somatic or sexual; and serious systemic or distant complications that do not respond to nonoperative measures. An indication for prophylactic operation is long-continued colitis, which carries a high risk of colonic cancer.

Preparation for operation, as time permits, is intensive and consists of blood and albumin transfusions to restore blood volume, hematocrit, and plasma proteins to normality; correction of electrolyte abnormalities; correction of avitaminoses; and preoperative broad-spectrum antibiotics. If the patient has received corticosteroids within the past year, a slow intravenous drip of 100 mg of hydrocortisone is given the night before operation and a similar infusion started in the morning prior to, and continued through, the operation. Steroids are gradually tapered off over several days postoperatively. An important part of preoperative preparation is a frank discussion with the patient and his family as to exactly what the procedure entails.

The definitive procedure of choice is total proctocolectomy and ileostomy. This is preferably done in one stage, though some surgeons prefer a subtotal colectomy at the first stage with removal of the rectal stump at a later date. Permanent urinary dysfunction and impotence are uncommon after proctectomy for ulcerative colitis, as compared to abdominoperineal resection for rectal cancer, because the dissection is kept close to the rectal wall.

Ileostomy was formerly made by simply exteriorizing the terminal several centimeters of the divided ileum. This was often followed by a stormy several months of ileostomy dysfunction while the ileostomy "matured." It is now known that the problems with the old form of ileostomy were caused by a local peritonitis on the short segment of exteriorized ileostomy. This trouble can be avoided by fashioning an immediately "matured" ileostomy. The mucosa of the exteriorized segment is turned back over the remainder, either with or without excision of a distal ring of the seromuscular layers, and sutured circumferentially to the skin (Fig. 28-2). The ileum should be brought out through a separate elliptical incision, not the operative

Fig. 28-2. Creation and maturation of ileostomy. *A.* Excision of distal ring of seromuscular layers. (1) Seromuscular layer dissected off distal ileum. (2) Remaining muscularis and mucosa turned back. (3) Sutures placed between mucosa and skin. *B.* Maturation without excision of seromuscular layers. (1) Inner layers everted. (2) Mucosa sutured directly to skin.

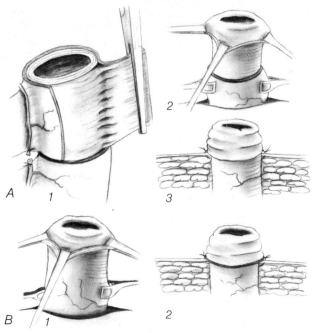

incision, so placed that the 10-cm disc of the ileostomy appliance will not encroach on the umbilicus or anterior superior iliac spine. The individually fitted ileostomy bag should be applied early in the postoperative period to avoid digestion and excoriation of the skin.

Kock has devised a "continent" ileostomy which, when successful, permits the patient to dispense with external appliances. An internal reservoir to hold 100 ml or more is made from a doubled loop of ileum just proximal to the cutaneous ileostomy. The ileostomy is made continent by intussuscepting a 5-cm segment of the distal limb back into the pouch. The internal pouch is emptied two or three times a day with a catheter and is continent not only of liquid but of gas as well. Revision procedures are necessary in about one-third of cases, but the procedure ultimately functions satisfactorily in about 80 percent of patients. Causes of failure are recurrence of inflammatory bowel disease, ileal stomatitis, and incontinence of the stoma.

Subtotal colectomy with ileoproctostomy has been championed by Aylett, but most surgeons are less enthusiastic about it. The procedure may be tried in patients who have refused operation because of the ileostomy if the rectal segment is not severely diseased or strictured, the sphincter function is not deficient, and there is no perianal infection. One-half to two-thirds of patients have acceptable results; the remainder have to be converted to total colectomy-ileostomy because of continuing severe ulcerative proctitis or because of cancer in the rectal stump.

The mortality rate for emergency operations for ulcerative colitis, including the fulminant type, is 15 to 20 percent; for elective operations, 3 to 5 percent. Morbidity is appreciable and is significantly higher in steroid-treated patients. Complications include severe wound infection, intraabdominal abscess, septicemia, wound dehiscence, retraction of mucous fistulas, severe electrolyte imbalance, hemorrhage, and postoperative psychosis.

The long-term outlook for patients with ulcerative colitis treated by proctocolectomy-ileostomy is quite favorable. Some 10 to 15 percent of these patients will require revision of their ileostomy, usually within the first year, and most of them have to watch their diets to avoid diarrhea of the ileostomy. But over the long term, fully 95 percent are in excellent or good health.

Crohn's Colitis

The disease that Crohn described in 1932 as "terminal ileitis" may also involve the colon either alone or in association with small bowel disease. Terminology has been confused, but there are now hopeful signs that consensus is close. Terms which have been used include granulomatous colitis, segmental colitis, Crohn's disease of the colon, regional colitis, cicatrizing colitis, regional enteritis of the colon, right-sided regional colitis, regional migratory ulcerative colitis, and transmural colitis. The preferred terminology for disease limited to the colon is Crohn's colitis; for disease of both small and large bowel, Crohn's enterocolitis.

INCIDENCE. Available information suggests that perhaps one-third of cases of primary ulcerative disease of the colon are Crohn's colitis; the remainder are idiopathic ulcerative colitis except for a small percentage that cannot be clearly classified. A recent report of colitis patients who had been operated upon revealed that 58 percent had Crohn's colitis and 32 percent, idiopathic ulcerative colitis; 10 percent could not be classified. This probably means that a larger percentage of patients with Crohn's colitis require surgical therapy and does not reflect the true incidence of the disease.

Most of the discussion of the etiology and pathogenesis of regional enteritis in Chap. 27 is applicable to Crohn's colitis and will not be repeated.

PATHOLOGY. The distribution of the disease is somewhat different in the two forms of primary ulcerative colitis. Total involvement of the colon is seen in both but is more frequent with idiopathic ulcerative colitis. With partial involvement, Crohn's colitis more often involves the right colon, while idiopathic ulcerative colitis generally affects the left colon and rectum. Rectal involvement is found in about 95 percent of patients with ulcerative colitis and in about 50 percent with Crohn's colitis. Ulcerative colitis involves the colon in continuity, whereas skip areas are common in Crohn's disease. The small bowel is involved, often extensively, in about one-half of patients with Crohn's colitis, i.e., enterocolitis, whereas "backwash ileitis" occurs in perhaps 10 percent of patients with idiopathic ulcerative colitis (Table 28-1).

The gross appearance of the colon is usually pathognomonic of Crohn's disease. The serosal surface is dull, thickened, hyperemic and granular, and fat partially envelops the bowel wall. Tiny, gray-white nodules may be visible in the subserosa. Shortening of the colon is minimal. The wall is thickened and rubbery hard—the fibrotic thickening of the wall producing stenosis of the lumen. The appearance of the mucosal surface of the opened specimen is also pathognomonic. In some areas, the mucosa, which appears knobby and swollen from lymphedema, remains intact. In other areas there are deep, serpiginous or undermined longitudinal furrow ulcerations with a characteristic shape—the "bear-claw" ulcer. Microscopically the two distinguishing features of Crohn's colitis are transmural inflammation and fibrous thickening of the bowel wall. This is due initially to submucous edema but later to extensive fibrosis. The inflammatory exudate consists of lymphocytes, often with prominent follicle formation; plasma cells; and sarcoidlike granulomas. Fully formed granulomas consist of collections of epithelioid cells, multinucleated giant cells predominantly of the Langhans type, but without any caseation. These granulomas are an important diagnostic feature when present but are not found in 20 to 25 percent of cases that otherwise fit the classification of Crohn's colitis.

CLINICAL MANIFESTATIONS. Symptomatically, the two types of colitis are similar—patients present with chronic diarrhea associated with abdominal cramps, fever, and weight loss. Grossly bloody stools which are the hallmark of idiopathic ulcerative colitis, however, are rarely seen in Crohn's colitis. The correct diagnosis may also be suspected at sigmoidoscopy—if the mucosa is essentially normal or just edematous but without bleeding, then the

presumptive diagnosis of Crohn's colitis is made, since this tends to spare the rectum.

The relative incidence of some complications also is quite different. Fistulas between the diseased colon and other segments of bowel, bladder, vagina, and skin as well as perianal fistulas are common in Crohn's colitis—more than 40 percent have perianal fistulas versus less than 10 percent in mucosal colitis. Fistulization except in the perianal area is rare in chronic ulcerative colitis. Carcinomas and toxic megacolon are seen much more often in ulcerative colitis. Gross hemorrhage is rarely a problem in Crohn's colitis, in contrast to ulcerative colitis.

The radiographic features usually serve to distinguish the two forms of ulcerative colitis (Figs. 28-1 and 28-3). In Crohn's colitis, shortening is not conspicuous, and there is often segmental involvement with intervening normal segments. Haustration is only partially obliterated; the wall is rigid and the lumen is stenotic. Fistulas are common. Intramural fissures or tracts appear as tiny radiating spikes extending from the lumen. The normal mucosal pattern is lost, replaced in some areas by gross ulcerations but in others by a coarse cobblestoning that can usually be distinguished from the irregular pseudopolyposis of ulcerative colitis.

Fig. 28-3. Barium radiograph of Crohn's enterocolitis with involvement of terminal ileum, cecum, ascending and transverse colon; left colon is normal. Colon is a little shortened, and haustra are present but abnormal. Mucosal pattern is altered but not destroyed.

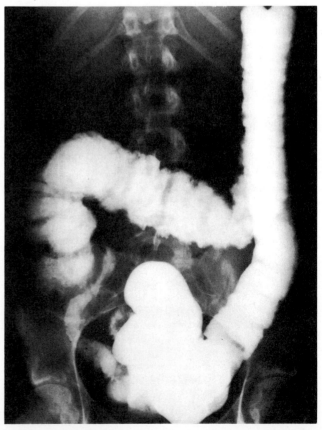

TREATMENT. Nonoperative therapy of Crohn's colitis is essentially the same as for idiopathic ulcerative colitis. The therapy, particularly corticosteroids, seems to be less effective in controlling Crohn's colitis or enterocolitis, with the result that a higher proportion require operative therapy. Azathioprine is also being tried for Crohn's colitis. Its use in this disease is certainly more justified than in ulcerative colitis. A curative operation is not available as it is in ulcerative colitis, and there is much less hazard of carcinoma. The principal use of azathioprine in Crohn's disease may well be in the postoperative patient to prevent recurrences.

In contrast to ulcerative colitis where ileostomy–total colectomy is clearly the procedure of choice, there is little unanimity of opinion as to the proper role of the various procedures that are available for the surgical therapy of the various problems encountered in Crohn's colitis.

Emergency operation is necessary much less frequently in Crohn's colitis than in ulcerative colitis; massive hemorrhage is rare, and toxic megacolon and free perforation are distinctly uncommon. The indications for elective operative therapy are also somewhat different for colonic disease than for Crohn's disease of the small intestine. Obstruction, abdominal abscess, or fistula formation are uncommon indications. The indication for most patients is chronic disabling symptoms that cannot be controlled by conservative means. Symptoms include chronic blood loss, hypoalbuminemia, chronic cramping abdominal pain and diarrhea, weight loss, and general ill health. Uncontrollable perianal disease is also a frequent indication.

With total involvement of the colon including the rectum most surgeons do a total proctocolectomy and permanent ileostomy. Reported recurrence rates vary from 3 to more than 50 percent. The reason for this wide variation is not apparent. The recurrence is nearly always just proximal to the stoma, and many but not all patients will require resection of the juxtastomal ileum and a new ileostomy. Oberhelman and Kohatsu, and others, have proposed the use of a diverting ileostomy without resection. The terminal ileum is transected and both ends brought out, the proximal as a functioning ileostomy and the distal as a defunctionalized mucous fistula. In many patients so treated the colonic disease becomes quiescent. A few patients have had intestinal continuity restored at a later time without exacerbation of the colonic disease; others have had flare-ups after restoration and have then required colectomy. Diverting ileostomy is also a useful first-stage procedure in patients whose conditions are so precarious as to preclude one-stage total colectomy. When general health has improved after diversion, colectomy can be done electively under more favorable circumstances.

When the colon is extensively diseased but without rectal involvement, total proctocolectomy and ileostomy are still preferred by most, but some would do total abdominal colectomy and leave the rectum. Ileoproctostomy can be done primarily or an ileostomy with oversewing the rectal stump, with expectation of restoring continuity at a later time. The recurrence rate after ileoproctostomy for Crohn's disease is about 50 percent.

Segmental colonic involvement would appear to invite segmental resection with primary anastomosis. Unfortunately, the extent of disease found at operation is often greater than appeared on barium enema. If disease is limited to the right colon, or right colon and terminal ileum, primary resection and ileo-transverse colostomy are preferred. If disease involves the left colon, proctocolectomy with ileostomy is advisable, since the results of left hemicolectomy have been poor.

The long-term outlook after definitive surgery in Crohn's colitis is less favorable than in ulcerative colitis. Recurrence of disease is a continuing problem and requires further surgery in about one-third of patients. Despite this, about 70 percent are sufficiently rehabilitated so that their health can be classified as excellent or good.

Ischemic Colitis

Although infarcts of the colon have been described from time to time, usually as single-case reports, only in the past decade has ischemic colitis emerged as a clearly defined clinicopathologic entity. Ischemic colitis is not primarily an inflammatory disease but is included in this section because of its importance in the differential diagnosis of inflammatory bowel disease as well as diverticular disease.

Ischemic colitis presents as three quite different clinical syndromes depending upon (1) the extent of the vascular occlusion, (2) the duration of the occlusion, (3) the efficiency of the collateral circulation, and (4) the extent of secondary bacterial invasion. With transitory impairment of arterial supply which is soon compensated by collateral flow there is a partial mucosal slough that is healed by mucosal regeneration within 2 or 3 days—reversible or *transient ischemic colitis* (Table 28-2). Gross impairment of arterial supply results in hemorrhagic infarction of the mucosa, which ulcerates, allowing invasion of bowel bacteria. Healing is by fibrosis, which often produces stenosis —*stricturing ischemic colitis.* With complete loss of arterial flow, there is full-thickness infarction, gangrene, and, if untreated, perforation with peritonitis and death—*gangrenous ischemic colitis.*

Early reports stressed that the splenic flexure is the most vulnerable segment, presumably because this is the area at the periphery of both superior and inferior mesenteric artery supply and because in this area the marginal artery of Drummond is at its greatest distance from the bowel wall. It is now clear, however, that ischemic colitis can affect any segment from the cecum to the rectosigmoid. Major vascular occlusion does not correlate with ischemic colitis; many patients, particularly those with abdominal aneurysms, have occlusion of the inferior mesenteric artery without bowel symptoms. Conversely, some patients with frank ischemic colitis have demonstrably patent major mesenteric arteries. Experimentally, ligation of the inferior mesenteric artery in the dog has no deleterious effect on the colon; it is only when the small vessels between the mesenteric arcade and the bowel are ligated that colonic ischemia is produced.

Most patients with ischemic colitis are in the older age group; it is rarely seen under age forty-five. The majority also have associated medical problems such as cardio-

Table 28-2. ISCHEMIC COLON DISEASE

	Form 1	*Form 2*	*Form 3*
Synonyms	Nonspecific colitis; ulcerative colitis of aged; reversible ischemia of colon	Ischemic stricture	Colonic infarction; necrotizing colitis; gangrene of colon; irreversible ischemia
Symptoms	Cramping abdominal pain; bloody diarrhea	Cramping abdominal pain; abdominal distension; decreased bowel movements	Diffuse abdominal pain; obtundation; bloody diarrhea
Signs	Localized tenderness; hyperactive intestinal sounds; mild pyrexia; leukocytosis	Abdominal distension, hyperactive intestinal sounds; normal temperature; normal white blood count	Diffuse direct and rebound tenderness; rigid abdomen; hypoactive or absent intestinal sounds; abdominal distension; pyrexia, leukocytosis, taciycardia, hypotension
Barium enema	Mucosal irregularity; thumbprinting; local narrowing	Stricture; intestinal obstruction	Mucosal irregularity; dilatation of colon; thickening of intestinal wall; perforation
Treatment	Medical	Resection of involved intestine	Correction of predisposing factors; immediate operation
Results	Resolution	Correction of symptoms	High mortality rate due to associated diseases or complications of colonic gangrene

SOURCE: From O'Connell, Kadell, and Tompkins, 1976.

vascular disease, rheumatoid arthritis, or diabetes. The onset of ischemic colitis is characteristically acute with mild to moderate generalized or lower abdominal cramping pain followed by passage of blood per rectum. Vomiting is uncommon. Further symptoms depend on which of the three types of ischemic colitis is developing. With the gangrenous type, the abdominal pain becomes more severe until it is constant. Systemic symptoms of an abdominal catastrophe ensue. On physical examination, abdominal tenderness is usually generalized but is often most marked over the ischemic segment. Voluntary guarding and involuntary spasm are present but are not marked. Bowel sounds, which are hyperactive early, gradually cease. Later, with progression of infarction to gangrene, necrosis, and perforation, the findings are those of spreading bacterial peritonitis and septic shock. Diagnosis can usually be made from the clinical picture alone. Sigmoidoscopy reveals only a normal distal segment with blood coming from above unless the rectosigmoid is the segment involved, in which case a blue-black, sloughing mucosa oozing blood is seen.

Barium enema is contraindicated in gangrenous colitis, and arteriography is unnecessary and delays proper treatment. Plain abdominal roentgenograms are often confirmatory and reveal adynamic ileus with the gaseous distension stopping at the involved segment. Occasionally small bubbles of gas may be detected in the wall of the infarcted bowel. Treatment is emergency operation as soon as the patient's condition is stabilized by vigorous preparatory therapy. Under favorable circumstances, the involved segment is resected and primary anastomosis performed.

More frequently, however, this disease in this age group dictates exteriorization of the involved segment.

With impairment but not complete loss of blood supply, the patient's symptoms do not progress, but neither do they disappear promptly. Mild to moderate abdominal pain continues, as does rectal bleeding, which, however, is usually not massive. There may also be symptoms and signs of partial intestinal obstruction. Barium enema radiography is diagnostic. Marginal "thumbprinting," or "pseudotumors," due to submucosal hemorrhage and pericolic fat inflammation is seen. Spasm and ulceration also may be present. Conservative therapy is indicated at this point since the process may be self-limited and reversible. Anticoagulants should not be used. After several days the barium enema findings revert toward normality, but repeat barium enema in a few weeks often reveals stricture formation at the ischemic site. The strictured colon should be electively resected with primary anastomosis.

In the transient or reversible form of ischemic colitis, symptoms are mild and last only 2 to 4 days. Barium enema, if done promptly, usually reveals thumbprinting or superficial ulceration but promptly reverts to normal. Follow-up barium enema is also within normal limits. No specific therapy is necessary.

Radiation Enterocolitis

That roentgen rays have deleterious effects on the intestine has been known since 1897, 2 years after their discovery, when Walsh described a self-limited instance of diarrhea and cramps which was resolved by placing a metal shield between the observer and the source of radiation. Radiation enterocolitis has become a major problem in recent years because of the higher radiation doses employed in the therapy of uterine, bladder, and prostatic malignancies and, perhaps, because the newer external radiation sources deliver large visceral doses with little or no skin reaction to alert the therapist.

The incidence of radiation injury to the bowel is very roughly dose-dependent. At tissue doses below 4,000 rads, significant bowel injury is quite uncommon. With 5,000 rads, essentially all patients will have some demonstrable damage; in 5 to 10 percent the damage will be significant and ongoing. Other factors that increase the likelihood of problems include asthenia, advanced age, hypertension, arteriosclerotic vascular disease, diabetes, and previous abdominal surgery with resulting adhesions that fix the bowel.

The rapidly proliferating intestinal epithelium is most sensitive to ionizing radiation and shows changes early in the course. There are mucosal hyperemia and edema, an extensive inflammatory cell infiltrate, and crypt abscesses. With higher doses there are areas of ulceration because of failure of epithelial regeneration. After cessation of therapy, reepithelization is the rule but with a thin mucosa with shortened villi. Of more serious import is the long-term effect of radiation on blood vessels. Beginning several weeks after radiation exposure and continuing for years is a progressive vasculitis, affecting principally the small arterioles in the submucosa with marked thickening of the vessel wall and leading to luminal occlusion and thrombosis. Large foam cells seen beneath the intima are said to be pathognomonic of radiation vasculitis. The progressive ischemia is accompanied by progressive thickening and fibrosis, principally of the submucosa. As ischemia progresses, ulceration supervenes. This in turn leads to abscess and fistula formation, also on an ischemic basis.

At least 75 percent of patients undergoing radiotherapy with exposure of the gastrointestinal tract will have nausea and vomiting, and often diarrhea with cramping. With high doses of radiation there may also be rectal bleeding and tenesmus. Most patients can be managed symptomatically, but in some the reaction is so severe that the therapy has to be stopped for a time or prolonged. These acute symptoms subside fairly promptly after completion of therapy.

Late symptoms of radiation damage to the intestines appear from several months to many years after exposure. The clinical presentation is determined by the segment of bowel involved as well as by the type of lesion: atrophic mucosa, ulcer, stricture, abscess, fistula, or perforation. The rectum is by far the most common site of involvement because of its proximity to the cervix and its fixed position. Rectal ulcers are most commonly seen on the anterior wall at 4 to 6 cm above the dentate line and cause the passage of bloody mucus and tenesmus. Symptomatic rectal strictures are usually found at the 8- to 12-cm level and produce the picture of partial colonic obstruction. A particularly distressing complication is a postradiation fistula from rectum into bladder or vagina producing feculent vaginal discharge or pneumaturia. With small intestine involvement, symptoms of malabsorption may be prominent. Extensive fibrosis also produces the bacterial stasis syndrome and intestinal obstruction.

Diagnosis may be difficult because of the difficulty in distinguishing between radiation changes and recurrent tumor. Barium contrast radiographic studies usually demonstrate rather characteristic changes, but these are not specific. Similarly, angiography also usually demonstrates changes that are characteristic of, but not specific for, radiation damage. Endoscopy with biopsy yields a specific diagnosis in some cases but not in all. If a positive histologic diagnosis is not possible prior to treatment, the patient should be given the benefit of the doubt and not denied maximal therapy because his lesion may be recurrent cancer.

Management of radiation injuries is difficult and often unsatisfactory. Conservative measures should be used as long as they are effective. Ischemic fibrotic tissues make for poor wound healing, anastomotic disruption, infection, and occult perforation. Morgenstern and associates have well summarized several caveats for the surgeon: (1) Avoid entry into the abdomen for radiation injury unless absolutely forced to operate. (2) Avoid extensive resections and multiple anastomoses. Short isolated segments are best resected, but long segments are most safely treated by side-to-side bypass. (3) Avoid extensive adhesiolysis. Lysis of adhesions in damaged intestine produces minute openings into the intestine which lead to postoperative perforation or fistulas. (4) Use frozen-section control of the intestinal ends to be anastomosed to rule out unsuspected radiation changes. (5) Protect anastomoses. Colon anastomoses should be protected with a proximal colostomy; small bowel anastomoses, with a long tube.

The outlook in radiation enterocolitis is grim. Many patients are spared this travail because they die of their primary diseases before radiation damage supervenes. But many more will die as a result of the treatment that cured their cancer. DeCosse and associates followed 94 patients with radiation enterocolitis. Of these, 27 were living, 28 died from cancer, 13 died from other causes, and 22 died from complications of radiation enterocolitis.

Pseudomembranous Enterocolitis

Shortly after the introduction of antibiotics, there were several reports of a presumably new syndrome that had occurred postoperatively in patients receiving antibiotics. These patients developed severe diarrhea, abdominal pain and distension, circulatory collapse, and death. Necropsy revealed severe enteritis with extensive pseudomembrane formation under which pure cultures of *Staphylococcus aureus* could usually be isolated. It was reasoned that the antibiotics had altered the normal flora of the bowel and allowed overgrowth of resistant pathogenic staphylococci. Doubt was soon cast on this hypothesis by finding that the syndrome had first been reported in 1893, noting that the syndrome sometimes occurred in patients who had not been operated upon and had not received antibiotics, finding patients with the syndrome whose stool culture did not grow staphylococci. Mucosal ischemia, rather than bacterial overgrowth, is currently the prime suspect in this condition.

PATHOLOGY. The intestine in pseudomembranous enterocolitis grossly resembles that found in uremia, bacillary dysentery, or heavy-metal poisoning. The entire gastrointestinal tract may be involved, or changes may be limited to one or more segments. In man the ileum is the most commonly affected part, followed by small and large bowel together, and by colon alone. The edematous bowel is usually distended with fluid and may contain as much as 5,000 ml. Serosa is hyperemic and edematous but otherwise not remarkable. The open bowel presents a shaggy yellow-green pseudomembrane, loosely adherent to the mucosa, and arranged in large patches or diffusely covering entire segments. The pseudomembrane consists of a fibrin mesh and mucus, containing inflammatory cells, and cellular debris of desquamated mucosal cells, leukocytes, erythrocytes, and bacteria. A severe inflammatory process affects principally mucosa and submucosa, occasionally extending into the muscularis. The inflammatory infiltrate consists chiefly of polymorphonuclear leukocytes, lymphocytes, and plasma cells. Necrosis of superficial mucosal cells is prominent. With deeper necrosis, mucosal ulcerations and fragmentation of villi are produced. Full-thickness necrosis with perforation of the bowel does not occur in pseudomembranous enterocolitis.

CLINICAL MANIFESTATIONS. Initial symptoms of pseudomembranous enterocolitis usually develop between the third and seventh postoperative days, and so may be masked by the general postoperative state. First noted are lethargy, weakness, and abdominal pain out of proportion to that usually due to the operative procedure. If diarrhea occurs, the diagnosis becomes obvious, but diarrhea is by no means a constant accompaniment of the enteritis. A valuable physical sign is abdominal distension despite audible peristalsis. The typical diarrheal stool is green and resembles rice water. The liquid stool contains suspended fragments, occasionally large sheets of pseudomembrane. If the disease pursues a severe course, then weakness, nausea, and mild abdominal distension are soon followed by vomiting, marked distension, copious diarrhea, tachycardia, fever to 40 or 41°C, disorientation, shock, and oliguria. The volume of stool passed in 24 hours may amount to 10,000 ml. Shock dominates the terminal phase, and death occurs in circulatory collapse. Less severe forms of the disease occur, but the incidence is not known, since the disease may not be recognized and mild forms may not be included in published reports. The incidence of circulatory collapse is low in the less severe forms.

TREATMENT. To be successful, therapy must be immediate and aggressive. The extensive water, electrolyte, and plasma deficits must be replaced rapidly, guided by monitoring vital signs and central venous pressure. All antibiotics that the patient has been receiving are immediately discontinued. Antibiotics specific for resistant staphylococci should be administered intravenously in large doses. Glucocorticosteroids in pharmacologic doses are given as in septic shock (Chap. 4).

The outcome is usually apparent within 24 or, at most, 48 hours. If the patient is going to respond to treatment, the response is rapid; if not, the continuing downhill course is also rapid.

CLINDAMYCIN-ASSOCIATED COLITIS

A condition related to but probably distinct from pseudo-membranous enterocolitis should be called *antibiotic-associated enterocolitis,* since it has been reported with aureomycin and other tetracyclines, streptomycin, chloramphenicol, ampicillin, and cephazolin as well as lincomycin and clindamycin. The reported incidence has been highest with the latter two agents; hence the name *clindamycin-associated colitis,* which is now in common usage.

In its mildest form, occurring in up to 20 percent of patients receiving lincomycin or clindamycin, there is bloodless, watery diarrhea without fever or leukocytosis. Proctoscopy reveals only some edema, hyperemia, and slight friability, but no ulceration or plaques. Bacteriological studies do not reveal single species overgrowth; the flora is qualitatively normal, though there is some quantitative reduction in anaerobes. The diarrhea subsides within a few days after administration of the antibiotic has been stopped, and only symptomatic treatment is indicated. The antibiotic need not be stopped if it is essential to the patient's care, but the patient's condition should be monitored by frequent proctoscopy to determine if progression to a more severe form of colitis is occurring which would require that the antibiotic be stopped.

In the severe forms, occurring in up to 10 percent of patients receiving lincomycin or clindamycin, there are severe diarrhea, abdominal cramping, high fever, and leukocytosis. Two different pictures are found on examination. In the more common one, proctoscopy reveals an erythematous friable mucosa studded with white-yellow plaques. The plaques when confluent form a pseudomembrane. Biopsy shows acute inflammation and microscopic ulceration covered by a layer of fibrin and mucus containing leukocytes and necrotic cells. Both in its symptoms and in the proctoscopic and barium enema radiographic findings, the less common form closely mimics an acute attack of idiopathic ulcerative colitis. In some patients the plain x-ray alone is adequate for diagnosis (Fig. 28-4). Bacteriologic studies of the colonic microflora in these severe forms have shown a striking decrease, both quantitatively and qualitatively, in the number of anaerobes present. The process is usually reversible, but recovery may be prolonged. The offending antibiotic must be stopped immediately and vigorous supportive therapy given. The role of corticosteroids is unclear; many feel they are beneficial but this is not based on solid evidence. A few patients have not responded to therapy: several have succumbed, and several more have required total colectomy-ileostomy.

Amebiasis

Amebiasis is an infection produced by the protozoan *E. histolytica,* involving the colon primarily and other organs secondarily, especially the liver. The infestation is an asymptomatic carrier state in most individuals with the incidence of carrier state ranging from about 10 percent

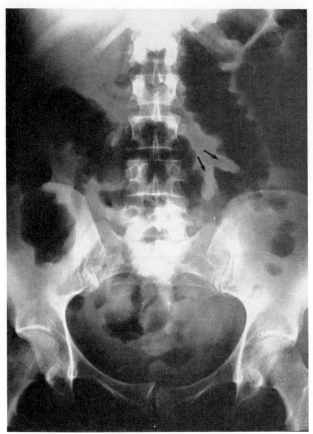

Fig. 28-4. Plain x-ray of the abdomen in a patient with fatal clindamycin colitis. Arrows point to "thumbprinting." Submucosal edema causes mucosal projections into the gas-filled lumen.

in the United States and Europe to over 60 percent in some undeveloped countries and some mental institutions.

ACUTE AMEBIC DYSENTERY

Acute amebic dysentery is unusual and is seen principally with massive contamination of the water supply. Onset is abrupt, with high fever, abdominal cramps, and profuse bloody diarrhea with tenesmus. Extensive ulceration of the rectum is usually seen at proctoscopy. Numerous trophozoites, containing ingested erythrocytes, can usually be found in warm saline preparations of fresh stool, exudate, or scrapings from the ulcers. Serological tests for *E. histolytica* antibodies should be used if the diagnosis is uncertain. It is imperative that amebic colitis be distinguished from idiopathic ulcerative colitis or Crohn's colitis, which it may closely resemble; because of systemic dissemination of the amebas, the usual corticosteroid therapy of these diseases can be lethal to the patient with amebic colitis. Administration of metronidazole, 750 mg three times daily for 10 days, is the preferred treatment. If the patient is unable to take oral medication, the conventional emetine-tetracycline-diiodohydroxyquin followed by chloroquin should be used.

Perforation of the colon is rare and is difficult to diagnose unless free intraperitoneal air is demonstrated, because acute amebic colitis is associated with diffuse abdominal tenderness often so severe that peritonitis is suspected. Exteriorization of the perforated segment is the preferred operation. Resection with primary anastomosis is dangerous because of the friability of the bowel.

CHRONIC AMEBIC DYSENTERY

Chronic amebic dysentery is the common form. Onset is gradual. There is usually intermittent diarrhea with two to four foul-smelling stools daily often containing blood and mucus, vague abdominal cramps, weight loss, and low-grade fever. Symptomatic periods may alternate with asymptomatic periods lasting for many weeks or months. Positive diagnosis may be difficult, since cysts or trophozoites are not always demonstrable in patients strongly suspected of having chronic amebiasis. The diagnostic yield is increased by looking for the organisms in rectal biopsies. Sigmoidoscopy is within normal limits in about 30 percent of cases, but organisms may be found in grossly normal mucosa. *E. histolytica* antibodies are detectable in the serum in over 90 percent of patients with active amebiasis. Asymptomatic or mild infestations should be treated with diiodohydroxyquin, 650 mg three times daily for 21 days. More severe infections are best treated by metronidazole followed by diiodohydroxyquin. Relapse is common; therefore monthly examination of stools should be carried out for at least a year, with retreatment as necessary.

Amebic abscess of the liver is the most common serious complication of amebic colitis. Hepatic abscesses may rupture into the pleura, pericardium, or peritoneum (see Chap. 30).

An uncommon complication of chronic amebic colitis of interest to surgeons is the ameboma, a mass of granulation tissue in the colon. Partial obstruction may be produced, and a tender, sausage-shaped mass is often palpable. Granulomas are most frequent in the cecum, where radiologic demonstration of ragged encroachment upon the lumen may lead to an erroneous diagnosis of carcinoma, tuberculosis, or actinomycosis. It is important therefore to search for amebas in the stools or rectal mucosa of patients with this finding. Surgical intervention in untreated ameboma can lead to peritonitis or to pericecal abscess and fecal fistula.

Actinomycosis

Actinomycosis is an uncommon suppurative infection produced by the anaerobic fungus *Actinomyces israelii,* a normal resident of the mouth. Clinical disease is characterized by chronic inflammatory induration and sinus formation. The cervicofacial area is the most frequently involved site, followed by thoracic and abdominal involvement.

The cecal area is most frequently the site of abdominal actinomycosis. An indurated, tumorlike pericecal mass sometimes develops. If the condition is untreated, abscesses develop and burst, forming indolent sinuses. More typically the history begins with an attack of acute appendicitis with perforation. After appendectomy, a persistent draining sinus forms, or, less commonly, an indurated mass forms under the incision which then results in a persistent sinus after surgical drainage.

The diagnosis of actinomycosis is made by demonstration of sulfur granules or the ray fungus in the purulent sinus discharge.

Treatment consists of surgical drainage and antibiotics. Both penicillin and tetracyclines are effective.

DIVERTICULAR DISEASE

Two types of diverticula of the colon are recognized: One is very common, an acquired disease which consists of multiple false diverticula principally in the left colon —*diverticulosis*. The other is very uncommon, is probably a congenital disease, and consists of a single true diverticulum of the cecum or ascending colon.

Diverticulosis Coli

INCIDENCE. The incidence of diverticulosis of the colon on barium enema examination or at necropsy is about 5 percent. Thus, about 11 million persons in the United States have the disease. Diverticulosis is rarely seen in persons under age thirty-five. The incidence rises with age, so at age fifty about 15 percent are affected; at sixty-five, about 35 percent; and at eighty-five, about 65 percent.

ETIOLOGY AND PATHOGENESIS. The sigmoid is the sole site of diverticula in about 50 percent of patients with diverticulosis; sigmoid and descending colon are the sites in 80 percent; sigmoid plus other colonic sites, in 95 percent. The cecum is involved in 2 percent; ascending colon and rectum, 4 percent each; and transverse colon, 10 percent.

Diverticula of the colon are herniations of mucosa and submucosa through the circular muscular layer and so are classified as false diverticula, since they lack a muscular coat. Diverticula characteristically break through the circular muscle on either side of the colon between the mesenteric and the respective antimesenteric taeniae. Radiographs of injected normal colon segments demonstrate a large circumferential vessel coursing around the bowel outside the muscular coat on each side with branches penetrating the muscularis on the mesenteric side of each antimesenteric taenia. This penetrating vessel is thought to create the *locus minoris resistentiae* through which mucosal herniation can occur. Injection studies of colon segments bearing diverticula also demonstrate that the penetrating vessel is in close relation to the neck of the diverticulum where it breaks through the circular muscle. The proximity of this vessel presumably accounts for the propensity of diverticula to bleed.

The mechanism(s) furnishing the pulsion force to herniate the mucosa through the weak spot in the circular muscle coat has not been clearly delineated. Contributing factors are thought to be chronic constipation, tissue degeneration associated with age and obesity, and an inherited predisposition. Hypertrophy of the bowel musculature is often demonstrable in diverticular disease but has been considered to be secondary to fully developed diver-

ticulitis. Morson has found hypertrophy of the sigmoid musculature in some specimens with only microscopic intrusions of mucosa—a prediverticular state—and suggests that the muscular abnormality is primary. Some investigators have confirmed this finding, but others have not. Painter et al. studied the colons of patients by means of simultaneous cineradiography and intraluminal pressure recordings. Contraction rings form in the sigmoid colon. These close the lumen, creating a series of "bladders" each of which has its outflow obstructed at each end. With contraction of the colonic muscle forming the wall of the segments, intraluminal pressures up to at least 90 mm Hg are generated. Contraction of these closed segments creates a pulsion force that was observed to distend existing diverticula. The investigators conclude that this mechanism may well be responsible for the initial mucosal herniation. Similar motility and pressure abnormalities have been demonstrated in the irritable colon syndrome, which is thought by some to predispose to diverticular disease.

Diet appears to play a prominent role in the causation of diverticulosis, since it is almost entirely a disease of industrial societies. Diverticulosis is rare in Asia and Africa but is relatively frequent among United States residents of African origin. Diverticulosis coli has been produced in the rat and rabbit by feeding a low-residue diet, a diet similar to that of industrial societies. Only four mammals have teniae coli—horse, guinea pig, rabbit, and man; three of these are herbivores. Was the human colon designed for a bulky herbivorous diet?

Diverticulosis per se does not cause symptoms. The majority of persons with this condition never have trouble enough to require medical attention. Only 1 in 70 will require hospital treatment, and only 1 in 200 will require operation for a symptomatic complication. Complications of diverticulosis are bleeding, and inflammation, i.e., diverticulitis.

BLEEDING IN DIVERTICULAR DISEASE

The reported incidence of bleeding in diverticular disease varies from 3 to 48.5 percent. This large variation is attributable to the following: (1) some writers have reported the incidence of bleeding in patients hospitalized for diverticular disease, whereas others have reported the incidence in all patients, clinic and hospital, in whom the diagnosis has been made; (2) some have included all bleeding, overt and occult, whereas others have reported only gross bleeding; and (3) until recently, many writers refused to believe that diverticulosis without frank diverticulitis could bleed. It is now recognized that gross rectal hemorrhage is caused more frequently by diverticulosis than by diverticulitis, that bleeding from diverticulosis is massive in about one-fourth of the patients, and that diverticulosis is responsible for about two-thirds of all cases of massive lower gastrointestinal bleeding. Colorectal carcinoma is the most frequent cause of rectal bleeding, but the bleeding is nearly always mild to moderate in degree, rarely severe and exsanguinating (see also Chap. 24).

DIAGNOSIS. Bleeding due to diverticular disease of the colon is characteristically sudden, unexpected, and often profuse from the onset, and occurs more frequently in older individuals and in those with arteriosclerotic and/or hypertensive cardiovascular disease. Bleeding is often the only symptom of diverticulosis. Many patients with massive rectal bleeding will have had a previous episode suggesting diverticulitis but usually do not have frank symptoms of inflammation at the time of the hemorrhage.

Some patients bleed so massively that immediate operation must be done to prevent death from exsanguination. Most, however, will respond, at least temporarily, to vigorous transfusion therapy. Every effort should be made, after the patient is clinically stable, to ascertain the nature of the bleeding lesion and its location. The known presence of diverticula does not guarantee that they are the source of the bleeding. The diagnostic steps to be taken are discussed in Chap. 24 under Lower Gastrointestinal Tract Bleeding. The use of selective angiography in recent years for detection of the bleeding point has demonstrated, unexpectedly, that although most diverticula are in the left colon, most major diverticular bleeding is from diverticula in the right colon. The use of aortography to demonstrate the bleeding point is illustrated in Fig. 28-5.

TREATMENT. The majority of patients with lower gastrointestinal hemorrhage will stop bleeding spontaneously with adequate transfusions and supportive therapy. Selective infusion of vasoconstrictive substances such as vasopressin into the visceral artery supplying the bleeding site, after identification by selective angiography, has been shown by several groups to be a quite effective and safe nonoperative method of controlling diverticular bleeding. In some patients the bleeding is controlled and does not recur; in others bleeding is only temporarily slowed or stopped but time is gained for a more orderly approach to the operative procedure. In a few, the selective infusion is completely ineffective and immediate operation is necessary. Adams has reported the use of the barium enema as therapy for massive diverticular bleeding; 47 of 49 bleeding episodes were arrested, possibly due to tamponade of the bleeding point by barium. If bleeding continues, after correction of hypovolemia, at a rate of more than 500 ml/8 hours or if massive hemorrhage recurs during the hospital course, then immediate operative therapy is indicated. Opinion is divided on whether a single massive hemorrhage in a patient who is found on work-up to have nothing but diverticulosis is sufficient reason for elective colon resection. Nearly all agree, however, that a second massive hemorrhage in such a patient is an indication for surgical intervention.

In elective operations for bleeding, the entire gastrointestinal tract should be minutely examined for lesions that might have been missed in the diagnostic work-up. If no other lesions are found, then all colon bearing diverticula is resected with primary anastomosis. This usually requires sigmoid or sigmoid and descending colon resection but may require removal of the entire colon down to the rectum. The mortality rate for elective resections is less than 5 percent.

Emergency surgical treatment for massive bleeding when the presumptive source of bleeding has not been identified preoperatively is often a frustrating, difficult

Fig. 28-5. Aortogram in bleeding diverticulosis. Arrow on left side of illustration points to the bleeding diverticulum in the right colon.

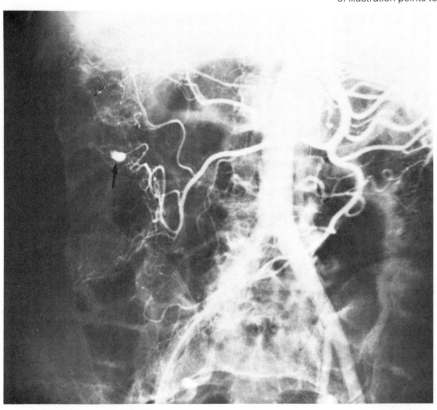

problem. The entire colon is usually grossly distended with blood, even though the bleeding point is in the sigmoid. Segmental colotomies with operative endoscopy is rarely rewarding. Isolation of segments with clamps is sometimes helpful. The colon is emptied of blood by "milking" it downward through a rectal tube; then several noncrushing clamps are applied to isolate the different colon segments. If active bleeding is present, the involved segment or segments will be seen to fill with blood, and the appropriate resection can then be done. For patients in whom the bleeding point cannot be located with assurance, total abdominal colectomy with ileoproctostomy is gaining favor as the procedure of choice. There is currently an unresolved difference of opinion between angiographers and surgeons as to the preferred operation when a bleeding diverticulum has been identified angiographically. Many surgeons feel that all diverticula-bearing colon should be resected. Angiographers, however, feel that this is unnecessarily radical. In their opinion a segmental resection of the bleeding area is sufficient, since they believe that the chance of bleeding from remaining diverticula is slight. The mortality rate of emergency surgical measures for massive rectal bleeding is over 20 percent.

DIVERTICULITIS

Inflammation is the most frequent complication of diverticulosis coli. Diverticulitis is more frequent in patients with widespread diverticulosis, and the frequency increases with age. The inflammation may remain localized as a simple diverticulitis or extend to produce secondary complications such as intestinal obstruction, confined perforation with abscess or fistula formation, free perforation with spreading peritonitis, and hemorrhage. These grave complications supervene in about 15 percent of patients with diverticulitis and usually require operative therapy.

PATHOGENESIS. Diverticula readily fill with colonic contents, as can be seen at barium enema examination, but emptying is often slow because of the narrow neck and the lack of musculature of the diverticulum. If an inspissated fecal plug obstructs the neck of the diverticulum, continued mucus secretion and proliferation of ever-present bacteria distend the flask-shaped diverticulum and produce inflammation at the apex. This focal diverticulitis often resolves by discharge of the contents into the colonic lumen, but if the obstructing plug remains in place, inflammation spreads to peridiverticular tissues. Initial spread is to the pericolic fat between the muscularis propria and serosa. Extension is usually longitudinal in this plane, giving rise to intramural fistulas, which are one of the diagnostic signs of diverticulitis on barium enema (Fig. 28-6). Diverticulitis is thought to start as inflammation of a single diverticulum; other diverticula may become secondarily involved as edema from the initial diverticulitis narrows their necks, preventing emptying and thus initiating another inflammatory focus. Berman and associates have presented evidence that actual perforation of a single diverticulum is the initiating event, followed by an inflammatory focus in the pericolic fat.

CLINICAL MANIFESTATIONS. The diagnosis of acute diverticulitis is aided by a history of previous demonstration of diverticulosis with barium enema radiography. The clinical picture of sigmoid diverticulitis so resembles appendicitis that it is often called "left-sided appendicitis." Pain is nearly always the most prominent symptom. It is mild to moderate and felt deep in the left lower quadrant or suprapubic area. The pain is usually dull, aching, and constant; less frequently, it is intermittent and crampy. Anorexia and mild nausea are common, but vomiting is uncommon. An associated change in bowel habits frequently is noted, i.e., diarrhea, constipation, or irregularity. Urinary symptoms are sometimes present as a result of inflammation close to bladder or ureter. On examination, low-grade fever and mild leukocytosis are usually found. Tenderness and some rigidity in the left lower quadrant and/or suprapubic area are the rule. A tender mass representing the inflamed, feces-filled colon may be palpable. Mild distension is common, but bowel sounds are usually within normal limits in uncomplicated diverticulitis. Sigmoidoscopy should be done if only to rule out other causes for the symptoms. Mucosal edema and erythema may be seen, but the most characteristic finding in acute diverticulitis is inability to introduce the scope beyond about 15 cm because of immobility of the bowel and fixed angulation at that point. It is advisable to defer the barium enema until the process has cooled off somewhat with conservative therapy. Barium enema then should be done, with caution, to attempt to differentiate diverticulitis from carcinoma of the colon, which can cause the same clinical picture. Differential diagnostic criteria are as follows: (1) Diverticulitis usually involves a long segment, carcinoma a much shorter one. (2) Normal bowel contour above and below diverticulitis tapers smoothly and gradually into the involved area to form a funnel-shaped transition; in carcinoma the transition is abrupt. (3) The bowel is spastic in diverticulitis. (4) The mucosa is intact, although it may show a picket-fence contour in diverticulitis, but it is destroyed in carcinoma. (5) Finally, diverticula in other areas of the bowel favor but do not prove diverticulitis, since carcinoma and diverticulosis may coexist. A typical radiograph of sigmoid diverticulitis is shown in Fig. 28-6 and of sigmoid carcinoma in Fig. 28-7.

TREATMENT. Nonoperative therapy should be tried for first attacks of acute uncomplicated diverticulitis. Operative therapy is indicated, if the patient does not respond promptly, for recurrent acute diverticulitis, for diverticulitis with complications, and if carcinoma cannot be ruled out. Initial nonoperative treatment consists of parenteral fluids, broad-spectrum antibiotics, and nasogastric suction. Pain is controlled with pentazocine or meperidine, but not morphine, to avoid increasing intracolonic pressure. Significant amelioration of all symptoms and signs should occur within 48 hours. If not or if symptoms progress, operation should be considered. After subsidence of acute symptoms, treatment is aimed principally at avoiding constipation. Bulk-forming hemicellulose laxatives are taken as needed to keep the stool soft and bulky. In the past, low-residue diets have been prescribed. It is now recognized that bulky high-residue diets should be advised since low-residue diets have been implicated in the etiology of diverticulosis coli.

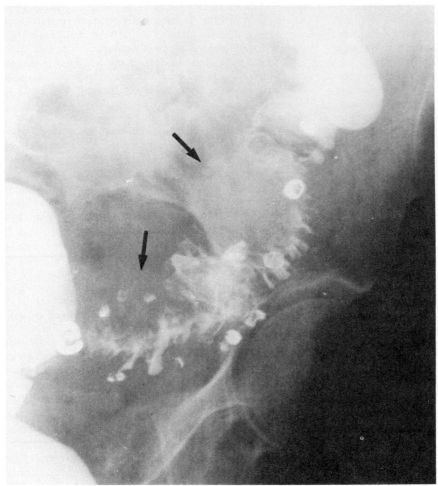

Fig. 28-6. Barium radiograph of diverticulitis of sigmoid colon. Note long length of involvement. Arrows point to intramural abscesses.

Fig. 28-7. Oblique view, barium radiograph of annular carcinoma of sigmoid colon. Note sharp transition from normal to abnormal area, short length of involvement.

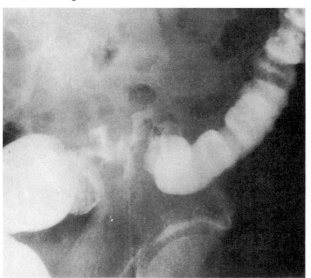

Colomyotomy has been advocated for the treatment of chronic persistent diverticular disease that is a nuisance to the patient but has not yet progressed to a complication that would require resective therapy. The operation interrupts the muscle coats of the colon by a longitudinal incision between the two antimesenteric teniae. It is designed to lower intraluminal pressure and thus diminish the threat of complications. Results to date are equivocal.

If attacks of diverticulitis recur despite medical therapy, elective resection is indicated. With proper preparation, single-stage resection of all diverticulum-bearing colon with primary anastomosis is usually possible.

Complications of Diverticulitis

Obstruction. Some degree of colonic obstruction occurs in about two-thirds of patients with acute diverticulitis. This is usually partial obstruction due to inflammation with spasm and edema, plus an element of adynamic ileus. Complete obstruction occurs in about 10 percent and is the second most frequent cause of acute colonic obstruction. Complete obstruction usually implies abscess formation with encroachment on the lumen or repeated episodes of diverticulitis with fibrosis and stenosis. Small bowel obstruction also occurs secondarily to involvement in an inflammatory mass or to adhesions. Clinical manifestations of intestinal obstruction are discussed in Chap. 24. Obstructive symptoms in diverticulitis usually respond fairly promptly to nonoperative therapy. Plain films of the abdomen are valuable to differentiate small and large bowel obstruction by delineation of the gas pattern. If there is doubt about the locus of the obstruction, barium enema, though somewhat hazardous in acute diverticulitis, should be done. Adynamic ileus secondary to free perforation and peritonitis must be kept in mind. If complete colon obstruction does not open up within a few hours, operative therapy is indicated lest cecal rupture occur.

Most surgeons still feel that the combination of acute inflammation and obstructed unprepared bowel interdict primary resection and consider diverting transverse colostomy to be the procedure of choice. A few advocate primary resection, feeling that the morbidity and mortality, though appreciable, is less than the combined morbidity and mortality of the two- or three-stage procedures. After colostomy, an interval of about 3 months is allowed for inflammation to subside before resection is done. If there is a question about the presence of carcinoma, however, the second-stage operation is done in 2 or 3 weeks. The colostomy may be closed at the time of the resection or may be left to decompress the colon anastomosis and closed later as a third-stage procedure.

Perforation. The inflammatory process of uncomplicated diverticulitis is confined to the colonic wall by the serosa; a breach in the integrity of this layer constitutes perforation. The inflammation is ordinarily localized to the area adjacent to the perforation by the body's walling-off mechanism, thus forming a pericolic abscess. The abscess may in turn burrow into one of the viscera contributing to the walling-off process with formation of an internal fistula. Less frequently, the pericolic abscess bursts into the free peritoneal cavity producing purulent peritonitis. Also infrequently, the initial perforation is not walled off, so that free communication is established between the colonic lumen and the peritoneal cavity with gross fecal spillage and generalized fecal peritonitis. About 10 percent of patients with diverticulitis requiring operative therapy have spreading peritonitis either from free perforation or from secondary rupture of an abscess. The clinical manifestations and the principles of management of peritonitis are discussed in Chap. 34. With small free perforations that appear to be walling off quickly, thus localizing the peritonitis, nonoperative therapy with very close observation is justified. Resectional therapy can then be done electively after subsidence of the acute inflammation. With spreading peritonitis or if a previously stabilized and subsiding abscess shows evidence of enlargement with increasing peritoneal signs, urgent operative therapy is mandatory.

There continues to be a difference of opinion as to which surgical procedure should be used. There is agreement that drainage alone, closure of perforation and drainage, or colostomy alone are inadequate. The procedure still preferred by many consists of closure of the perforation to prevent further peritoneal soiling, drainage, and proximal diverting colostomy. Three stages are required to complete the treatment—resection at the second stage and colostomy closure as the third stage. A more radical and direct approach consists of resection of diseased bowel and primary anastomosis, usually with a proximal decompressing colostomy. Primary resection has the advantage of being a two-stage procedure or even a single stage if colostomy has not been necessary at the time of resection. Enthusiasm for this approach seems to be waning as more surgeons realize that primary anastomosis in the presence of peritonitis is foolhardy.

A third approach (preferred by the authors) has the advantage of completing therapy in two stages but without the hazard of performing a colonic anastomosis in the presence of pus and feces. All diseased colon is mobilized and resected. The proximal bowel is brought out as an end colostomy. The distal bowel is brought out as a mucous fistula if this is possible, but if the distal segment is short, the end is closed and left in place (Hartmann procedure). The peritoneal cavity is copiously irrigated, the last wash containing cephalothin or kanamycin. Drains are placed in the pelvis and gutter. At a second stage, in 2 or 3 months, continuity is reestablished by end-to-end anastomosis.

Fistulas. In about 5 percent of patients with complicated diverticulitis fistulas develop between the involved segment of colon and adjacent organs, i.e., bladder, uterus, vagina, ileum, and ureter. Colocutaneous fistulas rarely occur spontaneously but are a common postoperative complication, discharging through the incision or drain site. Fistulas develop when adjacent organs wall off acute diverticulitis, with subsequent burrowing of the disease process into the lumen of the adjacent viscus. Urinary urgency and frequency, and dysuria occur with inflammation of the bladder or ureter before fistulization has occurred. After the process has broken through to form a fistula, pneumaturia and fecaluria are diagnostic. Chills and fever are also frequent. Sigmoidoscopy is of no value in demonstrating fistulas. Barium enema often, but not always, demonstrates the tract. Cystoscopy and cystography are also useful. If the actual opening is not demonstrated, its location can be suspected by finding localized edema, ulceration, and granulations. Fistulas into the uterus or vagina offer little difficulty—passage of flatus and feces per vaginam establishes the diagnosis; speculum examination, the location. Coloenteric fistulas may cause no symptoms in addition to those of the primary disease, or there may be fecal urgency and frequency.

The choice of operative procedure for diverticulitis complicated by fistula depends on the extent of the inflammatory process and whether the correct diagnosis has been made preoperatively. With proper preoperative preparation, a one-stage procedure is often feasible. Fistulas into the bladder are dissected out, the bladder wall closed, diseased colon resected with primary anastomosis, and suprapubic drainage instituted. Hysterectomy en bloc with involved colon is done for colouterine fistulas. Similarly, the involved ileal loop is resected en bloc with colon for coloenteric fistulas. If the inflammatory process is extensive or if the bowel has not been prepared, staged procedures are indicated. If possible, diseased tissue is resected, the proximal colon is brought out as an end colostomy, and the distal end is brought out as a mucous fistula or is dropped back as a Hartmann pouch. The anastomosis is done as a second stage. If inflammation is so extensive as to preclude resection, a diverting proximal colostomy only is done as the initial stage, with completion in one or two more stages.

Diverticulum of the Right Colon

The cecum and ascending colon infrequently are involved in diverticulosis coli. Even more uncommon is a solitary true diverticulum, usually called *cecal diverticulitis,* that is found only in the cecum and ascending colon. In contrast to the false diverticula of diverticulosis coli, solitary cecal diverticula contain all layers of the bowel wall and are, therefore, true diverticula. Because of this and because these lesions are found in younger individuals, they are considered to be congenital in origin.

Symptoms are produced in the same manner as in diverticulitis coli or acute appendicitis. The ostium of the diverticulum becomes obstructed by a plug of feces or fecalith, creating a miniature closed loop. Inflammation ensues from continued secretion within the diverticulum and infection by resident bacteria.

CLINICAL MANIFESTATIONS. Clinical manifestations of acute cecal diverticulitis are essentially identical to those of acute appendicitis. The true nature of the lesion may be suspected if there is a history of numerous frequent episodes of similar attacks. The correct diagnosis is made preoperatively in only about 5 percent of patients, nearly always by barium enema demonstration of the diverticulum. The preoperative diagnosis is acute appendicitis in about 80 percent, tumor in about 5 percent.

TREATMENT. The operative procedure is determined by the findings. If inflammation is limited to the diverticulum, then simple diverticulectomy with inversion of the stump is done as for appendicitis. Ruptured diverticulum with abscess is treated by drainage and removal of the diverticulum if it can easily be done; otherwise only drainage is performed, and interval diverticulectomy is carried out later. When inflammation involves the cecum also, resection of diverticulum and adjacent cecum is indicated if the cecal closure is through healthy tissue, and the ileocecal valve is not encroached upon. When the cecum is extensively involved, terminal ileum and cecum are resected with ileo-ascending colon anastomosis. If frank peritonitis is present, ileo-ascending colectomy, cutaneous ileostomy, and creation of a transverse colon mucous fistula should be done because of the risk of primary anastomosis in this situation. Chronic diverticular disease with extensive productive inflammation and fibrosis may be indistinguishable from neoplasm at the operating table. Right colectomy with ileo-transverse colostomy as for cancer is indicated.

No treatment is indicated for asymptomatic cecal diverticula that are an incidental finding on barium enema. Diverticula found incidentally at operation should be re-

moved if their removal does not add significantly to the risk of the primary procedure.

NEOPLASMS OF THE COLON AND RECTUM

Although a broad spectrum of neoplasms occurs in the colon and rectum, there are essentially only two important types of tumors: polyps, which may cause symptoms in themselves but more importantly may develop into, or be associated with, adenocarcinoma, and adenocarcinoma itself. Thus emphasis will be placed on these two lesions and their discussion followed by a brief discussion of some of the less common tumors. Neoplasms of the anus are quite different from those of colon and rectum and will be considered separately.

Polyps

The term *polyp* refers to any circumscribed mass of tissue that arises from mucosa and protrudes into the lumen of the gastrointestinal tract. It is a clinical term and should imply no histopathologic significance. After removal and histologic diagnosis, polyps are classified as: inflammatory—benign lymphoid polyps and pseudopolyps (ulcerative colitis); hamartomas—juvenile and Peutz-Jeghers polyps (Chap. 27); neoplastic—adenomatous (tubular) polyps, villous adenomas (papillomas); or unclassified—the hyperplastic (metaplastic) polyp.

JUVENILE POLYPS

This lesion, also called *mucous polyp* or *retention polyp,* technically should not be included under "neoplasms," since it is probably a hamartoma or possibly an inflammatory, polypoid, retention cyst.

INCIDENCE. As the name implies, juvenile polyps occur principally in children, but they also are found in young adults. They have not been reported in infants under age one. The peak incidence is about age five; they are uncommon after about age sixteen and very rare after age thirty-five. The incidence in children is probably about 1 percent. The polyps are single in 70 percent of patients. When multiple, there are usually only three or four polyps, but in rare instances the polyps may be so numerous that familial polyposis is simulated. This is now thought to represent an inherited polyposis syndrome. Inheritance is autosomal dominant with complete penetrance. Polyps are usually in the colon and rectum but may involve the small intestine and stomach. Some investigators consider these as variations of one syndrome, others divide them into juvenile polyposis coli and juvenile gastrointestinal polyposis.

PATHOLOGY. Grossly, juvenile polyps are nearly always pedunculated, rarely sessile, from 3 to 10 mm in diameter, smooth, spherical, reddish brown, and often covered with mucus. Histologically, the slender stalk is covered with essentially normal colonic mucosa that is continuous with adjacent mucosa. The bulbous portion is covered by a single layer of goblet cells, frequently with ulceration and chronic inflammation. In the tissue are numerous cystic spaces lined by mature, columnar, mucus-secreting cells, a heavy infiltration of leukocytes and plasma cells, and abundant granulation tissue. Strands of fibrous tissue from the stalk fan out into the bulbous portion.

CLINICAL MANIFESTATIONS. The usual symptom of colorectal polyps is blood streaking of the stool, less frequently rectal bleeding. Anemia is the presenting symptom in some patients. Rectal polyps may protrude through the rectum and be described as a small cherry by the parent. Rarely, a colonic polyp initiates intussusception. Diagnosis is by sigmoidoscopy, by air-contrast barium enema, or by colonoscopy for polyps beyond the reach of the sigmoidoscope.

TREATMENT. Treatment should take into account the fact that juvenile polyps have no malignant potential. All polyps within reach of the sigmoidoscope should be removed by excision biopsy, since this is so easily done. Polyps in the colon that would require laparatomy and colotomy for removal may be observed safely unless they are causing serious symptoms or unless they are so numerous that the possibility of familial polyposis exists. Autoamputation is common. New polyps, not recurrences, appear in about 10 percent after polypectomy.

HYPERPLASTIC POLYPS

These tiny mucosal excrescences—usually from 1 to 3 mm in diameter, very rarely over 5 mm, and never over 10 mm—can be found in 50 percent of adult colons if searched for diligently enough. Since they arise as the result of localized minor imbalances between cell division and desquamation (see Malignant Potential of Polyps, page 1214), the terms *hyperplastic* and *metaplastic* are appropriate. Hyperplastic polyps cause no symptoms and of themselves are of no consequence; they are important only because they arise in the same locations in the colorectum and in the same age groups as do neoplastic polyps. Removal is indicated only for histologic diagnosis. Distinction between adenomatous and hyperplastic polyps is usually easy. Differential features are summarized in Table 28-3.

ADENOMATOUS POLYPS

INCIDENCE. This is by far the most common neoplasm of the colon and rectum. Adenomatous polyps, except with familial polyposis, are rare under age twenty-one, and then the incidence gradually increases with age throughout life, perhaps indicating that the lesions do not spontaneously regress. The incidence in adults is variously reported as from 1 to 50 percent. There are several possible explanations for this great variation. Some writers include any and all lesions that are elevated above the surrounding mucosa, so that hyperplastic polyps and lymphoid polyps are counted. Others have reported only lesions found at sigmoidoscopy or on barium enema. The best available estimate is that about 5 percent of adults harbor at least one adenomatous polyp in the colon or rectum. There is also considerable variation in reports on the distribution of polyps within the different segments of the colon and rectum. In clinical studies, based on sigmoidoscopy and

Table 28-3. DIFFERENTIAL FEATURES OF ADENOMATOUS AND HYPERPLASTIC POLYPS

	Adenomatous polyp	Hyperplastic polyp
A. Tinctorial quality	Basophilic	Acidophilic
B. Glands per unit area	Greater than normal	Similar to normal
C. Cell number	Marked increase	Moderate increase
D. Papillary infolding of epithelium	Usually absent; gland lumen has smooth tubular profile	Present; lumen appears sawtooth, corkscrew, stellate
E. Cell crowding	Marked; narrowed, pencil-shaped cells	Minimal
F. Nuclei	Crowded, elongated, hyperchromatic	Inconspicuous, vesicular, basal
G. Cell types	Often only one type at any random level of adenomatous tubule	Usually two types: near-surface, absorptive cells adjacent to mature or distended goblet cells
H. Secretion	Unpredictable; may be absent; may be abundant, even in depth of tubule	Uniformly present in all tubules; generally most marked in upper one-half of gland
I. Over-all mitotic activity	Usually increased	Usually increased
J. Mitotic activity in:		
Surface	May be present	Absent
Neck and mouth of crypt	May be maximal	Absent
Midportion of crypt	Present	May be present
Depth of crypt	Present	Present
K. Thickness of basement membrane (collagen and mucopolysaccharide)		
Surface	Less than normal	Greater than normal
Depth of crypt	Minimal	Minimal

SOURCE: From Lane, Kaplan, and Pascal, 1971.

barium enema, about 73 percent are in the rectum, recto-sigmoid, and lower sigmoid within reach of the sigmoidoscope; 20 percent in the middle and upper sigmoid; 3 percent in the descending colon; 2 percent each in transverse and ascending colon. In autopsy studies, only 27 percent are found in the rectum and sigmoid, 11 percent in descending colon, 25 percent in transverse colon, and 37 percent in cecum and ascending colon.

PATHOLOGY. Adenomatous polyps are usually pedunculated firm tumors varying from 1 mm to several centimeters in diameter. Two-thirds are less than 1 cm. The bulbous head is irregularly lobulated. Microscopically, the vascular connective tissue stalk is covered by mucosa that appears to be an extension of the normal adjacent mucosa, suggesting that the stalk is not part of the neoplasia but rather a pedicle pulled out by traction exerted on the polyp by peristalsis. The microscopic characteristics are summarized in Table 28-3. About 15 percent of polyps demonstrate villous elements as well as the adenomatous or tubular architecture. The frequency of the villous admixture increases with the size of the polyp. Not infrequently, circumscribed areas of adenomatous polyps demonstrate the cytologic criteria of malignancy, i.e., marked pleomorphism and atypia of glands and cells, hyperchromatism, and frequent mitoses. This is carcinoma in situ. Truly invasive cancer can be diagnosed only if definite invasion beneath the muscularis mucosae is demonstrated. True invasion of the stalk or base by malignant glands is extremely rare; apparent invasion of the stalk may be seen when oblique sectioning of a polyp appears to project glands into the submucosa while actually they lie above the muscularis mucosae. Serial sectioning is necessary to clarify this pseudoinvasion.

CLINICAL MANIFESTATIONS. Adenomatous polyps may produce symptoms such as hematochezia, bleeding per rectum, anemia, prolapse of polyp through the anus, and, rarely, intussusception. Much more commonly they are asymptomatic and are an incidental finding by sigmoidoscopy, colonoscopy, or barium enema. Treatment is discussed below under Malignant Potential of Colorectal Polyps.

VILLOUS ADENOMA

These polypoid lesions, also called *papillary adenomas,* are so named because of their characteristic frondlike projections. The separation of villous adenomas from adenomatous polyps was first made in 1948 because of the marked difference in malignant propensity of the two lesions. It is now thought by many that they represent different points on the spectrum of abnormal cell division in the colonic mucosa.

INCIDENCE. Villous adenomas are found with about one-eighth the frequency of adenomatous polyps and represent from 1 to 3 percent of surgically removed neoplasms of the colon. One institution, however, reported that 10.3 percent of intestinal carcinomas in their material arose in villous tumors. About 60 percent of villous adenomas arise in the rectum, 20 percent in the rectosigmoid, 10 percent in the sigmoid, and 10 percent in all other segments of the colon. The average age of the patients is sixty-three;

for adenomatous polyp, fifty-four. Villous adenoma is rarely seen in patients under age forty-five.

PATHOLOGY. Grossly, villous tumors are poorly demarcated, bulky, broad-based lesions. They are smooth, soft, and velvety, and therefore are difficult to detect by palpation. Areas of firmness usually represent malignancy. On inspection, these polyps may be pale or may be similar in color to adjacent normal mucosa but can be detected because of the numerous characteristic frondlike projections. Microscopically, there are numerous long villous projections with narrow stroma covered by a single layer of cylindrical epithelial cells. The cells are elongated, with nuclei compressed and usually in a basal position, and contain less mucus than normal mucosal cells. The histologic abnormalities that characterize malignancy are often found. If subjacent tissues are included in the section and show invasion, the diagnosis of invasive villous adenocarcinoma is established. Invasive malignancy is present at the time of first treatment in about one-third of patients; cytologic evidence of malignancy but without frank invasion, in another one-third.

CLINICAL MANIFESTATIONS. Presenting symptoms are usually discharge of blood and mucus from the rectum and a feeling of incomplete evacuation. About one-half the patients have some obstruction with constipation and lower abdominal colic. A minority present with an interesting syndrome consisting of passage of numerous watery mucoid stools, severe muscle weakness, and weight loss. This is attributable to the secretion of very large quantities, i.e., up to 3 liters/day, of electrolyte-rich mucus by the tumor. Serum electrolyte determinations reveal a severe hypokalemia and hypochloremia, and often hyponatremia and uremia. Heroic therapy of this severe desalting water loss is necessary to prepare for operation. One writer has given as much as 1,000 mEq of potassium chloride daily, orally and parenterally, in order to restore normal values.

Diagnosis can be made in over 80 percent by sigmoidoscopy because of the usual fortuitous location of villous tumors. Several biopsies should be taken from several areas of the tumor including the base at the junction with "normal" colon in an attempt to establish histologically whether invasive cancer is present. Lesions above the sigmoidoscope can usually be seen on barium enema. They produce an irregular filling defect with wrinkled margins due to penetration of barium between the villous projections. Some alteration in shape is noted during compression or on the postevacuation film. Colonoscopic diagnosis has the advantage that the lesion can be biopsied.

TREATMENT. The operative procedure is determined by the location and size of the tumor and whether invasive malignancy is present. Colonoscopic removal is indicated for small tumors without invasive malignancy above the peritoneal reflection. Anterior resection is indicated for large tumors and for tumors of any size with demonstrated invasive malignancy located more than 7 cm above the dentate line. With lesions in the rectum proper, i.e., less than 7 cm above the dentate line, a combined abdominoperineal resection is done for those lesions with invasive cancer proved by biopsy. When invasive cancer is not demonstrable on biopsy, the lesion is locally completely excised after wide dilatation or division of the anal sphincter. The entire specimen is examined histologically. If invasive malignancy is not found, nothing further is done, but with demonstrable *invasive* malignancy, immediate abdominoperineal resection should be done. Frequent follow-up proctoscopy is mandatory after local excision; recurrence is common even though the lesion is histologically benign.

FAMILIAL POLYPOSIS

INCIDENCE AND PATHOGENESIS. This is a rare hereditary disease characterized by the appearance, early in life, of large numbers of adenomatous polyps in the colon and rectum. If untreated, it is almost invariably fatal because of carcinoma of colon or rectum. Estimates of the incidence vary from 1 in 8,300 live births to 1 in 29,000.

The mode of inheritance is not clear, though much of the evidence suggests a single dominant pleiotropic gene with variable penetrance. Males and females are equally affected, and either may transmit the disease. Marriage between a heterozygote (affected) and a homozygote (unaffected) results in one-half the children being affected, and only those who have inherited polyposis can transmit it to the next generation. Solitary, nonfamilial cases are probably a manifestation of gene mutation; these individuals can transmit the disease. The severity of the polyposis coli and the liability to carcinoma vary considerably in different families.

Colonic polyps are probably not present at birth but usually start appearing at about age thirteen, then appear with increasing frequency, until by about age twenty-one the entire colon and rectum are carpeted by hundreds—even thousands—of polyps ranging in size from 1 mm to several centimeters. The small bowel is not involved. The distal segments of the colon and the rectum are involved initially, and the polyps are mostly sessile in younger patients with a shift to pedunculated forms later. Though the above is the usual pattern, typical familial polyposis has been reported in 75 patients under age fourteen with the youngest a thirteen-month-old infant. The incidence of carcinoma in this group was 6.6 percent. Carcinoma of the colorectum will develop in essentially 100 percent of patients with familial polyposis unless treated or unless death from another cause supervenes. If untreated, most die of carcinoma before age fifty. The average age of death from cancer of the large bowel is 41.5 years, compared with 68 years of age for death from cancer of the large bowel in the general population. Cancer associated with familial polyposis is often multiple and presumably of multicentric origin.

Microscopically the polyps are adenomatous polyps that appear in no way different from the common adult-type single adenomatous polyp. Villous elements mixed with adenomatous glands—"intermediate" or "mixed" polyps—are seen, but true villous tumors are very rare.

It is logical to assume that carcinoma in familial polyposis arises in one of the myriad of adenomatous polyps; though the malignant potential of each individual polyp is very small, one chance in a thousand, if there are more than a thousand polyps in the colon, cancer is inevitable.

The association of polyps and cancer does not necessarily indicate a polyp-cancer sequence but may represent varying degrees of genetically dominated large bowel proneness both to cancer and to adenoma, so that an increased propensity to one may be reflected by an increased proclivity for the other.

CLINICAL MANIFESTATIONS. Symptoms may be absent or consist only of vague intermittent abdominal discomfort. In some, the first symptoms may be those of colorectal carcinoma. More commonly, however, rather marked symptoms develop consisting of frequent bouts of abdominal pain, passage of loose, blood-stained stools and much mucus, weight loss, anemia, and general debility. Occasionally, large polyps may prolapse through the anus, causing symptoms of intestinal obstruction, partial or complete, or initiate intussusception. Diagnosis is apparent on sigmoidoscopy and barium enema. Biopsy of one of the polyps, with histologic examination, should be done to be sure one is not dealing with multiple juvenile polyps. Any lesion in the rectum suspected of being malignant is also biopsied.

TREATMENT. If carcinoma is found in the rectum and is determined to be operable, total abdominal colectomy, abdominoperineal resection of rectum and anus, and terminal cutaneous ileostomy are done. Otherwise total abdominal colectomy with ileoproctostomy is usually done. After recovery from the operation, all polyps in the rectum are removed through the proctoscope, and the base is fulgurated. Proctoscopy at frequent intervals with removal of any polyps nearly always adequately controls the rectal polyposis. There are several reports of spontaneous regression of rectal polyps following subtotal colectomy. Some surgeons advise total coloproctectomy and cutaneous ileostomy for all patients with familial polyposis because of the possibility of cancer developing in the rectal stump.

The prognosis for patients with familial polyposis in whom invasive carcinoma of the colorectum develops is not good: the 5-year survival is probably about 20 percent compared to 40 percent for idiopathic colorectal carcinoma.

GARDNER'S SYNDROME

This inheritable disease, even more rare than familial polyposis, is characterized by polyposis coli, plus any combination of osteomas or exostoses, principally of the mandible, skull, and sinuses; multiple epidermoid or sebaceous cysts; desmoid tumors, principally in abdominal incisions; and postoperative mesenteric fibromatosis. The associated manifestations may appear before polyposis is present.

The intestinal polyposis pattern is somewhat different in Gardner's syndrome and familial polyposis. The colon polyps are more scattered in Gardner's syndrome, and polyps may occur also in the small bowel. Polyps may not develop in Gardner's syndrome until after age thirty or even forty years. The age of onset of colorectal cancer is also later in life. Possibly because of this, cancer has been found in only 36 percent of reported cases.

Gardner's syndrome is rather definitely thought to be determined by a single pleiotropic gene, transmitted as an autosomal dominant. This gene is thought to be distinct from that determining familial polyposis, but it is possible that it is all one syndrome with variable expressivity, and that patients with familial polyposis simply do not have the extracolonic abnormalities expressed. The Turcot syn-

Fig. 28-8. *A.* The normal colonic mucosa has a simple structure. There are no villi—only simple test tube glands (crypts of Lieberkühn). They contain fully differentiated goblet and absorptive cells. Cell division (shown in heavy shading) is restricted to the deepest third of the gland. *Mm,* muscularis mucosa; *Sm,* submucosa. *B.* In the hyperplastic polyp, excess cell production leads to crowding of cells, with resultant papillary infoldings of the epithelium. Full differentiation to goblet and absorptive cells also occurs. This combination of features imparts a distinctive and readily recognizable microscopic pattern. A key point indicating that this is a hyperplastic rather than a neoplastic process is that cell division remains restricted to the lower portion of the crypt (shaded area). *C.* In the adenomas, cell division is unrestricted, so that mitotic activity is observed at all levels of the adenomatous tissue (shaded area). This uncontrolled cell production elongates the crypts and, with further proliferation, leads ultimately to adenomas of all sizes and shapes. The unrestricted replication plus failure of orderly differentiation into mature goblet and absorptive cells indicate the neoplastic nature of this process. The resulting characteristic microscopic appearance of an adenoma is readily distinguishable from that of a hyperplastic polyp.

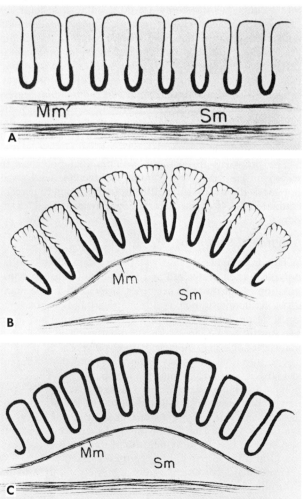

drome—central nervous system tumors and polyposis coli—may also be a variation of Gardner's syndrome.

The extraintestinal abnormalities of Gardner's syndrome are managed as they would be if they were idiopathic lesions. The treatment of the intestinal polyposis is essentially the same as outlined for familial polyposis.

MALIGNANT POTENTIAL OF COLORECTAL POLYPS

The hazard of malignancy in villous adenomas, familial polyposis, and Gardner's syndrome is clearly established, as described above, and generally accepted. Until 1958, it was nearly unanimously agreed that adenomatous polyps were also premalignant lesions. In 1958, Spratt and associates evaluated the evidence and concluded that "the theory of the origin of adenocarcinomas of the colon within adenomatous polyps has little to support it." Since then there has been a continuing vigorous controversy concerning the role of adenomatous polyps. Published conclusions have ranged from "Probably no benign process exists in which a greater incidence of malignant change occurs than that seen in colonic polyps. Eventually, 100 percent of these lesions become malignant" to "The adenomatous polyp is a lesion of negligible malignant potential."

Part of the difficulty is inherent in the available methods of study. It is impossible to examine a given tissue by present techniques without destroying its viability. A tissue that is excised, fixed, stained, and sectioned does not live out its natural course and disclose its destiny. Histologic examination of a polyp reveals only the situation obtaining at a given point in its development and maturation. Therefore what might have happened if the polyp had been left in place can only be surmised.

Studies of normal and abnormal cell division in the colonic mucosa have explained to the satisfaction of many investigators the natural history of neoplastic polyps. In the normal mucosa, cell division is restricted to the deepest one-third of the crypts of Lieberkühn (Fig. 28-8*A*). As the cells migrate up the crypt toward the surface, they differentiate into mature goblet and absorptive cells and after a life-span of 3 or 4 days are exfoliated from the free mucosal surface. Normally exfoliation just balances cell division. If exfoliation is slowed or cell division increased, cells will accumulate locally and form a protrusion. Both mechanisms are involved in the formation of a hyperplastic polyp.

In hyperplastic polyps there is a minor imbalance in the cycle of cell renewal. Cell division in the crypts is slightly expanded, but complete differentiation into goblet and absorptive cells occurs as the cells migrate to the surface (Fig. 28-8*B*). Migration of the cells is slower than normal, and desquamation from the surface is also delayed, leading some to call these polyps *hypermaturation* or *senescent* polyps. It is clear that these are not neoplastic lesions—cell division occurs only in its normal location, and there is complete cellular differentiation.

In neoplastic polyps, cell division is no longer restricted to its normal locus in the depths but is found at all levels in the crypts and on the mucosal surface as well (Fig. 28-8*C*). Cell differentiation into mature goblet and absorptive cells is incomplete. These are two of the hallmarks of neoplasia:

unrestricted cell division and incomplete cell differentiation.

The above-described mechanisms have been well worked out for adenomatous polyps. It is probable that villous adenomas arise in the same way, though there is much less evidence for this at present. Possible growth patterns are diagramed in Fig. 28-9.

There is still no agreement on the potential of adenomatous polyps to become carcinomatous. Morson says it is 5 percent; Grinnell and Lane, 2.9 percent; and Ackerman, from 0.2 to 0.8 percent. There is general agreement on the factors that correlate with incidence of malignancy in neoplastic polyps, however. These are size, histologic type, and epithelial atypia. Only 1 percent of adenomatous polyps under 1 cm are malignant; this rises to 10 percent for 1- to 2-cm polyps. Three histologic types are recognized: adenomatous polyp or tubular adenoma, villous adenoma, and an intermediate type which has an admixture of both. The malignancy rate for adenomatous polyps (all sizes) is about 5 percent; for villous adenomas, about 35 percent; and for the intermediate type, about 20 percent. Epithelial atypia is graded into mild, moderate, and severe. As might be expected, mild atypia is common in small adenomatous polyps and severe atypia in large villous adenomas.

Two clinical studies have shed some light on the polyp-cancer problem. Knoernschild followed the course of 213 patients with asymptomatic benign polyps by serial proctosigmoidoscopy for 3 to 5 years. A cytologic smear from the surface of the lesion was taken each time and the site of the lesion identified by a permanent tattoo mark. He showed that 18 percent of the lesions completely disappeared, 8 percent decreased in size, 70 percent showed no change, and 4 percent increased in size. Two polyps developed into histologically proved invasive carcinoma.

Gilbertsen has evaluated the role of proctosigmoidoscopy and polypectomy in reducing the incidence of lower bowel cancer. Over 18,000 patients participated in this 25-year study. During the years of the study, statistically 75 to 80 cancers could have been expected; only 11 were found.

It seems obvious that neoplastic polyps do become cancerous and so should be removed if this can be done safely. Colonoscopy has revolutionized the management of colonic polyps. In times past all polyps within reach of the sigmoidoscope were removed. Those above the reach of the scope were watched if they were less than 1.2 cm in diameter, since the risk of the operation was greater than the risk of cancer. Colonoscopic polypectomy can be done with a mortality of about 0.1 percent, a colonic perforation rate of 1 to 2 percent, and a serious hemorrhage rate of 2 to 4 percent. The most experienced colonoscopists report mortality-morbidity figures well below these levels. Large lesions and invasive carcinoma, whatever the size, should be removed at laparotomy after diagnosis is established by colonoscopic biopsy.

Carcinoma of the Colon and Rectum

INCIDENCE. Cancer of the colon and rectum is now the most common visceral cancer in the United States, exceeded in frequency only by skin cancer. In 1977, in about 101,000 Americans a diagnosis of colonic or rectal cancer was made for the first time, as mentioned earlier, and 51,300 died of the disease—13.3 percent of all cancer deaths. Lung cancer, with 98,000 cases in 1977, is the leading cause of cancer deaths in the United States, with 89,000 deaths in 1977, because the results of treatment of lung cancer are even poorer than the results for colorectal cancer. Cancer of the stomach, formerly the most common internal cancer and the leading cause of cancer deaths, has shown a steady significant unexplained decrease in incidence in both sexes since the early 1930s. Carcinoma of the lung has shown a steady increase in incidence in both sexes probably due to cigarette smoking. Colorectal carcinoma has shown a slight decrease in frequency in both sexes.

Females are affected by colonic cancer more than males in a ratio of 1.2:1; the sex ratio is reversed for rectal cancer with males predominating 1.1:1. Colorectal carcinoma is usually a disease of older persons with the peak incidence in the seventh decade. About 8 percent of colorectal cancers are diagnosed before age forty, however, and the disease is seen before age twenty, particularly in association with familial polyposis.

Fig. 28-9. Mechanism of carcinogenesis appears to involve induction of cell division in cells of the surface epithelium. Proliferating cells are seen on the periphery rather than in the depths of the crypts, indicating a centrifugal growth pattern. Increasing numbers of cells accumulate on the advancing edge of the tumor, but since not all are dividing at the same rate, lobulations may form and the same carcinogenic agent may produce different gross tumor forms, depending on the number of cells affected. A few cells protruding into the lumen could become pedunculated, but if a broad area is affected, a villous papilloma may develop.

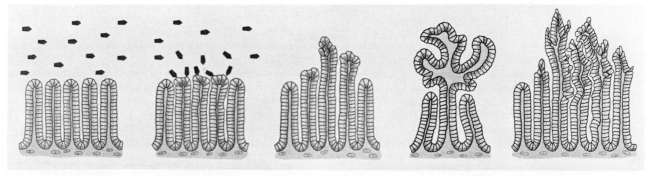

ETIOLOGY. Colorectal carcinoma develops in patients affected by familial polyposis, Gardner's syndrome, villous tumors, and chronic ulcerative colitis. The extent of the contribution of adenomatous polyps is still speculative. Genetic factors have been suggested because of a very high incidence of colorectal cancer in some families, but no convincing evidence for the hereditary transmission of the disease can be found in the vast majority. There are striking variations in the incidence of colorectal cancer in different parts of the world; the rate is very low in sub-Saharan Africa, low in Japan, and very high in the United States. Studies of migrant populations indict environmental factors, since colon cancer mortality in migrants shifts from the rate characteristic of the country of origin and tends to rise to the rate characteristic of their adopted country. Some epidemiologic data suggest a correlation between a high intake of fats and cancer of the colon. Metabolic products of bile acids or cholesterol are known to be carcinogenic in animals and are known to be degraded in the colon by certain bacteria, particularly a group of *Clostridia* and bacteroides. Populations with a high fat intake have a colonic bacterial flora of the type that metabolizes bile acids, and an increased fecal excretion of bile acid metabolites.

Burkitt has also implicated diet in the etiology of several colonic diseases. He has pointed out that rural blacks in Africa eat a diet of raw fruits and vegetables and unrefined grains, and produce large bulky stools with a rapid transit time. They have a very low incidence of polyps, cancer, and diverticulosis. Whites living in England consume a diet consisting largely of processed and refined foods and have much smaller stools and slower transit time. The English have a high incidence of polyps, cancer, and diverticulosis.

Recent animal studies tend to support the idea that ingestion of carcinogenic substances may be responsible for induction of colorectal cancer. Adenomatous polyps and adenocarcinoma of the colon can regularly be produced in laboratory animals by the administration of 4-aminobiphenyl derivatives or 1,2-dimethylhydrazine derivatives including the plant product cycasin.

PATHOLOGY. Carcinomas of the colon and rectum occur with different frequencies in the various segments of the colon. The relative segmental distribution is cecum, 11 percent; ascending colon, 9 percent; transverse colon, 12 percent; descending colon, 6 percent; sigmoid, 26 percent; rectosigmoid, 11 percent; and rectum, 25 percent. Thus 62 percent of colorectal cancer is found in the distal colon and rectum, with 25 percent of all cancers within reach of the examining finger and 50 percent within reach of the sigmoidoscope. A second or even a third primary colon carcinoma, either synchronously or metachronously, occurs in about 4 percent of patients with colorectal carcinoma. The incidence is higher in familial polyposis coli. Extracolonic malignant tumors also occur with increased frequency in patients with colorectal cancer.

Grossly, colorectal carcinomas are described as polypoid, nodular, ulcerating, scirrhous, or colloid. More than one descriptive term is often necessary, such as ulcerated, nodular carcinoma. Bulky exophytic tumors occur principally in the cecum. Colloid, or mucinous, carcinoma, which has a soft gelatinous consistency, occurs in the cecum, ascending colon, and rectum. Nodular and scirrhous tumors may be found anywhere in the colon but are more frequent in the left half. Scirrhous tumors are often associated with an exuberant desmoplastic reaction, as is seen in the napkin-ring lesion; they usually occur in the left colon and often produce obstruction. Gross characteristics do not correlate well with prognosis except for polypoid carcinomas on a stalk, which have a very good prognosis, and the rare linitis plastica type of infiltrating carcinoma, which carries a very poor prognosis.

Microscopically, colon carcinomas resemble the parent tissue in varying degrees, according to the degree of differentiation of the neoplastic cells. In well-differentiated tumors the cells are grouped in acinar clusters simulating normal glands. In poorly differentiated or anaplastic tumors, cells with little or no resemblance to colonic mucosa cells are dispersed in irregular sheets or cords with no suggestion of gland formation. Malignant cells are characterized by pleomorphism; hyperchromatism; large vesicular nuclei of various sizes, shapes, and position in the cytoplasm; and frequent mitoses, often with bizarre configurations. The Broders grading system classifies tumors numerically, based on increasing degrees of cytologic departure of individual cells from the glandular elements from which they derived. This system is of some value in predicting biologic behavior but does not correlate as well with prognosis as the Dukes system (see below).

Carcinoma spreads by direct extension, by lymphatic or bloodstream dissemination, by gravitational seeding, and by implantation at operation.

The significant extension by continuity is by penetration of the bowel wall. Some intramural extension, principally in the submucosa, may occur but is nearly always limited to less than 4 cm of grossly normal bowel distal to the tumor and 7 cm proximally.

Regional lymph node involvement is the most common form of metastasis in colorectal carcinoma. When carcinoma has extended through the bowel wall, lymph node involvement exceeds 90 percent; with lesions still confined to the bowel wall, the incidence of positive nodes is about 45 percent. Positive nodes are frequently found some distance from the primary site with normal nodes intervening. It is for this reason, rather than possible intramural extension, that long segments of colon are removed with accompanying blood and lymphatic channels in order to offer the best chance of eradicating the disease. The finding of retrograde nodal metastases due to lymphatic block in the normal drainage area is a grave prognostic sign; the 5-year survival rate is essentially zero.

Hematogenous metastases occur when tumor cells invade venous channels. The usual route is via the portal system to the liver. Lung and bone are next most frequently involved by metastasis, with cells reaching them either by passage through the liver into the inferior vena cava or by extension of tumor into tissues drained by systemic veins. Circulating tumor cells may be detected in the blood of some cancer patients, but the technique has not proved to be of significant value clinically either to diagnose malignancy or predict prognosis. The technique is hampered by the great difficulty in distinguishing between tumor cells and benign nucleated cells that are found normally in the bloodstream.

Gravitational metastases occur when the carcinoma has penetrated the bowel to involve the serosal surface; cells may become detached and seeded to distant points in the peritoneal cavity. Eventually peritoneal carcinomatosis results. Early sites of involvement by seeding are omentum and the rectovesical or rectouterine pouches with production of Blumer's shelf. Another frequent site is the ovary, occasionally resulting in large bilateral Krukenberg tumors. Bilateral oophorectomy should be a part of operations for colorectal cancer unless definitely contraindicated.

Recurrence after operations for carcinoma of the colorectum is frequently at or near the anastomosis even though the operation was considered to be curative and the cut ends of the resected specimen were histologically free of tumor. Recurrence is attributed to implantation of malignant cells spilled at operation. Newer operative techniques attempt to minimize this unfortunate complication.

The Dukes classification of colorectal cancer as modified by Astler and Coller is based on the extent of the malignant process and predicts prognosis reasonably well. It is particularly valuable to the surgeon, since he can perform the appropriate operation for the individual on the basis of findings at the operating table, which is not possible with grading systems based on gross configuration or degree of cellular dedifferentiation of the cancer. Dukes typing at the operating table is an approximation; final classification is done on the permanent histologic sections: Dukes type A, lesion confined to mucosa; type B-1, lesions extending into, but not through, muscularis propria, negative lymph nodes; type B-2, lesions penetrating the muscularis propria, negative nodes; type C-1, lesions limited to the wall, positive nodes; type C-2, lesions through all layers, positive nodes. There should also be added a type D, lesions with distant, unresectable metastases (liver, lung, spine).

Size of primary tumor does not correlate well with either incidence of metastasis or survival. Grinnell found a 23 percent incidence of metastasis from cancers 1.5 to 2.9 cm in diameter. The incidence rose to a peak of 53 percent in the 5 to 6.9-cm range and then decreased somewhat in larger tumors. Spratt and Ackerman found that single cancers of the colon are associated with the same frequency of metastasis to regional nodes whether they measure 2 to 3 cm in diameter or 7 to 12 cm in diameter. They also found that survival is independent of size with cancers larger than 1.5 cm in diameter. They made two significant observations: (1) even the very large colonic cancers are curable with a frequency comparable to that of small tumors provided that a circumscribing resection including contiguously involved organs together with the perirectal and mesocolic lymph nodes can be performed, and (2) the limited resection of a small invasive cancer is unwarranted, because 50 percent of the cancers of 3.12 cm diameter or smaller had lymph nodal metastases.

Despite advances in methods of diagnosis and techniques of treatment, the mortality rate in colorectal cancers has declined only very modestly over the past three decades. The chief cause of failure to achieve cure is presumed to be the occurrence of distant metastases beyond the area accessible to resection before the time of diagnosis and treatment. It is usually stated that the answer to the problem is earlier diagnosis—detection of malignant tumors prior to symptoms or signs which herald their presence. How much earlier would be early enough? When do distant metastases occur? How long are colon cancers present before they can be detected? Welin and associates determined the doubling time of colon tumors by serial barium enema radiography and found doubling times of colon cancer to range from 139 to 1,155 days. This probably gives a false impression, however, of the growth rate throughout the life of the tumor. The growth of microscopic tumors is thought to proceed exponentially until the tumor size approaches the limitations of nutrition, at which time apparent deceleration of net growth occurs. The doubling time of pulmonary metastases from colonic cancer may more closely reflect the true growth rate, since tumor necrosis is much less in the metastases than is often found in the primary growths. When the series of Welin et al. and of Collins were combined, the doubling time ranged from 34 days to infinity with a mean doubling time of 109 days. A minimum of 30 doublings is required for a single 10-μ malignant colonic mucosa cell to become a tumor 1 cm in diameter—the minimum size that can be detected clinically. Assuming a doubling time of 109 days, a 1-cm tumor would have been growing for over 9 years before detection as a small "early" cancer. Even the fastest growing tumor with a doubling time of 34 days would have been present for $2\frac{1}{2}$ years. The 1-cm nodule is small but not early. Tumors with long doubling times permit uncured patients to live clinically free of evidence of the disease and to contribute to "survival" figures.

CLINICAL MANIFESTATIONS. Symptoms of colorectal carcinoma depend on several factors including the anatomic location of the lesion, its size and extent, and the presence of complications such as obstruction, hemorrhage, or perforation. Some carcinomas are detected while patients are asymptomatic as part of a routine sigmoidoscopic and barium enema examination. Carcinomas arising in the right colon, left colon, and rectum produce characteristic, somewhat different symptom complexes.

The caliber of the cecum and ascending colon is about $2\frac{1}{2}$ times that of the left colon, and the fecal content is fluid. Thus obstructive symptoms are unusual despite the bulky polypoid lesions that are the most common type of tumor in this site. Dull, nagging, persistent right lower quadrant pain is frequent, as are symptoms of anemia. These include pallor, easy fatiguability, weakness, dizziness, dyspnea on exertion, and cardiac palpitation. Anorexia, indigestion, and weight loss are often presenting complaints. A mass in the right side of the abdomen is the first sign of disease in about 10 percent of patients with right colonic cancer. Obstructive symptoms are uncommon but do occur, particularly with hepatic flexure lesions. Severe symptoms such as excessive weight loss, cachexia, jaundice, and hepatomegaly usually imply far advanced cancer.

For purposes of grouping the symptom complexes of colorectal cancer, the left colon is considered to extend from the hepatic flexure to the rectosigmoid. The caliber of the lumen is smaller and the fecal content more solid in the left colon than the right. Cancers in the left colon are usually of the scirrhous or annular type, so that obstructive symptoms predominate. A change in bowel habits may be the first symptom noted with a progressive decrease in the caliber of the stools. Blood and mucus are seen in or on the stool. Severe anemia is uncommon but if present portends a poor prognosis. Tumors of the transverse colon and splenic flexure tend to invade adjacent structures. With gastric involvement, gastrocolic fistula may result. Complete intestinal obstruction may be the presenting picture in some patients.

Passage of bright red blood, often with mucus, is the most common symptom of rectal cancer. Since it frequently is the only symptom, the bleeding is often incorrectly attributed to hemorrhoids. With low rectal lesions there is often tenesmus and a feeling of incomplete evacuation. Obstructive symptoms are uncommon because of the large caliber of the rectal ampulla. Mild abdominal cramping may occur, but severe rectal pain usually means extensive local disease.

Examination of the abdomen of patients with colorectal cancer may disclose a palpable mass, extension to or involvement of the abdominal wall, umbilical metastasis, hepatomegaly, ascites, and a caput medusae. The general physical examination should include a thorough search for distant metastasis. If questionably involved nodes are found, they should be excised for histologic examination.

Digital examination of the rectum and sigmoidoscopy are done sequentially. If a rectal lesion is suspected, no preparation is indicated; for higher lesions, the colon is prepared as described later in this chapter. Carcinoma is usually easily diagnosed on digital examination because of the characteristic hard, rough, irregular surface. If no lesion is felt, the patient is asked to strain to bring higher lesions against the examining fingertip. Proctosigmoidoscopy is then done to the full length of the scope if possible. An adequate biopsy should be obtained from all suspicious lesions seen. Colitis cystica profunda may be confused with invasive carcinoma of the rectum, since mucus-filled glandular structures are seen microscopically in and below the muscularis. This rather rare entity, thought to be inflammatory but in any event not carcinomatous, occurs in a generalized form throughout the colon and in a localized form in the rectum.

DIAGNOSTIC STUDIES. Barium enema radiographic examination or colonoscopy is done next even though a lesion has been found on sigmoidoscopy, inasmuch as other lesions such as multiple polyps or a second primary tumor may be present at a higher level. Repeated examinations using air-contrast studies and oblique projections may be necessary. The "difficult" areas are the cecum, redundant sigmoid loop, and splenic flexure. A radiograph of a typical sigmoid carcinoma is shown in Fig. 28-7. The criteria for distinguishing carcinoma from diverticulitis are presented on page 1207. Colonoscopy has the advantage that a histologic diagnosis can be made by either biopsy or exfoliative cytology.

Patients with a histologic or clinical diagnosis of colo-

rectal cancer who are not categorically inoperable because of far advanced disseminated metastatic disease require further procedures to attempt to demonstrate any metastatic spread; to evaluate cardiac, pulmonary, and renal status; and to prepare the patient physically and mentally for operative therapy. The work-up should include determinations of serum electrolytes, plasma proteins and A/G ratio, blood urea nitrogen, 2-hour postprandial blood sugar, serum bilirubin, alkaline phosphatase, lactic dehydrogenase, and prothrombin time; radioisotope liver scan; electrocardiogram and radiography of the chest. Intravenous pyelography is done in patients with sigmoid colon lesions or any lesion elsewhere that is suspected of involving the urinary tract. Pulmonary function studies are done if indicated by clinical findings. Hemoglobin and plasma protein deficits are corrected by appropriate transfusion therapy.

TREATMENT. It is imperative that the surgeon have a frank discussion with the patient prior to operation, particularly if a colostomy will have to be done. A former patient who is well rehabilitated after cancer operation with colostomy can be very helpful.

Preoperative Preparation. There is unanimous agreement that preoperative mechanical cleansing of the gastrointestinal tract is important and desirable, and there is beginning to be some consensus on the role of preoperative intestinal antisepsis. Prospective, randomized, double-blind studies by Clarke, Condon, and associates, and by Washington and associates have clearly demonstrated that a preoperative oral antibiotic preparation significantly reduces the risk of septic complications after elective colorectal operations. Pseudomembranous enterocolitis from overgrowth of resistant species was not a problem. Many different antibiotic regimens are in use. One of the most popular consists of neomycin sulfate, 1 Gm, and erythromycin base, 1 Gm, at 1 P.M., 2 P.M., and 11 P.M. the day before operation.

Mechanical cleansing may be accomplished in 2 days unless significant obstruction exists. The patient is placed on a liquid or elemental diet, given a strong oral cathartic on each of two mornings before the operation, and given a saline enema the night before the operation. Nasogastric suction is usually not necessary.

Foley catheter drainage is instituted just prior to operation in all patients with lesions of the sigmoid or rectum. If ureteral involvement is suspected, then ureteral catheters may be inserted prior to operation, though this can be done during the procedure if it becomes necessary. The presence of the catheters facilitates identification of the ureters and thus avoidance of injury to them.

Operative Treatment. The abdomen is first thoroughly explored to determine the extent of intraabdominal spread if any. On the basis of these findings the decision is made as to whether a curative operation should be attempted.

After operability is determined, all lesions of the peritoneal colon are resected by the no-touch isolation technique with primary anastomosis (Fig. 28-10). This technique is designed to minimize hematogenous dissemination of cancers by the trauma of surgical removal. Turnbull and associates have reported a 5-year survival of 61 percent of patients resected for cure by this technique

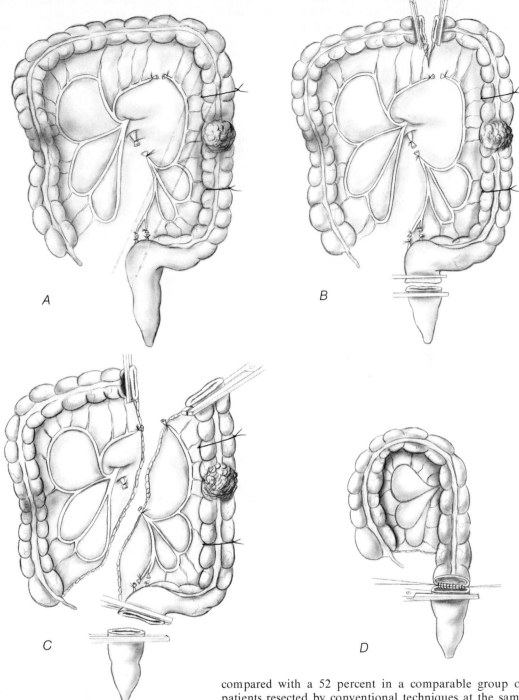

Fig. 28-10. No-touch isolation technique of anterior resection. *A.*
Major vascular pedicles are isolated and divided and tapes tied
tightly around colon and below lesion. *B.* Colon is divided at
elected sites of resection. *C.* Cancer-bearing segment is removed
last. *D.* End-to-end anastomosis is made. Posterior row is shown.
*(After R. B. Turnbull, K. Kyle, F. R. Watson, and J. Spratt, Ann
Surg, 166:420, 1967.)*

compared with a 52 percent in a comparable group of
patients resected by conventional techniques at the same
clinic. When corrected for age, the 5-year survival rate of
the patients of Turnbull and associates is 78 percent.

Recurrences due to implantation may be minimized by
the use of closed anastomosis, iodized suture, and copious
irrigation of the operative field with saline solution.

Extent of Resection. In an attempt to improve the results
of surgical therapy of colonic cancer, there was considerable enthusiasm in the late 1940s and early 1950s for
more radical operations. For example, radical left hemi-

colectomy instead of segmental resection was advised for left colon lesions. In this operation, the inferior mesenteric artery is divided at the aorta, thus achieving a wider resection of the lymph drainage area. The anticipated improvement was not forthcoming. Apparently, when metastases to lymph nodes near the origin of the inferior mesenteric artery has occurred, cancer cells have already spread beyond the reach of surgical procedures. Most surgeons then reverted to the former practice of segmental resection. There is now some renewed interest in wider resections, even subtotal colectomy, prompted by different considerations. First, a significant number of patients will have disease—second primaries, polyps, or diverticula—in segments other than that bearing the primary lesion. Second, Wright and associates found suture line recurrences in only 0.7 percent of patients with ileocolic anastomosis versus a 12 percent rate in patients with colocolic anastomosis. The mechanism is not known but may be related to the disappearance of rectal polyps after ileoproctostomy in patients with familial polyposis.

Now, more than ever, the well-worn cliché that the operation should be appropriate to the individual situation is applicable. The following list of resections applies to the majority of patients; greater or lesser procedures may be indicated in some patients. For cancers arising in the cecum, ascending colon, or hepatic flexure, the resection includes a short segment of terminal ileum, cecum, ascending colon, right half of the transverse colon, and ileocolic, right colic, and right branch of middle colic vessels with accompanying mesentery and greater omentum en bloc. Ileo-transverse colostomy restores gastrointestinal continuity.

Lesions in the mid-transverse colon are segmentally removed with the middle colic vessels. Both flexures must be mobilized to allow anastomosis. For cancers of the distal transverse colon or splenic flexure, the resection includes the transverse and descending colons along with middle colic and left colic vessels. The distal ascending colon is anastomosed to the proximal sigmoid colon. A more conservative resection would leave the right branch of the middle colic artery and join proximal transverse colon to distal descending colon.

For cancers of the descending colon, the segment supplied by the left colic vessels is removed, from distal transverse colon to proximal sigmoid colon.

For cancers of the sigmoid and most proximal rectosigmoid the resection includes distal descending colon, sigmoid and proximal rectosigmoid, with sigmoidal and superior hemorrhoidal vessels. The left colic vessels remain; the inferior mesenteric vessels are skeletonized to remove as much lymphatic tissue as possible. Distal descending colon is anastomosed to rectosigmoid. Mobilization of the splenic flexure may be necessary to be able to bring the ends together without tension. A temporary proximal colostomy or cecostomy is advisable when there is any question about a low anastomosis.

Emergency Operations. When surgical treatment must be carried out on unprepared bowel because of obstruction, perforation, or hemorrhage or when a colorectal cancer is encountered unexpectedly, most surgeons prefer to proceed with the definitive resection if the lesion is in the right half of the colon. Some surgeons are also doing emergency primary resections of left colon lesions. With lesions of the left half of the colon, most surgeons prefer to resect the lesion and bring both cut ends of the colon out—the proximal as an end colostomy, the distal as a mucous fistula. If the distal end is too short to exteriorize, the Hartmann procedure is used. Proximal diverting colostomy alone is the procedure of choice for obstruction in poor-risk patients. The 5-year survival rate is low in patients with perforating cancers in all segments and in those with obstructing cancers of the right colon.

Palliative Operations. If unresectable metastases preclude curative resection, a palliative resection should be done if the lesion is locally resectable. This does not lengthen survival but greatly improves the quality of survival. If the primary lesion is locally unresectable, a short-circuiting anastomosis around the lesion offers worthwhile palliation. Even a colostomy is usually preferable to death from intestinal obstruction.

Operations for Rectal Carcinoma. There is general agreement that lesions above the posterior peritoneal reflection, which is about 15 cm above the dentate line, can and should be treated by anterior resection with primary anastomosis (Fig. 28-10). There is also general agreement that lesions at or below 5.5 cm in women and 7 cm in men should be treated by the Miles procedure, combined abdominoperineal resection (Fig. 28-11). This is because it

Fig. 28-11. Abdominoperineal resection. *A.* Peritoneal cavity is entered through a paramedian or oblique incision. *B.* Lateral attachment of sigmoid colon is incised, taking care to avoid the ureter. *C.* Medial reflection of transverse mesocolon is incised. Inferior mesenteric artery and vein are transected. *D.* Peritoneal reflection between bladder and rectum is transected, and an anterior plane between these two organs is established. *E.* Posterior dissection is carried out in midline digitally. The finger establishes a plane just anterior to the anterior surface of the sacrum and continues the dissection as far caudad as possible. *F.* The lateral attachment of the rectum, including the middle hemorrhoidal vessels, is transected. These vessels are, at times, of sufficient size to require individual ligatures. G_1. Pelvic floor is reperitonealized. The distal colon and rectum are now caudad to the peritoneal floor. The proximal colon is mobilized so that a colostomy may be established without undue tension. G_2. Sagittal section demonstrating that distal colon resides below reperitonealized pelvic floor. *H.* With the patient in lithotomy position or on his side, the anal orifice is closed with a purse-string suture and a circumferential elliptical incision made in the perianal region. I_1. Dissection carried down to coccyx and the posterior dissection is continued until it communicates with the space anterior to the sacrum which has been established previously transabdominally. The levator muscles are then transected on each side. I_2. Distal colon is brought down into the anal wound and dissection carried between it and the prostate or bladder. *J.* Specimen resected and drain inserted into depth of wound. Multiple Penrose drains may be used, or a Foley catheter may be inserted and the deep tissues closed around it. K_1. Abdominal incision is closed and colostomy brought out through separate stab wounds. K_2. Perineal incision closed with Foley catheter brought out through depth of wound.

The abdominal and perineal portions of this operation may be carried out simultaneously with two teams. The patient is initially positioned on his back with the legs out in stirrups. This approach has resulted in a reduction in operating time and blood loss.

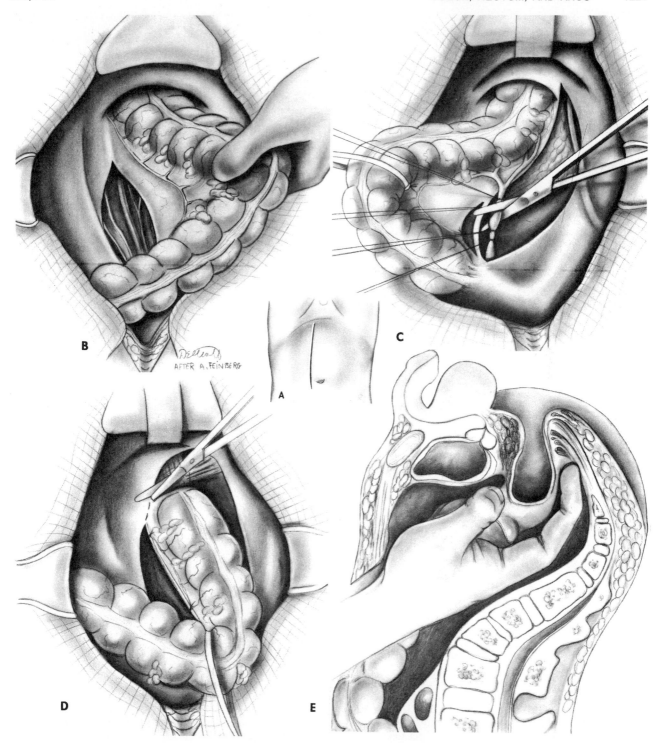

is not possible to resect with the mandatory 4-cm distal margin of normal tissue, perform an anastomosis, and have fecal continence postoperatively. Though abdominoperineal resection was first done by Czerny in 1883, it was Miles who perfected and popularized the procedure. It is the standard by which all other procedures for rectal cancer must be measured. The principal drawback is of course,

the permanent colostomy. It is also attended by a significant morbidity (see below). A simultaneous abdominal and perineal approach utilizing two surgical teams is widely used in England and is gaining favor in the United States, because it shortens operative time and also decreases blood loss. Abdominoperineal resection in the female should probably include in-continuity resection of the posterior

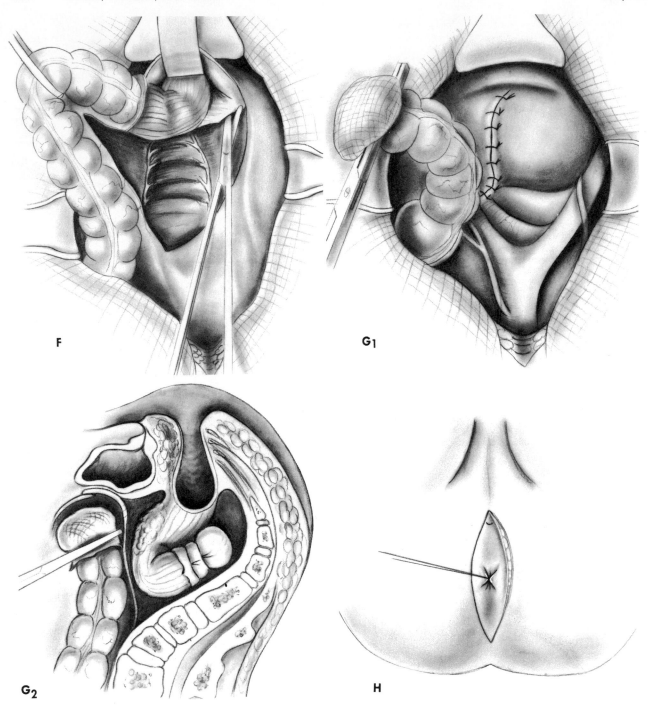

F

G₁

G₂

H

wall of the vagina, broad ligaments, cul-de-sac, uterus, tubes, ovaries, and cardinal ligaments, because of the abundant lymphatic connections from the rectum to the female genitalia.

Carcinoma of the rectum involving the lower urinary tract should be treated in good-risk patients by complete pelvic exenteration. The preferred procedure is left-sided colostomy and urinary diversion to an ileal segment draining through the right side of the abdomen. The mortality rate is under 20 percent; the 5-year survival rate is 30

percent in those surviving the procedure. Electrocoagulation has been advocated as an alternative to abdominoperineal resection for low-lying rectal cancer. Madden and Kandalaft have treated 77 patients by this method. The number followed for 5 years is too small to be significant, but earlier results at least equal and may surpass those of resection. Crile and Turnbull have carried on the electrocoagulation studies of Jones. Their 5-year survival rate is 68 percent in 62 patients, compared to 46 percent in a roughly comparable group treated by resection. Mucosal

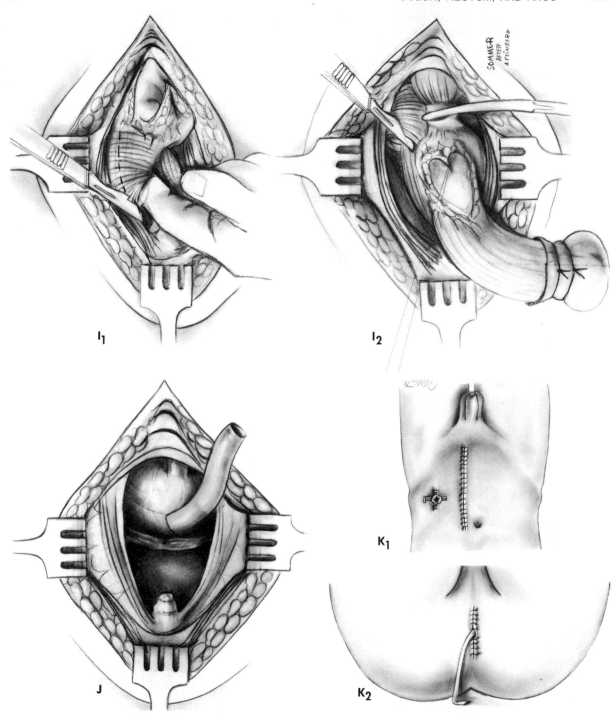

and polypoid lesions are most amenable to electrocoagulation. Anterior wall lesions in women should be resected because of the threat of rectovaginal fistula. Similarly, annular lesions are rarely controlled by local treatment, and stricture may result. If repeated electrocoagulation does not control the lesion within 6 months, abdominoperineal resection can still be done with as good prospects of cure as if it had been resected initially.

Radiotherapy administered directly to the lesion through a sigmoidoscope-like device has been used by Papillon. This technique is applicable as definitive therapy in small superficial lesions or as preoperative therapy in more invasive lesions.

The proximal rectum and the rectosigmoid lesions—from about 6 to 15 cm—constitute a gray zone where there is no unanimity of opinion as to the best operative procedure. Many surgeons still prefer abdominoperineal resection, feeling that the alternative procedures do not offer the patient an adequate "cancer operation." Statistical results do not confirm this; in general, the 5-year survival is about the same for low anterior resection and pull-through as for the Miles procedure.

Low anterior resection below the peritoneal reflection is technically difficult, particularly in the narrow male pelvis. The side-to-end technique described by Baker is often technically easier than end-to-end anastomosis. Aside from the technical aspects the principal drawback of low anterior resection is an incidence of anastomotic leak of about 25 percent; thus a proximal decompressing temporary colostomy is often advisable.

The pull-through operation has never attained popularity even though results equal the Miles procedure and permanent colostomy is avoided. A principal drawback is the fact that some patients do not regain fecal continence, and a perineal colostomy is much worse than an abdominal colostomy. Also, a surgeon who does not do a large volume of rectal surgery probably cannot attain the technical proficiency required to perform this procedure with consistent success. The modified Soave and Boley pull-through operation described by Gardner and associates may well prove to be the preferred pull-through technique.

Localio has described a combined approach to midrectal cancer. The abdominal dissection is done as in the Miles procedure. The rectum is then approached through a posterior transacral route. After resection of the lesion, the proximal colon is anastomosed primarily to the distal rectal stump. He has reported on 50 patients, with one operative death, seven anastomotic leaks, and fecal continence in all.

Several randomized, controlled prospective studies are now being conducted to evaluate the usefulness of preoperative radiation therapy in the treatment of carcinoma of the rectum. These studies were stimulated, in large part, by the report of a retrospective analysis of 971 patients who underwent resection for carcinoma of the rectum, one-half of whom had received from 1,200 to 2,000 rads, tissue dose of x-radiation, preoperatively. Patients with Dukes A and B lesions were not benefited; irradiated patients with Dukes C lesions had a 37 percent 5-year survival rate as compared to 23 percent for Dukes C controls. The same authors could not confirm this in a later randomized study.

A cooperative, prospective study by Higgins and collaborators randomized 700 patients with carcinoma of the rectum or rectosigmoid to be given either radiotherapy prior to operation (2,000 to 2,500 rads in 2 weeks) or the operation alone. Five-year survival was 48.5 percent in the radiated group, compared to 38.8 percent in controls. With low-lying lesions requiring abdominoperineal resection, survival was 46.9 in the treated group versus 34.3 percent in the controls. Although suggestive of a treatment benefit, neither finding is statistically significant.

There have been several trials of adjuvant chemotherapy with operation utilizing triethylenethiophosphoramide, 5-fluorouracil, or 5-fluorodeoxyuridine. No significant benefit was shown in any of the trials. Current trials of adjuvant therapy are evaluating combination drug therapy or combined postoperative radiotherapy-chemotherapy.

Mortality and Morbidity. The operative mortality of abdominoperineal resection varies in large reported series from 4 to 20 percent, with a mean of about 8 percent. The mortality of anterior resection is somewhat less, ranging from 2.4 to 20 percent, with a mean of about 5 percent. The morbidity of both procedures is formidable: from 25 to 68 percent for the Miles procedure, and from 15 to 56 percent for anterior resection. Morbidity in anterior resection is inversely proportional to the level at which it is done: the lower the resection, the higher the morbidity. It also correlates with whether or not proximal colostomy is done. Significant urinary tract obstruction or infection occurs in about 35 percent of patients after the Miles procedure, in about 15 percent after anterior resection. Aside from the cardiovascular and pulmonary complications that attend major surgery in this age group, septic complications loom large. The perineal wound is the principal site in the combined procedure, followed by the abdominal incision. Inadvertent perforation during the pelvic dissection contributes to the septic problems. Breakdown of the anastomosis is the principal source of sepsis after anterior resection. The incidence is higher than generally realized. Goligher and associates studied 73 patients in the early postoperative period by digital examination, sigmoidoscopy, and barium enema. Anastomotic dehiscence was detected in 40 percent after high anterior resection and in 69 percent after low anterior resection! Many of these were not serious, but Slanetz and associates had 35 symptomatic leaks in 247 patients after anterior resection—a rate of 17 percent. The use of drains near the anastomosis increases the incidence of dehiscence. Goldstein and Duff found an incidence of 23.1 percent in patients in whom the anastomosis was drained, but only 7.8 percent if no drain was used. Intestinal anastomoses must fulfill three criteria: no tension on the suture line, adequate blood supply, and minimal encroachment on the lumen. Whenever anastomosis is performed under less than ideal conditions, such as in the presence of infection or significant contamination, or low in the pelvis, a proximal decompressing colostomy or cecostomy should be done even though this means that another procedure may be necessary for closure. If anastomotic leak occurs or is strongly suspected, immediate reoperation is often indicated, though minor leaks may close with nonoperative therapy.

Pseudomembranous enterocolitis is an infrequent, serious complication. Preoperative bowel sterilization and systemic broad-spectrum antibiotics increase the hazard of this postoperative complication developing.

Wound complications, i.e., hemorrhage or hematoma, infection, and dehiscence, are fairly frequent. These may be minimized by meticulous hemostasis; changing gowns, gloves, drapes, and instruments before closing the incision; irrigating the wound, layer by layer, with a dilute antibiotic solution; and the use of retention sutures.

Urinary complications occur in at least 35 percent of patients after abdominoperineal resection. Nearly all have difficulty in voiding in the immediate postoperative period. After removal of the retention catheter, residual urine volume after voiding should be determined to make certain the bladder is emptying adequately. Transurethral resection is sometimes required if inadequate voiding persists. Most men are impotent after abdominoperineal resection for carcinoma secondary to injury of the autonomic nerve supply to the genital organs.

PROGNOSIS. The 5-year survival rates following curative resection are essentially the same for all segments of the colon. Rectal cancer has a somewhat lower overall survival rate because of a lower resectable-for-cure rate.

The 5-year survival rate in patients with carcinomas limited to the bowel wall and with no demonstrated metastases is 80 percent. The rate with disease extending through the bowel wall but with no evidence of metastasis is 71 percent. With disease in the bowel wall and lymph node metastases, the rate drops to 32 percent. With disseminated disease, only 1.2 percent live 5 years. Considering all stages of disease together, the absolute 5-year survival rate is 34 percent, and the determinate 5-year survival rate is 40 percent.

The above prognosis figures are from a compilation of published reports. They may be somewhat optimistic because of the human tendency to publish more favorable results.

Recurrent Disease. Since only 30 to 40 percent of patients with colorectal cancer are relieved of the disease by surgical therapy, it follows that 60 to 70 percent have recurrent disease. This is a very trying problem for patient and physician because of the often painful, debilitating, demoralizing symptoms produced by recurrent disease, and the lack of any really effective palliative therapy.

Wangensteen et al. and Griffen and associates have attempted to improve the outlook in colorectal cancer with lymph node metastases by routine abdominal exploration in asymptomatic patients at 6-month intervals. Seven percent of the patients found to have cancer at second-look operations were freed of the disease. However, the operative mortality (by patient) was also 7 percent, and there was often difficulty in detecting residual cancer.

Local recurrence in the bowel, usually at or near the anastomosis, can occasionally be resected with reanastomosis. Unresectable disease should be bypassed if possible; with distal lesions that preclude anastomosis below the lesion, proximal colostomy usually gives worthwhile symptomatic palliation.

The efficacy of the chemotherapeutic agents 5FU, 5FUDR, and methotrexate in the palliation of disseminated colorectal carcinoma has been evaluated by a cooperative group study. The results give small comfort. Requirements for admission to the study were stringent in order to obtain valid results, thus often excluding patients who most needed help. Overall response rate was about 15 percent with some very gratifying remissions. But drug toxicity was a major problem and was seen in 93 percent of the 134 patients, with seven fatalities. Furthermore, harm (in addition to fatality) may have been done to some of the 85 percent of the nonresponders. The response rates are just about as good and the toxicity much less on an ambulatory treatment schedule of one dose weekly. Current trials involve multiple drug therapy or combined chemotherapy-radiotherapy.

Metastases from colorectal carcinoma to the liver, too

extensive to be resected, have been treated with modest success by chronic infusion of 5FU into the hepatic artery.

Radiation therapy is usually not helpful in treating recurrences, because colorectal carcinomas are only moderately radiosensitive tumors whereas the liver and normal gastrointestinal mucosa do not tolerate radiation very well; anorexia, severe nausea, and diarrhea often result. Radiotherapy, however, sometimes gives good symptomatic relief in localized painful perineal recurrences after abdominoperineal resection and very often relieves pain in solitary skeletal metastases.

EARLY DETECTION. Sixty to seventy percent of persons who develop carcinoma of the colon or rectum will die of the disease. Most investigators agree that it is unlikely that changes in operative technique, chemotherapy, or radiotherapy will lead to a dramatic improvement in prognosis. But there is also agreement that improvement could be attained if presently available treatment modalities could be applied to localized disease, if the diagnosis could be made before clinical symptoms are obvious and the disease far advanced. Routine sigmoidoscopy of asymptomatic patients has been advocated; recent reports, however, are disenchanting. In seven published series, sigmoidoscopic examination of 50,727 asymptomatic patients detected invasive carcinoma in 0.11 percent. The incidence of polyps was 5 to 7 percent. If one holds that polyps have a negligible malignant potential, then it would appear that a yield of 1 cancer per 900 sigmoidoscopies would hardly justify the time, expense, and patient discomfort. If, however, one feels that all polyps will eventually undergo malignant change, then a 5 to 7 percent yield would certainly make the procedure worthwhile. On the basis of currently available evidence the authors feel that the use of sigmoidoscopy as a screening method is unrealistic. It should, however, continue to be done as an essential part of a complete physical examination for all patients over age forty.

Gold and Freedman in 1965 described an antigen present in the serum of patients with colorectal cancer, in extracts of the carcinomas and in fetal colonic mucosa, but absent from extracts of normal colonic mucosa. This carcinoembryonic antigen (CEA) can be detected in serum in the millimicrogram (nanogram) range by radioimmune assay. It was hoped that at last a blood test for colorectal cancer would be available. Gold and Freedman's findings have been confirmed by several groups, but the findings are not specific for colorectal cancer and not invariably positive in all patients with colorectal cancer. The results vary from about 20 percent positive with localized colorectal cancer to 100 percent with advanced metastatic cancer. Cancers of the pancreas, lung, breast, and other areas sometimes give positive results, certain nonneoplastic diseases such as uremia or cirrhosis also give some positive results, and, most significant, there have been some false positives in persons with no detectable disease. Thus the CEA cannot be used as a screening test because of the considerable number of false positives. Its principal use now is to monitor patients who have had a curative resection. Reversion to normal after operation is a hopeful sign that all tumor was removed. A rising CEA titer usually means recurrent disease. Serial determinations are of value in monitoring the efficacy of palliative therapy.

Chemical determination of occult blood in the stool is a simple, inexpensive screening method for lesions involving the gastrointestinal mucosa. If three consecutive stools are negative for occult blood in patients on meat-free, high-residue diets, nothing further need be done. All patients with positive reactions should undergo complete gastrointestinal work-up. Greegor, in a recent study, did stool studies for 900 patients, 5 percent of whom had positive stools. One percent of the entire group had an asymptomatic colon cancer, 2 percent had diverticulosis, and 1 percent had nonmalignant polyps. Greegor feels that every adult should have this screening test annually. The aesthetic problem of having patients bring stool specimens to the office is solved by the use of commercially available test slides that the patients can prepare at home and mail to the office. If properly done, stool examination is a much more realistic screening procedure for gastrointestinal carcinoma than is sigmoidoscopy.

Uncommon Neoplasms of the Colon and Rectum

CARCINOID

These interesting tumors are rare in the colon and uncommon in the rectum, about 2 percent of all gastrointestinal carcinoids occurring in the colon and 17 percent in the rectum. This probably does not represent true frequency, because small asymptomatic lesions are easily found in the rectum by sigmoidoscopy. Carcinoids of the colon and rectum very rarely cause the malignant carcinoid syndrome, which is usually associated with carcinoids of the ileum (Chap. 27).

Carcinoids smaller than 1 cm in diameter in the colon rarely cause symptoms, are very rarely malignant, and, because they are submucosal, rarely can be seen on barium enema. If found incidentally, they may safely be removed by wedge excision. The incidence of invasive malignancy in carcinoids, unlike adenocarcinoma of the colon, correlates well with size. Most carcinoids larger than 1 cm that produce symptoms are malignant, and more than half have nodal metastases at the time of diagnosis. Clinical and radiographic manifestations of symptomatic carcinoids are essentially the same as in adenocarcinoma of the colon. A definitive cancer resection is done if liver metastases are not demonstrable. Worthwhile palliation is often attained in patients with unresectable disease by resection of the primary. Some have lived in relative comfort for many years with residual disease.

Most rectal carcinoids are small, asymptomatic, yellow-gray nodules found incidentally at sigmoidoscopy. Larger lesions may bleed and cause rectal pain. Rectal lesions, unless frankly malignant clinically, should be completely excised transanally with the deep margin extending into the muscularis propria. The diagnosis of malignancy is based on invasion; cytologic criteria are unreliable. If invasive malignancy is found, abdominoperineal resection is indicated.

LYMPHOMA AND LYMPHOSARCOMA

Benign lymphoma occurs in the rectum and rectosigmoid as a polypoid circumscribed proliferation of the lymphoid tissue of the mucosa. These polyps, often mistaken grossly for adenomatous polyps, are generally single, but about 15 percent of patients have two or more. These lesions have no known malignant potential. Simple excision is adequate therapy.

Lymphosarcoma may involve the colon and rectum as part of generalized disease or as the dominant organ in "localized" disease. Reticulum cell and giant follicular lymphosarcoma predominate, though all cell types are seen. Longitudinal extent of involvement varies from a localized tumor to diffuse disease of the entire large bowel. Symptoms are abdominal pain, marked weight loss, and change in bowel habits. An abdominal mass is usually palpable. The radiologic diagnosis is frequently carcinoma unless involvement is extensive. If colonic involvement is part of widespread disease, no surgical therapy is indicated. The colonic lesions respond to irradiation and/or chemotherapy. Disease grossly limited to the bowel should be widely resected along with as much node-bearing mesentery as possible, since nodal involvement is common. The optimal timing for postoperative irradiation is not clear. Some feel that it should be given routinely in the immediate postoperative period; others prefer to wait. If and when the disease recurs, then irradiation therapy is given. The disease is unresectable for cure in the majority of patients, but when it is localized, the 5-year survival rate is about 50 percent.

LEIOMYOMA, LEIOMYOSARCOMA, AND OTHER TUMORS

Leiomyomas and leiomyosarcomas are very rare tumors of the colon and rectum, occurring much less frequently than in the stomach or small intestine. Leiomyomas are more frequent in reported series than their malignant counterpart by a 2:1 ratio. When symptomatic, they cause obstruction and bleeding. Deep ulceration with massive hemorrhage, such as occurs with lesions in the stomach or small intestine, has not been reported in lesions of colon or rectum. So few of these tumors are seen that rules of treatment are not yet formulated. Local excision of leiomyomas and small low-grade leiomyosarcomas is probably sufficient. Frank leiomyosarcomas are usually treated by the same procedures as carcinomas of the same area. The 5-year survival in lesions resected for cure is 30 to 40 percent.

Other rare sarcomas of the colon include rhabdomyosarcoma, fibrosarcoma, and hemangiopericytoma. Rare benign tumors include neurofibroma, eosinophilic granuloma, granular cell myoblastoma, lymphangioma, hemangioma, and lipoma. Their principal importance is that they may be mistaken for malignant lesions and are widely resected needlessly.

ENDOMETRIOSIS

Though not a neoplasm, endometriosis is included in this section because it may simulate cancer of the distal colon. The term *endometriosis* implies the occurrence of endometrial tissue at sites other than the lining of the corpus uteri. Ectopic endometrial tissue is found at the time of pelvic operation in 8 to 20 percent of women between the age of twenty and the menopause. The earliest reported case was in a sixteen-year-old; the oldest was seventy-eight years old. About 25 percent of patients with endometriosis have colonic involvement.

Endometrial ectopia is thought by most to result from influx of endometrial tissue through the fallopian tubes during menstruation. This hypothesis has been questioned, because menstrual endometrium may not be viable tissue—it has not been successfully transplanted. The hypothesis of lymphatic dissemination of endometrial emboli has some adherents. Others believe that serosal cells of the peritoneum, derived from the same embryonic tissue as the endometrium, undergo metaplasia and produce tissue identical with endometrium.

PATHOLOGY. The lesions of endometriosis, grossly and microscopically, essentially are identical to the normal uterine lining. These lesions also menstruate with the uterus, but since there is no cervix to drain off the effluvium, glands and cysts filled with menstrual blood are formed. Rupture of the cysts, with spillage of its irritating contents, produces dense reactive fibrosis. Spillage of viable cells produces new implants and spread of the fibroplastic process.

The frequency of endometrial implants varies with distance from the uterus. Most frequently and most heavily involved are external surface of the uterus, broad ligaments, ovaries, cul-de-sac, rectosigmoid, rectovaginal septum, rectum, and sigmoid colon. Colonic lesions may be a single discrete implant (endometrioma) in or on the wall of the bowel, or involvement may be diffuse and extensive, and completely surround the bowel.

CLINICAL MANIFESTATIONS. Symptoms may be present only at the time of menstruation or, if present throughout the cycle, are exacerbated at or just before the period. More common symptoms include gradually increasing dysmenorrhea, menstrual irregularities, rectal discomfort or pain on defecation, rectal tenesmus, lower abdominal cramps, constipation or diarrhea, abdominal distension, nausea, and dysuria. Less common are rectal bleeding and symptoms of intestinal obstruction, usually partial but occasionally complete. There is increased incidence of infertility in these patients.

Vaginal examination often reveals a general matting and nodular thickening of the pelvic organs. Speculum examination frequently discloses purplish submucosal nodules of varying size, which should be biopsied. Rectovaginal examination often demonstrates the same somewhat tender nodular thickening of the septum. On digital rectal examination, tenderness may be felt anteriorly at the fingertip, representing cul-de-sac lesions. Pelvic and rectal examinations should be repeated at different phases of the menstrual cycle, since cyclic changes in the findings help confirm the diagnosis.

Sigmoidoscopy is usually unrewarding except to note that the procedure causes more discomfort than usual and that intrinsic lesions are absent. It is usually impossible to introduce the sigmoidoscope beyond about 15 cm; some narrowing of the lumen may be seen.

The roentgenographic manifestations of endometriosis of the colorectum are not pathognomonic. Any lesion, benign or malignant, which seeds the pelvic peritoneum can mimic endometriosis. Changes in the rectosigmoid and sigmoid are those of extrinsic pressure with the picture of invasion of the outer layers without mucosal distortion or infiltration. A solitary endometrioma may be indistinguishable from neoplasm, particularly if located in a part of the bowel that is difficult to visualize adequately.

TREATMENT. If symptoms are mild, no treatment is necessary. With more severe symptoms, suppression of menstruation with gradually increasing doses of a combination birth-control pill, given continuously without cycling, for 6 to 9 months usually causes regression of the lesions and relief of symptoms. Exploratory laparotomy is indicated if the clinical evaluation does not exclude the possibility of neoplasm. Bowel resection is very rarely indicated. Solitary endometriomas that encroach on the lumen can be removed by anterior resection. If the disease is so severe and extensive that bowel function is compromised, a temporary colostomy is done and the patient placed on hormonal therapy as outlined above. After regression of lesions, the colostomy is closed. If lesions do not regress satisfactorily, however, then hysterectomy and bilateral salpingo-oophorectomy should be done. Abdominoperineal resection and permanent colostomy are not justified.

VOLVULUS

Volvulus of the colon results from rotation of a segment of bowel about its mesenteric axis sufficient to produce partial or complete obstruction of the lumen. Varying degrees of circulatory impairment of the twisted segment are produced by the twisting of the root of the mesentery and secondarily by progressive distension of the involved loop. Volvulus can occur only in a freely movable segment of bowel with its points of fixation in close approximation and thus is seen principally (90 percent) in the sigmoid colon, less frequently (10 percent) in the cecum. Volvulus of the transverse colon is very rare and usually a complication of megacolon. In the United States, volvulus is the third most common cause of colonic obstruction, is the leading cause of strangulated obstruction of the colon, and accounts for about 4 percent of all colonic obstructions.

Sigmoid Volvulus

A redundant sigmoid loop attached by a narrow mesenteric root is the *sine qua non* of sigmoid volvulus. In Eastern Europe, where volvulus is common, barium studies have shown that the sigmoid redundancy is present at an early age and so is presumed to be a congenital rather than an acquired condition. Congenital megacolon (Hirschsprung's disease), which is due to congenital absence of ganglion cells in the rectosigmoid, may be present in subclinical form throughout life. This probably accounts

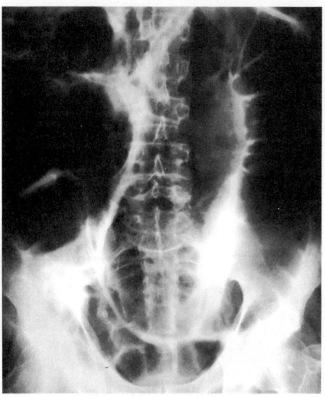

Fig. 28-12. Plain film of sigmoid volvulus, showing the greatly distended, horseshoe-shaped sigmoid loop (*right*) and distended cecum and ascending colon (*left*).

for only a small percentage of cases of sigmoid volvulus, however. In some parts of the world, acquired megacolon is a complication of Chagas' disease.

A history of severe chronic constipation can be elicited in nearly all patients with sigmoid volvulus in the United States. Dilatation and lengthening of the chronically destended colon occurs. This is most marked in the sigmoid colon. Chronic constipation of this magnitude and sigmoid volvulus are seen principally in two groups: The first includes patients of any age with severe psychiatric or neurologic diseases, such as parkinsonism; in some series, over one-half of the patients with sigmoid volvulus were inmates of mental institutions. The second group consists of the elderly, more often men than women, many with serious cardiovascular and pulmonary disease attendant upon their advanced age, who are now leading lives of inactivity. It is distinctly uncommon for sigmoid volvulus to occur in a person who leads an active life and who has no serious mental or physical illness.

CLINICAL MANIFESTATIONS. Symptoms of acute sigmoid volvulus are intermittent, cramping lower abdominal pain, progressive marked abdominal distension, complete obstipation, and absence of flatus. Nausea, vomiting, and dehydration occur after several hours. The majority of patients have had similar episodes in the past that spontaneously terminated by passage of large amounts of flatus and stool with relief of pain and distension. Marked abdominal distension and tympany are the most striking

physical findings. Respiratory embarrassment may be present because of extreme distension and elevation of the diaphram. Severe, constant abdominal pain and a shock syndrome usually mean strangulated obstruction.

DIAGNOSTIC FINDINGS. Plain film of the abdomen nearly always shows a spectacularly distended single loop occupying the left half of the abdomen with both ends in the pelvis and the bow at or near the diaphragm (Fig. 28-12.) This was called "bent inner-tube sign" before the advent of tubeless tires. The right half of the abdomen shows variable distension of the colon proximal to the obstruction and of small bowel, depending on the duration of the obstruction. Barium enema radiography is usually not necessary, unless the findings on plain films are atypical. The barium column ends at the level of the distal sigmoid torsion in a pathognomic twisted bird's beak or ace-of-spades deformity.

TREATMENT. General principles of management are discussed in Chap. 24. There are two specific problems in sigmoid volvulus: management of the acute episode and definitive management of the megasigmoid. Until about 1950, preferred management of nonstrangulated volvulus was operative detorsion of the sigmoid loop followed as soon as possible by elective sigmoid resection, because when only detorsion was performed, the volvulus recurred in up to 90 percent of patients. The combined mortality of the two-stage detorsion-resection management was 20 to 30 percent. Primary resection of sigmoid volvulus was tried by some but was attended by a mortality rate of at least 50 percent. Gradually, nonoperative detorsion followed by elective resection has emerged as the preferred management for nonstrangulated sigmoid volvulus. Sigmoidoscopy is done to visualize the site of distal sigmoid obstruction; only rarely is this beyond the reach of the 25-cm scope. If frank mucosal ulceration, or slough, or dark blood are seen, strangulation obstruction is probable, and emergency operative intervention is indicated. But if no signs of strangulation are seen, a well-lubricated long rectal tube is gently advanced via the sigmoidoscope through the obstructing twist into the distended sigmoid loop. Dramatic deflation usually results. (The sigmoidoscopist must be alert, or the result will be dramatic for him too!) The tube is secured in place in the loop by taping to the buttocks and left in place for 2 or 3 days, until bowel function resumes. Patients must be closely watched for signs of gangrenous bowel, which occasionally is present but unrecognized at the time of tube deflation. There is a small but definite risk of perforating the weakened sigmoid wall with the tube. Attempted tube deflation is successful in 80 to 90 percent of patients; the mortality rate is about 2 percent. Elective resection with primary anastomosis should be done as soon as the patient can be properly prepared, preferably within a week or so, because the risk of recurrent volvulus is so great. Not infrequently, the volvulus recurs while the patient is being prepared for elective resection. The mortality rate of elective resection is 8 to 10 percent. This higher rate for elective resection of volvulus than for other colonic problems is chiefly attributable to the age, debility, and concomitant disease that so many of these patients have.

When strangulation of the twisted loop exists or is suspected, emergency operation is required. If strangulation is not found, simple operative detorsion is done, but if strangulation is found, the nonviable bowel must be resected, and the proximal end brought out as a colostomy. When the distal limb is too short to allow exteriorization, a Hartmann procedure is preferred: normal bowel below the nonviable loop is divided, the distal end is oversewn and dropped back. The mortality rate for emergency resection of strangulated sigmoid volvulus is about 50 percent.

Cecal Volvulus

Volvulus of the sigmoid and of the cecum have in common only the pathogenetic mechanism of twisting of a mobile segment of bowel. Their etiology, clinical manifestations, and treatment are quite different.

Hypofixation of the cecum, terminal ileum, and proximal ascending colon is the prerequisite for cecal volvulus. Normally, the attachments to the posterior abdominal wall preclude volvulus. Rotation of the hypermobile cecum, usually 360° or up to 720° around the mesenteric pedicle of the ileocolic artery, produces a closed-loop obstruction. Circulatory impairment of the loop is frequent and occurs early in the course. A second mechanism has been suggested and may play a role in patients with partial intermittent cecal obstruction. This is a simple folding instead of twisting, with the mobile cecum pointing toward the left upper quadrant, producing partial obstruction of terminal ileum proximally and ascending colon distad.

Volvulus of the cecum is seen at all ages but is most frequent in the twenty-five to thirty-five age group.

CLINICAL MANIFESTATIONS. The clinical manifestations are essentially those of acute small bowel obstruction. Onset is rapid and characterized by severe midabdominal colicky pain, nausea, and vomiting, followed by moderate abdominal distension. The pain, intermittent and cramping early, may become a constant, severe burning pain within a few hours. Some gas and feces may be passed after onset of pain as the existing contents of the colon are eliminated, but complete obstipation and absence of flatus ensue. Physical findings may be only those of acute small bowel obstruction (Chap. 24), or there may be, in addition, hyperresonance of percussion in the right lower quadrant. Severe peritoneal signs indicate that strangulation is present.

DIAGNOSTIC FINDINGS. An abdominal plain film is often pathognomic but may be confusing unless one remembers that lack of lateral fixation allows the mobile cecum to be seen anywhere in the abdomen. Characteristically a large midabdominal ovoid dilated segment is seen, with distended small bowel loops and a relatively empty large bowel. Barium enema is usually not necessary and is not diagnostic, although it does indicate where the obstruction is located.

TREATMENT. Operation is indicated as soon as the patient can be prepared. Conservative measures cannot untwist the loop, and the hazard of strangulation in the closed-loop obstruction is great. Detorsion of the segment and suture fixation of the mobile cecum to the lateral gutter suffices if the cecum is viable. Right colectomy with ileo-

transverse colostomy is done for strangulation obstruction and for recurrent volvulus. Exteriorization obstructive resection is justified in moribund patients with gangrenous bowel.

The mortality rate for cecal volvulus is still about 10 percent, principally because of delay in diagnosis and treatment until strangulation obstruction with gangrenous bowel has supervened.

MEGACOLON

The term *megacolon,* meaning large colon, should also imply chronic dilation, elongation, and hypertrophy of the colon. Megacolon may be congenital or acquired. Acquired megacolon may be due to organic causes or may be idiopathic. The common denominator in megacolon is chronic partial colon obstruction with associated chronic constipation. In general the degree of megacolon is proportional to the duration of the partial obstruction. Megacolon is of interest to surgeons not only because many patients require surgical correction but also because of the propensity for volvulus in patients with megacolon.

Congenital Megacolon (Hirschsprung's Disease)

This disease is due to congenital absence of ganglion cells in the myenteric plexus of the bowel. The rectosigmoid is frequently involved, but the aganglionosis is sometimes more extensive, even involving the entire colon. The functional defect is the inability of the aganglionic segment to relax to allow a peristaltic wave to pass, thus producing a functional partial obstruction with proximal retention of feces, which in turn causes megacolon above the aganglionic segment. This is primarily a disease of infants and children (Chap. 39) but occasionally may not become manifest until later in life. It is therefore advisable, whenever performing operations for megacolon or volvulus, to have a frozen section of colon examined for ganglion cells.

A different form of megacolon that may be congenital has been reported to occur in certain areas of the world such as Eastern Europe and Okinawa where the vegetable diets are high in roughage and residue. It is not clear whether the unusually large, long colon is acquired by the individual as an adaptation of the high-residue diet or whether this is a hereditary characteristic that was selected in the evolutionary process because of its adaptive significance. It would be interesting to determine if children of immigrants to the United States from Eastern Europe have large colons when raised on the relatively low-residue diets of the United States.

Acquired Megacolon

Chagas' disease is caused by infection with a protozoan, *Trypanosoma cruzi,* and is endemic in South and Central America. Megacolon, one of the complications of the chronic form of the disease, is attributable to widespread destruction of the intramural nervous system. Surgical therapy is sometimes necessary for severe constipation, recurring fecal impaction, or volvulus. Subtotal colectomy with ileoproctostomy is probably the procedure of choice, though some surgeons prefer abdominoendoanal rectosigmoidectomy.

Acquired organic megacolon results also from partial mechanical obstruction of the lower colon, rectum, or anus. More common causes are postoperative anorectal stricture; lymphogranuloma venereum (lymphopathia venereum); endometriosis; radiation proctitis; and anorectal injury, either accidental or from sexual perversion. Treatment is aimed at the offending stricture; the secondary megacolon regresses toward, but not to, normal when the primary cause is removed.

Megacolon is also seen in association with neurologic disorders such as paraplegia or poliomyelitis. Constipation is a problem, because the contribution of the voluntary muscles to the defecatory act is lost. If constipation is avoided by the use of enemas and stool softeners, megacolon is avoided.

Acute dilatation of the colon, as seen in fulminating colitis, septic shock, prolonged adynamic ileus, or diabetes, has no relationship to chronic megacolon.

Megacolon is frequent in institutionalized psychotic patients. No organic cause has been found, so it is referred to as psychogenic or idiopathic megacolon. Severe constipation, because of extreme inactivity and perhaps voluntary inhibition of defecation, is presumed to be the principal cause. Better nursing care would avoid the problem if only it were possible to provide this. Psychogenic megacolon has also been seen in young children, presumably as an extension of problems with bowel training. Colectomy for megacolon is occasionally justified in these patients. If sigmoid volvulus occurs in patients with megacolon, subtotal colectomy to "straighten out" the colon is preferable to sigmoid segmental colectomy.

Fecal Impaction

Impaction is the arrest and accumulation of feces in the rectum or colon. Feces are progressively dehydrated by the colonic mucosa the longer they remain in the colon. When normal progression of feces does not occur, the hard dry fecal mass is increased in size as more feces are pushed downward from above. Retained barium after radiographic studies and calcium carbonate used as ulcer therapy frequently contribute to fecal impactions. With dehydration these substances attain a consistency resembling concrete.

Many of the patients with chronic constipation discussed above under Acquired Megacolon frequently have impactions. A frequent cause in otherwise healthy persons is an acute painful lesion of the anus—fissures, fistulas, thrombosed external hemorrhoid, or recent anorectal surgical therapy.

CLINICAL MANIFESTATIONS. The most common symptoms of a rectal impaction is the passage of frequent loose stools but without relief of the sense of rectal urgency and fullness. This is "overflow" evacuation around a partial obstruction. Marked rectal urgency but inability to defe-

cate is also common. In patients who have lost rectal sensation, as occurs in paraplegia or spina bifida, or in psychotics, there may be no symptoms of fecal impactions until a complication supervenes.

Infrequently, full-blown mechanical obstruction of the colon is the presenting picture. A fortunately rare but serious complication may occur when the fecal impaction does not obstruct completely and allows overflow evacuation to occur. The unmoving hard mass eventually erodes the mucosa with production of a stercoraceous ulcer. If the ulcer is in the rectum, serious bleeding may ensue; if in the abdominal colon, perforation with spreading fecal peritonitis. Management of this complication is the same as for perforated diverticulitis.

Diagnosis is usually easily made by digital rectal examination. If the impaction is higher, large, hard fecal masses can be palpated in the colon. These masses can also be seen on plain radiographs of the abdomen.

TREATMENT. Unless a complication is present, fecal impaction is treated by instillation of 5 ml of a 1% solution of dioctyl sodium sulfosuccinate in 60 ml of mineral oil into the rectum and left overnight. This will usually soften the stool sufficiently that it can be passed. If not, a saline enema may be given. If defecation still does not occur, then the impaction must be broken up and delivered digitally. It is helpful in female patients to exert gentle digital pressure on the rectal mass through the rectovaginal septum with two fingers in the vagina while the mass is delivered through the anus with the other hand. If a painful anal condition is present, hot sitz baths and an anesthetic ointment often relieve the spasm and permit defecation.

RECTUM AND ANUS

Anatomy

The rectum, measuring 12 to 15 cm, is the distal portion of the large intestine (Fig. 28-13), beginning at the level of the third sacral vertebra and ending at the anal canal. The rectum differs from the sigmoid colon in that it lacks haustra, teniae coli, and appendices epiploicae. The rectal valves of Houston represent folds of mucosa, submucosa, and circular musculature but contain no elements of longitudinal muscle. The upper one-third of the rectum is covered by peritoneum anteriorly and laterally; the middle one-third is covered anteriorly only; the lower one-third is devoid of peritoneum. On the average the anterior peritoneal reflection in the male is 7.5 to 8.5 cm from the anal verge, while in females it is 5.0 to 7.5 cm. The posterior peritoneal reflection is usually 12 to 15 cm from the anal verge.

The anal canal is the terminal portion of the large intestine. The "surgical anal canal" begins at the anorectal ring, terminates at the anal verge, and is about 4 cm long. The circular muscle of the large intestine continues downward and thickens to form the *internal sphincter.* The *external sphincter,* which is striated muscle, loops around the entire length of the anal canal. It has three components: the *subcutaneous, superficial,* and *deep portions.* Recently, it

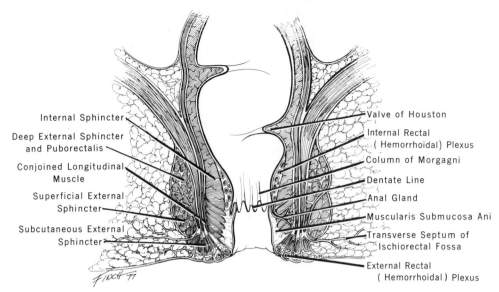

Internal Sphincter
Deep External Sphincter and Puborectalis
Conjoined Longitudinal Muscle
Superficial External Sphincter
Subcutaneous External Sphincter

Valve of Houston
Internal Rectal (Hemorrhoidal) Plexus
Column of Morgagni
Dentate Line
Anal Gland
Muscularis Submucosa Ani
Transverse Septum of Ischiorectal Fossa
External Rectal (Hemorrhoidal) Plexus

Fig. 28-13. Coronal section of the rectum and anal canal, showing sphincter muscles and the lining of anal canal.

was determined that the puborectalis is fused with the deep portion of the external sphincter and is not part of the levator ani muscles. Between the internal and external sphincter is the longitudinal smooth muscle. This muscle continues from the rectum to where it receives fibers from the levator ani and puborectalis muscles to form the *conjoined longitudinal muscle*. These muscle fibers pass down and break up into a series of septums and ultimately attach to the anal and perianal skin. Some of the longitudinal muscle fibers traverse the internal sphincter into the submucosa and are called *muscularis submucosa ani;* some fibers traverse the external sphincter to form the *transverse septum of the ischiorectal fossa*. The role of the longitudinal muscle is to affix the anal canal and to evert the anus during defecation.

The puborectalis, the deep part of the external sphincter, the longitudinal muscle layer, and the upper part of the internal sphincter form a palpable "anorectal ring."

ANAL SPHINCTER MECHANISM. The recent concept by Shafik of the anal sphincter as three distinct U-shaped loops simplifies the understanding of its mechanism (Fig. 28-14).

In the *top loop* the deep portion of the external sphincter and the puborectalis are fused into one muscle. This attaches to the lower part of the symphysis pubis and loops around the upper part of the anal canal with a downward inclination.

The *intermediate loop* is the superficial external sphincter which arises from the tip of the coccyx as a tendon and gives rise to strong muscle bundles passing forward to encircle the anal canal below the top loop.

The *base loop* is the subcutaneous external sphincter. It attaches anteriorly to the perianal skin in the midline and passes backward with an upward inclination to loop around the lower part of the anal canal.

During voluntary anal contraction the three loops contract in the direction of their origin. The top and the base

loops, innervated by the inferior hemorrhoidal branch of the pudendal nerve, will bring the posterior anal wall anteriorly, whereas the intermediate loop, supplied by the fourth sacral nerve, will pull the anal canal posteriorly. Thus, each loop is a separate sphincter and complements the other loops to maintain complete continence.

SURGICAL ANAL CANAL LINING (Fig. 28-13). The surgical anal canal is lined above by mucosa and below by anoderm, which is modified skin. The anal crypts are in the upper part of the anoderm. A line at the level of the crypts is the pectinate, or dentate, line. Above this line are a number of vertical mucosal folds, the columns of Mor-

Fig. 28-14. U-shaped anal sphincters.

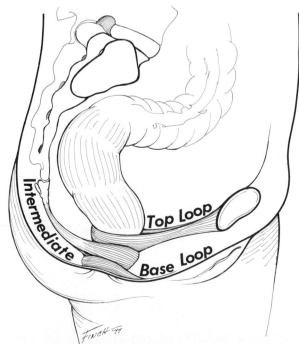

Intermediate
Top Loop
Base Loop

gagni, which overlie the internal hemorrhoidal plexus. Immediately above the dentate line is a zone of transitional epithelium, measuring 0.5 to 1.0 cm.

The pectinate, or dentate, line is an important landmark for surgeons. The epithelium above this line is supplied by sensory fibers from the autonomic nervous system and therefore is insensitive to painful stimuli such as cutting or cauterizing. The epithelium below this line is innervated by spinal nerves and has somatic sensation.

Anal glands are vestigial structures lined by stratified, mucus-secreting columnar epithelium and squamous epithelium. Normally there are 6 to 10 glands in the circumference of the anus. Each gland has a duct and discharges into an anal crypt at the dentate line. Some of the glands penetrate the internal sphincter, extending into the conjoined longitudinal muscle fibers, but not beyond them. Infection originating in these glands is the primary cause of perianal abscess and fistula-in-ano.

ARTERIAL SUPPLY OF THE RECTUM AND ANAL CANAL
(Fig. 28-15)

1. The superior rectal (hemorrhoidal) artery is the continuation of the inferior mesenteric artery and descends posteriorly to the rectum, where it bifurcates to supply the rectum and upper portion of the anal canal.
2. The middle rectal (hemorrhoidal) arteries arise from the internal iliac artery on each side and enter the lower portion of the rectum anterolaterly at the level of the levator ani muscle; they do not enter the lateral stalks, as previously believed. These arteries anastomose with the branches of the superior rectal artery.
3. The inferior rectal arteries arise on each side from the internal pudendal artery, a branch of the internal iliac artery, and traverse the ischiorectal fossa on each side to supply the anal sphincter muscles. There is no evidence of anastomosis between the superior and inferior rectal arteries.

4. The middle sacral artery provides an insignificant amount of blood supply to the rectum. It arises posteriorly, just above the bifurcation of the aorta, descends over the lumbar vertebrae, sacrum, and coccyx, and gives only small branches to the posterior wall of the lower portion of the rectum.

VENOUS DRAINAGE OF THE RECTUM AND ANAL CANAL
(Fig. 28-16). Return of blood from the rectum and the anal canal is via two systems: portal and systemic. The superior rectal (hemorrhoidal) vein drains the rectum and upper part of the anal canal into the portal system via the inferior mesenteric vein. Primarily, the middle rectal veins drain the lower part of the rectum and the upper part of the anal canal. They accompany the middle rectal arteries and terminate in the internal iliac veins. The inferior rectal veins, following the corresponding arteries, drain the lower part of the anal canal via the internal pudendal veins, which empty into the internal iliac veins. Dilatation of the inferior rectal veins leads to external hemorrhoids.

The superior, middle, and inferior rectal veins converge to form the internal rectal (hemorrhoidal) plexus in the submucosa of the columns of Morgagni. Dilatation of this plexus gives rise to internal hemorrhoids.

LYMPHATIC DRAINAGE OF THE RECTUM AND ANAL CANAL.
The lymph from the upper and middle parts of the rectum ascends along the superior rectal lymphatics and subsequently to the inferior mesenteric nodes. The lower part of the rectum and the upper part of the surgical anal canal drain cephalad via the superior rectal lymphatics and laterally via the middle rectal lymph vessels. The lymph from the anal canal, below the dentate line, can drain to the superior rectal lymph nodes, to the nodes on the lateral wall of the pelvis, or to the inguinal nodes.

Fig. 28-15. Arterial supply of the rectum and anal canal.

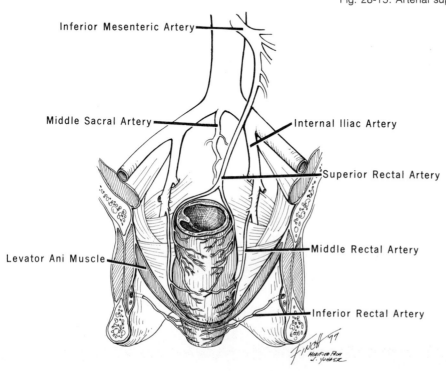

Inferior Mesenteric Artery

Middle Sacral Artery

Internal Iliac Artery

Superior Rectal Artery

Levator Ani Muscle

Middle Rectal Artery

Inferior Rectal Artery

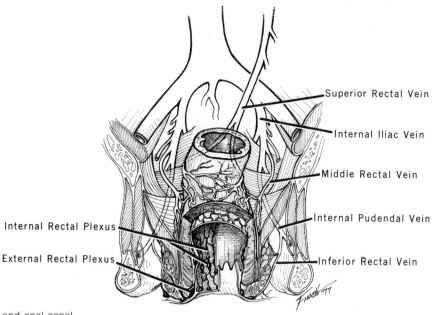

Fig. 28-16. Venous drainage of the rectum and anal canal.

PERIANAL AND PERIRECTAL SPACES (Figs. 28-17 and 28-18). Around the rectum and anal canal are several spaces filled with connective tissue or fat, which may become sites of abscesses. The *supralevator (pelvirectal) space* is situated on each side of the rectum above the levator ani. It is bound superiorly by the pelvic peritoneum, laterally by the pelvic wall, and medially by the rectum. The space is filled with fibroareolar tissue. The *retrorectal space* lies between the rectum and sacrum, above the levator ani muscles. It communicates with the supralevator space on each side. The *ischiorectal space* lies inferiorly to the levator ani muscle and is bound superiorly by the pelvic diaphragm (levator ani muscle), medially by the external sphincters, laterally by the pelvic wall, and inferiorly by the transverse septum of the ischiorectal fossa. It is filled com-

pletely with fat and contains the inferior rectal vessels and lymphatics. The space on each side communicates through the posterior space between the levator ani and tendinous portion of the superficial external sphincter (*deep postanal space*). With this communication, infection on either side of the ischiorectal space can lead to a horseshoe abscess or fistula. The *perianal space,* containing fat, inferior rectal vessels, and lymphatics, is located between the perianal skin and the transverse septum of the ischiorectal fossa. Posteriorly, this space lies inferiorly to the superficial external sphincter muscle and is called the *superficial postanal space.* The perianal space is the most common site of abscess in this region. The *intersphincteric space* lies within the conjoined longitudinal muscle between the internal and external anal sphincters. This space surrounds the anal canal.

Fig. 28-17. Coronal section of the perianal and perirectal spaces.

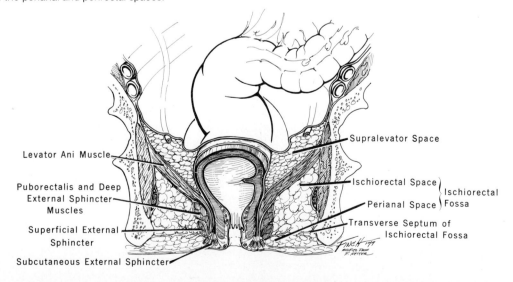

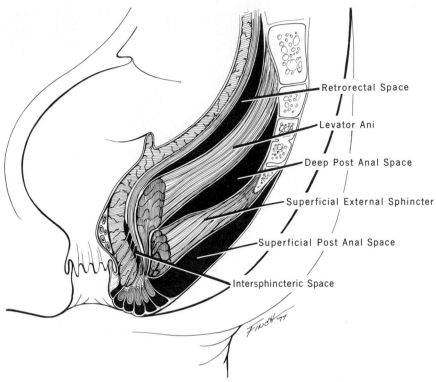

Retrorectal Space

Levator Ani

Deep Post Anal Space

Superficial External Sphincter

Superficial Post Anal Space

Intersphincteric Space

Fig. 28-18. Sagittal section of the perianal and perirectal spaces.

Examination

Patients with painful anal lesions are apprehensive about any examination; thus it is important they be approached gently and be informed of every step of the procedure. This "vocal anesthesia" should be applied to both digital and sigmoidoscopic examinations.

PREPARATION. Opinions vary with respect to the need for special preparation of the rectum prior to routine sigmoidoscopic examination. The most common preparation is one 4-oz packaged phosphate enema given 20 minutes prior to the examination. However, the majority of ambulatory patients can be examined adequately without prior enemas. This is particularly pertinent for the patient with a history suggestive of inflammatory bowel disease. In this circumstance, adding an irritating preparatory enema can often mask the salient early findings. Conversely, patients have been diagnosed as having inflammatory bowel disease when, actually, the mucous membrane appeared inflamed from the irritating enema. Evaluation of the patient with rectal bleeding should always be made without a preparatory enema in order to eliminate the possibility of washing away important clues such as bloody mucus streaked on the bowel wall, an indication of a lesion higher in the intestine. Proctosigmoidoscopic examination should not be carried out just prior to a barium enema unless there is an emergency, since the insufflation of air at the time of sigmoidoscopy can create artifacts simulating polyps or other filling defects on the barium enema examination.

SIGMOIDOSCOPIC EXAMINATION. This procedure can be performed on a proctosigmoidoscopic table which places the patient in an inverted position, allowing the viscera to slide cephalad and create a negative pressure, thus minimizing the need for insufflation to distend the bowel. Examination also may be carried out with the patient on a flat table in the prone or knee-chest position. In the latter position, the knees should be 6 to 8 in. apart to relax the gluteal musculature. For the elderly or seriously ill patient who cannot tolerate the knee-chest or prone positions, the lateral, or Sims' position may be used. After turning the patient on the side, the lower leg is extended while the upper leg is flexed at the knee and hip in order to spread the buttocks and lend some stability to the position. By positioning the buttocks 10 to 12 cm over the edge of the bed, a complete rotation of the sigmoidoscope is facilitated.

A variety of sigmoidoscopes is available. There are proximally lighted scopes, distally lighted scopes, and fiberoptic scopes. Advocates of the proximally lighted sigmoidoscopes claim that the distally lighted scopes become coated with bowel contents or blood, obscuring visibility. By contrast, advocates of the distally lighted scopes claim that better illumination is possible with this instrument. A recent advance in fiberoptics has led to the development of a flexible colonoscope which can be advanced throughout the entire colon in 70 to 90 percent of patients (Fig. 28-19). This instrument may be used diagnostically and therapeutically, since lesions throughout the colon may be biopsied and pedunculated polyps may be removed.

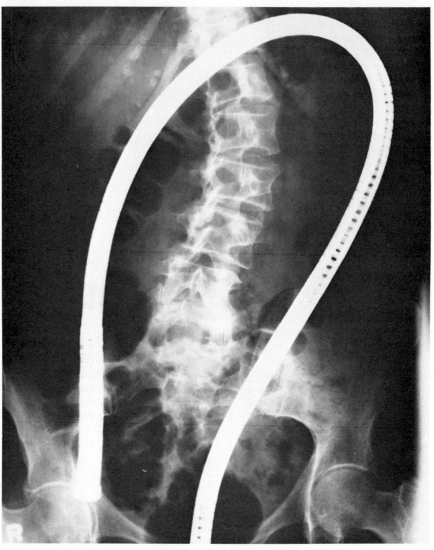

Fig. 28-19. Fiberoptic colonoscope introduced to the cecum.

Principles of Anorectal Surgery

PREPARATION. In preparing a patient for an anorectal operation, a general evaluation is mandatory. Proctosigmoidoscopy should be carried out preoperatively and is deferred only if the patient has an extremely painful condition, in which cases it is carried out under anesthesia. Contrast roentgenographic examinations of the large and small intestine are indicated when neoplastic lesions and/or inflammatory bowel diseases are suspected. Any patient presenting with a history of bleeding requires a complete roentgenographic assessment of the lower intestinal tract. If the patient gives a history of diarrhea or other symptoms suggestive of inflammatory bowel disease, both the small and large intestine should be studied roentgenographically prior to the performance of any anorectal operation. If a rectal lesion suggests the possibility of systemic diseases, such as leukemia, syphilis or Crohn's disease, these should be evaluated completely prior to surgery.

The preoperative preparation of the patient should take into consideration specific anxieties related to rectal surgery; these include fear of pain, incontinence, recurrence, and malignancy. Preparation of the bowel for most anorectal operations requires only a packaged phosphate enema the evening before and the morning of surgery. No specific antibiotic is given except when perforation of the bowel is a significant possibility, e.g., when sessile adenomas are excised from high in the rectum or a polyp in the sigmoid colon is snared with electrocautery. Laxatives or stool softeners are not administered routinely, although they are not contraindicated. No special diets are instituted preoperatively, since a bowel movement on the second or third postoperative day is desirable. Shaving the perianal skin, which has been a long-standing tradition, is totally unnecessary. Regrowth of hair adds to the postoperative pruritus and irritation, and the presence of hair does not complicate the healing process.

Most of the common rectal operations can be carried out under local anesthesia with regional field block, epidural anesthesia, spinal anesthesia or general anesthesia with or without endotracheal intubation, depending on the position of the patient. Many surgeons prefer to use supplemental local anesthesia combined with epinephrine solution to aid hemostasis and facilitate identification of the anatomy. Long-acting oil-soluble anesthetics have been used to assist in controlling postoperative pain, but these have been associated with a high incidence of postoperative suppuration.

TECHNIQUE. The three commonly used positions for anorectal operations are prone-jackknife, dorsal lithotomy, and Sims' position. The techniques should all be characterized by minimal handling of the tissue, sharp dissection, primary closure of wounds when possible, and the use of fine absorbable sutures *without tension* on the suture lines. In all circumstances, normal skin should be conserved, and injury to the sphincteric mechanism should be avoided.

POSTOPERATIVE CARE. Packing of the anorectum is rarely necessary to effect hemostasis, but some surgeons use a small amount of oxidized cellulose. Bulky, painful pressure dressings should be avoided so that spontaneous voiding can occur, and the need for catheterization is minimized. A bulk-producing compound and a lubricant are administered orally, starting on the day of operation. If the patient has not had a spontaneous bowel movement by the third postoperative day, a tap water enema is administered through a soft rubber catheter. Dilatation and irrigations of the anal canal are not used postoperatively. The patient is placed on a regular diet early in the postoperative course, usually on the first hospital day. Hospital dismissal is indicated following the first spontaneous bowel movement and when intramuscular injections of analgesics are no longer required. A psyllium seed bulk producer is prescribed, and the patient is instructed to keep a cotton dressing in the anal area to collect discharge and drainage. Sitz baths are encouraged as often as necessary for cleanliness and comfort. The patient is seen postoperatively approximately 10 days following hospital discharge and at regular intervals until complete healing has occurred.

COMPLICATIONS. Bleeding is one of the most common complications following anorectal surgery. This complication can be reduced by the use of electrocautery or suture ligature techniqe at the time of operation. In most instances, postoperative bleeding is related to either ineffective hemostasis at the time of operation or to heavy packing of the anal canal. The latter is unnecessary and should be discouraged, since it only adds to the patient's discomfort.

Direct suture of the bleeder is the treatment of choice to control postoperative hemorrhage during the first 24 hours. Thus, any patient who begins to bleed postoperatively and does not respond to light packing should be taken to the operating room, where, under the proper anesthetic, the site of bleeding can be demonstrated and sutured.

Secondary hemorrhage, or late bleeding, occurs in 1.0 to 1.5 percent of anorectal procedures. The most common time for this complication is the seventh or tenth postoperative day when the catgut suture is dissolved almost com-

pletely. The management is similar as for an acute bleeder, viz., examination under anesthesia, evacuation of clots, and suture of the bleeding point.

Abnormal pain accompanies a variety of complications related to rectal surgery. Pressure-like pain associated with fecal impaction must be differentiated from the usual postoperative pain related to the surgical procedure itself. This distressing complication can be avoided by or treated with simple tap water enemas administered through a soft rubber catheter. The pain associated with perianal suppuration, such as intersphincteric abscess, is usually described as a "toothache" type of pain and characteristically appears on the fourth or fifth postoperative day. The sharp, searing pain of an anal fissure, which persists long into the healing phase following rectal surgery, heralds the complication of anal stenosis. This usually occurs in the midline posteriorly or in one of the posterolateral quadrants and rarely responds to conservative management; a second operation is generally indicated. Similar pain may represent the first symptom of undiagnosed Crohn's disease. Approximately 20 percent of patients with Crohn's disease have, as their initial symptom, a fissure or suppurative process in the anorectum or a slowly healing anorectal wound.

Anal stricture is a dreaded complication of anorectal surgery. It is an infrequent complication of closed hemorrhoidectomy since this technique precludes the excessive removal of anoderm. Since treatment is difficult, efforts are best directed at prevention. Dilatation has been used for many years, but this is painful and often unsuccessful. The use of a bulk producer, such as psyllium seed compound, following rectal surgery is a simple and physiologic method for dilating the anal canal. It is far superior to forceful, painful dilatation with a finger or anal dilator. If stricture persists and is painful, anoplasty is indicated.

In certain anorectal operations, where the mucous membrane is advanced to form a new dentate line, an *ectropion* may result. This condition, in which the mucous membrane has been advanced beyond the anal verge, results in a "wet anus," and has been referred to as a *Whitehead deformity.* Ectropion is best treated by excision of the offending mucous membrane and application of a sliding skin graft.

Incontinence following anorectal procedures can arise from several causes. The most common cause, fecal impaction, allows liquid stool to bypass the impaction while the pressure of the impaction holds the sphinteric mechanism open. This may be corrected with tap water enemas. During the first few weeks following an anorectal operation, there may be some fecal staining, and the patient may report loss of ability to distinguish between flatus and feces. This is usually a temporary, self-limited situation due to the disruption of proprioceptive nerve endings in the anoderm. The use of large amounts of mineral oil compound to lubricate the stool following surgery results in a "leakage" of mineral oil which is often interpreted as incontinence. Severe forms of incontinence generally are related to division of the sphincteric muscles.

In operative procedures for anal fissures when a concomitant superficial partial sphincterotomy is carried out, a slight degree of fecal staining may result, but this is rarely permanent. In extensive fistula surgery, where a great deal of the sphincteric mechanism is transected, incontinence may persist; sphincteroplasty may be indicated if improvement is not effected with sphincteric exercises. Preservation of the sphincteric mechanism is a most important consideration in the treatment of deep or high fistulas and when fistulas involve the anterior sphincter mechanism, especially in females.

Anal pruritus is not a true complication of rectal surgery. Most patients notice a degree of anal pruritus during the healing phases, similar to that noted in the healing of any cutaneous wound. If anal pruritus persists, it may be a sign of an anal fissure or may be due to a particular sensitivity to one of the anesthetic ointments used following rectal surgery.

Urinary tract symptoms, particularly retention and infection, were frequent complications following anorectal operations in the past. The incidence of urinary retention recently has been reduced to 5 percent by decreasing fluid administration during operation and postoperatively, resorting to catheterization only when the patient is distended. When catheterization is to be repeated, the catheter should be left in place for several days.

Hemorrhoids

In the human being, the upper anal canal is lined by separate, bulky cushions of specialized submucosal vascular tissue, likened to erectile tissue, composed of a stroma of elastic connective tissue containing smooth muscle fibers derived from the outer longitudinal muscle coat of the colon. This supports the normally large and dilated veins of the internal hemorrhoidal venous plexus, which also have demonstrable arteriovenous shunts. Such cushions are discrete and separated so that the anal canal lumen is seen to form a triradiate slit. The stem of the "Y," so formed, invariably approaches the midline posteriorly, so that its arms separate three cushions lying in constant sites—left lateral, right anterior, right posterior. Secondary folds are present in each of these large cushions. This anatomical arrangement is remarkably constant; however, it bears no relationship, as previously thought, to the terminal branching of the superior rectal vessels, which is quite inconstant. That this arrangement of anal cushions is the normal state is borne out by its presence in children; it can also be demonstrated in the fetus and even in the embryo. The function of these cushions is speculative; however, many reasonable theories have been advanced. By their bulk, they must aid in anal continence, and, during the act of defecation when they become engorged with blood, they cushion the anal canal and support the lining. Being separate structures, rather than a continuous ring of vascular tissue, allows the anal canal to dilate during defecation.

ETIOLOGY. Hemorrhoidal disease exists only when this situation becomes exaggerated and the patient develops symptoms. Many factors have been implicated in the causation of hemorrhoids, including the erect position of the human being, the absence of venous valves, obstruction of venous return, and hereditary weakness of the vessels. Since these factors are all present in the normal physiologic status of the vascular arrangement of the anal canal, they bear no direct relationship to the disease state. Straining during defecation and the passage of hard, small-volume stools, however, results in tense engorgement of the anal cushions. This may cause injury to the mucous membrane, resulting in bright red bleeding from the capillaries of the lamina propria. With repeated straining, the anal cushions are damaged so that the normal supports are stretched and the tendency to prolapse outside the anal canal develops. Early in the evolution of the disease, the cushions reduce spontaneously; however, with repeated episodes, the situation becomes irreversible, so that manual replacement is necessary. In the prolonged state of the disease, the normally lax rectal mucosa above the anal cushions eventually is dragged with the prolapsing anal cushion so that it adds to the bulk of what now could be described as a classical hemorrhoid. The prolapsed hemorrhoids lying outside the normally contracted anal sphincter ring may become strangulated, with resulting thrombosis of the venous plexus. This, in turn, may result in gangrene and sloughing.

Recent epidemiologic studies have implicated the low-roughage "Western" diet as the cause of many diseases, including hemorrhoids. Adding bulk, in the form of cereal fiber or bulk-forming compounds, can prevent hemorrhoidal disease and, in many cases, reverse the early stages.

For clarity of surgical description, the various states of hemorrhoidal disease should be defined. *Internal hemorrhoids* are exaggerated vascular cushions, normally located above the dentate line, and are covered by the mucous membrane of the anal canal. *External hemorrhoids* are mainly the dilated venules of the inferior hemorrhoidal plexus, which are located below the dentate line and are covered by squamous epithelium. A *mixed hemorrhoid* is a combination of an external and internal hemorrhoid. *Prolapsing hemorrhoids* are internal hemorrhoids which protrude beyond the dentate line and lie outside the anal canal. They are always associated with redundant rectal mucosa. A *thrombosed hemorrhoid* is one in which the blood has clotted, both intravascularly and, to some degree, extravascularly. An *external skin tag* is an area of fibrous connective tissue, covered by skin, which is usually the result of a previously thrombosed hemorrhoid or anal surgery.

CLINICAL MANIFESTATIONS. External hemorrhoids are usually asymptomatic. Perianal irritation and pruritus rarely result from external hemorrhoids. The patient's first awareness of an external hemorrhoid may be the pain which accompanies thrombosis. Thrombosis may recur in the same or in a different hemorrhoidal complex. Internal hemorrhoids most commonly are manifested by painless, bright-red rectal bleeding associated with defecation. The patient commonly describes the bleeding episode by stating, "The blood drips into the toilet bowl." Prolapse of an internal hemorrhoid may be accompanied by a feeling of moisture in the anal region. Early in its course, the prolapse reduces spontaneously, but as the condition becomes chronic, the internal hemorrhoids prolapse permanently, a situation frequently accompanied by inflammation and thrombosis. Other sequelae of internal hemorrhoids are anemia, edema, suppuration, ulceration, fibrosis, strangulation, and, rarely, pylephlebitis with gangrene. Pain is not

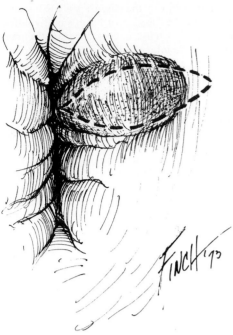

Fig. 28-20. Excision of thrombosed external hemorrhoid demonstrating elliptical skin incision.

a symptom of hemorrhoids, unless associated with thrombosis or infection, but indicates other anal disease which may accompany hemorrhoids; viz., anal fissure, proctalgia fugax, proctitis, or, occasionally, anal cancer. Likewise, discharge, with or without pruritus, is not a symptom of hemorrhoids unless chronic prolapse is present, but is indicative of other diseases, such as fistula, proctitis, procidentia, and neoplasm.

Uncomplicated internal hemorrhoids usually are not palpable, but having the patient strain at the completion of the digital examination will reveal prolapse of an internal hemorrhoid and the rectal mucosa. The anoscope is particularly suitable for viewing internal hemorrhoids, but proctosigmoidoscopy must be performed to rule out neoplastic or inflammatory disease, which may present with similar

Fig. 28-21. Ligation technique for internal hemorrhoids.

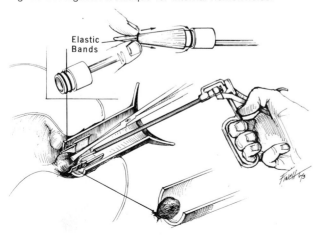

Elastic Bands

symptoms. In patients with an atypical history or in the older age group, a barium enema is mandatory to exclude colonic disease.

TREATMENT. Usually, the treatment of a painful thrombosed hemorrhoid is an outpatient procedure. Anesthesia is achieved by a subcutaneous injection of 3.5 ml of 1% procaine or lidocaine solution containing 1:200,000 epinephrine. Incision alone frequently does not suffice. It is preferable to excise the entire thrombosed hemorrhoid and electrocoagulate the bleeding points (Fig. 28-20). Adequate treatment by total excision of a single thrombosed external hemorrhoid prevents further thrombosis in that area and usually obviates the need for subsequent hemorrhoidectomy. If the thrombosed hemorrhoid is unassociated with pain, nonoperative therapy will suffice. Pain associated with thrombosis lasts only 2 to 3 days; resolution usually requires 10 to 14 days.

Initial treatment for bleeding internal hemorrhoids should be nonoperative, with emphatic dietary education of the patient to correct any underlying bowel disturbance attributed to constipating food, especially dairy products, inadequate hydration, and lack of high-fiber food, such as bran. The use of hydrophilic bulk stool–forming additives may be contemplated. Injection therapy of 5% phenol in vegetable oil or quinine urea hydrochloride to sclerose the submucosal tissue above the hemorrhoid may afford temporary, symptomatic relief but should be used only for uncomplicated bleeding internal hemorrhoids.

Another nonoperative technique is rubber band ligation of uncomplicated bleeding internal hemorrhoids. This is an effective, simple procedure and has gained in popularity, now superseding injection. In this outpatient procedure, a constricting rubber band is placed high in the anal canal on the most redundant portion of the rectal mucosa immediately above the internal hemorrhoid (Fig. 28-21). Incorporated tissue sloughs in approximately 7 days, leaving an area of inflammation which results in fibrosis and fixation. This technique does not require anesthesia. Any excessive discomfort indicates that the band has been placed too low and should be removed immediately. The technique provides a more permanent result than injection therapy, since there is precisely controlled loss of redundant mucosa. Repeated applications may be carried out at 6- to 8-week intervals until the patient's symptoms are improved. Occasionally, two to three areas can be banded per visit. The procedure has been performed without incident on patients receiving anticoagulant therapy. The contraindications are the same as for surgical hemorrhoidectomy, viz., inflammatory bowel disease, leukemia, and portal hypertension.

Hemorrhoidal tissue can be frozen with a specialized probe, activated by carbon dioxide, nitrous oxide, or, preferably, liquid nitrogen. With care, the final results of cryosurgery are anatomically satisfactory, and the procedure may be accomplished without anesthesia and with minimal discomfort to the patient. The aftertreatment period is characterized by profuse anal discharge and delayed wound healing, taking as long as 6 to 8 weeks for complete resolution. Moreover, a relatively high incidence of secondary hemorrhage is being reported. Because of these disadvantages and since the results of such treatment do not equal those of formal surgical hemorrhoidectomy, this technique has failed to gain widespread acceptance and use.

Hemorrhoidectomy. Principal indications for hemorrhoidectomy are prolapse, pain, bleeding, and large hemorrhoids associated with other anorectal pathologic conditions requiring operative management. In general, hemorrhoidectomy is reserved for patients having severe symptoms related to multiple thrombosed hemorrhoids or marked redundant protrusion which cannot be handled by the ligature technique. Hemorrhoidectomy may be indicated in the immediate postpartum period in women who have had difficulties prior to pregnancy and in whom prolapse of thrombosed hemorrhoids occurred at the time of delivery. In most instances, hemorrhoids which appear to intensify during delivery resolve, but there is a small group of women in whom the problem is of such magnitude as to indicate operation.

The principles for all operative procedures include removing diseased tissues (i.e., internal-external hemorrhoids and redundant rectal mucosa), leaving minimal scarring of the anal canal, avoiding interference with the sphincteric mechanism, and leaving an anal orifice ample for a normal bowel movement without discomfort. Although there are many variations, all hemorrhoid operations basically employ the ligature and excision technique; the method of handling the perianal skin differentiates various techniques. In some techniques, the mucous membrane is closed up to the dentate line, and the external wounds are left open. Other techniques employ primary closure of the hemorrhoidectomy wound.

The technique of *closed hemorrhoidectomy* offers (1) effective removal of hemorrhoidal tissue, (2) prompt healing of wounds, (3) elimination of mucous drainage by lining the anal canal with stratified squamous epithelium, (4) minimal inpatient and virtually no outpatient care, (5) less postoperative discomfort, (6) no loss of continence, and (7) no need for anal dilatation. An adequate dissection-type closed hemorrhoidectomy may be carried out on the acute, prolapsed, thrombosed, edematous hemorrhoid without fear of anal stenosis or stricture if meticulous dissection and preservation of anoderm are accomplished. This technique may be combined with other operative procedures, such as fissurectomy, internal sphincterotomy, fistulotomy, or excision of hypertrophied anal papillae.

Operative Technique (Fig. 28-22). The hemorrhoidal tissue and the extent of the redundant mucosa are demonstrated by grasping the redundant mucosa with tissue forceps. Although every case does not conform to the classic three-quadrant distribution, the most frequently involved quadrants are left lateral, right posterior, and right anterior. Removal of every hemorrhoidal plexus is unnecessary, since the symptoms usually are related to the prolapsing hemorrhoids.

After exposure is accomplished with an operating anoscope, dissection is started on the perianal skin, and the hemorrhoidal mass is dissected carefully off the sphincteric mechanism without injury to the internal sphincter. The redundant rectal mucosa is excised well above the internal hemorrhoid, to correct the redundancy. The mucous membrane and anoderm are elevated, and the hemorrhoidal tissue is dissected from beneath the flaps to remove the secondary hemorrhoidal complexes adequately. Anoderm is preserved, bleeding points are electrocoagulated or ligated with catgut sutures, and the mucous membrane is approximated and sutured to the underlying sphincteric mechanism with running fine chromic catgut suture. Edges of the perianal skin are trimmed, and the wound is closed *without tension.* This procedure is repeated in as many areas as necessary. At the completion of the operation it is imperative that the anal canal admit two fingers readily. An intraanal dressing is seldom used.

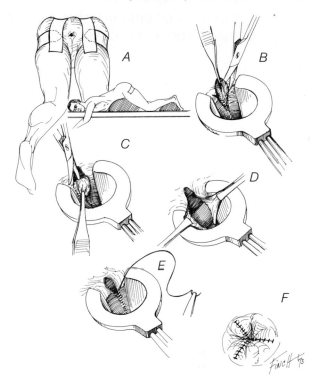

Fig. 28-22. Operative technique for a closed hemorrhoidectomy (see text for description).

PROGNOSIS. Symptoms rarely reappear following adequate hemorrhoidectomy. Reappearance of bleeding and prolapse following a hemorrhoidectomy is related to inadequate removal of redundant rectal mucosa or hemorrhoidal tissue. The opponents of primary closure technique express concern for the possible complications of infection and abscess formation, with consequent pain and stenosis. The postoperative infection rate for closed hemorrhoidectomy, as reported by Ferguson et al., was 0.2 percent, and postoperative bleeding occurred in 1.3 percent of patients.

Anal Fissure

Anal fissure is a tear of the skin-lined part of the anal canal. Distribution is equal between males and females. In 80 to 90 percent of the females and over 90 percent of the males, fissures occur in the posterior midline, and the remainder are in the anterior midline. The relatively im-

COMMON LOCATIONS OF CHRONIC ANAL FISSURE AND OTHER ANORECTAL CONDITIONS

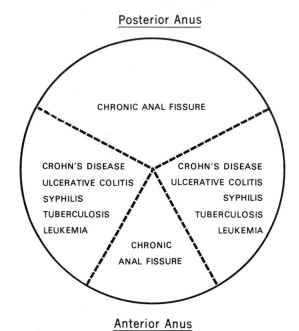

Fig. 28-23. Common locations of chronic anal fissure and other anorectal conditions.

mobile skin overlying the posterior area and the angulation of the anal canal cause the stool to traumatize the fissure-bearing area.

Acute fissure is invariably superficial and is extremely painful, especially during and after a bowel movement. Edematous skin edges and induration are absent. With proper conservative management, consisting of use of stool softeners and lubricants, most of these fissures will heal.

Chronic fissure is the result of repeated trauma to the fissure-bearing area. It is deep, with exposure of the underlying circular fibers of the internal sphincter muscle. The chronicity of anal fissure may be due to an abnormality of the internal sphincter. Anal pressure studies have provided conflicting findings. A tight anal sphincter observed in these patients makes it logical to assume that defecation stimulates the sensitive fissure and causes severe reflex spasm. This would draw the anal canal cephalad during anal contraction, and the stool traumatizes the fissure repeatedly.

Diagnosis of anal fissure presents no problem. The history of pain during and after defecation, bright spotted blood on the cleansing tissue after bowel movement, and the location of the fissure in the posterior or anterior midline are suggestive of the diagnosis. Indolent-looking fissures, or fissures located off the midline area, suggest possible inflammatory bowel disease. Anal fissure may represent the initial manifestation of Crohn's disease (Fig. 28-23).

Care should be taken to make the examination as painless as possible. It is advisable to apply a topical anesthetic to the fissure before examining the patient. Gentle spreading of the buttocks usually is all that is necessary to reveal the fissure. In some chronic cases, the triad consists of anal fissure, sentinel pile, or edematous skin tag, and hypertrophied anal papillae may be present.

Digital anoscopic proctosigmoidoscopic examination should be performed if this can be carried out without causing too much discomfort, mainly to exclude other lesions of the anal canal and rectum. In certain patients, excessive pain necessitates delayed examination, and an occasional patient may require examination under anesthesia.

The differential diagnosis for anal fissures includes:

1. Abrasion of the anal canal by trauma. This invariably heals with conservative management.

Table 28-4. ALTERNATIVE PROCEDURES FOR CHRONIC ANAL FISSURE

Type of procedure	Approximate days in hospital	Advantage	Disadvantage
Lateral sphincterotomy	1	Minimal operation	Skin tag remains, if present
Sliding V-flap	2–3	Eliminate skin tag Early primary healing	More extensive operation Possible slough of flap
Fissurectomy and sphincterotomy	3–5	None	"Key-hole" deformity Prolonged wound healing
Anal-sphincter stretching	1	No incision required	Uncontrolled tearing of sphincters Hematoma

2. Anal fissures secondary to ulcerative colitis and, more commonly, Crohn's disease. These are usually situated off the midline, frequently are multiple, and are more edematous or indolent in appearance. They should be treated conservatively. Definitive operation for these fissures should be deferred until the underlying condition has been quiescent for a long time.
3. Epidermoid carcinoma of the anal canal.
4. Tuberculous ulcer is a rare lesion. It is always associated with pulmonary tuberculosis.
5. Syphilitic fissure is usually a "mirror image" lesion which can be established by dark-field examination; serologic studies are necessary to confirm the diagnosis.
6. Leukemic infiltration of the perianal area is extremely painful. Treatment is drainage of the associated abscess.
7. Perianal fissuring, commonly associated with anal pruritus, responds to simple measures of anal hygiene.

TREATMENT. The objectives of treatment are to reduce pain and associated sphincter spasm. When this is accomplished, a superficial fissure will heal readily. Conservative treatment includes stool lubricants, preferably simple cocoa butter suppositories, bulk stool softeners, such as psyllium seed, and warm baths for comfort. To date, unequivocal studies establishing the advantage of steroid suppositories for this condition have not been conducted.

Anal fissures in children are generally superficial and rarely require an operation. Increased fluid intake and decreased consumption of dairy products are directed toward correcting the constipation problem. If these methods do not suffice, stool softeners and a sphincter stretch, without anesthesia, may be done.

Operative treatment of anal fissure is indicated if conservative measures fail (see Table 28-4). The concept of treatment is to enlarge the skin-lined portion of the anal canal and to relieve spasm during and after defecation. The classical fissurectomy and sphincterotomy at the posterior midline area should be avoided, since healing is delayed. Posterior sphincterotomy is associated with a high

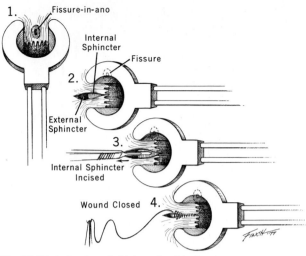

Fig. 28-24. Lateral partial internal sphincterotomy.

incidence of soiling from the "key-hole" deformity. Analsphincter stretching has been practiced since the nineteenth century and has become popular in the United Kingdom. The disadvantage of stretching is the uncontrolled amount of sphincter muscle torn. Additionally, it requires an anesthetic, during which a better-controlled internal sphincterotomy could be performed. Our treatment of choice is the lateral partial internal sphincterotomy (Fig. 28-24). If there is a redundant external skin tag, a partial internal sphincterotomy at the fissure site with a V-shaped sliding skin flap is used (Fig. 28-25). The procedure can be done under local, regional, or general anesthesia.

Perirectal Suppuration

Abscess formation in the tissues of the anal canal, rectum, and perirectal area is common. Most often no preexisting lesion can be found. The pathophysiology likely relates to abscess formation in the anal glands lying between the internal sphincter and the longitudinal inter-

Fig. 28-25. V-shaped sliding skin flap for anal fissure. 1 and 2. The 90° V-shaped flap with the apex at the fissure. 3. Full-thickness flap has been mobilized, the edges of the wound undermined, and the internal sphincterotomy made over the fissure. 4. The flap advanced to cover the entire wound.

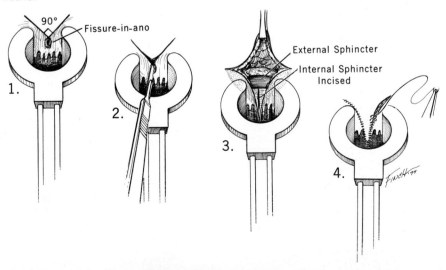

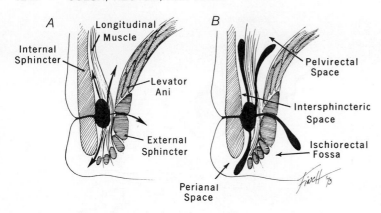

Fig. 28-26. Pathways of infection in perirectal spaces.

sphincteric muscle fibers. From this origin, the infection may spread downward, upward, circumferentially, or laterally to involve the various perianal and perirectal spaces (Fig. 28-26). At times, the cause of the infectious process is identifiable. These conditions include pilonidal abscess, hidradenitis suppurativa, infected sebaceous cyst, folliculitis, periprostatic abscess, Bartholin gland abscess, intraabdominal inflammatory disease with extraabdominal perforation, and, rarely, actinomycosis or tuberculosis.

Perirectal suppuration characteristically presents with pain, often with a palpable inflammatory process, and commonly with a high fever. The diagnosis of the more common perianal and ischiorectal abscesses is apparent. The throbbing pain in the perianal region is acute and aggravated by sitting, coughing, sneezing, and straining. Swelling, induration, and tenderness define the area of involvement. The horseshoe abscess, which begins in an infected, posterior midline anal gland and spreads to both ischiorectal spaces, presents with bilateral perineal findings. The infrequent intersphincteric abscess causes a dull, aching pain in the rectum rather than in the perianal region. There is no swelling or induration of the perianal skin, but excessive tenderness frequently precludes adequate examination without anesthesia. Rectal examination may reveal a soft, tender mass, and in the patient with a ruptured abscess, there may be passage of purulent material per rectum.

The rare supralevator abscess is difficult to diagnose. The patient may present with fever of unknown origin and no history of anal or rectal pain. Rectal or vaginal examination may reveal tenderness in the pelvis, and signs of peritonitis may be present, suggesting an intraabdominal process. In addition to extension of infralevator inflammatory processes, supralevator abscesses can result from a perforated intraabdominal viscus which has extended downward. Also, injudicious probing of a simple fistula-in-ano, creating a false infected passage in the previously uninfected supralevator space, accounts for some of these abscesses (Fig. 28-27).

TREATMENT. Standard treatment of perianal and perirectal suppuration is incision and drainage, even in the absence of evident fluctuation. Antibiotics should never represent principal therapy but may be used adjunctively. Drainage of most perianal abscesses using local anesthesia can be an outpatient procedure (Fig. 28-28). Many of these abscesses, properly drained, will heal primarily without subsequent formation of fistula-in-ano. Ischiorectal and horseshoe abscesses should be drained in the operating room under general or regional block anesthesia. Since a

Fig. 28-28. Drainage of perirectal abscess with cruciate incision.

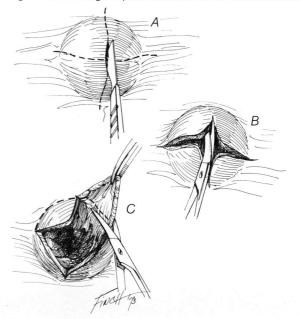

Fig. 28-27. Iatrogenic tract created by injudicious probing of a fistula-in-ano.

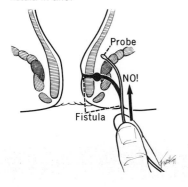

primary opening rarely can be defined, the initial approach should be limited to drainage. The presence of an acute process obviates definitive fistula operation (fistulectomy), since normal sphincter muscle may be sacrificed unnecessarily. A recent study by Scoma, Salvati, and Rubin documented primary healing in over one-third of 232 patients who had incision and drainage alone as their initial therapy for perianal suppuration.

The intersphincteric abscess is best treated in the operating room under general or regional anesthesia. The bulging area is visualized using an operating anoscope, and an internal sphincterotomy is performed directly over the abscess. Subsequent to incision, the abscess should be palpated digitally to establish complete drainage and to break up any loculations. Likewise, the supralevator or pelvirectal abscess should be treated in the operating room under anesthesia. The abscess may be drained through the appropriate ischiorectal space or through the rectum (Fig. 28-29). It is important that the aperture be enlarged to admit two fingers and to ensure continued drainage. A recent controlled study by Leaper et al. demonstrated excellent results in the treatment of idiopathic anorectal abscess by incision, curettage, and primary suture under systemic antibiotic cover. In selected patients, this technique offers shortened hospitalization and decreased morbidity.

Fistula-in-ano

Fistula-in-ano is an inflammatory tract with a *secondary* opening (external opening) in the perianal skin and a *primary* opening (internal opening) in the anal canal at the dentate line. The fistula originates in an abscess in the intersphincteric space of the anal canal. Goodsall's rule relates the location of the internal opening to the external opening (Fig. 28-30). If the external opening is anterior to an imaginary line drawn across the midpoint of the anus, the fistula usually runs directly into the anal canal. If the external opening is posterior to that line, the tract usually will curve to the posterior midline of the anal canal. An exception to this rule is an external opening anterior to this imaginary line and greater than 3 cm from the anus, in

Fig. 28-29. Proper route of drainage in supralevator abscess.

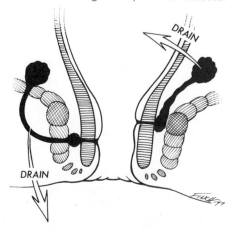

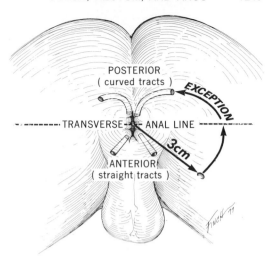

Fig. 28-30. Goodsall's rule.

which case the tract may curve posteriorly and end in the posterior midline.

A more precise classification of fistula-in-ano has been offered recently by Parks, Gordon, and Hardcastle. It consists of four categories: intersphincteric, transsphincteric, suprasphincteric, and extrasphincteric (Fig. 28-31).

Most patients present with previous history of anorectal abscess associated with intermittent drainage. Recurrence of a perianal abscess suggests the presence of a fistula-in-ano. The external opening is usually visible as a red elevation of granulation tissue with purulent or serosanguineous drainage on compression. In the simple or superficial fistula, the tract can be palpated as an indurated cord (Fig. 28-32). Deep, high, or horseshoe fistulas usually are not palpable.

Several disorders must be considered in the differential diagnosis of a fistula-in-ano. It is important to rule out fistulas associated with ulcerative colitis and Crohn's disease, in which case one would refrain from extensive operative procedures for fistula-in-ano because of poor secondary healing. This differential can be established by proctosigmoidoscopy, upper gastrointestinal examination with small bowel follow-through, and barium enema. Di-

Fig. 28-31. The four main anatomical types of fistula: (1) intersphincteric, (2) transsphincteric, (3) suprasphincteric, and (4) extrasphincteric.

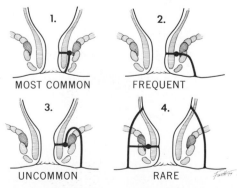

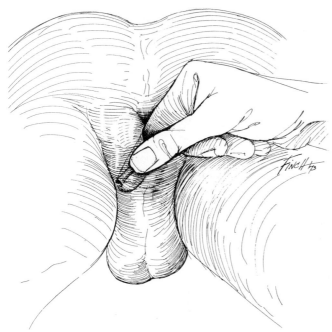

Fig. 28-32. Bidigital palpation for locating the indurated fistulous tract.

Fig. 28-33. Fistulotomy. 1. The probe is in the fistulous tract. 2 and 3. Unroofing of the fistulous tract over the probe. 4. Redundant skin is excised. 5. The wound is marsupialized.

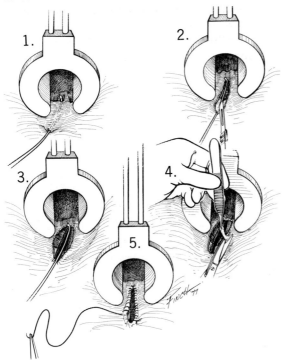

verticulitis of the sigmoid colon, with perforation and fistulization to the perineum, occurs rarely. Hidradenitis suppurativa is differentiated by the presence of multiple perianal skin openings. A pilonidal sinus with perianal extension and infected perianal sebaceous cysts must be considered. Rarely, carcinomas, mostly low-grade, may develop in long-standing fistulas. Low rectal and anal canal carcinomas rarely present as a fistula in the perineum.

TREATMENT. The first step in the management is the identification of the opening of the primary fistulous tract. About 50 percent of patients do not have clinically detectable openings. Positive identification is best accomplished in the operating room under anesthesia. Bidigital palpation, using the index finger and the thumb, delineates the indurated tract to the primary opening (Fig. 28-32). Probing the tract from the external opening is successful in 50 percent of cases, but care must be taken to avoid creating an artificial opening and seeding infected material into clean tissue, thus risking iatrogenic extensions above or beyond the original fistula (Fig. 28-27). The injection of methylene blue and/or other chemicals into the secondary opening is unsatisfactory and unnecessary. However, fistulography, utilizing water-soluble contrast solutions, is a valuable method to identify and to manage high, complicated fistulas. If definition of the primary opening is impossible at operation, the crypt-bearing area suspected of harboring the infected duct and gland must be excised.

The principles of fistulotomy include unroofing all fistulas, eliminating the primary opening (infective source), and establishing adequate drainage. The tracts are unroofed from the primary source at the dentate line through the secondary opening or openings by excising all overlying tissue, including sphincter (Fig. 28-33). Failure to unroof the entire tract and divide the necessary amount of sphincter may lead to recurrence. The wound is allowed to heal by secondary intention. Fistulectomy is the excision of the entire fistulous tract and is rarely necessary.

Occasionally, a patient may present with an acute perianal abscess associated with an obvious fistula-in-ano. Incision and drainage of the abscess and primary fistulotomy are indicated. If the fistula is high in relation to the anorectal ring, a two-stage procedure may be indicated. In the first stage, a seton of heavy black silk or a rubber band is placed loosely around the sphincter muscle as a marker (Fig. 28-34). This stimulates fibrosis adjacent to the sphincter muscle so that when the second stage, which involves laying open the intersphincteric portion of the fistulous tract, is completed, the sphincter will not gape. Incontinence is the most serious complication of operations for fistula. Concern that the patient may become incontinent postoperatively is the criterion for seton insertion.

Horseshoe fistula, an uncommon form of fistula-in-ano, is a direct extension of an intersphincteric abscess, and usually starts in the posterior midline. Radical unroofing procedures are seldom necessary. A posterior midline internal sphincterotomy combined with lateral tract curetting and drainage, as recommended by Hanley and Parks, has proved effective (Fig. 28-35).

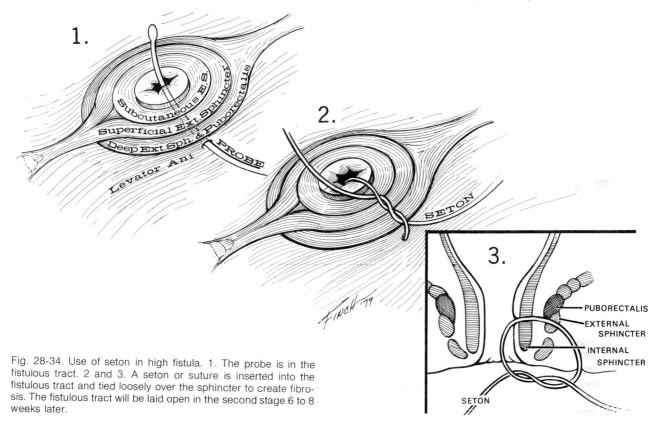

Fig. 28-34. Use of seton in high fistula. 1. The probe is in the fistulous tract. 2 and 3. A seton or suture is inserted into the fistulous tract and tied loosely over the sphincter to create fibrosis. The fistulous tract will be laid open in the second stage 6 to 8 weeks later.

Anal Incontinence

Anal incontinence results when there is loss of control of the anal sphincter. The term actually covers a broad spectrum of anal function impairment, ranging from simple involuntary passage of flatus to complete loss of sphincter tone with involuntary passage of formed stool.

The external sphincter and puborectalis muscles are primarily responsible for voluntary control. The internal sphincter muscle maintains continence at rest.

Total anal incontinence, with complete loss of sphincter muscle control, is due to physical loss of muscle mass, sensory innervation damage, or central nervous system disease.

Partial anal incontinence is intermittent soiling or passage of flatus involuntarily. This occurs if either the internal sphincter or the external sphincter muscle is defective. Trauma, obstetrical procedures, and anorectal surgery are the three main identifiable causes of partial incontinence. Other causes are inflammatory bowel disease, rectal carcinoma, or rectal prolapse.

Overflow anal incontinence is found in patients with fecal impaction or chronic constipation with prolonged laxative abuse. These patients are either the elderly (bedridden or chronically debilitated) or young children with acquired constipation and/or megacolon. The sphincter muscle mechanism is intact, but the large bolus of feces distends the rectal ampulla, causing relaxation of the internal sphincter, and is responsible for loss of the defecation reflex.

Correction consists of evacuation of the impaction with enemas and, occasionally, manually. Prevention is dietary alteration, the use of bulk-forming stool softeners, in-

Fig. 28-35. Internal sphincterotomy at the site of the intrasphincteric abscess and drainage of the limbs of a horseshoe abscess.

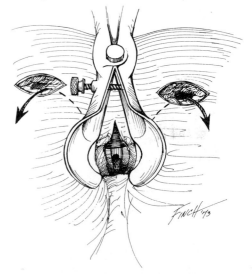

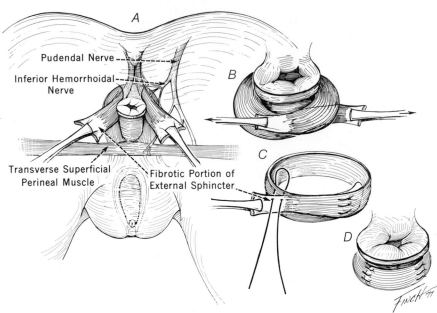

Fig. 28-36. Sphincteroplasty: *A.* The external sphincter muscle is mobilized along with the fibrotic ends. Care should be taken not to injure the inferior hemorrhoidal nerve. *B.* The well-mobilized external sphincter muscle is wrapped around the anal canal. *C.* Mattress sutures of 2-0 polyglycol inserted into the fibrotic ends. *D.* At completion, the anal canal should admit only an index finger.

creased fluid intake, and reestablishment of regular bowel habits. This may require the frequent use of enemas over a long period of time.

TREATMENT. Therapy must be based on consideration of the etiologic factors and judicious selection of patients for operative correction. Only patients with incontinence where there is a muscle defect secondary to trauma, obstetrical tears, or operative procedures should be treated operatively. There are varying types of sphincter repair, and the cause and extent of sphincter loss determine the procedure of choice.

Sphincteroplasty involves mobilization of the divided sphincteric muscle and reapproximation *without tension* (Fig. 28-36). This procedure has become the preferred treatment, because restoration of sphincter continence is achieved. In perineorrhaphy, the puborectalis sling is tightened by a row of sutures anterior or posterior to the rectum. Sphincter-reefing operations are designed to take a tuck in the sphincter to reduce patulousness. Fascial grafts

have been inserted as a sling around the anus to achieve some constriction. Also, the gracilis muscle has been transferred to encircle the anus in an attempt to substitute a segment of innervated muscle, which may be trained as a sphincter. The levator ani muscle group also has been substituted for the puborectalis sling in an attempt to gain voluntary control. Recently, electrical implants have been tried experimentally to provide exogenous electrical stimulation to atonic sphincter muscles. The results are not encouraging to date. Finally, if local operation is futile, a colostomy may be advisable, since an abdominal colostomy is more easily cared for than a "perineal colostomy."

Rectal Prolapse

Prolapse of the rectum is a rare condition in which some or all of the layers of the rectum extrude through the anus. There are two classes of prolapse: true procidentia and rectal mucosal prolapse (false procidentia). The true procidentia extrudes through the anus and is seen as concentric circular rings of mucosa (Fig. 28-37). Rectal mucosal prolapse is seen extruding through the anus in radial folds. True rectal prolapse can occur at any age; however, it seems to be prevalent in institutionalized patients with irregular bowel habits.

There are two predominant theories of the etiology of prolapse: sliding hernia and intussusception. Moschcowitz in 1912 put forth the theory that it is a sliding hernia of the peritoneum of the cul-de-sac of Douglas. The hernia slides through a defect in the pelvic diaphragm, invaginates the anterior wall of the rectum, and intussuscepts the rectum

Fig. 28-37. True rectal procidentia with concentric circular rings of mucosa.

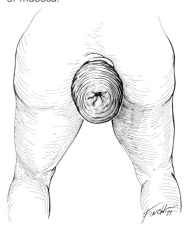

and the rectosigmoid, which protrudes through the anal sphincter. More recently, others have shown the prolapse is not a hernia but an intussusception of the rectosigmoid. It has been shown that the intussusception begins at the rectosigmoid junction. The intussusception pulls the rectosigmoid from its attachments, and, with repeated straining, the rectum pulls away distally. As the intussusception proceeds downward, it reaches the area of the lateral neurovascular stalks, where there are stronger fascial attachments, and hesitates for variable time periods. Eventually, repeated pressure from above, by straining, weakens this barrier and the bowel further descends and protrudes from the anus. In advanced cases, loss of sphincter tone may be due to a neuromuscular deficit. The anatomic defects associated with procidentia of the rectum are a diastasis of the levator ani muscles, weakened endopelvic fascia, loss of the normal horizontal position of the rectum, abnormally deep cul-de-sac, and a weak anal sphincter.

In all these theories, the common characteristic is marked redundancy of the rectosigmoid and loss of the normal angle the rectum makes with the puborectalis sling. Correction entails reestablishment of the proper angle, whether by closing the pelvic floor defect or securing the rectum to the hollow of the sacrum posteriorly.

TREATMENT. Irrespective of one's view of etiologic factors, the operative approach is to correct anatomic defects. Various technical aspects utilized in the repair are correction of the pelvic wall defect by endopelvic fascia repair, approximation of the levator ani muscles and the perineal body in the female, establishment of a normal angle between the rectum and anal canal by securing the rectum in the sacral hollow, obliteration of the cul-de-sac, and removal of the redundant sigmoid colon. The operative approach may be abdominal, abdominoperineal, perineal, or posterior to the rectum through the bed of the coccyx. Each and every procedure has advantages and disadvantages, and none is suitable for all patients.

Altemeier and associates employ resection via a perineal approach, thus avoiding an abdominal operation. This is surprisingly well tolerated in the elderly. It involves excising the protruding bowel, closing the pouch of Douglas as high as possible, and approximating the levator ani muscles anteriorly.

Thomas advocates another approach in which the deep cul-de-sac of Douglas is obliterated, the rectum is affixed to the sacral periosteum, and the mobile redundant sigmoid colon is resected through a sacral approach. This is a satisfactory procedure, but the morbidity and mortality are much higher than with Altemeier's technique.

Those who feel that prolapse is due to intussusception favor a technique by which the rectum is secured to the sacrum, thus restoring the normal horizontal position. Ripstein employs a sling of synthetic mesh to hold the rectum firmly in the sacral concavity and thus prevent prolapse. Beahrs feels that an anterior resection, removing the redundant sigmoid and rectosigmoid colon, produces the best results. He fully mobilizes the rectum to take advantage of the postoperative scarring that normally takes place, thereby securing the rectum to the sacrum and avoiding the use of a foreign material.

Goldberg and associates use an intraabdominal repair, fully mobilizing the rectum posteriorly but leaving the lateral stalks intact. The lateral stalks are sutured posteriorly to the sacral periosteum. A convenient sigmoid resection with primary anastomosis is performed to eliminate any redundant colon (Fig. 28-38).

In the elderly, if conditions preclude definitive repair, the Thiersch wire procedure may be used, i.e., the anus is encircled with wire or other suture material. The procedure is well tolerated, but success rate is poor, with a high incidence of fecal impaction and suture breakage.

Generally, an intraabdominal repair of anatomic defects is indicated whenever the patient can tolerate the procedure. Reported recurrence rates following the various operative procedures vary from 4 to 35 percent. The principal postoperative problem is anal incontinence. When compared with the perineal approach, the intraabdominal procedure to remove the redundant colon, combined with fixation of the colon to the sacrum, gives a better result, with a lower recurrence rate.

Pruritus Ani

Pruritus ani is a common problem, but a difficult one to solve. The perianal area is sensitive, and any condition causing soiling or moisture to the area can produce itching. The surgically correctable conditions contributing to this condition are prolapsing hemorrhoids, ectropion, anal fissure, fistula-in-ano, condylomata acuminata, and neoplasm of the anal canal and perineum. Other conditions include diabetes mellitus, dermatitis, jaundice, diarrhea, and leukorrhea. Fungous infections, most commonly due to *Monilia* and *Epidermophyton* organisms, are mainly secondary invaders. In children, *Enterobius vermicularis* (pinworm) is a common cause. When no specific causes are found, the pruritus is called "idiopathic" and can be very difficult to treat.

At the present time, there is no specific treatment for idiopathic pruritus ani. Anal hygiene, consisting of gentle cleansing of the anal canal with moist tissue or water, is the cornerstone of successful control. All other possible causes (e.g., sensitivity to toilet paper, various dyes in underclothing, allergy to soap, cream, and ointment) should be excluded. Hydrocortisone, 0.5% preparation, applied locally, gives temporary symptomatic relief. Topical fungicides have also been used successfully for symptomatic control of pruritus ani.

The undercutting operation described for idiopathic pruritus ani is to be condemned, since it provides only temporary relief. Similarly, the subcutaneous injection of alcohol, tattooing with mercury sulfate, and topical irradiation have been abandoned, since they are ineffective or achieve only transient relief.

Condylomata Acuminata

Anal condylomata acuminata, or warts, are caused by a papilloma virus. Condylomata occur in the perianal area or the squamous epithelium of the anal canal. Occasionally, the mucosa of the upper part of the anal canal or the lower

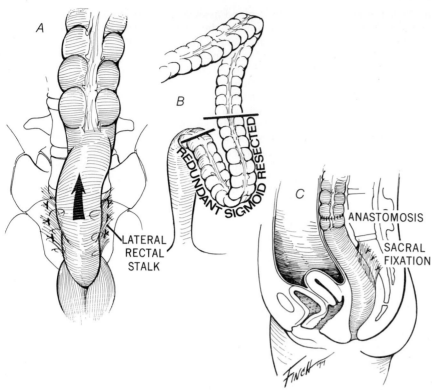

Fig. 28-38. Transabdominal repair of rectal prolapse. 1. Lateral stalks fixed to periosteum of sacrum with 2-0 silk, after rectum has been fully mobilized. 2. Resection of the redundant sigmoid colon. 3. Lateral view after completion.

part of the rectum is involved. The extent of the disease varies from a few small warts to an extensive mass, occluding the anal canal. Bleeding, itching, and irritation are common symptoms. The diagnosis is based on the characteristically soft, papillary appearance. Since most cases are transmitted by sexual contact, other coexisting venereal diseases, especially syphilis and gonorrhea, should be excluded. Multiple biopsies and histologic examination should be done in the extensive warts, since a few cases of squamous cell carcinoma arising from the condylomata acuminata have been reported.

TREATMENT. Small perianal warts can be destroyed by applying 25% podophyllin solution. Extensive warts in the perianal area or in the anal canal require fulguration and excision under anesthesia. Frequent postoperative follow-up is necessary, since recurrence is common. Recently, Abcarian reported encouraging results with immunotherapy, using autogenous wart tissue vaccine. This approach should be used with caution, since vaccines containing oncogenic viruses are potentially dangerous.

Gonococcal Proctitis

Gonococcal proctitis is found most commonly among homosexuals. In the female, the rectum may be infected by the spread of discharge from the gonococcal cervicitis or urethritis. Patients are generally asymptomatic but may have mild anal burning, pain, or discharge in the acute phase. Proctoscopic examination reveals hyperemic and edematous rectal mucosa with purulent discharge in the anal crypt. In the chronic phase, examination of the anal canal and rectum may show them to be normal. Diagnosis

is confirmed by gram smears of the discharge and culture in the appropriate media, Thayer-Martin or Stuart.

Penicillin remains the antibiotic of choice. Kanamycin is used if patients are sensitive to penicillin. Whether the cure is complete is determined by smears and cultures taken at regular intervals after treatment.

Lymphogranuloma Venereum

Lymphogranuloma venereum (lymphogranuloma inguinale) is either an acute or a chronic venereal disease caused by a minute chlamydial bacterium. Transmission of the disease is by intercourse or contact with contaminated exudate from active lesions. In the male, the most common sites are the coronal sulcus, prepuce, glans penis, and urethra. In the female, the primary lesion may appear on any part of the external genitalia, but the most common site is the posterior vaginal wall. The lesion usually is single, consisting of a small erosion, blister, or ulcer, without induration or infiltration. The primary focus is painless and so transient that few patients with lymphogranuloma venereum are aware of it. Adenitis develops in the lymphatic drainage area soon after the primary lesion disappears, although, at times, several months elapse.

Rectal stricture is the sequela to perirectal lymphatic involvement or direct anorectal mucosal infection. The stricture usually is several centimeters above the anal orifice and is 4 to 10 cm in length. Involvement of the perirectal tissues causes perirectal abscess or chronic anal fistulas. Diagnosis is confirmed by the Frei intradermal test and the lymphogranuloma venereum complement fixation test. A cross-reaction with organisms of psittacosis and other chlamydiae may take place. Once positive, the test remains positive for life, and a persistent negative result in the presence of the disease is rare.

Tetracycline or chloramphenicol is the drug of choice. In early stricture, dilatation by finger or dilator is recommended. Colostomy is indicated for complete obstruction. Biopsy for possible malignancy is mandatory.

Proctalgia Fugax

Proctalgia fugax is a severe, spasmodic rectal pain lasting a few minutes or longer. The exact cause is unknown, but the condition may be due to levator ani muscle spasm. The symptom generally occurs in patients who are anxious and overworked. The characteristic history is that of severe pain awakening the patient. The pain usually is located in the midrectum and disappears spontaneously without residual symptoms. Complete proctosigmoidoscopic examination should be performed to rule out anorectal disease.

Treatment to relieve the spasm during an acute attack consists of warm baths or a heating pad applied to the perineum. Since many of these patients are anxious and have cancer phobia, reassurance is an important aspect of therapy.

Neoplasms of the Anus

EPIDERMOID CARCINOMA

Epidermoid carcinoma of the anal canal is uncommon, representing 1 to 2 percent of rectal and colonic carcinomas. The two common varieties are squamous cell carcinoma and transitional cell carcinoma (cloacogenic, basosquamous or basaloid). Squamous cell carcinoma occurs both above and below the dentate line of the anal canal. Transitional cell carcinoma originates from the transitional zone above the dentate line. Since the clinical behavior and prognosis are similar to those of squamous cell carcinoma, transitional cell carcinoma is considered a variant of epidermoid carcinoma.

Early carcinoma of the anal canal presents as an indurated or ulcerated nodule. Rectal pain and bleeding are the most common symptoms. Many cases are misdiagnosed as benign anorectal problems, such as hemorrhoids and anal ulcers, and, consequently, treatment is delayed. Early diagnosis is made by careful examination of the anal canal and confirmed by biopsy.

TREATMENT. Carcinoma of the anal canal spreads to the superior rectal nodes, pelvic nodes, and inguinal nodes. Abdominoperineal resection, with wide excision of the perineal tissues, is the treatment of choice. In selected small tumors distal to the dentate line, local excisions have been adequate, provided the sphincter muscles are not involved. The 5-year survival of the operatively treated patients is 55 to 60 percent.

Recently, Papillon used radium implantation to treat epidermoid carcinoma of the anal canal. The 5-year survival, with no evidence of disease, was 68 percent. He selected patients who had no palpable nodes in the rectal wall. Those with clinically palpable nodes should have abdominoperineal resection. Modern techniques of supervoltage irradiation also offer good results. Williams treated 32 patients who were not suitable for surgery. The 5-year survival was 37.5 percent, and there was no irradiation necrosis. Prophylactic inguinal node dissection is not advisable. However, prompt radical groin dissection should be carried out when clinical metastases have developed. Frequent and careful follow-up examinations are essential, since the incidence of inguinal node involvement is 35 to 40 percent. Inguinal node metastases occur synchronously in 15 percent of patients and subsequently develop in 20 to 25 percent.

Generally, prognosis is poor in patients with anal epidermoid carcinoma with simultaneous groin metastases. Those with subsequent groin metastases have a much better prognosis. Stearns and Quan reported that 15 of 20 patients survived 5 years after groin dissection for subsequent metastases.

MALIGNANT MELANOMA

Melanoma, a rare malignant tumor of the anal canal, accounts for 0.5 to 1.0 percent of anal canal malignant tumors. The anal canal, however, represents the third most common site for melanomas, preceded only by the skin and eyes. Almost all the tumors arise from the epidermoid lining of the anal canal. Most melanomas occur adjacent to the dentate line, although there are a few reports of these tumors arising in the rectum.

Rectal bleeding is the most common symptom. Melanoma is suspected when a deeply pigmented lesion is noted, but this can be confused with thrombosed hemorrhoids. The majority of tumors, however, are pigmented lightly or nonpigmented, and they often are misdiagnosed as polyps or epidermoid carcinoma. In the amelanotic malignant melanoma, tissue biopsy can be misdiagnosed as an undifferentiated epidermoid carcinoma.

Anal canal melanomas have a marked tendency to spread submucosally into the rectum, but they rarely invade adjacent organs. Lymphatic spread to the mesenteric nodes occurs in about one-third of the patients; spread to the inguinal nodes is less common. Hematogenous spread to the liver and lung is early and rapid, accounting for most of the deaths.

Melanomas are radioresistant and do not respond well to chemotherapy. The only chance for cure, therefore, is early diagnosis followed by radical operation. Abdominoperineal resection represents the approach of choice, but the prognosis remains extremely poor.

References

Inflammatory Bowel Disease

Barker, W. F., Benfield, J. R., deKernion, J. B., Fonkalsrud, E. W., and Fowler, E.: "The Creation and Care of Enterocutaneous Stomas," *Curr Probl Surg,* Year Book Medical Publishers, Inc., Chicago, 1975.

Beahrs, O. H.: Creating an Ileal Reservoir with a Continent Ileostomy, *Contemp Surg*, **8:**43, 1976.

Binder, S. C., Patterson, J. F., and Glotzer, D. J.: Toxic Megacolon in Ulcerative Colitis, *Gastroenterology*, **66:**909, 1974.

Brooke, B. N. (ed.): Crohn's Disease, in "Clinics in Gastroenterology," vol 1, part 2, W. B. Saunders Company, Ltd., London, 1972.

Burch, P. R. J., DeDombal, F. T., and Watkinson, G.: Aetiology of Ulcerative Colitis: A New Hypothesis, *Gut*, **10:**277, 1969.

Buzzard, A. J., Baker, W. N. W., Needham, P. R. G., and Warren, R. E.: Acute Toxic Dilatation of the Colon in Crohn's Colitis, *Gut*, **15:**416, 1974.

Cave, D. R., Mitchell, D. N., and Brooke, B. N.: Evidence of an Agent Transmissible from Ulcerative Colitis Tissue, *Lancet*, **1:**1311, 1976.

Devroede, G., and Taylor, W. F.: On Calculating Cancer Risk and Survival of Ulcerative Colitis Patients with the Life Table Method, *Gastroenterology*, **71:**505, 1976.

Dissanayake, A. S., and Truelove, S. C.: A Controlled Therapeutic Trial of Long-Term Maintenance Treatment of Ulcerative Colitis with Sulphasalazine (Salazopyrin), *Gut*, **14:**923, 1973.

Eade, M. N., Cooke, W. T., and Brooke, B. N.: Liver Disease in Ulcerative Colitis: II. The Long-Term Effect of Colectomy, *Ann Intern Med*, **72:**489, 1970.

Esler, M. D., and Goulston, K. J.: Levels of Anxiety in Colonic Disorders, *N Engl J Med*, **288:**16, 1973.

Farmer, R. G., Hawk, W. A., and Turnbull, R. B., Jr.: Clinical Patterns in Crohn's Disease: A Statistical Study of 615 Cases, *Gastroenterology*, **68:**627, 1975.

Fawaz, K. A., Glotzer, D. J., Goldman, H., Dickerson, G. R., Gross, W., and Patterson, J. F.: Ulcerative Colitis and Crohn's Disease of the Colon—A Comparison of the Long Term Postoperative Courses, *Gastroenterology*, **71:**372, 1976.

Foglia, R., Ament, M. E., Fleisher, D., and Fonkalsrud, E. W.: Surgical Management of Ulcerative Colitis in Childhood, *Am J Surg*, **134:**58, 1977.

Gadacz, T. R., Kelly, K. A., and Phillips, S. F.: The Continent Ileal Pouch: Absorptive and Motor Features, *Gastroenterology*, **72:**1287, 1977.

Goodman, M. J., Kirsner, J. B., and Riddell, R. H.: Usefulness of Rectal Biopsy in Inflammatory Bowel Disease, *Gastroenterology*, **72:**952, 1977.

Greenstein, A. J., Sachar, D. B., and Kark, A. E.: Stricture of the Anorectum in Crohn's Disease Involving the Rectum, *Ann Surg*, **181:**207, 1975.

———, Sachar, D. B., Pasternack, B. S., and Janowitz, H. D.: Reoperation and Recurrence in Crohn's Colitis and Ileocolitis, *N Engl J Med*, **293:**685, 1975.

Keighley, M. R. B., Thompson, H., and Alexander-Williams, J.: Multifocal Colonic Carcinoma and Crohn's Disease, *Surgery*, **78:**534, 1975.

Kirsner, J. B.: Toxic Megacolon Complicating Ulcerative Colitis: Current Therapeutic Perspectives, *Gastroenterology*, **66:**1088, 1974.

———: Problems in the Differentiation of Ulcerative Colitis and Crohn's Disease of the Colon: The Need for Repeated Diagnostic Evaluation, *Gastroenterology*, **68:**187, 1975.

———, and Shorter, R. G.: "Inflammatory Bowel Disease," Lea & Febiger, Philadelphia, 1975.

Kock, N. G.: Present Status of the Continent Ileostomy: Surgical Revision of the Malfunctioning Ileostomy, *Dis Colon Rectum*, **19:**200, 1976.

Lefton, H. B., Farmer, R. G., and Fazio, V.: Ileorectal Anastomosis for Crohn's Disease of the Colon, *Gastroenterology*, **69:**612, 1975.

Margulis, A. R., Goldberg, H. I., Lawson, T. L., Montgomery, C. K., Rambo, O. N., Noonan, C. D., and Amberg, J. R.: The Overlapping Spectrum of Ulcerative and Granulomatous Colitis, *Am J Roentgenol Radium Ther Nucl Med*, **113:**325, 1971.

Mendeloff, A. I., Monk, M., Siegel, C. I., and Lilienfeld, A.: Illness Experience and Life Stresses in Patients with Irritable Colon and with Ulcerative Colitis, *N Engl J Med*, **282:**14, 1970.

Morson, B. C.: Rectal Biopsy in Inflammatory Bowel Disease, *N Engl J Med*, **287:**1337, 1972.

Mottet, N. K.: "Major Problems in Pathology," vol. II, "Histopathologic Spectrum of Regional Enteritis and Ulcerative Colitis," W. B. Saunders Company, Philadelphia, 1971.

Nugent, F. W., Veidenheimer, M. C., Meissner, W. A., and Haggitt, R. C.: Prognosis after Colonic Resection for Crohn's Disease of the Colon, *Gastroenterology*, **65:**398, 1973.

Rosenberg, J. L., Wall, A. J., Levin, B., Binder, H. J., and Kirsner, J. B.: A Controlled Trial of Azathioprine in the Management of Chronic Ulcerative Colitis, *Gastroenterology*, **69:**96, 1975.

Schachter, H., and Kirsner, J. B.: Definitions of Inflammatory Bowel Disease of Unknown Etiology, *Gastroenterology*, **68:**591, 1975.

Shorter, R. G., Huizenga, K. A., and Spencer, R. J.: A Working Hypothesis for the Etiology and Pathogenesis of Non-specific Inflammatory Bowel Disease, *Am J Dig Dis*, **17:**1024, 1972.

Sommers, S. C.: Mast Cells and Paneth Cells in Ulcerative Colitis, *Gastroenterology*, **51:**841, 1966.

Steinberg, D. M., Allan, R. N., Brooke, B. N., Cooke, W. T., and Alexander-Williams, J.: Sequelae of Colectomy and Ileostomy: Comparison between Crohn's Colitis and Ulcerative Colitis, *Gastroenterology*, **68:**33, 1975.

Teague, R. H., and Read, A. E.: Polyposis in Ulcerative Colitis, *Gut*, **16:**792, 1975.

Thayer, W. R., Jr.: Are the Inflammatory Bowel Diseases Immune Complex Diseases? *Gastroenterology*, **70:**136, 1976.

Tompkins, R. K., Weinstein, M. H., Foroozan, P., Marx, F. W., and Barker, W. F.: Reappraisal of Rectum-retaining Operations for Ulcerative and Granulomatous Colitis, *Am J Surg*, **125:**159, 1973.

Turnbull, R. B., Jr., Hawk, W. A., and Weakley, F. L.: Surgical Treatment of Toxic Megacolon, *Am J Surg*, **122:**325, 1971.

Veidenheimer, M. C., Nugent, F. W., and Haggitt, R. C.: Ulcerative Colitis of Crohn's Colitis: Is Differentiation Necessary? *Surg Clin North Am*, **56:**721, 1976.

Warshaw, A. L., Welch, J. P., and Ottinger, L. W.: Acute Perforation of the Colon Associated with Chronic Corticosteroid Therapy, *Am J Surg*, **131:**442, 1976.

Watt, J., and Marcus, R.: Progress Report. Experimental Ulcerative Disease of the Colon in Animals, *Gut*, **14:**506, 1973.

Watts, J. McK., and Hughes, E. S. R.: Ulcerative Colitis and Crohn's Disease: Results after Colectomy and Ileorectal Anastomosis, *Br J Surg*, **64:**77, 1977.

Wright, H. K.: The Functional Consequences of Colectomy, *Am J Surg*, **130:**532, 1975.

————, and Tilson, M. D.: A Method for Testing the Functional Significance of Tight Ileostomy Stomas, *Am J Surg,* **123:**417, 1972.

Yudin, I. Y., Sergevnin, V. V., Krasmova, A. I., and Ginsburg, S. A.: The Feasibility of Ileorectal Anastomosis for Nonspecific Ulcerative Colitis, *Contemp Surg,* **6:**73, 1975.

Ischemic Colitis

Marston, A. (ed.): Vascular Diseases of the Alimentary Tract, in "Clinics in Gastroenterology," vol 1, part 3, W. B. Saunders Company, Ltd., London, 1972.

O'Connell, T. X., Kadell, B., and Tompkins, R. K.: Ischemia of the Colon, *Surg Gynecol Obstet,* **142:**337, 1976.

Williams, L. F., Jr., and Wittenberg, J.: Ischemic Colitis: An Useful Clinical Diagnosis, but Is It Ischemic? *Ann Surg,* **182:**439, 1975.

Radiation Enterocolitis

Cram, A. E., Pearlman, N. W., and Jochimsen, P. R.: Surgical Management of Complications of Radiation-Injured Gut, *Am J Surg,* **133:**551, 1977.

DeCosse, J. J., Rhodes, R. S., Wentz, W. B., Reagan, J. W., Dworken, H. J., and Holden, W. D.: The Natural History and Management of Radiation Induced Injury of the Gastrointestinal Tract, *Ann Surg,* **170:**369, 1969.

Green, N., Iba, G., and Smith, W. R.: Measures to Minimize Small Intestine Injury in the Irradiated Pelvis, *Cancer,* **35:**1633, 1975.

Morgenstern, L., Thompson, R., and Friedman, N. B.: The Modern Enigma of Radiation Enteropathy: Sequelae and Solutions, *Am J Surg,* **134:**166, 1977.

Palmer, J. A., and Bush, R. S.: Radiation Injuries to the Bowel Associated with the Treatment of Carcinoma of the Cervix, *Surgery,* **80:**458, 1976.

Swan, R. W., Fowler, W. C., Jr., and Boronow, R. C.: Surgical Management of Radiation Injury to the Small Intestine, *Surg Gynecol Obstet,* **142:**325, 1976.

Pseudobranous Enterocolitis

Birnbaum, D., Laufer, A., and Freund, M.: Pseudomembranous Enterocolitis, *Gastroenterology,* **41:**345, 1961.

Gorbach, S. L., and Bartlett, J. G. (eds.): The Role of Clindamycin in Anaerobic Bacterial Infections. A Symposium, *J Infect Dis,* **135** (suppl), 1977.

Tedesco, F. J., Barton, R. W., and Alpers, D. H.: Clindamycin-associated Colitis, a Prospective Study, *Ann Intern Med,* **81:**429, 1974.

Amebiasis

Grigsby, W. P.: Collective Review: Surgical Treatment of Amebiasis, *Surg Gynecol Obstet,* **128:**609, 1969.

Mahmoud, A. A. F., and Warren, K. S.: Algorithms in the Diagnosis and Management of Exotic Diseases: XVII. Amebiasis, *J Infect Dis,* **134:**639, 1976.

Pittman, F. E., El-Hashimi, W. K., and Pittman, J. C.: Studies of Human Amebiasis. *Gastroenterology,* **65:**581, 1973.

Actinomycosis

Davies, M., and Keddie, N. C.: Abdominal Actinomycosis, *Br J Surg,* **60:**18, 1973.

Diverticular Disease

Adams, J. T.: The Barium Enema as Treatment for Massive Diverticular Bleeding, *Dis Colon Rectum,* **17:**439, 1974.

Athanasoulis, C. A., Baum, S., Rosch, J., Waltman, A. C., Ring, E. J., Smith, J. C., Jr., Sugarbaker, E., and Wood, W.: Mesenteric Arterial Infusions of Vasopressin for Hemorrhage from Colonic Diverticulosis, *Am J Surg,* **129:**212, 1975.

Behringer, G. E., and Albright, N. L.: Diverticular Disease of the Colon: A Frequent Cause of Massive Rectal Bleeding, *Am J Surg,* **125:**419, 1973.

Berman, L. G., Burdick, D., Heitzman, E. R., and Prior, J. T.: A Critical Reappraisal of Sigmoid Peridiverticulitis, *Surg Gynecol Obstet,* **127:**481, 1968.

Botsford, T. W., Zollinger, R. M., Jr., and Hicks, R.: Mortality of the Surgical Treatment of Diverticulitis, *Am J Surg,* **121:**702, 1971.

Canter, J. W., and Shorb, P. E., Jr.: Acute Perforation of Colonic Diverticula Associated with Prolonged Adrenocorticosteroid Therapy, *Am J Surg,* **121:**46, 1971.

Casarella, W. J., Kanter, I. E., and Seaman, W. B.: Right-sided Colonic Diverticula as a Cause of Acute Rectal Hemorrhage, *N Engl J Med,* **286:**450, 1972.

Classen, J. N., Bonardi, R., O'Mara, C. S., Finney, D. C. W., and Sterioff, S.: Surgical Treatment of Acute Diverticulitis by Staged Procedures, *Ann Surg,* **184:**582, 1976.

Colcock, B. P.: Diverticular Disease of the Colon, in "Major Problems in Clinical Surgery," W. B. Saunders Company, Philadelphia, 1971.

————, and Stahmann, F. D.: Fistulas Complicating Diverticular Disease of the Sigmoid Colon, *Ann Surg,* **175:**838, 1972.

Drapanas, T., Pennington, D. G., Kappelman, M., and Lindsey, E. S.: Emergency Subtotal Colectomy: Preferred Approach to Management of Massively Bleeding Diverticular Disease, *Ann Surg,* **177:**519, 1973.

Eng, K., Ranson, J. H. C., and Localio, S. A.: Resection of the Perforated Segment: A Significant Advance in Treatment of Diverticulitis with Free Perforation or Abscess, *Am J Surg,* **133:**67, 1977.

Fleischner, F. G.: Diverticular Disease of the Colon: New Observations and Revised Concepts, *Gastroenterology,* **60:**316, 1971.

Havia, T.: Diverticulosis of the Colon: A Clinical and Histological Study, *Acta Chir Scand [Suppl],* 415, 1971.

Magness, L. J., Sanfelippo, P. M., van Heerden, J. A., and Judd, E. S.: Diverticular Disease of the Right Colon, *Surg Gynecol Obstet,* **140:**30, 1975.

Meyers, M. A., Alonso, D. R., Gray, G. F., and Baer, J. W.: Pathogenesis of Bleeding Colonic Diverticulosis, *Gastroenterology,* **71:**577, 1976.

Miller, D. W., Jr., and Wichern, W. A., Jr.: Perforated Sigmoid Diverticulitis: Appraisal of Primary versus Delayed Resection, *Am J Surg,* **121:**536, 1971.

Morson, B. C.: Pathology of Diverticular Disease of the Colon, in A. N. Smith (ed.), "Clinics in Gastroenterology," vol 4, part 1, W. B. Saunders Company, Ltd., London, 1975.

Nahrwold, D. L., and Demuth, W. E.: Diverticulitis with Perforation into the Peritoneal Cavity, *Ann Surg,* **185:**80, 1977.

Nicholas, G. G., Miller, W. T., Fitts, W. T., and Tondreau, R. L.: Diagnosis of Diverticulitis of the Colon: Role of the Barium

Enema in Defining Pericolic Inflammation, *Ann Surg,* **176**:205, 1972.

Painter, N. S., Truelove, S. C., Ardran, G. M., and Tuckey, M.: Segmentation and the Localization of Intraluminal Pressures in the Human Colon, with Special Reference to the Pathogenesis of Colonic Diverticula, *Gastroenterology,* **49**:169, 1965.

Parks, T. G., and Connell, A. M.: The Outcome in 455 Patients Admitted for Treatment of Diverticular Disease of the Colon, *Br J Surg,* **57**:775, 1970.

Parsa, F., Gordon, H. E., and Wilson, S. E.: Bleeding Diverticulosis of the Colon, *Dis Colon Rectum,* **18**:37, 1975.

Ranson, J. H. C., Lawrence, L. R., and Localio, S. A.: Colomyotomy: A New Approach to Surgery for Colonic Diverticular Disease, *Am J Surg,* **123**:185, 1972.

Reilly, M.: Sigmoid Myotomy, in A. N. Smith (ed.), "Clinics in Gastroenterology," vol 4, part 1, W. B. Saunders Company, Ltd., London, 1975.

Rugtiv, G. M.: Diverticulitis: Selective Surgical Management, *Am J Surg,* **130**:219, 1975.

Walker, J. D., Gray, L. A., Sr., and Polk, H. C., Jr.: Diverticulitis in Women: An Unappreciated Clinical Presentation, *Ann Surg,* **185**:402, 1977.

Polyps and Polyposis

Alm, T.: Surgical Treatment of Hereditary Adenomatosis of the Colon and Rectum in Sweden during the Last 20 Years: II. Patients with Prophylactic Operations, Primary and Late Results, *Acta Chir Scand,* **141**:228, 1975.

Bussey, H. J. R.: "Familial Polyposis Coli," The Johns Hopkins University Press, Baltimore, 1975.

Cole, J. W.: Carcinogens and Carcinogenesis in the Colon, *Hosp Pract,* **8**:123, 1973.

———, and Holden, W. D.: Postcolectomy Regression of Adenomatous Polyps of the Rectum, *Arch Surg,* **79**:385, 1959.

———, and McKalen, A.: Studies on the Morphogenesis of Adenomatous Polyps in the Human Colon, *Cancer,* **16**:998, 1963.

DeCosse, J. J., Adams, M. B., and Condon, R. E.: Familial Polyposis, *Cancer,* **39**:267, 1977.

Erbe, R. W.: Current Concepts in Genetics. Inherited Gastrointestinal-Polyposis Syndromes, *N Engl J Med,* **294**:1101, 1976.

Fenoglio, C. M., and Lane, N.: The Anatomical Precursor of Colorectal Carcinoma, *Cancer,* **34** [suppl], 819, 1974.

Gilbertsen, V. A.: Proctosigmoidoscopy and Polypectomy in Reducing the Incidence of Rectal Cancer, *Cancer,* **34** [suppl], 936, 1974.

Knoernschild, H. E.: Growth Rate and Malignant Potential of Colonic Polyps: Early Results, *Surg Forum,* **14**:137, 1963.

Lane, N., Kaplan, H., and Pascal, R. R.: Minute Adenomatous and Hyperplastic Polyps of the Colon: Divergent Patterns of Epithelial Growth with Specific Associated Mesenchymal Changes. Contrasting Roles in the Pathogenesis of Carcinoma, *Gastroenterology,* **60**:537, 1971.

Lipkin, M.: Phase 1 and Phase 2 Proliferative Lesions of Colonic Epithelial Cells in Diseases Leading to Colonic Cancer, *Cancer,* **34** [suppl], 878, 1974.

Lynch, H. T., Harris, R. E., Organ, C. H., Jr., Guirgis, H. A., Lynch, P. M., Lynch, J. F., and Nelson, E. J.: The Surgeon, Genetics, and Cancer Control: The Cancer Family Syndrome, *Ann Surg,* **185**:435, 1977.

Moertel, C. G., Hill, J. R., and Adson, M. A.: Surgical Management of Multiple Polyposis: The Problem of Cancer in the Retained Bowel Segment, *Arch Surg,* **100**:521, 1970.

Morson, B. C., and Bussey, H. J. S.: Predisposing Causes of Intestinal Cancers, *Curr Probl Surg,* February, 1970.

Muto, T., Bussey, H. J. R., and Morson, B. C.: The Evolution of Cancer of the Colon and Rectum, *Cancer,* **36**:2251, 1975.

Nivatvongs, S., and Goldberg, S. M.: Results of 100 Consecutive Polypectomies with the Fiberoptic Colonoscope, *Am J Surg,* **128**:347, 1974.

Shinya, H., and Wolff, W.: Flexible Colonoscopy, *Cancer,* **37** [suppl], 462, 1976.

Spratt, J. S., Ackerman, L. V., and Moyer, C. A.: Relationship of Polyps of the Colon to Colonic Cancer, *Ann Surg,* **148**:682, 1958.

Watne, W. L., Lai, H.-Y., Carrier, J., and Coppula, W.: The Diagnosis and Surgical Treatment of Patients with Gardner's Syndrome, *Surgery,* **82**:327, 1977.

Welch, C. E., and Hedberg, S. E.: "Polypoid Lesions of the Gastrointestinal Tract," 2d ed., W. B. Saunders Company, Philadelphia, 1975.

Welch, J. P., and Welch, C. E.: Villous Adenomas of the Colorectum, *Am J Surg,* **131**:185, 1976.

Carcinoma

Bengmark, S., and Hafström, L.: The Natural History of Primary and Secondary Malignant Tumors of the Liver: I. The Prognosis for Patients with Hepatic Metastases from Colonic and Rectal Carcinoma by Laparotomy, *Cancer,* **23**:198, 1969.

Berge, T., Ekelund, G., Mellner, C., Pihl, B., and Wenckert, A.: Carcinoma of the Colon and Rectum in a Defined Population, *Acta Chir Scand* [suppl], 438, 1973.

Burkitt, D. P.: Large-Bowel Cancer: An Epidemiologic Jigsaw Puzzle, *J Natl Cancer Inst,* **54**:3, 1975.

Cass, A. W., Million, R. R., and Pfaff, W. W.: Patterns of Recurrence following Surgery Alone for Adenocarcinoma of the Colon and Rectum, *Cancer,* **37**:2861, 1976.

Clark, J., Hall, W. W., and Moossa, A. R.: Treatment of Obstructing Cancer of the Colon and Rectum, *Surg Gynecol Obstet,* **141**:541, 1975.

Clarke, J. S., Condon, R. E., Bartlett, J. G., Gorbach, S. L., Nichols, R. L., and Ochi, S.: Preoperative Oral Antibiotics Reduce Septic Complications of Colon Operations: Results of Prospective, Randomized, Double-blind Clinical Study, *Ann Surg,* **186**:251, 1977.

Cole, W. H.: Collective Review: The Mechanisms of Spread of Cancer, *Surg Gynecol Obstet,* **137**:853, 1973.

Collins, V. P.: Time of Occurrence of Pulmonary Metastases from Carcinoma of Colon and Rectum, *Cancer,* **15**:387, 1962.

Crapp, A. R., and Cuthbertson, A. M.: William Waldeyer and the Rectosacral Fascia, *Surg Gynecol Obstet,* **138**:252, 1974.

Crile, G., Jr., and Turnbull, R. B., Jr.: The Role of Electrocoagulation in the Treatment of Carcinoma of the Rectum, *Surg Gynecol Obstet,* **135**:391, 1972.

Ekelund, G. R., and Pihl, B.: Multiple Carcinomas of the Colon and Rectum, *Cancer,* **33**:1630, 1974.

Gardner, B., Kottmeier, P., and Harshaw, D.: The Surgeon at Work: A Modified One Stage Pull Through Operation for Carcinoma or Prolapse of the Rectum, *Surg Gynecol Obstet,* **136**:95, 1973.

Goldsmith, H. S.: Protection of Low Rectal Anastomosis with Intact Omentum, *Surg Gynecol Obstet,* **144:**585, 1977.

Goldstein, M., and Duff, J. H.: Reconsideration of Colostomy in Elective Left Colon Resection, *Surg Gynecol Obstet,* **134:**593, 1972.

Goligher, J. C., Graham, N. G., and DeDombal, F. T.: Anastomotic Dehiscence after Anterior Resection of Rectum and Sigmoid, *Br J Surg,* **57:**109, 1970.

Greegor, D. H.: Occult Blood Testing for Detection of Asymptomatic Colon Cancer, *Cancer,* **28:**131, 1971.

Griffen, W. O., Jr., Humphrey, L. J., and Sosin, H.: The Prognosis and Management of Recurrent Abdominal Malignancies, *Curr Probl Surg,* April, 1969.

Grinnell, R. S.: The Chance of Cancer and Lymphatic Metastasis in Small Colon Tumors Discovered on X-ray Examination, *Ann Surg,* **159:**132, 1964.

Herrera, M. A., Chu, T. M., Holyoke, E. D., and Mittelman, A.: CEA Monitoring of Palliative Treatment of Colorectal Carcinoma, *Ann Surg,* **185:**23, 1977.

Higgins, G. A., Jr., Conn, J. H., Jordan, P. H., Jr., Humphrey, E. W., Roswit, B., and Keehn, R. J.: Preoperative Radiotherapy for Colorectal Cancer, *Ann Surg,* **181:**624, 1975.

———, Humphrey, E., Juler, G. L., LeVeen, H. H., McCaughan, J., and Keehn, R. J.: Adjuvant Chemotherapy in the Surgical Treatment of Large Bowel Cancer, *Cancer,* **38:**1461, 1976.

Irvin, T. T., and Goligher, J. C.: A Controlled Clinical Trial of Three Different Methods of Perineal Wound Management following Excision of the Rectum, *Br J Surg,* **62:**287, 1975.

Johnson, R. J. R.: The Role of Radiation Therapy in the Management of Rectosigmoid Cancer, *Cancer,* **40:**595, 1977.

Keighley, M. R. B.: Prevention of Wound Sepsis in Gastro-intestinal Surgery, *Br J Surg,* **64:**315, 1977.

Lawrence, W., Jr., Terz, J. J., Horsley, S., III, Donaldson, M., Lovett, W. L., Brown, P. W., Ruffner, B. W., and Regelson, W.: Chemotherapy as an Adjuvant to Surgery for Colorectal Cancer, *Ann Surg,* **181:**616, 1975.

Localio, S. A., and Eng, K.: Malignant Tumors of the Rectum, *Curr Probl Surg,* September, 1975.

Lockhart-Mummery, H. E., Ritchie, J. K., and Hawley, P. R.: The Results of Surgical Treatment for Carcinoma of the Rectum at St. Mark's Hospital from 1948 to 1972, *Br J Surg,* **63:**673, 1976.

Madden, J. L., and Kandalaft, S.: Electrocoagulation in the Treatment of Cancer of the Rectum: A Continuing Study, *Ann Surg,* **174:**530, 1971.

Nadler, S. H., and Phelan, J. T.: The Surgeon at Work: Abdominoperineal Resection, *Surg Gynecol Obstet,* **128:**119, 1969.

Oh, C., and Kark, A. E.: The Transsphincteric Approach to Mid and Low Rectal Villous Adenoma: Anatomic Basis of Surgical Treatment, *Ann Surg,* **176:**605, 1972.

Papillon, J.: Intracavitary Irradiation of Early Rectal Cancer for Cure, *Cancer,* **36:**696, 1975.

Polk, H. C., Jr., Ahmad, W., and Knutson, C. O.: Carcinoma of the Colon and Rectum, *Curr Probl Surg,* January, 1973.

Reddy, B. S., Mastromarino, A., and Wynder, E.: Diet and Metabolism: Large-Bowel Cancer, *Cancer,* **39:**1815, 1977.

Schrock, T. R., Deveney, C. W., and Dunphy, J. E.: Factors Contributing to Leakage of Colonic Anastomoses, *Ann Surg,* **177:**513, 1973.

Silverman, D. T., Murray, J. L., Smart, C. R., Brown, C. C., and

Myers, M. H.: Estimated Median Survival Times of Patients with Colorectal Cancer Based on Experience with 9,745 Patients, *Am J Surg,* **133:**289, 1977.

Slanetz, C. A., Herter, F. P., and Grinnell, R. S.: Anterior Resection versus Abdominoperineal Resection for Cancer of the Rectum and Rectosigmoid, *Am J Surg,* **123:**110, 1972.

Spjut, H. J., and Noall, M. W.: Experimental Induction of Tumors of the Large Bowel of Rats, *Cancer,* **28:**29, 1971.

Tank, E. S., Ernst, C. B., Woolson, S. T., and Lapides, J.: Urinary Tract Complications of Anorectal Surgery, *Am J Surg,* **123:**118, 1972.

Turnbull, R. B., Jr.: The No-Touch Isolation Technique of Resection, *JAMA,* **231:**1181, 1975.

Wallack, M. K., Brown, A. S., Rosato, E. F., and Rosato, F. E.: Collective Reviews: The Treatment of Cancer of the Large Intestine, *Surg Gynecol Obstet,* **142:**97, 1976.

Washington, J. A., II, Dearing, W. H., Judd, E. S., and Elveback, L. R.: Effect of Preoperative Antibiotic Regimen on Development of Infection after Intestinal Surgery: Prospective, Randomized, Double-Blind Study, *Ann Surg,* **180:**567, 1974.

Weinstein, M., and Roberts, M.: Sexual Potency following Surgery for Rectal Carcinoma, *Ann Surg,* **185:**295, 1977.

Welch, J. P., and Donaldson, G. A.: Perforative Carcinoma of Colon and Rectum, *Ann Surg,* **180:**734, 1974.

Welin, S., Youker, J., and Spratt, J. S., Jr.: The Rates and Patterns of Growth of 375 Tumors of the Large Intestine and Rectum Observed Serially by Double Contrast Enema Study (Malmo Technique), *Am J Roentgenol Radium Ther Nucl Med,* **90:**673, 1963.

Whittaker, M., and Goligher, J. C.: The Prognosis after Surgical Treatment for Carcinoma of the Rectum, *Br J Surg,* **63:**384, 1976.

Winawer, S. J., Sherlock, P., Schottenfeld, D., and Miller, D. G.: Screening for Colon Cancer, *Gastroenterology,* **70:**783, 1976.

Wright, H. K., Thomas, W. H., and Cleveland, J. C.: The Low Recurrence Rate of Colonic Carcinoma in Ileocolic Anastomosis, *Surg Gynecol Obstet,* **129:**960, 1969.

Other Tumors

Freni, S. C., and Keeman, J. N.: Leiomyomatosis of the Colon, *Cancer,* **39:**263, 1977.

Gray, L. A.: Endometriosis of the Bowel: Role of Bowel Resection, Superficial Excision and Oophorectomy in Treatment, *Ann Surg,* **177:**580, 1973.

Orloff, M. J.: Carcinoid Tumors of the Rectum, *Cancer,* **28:**175, 1971.

Scott, J. E.: Carcinoid Tumours of the Colon, *Br J Surg,* **60:**684, 1973.

Wychulis, A. R., Beahrs, O. H., and Woolner, L. B.: Malignant Lymphoma of the Colon: A Study of 69 Cases, *Arch Surg,* **93:**215, 1966.

Volvulus and Related Problems

Andersson, Å., Bergdahl, L., and Van der Linden, W.: Volvulus of the Cecum, *Ann Surg,* **181:**876, 1975.

Arnold, G. J., and Nance, F. C.: Volvulus of the Sigmoid Colon, *Ann Surg,* **177:**527, 1973.

Caplan, L. H., Jacobson, H. G., Rubenstein, B. M., and Rotman, M. Z.: Megacolon and Volvulus in Parkinson's Disease, *Radiology,* **85:**73, 1965.

Childress, M. H., and Martel, W.: Fecaloma Simulating Colonic Neoplasm, *Surg Gynecol Obstet,* **142:**664, 1976.

da Silveira, G. M.: Chagas' Disease of the Colon, *Br J Surg,* **63:**831, 1976.

Fairgrieve, J.: Hirschsprung's Disease in the Adult, *Br J Surg,* **50:**506, 1963.

Flanigan, R. C., and Barry, F.: Dual Cecostomy as an Approach to Volvulus of the Cecum, *Surg Gynecol Obstet,* **141:**775, 1975.

Hines, J. R., Guerkink, R. E., and Bass, R. T.: Recurrence and Mortality Rates in Sigmoid Volvulus, *Surg Gynecol Obstet,* **124:**567, 1967.

Huttunen, R., Heikkinen, E., and Larmi, T. K. I.: Stercoraceous and Idiopathic Perforations of the Colon, *Surg Gynecol Obstet,* **140:**756, 1975.

Maglietta, E. D.: Congenital Aganglionic Megacolon in Adults, *Arch Surg,* **18:**598, 1960.

Peterson, H.: Volvulus of the Cecum, *Ann Surg,* **166:**296, 1967.

String, S. T., and DeCosse, J. J.: Sigmoid Volvulus: An Examination of the Mortality, *Am J Surg,* **121:**293, 1971.

Watkins, G. L., and Oliver, G. A.: Giant Megacolon in the Insane: Further Observation on Patients Treated by Subtotal Colectomy, *Gastroenterology,* **48:**718, 1965.

Rectum and Anus

Abcarian, H.: Lateral Internal Sphincterotomy—a New Technique for Treatment of Chronic Fissure-in-ano, *Surg Clin North Am,* **55:**143, 1975.

———: Acute Suppuration of the Anorectum, *Surg Annu,* **8:**305, 1976.

———, Smith, D., and Sharon, N.: The Immunotherapy of Anal Condyloma Acuminata, *Dis Colon Rectum,* **19:**237, 1976.

Abrams, A. J.: Lymphogranuloma Venereum, *JAMA,* **205:**199, 1968.

Alexander, R. M., and Cone, L. A.: Malignant Melanoma of the Rectal Ampulla: Report of a Case and Review of the Literature, *Dis Colon Rectum,* **20:**53, 1977.

Alexander, S.: Dermatological Aspects of Anorectal Disease, *Clin Gastroenterol,* **4:**651, 1975.

Alexander-Williams, J.: Fistula-in-ano: Management of Crohn's Fistula, *Dis Colon Rectum,* **19:**518, 1976.

———, and Crapp, A. R.: Conservative Management of Haemorrhoids. Part I: Injection, Freezing and Ligation, *Clin Gastroenterol,* **4:**595, 1975.

Altemeier, W. A., Culbertson, W. R., Schowengerdt, C., and Hunt, J.: Nineteen Years' Experience with the One-stage Perineal Repair of Rectal Prolapse, *Ann Surg,* **173:**993, 1971.

Ani, A. N., and Solanke, T. F.: Anal Fistula: A Review of 82 Cases, *Dis Colon Rectum,* **19:**51, 1976.

Barron, J.: Office Ligation Treatment of Hemorrhoids, *Dis Colon Rectum,* **6:**109, 1963.

Beahrs, O. H., and Wilson, S. M.: Carcinoma of the Anus, *Ann Surg,* **184:**422, 1976.

Bennett, R. C., and Goligher, J. C.: Results of Internal Sphincterotomy for Anal Fissure, *Br Med J,* **2:**1500, 1963.

Bevans, D. W., Jr.: Perirectal Abscess: A Potentially Fatal Illness, *Am J Surg,* **126:**765, 1973.

Block, I. R., and Enquist, I. F.: Lymphatic Studies Pertaining to Local Spread of Carcinoma of the Rectum in Female, *Surg Gynecol Obstet,* **112:**41, 1961.

———, Rodriquez M. S., and Calva P. C.: Levator Ani as Substitute Puborectalis Sling in Treatment of Anal Incontinence, *Surg Gynecol Obstet,* **141:**611, 1975.

Boxall, T. A., Smart, P. J. G., and Griffiths, J. D.: The Blood Supply of the Distal Segment of the Rectum in Anterior Resection, *Br J Surg,* **50:**399, 1962.

Brocklehurst, J. C.: Management of Anal Incontinence, *Clin Gastroenterol,* **4:**479, 1975.

Burkitt, D. P.: Hemorrhoids, Varicose Veins and Deep Vein Thrombosis: Epidermologic Features and Suggested Causation Factors, *Can J Surg,* **18:**483, 1975.

Catterall, R. D.: Sexually Transmitted Diseases of the Anus and Rectum, *Clin Gastroenterol,* **4:**659, 1975.

Cram, A. E., Pearlman, N. W., and Jochimsen, P. R.: Surgical Management and Complications of Radiation Injured Gut, *Arch Surg,* **133:**551, 1977.

Crapp, A. R., and Alexander-Williams J.: Fissure-in-ano and Anal Stenosis, *Clin Gastroenterol,* **4:**619, 1975.

DeCosse, J. J., Rhodes, R. S., Wentz, W. B., Reagan, J. W., Dworken, H. J., and Holden, W. E.: The Natural History and Management of Radiation Induced Injury of the Gastrointestinal Tract, *Ann Surg,* **170:**369, 1969.

Deveney, C. W., Lewis, F. R., and Schrock, T. R.: Surgical Management of Radiation Injury of the Small and Large Intestine, *Dis Colon Rectum,* **19:**25, 1976.

Douthwaite, A. H.: Proctalgia Fugax, *Br Med J,* **2:**164, 1962.

Duthie, J. L., and Bennett, R. C.: Anal Sphincteric Pressure in Fissure-in-ano, *Surg Gynecol Obstet,* **119:**19, 1964.

Editorial: To Tie; to Stab; to Stretch; Perchance to Freeze, *Lancet,* **2:**645, 1975.

Eisenhammer, S.: The Surgical Correction of Chronic Anal (Sphincteric) Contracture, *S Afr Med J,* **25:**486, 1951.

Ferguson, J. A., Mazier, W. P., Ganchrow, M. I., and Friend, W. G.: The Closed Technique of Hemorrhoidectomy, *Surgery,* **70:**480, 1971.

Fitzgerald, D. M., and Hamit, H. F.: The Variable Significance of Condylomata Acuminata, *Am J Surg,* **179:**328, 1974.

Frykman, H. M., and Goldberg, S. M.: The Surgical Treatment of Rectal Procidentia, *Surgery,* **129:**1225, 1969.

Gabriel, W. B.: Theirsch's Operation for Anal Incontinence, *Proc R Soc Med,* **41:**467, 1948.

Ganchrow, M. I., Bowman, E., and Clark, J. F.: Thrombosed Hemorrhoids: A Clinico-pathologic Study, *Dis Colon Rectum,* **14:**331, 1971.

———, Mazier, W. P., Friend, W. G., and Ferguson, J. A.: Hemorrhoidectomy Revisited: A Computer Analysis of 2038 Cases, *Dis Colon Rectum,* **14:**128, 1971.

Goldberg, S. M., and Gordon, P. H.: Treatment of Rectal Prolapse, *Clin Gastroenterol,* **4:**489, 1975.

Golden, G. T., and Horsley, J. S., III: Surgical Management of Epidermoid Carcinoma of the Anus, *Am J Surg,* **131:**275, 1976.

Goligher, J. C.: Cryosurgery for Hemorrhoids, *Dis Colon Rectum,* **19:**213, 1976.

———, Leacock, A. G., and Brossy, J. J.: The Surgical Anatomy of the Anal Canal, *Br J Surg,* **43:**51, 1955.

Gordon, P. H., and Hoexter, B.: Complications of Ripstein Procedure, Presented at 76th Annual Meeting, ASC&RS, Orlando, Fl, May 1977. To be published in *Dis Colon Rectum.*

Graham-Stewart, C. W.: The Etiology and Treatment of Fissure-in-ano, *Int Abstr Surg,* **115:**511, 1962.

Hagihara, P. F., and Griffen, W. O.: Delayed Correction of Ano-rectal Incontinence Due to Anal Sphincteral Injury, *Arch Surg,* **111:**63, 1976.

Hancock, B. D.: The Internal Sphincter and Anal Fissure, *Br J Surg,* **64:**92, 1977.

Hanley, P. H., Ray, J. E., Pennington, E. E., and Grablowsky, O. M.: Fistula-in-ano: A Ten Year Follow-up Study of Horseshoe Abscess Fistula-in-ano, *Dis Colon Rectum,* **19:**507, 1976.

Hawley, P. R.: Anorectal Fistula, *Clin Gastroenterol,* **4:**635, 1975.

Homan, W. P., Tang, C., and Thorbjarnarson, B.: Anal Lesions Complicating Crohn's Disease, *Arch Surg,* **111:**1333, 1976.

Jones, C. B., and Schofield, P. F.: Comparative Study of Methods of Treatment for Haemorrhoids, *Proc R Soc Med,* **67:**51, 1974.

Kheir, S., Kichey, R. C., Martin, R. G., MacKay, B., and Galla-gher, H. S.: Cloacogenic Carcinoma of the Anal Canal, *Arch Surg,* **104:**407, 1972.

Klein, E. J., Fisher, L. S., Chow, A. W., and Guze, L. B.: Ano-rectal Gonococcal Infection, *Ann Int Med,* **86:**340, 1977.

Klotz, R. G., Pamukcoglu, T., and Souilliard, D. H.: Transitional Cloacogenic Carcinoma of the Anal Canal, *Cancer,* **20:**1727, 1967.

Leaper, D. J., Page, R. E., Rosenberg, I. L., Wilson, D. N., and Goligher, J. C.: A Controlled Study Comparing the Conven-tional Treatment of Idiopathic Anorectal Abscess with That of Incision, Curettage and Primary Suture under Systemic Anti-biotic Cover, *Dis Colon Rectum,* **19:**46, 1976.

Lockhart-Mummery, H. E.: Anal Canal Perineal Ulceration in Crohn's Disease, *Proc R Soc Med,* **57:**897, 1964.

McColl, I.: The Comparative Anatomy and Pathology of Anal Glands, *Ann R Coll Surg,* **40:**36, 1967.

Mason, J. K., and Helwig, E. B.: Anorectal Melanoma, *Cancer,* **19:**39, 1966.

Morson, B. C.: The Pathology and Results of Treatment of Squa-mous Cell Carcinoma of the Anal Canal and Anal Margin, *Proc R Soc Med,* **53:**416, 1960.

———, and Volkstadt, H.: Malignant Melanoma of the Anal Canal, *J Clin Pathol,* **16:**126, 1963.

Moschcowitz, A. V.: The Pathogenesis, Anatomy, and Cure of Prolapse of the Rectum, *Surg Gynecol Obstet,* **15:**7, 1912.

Northman, B. J., and Schuster, M. M.: Internal Anal Sphincter Derangement with Anal Fissures, *Gastroenterology,* **67:**216, 1974.

Notaras, M. J.: The Treatment of Anal Fissure by Lateral Subcu-taneous Internal Sphincterotomy—a Technic and Results, *Br J Surg,* **58:**96, 1971.

O'Connor, J. J.: The Role of Cryosurgery in Management of Anorectal Disease: A Study of Cryosurgical Techniques, *Dis Colon Rectum,* **18:**298, 1975.

Oh, C., and Kark, A. E.: Anatomy of the External Anal Sphincter, *Br J Surg,* **59:**717, 1972.

Pack, G. T., and Oropeza, R.: A Comparative Study of Melanoma and Epidermoid Carcinoma of the Anal Canal: A Review of 20 Melanomas and 29 Epidermoid Carcinomas, *Dis Colon Rectum,* **10:**161, 1967.

Palmer, J. A., and Bush, R. S.: Radiation Injuries to the Bowel Associated with the Treatment of Carcinoma of the Cervix, *Surgery,* **80:**458, 1976.

Papillon, J.: Radiation Therapy in the Management of Epidermoid Carcinoma of the Anal Region, *Dis Colon Rectum,* **17:**181, 1974.

Paradis, P., Douglass, H. O., Jr., and Holyoke, E. D.: The Clinical Implications of a Staging System for Carcinoma of the Anus, *Surg Gynecol Obstet,* **141:**411, 1975.

Parks, A. G.: Anatomical Causes of Rectal Prolapse, *Proc R Soc Med,* **66:**26, 1975.

———: Fistula-in-ano: Perineal Fistula of Intra-abdominal or Intrapelvic Origin Simulating Fistula-in-ano—Report of 7 Cases, *Dis Colon Rectum,* **19:**500, 1976.

———, Goligher, J. C., Alexander-Williams, J., and Hanley, P. H.: Symposium (Moderator: S. M. Goldberg): Treatment of High Fistula-in-ano, *Dis Colon Rectum,* **19:**487, 1976.

———, Gordon, P. H., and Hardcastle, J. D.: A Classification of Fistula-in-ano, *Br J Surg,* **63:**1, 1976.

———, Porter, N. H., and Melyath J.: Experimental Study of the Reflex Mechanism Controlling the Muscles of the Pelvic Floor, *Dis Colon Rectum,* **5:**407, 1962.

Pilling, L. F., Swenson, W. M., and Hill, J. R.: The Psychologic Aspects of Proctalgia Fugax, *Dis Colon Rectum,* **8:**372, 1965.

Ripstein, C. B., and Lanter, B.: Etiology and Surgical Therapy of Massive Prolapse of the Rectum, *Ann Surg,* **157:**259, 1963.

Ross, S. T., and Bernstein, W. C.: The Role of Cryosurgery in Management of Anorectal Disease: The Loyal Opposition, *Dis Colon Rectum,* **18:**301, 1975.

Samson, R. B., and Stewart, W. R. C.: Sliding Skin Grafts in the Treatment of Anal Fissures, *Dis Colon Rectum,* **13:**372, 1970.

Schottler, J. L., Balcos, E. G., and Goldberg, S. M.: Postpartum Hemorrhoidectomy, *Dis Colon Rectum,* **16:**395, 1973.

Scoma, J. A., Salvati, E. P., and Rubin, R. J.: Incidence of Fistulas Subsequent to Anal Abscesses, *Dis Colon Rectum,* **17:**357, 1974.

Shafik, A.: A New Concept of the Anatomy of the Anal Sphincter Mechanism and the Physiology of Defecation:—The External Anal Sphincter: A Triple-loop System, *Invest Urol,* **12:**412, 1975.

———: A New Concept of the Anatomy of the Anal Sphincter Mechanism and the Physiology of Defecation: II. Anatomy of the Levator Ani Muscle with Special Reference to Puborec-talis, *Invest Urol,* **13:**175, 1975.

———: A New Concept of the Anatomy of the Anal Sphincter Mechanism and the Physiology of Defecation: III. The Lon-gitudinal Anal Muscle: Anatomy and Role in Anal Sphincter Mechanism, *Invest Urol,* **13:**271, 1976.

Sinclair, D. M., Hannah, G., McLaughlin, I. S., Patrick, R. S., and Slavin, G.: Malignant Melanoma of the Anal Canal, *Br J Surg,* **57:**808, 1970.

Slade, M. S., Goldberg, S. M., Schottler, J. L., Balcos, E. G., and Christenson, C. E.: Sphincteroplasty for Acquired Anal In-continence, *Dis Colon Rectum,* **20:**33, 1977.

Stearns, M. N., Jr., and Quan, S. H. Q.: Epidermoid Carcinoma of the Anorectum, *Surg Gynecol Obstet,* **131:**953, 1970.

Theuerkauf, F. J., Beahrs, O. H., and Hill, J. R.: Rectal Prolapse: Causation and Surgical Treatment, *Ann Surg,* **171:**819, 1970.

Thomson, W. H. F.: The Nature of Haemorrhoids, *Br J Surg,* **62:**542, 1975.

Wolfe, H. R. I., and Bussey, H. J. R.: Squamous Cell Carcinoma of the Anus, *Br J Surg,* **55:**295, 1968.

Chapter 29

Appendix

by **Edward H. Storer**

FUNCTION AND DEVELOPMENT

The human vermiform appendix is usually referred to as "a vestigial organ with no known function." This implies a more fully developed organ in an earlier stage of the individual or in earlier stages in the evolution of the species. There is little evidence that this is the case. On the contrary, currently available evidence suggests that the appendix is a highly specialized part of the alimentary tract. As the evolutionary scale is ascended, the lymphoid tissue of the large intestine becomes concentrated in the cecum, later in the apex of the cecum, and finally, in the higher anthropoids and man, as a vermiform appendix.

Lymphoid tissue first appears in the human appendix about 2 weeks after birth. The number of lymph follicles gradually increases to a peak of about 200 between the ages of twelve and twenty. After thirty there is an abrupt reduction to less than half and then to a trace or total absence of lymphoid tissue after sixty. Concurrent with lymphoid atrophy is fibrosis, which partially or totally obliterates the lumen in many older persons.

The role of the lymphoid aggregates in the appendix of higher mammals is still incompletely defined. Tonsils, Peyer's patches, and vermiform appendix together may well be the immunologic analog of the avian bursa of Fabricius and thus play an important role in immuno-globulin production.

A possible role for the appendix in human disease was suggested by McVay in 1964. In a retrospective study of necropsy data he found that the incidence of previous appendectomy in patients dying of carcinoma of the colon was significantly higher than in a comparable control group. He hypothesized that the appendix may act as a protective device against enteric viruses that may initiate malignant change in the colon and possibly at other sites.

He urged further studies since if his findings be confirmed, then incidental appendectomy in the course of another operation should not be proscribed. Several subsequent studies have been about evenly divided in supporting or denying an appendectomy-cancer relationship. All the above studies were designed to answer the question: "How many patients with cancer have had a previous appendectomy?" Moertel and associates designed a prospective study to answer the question: "In how many patients who have undergone appendectomy will cancer develop?" They studied 1,779 residents of Rochester, Minnesota, who had undergone appendectomy at the Mayo Clinic from 1925 through 1944, and a comparable control group. They found no evidence of a predisposition to cancer overall or to any specific cancer in patients who had undergone previous appendectomy, regardless of the age at which appendectomy was performed. Thus on the basis of currently available evidence, the practice of incidental appendectomy seems advisable since acute appendicitis and its complications continue to be significant sources of morbidity and mortality which removal of the appendix effectively prevents.

At birth the cecum and appendix have the so-called infantile contour—the appendix arising from the inferior tip of the cecum, which is shaped like an inverted pyramid. The cecum becomes bilaterally sacculated in early childhood but with the appendix still at the inferior tip. Further growth of the cecum is unequal, rapid growth of the right side and anterior aspects rotating the appendix to its adult position on the posteromedial aspect, below the ileocecal valve. The relation of the base of the appendix to the cecum is essentially constant, whereas the free end is found in a variety of locations—pelvic, retrocecal, retroileal, left lower quadrant, as well as right lower quadrant. The three taeniae coli meet at the junction of cecum with appendix and form the outer longitudinal muscle layer of the appendix. Thus the taeniae, particularly the anterior taenia, may be used as a landmark to identify an elusive appendix.

INFLAMMATION OF THE APPENDIX

Congenital defects of the appendix such as diverticula, duplication, or congenital absence are rare and of little clinical importance. The appendix occasionally gives rise to tumors, such as carcinoid or adenocarcinoma, and may be involved in inflammatory diseases of the cecum and ileum, such as tuberculosis, typhoid fever, or regional enteritis. However, by far the most important disease of the appendix is acute inflammation.

Acute Appendicitis

HISTORICAL BACKGROUND. There are isolated reports of appendectomy from 1736 on, when Amyand successfully removed from a hernial sac an appendix that had been perforated by a pin. There are also many reports, from 1581 on, of fatal suppurative disease of the cecal region, usually referred to, however, as "perityphlitis." The recognition of appendicitis as a clinical and pathologic entity for which surgical therapy is essential dates from 1886 when Reginald Fitz, Professor of Pathologic Anatomy at Harvard, gave a paper at the first meeting of the Association of American Physicians entitled "Perforating Inflammation of the Vermiform Appendix: with Special Reference to Its Early Diagnosis and Treatment." Soon thereafter McBurney described the clinical manifestations of early acute appendicitis prior to rupture, including the point of maximal abdominal tenderness, and an incision "made in the abdominal wall in cases of appendicitis."

INCIDENCE. Acute appendicitis is the most common acute surgical condition of the abdomen. The disease occurs at all ages but is most frequent in the second and third decades of life. It is quite rare in the very young, probably because the configuration of the appendix at this age makes obstruction of the lumen unlikely. There is a rough parallel between the amount of lymphoid tissue in the appendix and the incidence of acute appendicitis, the peak for both occurring in the middle teens.

The sex ratio in acute appendicitis is about 1:1 prior to puberty. At puberty the frequency in males increases, so that the male-to-female ratio is about 2:1 between the ages of fifteen and twenty-five, after which the male incidence gradually declines until the sex-related incidences are again equal.

The incidence of acute appendicitis requiring appendectomy has significantly decreased over the past 3 or 4 decades, and the trend appears to be continuing. The decline has been noted in many countries, particularly United States, Great Britain, and Scandinavia. Some of the decrease in the number of primary appendectomies is attributable to better diagnosis (and perhaps the advent of tissue committees): acute appendicitis is being reported in 75 to 80 percent of primary appendectomies in the 1970s, as opposed to 50 to 60 percent in the 1940s. But the declining incidence is much greater than can be accounted for by better diagnosis alone. No reason for the declining incidence of appendicitis has been established. Speculation has included changing dietary habits, changing intestinal flora, better nutrition, higher vitamin intake, antibiotics, and many other reasons.

ETIOLOGY AND PATHOGENESIS. Obstruction of the lumen is the dominant factor in the production of acute appendicitis. Fecaliths are the usual cause of appendiceal obstruction. Less common are hypertrophy of lymphoid tissue; inspissated barium from previous x-ray studies; vegetable and fruit seeds; and intestinal worms, particularly ascarids.

The frequency with which appendiceal obstruction is found is proportional to the diligence with which it is looked for. Only the more obvious obstructions are noted on "routine" surgical pathology reports. The frequency of obstruction also rises with the severity of the inflammatory process. Fecaliths are found in about 40 percent in simple acute appendicitis, in about 65 percent in gangrenous appendicitis without rupture, and in about 90 percent in gangrenous appendicitis with rupture.

The sequence of events following occlusion of the lumen is probably as follows: A closed-loop obstruction (Chap. 24) is produced by the proximal block, and continuing normal secretion of the appendiceal mucosa very rapidly produces distension. The luminal capacity of the normal appendix is only about 0.1 ml—there is no real lumen. Secretion of as little as 0.5 ml distal to a block raises the intraluminal pressure to about 60 cm H_2O. The human being is one of the few animals with an appendix capable of secreting at pressures high enough to lead to gangrene and perforation. Distension stimulates nerve endings of visceral afferent pain fibers, producing vague, dull, diffuse pain in the midabdomen or lower epigastrium. Peristalsis is also stimulated by the rather sudden distension, so that some cramping may be superimposed on the visceral pain early in the course of appendicitis.

Distension continues, not only from continued mucosal secretion, but also from rapid multiplication of the resident bacteria of the appendix. As pressure in the organ increases, venous pressure is exceeded. Capillaries and venules are occluded, but arteriolar inflow continues, resulting in engorgement and vascular congestion. Distension of this magnitude usually causes reflex nausea and vomiting, and the diffuse visceral pain becomes more severe. The inflammatory process soon involves the serosa of the appendix and in turn parietal peritoneum in the region, producing the characteristic shift in pain to the right lower quadrant.

The mucosa of the gastrointestinal tract, including the appendix, is very susceptible to impairment of blood supply. Thus its integrity is compromised early in the process, allowing bacterial invasion of the deeper coats. Fever, tachycardia, and leukocytosis develop as a consequence of absorption of dead tissue products and bacterial toxins. As progressive distension encroaches on the arteriolar pressure, the area with the poorest blood supply suffers most—ellipsoidal infarcts develop in the antimesenteric border. As distension, bacterial invasion, compromise of vascular supply, and infarction progress, perforation occurs, usually through one of the infarcted areas on the antimesenteric border.

This sequence is not inevitable—some episodes of acute appendicitis apparently subside spontaneously. Many patients who are found at operation to have acute appendicitis give a history of previous similar but less severe attacks of right lower quadrant pain. Pathologic examination of the appendices removed from these patients often reveals thickening and scarring, suggesting old healed acute inflammation. Presumable obstruction of the lumen when due to lymphoid hypertrophy or soft fecalith can be spontaneously relieved, allowing subsidence of appendiceal inflammation and attendant symptoms.

CLINICAL MANIFESTATIONS. Symptoms. Abdominal pain is the prime symptom of acute appendicitis. Classically the pain initially is diffusely centered in the lower epigastrium or umbilical area, is moderately severe, and is steady—sometimes with intermittent cramping superimposed. After a period varying from 1 to 12 hours, but usually within 4 to 6 hours, the pain localizes in the right lower quadrant. This classic pain sequence, though usual, is not invariable. In some patients the pain of appendicitis begins in the right lower quadrant and remains there. Variations in the anatomic location of the appendix account for many of the variations in the principal locus of the somatic phase of the pain. For example, a long appendix with the inflamed tip in the left lower quadrant causes pain in that area; a retrocecal appendix may cause principally flank or back pain; a pelvic appendix, principally suprapubic pain; and a retroileal appendix may cause testicular pain, presumably from irritation of the spermatic artery and ureter. Malrotation is also responsible for puzzling pain patterns. The visceral component is in the normal location, but the somatic component is felt in that part of the abdomen where the cecum has been arrested in rotation.

Anorexia nearly always accompanies appendicitis. It is so constant that the diagnosis should be questioned if the patient is not anorectic. Vomiting occurs in about 75 percent of patients but is not prominent or prolonged, most patients vomiting only once or twice.

Most patients give a history of obstipation from before the onset of abdominal pain, and many feel that defecation would relieve their abdominal pain. Diarrhea occurs in some patients, however, particularly children, so that the pattern of bowel function is of little differential diagnostic value.

The sequence of symptom appearance has great differential diagnostic significance. In over 95 percent of patients with acute appendicitis, anorexia is the first symptom, followed by abdominal pain, which is followed in turn by vomiting (if vomiting occurs). If vomiting precedes the onset of pain, the diagnosis should be questioned.

Signs. Physical findings are determined principally by the anatomic position of the inflamed appendix as well as by whether the organ has already ruptured when the patient is first examined.

Vital signs are not changed very much by uncomplicated appendicitis. Temperature elevation is rarely more than 1°C; the pulse rate is normal or slightly higher. Changes of greater magnitude usually mean that a complication has occurred or that another diagnosis should be considered.

Patients with appendicitis usually prefer to lie supine with the thighs, particularly the right, drawn up, because any motion increases pain. If asked to move, they do so slowly and gingerly.

The classic right lower quadrant physical signs are present when the inflamed appendix lies in the anterior position. Tenderness is often maximal at or near the point described by McBurney as being "located exactly between an inch and a half and two inches from the anterior spinous process of the ileum on a straight line drawn from that process to the umbilicus." Direct rebound tenderness

usually, and referred or indirect rebound tenderness frequently, are present and are also felt maximally in the right lower quadrant, indicating peritoneal irritation. Rovsing's sign—pain in the right lower quadrant when palpatory pressure is exerted in the left lower quadrant—also indicates the site of peritoneal irritation. Cutaneous hyperesthesia in the area supplied by the spinal nerves on the right at T_{10}, T_{11}, and T_{12} is a frequent but not a constant accompaniment of acute appendicitis. In patients with obvious appendicitis, this sign is superfluous, but in some early cases it may be the first positive sign. It is elicited either by needle prick or, better, by gently picking up the skin between forefinger and thumb. This ordinarily is not unpleasant but is painful in areas of cutaneous hyperesthesia.

Muscular resistance to palpation of the abdominal wall roughly parallels the severity of the inflammatory process. Early in the disease, resistance, if present, consists mainly of voluntary guarding. As peritoneal irritation progresses, muscle spasm increases and becomes largely involuntary—true reflex rigidity as opposed to voluntary guarding.

Variations in the position of the inflamed appendix produce variations from the usual in physical findings. With a retrocecal appendix, the anterior abdominal findings are less striking, and tenderness may be most marked in the flank. When the inflamed appendix hangs into the pelvis, abdominal findings may be entirely absent, and the diagnosis may be missed unless the rectum is examined. As the examining finger exerts pressure on the peritoneum of the cul-de-sac of Douglas, pain is felt in the suprapubic area as well as locally. Signs of localized muscle irritation may also be present. The *psoas* sign indicates an irritative focus in proximity to that muscle. The test is performed by having the patient lie on his left side; the examiner then slowly extends the right thigh, thus stretching the iliopsoas muscle. The test is positive if extension produces pain. Similarly, a positive *obturator* sign of hypogastric pain on stretching the obturator internus indicates irritation at that locus. The test is performed by passive internal rotation of the flexed right thigh with the patient supine.

LABORATORY FINDINGS. Moderate leukocytosis, ranging from about 10,000 to 18,000 per cubic millimeter and accompanied by a moderate polymorphonuclear predominance, is the rule in acute uncomplicated appendicitis. With normal total and differential white blood cell counts, the diagnosis of appendicitis is in question though not ruled out. If the white cell count is greater than about 18,000 per cubic millimeter or if the shift to the left is extreme, perforated appendicitis or an acute inflammatory disease of greater magnitude than appendicitis is probable.

Urinalysis, except for the high specific gravity of dehydration, is normal unless the inflamed appendix lies near the ureter or bladder, in which case white cells and occasionally even red cells may be seen. Bacilluria in a fresh catheterized urine is not seen in appendicitis, however, allowing differentiation from urinary tract infection.

Roentgenography. The diagnosis of acute appendicitis is usually based on history and clinical findings. X-rays are used, therefore, only in differential diagnosis and to demonstrate complications of appendicitis.

Plain films of the abdomen in acute appendicitis often reveal a distended loop or two of small bowel in the right lower quadrant, less often a distended cecum. Visualization of a gas-filled appendix usually, but not invariably, indicates acute appendicitis with proximal appendiceal obstruction. A radiopaque fecalith when present in the right lower quadrant is nearly always associated with gangrenous appendicitis. Barium enema examination may be helpful in selected patients, particularly children, in whom the diagnosis remains unclear and operation is thought to be hazardous. It is done cautiously and gently, without prior preparation of the colon and without external manipulation or pressure. Complete filling of the appendix and absence of mucosal changes in both the appendix and ileocecal region rule out acute appendicitis. Pathognomonic findings of acute appendicitis on barium enema consist of nonfilling of the appendix, mass effect on the medial and inferior borders of the cecum, and mass effect or mucosal irregularities of the terminal ileum.

Chest films are sometimes necessary to rule out disease in the right lower lung field, since lesions that irritate nerves at T_{10}, T_{11}, and T_{12} may simulate appendicitis.

COMPLICATIONS—APPENDICEAL RUPTURE. Though some patients with acute appendicitis have spontaneous subsidence of the acute process, there is no way of predicting in which patients this will occur. The only safe course of action in uncomplicated acute appendicitis is immediate appendectomy. Ideally, every patient would have the offending organ removed before complications, particularly rupture, supervene. Some progress has been made, but too many patients still are seen first only after rupture has occurred, and some physicians still are needlessly indecisive. The use of antibiotic therapy in an attempt to avoid or postpone operative therapy ignores the obstructive etiology of acute appendicitis, is dangerous, and is ill-advised.

Pathogenesis. Unrelenting obstruction of the appendiceal lumen leads inexorably to gangrene and rupture of the pus-filled organ. Among the sequelae are appendiceal phlegmon, abscesses, spreading peritonitis, suppurative pylephlebitis, and intestinal obstruction.

Rupture of the appendix nearly always is distal to an occluding fecalith. The contents of the distended distal appendix spill through the necrotic rent, but this is rarely more than a few milliliters because of the small capacity of the appendix. Retrograde spill of cecal contents is ordinarily prevented by the occluding fecalith, unless the fecalith becomes dislodged through the rupture site or the necrotic area involves the base of the appendix and contiguous cecum.

During the several hours elapsing between onset of acute appendicitis and rupture, nature's walling-off process is able to quarantine the inflammation in about 95 percent of patients and confine the spill to the periappendiceal area.

A phlegmon is produced consisting of a mass of inflamed, matted intestines and omentum but with little or no discrete collection of pus. This process may slowly resolve spontaneously or may be hastened in resolution by timely surgical intervention. In some patients, however,

a progressive suppurative process produces an expanding collection of pus contained by the walling-off process—a periappendiceal abscess.

If the walling-off process has not been completed by the time appendiceal rupture occurs, contamination spreads beyond the right lower quadrant. The two sites of predilection are the pelvic cul-de-sac via gravity drainage, and the right subhepatic space, which is reached via the right gutter (see also Chap. 34). With indiscriminate centrifugal contamination, virulent bacteria thus seeded initiate spreading diffuse peritonitis. An even more lethal form of peritonitis is produced by secondary rupture of intra-abdominal abscesses that were produced by ruptured appendicitis. Ascending septic thrombophlebitis of the portal venous system—pylethrombophlebitis—is a very grave but fortunately rare complication of gangrenous appendicitis. It is heralded by chills and spiking fever, followed by right upper quadrant pain and jaundice. Septic clots from the involved mesenteric radicles embolize the liver, producing multiple pyogenic abscesses (Chap. 30).

Incidence. The proportion of patients with acute appendicitis who already have ruptured appendicitis when they are first seen varies with the age of the patients and with the type of hospital reporting. Twenty-five to thirty percent of charity hospital patients have ruptured appendicitis on admission versus about 15 percent in private hospitals. The rupture incidence is also significantly higher in the pediatric and geriatric age groups.

Diagnosis. Diagnosis usually is not difficult after rupture has occurred. The patient is obviously quite ill, prostrated, toxic, dehydrated, and distended. Right lower quadrant pain increases in severity and spreads over a somewhat larger area. Abdominal pain has been said to lessen dramatically at the moment of perforation and to be diminished for a few hours thereafter. This was attributed to sudden relief of the pain-producing distension of the obstructed appendix. Temporary relief of pain is rarely seen, however, occurring in only 4 percent in one series. In the vast majority, pain continues unabated—apparently local peritonitis is as effective in producing pain as distension of the appendix.

Physical findings are also more definite after rupture. With periappendiceal phlegmon or abscess, a tender, boggy mass with ill-defined margins usually can be felt. Tenderness, which is fingerpoint with simple acute appendicitis, now encompasses the whole right lower quadrant. Rebound tenderness and muscular rigidity are usually marked and correspond in extent to the extent of the local peritonitis. As in simple acute peritonitis, however, physical findings depend on the position of the appendix. For example, the only physical finding with a pelvic abscess secondary to a ruptured pelvic appendix may be a boggy tender mass on rectal examination. With spreading peritonitis, the physical signs advance with the spread of the inflammation (see also Chap. 34). Abdominal distension and paralytic ileus roughly parallel the severity and duration of the inflammatory process.

Fever and pulse also parallel the severity of the process. The temperature, which is rarely over 38°C in simple acute appendicitis, rises to about 39°C with localized peritonitis and often spikes over 40°C with diffuse peritonitis. Leukocytosis increases to 20,000 to 30,000 per cubic millimeter with extreme polymorphonuclear predominance and marked shift to immature forms. Hemoconcentration and desalting are variable and reflect the amount of fluid sequestered in the inflamed area as well as loss of oral intake.

DIFFERENTIAL DIAGNOSIS. The differential diagnosis of acute appendicitis is essentially the diagnosis of the "acute abdomen" (see Chap. 24). This is because clinical manifestations are not specific for a given disease but are specific for disturbance of a physiologic function or functions. Thus an essentially identical clinical picture can result from a wide variety of acute processes within or near the peritoneal cavity that produce the same alterations of function as acute appendicitis.

Accuracy of preoperative diagnosis should be about 80 to 85 percent. If it is consistently less than 75 percent, some unnecessary operations are probably being done, and a more rigorous preoperative differential diagnosis is in order. On the other hand, an accuracy consistently greater than 90 percent should also cause concern, since this usually means that some patients with atypical but bona fide acute appendicitis are being "observed" when they should have prompt surgical intervention. There are a few conditions in which operation is contraindicated, but in general the disease processes that are confused with appendicitis are also surgical problems or, if not, are not made worse by operation. The more frequent error is to make a preoperative diagnosis of acute appendicitis only to find some other condition (or nothing) at operation; much less frequently, acute appendicitis is found after a preoperative diagnosis of another condition. Most common erroneous preoperative diagnoses—accounting for more than 75 percent—in descending order of frequency are acute mesenteric lymphadenitis, no organic pathologic condition, acute pelvic inflammatory disease, twisted ovarian cyst or ruptured graafian follicle, and acute gastroenteritis.

Differential diagnosis of appendicitis depends upon three major factors: the anatomic location of the inflamed appendix, the stage of the process—whether simple or ruptured, and the age and sex of the patient.

Diseases to be considered in the differential diagnosis of appendicitis in children include primary acute mesenteric lymphadenitis; acute gastroenteritis, usually "green-apple colic" or "viral" gastroenteritis but occasionally paratyphoid or typhoid infections; acute pyelonephritis; Meckel's diverticulitis; intussusception; regional enteritis; primary peritonitis; and Henoch-Schönlein purpura.

Acute Mesenteric Adenitis (Chap. 35). This is the disease most often confused with acute appendicitis in children. Almost invariably an upper respiratory infection is present or has recently subsided. The pain is usually less or more diffuse, and tenderness is not as sharply localized as in appendicitis. Voluntary guarding is sometimes present, but true rigidity is rare. Generalized lymphadenopathy may be noted. Laboratory procedures are of little help in differentiating, though a relative lymphocytosis, when present, suggests mesenteric adenitis. Observation for several hours to allow the clinical picture to clarify is in order if the diagnosis of mesenteric adenitis seems likely, since this is

a self-limited disease, but if the differentiation is in doubt, then immediate operation is the only safe course.

Acute Gastroenteritis. This is very common in childhood but usually can easily be differentiated from appendicitis. Viral gastroenteritis, an acute self-limited infection of diverse causes, is characterized by profuse watery diarrhea, nausea, and vomiting. Hyperperistaltic abdominal cramps precede the watery stools. The abdomen is relaxed between cramps, and there are no localizing signs. Laboratory values are normal.

Salmonella gastroenteritis results from ingestion of contaminated food. Abdominal findings are usually similar to those in viral gastroenteritis, but in some the abdominal pain is intense, localized, and associated with rebound tenderness. Chills and fever are common. Leukocyte count is usually normal. The causative organisms can be isolated from essentially 100 percent of patients, but this may take too long to help the clinician in differential diagnosis of abdominal pain. Similar attacks in other persons eating the same food as the patient greatly strengthen the presumptive diagnosis of salmonella gastroenteritis.

Typhoid fever is now a rare disease. This probably accounts for the frequency of missed diagnosis—it is rarely seen and rarely thought of. The onset is less acute than appendicitis, with a prodrome of several days. Differentiation is usually possible because of the prostration, maculopapular rash, inappropriate bradycardia, and leukopenia. Diagnosis is confirmed by culture of *Salmonella typhosa* from stool or blood. Intestinal perforation, usually in the lower ileum, develops in about 1 percent of cases and requires immediate surgical therapy.

Yersiniosis. Human infection with *Yersinia enterocolitica* or *Y. pseudotuberculosis,* though reported frequently in Europe, has only recently become generally recognized in the United States. It is probable that the recent increase in the incidence of *Yersinia* infections is attributable to increased awareness and laboratory skill, not to actual spread of the disease in human beings and animals. These zoonotic organisms are not members of the indigenous biota of man and are probably transmitted through food contaminated by feces or urine.

Yersinia infections cause a variety of clinical syndromes, including mesenteric adenitis, ileitis, colitis, and acute appendicitis. Many of the infections are mild and self-limited, but some lead to a systemic septic course with a high fatality rate if untreated. The organisms are usually sensitive to tetracyclines, streptomycin, ampicillin, and kanamycin. A preoperative suspicion of the diagnosis should not delay operative intervention, since appendicitis caused by *Yersinia* cannot be clinically distinguished from appendicitis of other causation.

Recent studies in Europe indicate that about 6 percent of cases of mesenteric adenitis and 5 percent of cases of acute appendicitis are caused by *Yersinia* infection.

Urinary Tract Infection (Chap. 40). Acute pyelonephritis on the right side particularly may mimic a retroileal acute appendicitis. Chills, right costovertebral angle tenderness, pus cells, and particularly bacteria in the urine usually suffice to differentiate the two.

Meckel's Diverticulitis (Chap. 39). This causes a clinical picture very similar to acute appendicitis. Preoperative differentiation is academic and unnecessary, since Meckel's diverticulitis is attended by the same complications as appendicitis and requires the same treatment—prompt surgical intervention. Diverticulectomy can nearly always be done through a McBurney incision, extended if necessary. If the base of the diverticulum is broad, so that removal would compromise the lumen of the ileum, then resection of the segment of ileum bearing the diverticulum with end-to-end anastomosis is done.

Intussusception (Chap 39). In contrast to Meckel's diverticulitis, it is extremely important to differentiate intussusception from acute appendicitis, because the treatment may be quite different. The age of the patients is important: appendicitis is very uncommon under age two, whereas nearly all idiopathic intussusceptions occur under age two. Intussusception occurs typically in a well-nourished infant who is suddenly doubled up by apparent colicky pain. Between attacks of pain the infant appears quite well. After several hours, the patient usually passes a bloody mucoid stool. A sausage-shaped mass may be palpable in the right lower quadrant. Later, as the intussusception progresses distad, the right lower quadrant feels abnormally empty. The preferred treatment of intussusception, if seen before signs of peritonitis supervene, is reduction by barium enema. Treatment of acute appendicitis by barium enema might well be catastrophic.

Regional Enteritis (Chap. 27). The manifestations of acute regional enteritis—fever, right lower quadrant pain and tenderness, and leukocytosis—often simulate acute appendicitis. Diarrhea and the infrequency of anorexia, nausea, and vomiting favor a diagnosis of enteritis but are not sufficient to exclude acute appendicitis without celiotomy. In an appreciable percentage of patients with chronic regional enteritis, the diagnosis has been first made at the time of operation for presumed acute appendicitis.

Primary Peritonitis (Chap. 34). This situation rarely mimics simple acute appendicitis but presents a picture very similar to diffuse peritonitis secondary to a ruptured appendix. The diagnosis is made by peritoneal aspiration. If nothing but cocci are seen on the Gram-stained smear, peritonitis is primary and treated medically; if the flora are mixed, secondary peritonitis is indicated.

Henoch-Schönlein Purpura. This syndrome usually occurs 2 to 3 weeks after a streptococcal infection. Abdominal pain may be prominent, but joint pains, purpura, and nephritis are nearly always present also.

Gynecologic Disorders. Diseases of the female internal generative organs (Chap. 41) that may be erroneously diagnosed as appendicitis are, in approximate descending order of frequency, pelvic inflammatory disease, ruptured graafian follicle, twisted ovarian cyst or tumor, endometriosis, and ruptured ectopic pregnancy.

Pelvic Inflammatory Disease ("Pus Tubes"). The infection is usually bilateral but if confined to the right tube may mimic acute appendicitis. Pain and tenderness are usually lower, and motion of the cervix is exquisitely painful. Intracellular diplococci may be demonstrable on smear of the purulent vaginal discharge.

Ruptured Graafian Follicle. Not uncommonly ovulation results in spill of sufficient blood and follicular fluid to produce brief, mild lower abdominal pain. If the fluid is unusually copious and from the right ovary, appendicitis may be simulated. Pain and tenderness are rather diffuse. Leukocytosis and fever are minimal or absent. Since this occurs at the midpoint of the menstrual cycle, it is often called *mittelschmerz*.

Ruptured Ectopic Pregnancy. This is manifested by lower abdominal pain and symptoms of hypovolemia. A tubo-ovarian mass is usually palpable on pelvic examination. Culdocentesis yields nonclotting blood.

Diseases of the Male. Two diseases of males (Chap. 40) must be considered in differential diagnosis of appendicitis, torsion of the testis and acute epididymitis, since epigastric pain may overshadow local symptoms early in these diseases. The correct diagnosis is easily made if one remembers to include the genitalia in the physical examination.

Other Diseases. Diseases occurring in patients of all ages and both sexes, not mentioned above, that must be considered in differential diagnosis are perforated peptic ulcer (Chap. 26); diverticulitis coli, particularly cecal (Chap. 28); perforating carcinoma of the colon, particularly cecal (Chap. 28); foreign body perforations of the bowel; closed-loop intestinal obstruction (Chap. 24); mesenteric vascular occlusion (Chap. 35); pleuritis of the right lower chest (Chap. 24); acute cholecystitis (Chap. 31); acute pancreatitis (Chap. 32); right ureteral calculus (Chap. 40); infarcted epiploic appendage (Chap. 35); hematoma of abdominal wall (Chap. 35); and many others too numerous and too rare to mention.

Perforated Peptic Ulcer. This closely simulates appendicitis if the spilled gastroduodenal contents gravitate down the right gutter to the cecal area and if the perforation spontaneously seals fairly soon, thus minimizing upper abdominal findings.

Diverticulitis or Perforating Carcinoma of the Cecum or of That Portion of the Sigmoid That Lies on the Right Side. These lesions may be impossible to distinguish from appendicitis. Extensive diagnostic studies in an attempt to make a preoperative differentiation are not warranted.

Ureteral Stone. If the calculus is lodged near the appendix, it may simulate a retrocecal appendicitis. Pain referred to the labia, scrotum, or penis, hematuria, or absence of fever or leukocytosis suggests stone. Pyelography usually confirms the diagnosis.

Epiploic Appendicitis. Epiploic appendicitis probably results from infarction of the appendage(s) secondary to torsion. Symptoms may be minimal, or there may be continuous abdominal pain in an area corresponding to the contour of the colon, lasting several days. Pain shift is unusual, and there is no diagnostic sequence of symptoms. The patient does not look ill, nausea and vomiting are unusual, and unlike in appendicitis appetite is commonly unaffected. Localized tenderness over the site is usual and is often marked on rebound but without rigidity. In 25 percent of reported cases pain has persisted or recurred until the infarcted epiploic appendages were removed.

TREATMENT. There is but one treatment for acute appendicitis and its complications. Thus the only question to be resolved is when—the timing of surgical intervention.

Immediate appendectomy is indicated in acute appendicitis without rupture just as soon as the minimal work-up compatible with good medical practice is completed. Ruptured appendicitis with local peritonitis or phlegmon formation also should be operated upon early in the hospital course. A brief period of preparation is advisable during which nasogastric suction is instituted and sufficient intravenous fluids, usually Ringer's lactate solution and 5% dextrose in water, are given to correct systemic fluid and electrolyte deficits. Systemic antibiotics in large doses are administered: since bacteroides organisms play such a major role in appendiceal infections, clindamycin should be one of the antibiotics used pending culture-sensitivity data. (See also Chap. 5.)

Patients with ruptured appendicitis producing spreading peritonitis should similarly be prepared with "all deliberate haste" for early surgical intervention. Preparation (Chap. 34) may take somewhat longer than with localized peritonitis because of the greater magnitude of the physiologic derangements caused by the more extensive process but rarely requires more than 3 or 4 hours. It is essential to remove the necrotic appendix to prevent continued contamination of the peritoneum.

There is general agreement on the timing of the operation for the three categories of appendicitis mentioned above—acute appendicitis without rupture, ruptured appendix with local peritonitis or phlegmon formation, and ruptured appendix with spreading peritonitis. There is still a difference of opinion, however, concerning the optimal timing of the operation for ruptured appendicitis with frank periappendiceal abscess formation. "Expectant treatment" was advocated by A. J. Ochsner in 1901. As now practiced this consists of intravenous fluids, nasogastric suction, and large doses of antibiotics. Vital signs, leukocytosis, and size of the mass are followed closely. If progression occurs, the abscess is drained. If the patient improves, conservative treatment is continued. With these measures the majority of appendiceal abscesses resolve satisfactorily, although many days of hospital treatment are required. An elective appendectomy 6 weeks to 3 months later is strongly advised, since the recurrence rate is very high. Proponents of conservative treatment feel that operation in the acute phase of the abscess is dangerous, because the protective walling-off barrier may be broken down by the procedure.

Advocates of prompt operation for ruptured appendicitis with abscess as soon as the patient can be prepared feel that, with the supportive measures now available, drainage of the abscess and removal of the appendix, if possible, can be done with a lower mortality and morbidity than with expectant treatment. They point out that the mortality rate following secondary rupture of a periappendiceal abscess is about 90 percent. Expectant treatment also necessitates two hospitalizations, the first often prolonged.

Nearly all surgeons favor prompt operation for all categories of acute appendicitis in children, since expectant treatment of ruptured appendicitis has been less successful than in adults.

Conduct of the Operation (Fig. 29-1). Many surgeons (including the author) prefer a McBurney incision in all patients with suspected appendicitis, while others use a McBurney incision in clear-cut appendicitis but use a right paramedian incision if the diagnosis is in doubt, particularly in females. The principal argument against the McBurney incision is that a second incision may be necessary if a procedure other than appendectomy has to be done. The principal argument against the paramedian incision is that if the patient does indeed have appendicitis, the diseased organ can be removed only by traversing the previously unsoiled peritoneal cavity.

When a periappendiceal abscess is suspected, paramedian incision is contraindicated. The abscess is approached from a laterally placed McBurney incision without entering the free peritoneal cavity. The abscess is evacuated, with care to avoid breaking down any of the walling-off process. Most surgeons attempt to remove the appendix in this situation. If the appendix is in the surgical field, it should be removed, but if extensive dissection is necessary to expose the organ, appendectomy is hazardous. Interval appendectomy should be done some weeks later.

There are several methods of managing the appendiceal stump. The traditional method of ligation-inversion has the advantage that peritonealization and hemostasis are secured, but the disadvantage of inverting an infected stump into a closed cavity is the risk of an intramural abscess of the cecum. However, if the ligation is done with fine plain catgut this risk is minimal. Inversion without ligation obviates the risk of abscess, but hemostasis of the intramural branch of the appendiceal artery may not be secure. Ligation without inversion avoids burying the stump and secures hemostasis but is unsurgical because there remains free in the peritoneal cavity a contaminated raw surface. Contamination of the peritoneal cavity may result from the ligated stump either from bacteria on the stump or from the slipping of the ligature or necrosis of the stump as a result of the ligation. Total inversion of the normal appendix after division of the mesoappendix has been revived recently as an alternative to stump closure at the time of incidental appendectomy. It is technically more difficult but has the advantage that the gastrointestinal tract is not opened. Intussusception of the cecum has not been a significant problem.

If appendicitis is not found, an orderly investigation for the cause of the symptoms must be done. This should include gross examination and immediate Gram stain of any peritoneal fluid or exudate. With the assistant elevating the anterior abdominal wall by retraction, the pelvic organs are examined. Next the gallbladder and gastroduodenal areas are visualized. The mesentery is examined for nodes. The small intestine is then "run" in a retrograde manner, starting at the cecum, looking particularly for regional enteritis and Meckel's diverticulum. Finally, palpation of the colon and kidneys is done as well as is possible through a McBurney incision. It is axiomatic that if the cause of the acute abdomen is found, exploration

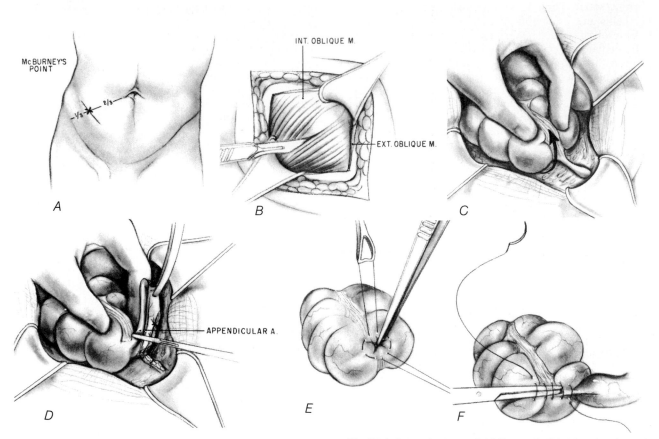

Fig. 29-1. Appendectomy. *A.* McBurney incision passing through McBurney's point, which is located one-third of the distance from the anterior superior iliac spine to the umbilicus. *B.* The incision has been carried through skin and subcutaneous tissue, and has divided the aponeurosis of the external oblique muscle in the course of its fibers. The internal oblique muscle is being separated in the direction of its fibers. *C.* The peritoneum has been incised and the peritoneal cavity entered. The appendix is delivered into the wound by rotation of the cecum up and out. *D.* The vessels within the mesoappendix have been doubly ligated and transected with particular attention directed toward the appendicular artery. A crushing clamp is applied to the base of the appendix and then moved distad (to dotted line), so that a ligature may be placed in the resulting groove. *E.* The stump of the appendix may or may not be tied with a ligature. It is customary to invert the stump and place a purse-string suture through the seromuscular layers of the cecum. *F.* An alternate method of inverting the appendiceal stump is demonstrated with a continuous seromuscular suture. A Z suture can also be used to achieve this end.

is terminated and appropriate therapy for the offending process undertaken.

The question of when to drain has been contentious for many years. Some have followed the dictum "When in doubt, drain." Others, with equal vehemence have said, "When in doubt, don't drain." The following is based on collected currently available evidence:

Drainage of localized collections of pus is indicated and should be done with one or more soft rubber drains to each collection, brought out through the McBurney incision. If a paramedian incision has been used, then a separate stab wound is preferred to avoid incisional hernia. A sump drain is more effective in large collections. Drainage of diffuse peritonitis is unwarranted, because it is physically impossible and physiologically undesirable. If an intact though inflamed appendix has been removed, all layers of the incision should be closed without drainage. However, if a ruptured appendix has been removed, then each anatomic layer is washed with a dilute antibiotic solution such as kanamycin or neomycin as it is closed. A small drain is placed in the subcutaneous tissues and the skin loosely approximated or left open for secondary closure in 4 or 5 days.

Appendicitis in the Young

Acute appendicitis is a more serious disease in infants and children than in adults, because the rupture rate is higher, which in turn produces higher morbidity and mortality rates.

Diagnostic accuracy for acute appendicitis is considerably lower than in adults. Contributing to this are a clinical picture that is less "typical"—a fever which is often higher and more vomiting; the unavoidable fact that infants cannot give a history of present illness; and the failure of physicians to consider appendicitis because of its relative infrequency in the very young.

The disease progresses more rapidly than in adults—

gangrene and rupture occur earlier in the course of acute appendicitis in children. The rupture rate varies from 15 to 50 percent in reported series. In preschool children it is even higher, ranging from 50 to 85 percent. Because of the frequency of "bellyaches" in children, parents may think that an attack of appendicitis is just another "bellyache" and not seek medical advice until after rupture has occurred and the child is obviously very ill. Too many parents still administer harsh cathartics to children with abdominal discomfort and/or constipation. The resulting increase in bowel motility hastens perforation.

Rupture of gangrenous appendicitis is more frequently followed by diffuse peritonitis and distant intraabdominal abscesses than in adults. The walling-off process is less efficient because of the small, incompletely developed greater omentum and because, as noted above, the interval between onset and rupture may be short. Cathartics are also implicated: the induced writhing of the bowel not only hastens rupture but after rupture smears contamination widely about the peritoneal cavity.

Appendicitis in the Elderly

Acute appendicitis in the older age group, as in the very young, is a much more serious disease. The mortality rate is many times that for younger adults. This is attributable to delay of definitive treatment, greater frequency of progressive uncontrolled infection, and a high incidence of concomitant disease.

Appendicitis is often very deceptive in the aged, because the clinical manifestations are much milder than might be expected from the gravity of the disease process. The usual symptoms are present but subtle and difficult to elicit; abdominal pain is often mild and causes little concern. Similarly, physical findings, with the exception of tenderness, may be minimal or absent. The fever and leukocyte response, which as a rule are very helpful in diagnosis, are less than expected and in some elderly patients are within normal limits. Because of the deceptively mild clinical course of the disease, from 67 to 90 percent of elderly patients are found to have a ruptured appendix at the time of operation.

Concomitant diseases, which dangerously lower physiologic reserve in this group, are present in significant degree in from one-half to two-thirds of the patients. These are principally cardiac disease, pulmonary insufficiency, pneumonia, and diabetes.

PROGNOSIS. Mortality. The mortality from appendicitis in the United States has steadily decreased from a rate of 9.9 per 100,000 in 1939 to 0.4 per 100,000 in 1975. Among the factors responsible are the significantly decreasing incidence of appendicitis; better diagnosis and treatment, attributable to the now available antibiotics, intravenous fluids, blood, and plasma, but particularly to the greatly improved training of most surgeons; and a higher percentage of patients receiving definitive treatment before rupture (though the rate of improvement is discouragingly slow).

Principal factors in mortality are whether or not rupture occurs prior to surgical treatment, and the age of the patient. The overall mortality rate in unruptured acute appendicitis is little higher than the rate for a general anesthetic (0.06 percent) and is now about 0.1 percent. The overall mortality rate in ruptured acute appendicitis is about 3 percent—a thirtyfold increase. The mortality rate of ruptured appendicitis in the elderly is about 15 percent—a fivefold increase from the overall rate.

Death is usually attributable to uncontrolled sepsis—peritonitis, intraabdominal abscesses, or gram-negative septicemia. Sepsis may impose metabolic demands of such magnitude on the cardiovascular or respiratory systems that they cannot be met, in which case cardiac or respiratory insufficiency is the direct cause of death. Pulmonary embolism continues to account for some deaths. Aspiration producing drowning in the patient's vomitus is a prominent mode of death in the older age group.

Morbidity. Morbidity rates parallel mortality rates, being precipitously increased by rupture of the appendix and to a lesser extent by old age. Most of the serious early complications are septic and include abscess (Chap. 34) and wound infection. Wound infection is common but is nearly always confined to the subcutaneous tissues and promptly responds to wound drainage, which is accomplished by reopening the skin incision. Wound infection predisposes to wound dehiscence also. The type of incision is relevant, since complete dehiscence rarely occurs in a McBurney incision.

Fecal fistula is an annoying but not particularly dangerous complication of appendectomy. This may be produced by sloughing of that portion of the cecum inside a constricting purse-string suture, by the ligature's slipping off a tied but not inverted appendiceal stump, by necrosis from an abscess encroaching on the cecum, or by a cecotomy produced by removing a cigarette drain that is adherent to the cecum—a cogent reason for removing the wick from the rubber drain before insertion.

Intestinal obstruction, initially paralytic but sometimes progressing to mechanical, may occur with slowly resolving peritonitis with loculated abscesses and exuberant adhesion formation.

Late complications are quite uncommon. Adhesive band intestinal obstruction after appendectomy does occur but much less frequently than after pelvic surgical therapy. Incisional hernia is analogous to wound dehiscence—infection predisposes to it, and it rarely occurs in a McBurney incision but is not uncommon in a lower right paramedian incision.

TUMORS

Neoplasms of the appendix are very uncommon and are usually diagnosed at operation or autopsy. Three histologic types of malignant tumors occur: carcinoid, adenocarcinoma, and malignant mucocele. Various benign tumors also occur but are of no clinical significance except as a very rare etiologic agent in the production of acute appendicitis from appendiceal obstruction. In a study of 50,000 appendices the incidence of carcinoid was 0.5 percent, primary adenocarcinoma 0.08 percent, and mucocele

0.2 percent. Carcinoid tumors of the gastrointestinal tract and the malignant carcinoid syndrome are discussed in Chap. 27.

Carcinoid

Forty-five percent of all reported carcinoid tumors of the gastrointestinal tract have been found in the appendix. The true incidence probably exceeds 75 percent, since carcinoids of the appendix are not sufficiently unusual to elicit the urge to publish while carcinoids elsewhere more often are. Although cytologic criteria of malignancy are not uncommonly present, biologic malignancy evidenced by mestastasis has been demonstrated in only 2.9 percent of appendiceal carcinoids. There are but six reported cases of malignant carcinoid of the appendix producing the malignant carcinoid syndrome.

Carcinoids of the appendix are typically small, firm, circumscribed, yellow-brown tumors. About three-fourths occur in the distal third of the appendix; less than 10 percent occur at the base. They are nearly always an incidental finding at the time of appendectomy (or autopsy), though rarely they may initiate acute appendicitis. Simple appendectomy with wide excision of the mesoappendix is adequate treatment unless invasion beyond the line of resection and/or nodal metastasis is demonstrated, in which case right colectomy with excision of the node-bearing mesentery is indicated.

Adenocarcinoma

This is often referred to as "colonic" type of carcinoma of the appendix because of the resemblance in behavior and in gross and microscopic appearance to colonic cancer. It also serves to distinguish it from the mucocele. Preoperative diagnosis may be based on the visualization of an extracecal mass on barium enema, but usually the appendiceal tumor is not suspected prior to operation, which is usually an appendectomy. In a few instances the lesion is unrecognized at appendectomy and is detected on pathologic examination of the specimen. Treatment is right colectomy including mesentery. The prognosis is probably about the same as for carcinoma of the cecum.

Mucocele

This is a cystic dilatation of the appendix containing mucoid material. Histologically, mucoceles are divided into a benign type, which results from noninflammatory occlusion of the proximal lumen of the appendix and thus is not a neoplasm, and a malignant type, which is a grade 1 mucous papillary adenocarcinoma. Appendectomy is adequate treatment, but care should be taken to avoid rupture, since pseudomyxoma peritonei has been reported to occur following rupture and peritoneal dissemination of the appendiceal contents.

References

Function and Development

Berry, R. J. A.: The True Caecal Apex, or the Vermiform Appendix: Its Minute and Comparative Anatomy, *J Anat Physiol,* **35:**83, 1900.

Buschard, K., and Kjaeldgaard, A.: Investigation and Analysis of the Position, Fixation, Length and Embryology of the Vermiform Appendix, *Acta Chir Scand,* **139:**293, 1973.

Mavligit, G. M., Jubert, A., Gutterman, J. U., Reed, R. C., and Hersh, E. M.: Subpopulations of Thymus Dependent and Thymus Independent Lymphocytes in Human Gut Associated Lymphoid Tissues, *Surg Gynecol Obstet,* **140:**397, 1975.

McVay, J. R. Jr.: The Appendix in Relation to Neoplastic Disease, *Cancer,* **17:**929, 1964.

Moertel, C. G., Nobrega, F. T., Elveback, L. R., and Wentz, J. R.: A Prospective Study of Appendectomy and Predisposition to Cancer, *Surg Gynecol Obstet,* **138:**549, 1974.

Perey, D. Y., Cooper, M. D., and Good, R. A.: The Mammalian Homologue of the Avian Bursa of Fabricius, *Surgery,* **64:**614, 1968.

Inflammation of the Appendix

Amyand, C.: Of an Inguinal Rupture with a Pin in the Appendix Caeci Encrusted with Stone: Some Observations on Wounds in the Guts, *Philosoph Trans,* **39:**329, 1736.

Bowers, W. F.: Appendicitis: With Special Reference to Its Pathogenesis, Bacteriology, and Healing, *Arch Surg,* **39:**362, 1939.

Burkitt, D. P.: The Aetiology of Appendicitis, *Br J Surg,* **58:**695, 1971.

Castleman, K. B., Puestow, C. B., and Sauer, D.: Is Appendicitis Decreasing in Frequency? *Arch Surg,* **78:**794, 1959.

Deschenes, L., Couture, J., and Garneau, R.: Diverticulitis of the Appendix, *Am J Surg,* **121:**706, 1971.

Fernel, J.: Universa Medicina, BK 6, 1554, in R. H. Major, "Classic Descriptions of Disease," Charles C Thomas, Publisher, Springfield, Ill, 1932.

Fitz, R. H.: Perforating Inflammation of the Vermiform Appendix: With Special Reference to Its Early Diagnosis and Treatment, *Trans Assoc Am Physicians,* **1:**107, 1886.

Gierup, J., and Karpe, B.: Aspects on Appendiceal Abscess in Children with Special Reference to Delayed Appendectomy, *Acta Chir Scand,* **141:**801, 1975.

Gilmore, O. J. A., Brodribb, A. J. M., Browett, J. P., Cooke, T. J. C., Griffin, P. H., Higgs, M. J., Ross, I. K., and Williamson, R. C. N.: Appendicitis and Mimicking Conditions. A Prospective Study, *Lancet,* **2:**421, 1975.

Grosfeld, J. L., and Solit, R. W.: Prevention of Wound Infection in Perforated Appendicitis: Experience with Delayed Primary Wound Closure, *Ann Surg,* **168:**891, 1968.

Haller, J. A., Jr., Shaker, I. J., Donahoo, J. S., Schnaufer, L., and White, J. J.: Peritoneal Drainage versus Non-drainage for Generalized Peritonitis from Ruptured Appendicitis in Children, *Ann Surg,* **177:**595, 1973.

Hobson, T., and Rosenmann, L. D.: Acute Appendicitis: When Is It Right to Be Wrong? *Am J Surg,* **108:**306, 1964.

Howie, J. G. R.: Death from Appendicitis and Appendectomy. An Epidemiological Survey, *Lancet,* **2:**1334, 1966.

Jepsen, O. B., Korner, B., Lauritsen, K. B., Hancke, A.-B., Andersen, L., Henrichsen, S., Brenøe, E., Christiansen, P. M., and Johansen, A.: *Yersinia enterocolitica* Infection in Patients with Acute Surgical Abdominal Disease, *Scand J Infect Dis,* **8:**189, 1976.

Jona, J. Z., Belin, R. P., and Selke, A. C.: Barium Enema as a Diagnostic Aid in Children with Abdominal Pain, *Surg Gynecol Obstet,* **144:**351, 1977.

Law, D., Law, R., and Eiseman, B.: The Continuing Challenge of Acute and Perforated Appendicitis, *Am J Surg,* **131:**533, 1976.

Leigh, D. A., Simmons, K., and Norman, E.: Bacterial Flora of the Appendix Fossa in Appendicitis and Post-operative Wound Infection, *J Clin Pathol,* **27:**997, 1974.

———, Pease, R., Henderson, H., Simmons, K., and Russ, R.: Prophylactic Lincomysin in the Prevention of Wound Infection following Appendicectomy: A double-blind study, *Br J Surg,* **63:**973, 1976.

Lewis, F. R., Holcroft, J. W., Boey, J., and Dunphy, J. E.: Appendicitis. A Critical Review of Diagnosis and Treatment in 1,000 Cases, *Arch Surg,* **110:**677, 1975.

Longland, C. J., Gray, J. G., Lees, W., and Garrett, J. A. M.: The Prevention of Infection in Appendicectomy Wounds, *Br J Surg,* **58:**117, 1971.

McBurney, C.: Experience with Early Operative Interference in Cases of Diseases of the Vermiform Appendix, *NY State Med J,* **50:**676, 1889.

———: The Incision Made in the Abdominal Wall in Cases of Appendicitis, *Ann Surg,* **20:**38, 1894.

McDonald, J. C.: Nonspecific Mesenteric Lymphadenitis: Collective Review, *Surg Gynecol Obstet,* **116:**409, 1963.

Magarey, C. J., Chant, A. D. B., Rickford, C. R. K., and Magarey, J. R.: Peritoneal Drainage and Systemic Antibiotics after Appendicectomy, *Lancet,* **2:**179, 1971.

Marchildon, M. B., and Dudgeon, D. L.: Perforated Appendicitis: Current Experience in a Children's Hospital, *Ann Surg,* **185:**84, 1977.

Mason, L. B., and Deyden, W. R.: Primary Appendectomy, *Am Surg,* **42:**239, 1976.

Meade, R. H.: The Evolution of Surgery for Appendicitis, *Surgery,* **55:**741, 1964.

Noer, T.: Decreasing Incidence of Acute Appendicitis, *Acta Chir Scand,* **141:**431, 1975.

Raftery, A. T.: The Value of the Leukocyte Count in the Diagnosis of Acute Appendicitis, *Br J Surg,* **63:**143, 1976.

Sherman, J. O., Luck, S. R., and Borger, J. A.: Irrigation of the Peritoneal Cavity for Appendicitis in Children: A Double-blind Study, *J Pediatr Surg,* **11:**371, 1976.

Thomas, D. R.: Conservative Management of the Appendix Mass, *Surgery,* **73:**677, 1973.

Thomas, E. J., and Mueller, C. B.: Appendectomy: Diagnostic Criteria and Hospital Performance, *Hosp Pract,* **4:**72, 1969.

Thorbjarnarson, B.: Acute Appendicitis in Patients over the Age of Sixty, *Surg Gynecol Obstet,* **125:**1277, 1967.

Wangensteen, O. H., and Dennis, C.: Experimental Proof of the Obstructive Origin of Appendicitis in Man, *Ann Surg,* **110:**629, 1939.

Weber, J., Finlayson, N. B., and Mark, J. B. D.: Mesenteric Lymphadenitis and Terminal Ileitis due to *Yersinia pseudotuberculosis, N Engl J Med,* **283:**172, 1970.

White, J. J., Santillana, M., and Haller, J. A., Jr.: Intensive In-hospital Observation: A Safe Way to Decrease Unnecessary Appendectomy, *Am Surg,* **41:**793, 1975.

Willis, A. T., Ferguson, I. R., Jones, P. H., Phillips, K. D., Tearle, P. V., Berry, R. B., Fiddian, R. V., Graham, D. F., Harland, D. H. C., Innes, D. B., Mee, W. M., Rothwell-Jackson, R. L., Sutch, I., Kilbey, C., and Edwards, D.: Metronidazole in Prevention and Treatment of Bacteroides Infections after Appendectomy, *Br Med J,* **1**(6005):318, 1976.

Tumors

Aho, A. J., Heinonen, R., and Laurén, P.: Benign and Malignant Mucocele of the Appendix. Histological Types and Prognosis, *Acta Chir Scand,* **139:**392, 1973.

Godwin, J. D., II: Carcinoid Tumors. An Analysis of 2837 Cases, *Cancer,* **36:**560, 1975.

Higa, E., Rosai, J., Pizzimbono, C. A., and Wise, L.: Mucosal Hyperplasia, Mucinous Cystadenoma, and Mucinous Cystadenocarcinoma of the Appendix: A Re-evaluation of Appendiceal "Mucocele," *Cancer,* **32:**1525, 1973.

Steinberg, M., and Cohn, I., Jr.: Primary Adenocarcinoma of the Appendix, *Surgery,* **61:**644, 1967.

Wilson, H., Cheek, R. C., Sherman, R. T., and Storer, E. H.: Carcinoid Tumors, in "Current Problems in Surgery," Year Book Medical Publishers, Inc., Chicago, 1970.

Wolff, M., and Ahmed, N.: Epithelial Neoplasms of the Vermiform Appendix (Exclusive of Carcinoid): I. Adenocarcinoma of the Appendix, *Cancer,* **37:**2493, 1976.

Wolff, M., and Ahmed, N.: Epithelial Neoplasms of the Vermiform Appendix (Exclusive of Carcinoid): II. Cystadenomas, Papillary Adenomas, and Adenomatous Polyps of the Appendix, *Cancer,* **37:**2511, 1976.

Chapter 30

Liver

by **Seymour I. Schwartz**

ANATOMY

The liver constitutes approximately one-fiftieth of the total body weight. Its size reflects the complexity of its functions. The anatomic division with respect to biliary drainage and vascular supply differs from the classic description in which the organ was divided into right and left lobes by the falciform ligament. True division is to the right of the falciform ligament, in line with the fossa for the inferior vena cava above and the gallbladder fossa below (Fig. 30-1). A right segmental fissure divides the right lobe into anterior and posterior segments, while the falciform ligament divides the left lobe into medial and lateral segments. The left lateral segment corresponds to the left lobe in the classic description. This segmental division can be observed only in cast specimens in which the Glissonian structures, i.e., hepatic artery, portal vein, and bile ducts, have been injected.

BILIARY DRAINAGE. Each segment is drained by a major segmental duct formed by the confluence of subsegmental draining structures. The anterior and posterior segmental ducts in the right lobe join to form the right hepatic duct, while the medial and lateral segmental ducts in the left lobe terminate in the left hepatic duct, which joins the right duct to form a common hepatic duct in the porta hepatis. This lies anteriorly in relation to other structures in the area. The common hepatic duct descends for a variable distance in the hepatoduodenal ligament and is joined by the cystic duct which enters from the right at an angle. These two structures and the liver form the cystohepatic triangle of Calot, which is extremely important surgically, since it frequently contains the cystic and right hepatic arteries as well as aberrant segmental hepatic arteries and ducts.

BLOOD SUPPLY. The afferent blood supply to the liver arises from two sources: (1) the hepatic artery, which carries oxygenated blood and accounts for approximately 25 percent of hepatic blood flow and (2) the portal vein, which accounts for approximately 75 percent of hepatic blood flow and drains the splanchnic circulation. The common hepatic artery originates from the celiac axis and, after contributing the right gastric artery, ascends in the hepatoduodenal ligament to the left of the common bile duct and anterior to the portal vein. It bifurcates into a right and left branch to the left of the main lobar fissure. The major right hepatic artery originates from the superior mesenteric artery in 17 percent of people. Intrahepatic anastomoses between the right and left hepatic arteries do not occur. The cystic artery is usually an extrahepatic branch of the right hepatic artery.

The portal venous system contains no valves (Fig. 30-2). It returns to the liver the blood that the celiac, superior mesenteric, and inferior mesenteric arteries supply to the gastrointestinal tract, pancreas, and spleen. The vessel is formed behind the pancreas, at the level of L_1 to L_2, by the confluence of the superior mesenteric and splenic veins and, at times, the inferior mesenteric vein. The portal vein resides posteriorly in relation to the hepatic artery and bile duct in the hepatoduodenal ligament but, in rare instances,

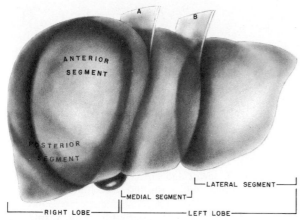

Fig. 30-1. Lobar and segmental divisions of the liver. *A.* Lobar fissure. *B.* Left segmental fissure. A right segmental fissure divides the right lobe into its anterior and posterior segments. (*From Seymour I. Schwartz, "Surgical Diseases of the Liver," McGraw-Hill Book Company, 1964.*)

is located anterior to the pancreas and first portion of the duodenum, in which circumstance it is frequently associated with a partial or complete situs inversus and is subject to injury during cholecystectomy or gastrectomy. In the porta hepatis the vein divides into two branches, which

Fig. 30-2. Anatomy of the extrahepatic portal venous system, anterior aspect. The termination of each vein is shown as it was encountered most frequently in 92 dissections. The pancreas is represented by the shaded area. *A.P.,* accessory pancreatic vein; *C.,* coronary vein; *Cystic,* cystic vein; *I.,* intestinal veins; *I.C.,* ileocolic vein; *I.M.,* inferior mesenteric vein; *I.P.D.,* inferior pancreaticoduodenal vein; *L.,* liver; *L.B.P.,* left branch of portal vein; *L.C.,* left colic vein; *L.G.E.,* left gastroepiploic vein; *M.C.,* middle colic vein; *O.,* omental vein; *P.,* pancreatic veins; *Pyloric,* pyloric vein; *R.C.,* right colic vein; *R.G.E.,* right gastroepiploic vein; *R.B.P.,* right branch of portal vein; *S.,* splenic vein; *S.G.,* short gastric veins; *S.H.,* superior hemorrhoidal vein; *S.M.,* superior mesenteric vein; *S.P.D.,* superior pancreaticoduodenal vein; *S.T.,* splenic trunks. (*From Douglass et al., Surg Gynecol Obstet, 91:562, 1950.*)

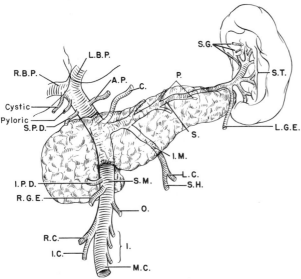

course to each lobe. The average length of the main portal vein is 6.5 cm, and the average diameter is 0.8 cm. Much has been written concerning the streaming phenomenon within the portal vein accounting for preferential metastases to the right and left lobe depending on the venous drainage of the primary site. Recent experimental and clinical findings have refuted this concept.

The hepatic venous system (Fig. 30-3) begins as a central vein of the liver lobule and represents the only vessel in man into which the sinusoids empty. The central veins unite to form sublobular veins, which in turn fuse to form collecting veins. The collecting veins gradually increase in size by joining other large intrahepatic collecting channels, which coalesce to form the three major hepatic veins. The hepatic venous tributaries occupy the fissures and are intersegmental in position. The major hepatic veins are classified as right, left, and middle. The right hepatic vein drains the entire posterior segment as well as the superior area of the anterior segment of the right lobe. The left hepatic vein drains the entire lateral segment and the superior area of the medial segment of the left lobe. The inferior areas of the medial and anterior segments of the two lobes are drained by the middle vein. In man there are no valves in the hepatic venous system, whereas the dog has a sphincteric action in the hepatic veins which constitutes an important difference experimentally. Total hepatic blood flow can be measured by means of hepatic vein catheterization and the use of the Fick principle. The average value is 1,500 ml/minute/1.73 m² of body surface.

LIVER FUNCTION

The liver consists of four physiologic-anatomic units which are interrelated:

1. The circulatory system. A dual blood supply nourishes the liver and acts as a vehicle for material absorbed from the intestinal tract to be utilized in the metabolic pool. Blood vessels are accompanied by lymphatics and nerve fibers which contribute to the regulation of blood flow and intrasinusoidal pressure.
2. Biliary passages. These serve as channels of exit for materials secreted by the liver cells, including bilirubin, cholesterol, and detoxified drugs. This system originates with the Golgi apparatus adjacent to the microvilli of the bile canaliculi and eventually terminates in the common bile duct.
3. The reticuloendothelial system. This system has 60 percent of its cellular elements in the liver and includes the phagocytic Kupffer cells and endothelial cells.
4. The functioning liver cells, which are capable of a wide variation of activity. The metabolic pool in the liver serves the needs of the entire body. The cell performs both anabolic and catabolic activities, secretes, excretes, and stores. The large amount of energies required for these transformations result from the conversion of adenosine triphosphate (ATP) to adenosine diphosphate (ADP). A second source is the aerobic oxygenation in the metabolic pool via the tricarboxylic acid cycle of Krebs.

Function Tests (Table 30-1)

The so-called liver "function" tests evaluate liver activity by assessing the degree of functional impairment. They do not provide a pathologic diagnosis, and the extreme functional reserve of the organ occasionally produces normal results in the face of significant lesions. Many of these tests do not measure a specific function of the liver, and other organ systems may be implicated. False positives for each of the tests are found in about 2.5 percent of normal controls and in about 10 percent of hospital controls. False-negative tests also occur in about 10 percent of most tests.

PROTEINS. Hepatic cells are responsible for the synthesis of albumin, fibrinogen, prothrombin, and other factors involved in blood clotting. A reduction of serum albumin is one of the most accurate reflections of the extent of liver disease and the effects of medical therapy. Because the half-life of albumin is slightly more than 10 days, impairment of hepatic synthesis must be present for over 2 weeks before abnormalities are noted. The correlation between total protein and disease of the liver is not as close as that between the serum albumin level and liver disease, since albumin is produced only by hepatic cells and a reduction is frequently compensated for by an increase in the level of globulin.

CARBOHYDRATES AND LIPIDS. Glycogenesis, glycogen storage, glycogenolysis, and the conversion of galactose into glucose all represent hepatic functions. Hypoglycemia is a rare accompaniment of extensive hepatic disease, but the amelioration of diabetes in patients with hemochromatosis is considered an indication of neoplastic change. The more common effect of hepatic disease is a deficiency of glycogenesis with resultant hyperglycemia. A hepatic enzyme system is responsible for the conversion of galactose into glucose, and abnormal galactose tolerance tests are seen in hepatitis and active cirrhosis. In rare instances, a familial deficiency in this enzyme system accounts for spontaneous galactosemia accompanied by an obstructive type of jaundice which appears after the first week of life and subsides when lactose is removed from the diet.

Synthesis of both phospholipid and cholesterol takes place in the liver, and the latter serves as a standard for the determination of lipid metabolism. The liver is the major organ involved in the synthesis, esterification, and excretion of cholesterol. In the presence of parenchymal damage, both the total cholesterol and percentage of esterified fraction decrease. Biliary obstruction results in a rise in cholesterol, and the most pronounced elevations are noted with primary biliary cirrhosis and the cholangiolitis accompanying toxic reactions to phenothiazine derivatives.

ENZYMES. The three enzymes which achieve abnormal serum levels in hepatic disease that have been widely studied are alkaline phosphatase, serum glutamic oxylactic transaminase (SGOT), and serum glutamic pyruvic transaminase (SGPT). The SGOT is present in the liver, myocardium, skeletal muscles, kidney, and pancreas. Cellular damage in any of the above-mentioned tissues results in elevation of the serum level. In reference to the liver, the most marked increases accompany acute cellular damage regardless of cause, and extremely high levels are noted in patients with hepatitis. The SGOT is only moderately increased in cirrhosis and biliary obstruction. The SGPT is more particularly applicable to the evaluation of liver disease, since the hepatic content greatly exceeds myocar-

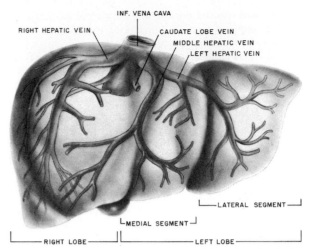

Fig. 30-3. Prevailing pattern of drainage of hepatic veins in the human liver. (*From Seymour I. Schwartz, "Surgical Diseases of the Liver," McGraw-Hill Book Company, 1964.*)

dial concentration. Elevations accompany acute hepatocellular damage. Lactic acid dehydrogenase (LDH) levels also may be elevated.

A variety of methods of assaying the serum alkaline phosphatase are currently in use, and in all notations of results normal values should be parenthetically indicated. Serum alkaline phosphatase provides an evaluation of the patency of the bile channels at all levels, intrahepatic and extrahepatic. Elevation is demonstrated in 94 percent of

Table 30-1. NORMAL VALUES FOR HEPATIC "FUNCTION" TESTS

Test	Normal value
Serum albumin	4.6–6.7 Gm/100 ml
Total protein	6.0–8.0 Gm/100 ml
Albumin/globulin	1.5–3.6
Cholesterol	135–325 mg/100 ml
Esters	65% of total
Alkaline phosphatase:	
Bodansky	1.5–4.0 units
King-Armstrong	3–13 units
Shinowara-Jones-Reinhart	2.8–8.6 units
Bessey-Lowry-Brock	1.8 × Bodansky units
Serum glutamic oxalacetic transaminase	40 units
Serum glutamic pyruvic transaminase	45 units
Lactic acid dehydrogenase	90–200 units
Bromsulphalein retention	0–6% at 45 minutes
Prothrombin time	90–100%
Fibrinogen	200–400 mg/100 ml
Blood "ammonia"	40–60 μg/100 ml
Icterus index	3–8 units
Serum bilirubin:	
Total	Less than 1.5 mg/100 ml
Direct	Less than 0.3 mg/100 ml
Indirect	Less than 1.2 mg/100 ml
Urinary bilirubin	0
Urobilinogen:	
Urinary	0.2–3.0 mg/day
Fecal	40–300 mg/day

patients with obstruction of the extrahepatic biliary tract due to neoplasm and 76 percent of those in whom the obstruction is caused by calculi. Intrahepatic biliary obstruction and cholestasis also cause a rise in the enzyme level. In the presence of space-occupying lesions such as metastases, primary hepatic carcinoma, and abscesses, the alkaline phosphatase is also increased. The overall correlation between metastatic carcinoma of the liver and an elevated enzyme level is as high as 92 percent. Sixty percent of patients with primary hepatic carcinoma also demonstrate a significant increase. Granulomatous and infiltrative lesions such as sarcoidosis, tuberculosis, and lymphoma are irregularly associated with mild to moderate increases in the alkaline phosphatase. Elevation of the serum level of this enzyme is also associated with diseases that have as a common denominator increased osteoblastic activity.

DYE EXCRETION. The hepatic removal of dyes from the circulation is dependent upon hepatic blood flow, hepatocellular function, and biliary excretion. Sulfobromophthalein (Bromsulphalein, or BSP) provides an assessment of hepatic function, although 20 percent is removed by an extrahepatic means. The presence of jaundice produces a disproportionate BSP retention, and fever, shock, hemorrhage, and recent surgical treatment may all result in increased levels. An increased retention is associated with acute cellular damage and is also noted in patients with cirrhosis, carcinoma, and chronic passive congestion. Since the rate of disappearance from the blood is constant, hepatic blood flow can be determined by injecting the dye at a rate which will maintain a constant blood level and applying Fick's principle to the blood removed from a catheterized hepatic vein.

Indocyanine green now is used more frequently to determine hepatic blood flow. More recently an intestinal xenon technique has been shown to provide an accurate method of measuring portal vein and total hepatic blood flow.

Rose bengal is another phthalein dye which, when labeled with radioactive iodine, has been useful in the evaluation of liver disease. Since all of this material is removed by the hepatic parenchymal cell, it provides a more accurate estimate of hepatic blood flow. Determination of the fecal excretion of the radioactive material has been applied to the differential diagnosis of obstructive jaundice, particularly in the establishment of the diagnosis of congenital atresia of the bile ducts.

COAGULATION FACTORS. In liver disease, multiple coagulation defects may occur. Two mechanisms contribute to the deficiency of coagulation factors: (1) in obstructive jaundice, the bile source required for the absorption of the fat-soluble vitamin K results in a decreased synthesis of prothrombin, and (2) hepatocellular dysfunction is accompanied by an inability of the liver to synthesize the prothrombin. Abnormal values for prothrombin time have been noted in a variety of hepatic diseases with parenchymal damage, and determination is particularly applicable in the evaluation of patients undergoing liver biopsy or surgical procedures. Values above 40 percent are generally not associated with excessive bleeding. An increase in prothrombin time subsequent to the injection of parenteral vitamin K is used as an indication of hepatic function and suggests obstructive jaundice. Decreases in factor V (proaccelerin), Christmas factor, factor VII (proconvertin), and fibrinogen have also been noted in hepatic disease.

BILE PIGMENT METABOLISM. See the section on Jaundice in Chap. 24.

SPECIAL STUDIES

NEEDLE BIOPSY OF THE LIVER. This is the one study which provides a pathologic diagnosis. It is dependent on an area of tissue measuring 1 to 4 cm in length and containing approximately 5 to 20 lobules representing a general anatomic change. Close to 100 percent accuracy has been demonstrated for both posthepatitic and postnecrotic cirrhosis. Intrahepatic cholestasis, hepatitis, and cellular degeneration resulting from toxicity are all diffuse lesions and readily diagnosed. Focal lesions, such as neoplasm, granulomas, and abscess may be missed, but the correlation between needle biopsy and operative and autopsy findings is high. A mortality rate of 0.08 percent has been determined, and pain, pneumothorax, hemorrhage, and bile peritonitis are the complications to be considered.

SCINTILLATION SCANNING. This technique has been used as a method of evaluating liver size, shape, and position, and also to determine the presence and location of intrahepatic neoplasms or focal lesions. Either ^{131}I-tagged rose bengal, which is absorbed and excreted by the parenchymal cells of the liver, or [198]Au or preferably technetium-sulfur colloid (^{99m}Tc), which is deposited in the reticuloendothelial system, may be utilized. The scan is limited in detection to small lesions. For lesions over 1.5 cm, the correlation with autopsy and operative findings is excellent and is over 83 percent for metastatic lesions.

ANGIOGRAPHY. Since hepatic tumors, both primary and metastatic, are dependent on an arterial circulation, unusual vascular patterns are also detected by injection of the hepatic artery with the radiopaque material. Unusual arrangements of the arteries and "tumor staining," analogous to that found in cerebral and osseous neoplasms, may be noted.

MEASUREMENTS OF PORTAL PRESSURE, SPLENO-PORTOGRAPHY, ISOTOPIC EVALUATION OF PORTAL CIRCULATION. See Portal Hypertension, later in this chapter.

TRAUMA

INCIDENCE. The liver ranks high on the list of intra-abdominal organs involved by injury (Table 30-2). The rapid increase in motor traffic has resulted in an increasing incidence and in a change of pattern from one with a predominance of penetrating wounds to the present higher incidence of blunt traumatic injuries. The frequency of traumatic rupture of the liver was 1 in 1,300 accident admissions to a general hospital. Seventy-four percent had additional abdominal organs involved, and 45 percent also had thoracic injuries.

Table 30-2. RELATIVE FREQUENCY OF VISCERAL INJURY FROM BLUNT TRAUMA

Viscera involved	Series I	Series II	Series III	Series IV	Series V	Series VI
Spleen	56	20	53	37	20	38
Intestine	14	3	27	13	4	19
Liver	6	9	45	5	14	19
Kidneys	8	25	Not incl.	26	27	91
Bladder	11	9	Not incl.	4		8
Others, including pancreas, the diaphragm, and mesentery . . .	46	8	8	39	7	25
Total	141	74	183	124	72	200

SOURCE: From McCort, *Radiology,* **78**:49, 1962.

Rupture of the liver also occurs spontaneously in pathologic organs. It occurs in approximately 8 percent of patients with primary carcinoma and has been reported with increasing frequency for benign hepatic adenoma and in association with toxemia of pregnancy. Rupture of the liver in the newborn infant is related to the trauma of birth and is more common in infants who are larger than average and classified as "postmature."

PATHOLOGY. Liver injuries are classified as transcapsular, subcapsular, or central (Fig. 30-4). When rupture of the liver extends through Glisson's capsule, extravasated blood and bile are found in the peritoneal cavity. If the capsule remains intact, the collection of blood between the capsule and parenchyma is usually found on the superior surface of the organ. Central rupture consists of interruption of the parenchyma of the liver. Blunt trauma may be associated with hepatic parenchymal emboli to the right heart and lungs, causing death.

Persons with injury about the hilus rarely survive long enough for surgical exploration. Nonpenetrating injuries result in a tear in the anteroposterior portion. The dome of the liver is frequently involved, particularly in older patients. With penetrating lesions of the lower thorax, the dome is also most frequently involved, and the ratio of right lobe to left lobe involvement is 7:1.

CLINICAL MANIFESTATIONS. These are determined by the pathologic types. With rupture of Glisson's capsule, signs and symptoms are related to shock and peritoneal irritation. Shock is present in over three-quarters of the cases, and abdominal pain, spasm, and rigidity are usual accompaniments.

DIAGNOSTIC STUDIES. Shortly after trauma, an increased leukocyte count is more consistent than a reduced hemoglobin. Hematuria is frequently coexistent. The SGOT and SGPT levels are elevated, but this usually occurs several hours subsequent to trauma. Infrequently mild elevation of the serum bilirubin level occurs on the third or fourth day. X-ray may reveal evidence of fluid in the peritoneum and pelvis or a wide right flank stripe indicating blood accumulated between the ascending colon and the peritoneal line. Paracentesis is useful in verifying the presence of hemoperitoneum, but a negative tap does not exclude the diagnosis. Celiac angiography may precisely define hepatic rupture and will distinguish between hepatic splenic rupture in a patient with a positive tap (Fig. 30-5).

TREATMENT. Shock is corrected and associated thoracic lesions are treated first. Surgical procedures are directed at the control of bleeding, the removal of necrotic devitalized tissue, and the establishment of external drainage. These should be initiated early, because time has proved to be a definite factor in morbidity and mortality statistics. With penetrating wounds of the liver, particularly knife wounds, the bleeding has usually stopped at the time of exploration and simple drainage is all that is required. Such is usually not the case with blunt trauma and shotgun wounds. Hemorrhages are controlled preferably by exposing individual bleeders within the parenchyma of the liver and ligating these vessels. The technique of placing a row of interlocking through-and-through mattress sutures parallel to the surfaces of the laceration should be avoided, since this adds to the amount of tissue necrosis. In general, hepatic resection is not carried out along precise anatomic lines

Fig. 30-4. Diagram of three types of liver rupture. *A.* Transcapsular. *B.* Subcapsular. *C.* Central. (*From Seymour I. Schwartz, "Surgical Diseases of the Liver," McGraw-Hill Book Company, 1964.*)

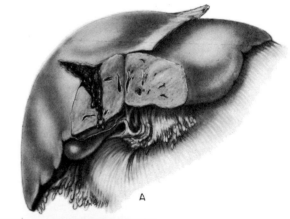

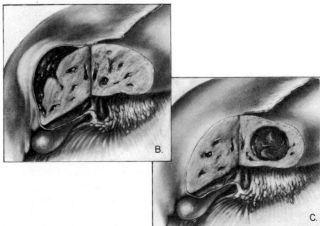

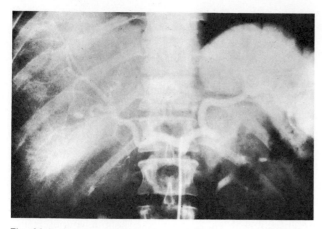

Fig. 30-5. Celiac angiogram demonstrating normal spleen and hepatic rupture.

Hematobilia

The pathologic *sine qua non* for this condition is free communication between a blood vessel and the biliary tree. It is a consequence of central or subcapsular hematomas and also capsular wounds which have been primarily closed or packed. The triad of abdominal injury, subsequent gastrointestinal hemorrhage, and colicky pain should raise a high index of suspicion. This may occur within few days after injury or, more characteristically, after a period of weeks. Multiple episodes of bleeding with some suggestion of periodicity occur. Melena is more frequent than hematemesis, and jaundice of mild to severe proportion is present in some cases. Diagnosis is established and the lesion located by angiographic techniques. Operations have been varied and have included resection of the lesion, which is preferable, debridement and unroofing, or ligation of the contributing hepatic artery.

Hepatorenal Syndrome

The term *hepatorenal syndrome* was introduced to describe the fatal combination of renal and hepatic dysfunction occurring in patients after biliary tract surgery. Shortly thereafter, the association of this syndrome with traumatic necrosis of the liver was proposed. It was theorized that the damaged liver cells released into the circulation a toxin capable of destroying kidney cells. There is no question that renal failure often is associated with massive hepatic injury, but the so-called "hepatic nephrotoxin" has not been identified. In this regard, recent animal experiments have demonstrated abnormal renal function and increased exchangeable sodium in animals subjected to hepatic damage.

PROGNOSIS. The improvement in mortality statistics accompanying hepatic injuries is evident from war experience. During World War II with the institution of routine drainage and the elimination of gauze packs the mortality rate dropped from 30 to 17 percent. During the Korean war, penetrating injuries were associated with a mortality rate of 14 percent, whereas in the Vietnam war a mortality rate of 4.2 percent has been reported for United States military personnel. The mortality rate associated with blunt trauma is consistently higher than that accompanying penetrating injuries. In a large series, extending from 1963 to 1971, the overall mortality was 13 percent. Blunt trauma and shotgun wounds had a significantly higher mortality rate than penetrating wounds. In patients requiring a sublobar resection the mortality rate was 47 percent; associated damage to the hepatic veins or inferior vena cava raised the rate to 85 percent.

MAJOR VASCULAR INJURIES. The effects of ligation of the major vessels are diagrammed in Fig. 30-6. When the common or proper hepatic artery is ligated, collateral supply is apparent roentgenographically within 4 hours and it is unusual for major dysfunction caused by hepatic ischemia to occur. However, primary repair of a surgically traumatized artery and restoration of flow are indicated.

Hepatic vein injuries represent a significant factor in the high mortality accompanying blunt liver trauma. Fifteen

unless the injury demands it. Most resections are best regarded as sublobar debridements, with as much tissue preserved as possible. All the devitalized tissue and markedly traumatized tissue is removed to avoid subsequent autolysis, abscess formation, and secondary hemorrhage.

Packing with gauze is contraindicated, since it is attended by a high incidence of secondary hemorrhage and infection. Recently, there has been enthusiasm for hepatic artery ligation to control bleeding. This is appropriate when it can be demonstrated that bleeding is reduced by temporarily cross-clamping the hepatic artery. In most circumstances of extensive bleeding, it is venous in character and requires a direct approach. The most vigorous bleeding associated with hepatic trauma is usually caused by deep lacerations of the posterior portions of the right lobe with involvement of the hepatic veins. The use of an internal stent passed either from the atrium down to the infrahepatic vena cava or from the infrahepatic vena cava up to the suprahepatic vena cava may facilitate control of the bleeding while maintaining caval flow.

External drainage should be carried out in almost all cases and is directed at the prevention of abscess and bile peritonitis. The drains are brought out from the subphrenic and subhepatic spaces, depending upon the lesion. There is controversy regarding the appropriateness of routinely draining the common bile duct. An increased complication rate has been reported for T-tube drainage in patients with hepatic trauma. This includes infections and an increased incidence of upper gastrointestinal bleeding. Although common duct drainage does not prevent the development of a hematobilia, it does permit postoperative cholangiography, which may aid in the diagnosis of this complication and which also can be used to determine the status of hepatic regeneration.

COMPLICATIONS. The incidence of complications is well over 50 percent and is related to the extent of injury to other organs. Hemorrhage is the most important cause of death, and recurrent bleeding may occur secondarily to necrosis and sequestration of infected tissue.

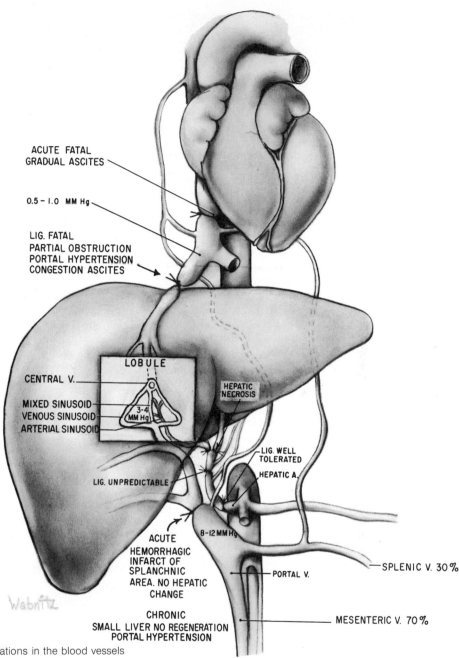

ACUTE FATAL
GRADUAL ASCITES

0.5 - 1.0 MM Hg

LIG. FATAL
PARTIAL OBSTRUCTION
PORTAL HYPERTENSION
CONGESTION ASCITES

LOBULE

CENTRAL V.

HEPATIC
NECROSIS

MIXED SINUSOID
VENOUS SINUSOID
ARTERIAL SINUSOID

3-4
MM Hg

LIG. WELL
TOLERATED

HEPATIC A.

LIG. UNPREDICTABLE

ACUTE
HEMORRHAGIC
INFARCT OF
SPLANCHNIC
AREA. NO HEPATIC
CHANGE

8-12 MM Hg

SPLENIC V. 30%

PORTAL V.

MESENTERIC V. 70%

CHRONIC
SMALL LIVER NO REGENERATION
PORTAL HYPERTENSION

Wabnitz

Fig. 30-6. Pressures and effects of ligations in the blood vessels of the liver. (*From H. Popper and F. Schaffner, "Liver: Structure and Function," McGraw-Hill Book Company, 1957.*)

percent of patients with blunt hepatic trauma have sustained injury to the hepatic veins, and most of these patients die from uncontrollable hemorrhage either in the operating room or prior to operation. Because the hepatic veins are multiple, often forming connecting channels, the safe approach is to expose all the veins and the entire retrohepatic inferior vena cava. Control of the bleeding vein or veins is best accomplished by occluding the porta hepatis and inserting a catheter via either the inferior vena cava or the right atrium in such a fashion that umbilical

tapes may be placed above and below the area of the hepatic veins. A review of portal vein injury reported that 16 of 17 patients survived ligation but that reconstruction should be attempted.

HEPATIC ABSCESSES

Hepatic abscesses are related to two distinct groups of pathogens, pyogenic bacteria and *Entamoeba histolytica*.

Distinctive features in the clinical manifestations and therapy of these two variations necessitate separate consideration.

Pyogenic Abscesses

INCIDENCE. The lesion is present in 0.36 percent of autopsies. Prior to the widespread use of antibiotic therapy, this incidence was 0.44 percent as contrasted with 0.28 percent in autopsies since 1945. The highest percentage of cases occur in the sixth, seventh, and eighth decade, and there is no predilection for either sex.

ETIOLOGY. Pyogenic abscesses of the liver result from (1) ascending biliary infection, (2) hematogenous spread via the portal venous system, (3) generalized septicemia with involvement of the liver by way of the hepatic arterial circulation, (4) direct extension from intraperitoneal infection, and (5) other causes, including hepatic trauma. Recently, the most frequent antecedent cause has been cholangitis secondary to calculi or carcinoma in the extrahepatic biliary duct system. The second most common cause is related to generalized septicemia, while the portal venous route of infection has decreased in importance. Pylephlebitis occurs in 0.05 percent of cases of acute appendicitis and 3 percent of patients with perforated appendicitis. No segment of the intestine drained by the portal venous system can be excluded as a possible cause, and the incidence associated with acute diverticulitis is as high as that of appendicitis. There has been an increase in the percentage in which no cause is apparent. In one series these accounted for over half the cases.

Positive cultures are obtained from pyogenic abscesses in only 50 percent of cases. *Escherichia coli* has been the only microorganism demonstrated in abscesses secondary to biliary tract infection and infection along the portal venous route. By contrast, the cocci, particularly *Staphylococcus aureus* and hemolytic streptococcus, are usually isolated from abscesses related to systemic infection. *Bacteroides* and other anaerobes have become increasingly prevalent as a cause, thus emphasizing the need to culture anaerobically at the time of drainage.

Pyogenic abscesses may be solitary, multiple, and multilocular. The greatest proportion are multiple small abscesses. When a single abscess is present, it is usually located in the right lobe.

CLINICAL MANIFESTATIONS. Since most pyogenic hepatic abscesses are secondary to other significant infections, it is difficult to delineate a pathognomonic symptom. Fever is the most common symptom, and a "picket fence" configuration of the temperature chart generally has been noted. Fever is frequently accompanied by chills, profuse sweating, nausea, vomiting, and anorexia. Pain is a late symptom and is more common with large solitary abscesses. Enlargement of the liver and tenderness have been considered almost constant findings. However, in more recent series liver enlargement was noted in 30 to 60 percent of cases. Hepatic tenderness was absent in one-third of the patients. Jaundice is a relatively uncommon finding.

DIAGNOSTIC STUDIES. Leukocytosis with white blood cell counts ranging between 18,000 and 20,000 is usual. Most patients are anemic. Positive blood cultures are demonstrated in approximately 30 percent of patients, the most significant yields accompanying abscesses secondary to systemic septicemia. Liver function tests are not diagnostic, but elevation of the alkaline phosphatase level is the most frequent abnormality. Hypoalbuminemia is common. Characteristically, x-rays reveal an elevation and immobility or restriction of motion of the right leaf of the diaphragm. There is also obliteration of the right cardiophrenic angle on the posteroanterior chest film and the anterior costophrenic angle on the lateral film. Abscesses produced by gas-forming microorganisms are associated with air-fluid levels in the liver. Cholangiography is of little value. The lesions generally can be defined by hepatic arteriography or ^{99m}Tc-sulfur colloid scan.

TREATMENT. This is based on appropriate antibiotic therapy combined with surgical drainage in selected cases. Either chloramphenicol or gentamycin should be given until cultures and sensitivities are reported. Drainage is particularly indicated for solitary abscesses or for large multiple abscesses. The route of access depends on the position of the abscess and may be transthoracic or transabdominal (Figs. 30-7 and 30-8). Because of the availability of antibacterial agents, transperitoneal drainage is no longer associated with prohibitive morbidity or mortality.

PROGNOSIS AND COMPLICATIONS. The prognosis is significantly better in patients with single or multilocular abscesses than in those with multiple abscesses. Similarly, there is a much higher mortality rate associated with patients in whom complications including subphrenic abscess, empyema, or pyopericardium have developed. The mortality rate approaches 100 percent in undrained patients; 66 percent of the drained patients survive, and over 90 percent of patients with a solitary abscess which is drained survive. Subphrenic abscess occurs in approximately 5 percent of cases, and rupture of the hepatic abscess into the free peritoneal cavity may cause a diffuse peritonitis.

Amebic Abscesses

INCIDENCE. *Entamoeba histolytica* has been found wherever surveys have been made on the human population from Northern Canada to the Straits of Magellan. It has been estimated that at least 10 percent of the population of this country is infected with the parasite. The incidence of amebic involvement of the liver is more difficult to assess. An average involvement of 3.6 percent of autopsy cases and 1 to 25 percent of clinical cases have been reported. Much of this disparity is related to the lack of clinical recognition. Amebic abscess of the liver is a

Fig. 30-7. Extraserous transthoracic drainage. *A.* Incision is made posteriorly over right twelfth rib. *B.* Latissimus dorsi muscle exposed. *C.* Periosteum of twelfth rib incised. *D.* Twelfth rib removed subperiosteally and bed incised. *E.* Diaphragm is detached and peritoneum is reflected from the inferior surface of diaphragm. *F.* Schematic drawing of position of drain. (*From Seymour I. Schwartz, "Surgical Diseases of the Liver," McGraw-Hill Book Company, 1964.*)

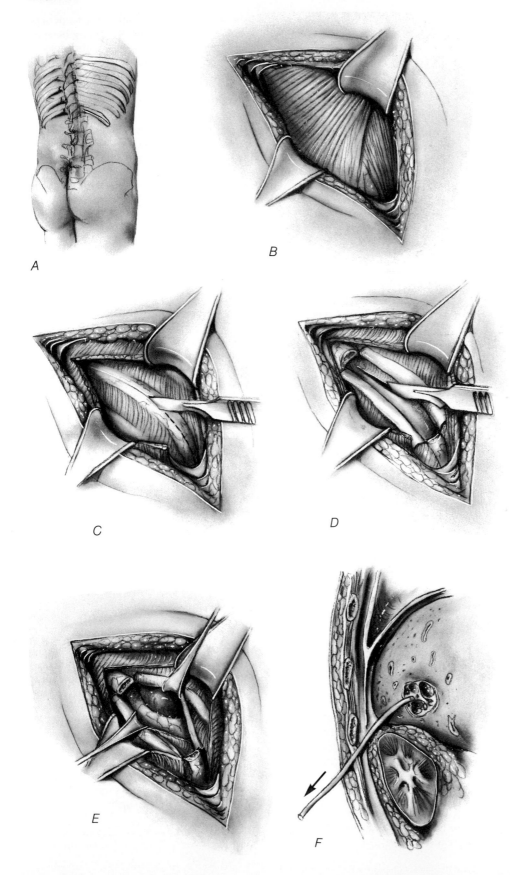

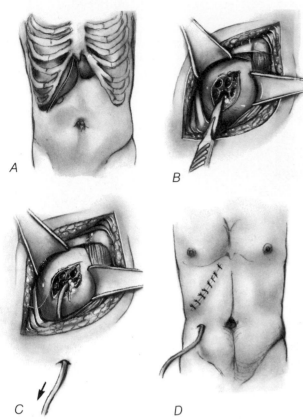

Fig. 30-8. Transabdominal drainage. *A.* Subcostal incision. *B.* Peritoneum has been entered and abscess incised. *C.* Drain is positioned in abscess and brought out through the stab wound. *D.* Closure of wound and position of stab wound. (*From Seymour I. Schwartz, "Surgical Diseases of the Liver," McGraw-Hill Book Company, 1964.*)

disease of the middle-aged adult and predominates in the male with a 9:1 ratio. The concept of racial immunity is no longer considered valid.

PATHOLOGY. Amebas reach the liver by way of the portal venous system from a focus of ulceration in the bowel wall. Hepatic involvement is usually a large single abscess containing liquefied material with a characteristic reddish brown "anchovy paste" fluid. The lesions are usually single and occur in the right lobe of the liver either near the dome or on the inferior surface in juxtaposition to the hepatic flexure. The wall is only a few millimeters thick and consists of granulation tissue with little or no fibrosis. Microscopically, three zones are recognized: a necrotic center, a middle zone with destruction of parenchymal cells, and an outer zone of relatively normal hepatic tissue in which amebas may be demonstrated. The concept of amebic hepatitis or presuppurative hepatitis has been challenged, since it is not certain that biliary abscesses or even larger central hepatic abscesses do not exist.

CLINICAL MANIFESTATIONS. Abscesses become evident when they cause generalized systemic disturbances coupled with symptoms and signs of hepatic involvement. The chief complaints are fever and liver pain. Pain is present in 88 percent of patients, and the pattern is related to the lo-

cation of the hepatic abscess. With pain and tenderness over the right lower intercostal spaces, there may be associated bulging and pitting edema of the subcutaneous tissue. Superior surface abscesses result in pain referred to the right shoulder, while abscesses in the bare area, which have no contact with the serosal surface, are latent as far as pain is concerned. Left lobe abscesses present as a painful epigastric swelling.

Fever accompanied by chills and sweating is present in over three-quarters of the patients, but the temperature does not reach the levels resulting from pyogenic abscesses unless there is secondary infection. One-third to one-half of the adults offer a history of antecedent diarrhea, while in children grossly bloody mucous stool occurs more frequently. Tender hepatomegaly is an almost constant feature. Clinical jaundice is relatively rare, and abnormal pulmonary findings are present in about one-quarter of the patients.

DIAGNOSTIC STUDIES. Patients with acute disease show no anemia but an appreciable degree of leukocytosis, whereas those with prolonged illness have anemia with less marked leukocytosis. Examination of the stool does not provide a high diagnostic yield. Although DeBakey and Ochsner demonstrated amebas in the stools of 47 percent of their own patients, these were found in only 15.4 percent of cases collected from the literature. Liver function tests are not helpful in establishing the diagnosis, although the BSP retention may be increased and the alkaline phosphatase level may be elevated. A specific complement-fixation test has been more reliable than a history of diarrhea, stool examination, and proctoscopy. However, a negative test does not exclude the diagnosis. Roentgenographic findings are similar to those described for pyogenic abscesses. Scintillography and angiography have also helped to localize the lesion.

Diagnosis is frequently established by aspiration of the abscess cavity, a relatively innocuous procedure. Although the "anchovy paste" aspirate is considered pathognomonic, the abscess content may be creamy white even though there is no secondary bacterial infection. Amebic trophozoites are demonstrated in the aspirate of fewer than one-third of the patients.

COMPLICATIONS. The most common complication is secondary infection, which occurs in approximately 22 percent of patients. Rupture of the amebic abscess accounts for the next most common group of complications. The direction of rupture is reproduced in Fig. 30-9. Pleuropulmonary complications occur in 20 percent of patients. This is usually the result of direct extension of the hepatic process. The most serious route of rupture is into the pericardial cavity, and this is usually secondary to extension of an abscess in the left lobe. Rupture into the peritoneal cavity or into an intraabdominal viscus occurs in 6 to 9 percent of the patients.

TREATMENT. This consists of administration of amebicidal drugs combined with aspiration or surgical drainage when indicated. The initial approach is usually conservative and directed toward eradicating the parasite from the intestinal tract, liver, and abscess itself. In general, the patient is not considered for surgical treatment until the intestinal phase is controlled. Metronidazole, which acts in both the hepatic and intestinal sites, has replaced emetine and chloroquine. Both the hepatic and intestinal infections have generally been cured by 400 mg three times a day for 4 days combined with closed aspiration. A single dose of 2.5 Gm combined with aspiration also has had dramatic results. Since both emetine, which may be cardiotoxic, and chloroquine act mainly on the hepatic phase, following completion of therapy with these drugs, intestinal amebicidals such as Diodoquin, chiniofon, and tetracycline must be administered to control the intestinal phase.

Surgical Procedures. The indications for aspiration are (1) the persistence of clinical manifestations following a course of amebicidal drugs, (2) clinical or roentgenographic evidence of a hepatic abscess, and (3) absence of findings which would suggest secondary infection of a liver abscess. Drug therapy should be instituted several days prior to aspiration. There is no indication for injection of any drug directly into the abscess cavity. In the absence of localizing signs, the preferred route is through the ninth or tenth interspace between the anterior and posterior axillary line. More recently, there has been renewed enthusiasm for frequent open drainage of amebic abscesses of the liver. Once an abscess has been demonstrated to be secondarily infected, open drainage is the treatment of choice. Although there is an obvious advantage to the extraserous approach, antibiotics have obviated the prohibitive mortality or morbidity associated with transserous drainage (Figs. 30-7 and 30-8).

PROGNOSIS. This is dependent upon the relative virulence of the organism and the resistance of the host, the stage of infection, the multiplicity of abscesses, and the presence of complications. In uncomplicated cases, the mortality rate is only 7 percent, whereas with complications a 43 percent mortality has been reported.

CYSTS AND BENIGN TUMORS

Nonparasitic Cysts

These lesions may be single, multiple, diffuse, localized, unilocular, or multilocular. They include (1) blood and degenerative cysts, (2) dermoid cysts, (3) lymphatic cysts, (4) endothelial cysts, (5) retention cysts, consisting of (*a*) solitary retention cysts and (*b*) multiple retention cysts (polycystic disease), and (6) proliferative cysts (cystadenomas). Autopsy incidences of approximately 0.15 percent have been reported. The clinically apparent cystic disease and nonparasitic solitary cysts occur more frequently in the fourth, fifth, and sixth decades, at an average age of fifty-three. Solitary cysts occur more commonly in females (4:1). Traumatic cysts are more common in children, whereas cystadenomas occur at an average age of fifty-two years. Polycystic hepatic disease also occurs much more frequently in the female.

PATHOLOGY. Solitary nonparasitic cysts are usually located on the anteroinferior surface of the right lobe of the liver. The cyst content is a clear, watery, yellowish brown material, and characteristically the cysts have a low inter-

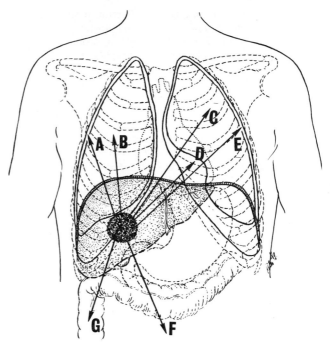

Fig. 30-9. Directions of rupture in 44 cases of amebic liver abscess: A. 8 cases, right pleural cavity. B. 13 cases, right lung. C. 4 cases, left lung. D. 7 cases, pericardium. E. 1 case, left pleural cavity. F. 10 cases, peritoneal cavity. G. 1 case, colon. (*After Lamont, Q J Med, 27:389, 1958.*)

nal pressure in contrast to the high tension in parasitic cysts. Polycystic disease of the liver has a honeycomb appearance with multiple cavities, and the lesions are commonly distributed throughout the entire liver, but at times one lobe, more frequently the right, is preferentially involved. Unlike the solitary nonparasitic cyst, polycystic disease of the liver is frequently associated with cystic involvement of other organs; 51.6 percent of polycystic livers are associated with polycystic kidneys. Conversely, the incidence of hepatic cysts in patients with known polycystic renal disease varies between 19 and 34 percent. Polycystic livers have been implicated as a rare cause of portal hypertension and also have been associated with atresia of the bile ducts, cholangitis, and hemangiomas.

Traumatic cysts are usually single, are filled with bile, and contain no epithelial lining. Cystadenomas are grossly smooth, encapsulated, and lobular, and contain a mucoid material. They are lined by a proliferative columnar epithelium.

CLINICAL MANIFESTATIONS. Both solitary and polycystic lesions grow slowly and are relatively asymptomatic. A painless right upper quadrant mass is the most frequent complaint, and when symptoms occur, they are usually related to pressure on adjacent viscera. Acute abdominal pain may accompany the complications of torsion, intracystic hemorrhage, or intraperitoneal rupture. Physical examination may reveal the mass, and the kidneys may be palpable. Jaundice is rare. Liver function tests are of little diagnostic aid. Scintillography and arteriography have been used to define the intrahepatic position of the mass, and peritoneoscopy may be diagnostic.

TREATMENT. With the exceptions of rupture, torsion, and intracystic hemorrhage, the treatment is elective. Ideally, complete extirpation is the treatment of choice, but few cysts are resectable. Solitary cysts which are superficial should be resected, but resection of a large cyst extending deep into the parenchyma may be hazardous. When the cyst contents are sterile and contain no bile, unroofing the cyst and establishing a free connection with the peritoneal cavity is satisfactory. When bile is present, internal drainage into a Roux en Y jejunal limb is preferable, while the presence of purulent contents indicates external drainage or marsupialization. With polycystic disease of the liver and serious renal involvement, excisional therapy for the hepatic cyst is contraindicated. Also, if the patient has been asymptomatic and excision is deemed to be technically difficult, resection should not be carried out. However, if the patient is in good health and there is a possibility of complete surgical extirpation, wide excision is justifiable.

PROGNOSIS. The prognosis of polycystic disease is essentially that of the accompanying renal disease. Hepatic failure, jaundice, and the manifestations of portal hypertension are rare. The mortality rate for surgically treated nonparasitic cysts of the liver is approximately 5 percent. The morbidity is usually related to the development of a persistent sinus.

Hydatid Cysts

Hydatid disease (echinococcosis) is characterized by worldwide distribution and frequent hepatic involvement. The incidence among human beings is dependent on the incidence in intermediate hosts including sheep, pigs, and cattle. The southern half of South America, Iceland, Australia, New Zealand, and southern parts of Africa are regarded as intensive endemic areas. Fewer than 1,000 cases have been reported in the United States, most of these occurring in immigrants.

PATHOLOGY. The most common unilocular hydatid cyst is caused by *Echinococcus granulosis,* while the alveolar type is caused by *Echinococcus multilocularis.* Approximately 70 percent of hydatid cysts are located in the liver, and in one-quarter to one-third of these cases there are multiple cysts. The right lobe is affected in 85 percent of patients. Cysts are usually superficial and are composed of a two-layer laminated wall, an inner germinative membrane, and an outer adventitia. The two membranes are in close contact with each other but are not linked. The fluid in the hydatid cyst has a high pressure of approximately 300 ml of water and is colorless, opalescent, and slightly alkaline. Inside the main hydatid vesicle daughter cysts are usually found. Extension is commonly into the peritoneal cavity, but progressive intrahepatic expansion may result in the replacement of liver parenchyma.

In contrast to the unilocular hydatid cysts, the alveolar hydatid is a growth without a capsule and with a tendency toward multiple metastases. As growth progresses, the center becomes necrotic, and the peripheral portion invades the blood vessels and lymph channels. The causative agent of this lesion is found more frequently in the colder regions of Alaska, Russia, and the Alps.

COMPLICATIONS. Intrabiliary rupture represents the most common complication and occurs in 5 to 10 percent of cases. Suppuration, the second most common complication, is caused by bacteria from the biliary tract. The formation of the purulent material results in the death of the parasite and conversion into a pyogenic abscess. Intraperitoneal rupture results in the showering of hydatid fluid, brood capsules, and scolices into the peritoneum, leading to transient peritoneal irritation of varying intensity. Usually, the reproductive elements survive and initiate the formation of new cysts, "secondary echinococcosis of the peritoneum." Cysts located in the superior portion of the liver tend to grow craniad into the pleural cavity and become intrathoracic. These can be differentiated from primary pulmonary cysts by the presence of daughter cysts and bile pigments. Empyema and bronchopleural fistula may result.

CLINICAL MANIFESTATIONS. Patients with simple or uncomplicated multivesicular cysts are usually asymptomatic. When symptoms occur, they are caused by pressure on adjacent organs. A tumor, which is palpable in 70 percent of the patients, or diffuse hepatic enlargement in a patient who has lived in an endemic region is cause for suspicion. The so-called "hydatid thrill" and "fremitus" are quite rare. Jaundice and ascites are uncommon. With secondary infection, tender hepatomegaly, chills, and spiking temperatures occur. Urticaria and erythema offer evidence of a generalized anaphylactic reaction. With biliary rupture, the classic triad of biliary colic, jaundice, and urticaria may be noted. Vomiting with passage of hydatid membranes in the emesis (hydatidemesia) and passage of membranes in the stool (hydatidenteria) may also occur. The complication of intraperitoneal rupture is heralded by abdominal pain and signs of anaphylactic shock. Intrathoracic rupture is associated with shoulder pain and cough initially productive of a frothy blood-stained fluid that subsequently becomes bile-stained. Membranes are intermittently expectorated in 80 percent of the cases.

DIAGNOSTIC STUDIES. Roentgenographically, an unruptured cyst presents as a round, reticulated calcified shadow in the liver (Fig. 30-10). Secondary infection with gas-producing organisms may demonstrate as daughter cysts. With intrabiliary rupture, gas is noted in the remaining cyst cavity. Liver scans furnish useful information and correlate well with operative findings. Eosinophilia is the least reliable of immunologic responses, being present in only 25 percent of all patients. Complement-fixation tests have been positive in up to 93 percent of patients with living cysts. This reaction becomes negative 2 to 6 months after removal of the cyst. Casoni's skin test is positive in approximately 90 percent of patients, and the reaction may be obtained years after surgical removal of the cyst or after the parasite has died. Diagnosis may also be made by demonstrating the elements of the hydatid cyst in the excreta or during biopsy.

TREATMENT. Small calcified cysts in patients with negative serologic test results need no treatment. Treatment is surgical, since there is no response to drug administration or radiation therapy. Therapy consists of removal of the cyst without contaminating the patient, followed by appropriate management of any remaining cavity. Since the hydatid fluid is under high tension, evacuation and sterilization are carried out initially using hydrogen peroxide or hypertonic saline solution. The classic approach using Formalin has fallen into disrepute. Removal of the parasite is accomplished by excision of the hydatid vesicle using the natural cleavage plane which exists between the germinative layer and adventitia. Total removal of the cysts, including the adventitial layer, may also be performed. Partial hepatectomy with controlled hepatic resection has been advised for larger and multiple cysts. When a hepatic cavity remains, this may be treated by (1) suture without drainage, (2) marsupialization and drainage, and (3) omentoplasty (Fig. 30-11). Omentoplasty is the treatment of choice in these cases since the incidence of biliary leakage is reduced. Marsupialization or partial hepatectomy are the alternatives for large or infected cysts. In uncomplicated cases, the results of surgical treatment are excellent, and the postoperative mortality is less than 5 percent. With intrabiliary rupture, marsupialization should be accompanied by drainage of the bile duct if there is associated obstruction. Rupture into the peritoneal cavity is treated by laparotomy and thorough cleansing, although it is frequently impossible to prevent secondary contamination. Intrathoracic, rupture generally can be controlled by evacuating and draining the hepatic cysts. Alveolar disease of the liver was inevitably fatal, but, more recently, satisfactory results have been obtained with extensive hepatic resection.

Benign Tumors

HAMARTOMA. Hamartomas are composed of tissues normally present in the organ but arranged in a disorderly fashion. The lesions vary from minute nodules to large tumors and are rarely of clinical significance. Grossly, the tumors are firm, nodular, and located immediately beneath the surface of the liver, and may be solitary or multiple. On cut section, they are grayish brown and frequently contain a central element of connective tissue arranged in a stellate fashion. With lesions of clinical significance, surgical excision is generally indicated. However, deeply located lesions should be left alone after histologic diagnosis has been established, since they do not grow rapidly and do not undergo malignant transformation.

ADENOMA AND FOCAL NODULAR HYPERPLASIA. In the past hepatic adenomas were extremely rare. In a 47-year-period only four cases were seen at the Mayo Clinic. In 1973 Baum and associates brought attention to a possible relationship between oral contraceptives and these tumors. Many subsequent reports have appeared, and an association with focal nodular hyperplasia also has been noted. Many of the reported patients with liver cell adenoma presented with massive intraperitoneal hemorrhage as an

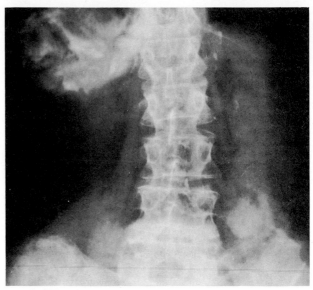

Fig. 30-10. Hydatid cyst of liver, demonstrating calcification. (*From Seymour I. Schwartz, "Surgical Diseases of the Liver," McGraw-Hill Book Company, 1964.*)

initial manifestation. This has not occurred in patients with focal nodular hyperplasia. A liver scan and arteriogram aid in diagnosis. Resection of the lesion and discontinuance of contraceptives are generally indicated. Recently regression of the lesions following cessation of contraceptives has been documented, and an operation may be avoided in a patient with a lesion which has not ruptured.

HEMANGIOMA. Hemangioma is the most common nodule in the liver, and the liver is the internal organ most frequently affected with this lesion. Of 126 benign tumors treated at Memorial Sloan-Kettering Cancer Center, 106 were hemangiomas. The tumor occurs five times more frequently in the female than in the male, and this has been related to the hormonal influence. There are two types, capillary and cavernous. Almost all liver lesions are cavernous. These are frequently associated with cysts of the liver and pancreas. Malignant degeneration does not occur, but the hemangioma must be distinguished from a hemangioendothelioma or diffuse hemangiomatosis. The latter consists of widespread multicentric lesions accompanied by vascular involvement of the skin and occurs in children with clinical manifestations in the first week of life.

When a mass is apparent, it is most commonly felt in the epigastrium or left upper quadrant, since the majority of lesions arise in the left lobe. A bruit is heard only rarely. Hepatic arteriography is frequently diagnostic. The major complication is rupture with intraperitoneal hemorrhage, which occurs more commonly in children. In this circumstance, the mortality rate has been over 80 percent. Large tumors in infants may be associated with high-output cardiac failure.

The management in infants is determined by the cardiac output. With high output and congestive failure, supportive therapy including steroids is effective and the lesions generally regress. In rare cases hepatic artery ligation may

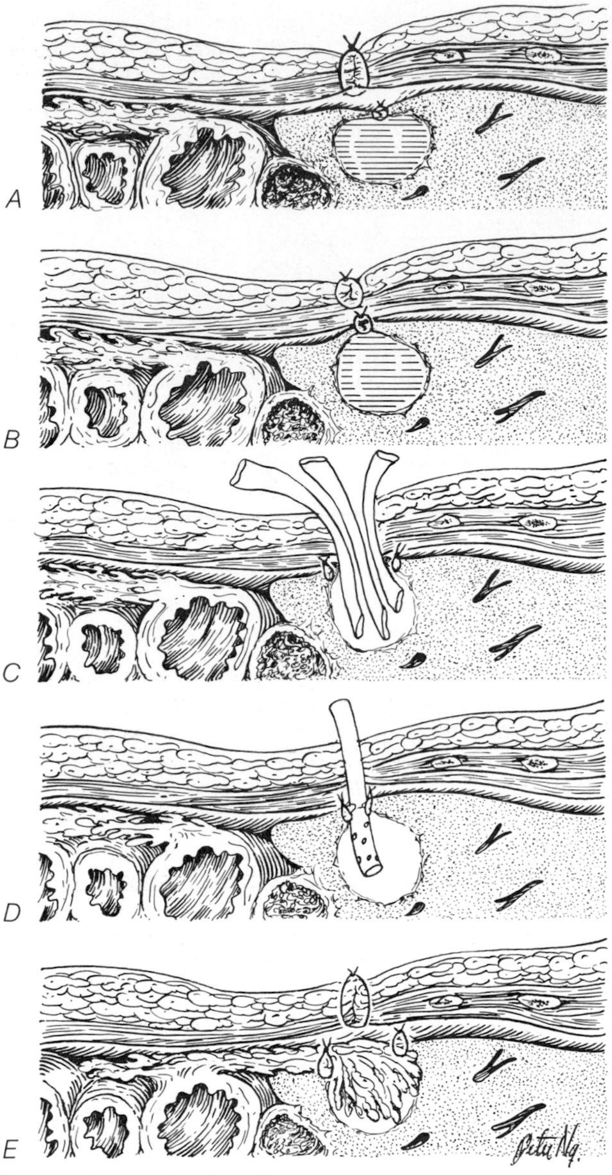

Fig. 30-11. Methods of handling residual hepatic cavity. *A.* Suture without drainage (capsulorraphy). Cavity is filled with sterile saline solution, and adventitia is closed without drainage. *B.* Same as *A* but peripheral peritoneum of anterior abdominal wall is sutured to periphery of capsule to facilitate extraperitoneal drainage of secondary infection, if one arises. *C.* Marsupialization. Edges of cavity are sutured to abdominal wall, and several drains are inserted into depths of wound. *D.* Variant of marsupialization. Catheter is inserted into cavity, and closed drainage is used. *E.* Omentoplasty. Omentum is used to fill remaining cavity and is sutured to periphery of fibrous capsule. Vascular omental pedicle absorbs effusion. (*From Seymour I. Schwartz, "Surgical Diseases of the Liver," McGraw-Hill Book Company, 1964.*)

be required to reverse the cardiac failure. Large lesions in any age group may necessitate resection, which is also indicated for a hemangioma with free intraperitoneal rupture. Radiation therapy using up to 2,000 rads in 15 days in adults and 600 rads in children may significantly reduce the size of the tumor.

MALIGNANT TUMORS

Primary Carcinoma

INCIDENCE. Although the disease is rare in people of Western Europe and North America, it is remarkably common among the aboriginal inhabitants of Africa and certain parts of Asia. Postmortem rates in the United States average 0.27 percent, whereas in Africa the postmortem rate is 1.1 percent, hepatic carcinomas representing 17 to 53 percent of all cancers.

Primary carcinoma of the liver occurs with greater frequency in the male sex. In the Caucasian it is rare before the age of forty, while in the African and Indonesian the affection is primarily one of youth, usually occurring before the age of forty. Although it has been suggested that the American Negro still exhibits a distinct predisposition toward the disease, recent statistics do not substantiate this. In contrast, a higher incidence is present in Chinese subjects even after they have changed their habitation. In children, the first appearance of the neoplasm is usually before the age of two, and primary carcinoma of the liver represents the most common carcinoma in the first few years of life.

ETIOLOGY. A variety of etiologic factors have been implicated. Aflatoxins of the mold *Aspergillus flavus* contaminate the diet in African and Asian communities with high incidences of hepatocellular carcinoma. Low protein intake and consequent kwashiorkor also may be factors. Just as almost every type of experimentally induced cirrhosis may be followed by carcinoma of the liver, so a definite association between cirrhosis and primary carcinoma has been noted in the human being. Postnecrotic cirrhosis is the type most commonly preceding hepatocellular carcinoma; cirrhosis is present in 60 percent of cases. Hepatic malignant tumors occur in 4.5 percent of cirrhotic patients, and the incidence is increased in patients with hemochromatosis. Parasitic infestation with the liver fluke *Clonorchis sinensis* has been considered a factor in the development of cholangiocarcinoma, but this is open to question. There is no increased risk for hepatic carcinoma following infectious hepatitis. In the pediatric age group cirrhosis is noted only rarely.

PATHOLOGY. Three types based on the prevalent cell have been defined: (1) liver cell carcinoma (hepatocellular), resembling the parenchymal cell and occurring most frequently, (2) bile duct carcinoma (cholangiocarcinoma), in which the cell is apparently derived from bile duct epithelium, and (3) a mixture of these two types. The term embryoma or hepatoblastoma has been used to represent an immature variant of the hepatic cell carcinoma.

Grossly, each of these types may present as a single large nodule, as extensive nodularity, or as a diffuse permeation throughout the organ. The hepatocellular carcinomas have a trabecular structure, and vascularity is a prominent feature. These lesions frequently invade branches of the portal vein and occasionally the hepatic veins. The formation of giant cells is a feature of hepatocellular carcinoma and aids in distinguishing this lesion from the secondary carcinoma of the liver. The cell type of the bile duct carcinoma is columnar, and its microscopic appearance may be impossible to distinguish from that of carcinoma of the gallbladder or extrahepatic biliary duct system. Bile is never seen in the acini or the cells, whereas mucus formation is common.

Hepatic tumors extend by four methods:

1. Centrifugal growth, which indicates nodular expansion leading to compression of the surrounding hepatic tissue.
2. Parasinusoidal extension, which refers to tumor invasion into the surrounding parenchyma, either through the parasinusoidal spaces or through the sinusoids themselves.
3. Venous spread, which is the extension of tumor from small branches of the portal system in a retrograde fashion into larger branches and eventually into the main portal vein. Invasion of hepatic vein tributaries is less common but may extend up to the inferior vena cava or right atrium.
4. Distant metastases, which are the result of invasion of lymph channels and vascular systems. The most frequently involved locations are regional lymph nodes and the lungs.

Metastases occur in 48 to 73 percent of cases.

CLINICAL MANIFESTATIONS. A correct antemortem diagnosis at one time was extremely rare, but recent figures represent significant improvement. Weight loss and weakness occur in 80 percent of cases, while abdominal pain is present in half. The pain is usually dull and persistent, but dramatic sudden onset may occur in patients with intraperitoneal hemorrhage secondary to rupture of a necrotic nodule or erosion of a blood vessel. This was the initial manifestation in 14 percent of one series. Bleeding varices are infrequent, but foreboding symptoms and delirium have almost always represented a terminal event (Table 30-3).

The liver is almost always enlarged but not tender. Splenic enlargement is present in one-third of the cases,

as are other signs of portal hypertension. The incidence of jaundice varies from 20 to 58 percent. Ascites develops in one-half to three-quarters of patients. A rapid increase in the symptoms and signs associated with cirrhosis or hemachromatosis is highly suggestive of superimposed hepatic carcinoma. In these cases, the amelioration of diabetes and occasional hypoglycemic intervals also indicate neoplastic change.

DIAGNOSTIC STUDIES. Erythrocytosis has been associated with hepatomas. The most consistently altered liver function tests are the BSP and alkaline phosphatase. An increase in alkaline phosphatase, in the absence of bone disease and significant hepatic dysfunction, is considered presumptive evidence of a liver tumor. The serum bilirubin level is usually normal, as are other liver function tests.

The demonstration of α-fetoprotein (AFP) in the serum by immunodiffusion, immunoelectrophoresis, and immunoassay techniques is useful in differential diagnosis and epidemiologic studies. This protein is normally present in the fetus but disappears a few weeks after birth. Positive AFP tests are noted in about 75 percent of Africans but in only 30 percent of patients in the United States and Europe. False-positive results occur with embryonic tumors of the ovary and testis. Resection of the tumor converts the test to "negative"; recurrence may be detected by the reappearance of AFP in the serum.

Selective hepatic arteriography has been utilized to demonstrate an arterial pattern within the tumor, characterized by pooling and increased vascularity (Fig. 30-12).

Fig. 30-12. Hepatic arteriogram demonstrating vascularity of hepatocellular carcinoma.

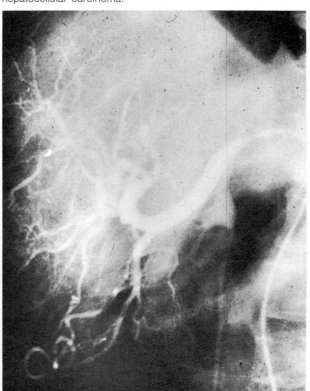

Table 30-3. PRIMARY EPITHELIAL CANCER IN ADULTS: 1974 LIVER TUMOR SURVEY— SYMPTOMS AND SIGNS ON HOSPITAL ADMISSION

Mass	60
Pain	51
Weight loss	29
Epigastric distress	16
Intraperitoneal hemorrhage	15
Hepatomegaly	14
Fever	9
Incidental at laparotomy for other disease	7
Diarrhea	6
Anorexia	6
Nausea and vomiting	6
Weakness, malaise	5
Misdiagnosis—cholecystitis	5
Endocrine symptoms	3
Pruritus	3
Jaundice	2
Calcification on x-ray	1
Needle biopsy for benign disease	1
Abnormal liver function tests	1
Abnormal scan	1

SOURCE: James Foster and Martin Berman, "Solid Liver Tumors," vol XXII, W. B. Saunders Company, Philadelphia, 1977.

Scintillation scanning may also identify the space-occupying lesion within the liver. A recent review has shown that even when angiography and scans are combined there are significant incidences of false positives and negatives. Percutaneous needle biopsy can provide a definitive diagnosis. Most investigators have been unable to find any evidence to support the view that the presence of hepatic tumor enhances the hazard of liver biopsy.

TREATMENT. The only definitive treatment is surgical excision. The criteria which should be met before resection include:

1. The carcinoma must be solitary or localized.
2. There must be no evident lymph node, blood vessel, or bile duct involvement.
3. There should be no distant metastases.

The recent appreciation of segmental anatomy of the liver coupled with improvements in surgical technique, anesthesia, and blood replacement have placed hepatic resection on an acceptable level. The overall operative mortality in a 1974 Liver Tumor Survey was 21 percent, with 12 percent in noncirrhotic patients.

Total hepatectomy with orthotopic liver transplantation has been performed in more than 48 patients. The results to date have not been encouraging, since only three patients survived longer than 1 year. Starzl's four patients with hepatoma who lived long enough to permit observation of the course of malignant disease all demonstrated diffuse metastases in addition to involvement of the homograft.

Radiation therapy is considered of little value, and extensive radiation damage to the liver, including suppurative cholangitis and abscesses, has been described. Systemic chemotherapy generally has not prolonged survival. However, one patient with disseminated hepatoma survived 10 years with continued 5-fluorouracil systemic therapy, and no tumor was noted at autopsy. Direct arterial infusion is reported to have obtained response in 25 percent of cases, but the response has been temporary. Hepatic artery ligation or more complete dearterialization has been applied, with minimal temporary success. Distal intraarterial infusion coupled with hepatic artery ligation has achieved similar results.

PROGNOSIS. The outlook for primary carcinoma of the liver is extremely poor, and the duration of the disease is rarely longer than 4 months from the time of onset of symptoms. Death is the result of cachexia, hepatic failure, sequelae of portal vein thrombosis, intraperitoneal hemorrhage, and metastases. In the 1974 Liver Tumor Survey 20 of 59 patients with epithelial liver carcinomas who survived the operative procedure lived 5 years or more. In children under age two years with hepatoblastoma, 21 of 27 who survived operation were alive and well with no evidence of disease for a mean of 53 months. In children over age two with the same lesion, 4 in 10 were alive without evidence of disease for a mean of 81 months. Five-year survival following dearterialization or chemotherapeutic regimens is extremely rare and difficult to evaluate, since spontaneous regression has been recorded.

Other Primary Neoplasms

A review in 1947 collected fewer than 100 cases of sarcoma of the liver. Twenty-five percent of these were combined with cirrhosis. The three major lesions are sarcoma, mesenchymoma, and infantile hemangioendothelioma. All hepatic mesenchymal lesions are considered malignant. Angiosarcoma is the most common primary sarcoma of the liver. Recently exposure to vinyl chloride has been implicated as an etiologic factor.

Angiosarcoma is characterized by short illness, jaundice, and coma progressing rapidly to death. Thorotrast also has been implicated as an etiologic factor. Infantile hemangioendotheliomas occur in children under the age of five and are associated with skin lesions and cardiac failure secondary to arteriovenous shunts within the tumor. Although most of these pediatric lesions are fatal, spontaneous regression has been recorded, as has success with partial hepatectomy.

Metastatic Neoplasms

These represent the most common malignant tumor of the liver. The liver is second only to regional lymph nodes as a site of metastases for tumors, and 25 to 50 percent of all patients dying of cancer have been found to have hepatic metastases. Fifty percent of patients with gastrointestinal tumors have hepatic metastases when autopsied. The relative proportion of primary to secondary neoplasms is estimated to be 1:20, and there is no statistical difference between those with and those without cirrhosis.

Metastatic neoplasms reach the liver by four routes: (1) portal venous circulation, (2) lymphatic spread, (3) hepatic arterial system, and (4) direct extension.

Metastases appear in the liver at varying times in relation to primary lesions: (1) Precocious metastasis is evident when the primary lesion is not suspected (carcinoid of the ileum). (2) Synchronous metastases occur when the hepatic neoplasm is detected at the same time as the primary lesion. (3) Metachronous metastasis is one in which appearance is delayed following the successful removal of a primary tumor (ocular melanoma). The growth pattern of the metastatic tumor is frequently more rapid than the original lesion, and the mitotic count of the metastatic hepatic neoplasms has been shown to be five times greater than that of the extrahepatic primary lesion.

CLINICAL MANIFESTATIONS. Symptoms referable to the liver are present in 67 percent of patients with proved metastases. These include hepatic pain, ascites, jaundice, anorexia, and weight loss. On examination, hepatic nodularity is apparent in half the cases, and a friction rub is audible in 10 percent. Jaundice, ascites, and the signs of portal hypertension are present in approximately one-quarter to one-third of the patients. With carcinoid tumors, hepatic metastases are of major importance in the pathogenesis of the flushing syndrome.

DIAGNOSTIC STUDIES. The BSP retention test and alkaline phosphatase level are the most sensitive indices of hepatic involvement. The former is increased in almost 100 percent of the patients, while the serum alkaline phospha-

Table 30-4. RESECTION OF METASTATIC CANCER—1974 LTS:
PRIMARY COLON AND RECTUM: OPERATION VERSUS SURVIVAL

Operation	Patients	Operative deaths	Survival*	
			Mean, mo	5-yr
Extended right lobectomy	4	1	70	1/2
Right lobectomy	25	4	29	2/16
Left lobectomy	10	0	9	0/8
Left lateral segmentectomy	20	0	24	3/12
Wedge	67	3	31	10/50

*Excludes operative deaths.
SOURCE: From James Foster and Martin Berman, "Solid Liver Tumors," vol XXII, W. B. Saunders
Company, Philadelphia, 1977.

tase is increased in over 80 percent of patients. The SGOT level is elevated in approximately two-thirds of the patients, but the serum α-fetoprotein determination is negative. Hepatic arteriography, biphasic splenoportography, and scintillation scanning may prove diagnostic. All are associated with significant incidences of false positives and negatives.

TREATMENT. This may be directed toward palliation or cure. Only surgical treatment has the possibility of curing. Encouraging results have been noted with involvement of the liver by direct extension from carcinoma of the stomach, colon, or gallbladder. Right hepatic lobectomy at the time of cholecystectomy has been advised for treatment of carcinoma of the gallbladder, but the data argue against a major hepatic resection, since cures are extremely rare. Surgical treatment of hepatic metastases should be considered only if (1) control of the primary tumor is accomplished or anticipated, (2) there are no systemic or intraabdominal metastases, (3) the patient's condition will tolerate the major operative procedure, and (4) the extent of hepatic involvement is such that resection and total extirpa-

tion of the metastasis is feasible. In a collective review, 21 percent of patients who survived curative resection of metastatic liver tumors lived 5 years. The results of resection of metastatic tumors in the liver are shown in Tables 30-4 and 30-5. Palliative surgical measures are indicated for marked pain associated with hepatic neoplasm and for the excision of metastases in patients with the flushing syndrome or carcinoid tumor.

Most tumors are not responsive to irradiation. The one exception is the neuroblastoma. Hepatic arterial infusion of chemotherapeutic agents, with or without dearterialization, has been applied to therapy of metastatic tumors. Although the response has been better than that noted for primary tumors of the liver (see above), improvement has been brief.

HEPATIC RESECTION

The present indications for hepatic resection include (1) trauma with resultant necrosis of hepatic tissue, (2) cysts,

Table 30-5. LIVER RESECTION FOR METASTATIC CANCER FROM PRIMARY
TUMORS OTHER THAN COLON AND RECTUM—1974 LTS: OPERATION
VERSUS SURVIVAL

	Patients	Operative deaths	Survival*		
			Mean, mo	Median, mo	5-yr
Extended right lobectomy	2	0	21	—	0/1
Right lobectomy . .	11	2	19	9	1/9
Left lobectomy . . .	2	0	6	—	0/2
Left lateral segmentectomy	9	3	13	8	0/4
Wedge	26	1	17	10	1/16
	50	6	17	9	2/32†

*Excludes operative deaths.
†Both 5-year survivors dead with disease at 105 months after liver resection.
SOURCE: From James Foster and Martin Berman, "Solid Liver Tumors," vol XXII, W. B. Saunders
Company, 1977.

(3) granulomas, (4) primary neoplasms of the liver, and (5) secondary malignant tumors which involve the liver either by direct extension or as metastatic lesions.

Up to 80 percent of the liver can be removed with little or no alteration in hepatic function. There is experimental evidence for hepatotropic substances in portal venous blood. Insulin may represent the major anabolic factor and may be counterbalanced by glucagon. Following excision of this amount, patients maintain normal blood ammonia levels and normal prothrombin times. Fibrinogen production is usually unimpaired, and clinical jaundice is a transient phenomenon. Immediately postoperatively, there may be an increase in alkaline phosphatase, transaminase, and BSP retention. However, by the fifth postoperative day, 95 percent of patients show clinical improvement in function, with the bilirubin and alkaline phosphatase returning to normal by the end of the third week. The most profound changes are noted in serum proteins, particularly the albumin fraction, which by the third week is usually restored to normal levels. Regeneration results from marked hypertrophy of the remaining lobe. The remaining portion of the liver responds as rapidly and completely after second and third partial hepatectomies as after an initial insult. It is now felt that portal venous blood flow is an important contributory factor in liver regeneration. Very little restoration occurs after partial hepatectomy of the cirrhotic liver.

MANAGEMENT OF THE PATIENT. Approximately 25 percent demonstrate significant dysfunction related to underlying cirrhosis or a critically positioned tumor. Preoperative therapy is directed at maintaining optimal liver function and correcting any defects which may be present.

Fig. 30-13. Nomenclature for hepatic resection.

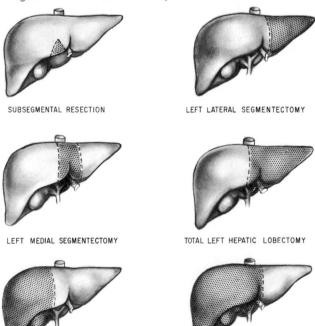

SUBSEGMENTAL RESECTION   LEFT LATERAL SEGMENTECTOMY

LEFT MEDIAL SEGMENTECTOMY   TOTAL LEFT HEPATIC LOBECTOMY

RIGHT LOBECTOMY   EXTENDED RIGHT LOBECTOMY

A diet high in calories, proteins, and carbohydrates is utilized, and the administration of serum albumin may be required to achieve normal levels. Vitamin K is given routinely until a normal prothrombin time results. In the presence of jaundice, other fat-soluble vitamins are added. Since many patients have a reduced hematocrit, transfusion with fresh whole blood rich in platelets and coagulation factors is indicated. Major hepatic resection is attended by a prohibitive mortality rate in the patient with BSP retention greater than 35 percent, a serum albumin level lower than 2.5 Gm, and an increased prothrombin time which does not respond to parenteral vitamin K.

Postoperatively, infusion of 10% glucose or fructose is continued until the patient maintains an adequate oral intake to obviate severe hypoglycemia, which has been reported. Daily administration of 25 to 50 Gm of albumin is usually required for 7 to 10 days to maintain the serum level above 3 Gm. Vitamin K and antibiotics which achieve a high biliary concentration are indicated. Analgesics and hypnotics which are detoxified by the liver are used only sparingly.

OPERATIVE PROCEDURES. Control of Bleeding. This may be accomplished by (1) compression of blood vessels within the substance of the remaining liver segment, (2) efforts directed at the raw surface, and (3) control of the main blood vessels entering the porta hepatis. Omental grafts, split-thickness grafts, peritoneal grafts, Gelfoam, micronized collagen, and rapidly polymerizing adhesives have been applied to the raw surface as local hemostatic agents. However, their effects are temporary, and generally are associated with high incidences of secondary hemorrhage and infection. Compression of the main vessels entering the liver facilitates the demonstration of bleeding sites along the raw surface. The hepatic artery and portal vein may be compressed for 15 minutes without affecting hepatic structure and function. Moderate hypothermia has extended the time safety factor.

Technique of Resection. On the basis of new concepts of segmental anatomy, the following classification of hepatic resection is applicable (Fig. 30-13): (1) Subsegmental or wedge resection is the removal of an area of the liver that is less than a segment and without an anatomic dissection plane. (2) Left lateral segmentectomy ("left lobectomy" in old nomenclature) is the excision of the liver mass to the left of the left segmental fissure along an anatomic plane. (3) Left medial segmentectomy is resection between the main interlobar fissure and the left segmental fissure. (4) Left lobectomy is the excision of all hepatic tissue to the left of the main lobar fissure. (5) Right lobectomy is the removal of the liver to the right of the main lobar fissure. (6) The extended right lobectomy is the excision of the entire right lobe plus the medial segment of the left lobe (trisegmentectomy), i.e., excision of all tissue to the right of the umbilical fossa, fossa for the ligamentum venosum, and the ligamentum teres.

Segmental resection is applicable for biopsy of the liver and for the removal of small localized benign tumors. Left lateral segmentectomy is performed for extensive trauma to that segment and for tumors or cysts confined to that portion of the liver. Left medial segmentectomy may be performed for benign tumors, particularly hemangiomas localized to this segment, and also as an en bloc dissection for direct extension of carcinoma of the gallbladder. Total left hepatic lobectomy is indicated for tumors of the left medial or lateral segments encroaching upon the lateral segmental plane and thus precluding a segmentectomy. Total excision of the right lobe of the liver is considered for massive injuries, large primary tumors residing in that lobe, metastatic tumors involving only the right lobe, and en bloc dissection of tumors extending from the gallbladder, colon, or stomach.

The liver is initially mobilized by dividing the appropriate ligamentous attachments, i.e., ligamentum teres and triangular ligament (Fig. 30-14A). It is then possible to rotate the liver to the side to expose its inferior surface at the porta hepatis. Dissection of the porta hepatis identifies the branches of the hepatic artery, portal vein, and biliary duct system supplying the segment or lobe to be removed (Fig. 30-14B). These are individually doubly ligated and transected. Glisson's capsule is then incised along the surgical plane (Fig. 30-14C), and the cleavage plane of the hepatic parenchyma itself is best established by means of a scalpel handle or finger to permit exposure of the larger ducts and vessels, which may be individually clamped and ligated as they are encountered. This incision is continued posteriorly until the major hepatic vein or veins are identified, doubly ligated, and transected. By rotating the liver, the hepatic veins may be isolated at their junctions with the inferior vena cava and ligated (Fig. 30-14D and E). The specimen is removed, and the duodenum area is covered with a flap of peritoneum provided by the transected ligament (Fig. 30-14F). The blood flow to and from the remaining segments of the liver must be carefully preserved.

The majority of lobar resections, even right lobe resections, can be carried out transabdominally, and it is not necessary to proceed along the outlined sequence of events for surgical excision. Finger fracture is employed for trauma but is also applied in many instances for tumor. One can reduce the blood flow into the liver by temporarily cross clamping the hepatoduodenal ligament; this procedure can be carried out for 20 minutes using a bulldog clamp intermittently. Glisson's capsule is then incised anteroinferiorly, and the incision is carried down to the region of the porta hepatis. The vessels in the porta hepatis are then picked up in the parenchyma as they enter the liver. The parenchymal dissection is continued along anatomic planes, picking up vessels and ducts as they traverse the liver, until the hepatic venous structures are also picked up in the hepatic parenchyma. The operative time is significantly reduced by this technique, and the blood loss is only moderately increased. Trisegmentectomy necessitates anatomic dissection in order to avoid interrupting veins from the remaining segment.

TRANSPLANTATION

Since the first orthotopic liver transplant was performed, approximately 13 years ago, about 275 patients have undergone the procedure. Of these transplants, 40 percent were carried out by Starzl and his associates. His last report indicates an overall 1-year survival of 29 percent, and half of all the 1-year survivors are still alive. There are four 5-year survivors.

Favorable indications for liver transplantation include biliary atresia, chronic aggressive hepatitis, inborn errors of metabolism, and certain other benign hepatic diseases. Alcoholic cirrhosis is regarded as a less favorable indication, and primary hepatic malignancy is now considered a relative contraindication. It is interesting that the immunologic criteria for donor recipients are less rigid than those for renal transplant. Biliary reconstruction at present is the principal technical problem encountered with orthotopic transplantation.

Another approach to the problem is the use of heterotopic (auxillary) liver transplantation. Fortner et al. have recently reported on six heterotopic liver transplants—three in patients with congenital biliary atresia, one with idiopathic cholestasis syndrome, and two with postnecrotic liver cirrhosis. One patient is alive and well 4 years after transplantation.

PORTAL HYPERTENSION

Hypertension within the portal vein and its tributaries may accompany hepatic disease or disturbance in the anatomy of the extrahepatic vascular system. As a consequence of this elevated pressure or in association with it, congestion of collateral pathways is established and may be manifested by esophagogastric varices, ascites, hypersplenism, or encephalopathy.

ETIOLOGY. The etiologic factors implicated in portal hypertension are listed in Table 30-6. Increased hepatope-

Table 30-6. ETIOLOGY OF PORTAL HYPERTENSION

A. Increased hepatopetal flow without obstruction
　1. Hepatic arterial–portal venous fistula
　2. Splenic arteriovenous fistula
　3. Intrasplenic origin
B. Extrahepatic outflow obstruction
　1. Budd-Chiari syndrome
　2. Failure of right side of heart
C. Obstruction of extrahepatic portal venous system
　1. Congenital obstruction
　2. Cavernomatous transformation of portal vein
　3. Infection
　4. Trauma
　5. Extrinsic compression
D. Intrahepatic obstruction
　1. Nutritional cirrhosis
　2. Postnecrotic cirrhosis
　3. Biliary cirrhosis
　4. Other diseases with hepatic fibrosis
　　a. Hemochromatosis
　　b. Wilson's disease
　　c. Congenital hepatic fibrosis
　5. Infiltrative lesions
　6. Venoocclusive diseases
　　a. *Senecio* poisoning
　　b. Schistosomiasis

tal flow is an infrequent cause of portal hypertension. Hepatic arterial–portal venous fistula has been reported 10 times and the diagnosis established by aortography. Successful treatment has been effected by ligation of the hepatic artery or aneurysmorraphy. Splenic arteriovenous fistula is also a relatively uncommon lesion. This has a predilection for females between the ages of twenty and fifty and may become symptomatic during pregnancy. Calcification in the left upper quadrant is suggestive, and aortography may be diagnostic. Resection of the fistula is therapeutic. An increase in forward blood flow in the portal venous system has also been proposed as the cause of portal hypertension in patients with Boeck's sarcoid, Gaucher's disease, and myeloid metaplasia. The pathophysiology is related to an intrasplenic arteriovenous fistula. A small group of well-documented cases of bleeding esophageal varices with portal hypertension in the absence of demonstrable intrahepatic or extrahepatic obstruction may be related to a similar intrasplenic pathology. These include tropical splenomegaly and represent the rare circumstances in which splenectomy alone may be therapeutic.

Since the hepatic veins constitute the sole efferent vascular drainage of the liver, obstruction or increased pressure within these vessels or their radicles results in an increased sinusoidal and portal pressure. This outflow obstruction (Budd-Chiari) syndrome is most frequently associated with an endophlebitis of the hepatic veins, which may be isolated or part of a generalized thrombophlebitic process. A web in the suprahepatic vena cava has been reported to cause the syndrome in Japanese people. The clinical picture depends on the rapidity and degree of venous

obstruction. With sudden and complete obstruction, the presentation is that of an abdominal catastrophe with severe abdominal pain, nausea, vomiting, and rapid enlargement of the abdomen by ascites. This rarely occurs. More commonly, obstruction to the hepatic venous tract appears to be gradual and is associated with mild to moderate abdominal discomfort and ascites. The therapy is a side-to-side portal systemic anastomosis, since the portal vein must act as an efferent hepatic conduit.

Portal hypertension secondary to impaired flow in the extrahepatic portal venous system is unique in that the hypertension usually is not complicated by hepatocellular dysfunction. Congenital atresia or hypoplasia, as an extension of the obliterative process of the umbilical vein and ductus venosus, is rare. More commonly, there is a cavernomatous transformation of the portal vein which probably represents organization and recanalization of thrombi within the vessel. The most common etiologic factor in the development of extrahepatic portal venous obstruction

Fig. 30-14. *A.* Right thoracoabdominal incision with division of right leaf of diaphragm is used. Ligamentum teres is transected and used for traction. *B.* After ligamentous attachments have been divided, dissection of hepatoduodenal ligament and porta hepatis is carried out. Cystic artery is traced to its origin from right hepatic artery, which is then doubly ligated and transected, and finally portal vein is treated in similar fashion. *C.* Glisson's capsule is incised and the hepatic parenchyma divided, ligating individual vessels and ducts. *D.* Right lobe is rotated clockwise, and inferior vena cava and right hepatic vein are demonstrated. *E.* Exposure of inferior vena cava with ligation of right hepatic vein and middle hepatic vein. *F.* Denuded surface of liver is covered by flap of falciform ligament. (*From Seymour I. Schwartz, "Surgical Diseases of the Liver," McGraw-Hill Book Company, 1964.*)

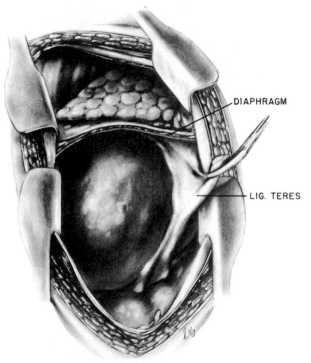

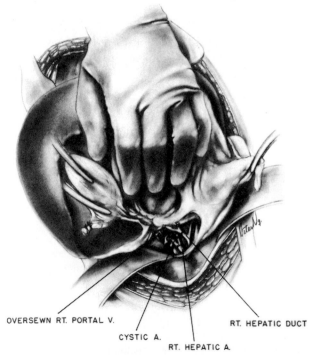

A

B

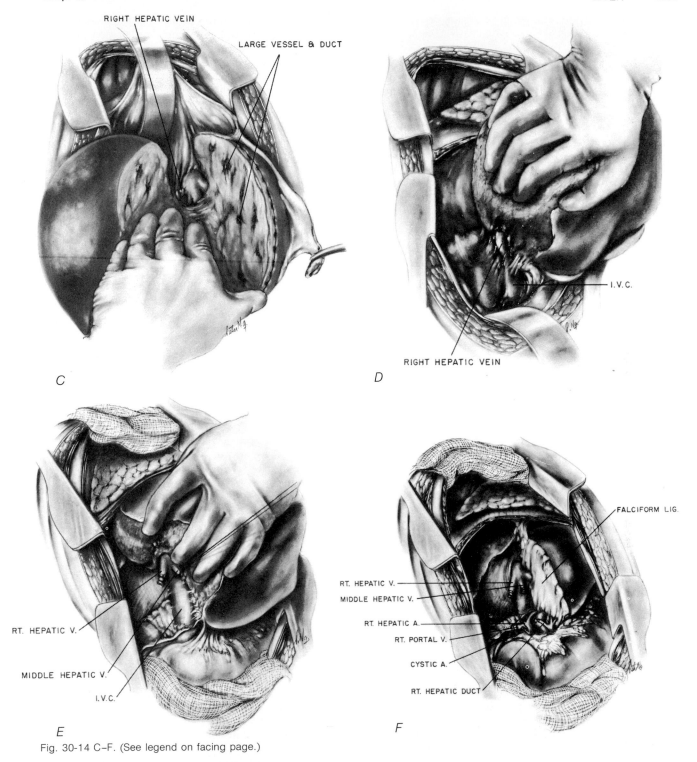

RIGHT HEPATIC VEIN

LARGE VESSEL & DUCT

C

RIGHT HEPATIC VEIN

I.V.C.

D

RT. HEPATIC V.

MIDDLE HEPATIC V.

I.V.C.

E

FALCIFORM LIG.

RT. HEPATIC V.

MIDDLE HEPATIC V.

RT. HEPATIC A.

RT. PORTAL V.

CYSTIC A.

RT. HEPATIC DUCT

F

Fig. 30-14 C–F. (See legend on facing page.)

in childhood may be some form of infection. Bacteria may be transmitted via a patent umbilical vein, but a history of neonatal omphalitis is rarely obtainable. Extrahepatic obstruction also may be secondary to trauma and extrinsic compression caused by adhesions, inflammatory processes, and tumors. Isolated splenic vein thrombosis, usually a consequence of alcoholic pancreatitis, may cause esophagogastric varices. In this case splenectomy cures the portal hypertension.

The overwhelming majority of cases of portal hypertension are related to an intrahepatic obstruction. This accounts for 90 percent of patients with portal hyper-

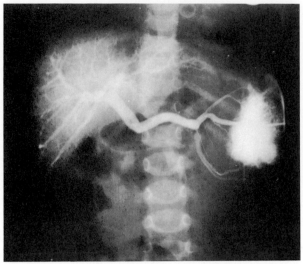

Fig. 30-15. Normal splenoportogram. Note site of injection in spleen and diffusion of radiopaque material through organ. Main splenic vein and two hilar veins are visualized. Portal vein, major branches, and intrahepatic arborization can be seen. No collateral veins are present. Note radiolucency at junction of splenic and superior mesenteric veins. (*From Seymour I. Schwartz, "Surgical Diseases of the Liver," McGraw-Hill Book Company, 1964.*)

Fig. 30-16. Splenoportogram: portal hypertension secondary to intrahepatic obstruction. Note large tortuous coronary vein and inferior mesenteric vein. Intrahepatic arborization is minimal. (*From Seymour I. Schwartz, "Surgical Diseases of the Liver," McGraw-Hill Book Company, 1964.*)

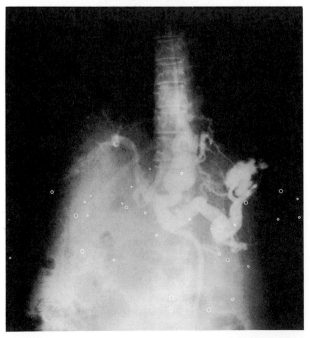

tension in most large series. A variety of hepatic diseases have been implicated, but no single explanation of pathogenesis has proved totally satisfactory. The implicated pathogenic factors include (1) hepatic fibrosis with compression of portal venules, (2) compression by regenerative nodules, (3) increased arterial blood flow, (4) fatty infiltration and acute inflammation, and (5) intrahepatic vascular obstruction. The hepatic diseases associated with portal hypertension include nutritional cirrhosis, postnecrotic cirrhosis, biliary cirrhosis, hemochromatosis, Wilson's disease, congenital hepatic fibrosis, and infiltrative lesions.

Nutritional cirrhosis is the most common and has a worldwide distribution. In the Western countries, it is frequently associated with chronic alcoholism. As is true with all intrahepatic lesions, with the exception of congenital hepatic fibrosis and schistosomiasis, the major resistance to the flow of portal blood is located on the hepatic venous side of the sinusoid (postsinusoidal). Postnecrotic cirrhosis accounts for 5 to 12 percent of the cases and represents progression of an acute viral hepatitis or toxic hepatic injury. Frequently a history of viral infection is not obtainable. Biliary cirrhosis may be due to extrahepatic obstruction and secondary cirrhosis or to a primary hepatic lesion. Advanced portal cirrhosis is an almost invariable feature of hemachromatosis. Wilson's disease (hepatolenticular degeneration) is characterized by alteration of hepatic function and structure and by mental deterioration. Congenital hepatic fibrosis is related to cystic disease of the liver. Clinical features include gross enlargement and firm consistency of the liver, accompanied by manifestations of portal hypertension. Hepatic function is not disturbed. As hepatic infestation with *Schistosoma mansoni* results in presinusoidal obstruction, there is no consequent impairment of hepatic function until late in the course of the disease.

PATHOPHYSIOLOGY. Portal hypertension refers to an elevated pressure within the portal venous system. This pressure reflects a dynamic, constantly fluctuating force. In addition to diurnal fluctuations, the pressure varies with changes of position, phases of respiration, and intraabdominal pressure. The normal portal pressure is less than 250 mm of water with a mean value of 215 mm of water. Portal pressure can be assessed by a variety of techniques. During an operative procedure, cannulation of an omental vein or the portal vein itself provides a direct recording. The pressure can also be determined by occlusive catheterization of a hepatic venule (OHVP). This procedure is analogous to determination of pulmonary capillary pressure, in that it is based on the assumption that the occluding catheter creates a static column of blood extending from the hepatic vein to the junction of the hepatic arterial and portal venous streams as they converge in the sinusoidal bed. The procedure is carried out by cardiac catheterization technique and is particularly valuable in the diagnosis of extrahepatic portal obstruction. In this situation, the presinusoidal obstruction is associated with a normal OHVP and an elevated splenic pulp pressure.

In all instances of portal hypertension, splenic pulp pressure is elevated. Intrasplenic pressure is essentially uniform throughout the pulp and is unrelated to the size of the organ. The pressure is usually 2 to 6 mm Hg higher than the pressure within the portal vein per se, a function of the direction of venous flow. Splenic pulp manometry is carried out under local anesthesia but is contraindicated in patients with a bleeding tendency or severe jaundice.

Splenoportography or the venous phase of celiac and superior mesenteric angiography defines the pathologic features of the portal circulation. The studies provide a demonstration of collateral veins, particularly esophagogastric varices. They also provide graphic demonstration of the site of obstruction, i.e., intrahepatic or extrahepatic. Under normal circumstances no collaterals are visualized and a good arborization is noted in the liver (Fig. 30-15). Whenever collaterals are apparent, the diagnosis of portal hypertension is suggested. Usually one can define the coronary vein contributing to esophageal varices by this technique (Fig. 30-16).

The umbilical vein also has been used to outline the portal system. In 80 percent of these cases the obliterated vein can be isolated and dilated to permit passage of a catheter and injection of radiopaque material into the left portal vein.

The injection of radioactive isotopes into the spleen with simultaneous external monitoring of the areas over the liver, right side of the heart, and esophagus have been used to define the dynamics of the portal circulation. The system employs the same equipment as that used for radioactive renography. Distinctive patterns for normal circulation, esophageal varices, portal vein thrombosis, and both natural and surgically created portal systemic shunts have been defined.

PATHOLOGIC ANATOMY. The collateral vessels (Fig. 30-17) which become functional in cases of portal hypertension are classified in two groups:

1. Hepatopetal circulation occurs only when the intrahepatic vasculature is normal and obstruction is limited to the portal vein. In this situation, the accessory veins of Sappey, the deep cystic veins, the epiploic veins, the hepatocolic and hepatorenal veins, the diaphragmatic veins, and the veins of the suspensory ligaments carry a limited amount of portal venous blood to the liver.
2. Hepatofugal flow is the type most commonly provided by the collateral circulation.

The vessels of the hepatofugal circulation include:

1. The coronary vein, which courses to the esophageal veins and thence to the azygos and hemiazygos veins with eventual termination in the superior vena cava.
2. The superior hemorrhoidal veins, which communicate by way of the hemorrhoidal plexus with hemorrhoidal branches of the middle and inferior hemorrhoidal veins and ultimately drain into the inferior vena cava.
3. The umbilical and paraumbilical veins, which communicate with superficial veins of the abdominal wall and anastomose freely with the superior and inferior epigastric veins. Dilatation occurs in 22 percent of patients with portal cirrhosis, and the advanced stage is known as the *caput Medusae*. The cephalad portion of the obliterated umbilical vein may remain patent in adult life or become recanalized, contributing to the Cruveilhier-Baumgarten syndrome.
4. Retroperitoneally, the veins of Retzius, which from an anastomo-

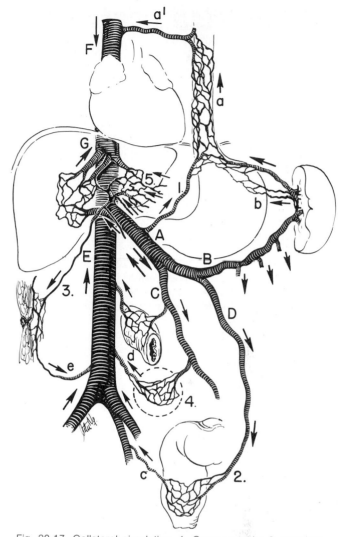

Fig. 30-17. Collateral circulation. 1, Coronary vein; 2, superior hemorrhoidal veins; 3, paraumbilical veins; 4, veins of Retzius; 5, veins of Sappey; A, portal vein; B, splenic vein; C, superior mesenteric vein; D, inferior mesenteric vein; E, inferior vena cava; F, superior vena cava; G, hepatic veins; a, esophageal veins; a¹, azygos system; b, vasa brevia; c, middle and inferior hemorrhoidal veins; d, intestinal; e, epigastric veins. (*From Seymour I. Schwartz, "Surgical Diseases of the Liver," McGraw-Hill Book Company, 1964.*)

sis between the mesenteric and peritoneal veins and empty directly into the inferior vena cava.

In general, the collateral circulation does not effectively decompress the portal system, and the amount of blood shunted is relatively insignificant. Assuming the cross-sectional diameter of the normal portal vein to be 2 cm, then, according to Poiseuille's law, over 4,000 collateral veins $\frac{1}{2}$ cm in diameter will be needed to provide equivalent flow. Collateral circulation in the veins of the portal system occurs in 97 percent of patients with elevated pressure, but this diversion does not produce any demonstrable alleviation of portal hypertension. On the contrary, the highest values of portal pressure are recorded in the group in which collateralization is more marked. In rare instances, spontaneous portal systemic shunts have effectively decompressed the portal system.

Esophagogastric Varices

As the veins become engorged, vessels in the submucosal plexus of the esophagus increase in size and become dilated. In the later stages, the overlying submucosa may disappear and the walls of the vein actually form a lining of the esophagus. The submucosal veins in the fundus and subfundal regions of the stomach also become varicose. Gastric varices occur predominantly in the cardiac end of the stomach but have also been found along the lesser curvature. Varices also have been demonstrated in the duodenum and ileum.

Although the presence of esophagogastric varices is, in itself, of minor consequence, rupture and bleeding from these vessels constitute the most alarming and serious complication of portal hypertension. The varices are almost always associated with portal hypertension but infrequently have occurred in patients with normal pressure. Ninety percent of adult patients demonstrate intrahepatic disease, whereas in childhood the varices are usually related to extrahepatic portal obstruction. Precipitation of the bleeding episode has been ascribed to two factors, increased pressure within the varix and ulceration secondary to esophagitis. Regurgitation of gastric juice into the esophagus has been implicated, and ulcers of the esophagus have been demonstrated in 25 percent of nonintubated and 50 percent of intubated patients. The frequency and severity of bleeding also is related to the degree of hepatic damage and ingestion of salicylates.

NATURAL COURSE. Bleeding is to be anticipated in approximately 30 percent of cirrhotic patients with demonstrable varices. The elapsed time from the diagnosis of varices to the first hemorrhage varies between 1 and 187 weeks. Almost all hemorrhages occur within 2 years of the initial observation. Survival of patients who have not bled at the time of discovery of varices is identical to the survival of the overall group of patients whose varices are discovered before death. Etiology is a prime consideration. Varices secondary to extrahepatic portal obstruction must be considered separately, since it is rare for these patients to die of hemorrhage. By contrast, the mortality risk of repeated hemorrhage in patients with esophageal varies secondary to cirrhosis is extremely high. Approximately 70 percent of these patients die within 1 year of the first hemorrhage. Sixty percent of cirrhotic patients who have hemorrhaged once rebleed massively within 1 year.

A prophylactic shunt is not advised for a patient with varices which have not bled, since one cannot predict which patients will bleed; the survival is not improved and encephalopathy may be induced.

ACUTE BLEEDING. In children, massive hematemesis almost always emanates from bleeding varices. Acute hemorrhage is usually the first manifestation of portal hypertension in children. Seventy percent of patients experience their first bleeding episode before the age of seven, and almost 90 percent hemorrhage before the age of ten.

In the adult, bleeding varices comprise one-quarter to one-third of the cases of massive upper gastrointestinal tract bleeding. In cirrhotic patients, varices are the source of bleeding in approximately 50 percent, whereas gastritis is implicated in 30 percent and duodenal ulcers in 9 percent. It is now felt that peptic ulcer does not occur more frequently in cirrhotic patients. Correlation of the lesion with the severity of bleeding reveals that in the majority of cases bleeding from varices is severe hemorrhage whereas bleeding from gastritis involves only mild to moderate blood loss.

Since the management of bleeding varices differs significantly from that of bleeding due to other causes, it is important to establish a diagnosis on an emergency basis. Physical examination may reveal the stigmata of cirrhosis. Splenomegaly is particularly suggestive of portal hypertension. Tests of hepatic function have been used but do not have uniform reliability. Abnormal BSP retention may be related to underlying liver disease or to shock from hemorrhage. A normal BSP value is more significant and in association with massive bleeding suggests that the liver is not responsible. The qualitative test for hyperammonemia is rarely performed, and pretreatment with antibiotics, glutamic acid, and arginine will negate the value of this test. The presence of any large portal-systemic collateral vessel will result in a positive test. Barium-swallow has a significantly high percentage of false-negative results. In a series of patients with proved varices, roentgenographic demonstration was present in only half. Selective angiography is replacing upper gastrointestinal series as a primary diagnostic procedure. Celiac angiography will rule out an arterial bleeding site, and the venous phase of the superior mesenteric arteriogram will demonstrate collateral venous circulation. Bleeding from a varix is not visualized. A 90 percent correlation has been reported for splenic pulp manometry, but there is a zone of splenic pulp pressures which may be characteristic of patients bleeding from varices or from other causes. The isotopic evaluation of the portal circulation has been applied with success to the differential diagnosis of acutely bleeding varices. Esophageal balloon tamponade has also been used as a diagnostic measure. However, varices are controlled in only two-thirds of the patients, and, moreover, peptic ulcer may stop bleeding after the gastric balloon is inflated. Esophagoscopy represents the single most reliable technique, since it alone defines the bleeding point. On the other hand, esophagoscopy may fail to reveal varices because of variations in transvariceal blood flow. In addition, there is a significant observer variation in the endoscopic evaluation of varices.

TREATMENT. The therapeutic regimen is directed at promptly controlling bleeding without further disturbing an already impaired hepatic function. Rapid control is critical in order to avoid the injurious effects of shock on hepatic function and also the toxic effects of absorption of blood from the gastrointestinal tract. The therapeutic approaches may be divided into methods which directly approach the bleeding site and techniques which act indirectly by decreasing portal pressure (Table 30-7).

Table 30-7. CONTROL OF ACUTE BLEEDING

A. Nonoperative
  1. Direct: control of bleeding site
    a. Tamponade
    b. Local hypothermia
    c. Esophagoscopic injection of sclerosing solution
    d. Transhepatic sclerosis of coronary vein
  2. Indirect: reduction of portal pressure
    a. Vasopressin
    b. Arfonad
    c. Paracentesis
B. Operative
  1. Direct: control of bleeding site
    a. Transesophageal ligation
    b. Esophageal transection
    c. Gastroesophageal resection: colon or jejunum interposition
  2. Indirect: reduction of portal pressure
    a. Portal-systemic shunt
    b. Drainage of thoracic duct ⎫
    c. Hepatic artery ligation   ⎬ No longer advised
    d. Splenectomy   ⎭

Balloon tamponade has been the most popular nonoperative method, and the Sengstaken-Blakemore tube has been used most frequently. This technique has reduced the mortality and morbidity from bleeding varices in good-risk patients, particularly those in whom the varices were secondary to extrahepatic portal hypertension or compensated cirrhosis. Little change has been noted in the mortality rate for poor-risk patients, and reports have indicated failure to control hemorrhage in 25 to 55 percent of cases. Increasing awareness of the complications associated with this technique, including aspiration, asphyxiation, and ulceration at the site of the tamponade, has reduced its use.

Hypothermia has been used, either in combination with tamponade or alone, to produce local vasoconstriction and thus control bleeding. Both general hypothermia and local gastric hypothermia have been employed. A special balloon with a long esophageal neck, which permits cooling of the distal half of the esophagus and the upper gastric fundus, has been devised for more effective application. Generalized hypothermia is ineffective, since it does not reduce hepatic flow until the core temperature drops below 35°C. Endoscopic injection of a sclerosing solution into varices has also successfully controlled bleeding. In a large series, bleeding was controlled in 93 percent of patients. Recently, transhepatic catheterization and obliteration of the coronary vein using thrombin, sclerosing solution, or microspheres have been applied to the control of bleeding.

Drug therapy to reduce portal hypertension has employed surgical vasopressin, which acts by constricting the splanchnic arterial circulation and consequently reducing portal pressure and flow by approximately 40 percent. The drug is contraindicated in patients with angina, since generalized vasoconstriction results. Effective control has accompanied direct infusion of vasopressin, 0.2 unit/ml/minute, into the superior mesenteric artery. Equal efficacy has been achieved with the same dosage administered into a peripheral vein. Isoproterenol may be given to reduce the hemodynamic hazards of vasopressin related to its potential effect on the cardiac output. Arfonad also has been used to induce a predictable decrease in portal hypertension by establishing a generalized arterial hypotension. Paracentesis in a patient with bleeding varices and tense ascites will immediately and significantly reduce portal pressure.

Surgical therapy includes transesophageal ligation, gastric resection, cannulation of the thoracic duct, and emergency portacaval shunt. The results of transesophageal ligation have not been uniformly encouraging, and in cirrhotic patients the procedure has been accompanied by a high incidence of recurrent bleeding. Other methods directed at the site of bleeding have been concerned with interrupting the blood supply of the esophagus by extensive gastroesophageal resection. Cannulation with drainage of the thoracic duct has also been applied as a method of reducing portal hypertension and controlling bleeding from the varices, but these effects have been inconsistent. Reduction of portal pressure by transumbilical decompression using an extracorporeal shunt has been applied with rare instances of success.

A more liberal use of emergency portacaval shunts to stop bleeding has been advised for the cirrhotic patients whose bleeding cannot be controlled by tamponade or vasopressin. The base figure which serves as a frame of reference for comparison is the mortality for patients with bleeding varices not subjected to emergency portacaval shunts, and this ranges between 66 and 73 percent. There is little question that an effective portal-systemic decompressive procedure almost always stops bleeding. A review of reported experiences indicates that so-called emergency shunts are associated with survival for immediate hospitalization in 50 to 71 percent of cases, despite a more liberal attitude toward acceptability of patients in reference to their liver profile. Orloff and his associates have reported an operative survival of 48 percent and an actuarial 7-year survival of 42 percent in consecutive, unselected patients with alcoholic cirrhosis and bleeding varices operated on within 8 hours of admission to hospital. In regard to selection of patients, reported results could not be correlated with the patient's liver function profile in some series. No significance could be attributed to the presence or absence of jaundice, but ascites, when present, was associated with a marked reduction of survival rate.

It is the author's personal opinion that in the absence of controlled and randomized trials an emergency portacaval shunt should be performed in selected patients, since it offers greater survival than a more conservative form of therapy. There has been a gradual liberalization of criteria for selection of patients, and there is an obvious advantage in the logistics of managing patients in reference to depletion of blood banks.

In the pediatric age group, despite the fact that the bleeding is often alarming, spontaneous cessation almost always occurs, and esophageal tamponade or vasopressin is rarely necessary. Hospitalization, bed rest, blood replacement, and sedation almost always suffice for patients with bleeding secondary to extrahepatic portal obstruction.

The majority of patients with acute bleeding varices are not in shock at the time of admission to the hospital, although the hematocrit is often reduced and blood replacement may be necessary. Fresh blood should be employed for transfusing cirrhotic patients. This provides the clotting factors which are frequently diminished in the presence of hepatic disease and avoids the increased ammonia content and diminished platelet and prothrombin supply characteristic of old bank blood. There is a linearly progressive daily increment of 35 $\mu g/100$ ml of ammonia nitrogen in banked blood, which can be responsible for exogenous hepatic coma. Therapy directed at preventing hyperammonemia and hepatic coma consists primarily of removing blood from the gastrointestinal tract. Catharsis, gastric lavage, and enemas are employed. If vasopressin has been administered, it will induce intestinal motility and effect a catharsis. A reduction in intestinal bacterial flora also contributes to the prevention of coma, and nonabsorbable antibiotic therapy is used to accomplish this.

Protocol for Acute Bleeding Episodes. *Treatment of Shock.* Intravenous administration of 10% dextrose in water and fresh blood are begun immediately.

Nursing Care. Special nursing care is advisable, particularly if balloon tamponade is employed. Repeated endotracheal suction is indicated, and tracheostomy may be necessary.

Control of Hemorrhage. A soft nasogastric tube is inserted into the stomach, or if the patient is in incipient or established coma or uncooperative, a gastrostomy tube is inserted under local anesthesia. Suction is established to monitor the extent of bleeding while the stomach is lavaged with iced saline solution. Vasopressin is administered via either the superior mesenteric artery or a peripheral vein. If bleeding is not controlled by these measures, balloon tamponade is applied. A conservative, nonsurgical regimen is relied upon to control bleeding in patients with a serum bilirubin level above 3 mg/100 ml, a serum albumin level below 2.5 Gm/100 ml, and a prothrombin time reduced to less than 30 percent of normal. Patients with minimally impaired liver function or portal hypertension secondary to extrahepatic obstruction who continue to bleed should be prepared for surgical intervention, and a portacaval shunt is performed as an emergency procedure.

Control of Hepatic Coma. Intestinal catharsis is accomplished by vasopressin or 15 ml of magnesium sulfate instilled via the nasogastric tube. Tap-water enemas are administered twice daily. Neomycin sulfate, 1 Gm every hour for 4 hours followed by 1 Gm every 4 hours, is administered via the nasogastric tube. Analgesics and hypnotics, which are detoxified by the liver, are avoided.

Diet. A diet high in carbohydrates and low in fat and protein with vitamin supplements, including vitamin K, is used. Atropine and antacids are administered to reduce gastric acidity.

Elective Surgical Treatment for Prevention of Recurrent Hemorrhage. The case for surgical intervention is based on the precept that a patient who has bled from esophageal varices is likely to rebleed and that subsequent bleeding episodes are associated with a higher mortality than an elective operative procedure. It is important to define the role of surgical procedure in relation to the factors implicated in the cause of portal hypertension.

A difference of opinion exists regarding the role of decompressive procedures in children with portal hypertension due to extrahepatic portal venous thrombosis. Some children can be treated satisfactorily and safely without operation despite repeated episodes of variceal bleeding. The results of operation in terms of survival are significantly more encouraging in this population than in adults. Therefore, most series have suggested an aggressive approach in children with recurrent bleeding episodes. The central splenorenal shunt or an anastomosis between the inferior vena cava and superior mesenteric vein is applicable to this group of patients. The incidence of postoperative encephalopathy has been negligible.

Presinusoidal obstruction (hepatic fibrosis, extrahepatic portal venous thrombosis, schistosomiasis) is characterized by portal hypertension and may be associated with normal hepatic function. In patients with hepatic fibrosis and extrahepatic portal venous obstruction the results are gratifying; the surgical procedure will generally prevent subsequent bleeding and provide the patient with an essentially normal life expectancy. The patients with schistosomiasis are a unique group in that they are extremely liable to postshunt encephalopathy.

Postsinusoidal portal hypertension is invariably complicated by impaired hepatic function. The role of decompressive procedures is least well defined for this group of cirrhotic patients. Elective procedure should be considered when the presence of an active intrahepatic process such as hyaline necrosis or acute fatty infiltration has been ruled out. Ascites which fails to respond to medical therapy, a prothrombin time which remains prolonged following parenteral administration of vitamin K, a serum bilirubin above 3 mg/100 ml, a BSP retention greater than 20 percent, and a serum albumin level less than 2.5 Gm/100 ml are all associated with a poor postoperative prognosis. In these patients there is immediate deterioration following portacaval shunting, but this is actually no greater than after other operations of comparable severity. Child's criteria and other assessments of hepatic function are not completely predictive.

Two randomized series have been reported. The Cooperative Study of the Veterans Administration randomized cirrhotic patients who had at least one major gastrointestinal hemorrhage and were considered suitable for an operative procedure. Increased survival rate was noted in the group of patients who were operated upon. By contrast, the Boston Interhospital Liver Group's study of patients on whom a therapeutic portacaval shunt had been performed showed that recurrent variceal bleeding could be prevented but that greater longevity could not be expected for these patients. Increased survival following shunting procedures in patients with a single major variceal hemorrhage remained a statistical possibility. Recently it has been shown that better results are to be anticipated in patients with biliary cirrhosis than in those with nutritional, alcoholic, or cryptogenic cirrhosis.

Ascites

ETIOLOGY. The mechanisms contributing to the formation of ascites are complex and incompletely understood.

Portal hypertension is regarded as a contributory but minor factor, since there is no correlation between the degree of portal hypertension and the extent of ascites. Ascites is not a usual accompaniment of extrahepatic portal venous obstruction but has been noted occasionally. Impairment of hepatic venous outflow with subsequent congestion of the liver is the experimental method most consistently used to produce ascites. This lesion is accompanied by an increase in the size of lymphatic vessels and increased production of hepatic lymph which extravasates through the capsule of the liver into the peritoneal cavity. In clinical cirrhosis, there is an increase in the size of hepatic channels and an augmented flow of thoracic duct lymph. Two distinct patterns of intrahepatic vasculature have been correlated with the presence or absence of ascites. With irreversible ascites, there is an absolute decrease in the hepatic venous bed and a concomitant increase in both the portal venous and hepatic arterial beds. By contrast, when cirrhosis is unaccompanied by ascites, there is a deficit in all vascular systems. Obstruction of the hepatic venous outflow fails to explain the development of ascites in patients with portal vein obstruction and also the relief of ascites following end-to-side portacaval shunt.

Reduced serum osmotic pressure related to hypoalbuminemia does exert some influence. However, the response of patients to albumin infusion is variable, and the reduced osmotic pressure may represent the result rather than the cause of fluid accumulation. The most profound biochemical change which accompanies the formation of ascites is the retention of sodium and water. There is evidence that the adrenal cortical hormone is a factor in the renal retention of sodium, and higher concentrations of antidiuretic substances have been noted in the urine of patients with cirrhosis and ascites.

TREATMENT. Bed rest is prescribed, since it reduces the functional demand on the liver. A diet high in calories with an excess of carbohydrates and proteins, supplemented by vitamins, is directed toward improving hepatic function, while low sodium (10 to 20 mEq daily) intake is essential. Fluid is usually not restricted, and potassium supplements are routinely provided to treat the potassium depletion which accompanies the formation of ascites. A negative sodium balance may be achieved by the use of ion-exchange resins. The administration of salt-poor albumin is directed at raising colloidal pressure. This may be provided by an intravenous infusion of antogenous ascitic fluid.

Chlorothiazide is usually used to initiate diuretic therapy, and approximately two-thirds of patients will respond to this medication. Potassium supplements are required, because the diuresis is accompanied by depletion. For patients refractory to chlorothiazide the aldosterone antagonists are employed, while for those patients with incipient or frank hepatic coma mercury diuretics are considered safer. Abdominal paracentesis as an initial procedure has diagnostic value, but repeated procedures are contraindicated, since they deplete the body of protein and contribute to the development of systemic hyponatremia. Furosemide (Lasix) and ethacrynic acid are recently introduced powerful diuretics.

Emphasis on the importance of obstruction of hepatic venous outflow led to the proposal of side-to-side portacaval shunts as a method of therapy. These procedures were based on the hypothesis of providing a second outflow tract with the portal vein acting as a hepatofugal conduit. At present, the operation is limited to those patients who cannot be managed on a strict low-sodium diet and diuretic therapy, an unusual circumstance. A variety of procedures has been proposed to augment internal drainage of the ascitic fluid. These include omentopexy, drainage into the subcutaneous tissue, drainage directly into the venous system, and ileoentectropy. None has been effective. Drainage of the lymph from the cannulated cervical thoracic duct also reduces the ascites, which reappears as soon as the drainage ceases. Bilateral adrenalectomy combined with sodium restriction has enjoyed some success. Recently Leveen and associates have reported success with a peritoneal-venous shunt which employs a one-way valve.

Umbilical herniorraphy in a cirrhotic patient with marked ascites presents a significant risk, with hazards of leakage of ascitic fluid, infection, necrosis of the abdominal wall, and variceal bleeding due to interruption of collateral veins.

Hypersplenism

Splenomegaly, with engorgement of the vascular spaces, frequently accompanies portal hypertension. There is little correlation between the size of the spleen and the degree of hypertension. When hematologic abnormalities occur, they have been related to sequestration and destruction of the circulating cells by immune mechanisms mediated by the enlarged spleen or secretion by the hyperactive spleen of a substance which inhibits bone marrow activity. The patient may demonstrate reduction of any or all of the cellular elements of blood. The usual criteria are a white blood cell count below 4,000 and a platelet count below $100,000/mm^3$. Schistosomal fibrosis frequently induces hypersplenism, which is best determined by the size of the spleen. No correlation exists between the degree of anemia or leukopenia and the 5-year survival rate in patients. Decompression of the portal venous system is rarely indicated for treatment of hypersplenism alone. Significant hypersplenism in a patient undergoing elective surgical treatment for bleeding varices favors a splenorenal anastomosis, but portacaval anastomosis has been accompanied by reduction of the spleen and correction of the hypersplenism in about two-thirds of the cases.

Hepatic Coma

The development of neuropsychiatric symptoms and signs is related to natural and surgically created portal-systemic shunts and is identified by the term *portal-systemic encephalopathy*. This rarely occurs in patients with obstruction of the extrahepatic portal venous system. The neuropsychiatric syndrome usually is associated with cirrhosis and occurs in patients with marked hepatic dysfunction. Hepatic coma or precoma is a clinical manifesta-

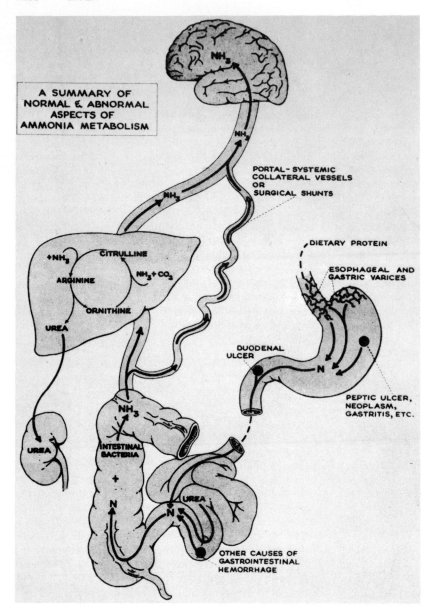

A SUMMARY OF NORMAL & ABNORMAL ASPECTS OF AMMONIA METABOLISM

Fig. 30-18. A summary of normal and abnormal aspects of ammonia metabolism. Dietary protein is the normal primary source of intestinal nitrogen. However, when gastrointestinal bleeding occurs, the blood that accumulates within the intestine may become an important source of intestinal nitrogen. Urea, which is excreted in part into the gastrointestinal tract, also adds to the intestinal nitrogen pool. All these nitrogen-containing compounds are converted into ammonia by the numerous bacteria within the colon. This ammonia is absorbed into the portal circulation and, under normal conditions, is rapidly removed in the liver by the formation of urea, which is excreted by the kidneys. This mechanism of detoxification of ammonia is so efficient that little or no ammonia can be found in the peripheral blood. Because of the important role of the liver in the detoxification of ammonia, (1) a decrease in hepatic function or (2) a bypass of the liver associated with (a) the development of portal systemic collaterals or (b) surgical shunting procedures will result in an increase in concentrations of ammonia in the peripheral blood, which will exert its toxic effects on the central nervous system. (*From Najarian et al., Am J Surg, 96:172, 1958.*)

tion in approximately two-thirds of patients with varices and is most prominent in cirrhotic patients who bleed. Coma and exsanguination are responsible for an almost equal percentage of deaths in cirrhotic patients with gastrointestinal varices. Operative procedures which decompress the portal system have also been associated with varying incidences of encephalopathy. With splenorenal anastomoses, the syndrome is demonstrated in 5 to 19 percent, while it has been reported in 11 to 38 percent following a portacaval anastomosis. The Warren distal splenorenal shunt has been associated with a negligible incidence of postoperative coma.

Hepatic coma has been related to hyperammonemia and ammonia intoxication (Fig. 30-18). Both exogenous and endogenous sources contribute to the blood ammonia level. Dietary protein is the usual source of intestinal am-

monia. In patients who bleed, blood within the intestinal tract is also converted into ammonia by bacteria. In the patient with hepatic disease, the ammonia formed within the intestine is carried to the liver but because of hepatic dysfunction cannot enter the Krebs-Henseleit (ornithine-citrulline-arginine) cycle. Endogenous urea produced within the gastrointestinal tract also represents an important source of ammonia, and gastric ammonia production from urea is a significant factor in patients with azotemia and cirrhosis. Galambos and associates have reported a randomized trial in which there was less deterioration of maximum urea synthesis following a selective splenorenal shunt than after total shunts.

In the cirrhotic patient with portal hypertension, the two factors implicated in the disturbed ammonia metabolism are impairment of hepatocellular function and portal-systemic collateralization. The blood ammonia level is raised by (1) ingested protein, (2) gastrointestinal bleeding, (3) increased ammonia production by the kidneys, and (4) increased ammonia production by muscles which are actively contracting during delirium tremens. The problem of an increased load is compounded by deficiencies in the removal mechanism caused by portal-systemic shunts which bypass the liver and hepatocellular disease which interferes with the functional activity of the liver. The neuropsychiatric manifestations involve the state of consciousness, motor activity, and deep tendon reflexes. These have been divided into three stages, delirium, stupor, and coma. In the early stages there is mental confusion and exaggerated reflexes. The characteristic "liver flap" may be elicited. In the second stage, there is an accentuation of muscular hypertonicity, to the extent of rigidity, and in the final stage there is complete flaccidity. The electroencephalogram is a sensitive indicator of portal-systemic encephalopathy, and the changes antedate clinical manifestations. Blood ammonia level does not define precisely the nature of material measured by standard tests. In patients with hepatic coma, the concentration of ammonia in the blood has correlated well with the clinical progress in over 90 percent of the cases. An elevated level, over 125 μg/100 ml, is usually associated with the clinical features of hepatic coma. Treatment with antibiotics negate the value of the test.

TREATMENT. Treatment is directed at (1) reducing nitrogenous material within the intestinal tract, (2) reducing the production of ammonia from this nitrogenous material, and (3) increasing ammonia metabolism. Since ammonia is an end product of protein metabolism, dietary protein must be drastically reduced to 50 Gm daily or less. Glucose is included in the diet, since it inhibits ammonia production by bacteria. Gastrointestinal hemorrhage frequently precipitates portal-systemic encephalopathy with blood acting as a source of ammonia. Therefore, a major factor in the prophylaxis of hepatic coma is prompt control of active bleeding. Potassium supplements are administered, particularly in patients who are receiving thiazide diuretics, since the rise in blood ammonia which accompanies diuresis has been related to hypokalemia.

The protein substrate on which bacteria can act may be initially reduced by using cathartics and enemas to purge the gastrointestinal tract. If active bleeding has occurred, infused vasopressin plays a dual role in temporarily stopping the bleeding as well as stimulating motility and evacuation of the intestine. Bacteria within the bowel are reduced by administering nonabsorbable antibiotics such as neomycin or kanamycin. In the presence of renal disease, kanamycin is preferred since there is less associated renal toxicity. For patients with severe renal impairment, chlortetracycline is more appropriate since it is not excreted primarily by the kidneys. Lactulose acts as a mild cathartic, and the products of its oxidation by bacteria include lactic and acetic acids, which lower the colonic pH and interfere with ammonia transfer across colonic mucosa. This drug has produced encouraging results in the treatment of hepatic encephalopathy.

Since the colon is the site of most ammonia absorption into the portal circulation, partial colectomy has been suggested as treatment of intractable encephalopathy. Resnick and associates studied a matched group of patients, randomly selecting half the group for colon bypass. The longevity figures for the two groups were identical, and the dietary protein tolerance and encephalopathy control only slightly favored the bypass group.

The possibility of stimulating the liver's intrinsic mechanism for detoxifying ammonia has fostered the use of glutamic acid and arginine. Although success has been reported, most studies have not been impressive. Recently, the pathophysiology of hepatic failure has been related to the accumulation of false neurochemical transmitters in the presynaptic storage sites of the peripheral and central adrenergic nervous system. L-Dopa, which represents normal precursor material in the central nervous system, is administered to permit restoration of central nervous system stores of norepinephrine and dopamine. An awakening effect of L-Dopa has been reported by Parkes and associates and by Fischer and James, but recent series have not been encouraging.

Attempts to dilute or remove toxic substances from the bloodstream will be discussed in the section on acute fulminant hepatic failure.

Surgery of Portal Hypertension

The surgical therapy of portal hypertension may be divided into two major categories: (1) procedures which directly attack a manifestation of portal hypertension, such as bleeding varices or ascites, and (2) procedures aimed at decreasing the portal hypertension and/or portal venous flow (Table 30-8).

TRANSESOPHAGEAL LIGATION OF VARICES. Using either a transthoracic or transabdominal approach, transesophageal ligation of varices and esophageal transection have been directed at controlling bleeding varices. The procedures do provide temporary control, particularly in children with extrahepatic portal block who are too small to be considered for splenorenal anastomosis. However, control is not prolonged. In patients without cirrhosis, recurrent bleeding has been reported in 28 percent, while among the cirrhotic group approximately 50 percent of survivors have recurrent bleeding. The operative mortality rate associated with this procedure is 43 percent, but it must be appreciated that the technique generally is applied to the poorest-risk patients.

Technique. Transthoracic ligation (Fig. 30-19) is performed through the eighth left intercostal space. The lower esophagus is freed, but the esophageal hiatus of the diaphragm is not disturbed. An umbilical tape is tightened around the esophagus just above the hiatus in order to minimize bleeding. A 7-cm longitudinal incision is made through all layers, and three tortuous columns of veins, coursing longitudinally and communicating with one another, are obliterated with continuous locking sutures of 3-0 chromic catgut. The esophagotomy is closed in two layers with interrupted silk sutures and the edges of the defect in the mediastinal pleura are reapproximated. Direct ligation of varices can be performed transabdominally.

Table 30-8. OPERATIVE PROCEDURES

I. Control of manifestation
   A. Bleeding varices
     1. Ligation of varices
       a. Transthoracic
       b. Transabdominal
     2. Transection procedures
       a. Gastric
       b. Esophageal
     3. Resection of varix-bearing area–esophagogastrectomy
       a. Roux en Y
       b. Jejunal interposition
       c. Colonic interposition
       d. Reversed gastric tube
   B. Ascites
     1. Crosby-Cooney button: subcutaneous drainage
     2. Ileoentectropy
     3. Peritoneal cavity–venous shunt
     4. Drainage of thoracic duct
     5. Adrenalectomy
II. Reduction of portal pressure and flow
   1. Splenectomy
   2. Hepatic and splenic arterial ligation
   3. Omentopexy
   4. Mediastinal packing
   5. Supradiaphragmatic transposition of spleen
   6. Portacaval shunt
     a. End-to-side
       (1) End-to-side shunt with arterialization of the portal
           vein stump
     b. Side-to-side
     c. Double end-to-side
   7. Splenorenal shunt
     a. End-to-end
     b. End-to-side
     c. Distal (selective)
   8. Superior mesenteric–inferior vena cava shunt

TOTAL OR NEAR-TOTAL GASTRECTOMY. This has been proposed in order to interrupt communication between the portal and esophageal veins and to remove the acid-peptic factor implicated in the initiation of bleeding from varices. To reduce the incidence of postoperative esophagitis, a variety of interposition procedures have been employed (Fig. 30-20). In the pediatric age group, esophagogastrectomy with colon interposition has successfully prevented recurrence of bleeding.

PROCEDURES FOR REDUCTION OF PORTAL PRESSURE. The operations directed at portal hypertension are based on the consideration that any reduction in portal pressure should decrease the potential for bleeding from varices. Splenectomy and hepatic arterial ligation have been offered as methods of reducing portal venous flow, but such an effect has not been documented. Splenectomy alone, unaccompanied by a concomitant splenorenal anastomosis, is now disapproved. Similarly, hepatic and splenic arterial ligation no longer enjoys a popularity. Reduction of portal pressure by diffuse shunts between a high-pressure portal venous system and low-pressure systemic circulation has also been attempted. These procedures include omentopexy, posterior mediastinal packing, and transposition of the spleen into the thoracic cavity. Encouraging results have been reported for the last procedure, but application of Poiseuille's law would suggest that

any diffuse shunting would be less effective than a major portal systemic shunt.

Functionally, portal-systemic shunts have been categorized as either totally or partially diverting portal venous flow away from the liver and also as decompressing or failing to decompress intrahepatic venous hypertension (Fig. 30-21). The end-to-side portacaval shunt prevents blood from reaching the liver by providing complete drainage of the splanchnic venous circulation to the vena cava. Controversy exists over whether this shunt deprives the liver of an important source of blood, and the associated alteration of hepatic blood flow is extremely variable, ranging from an increase of 34 percent to a decrease of 53 percent. This shunt also prevents the portal vein from serving as an efferent conduit from the liver. However, it has been shown that following the end-to-side shunt, the wedged hepatic vein pressure declined in all of a small series of patients. Proponents of the end-to-side shunt have indicated this as the best method of preventing recurrent bleeding from varices, since it most completely decompresses the portal venous system's splanchnic circulation. In refutation, it has been shown that end-to-side and side-to-side portacaval shunts demonstrate equal portal flow increases and equivalent reductions of portal pressure.

The concept that the side-to-side portacaval shunt provides the liver with portal venous flow is erroneous in most circumstances. Injection of radioisotope into the distal portal vein results in minimal recovery in the portal vein cephalad to a side-to-side anastomosis. Accumulated evidence indicates that the side-to-side portacaval shunt converts the cephalad portion of the portal vein to an outflow tract from the liver. Whether decompression of sinusoidal hypertension is greater with the side-to-side shunt than with the end-to-side shunt has not been defined. There is also concern whether the portal vein is beneficial or harmful as an efferent conduit, because of a possible siphon effect which may reduce the blood available to the hepatic cell.

The classic end-to-side splenorenal shunt using the central end of the splenic vein also prevents the flow of portal venous blood to the liver if it adequately performs its prescribed function of decompressing esophagogastric varices. In addition, the splenorenal shunt less completely decompresses portal venous hypertension. The other functional side-to-side shunts, including the end-to-side inferior vena cava–superior mesenteric shunt and the interposition of an H graft between these vessels, do not permit significant portal venous flow to enter the liver. This would be expected hemodynamically, since the flow within the cephalad portion of the portal vein should be away from high-pressure hepatic venous sinusoids into the low-pressure inferior vena cava if the functioning shunt is adequately decompressing esophagogastric varices.

The distal splenorenal shunt proposed by Warren and associates is the one procedure which can be classified as truly selective, because it decompresses esophagogastric varices while maintaining portal hypertension within the portal veins and hepatic sinusoids. Portal perfusion has been demonstrated in over 90 percent of patients with selective distal splenorenal shunts; the total hepatic blood

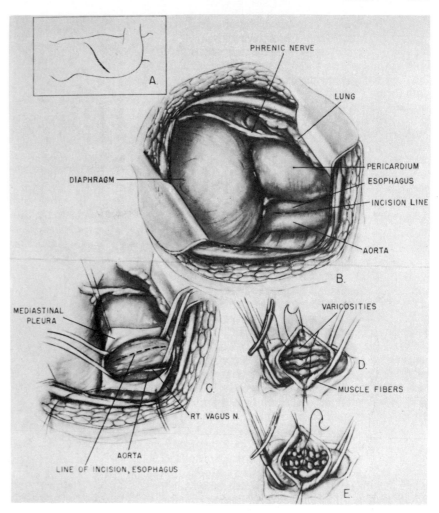

Fig. 30-19. Transthoracic transesophageal ligation. *A.* Left eighth intercostal space incision. Patient in right lateral decubitus position. *B.* Pulmonary ligament has been divided to permit retraction of lung, and line of incision in mediastinal pleura is outlined. *C.* Mediastinal pleura is incised, esophagus is mobilized, and line of incision in esophagus is outlined. *D.* Umbilical tape is tightened around esophagus just above hiatus to minimize bleeding, and edges of esophageal incision are retracted by stay sutures. *E.* The tortuous columns of esophageal veins are obliterated with continuous locked suture of 3-0 chromic catgut swaged on an atraumatic needle. (*From Seymour I. Schwartz, "Surgical Diseases of the Liver," McGraw-Hill Book Company, 1964.*)

flow has been shown to be unchanged, while the splenic venous circulation and esophagogastric veins have been reasonably decompressed.

Selection of Procedure. To date, selection of a surgical decompressive procedure has not been based on statistically valid data. Before performing a major shunt, the presence of portal hypertension should be defined manometrically, and a splenoportogram or a selective superior mesenteric arteriogram with a venous phase should be obtained to determine the status of the major veins. Portal vein thrombosis occurs as a complication in approximately 2 percent of the patients with portal cirrhosis. But lack of visualization of the portal vein in and of itself does not establish this diagnosis, and collateral veins of Sappey must be visualized. In order to obviate increasing hepatic dysfunction and portal-systemic encephalopathy, comparison with preoperative estimations of hepatic blood flow has been applied, but the estimations are fraught with errors in interpretation, particularly in cirrhotic patients. In reference to the role of blood flow and pressure determinations as factors in selection of the type of shunt, data can be offered to substantiate almost any argument. Large series have shown that pressure determinations and differentials within the portal venous system, measurements of the

estimated hepatic blood flow, and splenoportographic findings did not approximate true flow and these findings could not be related to the subsequent development of postshunt encephalopathy. Concerning the expressed advantage of side-to-side shunts for a cirrhotic patient in whom there is spontaneous reversal of flow in the portal vein, actual measurement in 273 cirrhotics showed no instance of spontaneous reversal. Recently, one factor, the increase in hepatic arterial flow subsequent to the creation of a portacaval shunt, has offered a hemodynamic correlate with the patient's prognosis.

The end-to-side portacaval shunt is the procedure most commonly performed, since it is technically easiest and has been associated with the lowest incidence of thrombosis. The presence of a large caudate lobe is less compromising to this procedure than to a side-to-side shunt. Rarely, a large caudate lobe encroaches upon the inferior vena cava and causes caval hypertension, which precludes any portal-systemic decompressive procedure. Therefore, the workup of the cirrhotic patient should include determination of infrahepatic caval pressure. For some patients with extensive adhesions from previous operative procedures in the right upper quadrant, the splenorenal and mesocaval shunts are preferred. Thrombosis with or without recanali-

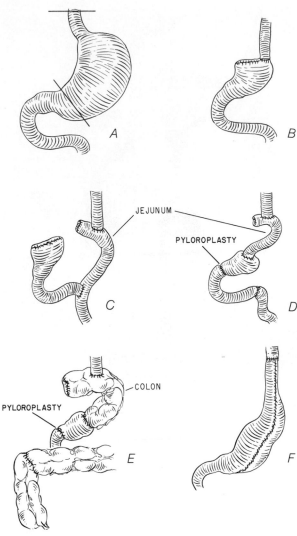

Fig. 30-20. Resection of varix-bearing area with or without inter-position. *A.* and *B.* Total or near-total gastrectomy with excision of distal third of esophagus. *C.* Roux en Y isoperistaltic esopha-gojejunostomy. *D.* Interposition of isoperistaltic isolated segment of jejunum. *E.* Interposition of segment of colon. *F.* Reversed gastric tube. (*From Seymour I. Schwartz, "Surgical Diseases of the Liver," McGraw-Hill Book Company, 1964.*)

zation of the portal vein (cavernomatous transformation) generally precludes a portacaval anastomosis. The Budd-Chiari syndrome, whether related to a web in the inferior vena cava or to endophlebitis of the hepatic veins, dictates a side-to-side shunt to decompress the liver.

To define whether the portal vein has been acting as a significant hepatic outflow, one can determine the portal pressure, apply a vascular clamp, and then remeasure the pressure on the cephalad limb. In the event that the portal vein is serving as a natural decompressive channel for the liver, the portal pressure in the cephalad limb would be significantly increased, but this is extremely rare.

In reference to the factor of ascites as a determinant of the decompressive procedure, Voorhees and associates indicated that 39 percent of patients with end-to-side

shunts who had preoperative ascites experienced postoper-ative relief; in 12 percent, ascites appeared after the shunt, while all patients with side-to-side shunts and ascites had permanent relief. Interestingly, the splenorenal shunt, which is a functional side-to-side shunt, failed to relieve ascites in 12 percent of the cases, and ascites appeared after the shunt in 16 percent. It is therefore felt that ascites per se cannot be considered a significant factor in determining the shunt to be performed. Similarly, whether previous encephalopathy or the presence of asterixis are important determinants of the type of shunt has not been resolved. The only procedures which specifically attack the problem of encephalopathy are the selective splenorenal shunt or the portacaval shunt with arterialization of the distal portal vein. In the case of the selective splenorenal shunt, coupled with ligation of the coronary vein, right gastroepiploic vein, and inferior mesenteric vein, randomized series have

Fig. 30-21. Diagrammatic representation of major portal-systemic shunts. (*From Seymour I. Schwartz, "Surgical Diseases of the Liver," McGraw-Hill Book Company, 1964.*)

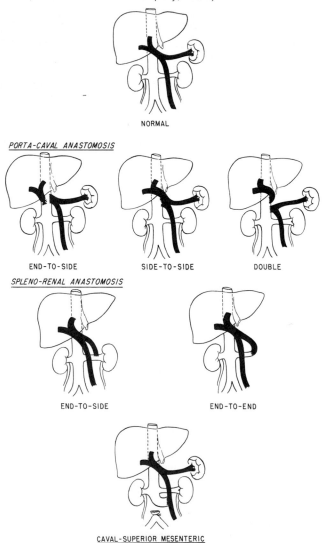

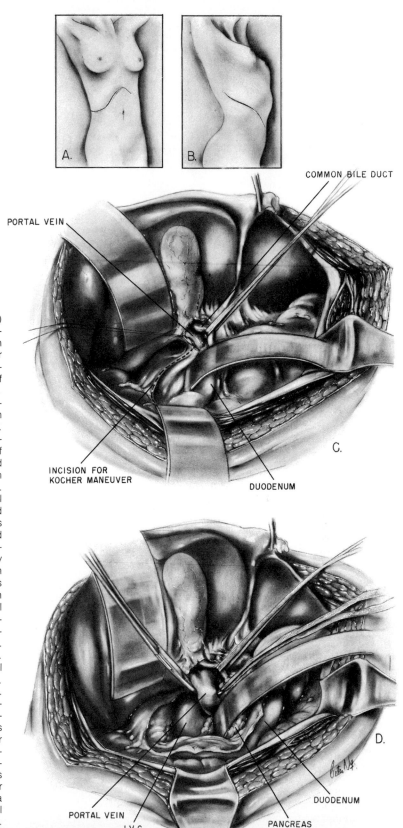

Fig. 30-22. Three kinds of portacaval shunt. (1) End-to-side portacaval shunt: *A.* Subcostal trans-abdominal incision. *B.* Thoracoabdominal incision over ninth intercostal space. *C.* Line of incision for Kocher maneuver. Initial dissection of hepatoduo-denal ligament, with isolation and retraction of common bile duct and exposure of portal vein. *D.* Completion of dissection of portal vein, with dem-onstration of bifurcation in porta hepatis. Dissection of retroperitoneum to clear inferior vena cava. *E.* Technique for end-to-side anastomosis. Note par-tially occluding clamp on anteromedial aspect of inferior vena cava. Atraumatic clamps are applied to proximal and distal portions of portal vein. *F.* An ellipse has been removed from inferior vena cava. This should measure $1\frac{1}{2}$ times diameter of portal vein. Portal vein has been transected. *G.* Distal end of portal vein has been oversewn with continuous silk sutures. (This may be handled by ligature and transfixion ligature.) Portal vein has been approxi-mated to stoma of inferior vena cava. Two stay sutures are initially tied, and posterior layer is in place. *H.* Placement of posterior layer of sutures is facilitated by passing cranial suture into lumen of portal vein and continuing this suture to caudal limb of portal vein, where it is then passed to out-side and tied. *I.* Closure of anterior row is accom-plished with interrupted horizontal mattress sutures. (A continuous suture may also be employed.) *J.* Completed anastomosis. (2) Side-to-side portacaval shunt: *K.* Beginning of side-to-side anastomosis. Use of rubber-shod bulldog clamps is preferable. An ellipse has been removed from both antero-medial aspect of inferior vena cava and anterolat-eral aspect of portal vein. Posterior row of sutures is shown in place. This is accomplished in a manner similar to that described for end-to-side anastomo-sis. *L.* Completed side-to-side anastomosis. Ante-rior row of sutures is placed in horizontal mattress fashion. (3) Double end-to-side shunt: *M.* Upper shunt is placed on anterior aspect of inferior vena cava; lower shunt is positioned on anteromedial aspect. Pancreas is split to facilitate lower shunt. (*From Seymour I. Schwartz, "Surgical Diseases of the Liver," McGraw-Hill Book Company, 1964.*)

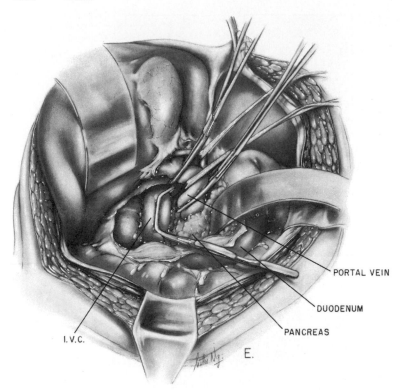

PORTAL VEIN

DUODENUM

PANCREAS

I.V.C.

E.

Fig. 30-22. Continued.

shown reduction in size of varices. The incidence of en-cephalopathy was less than that following total shunts. There are few long-term data for the arterialization proce-dure, and there is concern regarding the deleterious effects related to increased pressure.

Selection of Patients. Linton was one of the first to em-phasize the importance of the status of liver function on the patient's ability to tolerate portal-systemic decompres-sive procedures. Ascites which failed to respond to medical therapy, a prothrombin time which remained prolonged after parenteral administration of vitamin K, serum albu-min less than 3, serum bilirubin greater than 1, and BSP retention greater than 10 percent were all associated with poor postoperative prognosis. Child divided patients into three groups including those with good hepatic function (A), those with moderate hepatic function (B), and those with advanced disease and poor reserve (C). In group A are patients with a serum bilirubin below 2, albumin above 3.5, no ascites, no neurologic disorders, and excellent nu-trition. Patients in the B group have bilirubin between 2 and 3, albumin between 3 and 3.5, easily controlled ascites, minimum neurologic disorder, and good nutrition. In the C group, bilirubin is above 3, the albumin is below 3, and the ascites is poorly controlled with advanced coma and wasting. Operative mortality following portacaval shunts in the A group was zero, in the B group was 9 percent, and in the C group was 53 percent. There is general agree-ment that hepatic function is more important than the type of shunt in determining prognosis.

Portacaval Shunt Technique. This shunt (Fig. 30-22) gen-erally is performed through a subcostal incision, but in the presence of extreme hepatomegaly or obesity a thoraco-abdominal approach may be used. The liver is retracted craniad and a Kocher maneuver performed to permit mobilization of the duodenum. Dissection is begun in the hepatoduodenal ligament, and the portal vein, which re-sides posteriorly in relation to the common bile duct, is dissected free along the entire course. Small tributaries of the main portal vein may be encountered, and they are doubly ligated and transected. Attention is then directed to the dissection of the inferior vena cava. The incision in the retroperitoneum is extended, and the anterior and lateral aspects of the inferior vena cava are exposed from the renal veins inferiorly to the point where the vessel passes retrohepatically. Atraumatic clamps are applied to the portal vein just above its origin and just below its bifurcation, after which the vein is transected as far craniad as possible. The hepatic end is either ligated or oversewn. A sidearm, nonocclusive clamp is positioned along the anterior aspect of the inferior vena cava and an incision is made in the inferior vena cava wall. This should be approximately $1\frac{1}{2}$ times as long as the diameter of the portal vein. Employing vascular suture techniques, an anastomosis is made between the portal vein and the side of the inferior vena cava, utilizing a continuous suture which is interrupted at the two ends. After completing the anastomosis, the clamp is removed from the inferior vena cava, and then the clamp occluding the portal vein is

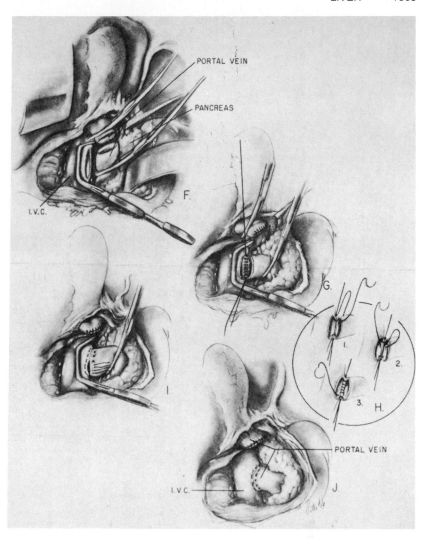

Fig. 30-22. Continued.

removed. Pressure should be recorded directly from the portal vein in order to define the efficacy of the shunt.

Splenorenal Shunt. In the cirrhotic patient with post-sinusoidal obstruction, the splenorenal anastomosis is not as hemodynamically efficient as the portocaval shunt and is associated with a higher incidence of recurrent bleeding. However, proponents of this procedure indicate that in their experience the prevention of recurrent bleeding is similar to that resulting from a portacaval shunt, and the incidence of portal-systemic encephalopathy and persistent hypersplenism is reduced. The operation is generally employed in patients with obstruction of the extrahepatic portal venous system in which the portal vein is not available for shunting. In the pediatric age group, it is preferable to postpone this procedure until the child is ten years old and the splenic vein is large enough to maintain its patency.

Technique (Fig. 30-23). An oblique subcostal incision or thoracoabdominal approach may be used. The transverse colon and splenic flexure are mobilized and retracted caudad, and the short gastric vessels are doubly ligated and transected. The splenophrenic and splenorenal ligaments are then transected and dissection continued in the hilus until an ultimate pedicle of splenic artery and vein remains. The splenic vein is freed as it courses along the pancreas. The posterior peritoneum is incised just medial to the hilus of the kidney and the left renal artery and vein dissected free. Tapes are passed around the main renal vein and the major branches in the hilus of the kidney. Traction on these tapes establishes control of bleeding and minimizes the number of clamps interfering with the anastomosis. The splenic artery is doubly ligated and transected, and an atraumatic clamp is applied to the central end of the splenic vein. The splenic vein is then transected as close to the hilus of the spleen as possible and brought down to an appropriate site on the anterosuperior aspect of the renal vein. The renal artery is occluded temporarily with a bulldog clamp, and an incision made in the renal vein.

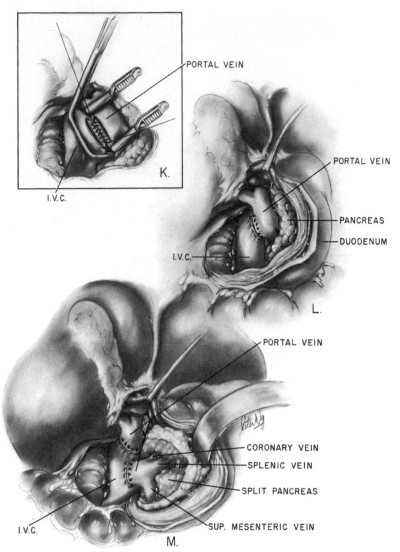

PORTAL VEIN

I.V.C.

K.

PORTAL VEIN

PORTAL VEIN

PANCREAS

DUODENUM

I.V.C.

L.

PORTAL VEIN

CORONARY VEIN

SPLENIC VEIN

SPLIT PANCREAS

I.V.C.

SUP. MESENTERIC VEIN

M.

Fig. 30-22. Continued.

An end-to-side anastomosis is performed by initially securing two stay sutures and completing the posterior layer as a continuous suture. Anastomosis of the anterior layer is accomplished with either horizontal mattress sutures or a continuous suture.

Superior Mesenteric–Inferior Vena Cava Shunt. This operation is generally employed for patients with extrahepatic vein obstruction and is particularly applicable to the patient in whom a previous splenorenal shunt failed or to a small child in whom a splenorenal anastomosis is doomed to failure because of the size of the splenic vein. The operation is also advised for patients with cirrhosis if there is associated thrombosis of the portal vein or extensive scarring in the right upper quadrant which precludes safe dissection of the portal vein or marked enlargement of the caudate lobe of the liver. Interruption of the inferior vena cava results in venous stasis in the lower extremity, and in the immediate postoperative pe-

riod the foot of the bed must be elevated to reduce potential edema. The procedure is well tolerated by young patients in whom postoperative chronic dependent edema of the legs is uncommon. In older patients, any edema may be readily controlled with elastic stockings. The report of prevention of recurrent bleeding in all 31 survivors of a large series has been encouraging.

Technique (Fig. 30-24). The peritoneal cavity is entered through a midline or right paramedian incision extending from the xiphoid process to well below the umbilicus. A branch of the superior mesenteric vein is cannulated and portal pressure determined manometrically. An operative phlebogram is then performed to define the patency of the superior mesenteric vein. Upward traction on the transverse colon exposes the superior mesenteric vessels. The peritoneum is incised in the region of the superior mesenteric arterial pulse, and the superior mesenteric vein is identified and dissected free. The lateral reflection of

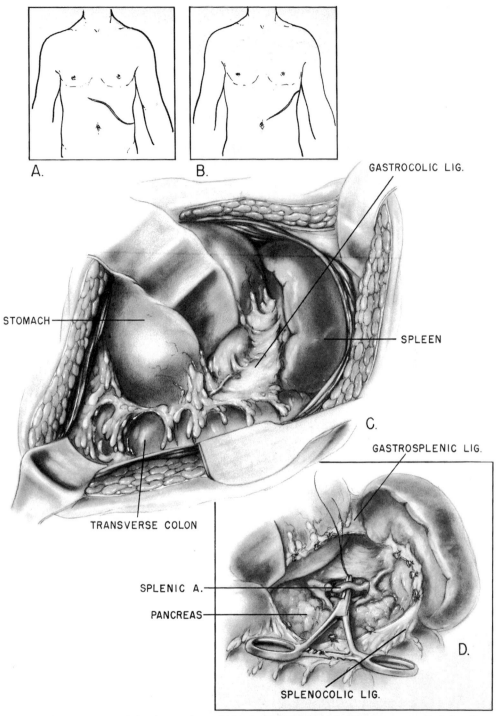

A.

B.

GASTROCOLIC LIG.

STOMACH

SPLEEN

C.

TRANSVERSE COLON

GASTROSPLENIC LIG.

SPLENIC A.

PANCREAS

D.

SPLENOCOLIC LIG.

Fig. 30-23. Splenorenal anastomosis. *A.* Subcostal transabdominal incision. *B.* Thoracoabdominal incision overlying ninth intercostal space. *C.* Retraction of stomach medially. *D.* Vasa brevia have been transected. Splenic artery is ligated. Gastrosplenic and splenocolic ligament are to be transected. *E.* Spleen is mobilized so that an ultimate pedicle of splenic vein remains. *F.* Retroperitoneum has been incised, and tapes are placed around renal artery and renal vein. *G.* Tapes are placed around major tributaries of renal vein within hilus of kidney and around main renal vein. Renal artery is occluded with bulldog clamp, and traction is applied to tapes around renal vein to secure control. An ellipse is then removed from anterosuperior aspect of renal vein. This should be $1\frac{1}{2}$ times diameter of splenic vein. Vascular clamp has been applied to splenic vein, and spleen is removed; as long a segment of splenic vein as possible is retained. *H.* Splenic vein is brought down and anastomosed to stoma which has been created in main renal vein. Occlusive tapes have been removed from splenic vein and renal artery. (*From Seymour I. Schwartz, "Surgical Diseases of the Liver," McGraw-Hill Book Company, 1964.*)

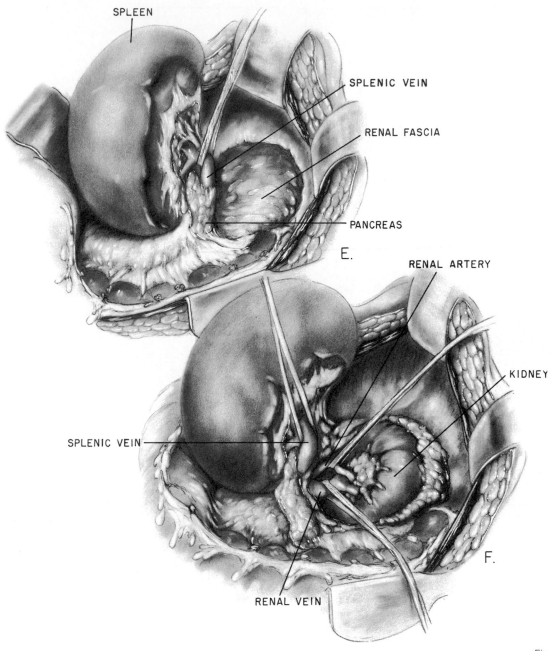

SPLEEN

SPLENIC VEIN

RENAL FASCIA

PANCREAS

E.

RENAL ARTERY

KIDNEY

SPLENIC VEIN

F.

RENAL VEIN

Fig. 30-23. Continued.

the ascending colon is then incised along its entire length to permit medial displacement of the transverse and ascending colons and the medial reflection of the ascending mesocolon. This exposes the inferior vena cava and the third portion of the duodenum. The inferior vena cava is mobilized from its origin up to the entrance of the right renal vein. The paired lumbar veins are ligated and transected. After the entire inferior vena cava has been freed, vascular clamps are applied immediately below the renal veins and at the junction of the iliac veins. The inferior vena cava is transected as far distad as possible and the

caudal stump ligated. The right iliac vein may be left attached to the vena cava to achieve greater length. A window is created in the mesentery of the small intestine between the ileocolic vessels and the origin of the main ileal trunk to permit approximation of the end of the inferior vena cava to the right posterolateral aspect of the superior mesenteric vein. The anastomosis between the inferior vena cava and the superior mesenteric vein is usually performed proximal to the right colic vein, utilizing a continuous arterial suture interrupted at both ends. Decompression also can be accomplished by the con-

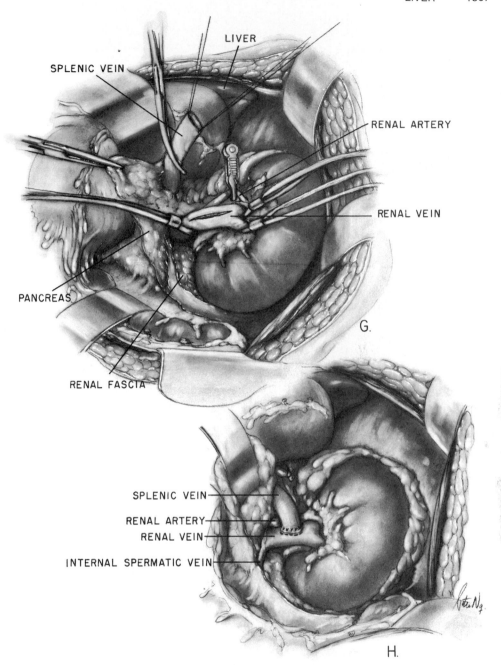

SPLENIC VEIN

LIVER

RENAL ARTERY

RENAL VEIN

PANCREAS

RENAL FASCIA

G.

SPLENIC VEIN
RENAL ARTERY
RENAL VEIN
INTERNAL SPERMATIC VEIN

H.

Fig. 30-23. Continued.

struction of an H-graft using a 19 to 22 mm prosthesis interposed between the superior mesenteric vein and the inferior vena cava (see Fig. 30-25).

Selective Splenorenal Shunt. The indications for the selective distal splenorenal shunt include a substantial portal venous flow to the liver, favorable anatomic features related to the site and patency of the splenic vein and the site and size of the left renal vein, and satisfactory liver function in the absence of ascites.

Technique. The operative procedure is shown in schematic fashion in Fig. 30-26. Decompression is effected

through the short gastric vessels in the spleen. The spleen is not removed, and the distal or splenic side of the splenic vein is used for an anastomosis to the left renal vein. This technique can be modified by transecting the left renal vein close to the hilus of the kidney, turning and anastomosing the caval side of the renal vein to the side of the splenic vein, and ligating the splenic vein close to the confluence with the superior mesenteric vein. Included in the procedure is ligation of the coronary vein and devascularization of the stomach by ligating of all vessels with the exception of the right gastric artery and the short gastric veins.

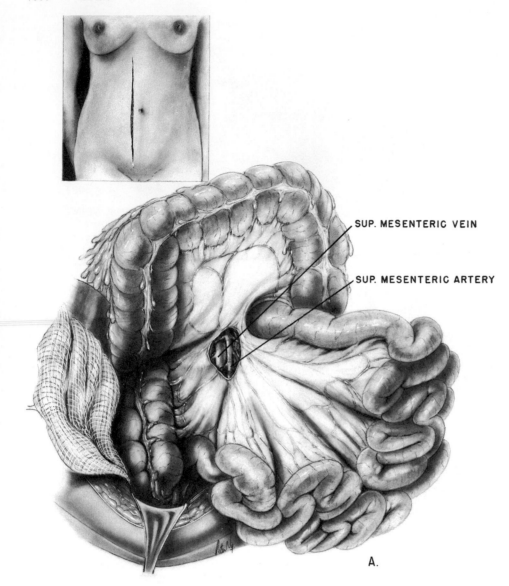

SUP. MESENTERIC VEIN

SUP. MESENTERIC ARTERY

A.

Complications of Portal-Systemic Shunts. The complications uniquely associated with portal-systemic shunting procedures occur intraoperatively or during the postoperative period. The intraoperative complications include bleeding and a nonshuntable situation, while the postoperative complications include rebleeding, hepatic failure, changes in cardiorespiratory dynamics, the hepatorenal syndrome, plus delayed complications of hemosiderosis, peptic ulcer, and portal-systemic encephalopathy.

The complication of intraoperative bleeding can be reduced by correction of coagulation defects and by continuing the infusion of vasopressin during the operative procedure. A nonshuntable situation may be related to extension of cavernomatous transformation of the portal vein to involve the superior mesenteric vein and the splenic vein. In these patients, the so-called makeshift shunt, using large collaterals, is generally doomed to failure. The circum-

Fig. 30-24. Superior mesenteric-inferior vena cava shunt, right route. *A.* Insert: right paramedian incision. Traction applied to transverse colon exposes superior mesenteric artery and vein. Peritoneum over vessels has been incised. Right side of superior mesenteric vein is dissected carefully to preserve colic branches. *B.* Lateral reflection of ascending colon has been incised, and colon is reflected medially. This has exposed inferior vena cava and third portion of duodenum. Inferior vena cava is mobilized from convergence of two common iliac veins up to entrance of right renal vein. In course of this dissection, paired lumbar veins are ligated in continuity and transected. *C.* Inferior vena cava has been transected. Stay sutures are inserted into adventitia of proximal vena cava, to be used for traction and orientation. Window has been created in small intestinal mesentery between ileocolic vessels and origin of main ileal trunk. *D.* Distal end of inferior vena cava has been oversewn. Proximal inferior vena cava is passed anterior to third portion of duodenum and through window in mesentery. Anastomosis is made between end of inferior vena cava and right posterolateral aspect of superior mesenteric vein. (*From Seymour I. Schwartz, "Surgical Diseases of the Liver," McGraw-Hill Book Company, 1964.*)

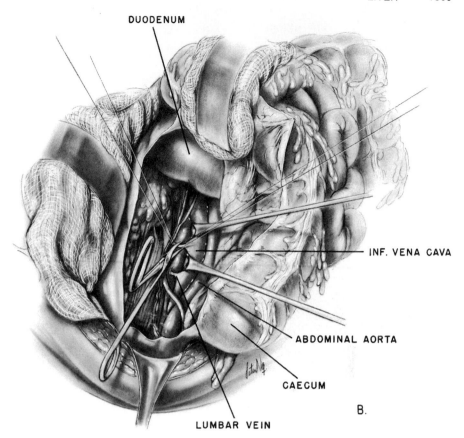

DUODENUM

INF. VENA CAVA

ABDOMINAL AORTA

CAECUM

LUMBAR VEIN

B.

Fig. 30-24. Continued.

stance of caval hypertension caused by hypertrophy and nodularity of the caudate lobe encroaching on the infra-hepatic vena cava has been referred to previously. Attempts have been made to shunt between the portal system and the pulmonary artery, but they have not provided long-term decompression.

Early postoperative bleeding is usually related to thrombosis of a reconstructed shunt. This can be defined by splenoportography in the case of a portacaval shunt. The rapid onset of ascites during the early postoperative period may be managed by restriction of sodium intake and the administration of diuretic agents. In this circumstance the early institution of a peritoneal-venous shunt has provided dramatic relief. Renal failure following a portal-systemic shunt is not predictable, and treatment consists of supportive measures. Recently the use of essential amino acids and hypertonic glucose hyperalimentation has added another factor in management. The early postoperative development of hepatic coma is an ominous sign, and the various treatments for fulminant hepatic failure are not applicable to these patients.

Portacaval Shunt for Glycogen Storage Disease and Hypercholesterolemia

In 1963, Starzl and associates performed a portacaval transposition on an eight-year-old child with type III gly-

cogen storage disease, which resulted in resumption of weight gain and growth rate. Since then, several investigators have reported clinical improvement following an end-to-side portacaval shunt in children with type I glycogen storage disease in which the enzyme glucose 6-phosphatase is deficient or absent. This represents the most severe and most common form of inherited disorders of glycogen metabolism. Intravenous hyperalimentation for 2 to 3 weeks prior to surgery is advised to reduce the liver size, restore the bleeding time to normal, correct acidosis and hypoglycemia, and promote a favorable outcome of the shunting procedure. Children who have undergone diversion of portal flow have shown no evidence of encephalopathy so far. Recently, portacaval shunts have been applied to a few patients with homozygous hypercholesterolemia.

FULMINANT HEPATIC FAILURE

This refers to the clinical syndrome characterized by sudden, severe impairment of hepatic function generally as a consequence of massive necrosis of liver cells. In most instances, the cause is acute hepatitis of viral origin. Massive necrosis and dysfunction have been reported with Reye's syndrome, as a rarity in pregnancy, and following exposure to drugs such as carbon tetrachloride and di-

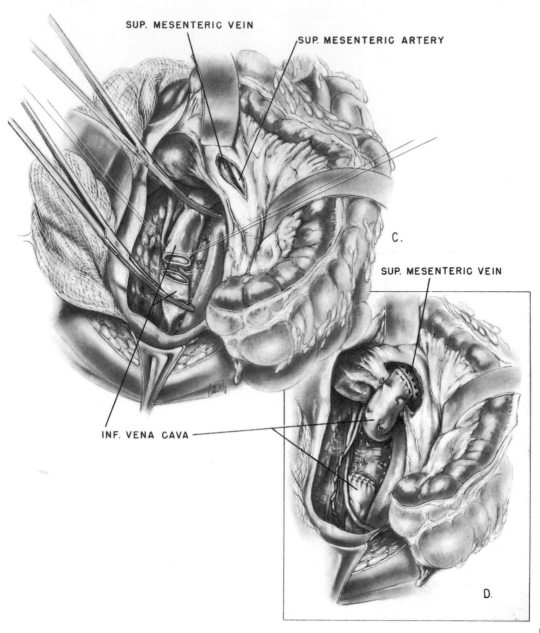

SUP. MESENTERIC VEIN

SUP. MESENTERIC ARTERY

C.

SUP. MESENTERIC VEIN

INF. VENA CAVA

D.

Fig. 30-24. Continued.

methyl nitrosamine. Circulatory necrosis of hepatic cells has been reported following vasopressor therapy and following the inadvertent intraarterial infusion of vasopressin into the hepatic artery. Halothane, particularly in cases of multiple exposures, has been indicted, but evaluation of its role awaits more statistically significant data.

The manifestations are essentially those described for hepatic encephalopathy, frequently accompanied by renal failure. The treatment can be considered in two major categories: The first is related to general supportive therapy plus regimens directed at reducing hyperammonemia which have been described in the section on encephalopathy, under Hepatic Coma, earlier in this chapter. The

second category consists of a series of intercessions, all aimed at removing so-called noxious elements from the affected patient and preserving life long enough for the liver to regenerate sufficiently. Included in this category are hemodialysis and peritoneal dialysis, exchange transfusion, plasmapheresis, asanguinous hypothermic total body perfusion, ex vivo perfusion of a liver of the same or different species, and cross circulation with a human being or a subhuman primate.

Patients in fulminant hepatic failure who are categorized at the comatose level with spasticity have a mortality of between 85 and 90 percent; this approaches 100 percent when the flaccidity stage is reached. The effect of any form

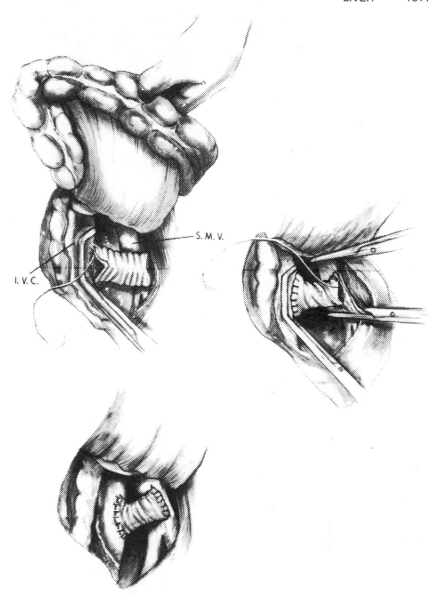

Fig. 30-25. H-graft (interposition mesocaval shunt). The transverse colon is elevated, and the superior mesenteric vein is dissected free at the route of the small bowel mesentery. A partially occlusive clamp is applied to the infrarenal vena cava, and an anastomosis is made between the vena cava and a 19- to 22-mm Dacron prosthesis. Occlusive clamps are then placed on the superior mesenteric vein, and the graft is anastomosed in an end-to-side fashion to the superior mesenteric vein. Heparinization is unnecessary.

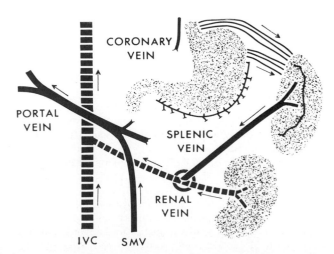

Fig. 30-26. Diagrammatic illustration of the selective distal splenorenal shunt. Note coronary vein ligation and gastric devascularization which protects the vasa brevia and other collateral vessels from esophagus and diaphragm. (*From A. A. Salam et al., Ann Surg, 173:827, 1971.*)

of therapy is difficult to evaluate since spontaneous recovery occurs in 10 to 20 percent of the cases. The difficulty in managing these patients is that recovery depends on hepatocyte regeneration, which usually takes several days, while the treatment only lasts for hours or fractions of days. To date, the results generally have been unsatisfactory.

References

General

Foster, J. H., and Berman, M. M.: "Solid Liver Tumors," W. B. Saunders Company, Philadelphia, 1977.

Popper, H., and Schaffner, F.: "Liver: Structure and Function," McGraw-Hill Book Company, New York, 1957.

Schwartz, S. I.: "Surgical Diseases of the Liver," McGraw-Hill Book Company, New York, 1964.

Sherlock, S.: "Diseases of the Liver and Biliary System," 5th ed., Blackwell Scientific Publications, Ltd., Oxford, 1977.

Anatomy

Douglass, B. E., Baggenstoss, A. H., and Hollinshead, W. H.: The Anatomy of the Portal Vein and Its Tributaries, Surg Gynecol Obstet, 91:562, 1950.

Dreyer, B.: Streamlining in the Portal Vein, Q J Exp Physiol, 39:305, 1954.

Healey, J. E., Jr., and Schroy, P. C.: Anatomy of the Biliary Ducts within the Human Liver: Analysis of the Prevailing Pattern of Branching and the Major Variations of the Biliary Ducts, Arch Surg, 66:599, 1953.

Michels, N.: The Hepatic, Cystic and Retroduodenal Arteries and Their Relations to the Biliary Ducts, Ann Surg, 133:503, 1951.

Liver Function

Faloon, W. W., Eckhardt, R. D., Murphy, T. L., Cooper, A. M., and Davidson, C. S.: An Evaluation of Human Serum Albumin in the Treatment of Cirrhosis of the Liver, J Clin Invest, 28:583, 1949.

Gutman, A. B.: Serum Alkaline Phosphatase Activity in Diseases of the Skeletal and Hepatobiliary Systems: A Consideration of Current Status, Am J Med, 27:875, 1959.

Leevy, C. M.: "Evaluation of Liver Function in Clinical Practice," The Lilly Research Laboratories, Indianapolis, Ind., 1965.

West, M., and Zimmerman, H. J.: Serum Enzymes in Disease. I. Lactic-Dehydrogenase and Glutamic Oxaloacetic Transaminase in Carcinoma, Arch Intern Med, 102:103, 1958.

Special Studies

Braunstein, H.: Needle Biopsy of the Liver in Cirrhosis: Diagnostic Efficiency as Determined by Postmortem Sampling, Arch Pathol, 62:87, 1956.

Greenway, C. V., and Stark, R. D.: Hepatic Vascular Bed, Physiol Rev, 51:23, 1971.

Nagler, W., Bender, M. A., and Blau, M.: Radioisotope Photoscanning of the Liver, Gastroenterology, 44:36, 1963.

Shizgal, H. M., and Goldstein, M. S.: Measurement of Portal and Total Hepatic Blood Flow by the Intestinal Xenon Technique, Surgery, 72:83, 1972.

Zamcheck, N., and Klausenstock, O.: Liver Biopsy (Concluded). II. The Risk of Needle Biopsy, N Engl J Med, 249:1062, 1953.

Trauma

Amerson, J. R., and Stone, H. H.: Experiences in the Management of Hepatic Trauma, Arch Surg, 100:150, 1970.

Brittain, R. S., Marchioro, T. L., Hermann, G., Waddell, W. R., and Starzl, T. E.: Accidental Hepatic Artery Ligation in Humans, Am J Surg, 107:822, 1964.

Carroll, C. P., Cass, K. A., and Whelan, T. J.: Wounds of the Liver in Vietnam: Critical Analysis of 254 Cases, Ann Surg, 177:385, 1973.

Crosthwait, R. W., Allen, J. E., Murga, F., Beall, A. C., Jr., and DeBakey, M. E.: The Surgical Management of 640 Consecutive Liver Injuries in Civilian Practice, Surg Gynecol Obstet, 114:650, 1962.

Fish, J. C.: Reconstruction of the Portal Vein. Case Reports and Literature Review, Am Surg, 32:472, 1966.

Koehler, R. E., Korobkin, M., and Lewis, F.: Arteriographic Demonstration of Collateral Arterial Supply to Liver after Hepatic Artery Ligation, Radiology, 117:49, 1975.

Lewis, F. R., Lim, R. C., Jr., and Blaisdell, F. W.: Hepatic Artery Ligation: Adjunct in Management of Massive Hemorrhage from the Liver, J Trauma, 14:743, 1974.

Lim, R. C., Jr., Knudson, J., and Steele, M.: Liver Trauma, Current Method of Management, Arch Surg, 104:544, 1972.

Lucas, C. E., and Ledgerwood, A. M.: Controlled Biliary Drainage for Large Injuries of the Liver, Surg Gynecol Obstet, 137:585, 1973.

——— and Walt, A. J.: Critical Decisions in Liver Trauma: Experience Based on 604 Cases, Arch Surg, 101:277, 1970.

McGhee, R. N., Townsend, C. M., Jr., Thompson, J. C., and Fish, J. C.: Traumatic Hemobilia, Ann Surg, 179:311, 1974.

Madding, G. F.: Injuries of the Liver, Arch Surg, 70:748, 1955.

Monafo, W. W., Ternberg, J. L., and Kempson, R.: Accidental Ligation of the Hepatic Artery, Arch Surg, 92:643, 1966.

Moss, L. K., and Hudgens, J. C., Jr.: Spontaneous Rupture of the Liver Associated with Pregnancy: Case Report and Review of the Literature, Am Surgeon, 26:763, 1960.

Trunkey, D. D., Shires, G. T., and McClelland, R.: Management of Liver Trauma in 811 Consecutive Patients, Ann Surg, 179:722, 1974.

Hepatic Abscesses

Altemeier, W. A., Schowengerdt, C. G., and Whiteley, D. H.: Abscesses of the Liver: Surgical Considerations, Arch Surg, 101:258, 1970.

Brodine, W. N., and Schwartz, S. I.: Pyogenic Hepatic Abscesses: Review of Representative Literature and Presentation of Ten Cases, NY State J Med, 73:1657, 1973.

Crane, P. S., Lee, Y. T., and Seel, D. J.: Experience in Treatment of 200 Patients with Amebic Abscess of the Liver in Korea, Am J Surg, 123:332, 1972.

DeBakey, M. E., and Ochsner, A.: Hepatic Amebiasis: A Twenty Year Experience and Analysis of 263 Cases, Surg Gynecol Obstet, 92:209, 1951.

Lee, J. F., and Block, G. E.: The Changing Clinical Pattern of Hepatic Abscesses, Arch Surg, 104:465, 1972.

Pitt, H. A., and Zuidema, G. D.: Factors Influencing Mortality in

Treatment of Pyogenic Hepatic Abscess, *Surg Gynecol Obstet,* **140:**228, 1975.

Powell, S. J., Wilmot, A. J., and Elsdon-Dew, R.: Further Trials of Metronidazole in Amoebic Dysentery and Amoebic Liver Abscess, *Ann Trop Med Parasitol,* **61:**511, 1967.

Rubin, R. H., Swartz, M. N., and Malt, R.: Hepatic Abscess: Change in Clinical, Bacteriologic and Therapeutic Aspects, *Am J Med,* **57:**601, 1974.

Cysts and Benign Tumors

Arce, J.: Hydatid Disease (Hydatidosis): Pathology and Treatment, *Arch Surg,* **42:**1, 1941.

Baum, J. K., Brockstein, J. J., Holtz, F., et. al: Possible Association between Benign Hepatomas and Oral Contraceptives, *Lancet,* **2:**926, 1973.

Christopherson, W. M., Mays, E. T., and Barrows, G. H.: Liver Tumors in Women on Oral Contraceptive Steroids, *Obstet Gynecol,* **46**(2):221, 1975.

Feldman, M.: Polycystic Disease of the Liver, *Am J Gastroenterol,* **29:**83, 1958.

Geist, D. C.: Solitary Nonparasitic Cyst of the Liver, *Arch Surg,* **71:**867, 1955.

Katz, A. M., and Pan, C.-T.: Echinococcus Disease in the United States, *Am J Med,* **25:**759, 1958.

Lewis, J. W., Koss, N., and Kerstein, M. D.: A Review of Echinococcal Disease, *Ann Surg,* **181:**390, 1975.

Longmire, W. P., Jr., Mandiola, S. A., and Earl, G. H.: Congenital Cystic Disease of the Liver and Biliary System, *Ann Surg,* **174:**711, 1971.

Magath, T. B.: The Antigen of Echinococcus, *Am J Clin Pathol,* **31:**1, 1959.

Melnick, P. J.: Polycystic Liver: Analysis of Seventy Cases, *Arch Pathol,* **59:**162, 1955.

Papadimitriou, J., and Mandrekas, A.: The Surgical Treatment of Hydatid Disease of the Liver, *Br J Surg,* **57:**431, 1970.

Park, W. C., and Phillips, R.: The Role of Radiation Therapy in the Management of Hemangiomas of the Liver, *JAMA,* **212:**1496, 1970.

Rake, M. O., Liberman, M. M., Dawson, J. L., Evans, R., Raftery, E. B., Laws, J., and Williams, R.: Ligation of the Hepatic Artery in the Treatment of Heart Failure Due to Hepatic Haemangiomatosis, *Gut,* **11:**512, 1970.

Sewell, J. H., and Weiss, K.: Spontaneous Rupture of Hemangioma of the Liver: A Review of the Literature and Presentation of Illustrative Case, *Arch Surg,* **83:**105, 1961.

Malignant Tumors

Adam, Y. G., Huvos, A. G., and Hajdu, S. I.: Malignant Vascular Tumors of Liver. *Ann Surg,* **175:**375, 1972.

Almersjö, O., Bengmark, S., Hafström, Lo., and Rosengren, K.: Accuracy of Diagnostic Tools in Malignant Hepatic Lesions: Comparative Study Using Serum Tests, Angiography, Scintiscanning and Laparotomy, *Am J Surg,* **127:**663, 1974.

Alrenga, D. P.: Primary Angiosarcoma of the Liver: Review Article, *Int Surg,* **60:**198, 1975.

Curutchet, H. P., Terz, J. J., Kay, S., and Lawrence, W., Jr.: Primary Liver Cancer, *Surgery,* **70:**467, 1971.

Edmondson, H. W., and Steiner, P. E.: Primary Carcinoma of the Liver: A Study of 100 Cases among 48,900 Necropsies, *Cancer,* **7:**462, 1954.

Fenster, L. F., and Klatskin, G.: Manifestation of Metastatic Tumors of the Liver: A Study of 81 Patients Subjected to Needle Biopsy, *Am J Med,* **31:**238, 1961.

Fortner, J. G., Mulcare, R. J., Solis, A., Watson, R. C., and Goiby, R. B.: Treatment of Primary and Secondary Liver Cancer by Hepatic Artery Ligation and Infusion Chemotherapy, *Ann Surg,* **178:**162, 1973.

Foster, J. H.: Survival after Liver Resection for Cancer, *Cancer,* **26:**493, 1970.

Gulesserian, H. P., Lawton, R. L., and Condon, R. W.: Hepatic Artery Ligation and Cytotoxic Infusion in Treatment of Liver Metastases, *Arch Surg,* **105:**280, 1972.

Kew, M. C., Dos Santos, H. A., and Sherlock, S.: Diagnosis of Primary Cancer of the Liver, *Br Med J,* **4:**408, 1971.

Lin, T.-Y., Chu, S.-H., Chen, M.-F., and Chen, C.-H.: Serum Alpha-Fetoglobulin and Primary Cancer of the Liver in Taiwan, *Cancer,* **30:**435, 1972.

Purves, L. R., Bersohn, I., and Geddes, E. W.: Serum Alpha-Feto-Protein and Primary Cancer of the Liver in Man, *Cancer,* **25:**1261, 1970.

Ramirez, G., Ansfield, F. J., and Curreri, A. R.: Hepatoma: Long-Term Survival with Disseminated Tumor Treated with 5-Fluorouracil, *Am J Surg,* **120:**400, 1970.

Rosenthal, S., and Kaufman, S.: Liver Scan in Metastatic Disease, *Arch Surg,* **106:**656, 1973.

Shallow, T. A., and Wagner, F. B.: Primary Fibrosarcoma of the Liver, *Ann Surg,* **125:**439, 1947.

Starzl, T. E.: "Experience in Hepatic Transplantation," W. B. Saunders Company, Philadelphia, 1969.

Warvi, W. N.: Primary Neoplasms of the Liver, *Arch Pathol,* **37:**367, 1944.

Hepatic Resection

Lin, T.-Y., and Chen, C.-C.: Metabolic Function and Regeneration of Cirrhotic and Non-cirrhotic Livers after Hepatic Lobectomy in Man, *Ann Surg,* **162:**959, 1965.

Starzl, T. E., Bell, R. H., Beart, R. W., and Putnam, C. W.: Hepatic Trisegmentectomy and Other Liver Resections, *Surg Gynecol Obstet,* **141:**429, 1975.

Transplantation

Fortner, J. G., Kinne, D. W., Shiu, M. H., Howland, W. S., Kim, D. K., Castro, E. B., Yeh, S. D. J., Benua, R. S., and Krimins, S.: Clinical Liver Heterotopic (Auxiliary) Transplantation, *Surgery,* **74:**739, 1973.

Putnam, C. W., Halgrimson, C. G., Koep, L., and Starzl, T. E.: Progress in Liver Transplantation, *World J Surg,* **1:**165, 1977.

Starzl, T. E.: "Experience in Hepatic Transplantation," W. B. Saunders Company, Philadelphia, 1969.

Portal Hypertension

Baggenstoss, A. H., and Wollaeger, E. E.: Portal Hypertension Due to Chronic Occlusion of the Extrahepatic Portion of the Portal Vein: Its Relation to Ascites, *Am J Med,* **21:**16, 1956.

Baker, L., Smith, C., and Lieberman, G.: The Natural History of Esophageal Varices, *Am J Med,* **26:**228, 1959.

Bauer, J. J., Gelernt, I. M., and Kreel, I.: Portosystemic Shunting in Patients with Primary Biliary Cirrhosis: A Good Risk Disease, *Ann Surg,* **183:**324, 1976.

Bismuth, H., and Franco, D.: Portal Diversion for Portal Hypertension in Early Childhood, *Ann Surg,* **183:**439, 1976.

Brown, H., Trey, C., and McDermott, W. V., Jr.: Lactulose Treatment of Hepatic Encephalopathy in Outpatients, *Arch Surg,* **102:**25, 1971.

Burchell, A. R., Moreno, A. H., Panke, W. F., and Nealon, T. F., Jr.: Hemodynamic Variables and Prognosis following Portacaval Shunts, *Surg Gynecol Obstet,* **138:**359, 1974.

Child, C. G. III: "Hepatic Circulation and Portal Hypertension," W. B. Saunders Company, Philadelphia, 1954.

Conn, H. O., Smith, H. W., and Brodoff, M.: Observer Variation in the Endoscopic Diagnosis of Esophageal Varices, *N Engl J Med,* **272:**830, 1965.

Eisenmenger, W. J., Blondheim, S., Bongiovanni, A. M., and Kunkel, H. G.: Electrolyte Studies on Patients with Cirrhosis of the Liver, *J Clin Invest,* **29:**1491, 1950.

Fischer, J. E., and James, H. J.: Treatment of Hepatic Coma and Hepatorenal Syndrome: Mechanism of Action of L-dopa and Aramine, *Am J Surg,* **123:**222, 1972.

Galambos, J. T., Warren, W. D., Rudman, D., Smith, R. B., III, and Salam, A. A.: Selective and Total Shunts in the Treatment of Bleeding Varices: A Randomized Controlled Trial, *N Engl J Med,* **295:**1089, 1976.

Garrett, J. C., Voorhees, A. B., Jr., and Sommers, S. C.: Renal Failure following Portasystemic Shunt in Patients with Cirrhosis of the Liver, *Ann Surg,* **172:**218, 1970.

Jackson, F. C., Perrin, E. B., Felix, W. R., and Smith, A. G.: A Clinical Investigation of the Portacaval Shunt: V. Survival Analysis of the Therapeutic Operation, *Ann Surg,* **174:**672, 1971.

Johnston, G. W., and Rodgers, H. W.: Review of 15 Years' Experience in Use of Sclerotherapy in Control of Acute Hemorrhage from Esophageal Varices, *Br J Surg,* **60:**797, 1973.

Langer, B., Stone, R. M., Colapinto, R. F., Meindok, H., Phillips, M. J., and Fisher, M. M.: Clinical Spectrum of the Budd-Chiari Syndrome and Its Clinical Management, *Am J Surg,* **129:**137, 1975.

Leveen, H. H., Christoudias, G., Ip, M., Luft, R., Falk, G., and Grosberg, S.: Peritoneo-Venous Shunting for Ascites, *Ann Surg,* **180:**580, 1974.

Linton, R. R.: The Selection of Patients for Portacaval Shunts, *Ann Surg,* **134:**433, 1951.

Lunderquist, A., and Vang, J.: Transhepatic Catheterization and Obliteration of the Coronary Vein in Patients with Portal Hypertension and Esophageal Varices, *N Engl J Med,* **291:**646, 1974.

Madden, J. L., Lore, J. M., Jr., Gerold, F. P., and Ravid, J. M.: The Pathogenesis of Ascites and a Consideration of Its Treatment, *Surg Gynecol Obstet,* **99:**385, 1954.

Maillard, J.-N., Rueff, B., Prandi, D., and Sicot, C.: Hepatic Arterialization and Portacaval Shunt in Hepatic Cirrhosis: Assessment, *Arch Surg,* **108:**315, 1974.

Malt, R. A.: Portasystemic Venous Shunts (First of Two Parts), *N Engl J Med,* **295:**24, 1976.

———: Portasystemic Venous Shunts (Second of Two Parts), *N Engl J Med,* **295:**80, 1976.

Merigan, T. C., Jr., Hollister, R. M., Gryska, P. F., Starkey, G. W. B., and Davidson, C. S.: Gastrointestinal Bleeding with Cirrhosis: A Study of 172 Episodes in 158 Patients, *N Engl J Med,* **263:**579, 1960.

Moreno, A. H., Burchell, A. R., Reddy, R. V., Steen, J. A., Panke, W. F., and Nealon, T. F., Jr.: Spontaneous Reversal of Portal Blood Flow: Case for and against Its Occurrence in Patients with Cirrhosis of the Liver, *Ann Surg,* **181:**346, 1975.

Nusbaum, M. S., Baum, S., Kuroda, K., and Blakemore, W. S.: Control of Portal Hypertension by Selective Mesenteric Arterial Drug Infusion, *Arch Surg,* **97:**1005, 1968.

Orloff, M. J., Charters, A. C., III, Chandler, J. G., Gordon, J. K., Grambort, D. E., Modafferi, T. R., Levin, S. E., Brown, N. B., Sviokla, S. C., and Knox, D. G.: Portacaval Shunt as Emergency Procedure in Unselected Patients with Alcoholic Cirrhosis, *Surg Gynecol Obstet,* **141:**59, 1975.

Owens, J. C., and Coffey, R. J.: Aneurysm of Splenic Artery including a Report of Six Additional Cases, *Surg Gynecol Obstet,* **97:**313, 1953.

Parkes, J. D., Sharpstone, P., and Williams, R.: Levodopa in Hepatic Coma, *Lancet,* **2:**1341, 1970.

Resnick, R. H., Chambers, T. C., Ishibara, A. M., Garceau, A. J., Callow, A. D., Schimmel, E. M., and O'Hara, E. T.: A Controlled Study of the Prophylactic Portacaval Shunt: A Final Report, *Ann Intern Med,* **70:**675, 1969.

———, Iber, F. L., Ishihara, A. M., Chalmers, T. C., Zimmerman, H., and the Boston Inter-Hospital Liver Group: Controlled Study of Therapeutic Portacaval Shunt, *Gastroenterology,* **67:**843, 1974.

Reynolds, T. B., Freedman, T., and Winsor, W.: Results of the Treatment of Bleeding Esophageal Varices with Balloon Tamponage, *Am J Med Sci,* **224:**500, 1952.

———, Redeker, A. G., and Davis, P.: Controlled Study of Effects of L-A ginine on Hepatic Encephalopathy, *Am J Med,* **25:**359, 1958.

Salam, A. A., Warren, W. D., and Tyras, D. H.: Splenic Vein Thrombosis: Diagnosable and Curable Form of Portal Hypertension, *Surgery,* **74:**961, 1973.

Schwartz, S. I.: Complications of Portal-Systemic Shunting Procedures, in H. Beebe (ed.), "Complications of Vascular Disease," J. B. Lippincott Company, Philadelphia, 1973.

———, Bales, H. W., Emerson, G. L., and Mahoney, E. B.: The Use of Intravenous Pituitrin in Treatment of Bleeding Esophageal Varices, *Surgery,* **45:**72, 1959.

——— and Greenlaw, R. H.: Evaluation of Portal Circulation by Percutaneous Splenic Isotope Injection, *Surgery,* **50:**833, 1961.

Sokhi, G. S., Morrice, J. J., McGee, J. O'D., and Blumgart, L. H.: Congenital Hepatic Fibrosis: Aspects of Diagnosis and Surgical Management, *Br J Surg,* **62:**621, 1975.

Starzl, T. E., Putnam, C. W., Porter, K. A., Halgrimson, C. G., Corman, J., Brown, B. L., Gotlin, R. W., Rodgerson, D. O., and Greene, H. L.: Portal Diversion for Treatment of Glycogen Storage Disease in Humans, *Ann Surg,* **178:**525, 1973.

Thompson, J. C.: Alterations in Gastric Secretion after Portacaval Shunting, *Am J Surg,* **117:**854, 1969.

Tisdale, W. A., Klatskin, G., and Glenn, W. W.: Portal Hypertension and Bleeding Esophageal Varices: Their Occurrence in the Absence of Both Intrahepatic and Extrahepatic Obstruction of the Portal Vein, *N Engl J Med,* **261:**209, 1959.

Turcotte, J. G., and Lambert, M. J., II: Variceal Hemmorhage, Hepatic Cirrhosis and Portacaval Shunts, *Am J Surg,* **126:**748, 1973.

Voorhees, A. B., Jr., Price, J. B., Jr., and Britton, R. C.: Portasystemic Shunting Procedures for Portal Hypertension: 26-

Year Experience in Adults with Cirrhosis of the Liver, *Am J Surg,* **119:**501, 1970.

Warren, W. D., Salam, A. A., Hutson, D., and Zeppa, R.: Selective Distal Splenorenal Shunt: Technic and Results of Operation, *Arch Surg,* **108:**306, 1974.

Glycogen Storage Disease and Hypercholesterolemia

Folkman, J., Philippart, A., Tze, W.-J., and Crigler, J., Jr.: Portacaval Shunt for Glycogen Storage Disease: Value of Prolonged Intravenous Hyperalimentation before Surgery, *Surgery,* **72:**306, 1972.

Starzl T. E., Brown, B. I., Blanchard, H., and Brettschneider, L.: Portal Diversion in Glycogen Storage Disease, *Surgery,* **65:**504, 1969.

Stein, E. A., Peltifor, J., Mieny, C., et al.: Portacaval Shunt, in Four Patients with Homozygous Hypercholesterolaemia, *Lancet,* **1:**832, 1975.

Fulminant Hepatic Failure

Abouna, G. M., Cook, J. S., Fisher, L. McA., Still, W. J., Costa, G., and Hume, D. M.: Treatment of Acute Hepatic Coma by Ex Vivo Baboon and Human Liver Perfusions, *Surgery,* **71:**537, 1972.

Klebanoff, G., Hollander, D., Cosimi, A. B., Stanford, W., and Kemmerer, W. T.: Asanguineous Hypothermic Total Body Perfusion (TBW) in the Treatment of Stage IV Hepatic Coma, *J Surg Res,* **12:**1, 1972.

Trey, C., and Davidson, C. S.: The Management of Fulminant Hepatic Failure, *Prog Liver Dis,* **3:**282, 1970.

Chapter 31

Gallbladder and Extrahepatic Biliary System

by **Seymour I. Schwartz**

ANATOMY

DUCT SYSTEM. The extrahepatic biliary system begins with the hepatic ducts and ends at the stoma of the common bile duct in the duodenum. The right hepatic duct is approximately 1 cm in length, while the left duct is somewhat larger. Both are approximately 3 mm in diameter. The two ducts join to form a common hepatic duct which resides in the porta hepatis and is 3 to 4 cm in length. It, in turn, is joined at an acute angle by the cystic duct from the gallbladder to form the common bile duct.

The common bile duct is approximately 8 cm in length and 6 mm in diameter. The upper portion is situated in the free edge of the lesser omentum, to the right of the hepatic artery, and anterior to the portal vein. The middle third of the common duct curves to the right behind the first portion of the duodenum, where it diverges from the portal vein and hepatic arteries. The lower third of the common bile duct curves more to the right behind the head of the pancreas, which it grooves, and enters the duodenum at the ampulla of Vater, where it is frequently joined by the pancreatic duct. The portions of the duct have also been named according to their relationships to intestinal viscera: the terms *suprapancreatic, intrapancreatic,* and *intraduodenal* have been applied.

The union of the bile duct and the main pancreatic duct follows one of three patterns. The structures may (1) unite outside the duodenum and traverse the duodenal wall and papilla as a single duct, (2) join within the duodenal wall and have a short, common, terminal portion, or (3) exit independently into the duodenum. The common channel has been considered important in permitting reflux from the pancreas into the biliary tract and the reverse. Separate orifices have been demonstrated in 29 percent of autopsied specimens, while injection into cadavers reveals reflux from the common bile duct into the pancreatic duct in 54 percent. Radiographically, reflux from the common bile duct into the pancreatic duct is present in about 16 percent of the cases. The sphincter of Oddi surrounds the common bile duct and pancreatic ducts at the papilla of Vater, and although some fibers are derived from the duodenal muscle, there are additional, intrinsic muscles of the duct in the ampulla. These provide a control of the flow of bile and pancreatic juice. An ampullary sphincter which is present in one-third of adults may produce a common channel effect.

GALLBLADDER. The gallbladder is located in the bed of the liver in line with the anatomic division of that organ into right and left lobes. It represents an outpouching of the extrahepatic biliary duct system and has an average capacity of 50 ml. It is a pear-shaped organ which is divided into four anatomic portions: fundus; corpus, or body; infundibulum; and neck. The fundus represents the rounded, blind end which normally extends beyond the liver margin behind the tip of the right costal cartilage. It may be unusually kinked and present the appearance of a "phrygian cap." It contains most of the smooth muscle of the organ, in contrast to the corpus, or body, which is the major storage area and contains most of the elastic tissue. The body tapers into a neck, which is funnel-shaped and connects with the cystic duct. The neck usually follows a gentle curve, the convexity of which may be distended into a dilatation known as the *infundibulum,* or *Hartmann's pouch.*

The wall of the gallbladder is made up of smooth muscle and fibrous tissue, and the lumen is lined with a high columnar epithelium which contains cholesterol and fat globules. The mucus secreted into the gallbladder originates in the tubular alveolar glands in the globular cells of the mucosa lining the infundibulum and neck.

The gallbladder is supplied by the cystic artery, which normally branches from the right hepatic artery behind the cystic duct. It is approximately 2 mm in diameter and courses above the cystic duct for a variable distance, until it passes down the peritoneal surface of the gallbladder and branches. Venous return is carried through small veins, which enter directly into the liver from the gallbladder, and a large cystic vein, which carries blood back to the right portal vein. Lymph flows directly from the gallbladder to the liver and drains into several nodes along the surface of the portal vein. The nerves of the gallbladder arise from the celiac plexus and lie along the hepatic artery. Motor nerves are made up of vagus fibers mixed with postganglionic fibers from the celiac ganglion. The preganglionic sympathetic level is at T_8 and T_9. Sensory supplies are provided by fibers in the sympathetic nerves coursing to the celiac plexus through the posterior root ganglion at T_8 and T_9 on the right side.

The gallbladder enters the common duct system by means of the cystic duct, which has a variable length, averaging 4 cm. It joins the common hepatic duct at an

Fig. 31-1. Variations of the cystic duct. *A.* Low junction between cystic duct and common hepatic duct. *B.* Cystic duct adherent to common hepatic duct. *C.* High junction between cystic and common hepatic duct. *D.* Cystic duct drains into right hepatic duct. *E.* Long cystic duct which joins common hepatic duct behind duodenum. *F.* Absence of cystic duct. *G.* Cystic duct crosses anterior to common hepatic duct and joins it posteriorly. *H.* Cystic duct courses posteriorly to common hepatic duct and joins it anteriorly. (*After W. H. Hollinshead, "Anatomy for Surgeons," vol. II, Hoeber Medical Division, Harper & Row, Publishers, Inc., New York, 1956.*)

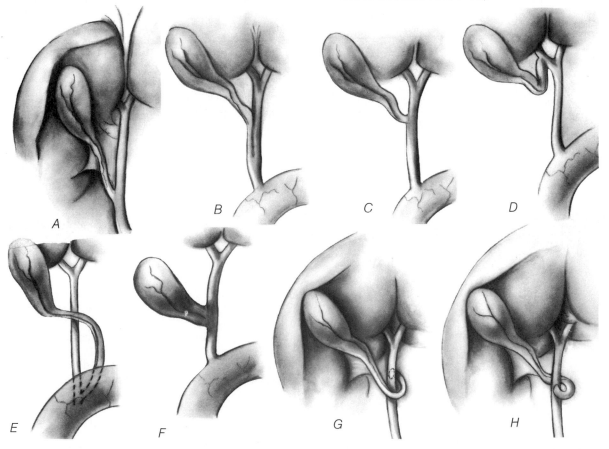

A   *B*   *C*   *D*

E   *F*   *G*   *H*

acute angle, and the right branch of the hepatic artery resides immediately behind it. Variations of the cystic duct are surgically important, relating to the point of union with the common hepatic duct (Fig. 31-1). The cystic duct may run parallel to the common hepatic duct and actually be adherent to it, or it may be extremely long and unite with the hepatic duct in the duodenum. On the other hand, the cystic duct may be absent or very short, and there may be an extremely high union with the hepatic duct. In some instances, the cystic duct may spiral either anteriorly or posteriorly in relation to the hepatic duct and join the common hepatic duct on the left side. The segment of the cystic duct adjacent to the gallbladder bears a variable number of mucosal folds which have been referred to as the "valves of Heister" but do not have valvular function.

Anomalies

The classic description of the extrahepatic biliary passages and their arteries applies in only about one-third of the patients. An appreciation of the great frequency of anomalies is critical to avoid errors in surgical technique. Important anomalies of the gallbladder relate to number, position, and form (Fig. 31-2). Isolated congenital absence of the gallbladder is extremely rare; autopsy incidences of 0.03 percent have been computed. Before the diagnosis is made, the presence of an intrahepatic vesicle or a left-sided organ must be ruled out. Duplication of the gallbladder with two separate cavities and two separate cystic ducts has an incidence of approximately 1 in 4,000. The accessory gallbladder may be situated on the left side, and its cystic duct may empty into the left hepatic duct rather than the common duct. Pathologic processes such as cholelithiasis and cholecystitis may involve one organ while the other is spared.

The gallbladder may be found in a variety of abnormal positions. The so-called "floating gallbladder" occurs when there is an increase in the peritoneal investment. The organ may be completely invested by peritoneum with no mesentery, in which case only the cystic duct and artery connect it to the liver. In other instances, the gallbladder may be suspended from the liver by a complete mesentery, or the neck may have a mesentery in which the cystic artery lies, while the fundus and body are free. This condition is relatively common, occurring in about 5 percent of the cases. This anomaly predisposes to torsion and resulting gangrene or perforation of the viscus. Left-sided gallbladder with the cystic duct entering directly into the left hepatic duct or common duct is extremely rare, as is the situation known as *retrodisplacement,* in which the fundus extends backward in the free margin of the gastrohepatic omentum. The gallbladder may also be totally intrahepatic, a situation occurring in many animals. In man, the partial or completely intrahepatic gallbladder is associated with an increased incidence of cholelithiasis.

The anomalies in the cystic duct have been referred to (Fig. 31-1). Accessory hepatic ducts are present in approximately 15 percent of cases. Large ducts are usually single and drain a portion of the right lobe of the liver joining the right hepatic duct, common hepatic duct, or infundibulum of the gallbladder. Small ducts (Luschka) may drain directly from the liver into the body of the gallbladder. It is the frequent incidence of the accessory hepatic ducts and the fact that they are overlooked during cholecystectomy that impel many surgeons to drain the hepatorenal pouch routinely following this operation.

Anomalies of the hepatic artery and cystic artery are very common (Fig. 31-3). The large accessory left hepatic artery, originating from the left gastric artery, occurs in about 5 percent of cases. In about 20 percent of cases, the right hepatic artery originates from the superior mesenteric artery, and in about 5 percent of cases there are two hepatic arteries—one originating from the common hepatic and the other from the superior mesenteric artery. The right hepatic artery is vulnerable during surgical procedures, particularly when it parallels the cystic duct and is adherent to it or when it resides in the mesentery of the gallbladder. In 10 percent of cases, the cystic artery originates from the left hepatic artery or from the junction of the left or right hepatic arteries with the common hepatic artery. In about 15 percent of cases, the cystic artery passes in front of the common hepatic duct, rather than to the right of or posterior to this duct. Double cystic arteries occur in about 25 percent of cases, and they may both arise from the right hepatic artery, or one may have an abnormal origin.

Fig. 31-2. Anomalies of the gallbladder. *A.* Double gallbladder with single cystic duct. *B.* Bilobed gallbladder. *C.* Intrahepatic gallbladder. *D.* Left-sided gallbladder.

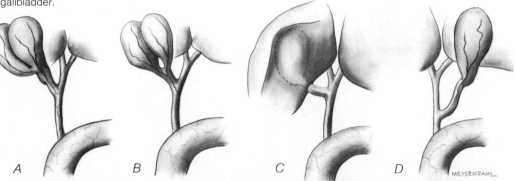

A   *B*   *C*   *D*   MEISENZAHL

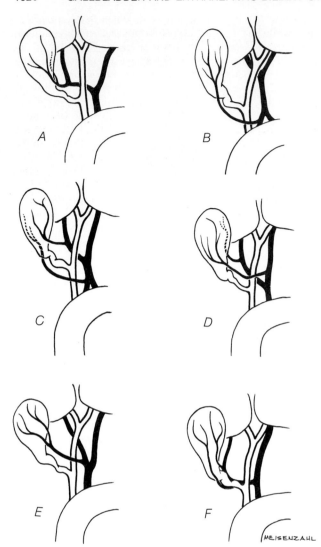

Fig 31-3. Anomalies of the arteries to the gallbladder. *A.* Cystic artery arises from right hepatic artery in 95 percent of cases. *B.* Cystic artery arises from gastroduodenal artery. *C.* Two cystic arteries, one arising from right hepatic artery and the other from common hepatic artery. *D.* Two cystic arteries. Abnormal one arises from left hepatic artery and crosses common hepatic duct anteriorly. *E.* Cystic artery arises from right hepatic artery but courses anterior to common hepatic duct. *F.* Two cystic arteries arising from right hepatic artery. Right hepatic artery is adherent to cystic duct and neck of gallbladder. Posterior cystic artery is very short (a common finding).

CYSTIC DISEASE OF THE EXTRAHEPATIC BILIARY TRACT (CHOLEDOCHAL CYST)

Congenital cystic abnormalities may occur throughout the entire biliary system, i.e., from intrahepatic biliary radicals to the terminal common duct. Intrahepatic cystic dilatation is discussed in Chap. 30, Liver. The present discussion is limited to extrahepatic cystic disease according to the original classification of Alonso-Lej et al. and the more recent classic review of Longmire et al.

Choledochal cyst (Alonso-Lej type A), the most common

congenital cyst of the extrahepatic biliary tract, occurs four times more frequently in females. There are three major varieties: cystic dilatation involving the entire common bile duct and common hepatic duct with the cystic duct entering the choledochal cyst; a small cyst usually localized to the distal common bile duct; and diffuse fusiform dilatation of the common bile duct. Over 30 percent of cases are diagnosed within the first decade of life. The clinical manifestations include pain, jaundice, and a palpable epigastric mass. The pain and jaundice are frequently intermittent and are generally progressive in severity. Diagnosis is occasionally established by cholangiography. But the highest diagnostic yield is associated with ^{131}I rose Bengal and other isotopic scans. Untreated cases may progress to complete biliary obstruction, cholangitis, secondary biliary cirrhosis, or spontaneous rupture, which occurs frequently during pregnancy. Early operation is therefore indicated.

A variety of operative procedures have been prescribed, but the preferable approach is cystojejunostomy, employing either a long antecolic limb with enteroenterostomy or the Roux en Y procedure (Fig. 31-4). Decompression may also be effected by a cystoduodenostomy (Fig. 31-5). Longmire et al. have advised cholecystectomy at the time of cyst drainage to obviate postoperative cholecystitis. Although a higher mortality rate is associated with the operation, some have advised excision of the cyst followed by hepatodochojejunostomy.

Congenital diverticulum (Alonso-Lej type B) is a rare disorder in which the cyst is connected by a stalk to the common duct, a hepatic duct, or the gallbladder and can be totally excised. The choledochocele (Alonso-Lej type C) is the least common cystic dilatation and involves only the intraduodenal portion of the common bile duct. Other cystic anomalies include multiple cystic dilatations of the common and hepatic ducts and unexplained diffuse ductal dilatations, usually manifested by repeated bouts of jaundice and cholangitis, pigment stones, and sludged bile. Choledochoduodenostomy has not been uniformly satisfactory, and at times hepaticojejunostomy may be required.

CONGENITAL BILIARY ATRESIA

Congenital atresia of the extrahepatic bile ducts is the most common cause of prolonged obstructive jaundice in the neonatal period. Although the entity was first described by Aristotle, it was not until 1916 that an operative approach was suggested.

INCIDENCE. It is estimated that biliary atresia may be expected to occur once in every 20,000 to 30,000 births. There are an equal number of males and females, and all races are represented in numbers proportional to their frequency in the population. A familial occurrence has been reported. Of 156 cases of prolonged obstructive jaundice seen at the Children's Medical Center in Boston from 1940 to 1951, 61 percent were due to biliary atresia.

PATHOLOGY. Coexistence of atresia of the extrahepatic and intrahepatic ducts supports the belief that a developmental anomaly is the basic defect. The developing bile ducts pass through a solid stage analogous to that of the intestine, becoming obliterated by epithelial concrescence or proliferation. In the course of normal development, this solid core becomes vacuolated, and the vacuoles coalesce to reestablish the lumen. The order of succession and appearance of the lumen is common bile duct, hepatic duct, cystic duct, and gallbladder. An arrest in this solid stage affords the best explanation for the malformation, and innumerable anomalies are possible (Fig. 31-6).

Stowens reported that 10 percent of the cases had complete absence of all extrahepatic ducts, 64 percent had partial absence, 11 percent had total atresia of the hepatic bile ducts associated with normal common ducts, 7 percent had atresia of the visible larger intrahepatic ducts, 5 percent had atresia of the intrahepatic bile canaliculi, and 3 percent demonstrated only stenosis. The atretic segment may not be identifiable or may appear as a thin, fibrous cord.

The obliterative process may involve the common duct, cystic duct, one or both hepatic ducts, and the gallbladder in a variety of combinations. With atresia of the distal portion of the common duct system, dilatation of the proximal portion and the gallbladder may be noted. The liver is usually enlarged, dark green, and in the late stages of disease diffusely nodular. Histologically, there is an increased amount of fibrous tissue in the periportal areas and proliferation of the bile duct with intraductal stasis. The signs of biliary cirrhosis may be apparent. Coexisting intrahepatic atresia is present in 3 to 5 percent of the cases. Approximately one-quarter of the patients have coincidental malformations including congenital heart disease, imperforate anus, duodenal atresia, mongolism, and, most commonly, urinary tract involvement.

CLINICAL MANIFESTATIONS. Jaundice, a constant finding, is usually present at birth or shortly thereafter but does not become marked until the child is two to three weeks old, after which it becomes progressively more intense. Initially, the growth and weight gains of the children are within normal limits, but in later stages of disease malnutrition and retarded growth may be apparent. Abdominal enlargement is frequent and may be related to hepatomegaly or, rarely, accumulation of ascites. In extended cases, the spleen may also be enlarged, and the anteroabdominal wall veins may be apparent, reflecting portal hypertension. Later in the course of the disease, the effects of limited absorption of fat-soluble vitamins may become apparent with bone changes and other signs of deficiency. Petechiae and subcutaneous hemorrhages are uncommon but suggest a reduction in prothrombin time secondary to vitamin K deficiency.

LABORATORY STUDIES. A mild anemia may be noted in the later course of the disease. The urine is dark and positive for bile, and contains no urobilinogen. The stools are acholic with pasty consistency. The initial stool may have a normal green color, since it is formed at the fourth month of fetal development and the obstruction of the biliary tract may occur after that time. Later, the occasional appearance of a yellow color in the stool and a positive test for bile may be explained by the excretion of small amounts of pigment by the glands of the intestinal tract. The serum bilirubin progressively increases with ultimate establishment of extremely high levels. Weekly determi-

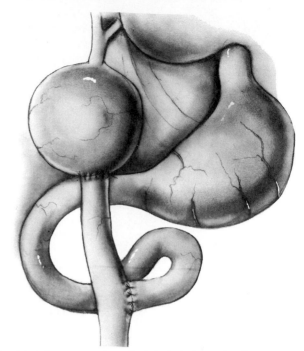

Fig. 31-4. Decompression of choledochal cyst by Roux en Y procedure.

nations for a period of 1 month is considered to be the single most valuable laboratory aid. High levels of alkaline phosphatase are common. Elevations in the serum transaminase levels with serum glutamic oxaloacetic transaminase (SGOT) between 400 and 500 have been reported.

DIFFERENTIAL DIAGNOSIS. Neonatal jaundice may also be due to (1) physiologic changes, (2) constitutional deficiency, (3) hemolytic disease, (4) sepsis, (5) neonatal hepatitis, or (6) the inspissated bile syndrome. Physiologic jaundice occurs in approximately two-thirds of full-term

Fig. 31-5. Decompression of choledochal cyst by cystoduodenostomy.

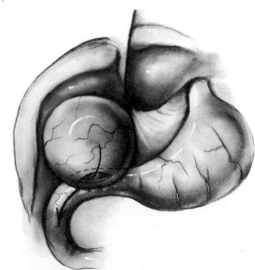

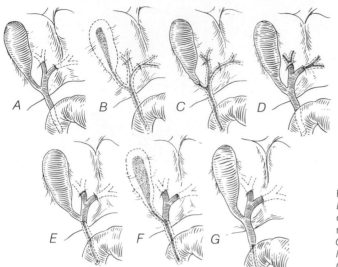

Fig. 31-6. Variations of extrahepatic bile duct atresia. *A.* Normal. *B.* Total atresia of all ducts. *C.* Atresia of all ducts with exception of gallbladder. *D.* Intrahepatic ductal atresia. *E.* Atresia of common bile duct. *F.* Atresia of common bile duct and gallbladder. *G.* Segmental atresia of distal common bile duct. (*From Seymour I. Schwartz, "Surgical Diseases of the Liver," McGraw-Hill Book Company, New York, 1964.*)

infants and more frequently in premature infants. It is due to the destruction of fetal red cells which are no longer required after birth and the normal functional immaturity of the liver at birth, which is unable to excrete the excessive load of pigment presented to it. The jaundice reaches its peak within 2 to 5 days after delivery and then gradually disappears. The serum bilirubin levels rarely exceed 10 mg/100 ml.

Of the constitutional deficiencies causing hyperbilirubinemia, only the rare Crigler-Najjar syndrome manifests itself early. The total serum bilirubin is usually over 10 mg/100 ml, and the greater proportion is unconjugated. There is always an associated hepatomegaly, and kernicterus is a common complication. The patients usually die early, although some may survive without neurologic deficit. Another hepatic disturbance with familial tendency is related to the ingestion of lactose in infants with galactosemia. An obstructive type of jaundice appears after the first week of life and subsides immediately when lactose is removed from the diet. If the lactose is not withheld, the jaundice spontaneously subsides over a period of several weeks. Examination of the urine for reducing substances provides the diagnosis.

Hemolysis due to blood grouping incompatibility between fetus and mother may result in neonatal jaundice. Jaundice may intensify until death ensues or until a gradual recovery takes place in several weeks. The increase in the bilirubin is in the unconjugated portion, the urine contains bilirubin and urobilinogen, and a positive Coombs test confirms the diagnosis for Rh incompatibility but may be negative with ABO incompatibility. Overwhelming sepsis can cause damage to the liver and jaundice. Recent interest has been directed toward cytomegalic inclusion disease with jaundice occurring in the first week or later and accompanied by hepatomegaly and splenomegaly, microcephaly and mental retardation, motor disability, and petechiae.

Twenty-five percent of cases of prolonged obstructive jaundice in infancy have been ascribed to neonatal hepa-

titis. The usual clinical picture is that of a fluctuating jaundice which appears during the early weeks of life. Liver function tests contribute little to the differential diagnosis, but liver biopsy may be diagnostic by demonstrating the microscopic picture of local necrosis and large multinucleated liver cells. Neonatal jaundice may also be caused by the "inspissated bile syndrome," which accounted for 15 percent of the cases in one large series. The term is applied to patients with normal biliary tracts who have had persistent signs of obstructive jaundice. Increased viscosity of bile and obstruction of the canaliculi are implicated as causes. Most cases are related to hemolytic disease, but in some instances no etiologic factor can be defined. It is now felt that many of the cases which were classified as the "inspissated bile syndrome" were, in fact, instances of prolonged hemolytic disease, hepatitis, cirrhosis, or cholangitis.

The clinical approach to persistent obstructive jaundice in infancy is directed at defining the cause and, more particularly, determining whether operative intervention is indicated and, if so, optimal timing. Several criteria are used to establish the diagnosis of biliary atresia. The conventional liver function tests are of little value, since they are normal in patients with either biliary atresia or "inspissated bile syndrome" and also frequently normal in patients with neonatal hepatitis. The alkaline phosphatase level is of little value, since it is elevated in all types of obstructive jaundice. Examination of the serum bilirubin level is helpful in that a slowly rising serum bilirubin level is to be expected with biliary atresia. Needle biopsy may be indicated to establish the diagnosis of neonatal hepatitis. The radioactive rose bengal test measuring the excretion of radioactivity in the stool has made it possible to differentiate between severe biliary obstruction of hepatitis and complete obstruction associated with biliary atresia. The maximal radioactivity consistent with the diagnosis of biliary atresia is between 2 and 4 percent. Higher levels may be reached with hepatitis. Determination of indocyanine green also has been used. Lipoprotein X is present in the serum of patients with cholestasis. An increase after administration of cholestyramine is evidence that an operation should be performed; a decrease suggests nonoperative management of the jaundice.

TREATMENT. Timing of the surgical operation is critical. This should be deferred if there is any evidence of bile in the duodenal fluid or stool or if the bilirubin has shown a tendency to decrease. However, surgical intervention is indicated if there is a consistent absence of bile in the stool, a continued rise in the serum bilirubin level, and no urobilinogen in the urine. Most investigators have advised early operative intervention, since biliary atresia may give rise to irreparable damage to the liver within $2\frac{1}{2}$ months. Well-established cirrhosis has been noted at six weeks, and almost all successfully treated patients have been operated on under the age of two months.

After the peritoneal cavity has been entered, liver biopsy should be performed, and a frozen section may be examined in order to rule out the possibility of intrahepatic bile duct atresia or neonatal hepatitis. Dissection is initiated in the region of the gastrohepatic ligament in an attempt to define the common hepatic ducts and/or atresic segments. If a proximal filled bile duct is not encountered, attention is directed toward the gallbladder. If the gallbladder contains a lumen, the fundus is opened to determine the characteristics of the fluid within (white bile indicates obstruction of the cystic duct; normal-appearing bile in the gallbladder implies that both the hepatic and cystic ducts are patent). The free flow of saline solution injected into the gallbladder suggests that the cystic and common duct are patent. An operative cholangiogram is useful in defining the pathologic anatomy in this situation. If no gallbladder is found, exploration is continued in the region of the porta hepatis with efforts directed at delineating the hepatic duct stump. During dissection possible residual or rudimentary structures which appear as tiny cords without lumens should be handled with great care

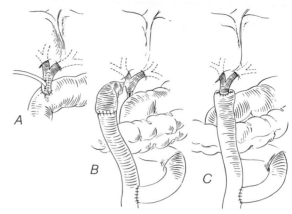

Fig. 31-7. Decompression of biliary tract. *A.* Choledochoduodenostomy. *B.* Cholecystojejunostomy (Roux en Y); *C.* Hepaticodochojejunostomy (Roux en Y). (*From Seymour I. Schwartz, "Surgical Diseases of the Liver," McGraw-Hill Book Company, New York, 1964.*)

and preserved, since there is evidence that bile ducts continue to grow after birth.

If a proximal segment of the extrahepatic bile duct system is patent, this can be decompressed by choledochoduodenostomy, cholecystojejunostomy, or hepaticodochoduodenostomy, depending on the circumstance (Fig. 31-7). In those cases without an identifiable extrahepatic biliary system, in which liver biopsy demonstrates the presence of intrahepatic ducts, transhepatic drainage should be attempted. Ksai has popularized the hepatic portoenterostomy with a double Roux en Y anastomosis, including an external vent to prevent ascending cholangitis. A single Roux en Y portoenterostomy is also used (Fig. 31-8).

A few patients who had been considered noncorrectible have been salvaged at a "second look" operation, since there is some evidence that the development of bile ducts is merely retarded and growth continues after birth, providing a situation which becomes correctible. Orthotopic total liver transplantation has been applied in patients with biliary atresia involving the intrahepatic duct, with result-

Fig. 31-8. Transhepatic drainage. *A.* Cholangiojejunostomy with partial left hepatic lobectomy. *B.* Cholangiojejunostomy through main interlobar plane. (*From Seymour I. Schwartz, "Surgical Diseases of the Liver," McGraw-Hill Book Company, New York, 1964.*)

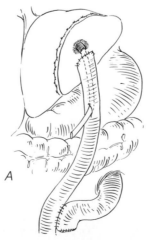

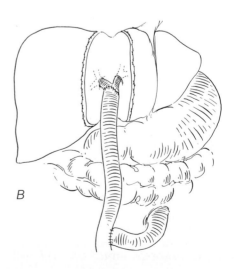

ant reduction in bilirubin levels and normal liver function extending for several years.

In general, the operative results have been poor. Even when good bile drainage has been established, cholangitis, cirrhosis, and portal hypertension eventually develop.

PHYSIOLOGY

BILE SECRETION. The normal adult with an intact hepatic circulation and consuming an average diet secretes from the hepatic cells 250 to 1,100 ml bile per day. This is an active process which is dependent upon hepatic blood flow and an oxygen supply available to the hepatic cell. The secretion of bile is responsive to neurogenic, humoral, and chemical control. Vagal stimulation increases secretion, whereas stimulation of the splanchnic nerves results in vasoconstriction and decreased bile flow. The release of secretin from the duodenum following the stimulus of hydrochloric acid, breakdown products of protein, and fatty acids results in an increased bile flow. Bile salts are very effective choleretics, acting directly on the liver to augment secretion.

COMPOSITION OF BILE. The main constituents of bile include electrolytes, bile salts, proteins, cholesterol, fats, and bile pigments. Sodium, potassium, calcium, and chloride have approximately the same concentration in bile as in plasma. There is a direct relation between the volume rate of secretion and the electrolyte concentration. As the former increases, there is an increase in bicarbonate and pH and a slight increase in chloride. The pH of liver bile, which usually ranges between 5.7 and 8.6, tending to the alkaline side, varies with the diet, an increase in protein ingestion shifting the pH to the acid side.

Bile salts act as anions which are balanced by sodium. The major salts, cholic, deoxycholic, and chenodeoxycholic acids, conjugate with taurine or glycine and are present in the bile in concentrations of 10 to 20 mEq/L. The bile salt anion has extremly weak osmotic activity because of its tendency to form large molecular aggregates. Proteins are present in lesser concentrations than in plasma, with the exception of mucoproteins and lipoproteins, which contribute to the composition of bile but are not present in plasma. Liver bile contains 0.6 to 1.7 Gm/L unesterified cholesterol, 1 to 5 Gm/L lecithin, and 3 Gm/L neutrofat, which in turn consists of palmitic, oleic, and linoleic acids. The concentrations of both cholesterol and phospholipids are lower in liver bile than in plasma.

The color of the bile secreted by the liver is related to the presence of the pigment bilirubin diglucuronide, which is the metabolic product of hemoglobin and is secreted into the bile in concentrations 100 times greater than that present in the plasma. After this pigment has been acted upon by the bacteria in the intestine and converted into urobilinogen, a small fraction of the urobilinogen is absorbed and also secreted into the bile. A variety of dyes foreign to the body, such as sulfobromophthalein (BSP), rose bengal, and indocyanine green, are removed from the blood by the liver, concentrated, and secreted into the bile.

GALLBLADDER FUNCTION. The gallbladder provides storage and concentration of bile, using the mechanisms of absorption, secretion, and motor activity. Sodium, chloride, and water are selectively absorbed, while the absorption of potassium and calcium is less complete and the concentration of bicarbonate in the gallbladder bile is twice that in plasma. This absorption of water and electrolytes results in a tenfold concentration of bile salts, bile pigments, and cholesterol in relation to levels present in liver bile. The gallbladder mucosa has the greatest absorptive power per unit area of any structure in the body, and this rapid absorption prevents a rise in pressure within the biliary system under normal circumstances.

Secretion of mucus in amounts approximating 20 ml/24 hr, protects the mucosa from the lytic action of bile and facilitates the passage of bile through the cystic duct. This mucus makes up the colorless "white bile" present in hydrops of the gallbladder resulting from obstruction of the cystic duct. The gallbladder also secretes calcium in the presence of inflammation or obstruction of the cystic duct.

Motor activity is a critical function, since the passage of bile into the duodenum requires the coordinated contraction of the gallbladder and relaxation of the sphincter of Oddi. In addition to rhythmic contractions occurring two to six times per minute and mediating of pressure less than 30 mm water, tonic contractions lasting 5 to 30 minutes increase the pressure within the gallbladder up to 300 mm water. Since the hepatic secretory pressure is 375 mm water and is greater than the maximal pressure mediated within the gallbladder, the passage of bile is dependent upon the relaxation of the sphincter of Oddi. The gallbladder empties following humoral or nervous stimulation. The main stimulus in man is cholecystokinin, which is released from the intestinal mucosa in response to food, particularly fat entering the duodenum. Following the intravenous injection of cholecystokinin, the gallbladder begins to contract in 1 to 2 minutes and is two-thirds evacuated within 30 minutes. Evacuation of the gallbladder occurs a half hour after a fatty meal. Cholecystokinin also relaxes the terminal bile duct, the sphincter of Oddi, and the duodenal musculature. Splanchnic sympathetic stimulation is inhibitory to the motor activity of the gallbladder, while the vagus stimulates contraction. Although vagotomy for duodenal ulcer will increase the size and volume of the gallbladder, the rate of emptying is unchanged. A gallbladder which contains calculi should be removed concomitantly with vagotomy in view of a significant incidence of early postoperative cholecystitis in this circumstance reported by Schein. Parasympathomimetic drugs such as pilocarpine and neostigmine contract the gallbladder, whereas atropine tends to relax the organ. Magnesium sulfate acts as a potent evacuator of the gallbladder. Hydrochloric acid and bile salts have little direct effect on motor activity.

The common bile duct was generally regarded as an inert tube until recent cineradiographic studies demonstrated waves of peristalsis. The sphincter of Oddi is a major factor in the evacuation of bile. During starvation, the sphincter maintains an intraductal pressure approximating the maximal expulsive power of the gallbladder, i.e., 300 mm water, and thus prevents evacuation. Following the ingestion of food, this is reduced to 100 mm water. When pressures within the biliary system are greater than 360 mm water, there is suppression of bile secretion. Following obstruction or occlusion of the common bile duct, the time required to reach this pressure level and to result in jaundice is dependent upon the presence and function of the gallbladder. When the gallbladder is absent, the bilirubin levels are raised within 6 hours of total occlusion, while with a functioning gallbladder jaundice may not occur for 46 to 48 hours.

Motor Dysfunction. Biliary dyskinesia, a term introduced by Westphal in 1923, lacks objective findings. It was originally used to describe functional disturbances of biliary tract motility which occurred in the absence of anatomic changes and were related to alterations in autonomic reflex activity. Subsequently, the term has been applied to both this primary condition and situations secondary to other biliary tract diseases, such as cholecystitis and cholelithiasis, and following biliary tract surgical treatment. However, the origin of biliary tract pain itself has not been precisely defined. Experiments inducing gallbladder contraction by fatty foods and cholecystokinin in the presence of a closed sphincter of Oddi have demonstrated that pain can result from motor incoordination. The factor of distension remains suspect, but this is difficult to implicate, since above pressures of 300 to 360 mm water bile secretion ceases. Acute distension of the common bile duct produced by inflation of a balloon-tipped catheter results in colicky pain. When identical pressures are used but dilatation is increased gradually, distress rather than colic results. Biliary tract pain has also been related to spasm of the sphincter of Oddi per se. Recently, Jutras has introduced the concept of hyperplastic cholecystoses, characterized by a functional abnormality manifested by hyperconcentrating and excessive emptying of the gallbladder on cholecystogram. Cholecystectomy is reported to be curative in symptomatic patients, but results are difficult to evaluate.

DIAGNOSIS OF BILIARY TRACT DISEASE

(See also Jaundice, in Chap. 24.)

Radiologic Studies

ROUTINE ABDOMINAL X-RAYS (Fig. 31-9). Plain films of the abdomen prior to the administration of any radiopaque material are indicated, since biliary calculi have been demonstrated in up to 15 percent of cases, and faintly calcified stones may be rendered invisible when contrast materials surround them. Demonstration of calculi on plain films is dependent upon the presence of calcium. Bile pigment calculi, which are characteristically associated with hemolytic disorders, are nonradiopaque, but in 10 percent of the cases they contain sufficient amounts of calcium to be noted on routine x-ray. Similarly, the pure cholesterol calculus is nonradiopaque, whereas calcium carbonate calculi are all visible. Gallstones formed in association with infection or inflammation are generally

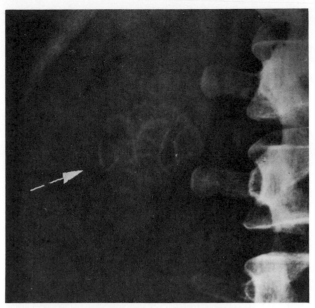

Fig. 31-9. Routine abdominal x-ray demonstrating radiopaque biliary calculi in gallbladder.

mixed and contain two or all elements. Their visibility is dependent upon the amount of calcium present.

CHOLECYSTOGRAPHY. In 1924, Graham and Cole introduced the use of contrast media for visualizing the gallbladder. There has been a gradual improvement in the radiopacity and toxicity of the contrast media, and the radiologic examination which was limited to the gallbladder has been extended to visualization of the bile ducts. In the 1950s, biligrafin and cholegrafin were administered intravenously to provide for rapid visualization of the biliary tract independent of the gallbladder's ability to concentrate. These drugs outline the major intrahepatic and extrahepatic ducts, and occasionally the gallbladder will visualize with cholegrafin after failure to do so with an orally administered agent such as Telepaque.

Successful visualization of the gallbladder by a radiopaque iodine-containing compound is dependent upon blood flow to the liver, functional ability of the liver cell to excrete the dye into the bile, patency of the hepatic and cystic duct system, and water absorption by the gallbladder to concentrate the excreted dye. Most diseases of the gallbladder reduce the absorptive capacity in the mucosa; an exception is cholesterosis, in which the dye may concentrate beyond normal. The primary examination of the gallbladder should be performed with an oral medium, while intravenous examination is used to define the common duct and extrahepatic bile duct, particularly in the absence of the gallbladder.

Oral Cholecystography. This procedure (Fig. 31-10) provides visualization of the normal gallbladder. Subsequent to the ingestion of a fatty meal, contraction begins promptly, and within 40 minutes the gallbladder should be reduced to at least one-third or one-fourth of its normal size. The abnormal cholecystogram may demonstrate poor visualization or nonvisualization of the gallbladder or may indicate the presence of filling defects such as calculi or

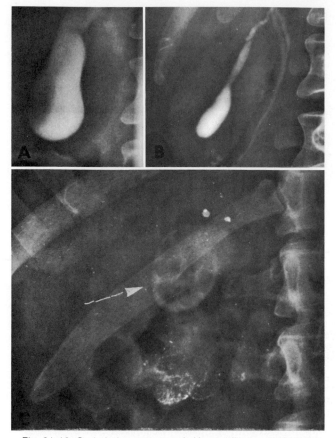

Fig. 31-10. Oral cholecystogram. *A.* Normal filled gallbladder. *B.* Normal emptying subsequent to fatty meal. This film also shows cystic duct and common bile duct and entrance of dye into duodenum. *C.* Calculi present in gallbladder as evidenced by radiolucent areas.

tumors. Reliability of the Telepaque examination has been reported as 98 percent accurate when compared with surgical findings. Nonvisualization with the use of the dye may be caused by failure to retain the oral medication, faulty absorption such as with pyloric obstruction, hepatic dysfunction, hepatic or cystic duct obstruction, loss of concentrating ability of the gallbladder mucosa, or faulty x-ray technique. Oral cholecystography is seldom effective if the serum bilirubin is over 1.8 mg/100 ml. Approximately 2 percent of nonopacifying gallbladders have been found to be normal at operation with no obvious reason for failure to concentrate the oral dye. Oral cholecystography is the best method of demonstrating calculi, either by direct visualization of filling defects or by demonstration of a nonopacifying gallbladder, which is associated with a 90 percent incidence of calculi. This technique has also been applied to the differential diagnosis of acute cholecystitis. If the gallbladder fills, the lesion can be excluded, but failure to fill is of little significance, since it may be related to vomiting and the patient's inability to retain or absorb contrast medium. Examination of the extrahepatic bile ducts by oral cholecystography can be accomplished in approximately 80 percent of patients whose gallbladders are visualized. Recently cholecystoki-

nin (CCK) cholangiography has been used to define gallbladder disease in patients with suggestive pain and a normal cholecystogram. 75 Ivy units of CCK are instilled intraduodenally or intravenously. The normal gallbladder will demonstrate a volume reduction greater than 50 percent in 20 minutes.

Intravenous Cholecystography. This technique (Fig. 31-11) is applied when there is failure of the gallbladder to visualize after oral cholecystography or there is inability of the patient to retain or absorb the orally administered medication. The technique is particularly applicable to the visualization of bile ducts in cholecystectomized patients, since oral administration of Telepaque results in demonstration of the ducts in only about 40 percent of the cases. The test is preferable to oral cholecystography to evaluate the status of the gallbladder in a patient with an acute condition in the abdomen. Intravenous cholecystography is of little value if the serum bilirubin is greater than 3.5 mg/100 ml, with the exception of the situation of hemolytic jaundice, in which case there is no impairment of gallbladder visualization. The standard dose of 20 ml of 52 percent Cholagrafin is associated with fewer adverse reactions than the infusion technique. The SGOT is elevated in 9 percent of patients receiving the single dose and in 18 percent of those receiving a double dose.

PERCUTANEOUS TRANSHEPATIC CHOLANGIOGRAPHY. See also Jaundice, in Chap. 24.

Fig. 31-11. Intravenous cholangiogram showing normal common duct and arborization of ducts in the liver. There is no evidence of ductal obstruction or choledocholithiasis.

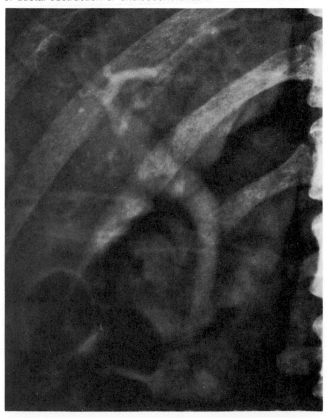

Operative Cholangiography (T-tube Cholangiography). This procedure (Fig. 31-12) is frequently performed in the operating room at the time of exploration of the biliary tract, with injection of radiopaque material either into the cystic duct or into the T tube placed in the common duct. The main application of cystic duct cholangiography is to avoid common bile duct exploration. It is also used to identify calculi which have escaped palpation in order to avoid a subsequent common duct exploration. The technique may contribute to confusion because of failure of the opaque medium to enter the duodenum despite the fact that there is no abnormality present in the sphincter of Oddi and no obstruction within the common duct. Postoperative cholangiography is usually performed in the x-ray suite prior to removal of a T tube to demonstrate the patency of the common duct, the absence of retained stones, and free passage of bile into the duodenum. The most rewarding technique employs 10 to 15 ml 50 percent Hypaque diluted to 30 ml with saline solution and administered slowly.

Isotopic Scans (Fig. 31-13)

A variety of isotopes which are secreted in the bile have been used to define gallbladder function and pathology. ^{131}I rose Bengal, ^{99m}Tc-dihydrothiotic acid, and ^{99m}Tc-pyridoxylideneglutamate are among the preparations employed. Accumulation of activity in the gallbladder has been recorded by a gamma camera. The isotopic technique has also been combined with computer axial tomography. The advantage of the technique is that the isotopes are administered intravenously and are not associated with the adverse reactions which occasionally accompany intravenous cholecystography. The absence of visualization of the gallbladder is highly suggestive of cholecystitis.

Cholangiomanometry

This procedure, which frequently combines determination of bile duct pressure (normal is 12 ± 3 cm) and flow of an infused solution (normal is 23.0 ± 7 ml/min), is widely used by the European surgeon but rarely used in North America. Proponents of the method suggest that the additional 5 minutes of operative time increases the yield for diagnoses of abnormalities in the common duct, stones in the distal end of the duct, and most particularly organic changes in the sphincter which cause functional changes.

TRAUMA

Penetrating and Nonpenetrating Injuries of the Gallbladder

Injuries of the gallbladder are uncommon, as evidenced by Penn's collective review of 5,670 abdominal injuries in which there was an incidence of 1.9 percent. However, in one series, an incidence of 8.6 percent was recorded for involvement of the gallbladder in war injuries of the abdo-

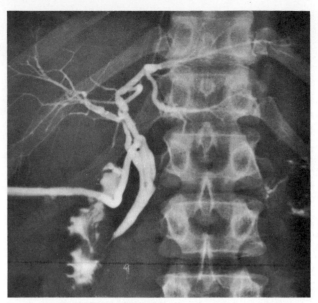

Fig. 31-12. T-tube cholangiogram demonstrating normal caliber of duct with absence of choledocholithiasis. Liver arborization is normal. Tapering at terminal portion of common bile duct is normal, and radiopaque material is noted in duodenum.

men. Penetrating injuries are usually due to gunshot wounds or stab wounds and occur rarely during attempted needle biopsy of the liver, particularly in patients with obstructive jaundice. Nonpenetrating injuries are most frequently caused by automobile accidents, kicks, blows, and falls. They are extremely rare; only about 50 cases have been reported. The associated visceral damage with both penetrating and nonpenetrating gallbladder injuries includes involvement of the liver in 72 percent, small bowel in 36 percent, colon in 32 percent, and in only 20 percent of the cases the gallbladder alone. Although it is very uncommon for the gallbladder to be the only organ involved with nonpenetrating injuries to the abdomen, isolated involvement of the gallbladder due to penetrating injuries is relatively frequent.

The types of injuries include (1) contusions, (2) avulsion, (3) rupture, and (4) traumatic cholecystitis. Contusion is difficult to verify but may be associated with vague or temporary symptoms which require no specific therapy. The contused area may undergo necrosis and perforate. Avulsion of the gallbladder from its liver bed occurs as a result of nonpenetrating injury. When the gallbladder's attachments are torn, the organ usually hangs by its neck but may be attached only by the cystic duct and artery. Volvulus of the gallbladder may result. Traumatic cholecystectomy, in which the cystic duct, cystic artery, and gallbladder attachments are transected, has been reported. An acutely inflamed gallbladder may be avulsed from the liver as a result of minor trauma. Laceration is the most common type of injury following penetrating wounds but also may result from blunt trauma. Cases of delayed rupture of the gallbladder occur days to weeks following injury. Traumatic cholecystitis is an unusual condition which occurs as a result of blunt trauma. Bleeding into

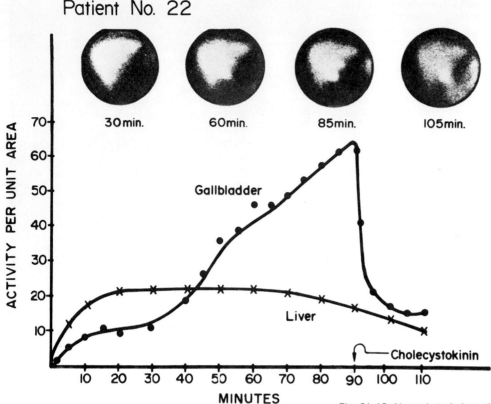

Fig. 31-13. Normal study in patient with pancreatitis. Thirty minutes before study, patient received 75 units of cholecystokinin. Then 150 uCi ^{131}I-rose Bengal was injected; sequential gamma camera images show accumulation, then slow decline of radioactivity in liver. Gallbladder is discernible by 60 minutes, providing evidence that cystic duct is patent. Some bowel activity is apparent by 60 minutes. At 90 minutes additional injection of cholecystokinin is associated with decrease in gallbladder activity and increase in bowel activity on images. Time-activity curves of liver and gallbladder are graphed below images. Characteristics of these curves varied from patient to patient but were unnecessary for diagnosis in this series. (*After Edward A. Eikman, Ann Int Med, 82:308, 1975.*)

the gallbladder, due to injury either of the gallbladder or of the liver, precipitates cholecystitis and, at times, gangrene of the gallbladder. The retained blood may clot and block the cystic duct, and the patient presents with the manifestations of hematobilia, including intermittent jaundice, colicky pain, hematemesis, and melena.

EFFECTS OF INTRAPERITONEAL BILE. Effects of extravasation of bile into the peritoneal cavity depend upon whether or not the bile is infected. When infected bile escapes into the peritoneal cavity, a fulminating and frequently fatal peritonitis results. On the other hand, when bile is sterile, it is well tolerated and results in a chemical peritonitis which may be relatively mild. In the majority of gallbladder injuries, the organ is normal and the bile is sterile. The fact that sterile bile is relatively innocuous is borne out by the very low mortality rate associated with nonpenetrating wounds of the gallbladder. Penetrating wounds are potentially more serious because of the danger of secondary infection. Continuous leakage of noninfected bile, however, is not innocuous. The extravasated bile may produce ascites or become encysted, and extensive chemical peritonitis causes an outpouring of fluid into the peritoneal cavity from the general circulation which may result in shock. There is also some evidence to indicate that absorption of large amounts of bile salts may be toxic.

CLINICAL MANIFESTATIONS. The diagnosis of involvement of the gallbladder or extrahepatic biliary tract is frequently entertained preoperatively in patients with penetrating injuries, in contrast to a low incidence of diagnosis associated with blunt trauma. Bile leakage through the penetrating wound suggests the possibility of damage to the biliary system, but duodenal laceration may have a similar manifestation. With blunt trauma, manifestations may be delayed for 36 hours or more. This has been related to the fact that there are other serious injuries which mask injury of the biliary tract and that the sterile bile causes only minimal symptoms. The presence of severe shock and pain in the right upper quadrant or lower part of the right side of the chest should make one suspicious. The manifestations of bacterial peritonitis may ensue, or if the bile leakage is minimal, the patient may recover only to subsequently develop ascites or an intraperitoneal cyst. The finding of bile-stained fluid during diagnostic paracentesis is suggestive, but a negative tap does not exclude gallbladder injury. In most instances, the diagnosis is made at laparotomy, emphasizing the necessity for careful examination of the biliary system following abdominal trauma.

TREATMENT. The injured gallbladder has been successfully treated by simple suture of the laceration, cholecystostomy, and cholecystectomy. In general, it is preferable to remove the traumatized gallbladder. Cholecystectomy is usually quite easy to perform, since the gallbladder is rarely diseased, and must be performed if the gallbladder has been avulsed or the cystic artery torn. In the severely ill patient, cholecystostomy may be used for treatment of the extensive laceration or traumatic cholecystitis in order to reduce the time of operative procedure and avoid injury to the common duct. Although suture of the clean laceration has been successfully used, this should be applied only infrequently. Prognosis is directly related to the incidence of associated injuries. In the Korean conflict of the 1950s there was no mortality in 33 cases of gallbladder injury.

Injury of the Extrahepatic Bile Ducts

Rare cases of solitary penetrating wounds involving the bile duct have been reported, but there is usually associated trauma to other viscera. Approximately 100 cases of traumatic rupture of the extrahepatic bile duct have been reported, and in 15 cases complete transection occurred. The clinical manifestations are similar to those described for gallbladder injury, and diagnosis is extremely difficult.

Treatment consists initially of meticulous exploration, particularly if injury to the gallbladder has been excluded and bile has been demonstrated retroperitoneally or within the peritoneal cavity. A Kocher maneuver should be performed to rule out perforation of the common duct behind the duodenum. The presence of hematoma in this region should make one suspicious. Complete transection by a knife of either the common hepatic duct or common bile duct is best treated by debridement and an end-to-end anastomosis over a T tube, which should be left in place for several weeks. If the lower end of the common bile duct is severely traumatized, and in most cases of blunt trauma, the proximal end of the duct should be anastomosed to a Roux en Y of jejunum. The patient should be placed on antibiotics, such as ampicillin or tetracycline, which achieve high levels in the bile.

Operative Injury of the Bile Ducts

The great majority of injuries of the extrahepatic biliary duct system are iatrogenic, occurring in the course of gallbladder surgical procedures. In a 15-year period, the Lahey Clinic managed 501 patients with stricture of the bile ducts subsequent to surgical treatment. In over 70 percent of the cases, the cholecystectomy had apparently been carried out without incident. In the remaining 30 percent, a variety of factors were implicated. These included cholecystectomy for contracted gallbladder, intimate association between the ampulla of the gallbladder and the common hepatic duct, massive hemorrhage at the time of operation with attempted "blind control," during which the duct was occluded and traumatized, and excessive tension when ligating a cystic duct. Lack of appreciation of anatomy and possible anomalies in the region increase the incidence of surgical trauma of the common duct.

DIAGNOSIS. In approximately 15 percent of the cases, ductal injuries are recognized and treated at the time of operation. The remaining 85 percent become manifest by either increasing obstructive jaundice or profuse and persistent drainage of bile through a fistula. Jaundice usually becomes manifest in 2 to 3 days but, in some instances, does not develop for weeks. It may be continuous or intermittent; if intermittent, it is frequently accompanied by attacks of chills and fever suggesting ascending cholangitis. Hepatomegaly almost always accompanies jaundice if it has been persistent for a period of time, and splenomegaly may also occur if secondary biliary cirrhosis has evolved. Some patients do not display the signs or symptoms of partial or complete blockage until months or years after surgical treatment. This is related to increasing fibrosis and narrowing of the channel and repeated episodes of cholangitis, which, in turn, leads to fibrosis. The intravenous cholangiogram usually fails to demonstrate the stricture. Percutaneous transhepatic cholangiography may clearly define the site of obstruction and is a helpful procedure. When this is performed on patients with prolonged extrahepatic obstructive jaundice, the bile should be removed before the radiopaque material is injected, and operation should be carried out shortly after the procedure to prevent the consequences of extravasated blood and bile.

TREATMENT. Patients with jaundice or persistent fistula require a vigorous preoperative regimen including a high-protein, low-fat diet and intravenous administration of fat-soluble vitamins, particularly vitamin K. If there is concomitant portal hypertension with bleeding varices, this preempts repair of the common duct, and the portal hypertension is usually best treated by a splenorenal shunt because of extensive scarring of the right upper quadrant. Sedgwick and associates have described 12 such patients, 5 of whom were salvaged.

Operative Approach. Injury of the bile duct recognized during surgical operation should be corrected with an immediate reconstructive procedure. Restoration of the continuity of the duct with an end-to-end anastomosis over a T tube may be feasible. Chronic strictures are also preferably treated by axial anastomosis to preserve sphincteric mechanism, employing a choledocho-choledochostomy or a hepaticocholedochostomy as indicated. However, direct anastomosis is usually impractical, in which case the proximal end of the duct should be anastomosed to a Roux en Y of jejunum. In most instances, the anastomosis is performed over a T or U tube which may be brought out through either the common duct or the intestine. The Longmire operation, with transection of the left lobe of the liver and anastomosis of the jejunum to a large intrahepatic bile duct, has been associated with discouraging results.

In general, the prognosis is good if the initial repair is carried out at the time of injury. The operative mortality of patients with chronic stricture is reported to be 8 percent, and approximately 10 percent of patients die of liver failure or its attendant complications after leaving the hospital. A satisfactory result is obtained in about 70 percent of patients after one or more operative procedures. If the patients are symptom-free 4 years after reconstruction, the cure is almost always permanent.

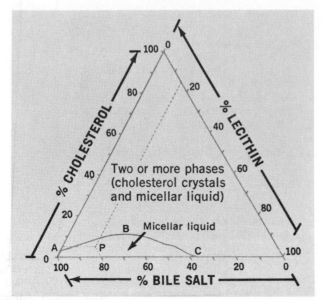

Fig. 31-14. Three major components of bile (bile salts, lecithin, and cholesterol) plotted on triangular coordinates. Point *P* represents bile consisting of 80 mol percent bile salt, 5 percent cholesterol, and 15 percent lecithin. Line *ABC* represents the maximal solubility of cholesterol in varying mixtures of bile salt and lecithin. Because point *P* falls below line *ABC* and within the zone of a single phase of micellar liquid, this bile is less than saturated with cholesterol. Bile with a composition that would place it above line *ABC* would contain excess cholesterol in supersaturated or precipitated form. (*After D. M. Small, Gallstones, N Engl J Med, 279:588, 1968.*)

GALLSTONES

COMPOSITION. The major elements involved in the formation of gallstones are cholesterol, bile pigment, and calcium. Other constituents include iron, phosphorus, carbonates, proteins, carbohydrates, mucus, and cellular debris. In Europe and the United States, most stones are made up of the three major elements and have a particularly high content of cholesterol, averaging 71 percent. These stones have a characteristic central nucleus which was initially thought to consist of epithelial desquamation from the inflamed gallbladder wall, but recently it has been shown that the constituents of the nucleus cannot be distinguished from the rest of the stone. Womack has demonstrated that a prosthesis of mucus is essential, and he suggests that crystal growth in gel may be critical. Surrounding the nucleus are layers of cholesterol and pigment. Most mixed stones are not radiopaque, and radiopacity is dependent upon the amount of calcium.

Pure cholesterol stones are uncommon, usually large with smooth surfaces, and solitary. Bilirubin pigment stones are also uncommon, with a characteristic smooth, glistening green or black surface. The pigment stones may be "pure" or consist of calcium bilirubinate. The "pure" pigment stones are usually associated with hemolytic jaundice or situations in which the bile is abnormally concentrated. Increased red blood cell destruction following cardiac valve replacement has resulted in production of

gallstones. Calcium bilirubinate stones are prevalent in Asia, where they constitute 30 to 40 percent of all gallstones. The bilirubinate content of these stones varies between 40 and 50 percent in contrast to the 0.2 to 5 percent bilirubin present in mixed stones. Cholesterol is also present in the calcium bilirubin stone in concentrations of 3 to 26 percent.

FORMATION. Gallstones form as a result of solids settling out of solution. The recent contribution of Small and his associates provides a working model of this process. The solubility of cholesterol (the predominant crystal in westernized countries) depends on the concentrations of conjugated bile salts, phospholipids, and cholesterol in bile. Lecithin is the predominant phospholipid in bile and, although insoluble in aqueous solutions, is dissolved by bile salts in micelles. Cholesterol is also insoluble in aqueous solution but becomes soluble when incorporated into the lecithin–bile salt micelle. By plotting the percentages of cholesterol, lecithin, and bile salts on triangular coordinates (Fig. 31-14), the limits of micellar liquid in which bile is less than saturated with cholesterol may be defined. Above these limits, the bile is either a supersaturated liquid or a two-phase system of liquid bile and solid crystalline cholesterol. When crystals achieve macroscopic size during a period of entrapment in the gallbladder, gallstones form.

Factors which have been implicated in the formation and precipitation of cholesterol include constitutional elements, bacteria, fungi, reflux of intestinal and pancreatic fluid, hormones, and bile stasis. Constitutional elements are best exemplified in the Pima Indians, of whom 70 percent of females by age 30 and 70 percent of males by age 60 have gallstones. The Masai of Africa, on the other hand, do not have gallstones. Evidence in favor of infection as a cause includes the isolation of such organisms as *Escherichia coli*, *Bacterium typhosum*, and *Streptococcus* from gallbladder walls and centers of stones in a high percentage of cases and the demonstration of slow-growing actinomyces recovered from over half the stones examined in one series. However, the development of gallstones in the absence of infection or inflammation argues against infection as a universal factor. In Oriental people, concretions are known to form about liver flukes and other parasites within the bile ducts.

The reflux factor receives support from the findings of Chaimoff and Dintsman, who demonstrated pancreatic enzymes in the gallbladders of patients with cholelithiasis. Trypsin disturbs colloidal balance, and pancreatic phospholipase A can convert lecithin into toxic lysolecithin. Hormones have been implicated in an unproved correlation between calculi and parity, diabetes, hyperthyroidism, and the predominance in females. It is known that prolonged administration of progesterone and estradiol to rabbits results in the formation of stones, and that symptoms frequently develop in patients during pregnancy.

Stasis, which includes temporary cessation of bile flow into the intestine and stagnation in the gallbladder, has also been assigned a major role. Temporary bile stasis may be due to functional disorders or to a mechanical blockage in the region of the choledochoduodenal junction or gallbladder. The interruption of bile flow to the intestine is associated with an interruption in enterohepatic circulation, which, in turn, is accompanied by a decrease in the output of bile salts and phospholipids, reducing the solubility of cholesterol. When over 20 percent of bile is diverted, the bile salt pool cannot be maintained. Bile salt secretion is also diminished by reduction of the distal third of the intestine, explaining the development of stones in patients with ileal resection or disease.

Solubility has been investigated as a possible regimen to prevent the development of stones in patients at risk and also to dissolve stones already formed. Chenodeoxycholic acid, which replenishes the bile acid pool and reduces cholesterol synthesis and secretion, administered to potential stone formers may return supersaturated bile to its normal composition, preventing stone formation. Oral administration of bile salts can be predicted to dissolve 15 small stones with a cumulative weight of 1 mg in 1 year and one large stone of similar weight in 3 years, according to Small. A question has been raised concerning hepatotoxicity, and the argument is advanced that even if stones disappear, a diseased gallbladder remains.

Asymptomatic Gallstones

Asymptomatic cholelithiasis is rare. Of 3,012 patients with cholecystitis and cholelithiasis, only 134 had no symptoms attributable to gallbladder disease. The liberal use of cholecystography has resulted in the diagnosis of calculi in patients without symptoms referable to the biliary tract. The question has been raised as to whether surgical intervention is indicated in this situation. In several large series of asymptomatic patients with gallstones who were followed without surgical treatment, symptoms developed in 50 percent, and serious complications occurred in 20 percent. An operative mortality of 0.7 percent has been reported for asymptomatic patients, in contrast with 5 percent in cases of acute cholecystitis. The relationship of cholelithiasis and carcinoma of the gallbladder is also of some significance. A review of several series showed that the incidence of calculi in cancer of the gallbladder varied between 65 and 100 percent with a mean of 90 percent. Conversely, the incidence of cancer of the gallbladder in patients with symptomatic gallstones ranged between 1 and 15 percent with a mean of 4.5 percent. However, Comfort et al. reported no carcinoma among 112 patients with asymptomatic cholelithiasis. Based on the high incidence of ultimate development of symptoms or complications and the small risk of carcinoma, it is generally felt that unless there is strong contraindication, the presence of cholelithiasis with or without symptoms is indication for cholecystectomy.

Cystic Duct Obstruction

Calculi, usually of the cholesterol type, may become impacted in the cystic duct or neck of the gallbladder, resulting in a hydrops. The bile is absorbed, and the gallbladder becomes filled and distended with mucinous material. The gallbladder is generally palpable and tender, and the impacted stone with the resulting edema may encroach upon the common duct and cause mild jaundice. Although hydrops may persist with few consequences, early cholecystectomy is generally indicated to avoid the complications of biliary tract infection or perforation of the gallbladder. In questionable cases, isotopic scanning of the gallbladder, following intravenous CCK (cholecystokinin) can define cystic obstruction or patency.

Choledocholithiasis

Common duct stones may be single or multiple and are found in approximately 12 percent of cases subjected to cholecystectomy. Most common duct calculi are formed within the gallbladder and migrate down the cystic duct into the common bile duct. Madden et al. have described stones which are thought to form within the ducts. In patients infected with tropical parasites such as *Clonorchis sinensis* and in other rare instances, stones may form within the hepatic ducts or the common bile duct itself. Although small stones may pass via the common duct into the duodenum, the distal duct with its narrow lumen (2 to 3 mm) and thick wall frequently obstructs their passage. Edema, spasm, or fibrosis of the distal duct secondary to irritation by the calculi contribute to biliary obstruction. The extrahepatic bile ducts become dilated, and there is evidence of laking in the biliary radicals of the liver. There is also thickening of the duct walls and inflammatory cell infiltration. Chronic biliary obstruction may cause secondary biliary cirrhosis with bile thrombi, bile duct proliferation, and fibrosis of the portal tracts. Also associated with chronic obstruction is the development of infection within the bile duct giving rise to ascending cholangitis and occasionally extending up to the liver, resulting in hepatic abscesses. The offending organism is almost always *E. coli*.

CLINICAL MANIFESTATIONS. The manifestations of calculi within the common duct are variable. Stones may be present within the extrahepatic duct system for many years without causing symptoms. Characteristically, the symptom complex consists of colicky pain in the right upper quadrant radiating to the right shoulder with intermittent jaundice accompanied by pale stools and dark urine. Biliary obstruction is usually chronic and incomplete but may be acute or complete. If obstruction is complete, jaundice progresses but is rarely intense. In contrast to patients with neoplastic obstruction of the common bile duct or ampulla of Vater, the gallbladder is usually not distended because of associated inflammation (Courvoisier's law). Liver function tests demonstrate the pattern of obstructive jaundice, and the alkaline phosphatase level usually becomes elevated earlier and remains abnormal for longer periods of time than the icterus index. The prothrombin time is frequently prolonged, because the absorption of vitamin K is dependent upon bile entering the intestine, but a normal level can usually be achieved with parenteral vitamin K. Tests of hepatocellular function are generally normal. In patients with ascending cholangitis, Charcot's intermittent fever accompanied by intermittent abdominal pain and jaundice is characteristic.

TREATMENT. The question of stones within the common bile duct is usually resolved surgically. When surgical operation is performed to establish the cause of obstructive jaundice, there is little question whether the duct should be explored, since there is dilatation and thickening of the duct and stones are usually palpable. Criteria for exploration of the common bile duct during cholecystectomy for cholelithiasis have been proposed. The three obvious indications are (1) palpable stones within the common bile duct, (2) dilated common bile duct, and (3) significant jaundice or a definite history of jaundice. Other indications are recurrent chills and fever suggestive of cholangitis, pancreatitis, multiple small stones within the gallbladder, and inflamed gallbladder which is empty of stones in a patient with biliary tract symptoms.

The optimal time for exploration of the common bile duct is during the initial procedure of cholecystectomy, provided acute inflammation does not obscure the anatomy. Recently one large prospective series showed that exploration of the common bile duct in the presence of acute cholecystitis carried no greater risk than during elective cholecystectomy. The higher the incidence of duct exploration at the time of cholecystectomy, the lower the incidence of residual stones but the higher the incidence of negative exploration. Considering all patients, including those with jaundice, the performance of a concomitant choledochostomy at the time of cholecystectomy increases the operative mortality by 0.2 to 1.2 percent. If one excludes the jaundiced patients, there is little difference in operative mortality between cholecystectomy alone and cholecystectomy plus concomitant choledochostomy. But there is a significant increase in postoperative morbidity and hospital stay. In order to avoid the negative duct explorations, an operative cholangiogram via a catheter inserted into the cystic duct has been used. This study will demonstrate the caliber of the duct, and a duct greater than 12 mm in diameter should be considered pathologic. The technique will also indicate the presence or absence of filling defects, in which case air bubbles within the ductal system must be differentiated before applying a diagnosis of choledocholithiasis. With this technique, the incidence of concomitant exploration of the common bile duct has been reduced from 65 to 29 percent, while the incidence of positive exploration has been increased from 23 to 66 percent in one large series. The treatment for stones within the common bile duct or hepatic ducts is surgical removal. Preoperatively, patients with common duct stones should be prepared with fat-soluble vitamins, particularly vitamin K, and if there is evidence of ascending cholangitis, a broad spectrum of antibiotics which achieve high levels in the bile should be administered. At the time of exploration, all stones and sludge should be removed, and free passage into the duodenum should be demonstrated. Removal of stones from the common and hepatic ducts may be facilitated by the use of balloon-tipped catheters. As instrumentation was refined, choledochoscopic techniques have been more widely applied. After exploring the common duct, a T tube is inserted prior to closure and drainage maintained for approximately 1 week, at which time a T tube cholangiogram is performed in order to demonstrate patency of the duct and absence of retained stones. If these criteria are met, the T tube then can be removed. If there is obstruction of the distal duct, transduodenal sphincteroplasty and

removal of the stone may be performed, or choledochoduodenostomy may be carried out. Choledochoduodenostomy has become increasingly popular for patients, particularly the elderly, with enlarged ducts and multiple retained stones. A wide sphincteroplasty is preferred by others.

RETAINED COMMON DUCT STONES. If stones are noted to be present when a T-tube cholangiogram is performed postoperatively, there are four general approaches which can be entertained. Small stones, particularly those located in the branches of the hepatic duct, may be disregarded since the majority will remain asymptomatic and if symptoms ensue, operative extraction is not associated with significantly increased morbidity. A second approach employs either flushing or chemical dissolution. Sodium cholate, 100 mmol in saline solution buffered to a pH of 7.5, is continuously infused into the T tube over a 14-day period at a rate of 30 ml/hour. Way and Dunphy have reported success in about two-thirds of the cases, but others have had less satisfying experiences. This approach is associated with diarrhea, which can be controlled by administering cholestyramine; there is also some suggestion of damage to the duct wall. Another approach of dissolution employs heparin, which acts by altering the zeta potential of particles. Heparin, 25,000 units in 250 ml saline solution, is infused every 8 hours as a continuous drip into the T tube. Complete dissolution of stones has been observed in a few cases within five days.

The most encouraging approach employs mechanical extraction of the retained stone under radiographic control. Mazzariello achieved success in 92.7 percent of 220 cases, while Burhenne and associates, reporting on 612 patients managed at 38 hospitals, reported no deaths and no significant complications, coupled with a 91 percent success rate. The T tube is generally left in place for at least 4 weeks after the operation; it is then extracted and a polyethylene catheter is used to instill radiopaque material into the common duct. A Dormia basket is then advanced through the catheter to entrap the stone (Fig. 31-15).

If the T tube had been removed and a common duct stone demonstrated cholangiographically, transduodenal papillotomy with extraction of the stone under endoscopic visualization has been reported. Operative intervention is indicated in some cases if there is evidence of obstruction and/or cholangitis, or if nonoperative methods fail.

Gallstone Ileus

Mechanical obstruction of the gastrointestinal tract caused by gallstones is a relatively infrequent occurrence. Gallstone ileus causes 1 to 2 percent of mechanical small intestinal obstructions and has been associated with high mortality rates. Recently, mortality rates of less than 10 percent have been reported.

Since cholelithiasis occurs three to six times more commonly in the female than in the male, the higher incidence of gallstone ileus in the female is to be anticipated. Preponderance in the female is actually higher than one would expect, and in several series all patients were female. It is characteristically a disease of the aged, with an average

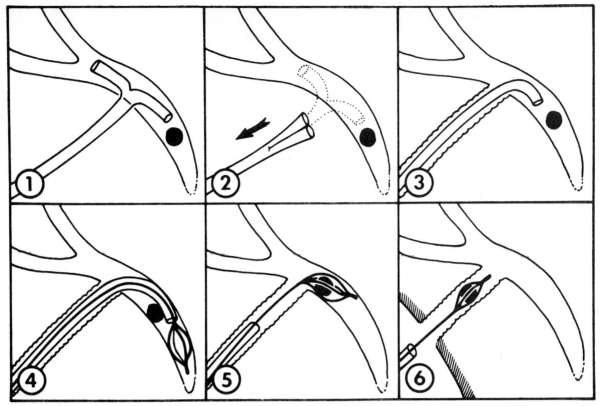

Fig. 31-15. Technical steps for retained common duct stone extraction. 1. Repeat T-tube cholangiogram is obtained on the day of stone extraction 4 to 5 weeks after choledochotomy. 2. After the location of the retained stone has been ascertained, the T tube is withdrawn. 3. Using the sinus tract of the T tube, the steerable catheter is guided into the bile duct, and its movable tip is advanced beyond the retained stone. 4. The basket is inserted through the steerable catheter, the catheter is withdrawn, and the basket is opened. 5. The open basket is withdrawn in order to engage the stone. The basket is only retracted, never advanced, outside the enclosure of the steerable catheter. 6. The stone is extracted through the drain tract. (*After H. J. Burhenne, Radium Therapy and Nuclear Medicine, Amer J Roentgenol, 117:388, 1973.*)

age of sixty-four, and is unusual under the age of fifty. Associated diseases are common, diabetes occurring in 50 percent and major cardiovascular disorders in 58 percent.

The process usually begins with formation of the stone within the gallbladder, but cases have been reported in which the gallbladder was not present, having been removed several years prior to the intestinal obstruction. After the gallstone has left the gallbladder, it may obstruct the alimentary tract in one of two ways: rarely, it enters the peritoneal cavity, causing kinking or inflammation and extrinsic obstruction of the intestine; more commonly, the blockage is caused by the entrance of the stone into the gastrointestinal tract, producing an intraluminal type of obstruction. The stone may enter the duodenum via the common duct, but this is unusual, and almost always the offending calculus enters through a cholecystoenteric fistula. The fistulous tract may connect the gallbladder with the stomach, duodenum, jejunum, ileum, or colon. In addition, internal biliary fistulas may communicate with

the pleural or pericardial cavities, tracheobronchial tree, pregnant uterus, ovarian cyst, renal pelvis, and urinary bladder. In a series of 176 fistulas caused by gallstones, the duodenum was involved in 101, the colon in 33, the stomach in 7, and multiple sites in 11.

The fistula probably originates with a stone obstructing the cystic duct, acute cholecystitis, empyema, and the formation of adhesions between the gallbladder and adjacent viscera. Perforation then occurs between the intimately adherent organs, and the stone traverses the fistula. The cholecystoenteric fistula then frequently closes, and only a fibrous remnant remains. Having entered the alimentary tract, the gallstone, which is usually single, may be vomited or passed spontaneously per rectum. The size of the stone is important, since stones smaller than 2 to 3 cm usually pass. When obstruction occurs, the site is usually at the terminal ileum, which is the narrowest portion of the small intestine. Of 154 collective cases, the duodenum was obstructed in 6, the jejunum in 14, the proximal ileum in 6, the middle ileum in 31, the terminal ileum in 88, the colon in 3, and the rectum in 2. When a gallstone blocks the small intestine, the morbid anatomic and physiologic effects of a mechanical obstruction pertain. There are extremely large losses of fluid into the intestine. Edema, ulceration, or necrosis of the bowel may occur, and perforation may result.

CLINICAL MANIFESTATIONS. A past history suggestive of cholelithiasis is present in 50 to 75 percent of patients. Symptoms of acute cholecystitis immediately preceding the onset of gallstone ileus are extremely uncommon, occurring in one-quarter to one-third of the cases. A history of jaundice is present in about 10 percent of the cases. Occasionally, there may be an initial episode of pain suggestive of biliary colic, but major pain is usually not experienced until the intestinal colic results. There is associated cramping, nausea, and vomiting which may be intermittent. When complete small intestinal obstruction occurs, the vomiting increases and the patient becomes obstipated. Analysis of the incidence of varying symptoms indicates that vomiting is present in almost 100 percent, cramps in 90 percent, distension in 90 percent, obstipation in 78 percent, and feculent vomiting in 67 percent. Serum electrolytes reveal the pattern of lower intestinal obstruction with marked hypochloremia, hyponatremia, hypokalemia, and an elevated carbonate level.

The correct preoperative diagnosis is infrequently made, ranging between 13 to 30 percent in several series. The usual diagnosis is that of intestinal obstruction of unknown cause. Radiologic examination may be diagnostic if air is demonstrated within the biliary tract (Fig. 31-16). Flat, upright, and lateral films plus spot films over the liver are indicated if the diagnosis is considered. The plain x-ray reveals the pattern of small intestinal obstruction, and in less than 20 percent of the cases a stone is visualized. The diagnosis has also been based on the migration of a previously observed radiopaque gallstone.

TREATMENT. The patient often requires vigorous fluid and electrolyte replacement in order to correct deficiency, and a nasogastric tube is used to decompress the stomach. Definitive therapy consists of locating the stone or stones, enterotomy proximal to the stone, and removing the offending calculi with closure of the intestine. The recurrence rate of gallstone ileus is 5 to 9 percent, and it is important

Fig. 31-16. Gallstone ileus. *A.* Radiopaque calculus present in right lower quadrant; suggestion of air in biliary tract within liver. *B.* Demonstration of air in intrahepatic biliary system.

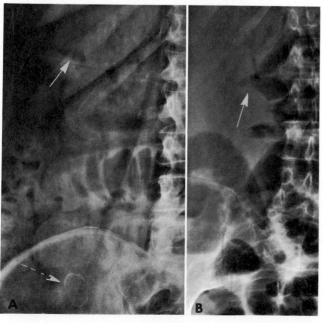

to palpate the intestine, gallbladder, and common duct for retained stones, particularly if the obstructing stone is faceted. Either concomitant or planned interval cholecystectomy and closure of the fistula, if patent, is indicated, since recurrent symptoms or complications develop in one-third of the patients and in eight cases carcinoma of the gallbladder was either present or developed 5 to 16 years after removal of the obstructing gallstone. Performance of concomitant cholecystectomy is determined by the patient's general condition, and since many of these patients are extremely ill and depleted, prolongation of the operative procedure is contraindicated.

INFLAMMATORY AND OTHER BENIGN LESIONS

Cholecystitis

In 85 to 95 percent of the cases, inflammation of the gallbladder is associated with calculi. Whether the stones represent cause or effect has not been defined, but they are generally implicated as a cause of the acute inflammatory process. Stasis of the gallbladder with consequent maintenance of contact between stagnant bile and the gallbladder wall is also considered a cause of cholecystitis. A bacterial cause of cholecystitis has been proposed, and positive bile cultures have been noted in 60 percent of patients with acute cholecystitis. A variety of organisms have been cultured both in acute and chronically inflamed gallbladders. *E. coli,* streptococci, *Aerobacter aerogenes, Salmonella,* and clostridia have all been implicated, but in many cases of both acute and chronic cholecystitis cultures of the bile are negative. In addition to bile, which in its concentrated or desiccated form is known to cause acute cholecystitis, pancreatic juice with its enzymatic properties is also considered a chemical irritant. Since pressures developed in the pancreatic duct are generally greater than those in the biliary tract, the presence of a common channel permits entrance of pancreatic juice into the gallbladder; the frequent finding of amylase in the bile supports this assumption.

ACUTE CHOLECYSTITIS

In the overwhelming majority of cases, acute cholecystitis is associated with an obstruction of the neck of the gallbladder or cystic duct due to stones impacted in Hartmann's pouch. Direct pressure of the calculus on the mucosa results in ischemia, necrosis, and ulceration with swelling, edema, and impairment of venous return. These processes, in turn, increase and extend the intensity of the inflammation. The ulceration may be so extensive that the mucosa is frequently hard to define on microscopic examination and there are segmented leukocytes infiltrating all layers. The results of necrosis are perforation with pericholecystic abscess formation, fistulization, or bile peritonitis. In the past, acute cholecystitis secondary to systemic infection occurred most commonly with typhoid fever, but this is now rare. Acute cholecystitis, due either to generalized sepsis or to stasis and/or impaction of a calculus, may occur while the patient is recovering from trauma or an operation. Among other causes of acute cholecystitis are the vascular effects of collagen disease, terminal states of hypertensive vascular disease, and thrombosis of the main cystic artery. Less than 1 percent of acutely inflamed gallbladders contain a malignant tumor which may play a role in causing obstruction. The incidence of common duct calculi is similar in acute and chronic cholecystitis, averaging 7 to 15 percent.

CLINICAL MANIFESTATIONS. Most attacks of acute cholecystitis occur in patients who give a past history compatible with chronic cholecystitis and cholelithiasis. Acute cholecystitis can occur at any age, but the greatest incidence is between the fourth and eighth decades, and patients over sixty comprise between one-quarter and one-third of the group. Caucasians are afflicted much more frequently than blacks.

The onset of acute symptoms is frequently related to a vigorous attempt of the gallbladder to empty its contents, usually after a heavy, fatty, or fried meal. Moderate to severe pain is experienced in the right upper quadrant or epigastrium and may radiate to the back in the region of the angle of the scapula or in the interscapular area. The patient is often febrile, and vomiting may be severe. Tenderness, usually along the right costal margin, often associated with rebound tenderness and spasm, is characteristic. The gallbladder is palpable in about one-third to three-quarters of the cases. Mild icterus may be present and can be related to calculi within the ampulla and edema encroaching upon the common duct. Moderate to marked icterus suggests the presence of associated choledocholithiasis but can occur with isolated cholecystitis.

The differential diagnosis includes perforation or penetration of peptic ulcer, appendicitis, hepatitis, myocardial ischemia or infarction, pneumonia, pleurisy, and herpes zoster involving an intercostal nerve.

The hemogram usually demonstrates leukocytosis with a shift to the left. Roentgenograms of the chest and abdomen are indicated to rule out thoracic processes. A radiopaque calculus is noted in less than 20 percent of the cases. The icterus index or serum bilirubin levels may determine the presence of common duct obstruction. Although the elevated amylase level is generally regarded as evidence of acute pancreatitis, levels as high as 1,000 Somogyi units have been associated with acute cholecystitis uncomplicated by pancreatitis. To rule out myocardial ischemia, an electrocardiogram should be made on any patient over the age of forty-five being considered for surgical treatment. However, acute cholecystitis may be responsible for some changes. Intravenous cholecystography and isotopic scans have been used diagnostically in patients presenting with acute abdominal pain. If the cholecystogram is normal, it is highly unlikely that cholecystitis is present. An abnormal oral cholecystogram is not necessarily diagnostic of biliary tract disease, since the oral Telepaque may not be absorbed in a patient with acute abdominal pain.

TREATMENT. Conflicting opinions concerning the management of acute cholecystitis, with particular reference to the optimal time for surgical intervention, persist. For the purpose of discussion, early operation is defined as one performed within 72 hours after the onset of the acute process; intermediate operation is one carried out between 72 hours and the cessation of clinical manifestations; delayed operative management permits the acute inflammatory process to subside; and scheduled elective surgery is performed at an interval of 6 weeks to 3 months.

The proponents of the conservative treatment, i.e., delayed operative management, base their thesis on the following premises: (1) Most cases of acute cholecystitis subside on conservative management without significant complications. (2) Surgery performed in the presence of inflammation with vascular congestion may be injurious as a result of spreading infection. (3) The acute inflammatory changes obscure the anatomy and lead to technical errors. In the presence of intense inflammatory process, exploration of the common duct for stones is compromised. (4) Many of the patients with acute cholecystitis have associated diseases and do not represent optimal risk for surgical intervention.

Nonoperative management is directed at creating a situation of functional rest for the gallbladder and upper gastrointestinal tract and relaxing spasm of the sphincter of Oddi. The regimen includes restriction of fluid and food intake and continuous nasogastric suction. Anticholinergic drugs are administered in an effort to decrease spasm of the sphincter. Pain is treated with small amounts of Demerol, while morphine is withheld, because it causes sphincteric spasm. Antibiotics which achieve high levels in bile are advised by many physicians.

The proponents of nonoperative management of acute cholecystitis argue against the importance of perforation and bile peritonitis. In one series of 679 patients subjected to laparotomy, although perforation was noted in 9 percent of the patients, only 3 percent demonstrated free perforation into the peritoneal cavity. In another series of 441 patients treated surgically, there were only 2 instances of free perforation, while 11 patients had pericholecystic abscesses. In several series, there was no serious morbidity associated with perforation.

The arguments for early or intermediate cholecystectomy point out that about 5 percent of patients fail to respond to medical management and more than half of the patients who respond initially experience an exacerbation. Unless there is a medical contraindication, eventual surgical intervention is indicated for almost all patients with cholecystitis and cholelithiasis. Low mortality rates have been reported for early cholecystectomy, and these rates are quite comparable with those reported for the elective procedure. The risk of operating in an area of inflammation, in the early stages of acute cholecystitis, is refuted. In the first 2 to 3 days after the onset of symptoms, although edema may be significant, there is usually little difficulty in displaying the duct system. If the structures can be safely defined, exploration of the common duct for stones can be carried out without increased risk. If early operation is performed and the inflammatory process has progressed to obscure the structures, cholecystostomy, which can be carried out with a low mortality rate, speeds the patient's recovery. Acute cholecystitis in the diabetic is associated with higher incidences of complications and

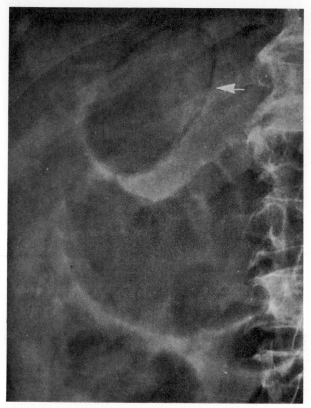

Fig. 31-17. Emphysematous cholecystitis. Gallbladder is shown as gas-filled organ.

mortality than in the nondiabetic. Schein reports significant improvement in these statistics with early cholecystomy.

In the United States the majority of surgeons favor early operation, whereas in Great Britain it is more customary to treat the condition conservatively, unless there is specific indication for surgical intervention.

The mortality rate for emergency cholecystectomy ranges from near zero to 5 percent and, in several series, is comparable to the mortality rate for elective cholecystectomy. In one series, the mortality rate for cholecystectomy was 3.9 percent, while the nonoperative patients had a mortality of 5.5 percent. In the first truly randomized series, van der Linden and Sunzel showed that early cholecystectomy was as safe as the nonoperative approach and that the period of morbidity and disability was shortened. Cholecystostomy for extremely ill patients was accompanied by a mortality rate of 15 percent in one series, in contrast to the 1.5 percent mortality rate reported by Dunphy and Ross.

Author's Approach. If the diagnosis of acute cholecystitis is relatively unequivocal and the patient presents within 3 days of the onset of symptoms, early operation is performed. Immediate *emergency* cholecystectomy is rarely indicated, and the patient should be thoroughly investigated and prepared prior to operation. If the patient is extremely ill with a palpable gallbladder, surgical treatment is usually carried out within 24 hours of admission.

If possible, cholecystectomy is performed. However, if the patient will not tolerate this procedure because of extreme toxicity or otherwise complicating medical illness, a cholecystostomy, under local anesthesia, is carried out. If a cholecystectomy has been planned but the inflammatory process is so marked that it compromises the dissection, cholecystostomy terminates the procedure. Patients whose symptoms continue to progress under medical management are operated upon. With associated cholangitis, a course of antibiotics is initiated, and early operation is performed for relief of obstruction. If the patient presents 72 hours after the onset of symptoms and shows signs of improvement during the early periods of hospitalization, surgical intervention is deferred, and an elective operation is planned in approximately 6 weeks in most instances, but there is no hesitation in operating after the "golden" 72 hours.

At the time of surgical treatment for acute cholecystitis, the indications for common bile duct exploration are the same as those which pertain during elective cholecystectomy. Patients with obstructive jaundice due to stones or ascending cholangitis require early surgical relief of obstruction and drainage of the common bile duct. Palpable stones and ductal dilatation demonstrated at operation constitute indications for common duct exploration. Pancreatitis is not, in itself, an indication in the presence of acute cholecystitis, since the yield is small, and it is best to leave a catheter in the cystic duct for future study. If indications for exploration of the common duct are present but the inflammatory process compromises dissection, cholecystostomy is performed and the stones are removed from the gallbladder. An attempt may be made to pass a catheter via the cystic duct into the common bile duct.

Emphysematous Cholecystitis. This is a rare form of acute, usually gangrenous, cholecystitis, caused by gas-forming organisms and characterized radiologically by the presence of gas in the gallbladder (Fig. 31-17). Approximately 100 cases have been reviewed in this century. Unlike ordinary acute cholecystitis, which is more prevalent among women, emphysematous cholecystitis is more often found in men, with a sex incidence of 75 percent for males and 25 percent for females. Pathogenesis is related to acute inflammation of the gallbladder, which often begins aseptically, complicated by a secondary infection with gas-forming bacilli. These may reach the gallbladder by bile ducts, bloodstream, or lymphatic channels and grow in an anaerobic environment. The clinical manifestations are similar to those present in acute cholecystitis. In approximately half the patients, a history of previous gallbladder attacks can be elicited. Cholelithiasis is also present in half the patients, who are frequently diabetic. The diagnosis is usually made on the basis of roentgenographic findings which show a globular shadow, distended with gas, in the region of the gallbladder. Later, intramural or submucosal gas may appear, and gas may also appear in the pericholecystic area denoting extension of the pathologic process outside the confines of the gallbladder. The treatment of choice is early operation, since the incidence of free perforation is reported to be 40 to 60 percent. Cholecystectomy is indicated, but if this is not feasible, cholecystostomy should be performed. In 9 percent of cases, choledocholithiasis is present, and exploration of the common duct may be required. Although positive bile cultures are found in only half the cases, antibiotics directed toward the clostridial and coliform organisms are indicated. The mortality rate is significantly greater than that for nonemphysematous cholecystitis.

CHRONIC CHOLECYSTITIS

Chronic inflammation of the gallbladder is generally associated with cholelithiasis and consists of round cell infiltration and fibrosis of the wall. Buried crypts of mucosa (Rokitansky-Aschoff sinuses) may be seen dipping into the mucosa (Fig. 31-18). Obstruction by gallstones of the neck of the cystic duct may produce a mucocele of the gallbladder (hydrops). The bile is initially sterile but may be secondarily infected with coliform bacilli, streptococci, and occasionally clostridia or *Salmonella* (typhoid). Secondary effects of cholecystitis include obstruction of the common duct, cholangitis, perforation of the gallbladder with formation of a pericholecystic abscess or a cholecystoenteric fistula, bile peritonitis, pancreatitis, and carcinoma of the gallbladder.

CLINICAL MANIFESTATIONS. The patients generally present with moderate intermittent abdominal pain in the right upper quadrant and epigastrium, occasionally radiating to the scapula and interscapular region. There is usually a history of intolerance of fatty and/or fried foods, and the patient may have noted intermittent nausea and anorexia. If the patient is not experiencing acute pain, there may be no diagnostic findings on physical examination. Occasionally tenderness is elicited over the gallbladder. This is usually maximal during inspiration. The diagnosis is usually established by an oral cholecystogram, which demonstrates either the absence of filling of the gallbladder or the presence of stones.

TREATMENT. The treatment of chronic cholecystitis and cholelithiasis is cholecystectomy, and the results are usually excellent. Early cholecystectomy is particularly important for the diabetic patient. Operative mortality of less than 1 percent has been reported for large series. Seventy-five percent of patients undergoing cholecystectomy for cholelithiasis are completely relieved of all preoperative symptoms, and the remaining 25 percent have only mild symptoms which are apparently unrelated to the biliary system.

POSTCHOLECYSTECTOMY SYNDROME. This ill-defined syndrome refers to symptoms which either develop subsequent to or continue in spite of cholecystectomy. In patients with abdominal symptoms subsequent to cholecystectomy for chronic cholecystitis and cholelithiasis, these symptoms are usually related to an extrabiliary cause such as hiatal hernia, peptic ulceration, or pancreatitis. However, symptoms may also be due to a residual stone in the common bile duct, residual cystic duct stones, or spasm of the sphincter of Oddi.

The *cystic duct stump* is rarely responsible for clinical manifestations similar to those of cholecystitis. It has been thought that the residual stump becomes a diseased gallbladder undergoing changes of inflammation and capable of forming calculi which may pass into the common duct.

However, cholangiographic studies have recently demonstrated that abnormalities in the insertion of the cystic duct are quite common, and it is probable that, in many instances, a significant length of cystic duct remains after cholecystectomy. Since many of the patients with the "cystic duct syndrome" have demonstrated calculi in the extrahepatic biliary system, it is difficult to determine which factor is responsible for postcholecystectomy symptoms.

ACALCULOUS CHOLECYSTITIS

Acute and chronic inflammatory disease of the gallbladder can occur without stones. Mackey reported recurrent symptoms after cholecystectomy in 36 percent of 264 cases in which stones were not present, while Glenn and Mannix reported poor results in 24 percent of patients from whom an acalculous gallbladder was removed. CCK-cholecystography has been helpful in determining which patients will benefit from cholecystectomy.

The incidence of acalculous cholecystitis is difficult to establish. It is present in over 50 percent of children and 35 percent of Nigerians with gallbladder disease, and the accepted incidence for adults in the United States is between 5 and 10 percent. Postoperative acute cholecystitis is frequently acalculous. Possible causes include (1) anatomic conditions such as kinking, fibrosis, and obstruction of the cystic duct due to tumor or anomalous vessels; (2) throm-

Fig. 31-18. Rokitansky-Aschoff sinuses presenting as a halo effect, a finding present in chronic cholecystitis.

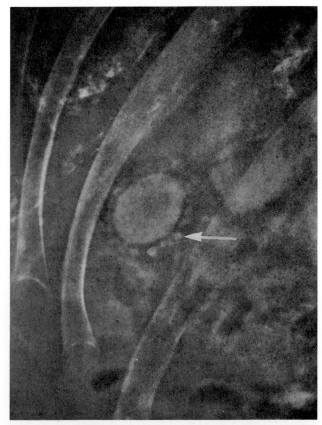

bosis of major blood vessels producing ischemia and gangrene; (3) spasm or fibrosis of the sphincter of Oddi in patients with a "common channel" with or without associated pancreatitis; (4) systemic diseases such as diabetes mellitus and collagen diseases; (5) specific infections such as typhoid fever, actinomycoses, and parasitic infestation; and (6) scarlet fever and a wide variety of febrile illnesses in young children.

TREATMENT. Cholecystectomy is generally carried out because of classic symptoms attributed to the gallbladder. An effort should be made to determine the presence of etiologic or associated conditions, and these should be corrected. The liver should be biopsied in any patient with a history of jaundice, and bacteriologic culture of the gallbladder wall should be carried out. Spasm or obstruction of the sphincter of Oddi due to papillitis or fibrosis should be ruled out. Postoperatively, the stool should be cultured for *Salmonella,* and serial estimations of the serum amylase level and a lupus erythematosus (LE) test are indicated.

Cholangitis

Infection within the biliary duct system is most frequently associated with choledocholithiasis but has also accompanied choledochal cysts and carcinoma of the bile duct, and has followed sphincteroplasty. Infection and inflammatory changes may extend up the duct system into the liver and give rise to multiple hepatic abscesses. Clinically, the condition is characterized by intermittent fever, upper abdominal pain, exacerbation of jaundice, pruritus, and at times rigor.

In patients with common duct stones in whom there is ascending cholangitis, a broad-spectrum antibiotic directed particularly at *E. coli,* which is the most common offending organism, should be given for several days prior to surgical treatment. Antibiotics usually control the infection, but if the temperature does not fall, surgical intervention should not be delayed. Occasionally, the patient may be so ill as to allow only insertion of a T tube into the common duct, and when cholangitis has subsided, a second operation can be performed to remove the stone.

ACUTE SUPPURATIVE CHOLANGITIS. Suppurative cholangitis, in which there is gross pus within the biliary tract, merits special consideration, since it constitutes one of the most urgent causes for laparotomy in patients with obstructive jaundice. The entity was first described in 1877 by Charcot, who suggested a diagnostic triad of jaundice, chills and fever, and pain in the right upper quadrant. To these, Reynolds and Dargan added shock and central nervous system depression as specific identifying features of the condition.

The disease occurs almost exclusively in patients over seventy years. All patients are febrile, and a majority are jaundiced. Hypotension, confusion, or lethargy occur in about 20 percent of cases. A white blood cell count of less than 12,000 has been reported in over half the patients, probably related to the age and lack of response. Bilirubin, SGOT, and alkaline phosphatase levels are characteristically elevated, but the serum amylase is usually normal. The correct diagnosis has been made in less than a third of the patients.

At operation, all patients demonstrate gross distension of the common bile duct, with frank pus, frequently under considerable pressure, and choledocholithiasis. If the gallbladder is present, it is invariably distended and inflamed. Spontaneous perforation of the bile ducts has been reported. Surgical treatment is directed at rapid decompression of the duct system and is combined with large doses of antibiotics, particularly those which achieve high levels in the bile. In a review of the literature, it was reported that all patients who were not operated upon died while mortality following surgical procedures ranged between zero and 88 percent, averaging 33 percent.

Cholangiohepatitis

Cholangiohepatitis, which is also known as "recurrent pyogenic cholangitis," is found almost exclusively among the Chinese, with the largest number of cases seen among Cantonese living in the Pearl River delta in China. In Hong Kong it is the most commonly encountered disease of the biliary passages and is the third most common abdominal emergency after appendicitis and perforated ulcer. It has also been encountered in Great Britain, in Australia, and in the Chinese population in the United States. Cholangiohepatitis occurs most frequently in the third and fourth decades but has been reported at all ages and has an equal sex frequency.

The etiology is summarized in Fig. 31-19. The pyogenic element probably originates from the bowel and is caused by *E. coli* or *Streptococcus fecalis.* In most instances, positive cultures are obtainable from the bile and portal venous blood. The Chinese liver fluke, *C. sinensis,* is thought to be an important contributing factor. Ova have been found in the feces or bile of 91 percent of cases, but in some instances there has been no evidence of infestation. It has been postulated that in the presence of the pyogenic infec-

Fig. 31-19. Schema of etiologic factors implicated in cholangiohepatitis. (*After F. E. Stock and J. H. Y. Fung, Oriental Cholangiohepatitis, in R. Smith and S. Sherlock, "Surgery of the Gall Bladder and Bile Ducts," Butterworth & Co. [Publishers] Ltd., London, 1964.*)

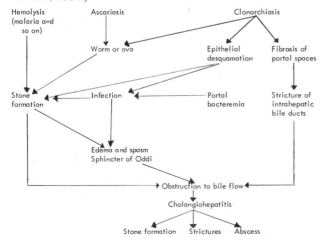

tion the fluke may die. *C. sinensis* has been shown to cause severe irritation of the bile passages and has been implicated as a cause of bile duct tumors. Other factors which have been implicated as contributing causes for cholangiohepatitis include ascariasis and hemolysis associated with malaria.

PATHOLOGY. The gallbladder is usually distended with viscous, dark bile. The wall is thickened but not grossly inflamed. The common bile duct is also usually grossly distended and contains large stones. The stones are produced by precipitation of bile pigments, desquamation of epithelium, and products of inflammation, and, not infrequently, the nucleus of the stone may contain an adult *Clonorchis* worm, an ovum, or an ascarid. Acute or hemorrhagic pancreatitis occurs in less than 1 percent of the cases. The most marked changes occur in the liver, where the intrahepatic bile ducts are both dilated and constricted. Inflammatory changes are present in the periductal tissue and may progress to frank abscess formation. With time, additional liver tissue is destroyed as abscesses are formed.

CLINICAL MANIFESTATIONS. In highly endemic areas, cholangiohepatitis is the first consideration in patients with jaundice, pain, and pyrexia. In almost all cases, pain is present at some stage and is frequently severe. It is usually located in the right upper quadrant and epigastrium and may be colicky or constant. As is typical with biliary tract disease, it radiates frequently to the back or shoulder tip. In most acute attacks, there is fever accompanied by chills and rigors, and 50 percent of the patients are jaundiced, while the remainder have an elevation of the serum bilirubin level. Recurrence of symptoms is one of the most characteristic features of the disease.

Most patients appear toxic, with temperatures up to 40°C. There is tenderness and guarding in the right upper quadrant. The white blood cell count is usually in about 15,000, and the serum bilirubin level is generally above 2 mg/100 ml with accompanying bilirubinuria. The alkaline phosphatase is increased, and there may be evidence of impairment of hepatocellular function. In the majority of cases calculi are not demonstrable on routine x-rays. An occasional finding of significance is the presence of air in the biliary tree, which may be due to a secondary gas-forming organism or a fistula between the duct and duodenum. Cholecystography and intravenous cholangiography rarely produce diagnostic findings. Endoscopic retrograde cholangiopancreatography (ERCP) may establish the diagnosis. Operative cholangiography also is helpful in revealing intrahepatic stones, constrictions of intrahepatic ducts, and small filling defects due to the liver fluke. Manifestations of portal hypertension may be present.

TREATMENT. Patients are generally prepared with antibiotics. Vitamin K should be administered, and anemia, if present, should be corrected. Surgical therapy, however, should not be delayed for the patient who is jaundiced and has pain and pyrexia.

Treatment is directed at providing an adequate permanent drainage of the biliary tree. Cholecystostomy is reserved for the seriously ill patient showing signs of rupture of the gallbladder. The definitive operative procedure, however, consists of removal of stones and debris from the extrahepatic bile ducts and providing an improved communication between the duct system and the intestine. Transduodenal sphincteroplasty has been performed in cases where the common duct was not grossly dilated, but wide choledochoduodenostomy is the treatment of choice. T-tube drainage represents a temporizing procedure, since obstruction frequently recurs after the tube has been removed. The gallbladder is usually removed, although it is rarely acutely inflamed and never represents the primary site of disease.

If large hepatic abscesses are noted, drainage should be performed. Left hepatic lobectomy has been carried out on occasion, when there has been gross dilatation of the ducts and abscess formation in the left lobe while the right was apparently normal.

The prognosis is generally guarded, since recurrence is not uncommon. In advanced cases, particularly with multiple abscesses, the prognosis is poor, and the patient eventually succumbs to liver failure, septicemia, or cholangiocarcinoma.

Sclerosing Cholangitis

Sclerosing cholangitis is an uncommon disease which involves either all or part of the extrahepatic biliary duct system and, occasionally, affects the intrahepatic biliary radicles. The disease has also been called *obliterative cholangitis* and *stenosing cholangitis*, in reference to a progressive thickening of the bile duct walls encroaching upon the lumen. It may be associated with gallstones, but several series have been presented in which there were no stones in either the gallbladder or the common duct. A significant number of cases have been associated with ulcerative colitis, Riedel's struma, retroperitoneal fibrosis, and porphyria cutanea tarda.

Schwartz and Dale reviewed the literature prior to 1958, and only 13 cases satisfied their criteria of generalized extrahepatic bile duct stenosis in the absence of previous biliary surgical treatment and gallstones. Manesis and Sullivan reviewed the literature for a 40-year period from 1924 to 1964 and found only 24 cases which they considered acceptable. By contrast, Warren et al. have been less restrictive in the diagnosis and reported a group of 42 cases seen at the Lahey Clinic including 15 with a history of gallstones or previous surgical treatment. A follow-up period long enough to exclude sclerosing carcinoma of the biliary tree is essential to the diagnosis.

Most patients present with symptoms during the fourth, fifth, and sixth decades of life, and the disease appears to occur more often in males, in contrast to acute cholecystitis.

The cause of sclerosing cholangitis is unknown. Histologic sections in several cases failed to reveal any granulomatous lesion, metaplasia, or neoplasia. In several series, none of the patients had had previous surgical treatment, and therefore trauma was excluded as an etiologic agent; irritation of the common duct by passage of calculi is refuted by the fact that there are usually no stones present either in the common duct or gallbladder. It has been suggested that the disease may be caused by local response to viral infection, since a relative lymphocytosis with atypical lymphocytes has been noted. Allergic reaction and collagen disease have also been considered as possible etiologic factors.

PATHOLOGY. Grossly there is diffuse thickening of the wall of the extrahepatic biliary tract with a concomitant encroachment upon the lumen, resulting in marked luminal narrowing. The duct system may be completely involved, or the hepatic ducts may be spared and the disease restricted to the entire length of the common duct. The gallbladder is usually not involved, but the lymph nodes in the region of the common duct and foramen of Winslow are usually markedly enlarged and succulent. Microscopic analyses of the affected duct show that the walls are as much as eight times thicker than normal. The areas of inflammation and fibrosis are in the submucosal and subserosal portions with an edematous field between them. The mucosa is intact throughout. Biopsy of the liver may reveal bile stasis or, in long-standing cases, biliary cirrhosis. The histologic evaluation is critical, since it is difficult to differentiate this disease from sclerosing carcinoma of bile ducts.

CLINICAL MANIFESTATIONS. The diagnosis is to be considered in patients, particularly those in middle age, with a clinical and laboratory picture of extrahepatic jaundice. Jaundice is usually associated with intermittent pain in the right upper quadrant, nausea, vomiting, and occasionally chills and fevers. In long-standing cases with biliary cirrhosis, the manifestations of portal hypertension, such as bleeding varices and ascites, may be apparent. The diagnosis has been established by ERCP. At operation a dense inflammatory reaction in the region of the gallbladder and gastrohepatic ligament is noted. Palpation of the duct reveals a cordlike structure which may feel like a thrombosed blood vessel, but the wall of the common duct is obviously thickened and cuts with difficulty. The edges of the incision characteristically pout out. Usually, only a fine

probe or small Bâkes dilator can be inserted into the lumen. Operative cholangiography may vividly demonstrate the extensive narrowing of the lumen (Fig. 31-20).

TREATMENT. Treatment has varied and is dictated by the extent of involvement of the extrahepatic biliary duct system. It is usually preferable to drain the common duct by means of a T tube. If the gallbladder is normal, it should not be removed, because it may be required subsequently to shunt bile from the biliary tract to the intestine. Postoperatively, the patient is treated with bile salts, such as dehydrocholic acid, to increase the fluidity of bile; a broad-spectrum antibiotic, which achieves a high level in bile; and corticoids. Prednisone (40 to 50 mg daily) is preferred for long-term use, since its anti-inflammatory effect is four to five times as great as that of cortisone with less salt-retaining potential. Recurrence of symptoms or icterus is indication for reinstitution of steroid therapy.

A T-tube drainage is maintained until a satisfactory lumen is demonstrated throughout the duct system by cholangiogram and it is apparent that the bile flows readily into the duodenum. The combination of surgical decompression of the biliary tract and administration of corticoids, bile salts, and antibiotics has reduced the overall mortality, but the prognosis is guarded because of the difficulty in differentiating primary sclerosing cholangitis from sclerosing carcinoma of bile ducts.

Fibrosis or Stenosis of the Sphincter of Oddi

In 1884, Langenbuch, only 2 years after reporting the first successful removal of a gallbladder, suggested trans-

Fig. 31-20. *A.* Operative cholangiogram of patient with sclerosing cholangitis showing markedly narrow common cystic and hepatic ducts. *B.* Cholangiogram on twenty-fourth postoperative day showing increased diameter of lumen of common, cystic and hepatic ducts in same patient. Patient had received cortisone from first postoperative day.

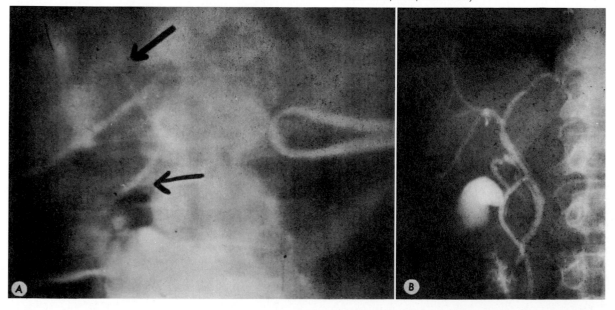

duodenal division of the "diverticulum" of Vater in cases of cicatricial stenosis for chronic inflammation. In 1901, Opie called attention to the "common channel" theory as the cause of pancreatitis, and in 1913 Archibald suggested sphincteroplasty as the treatment for pancreatitis.

The pathogenesis of fibrosis or stenosis of the sphincter of Oddi and the papilla of Vater is not fully understood. Long-standing spasm may play an important role, and infection of the biliary tract or pancreas have also been implicated. Irritation from stones within the common duct may also lead to fibrosis. In a series of 50 patients in whom sphincteroplasty was performed because of inability to pass a small Bâkes dilator, biopsies revealed no abnormalities in 18, while 18 showed inflammatory infiltration, 17 had minimal fibrosis, and 2 had diffuse fibrosis. Glandular dilatation was seen in seven cases, and squamous metaplasia and pyogenic granuloma were each seen in one case. No definite correlation could be found between the various manifestations of biliary tract disease and the histologic changes.

CLINICAL MANIFESTATIONS. The main symptom is abdominal pain, which is usually colicky and frequently associated with nausea and vomiting. The pain begins in the right upper quadrant and radiates to the shoulder, and it may be intermittent in nature. Over half the patients give a history of intermittent jaundice, and many indicate that they have had previous cholecystectomy without relief of symptoms.

TREATMENT. The diagnosis is generally made at operation when there is difficulty in passing a 3-mm Bâkes dilator through the ampulla of Vater into the duodenum. Operative cholangiography and pressure studies on the common bile duct have theoretical application but are generally not used. If a 3-mm dilator cannot be easily passed through the ampulla, a transduodenal exploration should be carried out. Thomas et al. compared the results of transduodenal sphincteroplasty and choledochoduodenostomy in 30 patients with stenosis or stricture of the sphincter. The procedures were equally and highly effective, and neither was associated with a significant incidence of subsequent cholangitis. Sphincteroplasty is preferable if the common duct is small, and a transduodenal approach is indicated if an ampullary tumor is suspected. Choledochoduodenostomy appears preferable if the stenosis is long, if it is difficult to identify the sphincter, or if exposure is difficult.

PAPILLITIS

In 1926, DelValle first described a benign inflammatory and fibrous process of the ampulla of Vater and indicated that it was a factor in producing stenosis. It was postulated that acute and subacute inflammatory changes occur and that stenosis is the final and irreversible result of these changes. Acosta and Nardi have presented 61 cases of papillitis, 21 of which were chronic ulcerative papillitis, 20 chronic sclerosing papillitis, 15 chronic granulomatous papillitis, and 5 chronic adenomatous papillitis. The acute stage, which is characterized by edema, papillary dilatation, hemorrhage, and infiltration, may be reversible, while sclerosing papillitis and chronic granulomatous papillitis

are considered irreversible in view of their inevitable evolution into scar tissue.

The clinical and pathologic features associated with papillitis include the postcholecystectomy syndrome in 30 percent, dilatation of the common duct in 50 percent, biliary disease without stones in 25 percent, obstructive jaundice in 60 percent, pancreatitis in 70 percent, and liver damage in 25 percent. There has been no correlation between the specific clinical syndromes and the pathologic changes. A pancreatic evocative test, utilizing morphine-prostigmine or secretin-CCK, has been used. Elevation of at least one serum pancreatic enzyme by a factor of 4 over the normal, coupled with reproduction of the patient's pain, is considered a positive test result. Since the majority of patients with papillitis have irreversible lesions, sphincteroplasty is generally employed.

TUMORS

Carcinoma of the Gallbladder

Carcinoma of the gallbladder represents the fifth most common type of carcinoma involving the gastrointestinal tract and accounts for 4 percent of all carcinomas. Its occurrence in random autopsy series averages approximately 0.4 percent, while approximately 1 percent of patients undergoing biliary tract operations are noted to have carcinoma. Approximately 80 percent of patients in most series are female. The lesion usually presents after the age of sixty.

PATHOLOGY. The relationship between gallstones and carcinoma has been emphasized for many years. Approximately 90 percent of patients with carcinoma have associated cholelithiasis. Five to ten percent of patients over the age of sixty-five with symptomatic gallstones have carcinoma of the gallbladder. However, it has been stressed that in patients with asymptomatic cholelithiasis the frequency of occurrence is extremely low.

Approximately 80 percent of the tumors are adenocarcinomas, while the remainder are either undifferentiated or squamous cell carcinomas. Of the adenocarcinomas, 70 percent are scirrhous, 20 percent are papillary, and 10 percent are mucoid. The routes of metastases include spread along the lymphatics to the choledochal and pancreatic or duodenal nodes, localized involvement of the venules and veins of the gallbladder, and invasion of the liver. In approximately one-third of the cases the disease spreads directly to the liver, an important consideration as far as therapy is concerned. In patients with metastases, the liver is involved in two-thirds of the cases, the regional lymph nodes in about one-half, and the omentum, duodenum, colon, or porta hepatis in about one-fourth. Pulmonary metastases are relatively uncommon.

CLINICAL MANIFESTATIONS. Signs and symptoms of carcinoma of the gallbladder are generally indistinguishable from those associated with cholecystitis and cholelithiasis. Most patients present with abdominal distress, epigastric and right upper quadrant pain, nausea, and vomiting. About half the patients are jaundiced, and in two-thirds there is a palpable right upper quadrant mass. Less than 10 percent present with normal findings on abdominal examination.

Laboratory findings are of little assistance. The liver function tests are diagnostic of obstructive jaundice, and the gallbladder is usually not visualized by cholecystography. A correct preoperative diagnosis has been made in less than 20 percent of patients, and in many patients the gallbladder carcinoma is found incidentally during routine cholecystectomy.

TREATMENT. Surgical treatment offers the only, albeit small, hope for cure. Most of the reported long-term survivors are patients who underwent surgical treatment for acute and chronic cholecystitis and in whom an incidental localized microscopic focus of neoplasia was detected in the specimen. The best results in patients with grossly visible carcinoma have been achieved with cholecystectomy and regional lymphadenectomy. When the lymph nodes are removed, the portal vein, hepatic artery, hepatic duct, and common bile duct should be skeletonized from the pylorus to the porta hepatis. The minimal liver resection which should be performed consists of removal of the wedge of hepatic tissue comprising the gallbladder bed. A formal right hepatic lobectomy has been suggested, but the 5-year survival rate has not been improved by this approach.

The prognosis for 5-year survival is extremely poor, however, approximating 2 percent. Ninety percent of patients die before the end of 1 year and 50 percent within 3 months.

Fig. 31-21. Transhepatic cholangiogram demonstrating a tumor of the common bile duct.

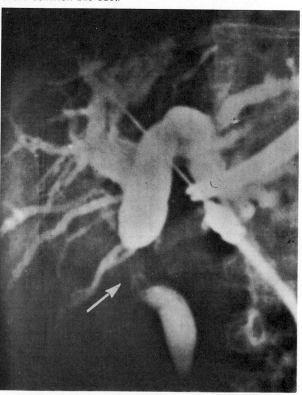

Carcinoma of the Extrahepatic Bile Ducts Exclusive of the Periampullary Region

This lesion has an average autopsy incidence of approximately 0.3 percent. The ratio of incidence of carcinoma of the extrahepatic bile duct exclusive of the periampullary region to that of carcinoma of the gallbladder ranges from 1:2 to 1:5 in various series, while the ratio of this lesion to carcinoma of the ampulla is 3:2. The tumor occurs more frequently in males and has the highest incidence in the sixth and seventh decades.

PATHOLOGY. The primary lesion is often small but so located as to cause symptoms early. Approximately one-third of the cases occur in the common bile duct, one-fifth are at the junction of the cystic and common hepatic ducts, and one-fourth are higher in the common hepatic duct. Ten percent occur in either the right or left hepatic duct, and about 13 percent are located in the cystic duct. The tumor usually involves the whole thickness of the duct, resulting in complete anatomic obstruction in about one-third of the cases. Grossly, the tumor presents as a firm, circumscribed, grayish tan mass which causes a "napkin ring" obstruction. In rare instances, the growth projects into the lumen of the duct in the form of a polypoid mass. Histologically, all lesions are adenocarcinomas. Metastatic spread has been reported in about three-fourths of autopsy cases, liver and regional lymph nodes being most frequently involved. Spread to adjacent structures accounts for 20 percent of metastases. Recently a series employing operative choledochoscopy has demonstrated that multicentric lesions in the duct are common. The extent of liver involvement is variable. In some instances there is severe bile stasis, while in others there are suppurative cholangitis and hepatic abscesses. The incidence of metastases at operation was reported to be approximately 50 percent.

Cholelithiasis has been implicated as a contributing factor just as in carcinoma of the gallbladder. However, the incidence of stones is not as high, ranging from 20 to 57 percent in several series. The incidence of calculi within the bile ducts themselves is extremely low.

CLINICAL MANIFESTATIONS. The symptoms are variable, and the correct preoperative diagnosis is seldom made. Characteristically, there is a rapid onset of jaundice, which is present in almost all patients. This is frequently preceded by pruritus. Nearly always there is weight loss, and abdominal pain occurs in over half the patients. The liver is palpable in about 80 percent of the cases and is usually nontender and rarely nodular. The gallbladder is palpable in about one-third of the patients who have not undergone previous cholecystectomy. The serum bilirubin is usually elevated, often to an extremely high level, and fluctuation of the bilirubin level has been recorded in about 60 percent of the cases. Intravenous cholangiography rarely visualizes the ducts because of the high degree of obstructive jaundice, but transhepatic cholangiography may provide a diagnosis (Fig. 31-21). At the time of surgical treatment, an operative cholangiogram is very helpful in establishing the diagnosis and choledochoscopy should be performed to assess multicentricity.

TREATMENT. The surgical procedure may be either a

potentially curative one or palliative and is dependent upon the location of the tumor. Tumors located within the common bile duct or common hepatic duct may be resected or bypassed by anastomosing the dilated proximal duct system to a segment of intestine, preferably by a Roux en Y procedure. Tumors occurring high in the hepatic duct system can rarely be removed, and palliative procedures are also difficult. The jejunum may be anastomosed to a dilated duct in the hilus or on the inferior surface of the left lobe of the liver. Recently Terblanche et al. have achieved prolonged palliation by decompressing the distended intrahepatic duct with a tube passed through the obstruction via the common duct and out the surface of the liver as a U tube (Fig. 31-22). The results either with or without surgical treatment are discouraging, and the patients survive an average of 4 months after operation or 6 months after the onset of their symptoms. Radical dissection has rarely proved curative and has been associated with a high operative mortality.

SCLEROSING CARCINOMA OF THE HILAR DUCTS

This lesion usually arises from the major hepatic ducts near the hilus of the liver and extends into the intrahepatic ducts, developing slowly and often mimicking a chronic inflammatory process. As the tumor obstructs the bile ducts, progressive jaundice, cholestasis, suppurative cholangitis, and hepatic abscess may result. The average age at diagnosis is about sixty-five, and the ratio of male to female has been reported at 8:1.

The signs and symptoms are variable. There is characteristically insidious and progressive jaundice, and there is usually associated marked weight loss. Fever is noted in over half the patients. The syndrome may progress to hepatic coma, renal failure, or septicemia. Laboratory and preoperative roentgenographic findings are inconclusive, but operative cholangiography has been helpful in establishing the diagnosis.

Surgical treatment is directed at establishing biliary drainage and has been accomplished by a T tube passed as a stent through the tumor, hepaticodochojejunostomy, and the Longmire procedure. If transhepatic cholangiography demonstrates high obstruction and no accessible segment for reanastomosis, percutaneous transhepatic catheter drainage can relieve the jaundice at least temporarily and at times for prolonged periods. In spite of the fact that metastases are frequently present in the regional lymph nodes, liver, and omentum, in several instances there has been a surprisingly long survival: the difficulty in establishing a diagnosis of sclerosing cholangitis is thus emphasized.

OPERATIONS ON THE BILIARY TRACT

ANTIBIOTIC THERAPY. The infectious complications after biliary surgery are more frequent in patients with infected bile than in those with sterile bile. It has been shown that patients over the age of seventy who have acute cholecystitis, common bile duct stones, jaundice, or diabetes have a significantly higher incidence of positive bile cultures and therefore are at risk for postoperative infec-

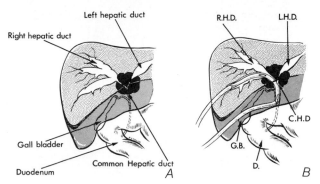

Fig. 31-22. The U-tube procedure. *A.* The carcinoma situated at the main hepatic duct junction. *B.* The U tube in situ after dilatation. (*From J. Terblanche et al., Surgery, 71:720, 1972.*)

tion. This group of patients should receive antibiotics preoperatively. In all cases, the gallbladder bile should be cultured at the time of the operative procedure. The selection of antibiotics should be based on appreciation of the fact that most organisms are *E. coli* or *Klebsiella*. One study has shown that half the bacteria cultured from the bile was resistant to ampicillin.

CHOLECYSTOSTOMY. The procedure accomplishes decompression and drainage of the distended, hydroptic, or empyematous gallbladder. It is particularly applicable if the patient's general condition is such that it precludes prolonged anesthesia, since the operation may be performed under local anesthesia. It is also performed for the situation in which marked inflammatory reaction obscures the anatomic relation of critical structures. Cholecystostomy may be a definitive procedure, particularly if a postoperative tube cholangiogram is normal.

Technique (Fig. 31-23). A circumferential purse-string suture is placed in the fundus of the gallbladder, and a small incision is made through the serosa within the suture. A trochar is inserted into the lumen of the gallbladder, which is then decompressed. After the gallbladder has been emptied, a stone forceps may be introduced to the junction of the ampulla and cystic duct, and obstructing calculi may be removed. A mushroom or Foley catheter is inserted into the lumen of the gallbladder, and a second purse-string suture is placed concentrically in relation to the first one. The sutures are tied, inverting the serosa. Unless a small, oblique incision was employed initially, the drainage tube should be brought out through a stab wound.

If the fundus of the gallbladder is necrotic, the gangrenous portion should be excised and the remainder of the gallbladder closed around the catheter, using purse-string sutures as previously described.

CHOLECYSTECTOMY. A principal aim of the technique is to avoid injury to the common duct while transecting the cystic duct close to its junction with the common bile duct to obviate a long cystic duct remnant.

Technique (Fig. 31-24). The gallbladder may be approached through an oblique right upper quadrant incision (Kocher or Courvoisier), through a vertical right paramedian incision, or through the upper midline. There are frequently adhesions between the gallbladder, particularly

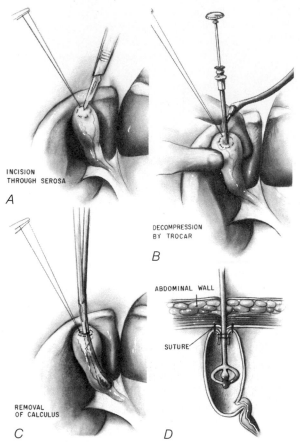

INCISION
THROUGH SEROSA

A

DECOMPRESSION
BY TROCAR

B

ABDOMINAL WALL

SUTURE

REMOVAL
OF CALCULUS

C   *D*

Fig. 31-23. Cholecystostomy. *A.* Placement of purse-string suture in fundus of gallbladder, and incision through serosa. *B.* Trochar decompression. *C.* Removal of calculus from ampulla. *D.* Sagittal section demonstrating two concentric purse-string sutures, intraluminal catheter, and suturing of serosa of gallbladder to peritoneum.

the ampulla, and the duodenum and colon. These should be lysed by sharp dissection. By applying traction laterally to the ampulla and retracting the duodenum medially, the veil of peritoneum running from ampulla to hepatoduodenal ligament may be accentuated and incised. The cystic duct is identified and a silk ligature passed around it. Traction is applied to the ligature to prevent passage of a stone down the cystic duct during dissection of the gallbladder. Dissection is then continued craniad in this peritoneal fold, and the cystic artery is identified. The course of this artery to the gallbladder should be demonstrated to avoid ligating the right hepatic artery. The cystic artery should be doubly ligated and transected. If bleeding occurs from the cystic artery, it is best controlled by applying pressure on the hepatic artery within the hepatoduodenal ligament. The artery is compressed between the index finger, which is inserted into the foramen of Winslow posteriorly, and the thumb anteriorly. The peritoneum overlying the gallbladder is then incised close to the liver, and dissection is begun from the fundus of the gallbladder down to an ultimate pedicle of cystic duct. During this dissection, blood vessels coursing from the liver may require ligation, and the gallbladder bed should be inspected

for large draining ducts, which should also be ligated. Attention is then directed toward visualization of the junction of the cystic duct with the common duct. The cystic duct is transected and ligated 3 mm from the common bile duct. It is not necessary to close the bed of the gallbladder, but a drain should be brought out from the hepatorenal pouch, which is the most dependent portion of the upper abdomen with the patient in the supine position, via a separate stab wound. Several series have shown that in the absence of specific indications, drainage is not required.

The above-described method is directed at facilitating demonstration of the junction between the cystic duct and common bile duct. The gallbladder may also be removed in a so-called "retrograde" fashion, in which the cystic duct is ligated close to the junction with the common duct as the initial part of the procedure. Then, after the cystic duct and artery have been transected, dissection is begun from the cystic duct and continued outward toward the fundus (Fig. 31-25).

OPERATIONS ON THE COMMON BILE DUCT. The situations necessitating operative procedure on the common bile duct include exploration for calculi, repair of a surgically interrupted or injured common duct, stenosis of the sphincter of Oddi, and bypass procedures for obstructive jaundice secondary to trauma, tumors, and atresia. The indications for concomitant exploration of the common bile duct during cholecystectomy have been enumerated in the section of choledocholithiasis.

Initial Exploration for Choledocholithiasis. When the procedure (Fig. 31-26) is being performed at the time of cholecystectomy, the cystic duct should be identified initially. Traction is applied to a ligature passed around this duct to avoid passage of stones from the gallbladder into the common duct. The gallbladder is generally removed after the common duct has been thoroughly explored and distal patency demonstrated. After the common duct has been visualized, aspiration with a fine needle provides confirmation. Two fixation sutures are placed distal to the junction of the cystic and common bile duct, and a vertical incision is made between these through the anterior wall. Calculi are removed by a combination of stone forceps, scoops, balloon-tipped catheters, and irrigation. These procedures should first be applied to the common bile duct toward the ampulla of Vater and subsequently to each of the main hepatic ducts. After the stones have been removed, a #6 Bâkes dilator should pass readily into the duodenum, and the tip of the dilator should be visualized through the wall of the intestine. After free passage of the dilator has been demonstrated, a T tube, with the ellipse removed from the junction of the horizontal and vertical limbs of the T to facilitate removal of the tube postoperatively, is inserted into the common duct. The limbs of the T should be short, so that the distal limb does not pass through the ampulla of Vater and the proximal limb does not obstruct either of the hepatic ducts. The common duct is then closed with interrupted sutures, and saline solution is injected into the T tube to demonstrate absence of leaks. At this stage an operative cholangiogram may be performed to rule out retained stones and demonstrate free passage of the radiopaque medium into the duodenum.

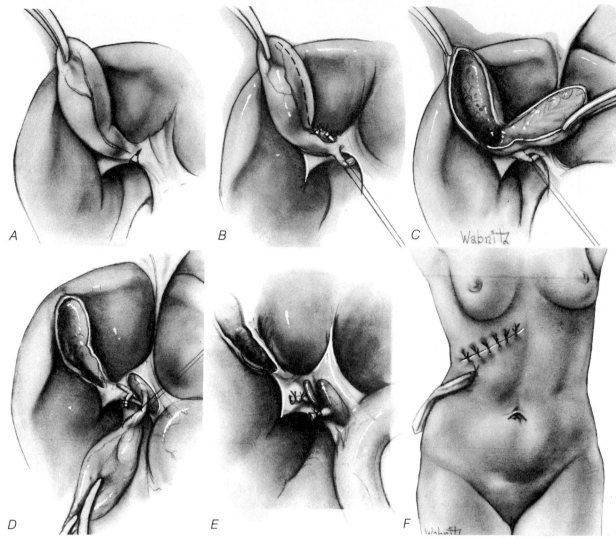

Fig. 31-24. Cholecystectomy (preferred approach.) *A.* Veil of peritoneum coursing from ampulla to hepatoduodenal ligament is transected, and cystic duct is identified. *B.* Ligature is passed around cystic duct and traction applied to prevent passage of calculi from gallbladder into common duct during the course of subsequent dissection. Dissection is continued along same fold of peritoneum, and cystic artery is doubly ligated and transected. Incision is made in peritoneum overlying gallbladder. *C.* Gallbladder is removed from its bed, and if large vessels or bile ducts are encountered, they are ligated. Dissection continues from fundus toward junction between cystic duct and common bile duct. *D.* Ultimate pedicle of cystic duct is established, and junction between cystic duct and common bile duct is defined. *E.* Cystic duct is ligated and transfixed and then transected approximately 3mm from its junction with the common bile duct. *F.* Drain is brought out via stab wound from the hepatorenal (Morison's) pouch.

The T tube should be brought out through a stab wound to prevent dislodgment when the major incision is dressed. If there is no evidence of choledocholithiasis or obstruction at the ampulla of Vater, some surgeons advise primary closure of the choledochotomy without T-tube drainage. Postoperative cholangiogram is performed on the seventh

to eighth day, and if absence of stones plus clear passage of radiopaque into the duodenum is demonstrated, the tube can be removed.

Transduodenal Choledochotomy: Sphincteroplasty (Fig. 31-27). In the event that a stone is impacted at the ampulla of Vater or that a Bâkes dilator cannot be passed into the duodenum thus suggesting fibrosis of the sphincter of Oddi, a duodenotomy is performed. The lateral peritoneal reflection of the second portion of the duodenum is incised (Kocher maneuver) to facilitate exposure. A longitudinal duodenotomy is performed on the anterior aspect of the duodenum and, with the Bâkes dilator in place in the common duct to facilitate demonstration of the sphincter, the sphincter is incised, and the impacted calculus is removed. If there is evidence of fibrosis of the sphincter, a V segment should be removed. Free passage of a #6 Bâkes dilator into the duodenum from the common bile duct should then be demonstrated and a T tube inserted into the common duct. The duodenotomy is preferably closed in two layers. The longitudinal incision may be converted into a transverse closure to prevent stenosis. The

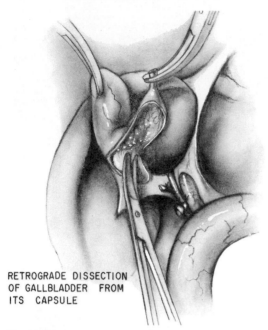

RETROGRADE DISSECTION
OF GALLBLADDER FROM
ITS CAPSULE

Fig. 31-25. Retrograde dissection of gallbladder. After cystic duct has been identified, its junction with common bile duct is defined, and cystic duct is transected. Cystic artery is also doubly ligated and transected, and gallbladder is removed from its bed with dissection progressing from the cystic duct and ampulla outward toward fundus.

procedure is also applicable to the problem of multiple or recurrent stones.

Operative Procedures for Recurrent Choledocholithiasis: Choledochoduodenostomy (Fig. 31-28). Common duct exploration is carried out as described above. If the surgeon is concerned about the possibility of subsequent reexplorations, either because of the patient's age or the fact that the surgeon is not totally satisfied that all stones have been removed, a choledochoduodenostomy may be performed.

The incision in the common duct should be enlarged, and after all apparent stones have been removed, a Kocher maneuver is performed on the duodenum, and a side-to-side anastomosis between the common duct and the duodenum is carried out. One or two layers may be used for this anastomosis, but it is imperative that the stoma be large enough so that subsequent scarring does not result in spontaneous closure.

Repair of Injured or Strictured Common Duct (Fig. 31-29). If transection of the common bile duct is noted at operation, an end-to-end anastomosis over a T tube stent is indicated. A single layer of sutures is sufficient, and the results are usually excellent.

If the stricture has developed subsequent to injury of the common duct, the preferable method of treatment is direct repair of the common bile duct over a T tube. The strictured area may be excised and the common duct mobilized so that an end-to-end anastomosis is possible. If the area of stricture is extensive and if the distal common bile duct cannot be identified, a proximal decompressive procedure is indicated.

Decompressive Procedures. A great variety of procedures are applicable, and the selection is primarily dependent upon the availability of the gallbladder or proximal ducts.

Fig. 31-26. Exploration of the common bile duct. *A.* Ligature has been placed around cystic duct to prevent passage of stones from gallbladder into common duct. After common bile duct has been identified by dissection and aspiration, two stay sutures are placed on either side. A longitudinal incision is made in the common duct. *B.* Duct is explored with stone forceps and scoops, and irrigated in both directions, i.e., toward liver and toward ampulla of Vater. Prior to insertion of a T tube, a #6 Bâkes dilator should pass readily into duodenum. *C.* An ellipse is removed from junction of horizontal and vertical limbs of the T tube, and a T tube is inserted into common duct via choledochotomy. Distal limb of T tube should be short and should not pass through ampulla of Vater. Proximal limb should also be short and positioned so that it does not obstruct either of hepatic ducts. *D.* Choledochostomy is closed tightly around T tube, which is irrigated to demonstrate absence of leakage.

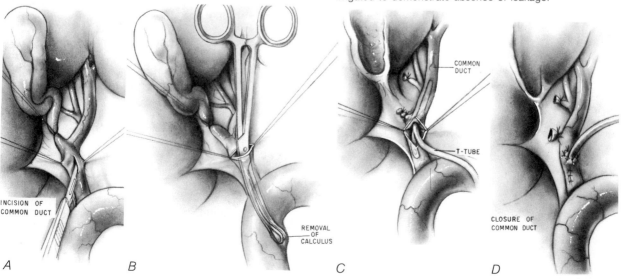

INCISION OF
COMMON DUCT

REMOVAL
OF
CALCULUS

COMMON
DUCT

T-TUBE

CLOSURE OF
COMMON DUCT

A   *B*   *C*   *D*

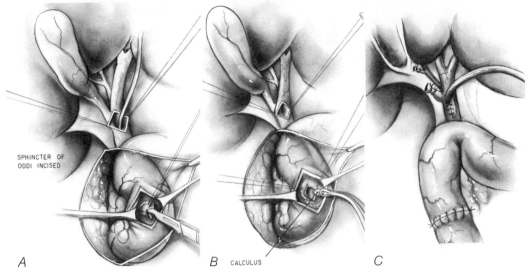

SPHINCTER OF ODDI INCISED

A

B CALCULUS

C

Fig. 31-27. Transduodenal choledochotomy: sphincterotomy. *A.* Kocher maneuver is performed on second portion of duodenum, and longitudinal duodenotomy is carried out. With Bâkes dilator inserted in common duct in order to define ampulla of Vater, stay suture is placed in ampulla, which is incised. *B.* Wedge of tissue should be removed from sphincter, and calculus impacted in this region can readily be excised. *C.* T tube is inserted into the common bile duct, and duodenotomy is closed transversely.

If obstruction is at the level of the distal common duct, an anastomosis between proximal common duct and intestine is indicated. The common duct may be anastomosed to the side of the jejunum or preferably to a Roux en Y jejunal segment 30 cm in length. The latter has the theoretic advantage of decreasing the incidence of ascend-

ing cholangitis. With obstruction of the proximal common bile duct, the gallbladder, if present, can be anastomosed to the jejunum (Fig. 31-7*B*), or the common hepatic duct may be anastomosed as a Roux en Y (Fig. 31-7*A*). If obstruction is at the confluence of the hepatic ducts, in the porta hepatis, decompression is more difficult, but a single hepatic duct may be anastomosed to the Roux en Y of the jejunum, or the liver may be split along its anatomic plane (Fig. 31-8*B*) and the confluence anastomosed to the intestine. With high ductal obstruction, the Longmire procedure, i.e., transection of the left lateral segment of the liver and identification of a duct with an anastomosis of the duct-bearing area of the liver to the side of the jejunum, has been applied (Fig. 31-8*A*). The results of this procedure have not been generally encouraging. The jejunal mucosal graft, as introduced by Smith (Fig. 31-30), and the U tube popularized by Terblance and associates (Fig. 31-22), have been applied with increasing frequency.

Fig. 31-28. Choledochoduodenostomy. *A.* Kocher maneuver is performed on second portion of duodenum, and common bile duct has been isolated. *B.* Seromuscular suture approximates duodenum to common bile duct. Longitudinal incision is made in distal common bile duct and in duodenum. *C.* Anterior row of anastomosis is completed, and wide stoma between duodenum and common bile duct is created.

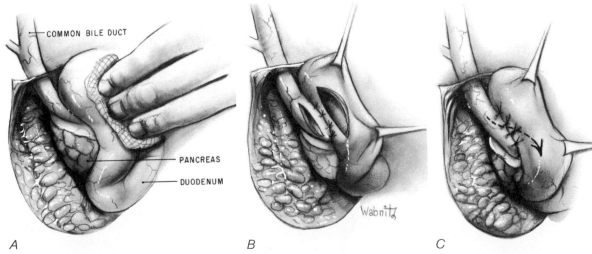

COMMON BILE DUCT

PANCREAS

DUODENUM

Wabnitz

A   *B*   *C*

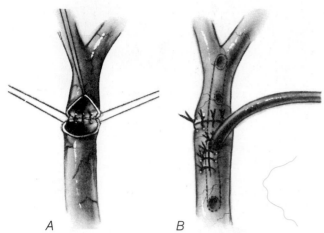

Fig. 31-29. Immediate repair of injured common duct. *A.* End-to-end anastomosis using interrupted suture is effected after cut ends of duct have been debrided. This procedure can also be carried out if there is stricture of common duct and both proximal and distal segments are identifiable. *B.* Anastomosis is complete, and T tube has been inserted as a stent via separate choledochostomy.

Fig. 31-30. Decompression of intrahepatic ducts by jejunal mucosal graft (Smith). *A.* Jejunal Roux en Y established and elipse of serosa removed. *B.* Catheter passed through liver parenchyma and into jejunal limb, where it is secured with catgut sutures. *C.* Jejunal limb pulled up so that mucosal patch abuts stoma of hepatic duct.

References

General

Glenn, F.: "Atlas of Biliary Tract Surgery," The Macmillan Company, New York, 1963.

Smith, R., and Sherlock, S.: "Surgery of the Gall Bladder and Bile Ducts," Butterworth & Co. (Publishers) Ltd., London, 1964.

Anatomy

Ahrens, E. H., Jr., Haris, R. C., and MacMahon, H. E.: Atresia of the Intrahepatic Bile Ducts, *Pediatrics,* **8:**628, 1951.

Alonso-Lej, F., Rever, W. B., and Pessagno, D. J.: Congenital Choledochal Cyst, with a Report of 2, and an Analysis of 94 Cases, *Surg Gynecol Obstet,* **108:**1, 1958.

Barlow, B., Tabor, Ed, Blanc, W. A., Santullo, T. V. and Harris, R. C.: Choledochal Cyst: A Review of 19 Cases, *J Pediatr,* **89:**934, 1976.

Benson, E. A., and Page, R. E.: A Practical Reappraisal of the Anatomy of the Extrahepatic Bile Ducts and Arteries, *Br J Surg,* **63:**853, 1976.

Bill, A. H., Brennom, W. S., and Huseby, T. L.: Biliary Atresia: New Concepts of Pathology, Diagnosis and Management, *Arch Surg,* **109:**367, 1974.

Boyden, E. A.: The Anatomy of the Choledochoduodenal Junction in Man, *Surg Gynecol Obstet,* **104:**641, 1957.

Campbell, D. P., and Williams, G. R.: Identification of the Jaundiced Infant Who Is Likely to Recover without Surgical Intervention, *Ann Surg,* **184:**89, 1976.

Gellis, S. S., and Hsia, D. Y.-Y.: Jaundice in Infancy, *Pediatr Clin North Am,* May, 1955, p. 446.

Hsia, D. Y.-Y., Patterson, P., Allen, F. H., Jr., Diamond, L. K., and Gellis, S. S.: Prolonged Obstructive Jaundice in Infancy: I. General Survey of 156 Cases, *Pediatrics,* **10:**243, 1952.

Ladd, W. E.: Congenital Atresia and Stenosis of the Bile Ducts, *JAMA,* **91:**1082, 1928.

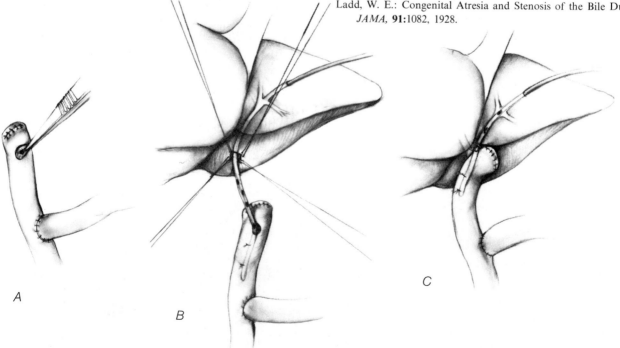

Leevy, C. M., Bender, J., Silverberg, M., and Naylor, J.: Physiology of Dye Extraction by the Liver: Comparative Studies of Sulfobromophthalein and Indocyanine Green, *Ann NY Acad Sci,* **111:**161, 1963.

Lilly, J. R., and Altman, R. P.: Hepatic Portoenterostomy (Kasai Operation) for Biliary Atresia, *Surgery,* **78:**76, 1975.

Longmire, W. P., Jr., Mandiola, S. A., and Gordon, H. E.: Congenital Cystic Disease of the Liver and Biliary System, *Ann Surg,* **174:**711, 1971.

Michels, N. A.: "Blood Supply and Anatomy of the Upper Abdominal Organs," J. B. Lippincott Company, Philadelphia, 1955.

Miyata, M., Satani, M., Ueda, T., and Okamoto, E.: Long-Term Results of Hepatic Portoenterostomy for Biliary Atresia: Special Reference to Postoperative Portal Hypertension, *Surgery,* **76:**234, 1974.

Odievre, M., Valayer, J., Razemon-Pinta, M., Habib, E.-C., and Alagille, D.: Hepatic Porto-enterostomy or Cholecystostomy in the Treatment of Extrahepatic Biliary Atresia. A Study of 49 Cases, *J Pediatr,* **88:**774, 1976.

Physiology

Davenport, H. W.: "Physiology of the Digestive Tract: An Introductory Text," The Year Book Medical Publishers, Inc., Chicago, 1961.

Ivy, A. C., and Goldman, L.: Physiology of Biliary Tract, *JAMA,* **113:**2413, 1939.

Jacobs, L. A., DeMeester, T. R., Eggleston, J. C., Margulies, S. I., and Zuidema, G. D.: Hyperplastic Cholecystoses, *Arch Surg,* **104:**193, 1972.

Johnson, F. E., and Boyden, E. A.: Effect of Double Vagotomy on Motor Activity of Human Gall Bladder, *Surgery,* **32:**591, 1952.

Jutras, J. A.: Hyperplastic Cholecystoses, *Am J Roentgenol Radium Ther Nucl Med,* **83:**795, 1960.

Kjellgren, K.: Persistence of Symptoms following Biliary Surgery, *Ann Surg,* **152:**1026, 1960.

Tanturi, C. A., and Ivy, A. C.: Study of Effect of Vascular Changes in Liver and Excitation of Its Nerve Supply on Formation of Bile, *Am J Physiol,* **121:**61, 1938.

Diagnosis of Biliary Tract Disease

Baker, H. L., Jr., and Hodgson, J. R.: Further Studies on the Accuracy of Oral Cholecystography, *Radiology,* **74:**239, 1960.

Eikman, E. A., Cameron, J. L., Colman, M., Natarajan, T. K., Dugal, P., and Wagner, H. N., Jr.: Test for Patency of Cystic Duct in Acute Cholecystitis, *Ann Intern Med,* **82:**318, 1975.

Freeman, J. B., Cohen, W. N., and Den Besten, L.: Cholecystokinin Cholangiography and Analysis of Duodenal Bile in Investigation of Pain in Right Upper Quadrant of the Abdomen without Gallstones, *Surg Gynecol Obstet,* **140:**371, 1975.

Graham, E. A., and Cole, W. H.: Roentgenologic Examination of Gallbladder: New Method Utilizing Intravenous Injection of Tetrabromphenolphthalein, *JAMA,* **82:**613, 1924.

Nora, P. F., Berci, G., Dorazio, R. A., Kirshenbaum, G., Shore, G. M., Tompkins, R. K., and Wilson, S. D.: Operative Choledochoscopy, *Am J Surg,* **133:**105, 1977.

Schein, C. J., and Beneventano, T. C.: Biliary Manometry: Its Role in Clinical Surgery, *Surgery,* **67:**255, 1970.

———, Stern, W. Z., and Jacobson, H. G.: The Common Bile Duct: Operative Cholangiography, Biliary Endoscopy and Choledocholithotomy," Charles C Thomas, Publisher, Springfield, 1966.

Scholz, F. J., Johnston, D. O., and Wise, R. E.: Intravenous Cholangiography: Optimum Dosage and Methodology. *Radiology,* **114:**513, 1975.

Shehadi, W. H.: "Clinical Radiology of the Biliary Tract," McGraw-Hill Book Company, New York, 1963.

White, T. T., Waisman, H., Hopton, D., and Kavlie, H.: Radiomanometry, Flow Rates, and Cholangiography in the Evaluation of Common Bile Duct Disease, *Am J Surg,* **123:**73, 1972.

Williams, J. A. R., Baker, R. J., Walsh, J. F., and Marion, M. A.: The Role of Biliary Scanning in the Investigation of the Surgically Jaundiced Patient, *Surg Gynecol Obstet,* **144:**525, 1977.

Trauma

Cattell, R. B., and Braasch, J. W.: General Considerations in the Management of Benign Strictures of the Bile Duct, *N Engl J Med,* **261:**929, 1959.

Cole, W. H., Ireneus, C., and Reynolds, J. T.: Strictures of the Common Duct, *Ann Surg,* **133:**684, 1951.

Diethrich, E. B., Beall, A. C., Jr., Jordan, G. L., Jr., and DeBakey, M. E.: Traumatic Injuries to the Extrahepatic Biliary Tract, *Am J Surg,* **112:**756, 1966.

Ellis, H., and Cronin, K.: Bile Peritonitis, *Br J Surg,* **48:**166, 1960.

Glenn, F.: Postoperative Strictures of the Extrahepatic Bile Ducts, *Surg Gynecol Obstet,* **120:**560, 1965.

Longmire, W. P., Jr.: Early Management of Injury to the Extrahepatic Biliary Tract, *JAMA,* **195:**623, 1966.

Manlove, C. H., Quattlebaum, F. W., and Ambrus, L.: Nonpenetrating Trauma to the Biliary Tract, *Am J Surg,* **97:**113, 1959.

Penn, I.: Injuries of the Gall-Bladder, *Br J Surg,* **49:**636, 1961–1962.

Rubenstone, A. I., Mintz, S. S., and Meranze, D. R.: Case of Fatal Bile Peritonitis following Liver Needle Biopsy, *Ann Intern Med,* **36:**166, 1952.

Schwartz, S. I., Adams, J. T., Cockett, A. T. K., and Morton, J. H.: Blunt Trauma to the Upper Abdomen, *Surg Annu,* **3:**273, 1971.

Sedgwick, C., Poulantas, J., and Kune, G.: Management of Portal Hypertension Secondary to Bile Duct Strictures: Review of 18 Cases with Splenorenal Shunt, *Ann Surg,* **163:**949, 1966.

Smith, S. W., and Hastings, T. N.: Traumatic Rupture of Gallbladder, *Ann Surg,* **139:**517, 1954.

Turney, W. H., Lee, J. P., and Raju, S.: Complete Transection of Common Bile Duct Due to Blunt Trauma, *Ann Surg,* **179:**440, 1974.

Gallstones

Adams, R., and Stranahan, A.: Cholecystitis and Cholelithiasis: Analytical Report of 1,104 Operative Cases, *Surg Gynecol Obstet,* **85:**776, 1947.

Bartlett, M. K., and Waddell, W. R.: Indications for Common-duct Exploration: Evaluation in 1,000 Cases, *N Engl J Med,* **258:**164, 1958.

Berliner, S. D., and Burson, L. C.: One-Stage Repair for Cholecyst-Duodenal Fistula and Gallstone Ileus, *Arch Surg,* **90:**313, 1965.

Bogren, H.: The Composition and Structure of Human Gallstones, *Acta Radiol Suppl,* 226, 1964.

Burhenne, H. J.: Complications of Nonoperative Extraction of Retained Common Duct Stones, *Am J Surg,* **131:**260, 1976.

Chaimoff, C., and Dintsman, M.: Presence of Pancreatic Juice in the Gallbladder of Patients with Cholelithiasis, *Isr J Med Sci,* **6:**313, 1970.

Colcock, B. P.: Stenosis of the Sphincter of Oddi, *Surg Clin North Am,* **38:**663, 1958.

———, Killen, R. B., and Leach, N. G.: The Asymptomatic Patient with Gallstones, *Am J Surg,* **113:**44, 1967.

Comfort, M. W., Gray, H. K., and Wilson, J. M.: Silent Gallstone: 10 to 20 Year Follow-up Study of 112 Cases, *Ann Surg,* **128:**931, 1948.

Cotton, P. B., Chapman, M., Whiteside, C. G., and LeQuesne, L. P.: Duodenoscopic Papillotomy and Gallstone Removal, *Br J Surg,* **63:**709, 1976.

Coyne, M. J., Bonorris, G. C., Chung, A., Goldstein, L. I., Lahana, D., and Schoenfield, L. J.: Treatment of Gallstones with Chenodeoxycholic Acid and Phenobarbital, *N Engl J Med,* **292:**604, 1975.

Day, E. A., and Marks, C.: Gallstone Ileus: Review of Literature and Presentation of 34 New Cases, *Am J Surg,* **129:**552, 1975.

Deckoff, S. L.: Gallstone Ileus, *Ann Surg,* **142:**52, 1955.

Degenshein, G. A.: Choledochoduodenostomy: An 18-Year Study of 175 Consecutive Cases, *Surgery,* **76:**319, 1974.

Fung, J.: Liver Fluke Infestation and Cholangio-Hepatitis, *Br J Surg,* **48:**404, 1961.

Henzel, J. H., and DeWeese, M. S.: Common Duct Exploration with and without Balloon-Tipped Biliary Catheters, *Arch Surg,* **103:**199, 1971.

Kleeberg, J.: Experimental Studies on the Colloid Chemical Mechanism of Gallstone Formation, *Gastroenterologia,* **80:**313, 1953.

Large, A. M.: On the Formation of Gallstones, *Surgery,* **54:**928, 1963.

Madden, J. L., Chun, J. Y., Kandalaft, S., and Parekh, M.: Choledochoduodenostomy: An Unjustly Maligned Surgical Procedure?, *Am J Surg,* **119:**45, 1970.

Maki, T.: Pathogenesis of Calcium Bilirubinate Gallstone: Role of *E. coli,* β-Glucuronidase and Coagulation by Inorganic Ions, Polyelectrolytes and Agitation, *Ann Surg,* **164:**90, 1966.

Merendino, K. A., and Manhas, D. R.: Man-Made Gallstones: New Entity following Cardiac Valve Replacement, *Ann Surg,* **177:**694, 1973.

Method, H. L., Mehn, W. H., and Frable, W. J.: "Silent" Gallstones, *Arch Surg,* **85:**338, 1962.

Räf, L., and Spangen, L.: Gallstone Ileus, *Acta Chir Scand,* **137:**665, 1971.

Rains, A. J. H.: Researches concerning the Formation of Gallstones, *Br Med J,* **2:**685, 1962.

Small, D. M.: Gallstones: Diagnosis and Treatment, *Postgrad Med,* **51:**187, 1972.

Thistle, J. L., and Schoenfield, L. J.: Lithogenic Bile among Young Indian Women: Lithogenic Potential Disease with Chenodeoxycholic Acid, *N Engl J Med,* **284:**177, 1971.

Thureborn, E.: Formation of Gallstone in Man, *Arch Surg,* **91:**952, 1965.

Van Der Linden, W.: Some Biological Traits in Female Gallstone-disease Patients, *Acta Chir Scand* [*Suppl*], vol. **269,** 1961.

Warshaw, A. L., and Bartlett, M. K.: Choice of Operation for Gallstone Intestinal Obstruction, *Ann Surg,* **164:**1051, 1966.

Way, L. W., Admirand, W., and Dunphy, J. E.: The Management of Choledocholithiasis, *Ann Surg.,* **176:**347, 1972.

Womack, N. A.: The Development of Gallstones, *Surg Gynecol Obstet,* **133:**937, 1971.

Zollinger, R. M., Boles, E. T., and Crawford, G. B.: The Diagnosis and Management of Biliary-Tract Disease, *N Engl J Med,* **252:**203, 1955.

Inflammatory and Other Benign Lesions

Acosta, J., and Nardi, G. L.: Papillitis of the Ampulla of Vater, *Arch Surg,* **92:**354, 1966.

Adams, J. T., Libertino, J. A., and Schwartz, S. I.: Significance of an Elevated Serum Amylase, *Surgery,* **63:**877, 1968.

Bartlett, M. K., and Dreyfuss, J. R.: Residual Common Duct Stones, *Surgery,* **47:**202, 1960.

Becker, W. F., Powell, J. I., and Turner, R. J.: A Clinical Study of 1,060 Patients with Acute Cholecystitis, *Surg Gynecol Obstet,* **104:**491, 1957.

Bisgard, J. D., and Baker, C. P.: Studies Relating to the Pathogenesis of Cholecystitis, Cholelithiasis, and Acute Pancreatitis, *Ann Surg,* **112:**1006, 1940.

Burnett, W.: The Management of Acute Cholecystitis, *Aust New Zeal J Surg,* **41:**25, 1971.

———, and Shields, R.: Symptoms after Cholecystectomy, *Lancet,* **1:**923, 1958.

Cattell, R. B., and Colcock, B. P.: Fibrosis of the Sphincter of Oddi, *Ann Surg,* **137:**797, 1953.

Charcot, J. M.: "Leçons sur les maladies du foie des voies filiares et des reins," Faculté de Médecine de Paris, 1877.

Chetlin, S. H., and Elliott, D. W.: Biliary Bacteremia, *Arch Surg,* **102:**303, 1971.

Colcock, B. P., and Perey, B.: Exploration of the Common Bile Duct, *Surg Gynecol Obstet,* **118:**20, 1964.

Danzi, J. T., Makipour, H., and Farmer, R. G.: Primary Sclerosing Cholangitis: A Report of Nine Cases and Clinical Review, *Am J Gastroenterol,* **65:**109, 1976.

DeCamp, P. T., Ochsner, A., Baffes, T. G., Bancroft, H., and Bendel, W.: Timing in the Surgical Treatment of Acute Colecystitis, *Ann Surg,* **135:**734, 1952.

Dunphy, J. E., and Ross, F. P.: Studies in Acute Cholecystitis, *Surgery,* **26:**539, 1949.

Ellison, E. H.: Early Operation for Acute Cholecystitis, in J. H. Mulholland, E. H. Ellison, and S. R. Friesen (eds.), "Current Surgical Management," W. B. Saunders Company, Philadelphia, 1957.

Friesen, S. R.: Management of Acute Cholecystitis by Selection of Patients for Early or Delayed Operation, in J. H. Mulholland, E. H. Ellison, and S. R. Friesen (eds.), "Current Surgical Management," W. B. Saunders Company, Philadelphia, 1957.

Garlock, J. H., and Hurwitt, E. S.: The Cystic Duct Stump Syndrome, *Surgery,* **29:**833, 1951.

Glenn, F.: Common Duct Exploration for Stones, *Surg Gynecol Obstet,* **95:**431, 1952.

——— and Moody, F. C.: Acute Obstructive Suppurative Cholangitis, *Surg Gynecol Obstet,* **113:**265, 1961.

——— and Whitsell, J. C., II: The Surgical Treatment of Cystic Duct Remnants, *Surg Gynecol Obstet,* **113:**711, 1961.

Goldstein, F., Grunt, R., and Margulies, M.: Cholecystokinin Cholecystography in Differential Diagnosis of Acalculous Gallbladder Disease, *Am J Dig Dis,* **19:**835, 1974.

Grage, T. B., Lober, P. H., Imamogly, K., and Wangensteen, O. H.: Stenosis of the Sphincter of Oddi, *Surgery,* **48:**304, 1960.

Haupert, A. P., Carey, L. C., Evans, W. E., and Ellison, E. H.: Acute Suppurative Cholangitis: Experience with 15 Consecutive Cases, *Arch Surg,* **94:**460, 1967.

Havard, C.: Non-malignant Bile Duct Obstruction, *Ann R Coll Surg Engl,* **26:**88, 1960.

Hinchey, E. J., Elias, G. L., and Hampson, L. G.: Acute Cholecystitis, *Surg Gynecol Obstet,* **120:**475, 1966.

Hoerr, S. O., and Hazard, J. B.: Acute Cholecystitis without Gallbladder Stones, *Am J Surg,* **111:**47, 1966.

Keighley, M. R. B., Lister, C. M., Jacobs, S. I., and Giles, G. R.: Hazards of Surgical Treatment Due to Microorganisms in Bile, *Surgery,* **75:**578, 1974.

Lindenauer, S. M.: Surgical Treatment of Bile Duct Strictures, *Surgery,* **73:**875, 1973.

McCubbrey, D., and Thieme, E. T.: Perforation of the Gallbladder, *Arch Surg,* **80:**204, 1960.

Mackey, W. A.: Cholecystitis without Stone, *Br J Surg,* **22:**274, 1934.

Mage, S., and Morel, S.: Surgical Experience with Cholangio-hepatitis (Hong Kong Disease), *Ann Surg,* **162:**187, 1965.

Manesis, J. G., and Sullivan, J. F.: Primary Sclerosing Cholangitis, *Arch Intern Med,* **115:**137, 1956.

Massie, J. R., Coxe, J. W., III, Parker, C., and Dietrick, R.: Gallbladder Perforations in Acute Cholecystitis, *Ann Surg,* **145:**825, 1957.

Mentzer, R. M., Jr., Golden, G. T., Chandler, J. G., and Horsley, J. S., III: Comparative Appraisal of Emphysematous Cholecystitis, *Am J Surg,* **129:**10, 1975.

Mulholland, J. H.: "Delayed Operative Management of Acute Cholecystitis," in J. H. Mulholland, E. H. Ellison, and S. R. Friesen (eds.), "Current Surgical Management," W. B. Saunders Company, Philadelphia, 1957.

Munster, A. M., and Brown, J. R.: Acalculous Cholecystitis, *Am J Surg,* **113:**730, 1967.

Ong, G. B.: A Study of Recurrent Pyogenic Cholangitis, *Arch Surg,* **84:**199, 1962.

Ostermiller, W., Thompson, R., Carter, R., and Hinshaw, D.: Acute Obstructive Cholangitis, *Arch Surg,* **90:**392, 1965.

Ottinger, L. W.: Acute Cholecystitis as a Postoperative Complication, *Ann Surg,* **184:**162, 1976.

Pheils, M. T., and Duraiappah, B.: Exploration of Common Bile Duct in Presence of Acute Cholecystitis, *Aust NZ J Surg,* **43:**136, 1973.

Reynolds, B. M., and Dargan, E. L.: Acute Obstructive Cholangitis, *Ann Surg,* **150:**299, 1959.

Rosoff, L., and Meyers, H.: Acute Emphysematous Cholecystitis: An Analysis of Ten Cases, *Am J Surg,* **111:**410, 1966.

Ruskin, R. B., Katon, R. M., Bilbao, M. K., and Smith, R.: Evaluation of Sclerosing Cholangitis by Endoscopic Retrograde Cholangiopancreatography, *Arch Intern Med,* **136:**232, 1976.

Schein, C. J.: "Acute Cholecystitis," Harper & Row, Publishers, Incorporated, New York, 1972.

Schwartz, S. I., and Dale, W. A.: Primary Sclerosing Cholangitis: Review and Report of Six Cases, *Arch Surg,* **77:**439, 1958.

Stefanini, P., Carboni, M., Patrassi, N., Basoli, A., Bernardinis, G. de, and Negro, P.: Roux en Y Hepaticojejunostomy: Reappraisal of Its Indications and Results, *Ann Surg,* **181:**213, 1975.

Stock, F. E., and Fung, J. H. Y.: Oriental Cholangiohepatitis, *Arch Surg,* **84:**409, 1962.

——— and Tinckler, L.: Choledochoduodenostomy in Treatment of Cholangiohepatitis, *Surg Gynecol Obstet,* **101:**599, 1955.

Ternberg, J. L., and Keating, J. P.: Acute Acalculous Cholecystitis: Complication of Other Illnesses in Childhood, *Arch Surg,* **110:**543, 1975.

Tinckler, L.: Primary Sclerosing Cholangitis, *Postgrad Med,* **47:** 666, 1971.

Van der Linden, W., and Sunzel, H.: Early Versus Delayed Operation for Acute Cholecystitis: Controlled Clinical Trial, *Am J Surg,* **120:**7, 1970.

Warren, K., Athanassiades, S., and Monge, J.: Primary Sclerosing Cholangitis: A Study of 42 Cases, *Am J Surg,* **111:**23, 1966.

Watkins, D. F. L., and Thomas, G. G.: Jaundice in Acute Cholecystitis, *Br J Surg,* **58:**570, 1971.

Welch, J. P., and Donaldson, G. A.: The Urgency of Diagnosis and Surgical Treatment of Acute Suppurative Cholangitis, *Am J Surg,* **131:**527, 1976.

——— and Malt, R. A.: Outcome of Cholecystostomy, *Surg Gynecol Obstet,* **135:**717, 1972.

Womack, N. A., and Crider, R. L.: Persistence of Symptoms following Cholecystectomy, *Ann Surg,* **126:**31, 1947.

Tumors

Altemeier, W. A., Gall, E. A., Culbertson, W. R., and Inge, W. W.: Sclerosing Carcinoma of the Intrahepatic (Hilar) Bile Ducts, *Surgery,* **60:**191, 1966.

Beltz, W. R., and Condon, R. E.: Primary Carcinoma of the Gallbladder, *Ann Surg,* **180:**180, 1974.

Brasfield, R. D.: Right Hepatic Lobectomy for Carcinoma of the Gallbladder: A Five-Year Cure, *Ann Surg,* **153:**563, 1961.

Comfort, M. W., Gray, H. K., and Wilson, J. M.: Silent Gallstone: A 10 to 25 Year Follow-up Study of 112 Cases, *Ann Surg,* **128:**931, 1948.

Donaldson, L. A., and Busuttil, A.: Clinicopathologic Review of 68 Carcinomas of the Gallbladder, *Br J Surg,* **62:**26, 1975.

Fahim, R. B., McDonald, J. R., Richards, J. C., and Ferris, D. O.: Carcinoma of the Gallbladder: A Study of Its Modes of Spread, *Ann Surg,* **156:**114, 1962.

Kirshbaum, J. D., and Kozoll, D. D.: Carcinoma of the Gallbladder and Extrahepatic Bile Ducts: A Clinical and Pathological Study of 117 Cases in 13,330 Necopsies, *Surg Gynecol Obstet,* **73:**740, 1941.

Kuwayti, K., Baggenstoss, A. H., Stauffer, M. H., and Priestley, J. T.: Carcinoma of the Intrahepatic and Extrahepatic Bile Ducts Exclusive of the Papilla of Vater, *Surg. Gynecol Obstet,* **104:**357, 1957.

Litwin, M. S.: Primary Carcinoma of the Gallbladder, *Arch Surg,* **95:**236, 1967.

Molnar, W., and Stockum, A. E.: Relief from Obstructive Jaundice through Percutaneous Transhepatic Catheter: New Therapeutic Method, *Am J Roentgenol Radium Ther Nucl Med,* **122:**356, 1974.

Mori, K., Misumi, A., Sugiyama, M., Okabe, M., Matsuoka, T.,

Ishii, J., and Akagi, M.: Percutaneous Transhepatic Bile Damage, *Ann Surg,* **185:**111, 1977.

Neibling, H. H., Dockerty, M. B., and Waugh, J. M.: Carcinoma of the Extrahepatic Bile Ducts, *Surg Gynecol Obstet,* **89:**429, 1949.

Pemberton, L. B., Diffenbaugh, W. F., and Strohl, E. L.: The Surgical Significance of Carcinoma of the Gallbladder, *Am J Surg,* **122:**381, 1971.

Quattlebaum, J. K., and Quattlebaum, J. K., Jr.: Malignant Obstruction of the Major Hepatic Ducts, *Ann Surg,* **161:**876, 1965.

Robertson, W. A., and Carlisle, B. B.: Primary Carcinoma of the Gallbladder: Review of Fifty-two cases, *Am J Surg,* **113:**738, 1967.

Sheinfeld, W.: Cholecystectomy and Partial Hepatectomy for Carcinoma of the Gallbladder with Local Liver Extension, *Surgery,* **22:**48, 1947.

Terblanche, J., Saunders, S. J., and Louw, J. H.: Prolonged Palliation in Carcinoma of the Main Hepatic Duct Junction, *Surgery,* **71:**728, 1972.

Thomas, C. G., Jr., Nicholson, C. P., and Owen, J.: Effectiveness of Choledochoduodenostomy and Transduodenal Sphincter-otomy in the Treatment of Benign Obstruction of the Common Duct, *Ann Surg,* **173:**845, 1971.

Thorbjarnarson, B.: Carcinoma of the Bile Ducts, *Cancer,* **12:**708, 1959.

Tompkins, R. K., Johnson, J., Storm, F. K., and Longmire, W. P., Jr.: Operative Endoscopy in the Management of Biliary Tract Neoplasms, *Am J Surg,* **132:**174, 1976.

Vaittinen, E.: Carcinoma of the Gallbladder: Study of 390 Cases Diagnosed in Finland, 1953–67, *Ann Chir Gynaecol Fenn,* Vol. 59, suppl, 168, 1970.

Whelton, M. J., Petrelli, M., George, P., Young, W. B., and Sherlock, S.: Carcinoma at Junction of Main Hepatic Ducts, *Q J Med,* **38:**211, 1969.

Operations on the Biliary Tract

Kambouris, A., Carpenter, W. S., and Allaben, R. D.: Cholecystectomy without Drainage, *Surg Gynecol Obstet,* **137:**613, 1973.

Wexler, M. J., and Smith, R.: Jejunal Mucosal Graft: Sutureless Technic for Repair of High Bile Duct Strictures, *Am J Surg,* **129:**204, 1975.

Chapter 32

Pancreas

by **William Silen**

ANATOMY

The pancreas extends transversely across the upper abdomen behind the stomach. The junction of the upper left portion of the head of the pancreas with the body is called the "neck," or "waist," a constricted and narrowed area rarely more than 3 to 4 cm wide. The superior mesenteric vein and artery lie just behind the neck and are enclosed behind by a posterior extension of the lower left portion of the head (uncinate process).

DUCTAL SYSTEM. The main pancreatic duct (duct of Wirsung) begins at the tail of the pancreas and extends to the right at, or slightly superior to, a point halfway between the superior and inferior borders of the pancreas. It lies somewhat closer to the posterior than to the anterior surface of the organ, and its tributaries enter almost at right angles along its entire course. In the head of the pancreas the major duct turns inferiorly and joins the common bile duct at the papilla of Vater. The minor duct, or duct of Santorini, lies in the head of the pancreas in a much more ventral plane and therefore in a surgically more vulnerable plane than the duct of Wirsung. This duct begins at its junction with the main duct in the neck of the pancreas and terminates in the minor papilla, located about 2 cm proximal to the major papilla and 7 cm distal to the pylorus. Tiny accessory ducts emptying directly from the pancreas into the intrapancreatic portion of the common bile duct have been described.

Many variations in the normal anatomy of the ductal system have been described (Fig. 32-1). Configuration of the ducts is "normal" in only 60 to 70 percent of the population. In about 30 percent of cases, although a duct of Santorini exists, it does not communicate with the duodenum. Reich has recently found that this anatomic arrangement is more frequent in patients with duodenal ulcer, and he has suggested that the lack of alkaline pancreatic juice in this region may make the duodenum more susceptible to peptic ulceration. In 5 to 10 percent of human beings, the duct of Santorini is the sole duct draining the pancreas into the duodenum. In such cases injury to the duct of Santorini, especially during gastrectomy, may cause severe hemorrhagic or recurrent pancreatitis. Since the gastroduodenal artery always passes behind the duodenum proximal to the minor papilla, this vascular landmark may be useful as an indication that further distal dissection of the duodenum may be extremely hazardous.

In the second decade of life the major pancreatic duct is 3 to 4 mm in diameter. As aging progresses, the ducts become larger, and in persons over the age of seventy, ducts 5 to 6 mm in diameter are commonly encountered in the normal pancreas.

BLOOD SUPPLY. The arterial supply to the pancreas is remarkably constant (Fig. 32-2). Anterior and posterior arcades supply the head of the pancreas; each arcade derives a superior component from the gastroduodenal artery and an inferior component from the superior mesenteric artery. The anterosuperior pancreaticoduodenal and anteroinferior pancreaticoduodenal arteries join to form the anterior arcade; the posterosuperior pancreaticoduodenal and posteroinferior pancreaticoduodenal arteries form the posterior arcade. This arrangement occurs in almost 100 percent of cases. The anterior arcade constitutes virtually the only major group of blood vessels on the anterior surface of the pancreas, an important surgical consideration.

The inferior pancreatic artery, which is nearly always constant, runs along the posteroinferior surface of the pancreas in intimate contact with the organ. Its origin is variable; it may start from the superior mesenteric artery, anterosuperior or anteroinferior pancreaticoduodenal artery, or superior pancreatic artery.

The superior pancreatic artery is present in from 50 to 90 percent of patients and arises from the splenic, hepatic, superior mesenteric, or celiac arteries. It lies along the posterosuperior portion of the neck and body of the pan-

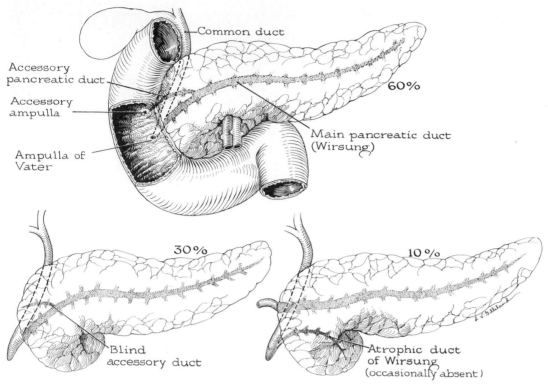

creas. The body and tail of the pancreas are also supplied by branches from the splenic and left gastroepiploic arteries.

The venous drainage of the pancreas follows the course of the arteries quite closely, but the veins lie superficial to their arterial counterparts. Anterior and posterior venous arcades are always present around the head of the pancreas. The confluence of the right gastroepiploic vein, anterosuperior pancreaticoduodenal vein, and middle colic vein forms the gastrocolic trunk, which empties directly into the superior mesenteric vein at the inferior border of

Fig. 32-1. Anatomic configuration of the intrapancreatic ductal system. Note the lack of communication between the two ducts in 10 percent of cases. (*From W. Silen, Surg Clin North Am, 44:1253, 1964.*)

the neck of the pancreas. This provides an important landmark for location of the superior mesenteric vein when the pancreas is mobilized to determine operability of pancreatic tumors.

From the surgical standpoint it is important to remem-

Fig. 32-2. Arterial supply and venous drainage of the pancreas. Note particularly the anatomic importance of the gastrocolic venous trunk in defining the inferior portion of the neck. (*From W. Silen, Surg Clin North Am, 44:1253, 1964.*)

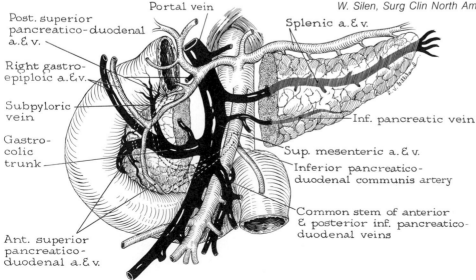

ber that occasionally the hepatic artery may arise from the superior mesenteric artery and pass behind the pancreas and common bile duct. An unusually long and tortuous hepatic artery may lie close to the superior border of the head of the pancreas, or in some cases it may be within the pancreas itself. Under these circumstances, the hepatic artery may be injured during resection of the body and tail of the pancreas and may require ligation. Pierson has pointed out that the distal duodenum and proximal jejunum receive their arterial supply from one of the inferior pancreaticoduodenal arteries, so that interruption of these vessels probably will necessitate resection of the proximal 3 to 5 cm of jejunum.

Anatomy textbooks usually state that the anterior surface of the superior mesenteric and portal veins is free of tributaries in the region of the pancreas. However, the superior pancreaticoduodenal vein often joins the portal vein at the anterior surface of the pancreas, and the gastrocolic vein almost always joins the anterior surface of the superior mesenteric vein inferior to the neck. Other small venous tributaries from the pancreas to the portal and superior mesenteric veins are often present, although hidden from view. The posterosuperior pancreaticoduodenal vein may be the source of severe hemorrhage during mobilization of the portal vein for portacaval shunt.

LYMPHATIC DRAINAGE AND NERVE SUPPLY. The lymphatic capillaries from the tail drain into the nodes at the hilus of the spleen. From the right side of the pancreas the lymphatics drain into the pancreaticoduodenal lymph nodes lying in the groove between the duodenum and pancreas and into the subpyloric nodes. Anteriorly the drainage is to the superior pancreatic, superior gastric, and hepatic nodes along the hepatic artery. Posteriorly the lymphatics pass to the inferior pancreatic, mesocolic, mesenteric, and aortic nodes.

The sympathetic nerve supply to the pancreas is derived from the greater, lesser, and lowest splanchnic nerves via the celiac ganglia and plexus. These fibers conduct the afferent pain fibers from the pancreas. The sympathetic nerves intermingle with branches of the right vagus nerve to form the splenic plexus from which most of the nerve supply to the pancreas emanates. The celiac branch of the right, or posterior, vagus nerve provides parasympathetic supply to the pancreas. This branch can be spared during selective gastric vagotomy for duodenal ulcer.

Annular Pancreas

Annular pancreas is a rare anatomic abnormality which results when two limbs of pancreatic tissue encircle the second portion of the duodenum because of incomplete migration of the ventral anlage of the gland. A variable degree of duodenal obstruction occurs, and associated anomalies, particularly complete atresia of the duodenum, are common. Histologically, the lesion presents as normal pancreatic tissue.

Frequently there are no symptoms, and the finding is incidental. When symptoms occur, they are related to acute and recurrent duodenal obstruction and include abdominal pain, nausea, and vomiting. The onset of symptoms ap-

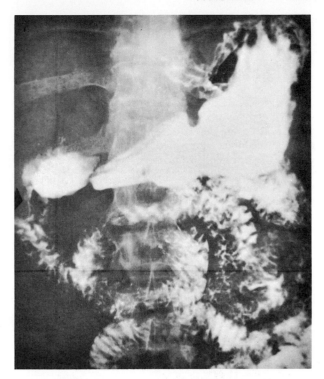
Fig. 32-3. Roentgenogram demonstrating annular pancreas.

pears at all ages, but one-third present under the age of one. The diagnosis is suggested by the roentgenographic finding of partial or complete duodenal obstruction with notching of the right lateral duodenal wall (Fig. 32-3). A variety of surgical procedures have been proposed, including partial resection of the annular portion of the gland or bypassing the area of obstruction. The former is frequently followed by pancreatic fistula, and it is the consensus that duodenojejunostomy is the least hazardous and most effective way of relieving the obstruction.

PHYSIOLOGY

Exocrine Pancreas

PANCREATIC JUICE. The human pancreas daily produces from 1,500 to 2,500 ml of a colorless, odorless fluid which has a pH of 8.0 to 8.3. Pancreatic juice is isosmotic with the plasma, and its osmolality is independent of the rate of flow, both in health and disease. The bicarbonate of pancreatic juice is secreted by an active transport mechanism, and as the solution moves down the collecting system, exchange with chloride ion takes place. The sum of the concentrations of bicarbonate and chloride is constant under all conditions of secretion, although bicarbonate concentration rises with increasing rates of secretion. The secretion of bicarbonate is under the catalytic influence of carbonic anhydrase. The isosmotic reabsorption of water and electrolytes from the ductal lumen may be governed by antidiuretic hormone. The concentration of sodium and potassium is similar to that in plasma, which indicates that these ions are moved passively rather than actively.

Pancreatic juice contains between 1 and 3 percent protein, 90 percent of which is enzymatic. Since the metabolic turnover of protein in the acinar cells of the pancreas is the highest of any cells in the body, the pancreas is dependent upon a constant supply of amino acids. It is not surprising, therefore, that protein deficiency may be associated with severe defects in exocrine pancreatic function, as in kwashiorkor. Proteolytic, lipolytic, and amylolytic enzymes are present in the pancreatic juice; the optimal pH for activity of all three enzyme systems is greater than 7. These enzymes are formed within the mitochondrial apparatus of the secreting cells, at the site of the attached ribosomes of the endoplasmic reticulum. Pancreatic trypsinogen and chymotrypsinogen are activated to trypsin and chymotrypsin by the intestinal enzyme enterokinase, as well as by trypsin itself. These enzymes hydrolyze proteins to peptones and peptides.

Recently, other proteolytic enzymes such as procarboxypeptidases, carboxypeptidase, ribonuclease, and deoxyribonuclease have been discovered in porcine and bovine pancreatic juice, and it is probable that at least some are present in human pancreatic juice. The fat-splitting enzymes of the pancreas are lipase, which splits fat into glycerol and fatty acids in the presence of bile salts; phospholipases A and B; and cholesterol esterase. Pancreatic amylase splits starch to dextrins and disaccharides, principally maltose.

CONTROL OF PANCREATIC SECRETION (Fig. 32-4). The vagus nerve is the secretory nerve to the pancreas and plays a role in the "cephalic phase" of pancreatic secretion somewhat analogous to its relationship to the cephalic phase of gastric secretion. Sham feeding of an unanesthetized dog causes a scant flow of juice rich in enzymes, beginning 1 to 2 minutes after feeding and lasting for 30 minutes, provided that gastric juice is prevented from entering the duodenum. This response is abolished by atropine or by vagotomy. Although the splanchnic nerves may contain secretory fibers to the pancreas, the importance of these fibers is probably minimal.

White et al. have presented evidence for the existence of a gastropancreatic reflex by demonstrating that distension of the fundus of the stomach increases the volume and enzyme output of pancreatic juice, but this reflex can be temporarily abolished by vagotomy. Further evidence is required before the existence of such a reflex is definitely

Fig. 32-4. Schema of neurohumoral influences on external pancreatic secretion.

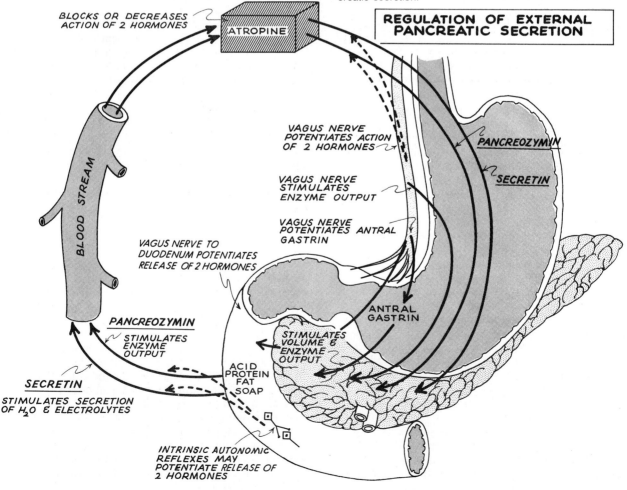

confirmed. Even though gastrin is capable of stimulating volume and enzyme output in the pancreatic juice of cats and dogs, it remains moot as to whether physiological amounts of gastrin can produce a humoral gastric phase of pancreatic secretion.

Quantitatively, the intestinal phase of pancreatic secretion is probably the most important. When gastric contents enter the duodenum, the volume and enzyme outputs of the pancreas greatly increase. This response is mediated by the release of secretin and cholecystokinin (pancreozymin) from the duodenal mucosa. These hormones may be produced in response to the introduction of a number of substances into the duodenum, including hydrochloric acid, acid peptone, sodium oleate, and a solution of amino acids. The release of secretin by intraduodenal acid has recently been shown to be directly related to the quantity of acid entering the duodenum per unit time. Small but significant amounts of secretin can be released even between pH 3.5 and 4.5 when the quantity of acid exposed to the duodenal mucosa per unit time is high.

Cholecystokinin potentiates pancreatic volume and bicarbonate output stimulated by small amounts of endogenous or exogenous secretin. The release of both secretin and cholecystokinin from the duodenal mucosa is now known to be substantially diminished by total abdominal vagotomy, although the response of the vagotomized pancreas to exogenous secretin is not altered.

The most important physiologic effect of secretin is stimulation of flow of water and electrolytes from the pancreas. There is a short latent period (about 20 seconds) between the injection of secretin or the instillation of acid into the duodenum and the onset of the secretory response. Cholecystokinin profoundly stimulates the output of enzymes; that is, its effects are similar to those of vagal stimulation. The response of the pancreas to both the intraduodenal instillation of hydrochloric acid and to secretin is considerably decreased by administration of anticholinergic drugs.

Pituitary and adrenal hormones affect pancreatic secretion, but their exact influence on the physiologic regulation of such secretion is not known. Serotonin seems to decrease food-stimulated pancreatic secretion and possibly that stimulated by secretin. Glucagon diminishes volume and bicarbonate output.

EFFECTS OF LOSS OF PANCREATIC JUICE. The functional consequences of loss of pancreatic juice may be considerable. Exclusion of pancreatic juice from the gastrointestinal tract by pancreatectomy, by ligation of the pancreatic ducts, or by total external pancreatic fistula results in severe impairment of the digestion and absorption of various foodstuffs, particularly fat. Excessive losses of fat in the stool occur in patients in whom pancreatic juice is completely excluded from the intestine. Yet, digestion is probably only slightly impaired if but a fraction of normal pancreatic juice enters the duodenum.

Profound gastric hypersecretion always occurs experimentally whenever pancreatic secretions are diverted from the intestine. It is likely that the absence of pancreatic juice from the intestine prevents normal fat inhibition by enterogastrone and that the nutritional consequences of inadequate digestion cause hepatic damage, which may also enhance gastric hypersecretion. Two conclusions of surgical importance can be reached: (1) if the head of the pancreas is resected, digestion is better, and the chances of marginal ulceration are less if the remaining pancreatic remnant is anastomosed to the gastrointestinal tract rather than being ligated; and (2) pancreatic extracts should be used freely whenever postoperative deficiency of external pancreatic secretion exists.

Impaired absorption of vitamin B_{12}, seemingly associated with a low duodenal pH, has been observed in patients with pancreatic insufficiency. Improved absorption of vitamin B_{12} occurred after administration of sodium bicarbonate, pancreatic extract, or both. Apparently, normal secretion of pancreatic juice is essential for unimpaired absorption of vitamin B_{12}. Conversely, pancreatic extracts may depress the abnormally high absorption of iron in hemochromatosis or pancreatitis. These findings provide further strong reasons for administering pancreatic extract to patients with pancreatic insufficiency.

PANCREATICOBILIARY PRESSURE RELATIONSHIPS. Studies of intrabiliary pressure in patients in whom T tubes have been placed in the common duct after cholecystectomy indicate that responses are similar to those observed in dogs. Menguy et al. have shown in dogs that resting pancreatic pressures consistently exceed those in the biliary tree, although the pressure in the bile duct rises after cholecystectomy. The pressure in both ductal systems rises after a meal. When the rate of flow of pancreatic juice is increased by injecting secretin, the pressure in the pancreatic ducts does not rise, although intravenous administration of sodium dehydrocholate definitely increases biliary pressure. Acid instilled into the duodenum causes little change in pancreatic intraductal pressure, in contrast to alcohol, which uniformly increases both pancreatic and biliary pressure. Morphine, codeine, and meperidine hydrochloride increase intrapancreatic pressure but raise biliary pressure only in the absence of the gall bladder. Atropine consistently lowers pancreatic intraductal pressure, and pilocarpine increases pressure. Infected bile, probably as a result of bacterial deconjugation of bile salts, causes a marked rise in resistance of the sphincter of Oddi.

Endocrine Pancreas

The internal secretions of the pancreas are formed by the islets of Langerhans, which approximate 1 million in number yet represent only about 1.5 percent of the normal pancreas by weight. The individual islets are 75 to 150 μ in diameter. The alpha cells are probably the source of glucagon. The beta cells manufacture, store, and secrete insulin, and comprise 60 to 80 percent of the cells of each islet. The function of C cells and delta cells is unknown, although gastrin-producing ulcerogenic tumors of the pancreas may arise from them. Delta cells may give rise to islet tumors which release VIP (vasoactive intestinal peptide).

Glucagon is composed of 20 amino acids arranged in a straight chain and has a molecular weight of 3,485. It causes glycogenolysis in the liver and release of glucose into the bloodstream. A decreased response to glucagon occurs in diseases of the liver. Purified glucagon, 1 mg given intravenously, will usually raise the blood sugar by 50 to 80 mg/100 ml, a gradual return to normal following in about 90 minutes. Glucagon is also secreted by the intestinal mucosa.

Insulin has a molecular weight of about 6,000 and consists of two polypeptide chains. The prime function of insulin is to promote the transfer of glucose and other sugars across certain cell membranes. The transfer of sugars into muscle cells, fibroblasts, and adipose tissue requires insulin, but neurons, erythrocytes, hepatic cells, and intestinal cells can accomplish this process without it. In the absence of glucose, fat is utilized, and ketosis and acidosis occur. Amino acids may be oxidized to provide energy and may cause a negative nitrogen balance when glucose is not being used properly. Insulin may also play a part in the conversion of glucose to glycogen in the liver.

Regulation of insulin secretion does not seem to depend upon trophic support, since neither vagotomy nor ablation of the anterior pituitary gland has an effect upon insulin secretion. The primary stimulus to the secretion of insulin is the blood sugar itself; an increase in blood sugar causes degranulation of the beta cells. Various hormones which increase the blood sugar, such as growth hormone, glucocorticoids, thyroid hormone, and epinephrine, may secondarily increase the secretion of insulin.

It has recently been demonstrated that all three of the major nutrient substrates, namely, glucose, amino acids, and fatty acids, stimulate varying degrees of insulin secretion. Gastrin, secretin, and cholecystokinin all produce a rise in insulin after injection, but the response to gastrin is quantitatively trivial while that to secretin is modest. Cholecystokinin elicits substantial release of both insulin and glucagon and augments the release of these two hormones by amino acids. Leucine and the sulfonureas used in the treatment of diabetes are known to produce their effects by releasing insulin from the beta cell granules.

It is possible that other humoral agents are produced by the islets of the normal pancreas. Certain islet-cell tumors produce gastrin, and others may secrete glucagon. Whether small amounts of gastrin are secreted by the normal pancreas remains conjectural, although gastrin-producing cells have now been identified in the normal pancreas by immunofluorescent techniques.

PANCREATITIS

Acute Pancreatitis

ETIOLOGY. There are two main types of pancreatitis, acute and chronic. Reference is frequently made in the literature to a form of "chronic relapsing pancreatitis" which is discussed as a third form of the disease. Most of these cases are actually recurrent attacks of acute pancreatitis or are simply acute exacerbations in the course of chronic pancreatitis.

Pancreatitis Associated with Gallstones. Approximately two-thirds of patients with pancreatitis in private hospitals have gallstones, but in charity hospitals only one-third or less prove to have gallstone pancreatitis. For many years, a common channel between the common bile duct and the duct of Wirsung was thought to be of great importance in the pathogenesis, not only of gallstone pancreatitis, but also of pancreatitis due to many other causes. It is true that, on occasion, a calculus impacted at the ampulla of Vater may produce pancreatitis. Yet this is a rare occurrence. Only about 18 percent of patients with gallstone pancreatitis have choledocholithiasis, and in only a small number of these is there impaction of a stone at the ampulla. Although a clear association exists between gallstones and acute pancreatitis and treatment of the biliary tract disease almost always cures the pancreatitis, the mechanism by which the pancreatitis is produced remains an enigma. Recent studies show that a high proportion of patients with gallstone pancreatitis have recoverable biliary calculi in the stools.

The classic experimental method for production of pancreatitis is injection of bile into the ductal system, but many facts militate against this mechanism in human gallstone pancreatitis. Continuous perfusion of the unobstructed pancreatic ductal system with bile in dogs and goats has not led to acute pancreatitis. In experimental biliary pancreatitis the bile is usually injected with sufficient pressure to rupture the pancreatic acini. The normal secretory pressure relationships argue against reflux, since pancreatic secretory pressure is generally higher than that of the liver. Radiocinemonometric studies have shown that contraction of the sphincter of Oddi often occludes both the biliary and the pancreatic ducts and isolates them from each other rather than producing an open common channel. Furthermore, reflux into the pancreatic duct occurs quite often during operative or T-tube cholangiography without apparent ill effects. Nevertheless, the bile factor cannot be discarded completely. Elliott et al. have shown that resistance to the flow of bile into the pancreatic duct greatly decreases after incubation of bile with pancreatic juice. Two components of bile, deconjugated bile salts and lysolecithins, have recently been found to be extremely toxic to the pancreas during experimental reflux. Deconjugated bile salts may be formed by bacterial action on conjugated bile salts, and lysolecithin results from the conversion of biliary lecithin by phospholipase A of pancreatic juice. It has been demonstrated that bile in the pancreas may cause vascular injury, stasis, and spasm, which may initiate pancreatitis.

Alcoholic Pancreatitis. About two-thirds of patients with pancreatitis in charity hospitals, but only one-third of such patients in private hospitals, have alcoholic pancreatitis. Alcohol is now known to cause an increase in protein concentration in pancreatic juice, precipitation of which may form a nidus upon which subsequent calcification occurs, and intraduodenal instillation of alcohol also causes a profound and sustained rise in pancreatic ductal pressure in dogs.

Duodenal inflammation may produce some degree of ductal obstruction in a gland actively secreting in response to the acid-secretin mechanism. Experimental ductal obstruction alone does not cause pancreatitis, but if hypersecretion induced by food, secretin, or vascular injury is also present, severe pancreatitis ensues. Persistent vomiting may cause regurgitation of duodenal contents into the pancreatic ducts. Dietary-induced hypertriglyceridemia has now been shown to produce a clinical syndrome of acute pancreatitis in about half of alcoholic patients who previously exhibited alcoholic pancreatitis. Pancreatic calculi and multiple stenoses within the ductal system late in the course of chronic pancreatitis are probably the sequelae of pancreatitis rather than the cause. As important as the mechanical factors may be, nutritional factors may ultimately prove to be more crucial. Since the turnover of protein by the pancreas is the greatest of any organ, it is not surprising that protein deficiency states have been associated with degeneration, atrophy, and fibrosis of the pancreas.

Postoperative Pancreatitis. Pancreatitis occasionally occurs after intraabdominal operations, especially those on the biliary tract and stomach. Rarely, it may develop after operations remote from the pancreas. It is clear that the pancreatitis which follows biliary operations occurs only when the common bile duct has been explored, especially if a long-armed T tube has been placed through the sphincter of Oddi. Pancreatitis is also likely to follow a gastrectomy in which the region of the head of the pancreas has been dissected. Direct ligation or laceration of the duct of Santorini may provide the insult that triggers the pancreatitis. Vascular injury, together with the damage to the duct, may set the stage for this serious disease. The interaction of obstruction and vascular factors is demonstrated by the development of experimental pancreatitis when the second part of the duodenum is converted into a closed loop. The clinical counterpart of this experiment is the occurrence of pancreatitis in a patient with afferent loop obstruction after a Billroth II gastrectomy. The mortality of postoperative pancreatitis is approximately 50 percent. After splenectomy, postoperative pancreatitis is usually the direct result of operative injury to the tail of the pancreas.

Metabolic Factors. An association exists between hyperparathyroidism and pancreatitis. Not only may repeated attacks of acute pancreatitis be one of the first signs of hyperparathyroidism, but occasionally a severe episode may follow removal of a parathyroid adenoma. Calcium markedly enhances the conversion of trypsinogen to trypsin, and its presence in high ionic concentration may produce a mass action effect that precipitates calcium phosphate in the ducts. Parathyroid function should always be investigated in any patient with pancreatitis of obscure cause.

A small group of patients with a hereditary type of pancreatitis have been described in whom aminoaciduria is a fairly consistent finding. Lysinuria and cystinuria are frequently observed, but the metabolic defect that produces the pancreatitis is not known. The disease usually begins in childhood, and inheritance follows the pattern of an autosomal gene. Some of these patients have calcification of the pancreas. The prognosis is generally good.

It has been known for many years that *transient* hyperlipemia may occur during the course of clinical and experimental acute pancreatitis. Release of an inhibitor of the

"clearing factor," lipoprotein lipase, by the diseased pancreas is the most likely cause of the hyperlipemia. This secondary type of hyperlipemia is to be distinguished from an idiopathic form in which the pancreatitis is probably caused by the hyperlipemia. In the idiopathic form, the neutral fats usually increase immediately before the onset of abdominal symptoms and return to normal when the attack is over. Klatskin and Gordon have suggested that the pancreatitis may be caused by fat emboli. The differentiation between the primary and secondary types of hyperlipemia is extremely important, because the attacks of pancreatitis may be prevented by a low-fat diet in the primary group. Dietary-induced hypertriglyceridemia can also cause attacks of acute pancreatitis in alcoholic patients.

Hemochromatosis has been thought to produce pancreatic fibrosis and atrophy because of the irritating properties of the deposited iron. However, iron absorption often increases after pancreatic damage caused by several diseases, and siderosis may in fact be secondary to the pancreatic disease.

Vascular, Toxic, Allergic, and Other Factors. Vascular stasis is an important factor in experimental pancreatitis. The process may be diffuse, probably at the arteriolar level, since ligation of major vessels to the pancreas alone causes only small infarcts. Occasionally, older patients who have widespread vascular obstruction are seen with severe hemorrhagic pancreatitis. The role of vascular spasm and obstruction in other forms of pancreatitis is not clear.

Various toxins, such as methyl alcohol, zinc oxide, cobaltous chloride, and chlorothiazide, have been known to produce pancreatic injury. Although Thal and others have implicated autoimmune mechanisms in the pathogenesis of pancreatitis, there is little evidence to suggest that these are of any particular importance in human pancreatitis.

Despite frequent reports of pancreatitis during mumps, no fatalities or complications have been recorded. The serum amylase may increase in patients with mumps, but whether this results from the parotitis or pancreatitis is unknown.

CLINICAL MANIFESTATIONS. Acute pancreatitis is sometimes divided into the acute edematous type and a hemorrhagic or necrotic form. This is a purely arbitrary distinction by the clinician which can be made only at operation or autopsy.

Attacks of acute pancreatitis often occur after a heavy meal or an episode of acute alcoholism. The pain usually begins suddenly but may start gradually. The pain is frequently located in the midepigastrium and often radiates to the back. The patient's discomfort is in many instances improved by sitting and aggravated by lying. The character of the pain is extremely variable, ranging from steady, knifelike distress to an agonizing intermittent cramping pain. Pain in the left or right upper quadrants is not uncommon and is caused by particularly severe involvement of the tail or the head of the gland.

Persistent and repeated vomiting without nausea but often to the point of extreme retching is common. The character of the vomitus is unremarkable, and the vomiting occurs with an empty stomach. Physical examination usually shows upper abdominal tenderness and guarding, sometimes far greater than what might be expected for the amount of pain the patient seems to have. About 90 percent of patients with proved pancreatitis have fever, tachycardia, and leukocytosis. Shock may be present, depending upon the amount of fluid and blood lost in the retroperitoneal area and peritoneal cavity, as well as the volume deficit incurred by persistent vomiting. Dissection of irritating exudate from the pancreas into the lower quadrants of the abdomen or even into the chest may produce signs and symptoms in these areas, as well as even greater volume deficits because of the local outpouring of fluid in response to the exudate. Adynamic ileus with intraluminal sequestration of fluid also contributes to extracellular fluid deficit. Lefer, with Wangensteen and others, has recently demonstrated a myocardial depressant factor (MDF) released from the pancreas during pancreatitis which may also contribute to the shock. Acute renal insufficiency often occurs in these patients. Mild jaundice occurs in 20 to 30 percent of the patients. This is partly due to swelling of the head of the pancreas and perhaps also to hemolysis of red blood cells, which become more fragile in acute pancreatitis. Carpopedal spasm may occur if enough fat necrosis is present in the abdomen and retroperitoneal area to remove large amounts of calcium from the blood to form calcium soaps. Recent studies indicate that an increased release of glucagon occurs in pancreatitis, which in turn stimulates the release of thyrocalcitonin, a factor which may also contribute to the development of hypocalcemia. It has been proposed recently that a substantial degree of hypocalcemia may be caused by the hypoalbuminemia found in patients with acute pancreatitis.

LABORATORY STUDIES. Acute pancreatitis is largely diagnosed by clinical history and findings rather than by laboratory studies. Disastrous outcomes have occurred when elevated serum amylase values have led the physician or surgeon immediately to eliminate from consideration any diagnosis but acute pancreatitis. Not only is simple elevation of the serum amylase level an inadequate diagnostic test of acute pancreatitis, but also there is ample evidence that serum amylase values of over 1,000 units are frequently caused by conditions other than acute pancreatitis. Blood drawn during the course of proved pancreatitis, when the amylase might be expected to be elevated, has indicated that approximately one-third of the patients had values of less than 200 Somogyi units, one-third had levels between 200 and 500 units, and one-third had more than 500 units.

Apart from acute pancreatitis, the most frequent causes of marked elevations of the serum amylase level are acute cholecystitis, common duct stone with or without cholangitis, perforated peptic ulcer, and strangulating obstruction of the small intestine. Other conditions in which the serum amylase level is elevated include acute alcoholism without pancreatitis, afferent loop obstruction after gastrectomy, ectopic pregnancy, perforated duodenal diverticulum, renal failure, carcinoma of the pancreas, and mumps. Although frequently claimed to have more diagnostic value than the serum amylase test, serum lipase not only

is a difficult determination to perform but also has proved to be disappointingly inaccurate.

Estimation of the total amount of amylase in a 2-hour urine sample is far more accurate than the concentration of the enzyme in the urine, blood, or the serum lipase. The number of positive diagnoses of pancreatitis is doubled when the amylase output in the urine exceeds 300 units in 1 hour. Recent studies show that the renal clearance of amylase in acute pancreatitis is much greater, relative to the creatinine clearance, than in any other condition. A ratio of amylase/creatinine clearance of >5 has recently been shown to be of greater diagnostic accuracy than either the serum or urinary amylase. Exceptions to this have been found in burned patients and in diabetic ketoacidosis. Elevated amylase values in pleural fluid are diagnostic of pancreatitis. Abdominal paracentesis may provide useful information, but increased amylase in abdominal fluid has been reported in other conditions as well. Estimations of trypsin levels in the blood and the separation of various organ-specific isoenzymes of the blood, especially those of amylase, seem to be encouraging but are not as yet sufficiently well evaluated to warrant widespread use.

Serum calcium values of less than 7.5 mg/100 ml generally indicate a poor prognosis and reflect the extensiveness of the disease process. Transient hyperglycemia and glycosuria have formerly been attributed to inadequate production of insulin by the injured pancreas, but recent work has shown that injection of amylase into the bloodstream converts glycogen to glucose in the liver, and that glucagon is released during the course of pancreatitis.

Radiologic examinations have only occasional value. The so-called "sentinel loop" of distended jejunum in the left upper quadrant is extremely nonspecific. Oral cholecystography during, or immediately following, an episode of acute pancreatitis frequently fails to produce visualization of the biliary tree, even when it is completely normal. Nonvisualization may persist for as long as 6 weeks after an attack. In contradistinction, intravenous cholangiography is often of great value in differentiating acute pancreatitis from acute cholecystitis, since the gallbladder can usually be visualized in most cases of acute pancreatitis.

The diagnosis of acute pancreatitis is usually made from clinical findings, although intelligent use of serum and urinary amylase tests and intravenous cholangiography may provide useful if not clearly diagnostic information. Frequent clinical reassessment of the patient is of the utmost importance. On occasion, laparotomy may be necessary in a carefully prepared patient as a purely diagnostic maneuver in order to avoid missing a strangulating obstruction of the small intestine or another potentially lethal but curable condition.

TREATMENT. Meticulous replacement of losses of colloid, fluid, and electrolytes, and adequate maintenance therapy are of the utmost importance. Constant attention to the urinary output, alterations in the hematocrit, blood volume, and central venous pressure, and estimation of the occult losses into the peritoneum and retroperitoneal area are mandatory. Blood transfusion may be required in hemorrhagic pancreatitis. Small doses of insulin may be necessary if hyperglycemia is marked and diabetic acidosis is imminent. Calcium gluconate should be given intravenously if the serum calcium level is depressed. Steroids should probably not be used, since they have been known to cause pancreatitis.

In addition to proper metabolic management, continuous aspiration of the stomach and withholding ingestion of food or fluids often relieves discomfort immediately. Parasympatholytic drugs may be used in moderate dosage. These maneuvers are designed to put the pancreas to rest by diminishing the acid-secretin mechanism of pancreatic stimulation, by eliminating gastric distension, which in turn invokes the gastropancreatic reflex and the production of antral gastrin, and by preventing the flow of pancreatic juice stimulated by foodstuffs in the duodenum. Adynamic ileus is also favorably affected by intubation. Such therapy is continued until the patient no longer has pain and tenderness. Suppression of pancreatic secretion by Diamox, propylthiouracil, or hypothermia has not been evaluated sufficiently in human pancreatitis to assess its true value. Trasylol, a trypsin inhibitor which also inhibits kallikrein, has received attention, but controlled clinical studies have not convincingly demonstrated the efficacy of this drug. Glucagon has recently been advocated in the treatment of acute pancreatitis, but no solid evidence to support its use has been forthcoming.

Although many authorities advocate the routine administration of antibiotics to patients with acute pancreatitis, we use these agents only in the occasional severe fulminating case, since these patients are the ones in whom secondary abscesses are most likely to develop. There is no evidence to support the belief that infection is an important contributing factor in the development of pancreatitis or that antibiotics can actually prevent the development of an abscess.

Meperidine is usually used to relieve pain, because it has less effect on the sphincter of Oddi than morphine and other opiates, although it does not relax this muscle, as was formerly believed. It is unnecessary to use paravertebral sympathetic blockade, since intubation usually provides marked relief of pain.

The patient with persistent or lingering acute pancreatitis secondary to acute or chronic biliary tract disease may require operation on the biliary tree with the expectation that the pancreatitis will subside. Recently Salzman and Bartlett have advocated transduodenal pancreatic duct exploration in certain patients with acute pancreatitis who did not respond to vigorous supportive measures. In fulminant hemorrhagic pancreatitis Watts and Smith have carried out total pancreatectomy with gratifying results, but the place of radical resection in the treatment of severe, acute pancreatitis is not yet clear. In some patients who fail to respond to all conservative means, it is probably more prudent to institute peritoneal lavage, which may produce profound improvement in selected instances.

COMPLICATIONS, MORBIDITY, AND MORTALITY. Pseudocyst is the most common complication of acute pancreatitis. Abscesses are rare but mortality is high, approaching 100 percent if clostridial organisms are the cause of the infection. Pseudocysts rarely appear before the second week of the disease and abscesses not usually before the third week. Obstruction of the common bile duct and duodenum is not common in the acute cases. The remaining complications of acute pancreatitis may be grouped together, since they are caused by the necrotizing effects of the process itself. These include rupture or thrombosis of the splenic, mesenteric, or portal vessels, necrosis and perforation of the common bile duct or colon, and perforation of the stomach and duodenum.

Just as important as the early complications of acute pancreatitis and perhaps even more so is the insidious development of sequelae of repeated attacks. Pancreatic calcification, secondary diabetes, and steatorrhea are far more common in alcoholic pancreatitis than in gallstone pancreatitis, in which these phenomena are almost nonexistent. Pseudocysts too are rarely encountered in the course of gallstone pancreatitis.

The overall mortality rate from acute pancreatitis in the past 10 years has been 10 to 15 percent. Twenty years ago most patients died during the first week of the disease, but now the vast majority do not succumb for several weeks after the onset, probably because of better early metabolic management. The mortality rate of alcoholic pancreatitis is approximately three times that of gallstone pancreatitis in most series, but reverse incidences have been recorded in a few reports. It is virtually impossible to determine the true mortality rate of hemorrhagic pancreatitis, since a clinical diagnosis may be impossible without operative or postmortem observation. Operation is generally regarded as detrimental to the outcome of the disease unless specific indications, as outlined above, are present. Paradoxically, operation has not increased the mortality rates in most reports. Secondary hemorrhage from major vessels, fulminating uncontrollable shock without hemorrhage, and infection are the most common causes of death.

Chronic Pancreatitis

This diagnosis usually refers to a clinical entity rather than a specific pathologic process. This is especially true during its early stages, when repeated attacks of acute pancreatitis of varying severity are likely to occur, whether alcoholism or biliary tract disease is the precipitating factor. As the disease progresses, however, the edges of the pancreas become rounded, and the organ becomes smaller, indurated, and nodular. Histologically, lobules of functional acinar and islet tissue are surrounded by thick bands of fibrous tissue. Alternating areas of stricture and dilatation of the main ductal system occur late in the disease. In the very last stages calcification occurs. It is almost always intraductal and rarely interstitial (Figs. 32-5 and 32-6). These severe changes are confined largely to patients with alcoholic pancreatitis and are extremely rare in gallstone pancreatitis. Calcification and ductal distortion have also been seen in familial or hereditary pancreatitis. Occasionally in chronic alcoholic pancreatitis, progressive fibrosis of the gland without ductal dilatation or calcification seems to be the primary pathologic process.

CLINICAL MANIFESTATIONS. The typical patient with

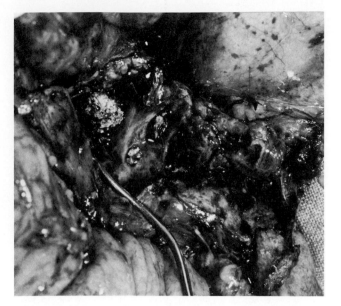

Fig. 32-5. Calcifications presenting within the duct of the opened pancreas. The guide probe is advanced into the head of the gland. Note alternate stenoses and dilatations of the main duct and the calcifications which occlude the ductal tributaries. (*From W. Silen, J. Baldwin, and L. Goldman, Am J Surg, 106:243, 1963.*)

chronic pancreatitis is in his late thirties or early forties and has a long history of alcoholism and repeated attacks of acute pancreatitis, often with delirium tremens. After approximately 10 years, the pain changes from intermittent to persistent and continuous. It is located in the epigastrium but radiates to the back and is often partially relieved if the patient sits in a hunched position. Anorexia and weight loss are common, and nausea and vomiting

Fig. 32-6. Example of amount of calcification removed from the ductal system of a patient with chronic pancreatitis.

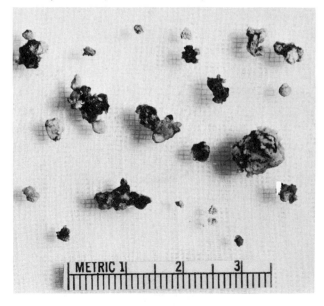

occur if an exacerbation has been precipitated by an acute bout of alcoholism. Diabetes and steatorrhea with foul, bulky, greasy stools are common. At this stage, addiction to narcotics as well as alcohol is extremely common. Strangely, cirrhosis of the liver and its stigmata are not often present. Pseudocysts are frequently found in these patients.

This picture is in sharp contrast to the patient who has recurrent pancreatitis in association with biliary tract disease. Such persons generally have episodic bouts of acute pancreatitis, sometimes in association with attacks of acute cholecystitis or cholangitis caused by common duct calculi. Severe pancreatic fibrosis and insufficiency almost never occur in association solely with biliary tract disease. Hyperparathyroidism is often associated with recurrent attacks of acute pancreatitis, as in patients who have severe ductal stenosis resulting from major trauma to the pancreas. Occasionally the picture of familial pancreatitis may be similar to that seen in alcoholic chronic pancreatitis, but these cases are rare, and at times severe damage to the pancreas and calcification may be present without any symptoms at all and in the absence of a known cause.

LABORATORY STUDIES. Many psychoneurotic patients with abdominal pains are labeled as having chronic pancreatitis without adequate substantiation for such a serious diagnosis. Documentation is difficult, but in these instances thorough roentgenologic examinations of the biliary tree and upper gastrointestinal tract are mandatory. The recent advent of endoscopic retrograde cannulation of the pancreatic duct has proved of great value in these cases, since abnormalities of the ductal system are readily detected. Determination of serum or urinary amylase or serum lipase may not be fruitful, especially if the pancreas has been seriously damaged. The presence of calcification in the pancreas virtually establishes the diagnosis.

TREATMENT. The wide variety of operative procedures devised for chronic pancreatitis are a reflection of the generally unsatisfactory results of treatment. However, some confusion has been created by our own inability, or refusal, to differentiate clearly among the various types of chronic pancreatitis.

It is evident that definitive and corrective biliary tract operations are almost always curative in gallstone pancreatitis. Whether this implies simple cholecystectomy or common duct exploration, with or without sphincteroplasty, is dictated by the local and cholangiographic findings at operation. Sporadic initial success with biliary operations led to their widespread, indiscriminate use without due regard for the precipitating cause of the pancreatitis. Large numbers of patients with alcoholic pancreatitis were subjected to cholecystectomy and a variety of other biliary tract procedures, only to find that relief was not obtained. Even when biliary calculi are present in the alcoholic patient, correction of the biliary tract disease will not alter the course of the pancreatic disease, especially if the ingestion of alcohol is continued.

In the case of chronic alcoholic pancreatitis, the only logical and effective therapy is complete abstinence from alcohol before the stage of fibrosis, calcification, steatorrhea, and diabetes is reached, but rarely can this be achieved. Once the severe complications of chronic pancreatitis has developed, consideration should be given to pancreaticojejunostomy, originally advocated by Puestow and Gillesby. This procedure is based on the fact that multiple areas of stricture within the pancreatic ductal system often occur in patients with severe chronic pancreatitis, so that simple retrograde drainage of the pancreas via its tail, as originally proposed by DuVal, does not adequately decompress the pancreatic ducts. The limb of jejunum may be anastomosed, side to side, to the pancreas after wide incision of almost the entire pancreatic duct but without removal of the spleen or mobilization of the pancreas (Fig. 32-7). This procedure can be carried out rather simply, with an extremely low mortality and little morbidity. The relief of pain is dramatic, particularly if the duct is dilated at operation. The most accurate preoperative indication of a dilated duct is the presence of calcification.

Lateral pancreaticojejunostomy also provides for the return of pancreatic juice to the intestine, offers the potential for pancreatic regeneration if it is to occur, and preserves pancreatic tissue. In addition, the adequacy of ductal exploration, removal of calculi, and drainage is far greater than that which can be accomplished through a transduodenal sphincterotomy, advocated by some. If the pancreatic duct is small, without evidence of stricture, yet severe chronic pancreatitis is present, the best procedure is that of 95 percent distal pancreatectomy, proposed by Fry and Child. This is associated with a high incidence of diabetes and exocrine pancreatic insufficiency, both of which may be excessively morbid in the nonresponsible alcoholic patient. Relief of pain occurs in the majority of patients.

Sphincterotomy, ligation of the pancreatic ducts, and lumbodorsal sympathectomy and splanchnicectomy have all failed to provide lasting relief in patients with chronic pancreatitis. On occasion, the Whipple pancreaticoduodenal resection may be indicated if stricture of the common bile duct or stenosis of the duodenum is the result of chronic pancreatitis localized to the head of the pancreas.

TRAUMA

MECHANISMS OF INJURY. Penetrating trauma, caused by gunshot or stab wounds, is more common than blunt injury to the pancreas and constitutes from 70 to 80 percent of pancreatic injuries, even in civilian practice. Penetrating injuries, especially knife wounds, usually cause less destruction and disruption of the organ than does blunt

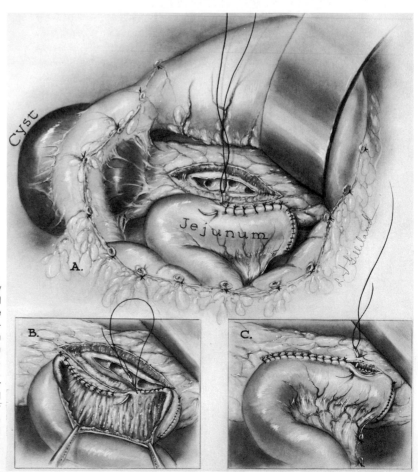

Fig. 32-7. Side-to-side pancreaticojejunostomy with preservation of the tail of the pancreas and spleen. An exploring needle is used to locate the dilated pancreatic duct, which is then incised. The end of the defunctionalized jejunum is closed and brought up for anastomosis with the opened pancreas in side-to-side fashion. The posterior row of sutures is placed first (A). The jejunum is then opened, and an inner layer of continuous sutures is placed, uniting jejunal mucosa and pancreatic duct (B). An anterior row of interrupted sutures completes the anastomosis (C). A Roux en Y is then constructed to complete intestinal continuity. (From W. Silen, J. Baldwin, and L. Goldman, Am J Surg, 106: 243, 1963.)

trauma. In gunshot wounds an area of contusion usually surrounds the track of the missile. Injury to adjacent structures is exceedingly common (70 to 96 percent). The stomach, liver, small intestine, spleen, colon, kidney, and duodenum are the most frequently wounded. These organs are usually the source of the most significant hemorrhage.

The immobility of the pancreas accounts for its vulnerability to blunt trauma, which may fracture it posteriorly across the rigid vertebral column. Usually the disruption occurs at the neck of the pancreas overlying the mesenteric vessels, although occasionally the gland may become completely separated from the duodenum. Associated injury to other organs is not as frequent as in penetrating trauma.

Although frequently referred to as "traumatic pancreatitis," the consequences of these injuries, such as fistula, pseudocyst, or death, are usually the result of disruption of the organ itself or its ductal system rather than pancreatitis per se. Crushing injury to the pancreas in itself does not seem to produce extensive inflammation in the remainder of the gland.

CLINICAL MANIFESTATIONS. It is significant that the interval between injury and surgical exploration is considerably longer after blunt trauma to the pancreas, often being many days. Adequate awareness of the possibility of this type of injury may shorten delay and reduce morbidity and mortality. Abdominal pain and findings on examination may be surprisingly minimal, which partly explains the frequent procrastination in undertaking laparotomy. Clinical and laboratory evidence of continuing hemorrhage makes the decision for operation an easy one. Continued abdominal pain, tenderness, fever, and ileus should immediately arouse suspicion of pancreatic injury.

Roentgenologic examinations, with or without contrast media, are rarely helpful. Paracentesis may provide a clear-cut indication for operation if the fluid is positive for blood or is rich in amylase, but a negative result should not deter the surgeon from exploration. Although frequently forgotten in cases of blunt trauma, serum amylase determination and amylase/creatinine clearance ratio may be of great help. These are elevated in over 80 percent of the patients with pancreatic injuries in whom they are measured. Possibly of greater surgical importance is the fact that persistent elevations of the serum amylase usually mean inadequate drainage of the injured pancreas.

TREATMENT. The high incidence of complications and the excessive mortality suggest that the treatment leaves much to be desired.

It is generally agreed that early operation is necessary in both penetrating wounds and in blunt injury.

Proper evaluation of the extent of the pancreatic injury is the key to adequate surgical therapy. It is impossible to explore the pancreas without widely exposing it by division of the gastrocolic omentum, as far as is necessary to provide adequate assessment of the major portion of the gland (Fig. 32-8). Care must be taken to protect the middle colic vessels during the procedure. If the injury is in the region of the head of the pancreas, the duodenum must be mobilized by the method of Kocher (Fig. 32-9) so that the full extent of the damage can be ascertained and the duodenum, common bile duct, and adjacent structures can be examined. If a hematoma is found over the pancreas, it should not be treated by drainage alone, but must be examined carefully, since it may hide major vascular or ductal injury. Vascular instruments should always

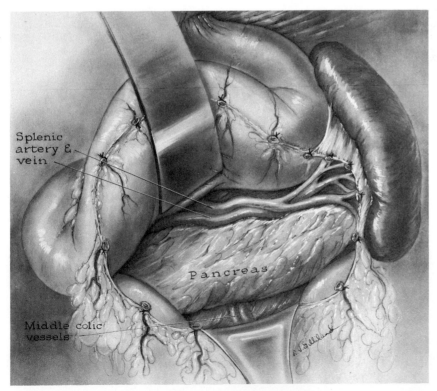

Splenic
artery &
vein

Pancreas

Middle colic
vessels

Fig. 32-8. Wide exposure of the pancreas obtained by the gastrocolic omental route. The middle colic vessels must be located and preserved. (*From W. Silen, Surg Clin North Am, 44:1253, 1964.*)

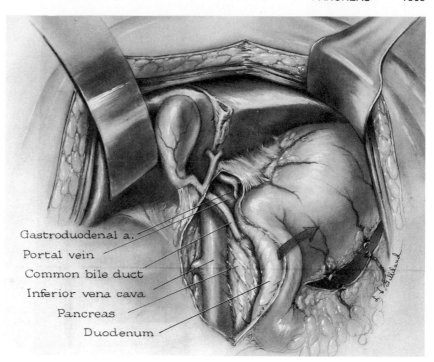

Gastroduodenal a.
Portal vein
Common bile duct
Inferior vena cava
Pancreas
Duodenum

Fig. 32-9. Operative exposure of the head of the pancreas after the Kocher maneuver. Note that portal or superior mesenteric veins are covered posteriorly by the uncinate process, preventing direct vision of these structures inferiorly. (*From W. Silen, Surg Clin North Am, 44:1253, 1964.*)

be readily available in the operating room when operations of this type are being performed.

During exploration of the hematoma, attention should be first directed toward hemostasis. Blind clamping in the depths of the pancreas or deep, carelessly placed sutures may injure the pancreatic ductal system, leading to pancreatitis or fistula. Damaged tissue should be thoroughly debrided; carefully placed nonabsorbable suture ligatures permit adequate hemostasis. If the ductal system is uninjured, these procedures, together with sump suction drainage, may be sufficient to treat small penetrating injuries. Complications with simple drainage or no drainage at all are considerably greater than when the more adequate sump drainage is used.

A much more aggressive approach is probably necessary when the pancreas is badly lacerated. Should the severely injured area involve only the tail or distal body of the pancreas, the simplest procedure is resection. Mobilization of the spleen and distal pancreas is easily carried out (Fig. 32-10). Since the gastrocolic omentum has already been opened, only a few vasa brevia remain to be ligated and divided; the distal pancreas and spleen can easily be delivered into the wound after division of the lienorenal and splenocolic ligaments and the thin posterosuperior and posteroinferior peritoneal attachments of the pancreas. After the splenic artery and vein are ligated and divided, the injured pancreas may be removed. The distal end of the pancreas remaining in situ should be carefully inspected for adequate hemostasis. If possible, the duct of Wirsung should be ligated with nonabsorbable sutures, and the area is then drained.

If the pancreas is transected near its neck or even farther to the right, preservation of pancreatic tissue may be important. The lacerated proximal segment is managed as outlined above. The distal transected portion of the organ can be anastomosed end to end with a Roux en Y limb of jejunum. Generally, the limb of jejunum is placed in a retrocolic position. The transected proximal pancreas can also be implanted into the same limb of jejunum used for the distal end, but this is unduly complicated and probably is not necessary.

Although these procedures might appear too involved to be used in seriously injured patients, less adequate therapy results in a high incidence of severe complications and death. Furthermore, ductal obstruction and the late development of chronic pancreatitis in inadequately recognized and treated injuries support an aggressive approach to such lesions. Thal and Wilson have recently proposed that pancreaticoduodenal resection be carried out for severe lesions of the head of the pancreas. Berne advocates distal Billroth II gastrectomy with careful local repair of the badly injured duodenum and pancreas, coupled with adequate drainage, for injuries of this area. The choice between this procedure and the Whipple operation is determined by the extent of the injury. Should the pancreas be sheared away from the duodenum, disrupting pancreatic and biliary ductal continuity, careful reanastomosis to the duodenum may be carried out if the blood supply to the pancreas and duodenum has not been disrupted. The importance of recognizing major ductal injury in any case of pancreatic injury cannot be overemphasized. Cannulation of the pancreatic duct can sometimes be facilitated by intubation through a transduodenal sphincterotomy, as suggested by Doubilet and Mulholland. Although drainage of the ductal system can undoubtedly be achieved in this manner, definitive therapy by splinting of the duct alone by this method will not prevent subsequent ductal stricture and pancreatitis.

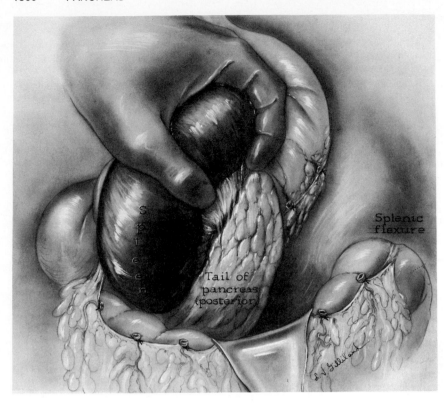

Fig. 32-10. Mobilization of tail and body of pancreas with spleen. (*From W. Silen, Surg Clin North Am, 44:1253, 1964.*)

MORBIDITY AND MORTALITY. The most serious complications of pancreatic injury are fistulization, pseudocyst formation, infection, and delayed hemorrhage. Fistula and pseudocyst are the result of disruption of a duct of significant size. Doubilet and Mulholland have suggested that the resistance to the flow of pancreatic juice into the duodenum by the duodenal musculature and sphincter of Oddi is sufficiently great so that in cases of injury the juice will preferentially flow into the retroperitoneal area. The incidence of complications in most series averages 30 percent. Pancreatic complications seem to occur much more frequently after blunt trauma than in penetrating injuries.

The overall mortality rate in recent years, like the complication rate, has averaged 20 percent. Usually the death rate after penetrating injuries is higher than that after blunt trauma, probably because adjacent organs are often injured. The most frequent causes of death are shock, renal failure, and sepsis.

CYSTS AND PSEUDOCYSTS

True cysts of the pancreas are filled with fluid and have an epithelial lining. These cysts are to be distinguished from the much more common pseudocysts, which have fibrous lining rather than epithelium.

True Cysts

A simple classification of true cysts of the pancreas is presented in Table 32-1.

Congenital cysts of the pancreas are extremely rare, and parasitic cysts of the pancreas have not been reported in the United States. Retention cysts are cystic dilatations of the pancreatic ducts and are almost always caused by pancreatitis. Although not as rare as the congenital cysts, neoplastic cysts of the pancreas are relatively uncommon. Cystadenoma and cystadenocarcinoma are important, since they may be confused with the much more common pseudocyst. The benign lesion (cystadenoma) is somewhat more common than its malignant counterpart.

CLINICAL MANIFESTATIONS. The benign tumors are very slow-growing, and even cystadenocarcinomas do not grow very rapidly. These tumors occur far more frequently in women than in men (9:1) and are most common in the sixth and seventh decades of life. They may be present for many years without causing symptoms. An abdominal mass is usually the only symptom. Minor discomfort,

Table 32-1. CLASSIFICATION OF TRUE CYSTS OF THE PANCREAS

A. Congenital
  1. Single cyst
  2. Multiple (polycystic disease)
  3. Dermoid cyst
  4. Fibrocystic disease
B. Acquired
  1. Retention cysts
  2. Parasitic cysts
  3. Neoplastic cysts
    a. Benign cystadenoma
    b. Cystadenocarcinoma

vague dyspepsia, and jaundice may be present. The diagnosis may be suggested if radiologic examination shows a mass in the region of the pancreas. Because of the profuse vascularity of these tumors, a loud bruit is occasionally heard over the lesion, and an arteriogram may visualize the profuse vascularity of the mass.

TREATMENT. Marsupialization or internal drainage are to be condemned. The tumor invariably recurs and presents far greater difficulties at a second operation. The importance of distinguishing between these lesions and pseudocysts becomes obvious. Whether the lesion is benign or malignant, complete excision is the preferred method. This is a simple matter when the lesion is located in the tail or body, since distal pancreatectomy, usually with splenectomy, is readily accomplished. If the lesion is in the head of the pancreas, simple resection of the lesion alone can be done if it has a small pedicle. However, pancreaticoduodenal resection may be necessary if the common bile duct is involved. Recurrences should not be anticipated if the entire lesion is removed.

Pseudocysts

More than three-quarters of all cystic lesions of the pancreas are pseudocysts. The fibrous wall of a pseudocyst surrounds a collection of pancreatic juice (with or without blood clot) and necrotic or suppurative pancreatic tissue. Most pseudocysts are unilocular and are located in the lesser sac. However, they occasionally occur within the pancreas (retention cysts), transverse mesocolon, or omentum and even more rarely may be found behind the pancreas or within the mediastinum. Since a pseudocyst usually results from disruption of the ductal system of the pancreas, the ultimate form and location of the lesion are dependent upon the position and the extent of pancreatic injury and the secretory pressure of the pancreas distal to the point of ductal damage. The fluid within a pseudocyst varies from clear and colorless to a brown or green murky material, depending upon the amount of blood or necrotic pancreas present.

Pancreatitis and trauma are the most important causes of pseudocysts, accounting for about 75 percent and 25 percent of cases, respectively. Neoplasm and parasites are extremely rare causes, and occasionally pseudocysts develop without any demonstrable cause whatever. In patients with pseudocysts caused by pancreatitis, alcoholism is more common than cholelithiasis. For this reason, pseudocysts appear most frequently in the fourth and fifth decades of life and are more common in men.

CLINICAL MANIFESTATIONS. The usual clinical findings in patients with pseudocysts are persistent pain, fever, and ileus, appearing 2 to 3 weeks after an attack of pancreatitis or trauma to the pancreas. Although a pseudocyst may develop after one attack of pancreatitis, the patient usually has had several previous attacks. Pain, in the epigastrium or the left upper quadrant with occasional radiation to the back, is the most common symptom. A mass, nausea, vomiting, and anorexia occur in approximately 20 percent of the patients. Rarely, gastrointestinal hemorrhage from gastroesophageal varices occurs from compression of the portal venous system by the pseudocyst. Narrowing of the common bile duct may cause jaundice.

A mass is found on physical examination in about 75 percent of patients and is usually nontender or only slightly tender. The amount of movement of the mass is variable, depending upon the degree of surrounding inflammatory reaction and fixation to adjacent structures. The mass often changes in size, probably because of partial drainage into the ductal system of the pancreas. The complete and prolonged disappearance of the mass in some patients may be explained by the fact that these masses develop after attacks of acute pancreatitis and may represent small fluid collections, matted omentum, and enlarged pancreas, all of which resolve after the acute attack has subsided. Occasionally the mass may be confused with an aortic aneurysm because of the pulsations transmitted by the aorta immediately posterior to the pancreas. Patients may present with pleural effusion as the sole finding, undoubtedly caused by transdiaphragmatic drainage of pancreatic lymph. Pleural or pulmonary manifestations are common.

The diagnosis of pseudocyst is not particularly difficult. In addition to persistent pain, fever, and ileus during or after an attack of pancreatitis, continued elevation of the serum amylase level should suggest the development of a pseudocyst. The most helpful radiologic examination is the upper gastrointestinal tract barium study, which usually shows an extrinsic mass displacing the stomach anteriorly and superiorly. Occasionally the lesser curvature of the stomach may be flattened by a high-lying pseudocyst (Figs. 32-11 and 32-12). If located in the head of the pancreas, the duodenal loop may be widened. Barium enema may show inferior displacement of the colon. Ultrasonography has recently been shown to be of value in detecting a pseudocyst, and endoscopic retrograde cannulation of the pancreatic duct may show either obstruction of the duct of Wirsung or extravasation of dye into the pseudocyst.

The development of a pancreatitic abscess is detected by accentuation of fever and toxicity, usually at least 3 weeks after the onset of an attack of acute pancreatitis. The presence of gas bubbles on a plain film of the abdomen and bacterial growth in the bloodstream may help establish the diagnosis. The clinician should also be alert to the syndrome of pancreatic ascites, which is caused by leakage of pancreatic juice from a pseudocyst or actual pancreatic ductal disruption. The demonstration of high amylase content of ascitic fluid which also has the characteristics of an exudate serves to differentiate this condition from ascites of hepatic origin.

TREATMENT. Surgical treatment is recommended for pseudocyst of the pancreas, for two reasons: first, complications such as secondary infection, severe hemorrhage, or rupture into an adjacent viscus or into the free peritoneal cavity may occur if a pseudocyst remains untreated; second, these lesions rarely resolve once a thick fibrous wall has developed. If a patient develops a mass during an attack of acute pancreatitis and his condition remains satisfactory, he should be observed for several weeks. Should the mass enlarge or the patient become more ill during this period, immediate operation is indicated. If

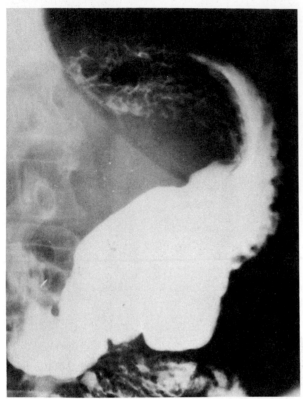

Fig. 32-11. Flattening of the upper portion of the lesser curvature of the stomach by a pseudocyst of the tail of the pancreas.

Fig. 32-12. Roentgenogram taken after injection of contrast material into the dilated and tortuous pancreatic duct. Note the large pseudocyst of the tail of the pancreas in communication with the ductal system which produced the compression of the lesser curvature seen in Fig. 32-11. There is a smaller pseudocyst in the head of the pancreas.

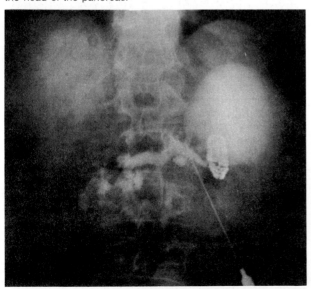

physical and radiologic examination show complete disappearance of the mass, operation may be postponed indefinitely. True intrapancreatic pseudocysts often vary greatly in size and frequently disappear completely only to reappear at a later date.

No single operative procedure is appropriate for every pseudocyst of the pancreas. Simple external drainage or marsupialization should be used in extremely ill patients requiring urgent drainage in whom more extensive procedures might endanger life. If the pseudocyst has a thin flimsy wall, external drainage may be the only means of treatment. The mortality rate of this procedure is low (about 4.5 percent), but the morbidity (prolonged drainage, loss of electrolytes, and a relatively high rate of recurrence) is about 17 percent. Extensive and early drainage is mandatory for pancreatic abscess. In these instances, the lesser sac should be opened widely and all necrotic areas should be debrided and widely drained. Repeated operations may be necessary to accomplish complete cure.

Extirpation theoretically is an ideal method of therapy. Yet only the rare, very small pseudocyst located in the distal pancreas and unattached to vital structures lends itself to excision. Extirpation is not recommended except in these special circumstances, since the mortality is high.

Internal drainage of some type is the best treatment for most pseudocysts. Transgastric cystogastrostomy when the lesion is adherent to the stomach or transduodenal cystoduodenostomy if the cyst is located in the head of the pancreas have produced mortality rates of 2.5 to 5 percent with approximately the same low rate of recurrence. They are almost as easily accomplished as external drainage is. Suturing of the edges of the stomach and cyst or excision of a large ellipse of tissue may predispose to regurgitation. Pancreatic abscesses and gastric ulcer have also been sequelae of cystogastrostomy, and therefore cystojejunostomy to a Roux en Y of jejunum is preferred. A small piece of the wall of the cyst should always be excised and submitted for microscopic examination to exclude the possibility of a neoplastic cyst. Anastomosis of a Roux en Y jejunum to the wall of the pseudocyst requires a thick fibrous wall and results in the same mortality and recurrence rates as cystogastrostomy or cystoduodenostomy.

Drainage through the duct of Wirsung after transduodenal sphincterotomy has been advocated by Doubilet and Mulholland, based on the principle that pseudocysts have major ductal communications. There is little question that drainage of the ductal system will accomplish decompression of most pseudocysts, but the procedures mentioned above would seem to be simpler and more direct in most cases. The primary indication for transphincteric drainage is in patients with gallstone pancreatitis who are undergoing corrective biliary tract operation. In these cases, common duct exploration is frequently performed, making transphincteric drainage a rather simple matter, and recurrence of the pancreatitis is unlikely.

For cases of pancreatic ascites, internal drainage of the offending pseudocyst or resection of the pancreas distal to a ductal disruption is curative.

TUMORS

Carcinoma of the Pancreas and Periampullary Area

The manifestations of carcinoma of the pancreas and other malignant tumors of the periampullary areas (see Chap. 31 for carcinoma of the bile ducts) are so frequently indistinguishable that it seems reasonable to consider these neoplasms as a group. The relative frequency of these lesions in a series of 159 patients is shown in Table 32-2.

The average age of patients with carcinoma of the pancreas, duodenum, and common bile duct is sixty years, but in carcinoma of the ampulla the average age is about five years less. Males are more frequently affected by all these lesions, but there is no special racial predilection. The cause is unknown. Biliary lithiasis has been suspected as a cause of carcinoma of the common bile duct, but not all such patients have cholelithiasis.

PATHOLOGY. Carcinoma of the pancreas arises from the ductal system in 90 percent of the cases and from the acini in the remainder. Adenocarcinoma is the predominant lesion, often accompanied by extreme fibrous connective tissue stromal proliferation. The lesion itself is frequently small, in many instances one-third to one-half of the bulk of the gross lesion, the remainder consisting of a zone of pancreatitis. These tumors are most frequently found within the head of the pancreas and compress the pancreatic and common bile ducts. The pancreatic duct may become extremely dilated and tortuous and is often easily palpable at operation, especially if the surrounding pancreas is somewhat atrophic and firmer than usual. Other adjacent structures, such as the portal vein, stomach, duodenum, and vena cava, may be invaded by tumor. Regional lymph node metastasis is present in 90 percent of patients, and perineural invasion is extremely common. About 80 percent of the patients have liver metastases.

Carcinomas of the ampulla of Vater and the duodenum are frequently impossible to differentiate. Grossly and microscopically, they are columnar cell adenocarcinomas. Frequently, a large area of pancreatitis in the head of the pancreas will not only obscure the small primary lesion but may also be erroneously interpreted as the primary neoplasm itself. Some tumors of the ampulla are so small that they are not readily detected at operation, since biliary obstruction may have occurred very early. In both these neoplasms, intermittent jaundice is caused by recurrent sloughing of the central portion of the tumor. The pattern of metastatic spread is similar to that of carcinoma of the pancreas. Carcinomas of the common bile duct occasionally are fleshy fungating growths but more frequently form a hard mass which may be mistaken for a stone or stricture. In the absence of previous operation, a stricture should be considered to be carcinoma even though biopsies may not initially confirm this. Metastases generally follow the same route as other tumors in this region.

CLINICAL MANIFESTATIONS. Weight loss is the single most common symptom in carcinoma of the pancreas, no matter where the lesion is located. Pain is extremely frequent (70 to 80 percent), although it is rarely of the dramatic type caused by biliary colic resulting from a stone in the common bile duct. The pain is usually dull and aching and is most often confined to the midepigastrium. Radiation to the back is frequent, although the pain may extend to both lower quadrants. A helpful diagnostic feature of the pain is that it is relieved by sitting in a hunched position and accentuated by lying supine. Eating may aggravate the pain, which often antedates jaundice by many weeks or months, depending upon the proximity of the primary lesion to the common bile duct. Distension of the common bile duct, and especially of the pancreatic duct, and perineural invasion by tumor, are usually responsible for pain in carcinoma of the pancreas.

Progressive jaundice occurs in about 75 percent of patients with carcinoma of the head of the pancreas; the incidence of jaundice decreases as the location of the lesion progresses to the left. Occasionally a tumor may deform the second part of the duodenum without obstructing the common bile duct. Anorexia and weakness are common (about 50 percent of cases). Diarrhea, constipation, nausea, and vomiting are inconstant symptoms. Chills and fever are rare. Pruritus is frequent and may be an extremely trying symptom for the patient. The liver is palpable in 50 to 70 percent of patients with carcinoma of the head of the pancreas, but the gallbladder can be palpated in only one-third to one-fourth of the cases. These findings are obviously much less frequent in lesions of the body and tail of the pancreas. An enlarged palpable gallbladder in a jaundiced patient without chills or fever is most certainly a reliable diagnostic criterion for malignant choledochal obstruction, but no diagnostic inference is justified if the gallbladder cannot be palpated. Tenderness, ascites, the presence of an abdominal mass, a rectal shelf, or Virchow's nodes are all less frequent findings.

Pancreatic malignant tumors occur at least twice as frequently in diabetic as in nondiabetic patients, but diabetes is rarely the first sign of pancreatic cancer. Approximately 10 percent of patients with carcinoma of the pancreas are overtly diabetic, and 20 percent have asymptomatic glycosuria or hyperglycemia. It has often been stated that because of the high incidence of thrombosis in carcinoma of the pancreas, it must be seriously

Table 32-2. RELATIVE FREQUENCY OF PERIAMPULLARY NEOPLASMS

	Percent
Pancreas	83
Ampulla of Vater	10
Duodenum	4
Common bile duct	3

SOURCE: Taken with permission from G. L. Jordan, Jr., Benign and Malignant Tumors of the Pancreas and the Periampullary Region, in J. M. Howard and G. L. Jordan, Jr. (eds.), "Surgical Diseases of the Pancreas," J. B. Lippincott Company, Philadelphia, 1960.

considered in all patients who have a spontaneous onset of venous or arterial thrombosis. In fact, clinically detectable thromboses are quite rare in patients with carcinoma of the pancreas.

The clinical signs of carcinoma of the ampulla of Vater, common bile duct, and duodenum are similar to those of carcinoma of the head of the pancreas. Yet, a few distinguishing features may allow differentiation of these lesions from carcinoma of the pancreas. Pain is somewhat less frequent; when present it is apt to be more colicky in nature than the pain of pancreatic cancer. The jaundice is usually less intense when the patient is admitted to the hospital and is more likely to be intermittent (25 percent). Chills and fever are also somewhat more common. In carcinoma of the duodenum, duodenal obstruction and gastrointestinal hemorrhage are more common than in carcinoma of the pancreas.

LABORATORY AND DIAGNOSTIC STUDIES. The most important laboratory studies in periampullary and pancreatic carcinoma are tests for obstructive jaundice. No great significance can be attached to the relationship between the direct and indirect fractions of bilirubin, since they are nearly equal even in only moderately advanced obstructive jaundice. The serum bilirubin almost never rises above 30 to 35 mg/100 ml in pancreatic cancer, whereas acute hepatic necrosis may be associated with much higher levels. The alkaline phosphatase is almost always increased, occasionally even before the onset of jaundice. Quantitative tests of fecal urobilinogen over a 72-hour period are valuable in demonstrating complete or almost complete biliary obstruction if less than 5 mg of urobilinogen is excreted per 24 hours. Impaired bilirubin excretion to this degree is almost never seen in intrahepatic jaundice. Serum transaminase is of value in ruling out hepatitis, since in this disease the serum transaminase often rises to more than 1,000 units. In mechanical biliary obstruction, values below 500 are the rule. Exfoliative cytology and the response of the pancreas to secretin and pancreozymin are time-consuming and rarely of real diagnostic help.

Fifty to sixty percent of patients with pancreaticoduodenal cancer will have some radiologic abnormality, such as distortion and flattening of the gastric antrum or second and third parts of the duodenum, anterior displacement of the stomach, gross distortion of the duodenum and "reverse 3" sign, or widening of the duodenal loop. Yet, the normal variation is so great and these findings are so nonspecific that a definitive radiologic diagnosis is usually impossible. Hypotonic duodenography may provide a more accurate assessment of the duodenal loop in some instances. Positive radiologic findings in a patient whose history and physical examination are compatible with a diagnosis of carcinoma should be considered as strong confirmatory evidence. The biliary ducts cannot be visualized on oral or intravenous cholangiography when the bilirubin exceeds 4 mg/100 ml, especially if it is rising, and these tests are of little value.

Transhepatic cholangiography using a fine needle has been proposed as a means of differentiating between carcinoma and calculus. Carcinoma produces a smooth, tapering, complete obstruction, but calculi cause a typical convex deformity. This technique may be extremely helpful, especially in poor-risk patients, when preoperative assessment might permit a more rapid and less manipulative procedure. However, since hemorrhage and bile peritonitis may occur, it should only be done when the patient is thoroughly prepared for operation. Retrograde cannulation of the common bile duct and pancreatic duct by means of an endoscopic approach has recently received a great deal of well-deserved acclaim and has entered into competition with transhepatic cholangiography.

Splenoportography, retroperitoneal gas insufflation, and celiac angiography do not provide sufficient information to warrant the added risk and discomfort to the patient except in very special circumstances.

DIAGNOSIS. In patients without jaundice, diagnosis of carcinoma of the pancreas may be virtually impossible, despite all possible radiologic and laboratory studies. Many of these patients are thought to be psychoneurotic and are sent from one physician to another, often ending up in the care of a psychiatrist. It is for these cases that angiography and retrograde cannulation may be of special value. The diagnosis of carcinoma of the head of the pancreas and other periampullary lesions, on the other hand, is far easier. Differentiation between the various types of pancreaticoduodenal carcinoma is an interesting intellectual exercise and is to be encouraged, but definitive diagnosis from clinical and laboratory examination may be impossible. Hepatitis can usually be excluded by its tendency to affect younger persons; the 1- to 2-week prodromal period of malaise, anorexia, and fever which precedes the onset of jaundice; the presence of diffuse hepatic tenderness; and a marked increase in serum transaminase. Profound weight loss in a jaundiced patient almost always means carcinoma. Cholestatic jaundice due to viral hepatitis or drugs may be difficult to differentiate from obstruction caused by tumors, because the hepatic function tests show similar abnormalities. In these instances, needle biopsy of the liver should be done and may be invaluable.

TREATMENT AND PROGNOSIS. Once the diagnosis of obstructive jaundice has been established, early operation is advised. Procrastination can only lead to further deterioration of hepatic function and increased operative risk as the patient continues to lose weight. Adequate nutrition and correction of anemia should be accomplished as rapidly as possible. Preoperative evaluation of renal function is essential, since postoperative renal failure is common in severely jaundiced patients. Adequate hydration immediately prior to operation is mandatory for the same reason.

The only definitive and potentially curative therapy for pancreaticoduodenal carcinoma is adequate surgical resection. This implies pancreaticoduodenal resection of the type first successfully performed by Whipple in 1935. During the early years after this formidable operation was first introduced, mortality and morbidity were extremely high, often 40 to 50 percent. Because of these dismal statistics, many surgeons developed a fatalistic attitude toward the therapy of pancreaticoduodenal carcinoma, regarding surgical treatment as merely palliative. Recent improvements in preoperative and postoperative care as well as meticulous attention to technical details have markedly reduced mortality rates, in one instance to 0 percent in forty-one consecutive cases, making this operation a feasible therapeutic technique.

Most surgeons agree that pancreaticoduodenectomy should be performed for localized carcinoma of the ampulla of Vater, duodenum, or common bile duct in good-risk patients who have not been jaundiced for prolonged periods. Although many surgeons do not advocate excision of primary carcinoma of the pancreas, if the lesion is relatively confined and there is no evidence of spread to the liver, resection should be carried out. Additional reasons for resection in those cases which are locally removable include the surgeon's inability to differentiate between a primary lesion of the head of the pancreas and a tumor of the ampulla or the lower end of the common bile duct and also a longer, more comfortable survival after resection even for those who ultimately succumb to their disease.

A 5-year survival rate as high as 18.2 percent has recently been reported after resection for carcinoma of the head of the pancreas, and the 5-year survival rate for carcinoma of the ampulla of Vater and the duodenum may be twice as high. Twenty-five percent of patients who survived resection for cancer of the head of the pancreas have lived for 5 years or more.

The major problem confronting the surgeon at operation is accurate diagnosis, especially before he embarks upon a procedure as large as pancreaticoduodenectomy. Carcinoma of the ampulla of Vater and duodenum can usually be diagnosed rather easily by biopsy of the lesion through a duodenotomy. Establishing the existence of carcinoma of the head of the pancreas or lower end of the common bile duct is often impossible; repeated biopsies not only may be hazardous but are usually unrewarding because of the inflammation surrounding the primary lesion. The decision for resection must be made on the basis of the clinical and operative findings of a mass in the region of the head of the pancreas in a patient in the sixth or seventh decade of life, very frequently with dilatation of the duct of Wirsung. If a calculus can be ruled out by exploration of the common bile duct and cholangiography, the surgeon can take solace in the fact that he will rarely be wrong in the diagnosis of malignancy. Furthermore, if pancreatitis has progressed to the point of obstructing the common bile duct and if the resection can be performed with a reasonably low mortality rate, then successful resection for this benign lesion cannot be too strongly criticized.

Although the resectability rate of carcinoma of the ampulla and duodenum is between 65 and 75 percent, only 10 to 15 percent of patients with carcinoma of the pancreas have resectable lesions. The surgeon's role in palliation is, therefore, an important one even though the average survival after diagnosis in patients with unresectable neoplastic obstructions of the biliary tract is approximately 6 months. Rarely do these patients live longer than 1 year. However, the relief of the jaundice, with its attendant pruritus, and possibly alleviation of obstruction, will often provide significant palliation for these unfortunate patients. A simple cholecystojejunostomy to a loop of jeju-

num without enteroenterostomy is easily performed and is rarely followed by cholangitis. Choledochojejunostomy may be necessary when the gallbladder is absent or the cystic duct is obstructed by tumor. Anastomosis of the biliary tree to the duodenum has been done successfully but is unwise if duodenal obstruction is likely. Invasion of the duodenum and stomach produces gastrointestinal obstruction in 20 percent of patients with carcinoma of the pancreas, and for this reason gastroenterostomy may be advisable.

Cattell and Warren advocate anastomosis of the dilated duct of Wirsung to the jejunum to improve digestion and possibly relieve the pain of ductal distension, but this adds to the extent of operation in an often already debilitated patient and may increase mortality and morbidity. Recently, Merendino has shown that vagotomy relieves the pain of pancreatic cancer. Combined radiation therapy and 5-fluorouracil have recently been shown to significantly prolong comfortable survival of patients with carcinoma of the head of the pancreas.

Pancreaticoduodenal Resection (Fig. 32-13). Pancreaticoduodenectomy is almost always performed in one stage. The two-stage procedure decreases the operative risk in only a small number of deeply jaundiced patients with prolonged obstruction and consequent hepatic injury.

A vertical or a transverse abdominal incision may be used, depending upon the habitus of the patient. The duodenum should have been thoroughly mobilized by the maneuver of Kocher, not only in its second part, but also in the third portion to the superior mesenteric vessels. This usually requires prior mobilization of the hepatic flexure. Gentle dissection between the vessels and the neck of the pancreas with a blunt-nosed clamp is performed once the gastrocolic trunk and pancreatic tributaries have been divided and the posterosuperior pancreaticoduodenal vein has been located. At this point, the surgeon may still turn back, before he has performed an irrevocable maneuver, but excellent assessment of the entire area is still available to him.

The gastrocolic omentum may also be divided at this point to allow better evaluation or so that resection can be continued. The right gastric, gastroduodenal, and descending branch of the left gastric arteries are divided and ligated. The stomach is transected between Payr clamps, leaving the entire antrum with the specimen. The pancreas is transected, usually at its neck. Large vessels are transfixed with fine nonabsorbable sutures. The uncinate process is mobilized by dividing numerous vessels to it between ligatures. Varying amounts of pancreas, or even the entire organ, may be removed with this procedure, at the discretion of the surgeon. The jejunal mesentery and jejunum are divided to allow removal of a few inches of jejunum distal to the ligament of Treitz; the jejunum is withdrawn from beneath the mesenteric vessels. The entire specimen may now be removed by division of the common bile duct. A concomitant cholecystectomy is not always necessary but is usually performed.

Many methods of reconstruction are available. The end of the jejunum is brought into the upper abdomen in a retrocolic position but anterior to the mesenteric vessels.

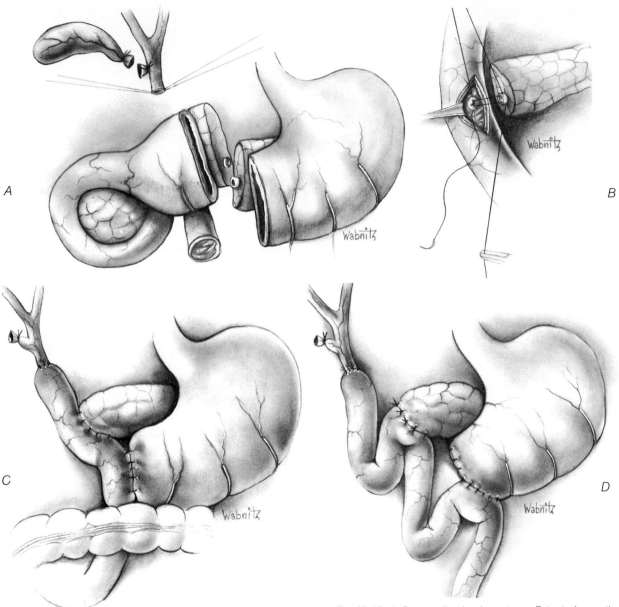

Fig. 32-13. *A.* Pancreaticoduodenectomy. Extent of resection. *B.* Anastomosis of pancreatic duct. *C.* Retrocolic method of reconstitution. *D.* Antecolic method of reconstitution.

Of prime importance is the anastomosis of the biliary and pancreatic ducts above, or proximal to, the gastrojejunal anastomosis, to prevent marginal ulceration. Vagotomy is not generally performed, although it has been recommended by some. If the common duct and jejunum are of equal size, they are joined end to end. When the jejunum is larger than the common bile duct, the end of the jejunum is closed, and end-to-side anastomosis is carried out. The pancreaticojejunostomy is performed between the end of the pancreas and the side of the jejunum several inches distal to the choledochojejunostomy, suturing the duct of Wirsung to jejunal mucosa, as suggested by Cattell and Warren. A gastrojejunostomy completes the operative procedure. A single soft Penrose drain is left in place close to, but not in apposition with, the pancreaticojejunal anastomosis.

Hemorrhage and renal failure are the most common complications in the early postoperative period. Meticulous hemostasis during operation and the administration of vitamin K will generally prevent hemorrhage and later renal failure. The importance of adequate replacement of blood, fluids, and electrolytes cannot be overemphasized. Pancreatic fistula is the third most common complication and is particularly apt to occur if the stump of the pancreas is closed. Careful pancreaticojejunostomy with anastomosis of the duct of Wirsung to the mucosa of the jejunum over a fine tube has largely obviated this complication. Should a pancreatic fistula occur, sump drainage should be instituted. The fistula will close in 2 to 3 weeks if adequate nutrition and electrolyte balance are maintained.

Metabolic Consequences of Pancreaticoduodenectomy.
Most patients tolerate pancreaticoduodenectomy relatively
well. Although some patients gain weight and thrive, the
majority tend to lose some weight and may have varying
degrees of malabsorption. The management of these problems is not unlike that in the postgastrectomy patient, but
exocrine pancreatic substitution therapy is often necessary.
Viokase in divided doses, up to 20 Gm daily, is preferred.
Whether resection of the head, uncinate process, and neck
of the pancreas or closure of the pancreaticojejunostomy
causes the pancreatic insufficiency often seen after pancreaticoduodenectomy is unknown.

The nutritional and metabolic picture is quite different
in the case of total pancreatectomy. The postoperative
diabetes, even though mild and rarely requiring more than
30 units of insulin daily, is exceedingly difficult to manage
because of the patient's extreme sensitivity to insulin.
Diabetic retinopathy and glomerulosclerosis have been
reported but are rare. Loss of nitrogen in the stool increases, and fat absorption is severely impaired. Iron
absorption is very poor, and negative calcium and phosphorus balance is common. Theoretically, total pancreatectomy should improve the results of surgical
therapy for carcinoma of the pancreas, since the tumor
may spread via the pancreatic duct; the lesion is often
multifocal; and the gross extent of the tumor may be
difficult to ascertain at operation. However, the extreme
metabolic derangements produced by total pancreatectomy
and the absence of data to indicate that this operation
increases survival in cancer of the pancreas make its use
debatable at the present time.

Islet-Cell Tumors and Hyperinsulinism

Roscoe Graham achieved the first recorded cure of organic hyperinsulinism by removing an islet-cell adenoma.
In a review of the literature published between 1929 and
1958, Moss and Rhoads found 766 cases, of which only
93 were malignant.

PATHOPHYSIOLOGY. The beta cells of the pancreatic
islets secrete insulin, and tumors that cause hyperinsulinism arise from these cells. Bioassays of these tumors have
usually shown large quantities of insulin, and recent studies of plasma insulin in patients harboring beta cell tumors
have indicated markedly elevated levels after islet-cell
stimulation by a variety of means.

The excessive circulating insulin causes profound hypoglycemia. Since the brain depends primarily on glucose
for its metabolism and cannot store either glucose or glycogen in significant amounts, the hypoglycemia may cause
convulsions, severe cerebral depression, and coma, which
if allowed to persist for a prolonged period will be followed by death within 3 to 20 days. Mental deterioration,
ataxia, hemiparesis, and a wide variety of neurologic sequelae may result from repeated minor hypoglycemic episodes. Early diagnosis and prompt treatment are of importance in the prevention of these irreversible changes.

Administration of glucose promptly reverses the hypo-

glycemia and relieves the symptoms. The spontaneous
recovery which is so frequent in patients with organic
hyperinsulinism has not been adequately explained. However, it has been suggested that hypoglycemia stimulates
the release of epinephrine and glucagon, which in turn
mobilize sufficient glycogen to elevate the blood sugar.

PATHOLOGY. Approximately 75 percent of patients with
pancreatic organic hyperinsulinism have benign adenomas; 12.9 percent have suspiciously malignant lesions, and
in 12.1 percent the lesions are clearly malignant. About
15 percent of the patients have multiple adenomas, but
only a few cases of diffuse adenomatosis involving the
entire pancreas have been described. Most of the adenomas measure between 1 and 3 cm, but the size of the tumor
seems to have little relationship to the severity of the
clinical symptoms. Metastases from malignant beta cell
tumors may be functional or nonfunctional.

CLINICAL MANIFESTATIONS. Most of the patients with
this syndrome are in the fourth to seventh decades of life.
The sex incidence is approximately equal. Functioning
islet-cell tumors are rare in childhood, but spontaneous
hypoglycemia occasionally occurs without tumor. This type
of hypoglycemia usually subsides spontaneously as the
child grows older; its cause is unknown.

The symptoms may take one of two general forms, but
between the two extremes many combinations of clinical
signs may occur. The absolute level of blood sugar often
bears little relationship to the severity or character of the
symptoms, even in the same patient on different days. If
the blood sugar falls rapidly, the primary symptoms may
be referable to the release of epinephrine caused by the
hypoglycemia. Sweating, hunger, weakness, tachycardia,
and "inward trembling" result from this mechanism. A
slower decrease in blood sugar produces "cerebral" symptoms, such as headache, mental confusion, visual disturbances, convulsions, and coma. Symptoms may last for a
few weeks or as long as 20 years. Signs and symptoms of
progressive muscular atrophy have been reported in these
cases. The widest possible variety of bizarre neurologic or
psychiatric disorders may be mimicked by organic hyperinsulinism. Fear of attacks leads many patients to consume
large quantities of food, especially carbohydrates, and they
often become extremely obese.

LABORATORY AND DIAGNOSTIC STUDIES. Whipple's
triad consists of (1) attacks precipitated by fasting or exertion, (2) fasting blood sugar concentrations below 50
mg/100 ml, and (3) symptoms relieved by oral or intravenous administration of glucose. These criteria should always be met before considering operation. Three types of
spontaneous hypoglycemia account for about 80 percent
of all such cases: (1) functional hyperinsulinism, (2) organic hyperinsulinism due to pancreatic islet-cell tumor,
and (3) hepatogenic hypoglycemia. Functional and alimentary hypoglycemia are usually easily ruled out, because
they never occur in the fasting state and invariably occur
2 to 4 hours after eating. Hepatogenic hypoglycemia may
be almost impossible to differentiate from insulinoma.
Abnormal hepatic function and a high-plateau type of
glucose tolerance curve which does not respond to a high-
carbohydrate diet are the keystones to diagnosis of hepato-

genic hypoglycemia. Abnormalities of the pituitary, adrenal, and central nervous system may also cause organic hypoglycemia but can usually be ruled out.

Apart from satisfying the conditions of Whipple's triad, prolonged fasting with or without exercise is the single most valuable test in the diagnosis of insulinoma. The blood sugar will invariably decrease to below 50 mg/100 ml under these circumstances, and fasting for longer than 30 hours is almost never necessary. Simultaneous measurement of serum insulin and blood sugar levels with the finding of an insulin level inappropriately high for the level of the blood sugar is diagnostic of insulinoma. Other aids to diagnosis are the response of the blood sugar to tolbutamide (oral or intravenous) and leucine. These drugs stimulate the release of insulin by the tumor; patients with insulinoma have a much greater and more prolonged depression in the blood sugar level than normal and for that reason these tests may be dangerous. The glucose tolerance test has been unduly deprecated because of the wide variation in the responses. However, if care is taken to restore the sensitivity of the islets in the nontumorous portion of the pancreas by feeding carbohydrates for a few days, the typical flat low curve will almost always be seen. Once the diagnosis has been established by biochemical means, pancreatic angiography may be extremely helpful in localizing the lesion for the surgeon, especially in patients who have undergone unsuccessful exploration before.

TREATMENT. Although dietary therapy has been attempted, the only permanent cure of organic pancreatic hyperinsulinism is by removal of the offending lesion. Streptozotocin, a potent antibiotic which destroys islets, is useful in treating patients with far-advanced metastatic islet-cell carcinoma but should be reserved for these patients because of the antibiotic's toxic side effects. The preoperative management is concerned mainly with the provision of adequate quantities of glucose, usually in the form of 10 percent dextrose solutions. ACTH and cortisone have been recommended, presumably to prevent hyperthermia during, or immediately after, operation. However, it is not necessary to use these drugs, and there is no sound physiologic reason for them.

Surgically, every portion of the pancreas must be carefully examined. The entire anterior aspect of the body, tail, and a portion of the head of the pancreas should be exposed. Then the entire body and tail of the pancreas with the spleen must be mobilized into the wound by division of the splenocolic and lienorenal ligaments and incision of the parietal peritoneum along the inferior and superior aspects of the pancreas. The entire posterior surface of the organ as far right as the superior mesenteric vessels may then be palpated and visualized. The head of the pancreas must be completely mobilized by the Kocher maneuver. Particular attention should be paid to exposure of the neck of the pancreas by division and ligation of the gastrocolic venous trunk and to the uncinate process. The latter is best seen after meticulous clearing of the superior mesenteric vessels. Adenomas in the stomach, duodenum, jejunum, ileum, mesentery, and omentum are aberrant locations in 1 to 2 percent of cases, and these areas should be carefully searched.

Simple excision of the adenoma is sufficient in most cases, since the majority are benign. If malignancy is suspected, a pancreatic resection should be done. Complete exploration should be performed even if a single tumor is found, since about 14 percent are multiple.

The greatest current controversy concerns proper procedure when the tumor cannot be found after thorough examination. Classically, a distal subtotal pancreatectomy to the left of the mesenteric vessels has been advocated under these circumstances, with the hope that a small adenoma might be present in this tissue (21 percent chance) or that hyperplasia of the islets might be ameliorated. It is doubtful whether there are any authenticated cases of hyperplasia of the islets in adults. Yet Moss and Rhoads have found that 42.6 percent of 129 patients were cured and 10.9 percent were improved after "blind" distal pancreatectomy when no tumor was found. The original diagnosis in those who were improved is questionable. Fonkalsrud et al. have suggested that pancreaticoduodenal resection with preservation of the tail of the pancreas should be done when the pancreatic tumor cannot be found after thorough exploration. These investigators feel that a small tumor is much more easily overlooked in the head and uncinate process than in the tail or body. They believe that distal pancreatectomy would be far easier technically after "blind" pancreaticoduodenectomy when no tumor has been found than the reverse sequence of operations. We are reluctant to advocate "blind" pancreaticoduodenectomy because of the higher morbidity and mortality and would still choose distal resection. The distal pancreatectomy can be extended to a 90 percent resection or more if necessary, more easily and with less morbidity than pancreaticoduodenectomy. However, it cannot be stressed strongly enough that all of the pancreas, and especially the head and uncinate process, must be seen and felt. A marked increase in blood glucose within 30 minutes of removal of tissue suspected of being responsible for the hyperinsulinism is confirmatory evidence that the disease has been eradicated. Subsequent determination of serum insulin levels on the same blood taken at operation will provide postoperative substantiation of cure.

The child with organic hypoglycemia can usually be managed with diet and ACTH or cortisone. If a response is not evident and if the patient seems to be deteriorating, operation is indicated, even though tumors are exceedingly rare in children. If no tumor is found, distal subtotal pancreatectomy in a child is much more logical procedure than in adults, since hyperplasia of the islets does occur and is responsive to partial resection.

The overall operative mortality for removal of a localized islet-cell tumor is 8.2 percent, and for partial resection (distal) of the pancreas it is 9.6 percent.

Ulcerogenic and Nonulcerogenic Tumors of the Islets

In 1955, Zollinger and Ellison reported two patients with coincidental fulminant peptic ulceration and non-beta cell tumors of the pancreas. Since then, many cases of ulcerogenic tumors of the pancreas have been described.

CLINICAL MANIFESTATIONS. The triad described originally by Zollinger and Ellison remains extremely useful today: (1) fulminant and often complicated peptic ulceration, frequently found in atypical locations, (2) extreme gastric hypersecretion, and (3) non-beta cell tumor of the pancreatic islets. The symptoms are similar to those caused by ordinary peptic ulceration. Some patients with this syndrome have had explosive and unrelenting ulceration from onset; others have had symptoms for several years which suddenly become fulminant. Perforation, hemorrhage, obstruction, internal fistulization, and intractability may occur. The ulceration, although often present in the first portion of the duodenum, occasionally is found in unusual locations, such as the third and fourth parts of the duodenum or the jejunum. Perforation or any other complication of jejunal ulceration should always make one suspect the presence of an ulcerogenic pancreatic tumor, since peptic ulceration of the jejunum rarely occurs when no tumor is present.

Fulminant ulceration often recurs within weeks after ordinarily effective surgical therapy. Subtotal gastrectomy with or without vagotomy, vagotomy with a drainage procedure, radiation therapy, and prodigious doses of alkalinizing and anticholinergic agents have generally been ineffective in controlling the ulcer diathesis. H_2 receptor antagonists have recently proved to be effective in selected patients who may have inoperable situations. Many patients have undergone several of these procedures before the true nature of the process was discovered.

The syndrome is slightly more common in males, the ratio being approximately 6:4. Most of the patients are in the third to fourth decade of life, although a few cases have occurred in the first decade and a rare case in the ninth. Two to three liters of fluid in a 12-hour nocturnal secretion is common even in the absence of pyloric obstruction. The overnight resting secretion often contains 200 to 300 mEq of free acid, although some patients have less than 100 mEq of free hydrochloric acid. Even the smallest remnants of gastric mucosa can cause extreme hypersecretion and recurrent ulceration in these patients. Since the secretory rates are already close to their maximum, further stimulation with histamine generally produces very little response. Marks et al. have suggested that a ratio of basal acid output to histamine-stimulated output of greater than 60 percent is virtually diagnostic of the Zollinger-Ellison syndrome, but exceptions are more common than generally recognized.

The extreme gastric hypersecretion is associated with distressing watery diarrhea in about a third of the reported cases. Some patients have excreted between 2 and 8 liters of liquid stool daily, and in many cases profound diarrhea has preceded the onset of peptic ulceration. In some cases in which diarrhea is the sole symptom, the patient has had gastric hypersecretion without peptic ulceration. Steatorrhea may also occur and probably is caused by three mechanisms: (1) inactivation of pancreatic and intestinal lipase by the abnormally acid environment of the upper small intestine, (2) precipitation of bile salts, and (3) irritative and inflammatory action of the acid environment upon the mucosa of the small bowel. Aspiration of the gastric secretion often temporarily relieves the diarrhea.

A sharp distinction should be made between the diarrhea of the Zollinger-Ellison syndrome and another syndrome of watery diarrhea and non-beta cell tumors of the pancreas which is much less common than the former, only about fifty cases having been reported. This latter group of patients is usually free from ulcers; gastric secretion is normal or low; the hypokalemia and alkalosis are almost always present. Hyperglycemia is common, and alternating hypercalcemia and normocalcemia are frequently encountered in the same patient. Total removal of the tumor results in cure of the disabling watery diarrhea, although steroid therapy may be temporarily beneficial for those with malignant tumors where all tumor could not be extirpated and the metastatic malignancy is functional. Although Kraft, Tompkins, and Zollinger originally proposed that secretin produced by the tumor was responsible for the observed effects, more recent studies indicate that the responsible agent is vasoactive intestinal peptide (VIP).

In addition to the usual radiologic findings of peptic ulceration, duodenal ileus with enlargement of rugal folds, hypertrophy of the gastric mucosa, and an abnormal feathery pattern of the small bowel are frequently found in patients with the Zollinger-Ellison syndrome.

PATHOLOGY AND PATHOPHYSIOLOGY. The origin of these tumors is as yet unknown, although histologic studies indicate that they do not arise from the alpha or beta cells of the islets. The typical tumor is composed of rather uniform cuboidal cells arranged mainly in strands and ribbons or occasionally in sheets and clumps. The nucleus is oval and has one or more round nucleoli. The cytoplasm usually contains fine stippling and irregular vacuoles, but no secretory granules have been identified. These tumors often bear a striking resemblance to argentaffin tumors (carcinoids) but do not react to silver stains. The growth pattern of these two tumors is remarkably similar in that both tend to grow slowly, metastasize late, and exhibit little correlation between the microscopic appearance and growth propensities. The patient with an islet-cell tumor often dies from the unremitting peptic ulceration rather than from metastasis, although recent long-term follow-up indicates an increasing and unexpected incidence of death from metastatic disease. Grossly, the tumors are slate gray to red-brown and vary from 2 mm to 10 cm. Most are solid, although a few cystic tumors have been reported.

In 249 collected cases, 61 percent of the patients had malignant tumors, and 44 percent of these had metastases, usually to the regional lymph nodes. The tumors are located with equal frequency in the head and tail of the pancreas. Diffuse microadenomatosis has been observed in 19 percent of the cases. A significant number of patients have had lesions in the duodenal wall. This is of particular interest because removal of the tumor alone in these cases has frequently sufficed to eradicate the disease, in contradistinction to the radical treatment by total gastrectomy usually advocated in this syndrome.

Associated endocrine disease has been found in 21 percent of the patients with the Zollinger-Ellison syndrome. This usually consists of adenomas of other endocrine glands, such as the pituitary, parathyroid, pancreatic islets (beta cells), and adrenal cortex, in that order of frequency. These patients usually do not have family histories of similar disturbances; therefore most of these cases can be distinguished from the group described by Wermer in 1954. He pointed out that some patients with polyendocrine adenomas and peptic ulceration often have giant gastric rugae (Ménétrier's disease) and that an abnormal gene may be responsible. Ellison and Wilson have found that only 3 percent of the patients with the Zollinger-Ellison syndrome fall into this classification. Gastrin is secreted by these tumors, and that extracted from tumors has physiologic effects identical to those of synthesized pure gastrin. Thus, the diagnosis can be substantiated by the detection of extremely high levels of gastrin in the serum. Sometimes the levels of serum gastrin are borderline elevated in patients with gastrinoma, especially if prior vagotomy without resection has been carried out. An exaggerated response of the serum gastrin to the intravenous infusion of calcium and a paradoxical rise of the serum gastrin level after intravenous infusion of secretin serve to elucidate the diagnosis in doubtful cases. These findings, together with the absence of a rise in serum gastrin level after a meal, are helpful in differentiating patients with gastrinoma from those who have the recently described antral G cell hyperplasia.

TREATMENT AND PROGNOSIS. It is attractive to hypothesize that removal of the pancreatic islet-cell tumor alone should suffice to alleviate the potent ulcerogenic stimulus in patients with this disease. Although a few patients with fulminant peptic ulceration have responded to removal of the pancreatic tumor alone or to excision of the tumor with concomitant subtotal gastrectomy, these procedures are usually destined for failure. The high incidence of malignancy with functioning metastases as well as the possibility of multiple pancreatic tumors or islet hyperplasia are responsible for these failures. Even the smallest amount of gastric mucosa is capable of secreting huge quantities of highly acid gastric juice in the presence of the ulcerogenic tumor. Thus, the safest and most conservative treatment of these patients is total gastrectomy, usually with Roux en Y jejunal reconstruction, and removal of the pancreatic tumor if possible.

Experience has repeatedly indicated that lesser operations or radiation therapy usually invite disaster in the form of recurrent ulceration, internal fistulization, hemorrhage, perforation, and death. The relatively protracted course of the tumor, even when it has metastasized, justifies the more radical procedure. Repeated determinations of serum gastrin levels may be of some prognostic value following total gastrectomy since disappearance of metastases and return of serum gastrin to normal have been reported in some cases. Persistently high levels of serum gastrin probably indicate lack of primary or metastatic tumor regression, whereas elevation of a posttherapeutic low level of serum gastrin suggests the development of metastatic disease. Oberhelman et al. have had good results from removal of the tumor alone without total gastrectomy when the tumor has been located in the wall of the duodenum. We have had similar results, but only in these cases would we consider procedures of less than total

gastrectomy. Whether these duodenal tumors differ materially from those in the pancreas is not known, although the microscopic appearance is similar.

References

Anatomy

Kleitsch, W. P.: Anatomy of the Pancreas: A Study with Special Reference to the Duct System, *Arch Surg,* **71:**795, 1955.

Payne, R. L., Jr.: Annular Pancreas, *Ann Surg,* **133:**754, 1951.

Pierson, J. M.: The Arterial Blood Supply of the Pancreas, *Surg Gynecol Obstet,* **77:**426, 1943.

Reemtsma, K.: Embryology and Congenital Anomalies of the Pancreas, in J. M. Howard and G. L. Jordan (eds.), "Surgical Diseases of the Pancreas," J. B. Lippincott Company, Philadelphia, 1960.

Reich, H.: Relation of the Duct of Santorini to the Pathogenesis of Duodenal Ulcer, *N Engl J Med,* **269:**1119, 1963.

Physiology

Albo, R., Silen, W., Hein, M. F., and Harper, H. A.: Relationship of the Acinar Portion of the Pancreas to Gastric Secretion, *Surg Forum,* **14:**316, 1963.

Christodoulopoulos, J. B., Jacobs, W. H., and Klotz, A. P.: Pharmacologic Inhibition of Humoral-stimulated Pancreatic Secretion, *Gastroenterology,* **40:**671, 1961.

Drapanas, T., Pollack, E. L., and Shim, W. K.: The Regulation of Pancreatic Secretion by Serotonin, *Arch Surg,* **83:**462, 1961.

Gregory, R. A.: "Secretory Mechanisms of the Gastro-intestinal Tract," The Williams & Wilkins Company, Baltimore, 1962.

——— and Tracy, H. J.: The Constitution and Properties of Two Gastrins Extracted from Hog Antral Mucosa, *Gut,* **5:**103, 1964.

——— and ———: A Note on the Nature of the Gastrin-like Stimulant Present in Zollinger-Ellison Tumors, *Gut,* **5:**115, 1964.

Janowitz, H. D., and Dreiling, D. A.: The Pancreatic Secretion of Fluid and Electrolytes, in *Ciba Found Symp Exocrine Pancreas Normal Abnormal Functions,* 1962.

Konturek, S. J., Radecki, T., Biernat, J., and Thor, P.: Effect of Vagotomy on Pancreatic Secretion Evoked by Endogenous and Exogenous Cholecystokinin and Caerulein, *Gastroenterology,* **63:**273, 1972.

McIlrath, D. C., Kennedy, J. A., and Hallenbeck, G. A.: Relationship between Atrophy of the Pancreas and Gastric Secretion: An Experimental Study, *Am J Digest Diseases,* **8:**623, 1963.

Menguy, R. B., Hallenbeck, G. A., Bollman, J. L., and Grindlay, J. H.: Intraductal Pressures and Sphincteric Resistance in Canine Pancreatic and Biliary Ducts after Various Stimuli, *Surg Gynecol Obstet,* **106:**306, 1958.

Meyer, J. H., Spingola, L. J., and Grossman, M. I.: Endogenous Cholecystokinin Potentiates Exogenous Secretin on Pancreas of Dog, *Am J Physiol,* **221:**742, 1971.

Meyer, J. H., Way, L. W., and Grossman, M. I.: Pancreatic Response to Acidification of Varying Lengths of Proximal Intestine in Dog, *Am J Physiol,* **219:**971, 1970.

Moreland, H. J., and Johnson, L. R.: Effect of Vagotomy of

Pancreatic Secretion Stimulated by Endogenous and Exogenous Secretin, *Gastroenterology,* **60:**425, 1971.

Perks, A. M., Schapiro, H., and Woodward, E. R.: The Influence of Antidiuretic Hormone on Pancreatic Exocrine Secretion, *Acta Endocrinol,* **45:**340, 1964.

Poncelot, P. R., and Thompson, A. G.: Role of Infected Bile in Spasm of Sphincter of Oddi, *Am J Surg,* **126:**387, 1973.

Routley, E. F., Mann, F. C., Bollman, J. L., and Grindlay, J. H.: Effects of Vagotomy on Pancreatic Secretion in Dogs with Chronic Pancreatic Fistula, *Surg Gynecol Obstet,* **95:**529, 1952.

Thomas, J. E.: Mechanism of Action of Pancreatic Stimuli Studied by Means of Atropine-like Drugs, *Am J Physiol,* **206:**124, 1964.

Unger, R. H., and Eisentraut, A. M.: Enteroinsular Axis, *Arch Intern Med,* **123:**261, 1969.

Unger, R. H., Ketterer, H., Dupre, J., and Eisentraut, A. M.: The Effects of Secretin, Pancreozymin, and Gastrin on Insulin and Glucagon Secretion in Anesthetized Dogs, *J Clin Invest,* **46:**630, 1967.

Veeger, W., Abels, J., Hellemans, N., and Nieweg, H. O.: Effect of Sodium Bicarbonate and Pancreatin on the Absorption of Vitamin B_{12} and Fat in Pancreatic Insufficiency, *N Engl J Med,* **267:**1341, 1962.

Wang, C. C., and Grossman, M. I.: Physiological Determination of Release of Secretin and Pancreozymin from Intestine of Dogs with Transplanted Pancreas, *Am J Physiol,* **164:**527, 1951.

Warshaw, A. L., and Lesser, P. B.: Amylase Clearance in Differentiating Acute Pancreatitis from Peptic Ulcer with Hyperamylasemia, *Ann Surg,* **181:**314, 1975.

White, T. T., Hayama, T., and Magee, D. F.: Alternate Nervous Pathways for the Gastropancreatic Reflex, *Gastroenterology,* **39:**615, 1960.

———, Lundh, G., and Magee, D. F.: Evidence for the Existence of a Gastropancreatic Reflex, *Am J Physiol,* **198:**725, 1960.

Acute Pancreatitis

Adams, J. T., Libertino, J. A., and Schwartz, S. I.: Significance of an Elevated Serum Amylase, *Surgery,* **63:**877, 1968.

Albo, R. J., Silen, W., and Goldman, L.: A Critical Clinical Analysis of Acute Pancreatitis, *Arch Surg,* **86:**1032, 1963.

Avioli, L. V., Birge, S. J., Scott, S., and Shieber, W.: Role of the Thyroid Gland During Glucagon-induced Hypocalcemia in the Dog, *Am J Physiol,* **216:**939, 1969.

Bernard, H. R., Criscione, J. R., and Moyer, C. A.: The Pathologic Significance of the Serum Amylase Concentration: An Evaluation with Special Reference to Pancreatitis and Biliary Lithiasis, *Arch Surg,* **79:**311, 1959.

Bradley, E. L., III, and Clements, L. J.: Spontaneous Resolution of Pancreatic Pseudocysts: Implications for Timing of Operative Intervention, *Am J Surg,* **129:**23, 1975.

Cameron, J. L., Zuidema, G. D., and Margolis, S.: Pathogenesis for Alcoholic Pancreatitis, *Surgery,* **77:**754, 1975.

Elliot, D. W., Williams, R. D., and Zollinger, R. M.: Alterations in the Pancreatic Resistance to Bile in the Pathogenesis of Acute Pancreatitis, *Ann Surg,* **146:**669, 1957.

Gambill, E. E., and Mason, H. L.: One-hour Value for Urinary Amylase in 96 Patients with Pancreatitis: Comparative Diagnostic Value of Tests of Urinary and Serum Amylase and Serum Lipase, *JAMA,* **186:**24, 1963.

Gross, J. B., and Comfort, M. W.: Hereditary Pancreatitis, *Proc Staff Meetings Mayo Clinic,* **32:**354, 1957.

Haverback, B. J., Dyce, B., Bundy, H., and Edmondson, H. A.: Trypsin, Trypsinogen, and Trypsin Inhibitor in Human Pancreatic Juice: Mechanism for Pancreatitis Associated with Hyperparathyroidism, *Am J Med,* **29:**424, 1960.

Howard, J. M.: The Causes of Death from Pancreatitis, in J. M. Howard and G. L. Jordan, Jr., "Surgical Diseases of the Pancreas," J. B. Lippincott Company, Philadelphia, 1960.

——— and Ehrlich, E. W.: The Etiology of Pancreatitis: A Review of Clinical Experience, *Ann Surg,* **152:**135, 1960.

Howes, R., Zuidema, G. D., and Cameron, J. L.: Evaluation of Prophylactic Antibiotics in Acute Pancreatitis, *J Surg Res,* **18:**197, 1975.

Kessler, J. I., Kniffen, J. C., and Janowitz, H. D.: Lipoprotein Lipase Inhibition in the Hyperlipemia of Acute Alcoholic Pancreatitis, *N Engl J Med,* **269:**943, 1963.

Klatskin, G., and Gordon, M.: Relationship between Relapsing Pancreatitis and Essential Hyperlipemia, *Am J Med,* **12:**3, 1952.

Lefer, A. M., Glenn, T. M., O'Neill, T. J., Lovett, W. L., Geissinger, W. T., and Wangensteen, S. L.: Inotropic Influence of Endogenous Peptides in Experimental Hemorrhagic Pancreatitis, *Surgery,* **69:**220, 1971.

Levitt, M. D., Rapoport, M., and Cooperbrand, S. R.: The Renal Clearance of Amylase in Renal Insufficiency, Acute Pancreatitis, and Macroamylasemia, *Ann Intern Med,* **71:**919, 1969.

Ranson, J. H. C., Rivkind, K. M., Roses, D. F., Fink, S. D., Eng, K., and Spencer, F. C.: Prognostic Signs and Role of Operative Management in Acute Pancreatitis, *Surg Gynecol Obstet,* **139:**69, 1974.

Robinson, T. M., and Dunphy, J. E.: Continuous Perfusion of Bile and Protease Activators through the Pancreas, *JAMA,* **183:**530, 1963.

Salzman, E. W., and Bartlett, M. K.: Pancreatic Duct Exploration in Selected Cases of Acute Pancreatitis, *Ann Surg,* **158:**859, 1963.

Schmidt, H., and Creutzfeld, W.: The Possible Role of Phospholipose A in the Pathogenesis of Acute Pancreatitis, *Scand J Gastroenterol,* **4:**39, 1969.

Smith, R. B., III, Warren, W. D., Rivard, A. A., Jr., and Amerson, J. R.: Pancreatic Ascites: Diagnosis and Management with Particular Reference to Surgical Technics, *Ann Surg,* **177:**689, 1973.

Watts, G. T.: Total Pancreatectomy for Fulminant Pancreatitis, *Lancet,* **2:**384, 1963.

Chronic Pancreatitis

Child, C. G., III, Frey, C. F., and Fry, W. J.: A Reappraisal of Removal of 95% of the Distal Portion of the Pancreas, *Surg Gynecol Obstet,* **129:**49, 1969.

Dreiling, D. A., and Janowitz, H. D.: Measurement of Pancreatic Secretory Function, in *Ciba Found Symp Exocrine Pancreas Normal Abnormal Functions,* 1962.

DuVal, M. K., Jr.: Caudal Pancreatico-jejunostomy for Chronic Relapsing Pancreatitis, *Ann Surg,* **140:**775, 1954.

Howard, J. M.: The Etiology of Acute Pancreatitis: Facts and Fancies, in J. M. Howard and G. L. Jordan, Jr. (eds.), "Surgical Diseases of the Pancreas," J. B. Lippincott Company, Philadelphia, 1960.

Joffe, B. I., Bank, S., Jackson, W. P. V., and Keller, P.: Insulin Reserve in Patients with Chronic Pancreatitis, *Lancet,* **2:**890, 1968.

Kalser, M. H., Leite, C. A., and Warren, W. D.: Fat Assimilation After Massive Distal Pancreatectomy, *N Engl J Med,* **279:**570, 1968.

Owens, J. L., and Howard, J. M.: Pancreatic Calcification: A Late Sequel in the Natural History of Chronic Alcoholism and Alcoholic Pancreatitis, *Ann Surg,* **147:**326, 1958.

Puestow, C. B., and Gillesby, W. J.: Retrograde Surgical Drainage of Pancreas for Chronic Relapsing Pancreatitis, *Arch Surg,* **76:**898, 1958.

Silen, W., Baldwin, J., and Goldman, L.: Treatment of Chronic Pancreatitis by Longitudinal Pancreaticojejunostomy, *Am J Surg,* **106:**243, 1963.

White, T. F., and Keith, R. G.: Long-term Follow-up Study of 50 Patients with Pancreaticojejunostomy, *Surg Gynecol Obstet,* **136:**353, 1973.

Trauma

Anderson, M. C., and Bergan, J. J.: An Experimental Study of Pancreatic Trauma and Its Relationship to Pancreatic Inflammation, *Arch Surg,* **86:**1044, 1963.

Baker, R. J., Dippel, W. F., Freeark, R. J., and Strohl, E. L.: The Surgical Significance of Trauma to the Pancreas, *Arch Surg,* **86:**1038, 1963.

Berne, C. J., Donovan, A. J., White, E. J., and Yellin, A. E.: Duodenal "Diverticulization" for Duodenal and Pancreatic Injury, *Am J Surg,* **127:**503, 1974.

Cleveland, H. C., Reinschmidt, J. S., and Waddell, W. R.: Traumatic Pancreatitis: An Increasing Problem, *Surg Clin North Am,* **43:**401, 1963.

Doubilet, H., and Mulholland, J. H.: Some Observations on the Treatment of Trauma to the Pancreas, *Am J Surg,* **105:**741, 1963.

Freeark, R. J., Kane, J. M., Folk, F. A., and Baker, R. J.: Traumatic Disruption of the Head of the Pancreas, *Arch Surg,* **91:**5, 1965.

Howard, J. M.: Pancreatic Trauma, in J. M. Howard and G. L. Jordan, Jr. (eds.), "Surgical Diseases of the Pancreas," J. B. Lippincott Company, Philadelphia, 1960.

Howell, J. F., Burrus, G. R., and Jordan, G. L., Jr.: Surgical Management of Pancreatic Injuries, *J Trauma,* **1:**32, 1961.

Stone, H. H., Stowers, K. B., and Shippey, S. H.: Injuries to the Pancreas, *Arch Surg,* **85:**525, 1962.

Thal, A. P., and Wilson, R. F.: A Pattern of Severe Blunt Trauma to the Region of the Pancreas, *Surg Gynecol Obstet,* **119:**773, 1964.

Cysts and Pseudocysts

Balfour, J. F.: Pancreatic Pseudocysts: Complications and Their Relation to the Timing of Treatment, *Surg Clin North Am,* **50:**395, 1970.

Cullen, P. K., Jr., ReMine, W. H., and Dahlin, D. C.: A Clinicopathological Study of Cystadenocarcinoma of the Pancreas, *Surg Gynecol Obstet,* **117:**189, 1963.

Doubilet, H., and Mulholland, H. J.: Pancreatic Cysts, *Surg Gynecol Obstet,* **96:**683, 1953.

Evans, F. C.: Pancreatic Abscess, *Am J Surg,* **117:**537, 1969.

Finley, J. W.: Respiratory Complications of Acute Pancreatitis, *Ann Surg,* **169:**420, 1969.

Jordan, G. L., Jr.: Pancreatic Cysts, in J. M. Howard and G. L. Jordan, Jr. (eds.), "Surgical Diseases of the Pancreas," J. B. Lippincott Company, Philadelphia, 1960.

Kaiser, G. C., King, R. D., Kilman, J. W., Lempke, R. E., and Shumacker, H. B.: Pancreatic Pseudocysts: An Evaluation of Surgical Management, *Arch Surg,* **89:**275, 1964.

Murphy, R. F., and Hinkamp, J. F.: Pancreatic Pseudocysts: Report of Thirty-five Cases, *Arch Surg,* **81:**564, 1960.

Piper, C. E., ReMine, W. H., and Priestley, J. T.: Pancreatic Cystadenomata: Report of 20 Cases, *JAMA,* **180:**648, 1962.

Polk, H. C., Zeppa, R., and Warren, W. D.: Surgical Significance of Differentiation Between Acute and Chronic Pancreatic Collections, *Ann Surg,* **169:**444, 1969.

Schindler, S. C., Schaefer, J. W., Hull, D., and Griffen, W. O., Jr.: Chronic Pancreatic Ascites, *Gastroenterology,* **59:**453, 1970.

Varriale, P., Bonanno, C. A., and Grace, W. J.: Portal Hypertension Secondary to Pancreatic Pseudocysts, *Arch Intern Med,* **112:**191, 1963.

Carcinoma of the Pancreas and Periampullary Area

Buckwalter, J. A., Lawton, R. L., and Tidrick, R. T.: Bypass Operations for Neoplastic Biliary Obstruction, *Am J Surg,* **109:**100, 1965.

Cattell, R. B., and Warren, K. W.: "Surgery of the Pancreas," W. B. Saunders Company, Philadelphia, 1954.

Eaton, S. B., Fleischli, D. J., Pollard, J. J., Nebesar, R. A., and Potsaid, M. S.: Comparison of Current Radiologic Approaches to the Diagnosis of Pancreatic Disease, *New Engl J Med,* **279:**389, 1968.

Guynn, V. L., Overstreet, R. J., and Reynolds, J. T.: Reduction of Mortality and Morbidity in Pancreatoduodenectomy, *Arch Surg,* **85:**260, 1962.

Howard, J. M.: Pancreatico-duodenectomy. Forty-one Consecutive Whipple Resections Without an Operative Mortality, *Ann Surg,* **168:**629, 1968.

Jordan, G. L., Jr.: Benign and Malignant Tumors of the Pancreas and Periampullary Region, in J. M. Howard and G. L. Jordan, Jr. (eds.), "Surgical Diseases of the Pancreas," J. B. Lippincott Company, Philadelphia, 1960.

———— and Grossman, M. I.: Pancreaticoduodenectomy for Chronic Relapsing Pancreatitis, *Arch Surg,* **74:**871, 1957.

Madden, J. L.: Technique for Pancreaticoduodenectomy, *Surg Gynecol Obstet,* **118:**247, 1964.

Merendino, K. A.: Vagotomy for the Relief of Pain Secondary to Pancreatic Carcinoma, *Am J Surg,* **108:**1, 1964.

Moertel, C. G., Reitemeier, R. J., Childs, D. S., Colby, M. Y., and Hallbrook, M. A.: Combined 5-fluorouracil and Supervoltage Radiation Therapy of Locally Unresectable Gastrointestinal Cancer, *Lancet,* **2:**865, 1969.

Monge, J. J., Dockerty, M. B., Wollaeger, E. E., Waugh, J. M., and Priestley, J. T.: Clinicopathologic Observations on Radical Pancreatoduodenal Resection for Peripapillary Carcinoma, *Surg Gynecol Obstet,* **118:**275, 1964.

ReMine, W. H., Priestley, J. T., Judd, E. S., and King, J. N.: Total Pancreatectomy, *Ann Surg,* **172:**595, 1970.

Silen, W.: Surgical Anatomy of the Pancreas, *Surg Clin North Am,* **44:**1253, 1964.

Warren, K. W.: The Surgical Exposure in the Differential Diagnosis of Pancreatic Disorders at Operation, *Surg Clin North Am,* **38:**799, 1958.

Islet Cell Tumors and Hyperinsulinism

Conn, J. W., and Seltzer, H. S.: Spontaneous Hypoglycemia, *Am J Med,* **19:**460, 1955.

Fajans, S. S., and Conn, J. W.: An Intravenous Tolbutamide Test as an Adjunct in the Diagnosis of Functioning Pancreatic Islet Cell Adenomas, *J Lab Clin Med,* **54:**811, 1959.

Flanagan, G. C., Schwartz, T. B., and Ryan, W. G.: Studies on Patients with Islet-cell Tumor, Including the Phenomenon of Leucine-induced Accentuation of Hypoglycemia, *J Clin Endocrinol Metab,* **21:**401, 1961.

Floyd, J. C., Fajans, S. S., Knopf, R. F., and Conn, J. W.: Plasma Insulin in Organic Hyperinsulinism: Comparative Effects of Tolbutamide, Leucine and Glucose, *J Clin Endocrinol,* **24:**747, 1964.

Fonkalsrud, E. W., Dilley, R. B., and Longmire, W. P., Jr.: Insulin Secreting Tumors of the Pancreas, *Ann Surg,* **159:**730, 1964.

Graham, R. R.: Quoted in G. Howland, W. R. Campbell, E. J. Maltby, and W. L. Robinson: Dysinsulinism: Convulsions and Coma Due to Islet-cell Tumor of the Pancreas, with Operation and Cure, *JAMA,* **93:**674, 1929.

Harrison, T. S., Child, G. C., III, Fry, W. J., Floyd, J. C., Jr., and Fajans, S. S.: Current Surgical Management of Functioning Islet Cell Tumors of the Pancreas, *Ann Surg,* **178:**485, 1973.

Moss, N. H., and Rhoads, J. E.: Hyperinsulinism and Islet-cell Tumors of the Pancreas, in J. M. Howard and G. L. Jordan (eds.), "Surgical Diseases of the Pancreas," J. B. Lippincott Company, Philadelphia, 1960.

Porter, M. R., and Frantz, V. K.: Tumors Associated with Hypoglycemia: Pancreatic and Extrapancreatic, *Am J Med,* **21:**944, 1956.

ReMine, W. H., Scholz, D. A., and Priestley, J. T.: Hyperinsulinism: Clinical and Surgical Aspects, *Am J Surg,* **99:**413, 1960.

Schnelle, N., Molnar, G. D., Ferris, D. O., Rosevear, J. W., and Moffitt, E. A.: Circulating Glucose and Insulin in Surgery for Insulinomas, *JAMA,* **217:**1072, 1971.

Whipple, A. O., and Frantz, V. K.: Adenoma of Islet Cells with Hyperinsulinism: A Review, *Ann Surg,* **101:**1299, 1935.

Ulcerogenic and Nonulcerogenic Tumors of the Islets

Ellison, E. H., and Wilson, S. D.: The Zollinger-Ellison Syndrome: Re-appraisal and Evaluation of 260 Registered Cases, *Ann Surg,* **160:**513, 1964.

Espiner, E. A., and Beaven, D. W.: Non-specific Islet-cell Tumor of the Pancreas with Diarrhea, *Q J Med,* **31:**447, 1962.

Friesen, S. R., Bolinger, R. E., Pearse, A. G. E., and McGuigan, J. E.: Serum Gastrin Levels in Malignant Zollinger-Ellison Syndrome After Total Gastrectomy and Hypophysectomy, *Ann Surg,* **172:**504, 1970.

Gjone, E., Fretheim, B., Nordoy, A., Jacobsen, C. D., and Elgjo, K.: Intractable Watery Diarrhoea, Hypokalaemia, and Achlorhydria Associated with Pancreatic Tumor Containing Gastric Secretory Inhibitor, *Scand J Gastroenterol,* **5:**401, 1970.

Hofmann, J. W., Fox, P. S., and Wilson, S. D.: Duodenal Wall Tumors and Zollinger-Ellison Syndrome: Surgical Management, *Arch Surg,* **107:**334, 1973.

Kraft, A. R., Tompkins, R. K., and Zollinger, R. M.: Recognition and Management of the Diarrheal Syndrome Caused by Nonbeta Islet Cell Tumors of the Pancreas, *Am J Surg,* **119:**163, 1970.

Oberhelman, H. A., Jr., Nelsen, T. S., Johnson, A. N., Jr., and Dragstedt, L. R., II: Ulcerogenic Tumors of the Duodenum, *Ann Surg,* **153:**214, 1961.

Silen, W.: Personal observations.

Singleton, J. W., Kern, F., Jr., Waddell, W. R.: Diarrhea and Pancreatic Islet-cell Tumor: Report of a Case with Severe Jejunal Mucosal Lesion, *Gastroenterology,* **49:**197, 1965.

Summerskill, W. H. J.: Malabsorption and Jejunal Ulceration Due to Gastric Hypersecretion with Pancreatic Islet-cell Hyperplasia, *Lancet,* **1:**120, 1959.

Wermer, P.: Genetic Aspects of Adenomatosis of Endocrine Glands, *Am J Med,* **16:**363, 1954.

Zollinger, R. M., and Ellison, E. H.: Primary Peptic Ulcerations of the Jejunum Associated with Islet-cell Tumors of the Pancreas, *Ann Surg,* **142:**709, 1955.

Chapter 33

Spleen

by **Seymour I. Schwartz**

ANATOMY

The spleen arises by mesenchymal differentiation along the left side of the dorsal mesogastrium in the 8-mm embryo. The weight of the spleen in the healthy adult ranges between 75 and 100 Gm, decreasing somewhat with age. The organ is located in the left upper quadrant, having a superior relationship to the under surface of the left leaf of the diaphragm and protected anteriorly, laterally, and posteriorly by the lower portion of the rib cage. Its position is maintained by several suspensory ligaments, the major ones being the splenophrenic, splenorenal, splenocolic, and gastrosplenic ligaments (Fig. 33-1). The gastrosplenic ligament normally contains the short gastric vessels, while the remaining ligaments are generally avascular, except in patients with portal hypertension and myeloproliferative disorders. Arterial blood enters the spleen via the splenic artery, a branch of the celiac artery. The major venous drainage courses through the splenic vein, which joins the superior mesenteric vein to form the portal vein.

Accessory spleens have been reported in 14 to 30 percent of patients, with a higher incidence occurring in patients operated on for hematologic disorders. These accessory organs, which receive their vascular supply from the sple-nic artery, are present, in decreasing order of frequency, in the hilus of the spleen, the gastrosplenic and splenocolic ligaments, the gastrocolic ligament, the splenorenal ligament, and the greater omentum (Fig. 33-2). They also may occur in the pelvis of the female, and functioning splenic tissue has been removed from the scrotum in juxtaposition to the left testicle.

The spleen consists of a capsule which is normally 1 to 2 mm thick and trabeculae which enclose the pulp. The pulp, itself, has conventionally been divided into three zones: white, marginal, and red. The white pulp consists of lymphocytes, plasma cells, and macrophages and is analogous to the lymph node, even to the extent that the follicles contain germinal centers. The marginal zone contains elements of blood plasma and also sequestered foreign material. The red pulp is made up of splenic cords and sinuses which interrelate to form a vascular space.

The spleen is the most vascularized organ in the body, and the splenic circulation has been the subject of disagreement for almost 300 years. Three major concepts of splenic circulation have been proposed. The "closed circulation" theory holds that the blood in the spleen follows endo-

Fig. 33-1. Ligaments of the spleen. (*From A. J. Erslev and W. F. Ballinger, II, Splenectomy, Curr Probl Surg, 1965. Copyright 1965, Year Book Medical Publishers, Inc., Chicago. Used by permission.*)

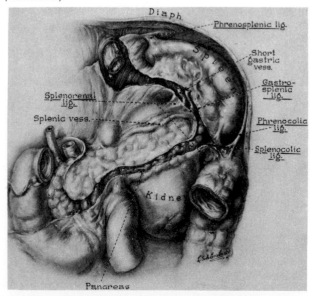

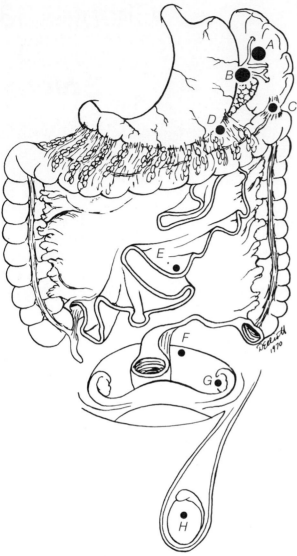

Fig. 33-2. Location of accessory spleens. *A.* Splenic hilus. *B.* Along splenic vessels; tail of pancreas. *C.* Splenocolic ligament. *D.* Greater omentum; perirenal regions. *E.* Mesentery. *F.* Presacral region. *G.* Adnexal region. *H.* Peritesticular region. (*From S. I. Schwartz, J. T. Adams, and A. W. Bauman, Splenectomy for Hematologic Disorders, Curr Probl Surg, May, 1971. Copyright 1971, Year Book Medical Publishers, Inc., Chicago. Used by permission.*)

thelialized pathways throughout. This theory generally has been abandoned because of the proven nature of the sinus walls, which as early as 1686 were shown by Malpighi to contain perforations in the finest ramifications of the intrasplenic veins. The "open circulation" theory, which can be credited to Billroth in 1860, suggests that the arteries empty into tissue spaces or that sheathed capillaries pour their blood directly into pulp cords from which the blood can then pass through sinus wall stomata and enter the veins. The theory of "divided circulation," as proposed by

Knisely, suggests that whole blood enters the sinuses from the afferent capillaries and that deplasmatization occurs through the sinus walls.

Electron microscopic studies have resolved some of the controversy. It has been established that blood which is brought to the spleen via the splenic arteries courses through branches, the trabecular arteries, which leave the trabeculae and enter the white pulp as central arteries (Fig. 33-3). These central arteries give off at right angles many arterioles, some of which terminate in the white pulp. Other branches cross the white pulp and end in the marginal zone or in the red pulp, itself. The branch of the central artery which terminates in the red pulp, known as the "artery of the pulp," breaks up into many arterioles or branches. Within the red pulp, the blood is collected in venous sinuses known as the "splenic sinuses." These large, thin-walled vascular spaces drain into the pulp veins which, in turn, drain into the trabecular veins and then into the main splenic veins to enter the portal circulation. Thus splenic pulp pressure reflects pressure throughout the portal venous system. The tissue between the splenic sinuses is a reticular, connective tissue meshwork which appears as cords on histologic section, hence designated the "splenic cords." Whether the splenic circulation is truly open or closed may not be of great importance with respect to functional capability since, even if the blood flows in a closed system, the presence of many fenestrations in the basement membranes facilitates passage from cord to sinus. Although these fenestrations are of small diameter (0.5 to 5.0 μ), they are traversed by normal red cells, which easily adjust to these dimensions. Under normal conditions, red cells pass from terminal arterioles directly into splenic sinuses (physiologic shunt) as well as from terminal arterioles into pulp cords and into splenic sinuses after traversing the cordal–sinus wall apertures.

PHYSIOLOGY AND PATHOPHYSIOLOGY

Galen is credited with the phrase "The spleen is an organ full of mystery"; to date this mystery has been only minimally unraveled. During the fifth to eighth month of fetal life, the spleen contributes actively to the production of both red cells and white cells which enter the circulation. This function does not continue in the normal adult, and both the qualitative and quantitative effects of splenic extramedullary hematopoeisis seen in myeloproliferative disorders have not been consistent. The role of the spleen in the immunologic processes of the body is discussed in Chap. 10, Transplantation. The splenic function, which is the focus of surgical attention, is determined by the organ's organization as a large mass of reticuloendothelial tissue which contributes to the removal of cellular elements from the circulating blood. Approximately 350 liters of blood pass through the spleen daily, and a variety of transsplenic circulation times have been demonstrated. Normally, cells pass through the spleen rapidly, but in the presence of splenomegaly and other disease states, the flow patterns become circuitous, contain more obstacles, and result in pooling of cells within the cords. Motulsky and associates, using ^{51}Cr studies, have demonstrated that the slow-circulating component may have a half-life of 30 minutes.

Abnormal and aged erythrocytes, abnormal granulocytes, normal and abnormal platelets, and cellular debris may be cleared by the spleen, which apparently is capable of discriminating between these and normal cellular components. In the normal adult, the spleen is the most important site of selective erythrocyte sequestration and, during its 120-day life cycle, the red cell spends an estimated minimum of 2 days within the spleen. The action of the spleen which results in the pathological reduction of circulating cellular elements of blood has been attributed to three possible mechanisms: (1) excessive splenic destruction of cellular elements, (2) splenic production of an antibody which results in the destruction of cells within the circulating blood, and (3) splenic inhibition of the bone marrow causing failure of maturation and cell release. The last proposal is not important in most circumstances. The production of antibodies may be important in certain circumstances, but, as this is not an exclusive function of splenic immunocytes, antibody production would continue in the absence of the spleen. Overactivity of splenic function leading to accelerated removal of any or all of the circulating cellular elements of the blood has been referred to as *hypersplenism*. This condition accounts for most of the splenic removal of apparently normal cells and may result in anemia, leukopenia, or thrombocytopenia, alone or in combination.

The normal adult spleen contains about 25 ml of red blood cells, but relatively few of these are removed during one passage through the organ. The spleen is capable of removing nuclear remnants from circulating erythrocytes (Howell-Jolly bodies) leaving the intact parent erythrocyte and cytoplasmic siderotic granules. The postsplenectomy blood smear may show the presence of circulating erythrocytes with Howell-Jolly bodies and Pappenheimer bodies (siderotic granules which stain with Wright's stain) as a result of the loss of the pitting function of the spleen. In addition, during the course of a day, approximately 20 ml of aged red blood cells are removed.

The alterations in the red cell which makes it sensitive to splenic destruction after 105 to 120 days in circulation have not been established with certainty. It appears that aging changes the biophysical properties of the red cell, making splenic entrapment more likely. In parallel, the enzyme activity and, therefore, the metabolic capacity of the red cell wanes with cell aging. Delay in splenic transit of aged or abnormal cells can lead to further cell injury because of the relatively hypoxic, acidotic, and substrate (glucose)-deprived environment which is present in congested splenic red pulp cords. These environmental conditions lead to further physical and chemical deterioration of the erythrocyte, making it more susceptible to phagocytosis by splenic macrophages and reticuloendothelial cells or to intrasinusoidal disintegration. The central event in cytolysis may be the fall in cellular adenosine triphosphate (ATP) to very low levels and the loss of vital cellular functions dependent on ATP, such as sodium and calcium

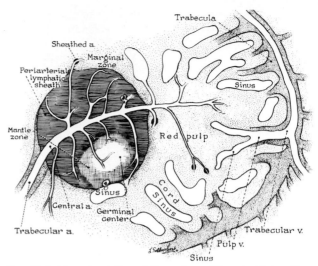

Fig. 33-3. Microcirculation of the spleen. (*From L. Weiss, The Spleen, in R. O. Greep (ed.), "Histology," McGraw-Hill Book Company, New York, 1966.*)

efflux, priming of glycolysis, and maintenance of membrane integrity. To what extent repeated passages through the spleen contribute to normal red cell aging is not certain, but evidence that the red cell loses surface area with aging, combined with the ability of the spleen to remove bits of red cell with surgical precision, raises this possibility. On the other hand, the presence of a normal red cell life span in splenectomized subjects suggests that red cell aging occurs independently of splenic presence and at approximately the normal rate. A variety of erythrocytes altered by intrinsic factors (membrane, hemoglobin, or enzymic abnormalities) or extrinsic factors (antibody and nonantibody injury) may be prematurely removed by the spleen. Severely damaged cells may be removed by the reticuloendothelial system at a variety of sites. Minimally altered erythrocytes may require the specific rigors of the splenic circulation for premature destruction and, therefore, may have normal or near-normal survival after splenic removal. In the dog and cat, unlike man, the spleen may contract significantly in response to hypovolemia or catecholamines, resulting in an autotransfusion; this is an important consideration in studies of experimental shock.

The neutrophil is removed from the circulation with a half-life of about 6.0 hours, hence 85 percent of neutrophils either emigrate at random into tissues or are destroyed within 24 hours. Although the role of the spleen in the destruction of neutrophils under normal conditions is not well quantified, in some hypersplenic states the spleen's role is augmented, with resulting neutropenia. This augmented removal can occur because of splenic enlargement and accelerated sequestration of granulocytes or because of enhanced splenic removal of altered granulocytes, as seen in immune neutropenias.

The platelet (thrombocyte), under normal circumstances, has a finite survival of about 10 days in the circulation. One-third of the total platelet pool is normally sequestered in the spleen, but the role of the spleen in the final removal of normal platelets has not been precisely defined. With splenomegaly, a larger proportion of platelets is sequestered in the spleen (up to 80 percent), and this and accelerated platelet destruction in the spleen account for thrombocytopenia. Splenectomy results in an increase in platelets, which at times reach levels greater than 1 million cells per cubic millimeter. Postsplenectomy thrombocytosis is often transient but may persist. This is particularly notable in congenital hemolytic states which do not respond well to splenectomy. In these circumstances, continued hemolysis in the absence of the splenic removal mechanism can lead to persistent, extreme thrombocytosis and intravenous thrombosis.

DIAGNOSTIC CONSIDERATIONS

EVALUATION OF SIZE. Normally the spleen is not palpable on abdominal examination, but the organ may be felt in about 2 percent of healthy adults. In healthy subjects, no significant dullness is elicited by percussion over the spleen either anteriorly or laterally. As the organ enlarges, dullness may be detected at the level of the ninth intercostal space in the left anterior axillary line especially on expiration. Thereafter, it becomes first percussible and then palpable below the left costal margin. With increasing splenomegaly, notching may be palpable on the anteromedial surface, distinguishing the spleen from other abdominal masses.

Routine radiologic examination of the abdomen usually provides an accurate estimate of the size of the spleen. Although splenomegaly may be suggested by medial or caudad displacement of the stomach bubble, frequently accompanied by caudad displacement of air in the splenic flexure, the organ's outline can often be clearly demarcated in the left upper quadrant, corroborating enlargement. Radioisotopic scanning of the spleen has provided a more precise method of outlining the organ and differentiating it from other masses in the left upper quadrant. The technetium (^{99m}Tc-sulfur colloid) scan (Fig. 33-4) is dependent upon the ability of the spleen to retain the radiocolloid; thus, "functional asplenia," in which vascular shunts allow blood to bypass splenic phagocytes, complicates radioisotopic estimate of splenic size.

EVALUATION OF FUNCTION. The functional abnormality of hypersplenism may be manifested by a reduction in the number of red cells, neutrophils, or platelets in the peripheral blood. An increase in the rate of red cell destruction will always result in a compensatory rise in the rate of production unless disease of the marrow coexists. The hallmark of increased red cell turnover (hemolysis) is reticulocytosis in the absence of blood loss. Other tests such as the plasma bilirubin, haptoglobin, and hemoglobin are less sensitive, dependent on the rate of hemolysis, the sites of hemolysis, and liver function, and are therefore only of adjunctive value.

Reduced red blood cell survival in patients with hemo-

Fig. 33-4. Scan of normal adult human spleen. (*Courtesy of Henry N. Wagner, Jr., M. D.*)

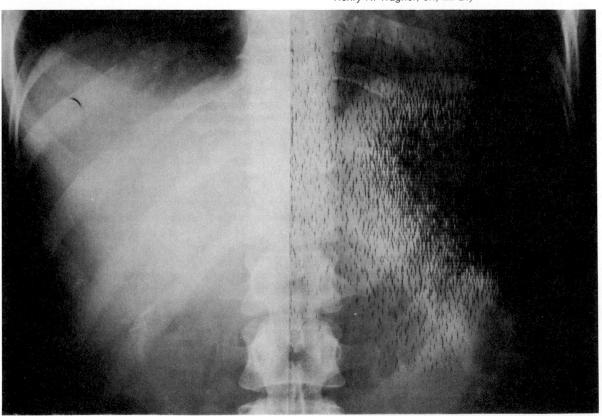

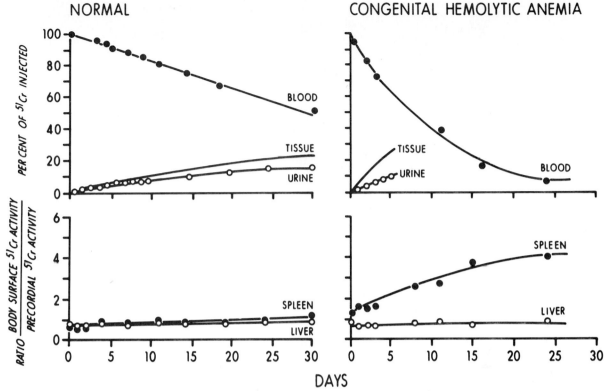

Fig. 33-5. ^{51}Cr-labeled red cell determination of hemolytic anemia and splenic sequestration. Top, disappearance of ^{51}Cr-labeled normal autogenous red cells from the bloodstream and accumulation by the tissues in normal subjects and in patients with hemolytic anemia. Bottom, accumulation of radioactivity in liver and spleen of normal subjects and patients with hemolytic anemia and splenic sequestration. (*After J. Jandl et al., J Clin Invest, 35:842, 1956.*)

lytic anemia may be more precisely demonstrated by measuring the disappearance of blood radioactivity after the patient's erythrocytes are labeled with $Na_2^{51}CrO_4$ (Fig. 33-5). With this technique, the normal half-life of the red cells is about 30 days, i.e., 50 percent of the cells remain in the circulation at that time. A half-life of 15 days or less indicates significantly increased hemolysis. The spleen's role in a hemolytic anemia may be assessed by determining the relative uptakes of ^{51}Cr-tagged erythrocytes by the spleen and the liver. A spleen/liver ratio greater than 2:1 indicates significant preferential splenic sequestration and anticipates a beneficial effect of splenectomy. Radioisotopic labeling also has been used to evaluate the survival of neutrophils and platelets. Presently there is no clinically practical method of assessing the decreased longevity of neutrophils or of measuring the role of the spleen in the destruction of these cells. The role of the spleen as a major offending organ has been precisely defined in patients with hypersplenism or immune thrombocytopenia. Platelet destruction in the spleen is such a common mechanism in thrombocytopenia that radioisotopic studies are not often done if the bone marrow aspirate indicates an abundance of megakaryocytes, suggesting adequate platelet production.

RUPTURE OF THE SPLEEN

The term "rupture" has been applied to splenic injuries in which there is disruption of the organ's parenchyma, capsule, or blood supply.

ETIOLOGY. The causes of splenic rupture include either transabdominal or transthoracic penetrating trauma, nonpenetrating trauma, operative trauma, and spontaneous rupture.

Penetrating Trauma. Rupture of the spleen may occur as a consequence of large gunshot wounds or small puncture lacerations due to stabbing or missiles traveling at high speeds. The trajectory of the penetrating wound may pass through the anterior abdominal wall, through the flank, or transthoracically, piercing the pleural space, the lung, and the diaphragm. Isolated splenic injury may be present. With penetrating trauma, the associated organs most frequently injured include the stomach, the left kidney, the pancreas, and vascular structures at the root of the mesentery. Percutaneous splenic puncture to perform splenic pulp manometry and splenoportography may be associated with persistent bleeding, but this is uncommon in patients whose platelet counts are above 70,000 and prothrombin times are greater than 35 percent.

Nonpenetrating Trauma. The spleen, alone or in combination with other viscera, is the most frequently injured organ following blunt trauma to the abdomen or the lower thoracic cage. Automobile accidents provide the predominating cause, while falls, sledding and bicycle injuries, and blows incurred during contact sports are frequently implicated in children. Splenic rupture which follows blunt trauma is an isolated event in only 30 percent of patients. The other organs which may be injured, in decreasing order of incidence, include (1) chest (rib fracture), (2) kidney, (3) spinal cord (fracture), (4) liver, (5) lung, (6) craniocerebral structures, (7) small intestine, (8) large intestine, (9) pancreas, and (10) stomach.

Operative Trauma. Operative trauma to the spleen most commonly occurs during operations on adjacent viscera. The spleen has been injured in about 2 percent of patients whose operations involved viscera of the left upper quadrant. Injury usually results from retractors placed against the organ in order to obtain exposure. This injury may permit repair or require splenectomy.

Spontaneous Rupture. Although spontaneous rupture of the normal spleen has been reported, it is a much more common event when the spleen is involved with a hematologic disorder. It is likely that the majority of patients classified as experiencing spontaneous rupture had trauma which was not appreciated. Spontaneous rupture or rupture associated with minor trauma is the most common cause of death for patients with infectious mononucleosis, which is second only to malaria as a cause of spontaneous splenic rupture. In patients with infectious mononucleosis, this complication occurs most frequently in the second to fourth weeks of the disease. Splenic rupture has also been reported in patients with sarcoidosis, acute and chronic leukemia, hemolytic anemia, congestive splenomegaly, and polycythemia vera.

Pathology. The spectrum of lesions associated with trauma to the spleen include linear and stellate lacerations, capsular tears secondary to traction from adhesions or suspensory ligaments, puncture wounds caused by penetrating objects or fractured ribs, subcapsular intrasplenic hematomas, avulsion of the organ from its vascular pedicle, and laceration of the short gastric vessels within the gastrosplenic omentum. In view of the extreme friability and vascularity of the organ, even minor trauma may result in significant bleeding, particularly if the spleen is enlarged or diseased.

Splenic rupture may be acute, delayed, or occult. *Acute rupture* which is attended by immediate intraperitoneal bleeding occurs in about 90 percent of the cases of blunt trauma to the spleen. *Delayed rupture,* with an interval of days or weeks between the injury and intraperitoneal bleeding, is reported in 10 to 15 percent of the cases of blunt trauma. The quiescent period, referred to as the "latent period of Baudet," persists for less than 7 days in half of these patients and less than 2 weeks in three-quarters of them. This is probably related to a temporary tamponade of a minor laceration or the presence of a slowly enlarging subcapsular hematoma which eventually ruptures. *Occult splenic rupture* is the term applied to traumatic pseudocysts of the spleen when injury to the organ previously has not been diagnosed. These appear in less than 1 percent of patients sustaining trauma and are generally caused by organization of an intrasplenic or parasplenic hematoma. Another pathologic lesion related to splenic trauma is *splenosis,* which is the result of autotransplantation of fragments of the traumatized spleen onto the peritoneal surfaces. Patients with splenosis are generally asymptomatic, but the lesions may stimulate adhesions which, in turn, lead to intestinal obstruction.

CLINICAL MANIFESTATIONS. The signs and symptoms produced by trauma to the spleen vary according to the severity and rapidity of intraabdominal hemorrhage, the presence of other organ injuries, and the interval between the injury and examination. The majority of patients present with some degree of hypovolemia, and tachycardia is almost always present. The latter is particularly evident when the pulse is recorded with the head of the patient elevated. A slight reduction of the blood pressure is characteristic. The patient usually complains of generalized upper abdominal pain, which in one-third of the cases is localized in the left upper quadrant. Pain at the tip of the shoulder (Kehr's sign) is evidence of diaphragmatic irritation but occurs in less than half the patients. If the patient is placed in the Trendelenburg position, left shoulder pain may be produced to accentuate it. Tenderness of the left upper quadrant or left flank is a frequent physical sign. A mass or a percussible area of fixed dullness in this region (Ballance's sign), secondary to subcapsular hematoma or omentum surrounding an extracapsular hemotoma, is rarely detected.

DIAGNOSTIC STUDIES. The hematocrit may be reduced if there is major bleeding, but the initial determination may be normal, emphasizing the fact that serial hematocrits are more meaningful. Increases of the white blood cell count to levels frequently greater than 15,000 per cubic milliliter are to be anticipated. Routine abdominal roentgenograms may demonstrate fractured ribs which should arouse suspicion of injury to the spleen. More specific findings which may be noted on abdominal films include: (1) elevated immobile left diaphragm, (2) an enlarged splenic shadow, (3) medial displacement of the gastric shadow with serration of the greater curvature due to dissection of blood into the gastrosplenic omentum, and (4) widening of the space between the splenic flexure and the properitoneal fat pad. Abdominal paracentesis yields a positive tap, i.e., return of blood which does not clot, in about 50 percent of the cases. A scan or celiac angiogram may define the lesion. The diagnosis may be established angiographically by visualization of (1) the disruption, (2) radiopacity in the peritoneal cavity, or (3) early filling of the splenic vein.

TREATMENT. Once the diagnosis of splenic rupture has been made, operation should not be delayed. Splenectomy is generally the recommended treatment, but efforts at preserving the spleen in children have become popular. An upper midline incision is generally preferred since this may be performed rapidly and can be extended to manage other intraabdominal injuries. The posterior approach to the splenic pedicle, emphasized by Dunphy, offers the most rapid means of controlling hemorrhage. Manual compression of the pedicle usually controls the bleeding and permits transection of the splenic ligaments and mobilization of the spleen forward and medially. Under adequate exposure lacerations may be sutured over omentum, oxidized cellulose, or micronized collagen. A damaged pole or segment may be excised and the raw edges compressed using sutures tied over the same hemostatic materials. The operative mortality for isolated penetrating injuries of the spleen is less than 1 percent. Operative mortality for blunt trauma to the spleen alone ranges between 5 and 15 percent, while the rates are between 15 and 40 percent when other serious concomitant injuries occur.

HEMATOLOGIC DISORDERS FOR WHICH SPLENECTOMY IS POTENTIALLY THERAPEUTIC

In 1887, Spencer-Wells performed a therapeutic splenectomy in a patient with what subsequently proved to be hereditary spherocytosis. Since then, as a consequence of appreciation of the physiology and pathophysiology of the spleen, the application of splenectomy for hematologic disorders has been extended.

Hemolytic Anemias

This category includes a broad spectrum of disorders in which there is accelerated destruction of mature red blood cells. Hemolytic anemias are generally classified as congenital or acquired. The congenital anemias are due to an intrinsic abnormality of the erythrocytes, and the acquired anemias are related to an extracorpuscular factor acting on an intrinsically normal cell. In both types of disorder, the reduced red blood cell survival may be demonstrated by measuring the disappearance of the patient's radioactive erythrocytes (labeled with ^{51}Cr), and the spleen's role may be evaluated by determining the relative uptakes of this radioactivity by the spleen and liver (Fig. 33-5).

HEREDITARY SPHEROCYTOSIS. Hereditary spherocytosis is transmitted as an autosomal dominant trait and is the most common of the symptomatic familial hemolytic anemias. The fundamental abnormality stems from a defective erythrocyte membrane which causes the cell to be smaller than normal, unusually thick, and almost spherical in shape. These cells also demonstrate increased osmotic fragility, i.e., lysis occurs at a higher concentration of sodium chloride than normal. The role of the spleen in this disorder is related to the inability of the spherocytic cells to pass through the splenic pulp. The cells that escape from the spleen are more susceptible to trapping and disintegration during each successive passage, until cell loss ensues. The precise pathogenesis of the cell injury may relate to a decreased availability of red cell ATP in the environment of the spleen, combined with a cell membrane which has been shown in in vitro studies to be more susceptible to reduction in ATP levels.

The salient clinical features of the disease are anemia, reticulocytosis, jaundice, and splenomegaly. It is unusual for the anemia to be extremely severe, and the jaundice usually parallels the severity of the anemia. Periodic and sudden increases in the intensity of the anemia and jaundice may occur, and rare, fatal crises have been reported. Cholelithiasis with gallstones of the pigmented variety has been reported in 30 to 60 percent of the patients but is rare in children under the age of ten. Leg ulcers, although emphasized in texts, are extraordinarily uncommon.

Diagnosis is generally established by the peripheral blood smear, which demonstrates the spherocytic-shaped erythrocyte with a mean diameter less than normal and a thickness greater than normal. The degree of spherocytosis varies from case to case, but usually more than 60 percent of the red cells demonstrate this characteristic. Increased osmotic fragility of the red blood cells provides diagnostic confirmation, but this test rarely is performed.

Splenectomy is the sole therapy for hereditary spherocytosis. It is generally recommended that the operation be delayed until the fourth year of life. Intractable leg ulcers indicate early splenectomy, as they heal only after the spleen is removed. The results of splenectomy have been uniformly good. Although an inherent membrane abnormality persists and the spherocytosis and increased osmotic fragility of the cells are not altered, in vivo hemolysis virtually ceases and, following removal of the spleen, the erythrocytes achieve a normal life span and the jaundice, if present, disappears. It is appropriate to perform an oral cholecystogram prior to splenectomy, and the gallbladder should always be examined at the time of operation. If gallstones are present, the gallbladder should be removed during the operation.

HEREDITARY ELLIPTOCYTOSIS. This usually exists as a harmless trait, but occasionally, when oval and rod-shaped forms constitute 50 to 90 percent of the red cell population, clinical manifestations indistinguishable from those noted with hereditary spherocytosis may occur. Splenectomy is indicated for all symptomatic patients since removal of the organ often is followed by decreased hemolysis and corrected anemia, although the morphologic abnormality of the red blood cell remains unchanged. Associated cholelithiasis should be managed as in hereditary spherocytosis.

HEREDITARY NONSPHEROCYTIC HEMOLYTIC ANEMIA. Included in this category are: (1) enzyme deficiencies in anaerobic glycolytic pathways, the prototype of which is the pyruvate-kinase deficiency (PK), and (2) enzyme deficiencies in the hexose monophosphate shunt, the prototype of which is the glucose-6-phosphate deficiency (G-6-PD). These deficiencies render the cells susceptible to increased hemolysis. Splenic enlargement occurs more frequently with PK deficiency, and the spleen is rarely enlarged in patients with G-6-PD deficiency. Specific enzyme assays are employed to define the deficiency.

The majority of patients maintain hemoglobins greater than 8 Gm/100 ml, are asymptomatic, and do not require therapy. With significant anemia, blood transfusions are indicated, and the transfused cells survive normally. ^{51}Cr-tagged red cell studies have demonstrated that the spleen serves as a major site for hemolysis in some patients with PK deficiency, and recent reports have suggested limited improvement following removal of the spleen from these patients. Splenectomy is not indicated for patients with G-6-PD deficiency.

THALASSEMIA. Thalassemia (Mediterranean anemia) is transmitted as a dominant trait and primarily derives from a defect in hemoglobin synthesis. The disease is classified as alpha, beta, and gamma types, determined by the specific defect in synthesis rate of the peptide chain. In the United States, most patients are of Southern European origin and suffer from beta thalassemia, i.e., a quantitative reduction in the rate of beta chain synthesis, resulting in a decrease in hemoglobin A (Hb-A). Thalassemia occurs in two major degrees of severity; homozygous thalassemia (thalassemia major), a severe disorder in which the affected child receives a gene for thalassemia from each parent, and heterozygous thalassemia (thalassemia minor), a mild disorder in which the affected child receives a gene from only one parent. Gradations of thalassemia range from heterozygous thalassemia (minor), often not detected until examination of the blood for an unrelated problem, to homozygous thalassemia, a severe, chronic anemia, with icterus, splenomegaly, and death early in life. In thalassemia minor, Hb-A_2 is always increased, and slight increases in Hb-F occur in 50 percent of patients. In both types of thalassemia, the hemoglobin-deficient cells are small, thin, and misshapen. These cells appear washed out and have a characteristic resistance to osmotic lysis.

The clinical manifestations of thalassemia major usually occur in the first year of life and consist of pallor, retarded body growth, and enlargement of the head. Intractable leg ulcers may be noted, intercurrent infections are common, and gallstones are reported in about 24 percent of patients. The manifestations of thalassemia minor may vary. Most patients with thalassemia minor lead normal lives, but some patients have a more severe expression of their disease (referred to as thalassemia intermedia) and generally present with signs and symptoms attributable to mild anemia, chronic mild jaundice, and moderate splenomegaly.

The diagnosis of thalassemia major is established by the smear revealing the hypochromic, microcytic anemia with markedly distorted red cells of various sizes and shapes. Nucleated red cells invariably are present, and the reticulocyte count is elevated, as is the white blood count. The characteristic feature of the disease is the persistence of Hb-F and a reduction in Hb-A, demonstrated by the alkali denaturation study. Importantly, both parents should have evidence of thalassemia minor.

Treatment is directed only at symptomatic patients. Transfusions are usually required at regular intervals, but as most patients accommodate to low hemoglobin levels, the transfusions should be directed at maintaining the hemoglobin level at 10 Gm/100ml. Although splenectomy does not influence the basic hematologic disorder, it may reduce both the hemolytic process and the transfusion requirements.

SICKLE CELL DISEASE. Sickle cell anemia is a hereditary hemolytic anemia seen predominantly in Negroes and characterized by the presence of sickle- and crescent-shaped erythrocytes. In this hereditary hemoglobinopathy, the normal Hb-A is replaced by the abnormal form of hemoglobin, sickle hemoglobin (Hb-S). Hb-F is also usually mildly increased. Combinations of Hb-S with other hemoglobin variants also occur as a result of an abnormal trait inherited from each parent, e.g., Hb-S/Hb-C or Hb-S/thalassemia.

Under conditions of reduced oxygen tension, Hb-S molecules undergo crystallization within the red cell, which elongates and distorts the cell. The sickling phenomenon occurs more readily with higher percentages of Hb-S, with a reduced pH, and under conditions of circulatory stasis which tend to exaggerate hemoglobin deoxygenation. The sickle cells, themselves, contribute to increased blood viscosity and circulatory stasis, thus establishing a vicious cycle. The primary consequence of this stagnation is thrombosis, which leads to ischemia, necrosis, and organ fibrosis.

The role of the spleen in this disorder is not clear. Early in the course of the disease, splenomegaly occurs, but following varying intervals in most patients, the spleen undergoes infarction and marked contraction with eventual autosplenectomy.

Although the sickle cell trait occurs in approximately 9 percent of the Negro population, the majority of patients are asymptomatic. However, sickle cell anemia has been observed in 0.3 to 1.3 percent of Negroes, who often show remarkable adaptation to the state of chronic anemia and jaundice. This adaptive state may be interrupted at intervals by acute symptoms or crises which are related to vascular occlusion. Depending on the vessels involved, the patient may have bone or joint pain, hematuria, priapism, neurologic manifestations, or ulcers over the malleoli. Abdominal pain and cramps due to visceral stasis are frequent, simulating an acute surgical abdomen. Thrombosis of the splenic vessels may result in an unusual complication of splenic abscess, manifested by splenomegaly, splenic pain, and fever. Most patients with sickle cell anemia die in the first decade of life, but a few survive to the fifth decade. Death may be the result of intercurrent infections or cardiac or renal failure.

The diagnosis is established by the presence of anemia, characteristic sickle cells on smear, hemoglobin electrophoresis showing 80 percent or more Hb-S, and the presence of the trait in both parents. Leukocytosis is often noted, and the platelets are frequently increased in number. There may be modest elevation of the serum bilirubin, and cholelithiasis is a frequent accompaniment.

For most patients only palliative treatment is possible. Recently, studies have shown that sodium cyanate will prevent sickling of Hb-S. Transfusions may be required to maintain adequate hemoglobin levels. Adequate hydration and partial exchange transfusion may help during a crisis. In the circumstance of splenic abscess, incision and drainage of the abscess cavity within the parenchyma of the spleen may be necessitated, since removal of the organ is hindered by marked inflammatory and adhesive processes. Splenectomy may be of benefit in a very few patients in whom excessive splenic sequestration of red cells can be demonstrated, although the operation does not affect sickling process. In general, splenectomy is most effective in children with large spleens but is not indicated for the trait.

IDIOPATHIC AUTOIMMUNE HEMOLYTIC ANEMIA. This is a disorder in which the life span of a presumably normal erythrocyte is shortened when exposed to an endogenous hemolytic mechanism. The etiology has not been defined, but an autoimmune process appears to be fundamental. In such patients, antibodies reacting with the patient's normal red cells have been defined, and there is evidence that the spleen may serve as a source of antibody. Both "warm" and "cold" antibodies have been described. Some "warm" antibodies have Rh specificity. Since most of these antibodies are hemagglutinins rather than hemolysins, the means by which hemolysis is initiated in vivo is not clear, but it is believed that the reticuloendothelial system traps and destroys the immunologically altered cells. Sequestration studies have demonstrated that this process sometimes occurs primarily in the spleen.

Although autoimmune hemolytic anemia may be encountered at any age, it occurs more frequently after the age of fifty and twice as often in females. Mild jaundice is often present. The spleen is palpably enlarged in half the cases, and gallstones have been demonstrated in a quarter of the cases. The extent of anemia varies, and hemoglobinuria and tubular necrosis have been reported in severe cases. In this circumstance, the prognosis is serious, as the mortality rate is 40 to 50 percent.

The diagnosis of hemolysis is made by demonstrating anemia and reticulocytosis accompanied by the products of red cell destruction in the blood, urine, and stool. The bone marrow is hypercellular with a predominance of erythroid precursors. A distinguishing feature of the disease is the demonstration by direct Coombs' test of an autoantibody on the patient's red cells.

In some patients, the disorder tends to run an acute, self-limiting course, and no treatment is necessary. If the anemia becomes severe, corticosteroids or blood transfusions may be required. Splenectomy should be considered in the following circumstances: (1) if steroids have been ineffective, (2) if excessive doses of steroids are required to maintain remission, (3) if toxic manifestations of steroids become apparent, and (4) if steroids are contraindicated for other reasons. Excessive splenic sequestration of ^{51}Cr-tagged red cells offers a guide for the selection of patients who may respond to splenectomy. A favorable response is to be anticipated in about 80 percent of selected splenectomized patients, with either complete hematologic remission or a significant decrease in the rate of hemolysis and alleviation of anemia.

Idiopathic Thrombocytopenic Purpura

Idiopathic thrombocytopenic purpura (immune thrombocytopenic purpura) (ITP) has no established etiology. Many cases are felt to represent the results of autoimmunity. The term ITP should be reserved for a hemorrhagic disorder characterized by a subnormal platelet count in the presence of bone marrow containing normal or increased megakaryocytes and in the absence of any systemic disease or history of ingestion of drugs capable of inducing thrombocytopenia. The spleen may be implicated either as a source of antibody production or as the major sequestering site for sensitized platelets.

Female patients outnumber males at a ratio of 3:1. The most common presenting signs are petechiae and/or ecchymoses. In the majority of patients, these signs are accompanied by one or several other symptoms which in order of frequency are: bleeding gums, vaginal bleeding, gastrointestinal bleeding, and hematuria. In some patients,

the clinical manifestations take an almost cyclic course with exacerbations occurring at the time of menses. The incidence of central nervous system bleeding ranges between 2 and 4 percent and usually occurs early in the course of the disease. The spleen is palpable in approximately 2 percent of cases, and its enlargement should evoke suspicion of the presence of another disease causing thrombocytopenia.

The characteristic laboratory findings include a platelet count generally reduced to 50,000 or less and at times approaching zero. Associated with reduced platelet count, the bleeding time may be prolonged, but the clotting time remains normal. There is usually no significant anemia or leukopenia. Platelet survival following the transfusion of ^{51}Cr-labeled normal platelets is short, but this test is not necessary for establishing the diagnosis of ITP. Bone marrow examination reveals megakaryocytes either normal or increased in number, with or without a relative increase in small forms. Qualitative changes in the megakaryocytes are characterized by degranulation of the cytoplasm, rounding of cytoplasmic edges, the disappearance of the usual pseudopodia containing granular-free platelets, and a varying degree of vacuolization of the cytoplasm.

Acute ITP has an excellent prognosis in children under the age of 16; approximately 80 percent of these patients will make a complete and permanent recovery without specific therapy. Much of the discussion regarding therapy for ITP centers around the relative values and disadvantages of steroid therapy and splenectomy. In 1916, Kaznelson, then a fourth-year medical student in Prague, suggested that splenectomy could induce an increase in circulating platelets and reported good results following splenectomy performed by Schloffer. The advent of steroid therapy provided the impetus for reevaluating the efficacy of splenectomy. In most series, the results achieved by splenectomy are significantly more impressive than are the responses to steroids (Fig. 33-6). Between 75 and 85 per-

Fig. 33-6. Idiopathic thrombocytopenic purpura. Comparative responses to steroids and splenectomy. (*From S. I. Schwartz, J. T. Adams, and A. W. Bauman, Splenectomy for Hematologic Disorders, Curr Probl Surg, May, 1971. Copyright 1971, Year Book Medical Publishers, Inc., Chicago. Used by permission.*)

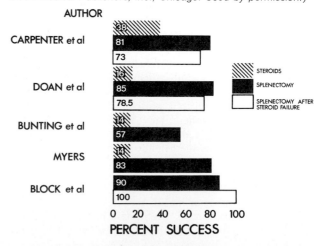

cent of the total number of patients subjected to splenectomy respond permanently and require no further steroid therapy. A long-term follow-up of splenectomized patients does not support the contention that disseminated lupus erythematosus develops after this procedure. Reported series disagree regarding a correlation between response to steroids and splenectomy.

At present, the generally accepted protocol for managing patients with diagnosed ITP includes an initial 6-week to 2-month period of steroid therapy. If the patient does not respond with elevation of the platelet count, splenectomy is performed. If the patient does respond, the steroid therapy is tapered off, and, if thrombocytopenia recurs, splenectomy is carried out. Any manifestation suggestive of intracranial bleeding demands emergency splenectomy.

The majority of patients are seen by the surgeon after they have been taking steroids for weeks or months. Consequently, these patients require a booster dose of cortisone acetate during the evening prior to the splenectomy and intravenous cortisone during the surgical procedure. For patients with platelet counts approaching zero, platelet packs should be available for the operative procedure but should not be administered preoperatively. Platelet transfusion is reserved for patients who continue bleeding following removal of the spleen. Occasional patients in whom signs of the disease recurred months or years following splenectomy achieved permanent cure following removal of an accessory spleen, the presence of which may be defined by technetium scan.

Thrombotic Thrombocytopenic Purpura

Although thrombotic thrombocytopenic purpura (TTP) is a disease of arterioles or capillaries, there are significant accompanying hematologic changes for which the response to splenectomy may be striking. The etiology has not been precisely defined, but immune mechanisms have been suggested. Approximately 5 percent of reported cases occurred during pregnancy. TTP in pregnancy must be distinguished from an idiopathic thrombocytopenia which may develop in the third trimester and is reversed by termination of the pregnancy. Histologically, there is widespread occlusion of multiple arterioles and capillaries by hyaline membranes, with minimal inflammatory change and limited infarction.

The pentad of clinical features of virtually all cases consists of fever, purpura, hemolytic anemia, neurologic manifestations, and signs of renal disease. The pertinent laboratory findings include anemia with reticulocytosis, thrombocytopenia, and leukocytosis, at times accompanied by elevated serum bilirubin, proteinuria, hematuria, casts, or azotemia. The peripheral blood smear reveals pleomorphic, normochromic red cells that are fragmented and distorted. The degree of thrombocytopenia varies during the course of the illness, but a profound decrease often develops within hours of onset. The bone marrow usually reveals erythroid and myeloid hyperplasia with a normal or increased number of megakaryocytes.

In the majority of cases, the disease has a rapid onset, fulminating course, and fatal outcome usually due to intracerebral hemorrhage or renal failure. Recovery has been reported for patients treated with heparin, exchange transfusion of fresh blood, dextran, antimetabolites, and massive doses of steroids. However, the combination of steroid therapy and splenectomy has achieved the highest degree of success. Of approximately 350 cases reported, 44 patients were alive at the time of reporting, and 65 percent of the survivals had been treated with steroid therapy and splenectomy.

Primary Hypersplenism

In 1939, Doan and Wiseman described a disease consisting primarily of splenomegaly and neutropenia for which splenectomy is curative. A few years later, the concept of splenic neutropenia was enlarged to include some patients with anemia, thrombocytopenia, or pancytopenia. The etiology has not been determined, but ^{51}Cr-tagged red cell sequestration studies indicate that the spleen is a major site of phagocytosis. In some patients, lymphoproliferation of the spleen is so marked as to suggest the development of premalignant lymphoma. The spleen is almost always enlarged and the histologic features vary.

The overwhelming majority of patients are female, and the clinical manifestations are related to the depressed cell type. Fever, frequent and recurring infections, and oral ulcerations may be noted with neutropenia. Petechiae and ecchymoses predominate with thrombocytopenia, and pallor may indicate depression of the red cells. The peripheral blood smear is devoid of any of the diagnostic features of leukemia or myeloproliferative disorders. The bone marrow reveals a pancellular hyperplasia. The diagnosis is essentially one of exclusion, confirmed by clinical response to splenectomy.

Corticosteroids rarely affect the disease process, but splenectomy facilitates hematologic improvement in almost all patients. Disturbingly, occasional patients followed for long periods of time have subsequently developed reticulum cell sarcoma or histiocytic lymphoma.

Secondary Hypersplenism

Pancytopenia, thrombocytopenia, and leukopenia or anemia may stem from portal hypertension due either to hepatic disease or extrahepatic portal vein obstruction. Splenomegaly with engorgement of the vascular spaces accompanies portal hypertension, and accelerated destruction of the circulating cells within the spleen results. The clinical manifestations of thrombocytopenia, i.e., petechiae and spontaneous bleeding, are extremely uncommon in patients with portal hypertension. As no correlation exists between the degree of anemia, leukopenia, or thrombocytopenia and the long-term survival of patients with cirrhosis, hypersplenism per se rarely indicates operative intervention in a patient with portal hypertension. Percutaneous transfemoral arterial embolization has been performed in some of these patients. Although splenic hyperfunction was controlled, the development of painful infarction of the spleen and septic splenitis suggests that such an approach has limited value. The more common surgical situation relates to the patient with bleeding esophagogastric varices accompanied by significant secondary thrombocytopenia. In the experience of Child and Turcotte with more than 300 shunts, it was necessary to perform only one splenectomy for persistent, clinically significant hypersplenism. Thrombocytopenia is generally improved by a portacaval shunt, and, in the few instances in which the platelet count does not return to normal, complications are rarely attributable to thrombocytopenia. Splenectomy alone should not be performed in a patient with portal hypertension and secondary hypersplenism as there is no long-term effect on the elevated portal pressure. In the rare circumstance that splenectomy is required for a severe degree of hypersplenism in such a patient, it should be combined with a splenorenal shunt to decompress the portal circulation.

Myeloid Metaplasia

Myeloid metaplasia is a panproliferative process manifested by increased connective tissue proliferation of the bone marrow, liver, spleen, and lymph nodes and simultaneous proliferation of hemopoietic elements in the liver, spleen, and long bones. The disease is closely related to polycythemia vera, myelogenous leukemia, and idiopathic thrombocytosis. The etiology remains unclear. The spleen may be markedly enlarged, and portal hypertension has been described in some patients, due either to hepatic fibrosis of sufficient degree to be obstructive to the portal circulation or to increased forward blood flow through the splenoportal system in the absence of hepatic involvement.

Clinical manifestations generally become apparent in middle-aged and older adults. The presenting symptoms usually are related to anemia and increasing splenomegaly. Symptoms related to the spleen include the intermittent pain of splenic infarction, generalized abdominal discomfort, and a feeling of fullness after meals. Other symptoms include spontaneous bleeding, secondary infection, bone pain, pruritus, hypermetabolism, and complications associated with hyperuricemia. The most common physical findings are pallor and splenomegaly. Hepatomegaly is present in about three-quarters of the patients.

The laboratory hallmark of myeloid metaplasia is the peripheral blood smear. The red cells are characterized by fragmentation and immature forms and poikilocytosis with numerous teardrop and elongated shapes. Characteristically, the patients have anemia of the normochromic type. The white blood count is under 50,000 in the majority of the cases but may reach extremely high levels. Immature myeloid cells are found in the peripheral smear. The platelet counts are normal in about a quarter of the patients, thrombocytopenia is present in about one-third, and marked thrombocytopenia is present in 5 percent. Thrombocytosis over 1 million per cubic millimeter is observed in one-quarter of the patients. The platelets frequently are enlarged and bizarre in appearance. The leukocyte alkaline phosphatase usually is high, and hyperuricemia frequently is present. Roentgenograms of the bone demonstrate increased density in approximately 50 percent of the patients, particularly in the pelvic region. Marrow biopsy sections show varying degrees of bone marrow replacement by fibrous tissue interposed with small foci of megakaryocytes, erythropoiesis, and myeloid cells. ^{51}Cr-tagged red cell scan may be used to indicate the degree of splenic sequestration and to evaluate the applicability of splenectomy.

Treatment is generally directed at the anemia and splenomegaly. It usually consists of transfusions, hormones, chemotherapy, and radiotherapy. Male hormone preparations may be of value in patients with anemia due to marrow failure. Alkalating agents may be effective in reducing splenic size and transfusion requirements as well as for patients whose predominant clinical problem is hypermetabolism. Busulfan is the most commonly used alkalating agent, but cyclophosphamide may also be used in thrombocytopenic subjects since it is less likely to suppress platelet production. Since patients with myelofibrosis are very sensitive to chemotherapy, such agents must be used very cautiously.

Although splenectomy does not alter the general course of the disorder, the procedure is indicated for control of anemia, thrombocytopenia, and for symptoms attributable to splenomegaly. Thrombocytopenia associated with sufficiently reduced megakaryocytes to contraindicate chemotherapy is also a frequent indication for splenectomy, as is the large spleen which causes digestive difficulties or is symptomatic because of multiple infarctions despite chemotherapy and/or local irradiation. In patients with esophagogastric varices portal pressures should be determined before and after splenectomy. In most instances splenectomy alone will effect significant reduction in pressure and obviate the need for a concomitant splenorenal or portacaval shunt.

Splenectomy rarely has a deleterious effect on the hematologic status of the patient, and the old concept that splenectomy resulted in the removal of a significant hemopoietic element does not pertain. The incidence of the mortality and morbidity rates for patients with myeloid metaplasia undergoing splenectomy are higher than those reported for other hematologic disorders. Postoperative thrombocytosis and/or thrombosis of the splenic vein extending into the portal and mesenteric vein occur more commonly in these patients. The incidence of this complication can be reduced by correction of the thrombotic state preoperatively using alkylating agents and the use of drugs to prevent platelet aggregation during the perioperative period.

Hodgkin's Disease, Lymphoma, Reticulum Cell Sarcoma, and Chronic Leukemia

Splenectomy for patients with these disorders has been recently brought into focus for two reasons: first, the need for a more aggressive therapeutic approach in patients with advanced disease and hypersplenism, and, second, the introduction of laparotomy, including splenectomy, as a method of staging Hodgkin's disease in order to determine appropriate therapy.

PALLIATIVE SPLENECTOMY. Chemotherapy and/or radiation therapy are the major approaches to the treatment of these disorders. Splenectomy may be considered for patients with symptomatic splenomegaly and/or hypersplenism. Many of the older series report extremely high mortality rates, but review of these cases indicates that the patients were in a terminal phase. Recent series have reported more favorable results, with improvement in hematologic pattern although the eventual outcome of the primary disease was in no way altered. Crosby and associates suggested that splenectomy should be performed at the first sign of hypersplenism with Hodgkin's disease, before the patient becomes a hematologic cripple.

The results associated with palliative splenectomy for patients with lymphoma and chronic lymphatic leukemia who have symptomatic hypersplenism and/or splenomegaly uniformly are more encouraging. The hematologic responses are favorable in the majority of patients, and many have long periods of survival.

A favorable hematologic response has been reported for about half the patients with chronic myelogenous leukemia, while the results for patients with reticulum cell sarcoma generally are poor.

SPLENECTOMY IN THE STAGING OF HODGKIN'S DISEASE AND NON-HODGKIN'S LYMPHOMA. The diagnosis of Hodgkin's disease is generally established by histologic evaluation of a clinically suspect area of lymphadenopathy or splenomegaly. Demonstration of the typical, large, multinuclear cell, the Sternberg-Reed cell, is regarded as essential for the diagnosis. However, these cells do not form the bulk of the tumor. Four major histologic types have been defined: lymphocyte predominance, nodular sclerosis, mixed cellularity, and lymphocyte depletion. Survival with Hodgkin's disease is related in part to the histologic type and also to the distribution of disease and the presence or absence of specific symptoms. Stage I disease is defined as limited to one anatomic region; Stage II disease is limited to two or more contiguous or noncontiguous regions on the same side of the diaphragm; Stage III disease refers to disease on both sides of the diaphragm with involvement limited to lymph nodes, spleen, and Waldeyer's ring; and Stage IV refers to involvement of the bone marrow, lung, liver, skin, gastrointestinal tract, and any organ or tissue other than the lymph nodes or Waldeyer's ring.

The application of laparotomy, splenectomy, liver biopsy, and retroperitoneal node biopsy as diagnostic tools is based on the following considerations: (1) the lesion generally begins as a single focus and spreads in a predictable manner along adjacent lymph channels, (2) prognosis is related to clinical stage, (3) therapy may be dictated by clinical stage, and (4) previous methods of evaluating the clinical stage, including the physical examination, laboratory studies, and roentgenographic studies have significant degrees of inaccuracy. The procedure begins with a wedge biopsy of the liver performed before retractors are applied to avoid confusion of white cell migration. Splenectomy is then performed, the entire periaortic chain of lymph nodes is examined, and representative nodes are removed. The sites of lymph node removal are chosen according to preoperative lymphangiogram and surgical evaluation. Examination of the upper aortic chain, facilitated by transecting the ligament of Treitz, has proved most rewarding in regard to positive lymph node findings. Representative mesenteric and hepatoduodenal nodes should also be biopsied. A liberal iliac crest marrow biopsy is generally included.

The concept of surgical staging as a routine procedure for untreated patients with Hodgkin's disease was initiated at Stanford University Medical Center in July of 1968. A collation of reported series is presented in Fig. 33-7. The error for patients with preoperative diagnoses of splenic involvement based on palpability, roentgenographic, and/or scintillation scan studies which suggested enlargement was 38 percent, while the error for patients with preoperative diagnoses of normal spleens was 36 percent. The liver is suspected of being infiltrated by Hodgkin's disease if there is evidence of hepatomegaly, if liver function tests demonstrate abnormalities, or if liver scans define a space-occupying lesion. Preoperative suspicion of Hodgkin's disease of the liver was incorrect in 45 percent of the cases, whereas clinical judgment that the liver was not involved was incorrect in only 4 percent. Abdominal lymphangiography has been shown to be superior to both inferior vena cavography and intravenous pyelography for defining retroperitoneal node involvement. Thirty percent of positive lymphangiograms were not confirmed by laparotomy, while 15 percent of patients whose lymphangiograms were considered normal were shown to have Hodgkin's involvement of the retroperitoneal nodes. Summary of the reported cases indicates that surgical staging upgraded the clinical stage in about 27 percent of cases and decreased it in 15 percent, for a total alteration of 42 percent.

The applicability of surgical staging in patients with Hodgkin's disease has not been resolved. It is generally agreed that the procedure is indicated for a patient with Hodgkin's disease who presents evidence or suggestion of disease in the upper part of the abdomen, providing that the patient is not jaundiced and does not have other evidence of significant hepatic dysfunction. Other generally accepted indications include the presence of systemic symptoms in clinical Stage I and II patients, and a mixed cellularity or lymphocyte depletion type of histology. By

Fig. 33-7. Correlation between operative staging and clinical assessment. (*From S. I. Schwartz and R. A. Cooper, Jr., Surgery in the Diagnosis and Treatment of Hodgkin's Disease, Adv Surg, vol 6. Copyright 1972, Year Book Medical Publishers, Inc., Chicago. Used by permission.*)

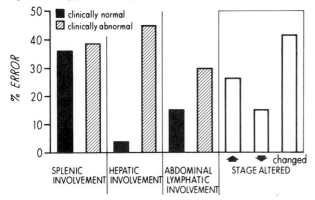

contrast, in patients with high cervical, lymphocyte-predominant lesions and no evidence of mediastinal involvement, staging is not indicated, since these lesions rarely involve the subdiaphragmatic nodes.

The argument regarding the role of staging centers around patients with clinical Stage I-A or II-A (asymptomatic). Those in favor base their opinion on negligible mortality and morbidity rates coupled with the additional "bonus" that splenectomy has facilitated radiation therapy and reduced the potential radiation pneumonitis and/or nephritis as well as leukopenia and thrombocytopenia which may complicate either radiotherapy or chemotherapy. The objections to routine staging in these patients relate to the facts that (1) some series do include perioperative deaths, and (2) the problem of susceptibility to infection subsequent to splenectomy has not been resolved. It has also been pointed out that ablation of the spleen can be accomplished by radiation therapy; many therapists advocate prophylactically treating all infradiaphragmatic areas in patients with Stage I and II Hodgkin's disease.

In reference to the routine staging for non-Hodgkin's lymphoma, a difference of opinion also pertains. Veronesi and associates conclude that diagnostic laparotomy and staging should be carried out in centers in which the information can be translated into aggressive treatment, but feel that it should not have the wide adoption which Hodgkin's staging has had. Chabner et al. reported that percutaneous and peritoneoscopically directed biopsies were reasonable alternatives to staging for non-Hodgkin's lymphoma and that the presence or absence of subdiaphragmatic disease could be established in over 80 percent of the patients by nonsurgical procedures, including lymphangiography, marrow biopsy, and percutaneous liver biopsy. The yield of staging procedures was highest in patients with nodular lymphomas and lowest in patients with histiocytic lymphomas.

Miscellaneous Diseases

FELTY'S SYNDROME. The triad of rheumatoid arthritis, splenomegaly, and neutropenia is referred to as Felty's syndrome. Mild anemia and/or thrombocytopenia have been noted in some cases, and gastric achlorhydria is common. An antibody specifically directed against neutrophil nuclei is nearly always demonstrable by fluorescent stains. Corticosteroids and splenectomy have been used to reverse the neutropenia in order to reduce susceptibility to infection. The response to steroids is usually not long-lasting, but the hematologic effects of splenectomy generally are excellent. There is a sharp rise in the total number of leukocytes in the first 24 hours, reaching a peak at about the third postoperative day. Although relative neutropenia may persist, the neutrophilic response to infection in the postsplenectomy state becomes normal. However, the clinical course of the arthritis is rarely altered.

SARCOIDOSIS. This disease affects young adults. There are few constitutional symptoms, and fever is unusual, although night sweats have been noted. Cough and shortness of breath may attend mediastinal or pulmonary involvement. Skin lesions appear in about 50 percent of

patients, and generalized lymphadenopathy is frequent. Involvement of the liver and spleen may produce hepatomegaly and splenomegaly in about 25 percent of the cases. About 20 percent of the patients with splenomegaly develop manifestations of hypersplenism, particularly thrombocytopenic purpura. Hemolytic anemia, neutropenia, pancytopenia, and spontaneous splenic rupture have all been observed.

There is no specific treatment, and spontaneous recovery can be anticipated in the majority of cases. Splenectomy should be considered for patients with splenomegaly when there are complications of hypersplenism, since the operation has been almost uniformly followed by correction of the hematologic abnormality.

GAUCHER'S DISEASE. This is a familial disorder characterized by abnormal storage or retention of glycolipid cerebrosides in reticuloendothelial cells. Proliferation and enlargement of these cells produces enlargement of the spleen, liver, and lymph nodes. The disease is generally discovered in childhood, but may become evident either early in infancy or late in adult life.

The sole clinical manifestation may be awareness of a progressively enlarging abdominal mass, primarily due to splenomegaly and, to a lesser extent, to hepatomegaly. The yellowish-brown pigmentation of the head and extremities occurs in about 45 to 75 percent of cases. Bone pain and pathologic fracture may develop in long-standing cases. Many patients develop the hematologic manifestations of hypersplenism as a result of excessive sequestration of formed blood elements. Moderate to severe thrombocytopenia and normocytic anemia are almost always present, and often there is mild leukopenia. In the patients with hypersplenism, splenectomy almost uniformly has been beneficial in correcting the hematologic disorder, but there is no evidence that the operation influences the course of the basic disease.

FANCONI SYNDROME (ANEMIA). This rare, hereditary condition is characterized by pancytopenia, bone marrow hypoplasia, and a variety of developmental abnormalities and is somewhat more common in males than in females. Anemia, often severe, is the most prominent of the hematologic abnormalities. Mild or moderate leukopenia and thrombocytopenia occur. The bone marrow is usually hypocellular and fatty but occasionally may be normal and even hypercellular.

Most patients die early in life. Splenectomy has been performed in a few patients with severe anemia and increasing transfusion requirements, but the results have been inconsistent.

PORPHYRIA ERYTHROPOIETICA. This is a congenital disorder of erythrocyte pyrrole metabolism which is transmitted as a recessive trait and characterized by the excessive deposition of porphyrins in the tissues. In the skin this results in pronounced photosensitization and severe bullous dermatitis. Premature red cell destruction within the spleen contributes to severe anemia. When the disease is complicated by hemolysis or splenomegaly, splenectomy is followed by marked improvement in the anemia and decreased concentrations of porphyrins in the red cells, bone marrow, and urine.

MISCELLANEOUS LESIONS

ECTOPIC SPLEEN. This unusual condition is ascribed to lengthening of the splenic ligaments which results in extreme mobility of the organ so that the spleen of normal size may be palpable in the lower abdomen or in the pelvis. In some cases, acute torsion of the pedicle occurs, necessitating surgical intervention.

SPLENIC ARTERY ANEURYSM. The splenic artery is the most common site of intraabdominal aneurysm other than the aorta. The incidence of splenic artery aneurysm ranges between 0.02 and 0.16 percent in autopsy series. The lesions occur more frequently in females, and the most common predisposing factor is atherosclerosis. Splenic artery aneurysms are usually discovered as incidental findings on an abdominal x-ray, and a bruit is rarely heard in the left upper quadrant. The frequency of rupture ranges between less than 10 percent to 46 percent, with about 20 percent of ruptures having occurred during pregnancy. Excision of the aneurysm, with or without splenectomy, is recommended for enlarging or symptomatic aneurysms, and in women in the child-bearing age. In many asymptomatic patients close observation is justified.

CYSTS AND TUMORS. Cysts of the spleen are unusual. Parasitic cysts are usually due to echinococcal involvement, while the nonparasitic cysts may be categorized as dermoid, epidermoid, epithelial, and pseudocysts. Pseudocysts occur after occult rupture of the spleen.

Primary and malignant tumors of the spleen are sarcomatous. Recent autopsy series have refuted the concept that metastases to the spleen are rare. However, laparotomy for undiagnosed splenomegaly which reveals unsuspected metastatic deposit in the absence of known generalized metastases is extremely uncommon.

ABSCESSES. Splenic abscess is an uncommon cause of abdominal sepsis. Primary splenic abscesses occur much more often in the Tropics, where they are frequently related to thrombosis of the splenic vessels with infarction in patients with sickle cell anemia. Clinical manifestations include fever, chills, splenomegaly, and left upper quadrant tenderness. Diagnosis may be established by scan or angiography. Removal of the spleen is the operation of choice, but some cases have been treated with splenotomy and drainage when there were gross adhesions or the condition of the patient did not permit splenectomy.

SPLENECTOMY

The operation for splenic rupture frequently requires the administration of whole blood. When elective splenectomy is performed for hematologic disorders, other specific considerations arise. Patients with malignant lymphoma and leukemia may develop cryoglobulinemia and, therefore, the blood should be administered at room temperature. For patients with thalassemia and, more particularly, acquired hemolytic anemia, typing and cross matching may be difficult, and sufficient time should be allotted during the preoperative period to accumulate the blood that may be required during the operation. For patients with marked immune thrombocytopenia (ITP), platelet packs are not usually administered preoperatively since the platelets are rapidly destroyed by the spleen and, therefore, not very effective.

TECHNIQUE. Although the midline incision is generally employed for a ruptured spleen, the left subcostal incision is preferred for elective resection. The spleen is mobilized initially by dividing the ligamentous attachments, which are usually avascular but may contain large vessels in patients with secondary hypersplenism and myeloid metaplasia. The short gastric vessels then are doubly ligated and transected, taking care not to traumatize the stomach itself. If compromise of blood supply to the fundic portion of the greater curvature of the stomach is a concern, enfolding of this area should be performed to prevent the development of a gastric fistula. This permits ultimate dissection of the splenic hilus with individual ligation and division of the splenic artery and vein. During the course of hilar dissection, care should be taken to avoid injury to the tail of the pancreas in order to obviate pseudocyst formation. The technique of initial ligation of the splenic artery by exposure through the gastrosplenic omentum is applicable to the small spleen but not appropriate when there is marked splenomegaly or when large lymphomatous lymph nodes encircle the splenic vessels. Whenever splenectomy is performed for hematologic disorder, a careful search should be made for accessory spleens. The splenic bed is not drained routinely, but drains are used in patients with myeloid metaplasia.

POSTOPERATIVE COURSE AND COMPLICATIONS. Following splenectomy, characteristic changes in blood composition occur. Howell-Jolly bodies are present in almost all patients, and siderocytes are common. Generally, leukocytosis and increased platelet counts are observed. In patients with marked thrombocytopenia, the platelet count often returns to normal within two days, but peak levels may not be reached for two weeks. The white blood cell count usually is elevated the first day and may remain persistently elevated for several months. The most frequent complication is that of left lower lobe atelectasis. Other complications include subphrenic hematoma and abscess, injury to the pancreas causing fistula, or pancreatitis. Excessively elevated platelet counts, particularly in patients with myeloid metaplasia, and increased platelet adhesiveness have been reported. Although these factors have been implicated in the greater incidence of thrombophlebitis following splenectomy, many series can show no good correlation between these complications and the platelet counts.

There has been increasing concern regarding infection and sepsis in splenectomized patients. In a large review Singer reported that deaths from sepsis in splenectomized patients were 200 times as prevalent as in the population at large. Eraklis and Filler felt that overwhelming infection in splenectomized patients was mainly related to the primary disease and that the higher risk of sepsis occurred in patients with thallasemia, malignancies, and aplastic anemia. When the risk of infection in childhood Hodgkin's disease was assessed in 181 consecutive, previously untreated patients, the episode did not correlate with splenectomy alone, but appeared to be related more to the treatment with chemotherapy and radiotherapy.

It has been shown that splenectomy results in a variety of immunologic defects, including a poor response to intravenous immunization with particulate antigens, a deficiency in phagocytosis-promoting peptide, decreased serum Igm, and decreased properdin. The organisms most frequently isolated from septic splenectomized children are those of diplococcus pneumonia and H-influenza. It is therefore reasonable to delay splenectomy for hematologic disorders in very young children, especially those under the age of two years, to attempt to preserve the traumatized spleen in the pediatric patient and to maintain patients with "at-risk" diseases on long-term oral antibiotic therapy.

References

General

Schwartz, S. I., Adams, J. T., and Bauman, A. W.: Splenectomy for Hematologic Disorders, *Curr Probl Surg,* May, 1971.

Anatomy

Burke, J. A., and Simon, G. T.: Electron Microscopy of the Spleen. I. Anatomy and Microcirculation. II. Phagocytosis of Colloidal Carbon, *Am J Pathol,* **58:**127, 1970.

Knisely, M. H.: Spleen Studies: I. Microscopic Observations of the Circulatory System of Living Unstimulated Mammalian Spleens, *Anat Rec,* **65:**23, 1936.

Weiss, L.: The Structure of Intermediate Vascular Pathways in the Spleen of Rabbits, *Am J Anat,* **113:**51, 1963.

Wennberg, E., and Weiss, L.: The Structure of the Spleen and Hemolysis, *Ann Rev Med,* **20:**29, 1969.

Physiology and Pathophysiology

Doan, C. A.: The Spleen: Its Structure and Functions, *Postgrad Med,* **43:**126, 1968.

Harris, J. W.: "The Red Cell: Production, Metabolism, Destruction, Normal and Abnormal," Harvard University Press, Cambridge, Mass., 1963. (Published for the Commonwealth Fund.)

Motulsky, A. G., Casserd, F., Giblett, E. R., Broun, G. O., and Finch, C. A.: Anemia and the Spleen, *N Engl J Med,* **259:**1164 and 1215, 1958.

Diagnostic Considerations

Jandl, J. H., Greenberg, M. S., Yonemoto, R. H., and Castle, W. B.: Clinical Determination of the Sites of Red Cell Sequestration in Hemolytic Anemias, *J Clin Invest,* **41:**1628, 1962.

Samuels, L. D., and Stewart, C.: Estimation of Spleen Size in Sickle Cell Anemia, *J Nucl Med,* **11:**12, 1970.

Wagner, H. N., Jr., McAfee, J. G., and Winkelman, J. W.: Splenic Disease Diagnosis by Radioisotope Scanning, *Arch Intern Med,* **109:**673, 1962.

Rupture of the Spleen

Ayala, L. A., Williams, L. F., Widrich, W. C.: Occult Rupture of Spleen: Chronic Form of Splenic Rupture, *Ann Surg,* **179:**472, 1974.

Burrington, J. D.: Surgical Repair of a Ruptured Spleen in Children, *Arch Surg,* **112:**417, 1977.

Cioffino, W., Schein, C. J., and Gliedman, M. L.: Splenic Injury during Abdominal Surgery, *Arch Surg,* **111:**167, 1976.

Dunphy, J. E.: Splenectomy for Trauma, *Am J Surg,* **71:**450, 1946.

Lieberman, R. C., and Welch, C. S.: A Study of 248 Instances of Traumatic Rupture of the Spleen, *Surg Gynecol Obstet,* **127:**961, 1968.

Orloff, M. J., and Peskin, G. W.: Collective Review. Spontaneous Ruptures of the Normal Spleen: A Surgical Enigma, *Intern Abstr Surg,* **106:**1, 1958.

Schwartz, S. I., Adams, J. T., Cockett, A. T. K., and Morton, J. H.: Blunt Trauma to the Upper Abdomen, *Surg Ann,* **3:**273, 1971.

Widman, W. D., and Laubscher, F. A.: Splenosis: Disease or Beneficial Condition? *Arch Surg,* **102:**152, 1971.

Hematologic Disorders

Adler, A., Stutzman, L., Sokal, J. F., and Mittelman, A.: Splenectomy for Hematologic Depression in Lymphocytic Lymphoma and Leukemia, *Cancer,* **35:**521, 1975.

Bernard, R. P., Bauman, A. W., and Schwartz, S. I.: Splenectomy for Thrombotic Thrombocytopenic Purpura, *Ann Surg,* **169:**616, 1969.

Bertino, J., and Myerson, R. M.: The Role of Splenectomy in Sarcoidosis, *Arch Intern Med,* **106:**213, 1960.

Cannon, W. B., and Nelson, T. S.: Staging of Hodgkin's Disease: A Surgical Perspective, *Am J Surg,* **132:**224, 1976.

Chabner, B. A., Johnson, R. E., Young, R. C., Canellos, G. P., Hubbard, S. P., Johnson, S. K., and DeVita, V. T., Jr.: Sequential Nonsurgical and Surgical Staging of Non-Hodgkin's Lymphoma, *Ann Intern Med,* **85:**149, 1976.

Cooper, I. A., Ironside, P. N. J., Madigan, J. P., Morris, P. J., and Ewing, M. R.: Role of Splenectomy in Management of Advanced Hodgkin's Disease, *Cancer,* **34:**408, 1974.

Dacie, J. V.: "The Haemolytic Anaemias, Congenital and Acquired," vol. 2, pt. 1, Grune & Stratton, Inc., New York, 1960.

DeWeese, M. S., and Coller, F. A.: Splenectomy for Hematologic Disorders, *West J Surg,* **67:**129, 1959.

Doan, C. A.: Hypersplenism, *Bull NY Acad Med,* **25:**625, 1949.

———, Bruce, M. D. and Wiseman, B. K.: Hypersplenic Cytopenic Syndromes: A 25 Year Experience with Special Reference to Splenectomy, in "Proceedings of the Sixth International Congress of the International Society of Hematology," Grune & Stratton, Inc. New York, 1958.

———, Bouroncle, B. A., and Wiseman, B. K.: Idiopathic and Secondary Thrombocytopenic Purpura: Clinical Study and Evaluation of 381 Cases over a Period of 28 Years, *Ann Intern Med,* **53:**861, 1960.

Fabri, P. J., Metz, E. N., Nick, W. V., and Zollinger, R. M.: A Quarter Century with Splenectomy: Changing Concepts, *Arch Surg,* **108:**569, 1974.

Gendel, B. R.: Chronic Leg Ulcers in Diseases of the Blood, *Blood,* **3:**1283, 1948.

Glatstein, E., Guernsey, J. M., Rosenberg, S. A., and Kaplan, H. S.: The Value of Laparotomy and Splenectomy in the Staging of Hodgkin's Disease, *Cancer,* **24:**709, 1969.

Gruenberg, H., and Penner, J. A.: Gaucher's Disease: Observations on Its Clinical Course, *Mich Med,* **74:**323, 1975.

Liebowitz, H. R.: Splenomegaly and Hypersplenism Pre- and Post-portacaval Shunt, *NY J Med,* **63:**2631, 1963.

Lipton, E. I.: Elliptocytosis with Hemolytic Anemia: The Effects of Splenectomy, *Pediatrics,* **15:**67, 1955.

Meilleur, P. A., and Myers, M. C.: Thrombocytosis: A Postsplenectomy Complication in Agnogenic Myeloid Metaplasia, *Am J Med Sci,* **241:**68, 1961.

Mitchell, R. I., and Peters, M. V.: Lymph Node Biopsy during Laparotomy for Staging of Hodgkin's Disease, *Ann Surg,* **178:**698, 1973.

Necheles, T. F., Allen, D. M., and Gerald, P. S.: The Many Forms of Thalassemia: Definition and Classification of the Thalassemia Syndromes, *Ann NY Acad Sci,* **165**(Art. 1):5, 1969.

O'Brien, P. H., Hartz, W. H., Derlacki, D., and Graulich, K.: Splenectomy for Hypersplenism in Malignant Lymphoma, *Arch Surg,* **101:**348, 1970.

O'Neill, J. A., Jr., Scott, H. W., Jr., Billings, F. T., and Foster, J. H.: The Role of Splenectomy in Felty's Syndrome, *Ann Surg,* **167:**81, 1968.

Reynolds, P. M., Jackson, J. M., Brine, M. A. S., and Vivian, A. B.: Thrombotic Thrombocytopenic Purpura—Remission Following Splenectomy, *Am J Med,* **61:**439, 1976.

Schwartz, S. I.: Myeloproliferative Disorders, *Ann Surg,* **182:**464, 1975.

———, Adams, J. T., and Bauman, A. W.: Splenectomy for Hematologic Disorders, *Curr Probl Surg,* May, 1971.

———, Adesola, A. O., Elebute, E. A., and Rob, C. B.: "Tropical Surgery," McGraw-Hill Book Company, Inc., New York, 1971.

——— and Cooper, R. A., Jr.: Surgery in the Diagnosis and Treatment of Hodgkin's Disease, in "Advances in Surgery," vol. 6, Yearbook Medical Publishers, Inc., Chicago, 1972.

Veronesi, U., Musumeci, R., Pizzetti, F., Gennari, L., and Bonadonna, G.: Value of Staging Laparotomy in Non-Hodgkin's Lymphomas (with Emphasis on the Histiocytic Type), *Cancer,* **33:**446, 1974.

Wintrobe, M. M.: "Clinical Hematology," 6th ed., Lea & Febiger, Philadelphia, 1967.

Yam, L. T., and Crosby, W. H.: Early Splenectomy in Lymphoproliferative Disorders, *Arch Intern Med,* **133:**270, 1974.

Miscellaneous Lesions

Chulay, J. D., and Lankerani, M. R.: Splenic Abscess, *Am J Med,* **61:**513, 1976.

Gadacz, T., Way, L. W., and Dunphy, J. E.: Changing Clinical Spectrum of Splenic Abscess, *Am J Surg,* **128:**182, 1974.

Saw, E. C., Arbegast, N., Schmalhorst, W. R., and Comer, T. P.: Splenic Artery Aneurysms, *Arch Surg,* **106:**660, 1973.

Splenectomy

Ein, S. H., Shandling, B., Simpson, J. S., Stephens, C. A., Bandi, S. K., Biggar, W. D., and Freedman, M. H.: The Morbidity and Mortality of Splenectomy in Childhood, *Ann Surg,* **185:**307, 1977.

Eraklis, A. J., and Filler, R. M.: Splenectomy in Childhood: A Review of 1413 Cases, *J Pediatr Surg,* **7:**382, 1972.

Glatstein, E., Vosti, K. L., Donaldson, S. S., et al.: Serious Bacterial Infections in Pediatric Hodgkin's Disease: Relative Risks of Radiotherapy, Chemotherapy and Splenectomy, *Proc Am Soc Clin Oncol,* **17:**252, 1976.

Haller, J. A., Jr., and Jones, E. L.: Effect of Splenectomy on Immunity and Resistance to Major Infections in Early Childhood: Clinical and Experimental Study, *Ann Surg,* **163:**902, 1966.

Olsen, W. R., and Beaudoin, D. E.: Increased Incidence of Accessory Spleens in Hematologic Disease, *Arch Surg,* **98:**762, 1969.

Singer, D. B.: Postsplenectomy Sepsis, in Perspectives in Pediatric Pathology. Chicago, Year Book Medical Publishers Inc., 1973, vol. 1, pp. 285–311.

CHAPTER 34

Peritonitis and Intraabdominal Abscesses

by **Robert E. Condon**

PERITONEUM

STRUCTURE. The peritoneum is a single layer of flat mesothelial cells resting on a bed of looser connective tissue containing fat cells, macrophages, and some collagen and elastic fibers. The parietal peritoneum lines all of the abdominal cavity, covering the abdominal wall, diaphragm, and pelvis. Parietal peritoneum everywhere is reinforced by the endoabdominal (transversalis) fascia, which lies external to it. The visceral peritoneum covers all the intraabdominal viscera and mesenteries, and is identical with the serosa or capsule of the several intraabdominal organs. Excepting the ends of the fallopian tubes, the peritoneum is a completely closed sac.

The abdominal cavity is divided into the general peritoneal cavity, or greater sac, and the lesser sac. The lesser sac arises in the upper half of the abdomen during fetal development because of persistence of the embryologic ventral mesentery and rotation of the upper abdominal viscera. As a consequence, the embryologic right upper peritoneal cavity becomes isolated from the remainder of the peritoneal cavity, remaining in communication only at the foramen of Winslow.

INNERVATION. The parietal peritoneum is innervated by both somatic and visceral afferent nerves and is quite sensitive, responding to various stimuli somewhat as the skin does. As is true of the skin, there are regional differences in ability of the peritoneum to localize pain. The anterior parietal peritoneum is the most sensitive, and the pelvic peritoneum is relatively the least sensitive. The ability to localize a noxious stimulus affecting the parietal peritoneum, particularly that of the anterior abdominal wall, underlies much of our ability to diagnose acute intraabdominal illness.

In addition to perception of pain as localized tenderness and rebound tenderness, local injury or inflammation of the parietal peritoneum leads to protective voluntary muscular guarding and then to reflex muscular spasm, signs which are very useful in determining the presence and state of progression of intraabdominal disorders.

In contrast to the parietal peritoneum, the visceral peritoneum receives afferent innervation only from the autonomic nervous system and is relatively insensitive. Stimuli are perceived as poorly localized pain, often with the character of a toothache or of colic. Visceral afferent nerves respond primarily to traction or distension, less well to pressure, and apparently have no receptors capable of mediating pain and temperature sensation.

The root of the small-bowel mesentery and the biliary tree are relatively better innervated, accounting for more intense and more localized responses to stimulation of these areas. The small bowel, itself, is not well innervated, so that stimulation of its visceral afferents produces only a vague, dull ache in the midabdomen. Somatic reflex responses to visceral peritoneal stimulation are uncommon, but with maximal stimulation may result in bradycardia or hypotension. By contrast, visceral reflex responses serve to produce ileus early after the onset of peritoneal inflammation or irritation.

MEMBRANE FUNCTION. The surface area of the peritoneum is nearly 2 m², approximately identical to the area of the skin, and is appreciably larger than the filtering surface area of the renal glomeruli. Unlike the skin, the peritoneum acts as a semipermeable membrane and permits bidirectional transport of water, electrolytes, peptides, and similar small molecules.

The peritoneal cavity normally contains only about 100 ml of fluid to serve as lubrication between the abdominal viscera and the parietes. Since the peritoneum permits bidirectional fluid movement, the peritoneal cavity functions as a part, albeit a small one, of the total body extracellular fluid compartment. Hydraulic and osmotic concentration forces control the movement and the direction of transport across the peritoneum. In addition to these passive processes, there is evidence that active absorption also occurs, both intercellularly and transcellularly across the peritoneum.

Fluid tagged with heavy water or another marker and placed in the peritoneal cavity rapidly equilibrates with the interstitial fluid and the plasma. Albumin, electrolytes, and urea are freely transported bidirectionally across the peritoneum. Antibiotics also are easily absorbed. Endogenous and exogenous toxic substances, including bacterial toxins, are freely absorbed as well, and may produce systemic effects. Because of the tremendous surface available, the bidirectional transfer of substances across the peritoneal membrane is rapid and potentially large in volume. The membrane transfer properties of the peritoneum are used to advantage in peritoneal dialysis for acute renal insufficiency, but also may be a fatal disadvantage if spill of toxic bowel content occurs, as in strangulation obstruction.

In addition to fluid exchange across the peritoneal membrane, transdiaphragmatic lymphatic channels also play a role in fluid transport from the peritoneal cavity. These lymphatic channels probably are responsible for the appearance of so-called sympathetic pleural effusions whenever an intraabdominal inflammatory process involves the undersurface of the diaphragm. These lymphatic channels also provide a route by which amylase-rich abdominal fluid is transported into the pleural space, particularly on the left side, in patients suffering from pancreatitis.

RESPONSE TO INJURY. The peritoneum heals very rapidly following injury. Even large defects can be restored in a matter of hours. Unlike the skin, which heals only by regeneration of epithelial cells from the margins of a defect, a peritoneal defect is restored everywhere simultaneously, usually without adhesion formation. The majority of cells involved in healing of a peritoneal wound are derived by differentiation of stem cells present within the subperitoneal tissues. Transperitoneal migration of mesothelial cells shed by intact peritoneum to implant in the area of injury, and ingrowth of mesothelial cells from the margins of a defect, are additional mechanisms which play a minor role in peritoneal healing.

If normal peritoneal healing is delayed or incomplete, adhesions form. The adhesions may be transient in nature, eventually resolving as delayed healing becomes complete, or they may be more permanent in nature. Fibrin elaborated from the inflamed peritoneal mesothelium is the scaffold upon which adhesions are built. Agglutination of fibrin strands during the course of acute peritonitis leads to the formation of soft, fibrinous adhesions. In most instances, deposited fibrin is absorbed if functioning and intact mesothelium is present in the immediately adjacent area. If the fibrinous adhesions are not absorbed for any reason, they are invaded by fibroblasts between 5 and 10 days after the initial insult. Fibroblast invasion is followed by ingrowth of capillaries and further organization into true fibrous tissue.

The factors which favor development of fibrous adhesions following peritonitis include continuing action of an intraperitoneal irritant, necrosis extending through the mesothelium to involve the subperitoneal tissues, and a predisposition in certain persons that is not well understood. Fortunately, even fibrous adhesions become attenuated and may disappear with time.

Formation of adhesions is both a protective response, helping to localize a peritoneal insult, and an adaptive healing response which helps to bring additional blood supply to ischemic injured areas of perineum. These beneficial effects of adhesions are sometimes overlooked by surgeons.

PERITONITIS: GENERAL CONSIDERATIONS

Peritonitis is inflammation of a portion or all of the parietal and visceral surfaces of the abdominal cavity. The classical division of peritonitis into primary and secondary forms has little clinical utility. When a surgeon refers to "peritonitis" without qualification, the clinical situation is acute suppurative bacterial peritonitis. Other forms of peritonitis are less common, although nonetheless important.

Every case of peritonitis, of whatever cause, initiates a sequence of responses involving the peritoneal membrane, the bowel, and the body fluid compartments, which then produce secondary endocrine, cardiac, respiratory, renal, and metabolic responses (Fig. 34-1). In certain forms of peritonitis, most notably acute suppurative peritonitis, additional responses due to the presence of infection also occur. The general responses, found to some degree whenever peritonitis occurs, are described here; additional reactions specific to the various forms of peritonitis are described later.

Primary Responses in Peritonitis

MEMBRANE INFLAMMATION. The peritoneum responds to insult with hyperemia followed by transudation. Edema and vascular congestion occur in the subperitoneal tissues immediately external to the peritoneal membrane. Absorption across inflamed peritoneum is somewhat impaired while at the same time the peritoneal membrane permits passage of larger molecules than when in its normal state. Transudation of fluid with a low protein content from the extracellular interstitial compartment into the abdominal cavity is accompanied by diapedesis of large numbers of polymorphonuclear leukocytes. During the early vascular and transudative phase of engorgement, the peritoneum acts as a "two-way street," so that toxins and other materials which may be present in peritoneal fluid are readily absorbed, enter the lymphatics and bloodstream, and may lead to systemic symptoms.

Transudation of interstitial fluid into the peritoneal cavity across the inflamed peritoneum is followed shortly by

GENERAL RESPONSES TO PERITONITIS

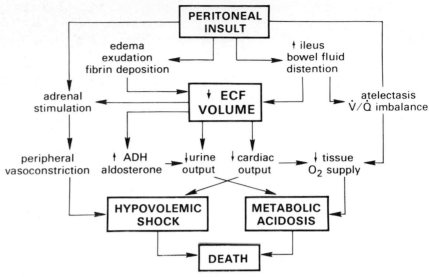

Fig. 34-1. The major general responses to peritonitis are mediated by a decreased extracellular fluid volume, which, if not corrected, leads to metabolic acidosis, hypovolemic shock, and death.

exudation of protein-rich fluid. The fluid exudate in the peritoneal cavity contains large amounts of fibrin and other plasma proteins in concentrations sufficient to bring about clotting, which, in turn, results in agglutination of loops of bowel, other viscera, and the parietes in the area of peritoneal inflammation. This response helps to confine the source of peritoneal contamination.

Dermal inflammation causes a rapid local decrease in the concentration of collagen and a marked increase in the concentration of hexosamine and noncollagenous nitrogen in the skin. The inflamed human peritoneum behaves in a similar manner. Within the peritoneal membrane, the concentration of uronic acids and noncollagenous nitrogen increases markedly in peritonitis, while the concentration of hydroxyprolene and the hydroxyprolene-nitrogen ratio decreases. The content of uronic acid in the peritoneum is proportional to the extent and severity of the peritonitis.

The RNA/DNA ratio, which is an index of the protein synthetic capability of tissue, is decreased in peritonitis, and the defect progresses if peritonitis persists for longer than 24 hours. These changes have not been fully elucidated but could be due to tissue hypoxia inhibiting the synthesis of collagen, the action of bacterial collagenase, or the release of proteolytic lysozymal enzymes. The increase in uronic acid concentration probably reflects increased formation of glycosaminoglycans because of activation of fibroblasts and mesothelial cells.

BOWEL RESPONSE. The initial response of the bowel to peritoneal irritation is transient hypermotility. After a short interval, motility becomes depressed and nearly complete adynamic ileus soon follows. The bowel distends, and both air and fluid accumulate in the lumen. The source of the accumulating gas is largely swallowed air. Fluid secretion (exsorption) into the bowel lumen is enhanced in ileus, while resorption (insorption) is relatively impaired, pro-

moting sequestration of fluid in the bowel lumen. If the patient continues to ingest food or fluid, vomiting eventually occurs.

HYPOVOLEMIA. As noted above, the peritoneum reacts to irritation by vascular dilation and an outpouring of plasmalike fluid from the extracellular vascular and interstitial compartments into the peritoneal space as an exudate. The loose connective tissue beneath the mesothelium of the viscera, the mesenteries, and the parietes traps extracellular fluid as edema. The atonic, dilated gastrointestinal tract also accumulates fluid in the bowel lumen which is derived from the extracellular fluid volume. This translocation of water, electrolytes, and protein into a sequestered "third space" functionally removes this volume temporarily from the body economy. The rate of functional extracellular fluid loss is proportional to the surface area of peritoneum involved in the inflammatory process. With extensive peritonitis, fluid translocation of 4 to 6 liters, or more, in 24 hours is not uncommon.

Secondary Responses to Peritonitis

ENDOCRINE RESPONSE. Peritonitis acts as a stimulus to many endocrine organs. There is an almost immediate adrenal medullary response, with an outpouring of epinephrine and norepinephrine, producing vasoconstriction, tachycardia, and sweating. The adrenal cortex is stimulated to increased secretion of cortical hormones during the first 2 to 3 days following peritoneal injury. Originally thought to be the cause of increased nitrogen excretion in peritonitis, it has now been shown that the increase in adrenocortical hormones persists only for about 72 hours. Circulating concentrations of these hormones have returned to normal long before nitrogen losses cease to occur.

Secretion of both aldosterone and antidiuretic hormone also is increased as a response to the hypovolemia of peritonitis, resulting in enhanced renal conservation of sodium and water. In fact, water retention may be greater than sodium retention, so that there is dilution of plasma sodium (hyponatremia). Thyroid metabolism probably is unaltered despite increased rates of energy utilization and increased heat production by the body during peritonitis.

CARDIAC RESPONSE. The effects of peritonitis on cardiac function are a reflection both of the decrease in extracellular fluid volume and of progressing acidosis. The volume deficit results in decreased venous return and diminished cardiac output. The heart rate increases in an attempt to maintain cardiac output, but compensation usually is incomplete. Progressing acidosis brings about secondary dysfunction in cardiac contractility and a further decrease in cardiac output that compounds the problem of maintaining adequate tissue perfusion and aerobic metabolism.

RESPIRATORY RESPONSE. Abdominal distension, primarily due to adynamic ileus, coupled with restriction of both diaphragmatic and intercostal respiratory movements, results in a decrease in ventilatory volume and the early appearance of basilar atelectasis. Early in the course of peritonitis, an increase in respiratory rate may be noted, stimulated both by the hypoxia of diminished ventilation and by beginning accumulation of acidic end products of anaerobic tissue metabolism. Ventilation-perfusion imbalances result from continued pulmonary perfusion of underventilated or nonventilated alveoli and produce functional intrapulmonary shunting of blood and peripheral hypoxemia.

RENAL RESPONSE. Hypovolemia, reduced cardiac output, and increased secretion of antidiuretic hormone and of aldosterone in peritonitis all act synergistically on the kidney. Renal blood flow is diminished, resulting in a decrease in the volume of glomerular filtrate and in tubular urine flow. Reabsorption of both sodium and water is increased, often in imbalance; potassium is wasted. Urine volume output is diminished, and renal capacity to handle excess solutes is impaired. A tendency to development of metabolic acidosis is enhanced.

METABOLIC RESPONSE. The metabolic rate generally is increased, with a corresponding increase in peripheral oxygen demand. Simultaneously, the capacity of the lungs and the heart to deliver oxygen is diminished. Poor circulation leads to a shift from aerobic to anaerobic metabolism in muscle and other peripheral tissues. As a result, anaerobic end products of carbohydrate metabolism accumulate and lactic acidosis begins to develop.

Under normal circumstances, local tissue perfusion is controlled by regional metabolic requirements. If anaerobic metabolic end products begin to accumulate, local arteriolar dilation occurs. Cardiac output, in the absence of hypovolemia, increases to maintain circulatory homeostasis. Perfusion in the periphery improves, the acidic metabolic end products are cleared, and the tissues return to aerobic metabolism. This fine balance is upset by circulatory insufficiency due to the hypovolemia which accompanies peritonitis. Cardiac output may be inadequate to maintain normal arterial blood pressure and to supply required perfusion of all body tissues.

Compensatory vasoconstriction results in increased total peripheral resistance, which, in turn, maintains essential perfusion to the heart and brain. The skin, muscles, the splanchnic bed, and, to some degree, the kidneys are denied a portion of their normal circulatory volume. As a result of decreased tissue perfusion and oxygenation, anaerobic glycolysis persists and leads to a progressive increase in lactic acid and other acidic metabolic end products. Decreased renal clearance of these acidic solutes, secondary to reduced renal perfusion, contributes to the metabolic acidosis. The body attempts to compensate with increased respiratory effort to excrete carbon dioxide, but the increased respiratory effort, in turn, places an additional demand on the already inadequate circulation to perfuse the muscles of respiration.

The appearance, in some cases of peritonitis, of lactic acidosis before systemic hypotension or hypoxemia suggests the existence of a primary cellular insult which makes cells unable to use available oxygen and substrate. This hypothesis was investigated in isolated hepatic mitochondria harvested following induction of peritonitis by cecal ligation. In these experiments, hepatic cellular hypoxia followed the development of peritonitis even while systemic oxygenation was adequate and hypotension had not yet developed. Mitochondrial respiration, however, was unaltered in these experiments, suggesting that primary cellular injury does not occur in peritonitis but that alterations in oxygen delivery are responsible for reduced oxygen consumption and lactic acidosis.

Hepatic glycogen stores are utilized promptly in peritonitis. Insulin secretion by islet cells increases, promoting mobilization of fat as an energy source. Nonetheless, relative insulin resistance to muscle utilization of glucose uptake is unchanged, and an energy deficit persists.

Protein catabolism begins early in peritonitis and becomes progressively more severe. However, some data indicate that the rate of synthesis of plasma proteins is increased in terms of concentration and turnover. Plasma proteins preferentially are synthesized while muscle proteins preferentially are catabolized. Weight loss of 25 to 30 percent of lean body mass can occur if peritonitis persists. Albumin synthesis also is apparently increased during peritonitis, as judged by increased uptake of radioactive label, but the increased synthesis occurs in the face of a decreasing concentration of circulating albumin. The reason for this disparity is that a considerable amount of albumin accumulates in the peritoneal cavity and thus is lost to the general circulation.

Clinical Manifestations

The appearance of a patient with advanced peritonitis was described by Hippocrates: ". . . hollow eyes, collapsed temples; the ears cold, contracted and their lobes turned out; the skin about the forehead being rough, distended, and parched; the color of the whole face being brown, black, livid, or lead-colored." Patients with peritonitis which is so advanced as to present this classic Hippocratic facies are usually in a preterminal state. But even much earlier in the clinical course of peritonitis, patients quite obviously are gravely ill. Characteristically, they lie quietly in bed, supine, with knees flexed and with frequent limited intercostal respirations since any other motion intensifies the abdominal pain.

Abdominal pain almost always is the predominant symptom, unless its perception is masked by the administration of anodynes or the presence of a fresh surgical wound. The pain may have been sudden in onset, associated with rupture of a viscus, or more insidious. When fully developed, pain is steady, unrelenting, burning, and aggravated by any motion. Pain usually is most intense in the area of most advanced peritoneal inflammation. Decreasing intensity and extent of pain with time suggest localization of the inflammatory process, while increasing intensity and extent imply the presence of a spreading peritonitis.

Anorexia almost always is present. Nausea is frequent and may be accompanied by vomiting. The patient usually complains of thirst and of feeling feverish, often with intermittent chills. Body temperature elevation in peritonitis usually is in the range of 38 to 40°C. Fever is usually higher and more spiking in character in younger and healthier patients, while older and debilitated patients may exhibit only a modest febrile response.

Tachycardia and a diminished palpable peripheral pulse volume are early signs of hypovolemia. The blood pressure is maintained in the early stages of peritonitis, but, as hypovolemia progresses, compensatory vasoconstrictive responses may be overcome, with the rapid appearance of hypovolemic shock. Respirations typically are rapid and shallow; rapid because of progressively greater tissue demands for oxygen and a need to correct developing acidosis, and shallow because deep respirations intensify the perception of abdominal pain.

The abdomen is distended, quiet to auscultation, and tender to palpation. Tenderness is present over the entire extent of the peritoneum involved in the inflammatory process. Maximal tenderness usually is noted in the region of the organ in which the process originated, but in some cases, maximal tenderness is found over the advancing edge of the peritoneal inflammation. Direct, percussive, and referred rebound tenderness confirms the presence of peritoneal irritation. Percussion tenderness sometimes is more accurate than direct palpation in locating the point of maximal tenderness as well as in delineating the extent of peritoneal irritation.

Rigidity of the abdominal muscles is produced initially by voluntary guarding and, following involvement of the parietal peritoneum by inflammation, also by reflex muscular spasm. As peritonitis advances, reflex spasm may become so severe that boardlike abdominal rigidity is produced. Hyperresonance due to accumulating gas in the paralyzed, distended intestines usually can be demonstrated easily by percussion. If a pneumoperitoneum has resulted from rupture of a hollow viscus, gas accumulating under the right side of the diaphragm may produce a decrease in the vertical extent of liver dullness to percussion.

Some bowel sounds may be audible on auscultation early in peritonitis, but as inflammation spreads, the nearly silent abdomen of adynamic ileus supervenes. Rectal examination and vaginal examination of female patients are essential steps in establishing the diagnosis. The location and extent of tenderness, and the possible presence of a pelvic mass, permit assessment of the degree of involvement of pelvic peritoneum. Vaginal examination of the cervix may provide clues to the origin of an inflammatory process within the female generative organs.

Leukocytosis is usual in acute peritonitis, but the total white cell count, taken alone without a differential count, can be very misleading. Massive peritoneal inflammation may mobilize sufficient numbers of leukocytes into the diseased area so that only 3,000 to 4,000 white cells per cubic millimeter remain behind in the circulating blood. The differential count shows a moderate to a marked left shift in peritonitis, and the predominance of polymorphonucleocytes in the differential provides evidence of the presence of inflammation even when the total leukocyte count is not markedly elevated. Blood chemistry determinations are quite variable but usually will reflect hemoconcentration due to dehydration (increased hematocrit) as well as metabolic acidosis.

The radiologic picture of generalized peritonitis is that of paralytic ileus with distension of both small intestine and colon. Inflammatory exudate and edema of the intestinal wall may produce widening of the spaces between adjacent bowel loops noted on a flat film of the abdomen. Peritoneal fat lines and the psoas shadows may be obliterated. Free air may be visible on an upright abdominal or lateral decubitus film if a ruptured viscus is the cause of peritonitis. Air beneath the diaphragm also may be noted on x-rays of the chest.

In general, the importance of laboratory work in the diagnosis of peritonitis has been overemphasized, a statement which also holds true for almost every other acute intraabdominal disease. Though laboratory determinations undoubtedly are of occasional help, the major emphasis in both the diagnosis and management of peritonitis should be on clinical examination of the patient. Amelioration of symptoms and restoration of the patient's physical state toward normal are the best indicators that treatment is effective. Laboratory and radiologic examinations should be employed only to help rule out other causes of abdominal pain such as pneumonia. In an occasional obscure case, confirmation of the presence of peritonitis may require such diagnostic measures as a peritoneal tap or lavage.

ACUTE SUPPURATIVE PERITONITIS

Any breach in the integrity of a hollow abdominal viscus or of the abdominal parietes which permits peritoneal contamination is a potential catastrophe. Loss of integrity may be due to direct contamination from a traumatic abdominal wound, to perforation of an inflamed or traumatized hollow abdominal viscus, to functional loss of bowel integrity secondary to ischemia; may occur retrogradely via the fallopian tubes in pelvic infections; or may be iatrogenic, such as an improperly executed bowel anastomosis.

While no longer the overwhelming clinical problem it once was, suppurative peritonitis still is the most common cause of death following an abdominal operation. The mortality risk of septic peritonitis ranges from 24 percent in acute perforated diverticulitis to 90 percent with acute perforated ischemic colitis, particularly if treatment is delayed. About half of all cases of septic shock which terminate fatally are secondary to peritonitis. In 5 to 7 percent of autopsies, peritonitis is the primary or a contributory cause of death.

Although there is some degree of peritoneal inflammation (from mechanical and desiccation injury of exposed peritoneum as well as intraoperative bacterial contamination from room air or spillage during manipulation of viscera and minor breaks in aseptic technique) every time the peritoneal cavity is entered surgically, such contamination usually is not so great that clinically significant peritonitis ensues. Peritonitis following an operation is due most commonly to bile leakage, less commonly to breakdown of an anastomotic suture line; on occasion it follows ill-advised attempts at peritoneal drainage. The integrity of an anastomosis is endangered by tension on the suture line, ischemia, hemorrhage, mucosal eversion, infection, or the presence of a drain in apposition to the suture line, as well as all the systemic factors which interfere with wound healing (see Chap. 8).

Perforated peptic ulcer is the most common cause of peritonitis due to visceral rupture. Appendicitis, formerly the most common cause, is now less frequent because of a recent overall decline in the incidence of appendicitis. Pancreatitis is a frequent cause of peritonitis in certain hospitals. Gangrene of the bowel from strangulation obstruction, acute mesenteric vascular occlusion, or nonocclusive, low-perfusion states involving the bowel also is an important cause of peritonitis. Other common visceral diseases that may lead to peritonitis due to rupture of an inflamed organ are acute gangrenous cholecystitis and colonic diverticulitis. Gonorrheal salpingitis is a common cause of pelvic peritonitis, although this disease does not often progress to a generalized peritonitis.

Trauma to the abdomen may produce peritonitis by contamination of the abdominal cavity with foreign material, such as shotgun wadding or clothing, or disruption of a hollow abdominal viscus as the result of severe blunt, nonpenetrating trauma or the penetrating trauma of a stab or gunshot wound. Blunt abdominal trauma also may disrupt the vascular supply to abdominal viscera, leading to gangrene or rupture of the involved organ.

Interactions of Bacteria and the Peritoneum

The presence of bacteria within the peritoneal cavity by no means invariably results in spreading diffuse peritonitis. On the contrary, peritoneal defense mechanisms contain the insult in most instances; invading microorganisms are destroyed, and the peritoneum is restored to a relatively normal state.

If peritoneal defenses are successful in localizing the infectious process but the interaction between invading microorganisms and body defense mechanisms does not result in early elimination of the bacteria, confined suppuration and abscess formation ensues (see further on). On occasion, however, initial defense reactions are insufficient

and a more diffuse peritonitis ensues. The general responses to peritonitis then follow. They are mediated largely by translocation of extracellular fluid into the peritoneal cavity, with both the local and systemic consequences enumerated above.

In suppurative peritonitis, in addition, a group of specific responses due to the presence of overwhelming numbers of bacteria is superimposed on the general responses to peritonitis (Fig. 34-2). The magnitude of the specific responses to generalized spreading peritonitis is, in part, determined by (1) the virulence of the contaminating bacteria, (2) the extent and duration of contamination, (3) the presence or absence of an adjuvant, and (4) the appropriateness of initial therapy. If treatment fails to bring about prompt control of peritoneal infection, endotoxemia and septic shock may ensue.

VIRULENCE OF CONTAMINATING BACTERIA. A mixed, or polymicrobial, bacterial flora usually is present in patients suffering acute suppurative peritonitis secondary to contamination of the abdominal cavity from the gastrointestinal tract. The most common offending organisms include aerobic coliform bacilli, anaerobic *Bacteroides* species, anaerobic and aerobic streptococci, enterococci, and *Clostridia* (Table 34-1). These bacteria are significant pathogens for human beings.

Experiments of Nichols and colleagues in which the entire range of peritonitis, from overwhelming sepsis to resolution with an abscess, was produced, indicate that mortality risk is a dose-related phenomenon and correlates directly with the total number of pathogenic bacteria present in the peritoneal cavity. Experimental evidence also indicates that the mixed fecal flora usually found in peritonitis acts synergistically, so that total virulence is greater than the sum of its parts. Experimentally, injection of massive numbers of single species of fecal pathogens may

Table 34-1. BACTERIA IN PERITONITIS

	Percent of recovery of organisms	
	Bartlett, 1977*	Lorber, 1975*
No. of patients studied . .	21	76
Aerobes		
Escherichia coli	100	57
Proteus	24	11
Klebsiella	24	8
Pseudomonas	24	3
Other bacilli	33	6
Streptococci	33	47
Staphylococci	0	0
Anaerobes		
Bacteroides fragilis	90	93
Other *Bacteroides*	24	59
Peptostreptococci	38	29
Peptococci	19	28
Fusobacteria	24	20
Clostridia	52	9
Other anaerobes	. . .	23

*First author; full citations will be found in the references at the end of the chapter.

not produce a fatality, whereas mixtures of organisms, in the same total numbers, particularly combinations of aerobes and anaerobes, result in overwhelming peritonitis and death. Further, there is evidence to indicate that apparently nonpathogenic microorganisms may increase the virulence of pathogenic bacteria with which they are associated.

Although the frequency with which anaerobic bacteria are present in peritoneal infections probably has not changed over the years, modern methods have greatly improved the rate at which these organisms are recovered. Thus, the importance of anaerobic bacteria in peritonitis recently has become more widely recognized. Years ago, Meleney and Altemeier emphasized the frequency of recovery of anaerobic organisms in peritonitis. Experimental evidence indicates not only that the presence of anaerobic microorganisms enhances the virulence of aerobic pathogens, but that it is the presence of anaerobes or their degradation products which is responsible for the resolution of acute peritonitis by formation of an abscess rather than by complete healing.

Stone and colleagues recently demonstrated in patients undergoing operation that the recoverability of anaerobic organisms from a soiled peritoneal cavity showed a progressive decline with the passage of time. If the abdomen was open for 3 hours or longer, anaerobes could no longer be recovered. Although Stone suggested that in some cases, exposure to room air might be sufficient to manage the anaerobic component of peritoneal sepsis, specific antibiotic therapy obviously is more certain therapy.

EXTENT AND DURATION OF CONTAMINATION. Massive sudden contamination, as from a burst carcinoma of the cecum, often disseminates bacteria rapidly throughout the peritoneal cavity. Dissemination occurs widely before localization mechanisms have time to be effective. Experimentally, bacteria or liquid radiopaque media injected intraperitoneally at one locus can be demonstrated to spread throughout the entire peritoneum within 3 to 6 hours. Spread is produced by normal intestinal and abdominal movements, by movement of the diaphragm during respiration (which establishes a cyclic negative pressure differential between the subphrenic space and the rest of the peritoneal cavity, promoting upward flow of fluid and particulate matter), and by the effect of gravity related to body position, which tends to promote flow into the pelvic cavity. Even though infection spreads diffusely throughout the peritoneal cavity, if the source is controlled by early surgical intervention, peritonitis usually responds to vigorous antibiotic and supportive therapy. On the other hand, if the source of contamination persists, death nearly always results because of continuing peritoneal soiling.

The severity and extent of peritonitis secondary to spontaneous or traumatic perforation of the gastrointestinal tract vary not only with the size of the perforation but also with its location. Spillage of distal ileal or cecal content is associated with greater morbidity than a perforation proximally or distally in the gastrointestinal tract. Proximally there are few bacteria; distally the fecal content is more solid and tends to be more easily localized. But ileal and cecal content is fluid and contains high concentrations of

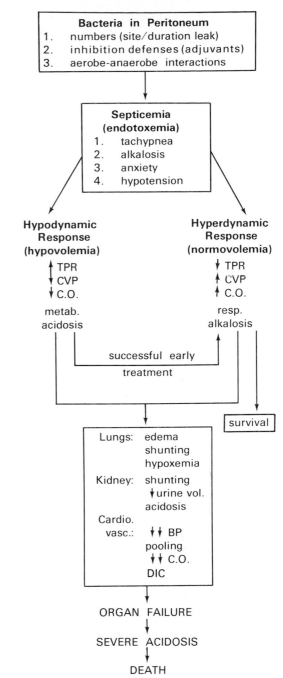

Fig. 34-2. The specific responses to suppurative peritonitis begin with septicemia, which initiates tachypnea, respiratory alkalosis, anxiety, and moderate hypotension in most cases. Continuing responses depend on the status of total body fluid volumes; in most cases of peritonitis, patients are hypovolemic and a hypodynamic response pattern is seen. Successful early fluid resuscitation may convert the hypodynamic response to a hyperdynamic one. If sepsis continues uncontrolled, major functional deficits appear in the vital organ systems which are essential to survival, and death ensues.

bacteria as well as residual active enzymes which increase the severity of peritonitis and prevent effective local sequestration.

INFLUENCE OF ADJUVANTS. The virulence of peritonitis not only is determined by the nature of the contaminating mixture of bacteria and the duration of peritoneal soiling, but is importantly influenced by the presence of adjuvant substances such as mucus and hemoglobin. Trauma or any foreign body will retard the clearance of bacteria from the peritoneal cavity and can act as an adjuvant. Foreign substances which are proteinaceous in nature seem to be particularly associated with enhanced virulence.

Experimentally, the presence of an adjuvant nearly always is necessary to produce lethal peritonitis. Intraperitoneal injections of bacteria can be made lethal by the addition of such foreign substances as bile salts, talc, gum tragacanth, gastric mucin, or blood. The enhancement of virulence is attributed to the adverse effect of these adjuvant substances on defense mechanisms, particularly phagocytosis. The body apparently does not differentiate between contaminating bacteria and the contaminating adjuvant, attacking both with vigor. The presence of the adjuvant dilutes the net effectiveness of phagocytosis, since a proportion of leukocytes is diverted to phagocytosis of the adjuvant, retarding clearance of bacteria from the peritoneal cavity.

Hemoglobin seems to be a particularly noxious adjuvant in both experimental and clinical peritonitis. Hemoglobin, certainly as is true of any adjuvant, retards clearance of bacteria from the peritoneal cavity. However, there also is evidence that hemoglobin exerts an additional toxic effect, possibly because of the action of pigments or of ferrous iron liberated when hemoglobin is degraded.

Experimentally, if a pure suspension of *Escherichia coli* containing 10^9 organisms per milliliter is injected intraperitoneally into experimental animals in a dose of 5 ml/kg, all animals survive. But if 3 to 4 mg/100 ml of hemoglobin is combined with the same dose of *E. coli* organisms, lethal peritonitis is produced in 90 percent of animals. These observations are pertinent to the problem of peritonitis in human beings, since hemoglobin frequently is present in peritoneal fluid in clinical peritonitis.

Recently, Hau and coworkers have shown that hemoglobin inhibits the normal chemotactic responses of polymorphonuclear neutrophils and, therefore, might inhibit either migration of polymorphs into the peritoneal cavity or their subsequent attachment to and lysis of bacteria.

INAPPROPRIATE THERAPY. Peritonitis may be spread by errors of omission as well as by errors of commission. A frequently fatal error of omission is failure to diagnose the presence of a ruptured viscus and to undertake surgical control of the source of contamination of the peritoneum in timely fashion. Another error of omission occurs in efforts to control a persisting or expanding intraabdominal infection by administration of antibiotics without adequate surgical debridement or drainage. Subsequent rupture of an undrained abscess will broadcast highly virulent contents throughout the abdomen, often with fatal consequences. Conversely, an error of commission may occur if laxatives or enemas are administered to patients suffering

abdominal pain. This practice seems to be on the wane, although occasional cases of injudicious catharsis are still seen. The bowel, stimulated to motility when otherwise it would be becoming quiescent, interferes with the walling-off process of localization which body defense mechanisms otherwise would dictate.

Pathophysiology of Sepsis

The presence of bacteria in suppurative peritonitis leads to a number of both local and systemic responses which are related directly to the effects of the microorganisms or their products. These responses are in addition to and superimposed on the general pathophysiologic responses which occur in all cases of peritonitis.

TOXIC ABSORPTION. The inflamed peritoneum acts as a bidirectionally permeable membrane, not only secreting fluid into the peritoneal cavity in the presence of peritonitis but also permitting ready absorption of both bacteria and bacterial toxins from peritoneal fluid. Endotoxins derived from the cell wall of aerobic gram-negative bacilli, such as *Escherichia coli,* are most frequently involved and are the most important in these systemic responses, although absorption of preformed exotoxins, elaborated by gram-positive organisms such as *Clostridia,* are the dominant influence in occasional cases.

Endotoxin is a lipopolysaccharide. It acts primarily on blood vessels, producing arteriolar and venular dilation and loss of endothelial integrity. Capillary leakage, accumulation of fluid in tissues, and intraorgan shunting are some of the consequences of endotoxin action which lead to the clinical features of septic shock. Exotoxins, in contrast, are proteins. They cause hemolysis of red cells or destruction of other body cells, or interfere with metabolic or other cellular processes. Exotoxins also cause peripheral arteriolar dilation, but the effects of exotoxins tend to be more cellularly specific and less totally pervasive compared with endotoxins.

Gram-negative sepsis of major proportions often begins with chills, rapid elevation of the temperature above 38.5°C, and moderate hypotension. Because of predominant peripheral vasodilation, the clinical picture often is characterized as "warm" shock unless the effects of hypovolemia predominate, in which case the clinical picture is of more typical "cold" shock.

The severity of septic shock varies depending on the amount and duration of exposure of body tissues to circulating gram-negative organisms and their endotoxins. Transient, self-limited bacteremia may produce minimal adverse systemic effects, whereas persisting or repetitive episodes of septicemia overwhelm the vital cardiorespiratory and renal support systems and, obviously, result in a much poorer prognosis. The presence of underlying disease of the cardiac, pulmonary, hepatic, or renal systems renders the patient more susceptible to development of septicemia and also impairs responses to the endotoxemic insult.

There are considerable species differences in the response to endotoxemia. Though the use of experimental animal models has contributed a great deal to our understanding of this entity, direct extrapolation of findings in animals to human septic shock cannot be made. For example, injection of lipopolysaccharide endotoxin in a dog causes splanchnic pooling as a consequence of hepatic venous constriction. Decreased venous return, reduction in cardiac output, and an abrupt fall in blood pressure follow immediately after injection of endotoxin. This pattern is very different from that seen in subhuman primates and in human beings, in whom injection of endotoxin produces chills, fever, transient vasoconstriction, then peripheral vasodilation; cardiac output initially rises and then declines.

There also are differences in response to experimental injection of preformed endotoxin as compared with septicemia produced by injection of live bacteria. Hypoglycemia and hypoinsulinemia are regularly observed after live *E. coli*-induced shock; hyperglycemia is a consistent hallmark in endotoxin-infused models. Renal fibrin thrombi (DIC) are present after live *E. coli* administration, while tubular necrosis is found following both organism and endotoxin infusions. Liver dysfunction is indicated by elevation of blood levels of hepatic enzymes and morphologic alterations in both models. The condition of the live *E. coli*-injected baboon appears to bear a closer similarity to the clinical entity of septic shock than does the endotoxin-treated animal.

Renal morphologic changes induced during experimental septic shock can be prevented by administration of heparin, although in all other respects, heparin-treated animals are identical to unheparinized animals in their reactions to injection of live organisms or endotoxin and suffer the same mortality risk. In particular, abnormal renal function, as reflected in rising BUN, creatinine, and uric acid levels, is not modified by administration of heparin.

INFLUENCE OF HYPOVOLEMIA IN SEPSIS. Septic shock in normovolemic patients begins with a hyperdynamic response associated with increased cardiac output, normal or high central venous pressure, low peripheral resistance, warm extremities despite a low blood pressure, hyperventilation, and respiratory alkalosis.

When sepsis is superimposed on hypovolemia, the typical situation in peritonitis, an initial hypodynamic pattern usually is present characterized by low cardiac output, low central venous pressure, vasoconstriction with high peripheral resistance, cold extremities, and low blood pressure. Expansion of venous capacitance vessels, together with the accumulation of fluid in the tissues as a result of capillary leakage (both effects of endotoxin), creates an additional functional "third-space" loss of fluid.

Hypovolemic septicemia is an unstable situation, since the peripheral vasoconstriction which is maintaining circulation to the heart and brain may, at any time, yield to the vasodilating effect of endotoxin, resulting in sudden loss of peripheral resistance and deep shock out of proportion to the degree of measurable hypovolemia. This form of combined shock does not respond completely to replenishment of fluid volume, but in the absence of overt cardiac failure, conversion to a hyperdynamic state despite continuing hypotension may be seen and is associated with a more favorable prognosis. If treatment is delayed or unsuccessful, circulatory failure, a low, fixed cardiac output, resistant metabolic acidosis, and death ensue.

RESPIRATORY RESPONSES IN SEPSIS. Compromise of vascular endothelial integrity in the lung as a consequence of the actions of endotoxin results in leakage of fluid from pulmonary arterioles and capillaries into the interstitial pulmonary space. The accumulating fluid makes the lungs stiffer (loss of compliance) and also results in pulmonary vascular hypertension. Interstitial edema also acts, in effect, as a barrier between pulmonary capillaries and adjacent alveoli, retarding uptake of oxygen and producing mild hypoxemia. Compensatory hyperventilation and respiratory alkalosis result. At this stage, there is little clinical or x-ray evidence of pulmonary compromise. It is worth emphasizing that the development of mild hyperventilation, respiratory alkalosis, and an altered sensorium may be the earliest signs of gram-negative sepsis; this triad may precede more obvious signs of sepsis or shock by many hours.

As pulmonary edema progresses, protein-rich fluid accumulates in alveoli. Directly or indirectly, endotoxemia also leads to a loss of pulmonary surfactant, promoting alveolar collapse and progressive pulmonary consolidation. The chest x-ray now shows patchy infiltrates diffusely in the lungs. Maintenance of circulation to areas of the lung which have lost effective capacity for oxygen uptake produces a ventilation-perfusion inequality. In addition, excessive beta-adrenergic stimulation is common in sepsis and causes opening of splanchnic and pulmonary arteriovenous shunts.

The effect of both functional and actual intrapulmonary shunting is entry of poorly oxygenated pulmonary blood into the general arterial circulation. This leads to tissue hypoxia, further compensatory hyperventilation, and respiratory alkalosis. "Respiratory distress syndrome," "septic lung," "shock lung," and "white lung" are some of the terms which have been used to describe the clinical and radiologic effects of this process. Subsequently, the picture frequently is one of rapid deterioration of pulmonary function, confluence of patchy infiltrates, and severe hypoxemia.

RENAL RESPONSE. The decrease in glomerular perfusion and filtration brought about by hypovolemia in peritonitis is reinforced by the endotoxin-induced opening of intrarenal shunts at the corticomedullary level. The blood circulating to the kidneys now preferentially perfuses more central renal tissues, while the cortex receives little blood flow at all. This phenomenon of "corticomedullary disconnection" produces a profound decrease in glomerular perfusion and results, when fully elaborated, in formation of little glomerular filtrate. As a consequence, urine flow is greatly diminished; this is recognized clinically by failure of urine output accompanied by progressive accumulation of unexcreted acidic end products of metabolism and metabolic acidosis. Recent evidence also indicates that prolonged sepsis in some cases may be accompanied by development of proliferative glomerulonephritis leading not only to acute renal failure but also to chronic renal insufficiency in survivors.

LEUKOCYTE FUNCTION. Both neutrophil and lymphocyte function are abnormal in patients suffering severe sepsis. Skin test anergy in septic patients is associated both with defects in cellular function and with the presence in serum of inhibitors of white cell function. These effects are reflected in abnormal neutrophil chemotactic responses and in decreased ability of lymphocytes to form rosettes. Severe infections also are associated with consumption of large amounts of antibody, decreases in concentration of complement in serum, and consumption of opsonic proteins which further hampers neutrophil responses to invading bacteria.

END-ORGAN FAILURE. The interaction of hypovolemia and endotoxemia in suppurative peritonitis is particularly vicious. Unless prompt and effective therapy is instituted, the multiple deleterious organ effects reinforce one another in a progressively worsening cycle of events. The elevated metabolic rate and great caloric expenditure, as well as local circulatory effects of extensive inflammation in peritonitis, contribute to a need for a greatly increased cardiac output. Increased respiratory efforts to correct acidosis are incapacitated by the inability of the already inadequate circulation to provide additional perfusion and oxygenation required by the muscles of respiration. Administration of fluid and electrolytes, respiratory support, reduction of body temperature, and maintenance of nutrition all may contribute to survival, but if these measures are not successful, pulmonary failure is followed rapidly by cardiorenal failure and death.

Clinical Manifestations

The patient with suppurative peritonitis presents all the features which characterize peritonitis in general: a distended, tender, painful abdomen; rapid, shallow respiration; fever; and tachycardia. The acute symptoms are of short duration and rapid progression, although occasional patients report symptoms suggesting past subacute or chronic disease.

The history and location of pain in the abdomen may provide clues to the possible organ source of peritonitis. Pain may increase or decrease at the time of viscus rupture. Thereafter, the story is one of progressively worse pain, initially diffuse but tending to localize if peritoneal defense mechanisms can contain the spillage. Tenderness increases, percussion tenderness appears or worsens, bowel sounds diminish and disappear, muscular rigidity replaces guarding, distension worsens. Leukocytosis with a left shift is usual but may not be marked in elderly or debilitated patients, or in patients with advanced peritonitis in whom trapping of neutrophils in the peritoneal cavity has occurred. Abdominal x-ray films may show paralytic ileus, free air, or atelectatic changes in the lung bases.

In some cases of septic peritonitis, fever may be misleading. Subnormal temperatures may occur, particularly later in the course of sepsis, because body compensatory mechanisms are unable to prevent hypothermia consequent upon peripheral vasodilation. Shock, due to accumulation of fluid in peripheral tissues as well as failure of compensatory vasoconstrictive mechanisms, is out of proportion to the degree of measurable hypovolemia.

In patients with generalized peritonitis, serum bilirubin and alkaline phosphatase levels demonstrate an irregular relationship. Sepsis is known to be associated with jaundice; it has been shown that some endotoxins inhibit mitochondrial respiration in human liver preparations. Among 44 fatal cases of peritonitis, 31 patients had an elevated bilirubin and 34 an elevated alkaline phosphatase level. When jaundice appeared after the ninth postoperative day or bilirubin exceeded 15.5 mg%, the outcome invariably was fatal. In 13 out of 14 patients, the reason for late onset of jaundice was traced to unsuspected peritoneal soiling from a leaking anastomosis. The presence of persisting or recurring hyperbilirubinemia is a warning sign of an intraabdominal abscess or leaking anastomosis.

Management

Initially, both therapeutic and diagnostic efforts are conducted simultaneously. Therapeutic efforts are directed to restoration of an effective total body fluid volume. Diagnosis is directed to the cause of the peritoneal sepsis. The objective is to determine the need for and the timing of operation.

Nonsurgical conditions simulating peritonitis should be considered and excluded. Pneumonia, particularly in the aged, often is accompanied by abdominal distension and ileus simulating a slowly progressive peritonitis. Diaphragmatic pleurisy may be associated with abdominal pain suggestive of acute cholecystitis or a perforated ulcer. Uremia commonly is associated with abdominal distension and ileus. A variety of other conditions, including acute gastroenteritis, ureteral calculi, and various female pelvic disorders such as twisted ovarian cyst, ectopic pregnancy, and ruptured ovarian follicle, may produce abdominal pain simulating early acute peritonitis.

PREOPERATIVE PREPARATION. The essential features of preoperative treatment of suppurative peritonitis involve (1) fluid resuscitation, (2) antibiotics, (3) oxygen and, if needed, ventilator support, and (4) nasogastric intubation, urinary catheterization, and monitoring of vital signs and biochemical and hemodynamic data. Additional measures which may need to be considered in an individual case are requirements for steroids, digitalis, and vasopressor drugs.

Patients are better served if major metabolic derangements and fluid deficits are corrected prior to operation, although inordinantly long periods of time cannot be taken in this exercise. Certain causes of peritonitis require more urgent intervention than others. For example, intestinal infarction demands nearly immediate intervention, whereas inflammatory perforation of the sigmoid colon with a developing fecal peritonitis will permit 1 or 2 hours of resuscitative effort prior to laparotomy.

Fluid Resuscitation. Large volumes of fluids may need to be administered very rapidly until blood volume and urine output are restored. In patients whose central venous pressure is less than 10 cm of water, fluid volume administration may go forward at as rapid a rate as can be achieved;

when the central venous pressure rises to 10 cm, the infusion rate can be slowed.

The most frequent mistake made in resuscitation of patients with advanced peritonitis and a major circulating blood volume deficit is that the rate of initial fluid administration is too slow. The slow rate is undertaken for fear of precipitating congestive heart failure. If the central venous pressure is monitored and the rate of infusion adjusted appropriately, congestive heart failure will not occur simply because initial fluid resuscitation is undertaken at rapid rates of administration. Fluids administered must include crystalloids for replacement of water and electrolytes functionally lost into "third-space" collections in the peritoneal cavity and bowel lumen. Whole blood or packed red blood cells are administered, if needed, to correct anemia and to maintain an adequate red cell mass (hematocrit, 30 to 35). The administration of colloid (albumin or plasma) is more controversial.

Crystalloid or Colloid. There is agreement that deficits in the interstitial fluid volume in patients with peritonitis should be replaced with a crystalloid solution, preferably Ringer's lactate. But controversy exists about replacement of the deficient plasma volume. Some authorities advocate administration of more crystalloid, others argue for administration of colloid.

The controversy over the relative merits of colloid versus large volumes of crystalloid solution as a replacement for plasma volume has raged for years. Proponents of each type of solution can cite evidence to support their view. The argument turns on the applicability of Starling's law to the pulmonary circulation, the liability to develop pulmonary edema, and the comparative efficiency of the two forms of therapy.

Though it is clear that albumin will restore an effective volume efficiently in terms of the total volume administered, the same end can be achieved if one gives three to four times as much crystalloid solution. The theoretical advantages of administering albumin in resuscitation of patients suffering peritonitis are that salt overload, peripheral edema, and weight gain are less likely. Administering balanced salt solutions in excess might result in interstitial fluid accumulation in the lung because of a reduction in the colloid osmotic pressure–pulmonary capillary wedge pressure gradient. This hypothesis is based on Starling's law of fluid movement across a semipermeable membrane, which, in essence, indicates that net movement of fluid is governed by the algebraic sum of the hydrostatic and colloid osmotic pressures on the two sides of the membrane.

However, it appears from experimental evidence that the oncotic pressure gradient as it relates to the alveolar-capillary membrane is not an important factor in the development of pulmonary edema. In studies in which pulmonary capillary wedge pressure has been measured, no relationship between colloid osmotic pressure or intrapulmonary pressure gradients and the development of pulmonary edema has been identified. Liability to development of pulmonary interstitial edema is related primarily to the degree of endothelial leakiness resulting from the actions of endotoxin, rather than being related to the type of resuscitation fluid. Colloid solutions are theoretically more efficient but also are more expensive and less readily available. Crystalloid solutions are readily available and more economical but require administration of a large volume excess which must later be excreted by the kidneys. Both types of solution are equally liable to be associated with pulmonary edema due to leakage from endotoxin-injured pulmonary capillaries; exclusive crystalloid resuscitation is more likely to be associated with pulmonary edema due to volume overload. We usually rely mainly on crystalloid solutions for resuscitation of most patients with septic peritonitis, but do employ partial colloid resuscitation in patients known to have preexisting cardiopulmonary disease.

Antibiotic Therapy. Although the actual organisms may not be known, intraabdominal infection should be presumed in every case of suspected septic peritonitis. Antibiotics which are effective against the full spectrum of aerobic and anaerobic gastrointestinal bacteria should be started as soon as feasible, either as a direct intravenous injection or rapidly instilled intravenously in a small volume of fluid from a subsidiary reservoir. Therapeutic levels of antibiotics should be present in the tissues at the time of operation. We currently administer gentamicin and clindamycin in full dosage to all patients suspected of having suppurative peritonitis.

Experimental evidence indicates that antibiotics which are effective against *Escherichia coli* are most important in reducing the mortality risk of experimental fecal septicemia. Drugs effective against *E. coli* include the cephalosporins, aminoglycosides, and chloramphenicol; tetracyclines and ampicillin also are active against many coliforms. Control of later liability to abscess formation, on the other hand, requires the additional administration of an antibiotic effective against anaerobic *Bacteroides fragilis*. Drugs effective against *B. fragilis* include clindamycin, chloramphenicol, metronidazole, and erythromycin; tetracycline and carbenicillin also may be active against this bacterium.

Oxygen and Ventilator Support. Oxygen is administered to help the response to the increased metabolic demands of peritonitis which are so often associated with impairment of pulmonary ventilatory function that mild hypoxia is common. A nasal catheter supplying oxygen at about 5 liters/minute usually is sufficient prior to induction of anesthesia. Assessment of respiratory function should be made clinically, noting apparent tidal volume and work of breathing. If impairment is suspected, measurement of ventilatory volume and arterial blood gases is indicated.

Ventilatory support, with an inspired gas concentration of 40 percent oxygen, should be initiated in patients whose arterial oxygen pressure falls below 70 mmHg. Addition of positive end-expiratory pressure (PEEP) to ventilator support is indicated in patients whose P_{O_2} is below 60 mmHg or who develop other evidence of more severe respiratory embarrassment. Efforts to maintain a normal or even rightward-positioned oxygen-hemoglobin dissociation curve are worthwhile, since red blood cell organic phosphates are reduced in sepsis.

Intubation, Catheterization, and Monitoring. Nasogastric intubation is performed to evacuate the stomach, prevent further vomiting, and, most importantly, reduce accumulation of additional air in the paralyzed bowel. Urinary catheterization is utilized to record initial volume and to monitor subsequent urinary output.

A central venous catheter should be placed to assess current hydration and intravenous replacement. Percutaneous subclavian vein catheterization is preferred except in infants, where it is easier and safer to place an internal jugular catheter. A chest roentgenogram after subclavian or jugular catheter placement is imperative to assure correct placement of the catheter tip and the absence of a pneumothorax or other complication. If pulmonary insufficiency or cardiac failure exists, placement of a Swan-Ganz catheter for direct measurement of pulmonary artery and wedge pressures is very helpful in precise fluid administration and avoidance of pulmonary edema.

Vital signs such as temperature, blood pressure, pulse and respiration rates are recorded every 4 hours, and more often if need be. Preoperative biochemical evaluation should include measurement of serum electrolytes, creatinine, glucose, bilirubin, and alkaline phosphatase, and a urinalysis.

Steroids. Administration of pharmacologic doses of steroids to septic patients has been advocated on the basis of experimental work in dogs but its advisability in the treatment of patients remains controversial. Recent clinical studies support the idea that large doses of potent steroids reduce the mortality risk in sepsis, particularly if given before or early after the onset of shock.

Steroids are not needed preoperatively in most cases of suppurative peritonitis. But if the patient's condition seems unstable or the symptomatic history is relatively long, consideration should be given to steroid administration. An initial intravenous dose of 30 mg methylprednisolone, or 5 mg dexamethasone, is given over 5 to 10 minutes, and may be repeated in 2 to 3 hours. If a beneficial response is obtained, additional injections usually are not needed. If no response is seen after two doses, continued administration of steroids is unlikely to have any effect.

Vasoactive Drugs. Experimentally, the effects of intraperitoneal injection of *E. coli* are not altered by the administration of alpha or beta blockers, phentolamine, propranolol, reserpine, or serotonin. By contrast, when *Staphylococcus aureus,* an exotoxin-producing organism, is used for challenge, administration of reserpine, serotonin, or the combination of phentolamine and propranolol significantly prolongs life.

Drugs with predominant alpha-adrenergic effects are of limited value in the treatment of sepsis secondary to peritonitis, since artificial attempts to maintain blood pressure by inducing vasoconstriction without thought to its consequences on tissue blood flow are potentially harmful. When volume replacement and other measures have failed to restore an adequate circulation, administration of isoproterenol may be helpful. Isoproterenol has potent inotropic and chronotropic effects on the heart. One or two milligrams of isoproterenol diluted in 500 ml of 5% dextrose in water may be administered by intravenous drip at a rate of 1 to 2 μg/minute, depending on the response. The infusion should be slowed or stopped completely if significant tachycardia (above 140 beats per minute) or cardiac arrhythmias occur. A fall in blood pressure in the absence of cardiac arrhythmia resulting from administration of isoproterenol indicates a need for additional volume replacement to maintain cardiac filling. The combination of isoproterenol stimulation of the heart together with effective volume resuscitation may restore tissue blood flow even though the blood pressure remains low.

Digitalis. Cardiac status should be assessed preoperatively in middle-aged or older patients by interpretation of a current electrocardiogram. Digitalis is not administered routinely. But gram-negative sepsis and shock frequently are superimposed on congestive failure in older patients or may precipitate early congestive failure in patients with limited cardiac reserve. In these instances, digitalis should be administered cautiously, with attention to its potential for toxicity if the patient is hypokalemic or also receiving isoproterenol.

Fever. A temperature above 38.5°C may be associated with difficulties in administration of anesthesia. Patients with such hyperthermia, and also those with hypothermia, should have their temperature corrected toward normal prior to operation. Administration of salicylates often will be effective in reducing fever. If not, or if the patient is hypothermic, a cooling-warming mattress should be employed.

Narcotics. Analgesic drugs should not be administered to patients with suspected peritonitis until a diagnosis has been made or, at least, a decision to operate has been made. The reason is that analgesia may obscure abdominal findings and hamper establishment of a diagnosis of peritonitis. Equally, once a decision to operate has been made, pain should be relieved with potent narcotics. Morphine is preferred to other drugs and should be given in small intravenous doses of 1 to 3 mg, frequently repeated, to maintain the patient's comfort. Small intravenous doses are safer than the traditional larger intramuscular doses, particularly in patients whose condition is unstable.

OPERATIVE MANAGEMENT. The incision of choice in adults is vertically in the midline. This incision can be extended from xiphoid to pubis, provides ready access to all quadrants of the abdomen, and is the quickest to open and to close. Transverse incisions are safer in patients under two years of age because of a propensity for postoperative dehiscence in infants. Another exception to the general recommendation for use of a vertical midline incision occurs in the presence of localized peritonitis, in which the objective is to open directly over the inflammatory process, avoiding contamination of other quadrants of the abdomen.

Objectives. The fundamental objective of the operation is to control the source of peritoneal contamination. The general principles of operative management include closure of perforations of the stomach and small bowel but exteriorization with fecal diversion of colonic perforations. As an example, management of acute perforated diverticulitis with generalized peritonitis by resection of the involved segment of sigmoid colon, temporary end colostomy, and peritoneal toilet is associated with survival of 9 of 10 patients. Alternative forms of management of this disorder, particularly attempts at a colonic anastomosis in the presence of peritonitis, are associated with a higher mortality risk.

Odor and Staining of Peritoneal Pus. Immediately on opening the abdomen, any odor should be noted and a representative sample of peritoneal pus sent for Gram stain and culture. An immediate report of the results of the Gram stain should be requested.

The odor of peritonitis pus is of diagnostic importance in relation to the bacteriology of suppurative peritonitis. Altemeier studied the ability of *E. coli* to produce a putrid odor when grown on sterile human pus and found that no odor resulted, although good growth of bacteria was obtained. On the other hand, when similar sterile pus was inoculated with anaerobic streptococci and *Bacteroides meleninogenicus,* a marked, penetrating foul odor was produced after 3 days of incubation under anaerobic conditions. In addition to these two organisms, other anaerobic bacteria, particularly members of the *Clostridium* group, recovered from pus of peritonitis are capable of producing strong odors.

The general rule is that aerobic infections do not produce a marked odor, whereas infections containing anerobes do. Combining information provided by the odor of the pus in peritonitis with the structure of bacteria noted on a Gram stain of the same material will permit a presumptive diagnosis of the infecting organisms.

Debridement of Exudate. All peritoneal pus, pseudomembranes, fibrin, and other exudates, as well as the content of any localized collections or abscesses, should be completely excised once the source of the peritonitis has been controlled. Gentle dissection of all adhesions and plications of bowel and mesentery should be done together with excision of pus and exudate from the subhepatic, subdiaphragmatic, and pelvic cavities. Although debridement has been a controversial issue, it is now clear that it has a salutary effect on mortality risk in peritonitis. For example, debridement was associated with no mortality in a group of 92 patients with peritonitis reported by Hudspeth.

Lavage. Debridement is followed by irrigation with saline solution of all parts of the peritoneal cavity until the effluent is clear. Washing the contaminated peritoneal cavity with large volumes of irrigant was first advocated by Price in 1905. The next year, Torek reported that the large-volume irrigation technique reduced mortality in general peritonitis following appendicitis to 14 percent, an extremely good experience at the time of this report. The procedure later fell into disrepute because of the fear, still widely held but never clinically proved, that lavage disseminates peritoneal contamination.

Burnett reintroduced peritoneal lavage in the management of suppurative peritonitis, and reported a two-thirds reduction in mortality. The modern concept of peritoneal lavage views the contaminated peritoneum in the same way as a contaminated dermal wound: copious irrigation is a major component of therapy and involves the use of large volumes, up to 10 liters, of saline solution and occasionally more, with the objective of diluting and removing all the contaminated peritoneal content.

Antibiotic Lavage. The addition of antibiotics to peritoneal lavage solutions is associated with decreased mortality and a lower incidence of infected wounds in cases of purulent peritonitis. Under usual circumstances, antibiotics are used only in the final "rinse" of the peritoneum, plain normal saline solution or Ringer's lactate being used for lavage to clear most of the peritoneal exudate. A variety of antibiotic solutions has been demonstrated to be effective. We prefer the kanamycin-bacitracin solution recommended by Noon and associates.

Reports concerning the effectiveness of noxytiolin or povidone-iodine solutions for peritoneal lavage have been mixed. The most recent controlled clinical studies indicate that neither agent is as effective as solutions containing antibiotics.

Patients with severe peritonitis who fail to improve despite correction of the source of infection and appropriate therapy with fluids and systemic antibiotics may benefit from postoperative peritoneal lavage with an antibiotic solution. Experience with multiple instillations of intraperitoneal kanamycin or cephalosporins in patients who had perforated appendicitis or generalized peritonitis confirms that this is a rational form of treatment.

Antibiotic lavage can be conducted using a single catheter for infusion and subsequent drainage, or an infusion catheter can be used simultaneously with another catheter or other drains to provide egress of lavage solution. Irrigation catheters should be placed during laparotomy if the need for postoperative antibiotic lavage can be anticipated. Lavage will result in absorption of some variable fraction of the antibiotic employed; this effect needs to be taken into account in managing overall antibiotic administration.

Closure. If a midline wound has been used, the fascia may be closed as a single layer with running monofilament suture (Prolene, nylon, or wire), taking generous bites of tissue on either side. Some surgeons recommend use of interrupted fascial suture technique and also favor placement of additional retention sutures; the reason advanced for recommending these more tedious suture techniques is a supposed reduction in the incidence of wound dehiscence. However, the occurrence of dehiscence in suppurative peritonitis is primarily due to infection in the wound; septic wounds are likely to fail to heal whatever suture technique is used for closure; interrupted or retention sutures will not prevent subsequent dehiscence.

The skin and subcutaneous portions of the wound usually should be left open. A few layers of fine gauze soaked in antibiotic irrigating solution are used to cover the subcutaneous tissues, but the wound should not be tightly packed. Dry gauze dressings then lightly cover the wound. All dressings, including those within the wound, are removed in about 48 hours and replaced with a simple covering bandage. Secondary closure with adhesive strips can be done 4 or 5 days later if the wound remains healthy.

POSTOPERATIVE MANAGEMENT. The general principles

of postoperative care include continued administration of intravenous fluids and antibiotics. Complications of sepsis —particularly respiratory failure, renal failure, and disseminated intravascular coagulation—should be expected and searched for continuously by monitoring ventilatory volumes, urine output, blood gases, serum creatinine, and coagulation factors. A rise in bilirubin level may indicate the presence of a persistent or recurrent intraabdominal abscess which requires prompt reoperation and drainage.

When the results of antibiotic sensitivity studies done on the operative specimen of peritoneal pus are available, consideration should be given to changing antibiotic therapy to the most specific and least toxic of the drugs which appear to be effective (see Chap. 5). Antibiotic treatment should not be stopped until the patient is clinically well enough to be consuming a regular diet, or other clinical evidence indicates that residual infection is unlikely.

ASEPTIC (CHEMICAL) PERITONITIS

This form of peritonitis develops whenever irritant materials gain entry into the peritoneal cavity, usually because of rupture of a solid or upper abdominal viscus. The soilage initially is sterile or nearly so, a feature by which chemical peritonitis differs from suppurative peritonitis. The aseptic inflammatory reaction gives rise to the general clinical symptoms and physiologic sequellae of peritonitis. Translocation of plasma volume into the peritoneal cavity with the secondary systemic responses to hypovolemia, discussed above under general responses to peritonitis, is the major initial reaction.

Secondary bacterial invasion commonly occurs, sometimes as early as 12 hours after the initial peritoneal insult, even when no bacteria enter the peritoneal cavity via a perforated viscus or from the environment through a traumatic wound. In fact, presumably because episodes of transient bacteremia are relatively common though ordinarily innocuous, an initially aseptic peritonitis cannot be expected to remain sterile. Most of the substances which cause aseptic peritonitis are capable of acting as adjuvants whenever secondary bacterial contamination occurs, promoting proliferation of microorganisms and, later, the onset of the systemic effects of suppurative peritonitis.

Symptoms typically are sudden, severe pain, and tenderness and rigidity of the abdominal muscles. Backache occurs if the retroperitoneal area is involved. During the next few hours, peritoneal fluid dilution and neutralization of the irritant may produce a deceptive sense of improvement. Leukocytosis is present. Plain abdominal and chest films are useful in showing specific injuries after trauma, bowel distension, and intraabdominal fluid accumulation. The most helpful diagnostic test in some situations, apart from exploratory laparotomy itself, is a peritoneal tap.

The principles of surgical management in cases of aseptic peritonitis include preoperative resuscitation with fluids and similar measures; control of the source of contamination during laparotomy by suture closure or excision, as appropriate; debridement of foreign substances; copious lavage; and administration of antibiotics to combat the risks of existing infection.

GASTRIC CONTENTS. Gastric juice is highly irritating to the perineum, not only because of its hydrochloric acid content but also because of the presence of mucin and digestive enzymes. If gastric juice gains access to the peritoneal cavity through a perforated duodenal ulcer, spilled material initially is sterile in the majority of cases because the normal "acid barrier" of the stomach effectively kills swallowed microorganisms. It must be remembered, however, that in cases of perforated gastric ulcer, in which a high proportion of patients have a defective gastric acid barrier to bacteria, the spilled gastric juice regularly is contaminated with swallowed aerobic and anaerobic organisms chiefly originating in the oral (mouth) flora.

In gastroduodenal perforation, the interval between the occurrence of the perforation and its closure is viewed by many surgeons as the primary determinant of postoperative morbidity and mortality. But Hamilton and Harbrecht, in a review of patients with perforated ulcer, found the degree of peritoneal contamination and the incidence of contaminating virulent pathogens greater when operation was performed 6 hours or less after perforation than in operations done after 24 hours. The incidence of negative cultures in this study (about 50 percent) was the same whether spillage was light or marked. Postoperative complications (64 percent of which were septic) were related only to the presence of marked spillage. This apparent paradox must be due partially to peritoneal fluid dilution which occurs during the initial inflammatory response to the peritoneal insult. Unfortunately, the use and duration of antibiotic therapy in these patients was not recorded.

The findings in this study are in contrast to the usually accepted surgical wisdom which indicates that the incidence of peritoneal contamination by virulent pathogens is less when operation is performed within 6 hours of perforation compared with later operative times. The important point illustrated by this study is that taking sufficient time preoperatively to complete fluid resuscitation and otherwise prepare the patient for operation is rewarded by a reduction in mortality risk.

PANCREATIC JUICE. Pancreatic secretions enter the peritoneal cavity during episodes of acute pancreatitis or following pancreatic trauma. If the mode of entry is due to rupture of a pancreatic duct or pseudocyst, with release of relatively large volumes of activated pancreatic juice, pancreatic ascites ensues. Because the pancreatic juice is diluted in the ascites, the overall peritoneal reaction varies considerably, from mild to relatively severe inflammation. Alternatively, pancreatic juice may transude through the retroperitoneum in acute pancreatitis. In these cases, typically, the volume of accumulating intraperitoneal fluid is less. If the pancreatic exudate is combined with blood and breakdown products of pancreatic necrosis, as is true in cases of hemorrhagic pancreatitis, secondary infection occurs in a higher proportion of instances.

BILE. Most commonly bile enters the peritoneal cavity as a result of leakage following exploration of the common bile duct or other operation on the biliary system. Rupture of the gallbladder during acute cholecystitis, perforation of a gallbladder carcinoma, or, infrequently, rupture of the common duct due to necrosis from a common duct stone also may lead to spill of bile into the peritoneal cavity. Although bile peritonitis follows rupture of an inflamed gallbladder, biliary peritonitis can occur without detectable gallbladder perforation. In such cases, presumably, the mechanism for leakage of bile involves transudation through an ischemic portion of the acutely inflamed gallbladder wall.

Sterile bile is a chemical irritant in its own right. Frequently, bacterial contamination, either associated with the rupture itself or having been acquired secondarily, leads to a particularly virulent form of septic biliary peritonitis. Experimental studies of bile peritonitis have shown that both inflammation and lethality in animals are reduced if therapeutic serum levels of antibiotics have been achieved at the time of biliary leakage.

URINE. Intraperitoneal rupture of the bladder usually is a sequella of severe trauma. Sterile urine is an extremely irritating substance, and the chemical insult frequently is followed by secondary infection. Spontaneous intraperitoneal perforation of the urinary bladder also occurs in neurologically handicapped patients. Necrosis of the bladder wall in these patients, secondary to chronic intramural infection, results in spill of infected urine into the peritoneal cavity.

ACUTE HEMOPERITONEUM (ABDOMINAL APOPLEXY). Intraperitoneal blood is not irritating at all. If red cells lyse, the released cell contents act as a mild hyperosmolar irritant. Blood can be transfused intraperitoneally; the rate at which red cells subsequently enter the general circulation is slow, but the fraction of a transfused unit of blood detectable in the circulating blood volume 48 to 96 hours after intraperitoneal injection is the same as after an intravenous transfusion. It is not blood, per se, which is of concern in relation to peritonitis, but the fact that blood or, more particularly, hemoglobin and ferrous iron act as adjuvants of a particularly noxious sort should subsequent bacterial infection of the peritoneal cavity occur.

Spontaneous rupture of a visceral artery, most frequently the splenic and less commonly a gastroepiploic artery, or rupture of the spleen, liver, or a hepatic tumor, may produce a massive acute hemoperitoneum. The clinical symptoms are of abdominal pain accompanied by tenderness, absent bowel sounds, and other clinical signs suggestive of peritonitis. The leukocyte count may be elevated. Treatment consists of early laparotomy and control of the bleeding source.

MECONIUM. Intrauterine perforation of the bowel with leakage of sterile meconium produces a marked sterile peritonitis, resulting in matted adhesive obliteration of the abdominal cavity. If the bowel perforation remains uncontrolled after birth of the infant, secondary bacterial infection is the rule; the outlook in such cases is grim (see Chap. 39).

CHYLE. Chronic chylous effusions either into the peritoneal cavity as chylous ascites or into the chest as chylothorax are not rare; acute symptoms are unusual. Acute chylous peritonitis, on the other hand, which results from a sudden outpouring of chylous fluid into the free peritoneal cavity may produce signs and symptoms suggestive of an acute abdominal catastrophe but is a distinctly rare clinical syndrome.

MUCUS AND SIMILAR SUBSTANCES. Mucus from intestinal secretions released in small-bowel rupture or the contents from a ruptured ovarian cyst induce a sterile inflammatory reaction of the peritoneum. Rupture of a dermoid cyst of the ovary can produce a severe peritonitis, presumably because of the cyst content of cholesterol, hair, and other irritant materials.

ENDOTOXIC PERITONITIS. Under certain circumstances, constriction or occlusion of intestinal vessels produces sufficient ischemia that there is increased permeability of the bowel wall, permitting transudation of preformed endotoxin generated by the intestinal flora within the bowel lumen into the peritoneal cavity. Transperitoneal absorption of endotoxin then produces systemic symptoms of gram-negative sepsis. The degree of peritoneal inflammation, per se, in such instances ordinarily is not great unless bowel wall necrosis or perforation ensues. The vascular obstruction leading to this syndrome can involve either large or small bowel and may be segmental or extensive. A history of symptoms or episodes suggestive of arrhythmia or heart failure should be sought.

Generalized crampy abdominal pain, tenderness, low-grade fever, mental apathy or agitation, abdominal distension, and bowel hypomotility may be accompanied by vomiting, anorexia, and mucoid or bloody diarrhea. Leukocytosis with a left shift is consistently present. The serum amylase level is elevated, since amylase also escapes from the bowel into the peritoneal cavity and is absorbed. Plain films of the abdomen show only ileus. When mesenteric occlusion is suspected, arteriography may establish the diagnosis and also permits intraarterial vasodilator perfusion before and during laparotomy.

Episodes of aseptic endotoxic peritonitis also have been reported among patients undergoing chronic peritoneal dialysis. These cases are due to contamination of dialysis fluid by preformed coliform endotoxin. Onset of symptoms occurs on the average 7 hours after initiation of dialysis with the contaminated fluids. Diffuse abdominal pain and rebound tenderness are the predominant findings; fever is present in only about half the patients. Discontinuation of dialysis usually relieves the pain promptly, and the symptoms rapidly clear.

FOREIGN BODIES. A foreign body may be deposited in the peritoneal cavity during an operative procedure (sponge or instrument inadvertently left behind) or may result from penetrating injuries, with the penetrating missile itself or material carried with it (clothing, earth) acting as a foreign body. Foreign bodies such as fish bones, wood splinters, needles, pins, and glass may perforate the gastrointestinal or genitourinary tracts to enter the peritoneal cavity.

The relative amounts of acute exudation and later fibrosis vary greatly depending on the nature of the foreign body and the degree of bacterial contamination which occurs in conjunction with it. A foreign body may lead to formation of an abscess with an interval course of fever, chills, and toxicity, and the eventual appearance of an intraabdominal mass. On the other hand, small foreign bodies, such as shrapnel, simply may be walled off by fibrous tissue and give rise to few if any significant clinical manifestations.

BARIUM. Barium may be spilled into the peritoneal cavity during radiologic investigation of perforated bowel disease. The barium is extremely irritating and sets up a granulomatous peritoneal reaction similar to that of talc (see below). Simultaneous bacterial contamination occurs in every case if the perforation is in the colon, and in many cases if the perforation is in the stomach or duodenum. The association of barium and bacteria is more deleterious than either alone. Viable bacteria tend to be caught up in the granulomatous peritoneal reaction to barium, resulting in persisting foci of sepsis. The presence of these microabscesses increases the density and number of adhesions. In addition, any one may act as a nidus for development of a larger abscess.

Some years ago, by means of a mail survey of approximately 100 teaching institutions, Zheutlin and colleagues collected 53 cases of peritoneal contamination by barium following rupture of the colon. They found a relatively high percentage of perforation in barium enema examinations performed via a colostomy, with use of an inflatable rectal balloon, or immediately after proctoscopic examination.

Because the barium crystals used for radiologic investigation are so fine, it is practically impossible to remove all spilled barium from the peritoneal cavity. The best therapy, as in other situations, is prevention. If a perforation is suspected and radiologic investigation is essential, the initial study should be made with soluble contrast media. If the soluble contrast examination shows no evidence of perforation, careful barium contrast examination may be undertaken. The examination should be terminated at the first sign of perforation and the residual barium within the gastrointestinal lumen aspirated to reduce further spill. The patient should undergo an urgent laparotomy to control the site of perforation by exteriorization or suture closure.

Nonoperative management of barium peritonitis recently has been suggested; it relies on administration of broad-spectrum antibiotics and vigorous fluid therapy. The rationale in recommending nonoperative management of barium peritonitis is that it is impossible to remove all the barium. However, the degree of peritonitis is related only in part to the barium present in the peritoneal cavity; the perforation through which the barium leaked also needs to be controlled. Therefore, laparotomy seems the more reasonable management for most patients suffering intraperitoneal rupture of the bowel and barium spill.

GRANULOMATOUS PERITONITIS

This group of diseases is characterized by a peritoneal reaction which includes formation of granulomas and is associated with a markedly increased incidence of adhesion formation compared with other forms of peritonitis.

TUBERCULOUS PERITONITIS. Formerly quite common, the incidence of tuberculous peritonitis has declined, as has the incidence of all forms of human tuberculosis over the past several decades. This now is a rare disease; it usually occurs in patients who are malnourished or who have cirrhosis. The primary focus from which secondary involvement of the peritoneal cavity occurs in tuberculous peritonitis may not be clinically apparent. Although nearly all patients dying with tuberculous peritonitis have a primary focus identified at autopsy, in only about a third of cases currently being seen clinically is the primary focus readily diagnosed. In cases in which the primary focus remains obscure, almost always it is later demonstrated to be in the lung. Most cases are due to reactivation of latent peritoneal tuberculosis which had been established by hematogenous spread from a pulmonary focus during an earlier episode of acute disease. In the past, the disease has been classified into wet and dry phases. The "wet" phase refers to the early, subacute, ascitic stage of the disease, while the "dry" phase refers to later resolution, during which dense adhesions are formed.

Clinically, tuberculous peritonitis is insidious, presenting with fever, anorexia, weakness, and weight loss. Ascites almost always is present, and more than half of affected patients have dull, diffuse abdominal pain. On examination, the abdomen is modestly tender, but the classically described "doughy abdomen" is rarely found today. Clinical manifestations of generalized tuberculous infection are seen in about one-third of patients, and include anorexia, weight loss, and night sweats.

Tuberculous organisms can be retrieved 80 percent of the time from ascitic fluid if more than 1 liter of fluid is cultured. The ascitic fluid has an increased protein concentration, lymphocytic pleocytosis, and a glucose concentration below 30 mg/dl. Blind peritoneal biopsy is positive in about 60 percent of cases. If these measures do not establish the diagnosis, peritoneoscopy and guided direct biopsy of the peritoneum are recommended. The peritoneoscopic appearance of tuberculous peritonitis is quite characteristic. Typical stalactite-like fibrinous masses hang from the parietal peritoneum in the lower part of the abdomen. A directed, percutaneous needle biopsy of a granulomatous lesion, as well as samples of peritoneal fluid for direct smear examination and injection into a guinea pig, is obtained. As a last resort, exploratory laparotomy may be undertaken to establish the diagnosis. If laparotomy is carried out, a peritoneal biopsy should be obtained; the placement of drains or the exteriorization of bowel should be avoided.

Tuberculous peritonitis, formerly frequently fatal as a manifestation of uncontrolled generalized tuberculosis, now is arrested in nearly all patients. Triple antituberculous drug therapy, instituted early in the course of the disease, is associated with a good prognosis. Chemotherapy should continue for at least 2 years after the patient becomes asymptomatic. Since tuberculous peritonitis may heal with formation of dense fibrous adhesions, patients suffering this disease always are liable to the future development of an intestinal obstruction. Treatment with prednisone during the initial few months of antituberculous drug therapy reduces the incidence of adhesion formation and the subsequent development of obstruction.

OTHER GRANULOMATOUS PERITONEAL INFECTIONS. These are excessively rare diseases and occur under special circumstances. The organisms involved may be *Candida* or *Histoplasma* (fungi), or amebas or *Strongyloides* (parasites). *Candida* peritonitis seems to be associated with prolonged administration of broad-spectrum antibiotics to extremely debilitated patients who also are receiving parenteral alimentation or who have a prosthetic cardiac valve. Amebic peritonitis usually follows rupture of a hepatic amebic abscess, but a few cases have been due to perforation of amebic colitis. The prognosis is grave, but operative debridement results in a better outcome than nonoperative management.

IATROGENIC GRANULOMATOUS PERITONITIS. Peritoneal inflammation, exudation, formation of granulomas, and healing by formation of dense adhesions all may follow contamination of the peritoneal cavity by glove lubricants (talc, lycopodium, mineral oil, cornstarch, rice starch), or cellulose fibers from disposable gauze pads, drapes, and gowns. The reaction, particularly that to rice starch, is largely a hypersensitivity response.

The clinical features include migratory abdominal pain, fever, physical signs of peritonitis and, often, the presence of an abdominal mass, all developing within 3 weeks after an otherwise uncomplicated abdominal operation. The surgical wound may appear normal or may be moderately indurated. Plain abdominal films are nonspecific. The total white blood cell count is normal; eosinophilia of 4 to 9 percent sometimes is identified.

Laparoscopy may be helpful in establishing the diagnosis. If recognized with assurance, reoperation should be avoided and corticosteroids administered. Eventually, the acute peritonitis resolves. If laparotomy is undertaken because the diagnosis is obscure, a thickened peritoneum studded by white nodules is found. Histologically, the nodules, which contain starch granules, are doubly refractile under polarized light and are surrounded by granulomatous foreign body inflammation.

The cornerstone of management of this problem is prevention. Current techniques of wiping and washing gloves do not remove all the starch from their surface. Nonetheless, gloves should be washed or wiped off before hands are put into the peritoneal cavity and care should be taken to avoid spillage of glove contents should a glove be torn during an operation. The search for an acceptable and risk-free glove lubricant continues. Sodium bicarbonate has been used successfully as a gloving agent, but requires special sterilization measures; silicones also have been suggested.

SPONTANEOUS (PRIMARY) PERITONITIS

Spontaneous, or primary, peritonitis is a diffuse bacterial peritonitis without any apparent intraabdominal source of infection. Although still uncommon, the incidence of spontaneous peritonitis seems to be increasing. The currently reported prevalence is 3 percent in hospitalized cirrhotics and 8 percent in ascitic cirrhotics in pre-coma or coma.

The spectrum of bacteria causing this syndrome and the population primarily affected have changed during the last decade or so. Formerly, this disease occurred primarily in children; today, adults more often are affected. Formerly, females developed spontaneous peritonitis four times as frequently as males; today, there is no differential sex incidence. Formerly, gram-positive organisms caused most of these infections; today, gram-negative bacteria predominate.

Children with nephrosis and adults with cirrhosis or systemic lupus are the populations primarily affected. It appears that impairment of body immunological defense mechanisms is related to development of spontaneous peritonitis. The mortality risk is of the order of 20 to 40 percent in cirrhotic adults but lower in children. The relevance of preexisting ascites is not clear; ascites certainly provides an ideal culture medium. Any abnormal fluid collection appears to be at risk to develop infection in patients who are constitutionally predisposed; both spontaneous empyema and pericarditis have been reported in association with spontaneous peritonitis. On the other hand, adult patients have been described who had no preceding ascites, and the great majority of patients who develop spontaneous peritonitis in childhood do not have ascites.

This form of peritonitis is a monomicrobial infection; i.e., there is only a single species of bacteria present, in contrast to the polymicrobial infection of typical suppurative peritonitis. Though pneumococci formerly were the most frequent infecting organisms, coliform organisms now are the chief pathogens, accounting for over half of cases. Streptococcal infections still occur but are uncommon. In an increasing number of current cases, no bacteria are recovered but high viral titers are found in the serum. The bacterial spectrum also is broadening, recent single cases due to *Hemophilus, Clostridia, Pasteurella,* and *Bacteroides* species having been recorded.

The route by which organisms are transmitted to the peritoneal cavity is not known. Evidence favoring transmural migration of bacteria from the intestine is derived from the fact that systemic endotoxemia and the presence of endotoxin in ascitic fluid can be demonstrated by limulus assay in many decompensated cirrhotics, even though no bacteria are present in the ascites and the patients do not have clinical evidence of peritonitis. Evidence favoring the hematogenous route stems from the frequent clinical association of spontaneous peritonitis with urinary tract infections harboring the same organism and from cases of simultaneous spontaneous empyema and pericarditis.

Clinical symptoms usually are of short duration in children; the onset of symptoms is more insidious in ascitic adults. Most patients complain of some abdominal pain and distension; vomiting, lethargy, and fever are more prominant in children. Diarrhea is usual in neonates but seldom seen in adults. Bowel sounds are variable. A brisk leukocytosis usually is present. No free air is seen on abdominal x-rays. All in all, the clinical picture may be quite desultory and never appears to be as severe as in suppurative peritonitis.

A peritoneal tap is the most useful diagnostic test. The ascitic fluid has the character of an "infected transudate," i.e., the protein content is not abnormally high, but the fluid does contain leukocytes. If more than 300 polymorphonuclear cells per cubic millimeter are seen, peritonitis of some variety is sure to be present. If the Gram stain shows gram-negative bacteria, the presence of a surgically correctable intraabdominal lesion cannot be excluded. If a Gram stain shows only gram-positive cocci, the presence of spontaneous peritonitis is possible; however, the fallacy of assuming that an apparent monomicrobial gram-positive infection always is spontaneous peritonitis is illustrated by a case reported by Dimond and Proctor in which pneumococcal peritonitis was secondary to rupture of an acute pneumococcal appendix.

Differentiation of truly spontaneous peritonitis, in which early operative intervention is unnecessary, from suppurative peritonitis, in which an early operation may be essential to a successful outcome, is the essential diagnostic exercise. Exploratory laparotomy should be undertaken, because, as a practical matter, in most cases the possibility of an intraabdominal lesion requiring surgical correction is sufficiently great and the relative risk of operation is sufficiently small. Little harm is done by a negative exploration in the presence of spontaneous peritonitis, and, in particular, the prognosis is not worsened. Only in a nephrotic child or a cirrhotic adult in advanced hepatic decompensation, in whom all diagnostic criteria for the presence of spontaneous peritonitis are present, should operation be withheld and antibiotic therapy alone undertaken.

Once the abdomen has been opened and the diagnosis of spontaneous peritonitis confirmed, a specimen of peritoneal exudate is obtained for Gram stain, culture, and sensitivity studies. Appendectomy, even in the presence of spontaneous peritonitis, does not increase morbidity or mortality risk and should be performed. Accomplishment of appendectomy will eliminate one source of diagnostic confusion, should recurrent episodes occur. Drains should not be placed because their presence retards resolution of the peritonitis.

OTHER FORMS OF PERITONITIS

SCLEROSING PERITONITIS (PRACTOLOL). During the past 4 years, a number of cases have been reported of patients who developed striking thickening of the visceral peritoneum weeks to months after treatment with the beta-blocking drug, practolol. The most frequent clinical presentation is with a typical small-bowel obstruction, often insidious in onset, associated with profound weight loss and with a prominent abdominal mass on physical examination. At laparotomy, the visceral peritoneum is greatly thickened and encases the small bowel, usually from the duodenojejunal flexure to the ileocecal valve. The operative findings are striking: the whole of the small bowel usually is caught up in a thick sac, which sometimes

can be lifted as a single mass from the peritoneal cavity. This agglomeration of small intestine produces the mass that is palpable preoperatively. Psoriasis-like skin lesions and conjunctivitis also have been reported to occur in association with administration of practolol.

OTHER DRUG-RELATED PERITONITIS. The sudden occurrence of severe acute abdominal symptoms as a manifestation of drug sensitivity is distinctly unusual. Isoniazid has been reported to cause such an acute syndrome, and erythromycin estolate has been reported on occasion to produce abdominal distress.

PERIODIC PERITONITIS. Recurrent episodes of abdominal pain, fever, and leukocytosis occur in certain population groups in and around the Mediterranean Basin, notably Armenians, Jews, and Arabs. The disease appears to be familial. The major point for the surgeon is that the episodes do not require laparotomy, so the diagnosis should be kept in mind if dealing with patients from the Levant. Laparotomy often is performed for the first episode, since an acute intraabdominal process requiring surgical cure cannot be ruled out. At operation, the peritoneal surfaces may be inflamed and there is free fluid, but smears and cultures reveal no bacteria. Even though it is normal, the appendix should be removed to eliminate the possibility of acute appendicitis in the differential diagnosis of future episodes. Colchicine is highly effective in preventing recurrent attacks, and, in fact, a favorable response to chronic administration of colchicine is a definitive diagnostic test.

INTRAABDOMINAL ABSCESSES

Intraabdominal abscesses are localized collections of pus walled off from the rest of the peritoneal cavity by inflammatory adhesions between the parietes, loops of bowel, other intraabdominal viscera, the mesenteries, or omentum. An abscess may be solitary or multiple and may be located within the peritoneal cavity proper, within a viscus, or in the adjacent retroperitoneum. Abscesses arise during resolution and healing of more generalized peritonitis, or during situations in which a perforation of the gastrointestinal or biliary tracts occurs which is successfully walled off in the acute state by peritoneal defense mechanisms. Abscesses within solid viscera usually arise following hematogenous or lymphatic dissemination of infection to these organs from a septic focus elsewhere in the body. Retroperitoneal abscesses typically arise as a consequence of primary infection or of inflammation of one of the retroperitoneal viscera followed by secondary bacterial contamination.

Resolution of peritonitis with formation of a pelvic or subphrenic abscess is a reflection of the anatomy of the peritoneal cavity (Fig. 34-3). The upper part of the abdomen is divided nearly in half by the vertebral column. Both the pelvis and the subphrenic spaces on either side form deep and dependent cavities into which infected material is directed by gravity. In addition, the suction effect of respiration tends to draw infected peritoneal fluid up under the diaphragm. In a clinical investigation conducted in patients

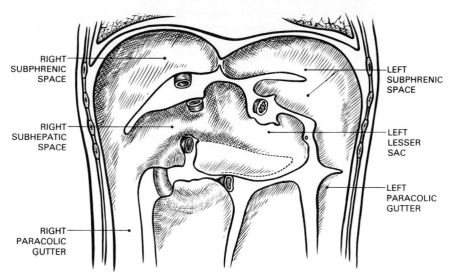

Fig. 34-3. The posterior attachments of the upper abdominal viscera subdivide the major right and left subphrenic spaces into a series of smaller spaces, as indicated by the labels.

undergoing cholecystectomy or appendectomy, Autio found that x-ray contrast media injected at the operative site became widely disseminated within a few hours after operation. Whether the contrast material originally had been placed in the upper or the lower part of the abdomen seemed to make little difference in its liability to spread; material was noted to move initially along the pericolic gutters in both directions and to collect primarily in the pelvis and in the subphrenic spaces.

Intraabdominal abscesses generally are polymicrobic (Table 34-2). Anaerobic organisms usually are the predominant flora, with bacteroides species and anaerobic streptococci being found most commonly. In part, the predominance of anaerobes in intraabdominal abscesses is

Table 34-2. BACTERIOLOGY OF
SUBPHRENIC ABSCESS

	Percent recovery of organisms	
	1950–1970 (60 patients)	1970–1975 (24 patients)
Aerobes		
E. coli	60	96
Streptococci	49	67
Staphylococci	31	8
Klebsiella	17	21
Proteus	11	38
Pseudomonas	8	8
Anaerobes		
Bacteroides spp.	11	83
Anaerobic cocci	0	50
Clostridia	6	50
Fusobacteria	0	38
Eubacteria	0	8

SOURCE: From Wang and Wilson, 1977.

related to the metabolic conditions existing within an abscess cavity, but also may be a reflection of the fact that aerobic organisms previously present in a more generalized peritoneal infection have been reduced in numbers or eradicated as a result of interactions of antibiotics and host defense mechanisms.

Symptoms of an intraabdominal abscess often are desultory, particularly early in the clinical course or with deep-seated infections. Recurring or persisting fever is seen in nearly all patients. Fever typically is intermittent or spiking in character at first, then becomes progressively more persistent as the abscess matures. The fever spikes, which often are accompanied by chills and tachycardia, are the result of transient episodes of bloodstream invasion from the abscess. On occasion, septicemia may be sufficiently persistent that septic shock ensues. Paralytic ileus, abdominal distension, and anorexia are frequent symptoms, and sometimes there is vomiting.

The intensity of symptoms may be modified by administration of antibiotics which tend to suppress the infection, although antibiotic therapy rarely cures an abscess once a phlegmonous infection has proceeded to the formation of fluid pus. Continued administration of antibiotics may only lead to a process which smolders for many weeks. Because continued administration of antibiotics may hamper diagnosis of an abscess, it often is preferable to discontinue antibiotic therapy when the presence of an intraabdominal abscess is suspected, and direct efforts toward establishing a precise diagnosis of the location of the abscess.

Abdominal tenderness and pain may be present with a visceral or midabdominal abscess, but are less commonly seen with subphrenic or retroperitoneal abscesses. Pain involving the anterior abdominal wall usually is absent with a pelvic abscess. When present, signs of pain and tenderness tend to be geographically related to the location of the abscess. Recurring or worsening jaundice also is an important clinical hallmark of the presence of an intraabdominal abscess.

Patients harboring an abscess invariably have leukocytosis accompanied by a left shift in the differential white cell count. The sedimentation rate is elevated, reflecting the presence of inflammation. Blood cultures will document septicemia and may identify one or several of the organisms involved in the abscess. Plain abdominal films may show localized gas bubbles or an air fluid level in the abscess. Barium contrast studies of the gastrointestinal tract may show organ displacement because of the abscess itself and, on occasion, may demonstrate a sinus tract or other extravasation which indicates the cause of the abscess. An intravenous pyelogram may indicate malfunction or displacement of genitourinary structures when the abscess is located in the retroperitoneum. Abdominal ultrasound scans are useful, particularly in thin patients, in localizing an abscess located in the upper part of the abdomen or retroperitoneum. Computer-assisted tomographic studies are most useful in patients who are moderately obese, since the presence of fat within the abdomen aids this examination in delineating the location of both normal and abnormal structures.

Diagnostic scans using gallium (^{67}Ga) also have been reported by some authors to be helpful in localizing an intraabdominal abscess. Radio-gallium collects and persists in areas of inflammation; in the presence of an intraabdominal abscess, the radioisotope tends to collect in the inflammatory membrane surrounding the abscess cavity. However, gallium scans are limited by the fact that the radioisotope also is excreted in the colon and the colon content must be evacuated before residual collections in the abdomen can be accurately localized. Because ileus so often accompanies an intraabdominal abscess, colonic emptying sometimes is incomplete or delayed, limiting the usefulness of this diagnostic test. Gallium scans, as is generally true of diagnostic scans directed at acute intraabdominal problems, have an indifferent record as regards accuracy, being subject to both false-positive and false-negative results in a significant proportion of cases.

The essential feature of surgical management of an intraabdominal abscess is to establish adequate drainage. Since many patients suffering an intraabdominal abscess are nutritionally depleted and septic, judicious, though urgent, preparation with attention to fluid resuscitation, parenteral nutrition, administration of antibiotics, and ap-

propriate monitoring measures should be instituted preoperatively. If the abscess is in contact with the abdominal parietes or the diaphragm, a direct and, insofar as possible, extraperitoneal approach is preferred. When the abscess is suspected clinically but cannot be accurately localized preoperatively, general abdominal exploration is needed. Abscesses in the lesser sac and in the midabdomen are best handled through transabdominal approaches. Abscesses in the pelvis, on the other hand, often can be drained through the rectum or vagina, obviating the need for an abdominal operation.

As the pyogenic membrane is encountered during exploration, confirmation of the presence of pus is obtained by needle aspiration. It is essential to obtain specimens of the abscess contents for Gram stain, culture, and sensitivity studies. All of the abscess contents should be evacuated by suction. The cavity should be thoroughly explored and all loculations within it broken down to create a single residual space. The cavity is irrigated and debrided of nonviable tissue. Multiple soft (Penrose) drains then should be brought from the abscess cavity to the exterior as directly and dependently as possible. If the abscess cavity is particularly large, or if thorough dependent drainage cannot be established, sump suction drains should be employed in addition to soft drains. Drains are left in place until external drainage stops or is clear; the drainage tract should then be irrigated, and a sinogram obtained to document collapse of the cavity before the drains are moved. It may take several weeks for a large cavity to become small enough to permit drains to be slowly advanced, allowing the drainage tract to seal as they are withdrawn.

Antibiotic therapy should be continued postoperatively, guided by the sensitivity studies obtained from the intraoperative specimen. Antibiotic administration should continue until all systemic signs of sepsis have been resolved and the patient's appetite and sense of well-being have returned. It is not, however, necessary to continue antibiotic therapy simply because drains remain in place.

Fig. 34-4. A combined liver-lung scan. Anterior view (*left*) suggests a defect laterally between the right lung and the liver. Lateral view (*right*) shows a posteriorly loculated abscess (arrow) with indentation of the liver and an increase in space between the liver and the lung. (*From White, Hayes, and Benfield, 1972.*)

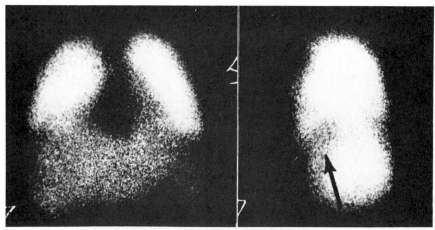

Recently there has been some recurrent enthusiasm for the management of suspected intraabdominal abscesses by antibiotic therapy without drainage. This form of therapy will be successful in a proportion of cases if instituted at the time when there is localized phlegmonous inflammation but before the appearance of fluid pus. But once a localized collection of pus is formed, it must be drained. If not, the risk of complications related to delayed rupture of the abscess cavity increases markedly. Such secondary abscess rupture may result in recurrent generalized peritonitis, dissection through the diaphragm with production of an empyema or bronchopleural fistula, rupture into an adjacent hollow or solid viscus with marked worsening of the clinical state of the patient, and, on occasion, necrosis of a major blood vessel with consequent rupture and exsanguination. Once an abscess forms, failure to drain only produces a prolonged course of illness that nearly always culminates in death of the patient.

Right Subphrenic Abscess

The right subphrenic space is only a potential space between the liver and the diaphragm, lying above the attachments of the coronary and triangular ligaments to the posterior parietes and extending anteriorly to the costal margin. Abscesses within this space are most frequently secondary to rupture of a hepatic abscess or to operations on the stomach or duodenum; less frequently, they are due to contamination of the subphrenic space during the course of a generalized peritonitis, and, least frequently, right subphrenic abscesses are related to operations on the appendix or biliary system. Because the potential space is so limited in vertical dimension, right subphrenic abscesses tend to be localized to only a portion of the total potential space, loculating either anteriorly or posteriorly.

Clinical signs and symptoms may be quite minimal. Pain is occasionally reported in the upper part of the abdomen or lower part of the chest, sometimes referred to the back or to the right shoulder. Chest x-rays show a pleural effusion or platelike atelectasis in the right lower lung in 9 out of 10 patients, and the diaphragm is elevated and shows reduced motion on sniffing in two out of three patients. An air fluid level can be demonstrated in about 25 percent of patients, and establishes the diagnosis. A combined liver and lung isotopic scan is an important diagnostic study with a high accuracy rate; it demonstrates an increase in space, which is occupied by the abscess, between the perfused lung, above, and the perfused liver, below (Fig. 34-4).

The surgical management of right subphrenic abscesses was confused for years by a misunderstanding of the relevant anatomy. Barnard (1907) had described the triangular and coronary ligaments of the liver as arising from the dome of the diaphragm. This error, perpetuated by surgical authors for the next half century, resulted in the recommendation that abscesses loculated in the posterior part of the right subphrenic space should be drained posteriorly through the bed of the twelfth rib. This anatomic error was corrected by Boyd, who pointed out that the coronary and triangular ligaments attach posteriorly rather than superi-

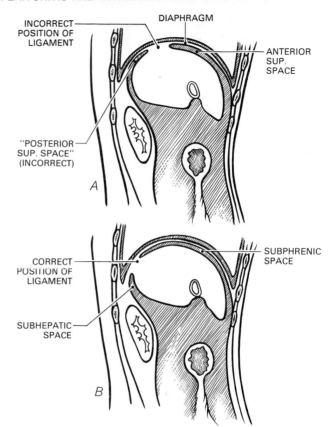

Fig. 34-5. *A.* The anatomic error that "created" a nonexistent postero superior subphrenic space was related to incorrect superior placement of the attachments of the liver (coronary and triangular ligaments) to the diaphragm. *B.* The correct anatomic relationships: the liver attaches posteriorly, separating the subphrenic from the subhepatic space.

orly (Fig. 34-5). It should be emphasized that abscesses in the right subphrenic space cannot be drained through a posterior approach unless the route of drainage transgresses the pleural space, a step which obviously is not desirable.

Right subphrenic abscesses preferably are drained using a lateral subcostal approach (Fig. 34-6). The incision is made beginning at the tip of the eleventh rib and carried obliquely anteriorly, paralleling the costal margin. The dissection is largely extraperitoneal until the abscess cavity, either anteriorly or posteriorly located, is approached. The advantage of the lateral approach is that it is possible to drain all the subphrenic and subhepatic spaces while avoiding contamination of the remainder of the peritoneal cavity.

Right Subhepatic Abscess

The right subhepatic space lies under the liver, is bounded inferiorly by the hepatic flexure and the transverse mesocolon, medially by the duodenum and hepatoduodenal ligament, and laterally by the body wall. The most posterior (deepest) part of this space is called *Morison's pouch*.

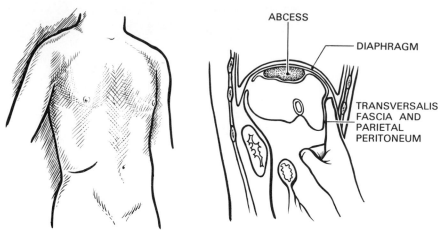

ABCESS

DIAPHRAGM

TRANSVERSALIS
FASCIA AND
PARIETAL
PERITONEUM

Fig. 34-6. Drainage of all subphrenic and subhepatic abscesses on the right side is done most easily through a lateral subcostal approach (DeCosse). *A.* The incision follows the costal margin anteriorly from the tip of the eleventh rib. *B.* The abscess is approached by blunt extraperitoneal dissection; the figure illustrates drainage of a high anterior subphrenic abscess; the arrows indicate the routes of approach to a posteriorly loculated subphrenic and to a subhepatic abscess. The principle of this approach also applies to drainage of a subphrenic abscess on the left side.

Gastric surgery, especially emergency operations for complications of ulcer disease, is the most common antecedent event. Biliary tract procedures are second in frequency. Appendicitis has now declined in importance and accounts for only 8 percent of cases of right subhepatic abscess. Complications of colonic surgery are increasing in importance. A right subhepatic abscess usually produces some tenderness in the right upper quadrant, and the patient may complain of pain, particularly exacerbated by coughing or similar activities which produce visceral motion in the region.

Halasz emphasized the serious problem of failure to recognize synchronous or multiple abscesses and recommended transperitoneal exploration for subphrenic abscess as preferable to more limited exploration. In his series of 43 patients, one-fourth had synchronous abscesses elsewhere in the abdomen. Failure to find and drain the concomitant abscess resulted in therapeutic failure. Our indications for use of a transabdominal exploration in the management of intraabdominal abscesses are limited to those situations in which the presence of an abscess in the midabdomen or in the lesser sac is suspected, and those situations in which the geographic location of the abscess is obscure. Whenever a well-localized pelvic, subphrenic, or subhepatic abscess is diagnosed, a direct approach for drainage should be made. The expectation is that the patient will promptly improve; should this not occur, consideration then should be given to transabdominal exploration to find and drain additional abscesses. Such a program will keep the risks of contamination of the general peritoneal cavity as a consequence of abscess drainage at a minimum, and yet should not result in excess mortality due to lingering, undrained, unrecognized abscesses.

Left Subphrenic Abscess

Formerly uncommon, these are now the commonest variety of upper abdominal abscess residual after peritonitis or leakage from a viscus. Left subphrenic abscesses follow splenectomy, particularly when the splenic fossa is drained; they also are a consequence of pancreatitis. The

physical signs are costal tenderness on the left, sometimes pain in the shoulder (Kehr's sign), the presence of a left pleural effusion, and limitation of diaphragmatic motion noted by x-ray. Unlike the subdiaphragmatic space on the right, which is divided by the liver into a suprahepatic (or subdiaphragmatic) space and a subhepatic space, on the left side all these areas are contiguous.

A left subhepatic abscess is best drained through a lateral extraserous approach, using fundamentally the same technique as recommended on the right side (Fig. 34-6). Alternatively, abscesses in the left subphrenic space may be drained posteriorly through the bed of the twelfth rib (Fig. 34-7). Via either route, the point at which the abscess is encountered during dissection is usually much deeper than might be expected. It is important in approaching a left subphrenic abscess to avoid injury to the spleen, should it still be present, and to ensure that the entire space has been explored by palpating the aorta, the esophagus and the region of the esophageal hiatus, the caudate lobe of the liver, and the anterior margin of the left lobe of the liver during exploration; such anatomic identification by palpation of the structures at the borders of the left subphrenic space will assure that no loculation of pus goes undrained to form a residual or recurrent abscess.

Lesser Sac Abscess

Technically, this is a variety of left subhepatic-subphrenic abscess, since the lesser peritoneal sac anatomically is a portion of the left subhepatic space. However, the anatomic features of this form of abscess, and the surgical maneuvers required for drainage, are distinctly different; hence its consideration as a separate entity. Lesser sac abscesses are unusual complications of diseases of the stomach, duodenum, or pancreas. The most common cause is a pancreatic abscess or a secondarily contaminated pancreatic pseudocyst which involves the lesser sac by direct extension. Perforation of a gastric ulcer or, less commonly, of a duodenal ulcer also may result in formation of a lesser sac abscess. Occasionally, rupture of an ulcerating malignant gastric tumor produces an abscess in the lesser sac.

Clinical diagnosis of a lesser-sac abscess can be extremely difficult, since much of this space is overlapped anteriorly by the liver. Tenderness to palpation in the midepigastrium usually is present but is such a nonspecific sign that it is not diagnostically very helpful. Ultrasonography is a most useful diagnostic test. Radiographic studies may show displacement of the stomach, but often appear quite normal; very occasionally, plain roentgenograms show fine gas bubbles within the lesser sac, indicative of the presence of purulent material.

Because of its anatomic location, extraperitoneal drainage of this variety of abscess is impossible. Lesser-sac abscesses should be approached through an upper abdominal incision, either vertical or transverse. If a transverse incision is chosen, it should be confined within the rectus sheath; rectus muscle should not be transected, only retracted. Drainage should be accomplished as dependently as possible. Theoretically, this would involve placement of drains inferior to the stomach, above the transverse mesocolon. However, it is usual for the lower portion of the lesser sac to be obliterated in cases of lesser-sac abscess, with the stomach densely adherent both to the transverse mesocolon and to the pancreas; attempts at dissection are

Fig. 34-7. Drainage of a left subphrenic abscess through the bed of the twelfth rib. Resecting the rib greatly improves exposure but is not essential; if the twelfth rib is not excised, the incision is carried deeply along its inferior margin. The pararenal space is entered and the dissection continued bluntly upward and medially on the undersurface of the diaphragm to locate and enter the abscess cavity.

fraught with considerable difficulty. The commonly utilized route of drainage is along the superior border of the antrum, the drains being exteriorized through the operative wound.

Interloop (Midabdominal) Abscess

These abscesses arise as loculations between loops of bowel, mesentery, the abdominal wall, and omentum. The right and left gutters also are common sites. The transverse mesocolon acts as a barrier to superior extension so that, as a group, interloop abscesses do not involve the upper part of the abdomen. Quite commonly, they may be associated with a simultaneous abscess in the pelvis.

Diagnosis of a midabdominal abscess is one of the most difficult exercises in abdominal surgery. There are no reliable symptoms or signs. Huge abscesses containing more than a liter of pus may occur without any significant physical findings. The surgeon must suspect the possible presence of an interloop abscess whenever the clinical context is appropriate, i.e., a preceding episode of peritonitis with incomplete clinical resolution and recurring signs of sepsis. Occasionally, abdominal films may show either edema in the wall of loops of bowel involved in the loculation, or separation or fixation of involved structures. Very occasionally an interloop abscess may produce a palpable, enlarging abdominal mass.

Midabdominal interloop abscesses are multiple more often than not. Because of the need for general exploration, and because extraserous drainage cannot be arranged in any case, transabdominal exploration is utilized. All abscesses should be opened, aspirated, and debrided. Unless the abscess cavity is in contact with the abdominal wall, insertion of drains is not indicated. Rather, reliance is placed on thorough debridement and irrigation of the peritoneal cavity with copious amounts of saline solution followed by antibiotic irrigation, as outlined above in the

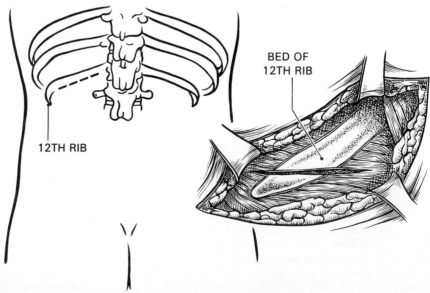

12TH RIB

BED OF 12TH RIB

management of suppurative peritonitis. Recurrence is common, and clinical evidence of such an event should be sought and treated vigorously.

Pelvic Abscess

These abscesses most often follow ruptured colonic diverticulum, pelvic inflammatory disease, ruptured appendix, or drainage into the pelvis during resolution of generalized peritonitis. Unless the abscess involves the anterior abdominal wall, few symptoms or physical signs are present on examination of the abdomen. The patient may complain of poorly localized, dull, lower abdominal pain. Irritation of the urinary system and the rectum produces symptoms of urgency and frequency or diarrhea and tenesmus.

Fortunately, localized purulent collections in the pelvis are the easiest of intraabdominal abscesses to diagnose. The abscess usually can be palpated directly by rectal or vaginal examination. The typical pelvic abscess bulges as a tender mass into the anterior rectal wall. It is important to distinguish between an inflammatory mass involving the pelvic organs and a true pelvic abscess. In general, pelvic inflammatory masses involving the fallopian tubes do not bulge into the rectum, and tend to become less tender and to resolve on serial examination, whereas a true pelvic abscess tends to enlarge and finally to rupture.

Drainage should be accomplished through either the rectum or the vagina. Incision for drainage should be delayed until formation of the pyogenic membrane has effectively excluded all of the small bowel and other intraabdominal viscera. If serial examinations have been done, readiness for drainage is apparent when the most prominent aspect of the abscess presenting vaginally or rectally begins to soften. Using a speculum or anoscope, the abscess should be exposed and the presence of pus confirmed by needle aspiration. The needle is left in place as a guide; sharp incision with a knife is made into the abscess cavity. The abscess cavity should be explored digitally, loculations broken down, and the cavity thoroughly irrigated. Drains are difficult to retain in a pelvic abscess cavity. To ensure continued drainage and obliteration of the cavity, daily dilations of the tract digitally or with an instrument should be done until the cavity becomes obliterated over the following few days.

Pancreatic Abscess

Acute pancreatitis is the antecedent cause of pancreatic abscess in the majority of cases. Secondary infection of a pancreatic pseudocyst is the only other important cause. Abdominal pain, nausea, vomiting, and swinging fever usually are present. Anterior abdominal tenderness may be present, although pain in the back is more common.

Pancreatic abscesses are polymicrobial in nature, the common organisms being aerobic representatives of the fecal flora, predominantly *E. coli* and aerobic hemolytic streptococci. Staphylococci usually are not involved in primary pancreatic abscesses but are frequently recovered

in those abscesses which follow inadvertent early abdominal exploration in the presence of pancreatitis.

Surgical drainage of a pancreatic abscess using large-bore sump suction and soft drains is the essential feature of therapy. This treatment should be supported by administration of appropriate antibiotics, fluids, and similar measures. The mortality is 26 percent with sump drainage; all alternative forms of treatment carry a higher mortality risk.

REFERENCES

Peritoneum

Allen, L., and Vogt, E.: Mechanism of Lymphatic Absorption from Serous Cavities, *Am J Physiol,* **119:**776, 1937.

Cascarano, J., Rubin, A. D., Chick, W. L., and Zweifach, B. W.: Metabolically Induced Permeability Changes across Mesothelium, *Am J Physiol,* **206:**373, 1964.

Courtice, F. C., and Simmonds, W. J.: Physiological Significance of Lymph Drainage of the Serous Cavities and Lung, *Physiol Rev,* **34:**419, 1954.

Raftery, A. T.: Regeneration of Parietal and Visceral Peritoneum. A Light Microscopical Study, *Br J Surg,* **60:**293, 1973.

———: Regeneration of Parietal and Visceral Peritoneum: An Electron Microscopical Study, *J Anat,* **115:**375, 1973.

General Responses in Peritonitis

Davis, J. H.: Current Concepts of Peritonitis, *Am Surg,* **33:**673, 1967.

Duff, J. H., Groves, A. C., McLean, A. P. H., LaPointe, E. R., and MacLean, L. D.: Defective Oxygen Consumption in Septic Shock, *Surg Gynecol Obstet,* **128:**1051, 1969.

Fry, D. E., Silver, B. B., Rink, R. D., and Flint, L. M.: Hepatic Mitochondrial Function in Intraperitoneal Sepsis, *Rev Surg,* **34:**214, 1977.

Kukral, J. C., Riveron, E., Tiffany, J. C., Vaitys, S., and Barrett, B.: Plasma Protein Metabolism in Patients with Acute Surgical Peritonitis, *Am J Surg,* **113:**173, 1967.

Renvall, S.: Peritoneal Reaction in Acute Appendicitis. A Biochemical Study, *Acta Chir Scand,* **142:**407, 1976.

Interactions of Bacteria and the Peritoneum

Altemeier, W. A.: The Pathogenicity of the Bacteria of Appendicitis Peritonitis, *Ann Surg,* **114:**158, 1941.

Bartlett, J. G., Miao, P. V. W., and Gorbach, S. L.: Empiric Treatment with Clindamycin and Gentamicin of Suspected Sepsis due to Anaerobic and Aerobic Bacteria, *J Infect Dis,* **135**(Suppl), 80, 1977.

Davis, J. H., and Yull, A. B.: Possible Toxic Factor in Abdominal Injury, *J Trauma,* **2:**291, 1962.

——— and ———: A Toxic Factor in Abdominal Injury, II. The Role of the Red Cell Component, *J Trauma,* **4:**84, 1964.

Filler, R. M., and Sleeman, H. K.: Pathogenesis of Peritonitis. I. The Effect of *Escherichia coli* and Hemoglobin on Peritoneal Absorption, *Surgery,* **61:**385, 1967.

Hau, T., Nelson, R. D., Fiegel, V. D., Levenson, R., and Simmons, R. L.: Mechanisms of the Adjuvant Action of Hemoglobin in Experimental Peritonitis. 2. Influence of Hemoglobin on

Human Leukocyte Chemotaxis in Vitro, *J Surg Res,* **22:**174, 1977.

Holland, J. W., Hill, E. O., and Altemeier, W. A.: Numbers and Types of Anaerobic Bacteria Isolated from Clinical Specimens since 1960, *J Clin Microbiol,* **5:**20, 1977.

Lorber, B., and Swenson, R. M.: The Bacteriology of Intra-abdominal Infections, *Surg Clin North Am,* **55:**1349, 1975.

Meleney, F. L.: Bacterial Synergism in Disease Processes, *Ann Surg,* **94:**961, 1931.

Nichols, R. L., Condon, R. E., Bentley, D. W., and Gorbach, S. L.: Ileal Microflora in Surgical Patients, *J Urol,* **105:**351, 1971.

———, Smith, J. W., and Balthazar, E. R.: Peritonitis and Intra-abdominal Abscess: An Experimental Model for the Evaluation of Human Disease, *J Surg Res,* accepted for publication, 1977.

Simmons, R. L., Diggs, J. W., and Sleeman, H. K.: Pathogenesis of Peritonitis. III. Local Adjuvant Action of Hemoglobin in Experimental *E. coli* Peritonitis, *Surgery,* **63:**810, 1968.

Sleeman, H. K., Diggs, J. W., Hendry, W. S., and Filler, R. M.: Pathogenesis of Peritonitis. II. The Effect of *Escherichia coli* and Adjuvant Substances on Peritoneal Absorption, *Surgery,* **61:**393, 1967.

Stone, H. H., Kolb, L. D., and Geheber, C. E.: Incidence and Significance of Intraperitoneal Anaerobic Bacteria, *Ann Surg,* **181:**705, 1975.

Weinstein, W. M., Onderdonk, A. B., Bartlett, J. G., and Gorbach, S. L.: Experimental Intra-abdominal Abscesses in Rats: Development of an Experimental Model, *Infect Immunol,* **10:**1250, 1974.

Pathophysiology of Sepsis

Alexander, J. W., McClellan, M. A., Ogle, C. K., and Ogle, J. D.: Consumptive Opsoninopathy: Possible Pathogenesis in Lethal and Opportunistic Infections, *Ann Surg,* **184:**672, 1976.

Beaufils, M., Morel-Maroger, L., Sraer, J.-D., Kanfer, A., Kourilsky, O., and Richet, G.: Acute Renal Failure of Glomerular Origin during Visceral Abscesses, *N Engl J Med,* **295:**185, 1976.

Berk, J. L., Hagen, J. F., and Dunn, J. M.: The Role of Beta-adrenergic Blockade in the Treatment of Septic Shock, *Surg Gynecol Obstet,* **130:**1025, 1970.

Clowes, G. H. A., Jr., Hirsch, E., Williams, L., Kwasnik, E., O'Donnell, T. F., Cuevas, P., Saini, V. K., Moradi, I., Farizan, M., Saravis, C., Stone, M., and Kuffler, J.: Septic Lung and Shock Lung in Man, *Ann Surg,* **181:**681, 1975.

———, Vucinic, M., and Weidner, M. G.: Circulatory and Metabolic Alterations Associated with Survival or Death in Peritonitis: Clinical Analysis of 25 Cases, *Ann Surg,* **163:**866, 1966.

Hill, H. R., Gerrard, J. M., Hogan, N. A., and Quie, P. G.: Hyperactivity of Neutrophil Leukotactic Responses during Active Bacterial Infection, *J Clin Invest,* **53:**996, 1974.

Hinshaw, L. B., Benjamin, B., Holmes, D. D., Beller, B., Archer, L. T., Coalson, J. J., and Whitsett, T.: Responses of the Baboon to Live *Escherichia coli* organisms and Endotoxin, *Surg Gynecol Obstet,* **145:**1, 1977.

Holcroft, J. W., Blaisdell, F. W., Trunkey, D. D., and Lim, R. C.: Intravascular Coagulation and Pulmonary Edema in the Septic Baboon, *J Surg Res,* **22:**209, 1977.

MacLean, L. D., Mulligan, W. G., McLean, A. P. H., and Duff,

J. H.: Patterns of Septic Shock in Man—a Detailed Study of 56 Patients, *Ann Surg,* **166:**543, 1967.

Meakins, J. L., Pietsch, J. B., Bubenrek, O., Kelly, R., Rode, H., Gordon, J., and MacLean, L. D.: Delayed Hypersensitivity: Indicator of Acquired Failure of Host Defenses in Sepsis and Trauma, *Ann Surg,* **186:**241, 1977.

Ollodat, R. M., Hawthorne, I., and Altar, S.: Studies in Experimental Endotoxemia in Man, *Am J Surg,* **113:**599, 1967.

Postel, J., and Schloerb, P.: Metabolic Effects of Experimental Bacteremia, *Ann Surg,* **185:**475, 1977.

Schumer, W., Das Gupta, T. K., Moss, G. S., and Nyhus, L. M.: Effect of Endotoxemia on Liver Cell Mitochondria in Man, *Ann Surg,* **171:**875, 1970.

Skillman, J. J., Bushnell, L. S., and Hedley-Whyte, J.: Peritonitis and Respiratory Failure after Abdominal Operations, *Ann Surg,* **170:**122, 1969.

Management of Suppurative Peritonitis

Altemeier, W. A.: The Cause of the Odor of Peritonitis Pus, *Ann Surg,* **107:**634, 1938.

Aune, S., and Notman, N. E.: Diffuse Peritonitis Treated with Continuous Peritoneal Lavage, *Acta Chir Scand,* **136:**401, 1970.

Burnett, W. E., Brown, G. R., Jr., Rosemond, G. P., Caswell, H. T., Buchor, R. B., and Tyson, R. R.: The Treatment of Peritonitis Using Peritoneal Lavage, *Ann Surg,* **145:**675, 1957.

Condon, R. E.: Rational Use of Prophylactic Antibiotics in Gastrointestinal Surgery, *Surg Clin North Am,* **55:**1309, 1975.

———: Management of the Acute Complications of Diverticular Disease: Peritonitis and Septicemia, *Dis Colon Rectum,* **19:**296, 1976.

Fowler, R.: A Controlled Trial of Intraperitoneal Cephaloridine Administration in Peritonitis, *J Pediatr Surg,* **10:**43, 1975.

Ger, R., Salazar, C., and Stratford, F.: Prognostic Factors in Generalized Peritonitis, *J R Coll Surg (Edinb),* **21:**173, 1976.

Halasz, N. A.: Wound Infection and Topical Antibiotics: The Surgeon's Dilemma, *Arch Surg,* **112:**1240, 1977.

Holcroft, J. W., Trunkey, D. D., and Carpenter, M. A.: Sepsis in the Baboon: Factors Affecting Resuscitation and Pulmonary Edema in Animals Resuscitated with Ringer's Lactate versus Plasmanate, *J Trauma,* **17:**600, 1977.

Hudspeth, A. S.: Radical Surgical Debridement in the Treatment of Advanced Generalized Bacterial Peritonitis, *Arch Surg,* **110:**1233, 1975.

Hunt, J. A.: An Assessment of Antibiotic Peritoneal Lavage in the Treatment of Severe Bacterial Peritonitis, *S Afr J Surg,* **14:**31, 1976.

Moss, G. S., Das Gupta, T. K., Newson, B., and Nyhus, L. M.: The Effect of Saline Solution Resuscitation on Pulmonary Sodium and Water Distribution, *Surg Gynecol Obstet,* **136:**934, 1973.

Nahrwold, D. L., and Demuth, W. E.: Diverticulitis with Perforation into the Peritoneal Cavity, *Ann Surg,* **185:**80, 1977.

Nelson, J. L., Kuzman, J. H., and Cohn, I., Jr.: Intraperitoneal Lavage and Kanamycin for the Contaminated Abdomen, *Surg Clin North Am,* **55:**1391, 1975.

Noon, G. P., Beall, A. C., Jr., Jordan, G. L., Jr., Riggs, S., and DeBakey, M. E.: Clinical Evaluation of Peritoneal Irrigation with Antibiotic Solution, *Surgery,* **62:**73, 1967.

Peloso, O. A., Floyd, V. T., and Wilkinson, L. H.: Treatment of

Peritonitis with Continuous Postoperative Peritoneal Lavage Using Cephalothin, *Am J Surg,* **126:**742, 1973.

Price, J.: Surgical Intervention in Cases of General Peritonitis from Typhoid Fever and Acute Gonococcus Infection, *Am Med,* **9:**769, 1905.

Robin, E. D., Cross, C. E., and Zelis, R.: Pulmonary Edema, *N Engl J Med,* **288:**239, 1973.

Schumer, W.: Steroids in the Treatment of Clinical Septic Shock, *Ann Surg,* **184:**333, 1976.

Smith, I. M., Kennedy, L. R., Regne-Karlsson, M. H., Johnson, V. L., and Burmeister, L. F.: Adrenergic Mechanisms in Infection. III. α and β-Receptor Blocking Agents in Treatment, *Am J Clin Nutr,* **30:**1285, 1977.

Torek, F.: The Treatment of Diffuse Suppurative Peritonitis following Appendicitis, *Med Rec,* **70:**849, 1906.

Tullis, J. L.: Albumin 1. Background and Use, *JAMA,* **237:**355, 1977.

Virgilio, R. W., Smith, D. E., Rice, C. L., Hobelmann, C. L., Zarins, C. K., James, D. R., and Peters, R. M.: Effect of Colloid Osmotic Pressure and Capillary Wedge Pressure on Intrapulmonary Shunt, *Surg Forum,* **27:**168, 1976.

Aseptic (Chemical) Peritonitis

Carter, R., and Gosney, W. G.: Abdominal Apoplexy: Report of 6 Cases and Review of the Literature, *Am J Surg,* **111:**388, 1966.

Cochran, D. Q., Almond, C. H., and Shucart, W. A.: An Experimental Study of the Effects of Barium and Intestinal Contents on the Peritoneal Cavity, *Am J Roentgenol,* **89:**883, 1963.

Dale, G., and Solheim, K.: Bile Peritonitis in Acute Cholecystitis, *Acta Chir Scand,* **141:**746, 1975.

Dinner, M.: Biliary Peritonitis due to Idiopathic Perforation of the Common Bile Duct, *S Afr J Surg,* **13:**207, 1975.

Gardiner, H., and Miller, R. E.: Barium Peritonitis, *Am J Surg,* **125:**350, 1973.

Garfinkle, S. E., Chiu, G. W., Cohen, S. E., and Wolfman, E. F., Jr.: Spontaneous Perforation of the Neurogenic Urinary Bladder, *West J Med,* **124:**64, 1976.

Hamilton, J. E., and Harbrecht, P. J.: Growing Indications for Vagotomy in Perforated Peptic Ulcer, *Surg Gynecol Obstet,* **124:**61, 1967.

Kent, S. J., and Menzies-Gow, N.: Biliary Peritonitis without Perforation of the Gallbladder in Acute Cholecystitis, *Br J Surg,* **61:**960, 1974.

Krizek, T. J., and Davis, J. H.: Acute Chylous Peritonitis, *Arch Surg,* **91:**253, 1965.

Michas, C. A., Pollack, E. W., and Wolfman, E. A., Jr.: Hemoperitoneum due to Spontaneous Gastroepiploic Artery Rupture, *JAMA,* **237:**2526, 1977.

Moore, T. C.: Massive Bile Peritonitis in Infancy due to Spontaneous Bile Duct Perforation with Portal Vein Occlusion, *J Pediatr Surg,* **10:**537, 1975.

Nahrwold, D. L., Isch, J. H., Benner, E. A., and Miller, R. E.: Effect of Fluid Administration and Operations on Mortality Rate in Barium Peritonitis, *Surgery,* **70:**778, 1971.

Westfall, R. H., Nelson, R. H., and Musselman, M. M.: Barium Peritonitis, *Am J Surg,* **112:**760 1966.

Zheutlin, N., Lasser, E. C., and Rigler, L. G.: Clinical Studies on Effect of Barium in the Peritoneal Cavity following Rupture of the Colon, *Surgery,* **32:**967, 1952.

Granulomatous Peritonitis

Bayer, A. S., Blumenkrantz, M. J., Montgomerie, J. Z., Galpin, J. E., Coburn, J. W., and Guze, L. B.: Candida Peritonitis. Report of 22 Cases and Review of the English Literature, *Am J Med,* **61:**832, 1976.

Cromartie, R. S., III: Tuberculous Peritonitis, *Surg Gynecol Obstet,* **144:**876, 1977.

Dimmick, J. E., Bove, K. E., McAdams, A. T., and Benzing, G., III,: Fiber Embolization—A Hazard of Cardiac Surgery and Catheterization, *N Engl J Med,* **292:**685, 1975.

French, M. L. V., Ritter, M. A., Eitzen, H. E., and Hart, J. B.: Microbial Evaluation of Reusable and Disposable Laparotomy Sponges, *Surg Gynecol Obstet,* **137:**465, 1973.

Lintermans, J. P.: Fatal Peritonitis, an Unusual Complication of *Strongyloides stercoralis* Infestation, *Clin Pediatr (Phila),* **14:**947, 1975.

Monga, N. K., Sood, S., Kaushik, S. P., Sachdeva, H. S., Sood, K. C., and Datta, D. V.: Amebic Peritonitis, *Am J Gastroenterol,* **66:**366, 1976.

Singh, M. M., Bhargava, A. N., and Jain, K. P.: Tuberculous Peritonitis: An Evaluation of Pathogenic Mechanisms, Diagnostic Procedures and Therapeutic Measure, *N Engl J Med,* **281:**1091, 1969.

Sturdy, J. H., Baird, R. M., and Gerein, A. N.: Surgical Sponges: A Cause of Granuloma and Adhesion Formation, *Ann Surg,* **165:**128, 1967.

Tinker, M. A., Burdman, D., Deysine, M., Teicher, I., Platt, N., and Aufses, A. H., Jr.: Granulomatous Peritonitis due to Cellulose Fibers from Disposable Surgical Fabrics: Laboratory Investigation and Clinical Implications, *Ann Surg,* **180:**831, 1974.

Warshaw, A. L.: Management of Starch Peritonitis without the Unnecessary Second Operation, *Surgery,* **73:**681, 1973.

Spontaneous (Primary) Peritonitis

Brown, R. L., and Peter, G.: Clostridial Spontaneous Peritonitis, *JAMA,* **236:**2095, 1976.

Conn, H. O., and Fessel, J. M.: Spontaneous Bacterial Peritonitis in Cirrhosis, *Medicine,* **50:**161, 1971.

Correia, J. P., and Conn, H. O.: Spontaneous Bacterial Peritonitis in Cirrhosis: Endemic or Epidemic?, *Med Clin North Am,* **59:**963, 1975.

Curry, N., McCallum, R. W., and Guth, P. H.: Spontaneous Peritonitis in Cirrhosis Ascites: A Decade of Experience, *Am J Dig Dis,* **19:**685, 1974.

Dimond, M., and Proctor, H. J.: Spontaneous Pneumococcal Appendicitis, Peritonitis, and Meningitis, *Arch Surg,* **111:**888, 1976.

Flaum, M. A.: Spontaneous Bacterial Empyema in Cirrhosis, *Gastroenterology,* **70:**416, 1976.

Fowler, R.: Primary Peritonitis: Changing Aspects, 1956–1970, *Aust Paediatr J,* **7:**73, 1971.

Gerding, D. N., Khan, M. Y., Ewing, J. W., and Hall, W. H.: *Pasteurella multocida* Peritonitis in Hepatic Cirrhosis with Ascites, *Gastroenterology,* **70:**413, 1976.

McDougal, W. S., Izant, R. J., Jr., and Zollinger, R. M., Jr.: Primary Peritonitis in Infancy and Childhood, *Ann Surg,* **181:**310, 1975.

Murray, H. W., and Marks, S. J.: Spontaneous Bacterial Empyema, Pericarditis, and Peritonitis in Cirrhosis, *Gastroenterology,* **72:**772, 1977.

Rubin, H. M., Balu, E. B., and Michaels, R. H.: *Hemophilus* and Pneumococcal Peritonitis in Children with the Nephrotic Syndrome, *Pediatrics,* **56:**598, 1975.

Taraok, S. O. K., Moroi, T., Ikeuchi, T., Suyama, T., Endo, O., and Fukushima, K.: Detection of Endotoxin in Plasma and Ascitic Fluid of Patients with Cirrhosis: Its Clinical Significance, *Gastroenterology,* **73:**539, 1977.

Targan, S. R., Chow, A. W., and Guze, L. B.: Spontaneous Peritonitis of Cirrhosis due to *Campylobacter fetus, Gastroenterology,* **71:**311, 1976.

————, ————, and ————: Role of Anaerobic Bacteria in Spontaneous Peritonitis of Cirrhosis: Report of Two Cases and Review of the Literature, *Am J Med,* **62:**397, 1977.

Other Forms of Peritonitis

Brown, P., Baddeley, H., Read, A. E., Davies, J. D., and McGarry, J.: Sclerosing Peritonitis, an Unusual Reaction to a Beta-Adrengeric-Blocking Drug (Practolol), *Lancet,* **2:**1477, 1974.

Eltringham, W. K., Espiner, H. J., Windsor, C. W., Griffiths, D. A., Davies, J. D., Baddeley, H., Read, A. E., and Blunt, R. J.: Sclerosing Peritonitis due to Practolol: A Report on 9 Cases and Their Surgical Management, *Br J Surg,* **64:**229, 1977.

Kvale, P. A., and Parks, R. D.: Acute Abdomen. An Unusual Reaction to Isoniazid, *Chest,* **68:**271, 1975.

Reimann, H. A.: Periodic Peritonitis—Heredity and Pathology. Report of Seventy-two Cases, *JAMA,* **154:**1254, 1954.

————: Colchicine for Periodic Peritonitis, *JAMA,* **231:**64, 1975.

Robinson, M. M.: Antibiotics Increase Incidence of Hepatitis, *JAMA,* **178:**188, 1961.

Intraabdominal Abscesses

Autio, V.: The Spread of Intraperitoneal Infection: Studies with Roentgen Contrast Medium, *Acta Chir Scand* **321**[Suppl]:5, 1964.

Barnard, H. L.: Address on Surgical Aspects of Subphrenic Abscess, *Br Med J,* **1:**371 and 429, 1908.

Boyd, D. P.: The Subphrenic Spaces and the Emperor's New Robes, *N Engl J Med,* **275:**911, 1966.

DeCosse, J. J., Poulin, T. L., Fox, P. S., and Condon, R. E.: Subphrenic Abscess, *Surg Gynecol Obstet,* **138:**841, 1974.

Halasz, N. A.: Subphrenic Abscesses: Myths and Facts, *JAMA,* **214:**724, 1970.

Laing, F. C., and Jacobs, R. P.: Value of Ultrasonography in the Detection of Retroperitoneal Inflammatory Masses, *Radiology,* **123:**169, 1977.

Monk, R. S., and Wilson, S. D.: The Abdominal Cavity: An Observation, *Am J Surg,* **111:**854, 1966.

Owens, B. J., III, and Hamit, H. F.: Pancreatic Abscess and Pseudocyst, *Arch Surg,* **112:**42, 1977.

Perez, J., Rivera, J. V., and Bermudez, R. H.: Peritoneal Localization of Gallium-67, *Radiology,* **123:**695, 1977.

Ransom, J. H. C., and Spencer, F. C.: Prevention, Diagnosis and Treatment of Pancreatic Abscess, *Surgery,* **82:**99, 1977.

Wang, S. M. S., and Wilson, S. D.: Subphrenic Abscess: The New Epidemiology, *Arch Surg,* **112:**934, 1977.

White, P. H., Hayes, M. H., and Benfield, J. R.: Combined Liver-Lung Scanning in the Management of Subdiaphragmatic Abscess, *Am J Surg,* **124:**143, 1972.

Chapter 35

Abdominal Wall, Omentum, Mesentery, and Retroperitoneum

by **James T. Adams**

ANTERIOR ABDOMINAL WALL

General Considerations

The abdominal parietes contain and protect the abdominal viscera. Topographically, the anterior abdominal wall is bounded by the flare of the costal margins and the xiphoid process of the sternum above and by the iliac crests, inguinal ligaments, and pubis below. The principal structures that comprise the anterior abdominal wall are the rectus, external and internal oblique, and transversus abdominis and lower intercostal muscles together with their enveloping fascial sheaths and aponeuroses. The linea alba, a tendinous raphe formed by a blending of the aponeuroses of the oblique and transversus muscles in the midline, divides the anterior abdominal wall into two parts and thus restricts the medial extension of pathologic processes that may arise within it. Deep to the muscles is the continuous transversalis fascia, considered to be the strongest layer of the abdominal wall, and peritoneum.

The blood supply is furnished by the superior and inferior epigastric, lower intercostal, lumbar, and iliac circumflex arteries. The venous drainage corresponds to the arteries. Lymphatics in the upper half of the abdominal wall drain to the axillary nodes and those in the lower abdomen to the inguinal and thence to the iliac nodes. Lymph flow around the umbilicus may also ascend around the ligamentum teres (obliterated umbilical vein) to reach the porta hepatis. The nerve supply is via the intercostal and upper lumbar nerves.

In addition to protecting the abdominal viscera, the muscles function as an accessory respiratory apparatus and also aid in defecation by increasing intraabdominal muscle pressure with contraction.

Surgical diseases of the anterior abdominal wall include (1) hernia, (2) infection, (3) primary and metastatic tumors of soft tissue and muscle, (4) rectus sheath hematoma, and (5) desmoid tumor. With the exception of rectus sheath hematoma and desmoid tumor, these conditions are covered in other chapters of this textbook.

Rectus Sheath Hematoma

Bleeding into the rectus sheath produces a clinical picture which may simulate the acute surgical abdomen. The bleeding is usually the result of rupture of the epigastric artery or veins rather than a primary tear of the rectus muscle fibers. In a review of the entity by Jones and Merendino in 1962, reports were found on only 250 patients. The condition is probably more common than this, however, since minor degrees of bleeding can occur without causing significant symptoms.

ANATOMY (Fig. 35-1). The rectus abdominis muscle is crossed by three transverse tendinous intersections on its anterior aspect, so that its contractile force is divided into

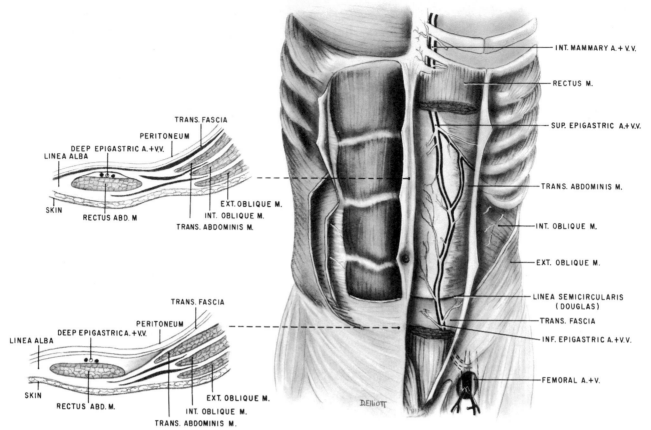

Fig. 35-1. Rectus abdominis muscle and rectus sheath. From the rib margin to a point midway between the umbilicus and the pubis (linea semicircularis of Douglas), the posterior sheath is made up of the posterior leaf of the internal oblique aponeurosis, the aponeurosis of the transversus abdominis muscle, and the transversalis fascia. Below this level, the posterior wall is formed by transversalis fascia alone. The deep epigastric arteries and veins course along the posterior surface of the rectus muscle so that below the linea semicircularis they are separated from the peritoneum by only transversalis fascia.

three parts. The lowermost part is the longest, and hence its shortening with contraction is the greatest. There may be a difference of as much as 18 cm in length between extreme contraction and relaxation.

A strong fascial sheath, made up of the aponeuroses of the oblique and transversus abdominis muscles and transversalis fascia, contains the muscle. Anteriorly, the sheath is complete throughout; however, midway between the umbilicus and the pubis, the posterior sheath ends, forming an arched border, the linea semicircularis (of Douglas). Cephalad to this level, the internal oblique aponeurosis splits into two leaves, one passing on either side of the rectus, while below it no such division takes place, and, together with the aponeurosis of the transversus abdominis, it passes anteriorly. This leaves the rectus muscle below the linea semicircularis separated from the abdominal viscera only by transversalis fascia and peritoneum. The anterior leaf of the sheath is adherent to the transverse tendons and also to the lateral and medial margins of the muscle, while posteriorly the rectus is free. As a consequence of this anatomic arrangement, when there is bleeding within the rectus sheath below the umbilicus, the free blood may lie against the peritoneum, producing irritation and pain suggesting an acute intraabdominal disease.

The blood supply to the rectus muscle is from the superior and inferior epigastric arteries. The superior epigastric enters the rectus sheath from above as a terminal branch of the internal mammary artery and passes caudad behind the muscle to anastomose with the larger inferior epigastric artery coming from below. The inferior epigastric artery, a branch of the external iliac artery, enters the rectus sheath just above the inguinal canal and courses upward along the posterior surface of the rectus muscle. Both arteries give off numerous muscular branches. Two veins accompany each artery. As the rectus muscle contracts, the epigastric vessels must glide beneath it to avoid injury.

ETIOLOGY. Rectus sheath hematoma may follow direct trauma to the epigastric blood vessels or occur spontaneously in association with several diseases. It has also been noted following a convulsive seizure. Spontaneous bleeding from the smaller muscular arteries has been reported in (1) infectious diseases, notably typhoid fever, (2) debilitating diseases, (3) collagen diseases, (4) blood dyscrasias such as hemophilia and leukemia, and (5) patients on anticoagulation therapy.

Frequently, however, bleeding occurs without obvious trauma or disease. In these patients the hematoma usually follows minor straining as in coughing or sneezing. Presumably the underlying factor is an inelasticity of the artery or vein which prevents the vessel from accommodating itself to the sudden marked variation in length which the rectus muscle undergoes during contraction and relaxation. Spontaneous rectus hematoma has also been described in pregnancy and in the puerperium. It is not known whether the hematoma is due to venous or arterial bleeding. However, stretching of the epigastric vessels by a distended abdomen during pregnancy or sudden relaxation after delivery are probably factors causing vessel injury. In the elderly, atheroma of an epigastric artery may predispose the vessel to rupture following minor exertion.

CLINICAL MANIFESTATIONS. Rectus sheath hematoma is three times more frequent in women than in men. The condition is rare in children and has a peak age incidence in the fifth decade. A prior history of trauma, sudden muscular exertion, generalized vascular disease, or anticoagulation suggests the diagnosis. Hematomas related to anticoagulation therapy usually become apparent 4 to 14 days after treatment is instituted. The first symptom is pain. This is sudden in onset, sharp, and progressively severe. The pain is felt in the side of the abdomen where the bleeding occurs and remains localized, since the hematoma in the rectus muscle is limited by the confines of its sheath. Usually this is the lower abdomen and more often on the right side. Anorexia, nausea but rarely vomiting, tachycardia, low-grade fever, and a moderate leukocytosis are frequent findings. With severe bleeding, signs of peripheral vascular collapse may develop. This is more apt to occur with bleeding below the linea semicircularis, where the peritoneum is only loosely adherent to the rectus muscle and thus cannot tampon the ruptured epigastric vessel. Tenderness and spasm are frequently present over the site of the hemorrhage. The bowel sounds are usually not altered. There may or may not be a palpable mass, depending on the extent of the bleeding. If present, the mass is tender, does not cross the midline, and remains palpable when the patient tenses the rectus muscle (Fothergill's sign). A bluish discoloration of the overlying skin is virtually diagnostic; however, this finding does not usually occur until 3 or 4 days after the patient is first seen.

The differential diagnosis may include almost every acute disease of the abdomen or pelvis. Notably, it has been mistaken for incarcerated interstitial hernia, acute appendicitis, acute cholecystitis, twisted ovarian cyst, diverticulitis, and ruptured aortic aneurysm. Teske, in a review of 100 cases, found that in only 17 percent was the correct diagnosis made preoperatively.

TREATMENT. If the correct diagnosis can be made and the rectus hematoma is small and not causing severe symptoms, the condition may be managed nonoperatively with bed rest and analgesics. Anticoagulants should be discontinued. It is rarely necessary to reverse a coagulation deficit when operation is not undertaken. Surgical intervention is necessary to rule out other, more serious diseases or to relieve symptoms of the hematoma. With a parame-

dian incision, the situation will become obvious as soon as the rectus sheath is opened and free blood is found. The hematoma may be diffuse throughout the rectus muscle or may be a localized clot. Bleeding arteries may or may not be present. Ideally, the hematoma is evacuated without entering the peritoneal cavity. Bleeding points are then ligated and the wound closed with or without drainage. The prognosis is dependent upon the underlying or concurrent disease but is generally good, and a full recovery can be anticipated. A poorer prognosis has been reported in pregnant patients in whom there is also a high fetal mortality.

Desmoid Tumor

Desmoid tumors are essentially benign, hard fibromas. It is probable, however, that they are not true neoplasms but an aggressive variant within a group of conditions referred to as "fibromatoses." The tumor is of aponeurotic origin and usually is found within or deep to the flat muscles of the anterior abdominal wall. Extraabdominal desmoid tumors involving skeletal muscles of the extremities, chest, and buttocks have also been reported but occur less frequently.

Desmoid tumors account for 3 to 4 percent of all tumefactions (7 percent of benign tumors) of the anterior abdominal wall. They usually occur in women in the childbearing age group, often after a recent gestation. Occasionally they are seen in children.

ETIOLOGY. The cause of the tumor is unknown. It has been thought to be the result of hemorrhage following muscular injury from external trauma or sustained during pregnancy or parturition. Desmoids have also been reported arising in laparotomy scars. However, microscopic evidence of previous trauma, such as hemosiderin pigmentation, is usually absent. The finding of a high assay of gonadotropic substance in the tumor has prompted a sex-linked concept in explaining its cause.

PATHOLOGY. Desmoids are benign tumors that have the malignant property of local invasiveness. They grow slowly but progressively and can reach huge proportions. Rarely, they may penetrate the abdominal cavity or retroperitoneum and may even invade the periosteum of the pelvic bones. With such aggressive growth, they may not be totally resectable. Occasionally the tumor undergoes malignant transformation to a low-grade fibrosarcoma, but metastases from desmoids have never been reported. A striking feature of the tumor is its tendency to recur following local excision. The incidence of local recurrence is particularly high after excision of extraabdominal desmoids.

Grossly, the tumor is circumscribed or diffusely infiltrating yet characteristically unencapsulated and it invades as well as compresses muscle. It has a hard rubbery consistency which cuts with a creaking sensation and has a glistening whitish pink color. The microscopic appearance varies from an acellular fibroma to that of a cellular, low-grade fibrosarcoma. Masses of fibrous tissue can be seen that infiltrate, compress, and often destroy muscle bundles. In this respect, the tumor differs from the more commonly occurring benign fibroma of soft tissue. The absence of mitotic figures and the well-differentiated fibrous tissue are features which differentiate it from the malignant fibrosarcoma.

CLINICAL MANIFESTATIONS. There are no special clinical features characteristic of desmoid tumors. They usually present as a painless, deeply situated mass that is solitary and may be fixed. Its deep location allows it to assume a large size before it is recognized. Usually the tumor is located in the lower abdomen and rarely crosses the midline. It must be differentiated from other tumors of soft tissue and muscle, particularly sarcomas.

TREATMENT. The ideal treatment of desmoid tumors is wide surgical excision. This often necessitates resection of a large portion of the abdominal wall including skin, muscle, and peritoneum. The resulting defect may require fascia, skin, or a sliding muscle graft for closure. The excision, however, should not sacrifice major blood vessels, nerves, or an extremity. Even though recurrences are frequent, they can still be successfully treated by reexcision. In spite of its tendency to recur, the tumor is rarely fatal. Drugs that affect the metabolism of cyclic 3′,5′-adenosine monophosphate, such as theophylline and chlorothiazide, have recently been shown to promote tumor shrinkage and may be worthy of use as an adjunct to surgery.

DISEASES OF THE OMENTUM

General Considerations

The greater omentum consists of a double sheet of flattened endothelium; between the folds the epiploic vessels, lymphatics, and nerves pass in areolar tissue enmeshed with a variable amount of fat. The structure hangs in a double fold, or sling, between the greater curvature of the stomach and the transverse colon. At birth, an agglutination of the two layers occurs, creating an apronlike shield overlying the intestinal coils. The right border attaches to the pylorus or first portion of the duodenum, while the left border forms the gastrosplenic ligament. The right side is usually longer and heavier and may possess tonguelike processes extending into the pelvis. Occasionally, accessory omenta exist attached to the main portion. The size of the greater omentum is related to the amount of fat which it contains, so that often it is huge in obese individuals and very thin and small in emaciated persons. The omentum in infants is usually underdeveloped and may be almost nonexistent. With growth of the individual, there is elongation and thickening of the organ due to the deposition of fat within its layers.

As a peritoneal fold, the omentum assumes the mechanical function of a mesentery, that is, the fixation of viscera and the transmission of a vascular supply. It is otherwise not a vital organ. Furthermore, it can be removed without appreciable disturbance to the individual.

It has long been held that the omentum possesses an inherent motility which allows it to seek out and arrest trouble that may arise within the peritoneal cavity. In this regard, it has been referred to as the "policeman of the abdomen." While it is true that the omentum is often found at the site of an intraabdominal pathologic condition, yet objective evidence, summarized by Rubin, shows that it has no spontaneous or ameboid activity and that displacement occurs as a result of intestinal peristalsis, diaphragmatic excursions, and postural changes of the individual. The areolar tissue is rich in macrophages which have been shown to rapidly remove injected bacteria or foreign particles. Draper and Johnston concluded that the usefulness of the omentum in inflammatory processes is related to its bactericidal and absorptive properties and also its ability to form adhesions.

Surgical diseases of the omentum include torsion, infarction, cysts, and solid tumors.

Torsion of the Omentum

Torsion of the omentum is a condition in which the organ twists on its long axis to an extent causing vascular compromise. This may vary from mild vascular constriction producing edema to complete strangulation leading to infarction and frank gangrene. For torsion to occur, two situations must exist: first, a redundant and mobile segment and, secondly, a fixed point around which the segment may twist.

ETIOLOGY. Omental torsion has been classified as primary or secondary. Primary, or idiopathic, omental torsion is relatively rare. It was first described by Eitel in 1899, and since then less than 200 cases have been reported in the literature. The cause is obscure. Leitner et al. group the causes of primary torsion into predisposing factors and precipitating factors. Among the suggested predisposing factors are a variety of anatomic variations including tonguelike projections from the free edge of the omentum, bifid omentum, accessory omentum, a large and bulky omentum with a narrow pedicle, and obesity associated with irregular distribution of fat within the organ. Venous redundancy relative to the omental arterial blood supply has also been cited as a predisposing factor. The omental veins are larger and more tortuous than the arteries, allowing venous kinking and thus offering a point of fixation around which twisting may occur. The higher incidence of right-sided omental torsion is related to the greater size and mobility of the right omentum.

Precipitating factors are those which cause displacement of the omentum. These include heavy exertion, sudden change in body position, coughing, straining, and hyperperistalsis with overeating. Primary omental torsion is always unipolar in that there is only one locus of fixation.

Secondary omental torsion is that which is associated with adhesions of the free end of the omentum to cysts, tumors, foci of intraabdominal inflammation, postsurgical wounds, or scarring, or to internal or external hernias. It is more common than the primary type and is usually bipolar; that is, torsion of the central portion occurs between two fixed points. About two-thirds of these cases are found in patients with hernias, usually of the inguinal variety. The precipitating factors which incite secondary torsion are the same as those for primary torsion.

PATHOLOGY. The omentum in both the primary and secondary varieties twists a variable number of turns around a pivotal point, usually in a clockwise direction (Fig. 35-2). Either the whole omentum or more often a small portion may undergo torsion. The right side is involved more frequently. Venous return is restricted, and the distal omentum becomes congested and edematous. Hemorrhagic extravasation results in a characteristic serosanguineous effusion into the peritoneal cavity. If the process is of sufficient duration, acute hemorrhagic infarction and eventual necrosis of the segment occur. If not excised, the mass becomes atrophied and fibrotic, and on rare occasions is autoamputated.

CLINICAL MANIFESTATIONS. The clinical features of primary and secondary omental torsion are similar. The condition usually occurs in the fourth or fifth decades of life. Males are affected twice as frequently as females. Pain is the initial and predominant symptom. The onset of pain is usually sudden, and it is constant with a gradual increase in severity. Occasionally the pain is first experienced in the periumbilical region or is generalized. However, invariably it becomes localized to the right side of the abdomen, usually the right lower quadrant. This is in keeping with the more frequent involvement of the right side of the omentum. Movement intensifies the pain. Nausea and vomiting occur in less than half the patients. There is a moderate leukocytosis and a fever which rarely exceeds a rise of 1°C. Tenderness is invariably present, and rebound tenderness and voluntary spasm are also frequent findings. A mass may be palpable if the involved omentum is sufficiently large.

The symptoms and signs are not usually sufficient to allow an accurate preoperative diagnosis. Secondary torsion of the hernial type, however, can be suspected if a tender mass is palpable in the groin. The clinical impressions, in order of frequency, are acute appendicitis, acute cholecystitis, and twisted ovarian cyst. Actually, a preoperative diagnosis is of academic interest only, since the clinical manifestations warrant exploration. The finding of free serosanguineous fluid at the time of laparotomy in the absence of a pathologic condition in the appendix, gallbladder, or pelvic organs should alert the surgeon to the possibility of omental torsion.

TREATMENT. Treatment consists of resection of the involved omentum. In patients with secondary torsion, the underlying etiologic condition, that is, hernia, cysts, adhesions, etc., should also be corrected. The operative mortality and morbidity are virtually nil.

Idiopathic Segmental Infarction of Omentum

Idiopathic segmental omental infarction is an acute vascular disturbance of the omentum of unknown cause. The criteria for diagnosis of this condition are that it not be accompanied by omental torsion, that there be no associated cardiovascular disease or local intraabdominal patho-

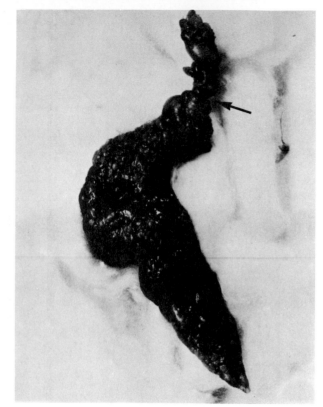

Fig. 35-2. Surgical specimen of primary torsion of the omentum. A small segment of normal-appearing omentum can be seen above the pivotal point (arrow), where it has twisted several times. The omentum below this is congested and hemorrhagic.

logic condition, and that there be no history of external abdominal trauma, situations which produce secondary omental infarction. The condition is rare, less than 70 cases having been reported.

ETIOLOGY AND PATHOLOGY. The condition is precipitated by thrombosis of omental veins secondary to endothelial injury. Halligan and Rabiah summarized the several proposed causes of endothelial damage and thrombosis. These include (1) stretching or primary rupture of the omental veins by a sudden increase in intraabdominal pressure as with coughing, sneezing, or lifting, especially after the ingestion of a heavy meal; (2) gravitational pull of an extremely fatty omentum on the omental veins, causing their rupture; and (3) an anatomic peculiarity of the venous drainage of the omentum which predisposes to thrombosis.

The right lower segment of the omentum, which is the most mobile and richest in fat, is the portion usually involved. The area of infarction may vary from 2 to 20 cm in its greatest diameter. Grossly, the involved segment is well demarcated, edematous, and hemorrhagic or gangrenous. It is usually closely adherent to the parietal peritoneum or adjacent abdominal viscera. A variable amount of serosanguineous fluid in the free peritoneal cavity is a constant finding. Microscopically, the picture is that of a hemorrhagic infarction with thrombosis of the omental veins and infiltration of the omentum with inflammatory cells.

CLINICAL MANIFESTATIONS. The majority of patients are young or middle-aged adults, and there is a 3:1 predilection for males. The clinical features are nonspecific. Most patients present with a gradual onset of abdominal pain which is steady and virtually always on the right side of the abdomen. Anorexia and nausea are frequent, but vomiting is rare. Diarrhea or constipation is unusual. There is always tenderness and often rebound tenderness over the region of infarction. Voluntary guarding and occasionally spasm are also common. The infarcted segment, if large enough, may be palpable. A slight fever (rarely over 38.5°C) and a moderate leukocytosis are usual.

TREATMENT. Treatment of this condition is resection of the infarcted area to prevent the possible complications of gangrene and adhesions. A correct preoperative diagnosis is unusual, and most patients are explored for acute appendicitis or acute cholecystitis. The finding of serosanguineous fluid in the abdomen and a normal appendix or gallbladder should make the surgeon suspect disease in the omentum. The operative mortality is nil.

Cysts of the Omentum

PATHOLOGY. Cysts of the omentum are rare. The pathogenesis of these lesions is unclear, but presumably most true cysts are caused by obstruction of lymphatic channels or by growth of congenitally misplaced lymphatic tissue that does not communicate with the vascular system. They contain serous fluid and may be unilocular or multilocular. The cysts have an endothelial lining similar to cystic lymphangiomas found elsewhere. Their size may vary from a few centimeters to over 30 cm in diameter. Dermoid cysts, which are very rare, are lined with squamous epithelium and may contain hair, teeth, and sebaceous material.

Pseudocysts of the omentum result from fat necrosis, trauma with hematoma, or foreign body reaction. These have a fibrous and inflammatory lining and usually contain cloudy or blood-tinged fluid.

CLINICAL MANIFESTATIONS. True omental cysts are discovered most frequently in children or young adults but have been reported in the aged. Small cysts are generally asymptomatic and discovered incidentally at laparotomy or at autopsy. Large cysts present as a palpable abdominal mass or produce diffuse abdominal swelling. These may cause symptoms of heaviness or pain or manifestations of possible complications of omental cysts such as torsion, infection, rupture, or intestinal obstruction. Complications are more frequent in children and often produce a clinical picture of an acute surgical condition of the abdomen. The uncomplicated omental cyst usually lies in the lower mid-abdomen and is freely movable, smooth, and nontender.

Plain roentgenograms sometimes show a circumscribed soft tissue haziness in the abdomen, or, following a barium meal, there may be displacement of intestinal loops with pressure on adjacent bowel. The presence of bone or teeth is diagnostic of dermoid cyst.

Differential diagnosis includes cysts and solid tumors of the mesentery, peritoneum, and retroperitoneal region. An absolute diagnosis can be made only at the time of exploratory surgical procedures. Treatment consists of local excision.

Solid Tumors of the Omentum

The most common solid tumor of the omentum is metastatic carcinoma, which generally involves the omentum by tumor implant. The primary source is usually the colon, stomach, pancreas, or ovaries. Frequently there is associated ascites, presumably from "weeping" of serous or blood-tinged fluid from the metastatic implants.

Primary solid tumors of the omentum are exceedingly rare. They may be benign or malignant. Stout et al. recorded only 24 seen over a 55-year period at a major tumor institution. Most are tumors of smooth muscle, and about one-third are malignant. Benign tumors consist of lipomas, leiomyomas, fibromas, and neurofibromas. The malignant tumors are leiomyosarcoma, fibrosarcoma, liposarcoma, and hemangiopericystomas. The malignant tumors spread by direct extension or tumor implants and kill by involvement of vital abdominal organs.

The only treatment is surgical excision. Primary malignant tumors are highly invasive and often require resection of adjacent organs as well as total omentectomy. The prognosis for these is very poor. Resection of benign tumors is curative, and recurrences have not been reported. Palliative omentectomy for metastatic tumor implants in the omentum has been suggested to control any associated ascites.

MESENTERY AND MESENTERIC CIRCULATION

Anatomy

The mesentery is essentially a reflection of the posterior parietal peritoneum onto the surface of the intestine, where it becomes visceral peritoneum. It connects the intestine to the posterior abdominal wall and carries blood vessels and nerves.

The mesentery proper serves primarily as a suspensory ligament of the jejunum and ileum. It is fan-shaped, its root extending downward and obliquely from the ligament of Treitz (duodenojejunal flexure) at the level of L_2 to the right sacroiliac articulation (ileocecal junction) (Fig. 35-3). The entire root is only about 6 in. long and allows free motion of the small intestine in any direction, limited only by the length of the mesentery. Within its two fused layers of peritoneum run the intestinal branches of the superior mesenteric artery and accompanying vein. It also contains lymph vessels, mesenteric lymph nodes, visceral nerve fibers, and a variable amount of adipose tissue.

Following the embryonic formation of a distinct intestinal loop, torsion of the loop takes place about the superior mesenteric artery. At about the third or fourth fetal month, posterior peritoneal fixation of the colon takes place. The leaves of the mesentery to the ascending colon fuse with

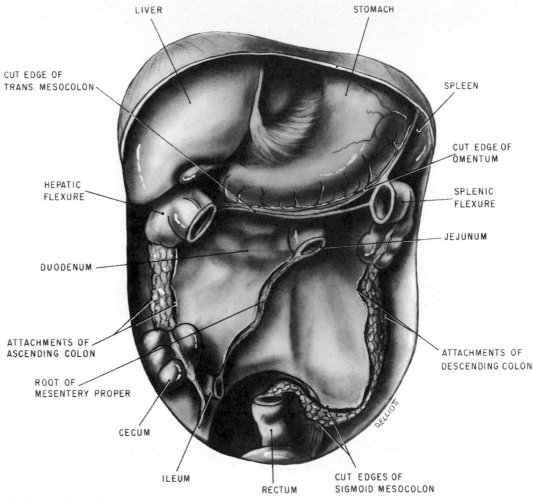

Fig. 35-3. Attachments of the mesenteries. The jejunum, ileum, and ascending, transverse, and descending colons have been removed.

the right parietal peritoneum, and those to the descending colon fuse with the left parietal peritoneum. The lateral posterior parietal peritoneum then passes directly from the abdominal wall over the ascending and descending colon respectively toward the midline and the root of the mesentery proper. For this reason, the mesentery to these portions of the large intestine is usually short or nonexistent. These fusions, however, form surgical cleavage plains allowing bloodless mobilization of the colon with its vascular supply. Within the embryonic mesentery to the ascending colon are the colonic arteries and veins from the superior mesenteric vessels, while those to the descending colon are derived from the inferior mesenteric vessels. On occasion, posterior fusion of the ascending or descending colon is incomplete or does not occur, leaving a well-developed mesentery and allowing free mobility of the bowel segment. This anomaly is more frequent with the right colon, thus predisposing to torsion with resulting intestinal obstruction.

The mesenteries of the transverse colon and sigmoid colon, in contrast to those of the ascending and descending colon, do not fuse with the posterior parietal peritoneum. These remain well developed and are referred to as the "transverse mesocolon" and "sigmoid mesocolon," respectively. The segment to the transverse colon extends obliquely across the posterior abdominal wall just below the pancreas, remaining fixed at the hepatic and splenic flexures of the bowel (Fig. 35-3). The fixation of the splenic flexure is higher than that of the hepatic flexure because of the presence of the liver on the right side. The mesocolon allows the transverse colon to hang over the small intestine. This sagging may be so marked that the transverse colon occasionally reaches the symphysis pubis. Within the transverse mesocolon run branches of the middle colic artery and accompanying vein. Fusion between the mesocolon and the undersurface of the greater omentum from the stomach offers stability which prevents the transverse colon from undergoing torsion.

The sigmoid mesocolon originates at the end of the descending colon in the left iliac fossa and has an inverted V-shape course (Fig. 35-3). It runs diagonally upward along the left iliac artery toward the aortic bifurcation and then bends directly downward into the pelvic fossa, where it is reflected off the rectum. It contains sigmoid vessels and branches of the superior hemorrhoidal vessels from the inferior mesenteric artery and vein. The length of the sigmoid mesocolon determines the location and mobility of the pelvic colon. If the sigmoid mesocolon is long, the bowel may cross the midline. Such a mobile pelvic colon may twist upon itself. The sigmoid colon is the most frequent site of torsion producing volvulus of the intestinal tract.

The lateral fixations of the ascending and descending colon and the superior origin of the transverse mesocolon serve to confine the small intestine within the midabdomen. The transverse mesocolon and greater omentum also restrict the small bowel from entering the upper abdomen to become adherent to inflammatory lesions of the stomach, duodenum, gallbladder, or liver.

Defects in the mesenteries are potential sites for internal hernia. Most defects are created inadvertently by the surgeon during the course of intraabdominal operations. On rare occasions congenital defects occur in areas of the mesentery that are thin and avascular. These are usually found in the mesenteries of the lower ileum, the sigmoid mesocolon, and the transverse mesocolon, the last through a wide avascular space just to the left of the middle colic artery (space of Riolan, Fig. 35-6).

The mesenteries share with the omenta bactericidal and absorptive properties as well as the ability to form adhesions. In this regard, they function to localize and combat intraperitoneal infection and to seal off intestinal perforations.

MESENTERIC CIRCULATION

In addition to serving as a system for the transport of nutriments, the mesenteric vascular bed is of major importance in the maintaining of bodily homeostasis. Under resting conditions, the splanchnic (visceral) vascular bed receives 25 to 30 percent of cardiac output and contains as much as one-third of total blood volume. It has been suggested that this reservoir of blood produces a mechanism for "autotransfusion" during periods of hypovolemia, when a relatively large volume of blood can be rapidly released into the circulation by active constriction of the splanchnic vessels. Control of the mesenteric vascular bed is primarily neural via sympathetic autonomic elements carried by the splanchnic nerves. These nerves accompany the celiac, superior mesenteric, and inferior mesenteric arteries which contain both alpha- and beta-adrenergic receptors. Stimulation of the splanchnic nerves produces vasoconstriction, with an increase in regional resistance. The mesenteric vasculature is also responsive to a number of pharmacological agents. Norepinephrine, an alpha-adrenergic stimulator, produces vasoconstriction, and epinephrine elicits a classic dose-dependent beta- or alpha-adrenergic response, low concentrations producing vasodilatation and higher concentrations producing vasoconstriction. Isoproterenol, a beta-adrenergic stimulator, effects a dilator response which can be blocked by propranolol. Tolazoline hydrochloride and papaverine hydro-

chloride elicit a direct vasodilatory effect, and the digitalis glycosides have been shown to produce mesenteric vasoconstriction, also presumably by a direct action on the mesenteric vasculature.

Knowledge of the anatomy of the mesenteric circulation is important in the performance of safe and adequate operations on the intestine and in the management of patients with occlusive mesenteric vascular disease and portal hypertension. In resections for malignant lesions, it is necessary to excise a wide segment of adjacent mesentery in order that real or potential sites of tumor spread to the mesenteric lymphatics and lymph nodes are removed.

ARTERIES. With the exception of the stomach and duodenum and the distal rectum, the arterial supply to the entire intestinal tract is derived from the superior and inferior mesenteric arteries.

The superior mesenteric artery arises from the aorta just below the celiac artery opposite the level of L_2. It passes behind the neck of the pancreas but in front of the uncinate process and crosses in front of the third portion of the duodenum to enter the root of the mesentery proper. The acute angle which the superior mesenteric artery makes at its origin from the aorta may compress the transverse portion of the duodenum between it and the aorta, causing partial intestinal obstruction, a condition referred to as the "superior mesenteric artery compression syndrome."

As the superior mesenteric artery continues downward between the two leaves of the mesentery, it gives off 12 or more major branches from its left side which supply the jejunum and ileum (Fig. 35-4). These jejunal and ileal arteries divide and then reunite within the mesentery to form groups, or arcades. Two to five such anastomotic arches are formed and allow collateral pathways for blood to reach the intestinal wall should occlusion of short arterial segments occur. The arcades become more numerous as the terminal ileum is reached. From the terminal arcades, straight branches (vasa recta) alternately pass to opposite sides of the jejunum and ileum. Within the intestinal wall, the vessels run parallel to the circular muscle coat and perpendicular to the direction of the lumen traversing successively the serous, muscular, and submucosal layers. Each of these terminal arteries supplies only 1 or 2 cm of bowel length. For this reason, they must be preserved as close to the cut margins of the intestine as is technically possible when performing a bowel resection to avoid necrosis and breakdown of the subsequent anastomosis. The terminal straight arteries do not anastomose until reaching the submucous plexuses, where their ramifications anastomose freely. This situation predisposes to serious compromise of the blood supply to the antimesenteric border of the intestine following segmental small bowel resection. Therefore, to ensure adequate circulation to the antimesenteric portion, it is customary to transect the small intestine obliquely rather than at a right angle (Fig. 35-5).

Arising from the right side of the superior mesenteric artery is the inferior pancreaticoduodenal artery and then successively, the middle colic, the right colic, and the ileo-

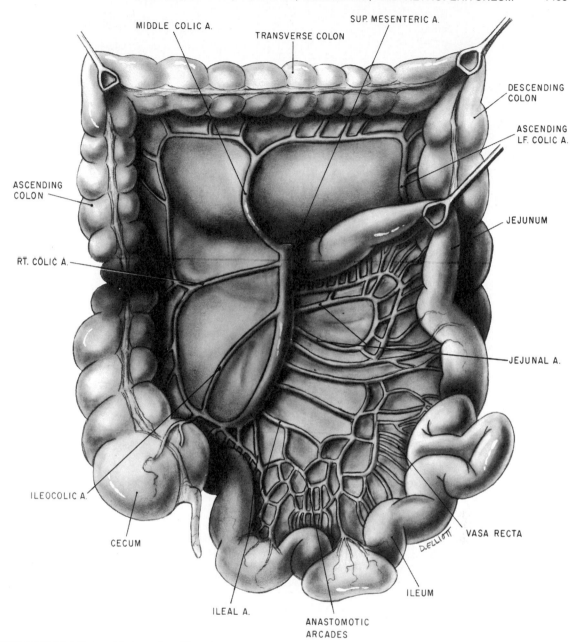

Fig. 35-4. Superior mesenteric artery and its branches. The artery supplies the distal duodenum, jejunum, ileum, ascending colon, and proximal two-thirds of the transverse colon.

colic arteries (Fig. 35-4). Except for the ileocolic artery, these vessels do not form anastomotic arcades until nearly reaching the bowel wall.

The middle colic artery arises below the pancreas, enters the transverse mesocolon, and passing to the right divides into a right and left branch. The right branch connects with the superior branch of the right colic artery and the left branch with the ascending branch of the left colic artery from the inferior mesenteric. It supplies the transverse colon. The location of the main arterial trunk to the right of the midline allows the left side of the transverse mesocolon to be opened through a relatively avascular area (space of Riolan) when performing a retrocolic gastrojejunal anastomosis.

The right colic artery arises just below the middle colic and passes to the right just behind the peritoneum. On reaching the mid-ascending colon, it divides into superior and inferior branches, which anastomose, close to the bowel wall, with branches from the middle colic and ileocolic arteries, respectively. The right colic artery supplies the ascending colon.

The ileocolic artery is the terminal branch of the superior mesenteric artery. It supplies the distal few inches of

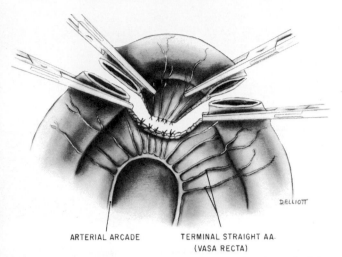

ARTERIAL ARCADE   TERMINAL STRAIGHT AA.
                              (VASA RECTA)

Fig. 35-5. Straight arteries (vasa recta) entering the wall of the small intestine perpendicular to the direction of its lumen. The arteries alternately pass to either side of the intestinal wall. In performing a segmental resection of the small intestine, transecting the bowel obliquely, as indicated, ensures an adequate blood supply to the antimesenteric border.

the ileum, the cecum, the appendix, and the lower portion of the ascending colon. It terminates by dividing into ascending and descending branches. The ascending branch anastomoses with the inferior branch of the right colic artery, while the descending branch forms secondary and tertiary arcades by anastomosing with terminal branches of the superior mesenteric artery within the mesentery proper. From these arcades arise the appendicular artery to the appendix, and cecal and ileal branches.

The superior mesenteric artery supplies the intestinal tract from the third portion of the duodenum to the midtransverse colon. Collaterals between the inferior pancreaticoduodenal artery and the superior pancreaticoduodenal artery from the gastroduodenal, a secondary branch of the celiac artery, enable the third part of the duodenum and proximal 4 or 5 in. of jejunum to survive when the superior mesenteric artery is occluded.

The inferior mesenteric artery supplies the left transverse colon, descending colon, sigmoid colon, and proximal part of the rectum. It arises from the anterior aorta opposite the body of the third lumbar vertebra and passes downward and to the left, entering the pelvis as the superior hemorrhoidal artery (Fig. 35-6). As it descends, it gives off the left colic and sigmoidal arteries. The left colic artery is the principal branch. It divides into ascending and descending limbs which anastomose with branches from the middle colic and sigmoid arteries, respectively. The sigmoid artery passes into the sigmoid mesocolon and divides into branches which anastomose with one another, forming several arcades. The lowest sigmoid arcade joins with arcades from the superior hemorrhoidal artery. The superior hemorrhoidal artery continues downward behind the rectum, where it communicates with branches from the middle and inferior hemorrhoidal arteries from the inter-

nal iliac artery, giving the rectum a dual source of arterial supply.

The anastomoses between primary branches of the superior and inferior mesenteric arteries form an arcade which passes along the margin of the colon and is referred to as the "marginal artery of Drummond" (Fig. 35-6). It is situated about $\frac{1}{2}$ in. from the margin of the bowel and extends from the end of the ileum to the end of the sigmoid colon. Through its anastomoses, it is capable of supplying the bowel even though one of the major arteries is ligated.

VEINS. The venous drainage of the small intestine and colon is through tributaries of the inferior and superior mesenteric veins, which in turn ultimately terminate in the portal vein (Fig. 35-7). The portal circulation begins within the mucosa of the intestine. Small venules coalesce, and the confluent veins pass through the wall of the intestine, emerging alternately in a similar manner to that of the straight arteries entering the bowel wall. These then converge to form a system of venous arcades within the mesentery from which blood enters the main tributaries to the superior and inferior mesenteric veins.

The inferior mesenteric vein is a continuation of the superior hemorrhoidal vein. It passes upward to the left side of the inferior mesenteric artery, receiving tributaries which correspond in name and location to the branches of the artery. However, the main trunk of the vein does not accompany the artery but rather courses over the duodenojejunal flexure just lateral to the ligament of Treitz and, passing over the body of the pancreas, joins with the splenic vein (Figs. 35-6, 35-7). It drains the left side of the large intestine from the upper rectum to the left midtransverse colon. A plexus of anastomoses around the midrectum between the superior hemorrhoidal vein and the middle and inferior hemorrhoidal veins to the internal iliac veins form a collateral pathway between the portal and systemic circulation.

The superior mesenteric vein runs within the mesentery proper lateral to the superior mesenteric artery. It receives tributaries which accompany corresponding branches of the superior mesenteric artery and which drain the entire small intestine and right half of the colon. As it passes over the third portion of the duodenum and behind the neck of the pancreas, it receives the confluence of the inferior mesenteric and splenic veins to become the portal vein (see Chap. 30).

The venous drainage from the entire gastrointestinal tract passes through the liver via the portal circulation before returning to the heart. Together with the mesenteric lymphatics, it represents the sole means by which ingested food products find their way into the circulation. The normal portal venous pressure is between 12 and 15 cm of water; that within the inferior vena cava (systemic pressure) varies between a positive pressure of about 3 cm during the expiratory phase of respiration to a negative pressure of 1 to 3 cm during inspiration. Like the vena cava, the portal system does not contain valves, and therefore the blood can flow in the direction of reduced venous pressure.

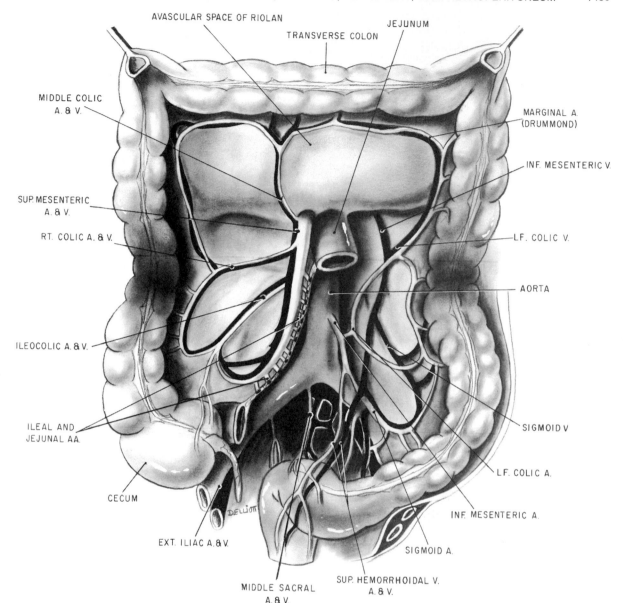

Fig. 35-6. Blood supply to the large bowel. An arterial arcade, formed by anastomoses between branches of the colic arteries, runs along the margin of the large intestine and is referred to as the *marginal artery of Drummond*. This vessel is the major collateral supplying blood to the colon when a main stem mesenteric or colic artery is occluded.

MESENTERIC LYMPHATICS AND LYMPH NODES. The lymph drainage of the small intestine and colon follow the course of the main blood vessels. Those accompanying the inferior mesenteric artery drain to periaortic nodes and thence to the superior mesenteric nodes before entering the cisterna chyli of the thoracic duct. Those accompanying branches of the superior mesenteric artery drain into the mesenteric glands within the mesentery proper, where they are closely related to the vascular arcades. The mesenteric nodes are distributed in three locations: (1) juxtaintestinal,

at the last anastomotic branch of the mesenteric arteries before they enter the intestines; (2) intermediate, in the region of the larger anastomosing branches; and (3) central, at the root of the mesentery near the origin of the main mesenteric artery. The nodes are more numerous in the right half of the mesentery, and they increase in size and number as they approach its root. These nodes are the usual site for mesenteric adenitis, tuberculosis, and other inflammatory as well as neoplastic conditions. From the mesenteric nodes, lymph drains into the superior mesenteric and celiac nodes and then to the thoracic duct.

Mesenteric Vascular Disease

Mesenteric vascular disease is not a single entity but rather a syndrome that includes (1) complete occlusion or

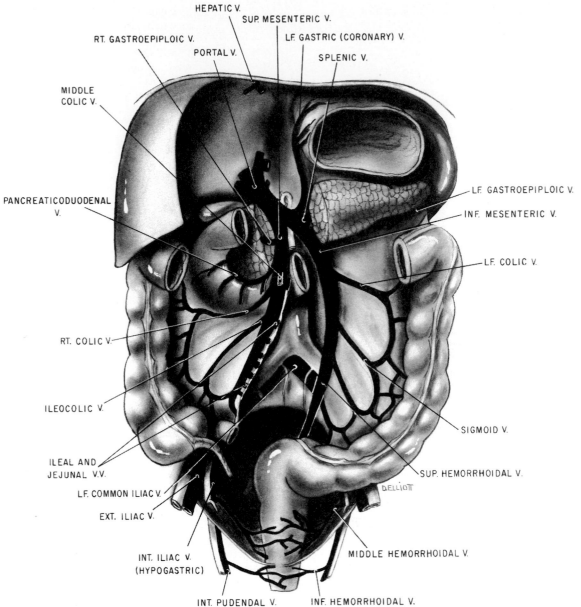

Fig. 35-7. Mesenteric (portal) venous circulation, showing the communication with the systemic circulation through the middle and inferior hemorrhoidal veins. A similar communication (not shown) exists between the left gastric vein and the azygos system of veins.

stenosis of mesenteric arteries by embolism, thrombosis, or obliterative disease; (2) thrombosis of mesenteric (portal) veins; (3) extraluminal obstruction of mesenteric arteries by aortic aneurysm, dissecting aneurysm, fibrous and ligamentous bands, or tumors; (4) spontaneous rupture of visceral blood vessels (abdominal apoplexy); and (5) traumatic injury to visceral vessels. These conditions produce vascular insufficiency or infarction of the affected intestine. Intestinal disease due to impaired circulation is relatively uncommon when compared to the more frequently occurring mechanical obstructions of the mesenteric vessels by adhesive bands, strangulated hernia, or intestinal volvulus.

Occlusions of the mesenteric arteries may be acute and complete (those due to emboli or thrombosis), gradual and partial (those due to obliterative arterial disease), or acute and complete superimposed upon a previously narrowed

or stenotic vessel. The superior mesenteric artery at its origin or close to the takeoff of its middle colic branch is the usual site of both acute and chronic mesenteric arterial occlusions. Complete occlusion of the inferior mesenteric artery usually produces symptoms only if there is compromise of collateral blood flow from the superior mesenteric or internal iliac (hypogastric) arteries. Clinically apparent venous occlusions are sudden and complete and invariably due to thrombosis. Partial mesenteric venous occlusion is usually due to external compression and is asymptomatic.

The relative incidence of mesenteric arterial as opposed to venous occlusions is not known. When intestinal infarction occurs, it is not unusual to find thrombosis of both sides of the splanchnic circulation at laparotomy or autopsy, since initial occlusion of one eventuates in clot formation in the other. Moreover, the clinical distinction between the two is often difficult. It has been variously estimated that 15 to 20 percent of all clinically significant mesenteric vascular accidents are due to primary venous thrombosis and approximately 50 percent to primary arterial occlusion. In the remaining cases, intestinal infarction occurs in the absence of major arterial or venous occlusion.

ACUTE OCCLUSION OF SUPERIOR MESENTERIC ARTERY

ETIOLOGY. Embolism. Sudden, complete occlusion of the superior mesenteric artery is due more often to an embolus than to thrombosis. The anatomic characteristics of this artery make it more susceptible than the inferior mesenteric artery to symptomatic embolic occlusion. Its main stem leaves the aorta at an acute angle which runs parallel to the aorta, thus maintaining a straight-line connection with the heart. Moreover, the smaller orifice of the inferior mesenteric artery allows only small emboli to enter it, and when this occurs, lodgment is more likely at a site beyond the division of the artery into its major branches.

Most emboli come from the heart, either from a mural thrombus in a patient with early postcoronary heart disease or from an auricular thrombus in a patient with atrial fibrillation. Less frequently, vegetative endocarditis, thrombi at the site of atheromatous plaques within the aorta, or dislodgment of atheromatous plaques during translumbar or retrograde femoral arteriography are the sources of the emboli. The embolus may occlude the main orifice of the artery, particularly if it has been previously narrowed by an atheromatous plaque. More often, however, it lodges near a major branch where the artery narrows, usually at the egress of the middle colic artery. It may then remain at its initial location or fragment and be carried more distad. The initial effect of the embolus on the artery is to cause spasm of its distal branches. This and the rapid closure of the main trunk do not usually allow time for the development of a collateral circulation. Secondary thrombosis of the distal artery then occurs, probably within a few hours. Frequently the artery proximal to the embolus dilates. Sudden occlusion of the main stem superior mesenteric artery produces ischemia of the entire small intestine distal to the ligament of Treitz and also ischemia of the proximal half of the colon. Only rarely, when there are exceptional collateral channels through the celiac axis and inferior mesenteric artery, does the bowel survive. Acute occlusion of short arterial segments or of smaller branches may or may not eventuate in infarction, depending on the status of the collateral circulation.

Thrombosis. Acute, complete thrombosis of the superior mesenteric artery nearly always occurs in an artery partially occluded by atherosclerosis. Less frequently, it is superimposed on a vessel narrowed by aortic aneurysm or involved by thromboangitis obliterans or periarteritis nodosa. A sudden decrease in cardiac output, as occurs in acute congestive failure or myocardial infarction, often precedes the final thrombotic episode. The extent of intestinal ischemia or infarction is dependent on the site of thrombosis and the status of collateral channels. Sudden thrombosis of the main stem artery, as in embolic occlusion, usually results in infarction of the entire small intestine and right colon. However, slowly developing stenosis may allow time for the development of adequate collaterals so that bowel viability is preserved when acute occlusion supervenes. In inflammatory vascular diseases, the smaller visceral branches are usually affected, and intestinal infarction occurs in shorter segments.

PATHOLOGY. Sudden, complete arterial occlusion first causes an ischemic infarct in which the bowel is pale. This is the result of intense vasospasm of the intramural vessels, and it produces mucosal ulceration. At this stage, the bowel becomes hypertonic and contracted. Within 1 to 2 hours, the initial vessel spasm subsides, and the capillaries in the anoxic bowel wall become engorged with blood. As subsequent thrombosis of the artery beyond the site of occlusion occurs, the intestinal musculature becomes fatigued, and contractility is lost. Thrombosis of the visceral veins follows, and the bowel wall becomes inert, boggy, and cyanotic as a result of regurgitant flow from the veins or seepage of blood into the mural tissues of the ischemic intestine. As the infarction progresses to full-thickness necrosis of the intestine, the bowel wall becomes blood-soaked and cyanotic, and "weeps" serosanguineous fluid into the peritoneal cavity. The appearance is that of hemorrhagic infarction and is the end result of either primary arterial or venous occlusion.

CLINICAL MANIFESTATIONS. Sudden, complete occlusion of the superior mesenteric artery presents as a surgical emergency with all the manifestations of paralysis of the peristaltic mechanism as well as loss of viability of the affected intestine. The result is a form of strangulated intestinal obstruction and includes all the hazards associated with this condition (see Chap. 24).

The clinical features are usually the same whether occlusion is the result of embolism or thrombosis. Males are affected more often than females. The peak age incidence is in the fifth and sixth decades. Frequently the patient has coronary artery disease, with or without atrial fibrillation, and other manifestations of generalized atherosclerosis. A prior history of repeated episodes of cramping abdominal pain following the ingestion of food (intestinal angina) may be elicited from as many as one-third of these patients.

The most striking and constant complaint is extreme abdominal pain, often unresponsive to narcotics and initially out of proportion to the physical findings. The pain comes on suddenly and is first colicky but soon becomes steady and continuous. The early localization of the pain is to the segment of bowel involved. With acute main stem artery occlusion, the pain is first experienced in the mid-abdomen or epigastrium but later becomes generalized. Vomiting follows, is protracted, and may contain blood. Diarrhea and later constipation occur, and often the stool contains occult or gross blood. A peculiar, mottled cyanosis of the abdomen and flanks has been observed in about one-fifth of patients, a manifestation of low cardiac output accompanying extensive bowel infarction. The abdomen does not usually become distended until late. Voluntary and involuntary muscle spasm will be present, but the rigidity is almost never boardlike. Tenderness and rebound tenderness become severe as intestinal infarction occurs and are most marked over the ischemic segment of bowel. The presence of a mass is more usual with infarction of short intestinal segments. Bowel sounds are at first hyperactive, but within a short time the abdomen becomes silent. At the onset, temperature, pulse, and blood pressure may not be significantly altered. However, as infarction of the intestine progresses, the patient becomes febrile, the pulse rate increases, and the patient becomes hypotensive. Not infrequently, main stem artery occlusion initially produces acute circulatory collapse which is readily reversible but then recurs as gangrene of the bowel with peritonitis supervenes. Once bowel necrosis and perforation occur, the findings are those of generalized peritonitis and sepsis.

A correct diagnosis is sometimes difficult to make, especially with occlusions of short arterial segments. The most important early diagnostic feature is the severity of the abdominal pain relative to the physical findings and its unresponsiveness to narcotics. This finding in a patient with a recent myocardial infarction or atrial fibrillation or in one who has previously suffered emboli to extremity arteries should make the physician highly suspicious of an acute mesenteric vascular accident.

DIAGNOSTIC STUDIES. The leukocyte count may be normal early in the course of the disease but is increased to over 20,000 as hemorrhagic infarction occurs. Most patients have normal or high hematocrit levels. Often the serum amylase level is elevated. This has been related to seepage of the enzyme through the ischemic bowel wall. Roentgenograms of the abdomen are not often of significant diagnostic value. Frequently they show moderate to slight distension of both small and large intestine. The presence of gas in the right half of the colon which stops abruptly in the midtransverse colon has been considered a valuable finding; however, this is infrequent and occurs late. An abdominal paracentesis may be helpful in making the diagnosis, anticipating the recovery of serosanguineous fluid in which staining does not reveal bacteria.

TREATMENT. The treatment of acute mesenteric vascular occlusion is emergency surgical intervention, preferably before necrosis and perforation of the bowel have occurred. Until recently, the only surgical procedure considered was resection of the involved intestine. This operation was first successfully performed by Elliot in 1895. It was not until over 50 years later, in 1957, that Shaw and Rutledge reported the first successful superior mesenteric artery embolectomy not requiring associated bowel resection. Yet, the number of patients who present with a situation amenable to arterial reconstruction is small. This is because embolectomy (or emergency thrombectomy) must be performed within a few hours after the acute occlusion, before irreversible bowel changes have occurred.

At laparotomy, the ischemic intestine will be pale and thin (anemic infarction) or more often in the stage of hemorrhagic infarction. In either case, the mesentery will be pulseless. If short segments are affected, they are best handled by resection with primary end-to-end anastomosis. From previous experience, it has been learned that as much as 70 percent of the small intestine can be removed without creating serious digestive disturbances. Such extensive resections are tolerated better by adults than children.

In the situation where the main stem superior mesenteric artery is occluded, the decision to reestablish arterial flow is based on whether the process in the ischemic intestine is reversible. Although outwardly appearing nonviable, the deeply cyanotic and dull surface of the intestinal wall is at times deceiving. An attempt should be made to stimulate peristalsis, since its presence is indicative of viable and potentially salvageable bowel. In the absence of peristalsis, the only surgical procedure which can be considered is removal of all infarcted intestine. This will usually require resection of the entire small intestine distal to the ligament of Treitz and resection of the right half of the colon. Although this extensive resection is associated with a high operative mortality and late morbidity, it is worthy of consideration in an otherwise hopeless situation.

If the ischemia of all or part of the intestine is felt to be reversible, an attempt at arterial reconstruction is indicated. The superior mesenteric artery is traced proximally, and the location of the embolus or thrombus determined by finding a bounding pulse proximal to the occlusion with no pulsations distad. The artery is isolated between clamps and the occluding lesion removed through a longitudinal arteriotomy incision. An embolus is usually easily extracted, while a thrombus in a sclerotic vessel will require thromboendarterectomy. Proximal "milking" of the distal vessels may be necessary if fresh thrombus is present. The incision in the artery is then closed, preferably using a patch graft of synthetic material or autogenous vein. With resumption of arterial flow, pulsations will be felt in the mesenteric vessels, and color will return to the bowel within a few minutes provided the ischemia is reversible. The intestine should be visualized for 10 to 15 minutes and all obviously nonvascularized segments resected. If there is any question about the viability of the intestine, it is best to leave it and then reexamine it at a second operation 24 to 36 hours later. The advantage of this two-stage procedure is that it conserves intestine by confining resection to those segments which are necrotic.

The preoperative preparation and postoperative care of patients with acute mesenteric infarction is particularly important. Most of these patients will have a depleted circulating blood volume resulting from loss of plasma and whole blood into the bowel lumen, bowel wall, and peritoneal cavity. This loss can be considerable, and rapid replacement should be started while readying the patient for operation. Added intravenous fluids are necessary postoperatively to combat the reactive hyperemia that occurs after revascularization of the intestine. Since the ischemic bowel wall allows passage of bacteria into the peritoneal cavity even before frank necrosis has occurred, broad spectrum antibiotics should be administered in large doses beginning preoperatively and continuing throughout the postoperative period. Anticoagulation, preferably with heparin, has been recommended for patients following arterial reconstructive procedures. Nasogastric decompression of the stomach and intestine are necessary until bowel function returns.

The overall mortality rate following sudden superior mesenteric artery occlusion varies between 65 and 85 percent. The cause of death is usually peritonitis with septicemia. Frequent atherosclerotic involvement of the heart, kidneys, and other organs contributes to the high mortality rates.

NONOCCLUSIVE MESENTERIC INFARCTION

ETIOLOGY. In about 20 percent of patients with mesenteric infarction, careful examination will reveal no gross arterial or venous occlusion. Ottinger and Austen found this situation to be the most frequent cause of intestinal gangrene on a circulatory basis. It produces diffuse intestinal necrosis and is invariably fatal. It has been related to a sustained decrease in cardiac output such as in prolonged circulatory collapse and hypoxic states that may accompany septicemia, congestive heart failure, cardiac arrhythmia, acute myocardial infarction, and profound hypovolemia. The common denominator appears to be a low cardiac output state. Very frequently it is a terminal event in these illnesses. Its occurrence has been explained on the basis of persistent compensatory splanchnic vasoconstriction which becomes intractable. Sludging of blood due to erythrocytic agglutination follows as blood flow through the small arterioles slows down, and ultimately intestinal anoxia and infarction occur. Vasopressor therapy for shock may prolong the vasoconstriction and hasten the onset of gangrene. Additionally, the majority of patients presenting with nonocclusive mesenteric infarction have received digitalis, an agent which has been shown to induce mesenteric vasoconstriction. The genesis of acute nonocclusive mesenteric infarction has been explained by applying the law of Laplace. According to this law, the tension in the wall of the vessel must be less than the hydrostatic pressure exerted by the column of blood, or the vessel will collapse. It has been shown in dogs that when the blood pressure in the vasa recta drops below 15 mm of mercury with a blood flow below 10 ml/100 Gm of intestinal tissue for 8 consecutive hours, irreversible intestinal ischemia develops.

PATHOLOGY. The gross pathologic picture seen in patients with nonocclusive mesenteric infarction is essentially that of hemorrhagic necrosis. The mucosa is ulcerated and edematous, and the submucosal vessels are grossly dilated and packed with erythrocytes. The outer surface of the bowel is initially mottled with segmental areas of cyanosis distributed throughout the length of the intestine. In the late stages of the disease, gangrenous changes become advanced and lead to perforation.

CLINICAL MANIFESTATIONS. The clinical picture may be identical to that of patients with acute arterial or venous mesenteric occlusions. The patients, however, are usually older, and the infarction develops slowly over a period of several days, during which time there may be prodromal symptoms of malaise and vague abdominal discomfort.

Associated congestive heart failure, with or without arrythmia, is frequent. An unusually large number of patients have been found to be overdigitalized. Infarction of the intestine is heralded by the sudden onset of severe abdominal pain and vomiting. The patient usually becomes acutely hypotensive and develops a rapid pulse. Watery diarrhea is frequent, and the stools may be grossly bloody. The abdomen becomes diffusely tender and rigid. Bowel sounds are diminished and later absent. Fever and leukocytosis are usual, and frequently there is a thrombocytopenia related to intravascular thrombosis. A characteristic early laboratory finding is a markedly elevated hematocrit, which is apparently due to "trapping" of serum in the bowel wall and seepage into the peritoneal cavity.

In disorders in which the sphanchnic circulation is thought to be diminished, unexplained abdominal signs and symptoms should be viewed with the possibility of mesenteric vascular insufficiency and intestinal necrosis in mind. The single most important aid in establishing the diagnosis is abdominal angiography. A diagnostic selective superior mesenteric arteriogram will demonstrate patent major vessels with multiple segmental areas of narrowing of both small and medium-sized branches and diminution or absence of a mural intestinal circulation.

TREATMENT. The initial approach to the treatment of this condition is to correct the underlying disorder producing the low flow state. At the same time, it has been suggested that an attempt be made to improve mesenteric artery flow. This can be accomplished by direct infusion of vasodilating drugs such as isoproterenol, tolazoline hydrochloride, or papaverine hydrochloride into a catheter positioned in the superior mesenteric artery, or by a continuous epidural block. The response can be assessed by obtaining sequential mesenteric angiograms. Antibiotics have been shown to delay or diminish loss of intestinal viability and should be administered early and in large doses.

If, despite mesenteric vasodilatation, the abdominal signs and symptoms persist or reappear, operation is mandatory. With intractable hypotension and congestive failure, the gangrenous changes in the bowel wall are usually segmental; areas of anemic infarction are found interspersed with those of hemorrhagic infarction. Pulses can be felt in the superior and inferior mesenteric arteries and their major branches extending almost to the bowel wall. Serosanguineous fluid is a constant finding in the peritoneal cavity. The process usually extends throughout the entire large and small intestine and may also involve the stomach. For this reason, resection is not usually feasible. With involvement of lesser portions of the intestine, primary resection with end-to-end anastomosis should be attempted, although too often the remaining intestine will subsequently become infarcted in the immediate postoperative period. Massive fluid replacement and support of cardiac function combined with interruption of splanchnic vasoconstriction by continuous epidural block have been recommended postoperatively to help prevent progression following intestinal resection. The reported mortality rates approach 100 percent, a reflection primarily of the frequent occurrence of this type of mesenteric infarction in terminal illnesses.

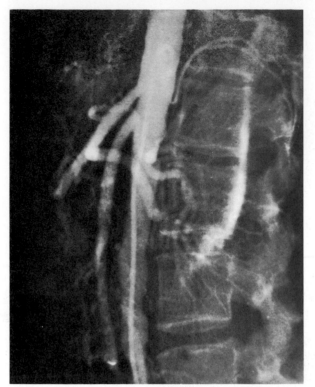

Fig. 35-8. Lateral view of a retrograde visceral arteriogram showing a normal celiac axis and superior mesenteric artery.

CHRONIC OCCLUSION OF VISCERAL ARTERIES (INTESTINAL ANGINA)

Three possible sequelae may follow gradual occlusion of the main stem visceral arteries: (1) establishment of an adequate collateral circulation; (2) intestinal infarction; and (3) intestinal ischemia without infarction, due to collateral blood supply sufficient for life but not for function of the affected bowel. The last of these three sequelae produces a now well-recognized syndrome termed "intestinal angina." This entity is analogous to angina pectoris and intermittent claudication due to, respectively, arterial insufficiency to the heart and to the extremities.

ETIOLOGY. Collateral anastomoses among the three main gastrointestinal arteries from the aorta (celiac axis, superior mesenteric, and inferior mesenteric) provide for maintenance of intestinal viability and function when one of these branches is gradually occluded (Fig. 35-6). For this reason, most patients with isolated chronic occlusion of the superior mesenteric artery are completely asymptomatic. However, when blood flow through one of the surviving vessels then becomes (or has been) compromised, the now relatively ischemic intestine is unable to respond to the demands of digestion for an increased blood supply. This explains the "food-pain" sequence that characterizes intestinal angina.

As a major visceral artery becomes critically narrowed, the others dilate in order to carry more blood. This finding is of practical significance when the inferior mesenteric artery must be sacrificed in patients undergoing surgical treatment for aortic aneurysm or colon resection for carcinoma. In these circumstances, patency of the superior mesenteric artery should be ascertained before an unusually large inferior mesenteric is sacrificed. Otherwise, infarction of the intestine may be precipitated when the latter vessel is ligated. This complication can be prevented either by reimplanting the inferior mesenteric artery into the aortic graft or by restoring blood flow through the superior mesenteric artery.

PATHOLOGY. Chronic occlusion of the visceral arteries is most often due to atherosclerosis. The atheromatous plaques are invariably located at or near the origin of these large vessels, thus in a segment which anatomically is suitable for arterial reconstruction. Most of these patients also have evidence of generalized arteriosclerosis. Less frequently, the stenosis is due to compression of the celiac axis by a celiac ganglion or arcuate ligament of the diaphragm, by involvement of the arteries in an expanding aortic aneurysm or dissecting aneurysm, or by thromboangiitis obliterans or periarteritis nodosa.

CLINICAL MANIFESTATIONS. The dominant clinical feature of intestinal angina is generalized cramping abdominal pain which comes on soon after eating and lasts as long as 3 hours. The severity and duration of the distress depends on the amount of food ingested. Occasionally it is merely a sense of distension, or bloating, with a constant abdominal ache. If the pain is severe, nausea and vomiting often occur. Initially the patient will complain of constipation and later of diarrhea. There is usually a steady progression in the frequency and duration of symptoms. The food-pain relationship soon leads to a reluctance on the part of the patient to eat. The subsequent rapid and severe weight loss characterizes the syndrome. As the intestinal ischemia progresses, a form of malabsorption syndrome occurs which contributes to the weight loss, and is manifest by bulky, foamy stools high in fat and protein content. Symptoms of intestinal angina may exist for months or years before the visceral circulation becomes critically curtailed. Morris et al. estimate that histories of prodromal symptoms of intestinal angina may be obtained from as many as one-third of patients with mesenteric infarction.

On physical examination, weight loss will be obvious. Usually there are varying degrees of disability associated with generalized arteriosclerosis. A bruit is often heard over the epigastrium, although this may be transmitted from the aorta or sites other than the stenotic visceral artery. Laboratory studies and routine roentgenographic studies are not often contributory except to rule out other abdominal conditions. The differential diagnosis includes peptic ulcer disease, cholecystitis, abdominal neoplasm, and pancreatitis.

An awareness of the syndrome is perhaps the most important factor in making the diagnosis, which is then best confirmed by a selective visceral angiogram using a Seldinger catheter (Fig. 35-8). Lateral views are essential, because the standard anteroposterior view does not show the origin of the celiac or mesenteric arteries. The catheter is passed via a left brachial or femoral artery puncture to a level just above the origin of the celiac axis. After a small test dose has established the proper position of the catheter, 30 to 40 ml of 50% Hypaque is injected rapidly while taking multiple films using a rapid cassette changer. This outlines both the celiac axis and superior mesenteric arteries. Diagnostic arteriograms will show stenosis or complete occlusion of one or both these vessels, usually within 1 cm of the aortic orifice (Fig. 35-9). The catheter is then repositioned just above the origin of the inferior mesenteric artery and the arteriogram repeated. The demonstration of a markedly dilated and elongated inferior mesenteric artery which fills the superior mesenteric through collaterals is indicative of a superior mesenteric artery occlusion (Fig. 35-10).

TREATMENT. Once stenosis of the celiac and mesenteric arteries has been demonstrated in a symptomatic patient, surgical correction is advised if the patient will tolerate the procedure. Arterial reconstruction not only corrects the symptoms of intestinal angina but also prevents the eventual progression to intestinal infarction. At laparotomy, critical stenosis of the involved arteries is obvious, because there will be no palpable pulsations distal to the stenosis. Surgical treatment may be one of three types: (1) thromboendarterectomy; (2) synthetic or autogenous vein bypass graft circumventing the stenotic segment; or (3) excision of the stenotic segment and reimplantation of the superior mesenteric artery into the aorta. Since exposure of the origins of the superior mesenteric and celiac arteries is difficult, Morris et al., Rob, and others prefer improving the circulation with a bypass graft. For a lesion in the celiac artery, the graft is inserted between a major branch of the celiac artery, usually the splenic, and the aorta. Occasionally, the splenic artery itself may be mobilized and anastomosed to the side of the aorta. Bypass of a

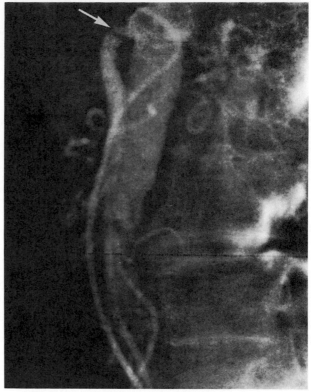

Fig. 35-9. Lateral view of retrograde visceral arteriogram showing a high-grade stenosis (arrow) of the superior mesenteric artery close to its origin from the aorta. (Compare with Fig. 35-8.)

superior mesenteric artery stenosis is best handled by inserting a graft to the side of the artery just beyond the egress of the middle colic artery and to the aorta below the origin of the renal arteries. When endarterectomy is performed, care should be taken to tack the distal intima to the artery wall in order to prevent dissection.

Fig. 35-10. Left: Retrograde inferior mesenteric arteriogram showing a prominent marginal artery of Drummond filling from a dilated and tortuous inferior mesenteric artery. Right: Later film showing filling of the superior mesenteric artery (arrow) through collaterals. The patient had complete occlusion of the celiac axis and superior mesenteric artery at their origins from the aorta.

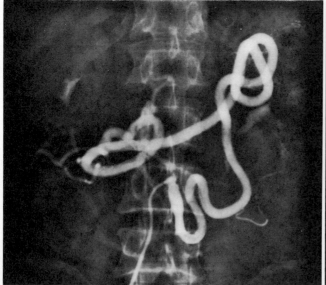
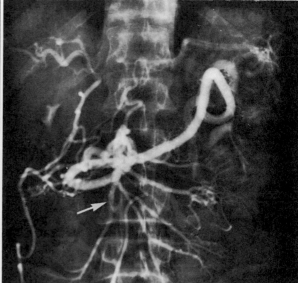

OCCLUSION OF INFERIOR MESENTERIC ARTERY

ETIOLOGY. Sudden occlusion of the inferior mesenteric artery is usually due to thrombosis superimposed on an atheromatous plaque and less often to embolism or a dissecting aneurysm. External compression by an expanding aortic aneurysm or involvement by atherosclerosis produces gradual occlusion. On occasion, obliterative arteritis, as associated with thromboangiitis obliterans and periarteritis nodosa, will involve the main artery or its branches.

Normally, the inferior mesenteric artery can be ligated at any point without interfering with bowel function or producing symptoms. This is because the extensive collateral circulation through anastomoses with branches of the middle colic artery (superior mesenteric) and lower hemorrhoidal arteries (internal iliac) are able to sustain the left colon (Fig. 35-6). When infarction of the descending colon follows thrombosis or ligation of the inferior mesenteric artery, there is almost always impairment of this collateral network. Usually this is due to advanced atheromatous narrowing or thrombosis of the superior mesenteric and internal iliac arteries. Such an event occasionally occurs when the inferior mesenteric artery is sacrificed during operations on the aorta for occlusive disease or aneurysm. Previous left colectomy with interruption of the marginal artery also predisposes to colon ischemia following occlusion of the inferior mesenteric artery.

CLINICAL MANIFESTATIONS. Circulatory infarction of the descending colon usually has a more insidious onset than infarction of other portions of the intestine. Since the inferior mesenteric supplies a shorter segment of bowel, occlusion produces less extensive disruption of circulating blood volume and fluid balance than when the superior mesenteric artery is occluded. Steady, slowly progressive lower abdominal pain is usually followed by loose, bloody stools and then constipation. The abdomen becomes distended and tender over the course of the descending colon. Occasionally a tubular mass may be felt in the left side of the abdomen. Some degree of circulatory collapse occurs. This is initially mild but becomes profound as the bowel becomes necrotic. The temperature and white blood cell count are only moderately elevated unless perforation has occurred. Roentgenograms of the abdomen may show an absence of gas in the descending colon, suggesting a mechanical obstruction of the transverse colon. Edema, cyanosis, and ulceration of the mucosal membrane of the sigmoid colon can often be detected by sigmoidoscopy. Unexplained diarrhea, with or without rectal bleeding, which comes on after operations on the abdominal aorta, suggests vascular impairment of the left colon and prompts immediate sigmoidoscopic evaluation.

TREATMENT. Early recognition of the intestinal ischemia and prompt surgical intervention is important for survival. Treatment consists of resection of the infarcted colonic segment. A temporary proximal end colostomy is safer than a primary anastomosis. The preexisting generalized arteriosclerotic disease afflicting most of these patients renders them poor operative risks. The overall mortality rate is about 70 percent.

MESENTERIC VENOUS OCCLUSION

ETIOLOGY. When occlusion of a visceral vein produces symptoms, they are almost always due to acute thrombosis. Mesenteric venous thrombosis may be idiopathic or evolve secondarily as a complication of several clinical disorders. The predisposing factors in secondary mesenteric venous thrombosis are (1) infection, usually intraabdominal suppuration such as appendicitis, diverticulitis, or pelvic abscess; (2) hypercoagulable states such as polycythemia vera and carcinomatosis; (3) local venous congestion and stasis, as with hepatic cirrhosis with portal hypertension or extrinsic obstruction of portal venous radicles by tumor masses; and (4) accidental or operative trauma to the mesenteric veins, particularly during or following a portacaval surgical procedure. In approximately 25 percent, no associated factor may be implicated; these cases are classified as primary, or idiopathic. A significant number of patients in this last group will give a past history of peripheral thrombophlebitis, suggesting a common cause.

PATHOLOGY. Sudden occlusion of the main stem superior mesenteric vein in the dog leads to rapid sequestration of splanchnic venous circulation, stagnation shock, and hemorrhagic infarction of the bowel progressing to necrosis and gangrene. However, in man, ligation of the portal vein or superior mesenteric vein does not produce infarction unless secondary thrombosis extends to the bowel wall and involves the venous arcades and vasa recta. Primary thrombotic occlusion of the visceral veins usually begins in the smaller tributaries. Depending on the extent and location of the propagating clot, the bowel lesion may be represented by small localized areas or extensive segments of infarction. With extensive venous occlusion, thrombosis of the arterial side of the splanchnic circulation often follows, so that it becomes impossible to determine accurately whether the occlusion was initially arterial or venous.

Phlebitis secondary to inflammatory diseases of the bowel may extend to involve the entire portal system (pyelophlebitis) or give rise to septic emboli that lodge within the liver, causing intrahepatic abscess. This complication of mesenteric venous thrombosis has become less frequent with the advent of antibiotics, and the bowel symptoms are usually overshadowed by those due to the infection.

Acute thrombosis of mesenteric veins is followed promptly by hyperemia, edema, and subserosal hemorrhages in the affected segment of intestine. The bowel wall becomes markedly thickened and cyanotic, and the lumen fills with dark bloody fluid. Serosanguineous fluid seeps from the surface of the congested mesentery and also from the intestinal loop. The picture is that of hemorrhagic infarction.

CLINICAL MANIFESTATIONS. The clinical manifestations are similar to those following acute visceral artery occlusion. Not infrequently, the patient complains of vague abdominal discomfort, anorexia, and change in bowel habits a few days or even weeks prior to the onset of severe symptoms. This prodromal period is more evident when the venous thrombosis is idiopathic. The early symptoms are then followed by sudden severe abdominal pain, vomiting, and circulatory collapse. Narcotics usually do not relieve the pain. Bloody diarrhea is more frequent than with arterial occlusions. The bowel sounds will be hypoactive or absent. Generalized abdominal tenderness, guarding, and distension are usual; however, true rigidity is not present unless gangrene and perforation of the bowel have occurred. A marked leukocytosis and elevated hematocrit are characteristic findings in venous thrombosis. The latter reflects the trapping of plasma in the occluded bowel segment as arterial blood continues to flow into a splanchnic bed without adequate venous drainage. Plain roentgenograms of the abdomen usually show dilated loops of small bowel with air fluid levels which, however, are not specific. Abdominal paracentesis invariably yields serosanguineous fluid, which, if foul-smelling, makes immediate laparotomy mandatory.

TREATMENT. The definitive treatment of mesenteric venous infarction is surgical. Without operation the mortality approaches 100 percent. Preparation of the patient for operation includes correcting the usually severe circulating volume deficit with blood and a balanced salt solution and decompression of the stomach via a nasogastric tube. Broad-spectrum antibiotics and penicillin in large doses should be started and should be continued in the postoperative period.

As soon as possible and when his condition permits, the patient is taken to the operating room. In contrast to acute mesenteric arterial occlusion, venous thrombosis tends to occur more frequently in peripheral tributaries than in the main stem vessel. For this reason, shorter segments of intestine are usually involved than if occlusion is primarily arterial. All devitalized intestine is resected and a primary end-to-end anastomosis performed. Frequently the thrombosis extends beyond the limits of gross infarction. Therefore, resection should include adjacent normal bowel and mesentery until all grossly thrombosed veins are encompassed. Otherwise, extension of residual clot postoperatively will lead to subsequent infarction. Intestinal infarction associated with acute thrombosis of the portal vein is usually not amenable to resection because of the wide extent of involved intestine.

Anticoagulation should be started 12 to 24 hours postoperatively. Naitove and Weismann reported no deaths in their cases of idiopathic mesenteric venous thrombosis in which anticoagulants were administered, in contrast to a 50 percent mortality in the group in which the drugs were not used. A second-look operation 24 to 36 hours later should be performed in this form of mesenteric infarction because of the frequent recurrence of thrombosis or extension of residual clots. In general, the prognosis is somewhat better than in mesenteric infarction due to arterial occlusion. This is probably a reflection of the shorter bowel segments usually involved, which make it more amenable to surgical treatment. The most important factor in prognosis is early operative intervention before extensive thrombosis has occurred throughout the splanchnic venous circulation.

MEDIAN ARCUATE LIGAMENT SYNDROME

In 1965, Dunbar and his associates reported 15 patients with abdominal complaints who were found to have partial occlusion of the celiac artery by fibers of the median arcuate ligament, since referred to as the median arcuate ligament syndrome. All of their patients had relief of symptoms following division of the diaphragmatic fibers which were compressing the artery. The basis of the constriction appears to be either a high origin of the celiac artery, with resultant compression as it passes through the aortic hiatus beneath the median arcuate ligament, or an abnormally low crossing of the ligament causing compression of a normally located artery. However, there are some who doubt whether the syndrome is a true clinical entity, because the arterial narrowing which is presumed to cause the syndrome is often encountered in patients without symptoms.

CLINICAL MANIFESTATIONS. The condition is most likely to occur in the fourth and fifth decades of life, with a three-to-one predominance of females. The principal and usually only symptom is abdominal pain which may vary from a vague periumbilical or epigastric aching discomfort to a severe postprandial pain. It has been inferred that the pain is related to intestinal ischemia, but true, chronic ischemia of the gastrointestinal tract generally requires interference with the blood flow in at least two of the three major visceral arteries. Irritation of visceral autonomic nerve fibers by the constricting fibers of the diaphragm has also been considered as the basis of the pain, but perivascular sympathectomy or ganglionectomy is not consistently palliative. Diarrhea and nausea with occasional vomiting also may occur, and weight loss because of voluntary avoidance of food is characteristic of patients with postprandial pain. A significant physical finding is a bruit invariably present in the upper midabdomen.

The diagnosis is made by arteriography demonstrating the entrapment of the celiac artery by the diaphragmatic fibers. The lateral film is the most reliable and, characteristically, will show eccentric compression of the celiac artery along its superior border with caudal displacement of the artery so that it lies adjacent to the superior mesenteric artery (Fig. 35-11). A presumptive diagnosis may be entertained if the selective superior mesenteric arteriogram demonstrates collateral filling of the celiac system. (In the true syndrome, both the superior mesenteric and inferior mesenteric arteries are of normal caliber radiographically.) Stanley and Frey believe that the demonstration of impaired absorption of xylose is useful in diagnosis as well as in selecting patients for surgery.

TREATMENT. Normal blood flow in the celiac artery can usually be restored by transecting the constricting median arcuate ligament. The results have generally been excellent: Marable et al. reported complete relief or marked improvement of symptoms in 24 of 30 patients following this operation. Direct arterial reconstruction may be necessary if the stenosis persists and the patient remains symptomatic after division of the ligament.

SPONTANEOUS RUPTURE OF VISCERAL BLOOD VESSELS (ABDOMINAL APOPLEXY)

The term "abdominal apoplexy" has been applied to the situation of massive abdominal hemorrhage from spontaneous rupture of visceral blood vessels. It is an unusual

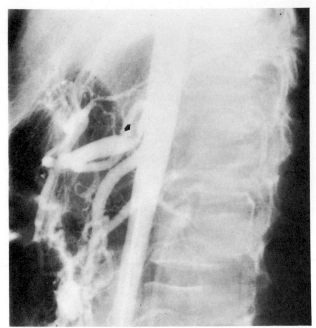

Fig. 35-11. Lateral abdominal aortography showing compression of the superior border of the celiac artery (arrow) by the median arcuate ligament.

and very rare form of mesenteric vascular disease that is the abdominal counterpart of cerebral hemorrhage. In a recent review of the literature, Kleinsasser noted only 83 patients whose diagnoses could be substantiated.

ETIOLOGY. The occurrence of abdominal apoplexy in older patients has been related to localized arteriosclerotic disease causing weakness or aneurysmal formation of mesenteric vessels which later spontaneously rupture. In younger patients, congenital defects in the medial coat of the visceral arteries and veins have been incriminated. Necrotizing arteritis associated with certain autoimmune diseases may on rare occasion be the etiologic factor. Most of the patients have hypertension, which is believed to be of etiologic significance.

PATHOLOGY. The bleeding comes from an arterial source far more frequently than from a venous one. Multiple sites of rupture have been reported. Although it does not fulfill the exact criteria for abdominal apoplexy, rupture of a splenic artery aneurysm is perhaps the best-known source. This usually occurs during pregnancy or the puerperium. Of the intestinal vessels, rupture occurs most often in the superior mesenteric artery or its major colic branches. Not infrequently, no site of bleeding can be found at laparotomy or autopsy despite the loss of several liters of blood.

Bleeding may initially be intraperitoneal or, by extending between the leaves of the mesentery, retroperitoneal. The latter situation often secondarily produces a tear in the peritoneum, thus giving the picture of both retroperitoneal and intraperitoneal bleeding. The severity of hemorrhage will depend on the size of the ruptured vessel.

CLINICAL MANIFESTATIONS. With confined retroperitoneal bleeding, the clinical features will include steady back or testicular pain, pallor, tachycardia, and occasional vomiting. When bleeding is into the peritoneal cavity, there is sudden, severe abdominal pain rapidly followed by circulatory collapse. The pain is generalized and often referred to the left shoulder. Abdominal distension, spasm, and generalized tenderness are present. Bowel activity will be depressed or absent. The temperature is usually normal, but generally the white blood cell count will be increased. The hematocrit may or may not be low, depending on whether hemodilution has taken place. The vital signs following the initial bleeding may improve for a period of several hours and then be followed by a second, usually massive episode of bleeding which is fatal without prompt surgical intervention.

The above clinical findings in an older patient with hypertension and generalized arteriosclerosis or in a pregnant patient should lead one to suspect abdominal apoplexy. It must be differentiated from such abdominal catastrophes as perforated peptic ulcer, hemorrhagic pancreatitis, strangulated intestinal obstruction, ruptured abdominal aneurysm, and mesenteric vascular occlusion. An abdominal paracentesis with the recovery of nonclotting blood is diagnostic of intraabdominal bleeding from any source. Selective mesenteric arteriography may help to localize the bleeding site, but usually surgery cannot be delayed.

TREATMENT. Treatment of abdominal apoplexy is immediate blood replacement and surgical intervention as soon as the patient's condition permits. At times the bleeding may be so brisk that it will be necessary to take the patient to the operating room while still in shock. However, the chances of finding an open vessel are better if the blood pressure can be elevated. Bleeding from the smaller visceral arteries and most venous bleeding are the best treated by ligation. Splenectomy will facilitate exposure for ligation of a ruptured splenic artery aneurysm. A ruptured hepatic artery or main stem superior mesenteric artery should be reconstructed, if possible. This will usually require excision of the segment and replacement with a graft, preferably of autogenous vein. Following ligation of visceral arteries or reconstruction of the superior mesenteric artery, adequate circulation to the bowel must be assured and all obviously ischemic intestine resected. If there is a question of viability of a long segment, a second-look operation in 24 to 36 hours may avoid an extensive resection. When it is necessary to ligate the hepatic artery, protection should be afforded the liver with large doses of broad-spectrum antibiotics postoperatively.

The outlook for recovery is good, even with massive bleeding, if the patient is operated upon early and a definite bleeding point located. The overall mortality rate in a collected review by Carter and Gosney was 47 percent. However, of those coming to the operating room, the rate fell to 15 percent when the ruptured vessel could be identified.

TRAUMA TO VISCERAL BLOOD VESSELS

ETIOLOGY. Mesenteric arteries and veins may be injured by either penetrating or nonpenetrating abdominal trauma or accidentally during abdominal operations. In most cases, the vessels are lacerated. Less frequently, contusion of an artery by blunt trauma eventuates in thrombosis or later aneurysmal formation with rupture.

Most penetrating injuries of the mesenteric vessels are due to stabbings or gunshot wounds. In these circumstances, associated injury to other organs is frequent. Isolated injury to mesenteric vessels following blunt abdominal trauma is rare and usually involves vessels in the mesentery proper or porta hepatis.

CLINICAL MANIFESTATIONS. Depending on the size of the vessel lacerated, the rapidity of the bleeding, and associated organ injury, the patient will present with varying degrees of shock, abdominal pain, tenderness, distension, and spasm. Pain referred to the left shoulder is a particularly valuable diagnostic symptom. X-rays of the abdomen are not helpful unless associated visceral rupture has occurred, in which case free air may be seen.

TREATMENT. It is generally held that all gunshot wounds of the abdomen and most stab wounds should be explored early regardless of the physical findings. In nonpenetrating injury, a paracentesis yielding nonclotting blood prompts early surgical intervention. Basically, treatment consists of controlling the bleeding vessel. Lacerations of the inferior mesenteric artery or smaller mesenteric arteries and most mesenteric veins can usually be successfully treated by ligation. In the past, few patients with injury to the main trunk of the superior mesenteric artery survived. Most died from infarction of the intestine or because of complications arising from associated organ injury. Today, if the patient can be resuscitated and reaches the operating room, then arterial repair may be possible. This can be accomplished by either primary suture or interposition of a vascular graft between the severed ends of the vessel. Every attempt should also be made to repair lacerations of the hepatic artery or portal vein. Whether treatment is by ligation or reconstruction, it is important that adequate circulation to the intestine be established and any obviously ischemic bowel resected before closing the abdomen. Long segments of small intestine that are of questionable viability are best left in place and reexamined at a second operation 24 hours later.

Nonspecific Mesenteric Lymphadenitis

Nonspecific mesenteric lymphadenitis is one of the common causes of acute abdominal pain in children. Its existence as a distinct clinicopathologic entity is now well accepted, although the condition received little attention in early medical texts following its initial description by Wilensky and Hahn in 1926. An extensive review of the disease has been reported by McDonald.

Since the condition is invariably self-limiting and can be accurately diagnosed only at laparotomy, its true incidence is unknown. Yet, it is probably the most common cause of inflammatory enlargement of abdominal lymph glands, far surpassing that due to tuberculosis, with which it has been confused in the past. Consideration of the disease is important because of its clinical similarity to several abdominal conditions requiring surgical intervention, notably acute appendicitis.

PATHOLOGY AND PATHOGENESIS. The lymph nodes primarily involved in nonspecific mesenteric lymphadenitis are those that drain the ileocecal region. Undoubtedly this is due to the concentration of mesenteric nodes in this area and because the most abundant lymphatic drainage in the intestinal tract is in the lower ileum. Moreover, stasis of intestinal contents in the terminal ileum favors absorption of toxic or bacterial products from the bowel lumen, agents which may have a bearing on the pathogenesis of the disease.

In the early stages, the juxtaintestinal glands are predominantly affected. Later, there is involvement of the intermediate and terminal or central glands at the root of the mesentery. The nodes are enlarged, discrete, and soft and pink at first; later they may become firm and white. It is uncertain whether calcification ever occurs in nontuberculous adenitis, and suppuration is rare unless specific bacterial infection is present. The gross appearance of the intestine and appendix is normal, although often there is slight vascular congestion of the mesentery. A small amount of clear serous fluid is frequently present within the peritoneal cavity. Histologically, the involved nodes present a pattern of reactive hyperplasia similar to that found in inflammatory and allergic affections of lymph nodes in other parts of the body. The nodes and free peritoneal fluid, with rare exception, prove to be sterile on culture or on animal inoculation.

Although the appearance of the glands grossly and histologically suggests a response to infection, experimental and clinical studies have failed to support a specific bacterial or viral agent as the causal factor. Occasionally, specific mesenteric adenitis due to beta hemolytic streptococcal infection occurs. In these instances, there is an acute febrile illness with signs of peritoneal involvement, and the organism can be cultured from the glands. Only rarely have coliform organisms been isolated. Parasitic mesenteric adenitis secondary to ascariasis occurs in endemic areas; however, the lymph nodes contain numerous eosinophils, and worms are present within the intestine. The disease is distinct from the mesenteric node enlargements which accompany bowel diseases in which there are associated changes in the intestine.

It seems likely that nonspecific mesenteric adenitis represents a reaction to some type of material absorbed from the small intestine. The stimulating substance could reach the nodes via either lymph channels or the bloodstream, although the usual absence of generalized lymphadenopathy would make the latter route unlikely. The possibility that the disease represents a hypersensitive reaction to a foreign protein has also been suggested.

CLINICAL MANIFESTATIONS. The disease most commonly occurs in patients under eighteen years of age. There is no sex predilection. The clinical signs and symptoms are not particularly characteristic. Very often there has been a recent sore throat or upper respiratory tract infection. Pain is usually the first symptom. It varies in intensity from an ache to a severe colic. The mechanism responsible for producing pain is not completely understood. Lymph nodes have not been shown to have sensory innervation, and therefore enlargement of the node by itself should not produce pain. It is probable that the pain is referred from the mesentery, which has an abundance of sensory end organs that are stimulated when the mesentery is stretched during peristalsis. The initial pain is usually in the upper abdomen, but it may also begin in the lower right quadrant or be generalized. Eventually the pain localizes to the right side; however, an important point in differentiating the disease from acute appendicitis is that the patient is unable to indicate the exact site of the most intense pain. Between spasms of colic, the patient feels well and moves about without difficulty. Nausea and vomiting occur in about one-third of patients, while malaise and anorexia are inconstant symptoms. A previous history of one or more similar attacks is frequently obtained from the patient or the parents.

The patient often appears flushed, and an associated rhinorrhea or acute pharyngitis is not unusual. Approximately 20 percent of patients will have lymphadenopathy elsewhere, most often in the cervical region. The usual finding on examination of the abdomen is tenderness in the lower aspect of the right side, which is somewhat higher and more medial and considerably less severe than in acute appendicitis. The point of maximal tenderness often varies from one examination to the next. An appreciable number of patients will have diffuse or periumbilical tenderness as well. Rebound tenderness may or may not be demonstrated. Voluntary guarding is sometimes present; however, true muscular rigidity is rare. The enlarged abdominal lymph glands are seldom palpable. On rectal examination, there may be tenderness on the right side of the pelvis. Early in the attack, the temperature is moderately elevated, to 38 or 38.5°C, and at least half of the patients will have leukocyte counts over 10,000 per cubic millimeter.

DIFFERENTIAL DIAGNOSIS. The disease is most often confused with acute appendicitis but must also be differentiated from regional enteritis, intussusception, specific bacterial and granulomatous adenitis, and other forms of mesenteric glandular enlargement such as with infectious mononucleosis or lymphoma. The clinical similarity to acute appendicitis is such that, in several large series, as many as 20 percent of patients coming to the operating room for appendectomy were found to have nonspecific mesenteric adenitis and a normal appendix. Important differentiating factors are the more localized and constant location of the pain and tenderness, the presence of muscle rigidity, and the frequent occurrence of nausea and vomiting in children with appendicitis.

Tuberculous mesenteric adenitis has been rare since the almost universal use of pasteurized milk and the advent of antituberculous chemotherapeutic drugs. It is most often due to ingestion of milk containing bovine tubercle bacilli, which gain entry to the lymph nodes by way of a Peyer patch, or lymph follicle, in the terminal ileum. The patient usually complains of a less constant aching pain; abdominal tenderness is slight; and enlarged, matted glands are usually palpable in the root of the mesentery. At operation, the diagnosis can be suspected if there are surface tubercles on the nodes which may be caseous. Biopsy of the node

and acid-fast stain or guinea pig inoculation will be diagnostic.

Differentiation from *acute regional ileitis* is at times difficult. Mesenteric adenitis is an almost constant feature of regional ileitis, and indeed the adenitis is often nonspecific in this disease. Inflammatory edema or induration of the serous coat of the ileum with thickening and induration of the mesentery are characteristic of regional enteritis.

The low incidence of lymphadenopathy in other parts of the body and the brief course of nonspecific mesenteric adenitis are factors in excluding lymphomas and infectious mononucleosis. A peripheral blood smear and a Paul-Bunnell test for sheep red cell agglutinins are also helpful.

TREATMENT. The prognosis of nonspecific mesenteric adenitis is excellent, and complete recovery from an individual attack can be expected without specific treatment. Death from the disease is extremely rare and occurs only when secondary specific bacterial infection, usually caused by hemolytic streptococci, causes suppuration of the nodes with rupture leading to abscess or peritonitis.

If the condition is mistaken for acute appendicitis, as it frequently is, laparotomy should be undertaken. In such an instance, it is far safer to find a normal appendix than to run the risk of allowing acute appendicitis to go on to rupture. The diagnosis is readily established at the time of operation with the finding of enlarged mesenteric nodes in the absence of disease in the appendix or elsewhere in the intestinal tract or abdomen. In view of the tendency for recurrence and the difficulty of differentiating it from appendicitis, appendectomy should be performed. Approximately 25 percent of patients will have further bouts of abdominal pain during the childhood years. Apparently, generalized involution of lymphoid tissue with maturity leads to atrophy of many of the nodes, accounting, perhaps, for the rarity of the disease in adult life.

Mesenteric Panniculitis

"Mesenteric panniculitis" is a term applied by Ogden et al. in 1960 to describe a process of extensive thickening of the mesentery by a nonspecific inflammatory process. It has also been variously designated "retractile mesenteritis," "mesenteric lipodystrophy," "lipogranuloma of the mesentery," and "mesenteric manifestations of Weber-Christian disease." Many consider it a variant of retroperitoneal fibrosis.

ETIOLOGY AND PATHOLOGY. The cause of the condition is unknown; however, the process apparently results from an insult to the fatty tissue of the mesentery. Trauma, allergy, and subacute infection have all been implicated. The process usually involves the mesenteric root of the small bowel. Grossly, the normal fat lobulations of the markedly thickened and firm mesentery are lost. Scattered throughout are irregular areas of discoloration, which vary from reddish brown plaques to pale yellow foci resembling fat necrosis. The superior mesenteric vessels, though surrounded by the tumorlike mass of tissue, pass through it unaltered. Histologic sections show inflammatory involvement of the fibroadipose tissue with round cells, foam cells, and giant cells and various degrees of necrosis, fibrosis, and calcification.

CLINICAL MANIFESTATIONS. Men are affected more often than women. It is rarely described in children, in whom mesenteric fat is usually scant. The clinical features are nonspecific. Recurrent episodes of moderate to severe abdominal pain, nausea, vomiting, malaise, and low-grade fever are the usual complaints. In over 60 percent of patients, there is a palpable tender mass, usually in the right side of the abdomen. Roentgenograms are helpful only if the mass displaces or compresses viscera.

TREATMENT. Laparotomy is necessary to establish the diagnosis and to rule out other tumefactions of the abdomen. The widespread involvement of the mesentery precludes doing more than obtaining a biopsy. Since neoplasms of the mesenteric lymph nodes may present a similar gross appearance, several biopsies from different sites should be obtained. Rarely, colostomy or bypass will be necessary to relieve symptoms of obstruction. Treatment of the disease with steroids and irradiation has been suggested. However, the benefits from these are difficult to evaluate, because the inflammatory process is self-limiting and seldom causes any serious complications.

Tumors of the Mesentery

Tumors originating between the leaves of the mesentery are quite rare. In contrast, malignant implants from intra-abdominal or pelvic tumors or metastases to mesenteric lymph nodes are relatively common. Tumors arising from mesenteric lymph nodes occur; however, these are not generally included in a discussion of primary mesenteric tumors.

Historically, primary mesenteric tumors were recognized as early as 1507, when Benivieni, a Florentine anatomist, described at autopsy a cyst originating in the small bowel mesentery. The first successful removal of a mesenteric tumor is credited to Tillaux in 1880. Isolated reports and a few large series have appeared in the literature subsequently. More recently, Rankin and Major, Hart, Fowler, and Yannopoulos and Stout have reviewed these tumors. Excepting tumors arising in lymph nodes, no more than 500 cases of primary mesenteric tumors have been described to date.

PATHOLOGY. Primary tumors of the mesentery may be cystic or solid. Of these, cystic growths occur more frequently than solid ones in a ratio of 2:1. A variety of tissues, including lymphatic, vascular, nervous, and connective tissue, are the source of these tumors. In addition, cystic tumors may arise from embryonic rests (enteroceles or dermoids), from developmental defects (chylous or serous retention cysts), or following trauma (hemorrhagic cysts). A classification of these tumors is shown in Table 35-1.

The majority of cystic mesenteric tumors are benign. Rare exceptions are lymphangiosarcomas, which are true neoplasms arising from lymph channels, and malignant teratomas arising from multipotential embryonic rests.

Table 35-1. CLASSIFICATION OF PRIMARY MESENTERIC TUMORS

Origin	Benign	Malignant
Cystic tumors:		
Developmental defects	Chylous cyst	
	Serous cyst	
Lymphatic tissue . . .	Lymphangioma	Lymphangiosarcoma
Trauma.	Traumatic cyst	
Embryonic rests	Enteric cyst	
	Dermoid	Malignant teratoma
Solid tumors:		
Adipose tissue	Lipoma	Liposarcoma
Fibrous tissue	Fibroma	Fibrosarcoma
Nerve elements	Neurilemoma	Malignant schwannoma
	Neurofibroma	
Smooth muscle	Leiomyoma	Leiomyosarcoma
	Fibromyoma	Fibromyosarcoma
Vascular tissue.	Hemangioma	Hemangiopericytoma

Rankin and Major contend that chylous or lymphatic cysts are the most frequently encountered benign mesenteric masses. These are thought to arise from developmental defects in mesenteric lymphatics creating closed spaces within which fluid accumulates. They may be unilocular or multilocular, have an endothelial lining, contain a grossly cloudy fluid resembling chyle, and often grow to extremely large size. A similar cause has been ascribed to serous cysts, which are differentiated from chylous cysts in that they contain clear fluid, are invariably unilocular, and may or may not have an endothelial lining. Lymphangioma of the mesentery is apparently a true neoplasm of lymphatics similar to those found in other parts of the body (cystic hygroma). Grossly and histologically, it is often difficult to differentiate this tumor from a chylous cyst, and in many series the two are grouped in a single category. Traumatic cysts follow external or surgical injury to the mesentery. They are lined with fibrous tissue and usually contain bloody fluid. It is probable that many serous retention cysts are in reality traumatic cysts which have evolved from disruption of mesenteric lymph channels. Enteric cysts are lined with intestinal mucosa and represent duplications of the intestinal tract that do not communicate with the bowel lumen. These and dermoid cysts of the mesentery are exceedingly rare.

Benign solid tumors of the mesentery are more common than malignant ones, and of these, lipomas and fibromas predominate. However, recurrence after incomplete excision of histologically benign mesenteric tumors has been reported and malignant degeneration also suggested. Moreover, histologically benign tumors can kill by local invasion with mechanical compression of adjacent viscera. The benign tumors of nerve elements and smooth muscles are uncommon. Vascular tumors of the mesentery are very rare, and of these, hemangiopericytomas dominate the picture. Ackerman states that liposarcoma is the most frequently encountered malignant tumor of this area,

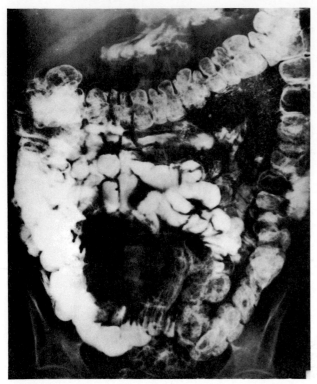

Fig. 35-12. Small intestinal series showing displacement of bowel loops by a mass lesion in the lower right side of the abdomen. The patient proved to have a large benign fibroma in the mesentery of the terminal ileum. (*J. Adams and F. Kutner, Am J Surg, 111:735, 1966.*)

whereas Yannopoulos and Stout report leiomyosarcoma to be the most frequent. Few malignant mesenteric tumors have embolic metastases until very late. They spread by local extension or by peritoneal implants, which occurs most often with leiomyosarcomas. As a rule, the malignant solid tumors arise near the root of the mesentery, whereas solid benign tumors have a greater tendency to develop peripherally near the intestine.

Approximately two-thirds of mesenteric tumors, either cystic or solid, are located in the mesentery of the small intestine, usually that of the ileum. Less frequently, they arise in the transverse or sigmoid mesocolon or in the gastrohepatic ligament. In the greater number of cases, the tumor is located peripherally in the mesentery, where it is often adherent to the adjacent intestine. The mobility of the mesentery permits both benign and malignant tumors to grow to very large sizes before causing symptoms.

CLINICAL MANIFESTATIONS. The early clinical features do not usually differentiate benign tumors from malignant ones. There is an equal sex incidence, although benign cystic tumors are somewhat more common in women and malignant tumors occur more frequently in men. These tumors have been described in children and also the very aged; however, the average age of patients with benign tumors is forty-five years, while those with malignant tumors average fifty-five years old.

The manifestations of mesenteric tumors are dependent upon the size, location, and mobility of the growth. In the vast majority of patients, symptoms are few or nonexistent, and the tumor is detected during a routine examination. Symptoms appear sooner when the tumor is situated in the periphery of the mesentery near the intestine than when located at its root. The patient may merely experience a sensation of fullness or pressure in the abdomen, particularly after eating. Less frequently, there are frank abdominal complaints. About one-half of patients with malignant tumors complain of abdominal pain, weakness, and weight loss, and one-third have diarrhea, cramps, anorexia, and nausea. Only rarely will the patient present with symptoms of complete intestinal obstruction or symptoms resulting from complications of the tumor per se such as torsion, hemorrhage, or infarction of the tumor mass. In the absence of intestinal obstruction or these complications, the sole clinical finding will be the presence of a nontender, intraabdominal mass, usually in the lower right part of the abdomen. The mass varies in size from a few inches in diameter to one which may literally fill the entire abdomen. The extremely large masses are usually cystic, in which case they are tense and fluctuant. Both cystic and solid tumors of the mesentery are mobile; they can be easily moved from side to side but only slightly in an upward and downward direction.

The differential diagnosis takes into consideration all tumefactions of the abdominal cavity and retroperitoneum. Roentgenograms are helpful only when the mesenteric mass is sufficiently large to cause compression and displacement of the bowel or ureters (Fig. 35-12). They do not differentiate a benign tumor from a malignant one, and in most instances the x-ray studies are not helpful. Calcification in the mass is suggestive of a dermoid or teratoma. Routine laboratory studies are usually uninformative.

Since there are no pathognomonic symptoms or signs, a high index of suspicion is necessary for the diagnosis to be made preoperatively. A mesenteric tumor may be suggested by a movable abdominal mass extrinsic to the gastrointestinal and urinary systems; however, final diagnostic confirmation can be made only during laparotomy.

TREATMENT. Surgical excision is the only treatment for both benign or malignant lesions. All mesenteric cysts of a size sufficient to be palpated should be removed if at all possible, since even benign lesions eventually cause pain and compression of neighboring structures. Benign cystic tumors can be removed by enucleation or local excision, although resection in continuity with the adjacent intestine is often necessary because of possible compromise to the vascularity of the bowel or difficulty in separating the tumor from the intestine. Wide excision together with resection of adjacent intestine are recommended for benign solid tumors, since these have a tendency toward local recurrence and malignant degeneration. Prognosis after adequate excision of both cystic and solid benign tumors of the mesentery is excellent.

The outlook for malignant mesenteric tumors is dependent upon whether complete removal is possible and is generally poor. Since malignant growths tend to occur in the root of the mesentery and often involve the great vessels and vasculature to most of the small intestine and colon, curative resection is usually prohibitive. Resectable lesions invariably will require removal of a portion of bowel; however, fewer than one-third of the malignant tumors are totally resectable. Nevertheless, since these growths may enlarge slowly and embolic metastases occur late, it is worthwhile to partially remove them to relieve obstructions, and prolonged survival has been recorded in a few instances. Irradiation therapy offers little if any benefit, since the tumors are invariably radioresistant. Few patients with malignant primary mesenteric tumors are alive after 5 years. Death results from invasion with obstruction of the gastrointestinal tract leading to perforation and hemorrhage or from metastases to liver and lung.

RETROPERITONEUM

General Considerations

The retroperitoneum consists of that portion of the body which is bounded anteriorly by the peritoneum, posteriorly by the spine and psoas and quadratus lumborum muscles, superiorly by the twelfth ribs and attachments of the diaphragm, and inferiorly by the brim of the pelvis. The lateral margins of the space correspond to the lateral borders of the quadratus lumborum muscles. These limits define both an actual and a potential space, the actual space containing solid organs and major blood vessels while the potential space includes soft tissues, nerve elements, and small blood vessels. Since there are no anatomic barriers in this area, pathologic processes may extend easily throughout it and therefore are often bilateral.

Contained within the retroperitoneum are the kidneys, ureters, adrenal glands, portions of the autonomic and peripheral nervous systems, pancreas, abdominal aorta, inferior vena cava, spermatic or ovarian vessels, lymphatics and lymph nodes, and certain portions of the intestinal tract, notably the duodenum. The space also contains fatty and areolar tissue and fibrous connective tissue.

The diagnosis of diseases involving the retroperitoneum has been enhanced by the application of such radiocontrast roentgenographic studies as pyelography, venography, arteriography, lymphangiography, and presacral air insufflation. Nevertheless, it remains an obscure area of the body, enabling pathologic processes to become advanced before producing symptoms.

The multiplicity of structures within the retroperitoneum gives rise to a variety of pathologic conditions. This chapter will deal with the relatively uncommon entities of (1) idiopathic retroperitoneal fibrosis and (2) primary tumors of the retroperitoneal space.

Idiopathic Retroperitoneal Fibrosis

Idiopathic retroperitoneal fibrosis is a nonspecific, nonsuppurative inflammation of fibroadipose tissue of unknown cause which produces symptoms by the gradual compression of the tubular structures in the retroperitoneal space. It is currently believed that the disease represents one of the manifestations of a widespread entity termed "systemic idiopathic fibrosis." Idiopathic mediastinal fibrosis, Riedel's struma, sclerosing cholangitis, mesenteric panniculitis, Peyronie's disease, pseudotumor of the orbit, and perhaps desmoid tumor are other fibromatoses which are considered to be localized forms of systemic idiopathic fibrosis. A factor common to all these diseases is an inflammatory fibrotic process involving areolar and adipose tissue.

Retroperitoneal fibrosis was first described in 1905 by Albarran, a French urologist, who performed ureterolysis for ureteral compression produced by the disease. The first report in English is credited to Ormond in 1948. It has since been referred to as Ormond's syndrome but has also been labeled "idiopathic fibrous retroperitonitis," "periureteritis plastica," and "sclerosing retroperitonitis." Retroperitoneal lipogranulomatosis (xanthogranulomatosis), which can produce a similar clinical picture, may be a granulomatous, prefibrotic stage of retroperitoneal fibrosis.

ETIOLOGY. Attesting to the obscure etiology of retroperitoneal fibrosis are the many theories which have been advanced to explain its origin. Hackett, in finding hemosiderin deposits in biopsy specimens, felt that the cause might be previous trauma that produced a retroperitoneal hematoma which subsequently underwent organization. The possibility that extravasated urine might cause a fibrotic reaction in the retroperitoneum was mentioned by Ormond, and both he and Hackett also suggested that an abortive infection elsewhere, only partially treated with antibiotics, might later start an inflammatory reaction in the lymphatic and perivascular tissues of the retroperitoneum. Others have speculated that the disease may be an autoimmune reaction to interstitial protein. Hache et al. proposed the concept that the fibrosis was the end result of an ascending lymphangitis, adenitis, or periadenitis in the retroperitoneum with the infection arising from chronic or recurrent genitourinary infections or inflammatory diseases of the gastrointestinal tract or pelvic organs. Reports of retroperitoneal fibrosis occurring in patients taking the antiserotonin drug methysergide for headache prompted the theory that the disease may be due to a hypersensitivity reaction to the drug. Suby reported a reversal of the fibrotic process after discontinuing the medication and speculated that other drugs may be similarly at fault.

It is probable that no single factor is responsible for causing the disease in all cases and that perhaps multiple factors may be implicated in any one case.

PATHOLOGY. The gross appearance of retroperitoneal fibrosis is usually that of a plaque of woody, white fibrous tissue which is distributed along the course of the periaortic lymphatics. In about one-third of the cases, it is bilateral. The diseased tissue, which may be 2 to 12 cm thick, extends from the sacral promontory to the renal pedicles and laterally to cover the iliopsoas muscles. It is sharply demarcated but not encapsulated. The mass surrounds and constricts but does not invade the regional structures in the retroperitoneum, primarily the blood vessels, nerves, and ureters to which it becomes adherent.

A localized form has been observed as a circumscribed fibrous reaction surrounding only the ureters, and exten-

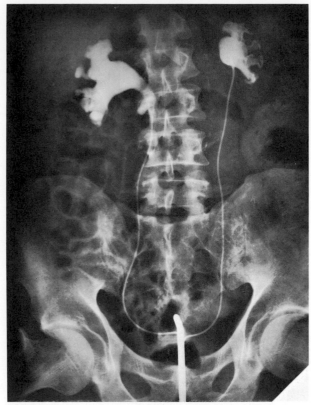

Fig. 35-13. Retrograde pyelogram in a patient with retroperitoneal fibrosis showing bilateral hydronephrosis without organic obstruction of the ureters. The medial displacement of the ureters is a characteristic roentgenographic finding which differentiates this disease from retroperitoneal tumefactions.

sive involvement of the entire retroperitoneum with compression of the duodenum, common bile duct, and pancreas has also been seen. A similar fibrotic process has been described penetrating the diaphragm along the great vessels into the mediastinum causing superior vena cava obstruction and also extending into the root of the mesentery, causing intestinal obstruction.

Microscopically, the pattern varies from a subacute cellular process with polymorphonuclear cells, lymphocytes, fibroblasts, and fat cells to a completely hyalinized, relatively acellular sclerosis. Eosinophils, foreign body giant cells, and small areas of calcification may also be present. Suppuration with abscess formation does not occur. The amount of fat and cellular infiltration and the degree of fibrosis vary between patients and in different biopsy specimens from the same patient. The more cellular picture is usually seen in the early stages of the disease, when there may be systemic signs of inflammation, whereas the dense fibrotic process is found late.

CLINICAL MANIFESTATIONS. Retroperitoneal fibrosis is two to three times more common among men than among women. It may occur in children and also the aged; however, about two-thirds of the patients are between forty and sixty years old.

The protean manifestations of the disease are related to the phase and extent of the process and the structures secondarily involved. Ormond divided the natural history of the disease into three periods: (1) the period of incidence and development; (2) the period of activity, that is, spread of the cellular and fibrotic process to envelopment of the retroperitoneal structures; and (3) the period of contraction of the fibrotic mass with compression of the involved structures. The disease is apparently self-limiting once the fibrotic stage is reached, a factor of major importance in considering types of therapy.

Early symptoms are vague and nonspecific, but the first complaint is invariably pain. This is dull, noncolicky, and insidious in onset. It usually originates in the flank or low back and often radiates to the lower abdomen, groin, genitalia, or anteromedial aspect of the thigh. The pain is unilateral at first but may become bilateral later, as the fibrotic process spreads. Anorexia, nausea, diarrhea, generalized malaise, and weight loss variably occur in the early and late phases of the disease. Features of a subacute inflammation such as lower abdominal or costovertebral tenderness, moderate fever, leukocytosis, and an elevated sedimentation rate are often present early. A transabdominal or pelvic mass is palpable in about one-third of the patients during some phase of the disease.

Symptoms due to compression of the tubular retroperitoneal structures may follow the initial complaints by 1 month to 2 years and reflect the late fibrotic phase of the disease with sclerotic contraction. The major structures involved are the ureters, aorta, and inferior vena cava. These all lie within the same fascial compartment. However, the aorta is resistant to compression, and the inferior vena cava has abundant collaterals, so that the symptoms are generally related to ureteral involvement. Partial or complete ureteral obstruction occurs in 75 to 85 percent of patients. The usual site of obstruction is in the lower third of the ureter. Excretory urograms will show a hydroureter and hydronephrosis on one or both sides with medial deviation of the ureter in contrast to lateral displacement that is characteristically associated with retroperitoneal tumors. Retrograde studies may be required if there is complete ureteral obstruction with nonfilling of the kidney (Fig. 35-13). The ureteral obstruction is usually functional, rather than organic, as a consequence of cessation of peristalsis in the incarcerated ureteral segment. In the majority of cases, a ureteral catheter can still be passed in a retrograde manner.

Dysuria, frequency of urination, and chills and fever occur with secondary infection of a hydronephrotic kidney. These symptoms may be intermittent for years, or a single attack may culminate in sudden anuria from bilateral obstruction. As many as 40 percent of patients will have oliguria or anuria with laboratory evidence of azotemia. Clinically, the enlarged kidneys may be palpable, and the urine, if infected, will contain white blood cells and bacteria. Hematuria, in the absence of infection, is rare.

Lower extremity edema, presumably from lymphatic as well as venous obstruction, occasionally occurs and may be unilateral. The level of obstruction in most cases will correspond to that of the ureteral obstruction and can be demonstrated on phlebograms.

Arterial insufficiency due to fibrous constriction of the aorta or iliac arteries is uncommon but can occur and may constitute the major problem. The intermittent claudication, rest pain, and limb ischemia are indistinguishable clinically and radiographically from those of atherosclerotic occlusion.

Rarely, the fibrotic process will involve the retroperitoneal duodenum and common bile ducts, causing duodenal and biliary obstruction. Mechanical or functional intestinal obstruction due to extension into the root of the mesentery or sigmoid mesocolon is also a rare manifestation.

The diagnosis of retroperitoneal fibrosis may be suspected from the clinical features and the contrast roentgenograms of the urinary and vascular systems. Intravenous pyelography is the most definitive noninvasive diagnostic test. The triad that is highly suggestive of retroperitoneal fibrosis is (1) hydronephrosis with a dilated, tortuous upper ureter; (2) medial deviation of the ureter; and (3) extrinsic ureteral compression. However, a variety of conditions can produce a similar picture, and final confirmation can be made only following exploratory surgical procedures and biopsy of the fibrotic mass. The differential diagnosis includes the primary retroperitoneal tumors, notably Hodgkin's disease, and metastatic tumor from the kidneys, pancreas, or pelvic organs. Inflammatory conditions to be excluded include tuberculosis, pancreatitis and intraabdominal inflammation of the intestine tract.

TREATMENT. Once the diagnosis is established, the patient should be carefully followed and surgical intervention timed properly. Improvement may be anticipated in some patients with supportive measures alone. However, with the onset of urinary infection or depression of renal function, surgical intervention becomes necessary.

The discontinuance of methysergide is sometimes followed by a reversal of the fibrotic process with an improvement in symptoms. Steroids, antibiotics, and x-ray therapy have been used with inconsistent results. The self-limiting nature of the disease and the reports of spontaneous resolution in untreated patients make it difficult to evaluate the results of any of these therapeutic modalities. Steroids are of theoretical use in the early inflammatory stages to diminish the generation of fibrosis or control a hyperimmune reaction if one exists. For patients in the prefibrotic stage of the disease with renal insufficiency and prominent constitutional symptoms, steroid-induced regression of the inflammatory edema may reestablish urinary patency and thus facilitate elective, rather than emergency, surgery. However, usually an advanced stage of fibrosis has been reached before the diagnosis is made.

Surgical treatment is directed toward relief of the tubular obstructions, which are usually urinary, less often vascular, and rarely intestinal. Since the disease is fundamentally a midline process which is often bilateral, a midtransabdominal approach offers the best exposure. Several deep biopsies of the mass should be obtained to rule out the possibility of an underlying neoplasm, since these may produce a similar picture, particularly tumors of lymphatic origin. The aorta, inferior vena cava, small bowel mesentery, and sigmoid mesocolon as well as the ureters should be adequately examined for possible involvement.

Ureterolysis with intraperitoneal transplantation is currently the most effective means of relieving obstruction of the involved ureter. This consists of freeing the ureter from the enveloping mass of fibrous tissue and transferring it into the peritoneal cavity, closing the posterior peritoneum behind it. Lateral reposition of the ureter within the retroperitoneal space has been reported to yield equally good results. A preliminary nephrostomy may be indicated if bilateral ureteral obstruction has resulted in severe renal impairment with uremia. On rare occasion, it will be necessary to reimplant the mobilized ureter into the bladder or to replace it with a vascularized segment of small intestine.

Aortic or iliac artery obstruction can be treated by arteriolysis or bypass with a synthetic vascular graft.

Symptoms due to venous obstruction are best treated with elevation and elastic support to the lower limbs until a sufficient collateral venous system develops. The extent of any permanent venous insufficiency will depend upon the availability of collateral pathways and the competency of deep vein valves. Release of the obstructed vein from its fibrous encasement may be difficult and hazardous, and bypass procedures for obstruction of the inferior vena cava have been uniformly unsuccessful.

The prognosis of the disease is generally good, provided that appropriate treatment has been instituted prior to the development of irreversible renal damage. Ormond, in 1960, reviewed 64 cases and reported 10 deaths, most from renal failure secondary to unrecognized obstructive uropathy which presumably could have been corrected with earlier diagnosis. In 1977 a combined series of 481 cases reported by Koep and Zuidema showed the cumulative mortality to be 9 percent.

Retroperitoneal Tumors

Primary tumors of the retroperitoneum include those neoplasms arising from tissues which occupy the potential retroperitoneal space. These tumors develop independently and have no apparent connection with any organs or major vessels except by areolar tissue. Tumors of the retroperitoneal solid organs, such as the pancreas, adrenal, or kidney, and tumefactions of the great blood vessels, therefore, are not included in this category.

The first description of retroperitoneal tumors is credited to Morgagni in 1761. Several large series have been reported by Ackerman, Braasch, Donnelly, Melicow, and Pack and Tabah. Although they are uncommon, nonetheless, they are not rare and must always be considered in the differential diagnosis of an unexplained abdominal mass. The majority occur in the fifth or sixth decades with a peak incidence at about sixty years, although approximately 15 percent are found in children under ten years of age.

PATHOLOGY. The several theories relating to the histogenesis of these tumors have been summarized by Donnelly and by Pack and Tabah. Tumors in this locale may arise from fat, areolar connective tissue, fascia, muscle, vascular tissue, somatic and sympathetic nervous tissue, and lymph vessels and lymph nodes. Less frequent neoplasms are smooth muscle tumors, complex teratomas, embryonal carcinomas, and certain bizarre cysts of unknown origin. These rarer tumors are believed to arise from remnants of the embryonal urogenital apparatus, which includes tissue of both epithelial and mesothelial origin. A classification of the benign and malignant tumors according to tissue type is given in Table 35-2. Malignant tumors outnumber those which are benign in a ratio of 4:1.

The tumors may be solid, cystic, or a combination of both. Their color varies from white (fibroma), yellow (lipoma), or pinkish to red (sarcoma), depending on the predominant tissue. They may be single or multiple and vary in size from small outgrowths to tumors weighing as much as 40 lb. As a rule, the predominantly cystic tumors are benign, whereas the solid tumors are usually malignant.

CLINICAL MANIFESTATIONS. Early symptoms of retroperitoneal tumors are characteristically vague or lacking. The loose retroperitoneal areolar tissue allows the tumor to grow unrestricted in all directions except posteriorly. For this reason, it may attain an extremely large size before producing symptoms. As the tumor grows, it compresses, obstructs, or invades adjacent organs or structures, so that the presenting symptoms are often referable to these organs.

The initial manifestations include an enlarging abdomen, backache, a sense of fullness or heaviness, and vague indefinite pain which later may become severe and radicular. Nausea, vomiting, change in bowel habits, and other symptoms suggestive of bowel obstruction result from compression of portions of the gastrointestinal tract. Later,

the malignant tumors cause anorexia, weight loss, weakness, fever, and, less frequently, hematemesis. Genitourinary complaints include hematuria, dysuria, and urgency and frequency of urination. Rarely, there is oliguria or anuria. Pain radiating into one or both thighs is usually late and due to involvement of lumbar and sacral nerve routes; it invariably denotes a malignant tumor. Swelling and varicosities of the lower extremities are usually due to obstruction of lymphatics and venous return. Hormonally active tumors of extraadrenal chromaffin tissue (pheochromocytoma) produce symptoms referable to hypertension. Rarely, hypoglycemia and its associated symptoms may be seen with retroperitoneal sarcomas.

The predominant physical finding is the presence of an abdominal mass. This is usually nontender and may fill the entire abdomen. A fixed, hard mass suggests malignancy, whereas a soft or tense and ballottable one may be a benign neoplasm or cyst. The mass usually occupies the midline and extends into one or both flanks or may be deep-seated in the pelvis, where it can be felt through the rectum. Ascites due to compression of the portal or hepatic veins, edema of the lower extremities, scrotal varicosities, and dilated superficial abdominal veins are infrequently present. Enlarged hemorrhoids or rectal tenesmus are symptoms in patients with presacral neoplasms.

The diagnosis of primary retroperitoneal tumors is mainly one of exclusion of other abdominal tumefactions. Differential diagnosis includes lesions of the kidney, such as hydronephrosis, polycystic disease, or hypernephroma; pancreatic cysts and tumors; splenomegaly; neoplasms of the liver; tumors of the gastrointestinal tract; ovarian tumors; abdominal aortic aneurysms; and cysts of the omentum and mesentery. To aid in this differentiation,

Table 35-2. CLASSIFICATION OF RETROPERITONEAL TUMORS

Tissue type	Benign tumors	Malignant tumors
Lymphatic tissue	Lymphangioma	Lymphangiosarcoma
Lymph nodes	. . . .	Lymphosarcoma
		Hodgkin's disease
		Reticulum cell sarcoma
Adipose tissue	Lipoma	Liposarcoma
Fibrous tissue	Fibroma	Fibrosarcoma
Smooth muscle	Lieomyoma	Lieomyosarcoma
Nerve elements	Neurilemoma	Malignant schwannoma
	Neurofibroma	
	Ganglioneuroma	Sympathicoblastoma (neuroblastoma)
		Chordoma
Striated muscle	Rhabdomyoma	Rhabdomyosarcoma
Mucoid tissue	Myxoma	Myxosarcoma
Vascular tissue	Hemangioma	Malignant hemangiopericytoma
Mesothelial tissue	. . . .	Mesothelioma
Mesenchyme	. . . .	Mesenchymoma
Extraadrenal chromaffin tissue	Benign pheochromocytoma	Malignant pheochromocytoma
Gland tissue	Adenoma	Carcinoma
Embyronic remnants	Nephrogenic cysts	Urogenital ridge tumor
Cell rests	Dermoid	Teratoma
Miscellaneous	Xanthogranuloma	Synovioma
		Dysgerminoma
		Undifferentiated malignant tumor

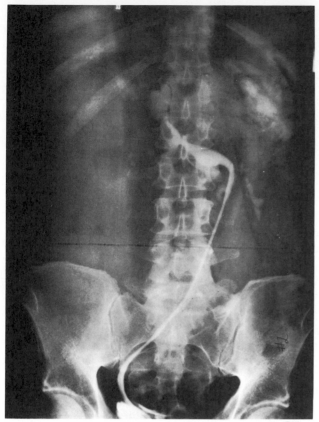

Fig. 35-14. Right retrograde pyelogram (anteroposterior film) showing displacement of the right kidney into the left side of the abdomen with distortion of the renal pelvis. At laparotomy, the patient was found to have a very large liposarcoma completely filling the right retroperitoneal space.

roentgenographic studies of the genitourinary and gastrointestinal tracts are particularly useful in addition to an ordinary flat plate of the abdomen, abdominal aortography, inferior vena cava phlebography, and special scanning techniques. The intravenous and retrograde pyelogram is the most valuable of these studies. Typically with malignant tumors, anteroposterior films will show distortion and displacement of the ureters laterally, partial or complete obstruction of the ureter, or distortion of the kidney pelvis (Fig. 35-14). Lateral films may demonstrate anterior ureteral displacement. Displacement of the ureter without distortion is seen with benign neoplasms (Fig. 35-15).

The main value of a gastrointestinal series and barium enema is the exclusion of gastrointestinal tumors. However, if the tumor is of sufficient size, it will show displacement or distortion of the stomach or intestines (Fig. 35-16). Calcification is not unusual in certain retroperitoneal tumors, while the finding of teeth or other recognizable bony structures is diagnostic of teratoma.

Lowman and associates reported in detail the diagnostic use of retroperitoneal angiography. The lumbar arteries supply a large segment of the retroperitoneal space, and stretching or displacement of these vessels or displacement of the aorta by the tumor mass can give precise localization of the tumor and exclude primary visceral tumors (Fig. 35-17). Neovascularity often indicates malignant disease, but most retroperitoneal tumors lack this feature.

Beta-scan ultrasonography is a safe, noninvasive technique which will differentiate solid tumors from cysts. Recently, computerized axial tomography has also been used for diagnosing retroperitoneal tumors. Retroperitoneal pneumography, although widely discussed in the literature, is now rarely used, having been replaced by safer diagnostic techniques.

Positive histologic diagnosis can be made only with biopsy of the tumor at the time of laparotomy. At least 75 percent of the malignant tumors are sarcomas. In order of frequency, these are malignant lymphomas, liposarcomas, leiomyosarcomas, rhabdomyosarcomas, and fibrosarcomas. Sympathicoblastomas or neuroblastomas also comprise a large group of the malignant tumors. The most frequent benign tumors are cystic and include lymphatic or chylous cysts, cysts of urogenital origin, dermoids, and enterogenous cysts. Other relatively common benign tumors are xanthogranulomas, lipomas, and benign pheochromocytomas.

TREATMENT. Some retroperitoneal tumors are benign and can be cured by simple excisions; some are histologi-

Fig. 35-15. Right retrograde pyelogram in a patient with a benign retroperitoneal neurofibroma causing partial obstruction of the kidney. The right ureter is displaced laterally, which is the usual finding with retroperitoneal tumors.

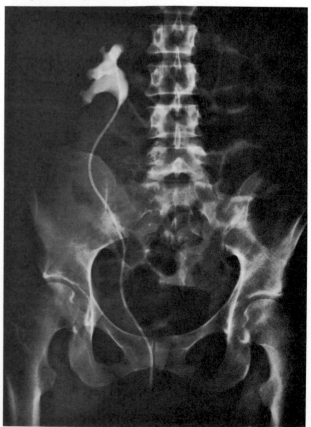

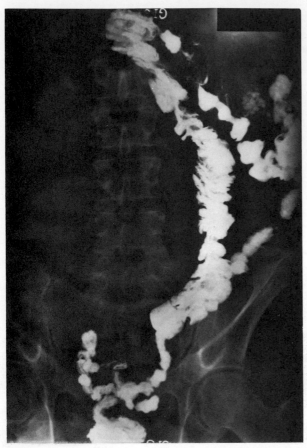

Fig. 35-16. Barium enema in the patient depicted in Fig. 35-14 showing marked displacement of the ascending colon to the left by the retroperitoneal tumor.

cally benign but clinically malignant; others grow slowly but tend to recur and invade locally; and still others are rapidly malignant from the start.

Treatment of these growths consists of surgical or irradiation therapy, or a combination of the two. With the exception of lymphomas, chemotherapy has only limited therapeutic application. Surgical treatment is the most effective and offers the greatest prospect for cure. In some cases, it is imperative because of intestinal or urinary obstructions or because of hemorrhage.

As many as one-third of patients with malignant tumors may be inoperable because of multiple peritoneal tumor implants or distant metastases to liver, lung, and bone, in order of frequency.

In operable patients, initial biopsy of the tumor with frozen section will usually determine its malignant or benign nature. A cure may be anticipated following complete resection of benign tumors. On occasion, however, a tumor previously considered benign will recur, and this is especially true of retroperitoneal lipomas, which may undergo sarcomatous change.

For a malignant tumor, the initial operation offers the best chance for cure. These tumors are quite invasive and often become adherent to vital organs or structures. Adequate exposure is extremely important to enable safe dissection of the tumor and avoid injury to major blood vessels. For this reason, a generous transperitoneal abdominal incision is preferred over an extraperitoneal flank approach. It is estimated that fewer than 25 percent of malignant tumors can be completely resected with anticipation of cure. Fixation of the tumor to the parietes does not contraindicate an attempt at resection, since partial excision can often give satisfactory palliation. At times, nephrectomy or partial intestinal resection may be required. Operative mortality is high, with reports varying between 10 and 25 percent.

Malignant retroperitoneal tumors have a high recurrence rate, from 30 to 50 percent in most large series. The tumors become more malignant with each recurrence, and reoperation becomes more hazardous. Nevertheless, long-term survival has been reported after multiple resections.

Radiotherapy, although rarely curative, may relieve pain, and obstruction and prolong life. As many as 75 percent of patients will benefit from irradiation therapy even though most retroperitoneal tumors are not radiocurative. Indications for irradiation include (1) inoperable tumors; (2) tumor recurrence following previous resection; (3) residual tumor following partial surgical resection; (4) certain radiosensitive tumors, particularly the malignant lymphomas; and (5) as an adjunct to surgery for some malignant tumors such as neuroblastomas, liposarcomas, rhabdomyosarcomas, and undifferentiated anaplastic sarcomas. Radiotherapy is the treatment of choice for malignant lymphomas, since the multicentric origin of these tumors makes surgical extirpation difficult.

The overall prognosis for malignant retroperitoneal tumors is poor. Five-year survival free of tumor is less than 10 percent and can be anticipated only in those patients in whom complete surgical removal is possible. Rare cures following irradiation therapy of neuroblastoma or lymphosarcoma have also been reported. However, since many of the tumors are slow-growing or responsive to irradiation, long-term survival with existing tumor is possible in as many as 15 percent of patients. Neuroblastoma and liposarcoma offer the best prognosis with average survivals of 4 and 5 years, respectively. Most patients with other malignant retroperitoneal tumors are dead in 2 years, death resulting from widespread metastases, intestinal or urinary obstruction, or hemorrhage from invasion of major blood vessels.

References

Abdominal Wall

Ackerman, L. V.: "Surgical Pathology," p. 964, The C. V. Mosby Company, St. Louis, 1964.

Brasfield, R. D., and Das Gupta, T. K.: Desmoid Tumors of the Anterior Abdominal Wall, *Surgery,* **65:**241, 1969.

Cullen, T. S., and Brodel, M.: Lesions of the Rectus Abdominus Muscle Simulating an Acute Intra-abdominal Condition, *Bull Johns Hopkins Hosp,* **61:**295, 1937.

Das Gupta, T. K., Brasfield, R. D., and O'Hara J.: Extra-

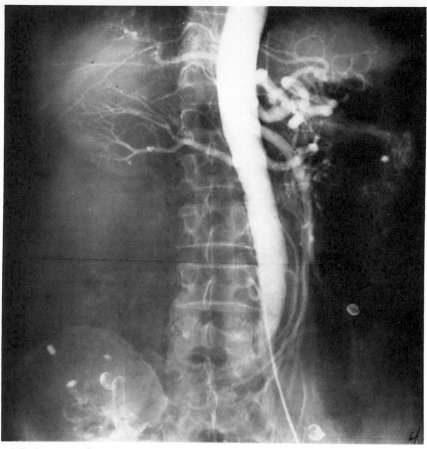

Fig. 35-17. Abdominal aortogram showing lateral displacement of the aorta and lumbar arteries by a large right retroperitoneal tumor.

abdominal Desmoids: A Clinicopathological Study, *Ann Surg,* **170:**109, 1969.

Geschickter, C. F., and Lewis, D.: Tumors of Connective Tissue, *Am J Cancer,* **25:**630, 1935.

Hildreth, D.: Anticoagulant Therapy and Rectus Sheath Hematoma, *Am J Surg,* **124:**80, 1972.

Jones, T. W., and Merendino, K. A.: The Deep Epigastric Artery: Rectus Muscle Syndrome, *Am J Surg,* **103:**159, 1962.

Pack, G. T., and Ehrlich, H. E.: Neoplasms of the Anterior Abdominal Wall with Special Consideration of Desmoid Tumors, *Surg Gynecol Obstet,* **79:**177, 1944.

Sheehan, V.: Spontaneous Hematoma of the Rectus Abdominis Muscle in Pregnancy, *Br Med J,* **2:**1131, 1951.

Stiles, Q. R., Raskowski, H. J., and Henry, W.: Rectus Sheath Hematoma, *Surg Gynecol Obstet,* **12:**331, 1965.

Stout, A. P.: Fibrosarcoma: The Malignant Tumor of Fibroblasts, *Cancer,* **1:**30, 1948.

Teske, J. M.: Hematoma of the Rectus Abdominis Muscle: Report of a Case and Analysis of 100 Cases from the Literature, *Am J Surg,* **71:**689, 1946.

Waddell, W. R.: Treatment of Intra-abdominal and Abdominal Wall Desmoid Tumors with Drugs that Affect the Metabolism of Cyclic 3′,5′-Adenosine Monophosphate, *Ann Surg,* **181:**299, 1975.

Omentum

Anton, J. E., Jennings, J. E., and Spiegel, M. B.: Primary Omental Torsion, *Am J Surg,* **68:**303, 1945.

Beahrs, O. H., Judd, E. J., Jr., and Dockerty, M. B.: Chylous Cysts of the Abdomen, *Surg Clin North Am,* **30:**1081, 1950.

Brown, H. J., and Noone, R. B.: Primary Omental Torsion, *J Okla State Med Assoc,* **64:**177, 1971.

Draper, J. W., and Johnston, R. K.: The Pathologic Omentum, *JAMA,* **88:**376, 1927.

Eitel, G. G.: A Rare Omental Tumor, *Med Rec,* **55:**715, 1899.

Halligan, E. J., and Rabiah, F. A.: Primary Idiopathic Segmental Infarction of the Greater Omentum, *Arch Surg,* **79:**738, 1959.

Leitner, M. J., Jordan, C. G., Spinner, M. H., and Reese, E. C.: Torsion, Infarction and Hemorrhage of the Omentum as a Cause of Acute Abdominal Distress, *Ann Surg,* **135:**103, 1952.

Mainzer, R. A., and Simoes, A.: Primary Idiopathic Torsion of the Omentum, *Arch Surg,* **88:**974, 1964.

Rubin, I. C.: The Functions of the Great Omentum, *Surg Gynecol Obstet,* **12:**117, 1911.

Stout, A. P., Hendry, J., and Purdie, F. J.: Solid Tumors of the Great Omentum, *Cancer,* **16:**231, 1963.

Walker, A. R., and Putnam, T. C.: Omental, Mesenteric and Retroperitoneal Cysts, *Surgery,* **178:**13, 1973.

Wrzesinski, J., and Firestone, S.: Primary Idiopathic Segmental Infarction of the Omentum, *Surgery,* **39:**663, 1965.

Mesentery

Ackerman, L. V.: "Surgical Pathology," The C. V. Mosby Company, St. Louis, 1964.

Adams, J. T., and Kutner, F. R.: Pure Fibroma of the Mesentery, *Am J Surg,* **111:**734, 1966.

Aird, I.: Acute Non-specific Mesenteric Lymphadenitis, *Br Med J,* **2:**680, 1945.

Anane-Safah, J. C., Blair, E., and Reckler, S.: Primary Mesenteric Venous Occlusive Disease, *Surg Gynecol Obstet,* **141:**740, 1975.

Beahrs, O. H., Judd, E. S., Jr., and Dockerty, M. B.: Chylous Cysts of the Abdomen, *Surg Clin North Am,* **30:**1081, 1950.

Bergan, J. J., Dean, R. H., Conn, J., Jr., and Yao, J. S. T.: Revascularization in Treatment of Mesenteric Infarction, *Ann Surg,* **182:**430, 1975.

Bernatz, P. E.: Necrosis of Colon following Resection for Abdominal Aortic Aneurysm, *Arch Surg,* **81:**373, 1960.

Berry, F. B., and Bougas, J. A.: Agnogenic Venous Mesenteric Thrombosis, *Ann Surg,* **132:**450, 1950.

Britt, L. C., and Cheek, R. C.: Nonocclusive Mesenteric Vascular Disease: Clinical and Experimental Observations, *Ann Surg,* **169:**704, 1969.

Carey, J. P., Stemmer, E. A., and Connolly, J. E.: Median Arcuate Ligament Syndrome, *Arch Surg,* **99:**441, 1969.

Caropreso, P. R.: Mesenteric Cysts, A Review, *Arch Surg,* **108:**242, 1974.

Carter, R., and Gosney, W. G.: Abdominal Apoplexy: Report of Six Cases and Review of the Literature, *Am J Surg,* **111:**388, 1966.

Connolly, J. E., Abrams, H. L., and Kieraldo, J. H.: Observations on the Diagnosis and Treatment of Obliterative Disease of the Visceral Branches of the Abdominal Aorta, *Arch Surg,* **90:**596, 1965.

Crile, G., Jr., and Newell, E. T., Jr.: Abdominal Apoplexy: Spontaneous Rupture of Visceral Vessel, *JAMA,* **114:**1155, 1940.

Donhauser, J. L.: Primary Acute Mesenteric Lymphadenitis, *Arch Surg,* **74:**528, 1957.

Dunbar, J. D., Molnar, W., Beman, F. F., and Marable, S. A.: Compression of the Celiac Trunk and Abdominal Angina: Preliminary Report of 15 Cases, *Am J Roentgenol Radium Ther Nucl Med,* **95:**731, 1965.

Dunphy, J. E.: Abdominal Pain of Vascular Origin, *Am J Med Sci,* **192:**109, 1936.

Durst, A. L., Freund, H., Rosenmann, E., and Birnbaum, D.: Mesenteric Panniculitis: Review of the Literature and Presentation of Cases, *Surgery,* **81:**203, 1977.

Fogerty, T. J., and Fletcher, W. S.: Genesis of Nonocclusive Mesenteric Ischemia, *Am J Surg,* **111:**130, 1966.

Fowler, E. F.: Primary Cysts and Tumors of the Small Bowel Mesentery, *Am Surg,* **27:**653, 1961.

Fry, W. J., and Kraft, R. O.: Visceral Angina, *Surg Gynecol Obstet,* **117:**417, 1963.

Grossman, L. A., Kaplan, H. J., Preuss, H. J., and Herrington, J. L., Jr.: Mesenteric Panniculitis, *JAMA,* **183:**318, 1963.

Habbooshe, F., Wallace, H. W., Nusbaum, M., Baum, S., Dratch, P., and Blakemore, W. S.: Nonocclusive Mesenteric Vascular Insufficiency, *Ann Surg,* **180:**819, 1974.

Handelsman, J. C., and Shelly, W. M.: Mesenteric Panniculitis, *Arch Surg,* **91:**842, 1965.

Hart, J. T.: Solid Tumors of the Mesentery, *Ann Surg,* **104:**184, 1936.

Jackson, B. B.: "Occlusion of the Superior Mesenteric Artery," Charles C Thomas, Publisher, Springfield, Ill., 1963.

Kleinsasser, L. J.: Abdominal Apoplexy: Report of Two Cases and Review of the Literature, *Am J Surg,* **120:**623, 1970.

Laufman, H., Nora, P. F., and Mittelpunkt, A. I.: Mesenteric Blood Vessels: Advances in Surgery and Physiology, *Arch Surg,* **88:**1021, 1964.

Levinsky, R. A., Lewis, R. M., Bynum, T. E., and Hanley, H. G.: Digoxin Induced Intestinal Vasoconstriction: The Effects of Proximal Arterial Stenosis and Glucagon Administration, *Circulation,* **52:**130, 1975.

Loeb, M. J.: Mesenteric Cysts, *NY State J Med,* **41:**1564, 1941.

McCort, J. J.: Infarction of the Descending Colon Due to Vascular Occlusion, *N Engl J Med,* **262:**168, 1960.

McDonald, J. C.: Nonspecific Mesenteric Lymphadenitis, *Surg Gynecol Obstet,* **116:**409, 1963.

Madore, P., Kahn, D. S., Webster, D. R., and Skoryna, S.: Nonspecific Mesenteric Lymphadenitis, *Can J Surg,* **5:**59, 1962.

Marable, S. A., Kaplan, M. F., Beman, F. M., and Molnar, W.: Celiac Compression Syndrome, *Am J Surg,* **115:**97, 1968.

Morris, G. C., Crawford, E. S., Cooley, D. A., and DeBakey, M. E.: Revascularization of the Celiac and Superior Mesenteric Arteries, *Arch Surg,* **84:**95, 1962.

—— and DeBakey, M. E.: Abdominal Angina: Diagnosis and Treatment, *JAMA,* **176:**91, 1961.

Naitove, A., and Weismann, R. E.: Primary Mesenteric Venous Thrombosis, *Ann Surg,* **161:**516, 1965.

Ogden, W. W., Bradburn, D. M., and Rives, J. D.: Mesenteric Panniculitis, *Ann Surg,* **161:**864, 1965.

Ottinger, L. W., and Austen, W. G.: A Study of 136 Patients with Mesenteric Infarction, *Surg Gynecol Obstet,* **124:**251, 1967.

Pierce, G. E., and Brockenbrough, E. C.: The Spectrum of Mesenteric Infarction, *Am J Surg,* **119:**233, 1970.

Rankin, F. W., and Major, S. G.: Tumors of the Mesentery, *Surg Gynecol Obstet,* **54:**809, 1932.

Reul, G. J., Jr., Wukasch, D. C., Sandiford, F. M., Chiarillo, L., Hallman, G. L., and Cooley, D. A.: Surgical Treatment of Abdominal Angina: Review of 25 Patients, *Surgery,* **75:**682, 1974.

Rob, C. G.: The Indications for Operation in Occlusive Disease of the Visceral Arteries, *J Thorac Cardiovasc Surg,* **3:**223, 1962.

——: Surgical Diseases of the Celiac and Mesenteric Arteries, *Arch Surg,* **93:**21, 1966.

Seldinger, S. I.: Catheter Replacement of Needle in Percutaneous Arteriography: New Technique, *Acta Radiol (Stockholm),* **39:**368, 1953.

Shaw, R. S., and Maynard, E. P., III: Acute and Chronic Thrombosis of Superior Mesenteric Arteries Associated with Malabsorption: Report of Two Cases Successfully Treated by Thromboendarterectomy, *N Engl J Med,* **258:**874, 1958.

—— and Rutledge, R. H.: Superior Mesenteric Artery Embolectomy in the Treatment of Massive Mesenteric Infarction, *N Engl J Med,* **257:**595, 1957.

Smith, R. F., Szilagyi, D. E., and Pfeifer, J. R.: Arterial Trauma, *Arch Surg,* **86:**825, 1963.

Stanley, J. C., Thompson, N. W., and Fry, W. J.: Splanchnic Artery Aneurysms, *Arch Surg,* **101:**689, 1970.

——— and Fry, W. J.: Median Arcuate Ligament Syndrome, *Arch Surg,* **103:**252, 1971.

Thorek, P.: "Anatomy in Surgery," 2d ed., J. B. Lippincott Company, Philadelphia, 1963.

Van Way, C. W., Brockman, S. K., and Rosenfeld, L.: Spontaneous Thrombosis of the Mesenteric Veins, *Ann Surg,* **173:**561, 1971.

Watson, W. O., and Sadikali, F.: Celiac Axis Compression: Experience with 20 Patients and a Critical Appraisal of the Syndrome, *Ann Intern Med,* **86:**278, 1977.

Wilensky, A. O., and Hahn, L. J.: Mesenteric Lymphadenitis, *Ann Surg,* **83:**812, 1926.

Yannopoulos, K., and Stout, A. P.: Primary Solid Tumors of the Mesentery, *Cancer,* **16:**914, 1963.

Retroperitoneum

Ackerman, L. V.: Tumors of the Retroperitoneum, Mesentery and Peritoneum, in "Atlas of Tumor and Pathology," Armed Forces Institute of Pathology, sec. VI, Washington, 1954.

——— and delRegato, J. A.: "Cancer: Diagnosis, Treatment and Prognosis," The C. V. Mosby Company, St. Louis, 1962.

Albarran, J.: Rétention rénale par périuretèrite libération externe de l'uretère, *Assoc Franc Urol,* **9:**511, 1905.

Armstrong, J. R., and Cohn, I.: Primary Malignant Retroperitoneal Tumors, *Am J Surg,* **110:**937, 1965.

Braasch, J. W.: Primary Retroperitoneal Tumors, *Surg Clin North Am,* **47:**663, 1967.

Donnelly, B. A.: Primary Retroperitoneal Tumors, *Surg Gynecol Obstet,* **83:**705, 1946.

Duncan, R. E., and Evans, A. T.: Diagnosis of Primary Retroperitoneal Tumors, *Urology,* **117:**19, 1977.

Gow, J. G.: An Appraisal of Inflammatory Strictures of the Ureter, *Ann R Coll Surg Engl,* **51:**177, 1972.

Hache, L., Utz, D. C., and Woolner, L. B.: Idiopathic Fibrosing Retroperitonitis, *Surg Gynecol Obstet,* **115:**737, 1962.

Hackett, E.: Idiopathic Retroperitoneal Fibrosis: A Condition involving the Ureters, the Aorta, and the Inferior Vena Cava, *Br J Surg,* **46:**3, 1948.

Harbrecht, P. J.: Variants of Retroperitoneal Fibrosis, *Ann Surg,* **165:**388, 1967.

Hewitt, C. B., Nitz, G. L., Kiser, W. S., Straffon R. A., and Stewart, B. H.: Surgical Treatment of Retroperitoneal Fibrosis, *Ann Surg,* **169:**611, 1969.

Hoffman, W. W., and Trippel, O. H.: Retroperitoneal Fibrosis: Etiologic Considerations, *J Urol,* **86:**222, 1961.

Koep, Lawrence, and Zuidema, G. D.: The Clinical Significance of Retroperitoneal Fibrosis, *Surgery,* **81:**250, 1977.

Longmire, W. P., Jr., Goodwirs, W. E., and Buckberg, G. D.: Management of Sclerosing Fibrosis of the Mediastinal and Retroperitoneal Areas, *Ann Surg,* **165:**1013, 1967.

Lowman, R. M., Peck, D. R., Love, L., and Dubash, D.: Lumbar Angiography in the Diagnosis of Primary Retroperitoneal Tumors, *Surg Gynecol Obstet,* **132:**597, 1971.

Melicow, M. M.: Primary Tumors of the Retroperitoneum, *J Intern Coll Surg,* **19:**401, 1953.

Mitchell, R. J.: Alimentary Complications of Non-malignant Retroperitoneal Fibrosis, *Br J Surg,* **58:**254, 1971.

Neistadt, A., Jones, T., and Rob, C.: Vascular System Involvement by Idiopathic Retroperitoneal Fibrosis, *Surgery,* **59:**950, 1966.

Ormond, J. K.: Bilateral Ureteral Obstruction Due to Envelopment and Compression by Inflammatory Retroperitoneal Process, *J Urol,* **59:**1072, 1948.

———: Idiopathic Retroperitoneal Fibrosis, *JAMA,* **174:**1561, 1960.

———: Idiopathic Retroperitoneal Fibrosis: Ormond's Syndrome, *Henry Ford Hosp Med Bull,* **10:**13, 1962.

Pack, G. T., and Tabah, E. J.: Primary Retroperitoneal Tumors, *Surg Gynecol Obstet,* **99:**209, 1954.

Ross, J. C., and Goldsmith, H. J.: The Combined Surgical and Medical Treatment of Retroperitoneal Fibrosis, *Br J Surg,* **58:**411, 1971.

Schneider, C. F.: Idiopathic Retroperitoneal Fibrosis Producing Vena Caval, Biliary Ureteral and Duodenal Obstructions, *Ann Surg,* **94:**316, 1964.

Suby, H. I., Kerr, W. S., Graham, J. R., and Fraley, E.: Retroperitoneal Fibrosis: A Missing Link in the Chain, *J Urol,* **93:**144, 1965.

Wagenknecht, L. V., and Auvert, J.: Symptoms and Diagnosis of Retroperitoneal Fibrosis, *Urol Int,* **26:**185, 1971.

Chapter 36

Abdominal Wall Hernias

by **John H. Morton**

DEFINITION

Although hernia is one of the most common ailments with which mankind is afflicted, there continues to be debate among physicians about many points ranging from etiology to proper management. Even the definition of a hernia remains a matter of discussion. Some writers define a hernia in terms of a weakness or abnormal opening in an enclosing layer. Others emphasize a protrusion through the opening rather than the opening itself. Still others stress a combination of both. Clearly, for herniation to occur there must be a defect in supporting structures through which a contained organ or tissue *may* protrude—but the organ need not be present within the weakness for a hernia to exist. The contents of many hernias will reduce readily when the patient is recumbent, but the basic anatomic defect persists. However, it is important to stress that a peritoneal diverticulum, such as a patent processus vaginalis, does not per se constitute a hernia. There must, in addition, be an associated weakness large enough to permit passage of a viscus into the sac before a hernia is truly present.

By far the larger number of hernias occur in the inguinal or femoral region, and these are usually classified together under the term *groin hernia.* If a contained viscus can be returned from the hernia to its normal domain, the hernia is *reducible.* A hernia from which a contained organ cannot be reduced is said to be *incarcerated;* this may be either an acute, painful condition or a long-standing, asymptomatic one. If, in addition to incarceration, there is a compromise of the blood supply of the contained organ, this is called a *strangulated hernia.* The term is a poor one since the contents of the hernia, not the sac itself, are strangulated. When a portion of the wall of the hernia sac is composed of an organ such as the cecum or the sigmoid colon, a *sliding hernia* is present. Rarely, the sac in a groin hernia spreads out between the layers of the abdominal wall instead of following the course of the inguinal canal. Under these circumstances the hernia is known as an *interparietal hernia.* These hernias may be preperitoneal, when the sac lies between peritoneum and transversalis fascia; interstitial, when it extends between the various muscle layers; or superficial, when it is found between external oblique aponeurosis and skin.

A *ventral hernia* occurs in the abdominal wall at some site other than the groin. The umbilical hernia and the incisional hernia, which develops in a previous laparotomy incision, are the most common ventral hernias. The epigastric hernia, another frequent ventral hernia, presents through a defect in the linea alba above the umbilicus. The linea semicircularis below the umbilicus marks the level below which the rectus abdominis muscle lies behind the aponeurosis of the oblique and transversus abdominis muscles rather than within the layers of the internal oblique aponeurosis. The point where the vertical linea semilunaris along the lateral border of the rectus muscle joins the linea semicircularis is a potential weak area. The rare hernia which protrudes at this site is known as a *Spigelian hernia.*

Hernias from the abdominal cavity may also develop through the lateral abdominal wall, the so-called lumbar hernias. The most common of these relatively unusual hernias is the postoperative hernia developing in an incision made to expose the kidney. The most frequent naturally occurring hernia in this area is the Petit's triangle hernia. Petit's triangle is bounded by the external oblique anteriorly, the iliac crest inferiorly, and the latissimus dorsi posteriorly. The internal oblique forms the floor of the triangle, and it must be weakened or absent for herniation to develop. Cystoceles, urethroceles, and rectoceles are common hernias in women, but perineal hernias through the levator ani area and sciatic hernias through either the greater or the lesser sciatic foramen are exceedingly rare. The obturator hernia is another rare defect, with herniation of a peritoneal sac into the medial thigh through the obturator foramen.

In addition to these abdominal wall hernias and to diaphragmatic hernias a number of internal hernias—all of them rare—may occur. In these instances a loop of intestine enters an opening, either congenital or acquired, and becomes obstructed. This may occur through the foramen of Winslow, at the junction of duodenum and jejunum, around the cecum or sigmoid colon in association with malrotation, through a defect in the mesentery following bowel resection, or between the urinary bladder and the anterior abdominal wall. These conditions are usually discovered during an exploration for intestinal obstruction. They are not true hernias in the sense of this discussion, and they will not be considered further here.

INCIDENCE

For several reasons the prevalence of abdominal hernias is difficult to estimate. If a hernia is small, it may not be readily detected on any one examination. If findings from anatomic dissections are used, the incidence will be higher than if figures are drawn from routine physical examinations. In certain borderline lesions, not all physicians will agree as to whether or not a hernia is present. For instance, some pediatric surgeons equate a patent processus vaginalis with an indirect inguinal hernia, but most surgeons and anatomists do not accept this proposition without qualification. However, it is generally agreed that the most common hernia in either sex is the indirect inguinal variety, that direct hernias are very unusual in females, that femoral hernias as a class are more common in females than in males, and that hernias in general are over five times more common in males. Summarizing available evidence, Zimmerman and Anson in their excellent monograph on hernias conclude that the frequency of hernia can be placed at 5 percent of the total male adult population. Regardless of the exact figure, the magnitude of the problem is readily appreciated.

ANATOMY

All hernias of the abdominal wall involve the same tissue layers. Under the skin lies the subcutaneous fat. In the inguinal area particularly, this fat includes a well-defined condensation of connective tissue, identified as *Scarpa's fascia*. Although this layer is not true fascia, the term is undoubtedly too ingrained in the literature to be altered. The external oblique, internal oblique, and transversus abdominis are encountered in order, either as muscle fibers laterally or as layers of aponeurosis medially. The longitudinal rectus abdominis muscle lies within layers of the aponeurosis down to the semilunar line and is placed entirely behind them in the lower abdomen. The important inner investing layer of the transversus abdominis, the

transversalis fascia, and parietal peritoneum complete the abdominal wall. With an abdominal hernia at any level, the parietal peritoneal sac either passes through a defect in some of the layers of the abdominal wall or is covered with attenuated remnants of these layers.

Inguinal Region

In the descent of the testicle from its original retroperitoneal site into the scrotum, it passes through the abdominal wall in the inguinal region. A diverticulum of parietal peritoneum, the processus vaginalis, accompanies the testicle, although normally this connection with the peritoneum is obliterated before birth or in early infancy. The spermatic cord contains layers representative of each abdominal wall layer as follows:

Abdominal wall layer	Spermatic cord layer
Parietal peritoneum	Obliterated processus vaginalis
Transversalis fascia ⎱	Internal spermatic fascia
Transversus abdominis ⎰	
Internal oblique	Cremaster muscle
External oblique	External spermatic fascia
Subcutaneous tissue	Dartos muscle (in scrotum)
Skin	Skin

The spermatic cord passes obliquely downward through the inguinal canal from the internal inguinal ring, an opening in the transversalis fascia and transversus abdominis aponeurosis where they extend onto the spermatic cord as internal spermatic fascia. The medial margin of the internal ring is defined by the inferior epigastric artery, coursing from the external iliac artery medially and superiorly into the rectus sheath. The cord lies superior to the inguinal ligament and anterior to the inguinal canal floor. After running obliquely downward, it emerges through the external inguinal ring, an opening in the external oblique aponeurosis just above the pubic spine, to pass into the scrotum. The tubular external spermatic fascia joins the cord at the external inguinal ring, the cremaster fibers having enveloped the cord along the course of the inguinal canal.

An indirect inguinal hernia (Fig. 36-1) leaves the abdominal cavity at the internal ring and passes with the structures of the spermatic cord either a variable distance down the inguinal canal or all the way into the scrotum. Thus the indirect hernia must lie within the fibers of the cremaster muscle. Except in infants an indirect hernia is associated with an enlargement of the internal ring. The opening in the transversus abdominis aponeurosis medial to the spermatic cord is dilated and the peritoneal sac enters the spermatic cord at this point. The edge of the sac is recognized as a readily defined grayish white membrane found inside these fibers, anteromedial to the vas deferens and the other structures of the cord. Should the hernia be of the sliding variety (Fig. 36-2), the intestinal component makes up a part or all of the posterior wall of the sac. A sliding hernia in the right groin may incorporate the cecum in this fashion. On the left, the lateral leaf of the meso-

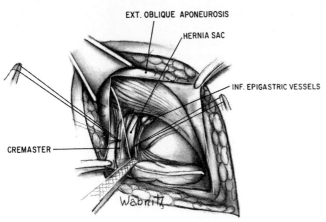

Fig. 36-1. Indirect inguinal hernia. Sac projects through internal inguinal ring anteromedial to vas deferens and inside cremaster fibers.

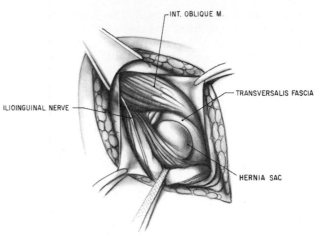

Fig. 36-3. Direct inguinal hernia. Weakness involves medial inguinal canal floor and lies behind structures of spermatic cord.

sigmoid and occasionally the sigmoid itself may be involved.

A direct hernia (Fig. 36-3) protrudes through the floor of the inguinal canal in Hesselbach's triangle, an area bounded laterally by the inferior epigastric artery, inferiorly by the inguinal ligament, and medially by the lateral margin of the rectus sheath. In Hesselbach's triangle the inguinal canal floor is formed by transversalis fascia reinforced by aponeurotic fibers from the transversus abdominis. In Hesselbach's triangle the aponeurotic reinforcement is discontinuous. Hence, the area is a potential site of weakness. When a direct hernia develops, either the entire canal floor in Hesselbach's triangle becomes attenuated and stretched out over the peritoneum, or, less commonly, a rent develops through the canal floor. Since the direct hernia projects through the medial canal floor, it cannot lie within the cremaster muscle fibers; rather, it is behind the cremaster and the rest of the spermatic cord. Thus this type of hernia is not guided through the external inguinal ring and is unlikely to reach the scrotum. On the rare occasion when a direct hernia does enter the scrotum, it must pass through the external ring separate from and behind the spermatic cord. In contrast to the other groin hernias, in which a diverticulum of peritoneum with a relatively nar-

row neck is present, the direct hernia usually presents as a diffuse weakness and general bulging in Hesselbach's triangle. The absence of this narrow neck makes incarceration unusual in direct inguinal hernia. When incarceration does occur, it is usually at the level of the external inguinal ring in those rare situations where a direct sac passes through this area. With a large direct hernia it is not unusual for a portion of the wall of the urinary bladder to be incorporated in a sliding fashion in the medial portion of the sac.

The third groin hernia, the femoral type (Fig. 36-4), also depends for its development upon a defect in the transversalis fascia in Hesselbach's triangle. In this type of hernia, however, there is a peritoneal sac which passes under the inguinal ligament into the femoral triangle rather than following the course of the direct hernia ante-

Fig. 36-4. Femoral hernia. Although sac projects beneath inguinal ligament into femoral triangle, basic defect making hernia possible is weakness in attachment of transversalis fascia and transversus abdominis aponeurosis to Cooper's ligament.

Fig. 36-2. Evolution of sliding hernia. A. Leading peritoneal sac "pulls" mobile cecum or sigmoid. B. Sliding hernia is established with colon or cecum as part of wall of sac.

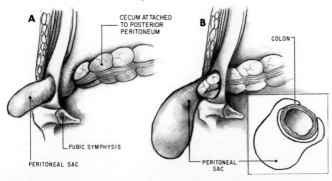

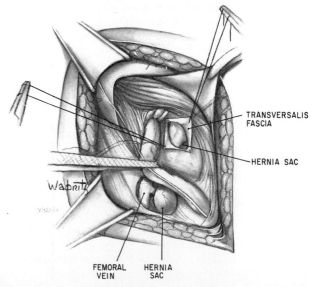

riorly into the inguinal canal. The inguinal ligament stretches as a tight band from the anterior superior iliac spine to the spine of the pubis, and beneath it the femoral vessels enter the thigh. Medial to the femoral vein is a small empty space through which a femoral hernia may project. The resulting sac will have, perforce, a very narrow neck. Once the sac enters the thigh, however, it may assume quite large proportions in the loose connective tissue. It may even double back on top of the external oblique aponeurosis, coming to lie over the groin, where it can be mistaken for an inguinal hernia. Because of the narrow neck in this type of hernia, incarceration with strangulation of the contents of the hernia is a strong possibility.

Umbilical Region

During the embryonic period before completion of intestinal rotation there is a herniation of abdominal contents through the umbilicus into the extraembryonic coelomic cavity. At about the tenth week of fetal life the viscera normally return to the abdominal cavity, the intestine completing its rotation in the process. The defect in the abdominal wall closes slowly during subsequent fetal development, until at birth only the space occupied by the umbilical cord remains patent. Following ligation of the cord, the umbilical stump heals by granulation and organization, with epithelialization from the margins of the defect. Abdominal wall closure at this level thus consists of the fusion of skin, a single fascial layer, and peritoneum.

At birth many infants will show a small umbilical hernia (Fig. 36-5) because this process has not been carried through to completion. In most of these children spontaneous closure of the fascial defect occurs within the first four years of life in a fashion identical with that described above. An umbilical hernia which is still present in a four-year-old will usually persist, but bowel strangulation in these congenital umbilical defects is unusual.

Occasionally, however, the process of abdominal wall closure is much less complete at birth, and several interesting congenital anomalies may be encountered. An omphalocele is present when at birth there is a defect at the umbilicus covered only by a peritoneal sac. Within such a sac virtually any abdominal organ may be encountered,

but small bowel, colon, and liver are the most common viscera present.

If the embryologic duct from small bowel to yolk sac remains attached to the umbilical cord at birth, it is likely to be included in the tie placed by the obstetrician. This duct, although extremely narrow, amounting to no more than a cord, may be lined with bowel epithelium. When the umbilical remnant sloughs later under these circumstances, a fistula into the small gut is created. This anomaly is known as a patent omphalomesenteric or viteline duct. On occasion the fibrous cord is not lined with epithelium, and the umbilicus then heals normally after ligation, usually without an umbilical hernia. The cord, however, may persist, connecting the umbilicus to the small gut, and it may be encountered in later life as one of the congenital bands leading to volvulus and intestinal obstruction. One patient in the author's experience was found to have a thin band of this type at abdominal exploration during adult life. The patient had never experienced drainage from the umbilicus, but the band was excised. A fecal fistula promptly developed. On further investigation it was evident that this band contained an epithelial lining at its intestinal end, although it had not extended far enough toward the umbilicus to create problems when cord ligature was performed following birth.

A sinus tract from the bladder, the urachus, enters the umbilical area from below, between the umbilical arteries, during fetal life. This tract, the remnant of the cephalic portion of the embryonic urinary bladder, is usually obliterated before birth, but should it remain patent, it may become incorporated in the umbilical cord ligature. Thus a later draining umbilical sinus may represent a patent urachus as well as a patent omphalomesenteric duct.

Umbilical hernias may also develop during adult life. This occurs more commonly in women, usually after childbirth. The hernia may become a large one, and strangulation of intestine or omentum within the defect is not uncommon.

ETIOLOGY

Hernias may result from congenital anomalies or may develop secondarily during later life. Although congenital

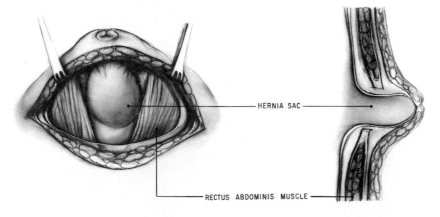

HERNIA SAC

RECTUS ABDOMINIS MUSCLE

Fig. 36-5. Umbilical hernia. Peritoneal sac is attached directly to underside of umbilical skin, with only thin attenuated fascia covering sac.

umbilical hernias are more common in black infants, other congenital hernias occur with equal frequency in blacks and whites. Inguinal hernias are more common in males, and femoral hernias occur primarily in females. When a hernia develops secondarily in later life, it is frequently the result of trauma. Hence it is compensable if the injury occurs when the patient is at work. It should be pointed out, however, that the traumatic explanation for these hernias is not entirely satisfying. In many instances, for example, the patient is not aware of any specific event which precipitated the hernia. Rather, a bulge develops gradually after years of hard work. In other circumstances, a similar hernia may develop in a sedentary individual who has not changed his habits before herniation occurred. In any case, many men never develop a hernia despite a lifetime of vigorous physical activity. In evaluating the direct hernia of later life, Zimmerman and Anson concluded that this lesion also results from a congenital anatomic defect—the absence of adequate muscular support for the lower portion of the inguinal canal. They find the lowermost fibers of the internal oblique lacking, so that a larger triangle without muscular reinforcement is present in the individual who is prone to hernia formation. As a result of his dissections Condon concluded that a direct hernia resulted from the lack of adequate reinforcement of transversalis fascia in Hesselbach's triangle.

In considering the development of a hernia in the groin during middle life, it is wise to remember that increased intraabdominal pressure is at least as important a predisposing factor as external trauma. Chronic cough or symptoms of genitourinary tract or gastrointestinal tract obstruction may precede herniation. Benign prostatic hypertrophy and carcinoma of the left colon are two important entities which should be considered in an adult seeking medical attention because of a hernia. Cirrhosis of the liver with ascites, massive splenomegaly, and uterine enlargement during pregnancy are other possible etiologic factors of this type.

Recently, several investigators have suggested that a connective tissue abnormality may be involved in adult-onset hernias. Abnormalities in the ultrastructure and the physicochemical properties of collagen in patients with direct hernias suggest that the hernia is one manifestation of a generalized abnormality in collagen metabolism.

From the legal point of view a hernia is an important condition about which a physician must frequently testify, and the wording or interpretation of a workmen's compensation law can be important. Many young adult males first discover a hernia after some vigorous physical labor; this type of hernia is usually indirect. The physician is aware that such a defect is almost always congenital, and it would be difficult to testify that the traumatic incident produced the hernia. On the other hand, it is hard to convince a young man that the hernia has been present all his life and that he was unaware of it because no intraabdominal organ had previously entered the sac. This uncomfortable situation is satisfactorily avoided in jurisdictions where exacerbation of preexisting disease is sufficient evidence of a compensable injury. In these circum-stances the surgeon can bear witness that a hernia is present and that its appearance may be related to the injury in question.

SYMPTOMS AND SIGNS

A hernia may be an asymptomatic defect, discovered incidentally during a routine physical examination. The individual may or may not have been aware of its presence. The usual reducible hernia produces no symptoms of importance other than pain. The type and degree of pain vary considerably from one individual to another. If the hernia is first recognized after an acute traumatic episode, local pain of a muscular type may be quite severe for several days. This pain occurs when, in the presence of a preexisting patent processus vaginalis, sudden enlargement of the internal inguinal ring permits development of a true hernia.

In a few days the discomfort subsides without specific treatment. In a long-standing hernia occasional twinges of local discomfort may be present, usually in association with straining or with the temporary entry of an intraperitoneal organ into the sac. Another type of discomfort may occur when a loop of small intestine enters the hernia. Epigastric or paraumbilical pain may then develop, representing visceral pain in the superior mesenteric distribution as a result of mesenteric stretching.

The physical signs of an uncomplicated hernia vary with the contents of the sac. When there are no peritoneal contents present, the sac is collapsed and its presence is difficult to identify. It is said that the opposing peritoneal surfaces may be rubbed one over the other to detect a sensation of gliding, but this is an unreliable sign. When an organ occupies the sac, the findings vary with the organ involved. If bowel is present, crepitation will be noted on palpation because of the presence of gas and fluid within the lumen. If a solid organ such as an ovary is present, a movable firm regular mass will be felt. When omentum is within the sac, an ill-defined irregular rubbery mass will be palpable. When an organ enters an inguinal hernia sac, reduction may be attempted by gentle pressure with a finger through the invaginated scrotal skin. This should be done with the patient supine and relaxed. If the organ is not readily reduced, a sliding hernia should be suspected, especially if the bulge is a large one.

A hernia may be particularly difficult to identify in an infant, who cannot cooperate during examination. If the mother gives a suggestive history and no hernia can be found, she should be instructed to bring the infant back when a bulge is obvious or to return later with the youngster for a second examination under any circumstance. If a hydrocele of the cord is present in an infant, an indirect hernia is almost invariably present as well, and it should be repaired at the time of hydrocelectomy.

If no hernia is obvious when examination is begun, one may become apparent if the patient is requested to strain. A sustained contraction of the muscles of the abdominal wall is more effective than the traditional cough as a method of raising intraabdominal pressure, thus demonstrating the hernia. Position during the examination is important. When a ventral hernia is suspected, the supine patient should be asked to raise head and shoulders from the bed. When a male is being examined for a groin hernia, he should be standing in a relaxed position, and the physician should invaginate the scrotum with the examining finger. The finger should be introduced through the external ring into the inguinal canal while the patient strains. It is harder to examine a female for a groin hernia. She should be standing and the labia majora examined while she strains. A definite bulge and mass should be palpated before the diagnosis of a hernia can be considered secure. The presence of a dilated external inguinal ring is of no significance per se as regards the presence of a hernia and does not predispose to the later development of a hernia. With groin hernias the location of the mass should be helpful in distinguishing the femoral hernia. However, an obese individual may be unaware of a mass in the groin, and the groin should be carefully palpated for evidence of an incarcerated hernia when a patient presents with intestinal obstruction.

The clinical distinction between direct and indirect hernia by physical examination is academic, since the operative approach for repair is the same for both. This is fortunate since accurate distinction is often difficult to make. When the examining finger has been advanced well into the inguinal canal, the indirect hernia should strike the fingertip and the direct hernia the ball of the finger—but this difference is frequently hard to appreciate. A thumb placed over the internal inguinal ring should keep an indirect hernia reduced when the patient strains while permitting a direct hernia to appear; again, it is not always possible to locate the internal ring accurately enough to make this technique foolproof.

The predominant finding with an incarcerated or strangulated hernia is a tender mass at one of the hernial sites.

Fig. 36-6. Richter's hernia. Strangulation of antimesenteric portion of the bowel may lead to abscess without intestinal obstruction.

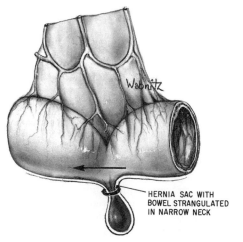

HERNIA SAC WITH BOWEL STRANGULATED IN NARROW NECK

A testicular torsion may be mistaken for an incarcerated inguinal hernia and an acute femoral lymphadenitis for an incarcerated femoral hernia.

COMPLICATIONS

The risk is that an intraperitoneal organ may become incarcerated or strangulated within the hernia sac. The small intestine is the organ most frequently affected, and acute incarceration or strangulation within a hernia sac remains one of the two most frequent causes for small bowel obstruction. This complication changes a simple situation into one which may prove fatal. A mass incarcerated in the inguinal hernia of a female infant is commonly an ovary, although incarceration of the appendix has been reported.

Occasionally only a portion of the antimesenteric wall of the intestine becomes strangulated within a hernia sac, producing a so-called Richter's hernia (Fig. 36-6). In this special situation there is not complete bowel obstruction, but the entrapped portion of bowel wall may become gangrenous. An abscess results if the strangulation is not recognized and treated early. An abscess of the medial thigh in an elderly female which, on incision and drainage, releases pus with a feculent odor suggests the presence of an obturator hernia with a partially strangulated bowel.

The development of complications in a hernia is not predictable. When complications do occur, an elective situation becomes an emergency, and a simple problem becomes more difficult. The rationale for elective herniorrhaphy is to prevent this situation.

TREATMENT

General

A hernia may be approached in three ways: expectantly, nonoperatively, or by surgical repair. Expectant treatment is based on the hope of spontaneous cure; in most situations this is not realistic. However, with the congenital umbilical hernia spontaneous cure does occur in most children before the age of four. This is a natural process which is not enhanced by the use of adhesive strapping. The physician should not advise operation until the patient reaches age four unless the hernia has incarcerated—a most unusual event in a hernia of this type—or unless it is a very large defect of the proboscis type. Expectant management of uncomplicated groin hernias is also reasonable in patients severely ill from some other cause. In most other circumstances an expectant attitude is not warranted.

The nonoperative treatment of a hernia involves the use of some external device or truss to maintain hernial reduction. These devices are a nuisance to the patient, and they are expensive to construct and to fit. In the groin they are almost universally unsuccessful in maintaining satisfactory reduction. A properly fitting corset may be an excellent remedy, however, for a ventral hernia, particularly when a large defect develops in an abdominal wound which became infected following initial laparotomy. Surgical repair of these defects is difficult, and a trial with external support is certainly justified before operation is recommended. With this exception external support has little to recommend it. The injection of sclerosing solutions into the tissues around a hernia, at one time a popular method of therapy, is mentioned only to be condemned.

Once the decision is made to perform an elective herniorrhaphy, it is a general rule that the operation should not be delayed. However, the presence of some other illness, such as an infection of the upper respiratory tract or a recent myocardial infarction, warrants delay. With premature infants it is wise to wait until the child is making satisfactory progress nutritionally so that the risk of anesthesia is decreased. With other infants many surgeons would prefer not to operate before the infant is ten weeks of age, since by this time the hemoglobin level is returning from its postnatal dip. Whenever operation is delayed for any reason, however, it should be realized that there is always the possibility of strangulation, which changes an elective situation into an emergency. Elderly patients with hernias are just as prone to strangulation as younger, more vigorous individuals, and old age per se should not be considered a contraindication to an elective herniorrhaphy.

When the patient has no systemic signs such as fever or leukocytosis, one preoperative effort to reduce an acutely incarcerated hernia is permissible. An ice bag should be applied to the local area and an appropriate dose of morphine given parenterally. With a groin hernia the patient should be placed in the Trendelenburg position as well. After 30 to 40 minutes, gentle sustained pressure over the mass may effect reduction without undue difficulty. The sensation that some gas has moved within the intestine frequently presages successful reduction. No more than one such effort should be attempted prior to emergency surgery—and the presence of systemic symptoms and signs contraindicates even this effort. Because of the small area below the inguinal ligament and medial to the femoral vein, reduction of an incarcerated femoral hernia is virtually impossible and should not be attempted. If these rules are followed, the reduction of a hernia en masse—that is, with the contained organ still strangulated—should not occur. The advantage of reducing an incarcerated hernia is that a repair 2 or 3 days later can be done at a time when edema has been reduced, thus permitting a better herniorrhaphy. Also, if other medical problems are present, the patient's general condition may be improved preoperatively, thus permitting a safer operative and postoperative course.

Operative Repair

PRINCIPLES. In any herniorrhaphy there are two essential steps to consider: (1) the management of the peritoneal sac and its contents, and (2) the repair of the fascial defect. If the sac is a narrow-necked diverticulum, it is usually

excised and the neck closed. If it is a broadbased bulge, the peritoneum is usually not opened; rather, it is reduced intact beneath the fascia and held there by the fascial repair. Management of the sac is complicated when a sliding hernia is present or when intraperitoneal organs are fixed within the sac by adhesions. If the latter situation is suspected, it is vital to make certain that the situation is not in reality a sliding hernia. Once the surgeon is convinced that adhesions are holding an organ *within* the peritoneal sac, these adhesions must be carefully divided to effect reduction of the incarcerated contents. The sac itself is then managed in the usual fashion. The presence of a sliding hernia requires that the organ forming part of the wall of the sac be returned to the abdomen before the sac is excised. If this condition is anticipated and recognized, direct reduction of the sliding organ from the groin through the fascial defect is usually possible. The peritoneal sac is then excised without injury to the bowel or its blood supply. Rarely, an adjacent separate incision into the peritoneal cavity may be required to reduce the viscus from above, but the need for this has been over-emphasized in the literature (Fig. 36-7).

Once the peritoneal sac has been satisfactorily managed, attention is turned to the associated fascial defect. When the patient is a youngster with a congenital indirect inguinal hernia, the opening in the transversalis fascia around the internal inguinal ring may not be dilated, and repair may not be required. In almost all other circumstances, however, closing or decreasing the size of this defect is vital. In certain circumstances the fascial margins of the defect can be approximated satisfactorily after adequate mobilization; this technique is applicable to most umbilical hernias, congenital or acquired, which require repair. In other instances an adjacent fascial relaxing incision makes possible a primary closure which would not otherwise be feasible. In some circumstances, especially when a large defect is present, repair will require the use of some substance introduced from elsewhere. An autogenous fascial graft, usually from the fascia lata, or an inert foreign body may be used for this purpose. A solid sheet of foreign material cannot be effectively organized by the body. Rather, it tends to become incorporated in a loose pocket or rejected altogether. Consequently, if an inert foreign material is selected, it should be in the form of a mesh which can be invaded and incorporated by the host's fibroblasts during the organization phase of wound healing. Screens of this type have been constructed of a metal such as tantalum or synthetic substances such as polypropylene (Marlex) or Dacron (Mersilene).

Following satisfactory repair of any hernia, it is traditional for the surgeon to advise against heavy lifting and other vigorous effort for 4 to 8 weeks. The rationale for this advice is to permit proper healing of the repaired tissues. Dunphy's studies indicate that collagen maturation and gain in tensile strength of the wound continue over many months, and this process is not complete within 4 weeks even under ideal circumstances. Studies by Lichtenstein and colleagues suggest that for at least the first 2 months strength of a repaired wound depends primarily

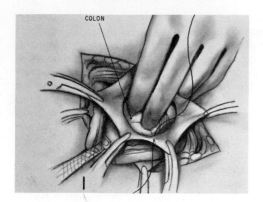

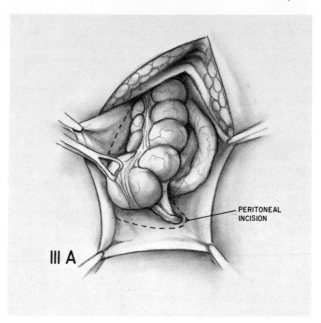

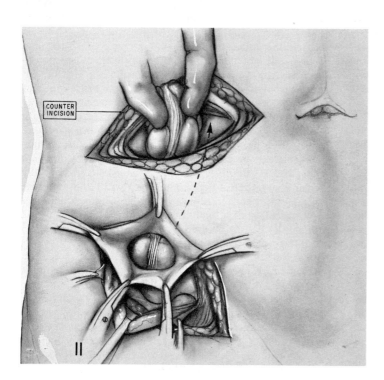

Fig. 36-7. Repair of sliding hernias. I. In simplest method, intestine, forming part of posterior wall of hernia sac, is directly reduced into abdomen, permitting closure of peritoneum and reconstruction of internal ring below it. II. Rarely, counterincision entering peritoneum above sac is needed to permit reduction of intestine by traction. III. *A,B,C.* Some surgeons free the sliding organ from the peritoneal sac (*A*). The posterior surface of the organ is then peritonealized (*B*), and the peritoneum is then closed at the internal ring (*C*). This procedure seems time-consuming and unnecessary.

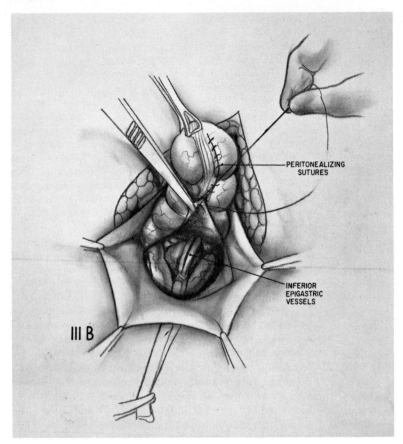

PERITONEALIZING
SUTURES

INFERIOR
EPIGASTRIC
VESSELS

III B

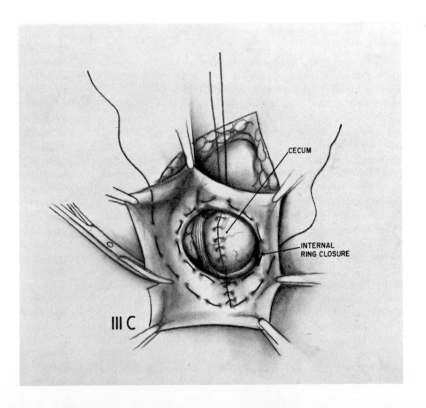

CECUM

INTERNAL
RING CLOSURE

III C

upon an intact suture line. In their experiments, the sutured wound showed 70 percent of intact tissue strength immediately, and there was no appreciable gain in strength during the next 8 weeks. The 4-week period of inactivity is perhaps a satisfactory compromise, postponing vigorous effort until some degree of healing has occurred, but it should be recognized that the basis for the recommendation is empiric rather than scientific.

STRANGULATED HERNIAS

When emergency operation is undertaken for a hernia with strangulated contents, it is vital that the operation be performed so that the contents of the sac can be inspected before reduction. To achieve this, it is necessary to open the sac early in the dissection and gain control of the structures within it. If operation has been done early enough, the prompt return of circulation to strangulated tissue indicates viability. Reduction is then effected and routine repair carried out. When gangrene has already developed, all gangrenous tissue must be resected. When strangulated intestine is present, this entails the construction of an anastomosis between normal bowel sections proximal and distal to the necrotic area. In some circumstances tissue viability is not so easily defined. Bowel of doubtful viability should be covered with a warm moist towel and reinspected after 5 minutes. Improved color of the bowel wall, passage of a peristaltic wave through the strangulated segment, or pulsation in the arcuate arteries usually indicate that the intestine will survive if returned to the peritoneal cavity. Intestine of questionable viability should be resected, since reduction of bowel which is not viable may lead either to early perforation with peritonitis or to late stricture. However, unnecessary intestinal resection increases morbidity and mortality.

GROIN HERNIAS

Many surgeons make the mistake of performing the same operation for all hernias in the groin. A proper evaluation of the anatomy in the area would make it evident that indirect, direct, and femoral hernias are different anatomic problems requiring different repairs.

Groin hernias can be successfully repaired with general, spinal, or local anesthesia. When local anesthesia is employed, the ilioinguinal and iliohypogastric nerves should be blocked just above and medial to the anterior superior iliac spine. The nerves lie deep to the external oblique aponeurosis at this level. In addition, subcutaneous infiltration of the incision site and deeper injection of the area around the pubic spine are required.

Certain authors suggest that the femoral hernia be repaired through a vertical incision over the femoral triangle. However, it is generally agreed that a better anatomic repair can be achieved through the groin. All groin hernias therefore should be approached through an incision above the inguinal ligament. Most frequently the incision is made above and parallel to the medial portion of the inguinal ligament; some surgeons extend this incision laterally almost to the iliac spine, but the lateral portion of the wound does not facilitate exposure and should be omitted. The subcutaneous tissue is incised and the external oblique aponeurosis exposed. The external oblique is then opened through the external inguinal ring, the ilioinguinal nerve being carefully identified and preserved. The nerve is most frequently adherent at the external ring; hence the aponeurosis should be opened from above downward to prevent nerve injury. The nerve is readily identified as a grayish white structure with a small red blood vessel on its surface, running roughly parallel to the external oblique fibers. Moosman and Oelrich have found that the nerve lies inside the cremaster fibers in direct contact with spermatic cord structures in 35 percent of patients. By dividing those cremaster fibers which join the spermatic cord from the inguinal ligament, the cord is freed from the inguinal canal floor and a tape passed around it at the level of the pubic spine. This step facilitates lifting the cord away from Hesselbach's triangle. The major portion of the cremaster muscle is then divided all the way around the cord at the internal inguinal ring, and it becomes possible to identify the type of hernia and isolate the structures required for fascial repair.

INDIRECT HERNIA. When an indirect hernia is present, the sac will be visible as a translucent white structure lying inside the cremaster fibers and anteromedial to the cord structures at the level of the internal inguinal ring. The sac may be obscured by a lobulated mass of fatty tissue, often incorrectly referred to as a "lipoma of the cord." In reality it represents a projection of fat from the retroperitoneal area. Typically the fat extends through the dilated internal inguinal ring lateral and inferior to the cord structures. Rarely, this retroperitoneal fat may be present without an associated peritoneal sac. In either instance it should be removed as part of the indirect hernia repair. Once the sac is identified, it is separated from the spermatic cord by sharp or blunt dissection back to the internal ring. The vas deferens, which is usually adherent to the sac at the level of the internal ring, is the only cord structure which does not separate easily once the proper plane for dissection is entered. When the sac is adequately freed, it can be opened and any intraperitoneal contents reduced, with lysis of adhesions as necessary. If the hernia has a sliding component, it will form part or all of the posterior wall of the sac. This component should be manually replaced into the abdominal cavity before the hernia sac is excised.

A palpating finger can then be introduced into the peritoneal cavity through the open sac. The finger is brought up beneath the inguinal canal floor in Hesselbach's triangle to test the possibility of an associated direct hernia. Palpation beneath the inguinal ligament medial to the femoral vessels will disclose a femoral hernia if one is present. Directly behind this area the obturator membrane can be felt and an obturator hernia sought where the obturator artery and vein leave the true pelvis.

The sac can then be transected at the level of the internal inguinal ring. In doing this it is well to remember that the parietal peritoneum is quite elastic and that by traction a good deal of peritoneum from the abdominal wall can be pulled through the ring. Depending upon the size of the peritoneal defect, it is closed with either a purse-string suture or a series of interrupted sutures of some nonabsorbable suture material.

Except in infants, in whom this step may be omitted because the internal ring is not dilated, the transversus abdominis aponeurosis below the spermatic cord should be reapproximated with a series of interrupted sutures (Fig. 36-8). This repair should be continued until it is barely possible to insert a small clamp through the internal ring alongside the cord. The external oblique muscle, subcutaneous tissue, and skin are then united over the cord, which occupies its usual location, passing obliquely through the inguinal canal. It is unnecessary to transplant the neck of the hernial sac up beneath the abdominal muscles and unwise to move the cord into a subcutaneous location by closing the external oblique aponeurosis underneath it. If the medial inguinal canal floor is strong, this area should not be repaired. Indeed, Glassow suggests that in women direct recurrences may result from unnecessary dissection in Hesselbach's triangle during the initial operation. In closing the external oblique aponeurosis it is important to avoid passing a suture around the ilioinguinal nerve. Incorporating the nerve in a suture may lead to the development of a troublesome, painful neuroma.

When an indirect hernia has been neglected for a prolonged period, it may become very large, and the inferior epigastric vessels may be displaced medially all the way to the pubic spine. In effect such a hernia is direct as well as indirect, and the area in Hesselbach's triangle should be managed in the manner adopted for a direct hernia. For large or recurrent indirect hernias it may be possible to achieve a more secure repair by dividing the cord at the internal ring and closing the defect completely at that level. Orchiectomy is usually performed along with cord transection. However, if the scrotum is not disturbed during operation and is handled gently after surgery, the testicle may be left in place with little likelihood that gangrene will occur.

SLIDING HERNIA. The most important step in operative management of a sliding hernia is recognition of the situation. On the right side the cecum and on the left the sigmoid colon may make up part of the posterior wall of an indirect sac, and failure to recognize this may lead to fecal contamination or to injury to colonic blood supply. The urinary bladder may be similarly involved in a direct sac, but since this type of sac is reduced unopened, the presence of bladder does not create a technical problem. Because a sliding component is present in only about 3 percent of groin hernias, the surgeon tends to forget the possibility. However, certain circumstances increase the likelihood of a sliding component, and the surgeon should be wary when dealing with any large indirect hernia, especially one of long standing in an elderly male.

Most sliding hernias can be managed without undue difficulty. The peritoneal sac is identified and opened anteriorly away from the bowel which makes up its posterior wall. The entire anterior portion of the sac is removed. Posteriorly as much sac as possible is removed without injuring the sliding bowel or its mesentery. The bowel is then reduced manually into its original retroperitoneal position and the defect in peritoneum closed. The defect in the transversalis fascia at the internal inguinal ring is then closed in the same manner used for any indirect

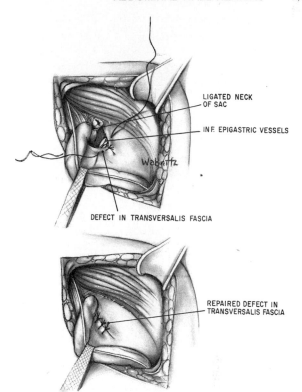

LIGATED NECK OF SAC

INF. EPIGASTRIC VESSELS

DEFECT IN TRANSVERSALIS FASCIA

REPAIRED DEFECT IN TRANSVERSALIS FASCIA

Fig. 36-8. Indirect inguinal hernia repair. High ligation of sac is followed by closure of defect in transversus abdominis aponeurosis at internal inguinal ring.

hernia, producing a snug internal ring. The herniorrhaphy is completed in whatever fashion is most appropriate to the remaining anatomic defect (Fig. 36-7I).

Rarely, when a large amount of colon is involved in the wall of the hernia, it may prove difficult to reduce the colon into its retroperitoneal position by manipulation from below. In these circumstances it is appropriate to enter the abdomen through a higher transverse incision so that the colon can be moved superiorly by traction from above, a procedure described by LaRoque. The abdomen may be entered through a fresh skin incision or by an extension of the groin incision, retracting the external oblique aponeurosis superiorly to facilitate the counterincision through the internal oblique, transversus abdominis, and peritoneum. In either event the colon is displaced from the internal ring by gentle traction and repair effected by excising the residual sac and carefully closing the internal ring (Fig. 36-7II).

Some surgeons consider it important to enter the abdomen in all cases and to dissect the herniated colon away from the peritoneal sac (Fig. 36-7III*A*). When the cecum is involved, these surgeons form a posterior peritoneal investment for this portion of the bowel by closing the margins of the peritoneal sac behind the cecum. In effect, this procedure makes an intraperitoneal organ out of one which previously lay retroperitoneally (Fig. 36-7III*B*). When the sliding hernia is on the left side involving the sigmoid, this procedure leaves a raw surface on the lateral aspect of the sigmoid mesocolon, and, again, closure of this

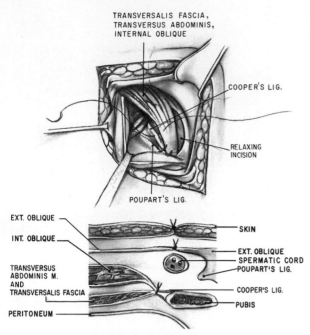

Fig. 36-9. Cooper's ligament repair. Cross section demonstrates level of repair; operative drawing shows placement of sutures in Cooper's ligament.

Fig. 36-10. Repair at level of inguinal ligament. Bassini operation remains standard against which other herniorrhaphies for direct inguinal hernia are judged; transversus abdominis aponeurosis as well as transversalis fascia should be incorporated in repair layer.

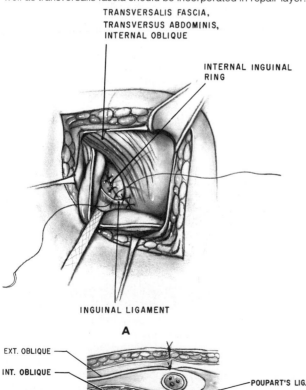

area is advised. In addition, surgeons who advocate an abdominal approach to sliding hernias sometimes fix this freed colon higher in the abdomen by some kind of colopexy. Both these procedures are designed to decrease the incidence of recurrence when this type of hernia is repaired. However, both procedures are cumbersome, the peritonealization of the posterior surface of the cecum is unsound anatomically, and the hernia should not recur in any case if the internal ring is properly closed (Fig. 36-7III*C*).

DIRECT HERNIA. When a direct hernia is present instead of or in addition to an indirect hernia, a different type of repair is required. Here the weakness lies in the inguinal canal floor medial to the inferior epigastric artery. In most instances there is a general ballooning out in the area, and the peritoneum should be reduced beneath the reconstituted inguinal canal floor without being opened. In the unusual instances where a narrow-necked diverticulum of peritoneum is present, it should be managed in the same way as an indirect sac.

To restore the inguinal canal floor requires removal of attenuated fascia and reconstruction with a new and stronger layer. In most instances this layer can be developed from the strong aponeurotic portion of the transversus abdominis muscle which is found just superior to the weakness in the inguinal canal floor. If a curved relaxing incision is made in the inner layer of the rectus sheath where the internal oblique and transversus abdominis form a fused aponeurosis, it is not difficult to bring the transversus abdominis aponeurosis down across Hesselbach's triangle. This layer can then be approximated to Cooper's ligament (Fig. 36-9), to the iliopubic tract, an aponeurotic band superficial to Cooper's ligament, or to the shelving edge of Poupart's ligament (Fig. 36-10), depending upon the preference of the surgeon. If Poupart's ligament is used for the repair, there are several levels at which the spermatic cord may be placed. The cord lies beneath the repaired inguinal canal floor as far as the external inguinal ring in the Ferguson repair (Fig. 36-11) and in the later technique described by Halsted. In the Bassini herniorrhaphy (Fig. 36-10*B*) the cord lies on top of the repaired canal floor. In the Andrews operation (Fig. 36-12) the superior leaf of the incised external oblique aponeurosis is sutured to Poupart's ligament beneath the cord to reinforce the repair of the inguinal canal floor, and the inferior leaf of the external oblique is then sutured up over the cord. In the original Halsted operation (Fig. 36-13) the external oblique aponeurosis is closed underneath the cord as far laterally as the internal ring, thus transplanting the cord into the subcutaneous tissue. Halsted himself later abandoned his technique, and most surgeons today employ some form of the Bassini operation. A properly done Bassini repair involves bringing transversus abdominis aponeurosis rather than muscle fibers from transversus abdominis and internal oblique down to Poupart's ligament. Bassini emphasized this point, although it has often been unwisely ignored by surgeons doing this type of repair. Bassini's technique—the first modern herniorrhaphy, originally described in 1887—has stood the test of time and remains today the standard against which the repair of direct inguinal hernias is judged.

McVay demonstrated that transversalis fascia normally attaches to Cooper's ligament, and theoretically transversalis fascia should be reapproximated to this ligament in direct hernia repairs. The procedure was first described by Lotheissen in 1898, and it is used in modified form by many surgeons today. However, this operation is technically more difficult than a repair to Poupart's ligament, and an adequate reconstruction based on Poupart's ligament will prevent recurrence of a direct hernia. Anatomically it is possible for a femoral hernia to develop below a Poupart's ligament repair, but if this actually occurs, it must be most unusual. If a Cooper's ligament repair is done, the surgeon is faced with a problem when he reaches the femoral vein, which passes in front of the ligament. From this point laterally the repair must be done at the more superficial Poupart's ligament level. Where the repair moves from Cooper's ligament to Poupart's ligament, there is a potential weakness, and recurrent herniation at this point is a distinct possibility. To prevent this weakness, McVay recommends suturing transversalis fascia to the medial side of the femoral sheath with one or two stitches as an intermediate step between the two levels of repair. The management of this area, and the greater danger of injury to the femoral vein with a Cooper's ligament repair, continue to be problems in the opinion of many surgeons. Hence the majority of surgeons continue to prefer repair at the level of the inguinal ligament, and many good results have been reported with this technique. Other surgeons feel that a Cooper's ligament repair for direct hernias is to be preferred whenever possible. A careful repair using strong tissue to cover the inguinal canal floor is probably more important than the level of the suture line. Glassow emphasized excision of all weak tissue from the inguinal canal floor and the construction of a multilayered, overlapping floor repair using continuous sutures of an inert material. He believed that recurrent hernias could develop between stitches if interrupted sutures were used for the herniorrhaphy.

Whichever level is selected for repair, it must be remembered that the hernia developed through a weakened transversalis fascia initially. Therefore, although McVay does nothing further to the canal floor, most surgeons agree that the newly constituted transversalis fascia repair should be reinforced in some manner. The technique suggested by Zimmerman and Anson, employing the inferior portion of the incised external oblique aponeurosis as a pedicle flap brought underneath the cord and sutured to transversalis fascia superior to the free edge of the internal oblique muscle, is probably the best anatomically. Another technique involves turning down a flap from the inner layer of the rectus sheath beneath the cord and uniting it to Poupart's ligament, thus reversing the procedure advocated by Zimmerman (Fig. 36-14). Still other surgeons prefer to place a free graft of autogenous fascia lata over the transversalis fascia repair. The graft is applied either as a single fascial sheet or as a mesh woven from fascial strips. In place of fascia lata, reinforcement can be done with a sheet of tantalum gauze or with a synthetic mesh sutured over the repaired Hesselbach's triangle beneath the cord. Because tantalum may break, leaving sharp metallic

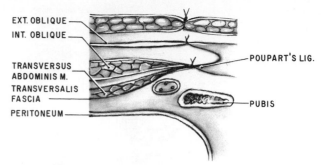

Fig. 36-11. Ferguson operation. Spermatic cord is placed deep to reconstructed inguinal canal floor.

ends to traumatize neighboring structures, a synthetic material is preferred. Once the inguinal canal floor is adequately repaired, the cord is replaced in the canal. External oblique aponeurosis, subcutaneous tissue, and skin are closed over it exactly as in the repair for indirect hernia.

FEMORAL HERNIA. The femoral hernia protrudes from the groin underneath the inguinal ligament between the

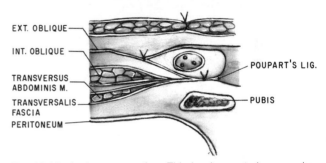

Fig. 36-12. Andrews operation. This involves suturing superior leaf of external oblique aponeurosis to shelving edge of Poupart's ligament beneath spermatic cord, with inferior leaf of external oblique sutured up over it.

lacunar ligament medially and the femoral vein laterally. If transversalis fascia is strongly attached to Cooper's ligament, as is normally the case, this creates a curtain which effectively prevents the peritoneum or any intraperitoneal structure from reaching the femoral ring. Thus the femoral hernia is a groin hernia and should be treated as such, with an incision above the inguinal ligament. When the inguinal

Fig. 36-13. Halsted's original repair. Spermatic cord is transplanted subcutaneously and inguinal canal closed beneath it. Halsted later abandoned this operation, and it is little used today.

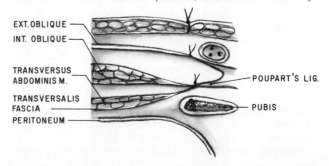

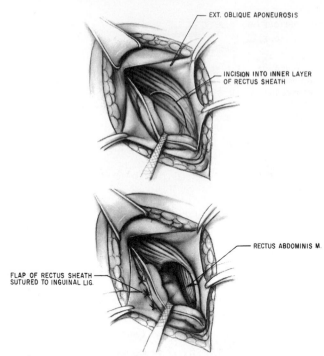

EXT. OBLIQUE APONEUROSIS

INCISION INTO INNER LAYER OF RECTUS SHEATH

RECTUS ABDOMINIS M.

FLAP OF RECTUS SHEATH SUTURED TO INGUINAL LIG.

Fig. 36-14. Reinforcement of canal floor repair using flap of rectus sheath. Some technique for reinforcement of Hesselbach's triangle should be part of any repair done for direct hernia.

canal is opened and the spermatic cord or the round ligament retracted, a bulge will be evident beneath the transversalis fascia near the pubic spine. When the transversalis fascia is incised, the peritoneal neck of the hernia sac will be visible, and the surgeon thus has control of the sac and its contents. This is important especially when there may be strangulation of bowel in the sac, for the hernia should not be permitted to reduce before the viability of its contents has been ascertained. Attention may then be turned safely to the femoral triangle, where the peritoneal sac is dissected free from the subcutaneous tissues. Once the sac is freed, it is frequently possible to reduce it beneath the inguinal ligament by traction from above. Since the neck of the sac is quite narrow, however, this reduction may not be possible without dividing the inguinal ligament transversely at the level of the hernia, thus releasing the sac. The continuity of the inguinal ligament is of little consequence, and it need not be restored.

After inspecting the contents of the sac and returning them to the peritoneal cavity, the sac itself is removed and its neck closed with a nonabsorbable purse-string suture. Anatomically, the best method of preventing recurrent herniation is to bring transversalis fascia down to Cooper's ligament exactly as described for the direct hernia. With the femoral hernia, repair must be at the level of Cooper's ligament rather than of the inguinal ligament, since herniation into the femoral triangle may recur beneath an inguinal ligament repair. Further reinforcement of the inguinal canal floor is then carried out, using the same approach described for the direct hernia.

Two other general methods for preventing recurrence

of a femoral hernia have been advocated. In the first of these, the Moschcowitz technique, the femoral ring is obliterated by suturing Poupart's ligament to Cooper's ligament. In the second a pedicle of aponeurosis from the inferior margin of the external oblique incision is sutured down to Cooper's ligament. Both these methods effectively obliterate the femoral ring, but they do not strengthen the inguinal canal floor, so that development of a direct hernia through the weakened floor remains possible. Strengthening the inguinal canal floor through a femoral triangle incision is difficult or impossible; hence the incision above the inguinal ligament is preferred.

BILATERAL HERNIAS. It is possible to operate on bilateral groin hernias through two separate groin incisions as described above. Most surgeons feel that in adults it is better to stage these operations, rather than doing both simultaneously. The recurrence rate when bilateral repairs are done simultaneously in adults seems unacceptably high. If both groins are to be repaired at one time, it is more expeditious to use a Cheatle-Henry incision. In this approach a vertical lower-midline incision is made and carried down to the peritoneum, which is then reflected away from the lower abdominal wall. By traction upward on the abdominal wall it is possible to dissect down to the inguinal triangle easily, and good exposure of Cooper's ligament is readily obtained. Transversalis fascia from the inner surface of the transversus abdominis can then be sutured down to Cooper's ligament under excellent direct vision to provide a satisfactory repair for either a direct or a femoral hernia. Reinforcement of the inguinal canal floor repair is not readily possible through this approach, and this represents a distinct disadvantage to its routine use. It is also somewhat more inconvenient, although not impossible, to deal with an indirect hernia. The major advantage of this approach is that bilateral hernias can be repaired much more rapidly. With a patient who is a poor anesthetic risk the resultant saving of time may be an important factor.

When an infant presents with a unilateral indirect inguinal hernia, there is perhaps 1 chance in 5 that a second undetected hernia is present on the opposite side. In the view of certain surgeons, this is sufficient reason for exploring the opposite side in all infants. Since right-sided hernias are somewhat more common than those on the left, this argument is advanced most strongly when a left-sided hernia is detected preoperatively. Since exploring the second side is a simple undertaking once the patient is under anesthesia, the argument seems superficially attractive. However, to carry out four negative explorations in the hope of finding one undetected hernia seems on reflection an unjustified meddling with normal tissues. Rather, a careful examination of both groins should precede any elective herniorrhaphy, and the second side should be explored only if there is reasonable suspicion of a defect on physical examination. It has been suggested recently that infant groin hernias may be identified preoperatively by injection of a radiopaque dye into the abdominal cavity followed by the exposure of an upright abdominal roentgenogram. If this technique proves safe and reliable, it will offer a reasonable solution to this debate.

UMBILICAL HERNIAS

When it has been decided that an umbilical hernia warrants surgical repair, a curved incision is made below the umbilicus and carried through subcutaneous fat to expose the anterior rectus sheath (Fig. 36-15). By dissecting toward the inferior margin of the defect, the surgeon delineates the peritoneal sac projecting through the fascial opening. Continued dissection at this level around the umbilicus defines the fascial defect and isolates the sac. The sac is then freed from the undersurface of the umbilical skin, and excess peritoneum is removed. Following closure of the peritoneum, the fascia above and below the defect is united by a series of nonabsorbable sutures. This repair is traditionally done by bringing the fascia above the defect down over the fascia from below to effect a two-layer closure—the so-called "vest over pants" type of repair (Fig. 36-16). These two fascial layers fuse, but there is no convincing proof that the resulting repair is any stronger than that produced by a careful approximation of fascial margins without undue tension. The umbilicus is then tacked down to the fascial repair and the skin incision closed. When a large hernia has been repaired in an obese adult, it is desirable to drain the resulting dead space to prevent formation of a seroma in the incision; otherwise drainage is not employed. Formerly it was customary to excise the umbilicus during umbilical herniorrhaphy. This is unnecessary except when a proboscis-type defect is present, and the loss of the umbilicus is psychologically disturbing to many children and even to some adults. When, for technical reasons, removal of the umbilicus is desirable, the patient should be clearly informed of this preoperatively.

VENTRAL HERNIAS

The hernia which develops in an old operative incision may present a vexing problem in repair; many hernias of this type can be successfully managed by a good external support. When operative repair is undertaken, the defect should be closed with local tissue if possible. The old operative scar can be excised or a fresh incision made perpendicular to it (Fig. 36-17A). In either event the first aim of the surgeon should be to dissect down to normal fascia all around the herniation. Dissection is then continued to separate the peritoneal sac from the margins of the fascial defect (Fig. 36-17B). The peritoneum is opened, the contents of the sac are appropriately managed, and excess peritoneum is removed. After closure of the incision into the peritoneum, the fascia is approximated to obliterate the hernia. If the initial defect was a small one, it may be possible to close it without undue tension by the use of interrupted sutures of some nonabsorbable material. With a larger defect, two relaxing incisions, one to either side of the original hernia, may make closure practical. This technique is particularly useful in the situation where the incisional hernia developed in a vertical midline or paramedian incision. The relaxing incisions are then made in the anterior rectus sheath, and midline approximation does not result in herniation laterally where the relaxing incisions were done (Fig. 36-17C). There is usually weak

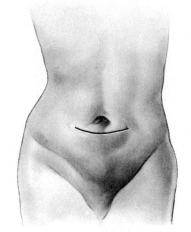

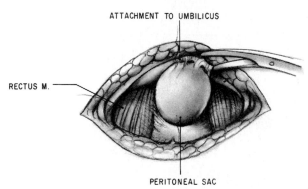

ATTACHMENT TO UMBILICUS

RECTUS M.

PERITONEAL SAC

Fig. 36-15. Umbilical hernia repair. Curvilinear incision below the umbilicus gives excellent exposure. Sac must be freed by sharp dissection from undersurface of umbilicus.

attenuated fascia surrounding the actual defect, and failure to extend the repair through this area is one of the common technical errors which frequently results in recurrence. When no local tissue can be found for this type of repair, an artificial substitute of metallic or synthetic mesh may be employed. Although Koontz has reported very good results

Fig. 36-16. Umbilical hernia repair. "Vest over pants" type of imbrication is traditionally used, but single layer, well opposed without imbrication, is equally effective.

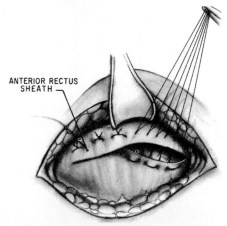

ANTERIOR RECTUS SHEATH

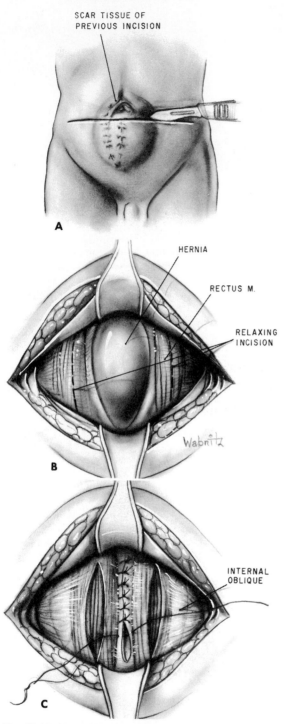

Fig. 36-17. Ventral hernia repair. *A.* It is frequently desirable to make fresh incision perpendicular to old hernia scar. *B.* Closure of fascial defect may be facilitated by making relaxing incision in rectus sheath to either side of hernia sac. *C.* Relaxing incisions permit good fascial approximation over defect without producing significant weakness in areas of relaxation.

from the use of tantalum for this purpose, most surgeons have not been happy with the use of any foreign material for these repairs.

RESULTS

Uncomplicated herniorrhaphies have a negligible operative mortality, and results must be evaluated in terms of recurrence rate. Acutely incarcerated or strangulated hernias remain even today significant causes for morbidity and mortality.

The literature gives no basis for dogmatic statements about the results of herniorrhaphy. Most hernias can be satisfactorily treated, but a small number of recurrences can be expected. If patients undergoing herniorrhaphy are followed carefully for a long enough period of time, the number of known recurrences will, of course, increase.

As a general rule, hernias treated early yield better results, and recurrence following repair of an indirect inguinal hernia in an infant is quite unusual. Indirect hernias at any age have a lower recurrence rate than direct or femoral hernias. A rather high recurrence rate is to be anticipated following repair of postoperative ventral hernias, because they usually develop following some wound complication such as infection or dehiscence, with consequent weakness of the tissues available for repair.

It is axiomatic that the first repair has the greatest chance of success and that recurrence is frequent following any secondary repair of a recurrent hernia. Glassow, reporting extensive experience at Shouldice Hospital in Toronto, indicates that the recurrence rate for primary inguinal or femoral hernias in women should be less than 1 percent. On the other hand, their rate for recurrent femoral hernias after secondary surgery in women was 6.5 percent. Since the most frequent cause for recurrence would appear to be improper technique during the original operation, the importance of a proper initial approach is obvious. All too frequently a hernia is treated by a junior member of the staff without adequate supervision. No surgeon should undertake herniorrhaphy until he is thoroughly conversant with the anatomy of the area and the theory behind the technique of repair.

Although McVay has reported recurrence rates as low as 0.6 percent for groin hernias, nationwide results do not approximate this degree of success. Zimmerman and Anson report from the literature recurrence rates varying between 2 and 30 percent for indirect hernias and between 4 and 33 percent for direct hernias. The recurrence rate for femoral hernias is harder to evaluate, but it probably approximates that for direct hernias. Certainly these results permit no ground for complacency. They emphasize the need for continued careful technique, with attention to detail and a proper evaluation of the type of repair appropriate for the hernia in question.

SUMMARY

Hernias are among the most common afflictions of mankind. Although the operative results are not perfect, repair of an uncomplicated hernia prevents the possibility of intestinal obstruction or gangrene secondary to hernial incarceration. Both these complications remain potentially lethal and entail a prolonged convalescence at best. Therefore it is a general rule that—save for the congenital umbilical hernias, which are likely to close spontaneously, and certain postoperative incisional hernias—all hernias of the abdominal wall should be subjected to prompt surgical correction. When it is elected for medical reasons not to repair other abdominal hernias, it must be remembered that, with a poor-risk patient, the danger of emergency surgery for strangulation is greatly increased. If good results are to be anticipated from operation, the surgeon must have a thorough knowledge of the involved anatomy and a respect for tissues. A repair which is appropriate to the type of defect present must be selected, and the patients must be followed carefully so that the surgeon can profit from his or her mistakes.

References

Carlson, R. I.: The Historical Development of the Surgical Treatment of Inguinal Hernia, *Surgery,* **39:**1031, 1956.

Condon, R. E.: Surgical Anatomy of the Transversus Abdominis and Transversalis Fascia, *Ann Surg,* **173:**1, 1971.

_____ and Nyhus, L. M.: Complications of Groin Hernia and of Hernial Repair, *Surg Clin North Am,* **51:**1325, 1971.

Dunphy, J. E.: Wound Healing, in C. Rob and R. Smith (eds.), "Clinical Surgery," vol. 1, pp. 219–232, Butterworth & Co. (Publishers), Ltd., London, 1964.

Glassow, R.: The Surgical Repair of Inguinal and Femoral Hernias, *Can Med Assoc J,* **108:**308, 1973.

Halverson, K., and McVay, C. B.: Inguinal and Femoral Hernioplasty: 22-Year Study of Authors' Methods, *Arch Surg,* **101:**127, 1970.

Heifetz, C. J.: Age and the Testis after Resection of the Spermatic Cord in the Repair of Inguinal Hernia, *Am J Surg,* **121:**634, 1971.

Koontz, A. R.: "Hernia," Appleton-Century-Crofts, Inc., New York, 1963.

Lichtenstein, I. L., Herzikoff, S., Shore, J. M., Jiron, M. W., Stuart, S., and Mizuno, L.: The Dynamics of Wound Healing, *Surg Gynecol Obstet,* **130:**685, 1970.

Margoles, J. S., and Braun, R. A.: Properitoneal versus Classical Hernioplasty, *Am J Surg,* **121:**641, 1971.

Mizrachy, B., and Kark, A. E.: The Anatomy and Repair of the Posterior Inguinal Wall, *Surg Gynecol Obstet,* **137:**253, 1973.

Moosman, D. A., and Oelrich, T. M.: Prevention of Accidental Trauma to the Ilioinguinal Nerve during Inguinal Herniorrhaphy, *Am J Surg,* **133:**146, 1977.

Ravitch, M. M., and Hitzrot, J. M., II: The Operations for Inguinal Hernia, *Surgery,* **48:**439, 1960.

Rowe, M. I., and Clatworthy, H. W., Jr.: The Other Side of the Pediatric Inguinal Hernia, *Surg Clin North Am,* **51:**1371, 1971.

Shackelford, G. D., and McAlister, W. H.: Inguinal Herniography, *Am J Roentgenol Radium Ther Nucl Med,* **115:**399, 1972.

Thompson, W., Longerbeam, J. K., and Reeves, C.: Herniograms, an Aid to the Diagnosis and Treatment of Groin Hernias in Infants and Children, *Arch Surg,* **105:**71, 1972.

Wagh, P. V., Leverich, A. P., Sun, C. N., White, H. J., and Read, R. C.: Direct Inguinal Herniation in Men: A Disease of Collagen, *J Surg Res,* **17:**425, 1974.

Zimmerman, I. M., and Anson, B. J.: "The Anatomy and Surgery of Hernia," The Williams & Wilkins Company, Baltimore, 1953.

Chapter 37

Pituitary and Adrenal

by **Richard M. Bergland and Timothy S. Harrison**

PITUITARY

(by Richard M. Bergland)

Historical Background

Harvey Cushing, near the end of his career, wrote:

I was once told by Professor Kocher, who I suppose had his experiences with the thyroid in mind, that no satisfactions in medicine were so great as those which came from concentration upon and the mastery of a small subject, and that this necessitated an approach from all aspects; diagnostic, experimental, pathological, and therapeutic, not the least important part of which at one time or another in the history of the subject was likely to be surgical.

Cushing must have heeded Kocher's advice and could surely have been satisfied with his lifelong productive involvement with the pituitary gland. He was the first to describe the syndrome of chiasmal compression, the first to demonstrate the usefulness of radiographs in the diagnosis of pituitary tumors, the first to emphasize that the pituitary holds the dominant position in the endocrine orchestra, the first to describe the hyposecretion associated with chromophobe tumors and the hypersecretion of both eosinophilic and basophilic tumors, and the first surgeon to operate successfully on a large series of patients with pituitary problems.

Remarkably, Harvey Cushing proposed in 1910 that pituitary secretions were released into the ventricle. This proposal has not been generally accepted, but Cushing maintained this belief throughout his career and in 1930 studied the physiological effects of pituitrin injected into the ventricles of humans. The discovery of the tanycyte ependyma, coupled to the reassessment of the vascular anatomy of the pituitary, lends credibility to Cushing's hypothesis. If pituitary secretions are indeed secreted directly to the brain, most of what we now know about the pituitary, and about the brain, will require rethinking.

Cushing's contributions to the understanding of the pituitary are of eternal significance; no other surgeon has made such a profound and lasting impact on any other organ system. The biography of this remarkable man should be read by every student of surgery; predictably some students reading this chapter will enter surgical research and carry on the rewarding tradition passed from Kocher to Cushing.

Gross Anatomy

The pituitary and its parts are schematically illustrated in Fig. 37-1. Unfortunately, pituitary nomenclature is not well standardized, but that of Wislocki is recommended. In his terminology, the *neurohypophysis* is composed of three parts: the infundibulum (which is often termed the median eminence), the infundibular stem (which is often termed the pituitary stalk), and the infundibular process (which is variably designated posterior lobe, posterior pituitary, or pars nervosa).

Wislocki separated the *adenohypophysis* into the pars distalis (often called the anterior lobe or anterior pituitary), the pars intermedia, and the pars tuberalis.

In clinical medicine the terms "median eminence," "pituitary stalk," "anterior pituitary," and "posterior pituitary" have gained general acceptance. But in basic research in other species, Wislocki's terminology is employed more often; an understanding of terms is essential if one is to apply laboratory observations to the understanding of clinical problems.

Fig. 37-1. A schematic illustration of the parts of the human pituitary, as well as the projection of parvicellular and magnocellular neurons into the neurohypophysis.

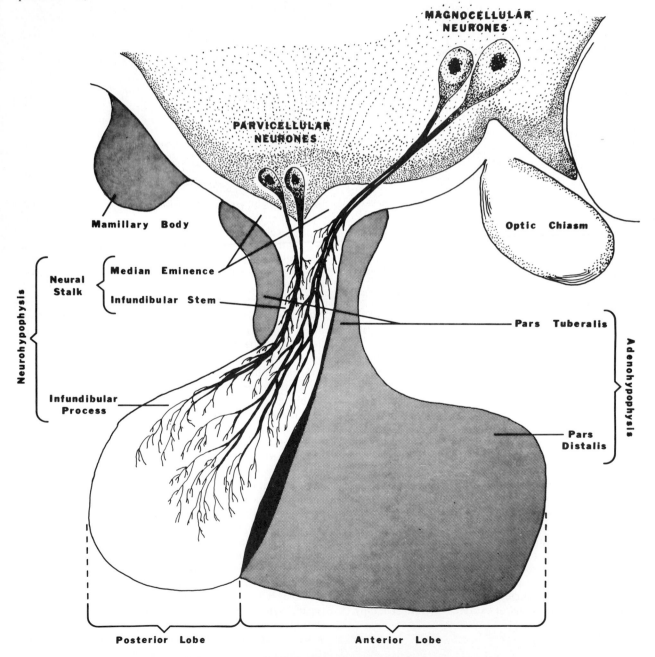

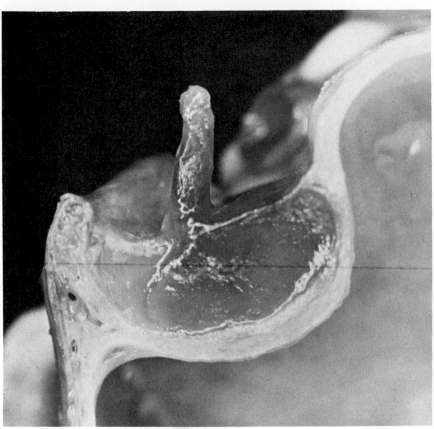

Fig. 37-2. A midline sagittal section of the human pituitary in situ within the sella. The height of the pituitary does not match the depth of the sella.

HUMAN ANATOMICAL VARIATIONS. The adult human pituitary does not have a distinct pars intermedia (Fig. 37-2); the basophils that invade the human posterior pituitary might be considered the functional counterpart of the pars intermedia found in other species.

The pars tuberalis varies in human beings; sometimes the entire pituitary stalk is surrounded by secreting adenohypophyseal cells, but in other instances, the surface of the stalk is totally devoid of adenohypophyseal cells.

In 50 percent of human beings, the sella turcica is covered by the dura of the diaphragma sella, and the intrasellar space is thus separated from the intracranial space. In 40 percent of human beings the opening in the diaphragma that surrounds the pituitary stalk is greater than 5 mm (Fig. 37-3), and in 10 percent of human beings the diaphragma is extremely thin. Without the sturdy barrier of the diaphragma sella, a pituitary tumor may preferentially extend into the suprasellar region; with a sturdy, complete diaphragma, a growing tumor will preferentially enlarge and balloon the sella.

The height of the human pituitary does not match the depth of the sella (Fig. 37-2), and the width of the pituitary does not match the width of the sellar floor (Fig. 37-4); thus plain x-rays permit assessment of the length of the pituitary but not of its height or its width.

Not infrequently the lateral margins of the pituitary are indented by the carotid arteries, and during stereotaxic pituitary procedures the carotids may be damaged. For this reason, some surgeons advocate carotid angiography before any stereotaxic procedure.

VASCULAR ANATOMY. The neurohypophysis is one of the five areas of brain that does not have a blood brain barrier. Its capillaries have a fenestrated endothelium (brain capillaries have no fenestrations) and are surrounded by a double basement membrane (brain capillaries have a single basement membrane). A distinct plane can be drawn between the neurohypophysis and the hypothalamus by the characteristics of the capillaries of each. No neuronal cell bodies are found within the neurohypophysis; all the axons projecting to the neurohypophysis are derived from hypothalamic neurons.

All the elements of the neurohypophysis (the median eminence, stalk, and posterior pituitary) are joined by a common capillary bed, and the direction of blood flow within that capillary bed is variable. The adenohypophysis does not receive a direct arterial supply; all blood reaching it must pass first through the capillary bed of the neurohypophysis.

Adenohypophyseal capillaries resemble those of the neurohypophysis. No nerves terminate within the adenohypophysis, but neurosecretory material is conveyed by pituitary portal vessels from the neurohypophysis to the adenohypophysis. Recently it has been established that some portal vessels carry adenohypophyseal secretions back to the neurohypophysis (Figs. 37-5 and 37-6).

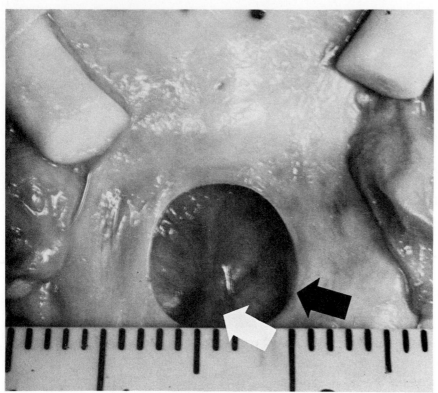

Fig. 37-3. The chiasm has been removed to expose the diaphragma sella. The opening in the diaphragm is about 7 mm in diameter (black arrow), much greater than the penetrating pituitary stalk (white arrow). In 40 percent of human beings, this opening is greater than 5 mm.

Fig. 37-4. A dissection of the human pituitary resting in situ on the floor of the sella. The width of the pituitary is greater than the width of the sella.

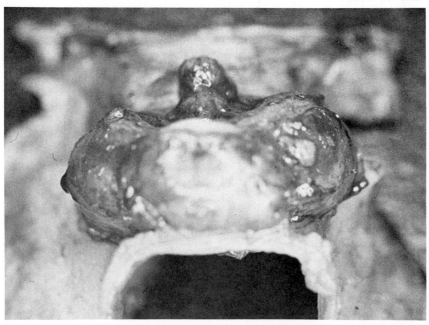

In other species the secreting cells within the pars intermedia have a limited capillary bed but are well innervated; in the human being those basophils that invade the posterior pituitary are also directly innervated.

The distortion of the normal vascular relationships of the pituitary by tumor growth may play an important role in the endocrine disturbances that develop with pituitary tumors, but the current techniques of angiography do not allow the visualization of pituitary vascular anatomy.

Cellular Physiology

THE NEUROHYPOPHYSIS

Hypothalamic neurons with large cell bodies (the *magnocellular neurons* of the supraoptic and paraventricular nuclei) project to the neurohypophysis, and most of them terminate near capillaries within the posterior pituitary (Fig. 37-1). The dense-core neurosecretory granules in these neurons measure about 2,000 Å in diameter and are

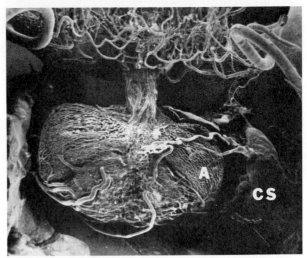

Fig. 37-5. A vascular cast of the monkey pituitary. Very few connections are found between the capillary bed of the adenohypophysis (*A*) and the cavernous sinus (*CS*). This suggests that some blood must exit from the adenohypophysis via other routes.

Fig. 37-6. The vascular relationships of the primate pituitary; arrows indicate the potential directions of blood flow. (1) In some portal vessels, flow may be *into* or *out of* the adenohypophysis. (2) Flow reversal may occur within the neurohypophysis. (3) Flow may occur from the posterior pituitary directly to the cavernous sinus. (4) Recent evidence suggests that flow reversal may occur in certain hypophyseal arteries. (5) Tanycytes may carry pituitary secretions into the ventricle. (6) Capillaries may carry hypophyseal blood directly to the hypothalamus. (7) Fenestrations within endothelial cells of the pituitary portal vessels may allow hormones access to the subarachnoid cerebrospinal fluid.

composed of octapeptides coupled to the carrier protein neurophysin. At the nerve terminals the octapeptides are uncoupled from neurophysin and released into the capillary bed of the neurohypophysis. Two kinds of octapeptides are present: vasopressin and oxytocin. Vasopressin has many systemic actions, but most interest has focused

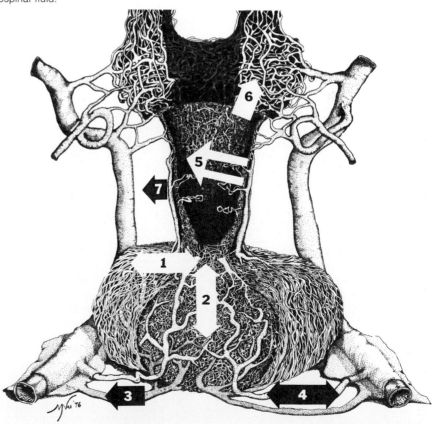

on its antidiuretic effect. Oxytocin has few established physiological effects in the human male, but a profound effect on the pregnant uterus. Like the octapeptides, the carrier protein neurophysin is released into the neurohypophyseal capillary bed, but its physiological role is uncertain.

Hypothalamic neurons with small cell bodies (the *parvicellular neurons* of the arcuate and other hypothalamic nuclei) project to the neurohypophysis, and most of them terminate near capillaries within the median eminence (Fig. 37-1). The dense-core neurosecretory granules in these neurons are smaller (about 800 to 1,000 Å in diameter) and are composed of releasing and inhibiting factors that are destined for the adenohypophysis. No carrier protein similar to neurophysin has been found for the releasing and inhibiting hormones. Many pituitary releasing and inhibiting substances have been isolated from hypothalamic extracts, and their chemical structure has been determined; three have been synthesized (TRH, somatostatin, and GNRH). By tradition, hypothalamic releasing and inhibiting substances have been called "factors" (such as prolactin-inhibiting factor, or PIF) until their chemical structure is identified; then they are termed "hormones" (such as thyrotropin-releasing hormone, or TRH).

Many other substances are found in the neurohypophy-sis. These include epinephrine, norepinephrine, dopamine, histamine, angiotensin, neurotensin, and substance P. Why these substances are released and/or stored in the neurohypophysis is uncertain; of the group, only dopamine has an established role in adenohypophyseal function.

THE ADENOHYPOPHYSIS

It is appropriate to recall that the chromophobe/eosinophil/basophil cellular classification was introduced in 1892, preceding the birth of endocrinology. There was no need at that time to link the histological appearance of pituitary cells to their secretory function, but as the several secretory functions of the adenohypophysis were established, an effort was made to link cell structure to cell function. For many decades, both histochemistry and electron microscopy were employed in an effort to determine which cells secreted which hormones. These techniques were not very successful and produced a nomenclature of such complexity that clinicians had little choice but to employ the chromophobe/basophil/eosinophil system of classification.

The development of immunohistochemistry brought order to the study of pituitary histology, and for the first time, pituitary cells could be described according to their secretory function (Fig. 37-7). Remarkably, this technique has established that some pituitary cells secrete more than one hormone. The use of the functional classification of pituitary cell types allows the simultaneous consideration of the biochemistry and physiology of each different trophic hormone.

GROWTH HORMONE CELLS (SOMATOTROPES). Growth hormone–secreting cells are found in the lateral aspect of the adenohypophysis; these cells appear eosinophilic with traditional stains. Growth hormone (GH) is a large peptide (190 amino acids) that effects the growth of bone, muscle, and visceral organs; it also elevates blood glucose level. GH is species-specific; human GH has not been synthesized and currently can be obtained only by extraction from human pituitaries recovered at autopsy.

Between 5 and 10 percent of the weight of the adenohypophysis is accounted for by GH; the pituitary glands of children and adults have a similar GH content. The resting level of serum GH is 1 to 5 ng/ml, but secretory surges occur six to eight times daily; the largest surge occurs during sleep in the early morning hours. During adolescence the total amount of GH secreted per 24 hours increases, largely because the secretory surges occur more frequently.

Secretions from the parvicellular hypothalamic neurons influence GH secretion; growth hormone–releasing factor (GRF) stimulates secretion, and growth hormone–inhibiting factor (somatostatin) limits secretion. GRF has been isolated from hypothalamic extracts, but its chemical structure has not been determined. Somatostatin, found during the search for GRF, has been isolated, chemically identified as a tetradecapeptide, and synthesized. Somatostatin has other biological effects, including the inhibition of glucagon release from the pancreatic islet cells and the inhibition of gastrin secretion from the stomach; somatostatin is produced in the pancreas and the intestine as well as within the hypothalamus.

Fig. 37-7. A schematic illustration of the Nakane horseradish peroxidase immunohistochemical staining technique. Antibodies to specific trophic hormones are produced in vivo, harvested, and conjugated with horseradish peroxidase. Serial sections of the pituitary are obtained, washed with the various antibody-horseradish peroxidase conjugates, and reacted with lead. The lead precipitate (brownish-black) is visible over the cell containing the appropriate antigen. The technique allows a functional designation of pituitary cells, i.e., somatotrophic cell, thyrotrophic cell, etc. Note that follicle-stimulating hormone (FSH) and luteinizing hormone (LH) are formed in a common "gonadotroph." This technique may be employed with the light microscope or the electron microscope. *GH*, growth hormone; *TSH*, thyroid-stimulating hormone; *ACTH*, adrenocorticotrophic hormone.

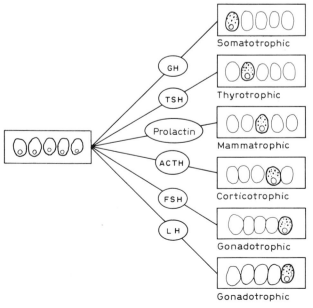

Exercise, stress, or hypoglycemia physiologically stimulate GH secretion. Insulin, arginine, epinephrine, L-dopa, and apomorphine can be infused pharmacologically to effect GH release.

PROLACTIN CELLS (MAMMOTROPES). Prolactin-secreting cells also are found in the lateral aspect of the adenohypophysis and also are eosinophils by traditional histochemical staining. Prolactin is a large peptide structurally similar in many ways to GH. In humans, prolactin promotes lactation, but in lower species the hormone has many different and profound effects on behavior. Synthetic prolactin is not available for therapeutic use.

The normal daytime levels of prolactin are 15 to 25 ng/ml; during sleep, prolactin levels increase two- or threefold by episodic surges of secretion. Men have circulating levels that equal those of nonpregnant women.

Hypothalamic control of prolactin secretion is achieved by the transport of prolactin-inhibiting factor (PIF) and prolactin-releasing factor (PRF) to the adenohypophysis. The net effect of the hypothalamic influence on prolactin secretion is inhibition. The chemical nature of PIF is not firmly established; some evidence suggests that dopamine may be PIF: for instance, L-dopa, the precursor of dopamine, limits prolactin secretion. No distinct prolactin-releasing factor (PRF) has been found, yet both TRH and somatostatin (along with their other established functions) increase prolactin levels, and either or both of them may serve as PRF.

Pregnancy, lactation, stress, and exercise are associated with high levels of prolactin; stimulation of the breast in both males and females activates reflex secretion of prolactin. Reserpine, synthetic TRH, and oral contraceptives all increase prolactin levels.

Prolactin levels are diminished by water loading and by the administration of L-dopa, apomorphine, and bromergocryptine.

THYROID-STIMULATING HORMONE CELL (THYROTROPE). The cells which make thyroid-stimulating hormone (TSH) are located in the central portion of the adenohypophysis and would be termed *basophils* by an older classification. TSH is a glycoprotein that increases thyroid growth and the synthesis of thyroid hormones.

Episodic secretory surges maintain a normal serum daytime level of TSH between 1 and 10 ng/ml; during the late stages of sleep (between 4 A.M. and 8 A.M.), a larger surge of secretion occurs which lasts 2 to 3 hours.

Hypothalamic control of TSH secretion is achieved in part by the delivery of thyrotropin-releasing hormone (TRH) to the adenohypophysis; TRH is a tripeptide (perhaps the smallest peptide) which effects TSH release. Thyroid hormones also inhibit TSH release by a direct effect on thyrotropes.

Cold, stress, and electrical stimulation of the hypothalamus cause TSH release; TRH administration has become a convenient pharmacological way to increase TSH levels and to test TSH secretory reserve.

Age, hyperthyroidism, L-dopa, adrenal steroids, somatostatin, and bromergocryptine all result in diminished TSH levels.

ADRENOCORTICOTROPIC HORMONE CELL (CORTICO-TROPE). Adrenocorticotropic hormone (ACTH) is formed by cells within the adenohypophysis as well as by those basophils which have invaded the neurohypophysis. ACTH is a peptide (39 amino acids) which promotes growth of the adrenal cortex and the synthesis of the adrenal steroid hormones.

The biological half-life of ACTH is about 10 minutes; throughout the day, from six to ten secretory surges occur, but circulating levels are highest during sleep. The nocturnal rise of ACTH is not the consequence of sleep and occurs in a circadian rhythm even in sleep-deprived subjects.

Hypothalamic stimulation, stress, fear, trauma, hemorrhage, and extreme cold cause ACTH release. The search for a hypothalamic corticotropin-releasing hormone (CRH) has to date been unsuccessful, but it is well established that the hypothalamus plays an important stimulatory role in ACTH release. Some investigators have postulated that vasopressin may function as CRH, since high levels of vasopressin cause ACTH release.

The feedback relationships between ACTH and the adrenal are discussed later in this chapter.

THE GONADOTROPES. Cells which produce follicle-stimulating hormone (FSH) and luteinizing hormone (LH) collectively have been termed *gonadotropes*. These cells would have been termed *basophils* by an earlier histological classification. Both FSH and LH are glycoproteins, and a single cell secretes both hormones. FSH promotes spermatogenesis in males and promotes the maturation of ovarian follicles and the production of ovarian steroids in females. LH stimulates the male's testes to produce testosterone and promotes the development of the corpus luteum in the female.

The basal levels of FSH and LH are maintained by small secretory surges that occur at hourly intervals. In the mid-cycle of menstruating women, a larger ovulatory surge of both hormones (the surge of LH is greater) occurs, which results in ovulation. During puberty, LH levels rise dramatically during sleep and are associated with REM (rapid eye movement) sleep.

The hypothalamus influences both FSH and LH secretion via a single releasing hormone which has been termed *gonadotropin-releasing hormone* (GNRH), a decapeptide which has been synthesized. Some have termed this substance *luteinizing hormone–releasing hormone* (LHRH), since its action is more pronounced on LH secretion than on FSH secretion.

The cyclical release of FSH and LH in females results from complex ovarian events, and although the hypothalamus controls gonadotropin release, the rhythm of the cycle is derived from cyclical changes in ovarian function.

Gonadotropin secretion is increased by electrical stimulation of the hypothalamus, stress, certain visual or olfactory stimuli, and castration; in lower forms, dopamine causes FSH and LH release, but this has not been demonstrated in human beings. Synthetic GNRH can be employed to stimulate gonadotropin release and to test gonadotropin reserve.

BETA-LIPOTROPIN CELLS. The pituitary produces beta-lipotropin (LPH), a peptide containing 91 amino acids. In other species this substance is found in both the pars intermedia and the pars distalis. The structural peptide sequence of LPH contains amino acid groups which are identical to ACTH, beta MSH, endorphine, and enkephalin; thus LPH may serve as a mother molecule which can be cleaved in various places to produce smaller peptides.

Melanocyte-stimulating hormone (MSH), one of the constitutents of LPH, is produced in the pars intermedia in other species and promotes melanin production by the melanophores in the skin; some evidence suggests that MSH functions as a neurotransmitter which enhances memory.

The endorphines (alpha and beta) are moderately large peptides which also are part of the LPH molecule; both have been found in brain and spinal cord. Endorphines are bound by the same opiate receptors that bind morphine, and their physiological effects are blocked by naloxone. There is increasing physiological evidence that these substances are involved in the modulation of pain perception.

Enkephalin is a pentapeptide that has part of the molecular sequence of LPH and some of the physiological properties of the endorphines; it too has been found in brain. The intraventricular injection of enkephalin into rats results in a catatonic stupor.

FOLLICULAR CELLS. The pituitary gland in many species, including the human, contains stellate-shaped cells which form PAS-positive follicles within the adenohypophysis. These cells are difficult to visualize with light microscopy, since their thin processes are below the level of optical resolution, but they are readily seen with the electron microscope.

To date, no function has been linked to follicular cells; they are the only cells within the pituitary that still must be designated by their structure rather than their function. Unfortunately, *follicular cells* (an anatomic designation) are often confused with *follicular-stimulating hormone cells* (a functional designation).

CELL RESTS. Frequently, large PAS-positive follicles or cysts are found in the cleft between the pars distalis and pars nervosa of the human pituitary; these cysts do not resemble the pars intermedia in lower species, and their function is unclear.

In the vicinity of the pars tuberalis, squamous cell rests are frequently found in the human being. These cells resemble those contained in a craniopharyngioma and may be the embryological remnant of Rathke's pouch.

Pituitary Disorders

TRAUMA

The pituitary stalk traverses the subdural space and may be partially or even totally disrupted during the deacceleration of head trauma. As many as 10 percent of patients with fatal head trauma have a divided pituitary stalk. Since the adenohypophysis derives all of its blood supply from the pituitary portal vessels and has no independent arterial supply, pituitary necrosis and panhypopituitarism result.

POSTPARTUM PITUITARY ISCHEMIA

During pregnancy the weight of the pituitary increases by as much as 50 percent, and should postpartum hemorrhage result in shock, the pituitary becomes necrotic. This syndrome, variously described as Sheehan's syndrome or Simmonds' disease, generally results in panhypopituitarism. Treatment must focus on prevention, but once present, the condition can be treated with endocrine substitution therapy.

CHROMOPHOBE ADENOMAS

Nonsecreting pituitary tumors, first described by Cushing, are the most common kind of pituitary tumor; these tumor cells have very few cytoplasmic granules and are commonly classified by the old nomenclature as *chromophobe adenomas.*

As chromophobe tumors enlarge, the adjoining secreting cells within the sella turcica are compressed, and diminished secretion results; most often growth hormone secretion is affected first, gonadotropic secretion next, thyrotropic secretion third, and ACTH secretion last. These functions are often lost in sequence, and patients who have lost adrenal function usually have had an earlier loss of thyroid and gonadal function. Despite the distortion of the

Fig. 37-8. *Left,* the normal arterial supply to the human optic chiasm. While the lateral portions of the chiasm receive a superior *and* an inferior arterial supply, the central portion of the chiasm receives only an inferior supply. *Right,* distortion of the inferior vascular supply by a pituitary tumor causes ischemia of the central portion of the chiasm, which results in a bitemporal hemianopsia.

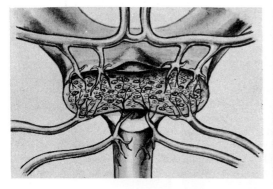
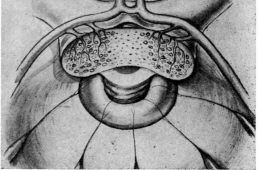

neurohypophysis that is caused by chromophobe adenomas, diabetes insipidus seldom occurs.

The visual system may be distorted by larger chromophobe adenomas, and typically a bitemporal hemianopsia develops. Although large tumors may compress the inferior aspect of the optic nerves, optic chiasm, and optic tract, a horizontal altitudinal defect rarely ensues; the peculiarities of the vasculature of the chiasm (Fig. 37-8) make the central portion of the chiasm (containing the crossing fibers from the mesial retina) more vulnerable.

Rarely, chromophobe adenomas may enlarge laterally to compress those cranial nerves within the cavernous sinus (the oculomotor, the trochlear, the first division of the trigeminal, and the abducent); this is more commonly noted when the tumors outgrow their vascular supply and "pituitary apoplexy" results. This sudden hemorrhage within the tumor occurs in 5 percent of chromophobe adenomas, usually in large tumors, and is associated with sudden visual loss, severe headache, hyposecretion of trophic hormones, and subarachnoid hemorrhage.

The largest of the suprasellar chromophobe adenomas will extend into the third ventricle to cause hydrocephalus and/or hypothalamic dysfunction.

Although radiotherapy is effective in treating chromophobe adenomas, surgical procedures (either via a transfrontal or transsphenoidal route) are generally indicated, both to decrease the bulk of the tumor and to verify the histopathology. Surgery can be accomplished with a mortality rate of 1 percent.

ACROMEGALY

The hypersecretion of growth hormone results in gigantism in adolescents (before the epiphyses have closed) and acromegaly in adults (after the epiphyses have closed). Growth hormone causes excessive bone growth, excessive muscle growth (with weight gain), diabetes (with elevation of blood sugar level), and organomegaly. Enlargement of the face, hands, and feet often permits a bedside diagnosis (Fig. 37-9). The enlargement of the heart may result in valvular dysfunction and cardiomyopathy; patients with acromegaly commonly die of cardiac complications.

Some hypersecreting growth hormone tumors are large and cause hypofunction of other secreting cells, visual symptoms, and hydrocephalus. Although the first tumors associated with acromegaly were small eosinophilic microadenomas, the majority of acromegalic pituitary tumors removed at surgery are chromophobe tumors, not eosinophilic tumors. Even so, immunohistochemical analysis of the chromophobe tumors found in acromegaly will demonstrate GH within the cytoplasm of the tumor cells (Fig. 37-10).

The goal of therapy in acromegaly or gigantism is a reduced level of GH. In smaller, well-circumscribed tumors, the so-called microadenomas (Fig. 37-11), this can be accomplished by tumor removal alone, but in larger tumors a radical hypophysectomy is necessary, with postoperative endocrine replacement therapy.

The development of the proton beam, which has added a new dimension to the therapy of acromegaly, may supplant invasive surgical approaches.

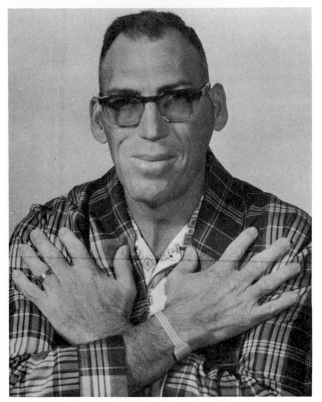

Fig. 37-9. Patient with acromegaly. Note the large broad hands, stubby thumbs, thick lips, and prominent jaw. The classic full-blown features of acromegaly are seldom seen at present, since treatment is instituted at a much earlier stage than formerly.

Fig. 37-10. Acidic-basic stains may show the tumor from an acromegalic patient to be chromophobic. The horseradish peroxidase immunohistochemical techniques can be used on serial sections of tumor tissue to reveal the presence of growth hormone within the cells. This allows a functional designation of the tumor, i.e., somatotrophic.

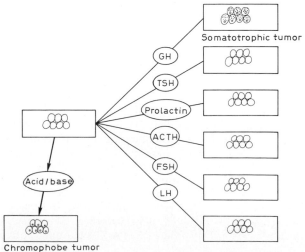

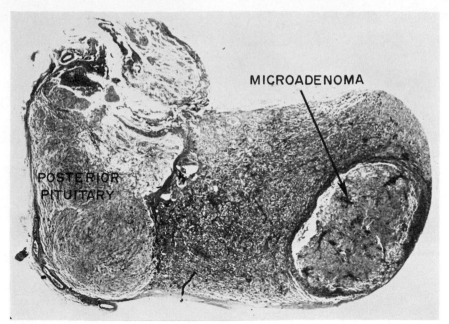

MICROADENOMA

POSTERIOR PITUITARY

Fig. 37-11. A microadenoma of the pituitary. (*Courtesy of Dr. J. Hardy.*) These tumors may secrete large amounts of hormones, yet not enlarge the sella. Their presence may be determined by radioimmune assay; they are perhaps best removed by the trans-sphenoidal approach.

CUSHING'S DISEASE

Hypersecretion of ACTH by the pituitary results in hypersecretion of steroid hormones from the adrenal cortex. Not all patients with excessive levels of adrenal steroid hormones have ACTH-producing tumors; the cause of the steroid excess can be determined only by the measurement of pituitary and adrenal secretions and by manipulating the pituitary/adrenal axis with dexamethasone and/or metapyrone.

Many of the ACTH-producing tumors are small, and a normal-sized sella turcica does not exclude the presence of a pituitary tumor; patients with the signs and symptoms of Cushing's disease must have a variety of hormone determinations before a pituitary tumor is excluded. Many small ACTH-producing tumors have been removed from normal-sized sella turcicas.

If excessive secretion of ACTH from a pituitary tumor is the cause of Cushing's disease, most investigators would agree that the pituitary tumor should be treated, rather than the adrenal hyperplasia.

The diagnosis and therapy of Cushing's disease is discussed more fully later in this chapter.

PROLACTIN-SECRETING TUMORS

Since a suitable assay for prolactin has been developed, it has been ascertained that 30 percent of all pituitary tumors originate in prolactin-secreting cells. Many of these grow to a large size and were previously termed *chromophobe adenomas,* but immunohistochemical analysis may demonstrate prolactin within the cytoplasm of the pale chromophobe cells.

In females, tumors which produce excessive prolactin cause amenorrhea as well as galactorrhea. The amenorrhea/galactorrhea syndrome (the "A/G syndrome") often results from microadenomas which do not enlarge the sella. With increasing frequency, surgeons are exploring the sella turcica to discover and remove small tumors that could not be visualized by radiography.

In males, excessive levels of prolactin may result in impotence; the removal of the offending prolactin-secreting tumor may return sexual function to normal.

Most patients with prolactin-secreting adenomas come to operation, and the surgical removal of a prolactin-secreting microadenoma can improve female fertility and give afflicted males a return of sexual vigor. Yet the systemic disturbances of prolactin excess are not known to be life threatening (in contrast to GH excess or ACTH excess), and a more conservative course often is indicated.

OTHER HYPERSECRETING TUMORS

Hypersecreting tumors of the gonadotropic cells or the thyrotropic cells are rare but have been reported.

CRANIOPHARYNGIOMAS

In both children and adults, remnants of Rathke's pouch may produce a squamous cell tumor of the pituitary, which has been termed a *craniopharyngioma.* Those tumors that develop within the sella turcica result only in hypofunction of the adenohypophysis, but the majority of craniopharyngiomas develop above the diaphragma sella and affect the neurohypophysis, the hypothalamus, the visual system, and the ventricular system. This tumor is a common cause of dwarfism. Many of these tumors are cystic, and many are calcified; not all these tumors are well encapsulated.

Once diagnosed, craniopharyngiomas may be totally

excised (if they are well encapsulated), but often cyst drainage with partial resection is preferable. Some degree of palliation may be achieved by radiotherapy.

OTHER TUMORS

Meningiomas of the tuberculum sella, ependymomas, gliomas, and pinealomas may distort the hypothalamus and/or pituitary and cause signs and symptoms not easily distinguished from those produced by primary pituitary tumors.

Metastases to the pituitary are not infrequent. Since all blood reaching the pituitary initially passes through the neurohypophysis, most metastases occur in the neurohypophysis, not the adenohypophysis.

Diagnostic Studies

RADIOLOGICAL PITUITARY STUDIES

Skull films should be obtained in patients whose signs and symptoms lead to the suspicion of a pituitary disorder. Lateral films will demonstrate the sagittal profile of the sella turcica, and anteroposterior films, properly taken, will demonstrate the floor of the sella. But only the posterior, anterior, and inferior aspects of the pituitary can be evaluated by these films. Tomograms provide a more certain assessment of the sella turcica and are especially helpful for the study of small microadenomas. The lateral aspect of the pituitary can be assessed only by angiography, and the superior aspect can be visualized only by pneumoencephalography. Since patients will often develop some degree of malaise following pneumoencephalography, angiograms usually are performed first. These radiological studies may be stressful, and patients with a disordered pituitary-adrenal axis should be protected with supplementary adrenal steroids during their radiographic studies.

Not all patients with enlargement of the sella turcica have pituitary tumors; fully 10 percent of this group have the empty sella syndrome, in which pneumoencephalography results in filling of the sella with air. The etiology of this syndrome is unclear. Should endocrine studies point to a hypersecreting tumor, the sella nonetheless should be explored as a moderate number of microadenomas have been removed from so-called empty sellas.

FUNCTIONAL PITUITARY STUDIES

Increasingly, endocrine studies of pituitary function are replacing anatomical studies in the diagnosis of hypersecreting tumors. Since patients with pituitary disorders may have hyperfunction of some cell populations and hypofunction of other cell populations, a full battery of assays is usually essential to understand the functional derangements caused by the tumor.

Therapeutic Modalities

TRANSCRANIAL SURGERY

Before the era of antibiotics, surgeons were reluctant to open the frontal sinus to reach the pituitary; the intracra-nial route was via a lateral subfrontal or temporal approach. Antibiotics made it possible for surgeons to remove the frontal bone and, if needed, to open the frontal sinus without fear of meningitis. Working through the frontal sinus (Fig. 37-12) permits less retraction of the frontal lobe and better exposure of the pituitary and chiasm; the unilateral anosmia that results is seldom noticed by patients.

Experienced surgeons can perform transfrontal pituitary surgery for hypophysectomy and for tumors with little morbidity or mortality. This approach allows the surgeon to visualize the anatomical variations that frequently surround the pituitary and to assay the distortions of the surrounding neural and vascular structures that result from tumor growth.

TRANSSPHENOIDAL APPROACHES

Early in the history of pituitary surgery, the advantages of the transsphenoidal approach to the pituitary were recognized; yet the high incidence of infection in the pre-antibiotic era worked against this approach. After opening the frontal sinus during pituitary surgery was proved safe, the transnasal approach through the sphenoid sinus was again employed (Fig. 37-13).

Although this approach does not allow the surgeon to visualize intracranial anatomical variations or the variable distortions that occur with large tumors, it is cosmetically superior, since the incision is hidden in the gingival mucosa of the upper lip. Experience has verified that this approach to the pituitary is safe, and in recent years it has supplanted the transfrontal intracranial approach in most clinics. This procedure demands an operative microscope and intraoperative fluoroscopy.

By this approach the normal sella turcica can be opened and microadenomas which were not visible by x-ray but whose presence was ascertained by functional endocrine assays can be removed. The sella turcica can be explored, much as the abdomen or chest is explored in troublesome diagnostic cases.

STEREOTAXIC TECHNIQUES

Because the sella turcica is such a convenient radiographic target, the pituitary has been treated by a variety of stereotaxic techniques. Many of these techniques were developed for the purpose of hypophysectomy in the treatment of metastatic cancer, but in selected cases, the same techniques have been employed in the treatment of pituitary tumors.

In most instances, the cannula employed in stereotaxic pituitary surgery is introduced by the transsphenoidal or transethmoidal route. Radiographic control is essential, but these procedures can be performed under local anesthesia.

Radioactive gold, radioactive yttrium, cryosurgery, and radiofrequency generators have been employed with good success to destroy the normal pituitary and to treat certain pituitary tumors. A major problem with stereotaxic procedures has been the high incidence of cerebrospinal fluid rhinorrhea.

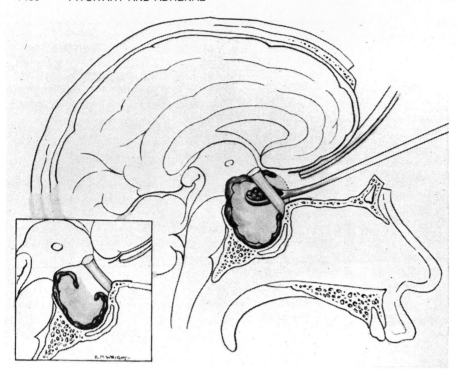

PROTON BEAM

The development of the linear accelerator led to efforts to treat certain pituitary diseases by the proton beam (only two clinics in this country have this capability). As in the stereotaxic procedures, the radiographic shadow of the sella turcica allows the surgeon to aim the proton beam at the pituitary and to destroy the normal pituitary or certain pituitary tumors. This procedure is performed without an incision and may be the first of many surgical procedures that will be done by noninvasive techniques.

Fig. 37-12. An illustration from Cushing of the transcranial approach to the pituitary. Note the unopened frontal sinus; Cushing's efforts preceded the development of antibiotics, and meningitis often ensued if the frontal sinus was opened. Modern surgeons often open the frontal sinus, since the lower exposure provides better visualization of the pituitary.

Fig. 37-13. Another illustration from Cushing of the transsphenoidal approach to the pituitary. Because of the high incidence of infection, Cushing gave up this approach. Since the advent of antibiotics, it has gained favor.

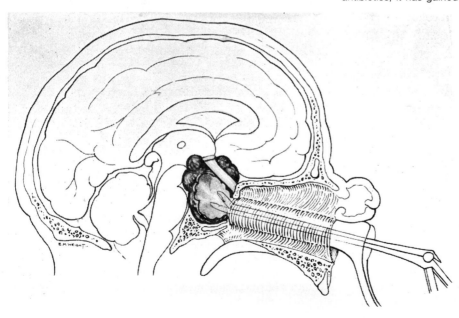

HYPOPHYSECTOMY

The beneficial effect of oophorectomy for patients with metastatic breast cancer was known before the discovery of the endocrine system. The discovery that ovarian function was largely controlled by the pituitary, coupled to the realization that some estrogen was formed by the adrenals, suggested that hypophysectomy might be a more effective method for treating patients with far-advanced breast cancer. Since hypophysectomy also causes hypoadrenalism, it could not be employed until 1952, when adrenal replacement therapy became available.

There is little doubt that hypophysectomy is effective in the palliation of metastatic breast cancer (and prostatic cancer), but not all patients achieve a beneficial response and none is cured. Perhaps 40 percent of patients with metastatic breast cancer are benefited; their objective remission is usually measured in months, not years.

The demonstration of estrogen receptor sites in the pathological evaluation of the cancerous breast tissue has aided in predicting which patients will benefit from hypophysectomy, but proper selection of patients is still critical in the recommendation of hypophysectomy for breast cancer.

Hypophysectomy has also been employed in the therapy of diabetic retinopathy; the serendipitous observation that retinopathy improved following postpartum necrosis of the pituitary led to this form of treatment. It has not been established which hormone is involved in the response, and selection of patients remains a problem; generally patients with hemorrhagic complications respond better than those with proliferative disease. It has been verified that the benefits of the procedure are enduring.

ADRENAL

(by Timothy S. Harrison)

Historical Background

ADRENAL CORTEX

Early confusion surrounding adrenal cortical hyperfunction has been largely resolved as the individual adrenal cortical hormones and their specific effects have been recognized. In this brief account early reports will be separated into the hormonal syndrome categories which they seem now in retrospect to have represented.

ADRENOGENITAL AND VIRILIZING. DeCrecchio in 1865 first reported congenital adrenal hyperplasia in a female pseudohermaphrodite. Phillips in 1887 reported four cases of female pseudohermaphroditism in one family, with adrenal hypertrophy and death, apparently from salt wasting. Marchand in 1891 suggested that the adrenal hyperplasia was the cause of pseudohermaphroditism, and Butler et al. in 1939 related the salt wasting to adrenal insufficiency. Fibiger in 1905 reported four siblings with the adrenogenital syndrome, including the first male, who apparently died of salt wasting. The first postnatal adrenogenital syndrome was reported by Cooke in 1811—in a four-year-old girl with marked virilization and some ele-

ments of Cushing's syndrome associated with an adrenal tumor. Linser in 1903 reported the first male, a five-year-old boy, with pseudoprecocious puberty and an adrenal tumor. Gallais in 1912 separated adrenal hyperplasia from virilizing tumors and tumors producing obesity and diabetes (Cushing's syndrome). Wilkins et al. in 1950 first demonstrated the therapeutic use of cortisone in congenital adrenal hyperplasia.

ESTROGEN-SECRETING TUMORS. Tilesius in 1803 described a four-year-old girl with pseudoprecocious puberty, breast development, hirsutism, and obesity with an adrenal carcinoma and metastases. This was probably an estrogen-secreting tumor with some cortisol secretion as well. Birtorf in 1919 reported the first case in an adult male, the most common circumstance with this tumor.

CUSHING'S SYNDROME. Guthrie and Emery in 1907 reported a boy of four with the clinical features of Cushing's syndrome and a large adrenal tumor, and a girl of three with an identical clinical picture and no endocrine abnormalities noted at autopsy. Apert in 1910 collected 31 cases from the literature with obesity, amenorrhea and hirsutism, often associated with adrenal cortical tumors, and Achard and Thiers in 1921 described a woman with Cushing's syndrome and adrenal hyperplasia.

Parkes-Weber in 1926 reported a case with the clinical findings of Cushing's syndrome and a basophil adenoma of the pituitary. Cushing gathered 12 cases from the literature with clinical features of the syndrome subsequently named after him. Eight of these cases had autopsies, but only two had basophil adenomas. Two others had chromophobe adenomas, but one of these had an adrenal adenoma as well. Moehlig and Bates in 1933 suggested that the pituitary changes were secondary. Oppenheimer et al. in 1935 and 1937 demonstrated that basophilic adenomas of the pituitary were associated with Cushing's syndrome only when adrenal hyperplasia was also present, and they felt that the adrenal changes were primary. Albright in 1942 suggested that Cushing's syndrome was due to an overproduction of "S hormone" while adrenal virilism was due to an overproduction of "N hormone." Crooke in 1935 thought that the hyaline changes of the basophils, present in all patients with Cushing's syndrome, were the cause of the syndrome, but Laqueur in 1950 showed that these changes were secondary to overproduction of corticosteroid.

Christy, Bornstein et al., Holub and Katz, and Meador et al. in 1961 first reported cases of Cushing's syndrome secondary to ectopic ACTH production by a nonadrenal carcinoma, and Marks et al. 1963 demonstrated the presence of corticotropic activity in the tumor and its absence in the pituitary.

ALDOSTERONISM. Greep and Deane in 1949 showed that hypophysectomy caused atrophy of the zona fasciculata and zona reticularis but not the zona glomerulosa (see under Anatomy, below) and postulated that the mineralocorticoids were made in the zona glomerulosa. Tait and Simpson identified aldosterone in 1952. The clinical syndrome of primary aldosteronism was first described in 1955 by Conn and by Foye and Feichtmeier and others.

ADRENAL MEDULLA

PHEOCHROMOCYTOMA. The first case of pheochromocytoma associated with hypertension was reported by Frankel in 1886. Manasse was the first, in 1896, to demonstrate the chromaffin reaction of the cells comprising the tumor. Kohn, in 1902, described the sites at which chromaffin tissue could be found in the body. Labbé, Tinel, and Doumer, in 1922, first described the typical paroxysmal attacks of hypertension and vasomotor phenomena in a twenty-eight-year-old woman found to have a pheochromocytoma at autopsy. The first pheochromocytoma to be removed at operation was in the case of Masson and Martin in 1923, but the patient died. The first clinical diagnosis was made in 1926 by Vaquez and Donzelot. The first successful removals of pheochromocytomas were by Roux in Lausanne in February, 1926, and by Charles Mayo in the United States in October of the same year, but in neither of these cases was a preoperative diagnosis made. Pincoffs, in 1929, made the first correct preoperative diagnosis of pheochromocytoma in a patient whose tumor

was successfully removed by Shipley on a second exploration.

The first patients in whom a pheochromocytoma was noted to be associated with sustained, as contrasted to paroxysmal, hypertension were those described by Binger and Craig and by Palmer and Castleman in 1938. Rabin, in 1929, demonstrated that a pheochromocytoma contained epinephrine in amounts greater than that seen in the normal adrenal medulla and suggested that this was the cause of the hypertension. Beer, King, and Prinzmetal, in 1937, first demonstrated a pressor agent, assumed to be epinephrine, in the blood of a patient with a pheochromocytoma during a hypertensive crisis. Holton, in 1949, reported the occurrence of norepinephrine in pheochromocytomas, and Engel and Von Euler, in 1950, demonstrated that large amounts of norepinephrine were secreted in the urine of two patients proved to have pheochromocytomas, in one of whom there was also an increased output of epinephrine.

Embryology

The adrenal cortex and medulla have separate embryologic origins. The medullary portion is derived from the chromaffin ectodermal cells of the neural crest. These cells are split off very early from the sympathetic ganglion cells, and migrate further ventrally, so as to lie ventrolateral to the aorta, where they form the paraganglia. Several such nodules near the cranial end of the gonads combine into a larger mass of cells lying between the dorsal aorta and the dorsomedial border of the mesinephros. Here they come into approximation with a group of mesodermal cells destined to become the adrenal cortex. These latter cells derive principally from a narrow strip of coelomic mesothelium lying between the dorsal mesentery and the genital ridge. These cells, arising in numerous places in the suprarenal ridge, lose their connection with the mesothelium and form a complete layer of mesoderm around the ectodermal cells derived from the sympathetic ganglia. The chromaffin cells thus become enclosed within the cortex to form the medulla.

In lower forms of vertebrates the adrenal cortex and medulla may remain completely separate. During the course of development medullary or cortical tissue may be left behind in various locations to form accessory collections of cells. The most common locations for this accessory tissue are shown in Fig. 37-14. Pheochromocytomas frequently develop in these accessory sites, particularly in the paraganglia around the aorta at the level of the kidney, anterior to the inferior aorta at the level of the organs of Zuckerkandl, in the mediastinum, in the bladder, and occasionally even in the neck or the sacrococcygeal, anal, or vaginal areas.

Adrenocortical rests are most commonly found close to the adrenal, within the kidney, in the ovarian pedicle, in the ovary itself, in the broad ligament, and in the testis. In the adrenogenital syndrome in the male there is often a well-developed adrenocortical rest in the testis that is sometimes mistaken for a normal-sized testis. Actually the

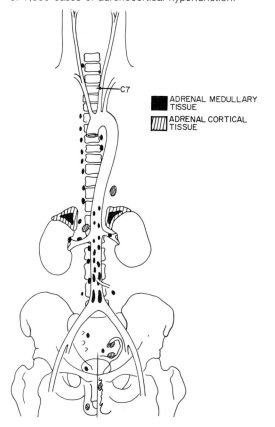

Fig. 37-14. Location of ectopic adrenal tissue. The location of ectopic adrenal medullary tissue is shown in black, while the cortical tissue is shown in the shaded areas. The incidence of extraadrenal medullary tissue is very high compared with the incidence of extraadrenal cortical tissue, and while functioning extraadrenal medullary tissue occurs in about 1 out of every 8 cases of medullary hyperfunction, it occurs in less than 1 out of 1,000 cases of adrenocortical hyperfunction.

■ ADRENAL MEDULLARY TISSUE

▨ ADRENAL CORTICAL TISSUE

testis is atrophic, and the adrenal cortical tissue is hyperplastic. Cushing's syndrome has resulted from the hyperplasia of an intrarenal rest and persisted after bilateral adrenalectomy. Adrenocortical rests are said to occur in 50 percent of newborn infants and to atrophy and disappear in a few weeks. Their persistence in the adrenogenital syndrome is due to continued ACTH stimulation.

It has been pointed out by Schechter that the anomalous locations of the adrenal cortex are clinically important for the following reasons: hyperplasia in the accessory adrenal tissue may produce continued adrenal activity after adrenalectomy for Cushing's syndrome or for metastatic cancer; adrenal insufficiency occasionally develops when misplaced normal adrenal glands are inadvertently ablated during nephrectomy; and neoplastic transformation of heterotopic or accessory adrenal tissue may take place.

Anatomy

The adrenal glands lie along the anteromedial border of the superior pole of the kidney reaching caudad at times almost as far as the renal vessels at the hilus of the kidney. The base of the gland is thicker and broader, while the apex of the gland is thin and narrow and along the diaphragm. The general anatomy of the gland is shown in Fig. 37-15.

The arterial blood supply of the glands is variable, although generally it comes from the three sources, the phrenic artery superiorly, the aorta medially, and the renal artery inferiorly. The extreme variability of the arterial supply of the glands has been recognized in recent years, since arteriography of the glands has been performed so frequently. Variation from the classic blood supply is said to be the rule rather than the exception. Some arteriograms of the blood supply of adrenal tumors are shown in Figs. 37-48 and 37-49.

The venous supply is more constant, there usually being one large vein on the left which drains into the left renal vein and a single vein on the right which drains into the inferior vena cava. There may occasionally be small accessory veins which drain into the inferior vena cava on the left and the renal vein on the right, but these are responsible for little of the circulation of the gland unless they increase in size and number, as with the development of an adrenal tumor. Coupland has emphasized the importance of the adrenal portal venous system. This delivers blood high in glucocorticoid content to the adrenal medulla, creating conditions favorable for the induction of the enzyme phenylethanolamine-*N*-methyl transferase (PNMT). PNMT is responsible for the methylation of norepinephrine to form epinephrine. This is why over 95 percent of epinephrine originates from the adrenal medulla.

Despite the vascularity of the adrenal the blood flow of the normal adrenal in man is only about 10 ml/minute. With large adrenal tumors, however, this blood flow is magnified many times. It has been assumed by some writers that constriction of the adrenal medullary blood supply takes place in trauma to provide a better blood

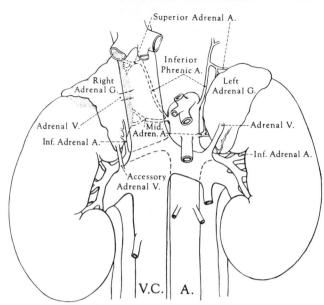

Fig. 37-15. Location and blood supply of the adrenal glands. There is great variation in the arterial blood supply of the glands, but this generally comes from three sources: a branch from the renal artery, a branch from the aorta, and a branch from the inferior phrenic artery. There is usually only one main vein on each side, the left adrenal vein opening into the left renal vein while the one on the right opens into the inferior vena cava. On occasion there may be very small accessory adrenal veins such as that illustrated for the right adrenal.

supply to the cortex. It was found by Kramer and Sapirstein in rats, however that the blood supply to both medulla and cortex increased under stress. ACTH produces an immediate marked increase in blood flow to the adrenal in dogs and man.

Microscopically the adrenal cortex is divided into three zones: the zona glomerulosa, or outer zone, the zona fasciculata—a wide intermediate zone—and the zona reticularis, a narrow inner zone closely applied to the medulla. The zona glomerulosa is responsible for the production of aldosterone, while the zona fasciculata and zona reticularis manufacture cortisol and other glucocorticoids. There is still some debate as to whether the androgens and estrogens are manufactured by cells distributed throughout the zona fasciculata and zona reticularis or whether their manufacture is primarily related to cells concentrated in or near the reticularis.

Adrenal Cortex

PHYSIOLOGY

The general structure of the steroids secreted by the adrenal cortex is shown in Fig. 37-16. The corticosteroids, or corticoids, include both the glucocorticoids and mineralocorticoids and are C-21 compounds, the androgens are C-19 steroids, and the estrogens are C-18 steroids.

The entire adrenal cortex normally contains 11- and 21-hydroxylating enzymes for the production of cortisol

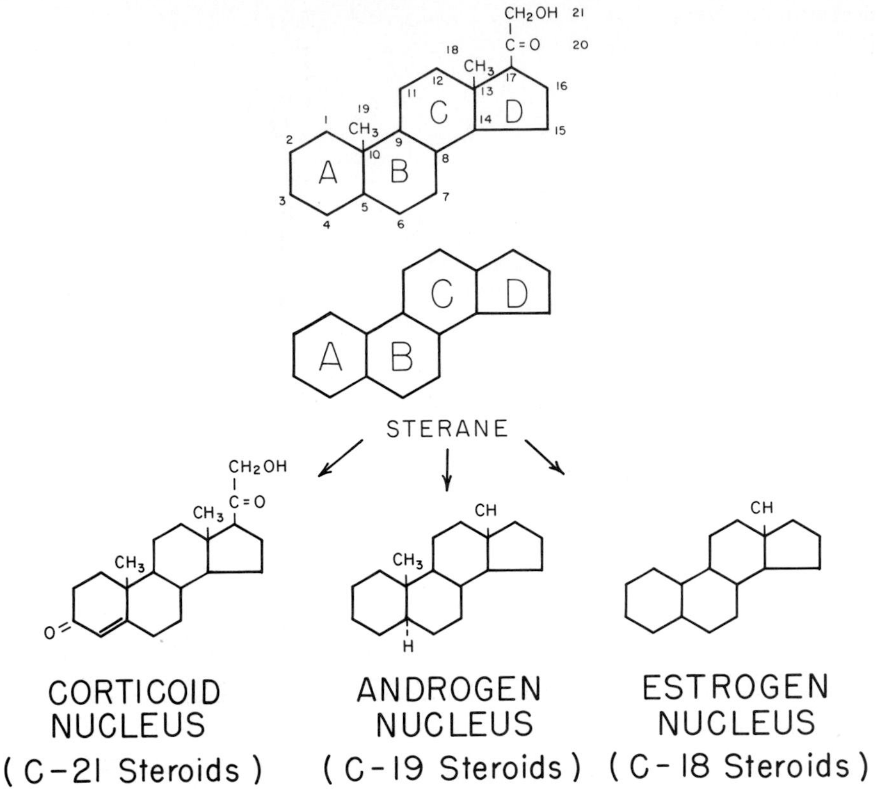

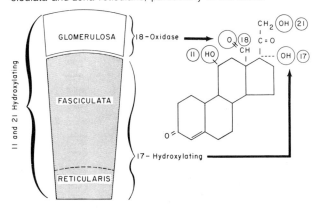

STERANE

CORTICOID
NUCLEUS
(C-21 Steroids)

ANDROGEN
NUCLEUS
(C-19 Steroids)

ESTROGEN
NUCLEUS
(C-18 Steroids)

and similar glucocorticoids, while only the zona glomerulosa contains 18-oxidase, an enzyme capable of oxidating the 18 carbon atom to produce aldosterone, the principal mineralocorticoid, as shown in Fig. 37-17. The principal active compounds of each class secreted by the adrenal are shown in Fig. 37-18. The relative secretion rates of the adrenal compounds are shown in Table 37-1. The two most important adrenal corticosteroids by far are cortisol, the major glucocorticoid, and aldosterone, the major mineralocorticoid.

Fig. 37-17. Enzymes of the adrenal cortex. The entire adrenal cortex contains 11- and 21-hydroxylating enzymes, while the zona fasciculata and zona reticularis contain 17-hydroxylating enzymes in addition. The zona glomerulosa lacks 17-hydroxylating but contains 18-oxidase, which is necessary for the formation of aldosterone. The androgens are also formed in the zona fasciculata and zona reticularis, particularly in the latter.

Fig. 37-16. Basic adrenal steroid structure. The numbering system for the carbon atoms in the steroid nucleus is shown at the top. The basic steroid nucleus (Sterane) is modified to form the C-21, C-19, and C-18 steroids, as shown in the lower line.

CORTISOL. Secretion. Normally the hypothalamus secretes CRF, which promotes the release of ACTH from the anterior pituitary. ACTH in turn stimulates the adrenal cortex to produce and release cortisol. Rising blood levels of cortisol then serve to inhibit the further release of CRF from the hypothalamus and thus effect a feedback regulatory mechanism (Fig. 37-19). After trauma this feedback

Fig. 37-18. Principal active compounds of the adrenal cortex. The structural formulas are shown for the principal glucocorticoids, mineralocorticoid, androgens, and estrogen.

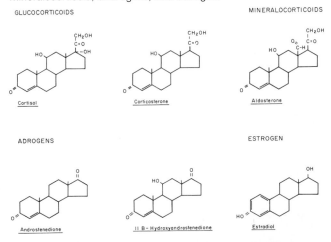

GLUCOCORTICOIDS   MINERALOCORTICOIDS

Cortisol   Corticosterone   Aldosterone

ADROGENS   ESTROGEN

Androstenedione   II B - Hydroxyandrostenedione   Estradiol

Table 37-1. SECRETION RATES OF ADRENAL
STEROIDS IN MAN

Compound	24-hour secretion
Cortisol	30 mg
Corticosterone	5 mg
Aldosterone	150 mg
Androstenedione	5 mg
11-β-Hydroxyandrostenedione	5 mg
Estradiol	Trace

SOURCE: From Forsham and Melmon, 1968.

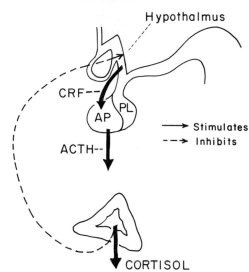

Fig. 37-19. Feedback regulation of cortisol secretion. CRF manufactured in the hypothalamus stimulates the anterior pituitary to release ACTH. ACTH stimulates the adrenal cortex to release cortisol and androgens. Cortisol, but not the androgens, act on the hypothalamus to inhibit release of CRF and thus of ACTH. In trauma the feedback mechanism is temporarily overcome as the hypothalamic centers secrete an increased amount of CRF leading to pituitary-adrenal stimulation and increased blood levels of cortisol.

mechanism is overcome by other central nervous system mechanisms, when CRF and ACTH are secreted in spite of rising levels of cortisol to bring about an acute increase in the blood level of cortisol. Normally there is a diurnal variation in the release of CRF, ACTH, and therefore cortisol. This diurnal variation, or circadian rhythm, is shown in Fig. 37-20. It occurs even in blind people or people who work at night and is independent of sleep. It shifts with changes in latitude but is not changed by travel from north to south. An important feature of Cushing's syndrome seems to be a failure of this diurnal variation, so that ACTH is secreted constantly around the clock, presumably in response to a continued CRF stimulus.

The normal feedback mechanism can be disturbed by metyrapone (Metopirone). This compound interferes with 11-β-hydroxylation in the adrenal cortex. The synthesis of cortisol therefore ceases, and there is thus no opposition to continued pituitary secretion of ACTH, as shown in Fig. 37-21. This is used as a test of pituitary activity, to determine whether the pituitary is capable of secreting increased amounts of ACTH. The 11-desoxycortisol which is produced instead of cortisol under these circumstances is incapable of inhibiting the release of CRF and ACTH. Since there is an oversecretion of ACTH, other adrenal substances such as the androgens are also produced in large quantities, since they are incapable of inhibiting the release of ACTH. This produces a situation similar to that seen in the adrenogenital syndrome.

Binding and Transport. Once secreted, the cortisol exists in three states in the blood—free, bound, and conjugated. In the free state cortisol is a metabolically active compound available to the tissues. For transport and protection from degradation it is bound to a substance known as corticosteroid-binding globulin (CBG), or transcortin, which is an α-globulin. This makes it somewhat more soluble and protects it from conjugation. When large amounts of cortisol are secreted, the binding sites become saturated, and the levels of free cortisol rise in the plasma. Under these circumstances some free cortisol will be excreted in the urine, although ordinarily only very tiny amounts of unconjugated cortisol appear in the urine.

Metabolism. Cortisol is metabolized in the liver by conversion to tetrahydrocortisol and conjugation with glucuronide and sulfate. Once the cortisol is conjugated, it becomes water-soluble and is easily excreted in the urine (Fig. 37-22*A* and *B*).

Fig. 37-20. Diurnal variation in cortisol plasma levels in response to a circadian hypothalamic rhythm. There is a daily variation in CRF and ACTH secretion which is reflected in the plasma cortisol levels. Thus blood cortisol (or ACTH) has its lowest rate of secretion around midnight with its highest secretion coming around 6 A.M. In Cushing's syndrome this rhythm is lost, and while the plasma cortisol level may not be greatly elevated beyond that seen in the normal patient in the early morning, it continues at the same level throughout the day and fails to show the decline in plasma cortisol levels seen normally during the late afternoon and evening. A good way to diagnose Cushing's disease is to compare the 12 midnight and 8 A.M. plasma cortisol levels. In Cushing's disease these are very nearly the same, while in normal patients the 8 A.M. level is two or three times as high as the midnight level.

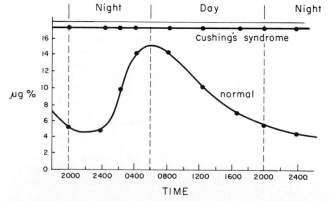

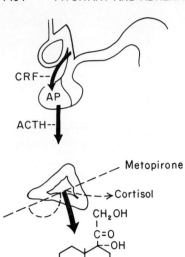

METABOLISM OF CORTISOL

CORTISOL

DIHYDROCORTISOL

TETRAHYDROCORTISOL

TETRAHYDROCORTISOL 3α GLUCURONIDE

A

Fig. 37-21. Effect of metyrapone (Metopirone, SU-4885) on ACTH secretion. Metyrapone interferes with 11-hydroxylation in the adrenal cortex, and 11-desoxycortisol is formed instead of cortisol. Since cortisol is not present in the plasma to inhibit the release of CRF from the hypothalamus, there is a markedly increased CRF and ACTH secretion which stimulates the adrenal cortex to secrete more and more 11-desoxycortisol. This substance is measured in the urine by methods designed to measure 17-hydroxycorticosteroids. An increase in these substances following the administration of metyrapone indicates a function of both the anterior pituitary and adrenal cortex. If there is a response to ACTH but not to metyrapone, this indicates a decreased pituitary reserve.

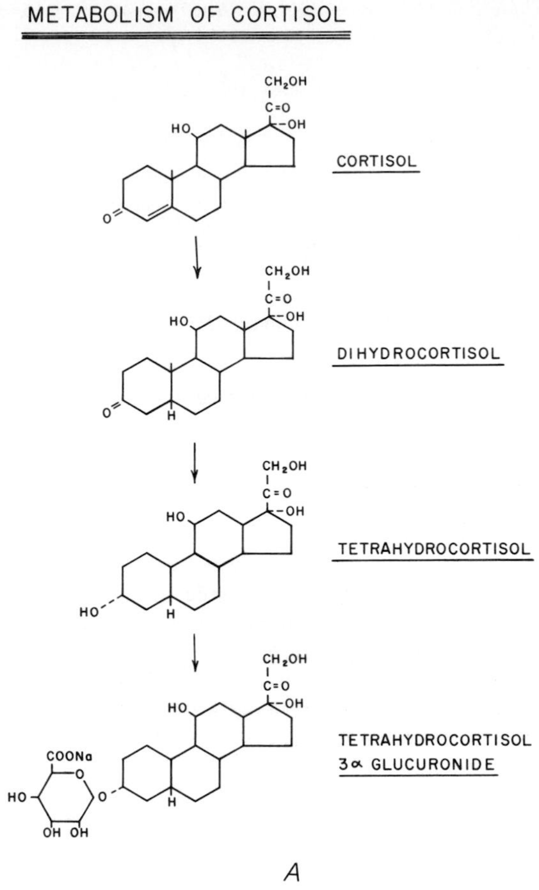

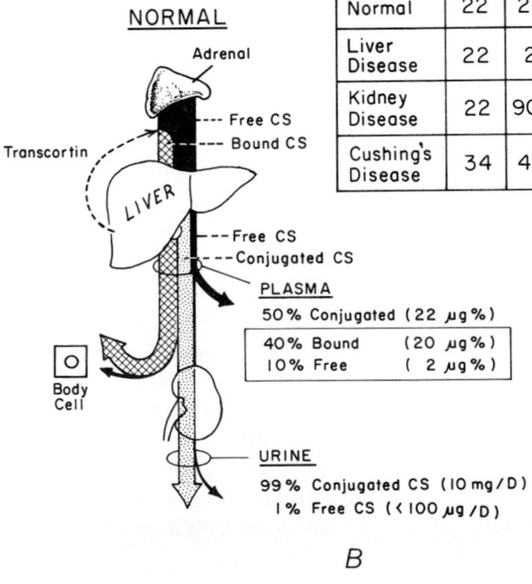

Fig. 37-22. Metabolism and excretion of cortisol. *A*. The degradation of cortisol takes place in the liver. In the first step dihydrocortisol is formed by a saturation of the double bond between carbons 4 and 5, adding a hydrogen to each of these carbon atoms. Further reduction takes place to the tetrahydrocortisol configuration by the substitution of a hydroxyl group for the ketone group on the 3 carbon atom. The tetrahydrocortisol is then conjugated with glucuronide through the hydroxyl group on the 3 carbon atom. Some conjugation with sulfates also takes place. The conjugated tetrahydrocortisol is then excreted in the urine. *B*. The free cortisol secreted by the adrenal cortex becomes largely bound to transcortin, an α-globulin manufactured in the liver. This carrier protein prevents the rapid breakdown of cortisol but makes it available to the tissues as needed. As the cortisol passes through the liver, it becomes reduced and conjugated and thus inactivated. The conjugated corticosteroids are water-soluble and are excreted in the urine. A small amount of free cortisol is also excreted in the urine. At any given time the peripheral blood contains free, bound, and conjugated cortisol. If there is a marked increase in cortisol secretion, the transcortin-binding sites become saturated, and the amount of free cortisol increases greatly. In renal failure the conjugated corticosteroids are not excreted normally, and they pile up in the bloodstream. In hepatic failure there is very little conjugation of the corticosteroids, and a proportionately greater amount of free cortisol is present in the plasma.

EXAMPLES

	PLASMA μg %		URINE mgm/D	
	Free + Bound	Conj.	Free + Bound	Conj.
Normal	22	22	10	0.1
Liver Disease	22	2	3	0.1
Kidney Disease	22	900	2	0
Cushing's Disease	34	45	20	0.3

NORMAL

Adrenal

Transcortin

LIVER

--- Free CS
--- Bound CS

--- Free CS
--- Conjugated CS

Body Cell

PLASMA
50% Conjugated (22 μg%)
40% Bound   (20 μg%)
10% Free   (2 μg%)

URINE
99% Conjugated CS (10 mg/D)
1% Free CS (<100 μg/D)

B

ANDROGENS. The androgens are conjugated and excreted in the same fashion as cortisol. While the androgens, like cortisol, are dependent upon ACTH secretion for their release, they are not capable of inhibiting ACTH secretion in a feedback fashion.

ALDOSTERONE. Secretion. Roughly 30 percent of aldosterone secretion is influenced by ACTH. The remainder depends primarily on the secretion of renin and angiotensin II for regulation. In response to a fall in blood volume there is a fall in pressure in the afferent renal arteriole. This produces a release of renin by the juxtaglomerular cells. The renin combines with angiotensinogen manufactured in the liver to form angiotensin I, which is converted by a converting enzyme in the pulmonary circulation into angiotensin II. Angiotensin II stimulates the zona glomerulosa of the adrenal cortex to release aldosterone. The feedback mechanism for the regulation of aldosterone production under normal circumstances depends upon the aldosterone-induced renal retention of sodium, which raises the blood volume and turns off the production of renin. This regulatory mechanism can be overcome by any situation in the kidney, e.g., renal artery stenosis, which produces a permanent fall in afferent arteriolar pressure. This gives rise to hypertrophy of the juxtaglomerular cells and a markedly increased secretion of renin, thus producing the increased aldosterone secretion which is seen in secondary aldosteronism. The normal mechanism for the regulation of aldosterone secretion is shown in Fig. 37-23.

The mechanism for aldosterone release is probably more complicated than this, but it seems certain that in man it proceeds without the stimulus of ACTH. Some experimental animals seem to require a pituitary factor other than ACTH for aldosterone release to be normally responsive to a fall in the plasma sodium level. In the rat this may be GH, whereas in the dog it may be some other, unnamed substance. Other workers have found that GH does not restore the response of aldosterone to hyponatremia in hypophysectomized rats and postulate an unnamed hormone in this species as well.

Because a low sodium intake stimulates an increased aldosterone production in the normal individual, it is essential that aldosterone excretion measurements to determine whether or not primary aldosteronism is present be made while the patients are on diets which are normal in sodium. Low-sodium diets appear to produce renal vascular constriction even when significant changes in serum levels are not seen, and this is postulated as one of the mechanisms whereby a low-sodium diet brings about renin release.

It is established that the sympathetic nervous system plays a role in aldosterone secretion. Plasma renin activity and aldosterone secretion in normal patients have been shown to increase in response to an infusion of catecholamines or electrical stimulation of the sympathetic nervous system. The stimulation of upright posture and of sodium depletion, which normally results in an increase of renin and aldosterone secretion, fails to do so when autonomic insufficiency is present. In such patients the injection of catecholamines produces an increase in the secretion of

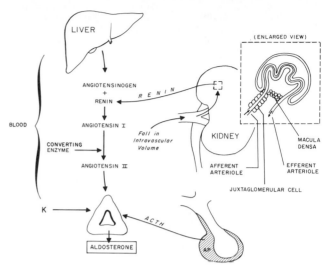

Fig. 37-23. Regulation of aldosterone secretion. A fall in blood volume, a fall in blood pressure, or vasoconstriction of the renal arteries due to norepinephrine produces a decrease in pressure in the afferent arteriole leading to a release of renin from the juxtaglomerular cells. The renin converts angiotensinogen manufactured in the liver to angiotensin I. This substance is further converted in the bloodstream by an enzyme in angiotensin II which stimulates the zona glomerulosa of the adrenal cortex to release aldosterone. Aldosterone, in turn, leads to sodium retention and a rise in blood pressure, which acts as a feedback mechanism to shut off the further release of renin. Secondary aldosteronism results when there is an obligatory secretion of renin as with an anatomic stricture of the renal arteries.

these two substances, presumably by producing renal afferent arteriolar constriction, thus leading to an increase in renin output. Renal transplantation with complete denervation of the kidney does not prevent the response to sodium depletion or the upright position, so that circulating, rather than locally formed, catecholamines may be responsible for this change. A review of this subject has been published by Gross. Marusic and Mulrow have studied isolated mitochondria from rat adrenal glands and have found that the mitochondria from rats on a low-sodium diet have a greater capacity for converting corticosterone to aldosterone than do mitochondria from rats fed a normal diet.

Metabolism. Aldosterone is metabolized in the same fashion as cortisol. Since it is such an active compound, it is excreted in the urine in minute quantities, and its chemical determination was, therefore, difficult until a radioimmunoassay for aldosterone became available.

SYNTHETIC ADRENOCORTICAL COMPOUNDS. Synthetic adrenocortical compounds are commonly used in clinical practice. Some common ones are shown in Fig. 37-24. Their relative potencies with respect to cortisol and aldosterone are shown in Table 37-2.

CUSHING'S SYNDROME

Cushing's syndrome refers to the changes seen with excess cortisol secretion. It may be produced as a consequence of excessive ACTH production either by the normal pituitary, presumably in response to a hypothalamic

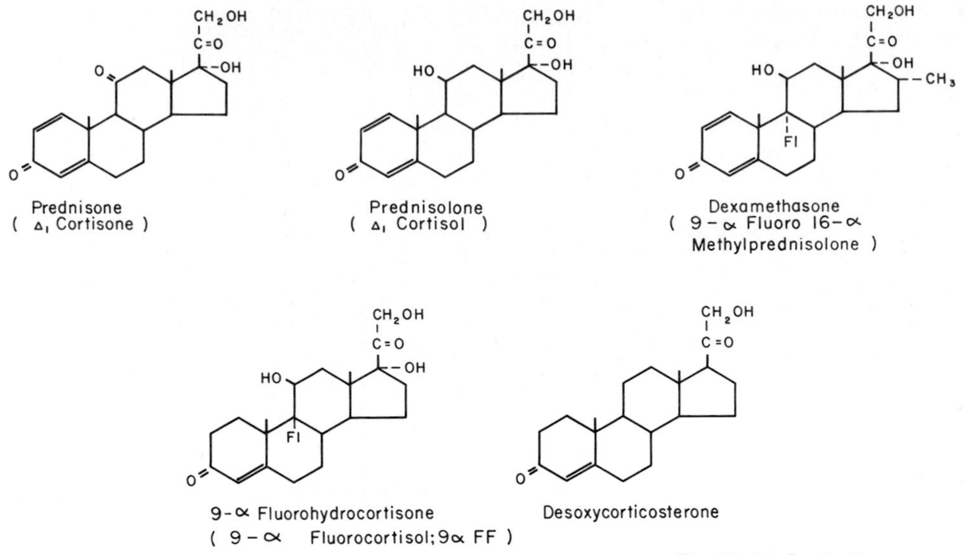

Prednisone
(Δ₁ Cortisone)

Prednisolone
(Δ₁ Cortisol)

Dexamethasone
(9 - α Fluoro 16-α
Methylprednisolone)

9- α Fluorohydrocortisone
(9 - α   Fluorocortisol; 9α FF)

Desoxycorticosterone

Fig. 37-24. Synthetic compounds. Structural formulas are shown for the synthetic glucocorticoids prednisone, prednisolone, and dexamethasone, and the mineralocorticoids, 9-α-fluorocortisol and deoxycorticosterone acetate (DCA).

stimulus, by a pituitary tumor, or by an ectopic ACTH-producing malignant tumor. Cushing's syndrome may result from increased cortisol production from an adrenal cortical carcinoma, an adrenal adenoma, or nodular hyperplasia of the adrenal cortex. Adrenal hyperplasia is the most common, followed by adrenal adenoma, adrenal carcinoma, an ectopic ACTH source, pituitary tumors secreting ACTH, and nodular dysplasia, in that order.

PATHOLOGY. The pathologic features of Cushing's syndrome vary, depending upon the cause, as shown in Fig. 37-25.

Hyperplasia, Adenoma, Carcinoma, Pituitary Tumor. Cushing in 1932 ascribed the syndrome to a basophilic adenoma

of the anterior pituitary. This is actually a very rare cause of this disease. Adrenal cortical hyperplasia, shown in Fig. 37-26 is the most common cause of Cushing's syndrome, and it is customary to refer to patients with adrenocortical hyperplasia as having Cushing's disease. Cushing's disease is due to increased production of ACTH, usually associated with loss of the normal diurnal variation of ACTH release.

Fig. 37-25. Causes of Cushing's syndrome. Hyperplasia of the adrenal cortex is brought about by an increased secretion of ACTH which may result either from a continual stimulation of the pituitary by CRF (1), an ACTH-secreting tumor of the anterior pituitary (2), or an ectopic malignant tumor secreting ACTH (3). The increased cortisol production can also come about as a consequence of an adrenal carcinoma (4), an adrenal adenoma (5), or nodular dysplasia (6).

Table 37-2. RELATIVE ANTI-INFLAMMATORY POTENCIES OF SOME THERAPEUTIC CORTICOIDS

Compound	*Relative potency compared to cortisol*	*Relative sodium-retaining activity*
Cortisol	1	+ +
Cortisone acetate	0.8	+ +
Prednisolone (1-2-dehydrocortisol) . .	4	+
Prednisone (1-2-dehydrocortisone) . .	3.5	+
Triamcinolone (9-α-fluoro-16-α-hydroxyprednisolone).	5	0
6-Methylprednisolone (9-α-fluoro-6-α-methylprednisolone)	5	0
Haldranolone (6-α-fluoro-16-α-methylprednisolone)	10	0
Betamethasone (9-α-fluoro-16-β-methylprednisolone)	25	0
Dexamethasone (9-α-fluoro-16-α-methylprednisolone)	30	0
9-α-Fluorohydrocortisone*	15	+ + + + +

*Used chiefly topically or as a sodium retainer.
SOURCE: From Forsham and Melmon, 1968.

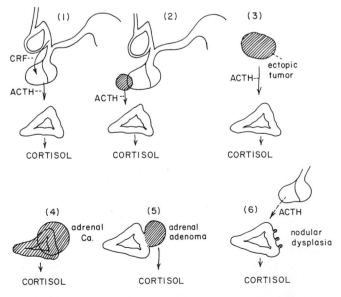

This in turn is presumed to be brought about by an increased hypothalamic stimulation of the pituitary. Cortical pathways subserving a wide variety of emotional and psychic stimuli can then influence the hypothalamic regulation of CRF and of pituitary ACTH release. Hyperplasia can also be caused by any excessive ACTH secretion either from a tumor of the pituitary or an ectopic tumor. Under any of these circumstances both adrenal glands are hyperplastic, and the usual sharp edge of the gland is rounded by the thickened cortices. Microscopically the widening of the cortex occurs primarily in the zona fasciculata. It may sometimes be difficult to distinguish hyperplasia, either grossly or microscopically, from the normal gland, but it is always easy to distinguish hyperplasia from an atrophic gland.

An adrenal adenoma causing Cushing's syndrome is shown in Fig. 37-27 and an iodocholesterol scan is presented in Fig. 37-28. The cortex of the remainder of the adrenal is extremely thin and atrophic, as was the cortex on the opposite side. This atrophy is due to inhibition of ACTH secretion by the large amounts of cortisol secreted by the autonomous tumor.

Adrenocortical carcinomas occur in about 10 percent of patients with Cushing's syndrome. They usually give rise to florid signs of the disease and sometimes occur in young children. Widespread metastases may occur, and the metastases are frequently hyperfunctioning.

It is sometimes difficult to make the diagnosis of malignancy in an adrenal cortical tumor, because the presence of bizarre cells and blood vessel invasion are not necessarily indicators of true malignancy. However, the histologic criteria which tend to suggest malignancy include pleomorphism, giant and bizarre nuclei, frequent and sometimes atypical mitoses, hemorrhage, necrosis, and calcification. The absolute criteria of malignancy are said by Heinbecker et al. to be invasion of veins, invasion into and through the capsule, and distant metastases.

Nodular Dysplasia. The syndrome of nodular dysplasia of the adrenal has been reported in recent years by Kirschner et al. and Meador et al., who named it. This strange type of hyperplasia, of which fewer than 10 cases

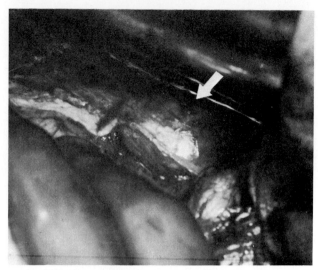

Fig. 37-27. Adrenocortical adenoma causing Cushing's disease. The oval-shaped adenoma can be easily seen beneath the retractor. Note the extreme thinning of the rest of the adrenal cortex. This severe adrenocortical atrophy is due to inhibition of ACTH release by the cortisol manufactured by the adenoma.

have been reported, behaves like an autonomous adenoma rather than hyperplasia, since the secretion is not suppressible with large doses of dexamethasone and does not respond to ACTH. Endogenous ACTH secretion is suppressed. The characteristic appearance on cut section is of numerous nodules 2 mm or less in diameter. Microscopically the nodules contain large oval or polyhedral

Fig. 37-28. An adrenal photoscan from a patient with Cushing's syndrome due to a hyperfunctioning adenoma of the right adrenal cortex. Viewed from the posterior aspect, the uptake seen is in a solitary lesion of the right adrenal gland. The remainder of the right adrenal and the entire left adrenal are suppressed by the exaggerated release of glucocorticoids and therefore do not take up the iodocholesterol.

Fig. 37-26. Adrenal cortical hyperplasia causing Cushing's disease. The cut section of the gland shows marked thickening of adrenal cortex.

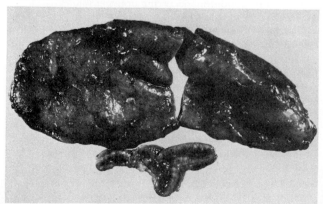

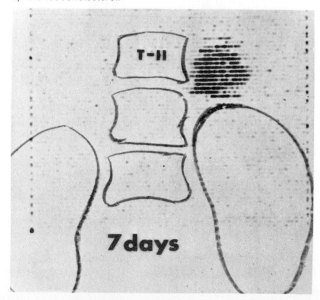

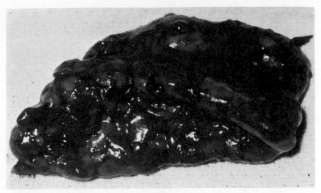

Fig. 37-29. Cushing's disease caused by nodular dysplasia: gross appearance of the gland.

cells with small, dark, round nuclei and slightly granular, heavily eosinophilic cytoplasm. In the case of Meador et al. the cells contained pigment and appeared black to the naked eye. The adrenal cortical cells adjacent to the nodules appear normal, not atrophic.

A gland involved in nodular hyperplasia is shown in Fig. 37-29. This case was complicated by the fact that bilateral adrenal hemorrhages developed following adrenal venograms. The patient made an uneventful recovery from surgical treatment.

Ectopic-ACTH Syndrome. It occasionally may be difficult

Fig. 37-30. Cushing's disease. *A.* Note the round face and the increase in preauricular fat pads. Despite the marked obesity and protuberance of the abdomen the extremities are disproportionately thin. There are a few striae over the lower abdomen. *B.* A side view of the same patient, again showing the marked protuberance of the abdomen and central fat, with thin extremities.

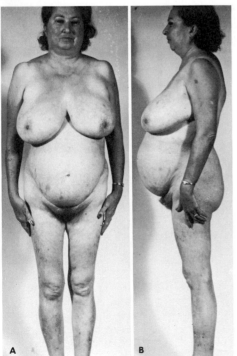

to make a definitive diagnosis of an ectopic ACTH-secreting tumor preoperatively. Clinically such patients often have chemically severe Cushing's syndrome without the typical distribution of fat, or even with weight loss. Chemically the diagnosis rests upon the demonstration of increased cortisol excretion, which is not suppressible with dexamethasone, coupled with elevated levels of ACTH in the plasma. Patients with the pituitary type of adrenal hyperplasia have ACTH in the plasma but generally show suppression of cortisol production with large doses of dexamethasone, while those patients with adrenocortical adenoma or carcinoma fail to show suppression of cortisol production by dexamethasone but have no measurable ACTH in the plasma. Since MSH is usually secreted in conjunction with ACTH, patients with ectopic ACTH syndrome may show hyperpigmentation, but this is usually not prominent until after adrenalectomy.

The primary source of these carcinomas is usually an oat cell carcinoma of the lung, but the syndrome has also been seen with tumors of the parotid, liver, pancreas, thymus, thyroid, esophagus, and the adrenal medulla.

General Considerations. Systemically, patients with Cushing's disease show marked muscle wasting and severe osteoporosis. There is disappearance of elastic fibers in the skin leading to thinning and fragility of the skin and production of striae. Marked atherosclerosis of the vessels occurs, and there may be nephrosclerosis of the kidneys and sometimes nephrocalcinosis. The ovaries and testes may show some atrophy, and the pancreas may show fatty necrosis and islet cell hyperplasia.

In the untreated case the cause of death is usually related to the sequelae of hypertension, but another common cause of death is infection, frequently with fungal organisms.

CLINICAL MANIFESTATIONS. Incidence. The peak incidence of Cushing's disease is found in the third and fourth decades. The syndrome has been known to occur in children less than a year of age and also to have its onset in patients as old as seventy. Some observers have been impressed that an experience with great emotional impact often precedes by several weeks the onset of Cushing's disease. Cushing's syndrome is considerably more common in women than in men, in a ratio of 4:1. Adenomas are also far more common in women than men, occurring particularly following pregnancy. Cushing's disease is a relatively rare condition, occurring in fewer than 1 of 1,000 autopsies.

Signs and Symptoms. The signs and symptoms of Cushing's syndrome are listed in Table 37-3. Most of these are due to an excess secretion of cortisol, and almost all of them, including hirsutism, hypokalemia, hypertension, and the typical moon face appearance, can be produced in normal patients by the exogenous administration of cortisol. At times, however, a tumor of the adrenal cortex may produce an increased secretion both of cortisol and of androgen, thus giving a mixed picture of Cushing's disease and the adrenogenital syndrome. This is discussed later on. The moon face, acne, hirsutism, striae, buffalo hump, ecchymoses, truncal obesity, and thin extremities are illustrated in Fig. 37-30*A* and *B*.

Table 37-3. SYMPTOMS AND SIGNS OF
CUSHING'S SYNDROME

Moon facies	Acne
Truncal obesity	Fungal infections
Hypertension	Back pain
Plethora	Headache
Amenorrhea or impotence	Emotional lability
Weakness and fatigue	Pathologic fractures
Hirsutism	Polyuria
Striae	Renal calculi
Easy bruising and ecchymoses	Hypokalemic alkalosis
Osteoporosis	Atherosclerosis
Edema	Possibly tumor shown on IVP
Diabetes, latent or overt	With malignant tumors, possibly metastases detected by x-ray
Supraclavicular fat pads	
Buffalo hump	
Muscle wasting	

As the disease progresses, the patients undergo marked muscle wasting and osteoporosis, with collapse of vertebrae, backache, buffalo hump, easy fatigability, and weakness. Spontaneous rib fractures may also occur. Arteriosclerosis develops, and the patients have a diabetic glucose tolerance curve, or occasionally frank diabetes. There is marked emotional lability or even frank psychosis.

Cushing's disease is potentially fatal, death usually occurring within 5 years of the first evidences of the disease.

DIAGNOSTIC FINDINGS. The diagnostic tests for Cushing's syndrome which have proved to be of most value are listed in Table 37-4.

Diurnal Variation of Blood Cortisol Levels. There is normally a diurnal variation in the blood ACTH and cortisol level, such that the cortisol level is at its highest around 6 A.M. and then gradually falls off during the day, hitting its lowest point around midnight (see Fig. 37-20). In some cases of Cushing's syndrome the blood cortisol level may not be elevated above normal, but the diurnal variation is gone, and the secretion of cortisol and ACTH remain constant throughout the day. Absence of the diurnal variation can easily be detected by taking blood samples for cortisol at midnight and at 8 A.M. The one taken at 8 A.M. should be two to three times as high as the one obtained at midnight. If they are the same, this is strong evidence for Cushing's syndrome. The normal values are listed in Table 37-5.

Diurnal Variation of Urinary Corticosteroid Levels. Vagnucci et al., Martin and Hamman, and Jefferies et al. have demonstrated a circadian cycle and characteristic patterns of urinary cortisol excretion which are helpful in

Table 37-4. TESTS FOR CUSHING'S SYNDROME

Diurnal variation of blood cortisol
Diurnal variation of urine cortisol
Blood cortisol response to ACTH with conjugates
Dexamethasone suppression
Rapid dexamethasone suppression
Metyrapone (Metopirone)
Blood ACTH measurement
Urinary, free cortisol, cortisol secretory tests, etc.
X-ray of sella turcica
Adrenal angiography
Iodocholesterol scan of the adrenal

Table 37-5. NORMAL STEROID VALUES

Steroid	Values
Plasma	
Cortisol:	
8 A.M.	6–28 µg/100 ml
Midnight	2–12 µg/100 ml
Urinary estrogens	
Ages 0–10 years	0–1 µg/day
Premenopausal females . . .	5–20 µg/day
Men	0.1–2 µg/day
Urinary pregnanetriol	
Ages 0–6 years	0.02–0.2 mg/day
Ages 7–15 years	0.6–1.2 mg/day
Over 16 years	0.5–2.5 mg/day

Urine	Male	Female
Urinary 17-OH corticoids	4–11 mg/day	3–11 mg/day
Urinary 17-ketosteroids	10–20 mg/day	5–15 mg/day

SOURCE: Modified from Forsham and Melmon, 1968.

the diagnosis of Cushing's disease. This is said to be useful in differentiating between hyperplasia, tumor, and normal adrenal cortical function.

Blood Cortisol Response to ACTH. Patients with adrenocortical hyperplasia have a greater responsiveness to ACTH than do normal patients. Thus the administration of ACTH intravenously over a 4- to 6-hour period produces a greater rise in plasma cortisol levels than one would expect in the normal patient. We have found it useful to measure the conjugated corticosteroids as well as the free, since the differential between adrenal cortical hyperplasia and the normal is even greater when the conjugated corticosteroids are measured. Patients with functioning adrenocortical adenomas as the cause of the Cushing's syndrome fail to show a rise in cortisol with ACTH administration, because the secretion is autonomous and not dependent upon ACTH production. This test is not always capable of differentiating between hyperplasia and tumor, since the adrenals of some patients with tumors will respond to ACTH stimulation, but it is usually possible to differentiate between the normal patient and one with Cushing's syndrome.

Dexamethasone Suppression Test. Dexamethasone is a synthetic corticosteroid of great potency. Small quantities of this drug are capable of blocking ACTH release in the normal patient, as demonstrated by a fall in urinary cortisol excretion (Fig. 37-31). The test, which was originally devised by Liddle et al., is usually done as follows: The patient is put on continuous 24-hour urinary collections for corticosteroids during the 6 days of the test. The first 2 days are control periods, the second two days the patient received 0.5 mg of dexamethasone by mouth every 6 hours for a total of 2 mg/day, and on the final 2 days the patient receives 2 mg of dexamethasone by mouth every 6 hours for a total of 8 mg/day. The normal patient will show a suppression of 17-hydroxycorticosteroid excretion of 50 percent or more on the 2 mg/day dose of dexamethasone. Patients with Cushing's syndrome do not. Patients with

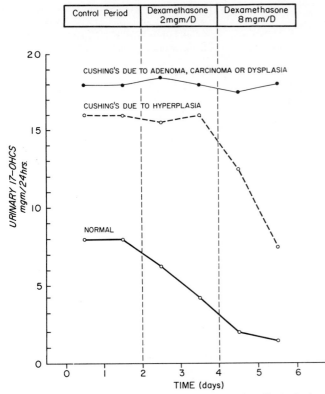

Fig. 37-31. Dexamethasone suppression test: the effect of a low and high dose of dexamethasone on urinary 17-hydroxycorticosteroid excretion. The normal patient shows suppression on both the low and the high dose, whereas in Cushing's disease due to hyperplasia there is no suppression with the low dose but there is suppression with the high dose. In Cushing's disease due to adenoma, cancer, or dysplasia, there is no suppression with either the low or the high dose.

Fig. 37-32. Metyrapone test. With adrenal cortical hyperplasia there is an increased urinary 17-hydroxycorticosteroid excretion in response to metyrapone, while there characteristically is no such response with adrenal cortical adenoma, dysplasia, or carcinoma.

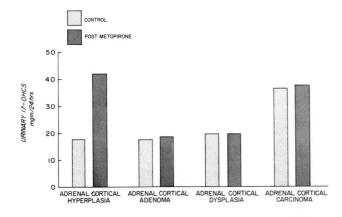

Cushing's disease due to bilateral adrenal hyperplasia show a suppression on 8 mg/day of dexamethasone, whereas those with an adrenal cortical adenoma or carcinoma do not. Unfortunately this test is not completely reliable, since it fails to show suppression in some cases of hyperplasia and does show suppression in some cases of cortical adenoma. It also fails to show suppression in patients with nodular adrenal dysplasia.

Rapid Dexamethasone Suppression Test. This test is better than the regular dexamethasone suppression test mentioned above and, along with the test for diurnal variation, is probably the best overall test for adrenocortical function. The test can be carried out either with plasma cortisol measurements or with urine corticosteroid and creatinine measurements. In the simplest form of the test the patient received 1 mg of dexamethasone by mouth at 11 P.M., and after adequate sedation with barbiturate a plasma cortisol sample is drawn the next morning at 8 o'clock. If the level of 17-hydroxycorticosteroids in the plasma is above $10\ \mu g/100$ ml, this suggests nonsuppressibility of ACTH secretion and is diagnostic of Cushing's syndrome. In the normal patient the level falls nearly to zero. In order to perform the test, the patient must not be taking birth control pills containing estrogen, since this raises the transcortin level and produces high levels of plasma hydroxycorticosteroids. It would be satisfactory to take two morning samples, one the day before and one the day after dexamethasone administration, since the normal patient even on birth control pills would be expected to show a very marked suppression of the cortisol level on the second day. The ratio of urinary corticosteroid to creatinine can be used in lieu of a plasma cortisol level to indicate suppression by dexamethasone.

Tucci et al. have extended the rapid dexamethasone suppression test by obtaining not only a plasma value the morning after the dexamethasone administration but also a 5-hour urinary collection from 7 A.M. until noon. Both 17-hydroxycortisteroids and creatinine are calculated. A steroid/creatinine ratio of less than 4 makes the diagnosis of Cushing's syndrome highly likely, whereas a ratio greater than 4 suggests either that the patient is normal or that further studies will have to be carried out to establish the diagnosis of Cushing's disease. Although the test is highly reliable, both false negatives and false positives have occasionally been found.

Metyrapone (Metopirone) Test. This test was devised by Liddle to test pituitary as well as adrenal function (Fig. 37-32). As noted previously, metyrapone blocks 11-β-hydroxylation in the adrenal cortex, resulting in a fall in cortisol production and therefore a release of ACTH inhibition. This leads to an increased output of ACTH in normal individuals, with an increased output of non-11-β-hydroxylated corticosteroids from the adrenal. Since these hormones are 17-hydroxycorticosteroids, they can be measured in the urine by the usual test. In patients with Cushing's disease due to adrenal hyperplasia there is a markedly increased output of corticosteroids in the urine, greater than that seen in the normal person. Patients with Cushing's syndrome due to autonomously functioning adrenal cortical adenomas do not show an increase. This test probably has no real advantage over ACTH stimulation in the detection of Cushing's disease, but it is very helpful in detecting inadequate pituitary reserve. Insulin and vasopressin can also be used to test pituitary adrenal cortical reactivity but are not of any value in diagnosing Cushing's disease.

Blood ACTH Measurements. The measurement of blood ACTH levels may be helpful in the diagnosis of Cushing's disease. The ACTH level is elevated in adrenal hyperplasia, and the characteristic diurnal variation of ACTH is absent. ACTH is absent in patients with adrenal adenomas, carcinomas, or nodular dysplasia. Thus the immunoassay of ACTH can be a helpful tool for the definitive diagnosis of Cushing's disease.

Other Tests. Various other tests may be useful in the diagnosis of Cushing's disease. Among these is the measurement of free cortisol. Although most of the urinary cortisol is conjugated, there is normally a very small amount of the free compound in the urine. The values in Cushing's disease increase from the normal level of 30 to 60 μg to levels of 200 or more per 24 hours. An increased cortisol secretion is diagnostic of Cushing's syndrome.

Some patients with a mixed syndrome will have a normal output of 17-hydroxycorticosteroids but an increased output of 17-ketogenic steroids. The measurement of 17-hydroxysteroids by the Porter-Silber method measures the usual conjugates of cortisol, but in some cases cortisol metabolism is greatly altered so that compounds are secreted that are not usually measured by the Porter-Silber method, largely cortolone. Cortolone and some of the other end products of corticosteroid metabolism are measured by the 17-ketogenic technique.

X-ray of the Sella Turcica and Angiography of the Adrenal. X-ray of the sella turcica should be made in all patients with Cushing's syndrome, particularly those with pigmentation, since a pituitary tumor is more likely under these circumstances. X-ray of the bones will frequently demonstrate pathologic fractures and osteoporosis.

Arteriograms or venograms of the adrenal are often used to localize adrenal tumors or to demonstrate hyperplasia of the adrenal in Cushing's syndrome. More recently [131]iodocholesterol emission photoscanning has been highly effective in demonstrating the adrenal lesion in Cushing's syndrome (Fig. 37-28). Occasionally an adrenal tumor can be seen on the intravenous pyelogram.

DIFFERENTIAL DIAGNOSIS. Obesity. Simple obesity can usually be differentiated from Cushing's disease because of the differences in the distribution of the fat, as shown in Fig. 37-30. Furthermore patients with Cushing's disease are seldom extremely obese; they rarely exceed 200 lb. Although obese people may have a slightly increased cortisol secretion, they show the normal diurnal variation, and their cortisol secretion is easily suppressed with dexamethasone.

Diabetes Mellitus and Hypertension. Patients with diabetes mellitus and hypertension may superficially resemble Cushing's syndrome but are easily differentiated by the various tests described above.

TREATMENT. Medical Treatment. The primary application of medical treatment in Cushing's syndrome is to inoperable carcinoma of the adrenal cortex with metastases. There may be an occasional patient, however, who is so sick that he would be an extremely poor surgical risk without a period of medical preparation.

At the present time there are four drugs which have received clinical trial. These are metyrapone, SU-9055, aminoglutethimide, and o,p'-DDD. The action of these drugs has been summarized by Lipsett.

When given by mouth in doses of 2 to 6 Gm/day in divided doses metyrapone is capable of lowering the plasma cortisol level considerably. This has been shown both for adrenocortical hyperplasia and for adrenocortical carcinoma. In metastatic adrenal cancer the response even to 6 Gm/day usually has not been good. There is relatively little toxicity. When present, the symptoms of toxicity have consisted of anorexia, nausea, and skin rash.

SU-9055 is a 17-hydroxylase and 18-hydroxylase inhibitor. It produces inhibition of aldosterone but has not been used clinically to inhibit cortisol production.

Aminoglutethimide is an anticonvulsant with the trade name of Elipten. It was withdrawn from the market because it tended to produce hirsutism and goiter. In patients with Cushing's syndrome doses of 1 to 2 Gm/day have caused significant decreases in cortisol secretion. The drug acts by blocking steroid synthesis at some point between cholesterol and pregnenolone. Benefit has also been observed in patients with Cushing's syndrome due both to adrenocortical carcinoma and to adenoma. It was not effective, however, in a case of Cushing's syndrome due to an ACTH-producing oat cell carcinoma. Fever, skin rashes, and somnolence may be permanent side effects.

The drug o,p'-DDD is unlike any of the previously mentioned drugs, since it is not an enzyme blocker and does not interfere with steroid synthesis but instead produces direct cellular damage to adrenocortical cells. There is marked species variation in the effectiveness of the drug, so that although it causes adrenocortical necrosis in the dog, it is inactive in the mouse, rat, monkey, and other animals. Some cytolytic changes have been observed in man. It has been used primarily to treat metastatic adrenocortical carcinoma. There has been some evidence of regression in 25 percent of the patients with steroid-producing carcinoma, and rarely in patients with nonfunctioning adrenocortical carcinomas.

O,p'-DDD is given in doses of 10 to 20 Gm/day for prolonged periods of time and has not produced a cure in any patient, although regressions of 3 to 5 years have been seen. The side effects of the drug are quite severe, including intolerable nausea, skin rashes, pigmentation, somnolence, nystagmus, blurring of vision, and slurring of speech. If the drug is effective in attacking the tumor, it may be necessary to give glucocorticoids to prevent adrenal insufficiency from developing. The drug has been used in doses of 2 to 5 Gm/day to treat Cushing's syndrome due to hyperplasia or adenoma.

Recently Krieger et al. have shown remission of Cushing's disease after treatment with the antiserotonin agent cyproheptadine. Effective in about 30 percent of the patients in whom it has been tried, cyproheptadine acts by inhibiting hypothalamic serotoninergic mechanisms which usually promote ACTH release.

Pituitary Irradiation. While the treatment of Cushing's disease due to adrenocortical adenoma or carcinoma is immediate surgical intervention, patients with adrenocortical hyperplasia and Cushing's syndrome may first be treated by pituitary irradiation. It is our feeling that unless the patient has a rapidly progressing Cushing's syndrome or is quite ill with hypotension (in which case immediate surgical treatment should be carried out), pituitary irradiation should be tried first. Pituitary irradiation takes at least 6 months to produce an effect, so the patient must be well enough to tolerate a 6- to 12-month wait, during or after which he may receive no benefit.

Since Cushing's syndrome due to adrenal hyperplasia is secondary to overproduction of ACTH, the objective of pituitary irradiation is to reduce ACTH secretion and perhaps prevent the development of pituitary tumors which sometimes follow bilateral adrenalectomy for Cushing's disease. The usual radiation dose is 4,000 to 5,000 r to the pituitary fossa using a ^{60}cobalt or other high-energy source. The remission rate with this technique has been variously stated to be from 10 to 60 percent but is probably somewhere in the neighborhood of 25 percent in most clinics. Proton beam irradiation has also been tried and may offer some advantages.

Fraser and Wright have recently summarized their experience with ^{90}yttrium implantation in the pituitary for Cushing's disease. Using doses up to 50,000 rads, they treated 18 patients, with death of 1 patient, satisfactory remission in 9, and partial remission in 8. Four of the eighteen patients needed a second implant. Long-term follow-up of these patients has not yet been achieved, however, and the likelihood that marked depression of other pituitary function will ensue lessens the appeal of this technique.

Since it seems probable that the increased ACTH secretion in this type of Cushing's disease comes about as a consequence of increased hypothalamic stimulus to the anterior pituitary, it is possible that in the future the disease will be treated by making discrete hypothalamic lesions in the CRF area or by increasing sophistication in the use of cyproheptadine.

At the present time it seems wise to use temporary medical management for those patients too sick to tolerate operation at once, to employ immediate surgical intervention for those patients with adenoma or nonmetastatic adrenal carcinoma, to administer ^{60}cobalt irradiation to the pituitary for those patients with adrenocortical hyperplasia in whom the disease is mild enough to tolerate a 6- to 12-month waiting period, to operate immediately on those patients with adrenocortical hyperplasia who are too sick to wait 6 months but not too sick to survive surgical treatment, and to operate on those patients who have been given a trial of x-ray therapy to the pituitary and have failed to respond. Many feel it is advisable to irradiate the pituitary following surgical treatment in all patients undergoing total bilateral adrenalectomy for Cushing's syndrome, without waiting for the possible development of a pituitary tumor. Those patients with metastatic adrenocortical carcinoma producing Cushing's disease should receive combined medical management, and those patients with ectopic tumors producing ACTH should have the tumor excised if possible. If this is not possible, adrenalectomy should be done. Patients with a pituitary tumor producing ACTH should have ^{90}yttrium or cold probe destruction of the tumor, or surgical excision of the pituitary.

Molinatti et al. have treated 24 patients with Cushing's syndrome by intrasellar implantation of ^{90}yttrium. He noted rhinorrhea in seven and fatal meningitis in two. Optic nerve injury, cerebral necrosis, and fibrosarcoma have also been noted following pituitary radiotherapy.

Preoperative Preparation. Preoperative preparation for Cushing's disease is unnecessary, as the patient already has an excess of cortisol. If the patient has received treatment with cortisol inhibitors prior to surgical treatment, it may be necessary to begin treatment with corticosteroids the night before the operation. Under ordinary circumstances, however, no particular preparation is necessary, except to correct hypokalemia if it exists. If bilateral adrenalectomy is carried out, intravenous cortisol administration is begun after removing the second adrenal, and postoperative therapy is given according to the schedule in Table 37-6.

Operative Technique. Although the transabdominal, back, and flank approaches have all been used to perform adrenalectomy for Cushing's syndrome, we prefer the posterior approach. It is our practice to take out the twelfth rib on the left and the eleventh rib on the right; this gives excellent exposure.

In most instances the presence of a tumor has been established preoperatively and has been localized by ap-

Table 37-6. SCHEDULE FOR INTRAOPERATIVE AND POSTOPERATIVE CORTICOSTEROID ADMINISTRATION AFTER ADRENALECTOMY

Day	Intravenous cortisol,* mg	Intramuscular cortisone,† mg	Oral cortisone,‡ mg
Day of operation .	300	100	
First day	200	100	
Second day	100	100	
Third day	. . .	100	50
Fourth day	. . .	50	50
Fifth day	. . .	50	50
Sixth day	. . .	. . .	75
Thereafter	. . .	. . .	50–37.5

*Intravenous cortisol given by continuous infusion through plastic cannula. On the operative day, 100 mg is given in the first 4 hours, 100 in the next 8 hours, and 100 in the next 12 hours.

†Intramuscular cortisone acetate given in two divided doses every 12 hours.

‡Oral cortisone given in divided doses every 12 hours. Reduction from 50 to 37.5 mg should be done slowly and cautiously. Some patients have to be maintained on 50 or even 75 mg/day.

propriate angiographic studies or by the radiocholesterol scan. The side where the tumor is located is operated upon, and the entire gland containing the tumor is excised. If the patient is thought to have bilateral adrenal hyperplasia, the left side is operated upon first, because exposure here is somewhat easier and faster. If the gland appears normal or enlarged, it is removed. If the gland appears atrophic, it is biopsied but is otherwise left undisturbed, and the wound is closed. This means that the diagnosis was incorrect and that the patient has adrenocortical adenoma or carcinoma on the opposite side. In either event a similar procedure is carried out on the second side. This is easy to do and has not led to any problems. When the second side is then exposed, if bilateral adrenal hyperplasia is present, the second adrenal is also totally removed. If an adrenocortical adenoma is present, the adrenal and the adenoma on that side are totally removed.

A great deal of controversy has evolved in the past about whether a subtotal adrenalectomy or total adrenalectomy should be done, but most people now feel that a total adrenalectomy is preferable in every case. The reasons for this are that with subtotal adrenalectomy there is a high recurrence rate, difficulty in adjusting the dose of steroid replacement therapy, a high incidence of failure to cure, uncertain function of the remnant, and a likelihood of development of adrenal insufficiency. In the Mayo Clinic series there was a recurrence rate of 30 percent after subtotal adrenalectomy, and in the Massachusetts General Hospital series of 30 patients having adrenal surgical treatment other than total adrenalectomy for adrenocortical hyperplasia 10 had no relief, and of the 20 who were relieved, 9 needed further surgical treatment for recurrence. Furthermore, adrenal insufficiency has developed in patients having subtotal adrenalectomy months or years after surgical treatment despite the presence of seemingly normal adrenal function early after surgical treatment.

As one might expect, the abnormal pituitary-adrenal relationship which gave rise to the adrenal hyperplasia in the first place still persists, and Drucker et al. have noted no ACTH response and no diurnal variation in plasma cortisol levels after subtotal adrenalectomy, the stage thus being set either for recurrent Cushing's disease or adrenal insufficiency during stress. Similar findings have been reported by Egdahl and Melby. Their patients were treated either by removal of the adrenal remnant or pituitary irradiation, which greatly facilitated the maintenance of the patients with exogenous steroid therapy.

Some surgeons have advised doing a subtotal adrenalectomy and making an adrenal autotransplant of the remaining fragment in some convenient location, such as the groin, so that the fragment can easily be removed if the disease recurs. Unfortunately the fragment usually fails to function, and this procedure, while ingenious, probably is not helpful in the treatment of Cushing's disease.

When the patient has a large adrenocortical carcinoma, it may be wise to use an abdominal approach to search for metastases and, if none is found, to extend the incision into a thorocoabdominal approach to achieve a wide margin around the tumor.

Operation for Ectopic-ACTH Syndrome. If the ACTH-producing tumor is resectable, this is the procedure of choice. If not, appropriate antitumor therapy should be carried out.

Postoperative Complications. Following bilateral total adrenalectomy for Cushing's syndrome due to adrenal hyperplasia, in about 10 to 15 percent of the patients an ACTH-secreting chromophobe adenoma of the pituitary develops. This is accompanied by marked hyperpigmentation and, if the adenoma becomes large, visual symptoms. The development of these tumors is usually seen about 3 years after surgical treatment. In order to attempt to avoid this difficulty some centers give 4,000 r of irradiation of the pituitary of all patients undergoing bilateral adrenalectomy for Cushing's syndrome, unless they have had irradiation prior to the operation. Once a tumor has developed, it may be treated by irradiation, cold probe hypophysectomy, ^{90}yttrium implantation, or surgical hypophysectomy.

Although it would appear that such tumors have arisen postoperatively *in response to* the bilateral adrenalectomy, they have occasionally been detected before the operation or after partial adrenalectomy. These tumors are accompanied by very high levels of blood ACTH, as shown in Fig. 37-33*A* and *B*, and the levels are usually not easily suppressible by the administration of large amounts of corticosteroids.

Patients with Cushing's disease are more prone to infection than the average patient, and wound infections must be guarded against. The patients are also particularly prone to fungus infection. Because of the involvement of the cardiovascular system and kidney from long-standing hypertension, failure of these systems may occur in the postoperative period.

As the corticosteroid replacement dose is gradually tapered, severe corticosteroid withdrawal symptoms will sometimes develop—including fever, depression, psychosis, and sometimes even suicidal attempts. These symptoms usually disappear after the patient becomes adjusted to the lower dosage level.

Patients having bilateral adrenalectomy for Cushing's disease usually require a higher maintenance level of corticosteroids than patients having adrenalectomy for carcinoma of the breast or for other conditions in which preexisting hyperfunction was not present.

Despite these potential complications the operative mortality in Cushing's syndrome is low, and unless metastatic neoplasm is present most patients do very well.

ADRENOGENITAL SYNDROME

The adrenogenital syndrome may appear at three different times in life—at birth, in childhood, or in adult life. The congenital adrenogenital syndrome showing symptoms at birth is by far the most common variety. Congenital adrenal hyperplasia in the female produces a pseudohermaphrodite, while in the male it produces macrogenitosomia praecox. The treatment is not operative, except for the occasional ultimate need to carry out plastic procedures on the genitalia of female pseudohermaphrodites.

The postnatal adrenogenital syndrome is usually the

result of an adenoma or carcinoma of the adrenal cortex. In the female it produces masculinization and in the male sexual precocity.

The adrenogenital syndrome appearing in adult life is usually due to a tumor and is much more common in

Fig. 37-33. Plasma ACTH levels in patients undergoing adrenalectomy. The technique used was a rather insensitive one, which is not usually capable of detecting levels in the unstressed normal individual or the patient with Cushing's disease prior to operation. *A.* There are uniformly low levels in the normal patient, in the patient undergoing adrenalectomy for carcinoma of the breast, and in Cushing's disease prior to operation. Following total adrenalectomy there was a marked increase in plasma ACTH levels, and this was particularly marked in those patients developing pigmentation postoperatively presumably on the basis of the development of the pituitary adenoma. The plasma ACTH levels in two patients having subtotal adrenalectomy for Cushing's disease was somewhat lower than those seen after total adrenalectomy, particularly for the patient who was pregnant. Pregnancy produces increased levels of corticosteroids, presumably because of the increased production of transcortin, which is produced in pregnancy, thus elevating the levels of bound cortisol. *B.* The plasma ACTH levels on a patient at various stages after total adrenalectomy. By 2 years postoperatively the patient had begun to develop pigmentation, presumably due to the formation of an ACTH-secreting chromophobe adenoma of the pituitary. This was accompanied by marked increases in the plasma ACTH level. These levels could be inhibited by the administration of intravenous cortisol but could not be inhibited by increasing the maintenance dose of cortisone from 37.5 to 50 mg/day.

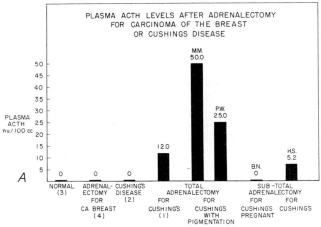

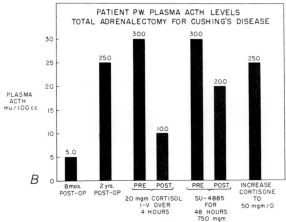

women than in men. In women it produces virilism with male habitus, with or without signs of Cushing's syndrome. In the male it produces feminization or Cushing's syndrome without virilism. Mixed patterns are very common in both sexes.

In broad terms the adrenogenital syndrome refers to any situation in which there is an overproduction of androgens resulting in virilization. For this reason the symptoms of the syndrome are much more marked and distressing in the female than in the male, with the solitary exception of the salt-losing form of the syndrome, which is often overlooked in males because of the apparent lack of physical stigmata of the syndrome.

CONGENITAL ADRENAL HYPERPLASIA. Congenital adrenal hyperplasia is thought to be familial, the inheritance being by an autosomal recessive gene. The incidence has been variously estimated at from 1:5,000 to 1:67,000.

Classification. There are six variants of congenital adrenal hyperplasia, although by far the most common type is that seen in patients with a block of C-21 hydroxylation. The defects present in the different types are shown in Fig. 37-34.

C-21 Hydroxylation Block. This is by far the most common type of congenital adrenal hyperplasia. It results in virilization due to androstenedione secreted by the adrenal cortex and converted into testosterone. In the incomplete syndrome female infants with C-21 hydroxylation defect are pseudohermaphrodites, while the males have macrogenitosomia praecox. In about a third of the cases the defect is more complete, and subnormal amounts of aldosterone are formed, leading to a salt-losing syndrome with vascular collapse and death unless treatment with mineralocorticoids is promptly stated.

C-11 Hydroxylation Block. This produces virilization with hypertension because of the production of 11-desoxycorticosterone and 11-desoxycortisol, in addition to adrenal androgens.

3-β-Hydroxysteroid Dehydrogenase Deficiency. This produces a male or female pseudohermaphrodite with adrenal insufficiency. Since both the adrenal and the gonads require 3-β-hydroxysteroid dehydrogenase for the synthesis of their active hormones, there is a defective production of androgen by the fetal interstitial cells. Females show less masculinization than with the preceding types of adrenal hyperplasia, but males exhibit varying degrees of male pseudohermaphroditism because of the lack of androgen. These patients frequently have severe salt losing, and most of them die in early life.

C-20 Block. This block prevents the production of any active steroids, and there have been no survivors. Males exhibit pseudohermaphroditism. The patients die from adrenal insufficiency, although it is possible that with the early institution of therapy survival might be achieved. The pseudohermaphroditism of the male is caused by the failure to produce any differentiation of the female external genitalia as a consequence of the lack of androgens. The adrenals characteristically show lipoid hyperplasia.

C-18 Hydroxylation Block. This produces severe salt losing because of the absence of aldosterone and is generally fatal.

C-17 Hydroxylation Block. This produces sexual infantilism, hypertension, and hypokalemic alkalosis. The patients are unable to make androgens, estrogens, or cortisol. The hypertension and hypokalemic alkalosis result from the secretion of large quantities of corticosterone and 11-desoxycorticosterone.

Clinical Manifestations. The first two types of congenital adrenal hyperplasia produce virilism, while the rest are usually fatal and do not produce virilism. In the male the virilism produces enlargement of the penis, usually with testicular atrophy and inhibition of spermatogenesis. Short stature due to closure of the epiphyses will occur unless treatment is instituted early. Adrenal rests are often present in the testes and are sometimes mistaken for Leydig cell adenomas. If early treatment with corticosteroids is instituted, normal sexual development will usually follow.

The female with a C-21 or C-11 defect is a pseudohermaphrodite. If the diagnosis is not made at birth, it can be made later on by the early appearance of pubic hair, clitoral hypertrophy, occasional presence of pigmentation due to the high ACTH levels, and an increase in 17-ketosteroids and pregnanetriol in the urine. Premature closure of the epiphyses will lead to dwarfism unless early treatment is instituted.

The cause of the virilism is the failure of the adrenal to produce cortisol, so that ACTH secretion is unopposed, thus causing adrenal hyperplasia and the production of large quantities of androgens.

The females have masculinization varying from simple enlargement of the clitoris to complete labioscrotal fusion with a normal appearing penis. However, the uterus, tubes, and ovaries are always normal. The problem is that the severely masculinized females are often mistaken for boys at birth and raised in this sex until the mistake is discovered. Before the advent of corticosteroids this was preferable, because the virilism persisted throughout adult life. It is impossible, of course, for the patient to function sexually as a male. With adequate substitution therapy the child can grow up as a perfectly adequate female capable of full sexual activity and procreation. It is thus mandatory that affected females be reared as girls. Female pseudohermaphrodites are much more apt to be tomboys than normal female infants and also tend to have higher intelligence than average. If corrective surgical treatment for clitoral hypertrophy is not undertaken at a very early age, the question in the child's mind as to whether she is a girl or a boy may be very difficult to resolve at a later date, and some of these children—though genetically and sexually female—may elect to remain males.

Differential Diagnosis. Female pseudohermaphroditism must be differentiated from true hermaphroditism where both ovary and testes are present. Determination of chromosomal sexing (Barr bodies) with a buccal smear will confirm the female genotype in female pseudohermaphroditism. A male pseudohermaphrodite with testes and female external genitalia may resemble this syndrome but can be differentiated by genotyping. An estrogen-secreting tumor of the adrenal occasionally will produce female genitalia in a male infant.

In the male, macrogenitosomia praecox must be differ-

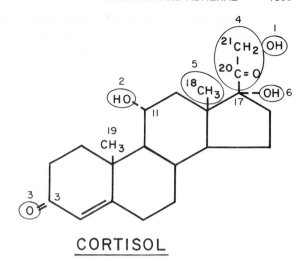

CORTISOL

Fig. 37-34. Alterations in the cortisol molecule seen in the adrenogenital syndrome. (1) C-21 hydroxylation block. A partial block produces simple virilization (female pseudohermaphrodite); a complete block produces virilization plus salt losing. (2) C-11 hydroxylation block. This produces virilization plus hypertension. (3) 3-β-hydroxysteroid dehydrogenase deficiency. This produces a male or female pseudohermaphrodite with adrenal insufficiency. (4) C-20 block. This produces a male pseudohermaphrodite with lipoid hyperplasia of the adrenal cortex, and no survivals. (5) C-18 hydroxylation block. This produces profound salt losing. (6) C-17 hydroxylation block. This produces sexual infantilism, hypertension, and hypokalemic alkalosis.

entiated from precocious puberty that is either idiopathic or secondary to a tumor around the third ventricle. Testicular biopsy will easily provide the differential, since in the child with precocious puberty the testicular tissue demonstrates early maturity whereas in macrogenitosomia praecox there is testicular atrophy or replacement of much of the testicular tissue with masses of adrenocortical cells.

Treatment. It is generally agreed that the child with female pseudohermaphroditism should be operated upon before she is four years of age and usually sometime after the first year. If the clitoris has not diminished significantly in size on medical management, the operation should be undertaken. It is preferable not to amputate the clitoris, although this has been advocated by some. A better procedure is to relocate it by removing the skin of the phallus, creating a tunnel leading to a buttonhole, severing the suspensory ligaments, pulling the phallus through the buttonhole, and suturing the skin around it to the edges of the hole. The skin defect at the base of the phallus is then closed over. Labioscrotal fusion is also corrected when present. The urogenital sinus is opened in the midline, the vaginal mucosa is freed on the rectal side, and the externalization of the vaginal orifice is completed by suturing the mucosa to the skin.

Even with early diagnosis by sex chromatin studies and immediate treatment with cortisone the clitoris still almost always requires plastic surgical procedures. The operation of recession and relocation of the enlarged clitoris was originally described by Lattimer and has been well illustrated by Seymour and Kinch.

POSTNATAL AND PREPUBERTAL ADRENOGENITAL SYNDROME. The postnatal and prepubertal adrenogenital syndrome is usually caused by an adenoma or carcinoma of the adrenal cortex. In the female masculinization occurs without change in the genitalia except for enlargement of the clitoris. Hirsutism, amenorrhea, short stature, and advanced bone age are characteristic. In the male pseudo-precocious puberty is seen. Signs include pubic hair, phallic enlargement, short stature, advanced bone age, and normal-sized testes, in contradistinction to congenital hyperplasia of the adrenal.

If the adrenogenital syndrome is produced by a tumor of the adrenal cortex instead of hyperplasia, there is a much-increased urinary 17-ketosteroid excretion, and this usually fails to be suppressed with corticoid administration. There is an excess production of urinary dehydroepiandrosterone rather than α-pregnanetriol, which is typical of congenital adrenal hyperplasia. No further increase in 17-ketosteroid excretion is usually seen with ACTH administration, since the tumor is already autonomous and functioning maximally.

ADULT ADRENOGENITAL SYNDROME. The adult form of the adrenogenital syndrome is usually produced by a tumor, although on occasion it may result from acquired hyperplasia. When a tumor is present, there is a large increase in the urinary excretion of 17-ketosteroids which is not suppressed with cortisol. The tumors can usually be distinguished from hyperplasia by the failure to respond to ACTH, the failure of 17-ketosteroid excretions to be suppressed by dexamethasone, and the preponderance of dehydroepiandrosterone rather than pregnanetriol in the urine. A single case has been reported in which an adult woman with a virilizing syndrome due to an adrenocortical tumor showed good suppression of 17-ketosteroid excretion by dexamethasone. The tumor was therefore dependent upon ACTH, unlike other reported cases.

In hyperplasia, ACTH produces a marked increase in 17-ketosteroid excretion in contrast to the findings when an adenoma or carcinoma is present.

The adult adrenogenital syndrome is much more common in women than in men. It produces virilism in the female, with or without some of the changes of Cushing's syndrome. Hirsutism, scanty or absent menses, decreased libido, atrophy of the breasts, male habitus, and hypertrophy of the clitoris are characteristic.

In the male the syndrome is very rare. It has been discovered only by chance and has been confirmed by the presence of an excess of androgen excretion, sometimes accompanied by testicular atrophy.

When the diagnosis of virilism due to an adrenocortical tumor is made, the tumor should be localized by arteriography, venography, and iodocholesterol scanning, and the adrenal on that side should be removed.

EXCESSES IN ANDROGEN PRODUCTION

There are a variety of situations in young women, including the Stein-Leventhal syndrome, in which there is a mild overproduction of androgens, leading to hirsutism, acne, and occasionally amenorrhea. There may be a slight increase in 17-ketosteroid excretion. Treatment is by the administration of corticosteroids or of estrogens.

ESTROGEN-SECRETING TUMORS

Feminizing adrenocortical tumors are rare. In the male the presenting sign is usually gynecomastia, occasionally with lactation. The prevalence of the various signs and symptoms are shown in Table 37-7.

The tumors are usually large and can be palpated in at least 50 percent of the cases. In the 52 cases of Gabrilove et al. there were 41 with carcinoma, 7 adenomas, and 4 of questionable nature.

The peak incidence for feminizing tumors is between ages of twenty-five and forty-five, and they occur only rarely in young boys. When the tumor occurs in young girls, it results in striking premature female sexual development. The signs of Cushing's syndrome are frequently present as well.

There is a marked increase in urinary estrogens, and often in 17-hydroxycorticosteroids and 17-ketosteroids as well. The steroids cannot be suppressed by dexamethasone or stimulated by ACTH in most cases.

In the adult male the testes show marked atrophy, and the diagnosis is based on gynecomastia and diminished libido, while in women the diagnosis is usually not apparent unless the patient has a mixed secretion and presents as a case of Cushing's syndrome.

The patient is treated by surgical excision as soon as the diagnosis is made, and this is followed by radiotherapy if the tumor is malignant. In most instances, in men, metastases are present by the time the patient is first seen, and the patient usually dies within a matter of 2 or 3 years. Metastases occur in the liver, lungs, bones, brain, and local lymph nodes and are usually hyperfunctioning. For a time after the operation libido and spermatogenesis return toward normal. Because estrogen-secreting tumors of the

Table 37-7. INCIDENCE OF SIGNS AND SYMPTOMS OF FEMINIZING TUMORS IN THE MALE (52 PATIENTS)

Sign or symptom	Percent
Gynecomastia	98
Palpable tumor	58
Atrophy of testis	52
Diminished libido and/or potency	48
Pain at site of tumor	44
Tenderness of breast	42
Pigmentation of areolae	27
Obesity	27
Feminizing hair change	23
Atrophy of the penis	20
Elevation of the blood pressure	16
Increasing skin pigmentation	12
Varicocele	11
Acne	8

SOURCE: From J. L. Gabrilove, D. C. Sharma, H. H. Wotiz, and R. I. Dorfman, *Medicine,* **44:**37, 1965.

adrenal cortex in men are so malignant and relatively insensitive to irradiation and chemotherapy, radical thoracoabdominal resection and lymphadenectomy have been advocated. Half the patients with this tumor are dead within 18 months, and the 3-year survival rate is only 20 percent. Stewart et al. pointed out that almost all the feminizing adrenal neoplasms in adult men have been malignant, whereas all those in children have been benign. However, malignant tumors occasionally have been reported in children. This is in sharp contrast to the general picture of adrenal tumors causing Cushing's syndrome, which are usually benign in adults and often malignant in children.

ADRENOCORTICAL CARCINOMAS AND TUMORS WITH MIXED SECRETIONS

MacFarlane has reported on 55 patients with adrenocortical carcinoma, and Lipsett et al. have reported on 38 such patients. In this latter series the patient's ages varied between twelve months and sixty-two years. Twenty-three of the thirty-eight patients were females, which is similar to the increased incidence of Cushing's syndrome in women. Of those adrenocortical carcinomas producing Cushing's syndrome in the adult 87 percent were in women. In the non-hormone-secreting tumors the incidence was higher in men (60 percent). Adrenocortical carcinoma occurs more often on the left side than on the right. The tumor is highly malignant, 50 percent of the patients dying within 2 years of the onset of symptoms.

The presenting complaints in most instances are those associated with virilization, Cushing's syndrome, or precocious puberty. Women usually complain of hirsutism, acne, virilism, truncal obesity, and menstrual irregularity. In patients without endocrine symptoms abdominal discomfort, pain, distension, and the presence of a mass lead to the diagnosis. Mixed pictures are common, particularly those of Cushing's syndrome and virilization. Only one woman had Cushing's syndrome alone. In addition to producing Cushing's syndrome and feminizing and virilizing syndromes adrenocortical carcinomas can produce hypokalemic alkalosis and hypoglycemia. Villee et al. reported a case of virilizing adrenocortical carcinoma in a sixteen-year-old girl which eventually produced overt Cushing's syndrome.

Adrenal cortical cancer is almost always accompanied by large amounts of 17-ketosteroids in the urine. This appears to be true whether the tumor causes Cushing's syndrome, virilization, or even feminization. It is often true even if the tumor does not have any obvious endocrine manifestations. Since excessive virilization is difficult to pick up in men, the tumor usually appears nonfunctioning in the adult male.

After surgical excision of the tumor it is important to follow the urinary excretion of steroids at frequent intervals, so that the metastases can be detected early and treatment instituted. Adrenocortical carcinomas have been treated with o,p'-DDD. Hutter and Kayhoe reported the results of the treatment of 138 patients with adrenocortical carcinoma with o,p'-DDD. A marked reduction in urinary hormone excretion occurred in 69 percent of the patients and was often associated with a reduction in endocrine symptoms. The mean duration of response was 4.8 months. Thirty-four percent of the patients had objective tumor regression, with a mean duration of about 7 months. It was felt that this type of chemotherapy should be instituted for both functioning and nonfunctioning adrenal carcinoma.

DISORDERS OF SEXUAL DEVELOPMENT

Feminizing and virilizing tumors of adrenal origin can sometimes produce changes which can be confused with disorders of sexual development. It is therefore wise to have some idea about the diagnosis of these disorders (see Chap. 41). A summary presented by Federman is reproduced in Table 37-8. Sexual development can be divided into three phases:

1. Intrauterine genital differentiation, in which an inducer of testicular origin causes the otherwise female genitalia to differentiate into the male form. In the absence of this inducer at the proper time embryologically, regardless of the genetic sex, the duct system will differentiate along female lines. Androgen, in the absence of the inducer, does not suppress the development of female structures and has an incomplete effect on male development.

Table 37-8. SUMMARY OF THE DISORDERS OF SEXUAL DEVELOPMENT

Disorders of gonadogenesis	Klinefelter's syndrome Turner's syndrome	Infertility without ambiguity
	True hermaphroditism Mixed gonadal dysgenesis Male pseudohermaphroditism (dysgenetic)	Infertility with ambiguity
Disorders of endocrinology: Androgen deficiency in the male	Male pseudohermaphroditism (familial)	
Androgen excess in the female	Female pseudohermaphroditism Congenital adrenal hyperplasia Others	Ambiguity with infertility

SOURCE: From D. D. Federman, Disorders of Sexual Development, *N Engl J Med,* **277:**353, 1967.

2. The gradual development of the secondary sex characteristics in the male brought about by androgens.
3. Fertility, which occurs at puberty.

The disorders of sexual development can be divided into three types: infertility without ambiguity in genital development, infertility with ambiguity in genital development, and ambiguity without fertility.

The patients with *Klinefelter's syndrome* are phenotypic males, with no obvious abnormality before puberty. At the time of puberty pubic hair and some body hair develops, but the beards are sparser than normal, and the patients usually have gynecomastia. The body build ranges from rather feminine to eunuchoid to normal male. A key to the diagnosis is that despite development of the pubic hair and penis, the testes are extremely small, 1.5 cm or less in longest diameter. The urinary 17-ketosteroids are normal, while the gonadotropins are increased. Plasma testosterone levels are lower than in normal males but higher than in females. The patients are almost always genotypic females with chromatin-positive nuclei. The patients with chromatin-positive Klinefelter's syndrome have at least two X chromosomes and a Y chromosome in at least some of their cells.

In *Turner's syndrome* the patients are phenotypic females with short stature, amenorrhea, lack of estrogen effect, congenital anomalies consisting of low-set ears and hairline, coarctation of the aorta, congenital lymphedema, and other changes. The patients have female external and internal genitalia, but the gonad is an undifferentiated "streak" without true germinal secretory elements. After puberty the urinary gonadotropins are increased. About 60 percent of the patients with Turner's syndrome are chromatin-negative like the normal male, but unlike Klinefelter's syndrome, where there are more chromosomes than normal, in Turner's syndrome there are fewer, usually only a single X without a Y and no second X. The remainder of the patients are chromatin-positive, but in many of these there are fewer of the female markers than one sees in the normal woman.

The *true hermaphrodites* have both ovarian and testicular tissue. They may have a testes on one side and an ovary on the other or an ova-testis on one or the other side, or combinations of these two. Both gonads are usually intraabdominal, but the testes occasionally descend toward a scrotal position. The true hermaphodite almost invariably has a uterus and at least one tube on the ovarian side, while the other side may have some male structures. Most of these patients have been raised as males, but external virilization is seldom complete, and hypospadias and cryptorchidism are clues to the diagnosis. Gynecomastia usually develops at puberty, and about two-thirds of the patients menstruate, and half of them ovulate. The ovarian function is more nearly normal than the testicular, and an occasional true hermaphrodite may be potentially fertile. Eighty percent of hermaphrodites are chromatin-positive, or genetic females. Some of them may have mixtures of normal male and female cells, and they apparently develop from a double fertilization of the ovum, wherein the patient represents a fused fraternal twin.

Those patients with *mixed gonadal dysgenesis* have a "streak" gonad on one side similar to that of the Turner's syndrome and a testis on the other side. Other patients have a testis or a "streak" on one side and a gonadal tumor on the other. All these patients have a uterus and at least one tube but may have some male structures as well. There is an extreme variation in external appearance. A few have been normal females, others have been females with enlargement of the clitoris, while still others have graded off into male appearances with hypospadias and cryptorchidism. A very few have had the male phenotype and are normal except for unilateral cryptorchidism. At puberty the patients undergo virilism, and breast development occurs only in those who have a gonadal tumor.

These patients are always chromatin-negative, or males, which makes it easy to differentiate them at an early stage from female pseudohermaphrodites secondary to the adrenogenital syndrome. The dysgenetic male pseudohermaphrodite has two testes but incomplete virilization. Since the testes are abnormal, they fail to suppress female development, and the result is a female, or inadequate male, phenotype.

The *familial male pseudohermaphrodites* are genetic and gonadal males, with a defect in genital virilization, so that the testes secrete estrogens. They are chromatin-negative male genotypes with normal-appearing female external genitalia and breast development. At puberty they get normal breast development but no menstrual period. The vagina ends blindly, and there is no uterus. If the testes are removed before puberty, normal female breast development does not occur, and urinary estrogen levels fall immediately after orchiectomy. A patient has been reported in whom the urinary estrogen output remained normal after orchiectomy, which was considered as evidence for adrenal origin of the estrogens. The testes probably should not be removed.

ADRENALECTOMY FOR METASTATIC CANCER OF THE BREAST OR PROSTATE AND FOR HYPERTENSION

Adrenalectomy for Metastatic Breast or Prostatic Cancer

Cancer of the breast is sometimes responsive to estrogenic stimulation, and when this is the case, oophorectomy may provide a prolonged remission. Although the ovaries are the principal source of estrogen, the adrenal cortex also manufactures estrogenic substances. For this reason Dao and Huggins proposed and carried out adrenalectomy for metastatic carcinoma of the breast and, because the adrenals also manufacture androgens, for metastatic carcinoma of the prostate in patients who had previously had an orchiectomy. Dao and Huggins in 1953 reported 100 cases of patients with metastatic breast cancer who had undergone bilateral adrenalectomy. Adrenalectomy has been reported to ameliorate symptoms from metastatic carcinoma of the male breast as well.

Symptomatic improvement in metastatic carcinoma of the breast following either adrenalectomy or hypophysectomy is about 30 percent. Patients with bony or skin metastases do the best, those with lung metastases do not fare quite so well, and those with liver metastases seem to do most poorly. Block et al. in 1959 suggested that patients with cancer of the breast be selected for bilateral adrenalectomy only if they did not have liver metastases, had had a previous response to oophorectomy, had a high estrogen secretion, and had a relatively prolonged duration of the primary disease, i.e., over 3 years. Several workers have since emphasized that better results are obtained with adrenalectomy if the patient has had a positive response to oophorectomy.

In recent years it has been helpful to measure estrogen binding in tumor cells of the breast carcinoma. Only those patients demonstrating binding of estrogen to receptors on the tumor cell should receive hormonal therapy. In those patients without estrogen receptor activity the results of hormonal manipulation have been poor.

Dao and Nemoto have advocated the use of adrenalectomy as the primary therapy in patients with disseminated metastases and have claimed that involvement of over 30 percent of the liver is necessary before bilateral adrenalectomy is contraindicated.

Fracchia et al. in a report of 500 consecutive cases of adrenalectomy for metastatic cancer of the breast achieved an objective remission of 35.6 percent of the cases for 6 months or longer. Again, those patients did better the longer the interval between mastectomy and recurrence, if they were premenopausal and had shown a previous response to oophorectomy or if they were postmenopausal and vaginal smears showed a high level of estrogenic activity.

Fig. 37-35. Comparison of primary and secondary aldosteronism. In primary aldosteronism there is an obligatory secretion of aldosterone, which produces sodium retention, increased plasma volume, increased renal artery pressure, and inhibition of renin secretion. In secondary aldosteronism there is a primary decrease in renal artery pressure which stimulates the juxtaglomerular cells to secrete an increased amount of renin, thus leading to the production of angiotensin and stimulation of the adrenal cortex to produce increased amounts of aldosterone.

Bilateral Adrenalectomy for Essential Hypertension

Bilateral adrenalectomy either alone or combined with splanchnicectomy or thoracoabdominal sympathectomy used to be advocated for the treatment of hypertension. This is seldom practiced any longer.

PRIMARY ALDOSTERONISM

Primary hyperaldosteronism is characterized by hypertension, ADH-resistant polyuria, and muscle weakness due to hypokalemic alkalosis. Secondary aldosteronism has some of the same features and must be differentiated from the primary disease. There is little doubt that ACTH plays a minor but interesting role in aldosterone secretion. The chief stimulus to aldosterone production is angiotensin II.

The hormone secretion patterns in primary versus secondary aldosteronism are shown in Fig. 37-35. In the typical cases the principal endocrinologic difference is an increased renin and angiotensin secretion in secondary aldosteronism and inhibition of renin and angiotensin secretion in primary aldosteronism.

PATHOLOGY. At least 90 percent of patients with primary aldosteronism have a benign solitary adrenocortical adenoma, more commonly on the left than on the right side. These adenomas are sometimes so small that they cannot be seen or felt until the gland is sectioned. Unlike hyperparathyroidism, where the size of the tumor is roughly proportional to the degree of hypersecretion, the size of the tumor in aldosteronism has very little relation to the degree of hypersecretion. Very small tumors sometimes produce a profound hypokalemia and hypersecretion of aldosterone. The adenomas are bilateral in 5 percent of the cases or less. Bilateral adrenal glomerulosa cell hyperplasia can cause primary aldosteronism, and in these patients with hyperplasia plasma renin activity tends to be normal, rather than suppressed as it is with aldosterone-secreting adenomas. Nodular hyperplasia has also been said to cause primary aldosteronism occasionally. Rarely, primary aldosteronism is produced by an adrenocortical carcinoma.

SECONDARY ALDOSTERONISM | PRIMARY ALDOSTERONISM

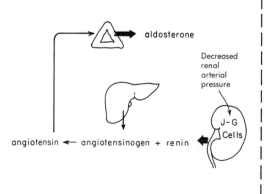

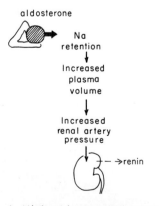

1. High aldosterone output

2. High renin output

1. High aldosterone output

2. Low renin output

A heterotopic adrenocortical adenoma has been reported to cause primary aldosteronism in one case. In a few cases mixed patterns of excessive aldosterone and excessive glucocorticoid or androgenic secretion have been observed. In some cases the excessive secretion of aldosterone can be inhibited by 2 mg/day of dexamethasone, suggesting that the stimulus to excess aldosterone secretion must have been ACTH in those patients.

Grossly the tumors are discrete, circumscribed, and sharply demarcated from the normal cortex. On cut section they are characteristically bright canary yellow. The normal cortex is not atrophic (Fig. 37-36). The microscopic pathologic features of primary aldosteronism have been summarized by Neville and Symington, who observed that the cells often do not look like the zona glomerulosa while at other times they are composed largely of zona glomerulosa–type cells. They are said to be composed of "hybrid" cells with the biochemical features of both the zona glomerulosa and the zona fasciculata. The normal zona glomerulosa is hyperplastic.

CLINICAL MANIFESTATIONS. The most common incidence is between the ages of thirty and fifty, but the disease has been seen in children as young as three and adults as old as seventy-five. It is twice as common in women. Conn originally thought that the incidence of the disease might be as high as 20 percent of patients with essential hypertension, but it is now clear that only about 1 to 2 percent of the hypertensive population have primary aldosteronism.

Kaplan studied 75 patients with thiazide-induced hypokalemia and hypertension and found that none of them had primary aldosteronism. Furthermore the content of aldosterone in small adenomas seen in some patients with essential hypertension is similar to that seen in normal adrenal tissue and much less than the amounts present in adenomas of patients with primary aldosteronism. It seems likely, therefore, that many of the incidental adrenal tumors which were found in patients with hypertension and which Conn speculated were the cause of the hypertension did not actually function. This contention is further borne out by an autopsy study of Kokko et al. indicating that the incidence of hypertension was the same in patients who had adrenal adenomas, adrenal hyperplasia, or no adrenal disease. Fishman et al. found that subnormal plasma renin was characteristic of certain patients with essential hypertension and that primary aldosteronism rarely occurred in hypertensive patients with normal serum potassium levels.

Fig. 37-36. Section cut through an aldosterone-producing tumor and a portion of the normal cortex. The tumor was a rather large one which was well circumscribed. The cut surface was bright yellow, and there was no atrophy of the normal adrenal cortex.

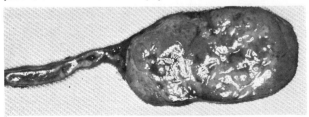

Table 37-9. SIGNS AND SYMPTOMS OF PRIMARY ALDOSTERONISM

Causes	Signs and symptoms
Hypertension and Na retention . .	Hypertension
	Headache
	Cardiac enlargement
Hypokalemia and K deficit	Muscle weakness and paralysis
	Tetany
	Paresthesias and muscle cramps
	Diabetic glucose tolerance curve
	Hypokalemic renal damage
Hypokalemic renal damage	Polyuria
	Polydipsia
	Nocturia
	Proteinuria
Hypernatremia	Increased blood volume (edema rare)

The symptoms and signs of primary aldosteronism are shown in Table 37-9, and the incidence of the major symptoms in Table 37-10. The most common symptoms and signs of primary aldosteronism are hypertension, muscle weakness, polydipsia, headache, nocturnal polyuria, and hypokalemic alkalosis.

Hypertension is frequently mild, and the retinal and renal changes of malignant hypertension are almost never seen. In contrast to pheochromocytoma, where there may be a contracted blood volume and severe, often episodic hypertension, in primary aldosteronism there is expanded blood volume and relatively mild sustained hypertension.

The disease is thus characterized by hypertension without grade IV retinopathy, hypokalemic alkalosis, overwhelming of the kidney's ability to conserve sodium, an increased aldosterone excretion, increased plasma aldosterone, decreased or undetectable levels of plasma renin, normal corticosteroid secretion, the absence of hyponatremia, and a normal renal arteriogram.

It is usually not difficult to differentiate secondary from

Table 37-10. FREQUENCY OF SYMPTOMS AND SIGNS IN CLASSIC PRIMARY ALDOSTERONISM

Symptoms and signs	Percent
Hypertension	100
Hypokalemia	100
High aldosterone	95
Polyuria	92
Polydipsia	84
Alkalosis	76
Albuminuria	68
Paresthesias	58
Periodic paralysis	38
Edema	Less than 10

SOURCE: After Conn.

primary aldosteronism, even though both may be accompanied by hypertension, increased aldosterone secretion, hypokalemia, and alkalosis. The plasma sodium level is usually lower in secondary hyperaldosteronism, the plasma renin levels are elevated rather than low, and a cause for the secondary aldosteronism—usually renal artery stenosis or malignant hypertension—can be demonstrated by the proper tests, including renal arteriograms.

A variant of classic primary aldosteronism has been described by Conn et al. under the title of "normokalemic primary aldosteronism." In these patients there is hypertension with increased aldosterone secretion and low plasma renin levels with normal serum potassium and cure of the hypertension by removal of an adrenal cortical tumor. This can be viewed as an early or prehypokalemic phase of the disease.

Proteinuria may be present as a consequence of the renal damage brought about by hypokalemia, and this is also the cause of the nocturnal polyuria.

There are some other rather rare variants of aldosteronism, including normotension with primary hyperaldosteronism in the early stages, and primary aldosteronism in patients who have become so potassium-depleted that they are secreting normal amounts of aldosterone. After restoration of normal potassium stores a very high level of aldosterone secretion can be demonstrated.

DIAGNOSTIC TESTS. The tests for primary aldosteronism may be divided into two categories, the first designed to establish the presence of hyperaldosteronism and the second to distinguish between primary and secondary hyperaldosteronism (Table 37-11).

Diagnostic Tests to Establish the Presence of Hypersecretion of Aldosterone. *Plasma Potassium and Sodium.* In primary aldosteronism there is typically a low potassium level and a high normal or elevated plasma sodium level, although normokalemic primary aldosteronism has been reported by Conn et al. The plasma potassium level is also low in secondary aldosteronism, but the sodium concentration is normal or low. Brown et al. found a good inverse correlation between plasma sodium and renin levels. Thus the greater the degree of secondary aldosteronism and renin secretion, the lower the sodium. Schacht and Frame have advocated the use of chlorothiazide to intensify the hypokalemia as a diagnostic aid. Chlorothiazide does produce more profound depression of the plasma potassium level in patients with primary aldosteronism than it does in other patients, and indeed in one of our patients it brought on paralysis, but Kaplan has shown that in many patients with essential hypertension hypokalemia develops on thiazide medication, and therefore it is probably not a discriminating test.

ECG. Severe hypokalemia produces *ECG* changes that may be helpful in establishing the diagnosis. The *ECG* changes in a patient with primary aldosteronism before and after operative removal are shown in Fig. 37-37. The changes characteristic of hypokalemia were present preoperatively and reverted to normal after removal of an aldosterone-secreting tumor.

Urinary Potassium (K) and Sodium (Na) Measurements. The patients suspected of having primary aldosteronism should be placed on normal sodium intake and taken off diuretics before coming into the hospital, since a low so-

Table 37-11. DIAGNOSTIC TESTS FOR ALDOSTERONISM

Test	Primary aldosteronism	Secondary (renal) aldosteronism	Normal or essential hypertension
To detect hyperaldosteronism:			
Serum K	3 mEq/100 ml or less	3 mEq/100 ml or less	Over 3 mEq/100 ml
Serum Na	High normal or high	Normal or low	Normal
Urine K on high-Na diet	Often exceeds intake <20 mEq/day rules out >30 mEq/day likely >50 mEq/day diagnostic	20–40 mEq/day	Less than intake, usually <20 mEq/day
Urine K on low-Na diet	Falls	Falls	Increases
Aldosterone excretion in urine	>10 μg/day, often 15–50 μg/day	>10 μg/day, often 25–100 μg/day	10 μg/day or less
Aldosterone secretion rate	>170 μg/day	>170 μg/day	60–170 μg/day
Spironolactone test	Rise in serum K 1 mEq/L or more	Rise in serum K 1 mEq/L or more	Low K does not rise
To differentiate primary from secondary hyperaldosteronism:			
Plasma renin on high-Na diet	Low or absent	High	Normal
Plasma renin on low-Na diet	Low or absent	Very high	High
Aldosterone response to DCA administration	No change	Falls	Falls
Renal vein renin	Low	High	Normal
Adrenal vein aldosterone	High on side with tumor	High both sides	Normal
Renal arteriography	Normal	Arterial lesion	Normal
Adrenal angiography	Tumor present	No tumor	No tumor
Angiotensin infusion	Blood pressure rises	No blood pressure change	Blood pressure rises

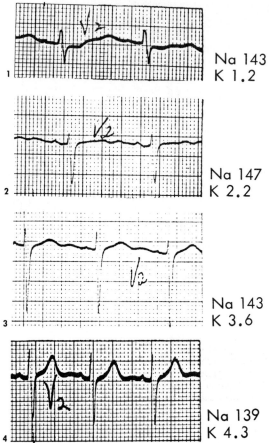

Na 143
K 1.2

Na 147
K 2.2

Na 143
K 3.6

Na 139
K 4.3

Fig. 37-37. ECG of a patient with primary aldosteronism. All the tracings are from lead V_2. The top strip was taken just after stopping the chlorothiazide diuretic which the patient had been receiving for some time. There are marked signs of hypokalemia including ST depression, inversion of the T wave, a prolonged ST interval, and U waves. The second strip was taken a week after cessation of the diuretic therapy and, despite some improvement in the plasma potassium level, still shows a markedly prolonged ST interval and well-developed U waves. The third strip shows tracing taken in the early postoperative period. There is marked improvement in the tracing with upright T waves, a shortening of the ST interval, and the absence of U waves. The last tracing was taken 10 days after the operation and is essentially a normal tracing.

dium intake will produce increased aldosterone secretion even in normal people. The patient with hyperaldosteronism and normal or elevated sodium intake loses excessive amounts of potassium in the urine, while salt restriction produces an immediate fall in urinary potassium excretion (Fig. 37-38). Postoperatively a high salt intake no longer produces excessive potassium loss. The patient should be on a constant potassium intake throughout the 6 days of the test, with 3 days of increased salt intake and 3 days of low salt intake.

Urinary Specific Gravity with Pitressin. Patients with hyperaldosteronism characteristically have large volumes of urine with a low specific gravity. This is resistant to ADH, so that the failure to increase the urinary concen-

tration with the administration of Pitressin can be used as a further diagnostic test.

Aldosterone Excretion in the Urine. If a patient has been on chlorothiazide diuretics or a low-sodium diet, these should be stopped for at least a month before measuring the urinary aldosterone excretion. Under circumstances of normal salt intake the normal patient will excrete less than 10 µg/day in the urine, while the patient with primary aldosteronism will excrete greater amounts, often between 15 and 50 µg/day. The patient with secondary aldosteronism will also excrete increased amounts of aldosterone, and often even greater amounts than are commonly seen in primary aldosteronism.

Espiner et al. have proposed the measurement of urinary aldosterone produced in response to an infusion of saline solution as a diagnostic test for aldosteronism. Patients are placed on a diet of 10 mEq of sodium and 60 mEq of potassium daily. After 5 days of this diet the patients are given 2,000 ml of physiologic saline solution over a 4-hour period on 2 consecutive days. Normal persons show a profound fall of aldosterone excretion, while patients with primary aldosteronism show only very small changes.

Induction of Hypokalemia by Oral Sodium Loading. It is helpful to give oral sodium chloride, 8 Gm/day for 4 days, to low-normokalemic patients suspected of having primary aldosteronism. At the end of this period the serum potassium may be distinctly low in the patients with hyperaldosteronism.

Aldosterone Secretion Rate. Although this test is still not available for general use, the rate of aldosterone secretion can be computed by giving the patient a small amount of radioactive aldosterone and measuring the amount of radioactivity and aldosterone excreted in the urine. The normal patient secretes between 60 and 170 µg/day, while patients with aldosteronism secrete greater amounts.

Spironolactone Test. The spironolactone test developed by Biglieri et al. consists of giving 100 Gm of Aldactone four times a day for 3 days while the patient is on normal sodium intake. The serum potassium level should rise by at least 1 mEq/L if aldosterone excess is present. Patients with hypokalemia from other causes will not show an increase. We have not found this to be a particularly useful test.

Tests to Differentiate Primary from Secondary Aldosteronism. Differentiation between primary and secondary aldosteronism is usually not difficult, since advanced renal disease is easy to detect and is usually accompanied by severe eye ground changes which are almost never seen in primary aldosteronism.

Plasma Renin Activity. Plasma renin levels are measured in the supine patient who is on a normal sodium intake. If primary aldosteronism is present, the values will be normal, low, or not measurable, while in secondary aldosteronism they will be high.

Aldosterone Excretion Response to DCA Administration. Biglieri et al. have developed a test in which the patient is given deoxycorticosterone acetate (DCA), 5 mg twice daily, for 3 consecutive days. If primary aldosteronism is

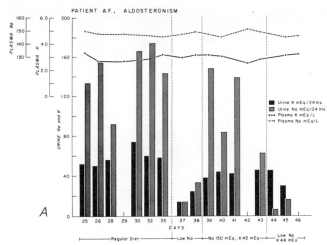

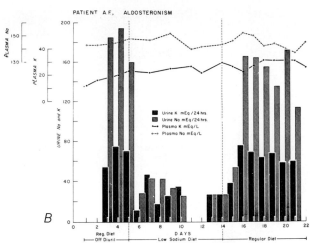

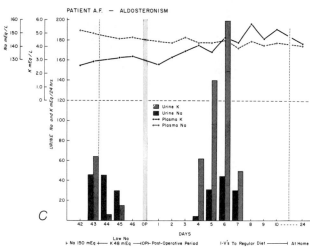

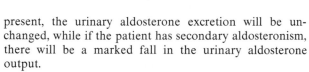

Fig. 37-38. The urinary and plasma sodium and potassium findings in primary aldosteronism. *A.* On a regular diet with an adequate intake of salt and potassium there is marked urinary potassium wasting, with daily urinary potassium excretions exceeding 50 mEq/L. When a low-sodium diet is instituted, there is an immediate sharp decline in urinary potassium excretion. On resumption of a normal sodium intake there is an immediate increase in urinary potassium excretion to levels which equal or exceed the intake. The plasma potassium level shows a fall during high-salt-intake periods and a rise during low-salt-intake periods. *B.* Same patient as in *A.* There is a striking urinary potassium wasting on a regular diet with a sudden and striking decrease on a low-salt diet. During the first period there is an increase in the plasma potassium level despite the high salt intake in response to stopping the diuretic. *C.* Same patient as in *A* and *B.* The patient was prepared for operation with a low-salt diet and adequate amounts of potassium. This produced a fall in the plasma sodium level and a rise in the plasma potassium level. Following excision of the adenoma there is a steady increase in the plasma potassium level.

present, the urinary aldosterone excretion will be unchanged, while if the patient has secondary aldosteronism, there will be a marked fall in the urinary aldosterone output.

Arterial and Venous Catheter Studies. Catheters may be inserted into the renal veins or into either adrenal vein. An elevated renin level in the renal venous blood establishes the diagnosis of secondary aldosteronism, and if the level is elevated on only one side, this pinpoints the site of the pathologic change. Catheterization of the adrenal vein reveals an elevated aldosterone level in primary aldosteronism. This is elevated only on the side of the tumor. In secondary aldosteronism levels may be elevated on both sides. In the instances of primary aldosteronism due to bilateral adrenal hyperplasia, elevated aldosterone levels will be found on both sides.

Angiography of the adrenal gland, both venous and arterial, can be used to demonstrate the location of the tumor. Venous angiography is not without hazard in hyperaldosteronism because the adrenal veins are notoriously fragile in this condition and adrenal hemorrhage may occur even with gentle retrograde injection of the contrast medium. Renal arteriography demonstrates the site of the lesion in renal artery stenosis and may demonstrate disease of the intrarenal vessels in malignant hypertension due to intrinsic renal disease.

[131]*Iodocholesterol Adrenal Scan.* Beierwaltes and his coworkers have recently developed a photoscan of the adrenals. This technique images tissue in which iodinated cholesterol is concentrated. The adrenal cortex is such a tissue. Conn et al. have applied this technique, with good success, to the study of patients with primary hyperaldosteronism. Hyperfunctioning aldosteronomas appear as "hot spots" which are not suppressed with dexamethasone; in patients in whom adrenocortical hyperplasia causes the hyperaldosteronism, iodocholesterol uptake will be suppressed with administration of dexamethasone (Fig. 37-39). Conn has recently shown clear separation of these two groups using this technique. As we shall see later, it is an important distinction to make.

Angiotensin Infusion. An indirect measurement of renin-angiotensin activity in plasma using an intravenous infusion of angiotensin has been developed. In patients with secondary aldosteronism and increased levels of renin and angiotensin in the plasma there will be no blood pressure response to the infusion of angiotensin, while in

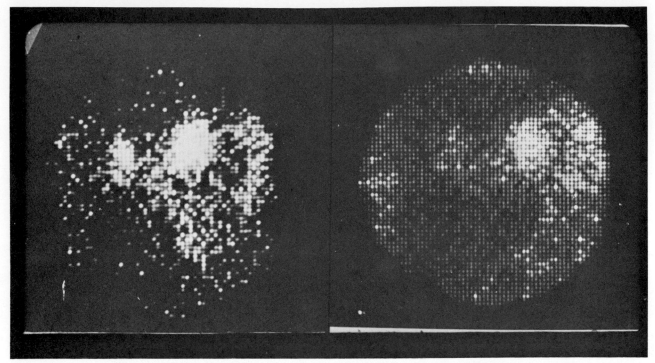

Fig. 37-39. A radio-cholesterol scan from a patient with primary hyperaldosteronism. In the right adrenal, imaged on the right side of the print-out, is an obvious area of focal increased uptake. The scan in the right half of the photograph was exposed after dexamethasone suppression. Normal adrenal tissue has been suppressed, but the increased uptake of the aldosterone-secreting tumor of the right adrenal persists.

patients with primary aldosteronism the infusion will produce a rise in blood pressure, as it will in the normal person.

SPECIAL CONSIDERATIONS. Normokalemic Primary Aldosteronism. This can be diagnosed with the routine tests used for any patient with primary aldosteronism, except that it is more difficult to recognize initially, and the urinary potassium studies are less apt to be diagnostic unless careful balance studies are done. These normokalemic patients characteristically have hypertension, increased aldosterone excretion, and suppressed plasma renin levels. Oral sodium loading, mentioned previously, may uncover their hypokalemia.

Bilateral Adrenal Hyperplasia. In a few cases typical primary aldosteronism is produced by bilateral adrenal hyperplasia. Adrenalectomy has not produced good resolution of the hypertension in the hyperplasia patients. For this reason many patients with hyperplasia are being treated medically with spironolactone, an aldosterone antagonist. In two cases of hyperplasia reported in a father and son, the entire clinical syndrome was relieved by the administration of 2 mg dexamethasone a day.

Normotensive Primary Aldosteronism. In the early phases of primary aldosteronism patients will sometimes be found who are hypokalemic and have all the other features of aldosteronism without hypertension. A high-sodium diet will sometimes reveal the hypokalemia.

Primary Aldosteronism with Normal Aldosterone Output. If the patient has undergone profound potassium depletion over a long period of time, aldosterone secretion may be diminished to normal levels. The diagnosis can be made by replenishing the potassium stores, after which markedly elevated levels of aldosterone can be detected.

Congenital Aldosteronism. There have been some patients described by Conn as having congenital aldosteronism who probably have malignant hypertension and secondary hyperaldosteronism. Some of these patients, however, may have bilateral adrenal hyperplasia.

DIFFERENTIAL DIAGNOSIS (Table 37-12). **Secondary Aldosteronism.** The differential diagnosis of secondary aldosteronism has been defined above. The differential can usually be established by plasma renin measurements.

Juxtaglomerular Cell Hyperplasia. Bartter et al. described the syndrome of juxtaglomerular hyperplasia with hyperaldosteronism and hypokalemia. At least 20 such patients have been detected. The cause of the syndrome is apparently impairment of the vascular response to angiotensin. The decrease in pulse pressure acts as a constant stimulus to the release of renin from the juxtaglomerular apparatus and leads to hypertrophy of these cells. Secondary aldosteronism develops as a consequence of the effects of angiotensin on the adrenal. Aldosterone levels are increased, the plasma renin level is markedly elevated, and the blood pressure is normal.

Cushing's Syndrome. Cushing's syndrome may be associated with hypertension and marked hypokalemia but can easily be differentiated by its physical features and the high levels of cortisol.

Potassium-wasting Renal Disease. Although many patients originally thought to have potassium-losing nephritis

Table 37-12. DIFFERENTIAL DIAGNOSIS OF ALDOSTERONISM

Clinical state	Aldosterone production	Plasma renin	Hypertension	Hypokalemia	Special features
Primary aldosteronism	High	Low	Yes—benign	Yes	
Normokalemic primary aldosteronism (Conn)	High	Low	Yes	No	High Na intake produces hypokalemia.
Normoaldosteronal primary aldosteronism (Biglieri)	Normal	Low	Yes	Severe	Aldosterone output increases with K replacement.
Normotensive primary aldosteronism	High	Low	No	Yes	
ACTH-dependent aldosteronism (Sutherland)	High	Low	Yes	Yes	Aldosterone output suppressed with dexamethazone.
Congenital aldosteronism (Conn)	High	....	Yes—usually malignant	Yes	Probably secondary to renal disease.
Secondary aldosteronism:					
Renal artery stenosis	High or normal	High	Yes—benign or malignant	Occasional	
Intrinsic renal ischemia	Usually high	High	Malignant	Frequent	
Juxtaglomerular hyperplasia (Bartter)	High	High	No	Yes	Impaired vascular response to angiotensin.
Secondary aldosteronism without renin (Laragh)	High	Low	Yes	Yes	Hypoplasia of juxtaglomerular cells. Nonrenin stimulus to aldosterone secretion.
Renal K wasting	Variable	....	No or benign	Yes	Acidosis, hyponatremia, hypovolemia.
With hypomagnesemia	Variable	High	No	Yes	Mg loss in urine.
With Na conservation	Low	Low	Yes	Yes	
Cushing's syndrome	Normal	Low or normal	Yes—benign	Occasional	Cortisol secretion increased.

have since been shown to have primary aldosteronism, there continue to be some patients who waste potassium because of a primary renal defect. The hypokalemia is associated with metabolic acidosis rather than alkalosis, hyponatremia rather than hypernatremia, and hypovolemia rather than hypervolemia. The production of aldosterone may be increased because of the impairment of the resorption of sodium. The plasma renin activity may be high.

Familial Disorders Mimicking Aldosteronism. Two familial disorders have recently been reported which could be confused with primary aldosteronism. In the first of these there is hypomagnesemia resulting from impaired conservation of magnesium by the kidney. These patients secondarily developed hypokalemia but are normotensive. The second disorder consists of a renal tubular defect characterized by increased reabsorption of sodium and thus excessive loss of potassium leading to hypokalemia. There is low renin activity in the plasma but decreased, rather than increased, production of aldosterone. These patients are hypertensive.

Other Causes of Hypokalemia. There are many other causes of hypokalemia including diarrhea, hypoparathyroidism, licorice addiction (the glycyrrhizic acid acts like aldosterone), small bowel fistula, chronic thiazide diuretic therapy, cirrhosis, and amyloidosis. The differentiation of primary aldosteronism from these causes is usually fairly easy.

TREATMENT. Medical Management. Spironolactone is an antagonist of aldosterone at the level of the kidney tubule but does not alter the production of aldosterone by the adrenal. The use of this substance to treat patients with primary aldosteronism has been summarized by Melby. As the spironolactone reduces serum sodium and elevates serum potassium levels, the hypertension is reduced. This substance does not have a similar effect in patients with secondary aldosteronism. The headaches and nocturnal polyuria vanish.

There are other drugs which act as antagonists to aldosterone, including progesterone and its derivatives. Recently a new heparinlike compound, heparinoid RO1-8307, has been utilized. This compound depresses aldosterone secretion rather than inhibiting its action on the kidney. Since surgical treatment in primary aldosteronism is primarily to correct the hypokalemia and thus prevent continuing damage to the kidney and other organs, these substances may find a place in the permanent treatment of this disease. At present it seems that their chief usefulness might be in patients with primary aldosteronism and mild hypertension who are found to have adrenal hyperplasia rather than a tumor. At the moment, however, the ideal treatment for an adrenal cortical adenoma producing primary aldosteronism is surgical removal, since this is safe and curative, and does not require substitution therapy.

Surgical Therapy. Preoperatively the patient with hyperaldosteronism should be placed on low-sodium, high-potassium intake. The serum potassium level should be raised to 3 mEq/L or more prior to surgical treatment.

Some have advocated the use of spironolactone as pre-operative preparation to aid in raising the plasma potassium level, though we have usually not found this necessary.

Operative Technique. Many prefer a simultaneous bilateral posterior approach for primary aldosteronism. The patients are usually thin, and exposure of the glands is easy. The adenomas are usually relatively small, discrete, smooth, and rounded. The entire gland is removed. The adenomas are seldom bilateral, but the other adrenal should be explored, with care not to injure its blood supply. On rare occasions a heterotopic adrenocortical adenoma causing primary aldosteronism may occur. One such case, in which the adenoma was located in the kidney, has been reported by Flanagan et al.

If no adrenal tumor is palpable at surgery, the adrenal which yielded the higher aldosterone content in its venous blood should be removed. Microscopic adenomas have been found in meticulous serial sections of such glands, and in one of our patients hypertension has resolved. If the sections should ultimately show hyperplasia, spironolactone therapy can easily be instituted.

The importance of obtaining adrenal venous blood samples for the localization of aldosteronomas has been stressed by Melby et al. Egdahl, Kahn, and Melby, using this technique, have been able to localize the site of the tumor in eight consecutive patients prior to operation and in two instances to localize two adenomas which were less than 0.3 cm in diameter. These were not palpable at operation, and could not be identified with certainty until the gland was sectioned after its removal. The increased rate of aldosterone production by these tumors was indicated by incubation studies after removal, which showed that the tumor was producing much more aldosterone than the normal zona glomerulosa of the remainder of the gland. This would certainly seem to be an important adjuvant to the surgical treatment of aldosteronomas, particularly in patients in whom the disease has been discovered very early in its course.

Postoperative Complications. Some writers have described hypoadrenocorticism after removal of one adrenal and exploration of the other. However, this can be avoided at operation by careful handling of the gland.

The blood pressure usually returns to normal in a matter of weeks unless severe renal changes have been present. The serum sodium levels may be low for a time in the postoperative period, but this can be counteracted by giving the patient large amounts of sodium immediately postoperatively (see Fig. 37-38).

ADRENOCORTICAL INSUFFICIENCY (ADDISON'S DISEASE)

Adrenocortical insufficiency is a relatively rare occurrence in the surgical patient, but since failure to recognize it may lead to the death of the patient, it is extremely important that it be kept in mind and recognized early.

ETIOLOGY. Classic Addison's disease in the past has frequently been due to bilateral adrenal tuberculosis, but in recent years with a general decline in tuberculosis bilateral atrophy is a somewhat more common cause. The most frequent cause for the atrophy is apparently an autoimmune mechanism which brings about a self-destruction of the adrenal cortex. Autoantibodies against adrenal tissue can usually be identified in this disease, and other glands are sometimes simultaneously involved with a similar process. There are also other agents which can bring about adrenal destruction, including fungus infection, amyloidosis, vascular lesions, and adrenal hemorrhage. Classic Addison's disease develops slowly and is usually not recognized until it has reached the chronic state.

The combination of Addison's disease and hypothyroidism, presumably on an immunologic basis, has been called "Schmidt's syndrome," although it was described many years earlier. The rather frequent coexistence of Addison's disease and diabetes mellitus has been thought to be due to antibodies to both the corticosteroid-secreting cells of the adrenal and the insulin-secreting islet cells of the pancreas. The frequency of extraadrenal endocrine deficiencies in patients with Addison's disease has recently been studied and in 32 patients was found to be 41 percent. Nineteen percent had diabetes, and 23 percent had primary gonadal disease. While this association is present in idiopathic adrenal insufficiency, presumably due to autoantibodies, it is not present in Addison's disease due to tuberculosis. Hereditary Addison's disease is sometimes associated with hypoparathyroidism or diabetes.

Hereditary, familial, and congenital Addison's disease has been reported, as has congenital absence or marked hypoplasia of the pituitary gland with secondary atrophy of the adrenal. Familial Addison's disease is sometimes associated with spastic paraplegia with or without gliosis of the cerebral hemispheres and with hypoparathyroidism, diabetes, and moniliasis. Hereditary familial adrenal atrophy and fibrosis also occur as an isolated autosomal recessive genetic defect. The adrenogenital syndrome is another congenital defect which may be associated with adrenal insufficiency.

Patients have been reported who show none of the usual stigmata of Addison's disease and who have relatively normal urinary 17-hydroxycorticosteroid excretion but who nonetheless fail to respond normally to ACTH. A 1-hour response of plasma corticosteroids to 25 units of ACTH has recently been reported as a method to detect such patients. A taste test has also been advocated to detect adrenal insufficiency. This is based on the fact that patients with Addison's disease are hypersensitive to the taste of salt and can detect the difference between a 1 mM/L saline solution and distilled water, whereas none of the normal subjects could detect less than 6 mM/L. The patients with Addison's disease also have a hypersensitivity to galvanic current applied to the tongue.

Isolated hypoaldosteronism, a reflection of a renin deficiency syndrome, has been reported by Schambelan et al. In these patients other aspects of adrenal cortical function were normal.

Some toxic substances, such as o,p'-DDD, interfere with adrenal production of corticosteroids and may produce adrenocortical insufficiency. Infection can cause adrenal insufficiency by hemorrhage into the glands or by tubular degeneration of the adrenals. Bilateral adrenal hemorrhage as a consequence of infection, the so-called Waterhouse-Friderichsen syndrome, is usually produced by meningococcal septicemia, and is usually seen in children under the age of two, although it has been described in adults. There is some question whether the patients actually die of adrenal insufficiency or of the effects of the meningococcal septicemia, the adrenal hemorrhage simply being a terminal manifestation of the disease. It seems likely that the latter is more often the case, the adrenal hemorrhage and consequent insufficiency developing so close to the terminal phase as to have little effect on the course of the disease. In adults with severe infection degeneration of the adrenal cortex can occur even without hemorrhage. This again is most commonly seen with meningococcal infections, but it is also occasionally seen with pneumococcal, streptococcal, and diphtherial infections. Adrenal insufficiency is occasionally seen in the severely burned patient with invasive sepsis.

There are four circumstances in which the adrenal can be occasionally destroyed by hemorrhage in addition to sepsis. Bilateral adrenal hemorrhage has been seen in the newborn infant as a consequence of asphyxia, syphilis, or eclampsia of the mother. Hemorrhage and necrosis of the maternal adrenals will occasionally occur during pregnancy, the cause being unknown. Bilateral adrenal hemorrhage has occurred as a consequence of anticoagulant therapy and in some instances has led to the death of the patient from adrenal insufficiency. It has been seen with both Coumadin and heparin. Hemorrhage into an adrenal tumor will occasionally produce destruction of the remainder of the gland; this can produce adrenal insufficiency if the opposite adrenal has been removed or is involved in a similar destructive process. Bilateral adrenal hemorrhage and adrenal insufficiency sometimes occur spontaneously for no discernible reason in patients with chronic illness or with cancer.

The adrenal is not infrequently the site of metastases, particularly from carcinoma of the lung or breast, but it is very rare for these metastases to produce sufficient destruction to lead to adrenal insufficiency.

Surgical excision of the pituitary or adrenal may lead to adrenal insufficiency if the patient's maintenance dose of corticosteroids is too low, if the patient forgets to take his medication, or if the patient is subject to an intercurrent infection or trauma without an increase in the maintenance dose. Patients with Cushing's disease and bilateral total adrenalectomy require more corticosteroid maintenance than patients who have had adrenalectomy for cancer of the breast. The development of adrenal insufficiency in patients who have had subtotal adrenalectomy for Cushing's disease, with uncertain or variable function of the remaining fragment, is one of the reasons why this operation has been largely abandoned in favor of total adrenalectomy with total replacement.

In bilateral pheochromocytoma, a fragment of one or both adrenal cortices, if left behind, will usually maintain the patient. However, temporary Addison's disease may develop until this occurs, and the patient has to be closely watched.

Pituitary insufficiency leads to secondary adrenal insufficiency which is not as severe as that seen in classic Addison's disease. Since aldosterone secretion depends only partially on ACTH stimulation, urinary salt wasting is less likely to occur in patients with pituitary insufficiency than in those with primary adrenal disease. Nevertheless these patients are often hypoglycemic, and they withstand trauma poorly without adequate adrenocortical support therapy. By far the most common cause of adrenal insufficiency at the present time is that secondary to the administration of adrenal corticosteroids. This suppresses the secretion of ACTH and leads to atrophy of the adrenal. After discontinuance of the corticosteroid therapy it may take a long time for adrenal reactivity to return. The patient may therefore have relative adrenal insufficiency if he is operated upon without supportive therapy. If operation is contemplated and the facilities are available, it is wise to carry out an ACTH stimulation test with plasma corticosteroid levels to determine whether the adrenal is reactive or not. If such facilities are not available, it is wise to put the patient on corticosteroid therapy during the acute phase of the operation.

CLINICAL MANIFESTATIONS. Adrenal cortical insufficiency may become apparent in any of four clinical patterns, depending on the time of development. The first of these is adrenal insufficiency appearing shortly after birth as a consequence of the salt-wasting variant of the adrenogenital syndrome. The insufficiency, of the salt-losing type, is manifested by fever, weight loss, vomiting, hyponatremia, shock, and marked salt loss in the urine. Symptoms often appear within the first week after birth and sometimes may not become noticeable for 5 or 6 weeks.

Chronic adrenocortical insufficiency due to classic Addison's disease which has been present for many months or years before operation or trauma is usually recognizable by the characteristic pigmentation, weakness, weight loss, hypotension, easy fatigability, and sometimes nausea, vomiting, abdominal pain, hypoglycemia, hyponatremia, and hyperkalemia. An x-ray of the abdomen may show adrenal calcification if the disease is caused by tuberculosis but will not be suggestive if the disease is due to an autoimmune mechanism. A chest x-ray will usually show reduced heart size. The diagnosis is confirmed by demonstration of reduced urinary corticosteroid excretion and the failure of plasma corticosteroids to increase in response to an infusion of ACTH. If such a patient is operated upon without establishing the diagnosis, death will usually occur within a matter of 3 to 6 hours.

The third form of adrenal insufficiency is acute Addisonian crisis. This may occur in response to injury or operative trauma, or it may occur spontaneously and mimic some other type of acute illness. It is accompanied by fever, shock, lethargy, somnolence or coma, nausea, vomiting, and abdominal pain. If unrecognized and untreated, it may lead to death in a short time. The diagnosis is confirmed by low levels of blood corticosteroid. Hypoglycemia, hyponatremia, and hyperkalemia will usually be present. The electrolyte changes are more apt to occur in the chronic Addisonian patient, whereas if the patient has adrenal insufficiency as a consequence of steroid administration ending in the recent past, the electrolyte changes and shock may not manifest themselves until the preterminal or terminal period.

The fourth type of adrenal insufficiency which is seen surgically is that of semiacute adrenal insufficiency. This is not present prior to operation but develops during surgery or in the immediate postoperative period. It has been seen when anticoagulants are begun in the immediate postoperative period producing bilateral adrenal hemorrhage which destroys the adrenals. It is also occasionally seen in the severely burned patient in whom invasive infection leads to adrenal insufficiency. When the adrenal insufficiency begins with, or immediately after, the operative insult, the symptoms are much slower to develop than when the patient has had preexisting adrenal insufficiency and is then operated upon. Instead of the patient's dying in a matter of hours, the development of symptoms takes place in a matter of days. Insufficiency is usually manifested in convalescence by weakness, abdominal distension, decreased peristalsis, anorexia, nausea, and general lassitude out of proportion to that expected. These symptoms usually begin to appear on the third or fourth postoperative day and gradually become worse during the next 3 or 4 days. If the condition is unrecognized and untreated, death is apt to ensue in about 7 to 10 days. There is a progressive hypoglycemia and hyponatremia, and the hyponatremia continues in spite of the intravenous administration of large amounts of saline solution. It is accompanied by massive urinary sodium loss. The diagnosis is made by measuring the 24-hour urinary sodium to document the marked salt wasting. This can be immediately corrected by deoxycorticosterone, and the response to this drug is a diagnostic finding. The further demonstration that the patient is unresponsive to ACTH clinches the diagnosis. The adrenal insufficiency is usually permanent.

Adrenal hemorrhage and infarction are sometimes seen as a consequence of adrenal vein thrombosis after adrenal venograms. A review of bilateral adrenal hemorrhage has been published by Jagatic and Rubnitz. The hemorrhages have occurred in response to involution and destruction of the glands in newborn babies, capillary wall damage, accompanying toxemia, various hemorrhagic disorders, adrenal vein thrombosis, electric shock therapy, pregnancy and delivery, anticoagulant therapy, exogenous corticosteroid therapy, and aortic aneurysms with arterial and venous thromboses of the adrenal vessels. The suggestion also has been made that irritation of the hypothalamus due to intracranial surgical procedures might lead to adrenal hemorrhage.

SURGICAL COMPLICATIONS
OF ADRENAL STEROID THERAPY

At the other extreme of the scale from Addison's disease are the problems that arise not from too little adrenal secretion but from the administration of excessive doses of adrenal steroids. The surgical complications of massive adrenal steroid therapy have been summarized by Glenn and Grafe. These writers reported 53 patients who required surgical treatment for a total of 109 complications. Rheumatoid arthritis, ulcerative colitis, and disseminated

lupus erythematosus were the most common diseases under treatment. Ten percent of the total did not have valid indications for adrenal steroid therapy.

Ulcers of the stomach and duodenum were the lesions most frequently encountered, 41 of the 53 patients having developed this complication. The ulcers were gastric in 23, of which 12 were single and 11 multiple. All occurred in the antrum. Eighteen patients had duodenal ulcers all in the first portion of the duodenum except for one. Fourteen females and nine males had gastric ulcers, and twelve males and six females had duodenal ulcers. There were 11 perforations of gastroduodenal ulcers, 2 of esophageal ulcers, 5 of small bowel ulcers, and 3 of large bowel ulcers. Acute pancreatitis was seen in two patients activation of pulmonary tuberculosis in two, and empyema in one. There were seven small bowel ulcers and three large bowel ulcers.

Although it has been claimed that the incidence of peptic ulcer is no higher in patients being treated with steroids for rheumatoid arthritis than it is in the general population, others have found a considerably higher incidence. This experience certainly points up the necessity for the withholding of corticosteroid therapy unless there is a specific well-established reason for it. It is of particular note that none of the patients in this series had complications within the first week of corticosteroid therapy.

Adrenal Medulla

The adrenal medulla gives rise primarily to two types of tumors, the pheochromocytomas, which are well differentiated, are metabolically mature, and occur primarily in adults, and the neuroblastomas, which are immature, are metabolically primitive, are virtually always malignant, and occur primarily in early childhood.

PHYSIOLOGY

Three catecholamines are found in adrenergically innervated human tissues—epinephrine, norepinephrine, and dopamine. These compounds are found in chromaffin cells of the sympathetic nervous system, which includes the adrenal medulla, aberrant tissue along the sympathetic chain, and paraganglia. Norepinephrine and dopamine are found at the endings of the postganglionic fibers of the sympathetic system and in the central nervous system. Dopamine is found in several other locations, notably the kidney, liver, and lungs.

In the embryo the chromaffin cells are widely distributed in the adrenal medulla, the sympathetic ganglia, the paraganglia, which lie along the sympathetic chain, and the organs of Zuckerkandl, which are paraganglia lying along the abdominal aorta with particular concentration in the region of the inferior mesenteric artery. The organs of Zuckerkandl usually degenerate shortly after birth. The fetal adrenal and the organs of Zuckerkandl contain norepinephrine only, epinephrine appearing some time after birth. In the adult the great majority of chromaffin cells are concentrated in the adrenal medulla, although small collections may be found along the aorta, particularly in the remnants of the organs of Zuckerkandl, in the walls of blood vessels, and scattered through various organs—especially the heart, prostate, and ovary. Aberrant collections of chromaffin tissue may persist in the adult and may be the site for the development of a pheochromocytoma.

The principal pathway for the production of epinephrine from phenylalanine and tyrosine is shown in Fig. 37-40. Norepinephrine is the immediate precursor of epinephrine and thus has a dual role, as a hormone and neurotransmitter and as an intermediate in the production of epinephrine. The proximity of adrenal cortex and medulla is functionally important. The N-methylation of norepinephrine to form epinephrine is promoted by the enzyme phenylethanolamine-N-methyltransferase (PNMT). PNMT requires adrenal steroids for its physiologic function. In man and in some other species there is an adrenal portal venous drainage system. This delivers large quantities of cortical steroids to the adrenal medulla. Norepinephrine and dopamine are therefore the catecholamines principally found in extraadrenal locations. Thus while norepinephrine is present in normal or slightly increased amounts in the urine of patients who have undergone bilateral adrenalectomy, epinephrine is markedly reduced. The epinephrine still present is presumed to come from chromaffin cells located in various organs and, over a period of time, can begin to produce increasing amounts of epinephrine as well as norepinephrine. Therefore, whereas the urine of patients who have undergone bilateral adrenalectomy is virtually devoid of epinephrine in the early postoperative period, it may contain appreciable but subnormal amounts of epinephrine from 6 months to 3 years later.

All three catecholamines are found in the adrenal medulla (epinephrine and norepinephrine being present usually in amounts of 0.5 to 1 mg/Gm of tissue) and physiologically are released in response to a wide variety of sensitive reflex stimuli, including body tilting, blood volume contraction, psychic arousal, and consciousness.

It has been recognized that when epinephrine and norepinephrine are injected intravenously, only small amounts appear in the urine, most of the urinary excretion consisting of various metabolites—primarily metanephrine, normetanephrine, and VMA (vanilmandelic acid, or 4-hydroxy-3-methoxymandelic acid). A simplified scheme of epinephrine and norepinephrine metabolism together with the relative amounts of these substances usually found in the blood and urine is shown in Fig. 37-41. Most commonly urinary catecholamines are measured for the diagnosis of benign pheochromocytoma. Epinephrine, norepinephrine, and VMA formerly were used for this purpose. More recently determinations of metanephrine and normetanephrine have been the most useful diagnostic adjuncts. Recently rare cases of pheochromocytoma have been found in which no convincing elevations of urinary catecholamine and metanephrine levels have appeared. Repeated study on different days, measurement of plasma norepinephrine and epinephrine before and after glucagon stimulation, and rarely abdominal exploration are necessary to resolve the problem.

While the metabolism of dopamine regularly leads to

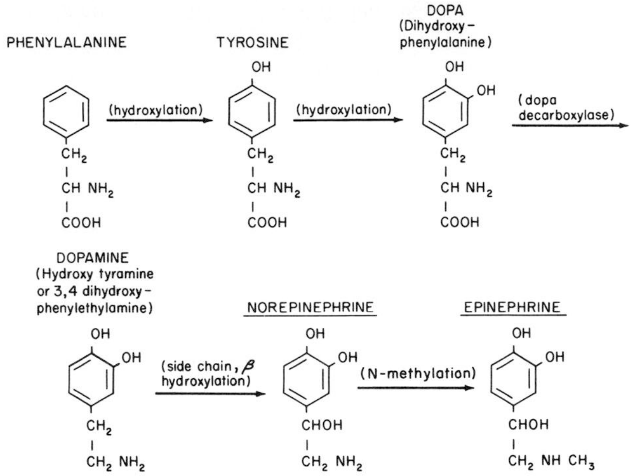

Fig. 37-40. Main pathway for the formation of epinephrine and norepinephrine. (*After Blaschko et al.*)

the production of norepinephrine, epinephrine, and their metabolites, an alternative route is available by means of which 3-methoxytyramine and homovanillic acid (HVA) are formed, as shown in Fig. 37-42. It was first suggested in 1956 that malignant pheochromocytomas may selectively secrete dopamine, though this was not confirmed by studies in 1961 of the primary growth of a malignant pheochromocytoma. Robinson et al. found large amounts of dopamine metabolites in the urine of a patient with a malignant pheochromocytoma. Increased secretion of dopamine metabolites was not found in patients with benign pheochromocytoma, and their presence was thought to be a valuable indication of malignancy. Subsequently many benign pheochromocytomas have been found to secrete dopamine and its metabolites.

Functionally active neuroblastomas secrete catecholamine metabolites which are very similar to those seen in the patient with the malignant pheochromocytoma, thus reflecting both their biochemical immaturity and their malignancy. These patients secrete large amounts of dopamine metabolites as well as norepinephrine metabolites. Neuroblastoma patients almost never form epinephrine in their tumors.

In addition to the well-known ability of epinephrine to promote glycogenolysis in muscle and liver it has a profound effect on lipid metabolism. Although the carbohydrate effects of catecholamines are limited primarily to epinephrine, both epinephrine and norepinephrine have the ability to release free fatty acids from adipose tissue by means of lipolysis, thus markedly increasing the blood level of nonesterified fatty acids. In patients with pheochromocytoma the blood levels of nonesterified fatty acids may be several hundred times normal, and serum cholesterol and phosphatide levels also may be high. The lipid-mobilizing effects of epinephrine and norepinephrine are opposed by the prostaglandins.

The effects of epinephrine on blood pressure, uterine motility, heat production, and glucose metabolism are all increased by thyroid hormone. The α- and β-adrenergic

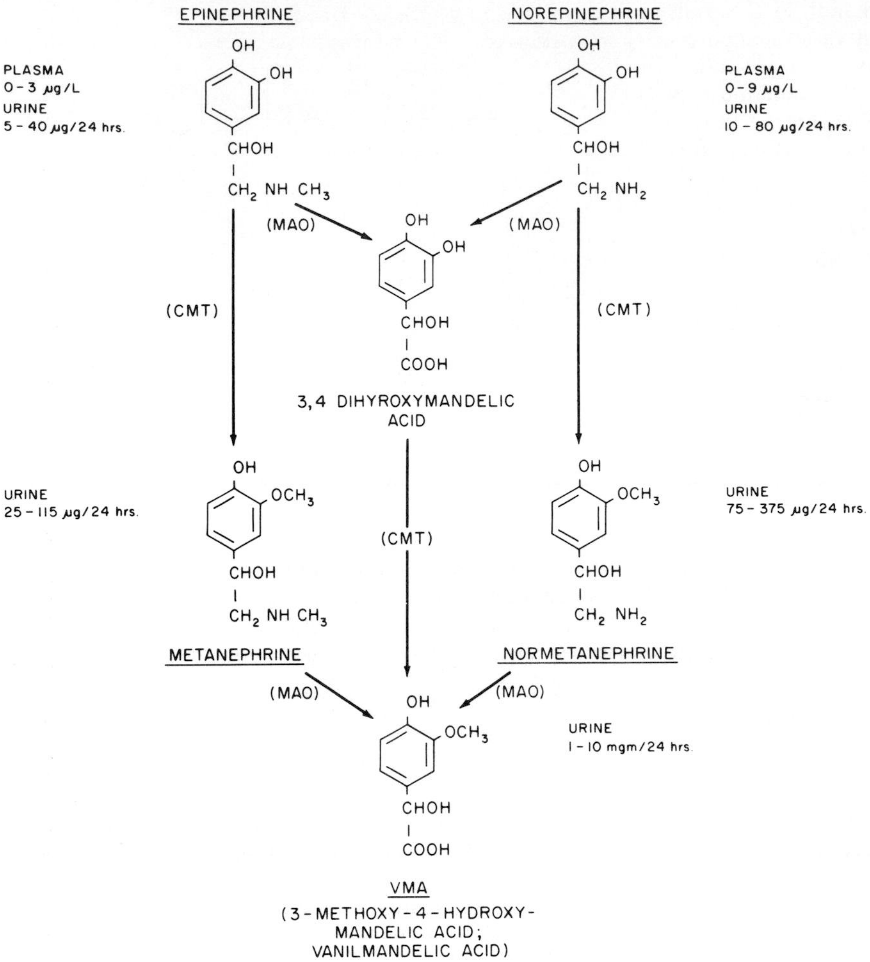

Fig. 37-41. Some of the principal metabolites of epinephrine and norepinephrine, with the urinary values for the commonly measured ones. MNO stands for monoamine oxidase, and CMT stands for catecholamine methyl transferase. (*After Kopin et al., Res Publ Assoc Res Nerv Ment Dis. 43:343, 1966.*)

effects of the catecholamines are outlined in Table 37-13. Some conditions characterized by altered sensitivities to catecholamines are shown in Table 37-14.

PHEOCHROMOCYTOMA

Pheochromocytomas are functionally active chromaffin tumors which may be located in the adrenal medulla or other sites where sympathetic ganglia or chromaffin tissue are known to exist. They are of particular interest because of their tendency to produce large amounts of catecholamines, primarily norepinephrine with or without epinephrine and, uncommonly, predominantly epinephrine.

CLINICAL PICTURE. Incidence. The incidence of pheochromocytoma in autopsy cases was reported by Minno et al. to be 15 out of 15,934, or 0.1 percent. In one study, eight unsuspected pheochromocytomas were found in the course of 1,700 splanchnicectomies performed for hypertension, an incidence of 0.7 percent. In three additional cases the diagnosis was made preoperatively. On the basis of this observation, Graham suggested that there should be about 600 to 800 new cases a year in the United States. Kvale et al. reported an incidence of 2 percent in 900 patients studied for hypertension and also reported the discovery of 51 patients with pheochromocytoma in 7,993 patients screened with pharmacologic tests and blood catecholamines for hypertension, an incidence of 0.64 percent. Hume found one pheochromocytoma in 317 hypertensive patients screened with urinary catecholamines, an incidence of 0.32 percent, and subsequent to this the incidence has been 0.4 percent, nine pheochromocytomas having been found in 2,386 patients screened for hypertension with urinary catecholamine determination (Table 37-15).

Folger et al. found 21 pheochromocytomas in 31,227 autopsies at the Johns Hopkins Hospital, an incidence of 0.07 percent. In Holland the autopsy incidence was found to be 0.02 percent, while the incidence in hypertensive patients was thought to be roughly 0.6 percent.

Pheochromocytomas have been reported in persons from five months to eighty-two years of age. The maximal incidence is between the ages of twenty and fifty. A pheochromocytoma should be suspected and searched for in hypertensive patients who show any of the findings listed in Table 37-16.

Location of Tumors. A predilection for the right adrenal

Table 37-13. CLASSIFICATION OF α- AND β-ADRENERGIC EFFECTS OF
CATECHOLAMINES

Effects	*Alpha** *(norepinephrine)*	*Beta†* *(isoproterenol)*	*Epinephrine*	*Dopamine*
Vasoconstriction	0	+	+	
Vasodilatation	0	+	−	+
Increase in systolic blood pressure . .	+	±	+	
Increase in diastolic blood pressure . . .	+	0	0	
Vascular:				
Increase in hepatic and muscle blood flow.	0	+	+	
Cardiac:				
Increase in coronary flow	+	+	0	
Increase in heart rate.	0	+	+	
Increase in atrial contracility and conduction rate	0	+	+	
Increase in conduction velocity of AV node.	0	+	+	
Increase in cardiac output	0	+	+	+
Pulmonary:				
Dilatation of bronchial musculature	0	+	+	
Metabolic:				
Increase in fasting blood glucose and free fatty acid levels	±	+	+	0
Increase in BMR	±	+	+	0

* α blockers: phenoxybenzamine (Dibenzyline), dibenamine, phentolamine (Regitine).
† β blockers: dichloroisoproterenol, pronethalol, and propranalol.

Table 37-14. SOME CONDITIONS CHARACTERIZED
BY ALTERED SENSITIVITY TO
CATECHOLAMINES

Conditions associated with increased sensitivity:
  Cardiomegaly
    Congestive heart failure
    Hypertrophy—secondary to physical obstruction or increase
      in peripheral vascular resistance
    Myocardiopathy of various causes
  Thyrotoxicosis
  Sympathetic denervation
    Diabetes mellitus
    Surgical or anesthetic procedures
    Orthostatic hypotension
  Nutritional abnormalities
    Scurvy
  Unclassified diseases
    β-Adrenergic hyperresponders
    Familial dysautonomia
  Drugs
    Imipramine
    Some antiadrenergic drugs (e.g., guanethidine and reserpine)
Conditions associated with decreased sensitivity:
  Acidosis—metabolic or respiratory
  Myxedema
  Adrenal insufficiency
Conditions associated with paradoxical effects:
  Diseases
    Carcinoid syndrome
  Drug administration
    Phenothiazine and congeners

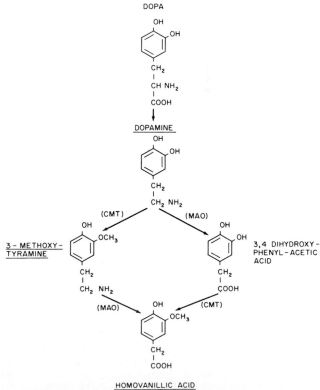

Fig. 37-42. Some of the metabolites of dopamine. MAO stands for monoamine oxidase, and CMT stands for catecholamine methyl transferase.

Table 37-15. MEAN FREE URINARY LEVELS IN NONPHEOCHROMOCYTOMA
HYPERTENSIVE PATIENTS AND IN PHEOCHROMOCYTOMA

	Normal (n = 100)	*Pheochromocytoma* (n = 63)
Norepinephrine	28.9* ± 29.0† (P < 0.001)	1250 ± 2456
Epinephrine	7.6 ± 7.4 (P < 0.001)	238 ± 408
	Normal (n = 37)	*Pheochromocytoma* (n = 29)
Normetanephrine	44.2 ± 38.9 (P < 0.001)	1127 ± 842
Metanephrine	32.9 ± 16.4 (P < 0.001)	1305 ± 1708

* All urinary values in micrograms per 24 hr.
† ± 1 Standard deviation.
SOURCE: From Freier and Harrison, *J Surg Res,* **14:**177, 1973.

is a constant finding. This predilection for the right side is even more pronounced in children, in whom the right adrenal is involved twice as often as the left.

Seven percent of tumors are bilateral in adults, while twenty-four percent are bilateral in children (Table 37-17). Nine percent of all tumors, in adults and children, are bilateral. When the familial cases are excluded (one-half are bilateral), only 5.3 percent are bilateral in adults. Abdominal pheochromocytomas are commonly located in the adrenal medulla, the extraadrenal paraganglia, the organs of Zuckerkandl, and the bladder, in that order. Extraabdominal tumors may be located in the thorax or neck (Fig. 37-43). The tumors range in size from tiny nodules up to 3,600 Gm. Some large tumors have relatively little function.

Malignant Pheochromocytomas. The incidence of malignancy in pheochromocytoma is about 10 percent or less. Many of these tumors appear malignant histologically, even with venous invasion, without ever subsequently demonstrating a true malignant potential. Some arise from multicentric though benign origins. The only acceptable criterion of malignancy, therefore, is definitive evidence of metastases to sites not usual for chromaffin tissue. Using

Table 37-16. CONDITIONS WHICH SUGGEST
PHEOCHROMOCYTOMA IF PRESENT IN
THE HYPERTENSIVE PATIENT

1. Any sort of "attack," with or without precipitating stress
2. Diabetes or elevated fasting blood sugar level, especially between the ages of twenty and fifty
3. An elevated BMR (and normal RAI)
4. Childhood—in the absence of renal disease or coarctation
5. Postural hypotension, excessive sweating, an elevated temperature, frequent headaches, or vasomotor phenomena
6. Pregnancy with sweating, vomiting, and headaches or shock or hypertension during delivery
7. Neurofibromatosis
8. Familial history of pheochromocytoma
9. A previously removed pheochromocytoma
10. Weight loss or failure to gain weight if patient is already thin
11. Recent onset of hypertension with severe retinopathy

this criterion the incidence has varied from 2.8 to 14.5 percent.

The metastases are frequently functional, and the symptoms of pheochromocytomas recur as the lesions spread. The metastases may be more primitive than the primary tumor and produce metabolic products of dopamine in addition to those of epinephrine and norepinephrine. The presence, therefore, of large amounts of 3-methoxytyramine and HVA in addition to VMA is highly suggestive of the presence of metastases.

The incidence of malignancy in childhood is not low, which is of interest in view of the almost complete restriction to childhood of neuroblastomas—a highly malignant neural crest tumor closely related to pheochromocytoma even in regard to the secretion of catecholamines or their metabolic products. Malignant tumors can occur in pheochromocytomas of the organs of Zuckerkandl or bladder as well as in those of adrenal origin and may be nonfunctioning. Malignant pheochromocytomas are relatively radioresistant, and prognosis is generally poor.

Signs, Symptoms, and Pathophysiology. The hypertension associated with pheochromocytomas may be paroxysmal, sustained, or absent. In adult patients the hypertension is sustained in about 65 percent, paroxysmal in about 30 percent, and absent in about 5 percent, whereas in children about 92 percent show sustained hypertension and 8 percent paroxysmal.

Typical paroxysmal attacks usually consist of severe headaches, palpitation, profuse sweating, nausea and vomiting, pallor, epigastric or substernal pain, dyspnea, vertigo, apprehension or fear of impending death, and visual difficulties, in that order. Sometimes only one or two of these symptoms are present.

A list of the symptoms and signs is shown in Table 37-18. The general symptom complexes with pheochromocytoma are shown in Table 37-19. Nausea, weight loss, abdominal pain, visual changes, and convulsions are more common in children. Attacks may last from a few moments to many hours, and they may occur several times a day or only once every year or two. They are often precipitated by emotional upsets, change in position, intercourse, physical

Table 37-17. LOCATION OF TUMORS

Location	Adult*		Child	
	No.	Percent	No.	Percent
Total cases	207		76	
Right adrenal	92	44.5	25	33
Left adrenal	70	33.8	11	14.5
Bilateral.	18	8.7	15	19.7
Bilateral plus extraadrenal	...	....	3	4.0
Right side, extraadrenal. .	7	3.4	1	1.3
Left side, extraadrenal . .	5	2.4	6	7.9
Adrenal and extraadrenal .	1	0.5	7	9.2
Multiple.	3	1.5	4	5.3
Aorta (organs of Zuckerkandl)	8	3.8	3	3.8
Intrathoracic	2	0.9	1	1.3
Celiac ganglion	1	0.5		

	Adult, percent	Child† percent	Familial† percent
Bilateral.	9 } 10.5	24 } 39	50
Multiple.	1.5	15	9
Extraadrenal	11.5	15	14
Total percent	22	54	73

Bilateral, familial, neurofibromatosis† (1960)

	Adult		Child	
	No.	Percent	No.	Percent
Total cases	543		83	
Bilateral.	38	7	18	24
Familial.	14	2.6	8	10
Familial bilateral	9	1.7	2	2.4
Bilateral, not familial . . .	29	5.3	16	21
Neurofibromatosis	26	4.8	1	1.4

*From J. B. Graham, Int Abstr Surg, **92:**105, 1951.
†See D. M. Hume, Am J Surg, **99:**458, 1960.

effort, trauma, sneezing, eating, urination, or anesthesia and operation. The attack often ends with profuse diaphoresis and a feeling of fatigue or even prostration. Attacks are usually accompanied by increases in blood sugar, body temperature, and blood and urinary catecholamines. The first sign may be sudden death, or the patient may have symptoms for as long as 32 years or more. Some patients with paroxysmal attacks early in their course may develop sustained hypertension later on or may continue to have only paroxysmal attacks for many years. If the hypertension is sustained, very advanced hypertensive retinopathy may develop.

There are other conditions which may produce paroxysms of hypertension not unlike those seen with pheochromocytoma. The most common among these include renovascular hypertension, angina pectoris, anxiety states, eclampsia, hysteria, migraine, neurosis, periarteritis nodosa,

thyroid crisis, toxemia, tumors of the brain, and diencephalic epilepsy. Recently monamine oxidase inhibitors have been shown occasionally to produce attacks simulating pheochromocytoma, including headaches, pallor, vomiting, and blood pressure elevation. These attacks are precipitated or exacerbated by cheese, which contains tyramine, a strong stimulant to catecholamine secretion, the effect of which is potentiated by monoamine oxidase inhibitors.

Most functioning pheochromocytomas secrete increased amounts of norepinephrine. About one-half of these secrete epinephrine as well. Uncommonly, most (80 percent) of the secreted catecholamine is epinephrine. These lesions are almost exclusively confined to the adrenal medulla.

Because epinephrine is a more metabolically active compound than norepinephrine, it has commonly been assumed that those patients with pheochromocytoma having marked metabolic manifestations and cardiac arrhythmias are epinephrine secretors. However, this assumption is incorrect. While the BMR is elevated in 50 percent of patients with pheochromocytoma, it is significant that Gifford et al. found it to be elevated nearly three times as

Fig. 37-43. Location of pheochromocytomas in ectopic sites. About 10 to 15 percent of pheochromocytomas are located in ectopic sites with principal concentration in the areas shown.

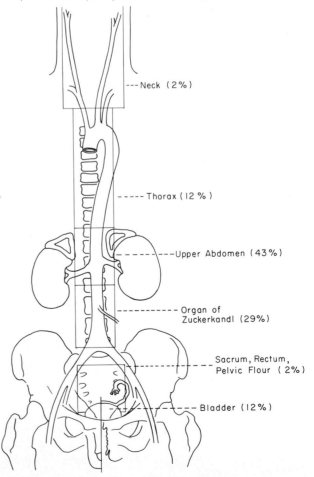

Neck (2%)

Thorax (12%)

Upper Abdomen (43%)

Organ of Zuckerkandl (29%)

Sacrum, Rectum, Pelvic Flour (2%)

Bladder (12%)

Table 37-18. SYMPTOMS AND SIGNS
OF PHEOCHROMOCYTOMA

	Approximate percent	
	Adult	*Child*
Symptoms:		
Persistent hypertension	65	92
Paroxysmal hypertension	30	8
Headache	80	81
Sweating	70	68
Palpitation, nervousness	60	34
Pallor of face	40	27
Tremor	40	
Nausea	30	56
Weakness, fatigue	25	27
Weight loss	15	44
Abdominal or chest pain	15	35
Dyspnea	15	16
Visual changes	10	44
Constipation	5	8
Raynaud's phenomenon	5	
Convulsions	3	23
Polydipsia, polyuria	..	25
Puffy, red, cyanotic hands	..	11
Signs:		
BMR over +20 percent	50	83
Fasting blood sugar over 120 mg/100 ml	40	40
Glycosuria	10	3
Eye ground changes	30	70

SOURCE: From D. M. Hume, E. B. Astwood, and C. E. Cassidy,
Grune & Stratton, Inc., 1968.

Table 37-19. SYMPTOM COMPLEXES
OF PHEOCHROMOCYTOMA

1. Symptom-free patients, with pheochromocytoma an incidental or accidental finding
2. Symptom-free patients who die suddenly after minor trauma
3. Patients with typical attacks
4. Patients with sustained hypertension indistinguishable clinically from essential or renal vascular hypertension
5. "Diabetics," with or without hypertension
6. Patients with headaches (migraine or other), fever, and nausea, or the metabolic changes of pheochromocytoma, without either sustained or paroxysmal hypertension
7. Patients who present with "hyperthyroidism," especially if BMR does not fall with treatment, RAI and PBI are normal, and patient has hypertension
8. Patients with unexplained shock during anesthesia or minor trauma
9. Patients with cardiac irregularities, tachycardia, or arrest with induction of anesthesia or beginning of operation
10. Patients whose symptoms simulate an acute anxiety attack
11. Patients who have attacks when voiding—occasionally occurs with pheochromocytoma in bladder

SOURCE: From D. M. Hume, E. B. Astwood, and C. E. Cassidy,
Grune & Stratton, Inc., 1968.

often in patients with persistent hypertension as in those with paroxysmal hypertension. Furthermore, children with pheochromocytomas, who usually have sustained hypertension and in whom the tumors are primarily norepinephrine-secreting, have an elevated BMR in 83 percent of cases. The PBI and uptake of radioiodine (RAI) are usually normal, even when the BMR reaches extremely high levels, and this can be an important diagnostic sign. The fasting blood sugar is elevated in 41 percent of the patients, while during an attack it is elevated in 75 percent. About 10 percent of the patients have frank "diabetes." On rare occasions the metabolic changes of a pheochromocytoma can occur in the absence of hypertension.

It is of note that pheochromocytoma patients demonstrate an increased release of catecholamines in response to the reflex stimulus of the tilt test (Fig. 37-44). We believe this represents release from adrenergic stores that contain greater than normal quantities of catecholamines because of increased uptake from prolonged elevations in circulating catecholamine levels which are seen in pheochromocytoma patients. Hepatic catecholamine content was significantly increased in four of five pheochromocytoma patients in whom we measured it when compared to the hepatic content of catecholamines in patients undergoing uncomplicated cholecystectomy.

From these facts one can form a dynamic picture in pheochromocytoma in which catecholamines are synthesized and released into the circulation with no restraint from the tumor. They are then taken up and stored in greatly increased quantities in adrenergic storage pools, from which they can be released in response to reflex stimulation (Fig. 37-45). The mechanisms no doubt account, at least in part, for the day-to-day variation in catecholamine excretion that occurs in many pheochromocytoma patients.

Patients with pheochromocytoma are usually thin or give a history of having recently lost weight. An occasional obese patient is noted, but this is almost always when paroxysmal rather than sustained hypertension is present.

DIAGNOSTIC FINDINGS. Prior to the advent of techniques for measuring urinary catecholamines several drug tests were developed for the detection of pheochromocytoma. These were based upon a fall in blood pressure with adrenolytic drugs and a rise in blood pressure with drugs which stimulated catecholamine release. For the most part these have been discarded. The phentolamine (Regitine) tests can be used only in patients with sustained hypertension. A positive test consists of a 35/25 mm Hg fall of pressure within 3 to 10 minutes after the intravenous injection of 5 mg of Regitine. False-positive reactions are common, and false-negative reactions are also seen. Deaths have been recorded in pheochromocytoma patients overreacting to the Regitine test.

The histamine test as it was originally described probably no longer has a place. A modification of this test to include the measurement of blood catecholamines is helpful in the rare patient with paroxysmal hypertension who does not have elevated levels of urinary catecholamines. The test is performed between paroxysms, when the blood pressure is fairly normal. After the intravenous injection

INCREASE IN FREE NOREPINEPHRINE EXCRETION AFTER TILT

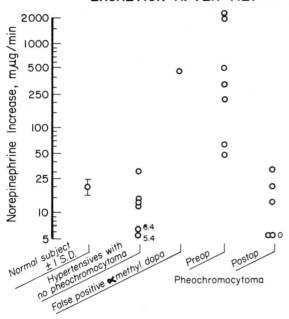

Fig. 37-44. Change in body posture with tilting is an easily reproduced reflex stimulus for catecholamine release. As is apparent in this study, the response is greatly exaggerated in pheochromocytoma. We believe this reflects release of catecholamines from increased peripheral adrenergic stores, and have demonstrated significant increases in hepatic catecholamines in four of five liver biopsies from pheochromocytoma patients. Of added interest is the exaggerated release of α-methyl norepinephrine in a patient receiving α-methyl-dopa treatment. (*By permission from the New England Journal of Medicine, 277:725, 1967.*)

of 0.025 to 0.050 mg of histamine base, blood samples are taken 4 and 6 minutes later. No increase in blood catecholamine levels occurs levels hypertensive patients, while a striking increase occurs in patients with pheochromocytoma. A stimulating test using tyramine has been advocated, but its error rate is unacceptably high. Tyramine proved to have fewer side effects than histamine, but to have only a disappointing 50 percent positive result in patients with pheochromocytoma and paroxysmal hypertension. A glucagon-provocative test advocated by Lawrence produced positive responses in 3 pateints with pheochromocytoma and negative responses in 126 hypertensive patients, but Sheps and Maher found positive responses in only 6 of 11 patients with pheochromocytoma.

It is far better to make the diagnosis of pheochromocytoma by measurement of urinary catecholamines or their metabolites. This was first demonstrated by von Euler, and since then a flood of articles has been published confirming his observations and developing scores of new ways to detect catecholamines in urine. The results of catecholamine determinations in screening hypertensive patients are shown in Table 37-15.

Because the amount of epinephrine and norepinephrine in the urine represents only 4 percent of the secretion of these substances and because in some cases of pheochro-

mocytoma the catecholamines are rapidly metabolized, methods have been developed for the measurement of the metabolites of catecholamines in the urine. α-Methyldopa (Aldomet) is a specific interfering drug in catecholamine determination and must be stopped for at least 3 weeks before collecting urine for analysis. It can interfere with metanephrine and normetanephrine measurements.

Urinary epinephrine and norepinephrine excretion remains a reliable method for the detection of pheochromocytoma, but less so for neuroblastoma or the occasional tumor in which the catecholamines are largely methylated in the tumor or consist principally of dopamine metabolites. The separate detection of urinary epinephrine and norepinephrine is diagnostically helpful and not difficult. The measurement of conjugated epinephrine and norepinephrine extends the usefulness of this determination, since some patients with pheochromocytomas excrete mainly conjugated catecholamines. Urinary VMA is less sensitive, is nonspecific for epinephrine and norepinephrine, requires strict dietary control to avoid interference,

Fig. 37-45. Findings from a pheochromocytoma patient with distinct elevations of urinary norepinephrine (NE) and epinephrine (E) secretion. The caval catheterization values show the highest NE content, 4.9 µg/liter, in the sample representing the tumor, and the highest E content, 4.8 µg/liter, from the left (normal) adrenal. The tumor itself contains only NE. After removal of the tumor, both NE and E excretion returned to normal, 17 and 7 µg/24 hours, respectively. The findings are compatible with release of NE from the tumor, uptake and methylation of NE to form E in the normal left adrenal gland, and subsequent release of increased quantities of E from the left adrenal gland into the circulation and ultimately to the urine. (*By permission from the Johns Hopkins Medical Journal, 139:137, 1976, The Johns Hopkins University Press, Md.*)

CAVAL CATHETERIZATION

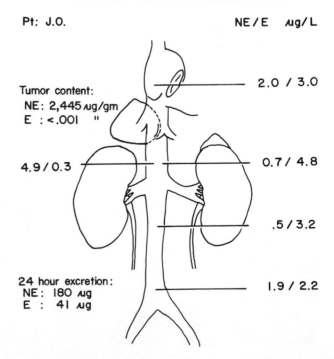

and gives rise to more equivocal results. Tumors other than pheochromocytomas or neuroblastomas can sometimes secrete catecholamines, and increased secretion of these substances may be seen in the absence of tumors. Thus elevated urinary excretion of VMA has been seen in ganglioneuroma, ganglioneuroblastoma, retinoblastoma, carotid body tumor, malignant carcinoid chemodectoma (a glomic tissue tumor which is a "nonchromaffin" paraganglioma), and acrodynia.

HVA, the major end product of dopamine metabolism, is useful primarily in the detection of malignant or dopamine-secreting pheochromocytoma or neuroblastoma. It may also be increased in ganglioneuroma, melanoma, Parkinson's disease, and Wilson's disease. Normal values are frequently found in pheochromocytoma. Elevated levels of metanephrine (M) and/or normetanephrine (NM) are a highly reliable sign of pheochromocytoma, and the measurement of conjugated metanephrines further improves the value of the test.

Although epinephrine, norepinephrine, metanephrine, normetanephrine, and 3-methoxy-4-hydroxyphenylglycol have been detected in tissue from pheochromocytomas, VMA has not, and studies by Sunderman suggest that the liver is the major site for the production of this metabolite.

Patients with neuroblastomas may not have hypertension, despite the excretion of large amounts of catecholamine metabolites. Although an occasional patient with nonmalignant pheochromocytomas will excrete dopamine metabolites, this is unusual, whereas the patients with neuroblastoma characteristically do. Furthermore the patients with neuroblastoma demonstrate a great fluctuation in day-to-day excretion rates, which may be related to the poorer function of cytoplasmic granules than is the case with pheochromocytomas. Gjessing and Hjermann have described three secretion patterns: (1) epinephrine and norepinephrine metabolites in benign pheochromocytoma, (2) dopamine metabolites in ganglioneuroma, and (3) dopa, dopamine, and norepinephrine-epinephrine metabolites in neuroblastoma, with increasing dopa metabolites excretion with increasing malignancy.

As mentioned earlier, a few cases have been reported of pharmacologically active pheochromocytomas in which the urinary epinephrine and norepinephrine, metanephrines, or VMA were near the upper limit of normal. Frequently this dilemma can be resolved by repeated study of resting urinary catecholamine and metanephrine excretion. Also, these patients usually exhibit paroxysmal hypertension and will nearly always show elevated catecholamine levels in plasma after histamine or glucagon stimulation. Forced ventilation will sometimes stimulate an increase in catecholamines, even under these circumstances.

In cases with minimally secreting tumors the excretion of free catecholamines may provide the greatest relative increase over normal values, while in patients in whom catecholamines are being methylated within the tumor metanephrines or VMA may show the greatest relative increase.

Localization. There are four circumstances in which localization of pheochromocytomas may be of importance: extraadrenal (or multiple) pheochromocytomas, which may be difficult to locate, tumors producing narrowing of the renal artery, extraabdominal pheochromocytomas, and functioning metastases.

Localization by retroperitoneal O_2 or CO_2 insufflation has been generally abandoned in the United States because of inconsistency of results, and the combination of this with aortography seems unnecessarily cumbersome. Retroperitoneal CO_2 insufflation with excretory nephrotomography is still used frequently in many European clinics. The intravenous pyelogram may occasionally show the tumor if it is in an adrenal location but is usually of no help in extraadrenal locations, unless the ureter is blocked by the tumor or stenosis of the renal artery results. Photoscanning with iodocholesterol has proved helpful in locating six adrenal pheochromocytomas recently under our care. The lack of uptake and dispersion of the adrenal cortical uptake on the involved side were clear (Fig. 37-46).

Fig. 37-46. *Left,* a typical retrograde venogram of an 11-year-old school boy with hypertension whose brother had multiple pheochromocytomas. This right adrenal tumor measured 5 cm in diameter. *Right,* a radio-iodocholesterol scan of the same patient. Because the image is made from a posterior orientation of the patient to the counter, the image of the right adrenal is that seen to the right of the photo. Dispersion of the adrenocortical tissue on the right indicates a mass in that adrenal which does not take up iodocholesterol. The image of the left adrenal gland is normal, indicating that physiological function of the left adrenal has been preserved.

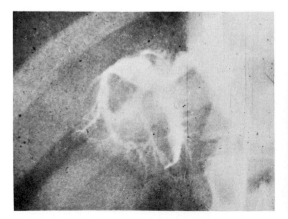
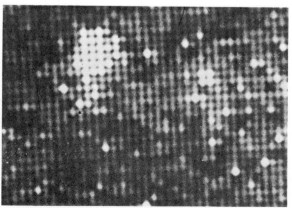

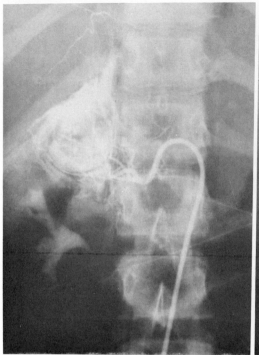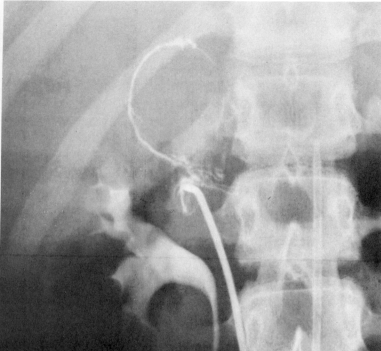

Fig. 37-47. A 16-year-old school girl with episodic hypertension. *Left,* a subselective middle adrenal arteriogram showing a lesion of the inferior portion of the adrenal which displaces the normal gland superiorly. *Right,* a retrograde venogram at a slightly higher magnification showing a beautifully delicate outline of the right adrenal tumor's venous silhouette. The lesion measured 4 cm in diameter and was removed without difficulty. The patient's attacks have completely subsided. (*By permission from T. S. Harrison, D. S. Gann, A. J. Edis, and R. H. Egdahl, "Surgical Disorders of the Adrenal Gland," p. 102, Grune & Stratton, Inc., New York, N.Y., 1975.*)

A chest x-ray will virtually always show the tumor if it is intrathoracic. The peculiar symptomatology of hematuria and hypertensive attacks with micturition may suggest the location of bladder pheochromocytomas, or they may be detected by cystoscopy. Occasionally a plain abdominal x-ray will show calcification in the tumor, or a venacavagram will show infringement by a bulky mass. A palpable mass may be noted in a few abdominal pheochromocytomas and may simplify the location of tumors in the neck. The first pheochromocytoma to be successfully removed (by Roux in February, 1926) was a palpable right adrenal mass the size of "a croquet ball."

It was originally suggested by von Euler that pheochromocytomas secreting epinephrine most likely were located in the adrenal, while those secreting norepinephrine were extraadrenal. Von Euler and Strom reviewed 35 cases of pheochromocytoma and noted several exceptions to this themselves. Actually, if the tumor is producing epinephrine as well as norepinephrine, it often will be located in the adrenal, the only exceptions being a rare epinephrine-producing tumor of the organs of Zuckerkandl, in the mediastinum, or pulmonary metastases secreting epinephrine. If it produces only norepinephrine, a pheochromocytoma will be located in the adrenal in about two-thirds

of the cases and extraadrenal (including the organs of Zuckerkandl) in about one-third. In about 6 percent it will be extraabdominal.

Localization of the primary tumor, recurrences, or metastases can sometimes be achieved by passing a catheter up the inferior vena cava and obtaining blood samples at various levels for catecholamine determination. The highest concentration is seen in relation to the tumor. This is not true for plasma VMA measurements, where the highest concentration is seen in relation to the hepatic veins, presumably because a large fraction of oxidative deamination of the catecholamines occurs in the liver.

Retrograde adrenal venography can often be done in conjunction with inferior vena caval sampling. Blood samples are taken first, and then 3 or 4 ml contrast medium is gently injected retrograde in the adrenal vein. The venous silhouette of the tumor is often clear. Ordinarily there is only a mild pressure response to the injection (Fig. 37-47).

Aortography, often with subtraction techniques, provides another means of localizing pheochromocytomas and has the advantage that it is equally as good for extraadrenal as adrenal tumors (Figs. 37-48 and 37-49). Although deaths have been reported with aortography, the newer methods, which include retrograde aortic catheterization, selective arteriograms, initial injection of small amounts of contrast material, and the availability of drugs to control a hypertensive reaction, appear to be safe in experienced hands.

SPECIAL CONSIDERATIONS. Familial Relationships. Some pheochromocytomas are definitely familial, being inherited by simple mendelian dominance with varying but usually high penetrance. Familial cases differ from sporadic ones in the following ways: They are much more

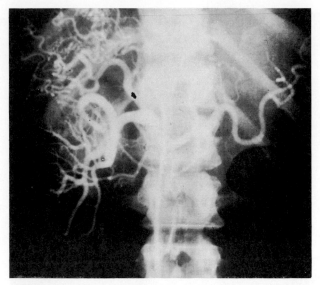

A

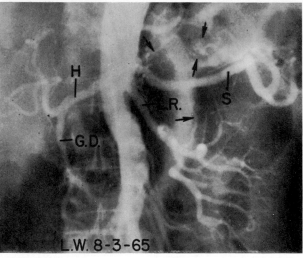

B

Fig. 37-48. Aortography for localization of pheochromocytoma. *A.* Retrograde femoral arteriogram in a patient with a pheochromocytoma of the left adrenal. There is a network of blood vessels supplying the tumor of the left adrenal gland and filling the space just above the left kidney, an arteriogram of which is also shown. *B.* A later picture of the same patient showing contrast material in vessels of the tumor as indicated by the arrows. The blood supply from the aorta and that from the left renal artery can be clearly seen. *S,* splenic artery; *L.R.,* left renal artery; *H,* hepatic artery; *G.D.,* gastroduodenal artery. The patient had congenital absence of the right kidney.

apt to be bilateral and multiple and somewhat more apt to be extraadrenal or extraabdominal (see Table 37-17). They affect children more frequently, and the mean age for familial cases is 26 compared to 37.1 years for sporadic cases. There is a striking predilection for the organs of Zuckerkandl in familial cases, several examples having been reported. Familial adrenal pheochromocytomas are more apt to be on the left, whereas sporadic ones are more

apt to be on the right. Familial cases are associated more frequently with neurocutaneous syndromes, other neural tumors, medullary carcinoma of the thyroid (Sipple's syndrome), and other polyglandular syndromes.

Pheochromocytoma in Pregnancy. Pheochromocytomas become symptomatic during pregnancy, about 80 cases having been reported. The symptoms appear as (1) severe or fatal preeclampsia; (2) typical attacks of paroxysmal hypertension with headache, restlessness, apprehension, sweating, and tachycardia; (3) headaches without hypertension; (4) sudden shock and death in the antepartum period; (5) hyperpyrexia after delivery; or (6) shock after delivery with or without previous symptoms, either spontaneous or induced by anesthesia or delivery.

A patient reported by Pickles had symptoms during three pregnancies, each time, and died immediately after the third delivery. In the patient of Parbossingh and Tate symptoms developed in the last trimester of her sixth pregnancy at twenty-five years of age. She aborted an incarcerated fetus and died. A previous successful pregnancy, with or without symptoms, does not, therefore, preclude the presence of a pheochromocytoma during a subsequent pregnancy. Patients with toxemia, preeclampsia, headaches, or unexplained attacks should be screened for the presence of a pheochromocytoma. Pregnancy per se does not increase urinary catecholamine excretion.

The outcome of pheochromocytoma in pregnancies has been poor, a 48 percent overall mortality being recorded. Walker reported four cases, all with survival of the mother and two with survival of the fetus as well. In three cases of 28, 29, and 30 weeks the tumor was removed during the pregnancy, and two of the patients went on to deliver normal infants by the vaginal route. The fourth patient had a Cesarean section with removal of the tumor. Walker feels that the tumor should be removed as soon as the diagnosis is made, instead of waiting if the diagnosis is made during the last trimester. An alternative approach is the intelligent use of α- and β-adrenergic receptor blockade through delivery until elective postpartum pheochromocytoma excision is carried out.

Barzel et al. measured norepinephrine in maternal and cord blood and noted results which suggested a placental barrier, presumably enzymatic, to norepinephrine transfer. Five times more VMA and ten times less norepinephrine have been noted in cord blood than in maternal blood. This also suggests that the placental barrier is enzymatic in nature, and, indeed, monoamine oxidase has been demonstrated in the human placenta.

Malignant tumors may occur in pheochromocytomas during pregnancy, and the tumors may be familial or bilateral. Several of the cases have been located in the organs of Zuckerkandl.

Neurocutaneous Syndromes. Multiple neurofibromatosis (von Recklinghausen's disease) occurs in about 5 percent of patients with pheochromocytoma. Other neurocutaneous syndromes are related to the occurrence of pheochromocytoma, including café au lait spots, tuberous sclerosis (Bourneville's disease), meningofacial angiomatosis (Sturge-Weber disease). Other neural tumors such as ependymoma of the cord, meningioma of the foramen magnum, and schwannoma have also been reported in patients with pheochromocytoma.

Shocket and Teloh reported a patient in whom there was an association of pheochromocytomas with several neural abnormalities including aganglionic megacolon, megalo-ureter, and neurofibroma. Megacolon has been seen by others. Williams and Pollack reported two cases with multiple unusual neuromas, pheochromocytoma, and thyroid cancer.

Congenital Heart Disease. Folger et al. first reported the association of pheochromocytoma and congenital heart disease, although the association of other endocrine tumors with congenital heart disease had previously been noted. They rejected a congenital cause for the pheochromocytomas associated with congenital heart disease on the basis that clinical manifestations of the tumor did not appear until the ages of twelve to forty-one years. However, there would seem to be strong evidence for a familial (genetic) rather than chronic stimulatory cause for these cases. This has been detailed by Hume.

Pheochromocytoma and Medullary Carcinoma of the Thyroid. In 1961 Sipple first published an article drawing attention to the association of pheochromocytomas with thyroid carcinoma—a syndrome now associated with his name. Since then other features of the syndrome have become apparent: (1) the thyroid cancer is virtually always a medullary cancer of the type described by Hazard et al.; (2) the adrenal tumors are frequently bilateral (65 percent), as they are in familial cases; (3) there is a strong familial history of pheochromocytoma (35 percent) and of medullary carcinoma of the thyroid (35 percent); (4) there is sometimes an association with multiple neural tumors or parathyroid adenomas, suggesting a relation to the multiple endocrine adenoma syndrome, although Williams points out that "multiple adenomas," which is taken to mean the association of pituitary, pancreatic, parathyroid, and occasionally adrenal cortical adenomas, have never been associated either with medullary carcinoma of the thyroid or pheochromocytoma. The parathyroid adenomas associated with thyroid carcinoma and pheochromocytoma do not, therefore, constitute a part of the former syndrome, which seems to originate from a diffuse neoplasia of the involved glands, with adenoma formation. In general the hyperparathyroidism of Sipple's syndrome (MEA-II) is milder than that seen in MEA-I.

Nourok found bilateral pheochromocytomas and medullary cancer in both mother and daughter, and Huang and McLeish reported three members of the same family with pheochromocytomas (two of them bilateral) and medullary thyroid cancer. Sapira et al. points out that the thyroid and adrenal medulla appear at similar periods, embryologically, and that both require tyrosine as the precursor of their respective hormones. The above findings taken together strongly suggest a common familial cause for medullary cancer of the thyroid and the associated pheochromocytoma.

It is felt by Schimke and Hartmann that the association of thyroid cancer and pheochromocytomas may depend upon a single gene, and the occasional additional association of parathyroid adenoma may represent pleiotropism.

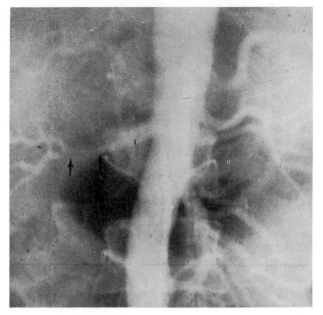

A

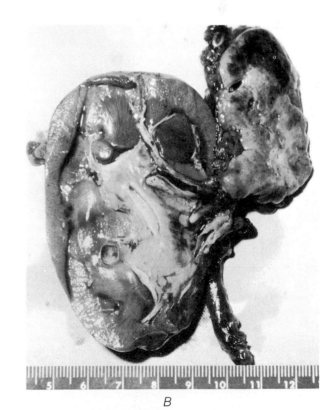

B

Fig. 37-49. Pheochromocytoma producing renal artery stenosis. *A.* Aortogram showing a marked constriction of the terminal portion of the right renal artery indicated between the two arrows. The patient had severe hypertension. *B.* Cut section of the kidney in pheochromocytoma showing the tumor closely applied to the terminal portion of the right renal artery.

These writers mention an unpublished case where bilateral pheochromocytoma, neurofibromatosis, and medullary cancer of the thyroid all coexisted, lending some credence to the genetic or embryologic theories.

Relation of Pheochromocytoma to Other Glands. Apart from the relation to thyroid cancer just discussed, pheochromocytomas may occasionally be associated with other endocrine abnormalities. Thus pheochromocytomas have been seen in association with acromegaly, adrenocortical hyperplasia, Cushing's disease and hyperaldosteronism, and parathyroid adenoma. Pheochromocytomas occasionally have been observed to produce cortisol, to inhibit insulin secretion, and to metabolize 17 β-estradiol.

Although the hypermetabolism seen in patients with pheochromocytoma is characteristically associated with an elevated BMR and normal RAI and PBI, a case has been reported in which the RAI was increased.

Pheochromocytoma, Cholelithiasis, and Increase in Free Fatty Acids. There have been a series of reports from the Mayo Clinic mentioning the high incidence (40 percent) of cholelithiasis in patients with pheochromocytoma. No explanation is offered, and this finding is not stressed by other writers. A possible explanation is that both epinephrine and norepinephrine stimulate the release of free fatty acids from adipose tissue, and elevated levels of free fatty acids are regularly seen in patients with pheochromocytoma. These elevations are directly correlated with the BMR.

Pheochromocytoma and Renovascular Hypertension. Extraadrenal pheochromocytomas, which constitute only 10 to 15 percent of the total group, are most commonly located in proximity to the kidneys, the organs of Zuckerkandl, the mediastinum, and the bladder, in that order. Those located on, or adjacent to, the renal artery may be associated with, or produce, renovascular hypertension. Harrison et al. reported a case in which renal hypertension persisted after excision of three pheochromocytomas, ultimately requiring a nephrectomy on that side for relief of hypertension. Rosenheim et al. reported two patients with unilateral renal ischemia due to compression of the renal artery by the pheochromocytoma. Both were treated by removal of the tumor and simultaneous nephrectomy. Hume had an identical case treated in the same manner (Fig. 37-49). Garret et al. reported a case treated by excision of the tumor and patch grafting of the renal artery stenosis, but there was no compression of the artery in his patient. It was postulated that the proximity of a norepinephrine-secreting tumor might have accounted for the changes in the arterial wall, though this seems somewhat unlikely, particularly in that case.

Straube and Hodges reported a case in which the tumor surrounded the renal artery. A portion of the artery was sacrificed and replaced by a Dacron graft. Kerzner et al. reported a patient treated by nephrectomy in an identical twin, the other twin being completely normal.

It is now established that plasma renin activity is raised in many pheochromocytoma patients who do not have renal artery lesions. This phenomenon is believed to be related to intense intrarenal vasoconstriction caused by high levels of circulating catecholamines. In one series renin elevation was most marked in patients with norepinephrine-secreting tumors and is decreased toward, but not all the way to, normal by α-adrenergic receptor blockade in pheochromocytoma patients. In a recent report from Germany, elevated plasma renin activity has been correlated with epinephrine-secreting lesions. In a case of malignant hypertension from pheochromocytoma we found the course of hypertension followed the plasma renin activity more closely than it did increased urinary norepinephrine excretion.

Hypotension, Shock, and Sudden Death. Some functional pheochromocytomas are characterized by lack of hypertension, hypotension, or shock and sudden death. These are usually epinephrine-secreting tumors.

In the case described by Parkinson the patient developed attacks of palpitations, headache, sweating, nausea, dyspnea, and abdominal pain on standing. Her initial blood pressure was 100/70, and this later declined to 70/50. She continued to be hypotensive with an occasional hypertensive episode, one of which was precipitated by metaraminol given to raise her blood pressure. At operation she was found to have a left adrenal pheochromocytoma containing large amounts of epinephrine and lesser amounts of norepinephrine.

In the case described by Richmond et al. the patient had recurrent attacks of *hypo*tension down to 70/0, associated with abdominal pain and vomiting. The attacks were preceded by aura of fear and apprehension, and accompanied by pallor and tachycardia, effects characteristic of epinephrine, rather than norepinephrine, excess. The patient had an epinephrine-secreting tumor of the right adrenal.

Abdominal pain and shock may occur as a consequence of sudden hemorrhage into a pheochromocytoma. Huston and Stewart reviewed the cases reported in the literature of four patients who died and one of their own who survived. There was no direct evidence of hyperfunction in this latter case, however, and the patient was obese, the tumor was located in the left paravertebral gutter, and the blood supply was thrombosed. There were no signs or symptoms to suggest functioning pheochromocytoma, except the degree of shock and the difficulty in maintaining blood pressure postoperatively. The other reported cases were all adrenal in origin. McAlister and Koehler reported a case of hemorrhage into a functioning right adrenal pheochromocytoma with shock, in a patient on anticoagulants. The patient was operated upon and survived.

In one group of hospitals two deaths have followed surgical treatment over a 10-year period (about 60,000 operations) in which the patients were found to have unsuspected pheochromocytomas, and these were the only two cases of pheochromocytoma found in those hospitals in that entire time. One patient was a forty-four-year-old thin woman with migraine (which might have been the clue) and a blood pressure of 120/80. She had a benign mass removed from her breast, using thiopentone and suxamethonium induction and nitrous oxide and halothane anesthesia. The pulse was 80, and the anesthesia and operation were uneventful. Fifteen minutes after the end of the operation she became restless and cyanotic, and marked tachycardia developed. Ten minutes later she was seen to be in collapse with pallor, sweating, dyspnea, dilated pupils, tachycardia, and pulmonary edema. Despite supportive measures she died 30 minutes later and was found to have a right adrenal pheochromocytoma at postmortem. An almost identical case has been reported in which the patient also had migraine, took ergotamine, had no hypertension, and died with dyspnea, tachycardia, pupillary dilatation, and peripheral vasoconstriction.

Two contrasting cases were reported by Crockett et al., in which marked hypertension and bradycardia developed upon induction, with subsequent tachycardia, shock, pulmonary edema, ventricular fibrillation, and death. Cyclopropane anesthesia was used for both cases. The pheochromocytoma was in the adrenal in each case.

Pheochromocytoma in Children. There have been about 140 cases of pheochromocytoma reported in children. Hypertension was sustained in 85 percent, the tumors were bilateral in 25 percent, and over 50 percent had bilateral, multiple, or extraadrenal tumors.

The high incidence of bilateral, multiple, and ectopic pheochromocytomas in children, the rapid and intense course often seen, and the preponderance of females (in adults the reverse is true), suggest a pathogenesis in childhood involving factors which are not operative in the adult. The most likely suspects are the advent of puberty and the influence of GH. The cases in females appear to be concentrated around the menarche, 62 percent occurring between the ages of eleven and fifteen, whereas in males the cases were more randomly distributed. Moon et al. injected GH into male rats over a 15-month period. They found that in 9 of 16 rats so injected pheochromocytomas developed, while this tumor was not seen in any of the controls. The tumor formation in the injected rats differed from the controls only with respect to the adrenal medulla. Of the nine pheochromocytomas, five were bilateral. Pheochromocytomas have been seen in association with acromegaly. Thus both the onset of puberty and the presence of GH may be factors leading to the appearance of pheochromocytoma in childhood. Ten percent of childhood cases are familial, while this is true for only 2.6 percent of adult cases (Table 37-17), so that a genetic cause is more commonly seen in the young.

Special Locations. There are four locations for pheochromocytoma about which specific references are often made: (1) bilateral, (2) intrathoracic, (3) the organs of Zuckerkandl, and (4) the bladder.

Bilateral Pheochromocytomas. Bilateral adrenal pheochromocytoma is an important entity because of its frequent occurrence in childhood (one-fourth of cases), its relatively high mortality, its familial relationship, and the surgical problems it poses, particularly the decision as to whether adrenal cortical substitution therapy is needed.

The hazards of bilateral pheochromocytoma are illustrated by two early papers reporting death from attempted aortography in one and death in a six-year-old boy from urethral dilation under anesthesia in the other. The operative mortality in bilateral pheochromocytomas in childhood was high, but this has been greatly improved with preoperative adrenergic receptor blockade, better anesthesia, and better operative methods, especially the abandonment of the flank approach for an abdominal exploration. Through the abdominal approach the second tumor can be easily detected and removed.

Successive bilateral pheochromocytomas have been detected by aortography, but strict precautions should be taken if this technique is utilized.

The anesthetic precautions referred to later should be particularly adhered to in operations for bilateral tumors.

Although some patients have been subjected to total adrenalectomy for bilateral pheochromocytomas, thus requiring lifetime corticosteroid administration, this is seldom necessary. A portion of the adrenal on both sides almost always can be left. Recurrent pheochromocytoma, although not uncommon (about 10 percent in our series), has not occurred in or near the adrenocortical remnant.

Hume had a case in which a total right adrenalectomy was done for a pheochromocytoma on that side. Several years later a large tumor developed in the left adrenal. A fragment of normal adrenal was left behind at the time that the tumor was removed, and its blood supply from the phrenic artery was left intact. An ACTH test postoperatively showed an excellent blood 17-OH corticosteroid response, and no replacement therapy was necessary. It may be necessary to use intravenous administration of cortisol during the operation if the blood supply of the fragment is in doubt and until its function can be demonstrated.

The Organs of Zuckerkandl. These vestigial organs are parananglia which lie on the aorta with greatest concentration in the region of the inferior mesenteric artery. Pheochromocytomas affecting these "organs" are found on the aorta from beneath the third portion of the duodenum to the bifurcation. They are important because they can be missed if the abdominal approach is not used. Tumors of the organs of Zuckerkandl tend to be familial and may on rare occasions produce epinephrine in addition to norepinephrine. On occasion the tumor will displace the duodenum and be visible by gastrointestinal series.

Pheochromocytoma of the Bladder. Pheochromocytomas of the bladder are often, though not always, characterized by hematuria, headache, and hypertensive attacks on micturition. Micturition may precipitate attacks, however, from pheochromocytomas not associated with the bladder. Bladder pheochromocytomas are usually benign but may be malignant and are apt to occur in childhood. They are sometimes seen on excretory urography and are usually confirmed by cystoscopy. They may block the ureteral orifice, producing a picture of hydronephrosis and nonfunction of the kidney. Partial cystectomy is the treatment of choice. One pheochromocytoma of the bladder produced some epinephrine as well as norepinephrine.

Intrathoracic and Mediastinal Pheochromocytoma. Intrathoracic pheochromocytomas are often not diagnosed prior to surgical intervention. Only 50 percent of these patients have elevated blood pressure, and some of these tumors are nonfunctioning. They generally occur in the sympathetic ganglia and may be malignant. They can always be found on chest x-ray, and when functioning the localization can be confirmed by vena cava catheter sampling for plasma catecholamines. Some intrathoracic and mediastinal pheochromocytomas have produced epinephrine.

TREATMENT. Medical Treatment. *α-Adrenergic Receptor Blockade.* Medical treatment of a patient with a pheochromocytoma is often employed in preparation for operation, for patients who have functioning metastases, or for patients who refuse surgical treatment.

The usefulness of the prolonged oral administration of phentolamine (Regitine) was first described by Iseri et al. It has been used for as long as eight years in one patient who refused surgical treatments. Despite control of symptoms on 25 mg every 3 hours this patient's blood pressure was not well controlled, and she had a marked hypertensive reaction to minor surgical treatment, followed by shock. The addition of reserpine was said to help control the hypertension, though other writers have failed to note an effect on blood pressure with this drug in patients with pheochromocytomas. Furthermore reserpine and guanethidine release peripheral stores of catecholamines and can precipitate hypertensive crises or arrhythmias.

More recently phenoxybenzamine (Dibenzyline), an α-adrenergic receptor blocking agent, has been used to achieve chronic blood pressure reduction in patients with pheochromocytomas, with excellent results. In one case of malignant pheochromocytoma α-methyldopa was tried without success.

β-Adrenergic Receptor Blockade. Recently the β-adrenergic receptor blocking agent propranolol has been used to prepare patients for surgical treatment or to treat malignant pheochromocytomas chronically. It provides control of the tachycardia and helps to prevent arrhythmias intraoperatively.

Propranalol can be a valuable asset but must be used carefully. We are aware of two preoperative deaths in pheochromocytoma patients in whom overdoses of propranalol were directly responsible for death. The dose necessary for effective preoperative β-adrenergic receptor blockade is generally around 60 mg/day by mouth in three or four divided doses. This is a smaller dose of propranalol than that used for indications other than pheochromocytoma. The end point of treatment is resolution of tachycardia to a pulse rate near 90 beats per minute.

Anesthesia and Surgical Therapy. Although pheochromocytomas have been successfully removed under adverse circumstances, there is sufficient operative risk, particularly in children with bilateral tumors, to justify attempts to provide an ideal anesthetic and operative environment. The intraoperative use of phentolamine, first described by Grimson et al., has markedly improved operative results.

Whether medical pretreatment is desirable is still being debated, the opponents pointing out that sometimes ineffective, detrimental, or even fatal results have followed the administration of phentolamine (Regitine). Furthermore, it is said that with pretreatment one cannot use the rise in blood pressure on palpation of a tumor to localize it. Actually this is seldom necessary and in fact can still be done whenever desired, even with pretreatment. It is further said that the pretreatment renders the patient un-

responsive to norepinephrine after the tumor is removed, although this is usually not true. This unresponsiveness can be overcome when present by using angiotensin II, a drug which is not affected by phentolamine. Furthermore, resistance to norepinephrine sometimes occurs even when phentolamine has not been used.

The advocates point out that the operative course is apt to be a great deal smoother with preoperative adrenergic receptor blockade. Epinephrine and norepinephrine reduce the blood volume by causing peripheral vasoconstriction, and plasma volume is decreased in many patients with pheochromocytoma. This is more apt to be true in some but not all patients with sustained hypertension. Therefore, preoperative vasodilatation with phenoxybenzamine will expand the blood volume and will help to correct the marked swings of blood pressure that characterize operation in the unprepared patient. The preparation of the patient may be further enhanced by the administration just prior to and during surgical treatment of β-receptor blockers, such as propranalol, to prevent or treat arrhythmias if such are present. Patients with very high plasma catecholamines or with very high basal metabolic rates are said to be the poorest anesthetic risks.

Premedication should consist of Demerol and a small dose of scopolamine, which is preferable to atropine because it produces less tachycardia. Furthermore atropine can produce arrhythmias and hypertension. Barbiturates are apt to cause arrhythmias in the presence of hypoxia.

The anesthetic agents to be avoided are cyclopropane, halothane, trichloroethylene, and chloroform. Halothane has been advocated as the anesthetic agent of choice by some because of its tendency to suppress circulating catecholamine levels. However, halothane may lead to arrhythmias in the presence of an excess of circulating catecholamine, and if used it should be in conjunction with a β-receptor blocker. We generally prefer not to use it. The safest anesthetic appears to be Pentothal-nitrous oxide-Demerol-muscle relaxant, preferably succinylcholine. The soda lime canister should be fresh and changed during the operation to provide for optimal absorption of carbon dioxide. Arterial and venous pressure monitors are helpful and an ECG monitor mandatory. Phentolamine or nitroprusside should be used to control hypertension, and blood and norepinephrine or angiotensin II to control hypotension after removal of the tumor. Postresection hypotension has been uncommon since the preoperative use of phenoxybenzamine has become widespread. Postexcision hypotension was apparently due to acute catecholamine withdrawal vasodilatation, chronically decreased blood volume, residual phentolamine effect, if this substance was used, and occasionally insensitivity to norepinephrine. Transfusion and vasoconstrictors are the treatment.

In addition to blocking the α receptors, inhibition of the β receptors during surgical treatment, as mentioned above, may be important to prevent cardiac arrhythmias—the usual cause of operative death. In patients whose increased catecholamine excretion is more than 80 percent epinephrine, we believe it is wise to use preoperative β-receptor blockade routinely. If a patient is receiving β-receptor blockade, it is wise to use α blockade as well, to diminish the vascular resistance against which the β-blocked heart is pumping.

Though the question of corticosteroid administration is often raised, the function of the adrenal cortex is usually normal, except in some cases of bilateral pheochromocytoma, where corticosteroids should be employed until the function of the adrenal fragment has been established.

It is generally accepted now that an abdominal approach with complete exploration is indicated in all cases (Fig. 37-50).

Despite the precision in diagnostic accuracy created by the advent of catecholamine measurements, cases are still occasionally missed for want of consideration of this diagnosis, and sudden death may eventuate. In recent years the operative mortality has been considerably reduced, but there remains the occasional case, especially in children, where survival may depend upon the employment of all possible adjuncts, particularly those designed to reduce the incidence of cardiac arrhythmias.

Recurrent Pheochromocytoma. Important but still underemphasized features of pheochromocytoma are the frequency and pathological diversity of recurrences after a seemingly successful primary operation.

In our total experience with 49 patients, 10 had recurrent disease. Six of those had been referred to us as having problems in recurrent pheochromocytoma, making the incidence of recurrence from our own primary operations approximately 10 percent. In three cases surgery could not be carried out. In the most extreme case under our care, 17 years elapsed before the recurrences became symptomatic.

They may be regional recurrences near the bed of the original tumor dissection, they may be diffusely occult occurrences in the lungs (as in two patients who died because we did not appreciate this), or the recurrences may be obviously malignant pheochromocytomas with metastases to bone, liver, and lung.

If the disease cannot be removed, effective palliation may be achieved with chronic α- and β-receptor blockade. Tyrosine hydroxylase inhibition, though theoretically appealing, has depended on agents such as α-methyl-paratyrosine which are too nephrotoxic to permit their extended use. Radiation therapy and chemotherapy have not been helpful to date.

NEUROBLASTOMA

Neuroblastomas are malignant tumors occurring primarily in children, usually under the age of five. They usually present with abdominal masses, often first noted by the mother or by the pediatrician on routine physical examination. The five recognized symptom complexes are shown in Table 37-20.

Neuroblastomas metastasize to bone (30 percent), regional lymph nodes (26 percent), liver (20 percent), skull or brain (11 percent), lungs (9 percent), or cervical lymph nodes (5 percent). They are more common on the left, as are adrenocortical carcinomas. While usually arising from the adrenal they can arise from the sympathetic chain or

Table 37-20. SYMPTOM COMPLEXES OF NEUROBLASTOMA

Abdominal mass and liver enlargement are the most common symptoms, with or without pallor, weight loss, diffuse adenopathy, leukocytosis, vomiting, and abdominal pain.
Swelling of head, exophthalmos with ecchymosis of eyelids, blindness, increased intracranial pressure, and palpable abdominal tumor.
Extensive bony metastases, pallor, and severe anemia, without other findings.
Abdominal distension and diarrhea with or without mass.
Hypertension may be an additional finding with any of the above.

paraganglia. On rare occasions they have been found in the pelvis or neck.

Liver function tests are usually not of great value even with hepatic metastases, because of the general unreliability of the liver function tests in very young children. There is often a severe anemia. The urinary excretion of catecholamines or the metabolites of catecholamines may be elevated. Since neuroblastomas are more embryonic than the better-differentiated pheochromocytomas, they tend to secrete epinephrine precursor rather than epinephrine itself. They may secrete large amounts of dopamine, and as a consequence the most common urinary metabolite to be found in neuroblastomas is HVA. The urinary VMA level is quite frequently elevated, whereas the urinary catecholamines are only occasionally increased. Postoperative elevation in level of those catecholamines or metabolites elevated preoperatively is often the earliest and most sensitive indicator of recurrence. When the urinary catecholamines are increased, hypertension may be present.

The great problem in operating for neuroblastoma is hemorrhage. These are extremely vascular tumors and very difficult to remove completely. Fresh blood should be available to help counteract the bleeding. Radiation should be given postoperatively, and Cytoxan has been added for the treatment of metastases. New combined chemotherapy protocols are under investigation now and give promise of more effective chemotherapeutic control of this tumor.

Familial neuroblastoma has been reported by Chatten and Voorhess. In this study neuroblastomas were observed in three of four siblings. During one pregnancy the mother was noted to be excreting abnormal amounts of urinary catecholamines during her sixth month of pregnancy. The infant born of this pregnancy was followed and became the fourth affected sibling, when she was discovered to have a mediastinal neuroblastoma at five months of age. The inheritance is thought to be by autosomal dominance. Despite this, there have been three examples of discordant twin pairs in which only one member of the pair had the disease. It is probable, therefore, that many sporadic cases arise by mutation and represent lethal genes or that the dominant gene has variable penetrance or expression. Neuroblastoma in situ is found in 1 in 200 autopsies on infants, while the incidence in live-born children is 1 in 10,000. Therefore, many in situ lesions may have regressed. While other congenital anomalies do not usually accom-

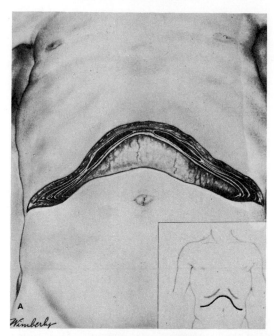

Fig. 37-50. Transabdominal exposure for operations for pheochromocytoma. *A.* A bilateral subcostal incision is made. A variety of other abdominal incisions can be used to good advantage depending on the patient's age, size, and abdominal configuration. *B.* The left adrenal gland is exposed by dividing the gastrocolic ligament and lifting the stomach upward. An incision is made in the posterior peritoneum along the lower border of the pancreas. *C.* The pancreas is elevated, exposing the renal and adrenal veins, and the adrenal gland is easily identified. *D.* An alternative exposure to the left adrenal can be obtained by dividing the peritoneum lateral to the splenic flexure of the colon and mobilizing the colon mediad. An incision is then made through the perirenal fascia, and the adrenal is exposed. *E.* Exposure of the right adrenal gland is obtained by doing a Kocher maneuver with a short lateral extension in the peritoneal incision. The liver is elevated upward, and the adrenal is exposed. The lateral border of the vena cava is rolled mediad to facilitate exposure of the gland, which is partially tucked under the vena cava.

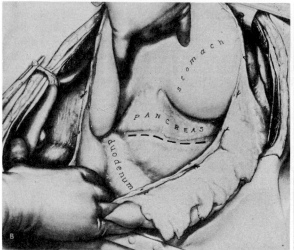

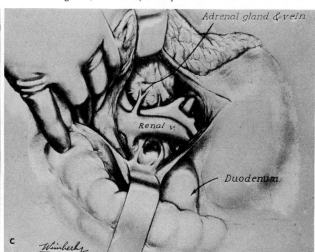

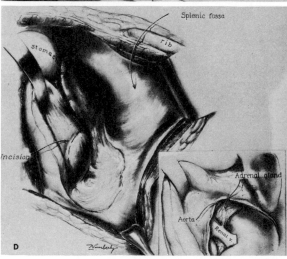

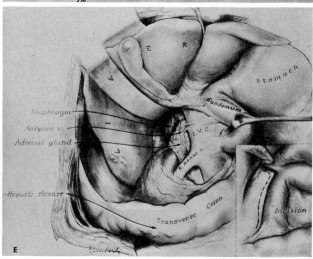

pany neuroblastoma, multiple developmental anomalies have been reported.

Although the mortality of neuroblastoma is high, there is a better prognosis if the diagnosis is made before the infant is one year of age, if the tumor is located in the mediastinum, if the tumor is more mature, and if metastases are not present at the time of treatment. Total removal followed by radiotherapy can be associated with an excellent prognosis.

The natural history of the disease and the results of treating 133 cases have been reported by Fortner et al. The degree of differentiation of the tumor is extremely important in the negative sense, in that without differentiation of the tumor beyond rosettes only one patient survived 5 years. Most of the patients in this series had advanced disease when first seen, only 4.5 percent of them having disease confined to the primary site. This has an extremely important prognostic implication, since in Gross' series 88 percent of patients whose tumors can be totally excised are cured while palliative excision resulted in a 64 percent cure rate and biopsy alone in 10 percent. In the patients of Fortner et al., many of whom had metastases when operated upon, there was a 36.3 percent 5-year survival rate in those with complete removal of the primary lesion and an 18.5 percent 5-year survival in those with partial removal. Because of the greatly improved prognosis with removal of the primary tumor, the writers advise reoperation after radiation therapy if the tumor is not removed when first explored. The exception to this is in those patients with a diffuse retroperitoneal spread of the malignancy over to the other side without massing of tumor at the primary site. This type is impossible to remove.

GANGLIONEUROMA

This is a rare tumor almost always occurring in the adult in contradistinction to neuroblastoma. It is benign and usually discovered as an asymptomatic incidental finding. There are no diagnostic laboratory findings.

References

PITUITARY

Historical Background

Bergland, R. M., Davis, S. L., and Page, R. B.: Pituitary Secretes to Brain, *Lancet,* **2:**276, 1977.

Cushing, H.: Basophil Adenomas of the Pituitary Body, *Bull Johns Hopkins Hosp,* **50:**137, 1932.

———: The Reaction of Posterior Pituitary Extract When Introduced into the Cerebral Ventricles, *Proc Natl Acad Sci,* **17:**163 and 239, 1931.

———: "Studies in Intracranial Physiology and Surgery," Oxford University Press, Fair Lawn, N.J., 1926.

———: The Functions of the Pituitary Body, *Am J Med Sci,* **139:**473, 1910.

———: "The Pituitary Body and Its Disorders," J. B. Lippincott Company, Philadelphia, 1912.

———: The Hypophysis Cerebri: Clinical Aspects of Hyperpituitarism and Hypopituitarism, *JAMA,* **53:**249, 1909.

——— and Davidoff, L.: The Pathological Findings in Acromegaly, Rockefeller Institute Monograph 22, pp. 1–131, 1927.

——— and Goetsch, E.: Concerning the Secretion of the Infundibular Lobe of the Pituitary Body and Its Presence in Cerebrospinal Fluid, *Am J Phys,* **27:**60, 1910.

Fulton, J.: "Harvey Cushing, A Biography," Charles C Thomas, Publisher, Springfield, Ill., 1946.

Henderson, W. R.: The Pituitary Adenomata, *Br J Surg,* **26:**809, 1939.

Page, R. B., Munger, B. L., and Bergland, R. M.: Scanning Microscopy of Pituitary Vascular Casts, *Am J Anat,* **146:**273, 1976.

Rodriguez, E. M.: Ependymal Specializations, *Z Zellforsch,* **102:**153, 1969.

Gross Anatomy

Bergland, R. M., Ray, B. S., and Torack, R. M.: Anatomical Variations in the Pituitary Gland, *J Neurosurg,* **28:**93, 1968.

Harris, G. W.: Neural Control of Pituitary Gland, *Physiol Rev,* **28:**139, 1948.

Lewis, D., and Lee, F. L.: On the Glandular Elements in the Posterior Lobe of the Human Hypophysis, *Bull Johns Hopkins Hosp,* **41:**240, 1927.

Oliver, C., Renon, S. M., and Parter, J. C.: Hypothalamic Pituitary Evidence Vasculature: Evidence for Retrograde Blood Flow in the Pituitary Stalk, *Endocrinol,* **101:**598, 1977.

Page, R. B., and Bergland, R. M.: The Neurohypophyseal Capillary Bed, *Am J Anat,* **148:**345, 1977.

Wislocki, G. B., and King, L. S.: The Permeability of the Hypophysis and Hypothalamus of Vital Dyes, *Am J Anat,* **58:**421, 1936.

Cellular Physiology

Bergland, R. M., and Torack, R. M.: An Electronmicroscopic Study of the Human Infundibulum, *Z Zellforsch,* **99:**1, 1969.

——— and ———: An Ultrastructural Study of Follicular Cells in the Anterior Pituitary, *Am J Pathol,* **57:**273, 1969.

Bloom, F., Segal, D., Ling, N., and Guillemin, R.: Endorphins: Profound Behavioral Effects in Rats Suggest New Etiological Factors in Mental Illness, *Science,* **194:**630, 1976.

deWied, D., and Bohus, B.: Retention of Continued Avoidance Response in Rats by Treatment with Pitressin or a-MSH, *Nature* (Lond.), **212:**1484, 1966.

Goldstein, A.: Endorphins in Pituitary and Brain, *Science,* **193:**1081, 1976.

Martin, J. B., Reichlin, S., and Brown, S.: "Clinical Neuroendocrinology," F. A. Davis Company, Philadelphia, 1977.

Nakane, P. K.: Classifications of Anterior Pituitary Cell Types with Immunoenzyme Histochemistry, *J Histochem Cytochem,* **18:**9, 1970.

Phifer, R. F., Midgley, A. R., and Spicer, S. S.: Histology of Human Hypophyseal Gonadotropin Secreting Cells, in "Gonadotropins," B. B. Saxena and C. G. Beling (eds.), John Wiley & Sons, Inc., New York, 1972, pp. 9–24.

Rasmussen, A. T.: The Percentage of Different Cells in Male Adult Human Hypophysis, *Am J Pathol,* **5:**263, 1929.

Schonemann, A.: Hypophysis and Thyreoida, *Arch Pathol,* **129:**310, 1892.

Snyder, S.: Opiate Receptors in the Brain, *N Engl J Med,* **296:**266, 1977.

Pituitary Disorders

Bergland, R. M., and Ray, B. S.: The Arterial Supply of the Human Optic Chiasm, *J Neurosurg,* **31:**327, 1966.

Ceballos, R.: Pituitary Changes in Head Trauma, *Alabama J Med Sci,* **3:**185, 1966.

Hardy, J.: Transsphenoidal Microsurgical Removal of Pituitary Micro-adenoma, *Prog Neurosurg* (Karger), **6:**200, 1975.

Hoff, J. T., and Patterson, R. H.: Craniopharyngiomas in Children and Adults, *J Neurosurg,* **36:**299, 1972.

Kjellberg, R. N., and Kliman, B.: Bragg Peak Proton Treatment for Pituitary-Related Conditions, *Proc R Soc Med,* **67:**32, 1974.

Malarkey, W. B., and Johnson, J. C.: Pituitary Tumors and Hyperprolactinia, *Arch Int Med,* **136:**40, 1976.

Ray, B. S., and Horwith, M.: Surgical Treatment of Acromegaly, *Clin Neurosurg,* **10:**31, 1964.

———— and Patterson, R. H.: Surgical Experience with Chromophobe Adenomas, *J Neurosurg,* **34:**726, 1971.

Rovitt, R., and Fein, J. M.: Pituitary Apoplexy: A Review, *J Neurosurg,* **37:**280, 1972.

Sheehan, H. L., and Whitehead, R.: The Neurohypophysis in Postpartum Hypopituitarism, *J Pathol Bacteriol,* **85:**145, 1963.

Teears, R. J., and Silverman, E. M.: Review of 88 Cases of Carcinoma Metastatic to the Pituitary Gland, *Cancer,* **36:**216, 1975.

Young, D. G., Bohn, R. C., and Randall, R. V.: Pituitary Tumors Associated with Acromegaly, *J Clin Endocrinol,* **25:**249, 1965.

Diagnostic Studies

Lee, W. M., and Adams, J. E.: The Empty Sella Syndrome, *J Neurosurg,* **28:**351, 1968.

Therapeutic Modalities

Beatson, G. T.: On the Treatment of Inoperable Cases of Carcinoma of the Mamma, *Lancet,* **2:**104, 1896.

Fraser, T. R., and Joplin, G. F.: Subtotal or Total Pituitary Ablation by Implantation of Radioactive Rods, *Mod Treat,* **3:**189, 1966.

Luft, R., and Oliverona, H.: Experiences with Hypophysectomy in Man, *J Neurosurg,* **10:**301, 1953.

Maas, H., et al.: Estrogen Receptors in Human Breast Cancer Tissue, *Am J Obstet Gynecol,* **113:**377, 1972.

Mundinger, F.: Interstitial Curie-Therapy in the Treatment of Pituitary Adenomas, *Prog Neurol Surg* (Karger), **6:**326, 1975.

Poulsen, J. E.: Recovery from Retinopathy in a Case of Diabetes with Simmonds' Disease, *Diabetes,* **2:**7, 1953.

Rand, R. W., Dashe, A. M., Paglia, D. E., et al: Stereotactic Cryohypophysectomy, *JAMA,* **189:**255, 1964.

Ray, B. S.: Intracranial Hypophysectomy, *J Neurosurg,* **28:**180, 1968.

———— et al.: Pituitary Ablation for Diabetic Retinopathy, *JAMA,* **203:**79, 1968.

Zervas, N.: Stereotaxic Thermal Hypophysectomy, *Prog Neurol Surg* (Karger), **6:**217, 1975.

Zimmerman, B. R., and Molnar, G. D.: Prolonged Followup in Diabetic Retinopathy, *Mayo Clin Proc,* **52:**233, 1977.

ADRENAL

General

Bajusz, E. (ed.), "An Introduction to Clinical Neuro-endocrinology," The Williams & Wilkins Company, Baltimore, 1967.

Blizzard, R. M.: in L. Wilkins (ed.), "The Diagnosis and Treatment of Endocrine Disorders in Childhood and Adolescence," Charles C Thomas, Publisher, Springfield, Ill., 1965.

Cope, C. L.: "Adrenal Steroids and Disease," J. B. Lippincott Company, Philadelphia, 1964.

Dorfman, R. I., and Ungar, F.: Metabolism of Steroid Hormones, Academic Press, Inc., New York, 1965.

Forsham, P. H., and Melmon, K. L.: The Adrenals, in R. H. Williams (ed.), "Textbook of Endocrinology," 4th ed., p. 287, W. B. Saunders Company, Philadelphia, 1968.

Soffer, L. J., Dorfman, R. I., and Gabrilove, J. L.: "The Human Adrenal Gland," Lea & Febiger, Philadelphia, 1961.

Van Wyk, J. J., and Grumbach, M. M.: Disorders of Sex Differentiation, in R. H. Williams (ed.), "Textbook of Endocrinology," 5th ed., p. 423, W. B. Saunders Company, Philadelphia, 1976, 1,138 pages.

Embryology

Schechter, D. C.: Aberrant Adrenal Tissue, *Ann Surg,* **167:**421, 1968.

Anatomy

Kramer, R. K., and Sapirstein, L. A.: Blood Flow to the Adrenal Cortex and Medulla, *Endocrinology,* **81:**403, 1967.

ADRENAL CORTEX

Physiology

Fraser, T. R., and Wright, A. D.: Treatment of Acromegaly and Cushing's Disease by ^{90}Y Implant for Partial Ablation of the Pituitary, in E. B. Astwood and C. E. Cassidy (eds.), "Clinical Endocrinology II," Grune & Stratton, Inc., New York, 1968.

Gordon, R. D., Kuchel, O., Liddle, G. W., and Island, D. P.: Role of the Sympathetic Nervous System in Regulating Renin and Aldosterone Production in Man, *J Clin Invest,* **46:**599, 1967.

Gross, F.: The Regulation of Aldosterone Secretion by the Renin-Angiotensin System under Various Conditions, *Acta Endocrinol* [*Suppl*] (*Kbh*), **124:**41, 1968.

Luetscher, J. A., and Cheville, R. A.: Measurement of Secretion Rates of Adrenal Cortical Hormones, in E. B. Astwood and C. E. Cassidy (eds.), "Clinical Endocrinology II," p. 444, Grune & Stratton, Inc., New York, 1968.

Marusic, E. T., and Mulrow, P. J.: Stimulation of Aldosterone Biosynthesis in Adrenal Mitochondria by Sodium Depletion, *J Clin Invest,* **46:**2101, 1967.

Palmore, W. P.: Control of Aldosterone Secretion by the Pituitary Gland, *Science,* **157:**1482, 1967.

Cushing's Syndrome

Pathology

Hyperplasia, Adenoma, Carcinoma, Pituitary Tumor

Chaffee, W. R., Moses, A. M., Lloyd, C. W., and Rogers, L. S.: Cushing's Syndrome with Accessory Adrenocortical Tissue, *JAMA,* **186:**799, 1963.

Heinbecker, P., O'Neal, L. W., and Ackerman, L. V.: Functioning and Nonfunctioning Adrenal Cortical Tumors, *Surg Gynecol Obstet,* **105:**21, 1957.

Hunder, G. G.: Pathogenesis of Cushing's Disease, *Proc Staff Meetings Mayo Clin,* **41:**29, 1966.

Neville, A. M., and Symington, T.: The Pathology of the Adrenal Gland in Cushing's Syndrome, *J Pathol Bacteriol,* **93:**19, 1967.

O'Neal, L. W.: Pathologic Anatomy in Cushing's Syndrome, *Ann Surg,* **160:**860, 1964.

Rovit, R. L., and Berry, R.: Cushing's Syndrome and the Hypophysis: A Re-evaluation of Pituitary Tumors and Hyperadrenalism, *J Neurosurg,* **23:**270, 1965.

Nodular Dysplasia

Cohen, R. B.: Observations on Cortical Nodules in Human Adrenal Glands: Their Relationship to Neoplasia, *Cancer,* **19:**552, 1966.

Kirschner, M. A., Powell, R. D., Jr., and Lipsett, M. B.: Cushing's Syndrome: Nodular Cortical Hyperplasia of Adrenal Glands with Clinical and Pathological Features Suggesting Adrenocortical Tumor, *J Clin Endocrinol Metab,* **24:**947, 1964.

Meador, C. K., Bowdoin, B., Owen, W. C., Jr., and Farmer, T. A., Jr.: Primary Adrenocortical Nodular Dysplasia: A Rare Cause of Cushing's Syndrome, *J Clin Endocrinol Metab,* **27:**1255, 1967.

Ectopic ACTH Syndrome

Feldman, F., Mitchell, W., and Soll, S.: Psychosis, Cushing's Syndrome and Hyperparathyroidism, *Can Med Assoc J,* **98:**508, 1968.

Gault, M. H., Bilefsky, R., Kinsella, T. D., and Aronoff, A.: Adrenocortical Hyperfunction Associated with Bronchogenic Carcinoma: Report of Five Cases, *Can Med Assoc J,* **93:**1243, 1965.

Goldberg, W. M., and McNeil, M. J.: Cushing's Syndrome Due to an ACTH-producing Carcinoma of the Thyroid, *Can Med Assoc J,* **96:**1577, 1967.

Harris, P. W. R., and El-Katib, M. B.: Cushing's Syndrome and Myelolipomatosis with Carcinoma of the Thymus, *Br J Surg,* **55:**472, 1968.

Hills, E. A.: Adrenocarcinoma of the Bronchus with Cushing's Syndrome, Carcinoid Syndrome, Neuromyopathy and Urticaria, *Br J Dis Chest,* **62:**88, 1968.

Liddle, G. W., Givens, J. R., Nicholson, W. E., and Island, D. P.: Ectopic ACTH Syndrome, *Proc Int Congr Endocrinol 2d London 1964,* International Congress ser., no. 83, 1965, pp. 1063–1067.

Marks, L. J., Russfield, A. B., and Rosenbaum, D. L.: Corticotropin-secreting Carcinoma, *JAMA,* **183:**115, 1963.

Sayle, B. A., Lang, P. A., Green, W. O., Jr., Bosworth, W. C., and Gregory, R.: Cushing's Syndrome Due to Islet Cell Carcinoma of the Pancreas: Report of Two Cases, One with Elevated 5-Hydroxyindole Acetic Acid and Complicated by Aspergillosis, *Ann Intern Med,* **63:**58, 1965.

Schteingart, E., Conn, J. W., Orth, D., Fox, J. E., Bookstein, J. J., and Harrison, T. S.: Secretion of ACTH and B/-MSH by an Adrenal Medullary Paraganglioma, *J Clin Endocrinol Metab,* **34:**676, April, 1972.

Strott, C. A., Nugent, C. A., and Tyler, F. H.: Cushing's Syndrome Caused by Bronchial Adenomas, *Am J Med,* **44:**97, 1968.

Biochemical or Physiological Diagnostic Tests

Baylink, D. J., and Hurxthal, L. M.: Assessment of Adrenocortical Function, *Postgrad Med,* **33:**20, 1963.

Cassidy, C. E., Rosenfeld, P. S., and Bokat, M. A.: Suppression of Activity of Adrenal Cortex by Dexamethasone in Cushing's Syndrome, *J Clin Endocrinol Metab,* **26:**1181, 1966.

Cope, C. L.: The Adrenal Cortex in Internal Medicine, pt. 1, *Br Med J,* **2:**847, 1966.

——— and Mattingly, D.: Some Recent Advances in Adrenal Diagnosis, *Postgrad Med J,* **44:**235, 1968.

Givens, J. R., Ney, R. L., Nicholson, W. E., Graber, A. L., and Liddle, G. W.: The Absence of a Normal Diurnal Variation of Plasma ACTH in Cushing's Disease, *Clin Res,* **12:**267, 1964.

James, V. H. T., Landon, J., and Wynn, V.: Oral and Intravenous Suppression Tests in Diagnosis of Cushing's Syndrome, *J Endocrinol,* **33:**515, 1965.

Jefferies, W. M., Michelakis, A. M., and Price, J. W.: Urinary Cortisol Metabolites in Adrenocortical Hyperfunction, *J Clin Endocrinol Metab,* **26:**219, 1966.

Liddle, G. W.: Tests of Pituitary-Adrenal Suppressibility in the Diagnosis of Cushing's Syndrome, *J Clin Endocrinol Metab,* **20:**1539, 1960.

———, Estep, H. L., Kendall, J. W., Jr., Williams, W. C., Jr., and Townes, A. W.: Clinical Application of a New Test of Pituitary Reserve, *J Clin Endocrinol Metab,* **19:**875, 1959.

Martin, M. M., and Hamman, B. L.: Patterns of Urinary Excretion of Steroids in Cushing's Syndrome, *J Clin Endocrinol Metab,* **26:**257, 1966.

Maynard, D. E., et al.: Rapid Test for Adrenocortical Insufficiency, *Ann Intern Med,* **64:**552, 1966.

Musa, B. U., and Dowling, J. R.: Rapid Intravenous Administration of Corticotropin as Test of Adrenocortical Insufficiency, *JAMA,* **201:**633, 1967.

Nelson, D. H., Sprunt, J. G., and Mims, R. B.: Plasma ACTH Determinations in 58 Patients before or after Adrenalectomy for Cushing's Syndrome, *J Clin Endocrinol,* **26:**722, 1966.

Paris, J.: On Diagnosis of Addison's Disease and Cushing's Syndrome by Laboratory Methods, *Proc Staff Meetings Mayo Clin,* **39:**26, 1964.

Tucci, J. R., Jagger, P. I., Lauler, D. P., and Thorn, G. W.: Rapid Dexamethasone Suppression Test for Cushing's Syndrome, *JAMA,* **199:**379, 1967.

Vagnucci, A. I., Hesser, M. E., Kozak, G. P., Pauk, G. L., Lauler, D. P., and Thorm, G. W.: Circadian Cycle of Urinary Cortisol in Healthy Subjects and Cushing's Syndrome, *J Clin Endocrinol Metab,* **25:**1331, 1965.

Angiographic or Vascular Catheter Studies

Kahn, P. C., and Nickrosz, L. V.: Selective Angiography of the Adrenal Glands, *Am J Roentgenol Radium Ther Nucl Med,* **101:**739, 1967.

Lagergren, C.: Angiographic Changes in the Adrenal Glands, *Am J Roentgenol Radium Ther Nucl Med,* **101:**732, 1967.

Starer, F.: Percutaneous Suprarenal Venography, *Br J Radiol,* **38:**675, 1965.

Selection of Treatment

Nelson, D. H.: Treatment of Cushing's Syndrome, *Mod Treat,* **3:**1421, 1966.

Soffer, L. J., Iannaccone, A., and Gabrilove, J. L.: Cushing's Syndrome: A Study of Fifty Patients, *Am J Med,* **30:**129, 1961.

Pituitary Irradiation

Levene, M. B.: Pituitary Radiotherapy, *Radiol Clin North Am,* **5:**333, 1967.

Molinnati, G. M., Massara, C. F., and Messina, M.: Implantation of the Sella Turcica with ^{90}Yttrium in the Treatment of Cushing's Syndrome of Pituitary Origin, *J Clin Endocrinol Metab,* **27:**861, 1967.

Medical Treatment

Coll, R., Horner, I., Kraiem, Z., and Gafni, J.: Successful Metyrapone Therapy of the Ectopic ACTH Syndrome, *Arch Intern Med,* **121:**549, 1968.

Hutter, A. M., and Kayhoe, D. E.: Adrenal Cortical Carcinoma: Results of Treatment with o,p'DDD in 138 Patients, *Am J Med,* **41:**581, 1966.

Krieger, D. T., Amorosa, L., and Linick, F.: Cyproheptadine-Induced Remission of Cushing's Disease, *N Engl J Med,* **293:**893, 1975.

Lipsett, M. B.: Rationale for Chemotherapy of Cushing's Syndrome, in E. B. Astwood and C. E. Cassidy (eds.), "Clinical Endocrinology II," p. 489, Grune & Stratton, Inc., New York, 1968.

Operative Approach and Results

Coone, H. W., and Humphreys, J. W., Jr.: Subtotal Adrenalectomy in Cushing's Syndrome, *Ann Intern Med,* **44:**188, 1956.

Drucker, W. D., Roginsky, M. S., and Christy, N. P.: Persistence of Abnormal Pituitary-Adrenal Relationship in Patients with Cushing's Disease Partially Corrected by Bilateral Subtotal Adrenalectomy, *Am J Med,* **38:**522, 1965.

Egdahl, R. H., and Melby, J. C.: Recurrent Cushing's Disease and Intermittent Functional Adrenal Cortical Insufficiency following Subtotal Adrenalectomy, *Ann Surg,* **166:**586, 1967.

Herrera, M. G., Cahill, C. F., Jr., and Thorn, G. W.: Cushing's Syndrome: Diagnosis and Treatment, *Am J Surg,* **107:**144, 1964.

Ledingham, J. G. G., Nabarro, J. D. N., and Le Quesne, L. P.: Adrenal Autografts in the Treatment of Cushing's Syndrome Caused by Adrenal Hyperplasia, *Br J Surg,* **53:**1057, 1966.

Raker, J. W., Cope, O., and Ackerman, I. P.: Surgical Experience with the Treatment of Hypertension of Cushing's Syndrome, *Am J Surg,* **107:**153, 1964.

Scott, H. W., Jr., Foster, J. H., Liddle, G., and Davidson, E. T.: Cushing's Syndrome Due to Adrenocortical Tumor: 11-Year Review of 15 Patients, *Ann Surg,* **162:**505, 1965.

———, Liddle, G. W., Harris, A. P., and Foster, J. H.: Diagnosis and Treatment of Cushing's Syndrome, *Ann Surg,* **155:**696, 1962.

Total Adrenalectomy for Treatment of Cushing's Syndrome, *JAMA,* **175:**130, 1961. (Editorial.)

Complications of Surgery

Montgomery, D. A. A., Welbourn, R. B., McCaughey, W. T. E., and Gleadhill, C. A.: Pituitary Tumors Manifested after Adrenalectomy for Cushing's Snydrome, *Lancet,* **2:**707, 1959.

Nelson, D. H., and Sprunt, J. G.: Pituitary Tumors Postadrenalectomy for Cushing's Syndrome, *Proc Int Congr Endocrinol 2d London 1964,* International Congress ser., no. 83, 1965, p. 1053.

Adrenogenital Syndrome, Feminizing Syndromes

Adrenocortical Carcinomas, and Inter-sex Problems

Adrenogenital

Congenital Adrenal Hyperplasia

Bongiovanni, A. M., and Root, A. W.: Adrenogenital Syndrome, *N Engl J Med,* **268:**1283, 1963.

Ehrhardt, A. A., Epstein, R., and Money, J.: Fetal Androgens and Female Gender Identity in the Early-treated Adrenogenital Syndrome, *Bull Johns Hopkins Hosp,* **122:**160, 1968.

Hamilton, W.: Surgical Procedures in Congenital Adrenal Hyperplasia, *Dev Med Child Neurol,* **10:**106, 1968.

Huffstadt, A. J. C.: Surgical Correction of Female Pseudo-hermaphroditism Due to Adrenal Hyperplasia, *Br J Plast Surg,* **20:**359, 1967.

Lattimer, J. K.: Relocation and Recession of the Enlarged Clitoris with Preservation of the Glans: An Alternative to Amputation, *J Urol,* **86:**113, 1961.

Seymour, R. J., and Kinch, R. A. H.: Recession and Relocation of the Enlarged Clitoris in Congenital Adrenogenital Syndrome, *Can J Surg,* **9:**365, 1966.

Postnatal

Cooper, J. D., Maldonado, L., and Earll, J. M.: Adrenocortical Carcinoma with Virilism in an Infant under 1 Year of Age, *Am J Dis Child,* **113:**730, 1967.

Adult

Brooks, R. V., Mattingly, D., Mills, I. H., and Prunty, F. T. G.: Postpubertal Adrenal Virilism with Biochemical Disturbance of the Congenital Type of Adrenal Hyperplasia, *Br Med J,* **1:**1294, 1960.

Gabrilove, J. L., Sharma, D. C., and Dorfman, R. I.: Adrenocortical 11β-Hydroxylase Deficiency and Virilism First Manifest in the Adult Woman, *N Engl J Med,* **272:**1189, 1965.

Hutter, A. M., Jr., and Kayhoe, D. E.: Adrenal Cortical Carcinoma: Clinical Features of 138 Patients, *Am J Med,* **41:**572, 1966.

——— and ———: Adrenal Cortical Carcinoma: Results of Treatment with o,p'DDD in 138 Patients, *Am J Med,* **41:**581, 1966.

Serge, E. J.: Androgens, Virilization and the Hirsute Female, Charles C Thomas, Publisher, Springfield, Ill., 1967.

Mild Excesses in Androgen Production

Jacobs, J. P.: Hirsutism and Benign Androgenic Hyperplasia of the Adrenals, *Am J Obstet Gynecol,* **101:**37, 1968.

Prunty, F. T. G.: Androgen Metabolism in Man: Some Current Concepts, *Br Med J,* **2:**605, 1966.

Estrogen-secreting Tumors

Gabrilove, J. L., Sharma, D. C., Woitz, H. H., and Dorfman, R. I.: Feminizing Adrenocortical Tumors in Male: Review of 52 Cases including Case Report, *Medicine,* **44:**37, 1965.

Stewart, W. K., Fleming, L. W., and Wotiz, H. H.: The Feminizing Syndrome in Male Subjects with Adrenocortical Neoplasms, *Am J Med,* **37**:455, 1964.

Adrenocortical Carcinomas and Tumors with Mixed Secretions

Lipsett, M. B., Hertz, R., and Ross, G. T.: Clinical and Pathophysiologic Aspects of Adrenocortical Carcinoma, *Am J Med,* **35**:374, 1963.

MacFarlane, D. A.: Cancer of the Adrenal Cortex, *Ann R Coll Surg Engl,* **23**:155, 1958.

Villee, D. B., Rotner, H., Kliman, B., Briefer, C., Jr., and Federman, D. D.: Androgen Synthesis in a Patient with Virilizing Adrenocortical Carcinoma, *J Clin Endocrinol Metab,* **27**:1112, 1967.

Disorders of Sexual Development

Federman, D. D.: Disorders of Sexual Development, *N Engl J Med,* **277**:351, 1967.

Adrenalectomy for Metastatic Cancer of the Breast or Prostate

Block, G. E., Jensen, E. V., and Polley, T. Z.: The Prediction of Hormonal Dependency of Mammary Cancer, *Ann Surg,* **182**:342, 1975.

————, Vial, A. B., McCarthy, J. D., Porter, C. W., and Coller, F. A.: Adrenalectomy in Advanced Mammary Cancer, *Surg Gynecol Obstet,* **108**:651, 1959.

Cade, S.: Adrenalectomy for Disseminated Breast Cancer, *Br Med J,* **2**:613, 1966.

Dao, T. L-Y., and Huggins, C.: Bilateral Adrenalectomy in the Treatment of Cancer of the Breast, *Arch Surg,* **71**:645, 1955.

———— and Nemoto, T.: An Evaluation of Adrenalectomy and Androgen in Disseminated Mammary Carcinoma, *Surg Gynecol Obstet,* **121**:1257, 1965.

Fairgrieve, J.: Selective Criteria for Surgical Removal of the Endocrine Glands in Advanced Breast Cancer, *Surg Gynecol Obstet,* **120**:371, 1965.

Fracchia, A. A., Randall, H. T., and Farrow, J. H.: The Results of Adrenalectomy in Advanced Breast Cancer in 500 Consecutive Patients, *Surg Gynecol Obstet,* **125**:747, 1967.

Huggins, C. B.: Adrenalectomy as Palliative Treatment, *JAMA,* **200**:973, 1967.

Nemoto, T., and Dao, T. L.: Significance of Liver Metastasis in Women with Disseminated Breast Cancer Undergoing Endocrine Ablative Surgery, *Cancer,* **19**:421, 1966.

Adrenalectomy for Hypertension

Sellers, A. M., Barrett, J. S., Wolferth, C. C., Sr., Lopez, R., Itskovitz, H. D., Blakemore, W. S., and Zintel, H. A.: Adrenalectomy and Sympathectomy for Hypertension, *Arch Surg,* **89**:880, 1964.

Smithwick, R. H.: Practical Treatment for Hypertension: Splanchnicectomy, Adrenalectomy and Nephrectomy, *Postgrad Med,* **34**:32, 1963.

Aldosteronism

Symptoms and Signs and Review

Conn, J. W.: Hypertension, the Potassium Ion and Impaired Carbohydrate Tolerance, *N Engl J Med,* **273**:1135, 1965.

————, Knopf, R. F., and Nesbit, R. M.: Clinical Characteristics of Primary Aldosteronism from an Analysis of 145 Cases, *Am J Surg,* **107**:159, 1964.

Kaplan, N. M.: Primary Aldosteronism, in E. B. Astwood and C. E. Cassidy (eds.), "Clinical Endocrinology II," p. 467, Grune & Stratton, Inc., New York, 1968.

Incidence

Conn, J. W., Rovner, D. R., Cohen, E. L., and Nesbit, R. M.: Normokalemic Primary Aldosteronism: Its Masquerade as "Essential" Hypertension, *JAMA,* **195**:21, 1966.

Fishman, L. M., Kuchel, Olo, Liddle, G. W., Michelakis, A. M., Gordon, R. D., and Chick, W. T.: Incidence of Primary Aldosteronism Uncomplicated "Essential" Hypertension, *JAMA,* **205**:497, 1968.

Kokko, J. P., Brown, T. C., and Berman, M. M.: Adrenal Adenoma and Hypertension, *Lancet,* **1**:468, 1967.

Pathology

Crane, M. G., Harris, J. J., and Herber, R.: Primary Aldosteronism Due to an Adrenal Carcinoma, *Ann Intern Med,* **63**:494, 1965.

Davis, W. W., Newsome, H. H., Wright, L. D., Hammond, W. G., Easton, J., and Bartter, F. C.: Bilateral Adrenal Hyperplasia as a Cause of Primary Aldosteronism with Hypertension, Hypokalemia and Suppressed Renin Activity, *Am J Med,* **42**:642, 1967.

Flanagan, M. J., and McDonald, J. H.: Heterotropic Adrenocorticol Adenoma Producing Primary Aldosteronism, *J Urol,* **98**:133, 1967.

Neville, A. M., and Symington, T.: Pathology of Primary Aldosteronism, *Cancer,* **19**:1854, 1966.

Biochemical or Physiologic Tests

Biglieri, E. G., Slaton, P. E., Jr., Kronfield, S. J., and Deck, J. B.: Primary Aldosteronism with Unusual Secretory Pattern, *J Clin Endocrinol Metab,* **27**:715, 1967.

————, ————, ————, and Schambelan, M.: Diagnosis of an Aldosterone-producing Adenoma in Primary Aldosteronism, *JAMA,* **201**:510, 1967.

Brown, J. J., Davies, D. L., Lever, A. F., and Robertson, J. I. S.: Plasma Renin Concentration in Human Hypertension: I. Relationship between Renin, Sodium, and Potassium, *Br Med J,* **2**:144, 1965.

Conn, J. W., and Cohen, E. L.: Primary Aldosteronism: Importance of the Level of Plasma Renin as an Adjunct in Diagnosis, in Bumpus, F. M., and Page, I. H., "Handbook of Experimental Pharmacology," Springer-Verlag, 1973.

Cope, C. L.: The Adrenal Cortex in Internal Medicine, pt. II, *Br Med J,* **2**:914, 1966.

Espiner, E. A., Tucci, J. R., Jagger, P. I., and Lauler, D. P.: Effect of Saline Infusions on Aldosterone Secretion and Electrolyte Excretion in Normal Subjects and Patients with Primary Aldosteronism, *N Engl J Med,* **277**:1, 1967.

Kaplan, N. M.: Hypokalemia in the Hypertensive Patient with Observations on the Incidence of Primary Aldosteronism, *Ann Intern Med,* **66**:1079, 1967.

Lauler, D. P.: Preoperative Diagnosis of Primary Aldosteronism, *Am J Med,* **41**:855, 1966.

Relman, A. S.: Diagnosis of Primary Aldosteronism, *Am J Surg,* **107**:173, 1964.

Salti, I. S., Stiefel, M., Ruse, J. L., and Laidlaw, J. C.: Non-tumorous "Primary" Aldosteronism: Type Relieved by Gluco-Corticoid, *Can Med Ass J,* **101:**1, 1969.

Schacht, R. A., and Frame, B.: Infusion of Chlorothiazide in a Patient with Primary Aldosteronism: Observations on Potassium Clearance, *JAMA,* **201:**323, 1967.

Localization Techniques

Conn, J. W., Beierwaltes, W. H., Liegerman, L. M., Ansari, A. N., Cohen, E. L., Bookstein, J. J., and Herwig, K. R.: Primary Aldosteronism: Preoperative Tumor Visualization by Scintillation Scanning, *J Clin Endocrinol Metab,* **33:**713, 1971.

Egdahl, R. H., Kahn, P., and Melby, J. C.: Unilateral Adrenalectomy for Aldosteronomas, Localized Preoperatively by Differential Adrenal Vein Catheterization, *Surgery,* **64:**117, 1968.

Melby, J. C., Spark, R. F., Dale, S. L., Egdahl, R. H., and Kahn, P. C.: Diagnosis and Localization of Aldosterone-producing Adenomas by Adrenal-Vein Catheterization, *N Engl J Med,* **277:**1050, 1967.

Sutton, D.: Diagnosis of Conn's and Other Adrenal Tumours by Left Adrenal Phlebography, *Lancet,* **1:**453, 1968.

Medical Treatment

Abbott, E. C., Gornall, A. G., Sutherland, D. J., Stiefel, M., and Laidlaw, J. C.: Influence of Heparin-like Compound on Hypertension, Electrolytes and Aldosterone in Man, *Can Med Assoc J,* **94:**1155, 1966.

Melby, J. C.: Aldosterone Inhibitors, in E. B. Astwood, and C. E. Cassidy (eds.), "Clinical Endocrinology II," p. 477, Grune & Stratton, Inc., New York, 1968.

Preoperative Treatment

Flanagan, M. J., Gantt, C. J., and McDonald, J. H.: Primary Aldosteronism, *J Urol,* **88:**111, 1962.

Mobley, J. E., Headstream, J. W., and Melby, J.: Primary Aldosteronism: Preoperative Preparation with Spironolactone, *JAMA,* **180:**1056, 1962.

Operative Technique and Results

Nesbit, R. M.: Primary Aldosteronism: Its Diagnosis and Surgical Management, *J Urol,* **97:**404, 1966.

Rhamy, R. K., McCoy, R. M., Scott, H. W., Fishman, L. M., Michelakis, A. M., and Liddle, G. W.: Primary Aldosteronism: Experience with Current Diagnostic Criteria and Surgical Treatment in Fourteen Patients, *Ann Surg,* **167:**718, 1968.

Silen, W., Biglieri, E. G., Slaton, P., and Galante, M.: Management of Primary Aldosteronism: Evaluation of Potassium and Sodium Balance, Technic of Adrenalectomy and Operative Results in 24 Cases, *Ann Surg,* **164:**600, 1966.

Smithwick, R. H., Harrison, J. H., Unger, L., and Whitelaw, G. P.: Surgical Treatment of Aldosteronism: Combined Experiences at the Massachusetts Memorial and the Peter Bent Brigham Hospitals, *Am J Surg,* **107:**178, 1964.

Complications and Postoperative Course

Bartter, F. C., Pronove, P., Gill, J. R., Jr., and MacCardle, R. C.: Hyperplasia of the Juxtaglomerular Complex with Hyper-aldosteronism and Hypokalemic Alkalosis: A new Syndrome, *Am J Med,* **33:**811, 1962.

Biglieri, E. G., Slaton, P. E., Jr., Silen, W. S., Galante, M., and Forsham, P. H.: Postoperative Studies of Adrenal Function in Primary Aldosteronism, *J Clin Endocrinol. Metab,* **26:**553, 1966.

Adrenocortical Insufficiency (Addison's Disease)

Autoimmunity in Idiopathic Addison's Disease, *Lancet,* **1:**1040, 1967.

Donnelly, W. J.: Unexplained Addison's Disease, *Postgrad Med,* **42:**339, 1967.

Jagatic, J., and Rubnitz, M. E.: Massive Bilateral Adrenal Bleeding: Five-Year Review of Cases, *Ill Med J.,* **132:**273, 1967.

Maynard, D. E., et al.: Rapid Test for Adrenocortical Insufficiency, *Ann Intern Med,* **64:**552, 1966.

Schambelan, M., Stockigt, J. R., and Biglieri, E. G.: Isolated Hypoaldosteronism in Adults, *N Engl J Med,* **287:**573, 1972.

Turkington, R. W., and Lebovitz, H. E.: Extra-adrenal Endocrine Deficiencies in Addison's Disease, *Am J Med,* **43:**499, 1967.

Surgical Complications of Adrenal Steroid Therapy

Glenn, F., and Grafe, W. R., Jr.: Surgical Complications of Adrenal Steroid Therapy, *Ann Surg,* **165:**1023, 1967.

ADRENAL MEDULLA

Pheochromocytoma

Glenn, F., and Mannix, H., Jr.: The Surgical Management of Chromaffin Tumors, *Ann Surg,* **167:**619, 1968.

Hume, D. M.: Pheochromocytoma in the Adult and in the Child, *Am J Surg,* **99:**458, 1960.

Scott, H. W., Riddell, D. H., and Brockman, S. K.: Surgical Management of Pheochromocytoma, *Surg Gynecol Obstet,* **120:**707, 1965.

Physiology and Pharmacology of Epinephrine and Norepinephrine

Axelrod, J.: Metabolism of Epinephrine and Other Sympathomimetic Amines, *Physiol Rev,* **39:**751, 1959.

———— and Weinshilboum, R.: Catecholamines, *N Engl J Med,* **287:**237, 1972.

Blaschko, H.: The Development of Current Concepts of Catecholamine Formation, *Pharmacol Rev,* **11:**307, 1959.

Von Euler, U. S. Noradrenaline: Chemistry, Physiology, Pharmacology and Clinical Aspects, Charles C Thomas, Publisher, Springfield, Ill., 1956.

Voorhess, M. L.: The Catecholamines in Tumor and Urine from Patients with Neuroblastoma, Ganglio-neuroblastoma and Pheochromocytoma, *J Pediat Surg,* **3:**147, 1968.

Wurtman, R. J., and Axelrod, J.: Control of Enzymatic Synthesis of Adrenaline in the Adrenal Medulla by Adrenal Cortical Steroids, *J Biol Chem,* **241:**2301, 1966.

Incidence

Graham, J. B.: Collective Review: Pheochromocytoma and Hypertension: An Analysis of 207 Cases, *Int Abstr Surg,* **92:**105, 1951.

Kvale, W. F., Roth, G. M., Manger, W. M., and Priestly, J. T.: Pheochromocytoma, *Circulation,* **14:**622, 1956.

Minno, A. M., Bennett, W. A., and Kvale, W. F.: Pheochromcytoma: Study of 15 Cases Diagnosed at Autopsy, *Proc Staff Meet Mayo Clin,* **30:**394, 1955.

Symptoms, Signs, and Pathophysiology

Harrison, T. S., Bartlett, J. D., Jr., and Seaton, J. F.: Exaggerated Urinary Norepinephrine Response to Tilt in Pheochromocytoma, *N Engl J Med,* **277:**725, 1967.

Vallance, W. B.: Sudden Death from an Asymptomatic Pheochromocytoma, *Br Med J,* **23:**686, 1957.

Simulation of Pheochromocytoma Attack

Plass, H. F.: Monoamine-Oxidase Inhibitor Reactions Simulating Pheochromocytoma Attacks, *Ann Intern Med,* **61:**924, 1964.

Location

Cahill, G. F.: Pheochromocytoma, *Bull NY Acad Med,* **29:**749, 1953.

Symington, T., and Goodall, A. L.: Studies in Pheochromocytoma: Pathological Aspects, *Glasgow Med J,* **34:**75, 1953.

Malignant Pheochromocytoma

Holsti, L. R.: Malignant Extra-adrenal Phaeochromocytoma, *Br J Radiol,* **37:**944, 1964.

Palmieri, G., Ikkos, D., and Luft, R.: Malignant Pheochromocytoma, *Acta Endocrinol, (Kbh),* **36:**549, 1961.

Diagnostic Tests

Bogaert, M. G., and Vermuelen, A.: Pheochromocytoma of the Urinary Bladder, with Inconclusive Chemical and Pharmacologic Tests, *Am J Med,* **53:**797, 1972.

Crout, J. R., Pisano, J. J., and Sjoerdsma, A.: Urinary Excretion of Catechol Amines and Their Metabolites in Pheochromocytoma, *Am Heart J,* **61:**375, 1961.

Engelman, K., Horwitz, D., Amerose, I. M., and Sjoerdsma, A.: Further Evaluation of the Tyramine Test for Pheochromocytoma, *N Engl J Med,* **278:**705, 1968.

Freier, D. T., and Harrison, T. S.: Rigorous Biochemical Criteria for the Diagnosis of Pheochromocytoma, *J Surg Res,* **14:**177, 1973.

Gifford, R. W., and Tweed, D. C.: Spurious Elevation of Urinary Catecholamines during Therapy with Alpha-Methyldopa, *JAMA,* **182:**493, 1962.

Gitlow, S., Mendlowitz, M., and Bertani, L. M.: The Biochemical Techniques for Detecting and Establishing the Presence of a Pheochromocytoma, *Am J Cardiol,* **26:**270, 1970.

Gjessing, L. R., and Hjermann, I.: Difficulties in Chemical Diagnosis in Phaeochromocytoma, *Lancet,* **2:**1014, 1964.

Lawrence, A. M.: Glucagon Provocative Test for Pheochromocytoma, *Ann Intern Med,* **66:**1091, 1967.

Robinson, R., Ratcliffe, J., and Smith, P.: A Screening Test for Pheochromocytoma, *J Clin Pathol,* **12:**541, 1959.

———, Smith, P., and Whittaker, S.: Secretion of Catecholamines in Malignant Phaeochromocytomas, *Br Med J,* **1:**1422, 1964.

Sheps, S. G., and Maher, F. T.: Histamine and Glucagon Tests in Diagnosis of Pheochromocytoma, *JAMA,* **205:**895, 1968.

Sunderman, G. W.: Measurements of Vanilmandelic Acid for the Diagnosis of Pheochromocytoma and Neuroblastoma, *J Clin Pathol,* **42:**481, 1964.

Wolf, R. L., Mendlowitz, M., Raboz, J., and Gitlow, S. E.: New Rapid Test for Pheochromocytoma, *JAMA,* **188:**859, 1964.

Localization

Epinephrine versus Norepinephrine

Von Euler, U. S.: Increased Urinary Excretion of Noradrenaline and Adrenaline in Cases of Pheochromocytoma, *Ann Surg,* **134:**929, 1951.

Inferior Vena Cava Sampling

Harrison, T. S., Seaton, J. F., Cerny, J. C., Bookstein, J. J., and Bartlett, J. D., Jr.: Localization of Pheochromocytoma by Caval Catheterization, *Arch Surg,* **95:**339, 1967.

Von Euler, U. S., and Strom, G.: Present Status of Diagnosis and Treatment of Pheochromocytoma, *Circulation,* **15:**5, 1957.

Arteriography and X-ray

Boijsen, E., Williams, C. M., and Judkins, M. P.: Angiography and Pheochromocytoma, *Am J Roentgenol Radium Ther Nucl Med,* **98:**225, 1966.

Kahn, P. C.: Radiologic Identification of Functioning Adrenal Tumors, *Radiol Clin North Am,* **5:**221, 1967.

Meaney, T. F., and Buonocore, E.: Selective Arteriography as a Localizing and Provocative Test in the Diagnosis of Pheochromocytoma, *Radiology,* **87:**309, 1966.

Meyers, M. A.: Characteristic Radiographic Shapes of Pheochromocytomas and Adrenocortical Adenomas, *Radiology,* **87:**889, 1966.

Rossi, Plinio, Young, I. S., and Panke, W. F.: Techniques, Usefulness and Hazards of Arteriography of Pheochromocytoma, *JAMA,* **205:**547, 1968.

Familial

Carman, C. T., and Brashear, R. E.: Pheochromocytomas as an Inherited Abnormality: Report of 10th Affected Kindred and Review of the Literature, *N Engl J Med,* **263:**419, 1960.

Tisherman, S. E., Gregg, F. J., and Danowski, T. S.: Familial Pheochromocytoma, *JAMA,* **182:**152, 1962.

Pregnancy

Barzel, U. S., Bar-Ilan, Z., and Rumney, G.: Pheochromocytoma and Pregnancy: Simultaneous Delivery by Caesarean Section and Resection of Tumor, *Am J Obstet Gynecol,* **89:**519, 1964.

Blair, R. G.: Phaeochromocytoma and Pregnancy: Report of a Case and Review of 51 Cases, *J Obstet Gynaecol Br Commonw,* **70:**110, 1963.

Parbossingh, I. S., and Tate, J.: Pheochromocytoma and Pregnancy: Case Report, *West Indian Med J,* **4:**265, 1955.

Pickles, B. G.: Phaeochromocytoma Complicating Pregnancy, *J Obstet Gynaecol Br Commonw,* **65:**1010, 1958.

Walker, R. M.: Phaeochromocytoma in Relation to Pregnancy, *Br J Surg,* **51:**590, 1964.

Neurocutaneous Syndromes

Shocket, E., and Teloh, H. A.: Aganglionic Megacolon, Pheochromocytoma, Megaloureter, and Neurofibroma: Co-occurrence of Several Neural Abnormalities, *Am J Dis Child,* **94:**185, 1957.

Williams, E. D., and Pollack, D. J.: Multiple Mucosal Neuromata with Endocrine Tumors: A Syndrom Allied to von Recklinghausen's Disease, *J Pathol Bacteriol,* **91:**71, 1966.

Congenital Heart

Folger, G. M., Jr., Roberts, W. C., Mehrizi, A., Shah, K. D., Glancy, D. L., Carpenter, C. C. J., and Esterley, J. R.: Cyanotic Malformations of the Heart with Pheochromocytoma, *Circulation,* **29:**750, 1964.

Lees, M. H.: Catecholamine Metabolic Excretion of Infants with Heart Failure, *J Pediat,* **69:**259, 1966.

Reisman, M., Goldenberg, E. D., and Gordon, J.: Congenital Heart Disease and Neuroblastoma, *Am J Dis Child,* **111:**308, 1966.

Pheochromocytoma and Thyroid Carcinoma

Hazard, J. B., Hawk, W. A., and Crile, G.: Medullary (Solid) Carcinoma of the Thyroid: A Clinicopathologic Entity, *J Clin Endocrinol Metab,* **19:**152, 1959.

Huang, S., and McLeish, W. A.: Familial Pheochromocytoma and Amyloid-producing Medullary Carcinoma of Thyroid, *Laval Med,* **39:**22, 1968.

Nourok, D. S.: Familial Pheochromocytoma and Thyroid Carcinoma, *Ann Intern Med,* **60:**1028, 1964.

Sapira, J. D., Althan, M., Vandyk, K., and Shapiro, A. P.: Bilateral Adrenal Pheochromocytoma and Medullary Thyroid Carcinoma, *N Engl J Med,* **273:**140, 1965.

Schimke, R. N., and Hartmann, W. H.: Familial Amyloid Producing Medullary Thyroid Carcinoma and Pheochromocytoma: Distinct Genetic Entity, *Ann Intern Med,* **63:**1027, 1965.

Sipple, J. H.: The Association of Pheochromocytoma with Carcinoma of the Thyroid Gland, *Am J Med,* **31:**163, 1961.

Williams, E. D.: A Review of 17 Cases of Carcinoma of the Thyroid and Phaeochromocytoma, *J Clin Pathol,* **18:**288, 1965.

Pheochromocytoma, Cholelithiasis, and Increase in Free Fatty Acids

Gifford, R. W., Jr., Kvale, W. F., and Maher, F. T.: Clinical Features, Diagnosis and Treatment of Pheochromocytoma: A Review of 76 Cases, *Proc Staff Meetings Mayo Clin,* **39:**281, 1964.

Pheochromocytoma and Renovascular Hypertension

Assaykeen, T. A., and Ganong, W. F.: The Sympathetic Nervous System and Renin Secretion, in W. F. Ganong and L. Martini (eds.), "Frontiers in Neuroendocrinology," Oxford University Press, New York, 1971.

Garrett, H. C., Scott, R., Jr., Howell, J. F., and DeBakey, M. E.: Pheochromocytoma and Renal Artery Stenosis: Surgical Treatment of Secondary Hypertension, Case Report, *Arch Surg,* **90:**97, 1965.

Harrison, J. H., Gardner, F. H., and Dammin, G. J.: Note on Pheochromocytoma and Renal Hypertension, *J Urol,* **79:**173, 1958.

Harrison, T. S., Birbari, A., and Seaton, J. F.: Malignant Hypertension in Pheochromocytoma: Correlation with Plasma Renin Activity, *Johns Hopkins Med J,* **130:**329, 1972.

Kerzner, M. S., Reeves, J. A., DeNyse, D., and Claunch, B. C.: Pheochromocytoma with Renal Artery Compression in an Identical Twin, *Arch Intern Med,* **121:**91, 1968.

Maebashi, M., Miura, Y., and Yoshinaga, K.: Plama Renin Activity in Pheochromocytoma, *Jap Circ J,* **32:**1427, 1968.

Rosenheim, M. L., Ross, E. J., Wong, O. M., Hudson, C. L., Davies, D. R., and Smith, J. F.: Unilateral Renal Ischaemia Due to Compression of Renal Artery by Phaeochromocytoma, *Am J Med,* **34:**735, 1963.

Straube, K. R., and Hodges, C. V.: Pheochromocytoma Causing Renal Hypertension, *Am J Roentgenol Radium Ther Nucl Med,* **98:**222, 1966.

Tanigawa, H., Allison, D. J., and Assaykeen, T. A.: A Comparison of the Effects of Various Catecholamines on Plasma Renin Activity Alone and in the Presence of Adrenergic Blocking Agents, in J. Genest and E. Koiw (eds.), "Hypertension—1972," Springer Verlag New York, Inc., New York, 1972.

Vetter, H., Vetter, W., Warnholz, C., Bayer, J.-M., Käser, H., Vielhaber, K., and Krück, F.: Renin and Aldosterone Secretion in Phenochromocytoma, *Am J Med,* **60:**866, 1976.

Hypotension, Shock, or Sudden Death

Hypotension or Shock

Huston, J. R., and Stewart, W. R.: Hemorrhagic Pheochromocytoma with Shock and Abdominal Pain, *Am J Med.,* **39:**502, 1965.

McAlister, W. H., and Koehler, P. R.: Hemorrhage into a Pheochromocytoma in a Patient on Anticoagulants, *J Can Assoc Radiol,* **18:**404, 1967.

Parkinson, T.: Phaeochromocytoma Presenting as Postural Hypotension, *Proc R Soc Med,* **57:**673, 1964.

Richmond, J., Frazer, S. C., and Miller, D. R.: Paroxysmal Hypotension Due to an Adrenalin-secreting Phaeochromocytoma, *Lancet,* **2:**904, 1961.

Sudden Death

Coates, P. A., and Rigal, W. M.: Post Anesthetic Death from Pheochromocytoma without Hypertension, *Lancet,* **1:**1374, 1961.

Crockett, K. A., Snow, E., and Rees, V. L.: Pheochromocytoma as Cause of Unexpected Operating Room Deaths, *Am Surg,* **27:**395, 1961.

Mitchell, L.: An Unusual Cause of Sudden Death, *Practitioner,* **193:**205, 1964.

Childhood

Insley, J., and Smallwood, W. C.: Pheochromocytoma in Children, *Arch Dis Child,* **37:**606, 1962.

Moon, H. D., Koneff, A. A., Li, C. H., and Simpson, M. E.: Pheochromocytomas of Adrenals in Male Rats Chronically Injected with Pituitary Growth Hormone, *Proc Soc Exp Biol Med,* **93:**74, 1956.

Stackpole, R. H., Melicow, M. M., and Uson, A. C.: Pheochromocytoma in Children: Report of 9 Cases and Review of the First 100 Published Cases with Followup Studies, *J Pediatr,* **63:**314, 1963.

Special Locations

Bilateral

Baker, N. H., Swindell, H. F., Rollins, L. T.: The Surgical Treatment of Bilateral Pheochromocytomas, *Ann Surg,* **159:**456, 1964.

Zuckerkandl

Van Zyl, J. J. W., van Zyl, F. D. dT, and Wicht, C. L.: Phaeochromocytoma of the Organ of Zuckerkandl, *Suid-Afrikaanse Tydskr Chir,* **4:**43, 1966.

Bladder

Besser, M. I. B., and Pfau, A.: Pheochromocytoma of the Urinary Bladder, *Br J Urol,* **40:**245, 1968.

Intrathoracic

Engelman, K., and Hammond, W. G.: Adrenaline Production by an Intrathoracic Phaeochromocytoma, *Lancet,* **1:**609, 1968.

Cervical

Fries, J. G., and Chamberlin, J. A.: Extra-adrenal Pheochromocytoma: Literature Review and Report of a Cervical Pheochromocytoma, *Surgery,* **63:**268, 1968.

Medical Treatment

Bellos, J.: Non Surgical Treatment of Pheochromocytoma, *JAMA,* **185:**601, 1963.

Crago, R. M., Eckholdt, J. W., and Wiswell, J. G.: Pheochromocytoma: Treatment with α- and β-Adrenergic Blocking Drugs, *JAMA,* **202:**870, 1967.

Egdahl, R. H., and Chobanian, A. V.: Acute Pheochromocytoma, *Surg Clin North Am,* **46:**645, 1966.

Harrison, T. S., Dagher, F. J., Beck, L., and Bartlett, J. D., Jr.: Rationale and Indications for Preoperative Adrenergic Receptor Blockade in Pheochromocytoma, *Med Clin North Am,* **53:**1349, 1969.

Iseri, L. T., Henderson, H. W., and Derr, J. W.: Use of Adrenolytic Drug, Regitine, in Pheochromocytoma, *Am Heart J,* **42:**129, 1951.

Surgical and Anesthetic Considerations

Buist, N. R. M., Mijer, F., and O'Brien, D.: Treatment of a Phaeochromocytoma with a β-Adrenergic Blocking Agent, *Arch Dis Child,* **41:**435, 1966.

Glenn, F., and Mannix, H. Jr.: The Surgical Management of Chromaffin Tumors, *Ann Surg,* **167:**619, 1968.

Grimson, K. S., Longino, F. H., Kernodle, C. E., and O'Near, H. B.: Treatment of a Patient with a Pheochromocytoma: Use of an Adrenolytic Drug before and during Operation, *JAMA,* **180:**1273, 1949.

Priestley, J. T., Kvale, W. F., and Gifford, R. W., Jr.: Pheochromocytoma: Clinical Aspects and Surgical Treatment, *Arch Surg,* **86:**778, 1963.

Schnelle, N., Carney, F. M., Didier, E. P., and Faulconer, A., Jr.: Anesthesia Surgical Treatment of Pheochromocytoma, *Surg Clin North Am,* **45:**991, 1965.

Recurrent Pheochromocytoma

Harrison, T. S., Freier, D. T., and Cohen, E. L.: Recurrent Pheochromocytoma, *Arch Surg,* **108:**450, 1974.

Neuroblastoma

Bohuon, C.: Catecholamine Metabolism in Neuroblastoma, *J Pediat Surg,* **3:**114, 1968.

Brown, W. G., Owens, J. B., Berson, A. W., and Henry, S. K.: Vanilmandelic Acid Screening Test for Pheochromocytoma and Neuroblastoma, *Am J Clin Pathol,* **46:**599, 1966.

Chatten, J., and Voorhess, M. L.: Familial Neuroblastoma, *N Engl J Med,* **277:**1230, 1967.

Fortner, J., Nicastri, A., and Murphy, M. L.: Neuroblastoma: Natural History and Results of Treating 133 Cases, *Ann Surg,* **167:**132, 1968.

James, D. H., Jr.: Proposed Classification of Neuroblastoma, *J Pediat,* **71:**764, 1967.

Keep, C. E.: The Role of Surgery in Resectable, and Metastatic Neuroblastoma, *JAMA,* **205:**57, 1968.

Rubin, P.: Urogenital Tract: Wilms' Tumor and Neuroblastoma, *JAMA,* **205:**153, 1968.

Chapter 38

Thyroid and Parathyroid

by **Seymour I. Schwartz and Edwin L. Kaplan**

THYROID

(by Seymour I. Schwartz)

Historical Background

The thyroid gland, previously referred to as the "laryngeal" gland, was so named by Wharton in 1646 because of either its own shieldlike (*thyreos,* shield) shape or the shape of the thyroid cartilage, with which it is closely associated. Classic descriptions of hyperthyroidism, or exophthalmic goiter, were presented by Parry (1825), Graves (1835), and von Basedow (1840), and hypothyroidism, or myxedema, was described by Curling (1850) and Gull (1875). Schiff, in the middle of the nineteenth century, conducted experiments demonstrating the importance of the thyroid. Excision in dogs resulted in fatality which could be prevented by a previous graft of the gland. In 1882, Reverdin produced experimental myxedema by total or partial thyroidectomy. In the 1890s, Murray and Howitz successfully treated myxedema with thyroid extract. Although Hedenus performed a total thyroidectomy for goiter in 1800, Theodor Kocher is regarded as the father of thyroid surgery. He was the first to successfully excise the thyroid for goiter (1878), and he performed this operation over 2,000 times with only a 4.5 percent mortality. He also described "cachexia strumipriva," i.e., myxedema, which he noted as a sequel in 30 of his first 100 thyroidectomies. For his pioneering efforts in the field of thyroid surgery, he received the Nobel prize in 1909. The first successful transplantation of thyroid was reported by Payr in 1906, who transplanted a portion of the gland from a woman into the spleen of a myxedematous daughter with "successful" results. Isolation of the hormone thyroxine (T4) was accomplished by Kendall in 1914.

Anatomy

The thyroid gland, which has an average weight of 20 Gm, is convex anteriorly and concave posteriorly as a result of its relation to the anterolateral portions of the trachea and larynx, around which it is wrapped and to which it is firmly fixed by fibrous tissue. The lateral lobes extend along the sides of the larynx, reaching the level of the middle of the thyroid cartilage. They reside in a bed between the trachea and larynx mediad and the two carotid sheaths and the sternocleidomastoid muscles laterally. The thyroid gland is enveloped by a thickened fibrous capsule which sends septa into the gland substance to produce an irregular and incomplete pseudolobulation. No true lobulation exists. The deep cervical fascia divides into an anterior and posterior sheath, creating a loosely applied false capsule for the thyroid. Anteriorly, the thyroids are in relation to the infrahyoid muscles. Situated on the posterior surface of the lateral lobes of the gland are the parathyroid glands, which reside within the surgical capsule, and the recurrent nerves, which lie in a cleft between the trachea and esophagus just medial to the lateral lobes. The lateral lobes are joined by the isthmus which crosses the trachea. The pyramidal lobe is a long, narrow projection of thyroid tissue extending upward from the isthmus lying on the surface of the thyroid cartilage usually to the left of the prominence of that structure. It represents a vestige of the embryonic thyroglossal duct and can be demonstrated in about 80 percent of patients at operation.

The thyroid has an abundant blood supply with a normal flow rate of about 5 ml/Gm/minute. The four major arteries are the paired superior thyroid arteries, which arise from the external carotid arteries and descend several centimeters in the neck to reach the upper poles of the thyroid glands, where they branch, and the paired inferior thyroid arteries, which arise from the thyrocervical trunks of the subclavian arteries and enter the lower poles from behind. A fifth artery, the thyroidea ima, arises from the arch of the aorta and enters the thyroid in the midline. A venous plexus forms under the capsule and contributes to confluences forming the superior thyroid vein at the upper pole and the middle thyroid vein at the lower pole, both of which enter the internal jugular vein. Also occasionally arising from the lower pole are the inferior thyroid veins, which drain directly into the innominate vein.

The gland receives its innervation from sympathetic and parasympathetic divisions of the autonomic nervous system. The sympathetic fibers arise from the cervical ganglion and enter with blood vessels, while the parasympathetic fibers are derived from the vagus and reach the gland via branches of the laryngeal nerves.

Microscopically, the thyroid is composed of follicles, or acini. The follicles are roughly spherical and have an average diameter of 30μ. They represent storage depots which receive and store the products of the lining epithelial cells. These are usually cuboidal. Under the influence of thyrotropin stimulation, the height of the cells increases, changing the shape to a columnar one, and the lumen decreases proportionately.

The thyroid gland's relation to the recurrent laryngeal and external laryngeal nerves is of major surgical significance. Riddell indicated that among cases in which surgeons "avoid" rather than expose the recurrent laryngeal nerve there is a 4 percent incidence of vocal cord damage. Hunt et al. reported the anatomy of the recurrent laryngeal nerves in 100 cases. The right recurrent laryngeal nerve resided in the tracheoesophageal groove in 64 percent of cases, whereas the left nerve was similarly located on the left side in 77 percent of cases. The nerve was lateral to the trachea in 33 percent of cases on the right side and 22 percent on the left side. In six cases on the right side and four on the left, the nerve was anterolateral to the trachea and in danger of division during subtotal lobectomy. On one occasion, a direct recurrent laryngeal nerve was given off in the neck without looping around the subclavian artery. The inferior thyroid artery is often used as a landmark for demonstration of the recurrent laryngeal nerve. The vessel was absent in five instances on the left and twice on the right in the above series. The recurrent laryngeal nerve passed anterior to the inferior thyroid artery in 37 percent of cases on the right side and 24

percent on the left. In 50 percent of cases, the nerve was embedded in the ligament of Berry, which is of importance because traction on the gland would put the nerve on stretch and make it subject to section. Damage to the recurrent laryngeal nerve results in paresis or paralysis of the intrinsic musculature of the larynx.

The superior laryngeal nerves innervate the cricothyroid muscle. There is dispute as to whether the innervation of the interarytenoid muscle is supplied by the superior or inferior laryngeal nerves. In 85 percent of cases, the superior laryngeal nerves lie immediately adjacent to the vascular pedicles of the superior poles of the thyroid glands, requiring that the vessels be ligated with care to avoid injury. In 18 percent of cases, the nerve is intimately related to the vessels lying parallel and just deep to them in the pretracheal fascia. In 7 percent, the nerve passes through the division of the superior thyroid vessels, coursing over the anterosuperior portion of the gland. In only 15 percent of cases does the superior laryngeal nerve enter the thyropharyngeal muscle before reaching the region of the superior pole of the thyroid gland, thus protecting it from manipulation by the surgeon.

ANOMALIES

The thyroid is embryologically an offshoot of the primitive alimentary tract, from which it later becomes separated. A median anlage arises from the pharyngeal floor in the region of the foramen cecum of the tongue. The main body of the thyroid descends into the neck from this origin and is supposedly joined by a pair of lateral components originating from the ultimobranchial bodies of the fourth and fifth branchial pouches. The contribution of these lateral components presently is considered to be small.

The median thyroid anlage may fail to develop, with the rare situation of athyreosis as a result, or it may differentiate in abnormal locations. The most common of these is the pyramidal lobe, which has been reported in as many as 80 percent of patients in whom the gland was surgically exposed. Other variations involving the median thyroid anlage represent an arrest in the usual descent of part or all of the thyroid-forming material to its normal location in front of the second to sixth tracheal rings. These include the development of a lingual thyroid, suprahyoid, infrahyoid, and prethyroid tissue, and persistence of the thyroglossal duct, which is the most common of the clinically important anomalies of thyroid development (see Chap. 39). Infrequently, the entire gland or parts of it descend more caudad, which results in thyroid tissue located in the superior mediastinum behind the sternum, adjacent to the aortic arch or between the aorta and pulmonary trunk, within the upper portion of the pericardium, and even in the interventricular septum of the heart. Most intrathoracic goiters, however, are not true anomalies but rather extensions of pathologic elements of a normally situated gland into the superior or posterior mediastinum.

LATERAL ABERRANT THYROID RESTS. True lateral aberrant thyroid tissue is rare, since the lateral anlagen are normally incorporated into the expanding lateral lobes of the median thyroid anlage. Lateral aberrant thyroid tissue has not been shown to function in man. It is now felt that the so-called "lateral aberrant thyroid" is a metastasis from the gland proper. Carcinoma, which has been noted so frequently in "lateral rests," actually represents metastatic disease within cervical lymph nodes from a primary site and does not arise independently.

LINGUAL THYROID. Lingual thyroid is relatively rare and estimated to occur in 1 in 3,000 cases of thyroid disease. It does, however, represent the most common form of functioning ectopic thyroid tissue which achieves clinical significance. Lingual thyroids are associated with cervical athyreosis in 70 percent of cases and occur much more commonly in females.

Clinical Manifestations. The diagnosis may be made by discovery of an incidental posterior lingual mass in an asymptomatic patient. The mass may enlarge and cause dysphagia, dysphonia, dyspnea, or sensation of choking. Lingual thyroid has been known to cause complications during induction of anesthesia. Hypothyroidism is frequently present, but hyperthyroidism, which is unusual, can occur. The incidence of malignancy is extremely low, occurring in 4 of 144 patients with symptomatic lingual thyroid. The diagnosis should be suspected when a mass is detected in the region of the foramen cecum of the tongue. The diagnosis is readily established by scanning with [131]I.

Treatment. Unless there is immediate surgical indication, treatment should be instituted with replacement thyroid hormone to suppress the lingual thyroid and reduce its size. Radioactive ^{131}I may also be used to reduce the size and is particularly appropriate if there is associated hyperthyroidism.

Indications for surgical intervention include difficulty in swallowing, speech, or breathing; hemorrhage; degeneration and necrosis; uncontrolled hyperthyroidism; and, occasionally, the suspicion of malignancy. A preliminary tracheostomy may be indicated with large or hemorrhagic lesions to obviate the consequences of postoperative tracheal edema. The lingual thyroid may be removed by an intraoral route, by drawing the tongue forward and incising directly over the growth, which is completely or partially removed. Lateral pharyngotomy, in some instances, may represent a preferential approach. Autotransplantation of the excised lingual thyroid has been recommended to avoid the development of hypothyroidism, and success has been reported by several writers.

Physiology

The function of the thyroid gland is to synthesize and secrete thyroid hormone, which is necessary for overall metabolism. This function is dependent upon an interplay between several processes, including (1) iodine metabolism, (2) the production, storage, and secretion of thyroid hormone by the thyroid gland, and (3) the effects of this hormone on various organ systems. The production of thyroid hormone is influenced by intricate regulatory mechanisms and responds to multiple and diverse physiologic, pathologic, and pharmacologic alterations.

IODINE METABOLISM. The formation of thyroid hormone depends upon the availability of exogenous iodine which is normally satisfied by dietary sources and is thus dependent upon the iodine content of water and soil. Ingested iodine is rapidly absorbed from the gastrointestinal tract, usually within 1 hour. It is then distributed through the extracellular space in the form of iodides and is progressively extracted from the plasma both by the thyroid and kidneys until essentially all the iodine is either bound in organic form within the thyroid or excreted as urinary iodides (Fig. 38-1). Ninety percent of the body iodine stores are present within the thyroid, predominantly in the organic form. Studies employing labeled iodine have demonstrated that approximately two-thirds of the administered dose ultimately appears in the urine, while the thyroid collects the remaining third. The partitioning of the ingested iodide between thyroid and kidney is complete within 48 hours, and the plasma and tissues are almost cleared of iodide. The subsequent appearance of labeled iodine within the circulation is the result of the secretion of thyroid hormone and is concomitant with a decrease in activity within the thyroid gland. A small fraction of the iodine which had been removed from the extracellular fluid by the thyroid gland is ultimately secreted back into the circulation as inorganic iodide. Renal disease such as nephrosis and marked proteinuria may be associated with a significant urinary loss of iodide affecting the body economy. Gastrointestinal malabsorption may be accompanied by significant augmentation of the usually small amounts of iodine lost in the stool.

SYNTHESIS AND SECRETION OF THYROID HORMONE. The steps in the synthesis of thyroid hormone are (1) the concentration of iodide within the gland, (2) the formation of precursor amino acids, 3-monoiodotyrosine (MIT) and 3-5-diiodotyrosine (DIT), (3) the coupling of these inactive iodotyrosines to form the hormonally active iodothyronines, triiodothyronine (T3) and thyroxine (T4).

The production of thyroid hormone begins with the active transport of iodine from the plasma into the thyroid cells. The iodine transfer mechanism is influenced by thyroid-stimulating hormone (TSH), which stimulates every step in thyroid hormone synthesis and secretion, and is also modified by an internal autoregulatory system so that its responsiveness to TSH stimulation varies inversely with the glandular content of organic iodine. When iodine transport is defective, because of either pharmacologic inhibitors or spontaneous disease, goiter and/or hypothyroidism results. However, this can be overcome by increasing the plasma iodine concentration and allowing quantities to enter the gland by diffusion.

The iodide which enters the thyroid remains in its free state only briefly before it is further metabolized. It is rapidly incorporated into thyroglobulin, and it has been shown that 24 hours after administration of labeled iodine, 99 percent is bound to protein. Tyrosine radicals of protothyroglobulin molecules are iodinated to form MIT and DIT. Organic iodinations are conditioned to some extent by the stimulation of TSH and may be inhibited by a great number of pharmacologic agents, including the usual antithyroid drugs, or by defects in the organ-binding mechanism with resultant hypothyroidism and/or goiter. The

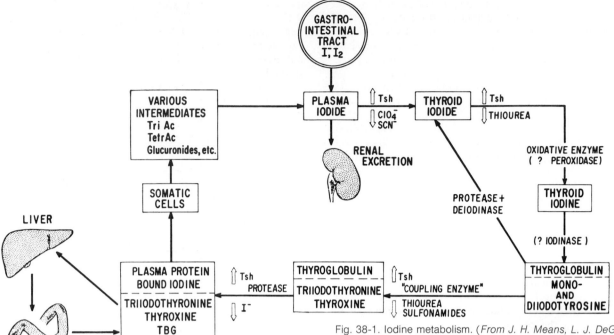

Fig. 38-1. Iodine metabolism. (*From J. H. Means, L. J. DeGroot, and J. B. Stanbury, "The Thyroid and Its Diseases," 3d ed., chap. 2, McGraw-Hill Book Company, New York, 1963.*)

coupling of two iodotyrosine molecules leads to the formation of iodothyronine, a process in which a variety of enzymatic systems have been implicated. T4 is formed by the coupling of two DIT radicals, while T3 is formed by the coupling of one MIT and one DIT radical. The proportion of T3 to T4 synthesized and secreted is dependent on the degree of iodination of intrafollicular thyroglobulin.

STORAGE, SECRETION, AND METABOLISM OF THYROID HORMONE. The hormonally active iodothyronines, T4 and T3, are held in peptide linkage with a specific thyroprotein, thyroglobulin, which forms the major component of intrafollicular colloid. The storage is of such magnitude that the administration of antithyroid blocking agents for as long as 2 weeks results in only minimal decrease of T4 and T3. The normal human thyroid gland contains enough preformed T4 to maintain the euthyroid state for 2 months without synthesis, thus forming an excellent buffer against the changes in dietary intake of iodine.

Release of the active hormones into the circulation involves hydrolysis of the thyroglobulin by proteases and peptidases, resulting in T4 and T3. The activity of these enzymes is enhanced by the administration of TSH. At the same time, some metabolically inert iodine amino acids enter the circulation and are deiodinized, and the iodine is reutilized in the metabolic cycle. The active thyroid hormones become attached to plasma protein, the best known of which is the thyroxine-binding globulin (TBG) and the more recently recognized thyroxine-binding prealbumin (TBPA).

Disorders related to the storage-and-release mechanism occur in subacute thyroiditis, in Hashimoto's disease, and after surgical manipulation of the gland. Also, iodides and iodotyrosines may be found in the blood, associated with several types of nontoxic goiter and hyperplastic tissue.

In the plasma, the ratio of T4 to T3 is 10–20:1. T3 is bound less firmly to protein and thus enters the peripheral tissues more rapidly. It is three to four times more active than T4 per unit weight and accounts for approximately half the metabolic effect of the secreted hormone. The free hormone available to the tissue is responsible for its metabolic action. The half-life of T3 is 2 to 3 days, while the half-life of T4 is 6 to 11 days, and both hormones leave the blood in an exponential fashion. A significant amount of T4 is converted to T3, which may be the only active hormone intracellularly. As they lose iodine atoms, the iodine returns to the blood to reenter the metabolic pool. T3 and T4 are conjugated in the liver with glucuronic acid and excreted into the bile. In the intestine, these conjugates are disrupted, and a portion of the free hormones is reabsorbed. In man, less than 5 percent of the circulating T4 is involved in the enterohepatic circulation. In acute hepatitis, the functional hepatic turnover of T4 is retarded, while in chronic diarrhea and nephrosis there may be excessive loss. Large amounts of hormone and iodide may appear in the milk of lactating females.

The metabolic impact of thyroid hormone on peripheral tissue is widespread and accompanied by an increased oxygen consumption and calorigenesis. Thyroid hormone stimulates protein synthesis and affects all aspects of carbohydrate metabolism, regulating the magnitude of the glycogenolytic and hyperglycemic effects of epinephrine and potentiating the effects of insulin on glycogen synthesis and glucose utilization. Thyroid hormone also influences the processes of lipid metabolism, as evidenced by the fact that the serum cholesterol and phospholipid vary inversely with the state of thyroid function.

REGULATION OF THYROID ACTIVITY. The function of the thyroid gland is closely regulated by the central nervous system and by the level of circulating iodine. As a consequence of these regulatory mechanisms, thyroid activity responds to a variety of physiologic and pathologic changes as well as pharmacologic agents.

The suspicion that the central nervous system is involved in the stimulation and inhibition of thyroid hormone is an old one, but scientific support is relatively recent. The anterior pituitary basophil cells secrete TSH, which regulates thyroid function. Absence or reduction of TSH secretion is accompanied by decreased synthesis and secretion of thyroid hormone, flattening of the thyroid epithelium, and reduction in vascularity of the gland. Conversely, increased TSH secretion accelerates the production and release of thyroid hormone while anatomically increasing the cellularity and vascularity of the thyroid gland. TSH stimulates all processes leading to the synthesis and secretion of thyroid hormone. When the target gland is responsive, the basal metabolic rate (BMR) is increased within a few hours of TSH administration, and there is an associated increase in the T4 and T3.

It is now felt that the cerebral cortex acts on the hypothalamus, which secretes a thyrotropin-releasing hormone (TRH), which in turn acts on the pituitary and induces the release of TSH. The secretion of TSH is also controlled in a "feedback" manner by the level of thyroid hormone in the blood (Fig. 38-2). TSH secretion is inhibited by an excess of circulating thyroid hormone and augmented by thyroid hormone deprivation. When antithyroid substances of the thiourea type cause hypothyroidism, the pituitary responds by increasing TSH secretion with resultant hyperplasia and increased vascularity of the thyroid gland.

The concentration of intrathyroidal iodide inversely influences responsiveness to TSH, thus effecting an intrinsic regulatory system. When small doses of iodine are administered, there is an increase in thyroid hormone synthesis for a short time. With progressively larger doses, there is a biphasic response, at first increasing and then decreasing, due to a relative blockade in organic binding. With moderate or large doses administered repeatedly, the relative inhibition of organic binding eventually escapes, representing an adaptation phenomenon. Pharmacologic doses of iodide decrease the rate of release of glandular iodine and the formation of active hormone. Concentration of T4 in the serum is reduced, and thyrotoxicity in patients with diffuse toxic goiter is rapidly relieved. The vascularity and hyperplasia of the gland are reversed through the action of iodine on TSH, thus facilitating surgical excision.

In addition to these pharmacologic effects of iodine, the biosynthesis of thyroid hormone may be altered by agents known as *antithyroid drugs*. There are two major categories: The first, represented by perchlorate and thiocyanate, prevent the concentration of iodine by the thyroid. In the presence of high iodine intake, however, the blood iodine can rise to a level at which the concentrating mechanism

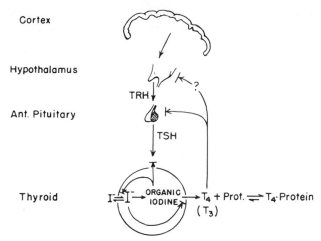

Fig. 38-2. Schema of the homeostatic regulation of thyroid function. Secretion of TSH is regulated by a negative feedback mechanism acting directly on the pituitary and is normally inversely related to the concentration of unbound hormone in the blood. Release of TSH is induced by TRH, secretion of which appears to set the level of the pituitary feedback mechanism. Factors regulating secretion of TRH are uncertain but may include the free hormone in the blood and stimuli from higher centers. Auto-regulatory control of thyroid function is also shown. High concentrations of intrathyroidal iodide decrease the rate of release of thyroidal iodine. In addition, the magnitude of the organic iodine pool inversely influences the iodide transport mechanism and the response to TSH. [*From S. H. Ingbar and K. A. Woeber, The Thyroid Gland, in R. H. Williams (ed.), "Textbook of Endocrinology," 4th ed., W. B. Saunders Company, Philadelphia, 1968.*]

is not required and the drugs lose their effect. The second group of antithyroid drugs include organic substances which prevent the binding of iodine to tyrosine radicals. The best known of this group are the thiourea derivatives. The action of this group of drugs is characteristically independent of the level of blood iodide.

The regulatory mechanisms contribute to the alterations in thyroid function associated with physiologic and pathologic changes in the organism. From childhood through senescence, the T4 and T3 are essentially unchanged, while the thyroidal ^{131}I uptake, clearance, and turnover rate tend to decrease slightly with age. In pregnancy, the thyroid becomes enlarged, and there is evidence of increased vascularity. Thyroidal uptake is increased, and the T4 and T3 levels rise and remain elevated until after delivery. All changes in thyroid function which accompany normal pregnancy are exaggerated in molar pregnancy, which may be associated with excess "placental thyrotropin." Ectopic TSH activity also has been described with choriocarcinomas. However, in general, thyroid function in human beings appears to be independent of sex. In women thyroid disorders do occur more frequently during puberty, pregnancy, and the menopause. ACTH and cortisone reduce thyroidal iodine uptake and slightly decrease the T4 and T3, while epinephrine and norepinephrine increase the BMR in thyrotoxic patients unassociated with a measurable alteration in T4 and T3.

Since the hepatobiliary system is an important site for

degradation of thyroid hormone, liver disease may cause an alteration in protein-bound iodine (PBI). With infectious hepatitis and obstructive jaundice, there may be an associated increase in PBI due to regurgitation of iodine from the bile to the blood. With cirrhosis there is a decrease in PBI and an increase in the proportion of the free T4 and T3, and the ^{131}I uptake is often increased. With reduced glomerular filtration and cardiac disease, there is an elevation in the PBI level and a lowered rate of thyroidal clearance of ^{131}I. A nephrotic syndrome may be associated with the stigmata of hypothyroidism, while in cardiac failure the increased work in breathing results in an elevated basal metabolic rate. Several anesthetic agents, particularly ether, increase the circulating thyroid hormone, and surgical treatment may be associated with an increased concentration of free T4 in the plasma due to a decrease in the binding by protein.

Evaluation of Patients with Thyroid Disease

Interview of the patient is directed at determining whether there is evidence of hyperfunction or insufficient function of the thyroid gland. Symptoms in this regard include gross changes in appearance, skin texture, hair, temperature tolerance, and perspiration. Inquiry should also evaluate changes in mental activity, irritability, emotional lability, lethargy, muscular strength, and endurance. Other evidences of abnormal thyroid activity include change in sleep habits, weight, appetite, bowel habits, and muscular strength. The specific signs and symptoms of thyrotoxicosis and myxedema will be presented in subsequent sections of this chapter.

Symptoms related to pressure of the thyroid on neighboring structures in the neck include dysphagia, dysphonia, dyspnea, and a choking sensation. When a thyroid mass is apparent, the duration, rate of growth, and presence of accompanying pain should be determined. A history of exposure to ionizing radiation is pertinent. In the patient with a nontoxic goiter, diet, possible ingestion of goiterogenic drugs, and family history are all relevant.

Physical examination requires a precise evaluation of the thyroid gland and adjacent cervical structures. The neck should be inspected while it is slightly extended. In thin patients, a normal thyroid, particularly in the region of the isthmus, may be visible. If the thyroid is visible, it will rise with deglutition unless it is adherent to adjacent structures because of invasive malignant disease or thyroiditis. A goiter which fills the suprasternal notch may be seen to rise out of the chest with swallowing. Asymmetry and large masses within the gland may be apparent. Palpation should be performed from two vantage points, in front of and behind the seated patient, applying the tips of the fingers in a gentle fashion. In most thin people, it is possible to outline the gland, whereas the normal thyroid is not palpable in obese individuals and in those with short necks. Palpation of the cricoid cartilage serves to orient the examiner, since the superior border of the isthmus lies just below this level.

The normal gland has a rubbery consistency. The diffuse goiter and hyperplastic gland is softer. In Hashimoto's disease the gland is firmer, while with carcinoma or Riedel's struma the thyroid may be stony hard. Nodules may be identified, and transillumination should be used to distinguish between cystic and solid masses. The thyroid should be auscultated to identify bruits which are indicative of a hyperactive gland but must be differentiated from murmurs transmitted from the base of the heart and venous hums. The regional lymph nodes should be examined in the anterior triangles of the neck. A node, known as the Delphian node, may be palpable on the trachea just above the thyroid isthmus. This is frequently associated with malignant disease or thyroiditis. If there is suggestion of retrosternal goiter, the arms should be raised in an attempt to elicit respiratory distress.

Radiologic examination of the upper neck and mediastinum may demonstrate evidence of compression or displacement of the trachea. Miliary calcification may be noted in papillary carcinoma, while more extensive calcification is suggestive of nodular goiter. An electrocardiogram is indicated if there is suggestion of thyrotoxicosis. If carcinoma is considered, the vocal cords should be visualized for mobility.

THYROID FUNCTION TESTS

A variety of laboratory tests have been developed to assess thyroid function and thyroid lesions. Each test has specific indications, none is uniformly reliable, and all are subject to alteration by exogenous and endogenous factors.

RADIOACTIVE ISOTOPE STUDIES. These are widely employed to evaluate the state of thyroid function and hormonal synthesis. Several radioactive isotopes of iodine, ^{131}I, ^{132}I, and ^{125}I, are available. ^{131}I is the most widely used, but ^{132}I is particularly applicable when repeated doses are required, because it has a shorter half-life. By contrast, ^{125}I is recommended for localization of functioning thyroid tissues with scanning procedures. Recently ^{99m}Tc has been used for scanning, since a reduced radiation is used and a more rapid readout is possible.

Thyroidal Uptake and Urinary Excretion. When iodine isotopes are administered either orally or intravenously, they are cleared by the thyroid and kidney. Within 24 hours, the mean value in the plasma is extremely low, and it is essentially undetectable by 72 hours. Measurements of the percentage of thyroidal uptake of radioactive iodine are therefore generally made at 24 hours and are directed at establishing or excluding a diagnosis of hyperthyroidism or hypothyroidism. When doses of 2 to 50 μc are given orally, the normal mean 24-hour thyroidal uptake is 25 percent, with a range of 9 to 35 percent. Values lower than 8 percent indicate hypothyroidism, while values higher than the normal range indicate hyperfunction. In states of severe hyperfunction the thyroidal uptake peak may be reached within a few hours, and it may be appropriate to measure the uptake several hours after administration. The normal uptake at 3 hours rarely exceeds 25 percent.

The expansion of the body stores of iodine is probably the most common exogenous cause of lowering of thyroidal ^{131}I uptake. This is seen following the administration of organic iodinated dyes as used in radiologic studies such as pyelography and cholecystography. While the dyes employed in pyelography are usually cleared rapidly, those used for cholecystography may last for several months. The reduction in renal iodide clearance may be due to renal failure or cardiac failure. Decreased thyroidal iodine accumulation follows the administration of replacement doses of thyroid hormone which suppress the secretion of TSH and also occurs in patients with nephrosis and excessive hormonal loss in the urine.

Thyroid Scanning. Scintillation scanning localizes the site of radioiodine accumulation in the thyroid gland or in ectopic thyroid tissue. ^{131}I is the time-honored isotope which has been utilized, but more recently ^{125}I with a softer gamma energy appears to be superior in resolving small areas and in defining some "cold" nodules. ^{125}I is inferior to ^{131}I when part of the thyroid is retrosternal because of the significant absorption of the soft radiation by the overlying bone. The technique employs a mechanical device which moves a columnated detector back and forth and determines the location of activity (Fig. 38-3).

The indications for thyroid scanning can be divided into three general categories: (1) patients with solitary or multiple nodules in whom clinical findings are insufficient, (2) thyrotoxicotic patients, and (3) patients with suspected or proved cancer of the thyroid. Nodules of the thyroid may be classified as hyperfunctional, that is, with more radioactivity than the normal portion of the gland (Fig. 38-4); functional, that is, nodules which concentrate radioactivity equal to the remainder of the gland (Fig. 38-5); hypofunctional, or nodules which concentrate less activity than the remainder of the gland; and finally nonfunctional, or "cold" nodules, which concentrate no radioactivity (Fig. 38-6). Caution must be exercised in interpreting the scintillation scan of nodules less than 1.5 cm in diameter. In hyperthyroidism, the scintillation scan may be of value in determining the presence of abnormally positioned hyperfunctioning tissue, such as substernal thyroid (Fig. 38-7) or lingual thyroid. In patients with recurrent thyrotoxicosis following thyroidectomy, remnants which are not palpable may be visualized by the scan.

Many feel that a scintogram should be routine before an operation on the thyroid is performed because of suspicion of carcinoma. A preoperative scan is of value in differentiating functioning metastatic carcinoma (Fig. 38-8). However, in patients with metastatic disease from an unknown primary lesion, the results are rarely helpful, because metastases from thyroid glands fail to pick up ^{131}I when normal thyroid is present.

T4 AND T3 DETERMINATIONS. The old standard measurement of PBI and butanol-extractable iodine in patients receiving large amounts of iodine has been replaced by specific measurements of T4 and T3. The PBI has been compromised by the widespread use of estrogen-containing oral contraceptives, which increase binding power, and also by the contamination of our environment with iodine, as well as the liberal use of iodinated compounds for radiologic procedures.

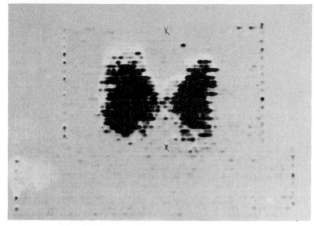

Fig. 38-3. ^{131}I scintillation scan. Normal thyroid.

The competitive binding (Murphy-Pattee) method measures T4 specifically and is unaffected by iodine-containing substances. However, oral contraceptives increase TBG and, therefore, increase total serum T4, while testosterone and anticonvulsants decrease this level. An absolutely free T4 test is uninfluenced by binding proteins or iodine, but it is too complex and not widely available. T3 resin uptake is readily determined and has been combined with the PBI to result in normal values in euthyroid patients with abnormal levels of binding proteins. Also, the serum T4 determination has been combined with a resin uptake test using labeled T4 to define the absolute free T4 value. Kits are available for these studies. Methods for determining T3 are also available commercially.

Normal ranges for these determinations are:

Total T4—4 to 11μg/100 ml
Free T4—0.8 to 2.9 mg/100 ml
     T3—160 to 320 mg/100 ml

Fig. 38-4. ^{131}I scintillation scan. Hyperfunctional nodule, left lobe. (Palpable mass enclosed in circle.)

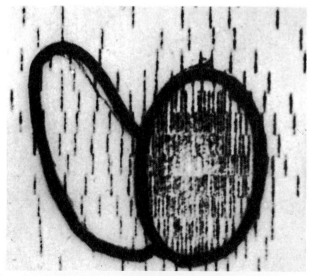

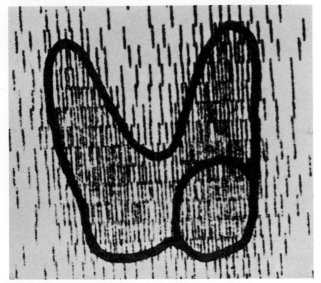

Fig. 38-5. ^{131}I scintillation scan. Functional nodule, left lobe. (Palpable mass enclosed in circle.)

Simplistically, the patient's T4/normal × patient's T3/ normal = 1. For euthyroid state

$$>1.2 = \text{hyperthyroidism}$$
$$<0.8 = \text{hypothyroidism}$$

TESTS OF REGULATION. Autonomy of thyroid function may be demonstrated by lack of suppression when T3 is administered in amounts to meet peripheral requirements. One hundred micrograms of T3 are given for 5 days. Lack of suppression is manifested by no decrease of thyroid-labeled iodine uptake. An abnormal suppression test oc-

Fig. 38-6. ^{131}I scintillation scan. Nonfunctional (cold) nodule, right lobe.

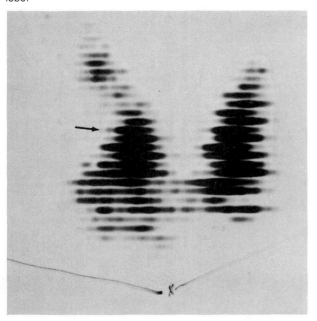

curs in thyrotoxicosis, since there is a disruption of the normal homeostatic mechanism. An abnormal suppression test in the absence of thyrotoxicosis is indicative of diffusely active goiter with opthalmopathy (Graves' disease). Recently, euthyroid patients with Graves' disease have shown a failure of serum TSH to increase in response to TRH. Tests of TSH stimulation have been supplanted by radioimmunoassay for TSH in serum.

BMR AND SERUM CHOLESTEROL. These determinations are directed at assessing the metabolic response to circulating thyroid hormone. They are particularly applicable when other indices are complicated by iodine injection and for patients on therapy.

The BMR is a measure of the calorigenic effect of thyroid hormone and the associated energy expenditure in heat production. The test specifically measures oxygen consumption, and standard values have been established for surface areas of normal patients of varying ages and sexes. The normal range of the BMR is −10 to +10 percent. The evaluation of the result is dependent upon the patient's being in a truly basal state, having fasted for at least 12 hours. The BMR is elevated with thyrotoxicosis and reduced during hypothyroidism. Extrathyroidal factors which increase the BMR include anxiety, food ingestion, smoking, perforated eardrums, and mechanical errors of testing such as leakage of oxygen. The BMR is also elevated in cardiovascular disease, leukemia, lymphoma, pheochromocytoma, adrenal hyperfunction, pregnancy, starvation, malnutrition, shock, skin diseases associated with increased heat loss, and fever.

The serum cholesterol is usually increased in primary myxedema, while the value is characteristically normal when hypothyroidism is due to pituitary failure. The concentration is influenced by age, sex, and dietary intake, but measurements are helpful in determining the response to therapy.

CIRCULATING ANTITHYROID ANTIBODIES. The work of Witebsky and associates has focused attention on the antigenic properties of thyroid protein and the importance of autoantibodies in the development of certain types of thyroid disease. Antibodies have been demonstrated in patients with Hashimoto's thyroiditis and spontaneous hypothyroidism. Circulating antithyroid antibodies are often found in high titers in patients with Graves' disease and in their relatives. Long-acting thyroid stimulator (LATS) is an immunoglobulin (IgG) with many qualities of an antibody.

THYROID BIOPSY. Biopsy of the thyroid is useful in establishing a diagnosis of thyroiditis and differentiating between nodular goiter and carcinoma. Histologic evidence of glandular hyperplasia can also result. Biopsy may be performed with a Vim-Silverman needle for diffuse disease, but if the diagnosis of malignancy is entertained, it is felt that excisional biopsy is preferable.

Thyrotoxicosis

Thyrotoxicosis refers to a spectrum of clinical manifestations which are related to primary excess secretion of active thyroid hormone or increased secretion of hormones

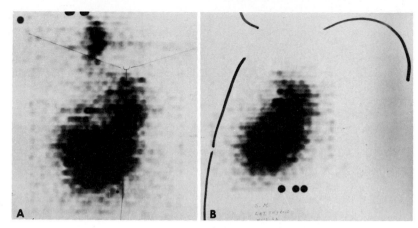

Fig. 38-7. ^{131}I scintillation scan. Substernal thyroid. *A.* Anteroposterior. *B.* Lateral.

which act on the thyroid to stimulate secretion. There are three types of pathologic processes associated with thyrotoxicosis: Graves' disease (toxic diffuse goiter), toxic multinodular goiter, and a single toxic adenoma. In rare instances, the pathologic process is located in ectopic thyroid tissue such as lingual thyroid or struma ovarii. Since the distinctions between these three pathologic processes are not absolute, thyrotoxicosis will be considered as an inclusive entity, and characteristic features of each of the three pathologic types will be presented.

ETIOLOGY AND PATHOLOGY. Graves' Disease. The cause of Graves' disease is unknown. In general, hyperthyroidism is currently regarded either as an autoimmune cell-mediated delayed hypersensitivity induced by thymic-dependent lymphocytes situated within the thyroid and acting directly on thyroid cells or as an intrinsic thyroid cellular disorder with secondary autoimmune phenomena as contributory factors. An LATS has been shown to be capable of inducing thyroid hyperplasia and increased

iodine accumulation independent of the pituitary gland. LATS is now thought to play an important role in the pathogenesis of Graves' disease, even though the titer in the serum does not correlate closely with the severity of thyrotoxicosis and LATS may be present when the thyrotoxicotic state has been relieved. Contributory factors include heredity, sex, and emotional disturbances. There is a tendency for Graves' disease to be present in several members of the same family, and the incidence of thyroid disorders other than Graves' disease, particularly Hashimoto's thyroiditis, is also increased in these families. Abnormalities of iodine metabolism have been demonstrated in euthyroid relatives of patients with Graves' disease. The proportion of nontasters of phenylthiourea is very low among patients with Graves' disease and families of these patients, which suggests an inherited predisposition. The incidence of females to males affected by Graves' disease is 6 : 1 to 7 : 1. The psychosomatic aspects have been stressed in many series, but although they modify the manifestations, their etiologic importance has not been defined.

Fig. 38-8. ^{131}I scintillation scan. Functional thyroid pulmonary metastases not demonstrated roentgenographically.

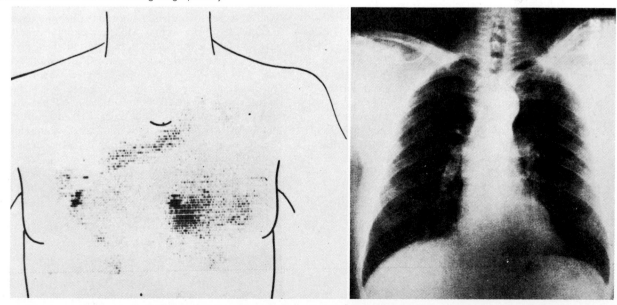

The term "Graves' disease" has been extended to include patients showing certain extrathyroid manifestations, even if goiter and/or hyperthyroidism are absent. In general, however, the thyroid of the patient with Graves' disease is enlarged and uniformly affected, and the surface is characteristically smooth but may be slightly nodular. Microscopically, the thyroid is hyperplastic, the epithelium is columnar, and only a minimal amount of colloid is evident in the gland. The nuclei may exhibit mitoses, and papillary projections of the hyperplastic epithelium are common. There may be aggregates of lymphoid tissue, and vascularity is markedly increased. These pathologic characteristics are associated with an overproduction of thyroid hormones, hypersecretion, an increased clearance of thyroidal iodine, an enhanced uptake of iodine, and an increased turnover of iodine. The thyroid hormone-protein interaction is also disturbed, and there is an increase in unbound circulating T4.

Toxic Multinodular Goiter. This is usually superimposed on a long-standing nontoxic multinodular goiter. The factors leading to alteration in function are unknown, but the hyperfunctioning cells are probably a somatic mutation resulting in units which function and grow unrelated to TSH. Genetic studies suggest a distinction between Graves' disease and toxic nodular goiter. Grossly, the gland contains multiple nodules, many of which contain aggregates of irregularly large cells and scant amount of colloid. These areas are capable of function independent of stimulation by TSH. The amount of overproduction of thyroid hormone is characteristically less than that associated with Graves' disease.

Toxic Adenoma. The solitary toxic adenoma is a follicular tumor of unknown cause. Like the multinodular toxic adenoma, it is capable of function independent of TSH and LATS, and the administration of exogenous thyroid fails to suppress the secretion of T3 and T4.

CLINICAL MANIFESTATIONS. The clinical manifestations of excessive secretion of thyroid hormone will be considered initially, since these pertain to Graves' disease, toxic multinodular goiter, and toxic adenoma, with minor individual variations. Subsequently, thyroidal and specific extrathyroidal manifestations of these three pathologic processes will be considered.

Hyperthyroidism. The onset of symptoms and signs related to an excess amount of circulating thyroid hormone differs for the three pathologic processes. Graves' disease most commonly becomes clinically apparent in patients in the third to fifth decade of life in the United States, but the age group with the highest prevalence in Great Britain is forty-five to sixty-five years. Although the disease can occur at all ages from infancy on, it is rare before the age of ten and in the elderly patient. The male/female ratio of 1 : 6 pertains in all geographic areas. The thyrotoxicosis of toxic multinodular goiter usually becomes manifest after the age of fifty and is more common in women than men. Toxic adenoma occurs in a younger age group, usually in the thirties to forties.

Many of the characteristic features of thyrotoxicosis in the adult are related to increased calorogenesis. The patient feels warmer than other people in the same environment and becomes intolerant of heat. There may be minimal to moderate temperature elevations, depending on the degree of thyrotoxicosis, and there is increased sweating and consequent thirst, due to the need of dissipating the excess heat. As a result of increased calorogenesis, weight loss associated with an increased appetite is generally noted. At times the intake of food may be sufficiently increased to prevent this loss. Increased appetite is more characteristic of younger patients, while anorexia is frequently noted in the elderly patients. These manifestations of increased calorogenesis are more marked in patients with Graves' disease than in those with toxic multinodular goiter or toxic adenoma.

By contrast, the cardiovascular manifestations of thyrotoxicosis are more prominent in patients with toxic adenomas. These include marked tachycardia, frequent atrial fibrillation, congestive heart failure, and poor response to digitalis. Hyperthyroidism increases the force and rate of the heartbeat, but this is probably related to the body's attempt to meet the general metabolic needs rather than a direct action. Sleeping pulse rate is characteristically over 80, and marked tachycardia may be apparent during the physical examination. Patients commonly experience palpitations. The marked cutaneous and peripheral vasodilatation results in an increased pulse pressure. Atrial fibrillation initially may be paroxysmal but eventually becomes continuous and is a common finding among older patients. In this group, it may be the only clinically detectable sign of hyperthyroidism. Congestive heart failure with ankle edema and dyspnea is seldom seen unless there is an underlying heart disease, which explains the increased incidence of these manifestations in patients with toxic nodular goiter who represent an older age group.

Patients with thyrotoxicosis frequently are extremely excitable, restless, hyperkinetic, and emotionally unstable, and complain of insomnia. Frank psychosis may develop, but this is not specific, and depression is as common as mania. The response of psychosis to therapy directed at relief of hyperthyroidism is unpredictable, and about half the cases return to normal. Muscle wasting, muscle weakness, and fatigue are common manifestations of thyrotoxicosis. There is usually no objective evidence of local disease of the muscle. Myopathy affects men more frequently, and the clinical picture may be confused by the fact that thyrotoxicosis occurs in 3 to 6 percent of patients with myasthenia gravis. The muscle weakness is most evident in the proximal limb muscles. Physical examination of patients with hyperthyroidism may demonstrate a tremor of the extended and abducted fingers and hyperactive Achilles tendon reflex. The emotional, neurogenic, and myopathic manifestations are more marked in patients with Graves' disease.

The changes of the skin and its appendages related to thyrotoxicosis include warm, moist skin, facial flushing, and perspiration. There also may be nail changes, which include softening, increased fragility, and separation of the distal margins from the nail bed. With advanced thyrotoxicosis and Graves' disease, clubbing of the fingers may become apparent. The hair is fine and readily falls out with combing. Pretibial myxedema occurs in 3 to 5 percent of patients with Graves' disease, is frequently present when the patient is euthyroid, and is almost always associated with eye signs. Gynecomastia occurs in 3 to 5 percent of males. Breast enlargement may be noted in females with diffuse toxic goiter. This has been related to hepatic dysfunction and incomplete metabolism of circulating estrogen. Menstrual periods are often scant or absent but return when thyroid function is controlled. Libido may be increased, but fertility is reduced, and the rate of miscarriages is reportedly high.

The effects on the gastrointestinal tract are variable. Diarrhea or increased frequency of defecation is the most characteristic symptom and may occur intermittently or chronically. Increased secretion of thyroid hormone results in increased excretion of calcium in both the feces and urine, with consequent diminution of the radiologic density of bones. There is no increased incidence of renal calculi. The relations between the thyroid gland and bone and mineral metabolism is complex. Although the thyroid gland secretes the hormone thyrocalcitonin, which is antagonistic to parathyroid hormone, alterations of thyrocalcitonin in thyrotoxicosis have not been established.

Graves' Disease. Clinically, Graves' disease is characterized by the classic triad of goiter, thyrotoxicosis, and exophthalmos. These features may occur singly or in any combination. The thyroid is nearly always diffusely enlarged and symmetric; the pyramidal lobe may be enlarged to the extent of becoming readily palpable. The gland is characteristically smooth but may be irregular. The extreme vascularity is evidenced by an audible bruit, best heard over the superior poles on either side. Obstructive symptoms, related to the size of the gland or encroachment on the trachea or esophagus, are rare. In about 3 percent of the patients with Graves' disease and thyrotoxicosis, the thyroid is normal in size. The eye signs vary from minimal to severe and, fortunately, are mild in most patients. Excess thyroxine per se will not produce exophthalmos. Severe thyrotoxicosis may be unaccompanied by exophthalmos, and, conversely, exophthalmos may be the only manifestation of Graves' disease. In about one-third of the cases, the ocular manifestations and the signs and symptoms of thyrotoxicosis begin coincidentally. Exophthalmos infrequently progresses after thyrotoxicosis has been relieved by surgical treatment or radioactive iodine.

The eye signs of Graves' disease include (1) spasm of the upper lid with lid retraction, (2) external ophthalmoplegia, (3) exophthalmos with proptosis, (4) supraorbital and infraorbital swelling, and (5) congestion and edema. Spasm of the upper lid may be manifested by lid lag and excessively apparent sclerae. Weakness of the extrinsic ocular muscles is present in about 40 percent of patients with Graves' disease. Upper rotation is the most common abnormality, while lateral rotation also occurs frequently. The extent of exophthalmos, or proptosis, can be measured with an exophthalmometer, which provides determination of the distance in a horizontal plane between the anterior convexity of the cornea and the bony margin of the orbit.

The appearance of venous congestion and edema is a sign of severity and has been described as "malignant exophthalmos." It occurs more commonly in the male and is associated with increased lacrimation and pain in the eye. In extreme cases, the eyesight may be lost.

Toxic Multinodular Goiter. The thyroid in these patients contains several palpable nodules, and in some instances the rings of the trachea may be felt because of the involution of the overlying glandular tissue. On palpation, the characteristics of the goiter cannot be distinguished from those of nontoxic multinodular goiter. Symptoms related to obstruction of the trachea and/or esophagus occur more commonly than with Graves' disease. Exophthalmos is rarely present.

Toxic Adenoma. There is frequently a history of a long-standing, slowly growing mass in the neck. Recent rapid growth may be associated with central necrosis and hemorrhage. Palpation reveals a solitary tumor within the thyroid. Thyrotoxicosis is uncommon unless the lesion is at least 3 cm in diameter. A toxic adenoma which undergoes hemorrhagic necrosis may be accompanied by spontaneous remission of the manifestations of thyrotoxicity. With larger lesions, cervical compression symptoms may be present. Exophthalmos is absent. As in the case of toxic multinodular goiter, no bruit is discernible.

DIAGNOSTIC FINDINGS. Thyrotoxicosis is characterized by an elevated T4 and/or T3 level (see the preceding section, Thyroid Function Tests).

Graves' Disease. The thyroidal ^{131}I uptake is characteristically markedly elevated with 45 to 90 percent of the administered dose localizing in the gland. If the thyroidal ^{131}I studies are equivocal, a 2-hour ^{132}I uptake with greater than 25 percent of the administered dose demonstrable in the gland confirms the diagnosis. The T3 suppression test is also applicable to the patient with an equivocal diagnosis. In normal patients the radioactive iodine uptake is decreased by 80 percent, and, for practical purposes, if the decrease is 50 percent or less, the diagnosis of hyperthyroidism can be made. The urinary excretion of nitrogen, phosphorus, calcium, and creatine is increased. The BMR is generally markedly elevated to levels of +35 to +70 percent. With severe thyrotoxicosis, hepatic dysfunction may be marked, in which case there will be associated hypoproteinemia, Bromsulphalein (BSP) retention, and increased serum alkaline phosphatase. About 1 percent of patients with Graves' disease have pernicious anemia, and 30 percent are reported to have circulating antibodies against gastric parietal cells. A high titer of thyroid autoantibodies is also found in about one-third of patients with Graves' disease.

Toxic Multinodular Goiter and Toxic Adenoma. In these patients, the thyroidal ^{131}I uptake is generally less than that in Graves' disease, 40 to 55 percent localizing in the functioning tissue. The BMR is elevated to +25 to +30 percent. The increase in urinary excretion of nitrogen, phosphorus, calcium, and creatine is less significant than that noted in patients with Graves' disease. In the case of a multinodular gland, ^{131}I thyroidal uptake and T4 and T3 determinations may be of little value unless they are distinctly elevated. The thyroid suppression test may provide the diagnosis but should not be performed in a patient with overt heart disease. In some instances, a therapeutic trial with an antithyroid agent constitutes the diagnostic test.

In the case of a toxic adenoma, much of the laboratory data also is determined by the extent of thyrotoxicosis. When thyrotoxicosis is clinically manifest, the thyroidal ^{131}I uptake and T4 and/or T3 are usually greatly increased. The scintillation scan is particularly critical, since it will indicate the functional status of the nodule (see Fig. 38-4).

TREATMENT. Definitive treatment may be effected with antithyroid drugs, radioactive iodine, or surgical excision of thyroid tissue. The approach to a given patient must be individualized and depends on the patient's age, general health, and the pathologic process involved.

Antithyroid Drugs. The majority of the presently employed antithyroid drugs interfere with the organic binding of thyroidal iodine and inhibit the coupling of iodotyrosines. They have no effect on the underlying cause of disease, and the thyroidal ^{131}I uptake remains elevated during treatment and when there is return to a euthyroid state. The drugs cross the placenta and inhibit fetal thyroid function and are also excreted in breast milk. Usually, some improvement in the degree of thyrotoxicosis is noted within the first 2 weeks of therapy, and a euthyroid thyroid state can be restored in 6 weeks. Treatment is generally regulated on a clinical basis, following the patient's weight and pulse. The size of the goiter and the eye changes should be recorded. The T4 and/or T3 levels and BMR may be helpful in assessing treatment, while radioiodine tests offer no guide.

The majority of patients are treated in the hope that a natural remission will occur within 1 to 2 years, at which time drug therapy can be stopped. A normal suppression test indicates that the disease is inactive. In Trotter's experience, one-third of the patients had remission lasting 10 years or more following a course of treatment with drugs of not more than 2 years' duration. The patients' response could not be identified prospectively. It has been reported that 54 percent of patients with diffuse or multinodular goiter had remissions lasting 10 to 20 years and no significant difference was noted in respect to the drugs which are commonly applied at the present time, i.e., propylthiouracil and methimazole (Tapazole).

Methimazole has a potency about 10 times that of propylthiouracil, and therefore one-tenth the dose is required: 100 to 300 mg of propylthiouracil every 6 to 8 hours or 10 to 40 mg of methimazole every 12 hours. The side effects of drug therapy include skin rash, fever, peripheral neuritis, and polyarteritis. Propylthiouracil has been associated with prothrombin deficiency responsive to vitamin K therapy. The serious complications of antithyroid drugs are agranulocytosis and aplastic anemia, which occur in less than 1 percent of the treated cases. Leukocyte counts are of little help, since agranulocytosis comes on so rapidly. When a significant reduction in the white blood cell count is noted, the drug should be stopped promptly, and the prognosis is good. Aplastic anemia is a much rarer complication, and the prognosis is poorer.

Antithyroid drugs are also employed in the preparation of thyrotoxicotic patients for surgical treatment. Propylthiouracil or methimazole is administered to establish a normal metabolic state. These drugs, however, increase the vascularity of the thyroid gland. Therefore, in order to facilitate surgical excision, iodine, in the form of Lugol's solution or potassium iodide, is added for a period of 10 days to 2 weeks immediately prior to the operation. Iodine inhibits hormonal release and results in a firmer and less vascular gland. Historically, iodine was used as a major chemotherapeutic agent, but since escape from its effects occurs in 2 to 3 weeks, long-term therapy is not advisable. In addition to the application of iodine in the preoperative preparation of the patient, the drug is used as treatment for impending or established thyroid storm.

Radioactive Iodine. This represents the treatment of choice in many large series. The average dose for diffuse toxic goiter was 7 to 9 mc of ^{131}I and for toxic nodular goiter 12 to 15 mc. This is intended to deliver approximately 8,500 rads to the thyroid. About 20 percent of patients treated with ^{131}I will require more than one dose. The advantages of radioactive therapy are the avoidance of a surgical procedure, with its attendant rare complications of recurrent nerve paralysis or hypoparathyroidism, and reduced cost. The major disadvantages of radioactive iodine treatment are the time required to gain control of the disease, the incidence of permanent myxedema, and the development of nodules. Remission rates ranging from 80 to 98 percent have been reported. Exacerbations are extremely uncommon. In most series, the results have been less satisfactory for hyperthyroidism associated with nodular toxic goiter than with diffuse toxic goiter. T4 and T3 determinations are less valuable in assessing thyroid functions after radioactive iodine therapy. Clinical criteria and BMR correlate better. Nofal et al. indicated a 70 percent incidence of hypothyroidism at the end of 10 years. The absence of a plateau in the slope of the curve suggests that hypothyroidism is a potentiality in almost 100 percent of the patients if they live long enough subsequent to therapy.

An objection to radioactive iodine therapy in the young patient is based on a subsequent development of carcinoma or leukemia. Many reports have indicated an increased incidence of benign and malignant tumors of the thyroid in patients subjected to irradiation of the thymic area or cervical lymphatics during infancy. Although there is a tendency for thyroid nodules to develop following radioactive iodine therapy, the incidence of thyroid carcinoma is not increased. Most centers have restricted the use of radioactive iodine to adults over the age of thirty-five and will not treat pregnant women or nursing mothers, since the isotope crosses the placenta and enters the milk. Review of the expected incidence of leukemia in the general population as compared to its occurrence in patients treated with radioactive iodine has led to the conclusion that the incidence of leukemia is little, if at all, increased by this therapeutic modality.

Subtotal Thyroidectomy. Prior to the advent of radioactive iodine, subtotal thyroidectomy was accepted as the treatment of choice for thyrotoxicosis. The operative procedure, which is generally planned to leave a remnant of 3 to 6 Gm, eliminates both the hyperthyroidism and the goiter. Patients with active hyperthyroidism require preoperative preparation. Antithyroid drugs are used initially in order to establish a euthyroid state. Iodine is added to the regimen 10 days to 2 weeks prior to the operation, to decrease the vascularity of the gland.

The mortality rate associated with the procedure is extremely low. Gould et al. reported 1,000 thyroidectomies for all causes with no deaths, while Colcock and King reported 1,246 consecutive thyroidectomies with no mortality. In a collected review of major series, the mortality rate was less than 0.1 percent. Subtotal thyroidectomy provides rapid correction of the thyrotoxicotic state in about 95 percent of patients.

The incidence of complications varies with the series. Permanent recurrent laryngeal nerve paralysis has been reported in 0 to 3 percent of the cases. Damage to the parathyroid gland resulting in tetany has been reported in about 3 percent of patients subjected to thyroidectomy for thyrotoxicosis. In 4 to 9 percent of patients subjected to thyroidectomy for thyrotoxicosis permanent hypothyroidism developed, while in 2 to 12 percent hyperthyroidism recurred. Thus, the major advantages of surgical therapy are prompt control of disease and a lowered incidence of myxedema as compared with radioactive iodine therapy. Surgical thyroidectomy also makes possible the simultaneous removal of an incidental papillary carcinoma, which was noted in 2 percent of the cases in one series. The patients usually leave the hospital within 4 to 5 days and resume work within 6 weeks.

Selection of Therapy. In patients with Graves' disease (diffuse toxic goiter) either antithyroid drug therapy or radioactive iodine is used initially. Antithyroid drugs are used in the younger age group and in pregnant or lactating females. Radioactive iodine is employed in patients over the age of thirty-five. If prolonged drug therapy is required, i.e., for more than 2 years, or if recurrence of thyrotoxicosis follows the discontinuance of drugs, thyroidectomy or radioactive iodine is used. Subtotal thyroidectomy occasionally represents the treatment of choice in young adults with severe disease and large goiters or in patients in whom a rapid response is desirable. Radioactive iodine is the treatment of choice in most patients with toxic multinodular goiter, but in regions where goiter tends to be endemic, such as the Great Lakes, there is an increased resistance to radioactive iodine therapy. In these regions, subtotal thyroidectomy may represent the procedure of choice. The preferable treatment for hyperfunctioning adenoma is surgical excision.

Because of the questionable carcinogenic potential of radioactive iodine in childhood, the choice of treatment is between surgical excision and antithyroid therapy. However, there is usually a lower incidence of remission following antithyroid therapy in adults, and recurrences are frequent. If sustained remission does not follow a 2-year course of antithyroid therapy in a child, surgical intervention is indicated. Thyrotoxicosis in pregnancy is best treated with antithyroid drugs. Surgical therapy may be required, but it is best not to use iodine in preparation because of the likelihood of an induced goiter in the fetus.

Hyperfunctioning thyroid tissue in the ovary should be treated by oophorectomy. Hyperfunctioning tissue within aberrant thyroid tissue, such as a lingual thyroid, may be treated by radioactive iodine or surgical excision. The uncommon situation of metastatic tumor with hyperfunctioning tissue is best treated by radioactive iodine.

RESULTS. Antithyroid drugs effect a remission of 10 years or more in one-third to one-half of the patients with diffuse or multinodular goiter. Radioactive iodine effectively controls hyperthyroidism in about 90 percent of patients, although some require one or more subsequent doses. Failure to control the hyperthyroidism occurs more frequently with nodular toxic goiter as compared to diffuse toxic goiter. This modality of therapy is associated with a high incidence of myxedema, which is greater than 60 percent at 10 years and increases each year by an additional 2 to 3 percent. Subtotal thyroidectomy is also associated with 90 percent good results in respect to control of thyrotoxicosis. In 2 to 12 percent of the patients, goiter and/or hyperthyroidism recurs at some time following the operation. In this group of patients, radioactive iodine is indicated. Permanent hypothyroidism occurs in 4 to 18 percent of the patients following subtotal thyroidectomy. Unlike the situation with radioactive iodine therapy where there is a continuous increase with time in the percentage of hypothyroid patients, hypothyroidism following subtotal thyroidectomy occurs within 1 year.

The effects of treatment on the eye signs are variable. The stigmata of exophthalmos may gradually improve or may deteriorate as the thyrotoxicosis is controlled. In general, the changes in the eye signs are biphasic. During the acute phase lasting some months, the signs progress fairly rapidly. Following this, there is a chronic phase lasting years during which the lid retraction tends to disappear while the exophthalmos increases slightly. The treatment of hyperthyroidism affects this pattern. The lid retraction disappears in about two-thirds of the patients who become euthyroid, while the exophthalmos increases by an average of 1 mm, partly because of the gain in body fat, when hyperthyroidism is removed. In most instances, treating the thyrotoxicosis improves the eye signs. In those instances in which the treatment seems to precipitate rapid deterioration of the eyes, this may represent the acute phase or the development of exophthalmos and should not necessarily be attributed to the therapy.

TREATMENT OF EXOPHTHALMOS. The severe form of exophthalmos is fortunately rare. The control of thyrotoxicosis has no appreciable effect on the progression of eye signs. The earliest symptom of development of the so-called "malignant exophthalmos" is increased lacrimation. The earliest signs consist of venous congestion and chemosis. Treatment is essentially symptomatic, since no therapeutic measure has been demonstrated to have a decisive influence on the progression of the disorder. The eyes should be protected against the wind and sun. The patients should sleep in a sitting position to reduce venous congestion. If chemosis is severe, tarsorrhaphy to oppose the lids and prevent corneal ulceration may be indicated. If the intraorbital tension increases to the extent of threatening vision, a trial of massive doses of prednisone (120 to 140 mg daily) is indicated. Steroids have been particularly effective in managing pain, tearing, and irritation. Other methods of therapy include external irradiation to the orbit or the pituitary gland, implantation of ^{90}yttrium into the pituitary, stalk section, or cryosurgical treatment of the pituitary gland. In cases where the intraorbital pressure immediately threatens vision, lateral decompression was generally used in the past, but the results were disappointing in that only half the patients were improved. Transfrontal craniotomy and transantral decompression have provided good results.

Hypothyroidism

Hypothyroidism is the term applied to a failure of the thyroid gland to maintain an adequate plasma level of hormone. A brief discussion is included in this chapter for three reasons: (1) the treatment of hyperthyroidism by subtotal thyroidectomy and, more commonly, by radioactive iodine represents one of the causes of hypothyroidism, (2) some of the clinical manifestations of hypothyroidism mimic a variety of surgical diseases, and (3) a recognition of the hypothyroid state in the preoperative patient is important, since major surgical treatment in the hypothyroid patient is associated with an increased mortality. The reader is referred to the general texts listed in the references for a more complete consideration of hypothyroidism.

ETIOLOGY. Spontaneous hypothyroidism, or myxedema, may result from aplasia of the thyroid or replacement of the gland by nonfunctional goiter, adenoma, or thyroiditis. In the presence of functioning thyroid tissue, hypothyroidism may be secondary to hypopituitarism. This is termed *pituitary myxedema.* Hypothyroidism following subtotal thyroidectomy or radioactive iodine therapy for hyperthyroidism accounts for about one-fourth of cases. Kocher recognized the importance of this disorder and referred to it as "cachexia strumipriva." In 4 to 18 percent of patients subjected to thyroidectomy hypothyroidism develops. The occurrence is related to the histologic state, being more common in patients with Hashimoto's disease and lymphadenoid changes. However, as far as absolute figures are concerned, postoperative hypothyroidism most frequently follows subtotal resection of a diffuse goiter in a patient with Graves' disease. Autoantibodies against thyroid cytoplasm are frequently present in patients who become hypothyroid. The incidence varies inversely with the incidence of recurrent hyperthyroidism. In most of these patients, the hypothyroidism becomes manifest during the first year after the operation, usually within the first few months. Following ablation of diffuse toxic goiter using radioactive iodine, there is a progressive rising incidence of hypothyroidism.

CLINICAL MANIFESTATIONS. Functional failure of the thyroid in the newborn is termed *cretinism.* This is not seen at birth because of the transplacental passage of hormone and becomes manifest later in infancy. Mental retardation is marked and frequently irreversible. Children demonstrate a poor growth pattern, are difficult to nurse, and

present with a typical appearance which must be distinguished from mongolism and dwarfism. The remaining manifestations are similar to those which will be described below for adult hypothyroidism but are more pronounced.

Thyroid failure during childhood or adolescence is known as *juvenile hypothyroidism,* and the extent and degree of symptoms and signs are intermediate between cretinism and adult hypothyroidism. The child appears younger than his chronologic age. Intellectual performance is poor, but severe mental deficiency is not present. In children, abdominal distension, umbilical hernia, and prolapse of the rectum are all common.

Spontaneous hypothyroidism in the adult is a rare disease. About one case of adult hypothyroidism is admitted for every eight cases of thyrotoxicosis. Eighty percent of adults with spontaneous hypothyroidism are female. Both spontaneous hypothyroidism and hypothyroidism which follows ablative procedures on the thyroid gland have an insidiously progressive course in the adult, with protean manifestations. There is increasing fatigue and apathy. Mental and physical processes are generally slowed. Intellectual function and speech may be impaired. Headaches occur frequently and dementia may develop. Weight gain is a characteristic feature. The skin becomes thickened and puffy; the nonpitting bogginess of the skin is most apparent around the eyes, hands, and feet. The secretion of sweat glands is reduced. The hair becomes dry and brittle, and tends to fall out. The tongue is enlarged and tends to fill the mouth, and the voice is hoarse. Muscle cramps are common and represent one of the early symptoms of hypothyroidism following ablative therapy. The cramps may be precipitated by slight motion, such as turning in bed or lifting of the arms, and may be accompanied by paresthesias.

The cardiovascular manifestations are related to a reduced cardiac output and hemodynamic alterations which resemble those of congestive heart failure. There is a narrowing in pulse pressure, a prolonged circulation time, and a decrease in cutaneous circulation resulting in coolness and pallor of the skin and intolerance to cold. There is widening of cardiac dullness due to dilatation of the heart or pericardial effusion, and the heart sounds are distant. The resting pulse is slow, and at times the blood pressure is elevated to hypertensive levels. As the disease progresses, shortness of breath and pulmonary effusions become more common.

Abdominal symptoms may represent the outstanding complaint. Most frequently, these consist of constipation and changes in bowel habits. Abdominal distension due to intraintestinal gases or ascites may be present. When pain is present, it is generally of a dull, nonperistaltic character and occasionally colicky. Achlorhydria occurs in about half the patients, and there is also an impairment of absorption of vitamin B_{12}. Pernicious anemia may be present in 12 percent of the cases.

In women, diminished libido, failure of ovulation, and menorrhagia may occur, and in men there may be decreased libido, impotency, and oligospermia.

DIAGNOSTIC FINDINGS. The hemogram may demonstrate anemia. The electrocardiogram is characterized by sinus bradycardia, diminished voltage, and inverted or flattened T waves; the electroencephalogram shows slow alpha activity and loss of amplitude. The tests of thyroidal function and the effects of thyroid hormone may be variable and contradictory. In general, the BMR and ^{131}I uptake are decreased in proportion to the extent of the disease. Early in the course of the disease, the BMR is only moderately lowered and with progression falls to about −35 to −45 percent. There is a decreased serum T4 and/or T3, and the serum cholesterol is frequently in excess of 300 mg/100 ml.

TREATMENT. Treatment of adult hypothyroidism is extremely effective and is directed at producing a normal metabolic state with the smallest possible dose of drugs. The choice of therapeutic agent is most frequently determined by the preference of the physician, and either synthetic hormones or thyroid extracts from animal glands may be employed. The approximate equivalence of biologic potency for the commonly used medications is 60 mg of thyroid extract = 100 µg of l-thyroxine = 25 µg of l-triiodothyronine.

The untreated patient with hypothyroidism is sensitive to small doses, and therefore caution is exercised in initiating replacement therapy. Treatment may be begun with 15 to 30 mg of thyroid extract daily, and the dose is increased by 15 to 30 mg at 2-week intervals until a satisfactory metabolic rate is obtained. The replacement therapy is augmented slowly to avoid cardiac problems related to an increased demand on the myocardium. Most patients perform well with a BMR of −20 to −10. The maintenance dose for thyroid extract is usually 60 to 120 mg. The maintenance dose for l-thyroxine is approximately 300 µg daily, and the maintenance dose for l-triiodothyronine is about 75 µg daily. In the infant or child, treatment may be begun with 25 µg of l-thyroxine (or its equivalent) and increased by 25 µg at weekly intervals, so that a daily dose of 100 µg is achieved in 3 to 4 weeks. Thereafter the dose is increased slowly in order to keep the total T4 at about 10 µg/100 ml.

Thyroiditis

Inflammatory processes of the thyroid may be acute or chronic. Acute thyroiditis is further subdivided into the suppurative and nonsuppurative varieties. Chronic thyroiditis includes Hashimoto's disease, granulomatous (giant cell) thyroiditis, and Riedel's thyroiditis.

ACUTE SUPPURATIVE THYROIDITIS

Acute suppurative thyroiditis is the most uncommon form of thyroiditis. Hendrick reviewed 1,309 consecutive operations on the thyroid of which 117 were on patients who had thyroiditis of various forms. Twenty-eight patients were classified as having acute thyroiditis, and of these only six had the suppurative form. Acute suppurative thyroiditis, with abscess formation, almost invariably follows an acute upper respiratory tract infection. The disease is characterized by the sudden onset of severe pain in the thyroid and anterior neck, accompanied by dysphagia, fever, and chills. The suppurative process usually remains unilateral, but there may be extension into the deep spaces of the neck with invasion of the trachea and/or esophagus, or tracking into the chest. Treatment consists of drainage of the abscess. There is no persistent effect on thyroid function.

HASHIMOTO'S DISEASE (LYMPHADENOID GOITER)

Hashimoto's disease is the most common form of chronic thyroiditis, and the incidence apparently has been increasing. The frequency with which this lesion is identified in specimens of removed thyroid glands varies with geographic location. In England, 1.5 percent of thyroidectomies demonstrate Hashimoto's disease. In the United States, in the Southern Gulf states 11 percent of glands contain the lesion, whereas in New England lymphadenoid goiter is present in only 0.3 percent of thyroidectomies. An increasing frequency which is greater in younger age groups recently has been reported in Minnesota. The disease occurs at least five to ten times more frequently than subacute thyroiditis.

ETIOLOGY. Hashimoto's disease is an autoimmune process in which the thyroid gland is sensitive to its own thyroglobulin. In 1957, Doniach and Roitt first discovered antithyroid antibodies in the serum of most patients with this disease. Four autoantigens have been detected: thyroglobulin, nonthyroglobulin colloid, thyroid cell microsomes, and nuclear component. Thyroglobulin antigen may be demonstrated by a precipitant test or agglutination of specifically treated red cells. Autoantibodies formed against nonthyroglobulin colloid may be demonstrated by the fluorescent technique of Coons and Kaplan. This technique can also be applied to the demonstration of antibody to thyroid intracellular microsomes and antinuclear antibody. The sera of patients with Hashimoto's disease also contain an abnormal iodinated protein distinct from thyroglobulin and apparently related to albumin. This is used as a diagnostic test. There is some evidence of genetic predisposition for Hashimoto's disease. Members of the family of patients with this disease have an increased incidence of Hashimoto's disease, goiter, spontaneous hypothyroidism, and thyrotoxicosis.

A statistically significant relationship has been demonstrated for the coexistence of papillary carcinoma of the thyroid and Hashimoto's disease. The data of Hirabayashi and Lindsay suggest that chronic thyroiditis occurs secondarily with papillary carcinoma and that there is a possibility that antigens from the neoplasm may be implicated in the formation of thyroiditis. In 92 percent of the specimens of papillary carcinoma which Hirabayashi and Lindsay studied, thyroiditis was found in the neoplasm, in the remaining thyroid parenchyma, or in both regions. The presence of thyroiditis was uncommon with other forms of thyroid carcinoma.

PATHOLOGY. In 80 percent of the cases, the thyroid is symmetrically enlarged, pale, and semifirm. In the remaining cases, the enlargement may be asymmetric, and the nodularity and firmness suggest colloid goiter and, at times, carcinoma. The disease is focal in the beginning but extends to involve one or both lobes and the isthmus. Lymphoid tissue predominates (Fig. 38-9). There is dis-

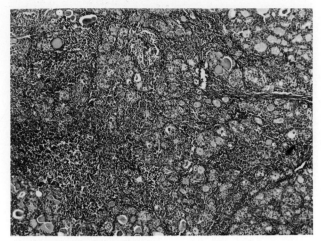

Fig. 38-9. Hashimoto's disease.

ruption of epithelial cells with degeneration and fragmentation of the follicular basement membrane. The remaining epithelial cells are larger and demonstrate oxyphilic changes (Askanazy cells). The lymphocytic infiltration may be focal or diffuse, and as the disease progresses, the thyroid tissue may degenerate or be replaced by fibrous tissue.

CLINICAL MANIFESTATIONS. The overwhelming majority of patients are women, and the disease occurs from age twenty to sixty-nine, with an average of fifty years. The most frequent complaints are enlargement of the neck with pain and tenderness in the region of the thyroid. There may be associated difficulty in breathing and swallowing caused by compression of the trachea and esophagus. Coughing is a common symptom. Shortness of breath, increasing fatigue, and increase in weight are related to a hypothyroid state when this is present. In the series reported by Linden and Clark, 22 percent presented with symptoms of hyperthyroidism, while 4 percent were myxedematous. Palpation generally reveals a diffusely enlarged gland, and enlargement of the pyramidal lobe is common. In about 20 percent of cases, the gland is nodular rather than diffusely enlarged.

Several investigators have indicated an increased incidence of autoimmune diseases such as rheumatic fever and rheumatoid arthritis, disseminated lupus, hemolytic anemia, purpura, myasthenia gravis, and pernicious anemia in these patients. On occasion Hashimoto's disease is part of a generalized endocrine organ failure syndrome which may include idiopathic Addison's disease, diabetes mellitus, and ovarian or testicular insufficiency. In contrast, Mulhern et al. could demonstrate no association between Hashimoto's disease and other autoimmune disorders, with the possible exception of rheumatoid arthritis and the presence of false-positive tests for syphilis.

DIAGNOSTIC FINDINGS. Early in the course of the disease, tests of thyroidal function occasionally indicated thyroidal hyperfunction without overproduction of metabolically active hormones. The thyroidal ^{131}I uptake may be increased. As the disease progresses, the thyroidal uptake and T4 reach subnormal levels, and the response to TSH reveals diminished thyroid reserve. In a majority of patients, however, tests of thyroidal function and clinical manifestations suggest a euthyroid state. Diagnosis is confirmed by demonstrating high titers of thyroid antibodies in the serum. Almost all patients with Hashimoto's disease have circulating antibody as determined by the tanned red cell agglutinin and complement-fixation tests. The various immunologic tests are not specific for Hashimoto's disease and occur in other disorders of the thyroid gland, such as spontaneous myxedema, hyperthyroidism, nontoxic goiter, and thyroid carcinoma.

Biopsy may be indicated in the case of asymmetric and nodular glands, to rule out the diagnosis of carcinoma. Crile and Hazard performed needle biopsy in 119 patients with Hashimoto's disease, and only one patient subsequently proved to have a malignant tumor, a reticulum cell sarcoma. Beahrs et al. also feel that needle biopsy of the thyroid has a role in the diagnosis and management of Hashimoto's disease. By contrast, others, for example Block et al., feel that whenever a nodule is suspicious, excisional biopsy is indicated.

TREATMENT. There is almost universal agreement that if the thyroid is symmetric and nonnodular and if there are no symptoms of compression, the patient should be managed with suppressive doses of thyroid hormone. Three hundred milligrams of thyroid extract may be required, and triiodothyronine in daily doses of 75 to 100 µg is also effective. Surgical intervention is indicated if there are marked pressure symptoms, such as difficulty in swallowing, for suspected malignant tumor, and for cosmetic reasons, in the case of an extremely enlarged gland. The surgical procedure usually performed consists of near-total thyroidectomy with clearing of the trachea. The treatment of a nodular form of Hashimoto's disease is controversial. Most writers prefer the use of suppressive hormone. Block et al. represent the other approach, which consists of surgical excision. They feel that if nodules are present in one lobe, lobectomy, isthmusectomy, and superficial contralateral lobectomy should be performed. Nodules within the isthmus should be treated by resection of the isthmus and the superficial portion of both adjacent lobes. Since most carcinomas associated with Hashimoto's disease are of the papillary type, concomitant radical neck dissection is not indicated. Suppressive therapy with thyroid hormones should be continued postoperatively.

SUBACUTE THYROIDITIS

In 1904 de Quervain described the pathology (Fig. 38-10) of subacute thyroiditis and reviewed the literature. Many synonyms, including granulomatous (giant cell), epidemic, and de Quervain's thyroiditis, have confused the diagnosis. In 1948, Crile clearly established subacute thyroiditis as an entity separate from Hashimoto's thyroiditis and Riedel's struma.

The disease occurs widely in over half of the United States but infrequently along the Eastern seaboard, in England, and in Japan. The age of onset ranges from three to seventy-six, with a mean in the forties. Females outnumber males in every series, the proportion varying between 60 and 100 percent.

Subacute thyroiditis is generally not felt to be of viral origin, but there is no definitive proof, and no epidemiologic pattern has been demonstrated. Recent studies have led to the conclusion that the disease is not autoimmune.

The gland is usually adherent to surrounding tissues but, unlike Riedel's struma, can be dissected free without difficulty. There is enlargement of the follicles with infiltration by large mononuclear cells, lymphocytes, and neutrophils. Giant cells of the epitheloid foreign body type containing many nuclei characterize the lesion.

Volpé et al. classified subacute thyroiditis into four stages:

Stage I—acute toxicity with a painful, swollen gland and thyrotoxic symptoms lasting 1 to 2 months.
Stage II—the transition or euthyroid stage with an enlarged, hard, nontender gland. The BMR is normal, but the sedimentation rate is still elevated.
Stage III—the compensation or hypothyroid phase, occurring 2 to 4 months after onset.
Stage IV—remission or recovery, which may occur in 1 to 6 months.

Almost all patients manifest thyroid swelling and pain which may radiate to parts of the head, neck, or anterior chest. The onset is usually sudden. About two-thirds of patients are febrile, and fatigue, weakness, malaise, menstrual irregularities, and weight loss are characteristic. White blood cell counts usually are normal, but the erythrocyte sedimentation rate (ESR) is almost always elevated during the first month. α_2- and γ-globulin levels are elevated. The latter is also elevated in Hashimoto's disease, but the colloidal gold reaction which is positive in Hashimoto's disease is negative in subacute thyroiditis. In the acute stage there is a characteristically low ^{131}I uptake. Needle biopsy may aid in establishing the diagnosis, as may cytodiagnosis by aspiration, but these techniques are not always reliable.

ACTH and corticosteroids effectively relieve the symptoms but do not alter the disease. Therapy should be initiated with 40 mg of prednisone daily, tapering the drug over 1 to 2 months. Radiation in doses of 200 to 400 rads has been used to treat thyroid pain, but steroids are generally more effective. Salicylates and desiccated thyroid (1 to 3 Gm daily) have provided successful therapy. Thyroidectomy is not applicable because of the high incidence of postoperative myxedema.

RIEDEL'S (STRUMA) THYROIDITIS

Riedel's thyroiditis is a rare chronic inflammatory process involving one or both lobes of the thyroid, frequently extending to the surrounding fascia, trachea, muscles, nerves, and blood vessels. It was formerly thought to be a terminal stage of Hashimoto's disease or granulomatous thyroiditis, but this thesis is no longer popular.

Microscopically, the follicles are small and few in number, and a dense fibrous tissue permeates the gland (Fig. 38-11). There is firm attachment to the trachea by scar tissue, resulting in constriction and narrowing of the tracheal lumen.

When involvement is unilateral, the disease is clinically indistinguishable from carcinoma. The disease occurs more

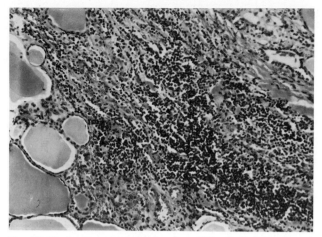

Fig. 38-10. Acute nonsuppurative thyroiditis. Note infiltration of inflammatory cells.

frequently in women but not to the same extent as Hashimoto's disease. The average age of patients is about fifty. Symptoms are generally due to compression of the trachea, esophagus, and recurrent laryngeal nerve. Consequently, there is difficulty in swallowing and hoarseness. Vocal cord paralysis may be demonstrable on indirect laryngoscopy. Thyroidal ^{131}I uptake may be normal or depressed, and in advanced disease tests of thyroidal function may indicate hypothyroidism. Some patients have circulating thyroid autoantibodies, but this occurs less frequently and in lower titers than in patients with Hashimoto's disease.

Treatment consists of thyroid hormones. Surgical intervention is justified to relieve symptoms of tracheal or esophageal constriction. The operation may be dangerous, resulting in damage to the trachea, carotid sheath, or recurrent laryngeal nerve. When only one lobe is involved, unilateral lobectomy and isthmusectomy are indicated. When there is bilateral involvement, the technique advocated by Lahey is applicable. This consists of removal of

Fig. 38-11. Riedel's thyroiditis.

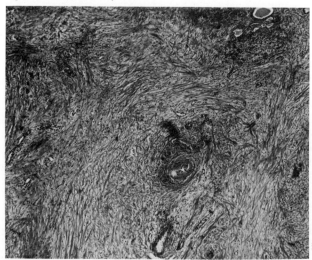

the isthmus and as much of each lobe as possible. The prethyroid muscles are sutured to the lateral wall of the trachea to cover the severed ends of the lobe and prevent fibrous thyroid tissue from uniting. The medial borders of the "strap" muscles are then sutured together to prevent the trachea from becoming adherent to the skin.

Goiter

The term *goiter* is derived from the French word *goitre,* which in turn comes from the Latin *guttur,* meaning "throat." In general, the term is applied to benign enlargement of the thyroid gland, usually associated with a normal production of thyroid hormone.

ETIOLOGY. The development of a goiter may be related to a variety of factors, including inherited enzyme defects and extrinsic causes, or it may be idiopathic. Goiters associated with thyrotoxicosis, thyroiditis, and benign and malignant neoplasms are excluded from this discussion.

Familial Goiter. Goiters caused by inherited enzyme defects are usually associated with hypothyroidism, but many patients remain euthyroid. The inborn error in metabolism is generally inherited as an autosomal recessive trait, but inheritance as a dominant characteristic also has been reported. The metabolic defect may impair iodine accumulation organification, coupling of iodotyrosine into iodothyronine, or dehalogenation of iodotyrosine, or it may be related to a disorder affecting the serum iodoprotein.

Endemic Goiter. The distinction between endemic and "sporadic" goiter is statistical and arbitrary. Endemic goiter is defined as thyroid enlargement affecting a significant number of inhabitants of a particular locale. Most major countries have goiter belts. In the United States, the prevalent regions are in mountainous areas, the upper Northwest, and around the Great Lakes. The extrinsic factors implicated in the etiology include iodine deficiency and the ingestion of goitrogens. Genetic factors may play a contributory role. Iodine deficiency is particularly important, and in the endemic areas the iodine content of the drinking water is extremely low. Surveys of patients in endemic goiter regions have demonstrated an augmented average uptake of radioiodine. No clearly defined biochemical abnormalities have been detected in the thyroid glands of these patients. The administration of iodine as prophylaxis prevents endemic goiter, and the preferable method has been iodination of table salt. Excess iodide ingestion may lead to goiter with hypothyroidism. Some opponents of this measure have suggested that it has also led to a higher incidence of toxic goiter. In patients with endemic goiter who receive daily supplemental doses of iodine, the adjustment period is slow. It takes several weeks for the level of iodine balance to be achieved and the thyroidal avidity for radioiodine to return to normal. Experiments in animals have demonstrated a goitrogenic property of yellow turnips, cabbage, kale, and other vegetables. However, the final proof implicating the goitrogenic factors in the etiology of endemic goiter in human beings is still lacking on epidemiologic grounds. Certain proprietary medications such as Felsol and therapeutic drugs such as paraaminosalicylic acid are goitrogenic. Patients administered very large doses of iodide daily may develop goiter with thyrotoxicosis, known as "jodbasedow" disease.

Sporadic Goiter. This term is applied to an enlargement of the thyroid for which a definite cause cannot be established. The diagnosis is one of exclusion in which thyroiditis and tumor and the possibility of endemic goiter are ruled out. It is thought that the goiter represents a compensatory response to an impaired efficiency of the thyroid gland. Hypersecretion of TSH may lead to stimulation of glandular growth and morphologic changes.

PATHOLOGY. The thyroid gland may be diffusely enlarged and smooth, or it may be grossly nodular. In the early stages of development, the gland is hyperplastic. The hyperplastic state may be reversed by the ingestion of iodine. Subsequently, hyperinvolution occurs forming enlarged follicles filled with colloid. At this stage, the administration of iodine fails to have an effect, but thyroid or thyroxine in replacement doses may cause reduction in size of the gland.

The nontoxic nodular goiter is grossly a multinodular structure in which the nodules vary in number and size. There is also variation in the extent of encapsulation, from sharp to poorly defined margins, and in the histology, from nonfollicular areas to gelatinous colloid-rich nodules. Scattered between the nodules are areas of normal thyroid tissue and focal areas of lymphocytic infiltration. There may be gross or microscopic evidence of degeneration of the nodules with cyst formation, recent or old hemorrhage, or calcification.

CLINICAL MANIFESTATIONS. In totally goitrous endemic regions, there is no difference in incidence related to sex. However, as one proceeds to areas diminishing in intensity, the ratio of females to males increasingly rises until in mildly endemic areas the ratio is 8 : 1. The age incidence varies with the amount of iodine available in the diet. Goiter may be observed in 20 percent of children at age five to six in some regions, while in others almost 100 percent of children have thyroids two to three times normal size. In females, the size increases up to age seventeen or eighteen, and although some glands become smaller, few disappear. In males, the number of presenting goiters declines after the age of fourteen, and there is a higher incidence of significant decrease in size and disappearance. In women, an increase in size may be noted during pregnancy with reduction in size after delivery to the antepartum level.

Most patients with goiter are asymptomatic and do not consult a physician. Those patients who are referred to the hospital, therefore, represent a selected group. The manifestations of hospitalized patients are related to the physical effects of the goiter, associated symptoms, or psychologic effects.

The most common symptom related to the thyroid gland itself is an awareness of increasing size of the neck or the presence of a mass. Pressure effects may cause embarrassment of the respiration with tracheal compression or dysphagia due to pressure on the esophagus. The tracheal compression is frequently associated with a goiter extending into the thorax. Distension of the jugular veins in these cases, indicative of impedance of return of blood, may be noted by the patient. The patients may achieve relief by flexing the neck to relieve the pressure on the trachea. Paralysis of the recurrent laryngeal nerve rarely is due to stretching across the surface of an expanding goiter and is more frequently related to a malignant tumor. Similarly, pressure on the superior sympathetic ganglion may produce a Horner's syndrome, but this is more suggestive of involvement by a neoplastic lesion. The patients may experience sudden pain in the neck associated with a rapid increase in size. This is generally related to hemorrhage into part of the goiter, either a cyst or a degenerating lesion. These symptoms usually subside spontaneously, and the gland reverts to its previous size. In rare instances, with large hemorrhage, the resulting pressure may obstruct the airway and be life-threatening.

The characteristic physical finding associated with an enlarged thyroid is a palpable mass which moves on swallowing. If the thyroid fails to move on swallowing, this suggests either goiter with intrathoracic extension, carcinoma of the thyroid with invasion of surrounding tissues, or thyroiditis extending into adjacent structures. An enlarged thyroid in a patient who is euthyroid generally is softer than the gland in a patient with Graves' disease. Marked discrepancy in the size of the two lobes of the gland is presumptive evidence that the goiter is nodular. The distinct presence or absence of nodularity and whether there is a single nodule or multiple nodules is frequently difficult to determine. Tracheal compression is difficult to recognize clinically. It may be detected by listening to the patient as he breathes with the mouth open, or displacement of the trachea may be apparent on inspection or palpation.

The history of a goiter and hypothyroidism which is manifest at birth or in childhood is evidence that some kind of inherited defect is present. In these patients, a family history is important. If the patient has been deaf since birth and goitrous since infancy or middle childhood, the diagnosis of a genetic entity known as *Pendred's syndrome* can be made. In this group of patients, the audiogram reveals a characteristic loss of hearing for high tones in those who are not totally deaf, and the diagnosis is confirmed by showing that perchlorate will result in a discharge of the radioiodine accumulated within the thyroid during the first few hours after administration.

One-third of patients with endemic cretinism have appreciable enlargement of the thyroid gland. Some children are born with marked enlargement. Endemic cretins are usually not deaf-mute but are more likely to suffer from neurologic disorders causing spasticity.

Simple and nontoxic nodular goiters rarely progress to hypothyroidism. By contrast, thyrotoxicosis develops in a large percentage of patients with a long-standing history of goiter. In the series at the Mayo Clinic, 60 percent of patients with nodular goiter over the age of sixty were thyrotoxicotic. The average duration of goiter before the onset of thyrotoxicosis was seventeen years. As indicated in the discussion of thyrotoxicosis, exophthalmos is a rare manifestation of toxic nodular goiter, whereas congestive heart failure and atrial fibrillation may dominate the picture.

DIAGNOSTIC FINDINGS. A radiogram of the chest and neck is important to visualize the trachea in order to establish its position and the diameter of the lumen. The study will also reveal whether the goiter has extended into the thorax. Barium swallowing is indicated only if the patient has dysphagia. In most patients with simple or endemic goiter, the thyroidal ^{131}I uptake, T4, and T3 are normal. The thyroidal iodine uptake may be increased if there is iodine deficiency. In patients with familial and drug-induced goiters, the 2-hour radioiodine uptake is in the hyperthyroid range, even though the patient is clinically euthyroid or hypothyroid. Since the iodine leaves the thyroid rapidly, the 24-hour uptake is lower than normal. When the goiter is caused by excess iodide or iodopyronine, the thyroidal 2-hour uptake of radiolodine is low. Return to normal can be effected by stopping the preparation and repeating the test in 1 week. At this stage, the thyroidal radioiodine uptake at 2 hours will be in the hyperthyroid range. A goiter retains its capacity to respond to TSH, indicating that the gland is not under maximal stimulation.

Differentiation from diffuse thyroiditis may be established by needle biopsy. The diagnostic findings in patients with goiters becoming hyperthyroid are discussed in the section on Thyrotoxicosis. Consideration of the differential diagnosis of the nodular thyroid is presented in the section on treatment that follows.

TREATMENT. The therapeutic approach to a patient with a goiter takes into account the etiology, symptoms, and the presence or absence of nodularity.

Diffuse (Nonnodular) Goiter. Goiters caused by inherited enzyme defects characteristically respond well to the administration of thyroxine. The drug eliminates hypothyroidism, if present, and diminishes the size of the gland by depressing TSH stimulation. The required dosage may be established by trial and error using ^{132}I thyroidal uptake as a method of control. The minimal dose needed to abolish ^{132}I uptake is employed, and treatment is continued indefinitely. Patients with Pendred's syndrome usually manufacture an adequate or nearly adequate amount of hormone. They have normal physical and mental development, but thyroid hormone should be administered to prevent growth of goiter.

Treatment of drug-induced goiter requires the discontinuance of the offending drug, if possible. If continued drug therapy, such as para-aminosalicylic acid for tuberculosis, is required, thyroxine should be administered. Occasionally goiters in newborn children can be attributed to drugs taken by the mother during pregnancy. The enlargement disappears spontaneously during the first months of life. Endemic goiter is prevented by the administration of iodine. Occasionally, when an endemic goiter is in a hyperplastic state, iodine therapy results in decrease in size. After hyperinvolution or colloid accumulation has occurred, the administration of iodine therapy fails to have an effect. Desiccated thyroid or thyroxine in replacement doses may result in a dramatic decrease in size. This is particularly true of the diffusely enlarged, nonnodular gland.

The possible coexistence of thyroid carcinoma is not a significant problem in the nonnodular goiter. The indications for operation are (1) signs and symptoms of pressure effects, (2) pain and rapid increase in size of the gland related to intraglandular bleeding, and (3) cosmetic needs. Low-lying goiters, intrathoracic goiters, and goiters which encircle the trachea are most likely to produce symptoms of respiratory obstruction. The rare circumstance of tracheal obstruction caused by congenital goiter in the newborn is best treated by resection of the thyroid isthmus rather than tracheostomy. Hemorrhage or rapid development of an intrathyroidal cyst may cause pain and an alarming mass. Crile has reported 50 patients treated with aspiration followed by administration of desiccated thyroid. There were only three failures. Others prefer surgical excision of the cyst and a rim of surrounding tissue. Surgical procedures for cosmesis must be individualized, but it is to be emphasized that partial thyroidectomy further restricts the ability of the gland to meet hormonal requirements. Therefore, whenever a significant segment of goiter is removed, supplemental hormone therapy is indicated.

Multinodular Goiter. The results achieved by suppressive therapy, 120 to 180 mg of thyroid extract or its equivalent daily, are variable. Astwood and associates noted reduction in size of multinodular goiters in over 50 percent of their cases, whereas most other investigators report favorable effects in less than one-quarter of the patients. In most instances, although there is a decrease in overall size, the nodularity remains unchanged. The indications for operation, which have been considered in the treatment of nonnodular goiter, pertain to the nodular gland. The major argument concerning the management of the nodular thyroid is related to the likelihood that carcinoma is present within the gland and the effects of excision on the course of the disease.

It is estimated that 4 percent of inhabitants of the United States have nodules which are clinically detectable, i.e., greater than 1 cm. In Boston, routine postmortem examinations demonstrated that 8 percent of the population had one or more nodules at least 1 cm in diameter, and in women over the age of fifty a 15 percent incidence was noted. Most series have demonstrated that benign nodular goiter occurs nine times more frequently in females than males and generally becomes manifest after the age of forty.

The incidence of malignant tumors within nodular goiters ranges between 4 and 17 percent. Cole et al., evaluating a large series of thyroidectomy specimens, noted that cancer was found in 24 percent of glands with solitary nodules as compared with 10 percent in those with multiple nodules. The distinction between uninodular and multinodular goiters is extremely difficult, and it has been shown in several series that at least 50 percent of cases diagnosed preoperatively as a single nodule proved to be multinodular at the time of surgical exploration. The incidence of carcinoma within nodular thyroids varies with criteria used by pathologists and the selection of patients. The incidence of malignant thyroid tumors is related to the incidence of goiter in that area. A particularly pertinent but unresolved question is: "What percentage of lesions which satisfy the criteria for malignancy are potentially lethal?"

The mortality for thyroid cancer in 1955 was five per million for men and eight per million for women. In England and Wales, carcinoma of the thyroid accounts for 0.2 and 0.5 percent of all cancer deaths in males and females respectively. These figures emphasize the discrepancy between the mortality from thyroid carcinoma and its reported incidence in surgical specimens of multinodular goiters. The discrepancy is in part related to the factor of selectivity of patients. Those patients with multinodular goiter subjected to surgical treatment represent a group in which clinically there is a greater likelihood of carcinoma. In the experience of Shimaoka et al., which is representative of other specialty clinics, the overall incidence of carcinoma in surgical specimens was approximately 7 percent. Fifteen percent of 235 patients were suspected of having a malignant lesion preoperatively, and 40 percent proved to have thyroid carcinoma. Only 2 percent of those classified as benign preoperatively proved to be malignant.

The possibility that a multinodular goiter contains carcinoma is difficult to exclude, but there are certain criteria which increase the diagnostic accuracy. The incidence of carcinoma within a multinodular gland is greater in patients less than forty years of age and in men. The increased incidence in truly solitary nodules has been referred to. Fixation of the gland, vocal cord paralysis, Horner syndrome, and involvement of the cervical nodes are suggestive of carcinoma. A history of recent rapid and painless growth also increases the index of suspicion. A roentgenogram of the neck may reveal localized deposits of calcium arranged in concentric layers (psammoma bodies). These are characteristics of papillary carcinoma. They also have been seen subsequent to hemorrhage in a benign lesion. Radioiodine scintillation scan of the thyroid gland may contribute to the diagnosis. Nodules in which the concentration of iodine is greater than, or equal to, the remainder of the gland are less likely to harbor malignant disease. "Cold" nodules with decreased concentration of iodine have a high incidence of malignancy. In operative cases, Robinson et al. reported an incidence of carcinoma for warm or hot nodules of 6.8 and 6.4 percent, respectively, while 31.5 percent of the cold nodules contained malignant tumor.

Therapeutic Approach. Operation is indicated if there is a high index of suspicion of carcinoma based on clinical findings or diagnostic studies. Solitary nodules in patients of either sex under the age of forty and particularly in children should be removed. Solitary nodules in men over forty should also be removed. In women over forty, if the nodule is functioning as evidenced by radioiodine scan, a trial of suppressive drug therapy may be undertaken. If this induces regression, drug therapy should be continued indefinitely. If the nodule fails to regress after several months or enlarges, surgical intervention is indicated. It is also indicated if there is evidence of thyrotoxicosis associated with the nodule.

The above-mentioned criteria pertain if two or three nodules are felt. If the gland obviously contains many nodules and the patient is asymptomatic, treatment with thyroid hormone in suppressive doses is indicated.

When an operation is performed for excision of nodular goiter and only one lobe is affected, a lobectomy and isthmusectomy is the procedure of choice. Frozen section should be performed to define any questionable lesion. The treatment of proved carcinoma is discussed later in this chapter. Following surgical treatment for nodular goiter, patients are placed on replacement doses of thyroid hormone to depress TSH production and prevent regeneration. The incidence of recurrence of benign nodules varies from 5 to 15 percent depending on the period of follow-up. Subtotal thyroidectomy for nodular goiter should not be regarded as prophylaxis against carcinoma of the thyroid, since abnormal tissue is left in the neck and has a tendency to grow.

Benign Tumors

Benign tumors of the thyroid are classified as embryonal, fetal, follicular, Hürthle cell, and papillary adenomas according to their predominant histologic pattern. Grossly, the lesions are enveloped by a discrete capsule surrounded by a thin zone of compressed thyroid tissue. Microscopically, the architecture is orderly, mitoses are rare, and there is no lymphatic or blood vessel invasion. In some series, papillary adenoma is considered as a low-grade carcinoma. Several series have indicated that 80 percent of surgical specimens which proved to contain a solitary nodule are benign tumors, while 20 percent are malignant growths.

CLINICAL MANIFESTATIONS. Patients usually present with a history of a slowly growing mass which must reach the size of 1 cm to be palpable. The lesions are rarely symptomatic. Bleeding into the mass is manifested by sudden onset of localized pain. There is no evidence of cervical node involvement. Radiogram of the neck may demonstrate encroachment on the trachea. Radioiodine may indicate concentration of iodine equal to, greater than, or less than normal thyroid tissue. The criteria of differential diagnosis from malignant lesion have been referred to under Multinodular Goiter.

TREATMENT. Although some writers report treatment of solitary nodules with thyroid hormone, the majority have had no success with this approach. Since malignancy cannot be ruled out, excisional biopsy is indicated. The lesion and a margin of normal tissue should be removed and a frozen section performed to establish the diagnosis. Excision is usually achieved by subtotal or total lobectomy and isthmusectomy. The postoperative mortality approaches zero; the hospitalization is 3 to 5 days, and the postoperative morbidity is extremely low.

Malignant Tumors

GENERAL CONSIDERATIONS

INCIDENCE. The number of new cases of thyroid cancer in the United States has been estimated as 25 per 1 million population. Annual mortality from thyroid cancer is five deaths per 1 million men and eight deaths per 1 million women. The incidence of malignant tumor within the thyroid observed at routine autopsy ranges between 0.08 and 0.11 percent. There is a disputed slight association of follicular carcinoma with endemic goiter, but this does not pertain for papillary carcinoma. Ionizing radiation in childhood, usually directed at the thymus or cervical lymph nodes, has been shown to be definitely carcinogenic for the human thyroid. There is no firm evidence of increased incidence of thyroid cancer in autoimmune thyroiditis.

Clinically significant thyroid carcinoma is two to four times more common in females than in males. This sex discrepancy is less marked than that noted for other thyroid diseases. The lesions can occur at any age. The mean age for men is fifty-three years and for women forty-eight years. There has been an increasing incidence in children related to ionizing radiation in childhood, as mentioned above.

PATHOLOGY. The American Thyroid Association has accepted the classification proposed by Hazard and Smith. The four major classes are (1) papillary adenocarcinoma, (2) follicular adenocarcinoma, (3) medullary adenocarcinoma or solid adenocarcinoma with amyloid stroma, and (4) anaplastic adenocarcinoma. In addition, the thyroid may be involved with lymphosarcoma and metastatic carcinoma.

CLINICAL MANIFESTATIONS. Patients generally present with enlargement or nodularity of the thyroid. Direct questioning should determine if there is a history of irradiation to the thymus or radiation therapy for cervical adenitis in infancy. Occasionally there is a history of recent rapid growth of the lesion. Hoarseness, dysphagia, and dyspnea are late symptoms. Physical examination in the case of an early lesion frequently reveals only a thyroid mass. This may be a diffusely enlarged firm gland, a discrete nodule, or an unusually hard and dominant nodule in a multinodular gland. Regional lymph nodes may be enlarged and firm, which is suggestive of metastatic involvement. Horner's syndrome may be present, and indirect laryngoscopy may reveal paralysis of the vocal cords in advanced cases. Limitation of movement of the thyroid on swallowing suggests fixation and extension of the tumor through the capsule. Most early lesions cannot be differentiated from nodular goiter.

In general, patients with thyroid carcinoma are euthyroid, and the indices of function are normal. However, an incidence of thyroid carcinoma in Graves' disease of 9 percent has been reported. The lesions may secrete an abnormal iodoprotein with the properties of serum albumin. A similar protein has been found in other types of thyroid disease, such as thyrotoxicosis and thyroiditis. Thyroid carcinomas, in general, lose their ability to accumulate iodide as evidenced by the scintiscan, which demonstrates a reduction or absence of radioiodine in the region of the lesion. Follicular carcinomas tend to retain the ability to accumulate iodide more completely than other tumors, and radioiodine scanning is therefore less diagnostic in these cases.

An association between thyroid carcinoma and other endocrine abnormalities has been noted. The medullary-type tumor of the thyroid may occur concomitantly with pheochromocytoma. Solid carcinomas with amyloid stroma also have been associated with Cushing's syndrome due to overproduction of ACTH and symptoms of the carcinoid syndrome. An increased incidence of thyroid cancer also has been reported in patients with hyperparathyroidism.

The differential diagnosis includes the thyroidites, benign adenomas, and nodular goiter. Although needle biopsy of the thyroid has been applied to establish the diagnosis, it is not generally recommended, since a negative biopsy may not be representative.

TREATMENT. Treatment generally consists of surgical excision of the lesion. There is a great difference of opinion concerning the extent of the procedure. This will be expanded in the discussion of the therapy of the various types of pathologic lesions. Radioiodine has been employed, but effectiveness is limited by the fact that almost all cancers of the thyroid have a relative to absolute lack of avidity for iodine. High-voltage and supervoltage local radiation therapy is used in some instances when the tumor is obviously not resectable.

PAPILLARY CARCINOMA

Papillary carcinoma is the most common of the malignant tumors of the thyroid. It accounts for approximately half the thyroid malignant tumors in adults and three-quarters of those in children. Over half the cases are clinically manifest before the age of forty, with a peak incidence in the third and fourth decades. The tumors occur three times more frequently in females than males. In some patients, radiation therapy which was administered during childhood for cervical lymphadenitis or thymic enlargement has been implicated. As papillary carcinoma grows slowly, follow-up periods of at least 10 years are required to assess mortality rates.

PATHOLOGY. Papillary carcinoma is composed of columnar thyroidal epithelium arranged in papillary projections with connective tissue and vascular stalks. Outside the papillae, there may be a homogeneous material resembling colloid. The tumor may contain localized deposits of calcium arranged in concentric layers (psammoma bodies). The papillary pattern may predominate in mixed lesions containing follicular elements, and, at times, Hürthle cells.

Papillary carcinoma is the most slowly growing of the malignant tumors of the thyroid and has a tendency to become more malignant with advancing age. It has been suggested that anaplastic carcinoma may develop from a preexisting low-grade papillary carcinoma. There is some evidence that the growth of papillary carcinoma is dependent on TSH stimulation. Spread of the lesion is usually intraglandular and via pericapsular regional lymph nodes, where it may remain localized for a long period of time. This spread, overshadowing the primary lesion, may occur when a primary tumor is of microscopic size, a circumstance now felt to be responsible for the so-called "lateral aberrant thyroid rest." The acceptable terminology is now *occult papillary carcinoma,* referring to small papillary tumors with or without deposits in cervical lymph nodes. Within the thyroid gland itself, the tumor is multicentric in about 20 percent of the cases. Although the carcinoma may persist in the neck for decades without further spread, distant metastases may occur. These are potentially functional and may accumulate radioiodine, particularly if there is a follicular element.

CLINICAL MANIFESTATIONS. The lesion usually presents as an asymptomatic nodule within the thyroid gland or as enlargement of the regional lymph nodes. Fixation of the thyroid, manifestations of pressure on adjacent structures, and distant metastases all occur late. A radiogram of the neck may reveal calcium flecks suggesting psammoma bodies. Radioiodine scan of the palpable nodule frequently demonstrates a lack of iodine uptake.

TREATMENT. All agree that the treatment of choice for contained lesions is surgical excision, but debate centers around the extent of resection. Most feel that if the tumor is apparently contained within the thyroid and there are no obvious cervical lymph node metastases, the entire lobe containing the tumor and the isthmus should be removed. Others feel that more radical surgical treatment is indicated. The latter thesis is based on the fact that several investigators have demonstrated that as many as two-thirds of the patients without clinical evidence of metastatic adenopathy have histologically apparent lymph node involvement. In addition, the multicentric origin of some of the papillary carcinomas suggests that the thyroid resection should be more extensive. In rebuttal to these histologic findings, definite proof that radical neck dissection or extensive thyroidectomy increases survival is difficult to obtain. Medina and Elliott demonstrated that more radical procedures, including neck dissection, produced no greater survival than lobectomy with or without excision of the opposite lobe. On the other hand, the more extensive procedures were associated with a higher incidence of serious complications including hypoparathyroidism, recurrent nerve injury, and airway obstruction. Crile has emphasized the fact that thyroidectomy and radical neck dissection does not meet the criteria for en bloc continuity, since the thyroid lies in the visceral compartment of the neck. In appreciation of this fact, Crile and others advise excision of cervical nodes only when they are apparently involved. Marchetta and Sako advise a modified neck dissection which preserves the sternocleidomastoid muscle, spinal accessory nerve, and internal jugular vein.

Our approach to papillary carcinoma of the thyroid is determined by the extent of the lesion. If the diagnosis of papillary carcinoma is made on frozen section and there is no apparent extension to cervical lymph nodes, a total lobectomy of the involved lobe plus isthmusectomy with subtotal lobectomy on the opposite side is performed. The node-bearing tissue adjacent to the gland is removed, and enlarged lymph nodes are excised. If there is bilateral involvement but no apparent extension outside the gland, a total thyroidectomy is performed. Solitary cervical node metastases at a distance from the gland are removed individually. If multiple nodes are involved on one side, a modified neck dissection which preserves the sternocleidomastoid muscle, spinal accessory nerve, and internal jugular vein is performed.

The prognosis for advanced lesions is usually not improved by extensive surgical treatment. Because of the chronic course of many of these tumors, solitary distant metastases, particularly in the mediastinum, which can be removed surgically should be so treated. If multiple metastases occur, treatment with radioactive iodine may be employed, but the results are frequently disappointing. Response to radioiodine therapy is more favorable when the lesion consists of an orderly arrangement of cells in the direction of an acinar pattern. Accumulation of radioactive iodine by metastases can be enhanced by total thyroidectomy or by the administration of thyroid hormone coupled with large doses of TSH. The administration of mannitol to induce acute iodine depletion has also increased the radioactive iodine uptake of metastases. Since many of the follicular carcinomas are TSH-dependent, suppressive doses of thyroid hormone should be administered to all patients with metastatic disease or locally invasive involvement on a long-term basis.

PROGNOSIS. The prognosis for long-term survival of patients with papillary carcinoma is excellent. In Crile's experience of 307 patients followed for at least 5 years 16 patients died of cancer. The prognosis is definitely worse in patients older than forty years of age. In this series, total thyroidectomy was employed only in patients with gross involvement of both lobes, and no clinically apparent cancer developed in the remaining contralateral lobe. There were no prophylactic neck dissections in patients who did not have gross evidence of nodal involvement. Black et al. analyzed 418 cases of papillary carcinoma. The 10-year survival rates for occult and contained intrathyroidal lesions were 89.5 and 83.9 percent respectively. None of the patients with occult lesions had metastases to distant sites or died of thyroidal cancer. Of 270 patients with clinically apparent but contained intrathyroidal cancer 6 died. Some patients with papillary carcinoma will die of the disease. In these cases, the originally dominant papillary elements become less prominent, and the histologic appearance becomes more anaplastic. Hirabayashi and Lindsay reported that 11 percent of their patients died of disease and that 40 percent of the deaths resulted from uncontrollable disease within the neck. Since many of the patients with papillary carcinoma are young, the effects of pregnancy on the prognosis has been of some concern. Hill et al., analyzing 70 patients, could demonstrate no difference in the overall recurrence rate subsequent to pregnancy and concluded that pregnancy had no effect on the course of disease.

FOLLICULAR CARCINOMA

Follicular carcinoma is the predominant element of one-quarter of malignant tumors of the thyroid. The lesion tends to occur in older age groups, with a peak incidence in the fifth decade. It is three times more common in females than in males.

PATHOLOGY. Grossly, the tumor may appear encapsulated. Histologically, the lesion resembles the acinar structure of normal thyroid tissue and is recognizable as an adenocarcinoma. The lumen of the acini may be devoid of colloid. The lesions contain varying numbers of large eosinophilic cells arranged in columns, Hürthle cells. The malignant potential exceeds that of papillary carcinoma. Although there may be spread to regional lymph nodes, hematogenous spread to distant sites such as bone, lung, and liver predominates and often occurs early. Occasionally, a follicular tumor with an extremely benign histologic appearance is coupled with distant metastases resembling normal thyroid. The term *benign metastasizing goiter* has been applied to these lesions.

CLINICAL MANIFESTATIONS. In many patients there is a long history of goiter with recent change in the gland, such as diffuse enlargement or the development of a single firm nodule. Pain and invasion of adjacent structures are late manifestations. Regional lymph nodes are seldom enlarged, but distant metastases are frequent. In the Massachusetts General Hospital series, one-half of the patients had evidence of distant metastases at the time that the diagnosis was established. Pulmonary and bony lesions, which are usually osteolytic, represent the most frequent sites of metastases. The metastases may possess an ability to retain iodine but are rarely responsible for thyrotoxicosis.

TREATMENT AND PROGNOSIS. In the case of an apparently contained lesion, hemithyroidectomy and isthmusectomy are usually the procedures employed. If local metastases are apparent, dissection includes these nodes. Since lymph node metastases are less common than hematogenous spread, concomitant radical neck dissection is rarely indicated. Metastases sometimes regress under the influence of suppressive thyroid hormone. Radioiodine may accumulate within the metastases and have a therapeutic effect. Total thyroidectomy has been performed in order to increase the avidity of metastases for radioiodine. Isolated metastases may be removed surgically.

Follicular tumors have the biologic behavior of a low-grade malignant tumor. The histologically more benign lesions (benign metastasizing goiter) have a better prognosis. The prognosis of follicular tumors in which the Hürthle cell predominates is similar to other follicular tumors but has a stronger propensity for recurrence. Black et al. reported 10-year survival rate of 72 percent for follicular tumors. In those lesions without marked invasiveness, the 10-year survival rate was 86 percent, whereas when invasiveness was apparent, the 10-year survival rate was 44 percent.

MEDULLARY CARCINOMA

PATHOLOGY. These lesions comprise about 7 to 10 percent of the cases of thyroid carcinoma and usually occur after the age of fifty. The diagnosis is based on specific microscopic features. The cell type varies from small and round to large and ovoid or polyhedral. At times, spindle cells are palisaded and show pleomorphism. Mitotic figures are not conspicuous. The stroma contains greater or lesser amounts of amyloid which may dominate the picture. The tumor tends to spread via the bloodstream to distant sites, particularly lung, bone, and liver. In some instances, medullary thyroid carcinoma can simulate papillary carcinoma with predominant cervical node metastases. Sixty to seventy-five percent of cases have cervical node metastases, and in thirty-eight percent mediastinal nodes are involved.

CLINICAL MANIFESTATIONS. The lesions are slightly more common in women. The first manifestation may be a hard nodular mass in the thyroid, at times accompanied by enlargement of the lymph nodes. Occasionally, symptoms attributable to a distant metastasis constitute the chief complaint. Both lobes of the thyroid are usually involved. Pain and tenderness may be severe. Thyroidal radioiodine scan demonstrates that the lesions accumulate iodine poorly. Clinically apparent regional lymph node metastases are present in over half the patients.

The lesion has evoked a great deal of interest because of its association with other endocrine abnormalities and is part of the multiple endocrine neoplasia (MEN-II) syndrome. The most commonly associated lesion is pheochromocytoma. This is thought to have a genetic basis in view of its familial occurrence. Block et al. reported personal experience with 18 patients, 10 of whom were members of two families. Either lesion, i.e., the medullary carcinoma or the pheochromocytoma, may predominate. Nonfamilial coexistence of these lesions also occurs. The frequency of bilateral thyroidal lesions in patients with medullary carcinoma combined with pheochromocytoma is greater than in those patients without pheochromocytoma (80 versus 8 percent). Other abnormalities occurring in families exhibiting the medullary carcinoma–pheochromocytoma syndrome include hyperparathyroidism, Cushing's syndrome, diabetes mellitus, carcinoid syndrome with flushing, mucosal neuromas, and unexplained diarrhea. It is thought that the syndrome may represent a disturbance in amine metabolism, and elevated serotonin calcitonin, and prostaglandin levels have been demonstrated in these patients. The diagnosis can be made by demonstration of hypocalcemia and assay of calcitonin. Determination of peak thyrocalcitonin response to pentagastrin provides a method for diagnosing medullary carcinoma in asymptomatic family members who are related to a patient with the MEN-II syndrome. Pheochromocytoma diagnostic studies must be performed in all patients with suspected medullary carcinoma.

TREATMENT AND PROGNOSIS. Pheochromocytomas, if present, should be removed first. The frequent involvement of both lobes of the thyroid and cervical lymph nodes makes an extensive excision advisable. Total or near-total thyroidectomy and modified neck dissection on one or both sides are justified if metastases are suspected. In some cases, pain emanating from the thyroid gland is so severe as to warrant palliative resection.

During the thyroid operation the parathyroid glands should be explored. If there is hypocalcemia or normocalcemia, the parathyroids should be left intact. If there is hypercalcemia, a single large gland should be removed if the remaining three are normal. This is the most common circumstance when there is hyperparathyroidism. If more than one gland is enlarged, the three largest glands and part of the fourth should be removed. Subtotal parathyroidectomy should not be routine in these patients, since hyperparathyroidism does not always occur and when present is mild.

The tumor does not respond to treatment with radioactive iodine, external radiation, or thyroid hormone. The prognosis is poorer than that noted for papillary and follicular carcinoma. Black et al. reported a 61 percent 10-year survival rate in 49 patients who underwent resection. Thirteen of twenty-five patients without involvement of the lymph nodes died during the follow-up period. However, the ultimate outcome appeared to depend more on the extent of disease than on the surgical procedure. In the experience of Black et al., recurrences within unresected remnants of the thyroid were not found.

ANAPLASTIC CARCINOMA

Undifferentiated carcinomas make up about 10 percent of malignant tumors of the thyroid and usually occur after the age of fifty. In some instances, the lesion represents a transformation of a low-grade differentiated tumor. Frazell and Foote reviewed 393 papillary tumors and reported 6 in which such a transformation occurred. Wychulis et al. reported 16 patients with mixed anaplastic and papillary carcinoma. The ratio of men to women is 1.3 : 1, and 50 percent are in the seventh and eighth decades of life, with an average age of sixty-six years.

Grossly, the tumor is unencapsulated and may extend widely outside the confines of the gland, invading adjacent structures. Histologically, the cell structure is variable, ranging from spindle-shaped to multinucleated giant cells. There are numerous mitoses, and the appearance is similar to that of a lymphosarcoma. In some cases, areas of follicular or papillary carcinoma may be present.

Patients generally present with painful enlargement of the thyroid, which is often fixed and moves poorly on swallowing. Regional lymph nodes are frequently enlarged, and signs and symptoms of pressure effects are common. Metastases are usually located in the lungs rather than the bones. The disease is characterized by an extremely rapid progress. Total thyroidectomy and modified neck dissection is the treatment of choice, but in many patients the lesion is not resectable. In one series of 130 cases, resection was attempted in only 49, and only one patient was known to be alive at the time of the report. Seventy-five percent of the deaths occurred within 1 year. External radiation may afford palliation for pain. Radioactive iodine is ineffective, since the tumors do not concentrate the material.

LYMPHOMA AND SARCOMA

The thyroid is a rare site for primary lymphoma. Mikal, in a review of the literature, indicated that 165 cases had been reported, with tumors arising from reticular cells, lymphoblasts, and lymphocytes. Only 13 cases of Hodgkin's disease arising primarily in the thyroid have been documented. At times the lesions are difficult to differentiate from Hashimoto's disease.

Treatment is determined by the extent of disease. When the tumor is localized, a total or near-total thyroidectomy followed by deep x-ray therapy to the cervical nodes is indicated. If the disease has metastasized to cervical nodes or invaded the capsule, a total thyroidectomy and radical neck dissection should be performed and followed by radiation. Disseminated lymphoma may be treated by Cytoxan or chlorambucil, or prednisone may be used in patients who cannot tolerate chemotherapy because of bone marrow depression. The 5-year survival rate is approximately 50 percent.

METASTATIC CARCINOMA

Metastases are present in the thyroid in 2 to 4 percent of the patients dying of malignant disease. Bronchogenic carcinomas account for 20 percent of secondary thyroid metastases. Three percent of all bronchogenic carcinomas autopsied demonstrate metastases to the thyroid. Wychulis et al. reported that among more than 20,000 surgical specimens 10 represented metastatic involvement of the thyroid gland. The most common primary lesion in that series was hypernephroma, with the average age of the patient fifty-six years. Freund reported two 5-year survivals following thyroidectomy in which there were metastatic lesions from bronchogenic carcinoma and lipomyxosarcoma.

Surgery of the Thyroid

Surgical treatment of the thyroid is performed (1) to establish the diagnosis in a patient with diffuse enlargement of, or a mass within, the thyroid gland; (2) to remove benign and malignant tumors; (3) as therapy for thyrotoxicosis; and (4) to alleviate pressure symptoms attributable to the thyroid. Preoperative preparation of patients with thyrotoxicosis is important to obviate the complication of thyroid storm during the operation and in the immediate postoperative period. The patients should be made euthyroid by the administration of an antithyroid drug. Seven to ten days prior to the operative procedure, potassium iodide or Lugol's solution is administered to decrease the vascularity and cause involution of the gland. Propanalol provides an alternative method of preparation.

OPERATIVE TECHNIQUE. The procedure (Fig. 38-12) is almost always performed under endotracheal anesthesia, although there was a time when local anesthesia was popular in some clinics. The patient's neck is extended by inflating a pillow beneath the shoulders. An equilateral low collar incision is made in the line of a natural skin crease approximately 2 cm above the clavicle. The incision is carried through skin, subcutaneous tissue, and platysma down to the dense cervical fascia that overlies the pretracheal muscles and anterior jugular veins. The upper flap is raised to the level of the thyroid cartilage, with care to avoid cutting sensory nerves, in order to obviate unnecessary paresthesias during convalescence. The lower flap is elevated to the level of the manubrial notch. If dissection of the flap is performed in the plane between the platysmal

muscle and the fascia overlying the strap muscles, the bleeding is minimal. The cervical fascia is then incised vertically in the midline from the upper margin of the thyroid cartilage to the manubrium.

Exposure of the superior and lateral aspects of the thyroid gland generally is achieved by retracting the sternohyoid and sternothyroid muscles or by dividing these muscles. Division of these muscles is associated with little or no disability, but is not necessary unless the gland is markedly enlarged. High transection is preferable, since the ansa hypoglossi nerve innervates the muscles from below. This diminishes the amount of muscle paralyzed.

Digital dissection frees the thyroid from surrounding fascia. We then prefer to rotate one lobe medially in order to identify the middle thyroid veins, which vary in number. These are doubly ligated in continuity and transected. This maneuver facilitates exposure of the superior and inferior poles of the thyroid. The suspensory ligaments are transected craniad to the isthmus, and the cricothyroid space is opened in order to separate the superior pole from surrounding tissue. During dissection of the superior lobe care is taken to avoid injury to the superior laryngeal nerve. The internal branch of the nerve, which provides sensory fibers to the epiglottis and larynx, is rarely in the operative field. It is the external branch, which supplies motor innervation to the inferior pharyngeal constrictor and cricothyroid muscles, which must be protected. This is accomplished by dissecting the nerve away from the superior pole vessels, which are then clamped and ligated separately.

The lobe is then retracted mediad to permit identification of the inferior thyroid artery and the recurrent laryngeal nerve. The inferior thyroid artery is isolated to avoid trauma to the recurrent laryngeal nerve and doubly ligated in continuity as it passes beneath the common carotid artery. The recurrent laryngeal nerve is identified along its course. At the junction of the trachea and larynx, it is in its most anterior position and relatively fixed. At this point, the lobe may be totally mobilized, as is indicated for tumor and *recurrent* hyperthyroidism, or a remnant of approximately 1 to 2 Gm of posterior thyroid tissue may be left in those patients in whom the operation is being performed for primary hyperthyroidism.

During exposure of the posterior surface of the thyroid gland, the parathyroids should be identified and preserved along with their vascular pedicle. Using sharp dissection, the lobe is then dissected clear from the lateral aspect of the trachea, and dissection is continued in order to separate the isthmus from the anterior trachea. If a pyramidal lobe is present, it is removed at this time. It is important that the entire anterior trachea be cleared in order to avoid development of a mass due to hypertrophy of the thyroid in this region. When the operation is being performed for a unilateral lesion, it is terminated at this point by approximating the anterior and posterior aspects of the cut end of the medial portion of the remaining lobe. When subtotal or total thyroidectomy is performed, the remaining lobe is removed in the same manner.

The remnants of thyroid are folded in and sutured to the trachea to complete hemostasis. The entire wound is

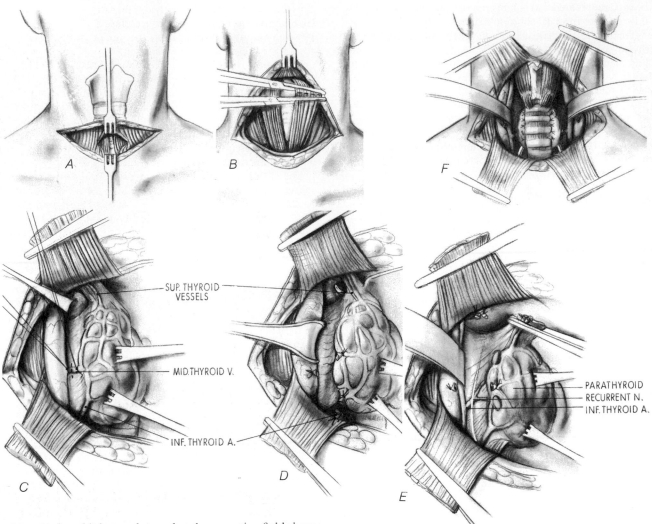

Fig. 38-12. Thyroidectomy. *A.* Collar incision made. Subplatysmal flaps developed. *B.* High transection of strap muscles (optional). *C.* Middle thyroid vein divided. *D.* Superior and inferior pole vessels divided. *E.* Identification of recurrent laryngeal nerve and parathyroids. *F.* Remnants of thyroid sutured to trachea to effect hemostasis.

inspected, and it is mandatory that the operative field show no evidence of bleeding. Some surgeons prefer to drain the bed of the thyroid lobes, employing a small, soft rubber drain which is split at one end to achieve a "Y" effect with the drain brought out through the incision. Others feel that little is accomplished by this maneuver, since rapid bleeding leading to respiratory distress cannot be decompressed by the small drain. The midline fascial incision is closed, and if the sternothyroid and sternohyoid muscles have been transected, they are reapproximated. The platysma and superficial fascia are then sutured with fine silk, and skin closure may be accomplished with fine silk or clips.

A tracheostomy set is left at the patient's bedside for 24 hours, so that the wound can be opened rapidly if there is significant distension, or a tracheostomy can be performed if there is evidence of respiratory obstruction.

Intrathoracic Goiter. In about 1 percent of patients undergoing thyroidectomy part or all of the thyroid tissue is intrathoracic. Intrathoracic goiter usually represents the extension of cervical thyroid tissue into the chest rather than aberrant glandular tissue. Since the lesion usually retains its connection to the cervical thyroid and receives its blood supply from the inferior thyroid artery, it generally can be removed through the conventional collar incision described above. In the case of a very large mass the semiliquid colloid and degenerated portions may be evacuated to permit delivery of the remainder of the tissue and the capsule in the neck. The indications for transsternal or transpleural thyroidectomy include (1) an inability to remove the tumor totally through a cervical approach, (2) large masses with extensive blood supply within the mediastinum, (3) evidence of superior vena cava obstruction, and (4) undiagnosed superior mediastinal lesions.

Transsternal thyroidectomy (Fig. 38-13) can be performed as an extension of a cervical exploration by "T-ing" the cervical incision over the sternum. The sternum is transected horizontally at the level of the third interspace and vertically from the suprasternal notch down to the level of the horizontal transection. This permits extrapleural resection of the gland and provides excellent visualization of the recurrent laryngeal nerves and the vascular supply.

A thoracic extension of a cervical goiter may also be removed through a combined cervical-anterior thoracic approach using two incisions, the standard cervical incision and an incision in the second interspace. In the case of an intrathoracic goiter in the posterior portion of the mediastinum, some have advised a posterolateral thoracotomy. The disadvantage of this approach is that the position of the recurrent laryngeal nerve is difficult to determine and the major blood supply from the inferior thyroid artery is harder to control.

COMPLICATIONS

The mortality rate accompanying thyroidectomy is very low. Gould et al. reviewed 1,000 patients, operated on consecutively by a large group of surgeons over a 5-year period, and reported no hospital deaths. The mortality rate reported by Colcock was 0.12 percent, with no deaths since 1954. The morbidity is about 13 percent when all complications, including those of the most minor types, are considered. Pulmonary problems and infections are relatively uncommon. Four major complications classically have been associated with thyroidectomy. These include (1) thyroid storm, which is related to the patient's thyrotoxicosis, (2) wound hemorrhage, (3) recurrent laryngeal nerve injury, and (4) hypoparathyroidism. The latter three are regarded as complications of technique.

THYROID STORM. Thyrotoxicotic storm occurs in patients with preexisting thyrotoxicosis who either have not been treated at all or have been treated incompletely. It usually occurs in patients with Graves' disease but may be related to toxic multinodular goiter. In the past, before adequate preparation with antithyroid drugs, surgical treatment was the most common precipitating factor. Presently thyrotoxicotic crisis is a rare complication of surgical treatment and is more frequently precipitated by trauma, infection, diabetic acidosis, or toxemia of pregnancy.

When thyroid storm is related to surgical treatment, the manifestation may develop during the operative procedure or in the recovery room. The patient becomes markedly hyperthermic with profuse sweating and tachycardia. Nausea, vomiting, and abdominal pain are common. Initial tremor and restlessness may progress to delirium with eventual coma.

Treatment is directed at inhibiting the production of thyroid hormone and antagonizing effects of the hormone. Large doses of sodium or potassium iodide, i.e., to 1 to 2.5 Gm, should be administered intravenously and supplemented with 100 mg of cortisol. Oxygen and large amounts of glucose should be administered intravenously as therapy for the hypermetabolic state. Fluid and electrolytes must be maintained in view of the losses. A hypothermia blanket may be applied to reduce the temperature. Propranolol has replaced guanethidine and reserpine to antagonize

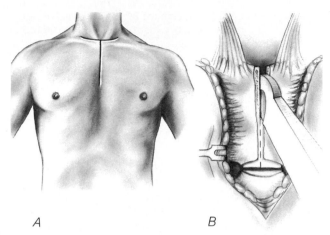

Fig. 38-13. Transsternal thyroidectomy. *A.* Incision. *B.* Transection of sternum. "T-ing" incision into second interspace.

sympathetic effects, since it is not complicated by congestive heart failure. Exchange transfusion is a last, but perhaps effective, resort. The mortality rate for this complication is approximately 10 percent.

WOUND HEMORRHAGE. This is a problem of the early postoperative period, i.e., within the first few hours. It has been reported in 0.3 to 1 percent of consecutive thyroidectomies. Hemorrhage in the neck is a significant problem, since small amounts of blood may obstruct the airway and result in respiratory death. The complication is usually caused by bleeding from branches of the inferior thyroid or superior thyroid artery, and the rate of bleeding is such that the commonly employed drains do not afford protection. Holl-Allen has reported four cases of postthyroidectomy hemorrhage due to hypoprothrombinemia with deficiency of factors VII and X. The deficiency was ascribed to carbimazole therapy for thyrotoxicosis. These patients required reoperation despite routine drainage at the time of the initial procedure, and vitamin K_1 corrected the deficiency.

The patients are rarely in shock. The initial manifestation is swelling of the neck and bulging of the wound, which demands immediate attention. If untreated, respiratory obstruction due to compression eventually ensues. Treatment consists of opening the incision, evacuating the clot, and securing the bleeding vessel. This constitutes an emergency procedure and frequently should be performed at the patient's bedside. Tracheostomy is not required, and is in fact contraindicated, if the wound is decompressed early. Only if there is a question of severe and potentially prolonged tracheal compression should tracheostomy be performed. Hemostasis should be complete prior to the tracheostomy to obviate bleeding into the tracheostomy tube and encrustation.

RECURRENT LARYNGEAL INJURY. Damage to the recurrent laryngeal nerve may be unilateral or bilateral and temporary or permanent. Injury occurs more commonly when thyroidectomy is being performed for malignant disease. In a series of 1,011 thyroidectomies there were 28 examples of vocal cord paralysis, three of which proved to be permanent. The incidence of recurrent nerve injury in another series of 1,000 patients reported by Gould et al. was 0.2 percent. Colcock and King, evaluating 1,246 thyroid operations, noted one bilateral recurrent laryngeal nerve paralysis. Recently Thompson and Harness reported an incidence of 4.8 percent for accidental unilateral nerve injury in total thyroidectomy for carcinoma.

Loss of function of the recurrent laryngeal nerve may result from excessive trauma to the nerve during exposure, inclusion of the nerve in a ligature, or an inadvertent sectioning of the nerve. Recurrent laryngeal nerve injury produces an abductor laryngeal paralysis, and the vocal cord assumes a median or paramedian position, which is identifiable on postoperative laryngoscopy. The involved cord or cords are initially flaccid, but with the passage of time the flaccidity is replaced by spasticity. If the injury is related to dissection and the nerve is intact, function should return usually within 3 months and invariably within 9 months. In the immediate postoperative period, cord paralysis results in narrowing of the glottic aperture, but this is not sufficient to produce obstruction of the airway unless it is accompanied by glottic edema due to hematoma in the cervical space or trauma to the larynx, or related to the cuffed endotracheal tube. Because of the initial flaccidity, bilateral or cord paralysis may not be apparent for several hours. As the laryngeal muscles atrophy, the cords contract and the glottic aperture narrows, causing airway obstruction. Paralysis of one cord results in disturbance of the voice with varying degrees of hoarseness.

The incidence of this complication can be markedly reduced by identifying the nerve or nerves routinely during thyroidectomy. The recurrent laryngeal nerve is in greatest jeopardy at the level of the two upper tracheal rings, where the middle third of the thyroid lobe is in closest contact with it. The lobe is attached by a strong process of pretracheal fascia (the suspensory ligament of Berry) to the cricoid cartilage and trachea, which must be severed before it can be removed. Although the recurrent laryngeal nerve usually runs posteriorly to this adherent connective tissue zone, in 25 percent of patients it courses through the ligament of Berry. Asymptomatic paralysis does not require treatment. In some instances, reexploration of the wound is indicated, since removal of a ligature often reestablishes function. Once the diagnosis of bilateral cord paralysis, a rarity, is established, tracheostomy should be performed, since airway obstruction eventually occurs, frequently related to a respiratory tract infection. Subsequently the glottic aperture can be widened by arytenoidectomy or arytenoidopexy, which displaces the posterior portion of the vocal cord laterally. These procedures provide an adequate airway but cause further deterioration of the voice. Six to nine months should be allowed to pass between the time of thyroidectomy and these procedures in order to be certain that there is no returning function. Direct repair of the transected recurrent laryngeal nerve as late as 2 to 3 months postinjury has been successful in some cases. Splitting the vagus nerve and anastomosing it to the distal end of the recurrent laryngeal nerve or burying the nerve in the posterior cricoarytenoid muscle are being evaluated.

HYPOPARATHYROIDISM. Overt manifestations of hypoparathyroidism occur in 2 to 3 percent of patients following thyroidectomy. This is usually a temporary syndrome related to dissection in the region of the parathyroid glands. There is an increased incidence of temporary hypoparathyroidism following thyroidectomy for hyperthyroidism. It is necessary to leave only one gland in situ with an adequate blood supply to avoid the complication. Postoperative permanent hypoparathyroidism occurred in 0.6 percent of the 1,000 thyroidectomies reviewed by Gould et al. and in 2.8 percent of the total thyroidectomies in that series. Persik and Catz, in a review of 210 consecutive total thyroidectomies, noted that permanent hypoparathyroidism resulted in none of the patients with nonmalignant disease and in 9 percent of those with malignant disease. In the series of Thompson and Harness permanent hypoparathyroidism occurred in 5.4 percent of all patients undergoing total thyroidectomy for carcinoma, in 1.6 percent of those having primary procedures, and in 7.4 percent of those having secondary operations. An incidence of 8.2 percent was noted when there was an associated neck dissection.

Postthyroidectomy hypoparathyroidism may be due to the inadvertent removal of the parathyroid glands but more frequently is caused by damage to the blood supply. The parathyroid end arteries have to be damaged in order to infarct the gland. The anastomotic arterial network is so extensive that if proximal arteries are injured, there is sufficient collateralization. The clinical manifestations usually occur within the second 24 hours after operation and almost invariably within the first week. The initial symptoms are circumoral numbness, tingling, and intense anxiety. The Chvostek sign appears early, followed by Trousseau's sign and carpopedal spasm. As the disease progresses, muscle cramps and frank tetany develop. Prolonged hypoparathyroidism may cause cataracts, convulsive episodes, and psychoses. The diagnostic findings consist of reduced serum calcium, increased serum phosphorus, and decreased or absent calcium in the urine as evidenced by the Sulkowitch test.

Recently an occult type of hypoparathyroidism has been described. The symptoms are those of general ill health and mental depression. The serum calcium is within normal limits, but there is a lack of parathyroid reserve which can be demonstrated by the calcium deprivation test. When the serum calcium is depressed in the normal patient, the parathyroid glands are stimulated to increase secretion of parathyroid hormone in order to restore the calcium to normal levels. In patients with occult hypoparathyroidism this response is inadequate. EDTA (edetic acid) is infused for 2 hours, and the serum calcium level falls in both normal and abnormal cases. In normal patients a rise to 8.5 mg occurs within 24 hours, while the rise is markedly delayed in patients with occult hypoparathyroidism. Abnormal response to calcium load also has been observed in patients following a thyroid operation with extensive removal of tissue. This has been interpreted as evidence of calcitonin deficiency, but no clinical significance has been ascribed to this situation.

Postoperative hypoparathyroidism must be differentiated from tetany caused by alkalosis associated with anxiety and hyperventilation. This causes a reduction in ionized calcium, but the manifestations can be promptly reversed by inhalation of carbon dioxide or breathing through an increased dead space.

The treatment of hypoparathyroidism should be initiated promptly. When the diagnosis has been made, 10 ml of a 10 percent solution of calcium chloride or gluconate should be administered intravenously and usually results in immediate improvement of symptoms. Continued therapy includes 5 to 15 Gm of calcium lactate powder daily or calcium syrup, and 50,000 to 200,000 units of vitamin D_2 daily. The dosage of these drugs is regulated by following the patient's clinical course and serum calcium and phosphorus levels. The intake of certain meat, fish, and dairy products which are high in phosphorus should be limited, since it results in a depression of serum calcium levels. Parathyroid hormone (PTH) and dihydrotachysterol (AT 10) should be reserved for the exceptional case when usual measures fail. Watkins et al. have employed autotransplantation of parathyroid tissue at the time of operation with questionable evidence of take. Because of the factor of vascular deficiency these writers employed aortic vascular pedicle transplantation of neonatal parathyroid tissue in eight patients. Clinical improvement was noted despite histologic evidence of graft rejection. The efficacy of parathyroid transplantation in this situation remains to be proved.

PARATHYROID

(*by Edwin L. Kaplan*)

Historical Background

HYPERPARATHYROIDISM. Von Recklinghausen, in 1891, first described the fibrocystic disease of bone produced by hyperparathyroidism but did not recognize the association. In 1903 Askanazy suggested a relation between tumors of the parathyroid and the bone disease described by von Recklinghausen. Erdheim in 1907 correctly surmised that parathyroid enlargement in osteomalacia, rickets, and pregnancy was *secondary* to the bone changes, and from this observation the concept grew that parathyroid enlargement was secondary in other types of bone disease as well. Schlagenhaufer in 1915 suggested that the parathyroid enlargement might be the cause of the bone disease and recommended excision of the parathyroid tumor as the treatment. The first parathyroidectomy was carried out by Mandl in Vienna in 1925 in a patient with classic von Recklinghausen's disease of bone. The patient's calcium level fell abruptly, and the bone lesions improved.

In 1926 a case referred by Du Bois for study by Aub at the Massachusetts General Hospital was diagnosed as probable hyperparathyroidism, and the neck was explored on two occasions, but no parathyroid tumor was found. These workers were at this time unaware of Mandl's experience, which had not yet been published. A third unsuccessful operation was carried out in New York. The patient ultimately returned to Boston, where, in 1932 at his seventh

operation, the adenoma was found in the mediastinum. The patient died 6 weeks later in tetany after another operation for a renal stone producing anuria. The first successful operation in America was that reported by Barr and Bulger in 1930.

The bone tumors of hyperparathyroidism were emphasized by Hunter and Turnbull, who called them "osteoclastomas" and in 1931 reported a case of successful removal of a parathyroid adenoma.

Hall and Chaffin reported the first parathyroid carcinoma in 1934. Water-clear cell (*wasserhellen Zellen*) hyperplasia was first described by Albright et al. in 1934 and primary chief cell hyperplasia by Cope et al. in 1958. Secondary chief cell hyperplasia in renal disease had been described by Pappenheimer and Wilens in 1935.

Albright recognized the association between parathyroid adenomas and renal stones, and in August 1932 the first patient to undergo excision of a parathyroid adenoma for renal stones without bone disease was operated upon. Albright emphasized that hyperparathyroidism was much more common than previously supposed, and often associated with renal stones. The frequency of the disease was further underscored by Cope, who in 1942 published a series of 67 cases from the Massachusetts General Hospital.

The association of hyperparathyroidism with peptic ulcer was first described by Rogers et al. (1946–1947) and the association with pancreatitis by Cope et al. (1957).

HYPOPARATHYROIDISM. Sanström (1880) first described the parathyroid glands. Gley (1891) showed that tetany following thyroidectomy in the dog was due to parathyroid removal. Vassale and Generali (1900) removed the parathyroids in the dog and produced tetany. Loeb (1901) showed that the injection of agents which bound calcium produced tetany. MacCallum and Voegtlin (1908) recognized that the function of the parathyroids was to regulate calcium metabolism and were able to relieve the tetany which followed parathyroidectomy by the administration of calcium.

Hanson (1924) and Collip (1925) prepared the first stable crude parathyroid hormone extracts. Collip (1926) correctly observed that parathyroid hormone (PTH) acted directly on bone to increase resorption. This view was challenged by Albright and Ellsworth (1929), who thought the bone effect was secondary to the effect of PTH on renal phosphate excretion. It is now clear that PTH acts both on bone and kidney.

Embryology

The upper parathyroids arise embryologically from the fourth branchial pouch along with the anlage of the thyroid (Fig. 38-14). They descend only slightly during embryologic life along with the thyroid and continue to remain in close association with the upper portion of the lateral thyroid lobes. Because of their relatively circumscribed migration their position in adult life remains quite constant. When they become adenomatous, they enlarge and tend to be displaced downward somewhat, dragging their blood supply with them. They may on occasion descend as far down as the superior portion of the posterior mediastinum. When they do descend into the mediastinum, they tend to be more posterior than the lower parathyroids.

The lower parathyroids arise from the third branchial pouch along with the thymus and descend with the thymus (Fig. 38-15). Because they travel so far in embryologic life, they have a very wide range of distribution in the adult. They may be found all the way from just beneath the mandible to the pericardium. When the lower parathyroid does descend into the mediastinum, it is almost always anterior and usually supplied by the inferior thyroid artery, which is dragged behind it (Fig. 38-16). A mediastinal parathyroid gland can be found by tracing the branch of the inferior thyroid artery which supplies it even in its abnormal location.

Anatomy

Gilmour, in a study of 527 autopsies, found that roughly 80 percent had four glands, 6 percent had five, and 13 percent had three. Two glands or six glands were present very rarely. These data are shown in Table 38-1.

In 1938 Gilmour described the position of the glands in 787 autopsy cases. The locations with the relative percentages found are shown diagrammatically in Figs. 38-17 and 38-18. In nearly 75 percent of the cases the upper gland lay on the posterior portion of the middle third of the thyroid, usually toward the superior part of this area, either in a groove on the thyroid or on a projecting nodule. It usually lay above the inferior thyroid artery but occasionally behind it or between it and the thyroid gland.

The inferior parathyroid glands were of course more

Fig. 38-14. Embryology of the parathyroid glands. The upper parathyroid has its origin in the fourth branchial pouch and moves to a position in adult life adjacent to the middle third of the lateral thyroid lobe. It thus travels little from its site of embryologic origin. The lower parathyroid, by contrast, arises from the third branchial pouch and travels down past the upper parathyroid to come to rest opposite the lower pole of the thyroid. Because of this embryologic mobility the lower parathyroid is more likely to lie in some ectopic location, either left behind high up in the neck or moving far down past the upper parathyroid into the mediastinum along with the thymus.

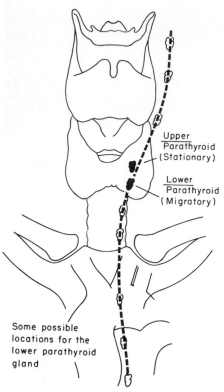

Upper Parathyroid (Stationary)

Lower Parathyroid (Migratory)

Some possible locations for the lower parathyroid gland

Fig. 38-15. Descent of the lower parathyroid. While the upper parathyroid occupies a relatively constant position in relation to the middle or upper third of the lateral thyroid lobe, the lower parathyroid normally migrates in embryonic life and may end up anywhere along the course of the dotted line. When this gland is in the chest, it is nearly always in the anterior mediastinum.

variable. In somewhat more than 50 percent of the cases the lower parathyroid was found on the lateral or posterior surface of the lower pole of the thyroid gland, or not more than 0.5 cm below the lower pole. The next most common location, in 12.8 percent, was 1 cm below the lower pole of the thyroid.

Gilmour, while examining 1,713 parathyroid glands in 428 patients, found that the parathyroids were occasionally included within the thyroid capsule or lay beneath it and

Table 38-1. NUMBER OF PARATHYROIDS
IN 527 AUTOPSY CASES

Number of parathyroid glands	Number of patients	Percentage of patients with this number
6	2	0.4
5	31	5.9
4	419	79.5
3	69	13.1
2	6	1.1
Total.	527	100

SOURCE: Gilmour, 1937.

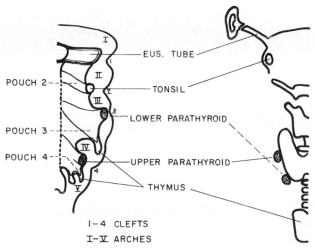

EUS. TUBE

POUCH 2

TONSIL

LOWER PARATHYROID

POUCH 3

POUCH 4

UPPER PARATHYROID

THYMUS

I-4 CLEFTS
I-V ARCHES

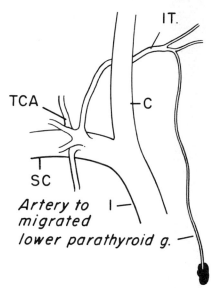

Fig. 38-16. Migration of the adenomatous parathyroid gland. If an adenoma develops in the parathyroid gland, the gland may gradually descend into the chest. Under these circumstances, it is always supplied with blood from the inferior thyroid artery. If the lower parathyroid has descended into the mediastinum during embryonic life, it may then receive its blood supply from the branches of the thymic arteries. *C*, carotid artery; *SC*, subclavian artery; *I*, innominate artery; *IT*, inferior thyroid artery.

that they were sometimes carried partially into the substance of the thyroid by the thyroid vessels but that they were never completely covered by thyroid tissue. In two other dissections, however, he did find a parathyroid completely covered by the thyroid, and in both instances these were the inferior parathyroid glands. Other writers have described normal parathyroids lying within the thyroid. Not only have we seen instances in which the normal gland has been entirely within the thyroid, but we have seen a parathyroid adenoma or a hyperplastic parathyroid gland which lay completely within the thyroid. This has been reported by others.

The upper parathyroids have been shown to be slightly larger than the lower in some studies. The average weight of a normal parathyroid gland is about 30 mg, but some authors think that normal glands may be heavier if they contain a great deal of fat. The total weight of four normal parathyroids is about 120 to 140 mg.

The usual positions for the superior and inferior thyroid arteries, the recurrent laryngeal nerve, and the parathyroids are shown in Figs. 38-51 and 38-52. The superior gland is usually supplied by the superior thyroid artery, while the inferior gland is almost always supplied by the inferior thyroid artery, though in rare instances it may be supplied by the superior thyroid artery. The inferior gland which descends into the mediastinum because of the development of an adenoma is always supplied by the inferior thyroid artery, while an adenoma which develops in a gland that has come to be located in the mediastinum embryologically may be supplied by branches from the internal mammary or thymic vessels, or rarely from the aorta.

Physiology

CALCIUM METABOLISM. The body contains somewhat over 1,000 Gm of calcium, of which 1 Gm is in the extracellular fluid, 4 Gm is exchangeable in bone, 1,000 Gm is stable in bone, and 11 Gm is in cells. The average daily dietary intake is 0.5 to 1 Gm. Urinary calcium excretion varies with the dietary calcium intake and may be as high as 300 to 400 mg/day on an unrestricted diet. Usually, however, it is about 100 to 200 mg/day. On a low-calcium diet containing 200 mg calcium, less than 175 mg calcium should be excreted in the urine. Small amounts of calcium, up to 100 mg/day, are also excreted in sweat; the remainder is excreted in the feces. About 600 mg of calcium is secreted into the intestines from various glands and most of it is resorbed. Calcium absorption takes place principally in the duodenum and upper jejunum. It is an active process involving vitamin D metabolites.

In plasma about 47 percent of the calcium is ionized, 47 percent is protein-bound, and the remainder is complexed to organic anions such as citrate and phosphates.

The ionized calcium is the important one physiologically. It is well known that calcium ion plays a critical role in determining the excitability of nerve function and in the contractility of skeletal and cardiac muscle. More

Fig. 38-17. Most frequent locations for the normal parathyroid (anterior view). The locations for the upper parathyroid are shown at the left and for the lower at the right. The relative frequency with which the glands are found in the various locations is indicated on the diagram. (*From J. R. Gilmour, J Pathol, 45:507, 1937.*)

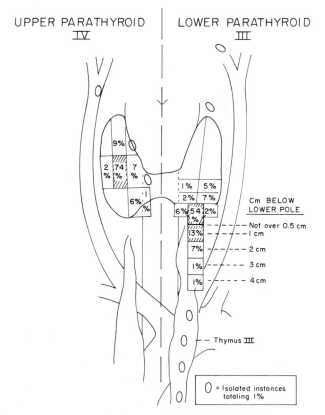

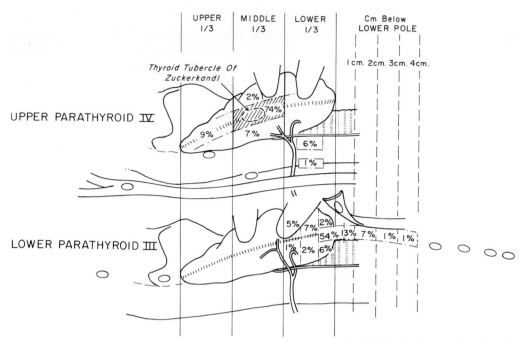

Fig. 38-18. Most frequent locations for normal parathyroid glands (lateral view). (*From J. R. Gilmour, J Pathol, 45:507, 1937.*)

recently it has been demonstrated that calcium ion is important in the structure and function of cell membranes and organelles, and in numerous cellular metabolic events including hormone release. In fact, it is postulated by Rasmussen that there is a close relation between calcium ion and the actions of cyclic adenosine monophosphate (cAMP). Ideally we would like to measure the ionized calcium concentration in serum. Since this is difficult to determine, we utilize the total serum calcium concentration, instead. Total serum calcium concentrations correlate

Fig. 38-19. The relationship of total calcium, ionized calcium, and protein-bound calcium in the serum. *A.* Normal serum. *B* and *D.* An elevated total calcium, due to an increase of ionized calcium, as found in cases of primary hyperparathyroidism. *C.* An elevated total calcium concentration due to an increase of serum proteins and hence of protein-bound calcium. This may be incorrectly interpreted as compatible with primary hyperparathyroidism if serum proteins are not determined.

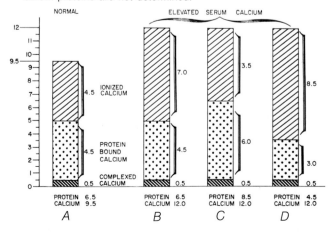

very well clinically as long as the serum protein concentrations are normal. However, in abnormal states, the total calcium must be considered in relation to plasma protein levels, especially albumin. Though there is not an invariable relationship between the amount of protein-bound calcium and total protein levels, in general for each gram of alteration of total protein above or below 6.5 Gm/100 ml there is an 0.8- to 1-mg/100 ml increase or decrease in protein-bound calcium and hence in total serum calcium as well (Fig. 38-19). Normal total serum calcium concentration ranges from 9 to 10.5 mg/100 ml in many laboratories, but this varies with the technique used.

The calcium in the extracellular pool exchanges forty to fifty times a day with that in the intracellular fluid, the glomerular filtrate, and the exchangeable bone (Fig. 38-20). The kidneys normally resorb 99 percent of the filtered calcium. Even with marked hypercalcemia the urinary calcium excretion rarely exceeds 500 mg/day. With rapid bone destruction from metastatic tumor or increased secretion of PTH the kidney is unable to excrete enough calcium to keep up with the rising serum levels, particularly if some renal damage is present, and a state of serious or fatal hypercalcemic crisis may ensue.

PHOSPHORUS METABOLISM. The body contains about 500 Gm of phosphate, the extracellular fluid 0.4 Gm, the bone 425 Gm, and the cells about 75 Gm. The diet contains about 1,000 mg/day.

In plasma about 15 percent is protein-bound, and a considerable amount exists as complexes with monovalent and divalent cations. In contrast to calcium, the serum phosphate value changes markedly with diet, age (it is higher in children), and hormone secretion (other than

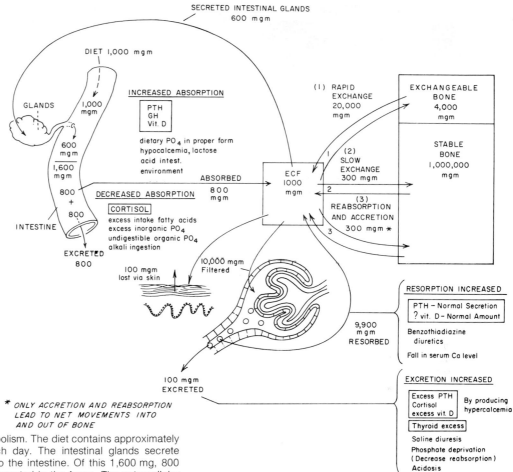

Fig. 38-20. Calcium metabolism. The diet contains approximately 1,000 mg of calcium each day. The intestinal glands secrete approximately 600 mg into the intestine. Of this 1,600 mg, 800 is absorbed, and 800 is excreted in the feces. The extracellular fluid contains about 1,000 mg of calcium. This is constantly being exchanged with calcium in other pools. Each day 10,000 mg are filtered through the glomerulus, and 9,900 mg of this are resorbed. There is a slow exchange from stable bone and a rapid exchange from exchangeable bone. Calcium is constantly being resorbed and added to bone, and this activity is under hormonal control.

PTH). The serum value varies between 3 and 4.5 mg/100 ml in adults and between 5 and 6 mg/100 ml in children.

About 70 percent of the dietary phosphate is absorbed from the intestine, the absorption primarily taking place in the midintestine. Absorption is increased by PTH, growth hormone (GH), vitamin D, and a low-calcium diet. It is decreased by a high calcium intake, beryllium poisoning, aluminum hydroxide ingestion, and factors which diminish calcium absorption.

Almost all of the absorbed phosphate is excreted in the urine. With a 1,000-mg diet 700 mg will be absorbed and 670 mg excreted in the urine. Urinary excretion is increased in hyperparathyroidism, vitamin D excess, vitamin D deficiency with secondary hyperparathyroidism, osteoporosis, bone metastases, sarcoidosis, acidosis, and various renal tubular disorders. It is decreased by GH, hypoparathyroidism, Addison's disease, chronic renal failure, lacta-

tion, dietary phosphate deficiency, osteopetrosis, and osteoblastic tumors of bone.

MAGNESIUM METABOLISM. The body contains about 200 mEq of magnesium. Half of this is in the skeleton, and most of the rest is intracellular, only 1 percent being in the extracellular fluid. The normal serum magnesium level is 1.6 to 2.5 mg/100 ml in our laboratory.

The daily dietary intake is about 25 mEq. About 8 to 10 mEq is absorbed and excreted in the urine. Absorption is increased by vitamin D and decreased by calcium. The renal excretion of magnesium closely follows that of calcium, and PTH increases the resorption of both.

The various factors regulating magnesium metabolism are not well known, but PTH certainly plays a role. Hypomagnesemia occurs in hyperparathyroidism, alcoholism, malnutrition, and chronic intravenous hyperalimentation if magnesium is not added to the feeding regimen. A low plasma magnesium level stimulates the secretion of PTH and an elevated level inhibits it, as with calcium. Plasma magnesium is also decreased in hyperthyroidism and increased in hypothyroidism.

While hypomagnesemia is present in many patients with hyperparathyroidism, the plasma levels may be normal if the dietary intake is good and intestinal absorption is not

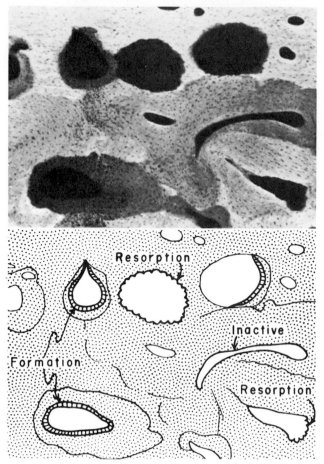

Fig. 38-21. Microradiograph of a cross section of a normal human cortical bone, showing regions of resorption, formation, and inactivity. (*Taken from J. Jowsey, Am J Med, 40:485, 1966.*)

interfered with by anorexia or vomiting. After resection of the parathyroid adenoma temporary hypomagnesemia frequently occurs even when the plasma level has been normal preoperatively. The serum magnesium level rises to normal values in a few days because of the marked increase in tubular resorption of this ion after parathyroidectomy. The variation in the magnesium balance probably relates to (1) variations in dietary intake, to which magnesium levels are very sensitive, (2) the degree of bone disease present—significant bone disease increasing the likelihood that postoperative hypomagnesemia will occur, and (3) the marked increase in renal magnesium resorption which occurs after removal of the adenoma. Some cases of tetany are caused by hypomagnesemia and cannot be corrected until serum magnesium levels are returned to normal.

HYDROXYPROLINE. Bone matrix is made up largely of collagen, which is the only major source of hydroxyproline in the body. When collagen is destroyed, most of it is hydrolyzed to amino acids or further degraded and then reused. However, about 5 to 8 percent of it is only partially degraded to hydroxyproline-containing peptides which are excreted in the urine. The urinary hydroxyproline content

thus serves as an index of the degree of bone resorption taking place. Hydroxyproline is not a perfect indicator of bone resorption, however, because not all collagen is in bone and various rate-limited factors affect hydroxyproline metabolism before it is excreted.

PTH increases degradation of collagen and increases urinary hydroxyproline excretion. Calcitonin decreases bone resorption in patients with Paget's disease of bone. A decrease in urinary hydroxyproline accompanies this response.

BONE. Bone is made up of a matrix (osteoid) which is nearly all collagen, and inorganic crystals of hydroxyapatite $[Ca_{10}(Po_4)_6(OH)_2]$. The matrix makes up 30 percent and the mineral 70 percent of the dry weight.

The metaphysis of the bone is the most active part metabolically and the first to respond to PTH excess.

The collagen matrix of the bone is covered by a layer of bone cells, some of which are engaged in osteoblastic activity, laying down new bone, and some in osteoclastic activity, resorbing bone. Osteocytes, which are located within the substance of compact cortical bone, have been demonstrated by Belanger also to be important in bone resorption. This process, called *osteocytic osteolysis*, may be the principal mechanism for rapid mobilization of calcium from bone particularly in response to the initial action of PTH. The osteoclast may be more important in bone remodeling and also in the chronic stimulation of bone resorption in hyperparathyroidism. Some measure of the metabolic activity of the bone has been gained by a study of the number and appearance of these cells. Recently, however, new techniques have permitted a quantitation of bone activity by a study of the bone tissue itself, in a calcified state, rather than of the cells which make or destroy it.

Microradiography has been used by Jowsey and others to avoid some of the difficulties inherent in other methods. This technique is used to study the distribution of minerals in bone. A section of bone is ground down, and an x-ray is made of the section with a low-energy beam and fine-grain film. The x-ray film (rather than the section) is then examined under the microscope, as shown in Figs. 38-21 and 38-33. Areas of active resorption and formation can be delineated and measured, to quantitate bone turnover. The percent of the total area of the section undergoing resorption and that undergoing bone formation are calculated.

Additional information concerning bone formation may be obtained by tetracycline labeling. When tetracycline is administered, it is incorporated in osteoid at the site of new mineral deposition. The tetracycline is located by its characteristic fluorescent emission. A rate of bone formation may be obtained by giving two doses of tetracycline at intervals of several weeks. Two discrete lines of deposition may be determined in subsequent biopsy specimens, and a measurement of the area between the lines gives a measure of growth rate.

The rates of bone formation and resorption are normally equal and low, and do not change significantly between the ages of twenty and forty. In young growing people the rates of formation and resorption are high, while in older people the rate of resorption increases, and the rate of formation remains the same as in the young adult, with a resultant net loss of bone.

Jowsey has compared bone taken in disease states to normal individuals of the same age and charted the results on the basis of the number of standard deviations from the normal for that age. In hyperparathyroidism (Fig. 38-22) the amount of resorption was increased to over 2 standard deviations above normal in all but one case—presumably because of the stimulation of the osteoclasts by PTH. This was true even when the bones appeared perfectly normal on standard skeletal x-rays. In three cases bone formation was also increased, which may account for the absence of gross bone changes. In hypoparathyroidism both formation and resorption are reduced.

In osteoporosis there is loss of bone mass. Osteoporosis may be primary (idiopathic) or secondary to hyperparathyroidism, hyperthyroidism, Cushing's syndrome, or many other causes. In primary osteoporosis there is an increase in bone resorption, while bone formation remains normal. In Cushing's syndrome there is a marked increase in bone resorption accompanied by a decrease in bone formation.

Bed rest reduces bone formation, while resorption is increased more in the osteoporotic patient than in the normal. In Paget's disease both resorption and formation are high, the first somewhat more than the second, while in hyperthyroidism there is also increased resorption and formation, but to a lesser degree. In osteomalacia and rickets little or no bone formation occurs.

PARATHYROID HORMONE, VITAMIN D, CALCITONIN.
Parathyroid Hormone. In recent years, PTH has been purified from bovine and porcine parathyroid glands. The amino acid sequence of both molecules has been determined; the bovine molecule is shown diagrammatically in Fig. 38-23. Both molecules have a molecular weight of about 9,500 and contain 84 amino acid residues. Synthesis of a biologically active fragment of the bovine molecule containing the 1 to 34 residues from the amino terminal has now been achieved. Purification of human glandular PTH has been hampered by the relatively small amount of human parathyroid tissue available for study. Recently, Brewer et al. purified human PTH from parathyroid adenomas and have determined the sequence of the 34 amino acids at the amino terminal of the molecule; this fragment has been shown to be biologically active. A comparison of the structure of these human and animal N-terminal fragments of PTH is shown in Fig. 38-24.

Within the parathyroid glands, larger precursor molecules of parathyroid hormone have now been identified. These are called *pro PTH* and *pre-pro PTH* (Fig. 38-25). It seems unlikely, at this time, that these larger molecules circulate in peripheral blood.

Vitamin D. Largely due to the work of DeLuca and associates many significant advances in vitamin D metabolism recently have been made. The natural form of vitamin D is called vitamin D_3, or cholecalciferol (Fig. 38-26). It is produced by the irradiation of 7-dihydrocholesterol in the skin. To be metabolically active D_3 is first hydroxylated in the liver to 25-hydroxyvitamin D_3 (25-OH D_3). The 25-OH D_3 is further hydroxylated in the kidney to 1,25-dihydroxy-

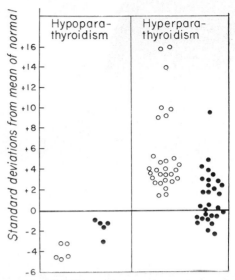

Fig. 38-22. Bone turnover in hypoparathyroidism and hyperparathyroidism. Open circles indicate resorption; solid circles indicate formation. (*From J. Jowsey, Am J Med, 40:485, 1966.*)

vitamin D_3 [1,25-$(OH)_2D_3$]. This latter metabolite is believed to be the metabolically active form of vitamin D which carries out the well-known functions of this substance—namely, mobilizing calcium and phosphorus from bone and enhancing intestinal absorption of calcium and phosphorus. Nephrectomized animals and human beings, for example, are insensitive to administration of both vita-

Fig. 38-23. Amino acid sequence of bovine parathyroid hormone. (*From J. T. Potts, Jr., et al., Am J Med, 50:639, 1971.*)

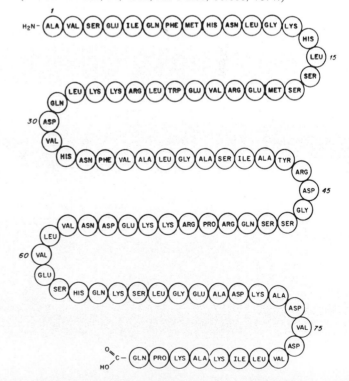

HUMAN PARATHYROID HORMONE

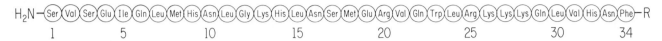

H₂N—(Ser)(Val)(Ser)(Glu)(Ile)(Gln)(Leu)(Met)(His)(Asn)(Leu)(Gly)(Lys)(His)(Leu)(Asn)(Ser)(Met)(Glu)(Arg)(Val)(Gln)(Trp)(Leu)(Arg)(Lys)(Lys)(Lys)(Gln)(Leu)(Val)(His)(Asn)(Phe)—R

1   5   10   15   20   25   30   34

BOVINE PARATHYROID HORMONE

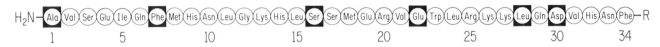

H₂N—[Ala](Val)(Ser)(Glu)(Ile)(Gln)[Phe](Met)(His)(Asn)(Leu)(Gly)(Lys)(His)(Leu)[Ser](Ser)(Met)(Glu)(Arg)(Val)[Glu](Trp)(Leu)(Arg)(Lys)(Lys)[Leu](Gln)[Asp](Val)(His)(Asn)(Phe)—R

1   5   10   15   20   25   30   34

PORCINE PARATHYROID HORMONE

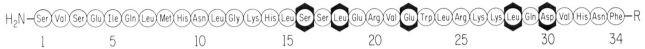

H₂N—(Ser)(Val)(Ser)(Glu)(Ile)(Gln)(Leu)(Met)(His)(Asn)(Leu)(Gly)(Lys)(His)(Leu)⟨Ser⟩(Ser)⟨Leu⟩(Glu)(Arg)(Val)⟨Glu⟩(Trp)(Leu)(Arg)(Lys)(Lys)⟨Leu⟩(Gln)⟨Asp⟩(Val)(His)(Asn)(Phe)—R

1   5   10   15   20   25   30   34

Fig. 38-24. Comparison of the amino acid sequence of the amino terminal 34 residues of human, bovine, and porcine PTH. (*From H. B. Brewer, Jr., et al., Proc Natl Acad Sci USA, 69:3585, 1972.*)

min D_3 and 25-OH D_3, since they cannot convert this to the active $1,25\text{-}(OH)_2D_3$ form.

It is now suggested that vitamin D acts as a physiologic hormone which has feedback control mechanisms in animals and human beings. In the presence of parathyroid hormone, when serum calcium or serum phosphorus levels are low, there is an increased synthesis of $1,25\text{-}(OH)_2D_3$, which then makes calcium and phosphorus available from the bone and intestines. Thus the serum calcium concentration returns toward normal. When the serum calcium concentrations are normal, less $1,25\text{-}(OH)_2D_3$ and more $24,25\text{-}(OH)_2D_3$ are produced. This latter metabolite is relatively inactive, and therefore less calcium and phosphorus are mobilized.

These findings not only are of interest physiologically but may be important clinically in the treatment of renal osteodystrophy and hypoparathyroidism. In both these conditions, microgram quantities of $1,25\text{-}(OH)_2D_3$ or its analogue, 1 α-hydroxy vitamin D_3, have proved effective. When they become available, they may well be the treatment of choice for these and other conditions, such as malabsorption states.

Recently, methods for measurement of serum 25-OH D_3 and $1,25\text{-}(OH)_2D_3$ in human beings have become available. These should lead to a better understanding of normal and abnormal states of vitamin D metabolism.

Calcitonin (Thyrocalcitonin). Calcitonin, a calcium-lowering polypeptide, was originally described by Copp (1962) and Hirsh and Munson (1963). It was originally shown to be present in the epifollicular or parafollicular cells of the mammalian thyroid gland. These cells are now commonly referred to as *C cells.* It has now been demonstrated that C cells come from the neural crest and are part of the APUD system of peptide- or amine-secreting cells described by Pearse. They migrate to the ultimobranchial bodies, glandular structures derived from the lowest branchial pouches embryologically. In man and other mammals these structures are vestigial; they fuse with and are incorporated into the lateral thyroid lobes during embryologic development. In lower animals C cells are found within the ultimobranchial bodies which remain as separate structures. Medullary carcinomas of the thyroid gland are C cell, calcitonin-producing tumors.

Calcitonin has been purified from the thyroid glands of pigs, sheep, and cows, from medullary carcinomas in man

Fig. 38-25. Partial amino acid sequence of bovine pre-proparathyroid hormone (Pre-proPTH). In the parathyroid glands, preproPTH, a molecule containing 115 amino acids, is converted to proPTH, a 90–amino acid molecule. Then six additional molecules are cleaved, leaving the 84 amino acids of PTH. PTH = amino acids 1 to 84. ProPTH = 6 amino acids added to the NH₂ terminus of PTH: −6 to 84. Pre-proPTH = 25 amino acids added to the NH₂ terminus of proPTH: −31 to 84. (*From B. Kemper et al., Biochemistry, 15:15, 1975.*)

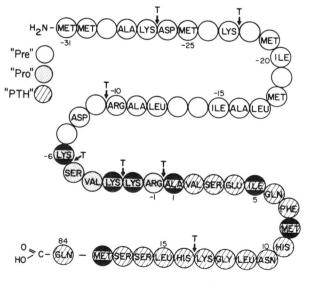

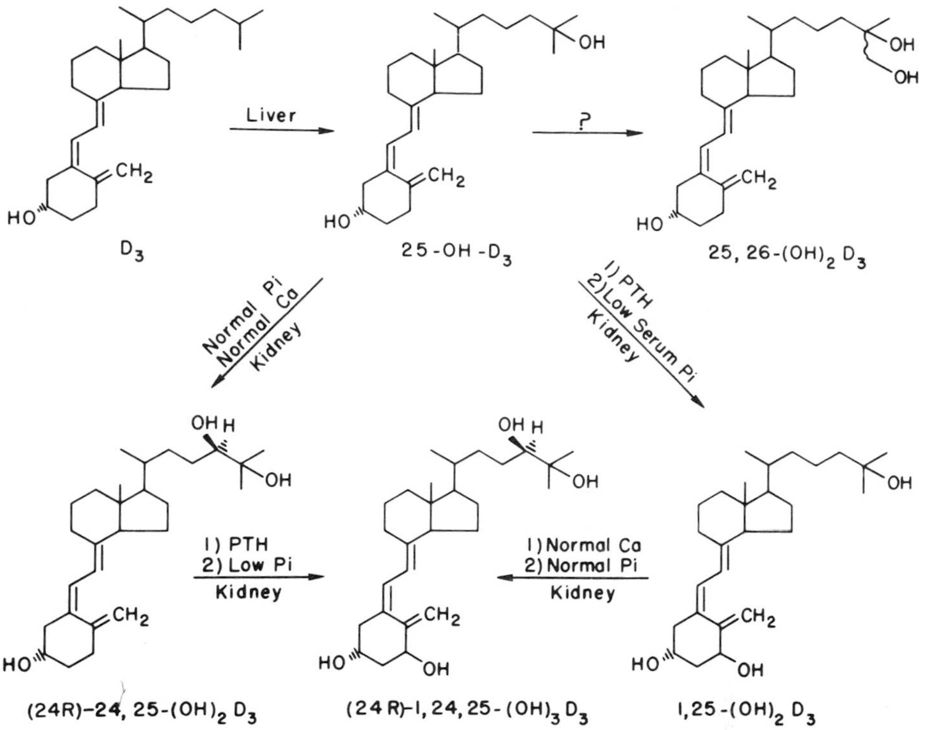

Fig. 38-26. Summary of vitamin D metabolism. (*From H. F. DeLuca, Ann Intern Med, 85:367, 1976.*)

(called *calcitonin M*), and from salmon ultimobranchial glands. Each of these has a molecular weight of 3,500 and 32 amino acids, and they have the same molecular configuration. However, as shown in Fig. 38-27, wide variations of amino acid sequences occur within these molecules. Radioimmunoassay systems for measurement of the different calcitonins have added greatly to our knowledge of the physiology of calcitonin and are important in the diagnosis of occult medullary carcinoma of the thyroid in man.

Calcitonin lowers the serum calcium concentration by inhibiting bone resorption. In pharmacologic doses, salmon calcitonin has been successfully utilized in the treatment of Paget's disease of bone.

Serum Calcium Homeostasis

Serum calcium concentration in man has long been recognized to vary only minimally from day to day (Fig. 38-28). Its regulation is primarily by the parathyroid glands through a negative feedback system. A fall in serum calcium (or serum magnesium) concentration stimulates secretion of PTH which then acts peripherally to raise the serum calcium concentration to normal. Hypocalcemia also results in increased formation of $1,25\text{-}(OH)_2D_3$.

An elevation of the serum calcium level reduces both PTH secretion and also the formation of $1,25\text{-}(OH)_2D_3$. Both effects tend to lower serum calcium concentration. Calcitonin may also be important in the control of hypercalcemia, especially in animals. In mammals other than man in whom it can be measured, secretion of calcitonin is

directly related to the serum calcium concentration. Hypercalcemia results in increased calcitonin release from the thyroid gland. Calcitonin lowers both the serum calcium and serum phosphorus concentrations primarily by an inhibition of bone resorption. Thus it seems to play an important protective role against hypercalcemia in these animals. Arnaud et al. hypothesize that in mammals calcitonin acts as a potent rapid-acting factor suppressing oscillations in the serum calcium *above* physiologic levels and that PTH acts as the major controlling factor of serum calcium *below* physiologic levels. In normal man, however, there is little or no evidence that calcitonin functions as a physiologic hormone responsible for regulation of serum calcium homeostasis.

The infusion of PTH into experimental animals or man results in hypercalcemia, hypophosphatemia, and phosphaturia. These effects are the result of three mechanisms:

1. Direct action on bone leading to increased bone resorption
2. Increased calcium absorption from the intestine
3. Decreased tubular resorption of phosphate (TRP) and increased tubular resorption of calcium by the kidney

In addition, PTH effects on the kidney lead to increased excretion of potassium, bicarbonate, amino acids, and, under some circumstances, sodium, while decreasing the excretion of magnesium, ammonia, and titratable acid. Vitamin D and its metabolites are not necessary for the renal tubular effects of PTH. However, vitamin D is necessary for the action of PTH on bone. Vitamin D also appears to have a direct action on bone resorption as well. Finally a major action of vitamin D is intestinal absorption of calcium. Recent studies suggest that $1,25\text{-}(OH)_2D_3$ plays

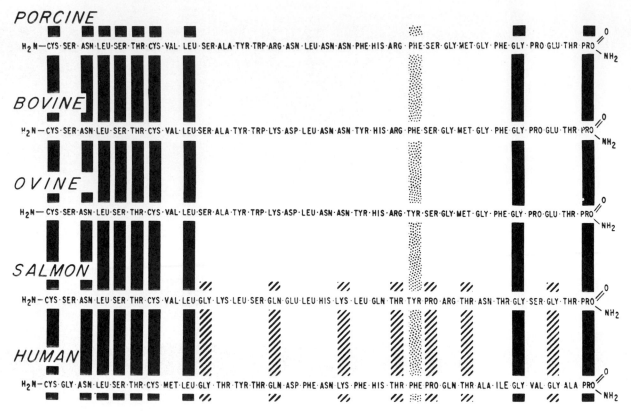

Fig. 38-27. Comparison of amino acid sequences of porcine, bovine, ovine, salmon, and human calcitonin. Solid bars indicate sequence positions homologous among all five molecules; cross-hatched bars indicate salmon and human calcitonin. [*From J. T. Potts, Jr., et al., in R. V. Talmage and P. L. Munson (eds.), "Calcium Parathyroid Hormone and the Calcitonins," Proceedings of Fourth Parathyroid Conference, Excerpta Medica, Amsterdam, 1972.*]

the most important direct role in intestinal absorption of calcium; PTH may act by regulating the formation of this metabolite.

The action of PTH on kidney and bone has been demonstrated to be mediated through the adenyl cyclase system. PTH stimulates adenyl cyclase activity and raises cyclic 3′, 5′-AMP levels in bone and kidney. Urinary excretion of cyclic AMP is a potentially useful test of parathyroid function.

Primary Hyperparathyroidism

PATHOLOGY. Parathyroid. Primary hyperparathyroidism may be due to a parathyroid adenoma, hyperplasia of the parathyroid glands, carcinoma, or a nonparathyroid tumor which is producing a parathyroidlike substance. The symptoms are similar whatever the actual cause of the primary hyperparathyroidism. It is also possible for a patient with secondary hyperparathyroidism due to renal, bone, or metabolic disease to develop hypercalcemia without any therapy. This condition is referred to as *tertiary hyperparathyroidism*.

The relative frequency of entities producing primary hyperparathyroidism is shown in Table 38-2. Several points are important to note. Primary chief cell hyperplasia was described by Cope in 1958. Hence studies which include data prior to 1958 can be misleading. Cope, for example, who reviewed his data of 343 cases at the Massachusetts General Hospital in 1966, carefully pointed out that in his

last 100 cases 25 percent had hyperplasia. This apparent trend toward increased primary chief cell hyperplasia is thought by some to be due in part to the fact that primary hyperparathyroidism is diagnosed and operated upon at a much earlier stage today. Several other trends are also evident. Water-clear hyperplasia is rarely diagnosed any longer. Multiple adenomas are less frequently diagnosed at the present time. More often these are thought to be part of chief cell hyperplasia. Finally, the incidence of carcinoma of the parathyroid glands is misleading when one is looking only at the larger referral series. As described below, carcinoma of the parathyroid makes up 1 percent or less of all cases of primary hyperparathyroidism.

It is apparent that the frequency of adenoma versus hyperplasia varies greatly in these series. Goldman, for example, reported that single glands were diseased in 92 percent of his patients, while Paloyan and coworkers found that almost two-thirds of all patients had more than one gland involved.

These discrepancies undoubtedly are due to several factors—the operative approach, the pathologic interpretation of the glands, and the incidence of patients with familial hyperparathyroidism or multiple endocrine adenomatosis in each series.

Paloyan performs a subtotal parathyroidectomy so that each gland can be examined. Others remove only any enlarged gland which is encountered. When a single enlarged gland is sent to a pathologist it is most likely to be called an adenoma. However, there is no uniform agreement among pathologists at this time as to what constitutes an adenoma and what represents chief cell hyperplasia. The condition described by the classical definition of an adenoma—an enlarged gland with a rim of normal tissue—is found in cases of hyperplasia as well. Roth and other pathologists state that they can not tell the difference between hyperplasia and adenoma from looking at only one gland. The greatest differences of opinion relate to what constitutes *mild* hyperplasia. Some pathologists feel that normal-sized or mildly enlarged glands are hyperplastic if they do not contain enough fat. Others do not feel that these glands are abnormal. Knowledge of the normal development of parathyroid glands is imperative.

From birth through three months of age, mean weight of the four parathyroid glands is 5 to 9 mg. There is then an almost linear increase in mean total parathyroid gland weight until the third to fourth decades, when it levels off at a mean of 117.6 mg for males and 131.3 mg for females. These changes in weight are accompanied by changes in histology of the gland. In children the gland is composed of fairly uniform sheets and cords of chief cells. The stroma has little or no mature fat cells, and oxyphil cells are absent. At puberty some mature fat cells appear. These increase in number through the remainder of life, and in older persons they may occupy 60 to 70 percent of the gland volume. Obese individuals have larger numbers of fat cells than one would expect for their age. Oxyphil cells also appear at puberty and show an increase with age. Chief cells and water-clear cells are thought to actively secrete PTH. Oxyphil cells are thought of as inactive but have been shown to be rich in mitochondria.

Thus to evaluate whether or not a parathyroid gland is normal, one must evaluate its size and weight, the number of chief cells, and the amount of fat which it contains in relation to the age of the individual.

The major problem for both the surgeon and the pathologist is to differentiate an adenoma caused by chief cell hyperplasia or single gland disease from multiglandular disease of the parathyroids. Perhaps the ultimate proof that a lesion is an adenoma is the lack of recurrence of hyperparathyroidism after its removal.

Adenomas. The sine qua non for the diagnosis of a parathyroid adenoma has been the presence of an enlarged parathyroid gland with a rim or fragment of normal parathyroid which is being compressed by the adenoma. This is shown in Fig. 38-29. Another previously demanded criterion was the presence of a normal or atrophic parathyroid elsewhere. However, since we now know that parathyroid adenomas and hyperplasias can coexist and that hyperplasia occasionally appears to spare one gland, this criterion no longer seems to be absolute. Furthermore, as Black has shown, chief cell hyperplasia may give the appearance of compression of normal gland beneath the capsule. Thus an

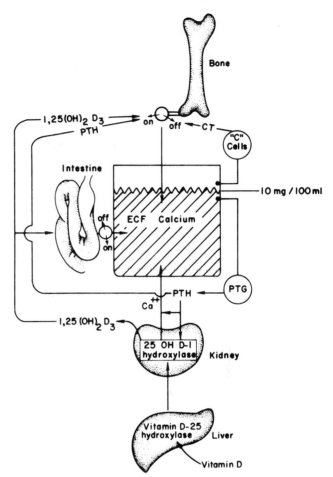

Fig. 38-28. Mechanism of calcium homeostasis. *Hypocalcemia* results in increased parathyroid hormone (PTH) secretion from the parathyroid glands (PTG). PTH acts directly on bone and on the kidney. PTH also results in an increase in the formation of 1,25-$(OH)_2D_3$ by the kidney, which acts on bone and promotes intestinal absorption of calcium as well. Each of these effects tends to raise the serum calcium concentration toward normal. *Hypercalcemia* results in a decrease in PTH secretion, a lesser production of 1,25-$(OH)_2D_3$, and an increase in calcitonin (CT) secretion. Calcitonin inhibits bone resorption and is important in animals other than human beings. These changes tend to decrease serum calcium levels to normal. (*From H. F. DeLuca, Ann Intern Med, 85:367, 1976.*)

adenoma should be diagnosed only when one or, rarely, two glands are enlarged, the others being normal in size and on histologic section. Any gland larger than 40 to 60 mg should be suspected of being abnormal.

Grossly adenomas are usually reddish brown, though they may be yellow-brown, particularly in older people. At times they may be very difficult to distinguish grossly from thyroid tissue, particularly when imbedded in the thyroid. They are usually soft and smooth, and the surface is very vascular, bleeding easily when rubbed. They are generally not adherent to the surrounding structures. On occasion they contain cysts, hemorrhage, or areas of calcification. Areas of necrosis are sometimes seen. The location of the tumors is given later under Operative Technique.

Table 38-2. RELATIVE FREQUENCY (PERCENT) OF ENTITIES PRODUCING HYPERPARATHYROIDISM

Author	Date	Institution	Adenomas		Hyperplasia		Carcinoma	Unknown	Total cases
			1 adenoma	*2 or more adenomas*	*Chief cell**	*Water-clear*			
Norris	1947	Collected	94	6	...	...	...	...	322
Cope et al	1958	Massachusetts General Hosp.	76	5	4	7	4	4	206
Black, B. M.	1961	Mayo Clinic	92	2.5	...	5	0.5	...	385
Cope	1966	Massachusetts General Hosp.	77	4	11	4	4	...	343
Straus and Paloyan	1969	University of Chicago	46	7	10	9	4	...	58
Haff et al	1970	Washington Univ., St. Louis	41	Mixed adenoma and hyperplasia—24	49	...	...	11	47
Goldman et al	1971	Univ. of Calif., San Francisco	92	4	3	...	<1	...	300
Paloyan et al	1973	University of Chicago	33	Multiglandular disease—65‡	...		2	...	84
Wang et al	1975	Massachusetts General Hosp.	81	2	12	2	3	...	525

*Since chief cell hyperplasia was described by Cope in 1958, there are no reports of this entity before that date.
†Of his last 100 cases, 25% had chief cell hyperplasia.
‡More than one gland involved with disease.

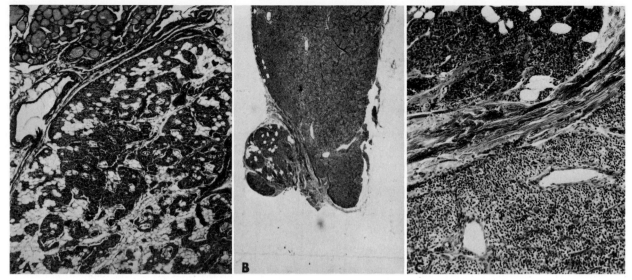

Fig. 38-29. Normal parathyroid compared with a chief cell adenoma. *A*. Photomicrograph of a normal parathyroid, below, adjacent to the thyroid gland, shown above. Note the abundant fat present in the normal gland. (×75.) *B*. Photomicrograph of a chief cell adenoma compressing the normal parathyroid beneath the capsule. The adenoma is the large mass shown to the right. The open spaces are blood vessels. The normal gland is the small rounded object shown to the left. The open spaces are fat cells. (×35.) *C*. Photomicrograph of a parathyroid adenoma shown below with the capsule separating it from the rim of normal parathyroid shown above. Note the fat in the normal parathyroid and the absence of fat cells in the adenoma. (×150.)

Microscopically chief cell adenomas are composed of closely packed small cells which resemble the cells of the normal parathyroid except that they are more tightly packed and there is little or no fat seen. The chief cells are of two types: the light cells, which are rich in glycogen and are thought to be inactive, and the dark cells, which are poor in glycogen and rich in secretory granules with a prominent Golgi apparatus and endoplasmic reticulum. The dark cells are thought to be the main source of PTH. A glandular pattern is sometimes seen with small uniform acini whose lumina are empty or filled with acidophilic colloid. These adenomas sometimes resemble fetal adenomas of the thyroid gland.

The water-clear, or *wasserhellen,* adenomas have large vacuolated cells with clear cytoplasm arranged in a uniform pattern. In the rare oxyphil adenomas the cells have a pink cytoplasm. Undoubtedly oxyphil cells can also secrete PTH, since adenomas of oxyphil cells, while rare, can also cause hyperparathyroidism.

The chief importance for the histologic differentiation into adenoma or hyperplasia has to do with what operation is performed. If one adopts the policy of exploring all four parathyroids in each case, the microscopic differentiation between adenoma and hyperplasia in a single gland becomes far less important.

Carcinoma. Carcinoma of the parathyroid is rare. Many cases which have originally been thought to represent carcinoma have been discarded on review, since benign adenomas can sometimes have cells with bizarre nuclear patterns. Black reviewed the literature to the end of 1953 and found only 20 cases which he thought were acceptable, using the diagnostic criteria of hyperfunction with local tissue invasion or metastases. Rapaport et al. in 1960 collected 8 more cases to make a total of 28 and found records of only 8 with visceral metastases. Holmes et al. found 46 cases of hyperfunctioning parathyroid cancer and 4 cases of apparent nonfunctioning cancer when they reviewed the literature in 1969. In these 50 patients, 85 percent presented with hypercalcemia. Bone disease was present in 73 percent, a palpable neck mass in 52 percent, and renal disease in 32 percent. Thus, hypercalcemia and a palpable neck mass should alert one to the possibility of parathyroid carcinoma. Cervical metastases were found in 32 percent and distant metastases (liver, lung, bone, pancreas, and adrenal) in 21 percent. Cervical recurrences following surgery occurred in 65 percent of patients. Typically hypercalcemia recurred several months after surgery in many instances and was the first sign of recurrent tumor.

It is apparent that a diagnosis of malignant disease cannot be made by the histologic features of the tumor, a situation which also obtains in pheochromocytoma. Very wild-looking tumors may pursue a completely benign course. The reverse is also true, as exemplified by a case reported by Rapaport et al. in which histology of the original tumor appeared to be that of an adenoma but in which the tumor recurred 22 months after operation, with pulmonary metastases confirmed at autopsy. Capsular infiltration is a particularly inadequate sign of malignancy, since this is often seen in benign adenomas and even the neoplastic cells can occur within blood vessels in benign tumors. The only completely acceptable criteria for malignancy are recurrence of the tumor following removal, distant metastases, or invasion of adjacent structures. Some carcinomas can be identified grossly because they are attached to adjacent tissues by a thick fibrous capsule which gives the gland a whitish hue. Fifty percent of reported cases were adherent to or invading into adjacent structures at the time of surgery.

Though some individuals die because of tumor growth and spread, more commonly morbidity and mortality are related to the complications related to the persistent and progressive hypercalcemia, which is very difficult to control chronically. Schantz and Castleman collected 70 cases of proved parathyroid carcinoma in their review in 1973.

Hyperplasia. Although it is stated in most older texts that the most common type of hyperplasia is the water-clear cell type, this no longer is true. Almost all incidences of hyperplasia in our experience have been of the chief cell type. Primary chief cell hyperplasia cannot be differentiated by light microscopy from the chief cell hyperplasia which is always present in secondary hyperparathyroidism, although there are ultrastructural differences. It seems likely that a number of instances previously thought to be multiple adenomas because of their predominant chief cell structure were in fact instances of chief cell hyperplasia.

Grossly the glands with *water-clear cell hyperplasia* show diffuse enlargement and are usually unequal in size. The color is a striking chocolate brown, and the parathyroids are often very large. They tend to be lobulated and irregular in shape, with pseudopods extending from the surface, in contrast to the generally smooth contour of adenomas or glands with chief cell hyperplasia.

Histologically they are composed of large clear cells arranged in a relatively uniform alveolar or acinary pattern.

The glands may be very large in water-clear hyperplasia, the total weight of all four glands ranging up to as much as 70 Gm. Their huge size plus the striking color and characteristic appearance makes them very easy to recognize.

Primary Chief Cell Hyperplasia. This condition was first described by Cope et al. in 1958. The incidence of this disease entity is becoming more common as it is being recognized that many cases thought to be multiple parathyroid adenomas are in reality chief cell hyperplasia. This disease entity is almost invariably encountered when surgical treatment of the parathyroid glands is carried out in patients with familial hyperparathyroidism and in patients with multiple endocrinopathies.

It may sometimes be extremely difficult to differentiate chief cell hyperplasia from the typical parathyroid adenoma if only one gland is examined (Fig. 38-30). Roth and other pathologists believe that grossly and histologically a single hyperplastic gland is *indistinguishable* from an adenomatous gland. Classically, one expects each of the glands to be enlarged; however, it is known that the size of glands may be very asymmetrical, and one or more glands may appear relatively normal. It is frequently stated in the literature that the presence of a single normal parathyroid is diagnostic of a parathyroid adenoma, since hyperplasia always involves all four glands. This is not true, however, because we and others have seen instances in which one gland was the site of a very clear-cut parathyroid adenoma, while two other glands showed hyperplasia and the fourth appeared normal. It is true, however, that the presence of a single normal parathyroid *usually* indicates that the enlarged gland represents an adenoma rather than hyperplasia.

Microscopically the cells appear identical to those of an adenoma (Fig. 38-31). There is a greater tendency, however, toward the appearance of many fibrous tissue septa, and the gland appears to have been composed of a number of nodules coalescing with each other. There are very few fatty cells, which are common in the normal gland. Although parathyroid adenomas are characterized by having a well-developed capsule and by the presence of an area where normal gland is compressed by the developing adenoma, a very similar appearance can be seen in chief cell hyperplasia. It is said that this develops when a hyperplastic area of the gland grows out into the surrounding fat and appears to be compressed normal gland or when one portion of the gland is simply separated from the rest of the gland by a well-developed septum in the course of development of nodular hyperplasia. It has been stressed

Fig. 38-30. Comparison of adenoma and hyperplasia. *A.* Detail of a chief cell adenoma adjacent to the capsule. Note the solid grouping of uniform chief cells, with absence of fat. (×200.) *B.* Chief cell hyperplasia. The cellular morphology is similar to that of the adenoma. Note the small focus of water-clear cells in the left central portion of the field. (×150.) *C.* Chief cell hyperplasia. Note the cords and small acinary groupings. (×200.)

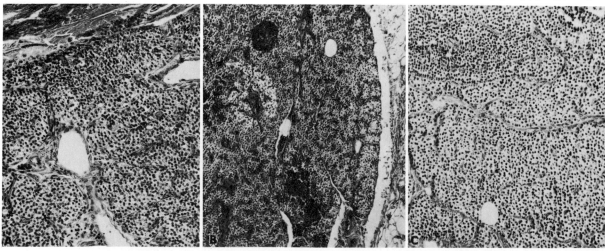

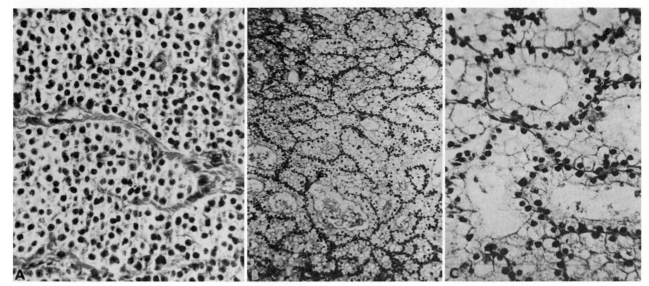

Fig. 38-31. Comparison of water-clear and chief cell hyperplasia. *A.* Chief cell hyperplasia. The cells are small and uniform, with finely granular and transparent cytoplasm. (×400.) *B.* Water-clear cell hyperplasia. The tubules are well formed, and the cells are large and clear. (×200.) *C.* Water-clear cell hyperplasia: a higher magnification of *B.* (×400.) (*Photograph courtesy Saul Kay.*)

by Black and Utley that the final diagnosis of adenoma or chief cell hyperplasia can sometimes be made only several years after the original operation and will occasionally have to be based on the subsequent course of the patient rather than on any absolute histologic diagnostic criteria. They feel, however, that the presence of a single normal or atrophic parathyroid is diagnostic of an adenoma, but, as mentioned above, this is not necessarily so. Although the differential diagnosis between chief cell hyperplasia and parathyroid adenoma is an extremely interesting and somewhat important one, its importance is diminished by inspecting all four parathyroid glands at operation for hyperparathyroidism, which is our practice. The difficulty in distinguishing between the two does add considerable impetus to the adoption of this practice.

While the chief cell is the predominant cell type in chief cell adenomas and in chief cell hyperplasia, the other cell types are frequently represented. In chief cell adenomas a mixture of water-clear and oxyphil cells is frequently seen, while in chief cell hyperplasia the oxyphil cell is the second most frequent type of cell seen. Occasional water-clear cells may also be seen, however, and multinucleated giant cells are occasionally present.

Hypercalcemia Associated with Nonparathyroid Malignancies. It has long been known that on occasion neoplasms can produce a variety of polypeptide hormones identical or biologically similar to ACTH, melanocyte-stimulating hormone (MSH), follicle-stimulating hormone (FSH), antidiuretic hormone (ADH), insulin, and chorionic gonadotropin. It is now clear that some tumors also produce PTH-like circulating hormones or prostaglandin E_2, each of which may result in hypercalcemia.

The most common cause of hypercalcemia of malignant disease is osseous metastasis. Normal radiographs do not always exclude the presence of bone metastases. Bachman and Sproul in a series of autopsies found that only one-half of the cases with histologically documented skeletal metastases had radiographic findings indicative of metastatic cancer. One hopes that the use of bone scans will help to diagnose some of these occult metastases.

Recent studies have shown that one cause of hypercalcemia associated with malignant tumor without apparent skeletal metastases is the synthesis and secretion of a PTH-like substance by the malignant tumor. This clinical syndrome of a nonparathyroid tumor associated with hypercalcemia and hypophosphatemia has been referred to as *pseudohyperparathyroidism,* or *ectopic hyperparathyroidism.*

Goldberg et al. in 1964 found reports in the literature of 18 patients with hypercalcemia associated with neoplasm in the absence of bony metastases. They explored the neck of one patient with hypercalcemia and found only atrophic parathyroid glands. At autopsy this was confirmed, and the patient was found to have a hypernephroma. Bioassays of both the tumor and a pulmonary metastasis revealed a substance indistinguishable from PTH. The removal of tumors of this type has been associated many times with a prompt fall of serum calcium concentration to normal as demonstrated in the case of hypernephroma reported by Plimpton and Gelhorn. The reappearance of metastases may be associated with an elevation of the serum calcium level.

Although a number of tumors can produce ectopic hyperparathyroidism, the most common are squamous cell and small cell carcinomas of the lung, and hypernephromas. Other less common neoplasms include hepatoma and cancer of the ovary, stomach, pancreas, parotid gland, and colon.

The hypercalcemia of breast cancer has not been demonstrated to be due to ectopic hyperparathyroidism. It has been postulated, but never proved, that a *vitamin D–like sterol* is responsible for hypercalcemia in patients with this tumor in whom no bone metastases are found. Most cases of hypercalcemia of breast cancer do not have hypophosphatemia. When a low serum phosphorus level is present with hypercalcemia, one should consider the possibility of a coincident parathyroid adenoma. Samaan and coworkers recently reported that 35 percent of patients with different types of malignancy and hypercalcemia were subsequently proved to have *coexistent primary hyperparathyroidism.* Thus, this diagnostic possibility should not be excluded because the patient has a malignancy.

In addition to ectopic PTH secretion, several other humoral factors have been associated with the hypercalcemia of some malignancies. Tashjian has demonstrated that *prostaglandin E_2* infused into animals causes hypercalcemia. In a rat sarcoma system, he has demonstrated that metabolites of prostaglandin increased before hypercalcemia occurred, and thus appeared to be the cause of the increased serum calcium concentrations. Seyberth and associates demonstrated that patients with various malignant tumors and hypercalcemia had elevated concentrations of metabolites of prostaglandins. In several of their patients, treatment with aspirin or indomethacin (which decreases prostaglandin production) resulted in a lowering of the serum calcium levels to normal. Prostaglandin E_2 appears to result in hypercalcemia by stimulating bone resorption. These data suggest that prostaglandin E_2 may be an important causative agent for the hypercalcemia of malignancy in some patients.

Finally, Mundy and associates have described a factor which they call *osteoclast activating factor* (O.A.F.). This is produced by myeloma and other lymphoid cells and causes bone resorption. It may be the cause of hypercalcemia in some patients with hematologic diseases. A great deal of investigation is continuing in the area of hypercalcemia in neoplastic diseases.

The differentiation of ectopic hyperparathyroidism from primary hyperparathyroidism due to parathyroid gland disease is often difficult. Lafferty suggests that ectopic hyperparathyroidism is more likely when the serum calcium concentration exceeds 14 mg/100 ml, when serum alkaline phosphatase activity is increased, when osteitis fibrosa is absent, and when there is a significant degree of anemia. Conversely, primary hyperparathyroidism is more likely with a long-standing history of repeated renal lithiasis or with radiographic evidence of osteitis fibrosa.

Skeletal Changes. The full-blown skeletal changes of hyperparathyroidism are rarely seen today, since most patients are operated upon at an early stage before such changes have had a chance to develop. The principal skeletal pathologic changes consist of osteitis fibrosa cystica, cysts, giant cell tumors, and osteoporosis.

When the skeletal changes become sufficiently pronounced, they can be detected by conventional x-rays, although it seems likely from recent studies that the skeleton is always involved even when the x-rays reveal no detectable change. The skeletal changes can be most easily demonstrated in the long bones, spine, skull, pelvis, hands, clavicles, and jaw.

Osteitis fibrosa cystica is brought about by an overactivity of the osteoclasts which causes resorption of cortical and cancellous bone. The bone is replaced by vascularized cellular connective tissue in which there may be abortive bone formation. As the condition progresses, there is an increasing loss of mature bone with the development of multiple soft cystic areas. These changes are histologically entirely similar to those seen in fibrous dysplasia.

The bone cysts may be small or large, single or multiple; they may have a solitary cavity or be multilocular. They contain brownish fluid or mucoid material and are lined by connective tissue. The giant cell tumors, or brown tumors, are frequently partly cystic and are brown or reddish on section. Histologically they consist of numerous large osteoclasts in a cellular stroma. They are commonly found in the long bones and in the jaw, where they may constitute the presenting symptom. In the jaw the lesion consists of an area of bony destruction with an expansion of the cortical contour of the bone which may erupt beneath the gum and is often confused with an epulis. Hemorrhage into the area may occur, followed by the appearance of multinucleated giant cells and organization of the area with the formation of delicate trabeculae of osteoid tissue. The brown tumors therefore grossly and microscopically resemble the osteoclastomas which are not of parathyroid origin.

CLINICAL MANIFESTATIONS. Incidence. Hyperparathyroidism very rarely occurs under the age of puberty, although a very few instances of neonatal familial hyperparathyroidism have been reported. Of those cases which were not familial the youngest to have been diagnosed and operated upon was a boy aged three. The most common age is between thirty and sixty. Those having prominent skeletal lesions tend to develop the disease at an earlier age, usually between ten and thirty, while those with renal calculi alone are much more common in the thirty-to-sixty age group. Hyperparathyroidism in children and in neonates is discussed in later sections.

Hyperparathyroidism is more common in women than in men, in a ratio of 2:1.

The incidence of skeletal and renal changes in patients with hyperparathyroidism reported prior to 1965 is shown in Table 38-3. It is interesting to note that in the earlier series of Norris, in 1947, when all cases of hyperparathyroidism that had been reported to that date were collected, only 5 percent of the patients had renal changes without skeletal changes while 61 percent of the patients had skeletal changes only. In a more recent series of published cases up to 1965 it was found that 59 percent had renal changes only while 16 percent had skeletal changes only. Thus 78 percent of all cases had renal involvement, and 35 percent of all cases had skeletal involvement. Ninety-four percent had renal or skeletal involvement, while only six percent had neither renal nor skeletal involvement.

Since 1965 marked changes in our understanding of the incidence and symptomatology of primary hyperparathyroidism have occurred. These changes are due largely to the fact that primary hyperparathyroidism is being diagnosed in many relatively asymptomatic individuals who are found to have an elevated serum calcium level on routine multiphasic serum chemistry screening programs which are being carried out in most hospitals today. The efficacy and importance of this screening can be seen in the

Table 38-3. INCIDENCE OF RENAL AND OSSEOUS INVOLVEMENT
IN EARLIER COLLECTED SERIES

	Skeletal only	*Skeletal plus renal*	*Renal only*	*No skeletal or renal*	*Total*
Norris (1947).......	191 (61%)	101 (32%)	17 (5%)	5 (2%)	314
1953–1965.........	83 (16%)	99 (19%)	308 (59%)	31 (6%)	521

	Percent
Renal only	59
Renal and osseous............................	19
Total renal involvement	78
Osseous only	16
Renal and osseous............................	19
Total osseous involvement	35
Renal *or* osseous involvement	94
Neither renal nor osseous involvement	6

following study conducted by a Mayo Clinic team. Automated screening of serum calcium resulted in the diagnosis of as many new cases of proved primary hyperparathyroidism in residents of the Rochester, Minnesota, area during a $1\frac{1}{2}$-year period (1974–1975) as had occurred during the previous $9\frac{1}{2}$ years. The minimum incidence of primary hyperparathyroidism in this geographical area now exceeds 0.1 percent of the population. In other series, an incidence of primary hyperparathyroidism as high as 0.5 percent of the general population has been noted. Many patients in this recent group have only mild symptoms.

The incidence of hyperparathyroidism in patients who have had urinary calcium stones is variously estimated to be between 2.5 and 15 percent. The mean figure is somewhere around 5 percent.

Symptoms. When the disease of hyperparathyroidism was first recognized, it was thought to be a skeletal disease, and it was not until 7 years after the first patient had been operated upon that it was recognized that the disease could occur only with renal manifestations. Now the disease is seldom seen with marked skeletal involvement, because it is usually recognized long before this occurs. Today the disease is sometimes diagnosed and treated in the absence of either skeletal or renal involvement. With the widespread application of multiphasic blood screening such as the SMA-12, more asymptomatic or mildly symptomatic (anxiety, depression, abdominal pain) patients are being discovered. In the Rochester, Minnesota, group, 49 percent had one or more of these serious complications possibly attributable to primary hyperparathyroidism: hypertension, 35 percent; renal stone disease, 25 percent; psychiatric symptoms, 21 percent; decreased renal function, 16 percent; and subperiosteal bone resorption, 5 percent.

Though some patients with only mild disease will be diagnosed as having primary hyperparathyroidism, it is important that the symptoms and signs of the classical clinical presentation of this disease be recognized. The clues which first led to the diagnosis in 343 cases of the Massachusetts General Hospital series are shown in Table 38-4. As expected, renal stones head the list, with bone disease a distant second. Peptic ulcer and pancreatitis

form a small but important minority, while 20 of the patients complained only of fatigue, mental disturbance, or central nervous system signs. Familial cases are sometimes diagnosed after diagnosis of one member of the family and subsequent screening of the kindred, and some cases are discovered through routine laboratory tests. A careful study of patients who are recurrent renal stone formers will establish the diagnosis of hyperparathyroidism in 2.5 to 12.5 percent of the cases. The causes of the symptomatology of hyperparathyroidism are shown in Table 38-5.

Symptoms Related to Hypercalcemia. Since virtually all the patients with hyperparathyroidism demonstrate hypercalcemia, it is not surprising that many of the symptoms and signs relate directly to this alteration.

Renal Damage. The renal damage which occurs in this disease is a consequence both of the hypercalcemia and of the increased secretion of PTH. Hypersecretion of PTH results in increased excretion of phosphate and in relative urinary alkalosis, both of which may predispose to calcium precipitation. Renal damage can occur, however, as a consequence of hypercalcemia from any source. The length

Table 38-4. CLUES TO THE DIAGNOSIS OF
HYPERPARATHYROIDISM IN THE FIRST
343 CASES AT THE MASSACHUSETTS
GENERAL HOSPITAL

Clue	*Number of cases*
Renal stones	195
Bone disease	80
Peptic ulcer..........................	27
Fatigue	10
Pancreatitis	9
Central nervous system signs	7
Hypertension	6
Mental disturbance	3
Multiple endocrine abnormalities	3
No symptoms (routine laboratory test)	2
Lump in neck	1

SOURCE: From Cope, 1966.

Table 38-5. CAUSES OF SYMPTOMS OF HYPERPARATHYROIDISM

Cause	*Symptoms and signs*
Hypercalcemia	Renal damage
	Mental: Depression, fatigue, delerium, coma
	Muscle: General muscle weakness, and hypotonia, walking with cane, hypoactive reflexes
	Gastrointestinal: Peptic ulcer, constipation, gastric disturbance, loss of appetite, pancreatitis (?)
	Eye changes: Band keratitis, calcium in palpebral fissure
	Ectopic calcification
	Hypercalcemic crisis: Profound muscle weakness, nausea and vomiting, lethargy and drowsiness, confusion, bone pain, abdominal pain, thirst, polyuria, constipation, coma, hypertension, fever, ECG changes, short Q-T interval and nearly absent ST segment, azotemia with increased PO_4, hypokalemia
Increased urinary calcium	Polyuria, polydipsia, and hypokalemia
Hypomagnesemia	Paresthesias, hyperreflexia
Direct action of PTH	Demineralization of the skeleton due to bone resorption: Bone pain, cysts, known tumors, fractures
	Renal damage
	Peptic ulcer (?)
	Pancreatitis (?)
Renal damage	Hypertension
	Renal stones, nephrocalcinosis

of time required for hypercalcemia to produce renal damage depends upon the degree of hypercalcemia. The renal damage is worse in those patients who have skeletal changes demonstrable by x-ray and in those patients with nephrocalcinosis than in those with renal calculi alone.

Mental Changes. Patients with hypercalcemia frequently complain of mental symptoms consisting of depression, fatigue, listlessness, and occasionally confusion. The patients may be irritable or regressive, subject to crying spells, or simply depressed. In some individuals with severe hypercalcemia, delirium and even coma may occur, while others tolerate the same increase in serum calcium with few symptoms. Correction of the hyperparathyroidism and hypercalcemia results in a reversion to a normal mental state in many but not all persons.

Muscle Weakness. Generalized muscle weakness is common in hypercalcemia and is associated with hypotonia and hyporeflexia. The joints are often extremely flexible, and the weakness may lead to difficulty in walking.

Gastrointestinal Symptoms. Some type of gastric disturbance, loss of appetite, nausea, vomiting, and/or constipation are common in hypercalcemia. There is a questionable increased incidence of peptic ulcer in patients with hyperparathyroidism, and this is probably related to the hypercalcemia, though direct action of PTH on the gastric mucosa may contribute as well. Duodenal ulcer is much more common than gastric ulcer. This entity will be discussed more fully below, under Peptic Ulcer. Pancreatitis may also be related to hypercalcemia, though direct action of PTH on the pancreatic cells may be more likely. Calcium salts are apt to be precipitated out in the pancreatic ducts in the presence of hypercalcemia, and this may contribute to pancreatitis. The increased calcium in the pancreatic juice which is present in hypercalcemia is said to accelerate the conversion of trypsinogen to trypsin, and the activated

enzyme may lead to pancreatitis. Pancreatitis has been noted only rarely in patients with hypercalcemia from causes other than hyperparathyroidism.

Eye Changes. Band keratitis and calcium in the palpebral fissure are seen in hypercalcemia of various causes.

Ectopic Calcification. Ectopic calcification occasionally occurs in primary hyperparathyroidism, almost always in association with gross pathologic changes in bone. It occurs in only a small percentage of patients and is not a particularly valuable sign of this disease.

Hypercalcemic Crisis. This is sometimes called "acute hyperparathyroidism," but since the signs and symptoms are common to those of hypercalcemia of any origin (for example, breast cancer), it seems best to refer to it as *acute hypercalcemic crisis.* In hyperparathyroidism this usually does not eventuate until the serum calcium level rises to 16 mg/100 ml or above. It is equally common in males and females, while hyperparathyroidism itself is twice as common in females as in males. It is much more apt to occur in the presence of severe renal damage, and at least 90 percent of the patients have some degree of renal failure. The patient has usually had a long-standing history of skeletal or renal involvement with more recent symptoms of loss of appetite and weight, nausea and vomiting, constipation, thirst and polyuria, and generalized muscular weakness. The relative frequency of the symptoms is shown in Table 38-6.

If the early symptoms of hypercalcemic crisis are ignored, they may progress to the more serious ones of lethargy and drowsiness, confusion, severe muscular weakness, prostration, and coma. The electrocardiographic changes of hypercalcemia do not usually make their appearance until the calcium levels are quite high, but they may be seen in hypercalcemic crisis and consist of a short Q-T interval and a nearly absent ST segment. Fever and tachycardia may be present. O_ ___nally there is an association of acute pancreatitis wit. __ypercalcemic crisis. A rising blood urea nitrogen (BUN) level is common.

In hypercalcemic crisis due to hyperparathyroidism there is a very high incidence of renal failure, nearly 90 percent, and a much greater percentage of the patients have bone involvement, nephrocalcinosis, and peptic ulcer than is true for hyperparathyroidism in general.

Hypercalcemic crisis was reviewed by Lemann and Donatelli, who collected 42 cases in 1964. Some of their findings are reproduced in Table 38-6. Payne and Fitchett collected 70 cases in 1965 in a review of the literature, and 16 cases were added by MacCleod and Holloway in 1967, including one of their own. In these 86 cases the age range was from five to seventy-seven years with a median age of fifty-one. The greatest incidence occurred in the three decades between forty and sixty-nine. Forty percent of the patients survived, and sixty percent died. Of the 45 patients undergoing operation, 33 survived. All patients not operated upon died, except for one who was a five-year-old child in whom the crisis was precipitated by injections of PTH. The crisis abated when the PTH was stopped. Since 1967, the medical treatment of hypercalcemia has improved greatly. Now parathyroidectomy as initial treatment is rarely indicated, even when primary hyperparathyroidism is diagnosed as the probable cause of the hypercalcemic crisis. The drug regimens which are useful in treating acute hypercalcemia will be discussed later in this chapter.

Symptoms Related to Increased Urinary Calcium. The symptoms of hyperparathyroidism due to increased urinary calcium loss are those of polyuria and polydipsia. The hypokalemia which is sometimes seen in this disease, particularly in cases of hypercalcemic crisis, is apparently due to excessive potassium loss in the urine, which may be related to the increased urinary calcium loss. Hypomag-

nesemia is sometimes seen in hyperparathyroidism. This appears to be more common when the serum calcium level is very high or when the intake of magnesium has been poor because of gastrointestinal disturbances. When present this may give rise to paresthesias or hyperreflexia.

Symptoms Related to Direct Action of PTH. *Demineralization of the Skeleton.* As a consequence of the increased bone resorption brought about by PTH the skeleton becomes demineralized and bone cysts, brown tumors, and pathologic fractures eventuate. The recent microradiographic studies of Jowsey and others have suggested that some degree of pathologic change in bone is present in virtually every case of hyperparathyroidism. This is frequently not detectable by the usual clinical means, however, and in many instances the patients do not have symptoms relating to the bones. The presence of demonstrable bony changes relates more to the severity of the disease, the duration of the disease, and the size of the adenoma than to anything else.

Cysts and tumors of the jaw are sometimes the presenting complaint. This appears as a swelling of the gum very similar to that seen with epulis and usually brings the patient to the dentist. Vague pains in the back, hip, or shoulder, often thought by the patient to be arthritis, are sometimes present, while in other instances the pain may be quite marked and related to a particular bone which is tender on palpation. In the more long-standing cases the stature may decrease, and a bowing of the spine may be apparent to the patient and his relatives. Sometimes local swelling of the bone or deformity of the bone may be noted. A pathologic fracture may be the first bone symptom of which the patient complains.

Renal Damage. Some of the renal damage in hyperparathyroidism is due to a direct effect of the PTH on the proximal tubular cell and is not related specifically to hypercalcemia. The most common symptom of renal

Table 38-6. SYMPTOMS AND SIGNS IN 42 PATIENTS WITH HYPERCALCEMIC CRISIS DUE TO HYPERPARATHYROIDISM

Symptoms	Percent of cases	Signs	Percent of cases
Muscular weakness	80	Hypotonia	44
Nausea and vomiting . . .	80	Neck mass	42
Weight loss	65	Hypertension	35
Fatigue	65	Dehydration	31
Lethargy and drowsiness .	65	Tachycardia	26
Confusion	57	Fever	22
Bone pain	55	Abdominal tenderness and distension . .	15
Abdominal pain	48	Band keratopathy	9
Polyuria	40	Tracheal deviation	4
Constipation	37		
Coma	26		
Polydipsia	24		
Renal colic	22		
Neck swelling	9		
Dysphagia and neck pain	4		

SOURCE: From Lemann and Donatelli, 1964.

damage is the presence of renal calculi. Symptoms related to the renal calculi are by far the most common presenting complaint of patients with hyperparathyroidism.

Peptic Ulcer (Questionable). Though it was originally thought that patients with primary hyperparathyroidism have a greatly increased incidence of peptic ulcers, this view has been recently challenged. It is well known that patients with severe ulcer diatheses and hyperparathyroidism are often markedly improved by parathyroidectomy and the return of their serum calcium level to normal. In these patients after parathyroidectomy, the gastric acid secretion falls dramatically and the ulcer may even heal. However, many of these individuals later prove to have a Zollinger-Ellison syndrome (gastrinoma) and their hyperparathyroidism is part of the multiple endocrine neoplasia, type 1, syndrome. If this group of Zollinger-Ellison patients with hypercalcemia is eliminated from consideration, it is difficult to demonstrate a truly increased incidence of peptic ulcer disease in patients with primary hyperparathyroidism.

Recent studies have demonstrated that calcium infusion with production of hypercalcemia results in (1) a small rise of basal gastric acid secretion in about one-half of normal patients, (2) a mean rise in basal acid in duodenal ulcer patients to about 30 percent of maximal Histalog (betazole) stimulation, and (3) a rise of gastric acid output in Zollinger-Ellison patients equal to that produced by maximal stimulation by Histalog. These changes are accompanied by a statistically significant increase in circulating gastrin in duodenal ulcer patients and a marked increase of serum gastrin in most patients with Zollinger-Ellison syndrome. To date, in fact, calcium infusion with measurement of gastrin and gastric acid output is one of the most reliable provocative tests for Zollinger-Ellison tumors. Calcium ion appears to play a significant role in release of gastrin and other polypeptide hormones.

Patients with parathyroid disease and hypercalcemia without the Zollinger-Ellison syndrome have been demonstrated to have mildly elevated serum gastrin concentrations which return to normal after parathyroidectomy and restoration of normocalcemia. On the other hand, it has *not* been conclusively demonstrated that patients with primary hyperparathyroidism have statistically increased acid secretion as a group. We and others have noted basal achlorhydria, in fact, in some of these patients. Some patients with severe chronic renal disease and secondary hyperparathyroidism have been shown to have increased serum gastrin levels as well, which appears to be due to the fact that the kidneys play an essential role in the metabolism of gastrin.

The incidence of peptic ulcer and hyperparathyroidism is probably somewhere around 10 percent. Incidences as high as this have been reported in some groups of normal population, and doubt has been expressed as to whether there really is an association between peptic ulcer and hyperparathyroidism.

Our view is that it is uncertain that hyperparathyroidism directly causes duodenal ulcer disease. In individuals who have an ulcer diathesis, however, this may be worsened by the hypercalcemia of parathyroid disease. Because of the fact that 20 percent of patients with Zollinger-Ellison syndrome have associated parathyroid gland abnormalities, this islet cell tumor must be ruled out in any hypercalcemic individual with an ulcer by obtaining a serum gastrin determination and making other appropriate tests. In both routine duodenal ulcers and those associated with the Zollinger-Ellison syndrome parathyroidectomy may be of benefit if primary hyperparathyroidism is present.

Pancreatitis (Questionable). The relation between hyperparathyroidism and pancreatitis seems less secure. If the relationship does exist, it is probably due either to the effect of hypercalcemia or of PTH on the precipitation of calcium salts from the pancreatic juice. Although calcification of the pancreas occurs in some patients with hyperparathyroidism, it is frequently only an incidental finding. Pyrah et al. suggest that the cases in which pancreatitis and hyperparathyroidism are associated fall into six groups:

1. One or more attacks of acute pancreatitis following which the diagnosis of hyperparathyroidism is established. With removal of the parathyroid adenoma there are no further attacks of pancreatitis, and the serum amylase returns to normal.
2. Acute pancreatitis occurring as a complication of operation for the removal of a parathyroid adenoma.
3. Acute pancreatitis occurring as a complication of some unrelated operation in a patient with hyperparathyroidism, as, for example, the removal of a renal calculus.
4. Acute pancreatitis occurring as a complication of acute hypercalcemic crisis due to hyperparathyroidism.
5. Chronic pancreatitis manifested by recurring attacks of abdominal pain and associated with pancreatic calculi in patients with hyperparathyroidism.
6. Development of hypercalcemia (tertiary hyperparathyroidism) in a patient with known chronic pancreatitis, steatorrhea, and secondary hyperparathyroidism.

One might add to the list above hereditary pancreatitis associated with familial hyperparathyroidism.

Paloyan et al. have demonstrated an increase in circulating glucagon in acute pancreatitis and postulate that this may be the cause of the hypocalcemia which frequently accompanies this disease. Glucagon infusions result in hypocalcemia in experimental animals and increased serum PTH in man. Thus it is possible but not yet proved that secondary hyperparathyroidism may occur in patients with pancreatitis and that hypercalcemia in these individuals may represent a form of tertiary hyperparathyroidism.

The incidence of pancreatitis associated with hyperparathyroidism has not been definitely established, but in the series reported by Mixter et al. it was about 7 percent. In carcinoma of the parathyroid and familial hyperparathyroidism the incidence of pancreatitis is somewhat higher.

Symptoms Related to Renal Damage. *Hypertension.* Although the association of hypertension with hyperparathyroidism is well known, it is likely that in almost all instances this is due to the renal damage brought about by the disease and not to any direct effect of PTH itself. In the study by Hellstrom et al. of 95 cases of hyperparathyroidism submitted to parathyroidectomy and followed afterward, 44 patients had a normal blood pressure preoperatively, but in 15 of them hypertension developed postoperatively. Forty-seven patients had preoperative hypertension, and in seventeen of these the blood pressure returned to normal following parathyroidectomy, but it remained elevated in thirty. Furthermore, the patients in whom the blood pressure became normal after the operation with a single exception had had only moderate hypertension preoperatively. In many patients with only moderate hypertension preoperatively increasing hypertension had developed in the postoperative period. There was a lower incidence of hypertension in those patients with renal stones or nephrocalcinosis only than in those patients who had bone changes preoperatively. There was a good correlation, however, between the degree of hypertension and the degree of renal damage. Hypertension and cardiac failure are important causes of death in hyperparathyroidism.

A role of serum renin in the pathogenesis of the hypertension of primary hyperparathyroidism has also been postulated.

Renal Stones, Nephrocalcinosis. Renal colic, of course, is frequently seen in patients with hyperparathyroidism. Nephrocalcinosis does not usually produce any symptoms. Hellstrom and Ivemark showed that the incidence of renal damage was high in patients with gross skeletal changes and in patients with nephrocalcinosis but much less so in patients with renal calculi alone. In a high proportion of patients there is an inability to concentrate the urine normally which is probably due to a direct physiologic action of PTH rather than to anatomic calcification.

Nephrocalcinosis refers to diffuse calcification of the kidney as demonstrated roentgenographically. These collections of radiopaque material are usually in the renal pyramids and the medulla. There are many other conditions which can give rise to nephrocalcinosis besides hyperparathyroidism. If one examines all cases of nephrocalcinosis, only about 20 percent or less are due to hyperparathyroidism, the next most common causes being tubular acidosis, medullary sponge kidney, and idiopathic causes. The patient with nephrocalcinosis usually has renal stones as well, so that renal colic or hematuria is a frequent complaint. Lumbar pain or aching may also be present. The nephrocalcinosis does not improve after removal of the parathyroid adenoma.

Other Manifestations. In some patients hyperparathyroidism manifests itself primarily in terms of mental changes consisting of depression, irritability, forgetfulness, confusion, and vague complaints. The diagnosis under these circumstances may be very difficult to make unless one is thinking of it.

Patients with nonparathyroid PTH-secreting tumors may have any of the usual symptoms of hyperparathyroidism due to parathyroid disease. Since these tumors are frequently malignant, they may have symptoms relating to the local or distant spread of the disease. Because of the rather frequent, and sometimes fatal, elevation of serum calcium levels in patients with malignant tumors with or without bone metastases, it is extremely important to follow blood calcium and phosphorous levels in such patients.

Physical Findings. Some of the physical findings and signs were discussed in the preceding section on symptoms, and others will be mentioned under diagnostic tests.

Hypotonia of the muscles can be detected in many patients. This hypotonicity leads to flexibility of the limbs, which develops to a marked degree in some patients. A decreased excitability of the neuromuscular apparatus can be demonstrated by nerve stimulation. It takes about twice as much galvanic current to stimulate the nerve in hyperparathyroidism as in the normal state. There is a decrease in auditory sensitivity, and some patients are quite deaf. The eyes show calcium phosphate crystals in the palpebral fissure, and band keratitis can be demonstrated with a slit lamp. There is sometimes difficulty in focusing the eyes. Metastatic calcification is rare, in contrast to the situation seen in secondary hyperparathyroidism and vitamin D intoxication, where it is quite common.

It is seldom possible to palpate the parathyroid adenoma, except in patients with hypercalcemic crisis, where the adenoma is usually very large and can be felt in 40 percent of the cases. Apart from this circumstance, the adenoma can be felt in only about 5 percent of the cases or less. A large parathyroid malignant tumor may be palpable.

When bone disease is present, it may be possible to detect bending of the long bones, vertebral deformity, a decrease in stature, fractures of the bones, or the appearance of an epulislike growth in the lower gum.

DIAGNOSTIC FINDINGS. Calcium, Phosphate, Alkaline Phosphatase, and Chloride Measurements. The diagnosis of hyperparathyroidism in most cases rests upon biochemical determinations. The most important of these is the *serum calcium level.* The normal range varies in different laboratories depending on the techniques used. In our own normal range is generally considered to be between 8.5 and 10.5 mg/100 ml. There are some cases of early hyperparathyroidism in which the calcium level may be very close to the normal range or may fluctuate from the normal levels to slightly elevated levels. Although some writers have stated that a single normal value, if obtained with proper techniques, makes a diagnosis of hyperparathyroidism unlikely, others, including McGeown and Morrison, have suggested that measurements should be repeated over a period of months or even years in borderline cases. Our own experience would fit with this latter concept. Hodgkinson and Edwards found that large fluctuations in serum calcium levels were not common but that variations of 1 to 2 mg/100 ml did occur occasionally over a period of weeks or months and that this could be misleading when the calcium level was only slightly elevated. They felt that such patients should be reexamined at intervals of several weeks until the diagnosis is firmly established (Fig. 38-32). Bartter and associates have popularized the concept of "normocalcemic hyperparathyroidism" in which renal stones occur in patients with borderline or totally normal serum calcium concentrations. Whether or not these patients have *primary* hyperparathyroidism has not yet been resolved.

An additional reason for following the blood calcium and phosphorous levels in patients who are suspected of having or who have once had the disease is shown in Fig. 38-54. This patient had three separate episodes of hypercalcemia and hypophosphatemia covering a 9-year period. The interim values were normal. While this was originally

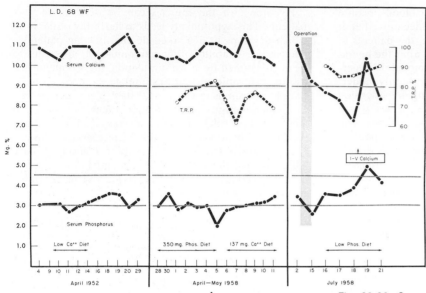

A

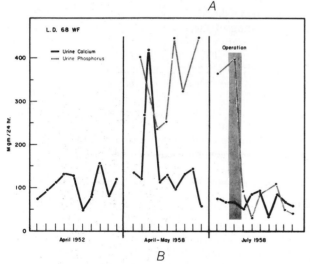

B

Fig. 38-32. Serum calcium and phosphate values. *A*. Serum calcium and phosphate values before and after excision of a parathyroid adenoma. The serum calcium values were only minimally elevated. The tubular resorption of phosphate (TRP) was depressed preoperatively and rose following the operation. Postoperatively the serum calcium level fell to the point where the patient required a brief intravenous treatment with calcium. *B*. Urine calcium and phosphate values of the same patient. During 1952, the patient was on a low-calcium diet, and urinary calcium excretion was never very high. In April-May, 1958, the patient was on a 350-mg calcium diet for the first half of the period charted and a 137-mg calcium diet for the second half. Apart from two determinations in the early part of this period the calcium excretion was never strikingly increased. The calcium excretion did not change appreciably following excision of the parathyroid adenoma, while the phosphate excretion decreased strikingly.

thought to represent the formation and removal of three separate parathyroid adenomas, it is much more likely that this represents unrecognized parathyroid hyperplasia treated by removal of a single grossly enlarged gland on each occasion.

In order to interpret the calcium level adequately it is helpful to get a serum total protein determination and electrophoretic pattern. Since it is only the *ionized calcium* which is physiologically active, it has been suggested that measurements of the ionized calcium would be more valuable than measurements of the total calcium. Ionized calcium recently has become much easier to measure because of the new electrode systems which are available. Ionized calcium concentrations are occasionally elevated in primary hyperparathyroidism when total calcium is normal. It is of course essential to rule out other possible causes for the elevated serum calcium level before concluding that the patient has hyperparathyroidism.

The *serum phosphate level* is a somewhat less reliable guide to the diagnosis of hyperparathyroidism. A normal

value does not rule out primary hyperparathyroidism. Low values may occur in several other diseases, e.g., idiopathic hypercalcinuria and renal calculi. Furthermore, it may rise considerably in patients with hyperparathyroidism in whom significant renal damage has developed. Nonetheless it remains a valuable test and in light of our experience should be taken cognizance of when it consistently runs below 3 mg/100 ml, especially if occasional values are below 2.5 mg/100 ml.

The *serum alkaline phosphatase level* usually is elevated in hyperparathyroidism only when there is x-ray evidence of bone disease, and it is frequently elevated in other conditions. This has not proved to be a helpful diagnostic test in our experience.

Wills and McGowan have reported that the *plasma chloride level* is elevated in patients with primary hyperparathyroidism. It was found to be higher than 102 mEq/L in all except 1 of 33 patients with hyperparathyroidism, whereas it was less than 102 mEq/L in all 28 patients with hypercalcemia due to other causes. Pyrah et al. surveyed their cases and confirmed this finding. Rasmussen has also noted an elevated chloride level in hyperparathyroidism but finds that it may be elevated in vitamin D intoxication and osteomalacia as well, although not as consistently so. It is probably a valuable additional test to determine.

Determination of *arterial pH* also may be helpful diagnostically. Barzel has demonstrated that patients with primary hyperparathyroidism have a hyperchloremic metabolic acidosis while those with hypoparathyroidism are slightly alkalotic. Hypercalcemia of nonparathyroid hormone origin results in suppression of the parathyroid glands and a mildly alkaline arterial blood pH.

Urinary Hydroxyproline and Calcium Excretion. The *urinary hydroxyproline level* is a rough measurement of collagen breakdown, and since most collagen is contained in bone, it is to that extent a measure of bone destruction. It is elevated in hyperparathyroidism but also in many other conditions. In general urinary hydroxyproline determinations have not been of much value in establishing the diagnosis of hyperparathyroidism. An elevated *urinary calcium level* may suggest a diagnosis of hyperparathyroidism but is certainly not diagnostic of it. Furthermore hypercalcinuria is not a constant finding in this disease, as may be seen in Fig. 38-32.

Tubular Resorption of Phosphate (TRP) Tests. Since one of the actions of PTH is to decrease the tubular absorption of phosphate, the TRP would seem to be a valuable determination to help establish the diagnosis of hyperparathyroidism. However, the test has not proved to be as useful as it was hoped. The formula for computing the TRP is

$$1 - \frac{UP \times SC}{SP \times UC} \times 100 = TRP$$

where UP = urinary phosphorus
SC = serum creatinine
SP = serum phosphorus
UC = urinary creatinine

The normal value is somewhere between 85 and 95 percent, whereas with hyperparathyroidism it falls to 35 to 85 percent. Although the TRP test is certainly not without error, it provides additional information which may help to confirm the diagnosis. Following a successful parathyroidectomy and correction of the hyperparathyroid state, the urinary excretion of phosphate decreases markedly and the tubular resorption of phosphate rises to normal (Fig. 38-32).

Cortisone Administration (Dent Test). The oral administration of 150 mg of cortisone daily for 10 days was found to reduce the serum calcium to normal levels in patients with hypercalcemia due to vitamin D intoxication or sarcoidosis, whereas the hypercalcemia of hyperparathyroidism was often unaltered. Cortisone also usually reduces the hypercalcemia due to carcinomatosis, multiple myeloma, and the milk-alkali syndrome, but this is not always the case, and hypercalcemia has been reduced in several patients with hyperparathyroidism. Although the test has its limitations, it may be of some value in differentiating between the various causes of hypercalcemia.

Strott and Nugent have emphasized that none of these indirect measurements of PTH hypersecretion is diagnostic of hyperparathyroidism with an accuracy greater than 88 percent.

Bone Biopsy. Even when no gross bone changes are discernible on x-ray, changes in the bone in hyperparathyroidism can almost always be detected by microradiography. These changes have been discussed in an earlier section. A bone biopsy specimen can be taken out of the iliac crest under local anesthesia and subjected to microradiography (Fig. 38-33). The findings, while not completely diagnostic, may help to establish the diagnosis when added to all other evidence.

Bone Densitometry. Cameron and Sorenson recently introduced photon beam scanning of bone. This method appears to be very promising and is being tested in a number of centers. Changes in bone density as small as 5 to 10 percent may be measured by this means. In hyperparathyroidism there is frequently a loss of bone density which returns to normal after parathyroidectomy.

Plasma PTH Measurements. Measurement of PTH in serum by radioimmunoassay has been one of the most exciting recent developments. It has been shown to be the most important and valuable tool for the diagnosis of hyperparathyroidism, since it provides a direct measurement of the hormone whose hypersecretion causes the disease.

Measurement of PTH by immunoassay has proved to be more difficult than that of most other polypeptides. Very useful assays have been developed in the laboratories of Arnaud, Potts, Reiss, and others. However, some results appear to differ from one laboratory to another. The reasons for these difficulties are now beginning to emerge. Circulating PTH in hyperparathyroidism is heterogeneous. At least three distinct fragments of PTH ranging in molecular weight from 4,000 to 10,000 have been identified. The various antisera used in detecting PTH at this time have been produced by injection of bovine or porcine PTH into animals. Different antisera detect different parts of the PTH molecule and hence measure all or only some of these PTH fragments; hence the differences in results. The

Fig. 38-33. Microradiography of a bone biopsy specimen in a patient with hyperparathyroidism due to an adenoma. The area labeled *S* is a static bone surface, the one labeled *F* is a bone formation area, and those labeled *R* are bone resorption areas. There is markedly increased bone resorption. (*Courtesy R. W. Bright.*)

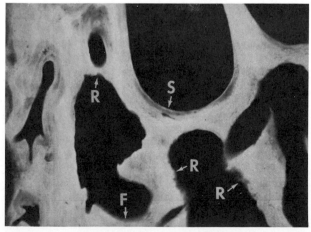

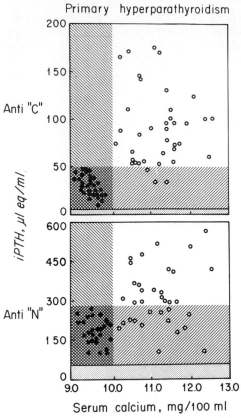

Fig. 38-34. Relationships between serum calcium and serum ⁱPTH values in normal subjects (●) and patients with proved primary hyperparathyroidism (○) using GP IM (anti-C) and CH 14M (anti-N) antisera. (*From C. D. Arnaud et al., Am J Med, 56:785, 1974.*)

amino (NH_2) terminal end of the PTH molecule (Fig. 38-24) confers the biological effects of parathyroid hormone. Antisera directed against this part of the molecule measure physiological secretion rates. However, it has been clearly demonstrated that antisera directed against the carboxyl fragments (C-terminal) of PTH are much better for diagnosing clinical primary hyperparathyroidism. In Fig. 38-34 the same blood samples from normal and hyperparathyroid patients were examined; the anti-C assay discriminates very well between normal subjects and patients with hyperparathyroidism, while in the anti-N assay there is a considerable overlap between these groups. Thus, C-terminal assays for PTH are excellent and aid greatly in our ability to diagnose primary hyperparathyroidism.

Another example of the value of direct measurement of plasma PTH is demonstrated in Fig. 38-35. Reiss and Canterbury were able to differentiate normal patients from those with primary hyperparathyroidism and others with hypoparathyroidism. In secondary hyperparathyroidism the serum PTH level is also elevated. In chronic renal failure, for example, circulating PTH varies inversely with the creatinine clearance; as renal function deteriorates, the PTH level rises. Therefore, one must know the serum calcium and serum PTH concentrations and correlate these two parameters. Elevation of both the serum calcium and PTH levels is diagnostic of primary or tertiary hyperparathyroidism or less commonly of ectopic secretion of PTH from a tumor; all other causes of hypercalcemia are associated with low PTH concentrations.

Other tests utilizing the measurement of PTH may have diagnostic applicability in primary hyperparathyroidism.

Calcium, EDTA, and sodium bicarbonate infusions have been utilized to try to differentiate adenomas from hyperplasia preoperatively. An adenoma, it was thought, would be autonomous and not change its PTH secretion when the serum calcium was raised or lowered. Since hyperplasia is

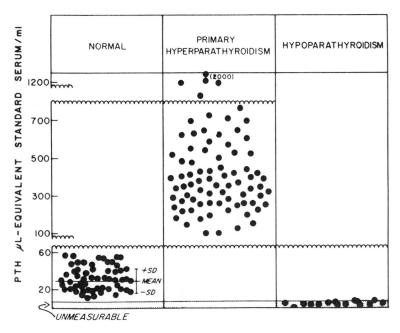

Fig. 38-35. Results of radioimmunoassy of PTH in normal subjects and patients with primary hyperparathyroidism and with hypoparathyroidism. The units of PTH in this figure relate the potency of test serums to that of an arbitrarily selected hyperparathyroid serum. In the hyperparathyroid group, the presence of disease was confirmed surgically in all instances. (*From E. Reiss and J. M. Canterbury, Am J Med, 50:679, 1971.*)

not a neoplasm, these parathyroid glands would be responsive to serum calcium changes, it was postulated. Unfortunately this differentiation has not proved to be as complete as originally thought. Many adenomas have been demonstrated to resemble hyperplasia in secreting more PTH when the calcium ion is lowered and in suppressing their secretion of PTH when serum calcium is elevated. Thus, it is difficult to differentiate adenomas from hyperplasia physiologically as well as histologically.

Roentgenography of Bones. The x-ray appearance of advanced hyperparathyroidism is characteristic. At times this will greatly aid in the diagnosis of primary hyperparathyroidism. X-rays of the skull may show the typical "moth-eaten" ground-glass skull of hyperparathyroidism, with either a thin or thick calvarium (Fig. 38-36). In osteogenesis imperfecta there is a thin, well-calcified skull, while in Paget's disease there is an overgrown fuzzy skull. In multiple myeloma there are many sharp, punched-out areas, and metastatic cancer, especially that from the breast, can give a similar appearance (Fig. 38-37). X-rays of the lamina dura are best taken on dental film. The lamina dura is frequently absent in patients with hyperparathyroidism, but it may also be absent in other conditions and present in hyperparathyroidism. Furthermore it is of no use in the edentulous patient. It is no longer regarded as a very valuable sign.

Chest x-rays may show multiple bony lesions (Fig. 38-38A). X-rays of the clavicle are sometimes helpful, since in hyperparathyroidism there is often a marked absorption of the distal third of the clavicle (Fig. 38-38B). The spine may show marked decalcification and wedging of the vertebrae (Fig. 38-39). The jaws are a favorite place for the development of bone tumors (Fig. 38-40A), and these may be seen in the metacarpals, metatarsals, and the ends of the long bones (Fig. 38-40B). On x-ray a bone tumor and a cyst look the same.

X-rays of the hands are particularly useful in diagnosis of hyperparathyroidism, since they may show the characteristic subperiosteal bone resorption in the middle and terminal phalanges of the fingers (Fig. 38-41). An x-ray of the pelvis may show the presence of metastatic malignancy, the decalcification of primary hyperparathyroidism, bone cysts in the femur, pathologic fractures, or other changes.

X-rays of the bones may show soft tissue calcification, which is much more common in secondary than in primary hyperparathyroidism and still more common in vitamin D intoxication (Fig. 38-42). It is uncommon in primary hyperparathyroidism.

In summary, in primary and secondary hyperparathyroidism bone changes may occur. Subperiosteal bone resorption of the middle and distal phalanges of the fingers and resorption of the distal end of the clavicle are the most common and useful diagnostic abnormalities noted. To be useful, hand films must be taken on high-grade industrial-type film. These abnormalities are pathognomonic of PTH excess.

Roentgenography of the Kidneys. A plain film of the kidneys will sometimes show renal calculi or nephrocalcinosis. Staghorn calculi may be present, as shown in Fig.

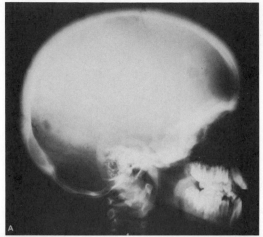
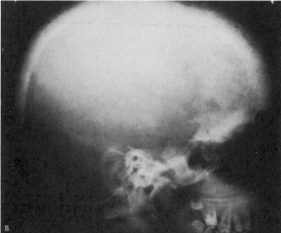
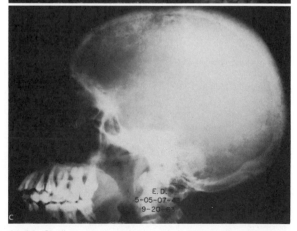

Fig. 38-36. Skull x-rays in patients with hyperparathyroidism. *A.* Lateral view of the skull in a child with secondary hyperparathyroidism due to renal failure. Note the punched-out lesions resembling multiple myeloma. *B.* Secondary hyperparathyroidism. Note the moth-eaten appearance of the skull. *C.* Primary hyperparathyroidism. Note the similarity between this and the patients with secondary hyperparathyroidism.

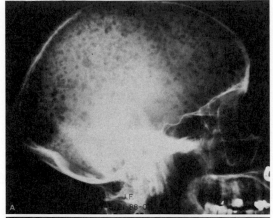

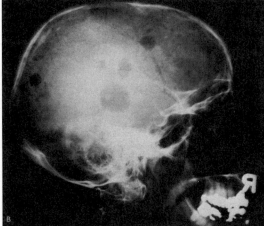

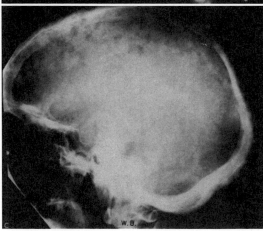

Fig. 38-37. Skull x-rays in patients with hypercalcemia but without hyperparathyroidism. *A*. This patient was admitted in a semi-comatose state with a serum calcium level of 21 mg/100 ml. The x-ray shows multiple small metastatic lesions. A bone biopsy showed metastatic squamous cell carcinoma. The metastases were ultimately demonstrated to have come from a squamous cell carcinoma of the esophagus. *B*. Skull metastases in carcinoma of the breast. *C*. Paget's disease. This disease is most often confused with hyperparathyroidism because of the bone changes. It can on occasion produce hypercalcemia.

38-39. An example of nephrocalcinosis is shown in Fig. 38-43. An intravenous pyelogram may confirm this diagnosis and may also give some idea as to the functional capacity of the kidney and the presence or absence of hydronephrosis. An intravenous pyelogram may also reveal the presence of a renal neoplasm producing the hypercalcemia, just as x-ray of the chest may reveal metastatic cancer or the presence of a mediastinal parathyroid adenoma.

Localization of Hyperfunctioning Parathyroid Glands. A parathyroid adenoma is rarely palpable preoperatively. In about 5 percent of patients the hyperfunctioning gland is found in the chest, not in the neck at all. Furthermore, occasionally an enlarged parathyroid gland is difficult even for the experienced neck surgeon to find. For these reasons many attempts have been made to localize the enlarged overactive parathyroid gland or glands before operation. Until recently, most attempts have met with little success.

A chest x-ray will occasionally be helpful by demonstrating a mass in the mediastinum. On very rare occasions a barium swallow may demonstrate an indentation due to an enlarged parathyroid gland. Thermography, ultrasonography, and computerized tomography have had only limited trials and limited success thus far. An isotope scan is an attractive idea; however, the use of ^{75}selenium methionine scanning, either preoperatively or at the operating table, has not proved to be of great value. We have recently visualized an oxyphil adenoma using a gallium scan. Further tests are necessary to determine if this technique has greater applicability; however, other procedures utilizing PTH secretion have been of considerable help in some instances. Reiss has described the *parathyroid squeeze test*. Massage of the side of the neck harboring the parathyroid adenoma results in a rise of the peripheral serum PTH level. Massage of normal glands results in no change in serum PTH. In the presence of hyperplastic glands, a rise in peripheral serum PTH follows the massage of both sides of the neck, since this disease is bilateral. Catheterization of the large veins of the neck and mediastinum (the jugulars, innominate, and superior vena cava) with sampling of blood for serum PTH from various sites has successfully localized the site of abnormal parathyroid glands in some patients (Fig. 38-44). The serum PTH level will be highest at the site of drainage from a hyperfunctioning gland or glands.

A recent modification of this technique is more efficacious. The small veins draining the thyroid gland, as well as the large veins of the neck and chest, are catheterized and sampled for serum PTH (Fig. 38-45). An elevation of serum PTH on one side of the neck signifies an adenoma, while a gradient of PTH on neck veins of both sides signifies the presence of bilateral hyperplasia. Often this examination has been performed with arteriography (Fig. 38-46). Arteriography by itself may be helpful in localizing an enlarged parathyroid gland, since in some cases a vascular tumor blush is seen, or one inferior thyroid artery may be deviated from its normal position or may be larger than the other. However, several cases of hemiplegia and quadriplegia have followed highly selective inferior thyroid artery arteriography, presumably because of spinal

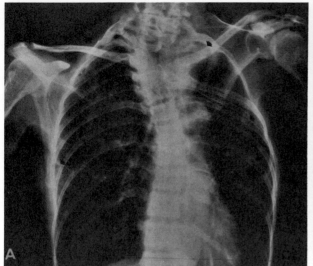
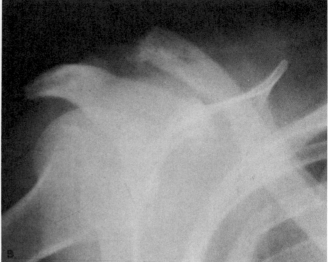

Fig. 38-38. Typical lesions of hyperparathyroidism. *A.* Multiple lesions of bones demonstrated on chest x-ray. *B.* Resorption of the outer end of the clavicle in a patient with secondary hyperparathyroidism. Similar lesions are seen in the primary disease.

cord injury. Hence, this technique should be used with the utmost of caution and only after careful consideration of alternative approaches.

Most endocrinologists and surgeons agree that venous catheterization studies should *not* be done routinely on all patients before their initial parathyroid exploration. We reserve the use of this procedure for patients who have already had a negative neck exploration performed by a highly competent parathyroid surgeon. Its greatest potential usefulness is in the preoperative localization of a mediastinal parathyroid adenoma.

SPECIAL CONSIDERATIONS. Familial Hyperparathyroidism. The familial occurrence of hyperparathyroidism was first reported by Goldman and Smyth in 1936, who described a case in siblings. All told, at least 15 families have been reported in which more than one member has had hyperparathyroidism. A distinction is made between these families and those in whom tumors of multiple endocrine glands have been encountered. This latter group of familial endocrinopathy is discussed later. Although the mode of inheritance has not been completely worked out, it has been assumed to be one of autosomal dominance with incomplete penetrance.

In familial hyperparathyroidism there is a high incidence of involvement of the glands by chief cell hyperplasia, and recurrence of the disease after operation is quite common. In the four cases reported by Stevens et al., however, the parathyroid involvement was by solitary adenomas in each case.

Familial hyperparathyroidism has been reported in conjunction with pancreatitis and with peptic ulceration. In one of the most convincing instances of familial hyperparathyroidism Cutler et al. reported a kindred involving 11 patients with hyperparathyroidism in two families in which the mothers were sisters and the fathers were brothers. Hillman et al. reported neonatal familial hyperpara-

thyroidism in two siblings born to first-cousin parents. One child died and the second was successfully operated upon.

Several of the cases of familial hyperparathyroidism have been asymptomatic, having been discovered when the members of an affected family were screened for hyper-

Fig. 38-39. X-ray of the abdomen of a patient with primary hyperparathyroidism, showing bilateral staghorn calculi with severe osteoporosis, scoliosis, and splenic calcification. The patient's chemical studies are shown in Fig. 38-32. A parathyroid adenoma was removed, and this was followed by chemical and clinical improvement.

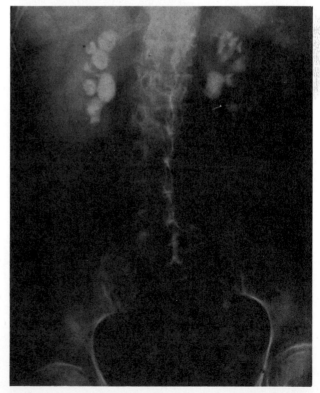

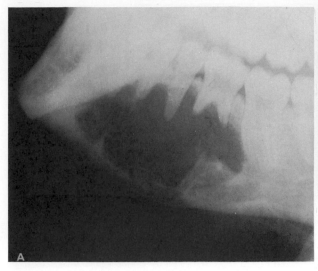

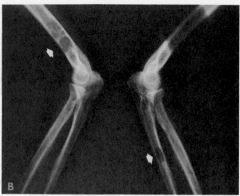

Fig. 38-40. Bone cysts and tumors in hyperparathyroidism. *A.* Bone cyst of the lower jaw. *B.* Cysts of long bones.

calcemia. In a recent study, in 11 percent of families, other members were proved to have primary hyperparathyroidism as well. Thus, a familial occurrence of primary hyperparathyroidism may be more common than previously considered.

Hyperparathyroidism in Children. Hyperparathyroidism is a rare occurrence before puberty. A few such cases have been reported, including the neonates mentioned above under Familial Hyperparathyroidism.

Fig. 38-41. X-rays of the fingers in primary and secondary hyperparathyroidism. *A.* Secondary hyperparathyroidism. Note the intense subperiosteal resorption of bone. This usually is most prominent on the radial side of the middle and distal phalanges of the index and middle fingers. *B.* Primary hyperparathyroidism. Many patients with primary hyperparathyroidism have normal hand films with conventional radiographic techniques. With *fine-detail* radiography, subtle cases of subperiosteal bone resorption can be recognized. Mild subperiosteal bone resorption (arrows) of middle phalanx in a patient with a parathyroid adenoma. (*From H. K. Genant et al., Radiology, 109:513, 1973.*)

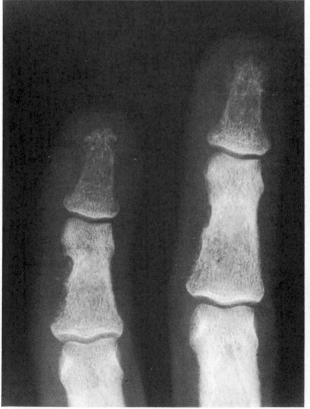

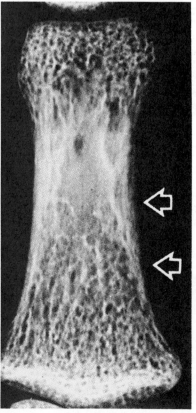

A   *B*

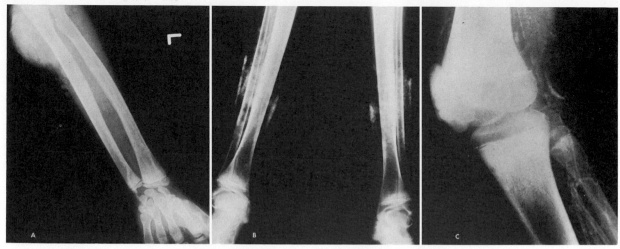

Fig. 38-42. X-ray studies of a child with chronic renal failure and vitamin D intoxication. Note the severe ectopic calcification in the soft tissues. *A.* The olecranon bursa and subcutaneous tissues of the left arm. *B.* The subcutaneous tissues and muscle of the lower leg. *C.* The patellar bursa and the popliteal and tibial arteries.

Apart from the neonates, there have been over 35 cases of hyperparathyroidism in children reported in the literature. The ages have ranged from three to sixteen. Over 80 percent of them have been between the ages of ten and fourteen, the disease being very rare before the age of ten.

The symptoms are the same as those recorded in the adult, including those referable to severe bone involvement. Duodenal ulcer has been reported, and joint abnormalities have occurred in 17 percent of the patients. Blindness was recorded in one case.

Acute hypercalcemic crisis has been recorded in neonates and in older children, with serum calcium values of over 20 mg/100 ml. The serum calcium values in children have generally been somewhat higher than those seen in adults.

Pregnancy. Fertility does not seem to be greatly depressed in hyperparathyroidism, and labor and delivery are not influenced by it. The birth weight of infants born to mothers who are suffering from hyperparathyroidism is low, being less than 3,000 Gm in 50 percent of the cases. There is a high frequency of stillbirth, neonatal death, and neonatal tetany.

In 1962, Ludwig reviewed the literature and described the clinical course of 40 gestations of the 21 women who were recognized at that time as having primary hyperparathyroidism while they were pregnant. Serious fetal complications were noted in half these pregnancies. Stillbirths, spontaneous abortions, and neonatal deaths occurred in 31 percent and neonatal tetany in 19 percent of these instances. Delmonico and associates, analyzing the 15 pregnancies of 13 hyperparathyroid women reported since that time who were not operated upon, found that 80 percent of these gestations were complicated. Spontaneous abortions and neonatal deaths occurred in 27 percent; 55 percent of the newborns suffered significant hypocalcemia soon after birth.

It appears that the diagnosis of primary hyperparathyroidism associated with pregnancy is rarely made. It is not uncommon, in fact, for this disease to be recognized in the mother only retrospectively following the appearance of hypocalcemia in the newborn infant. A potential difficulty in diagnosis may be the fact that during the normal pregnancy a physiologic decrease of maternal serum calcium concentration occurs. Thus, even borderline high values of serum calcium obtained from the pregnant woman should be considered to be of utmost significance.

Perhaps of even greater importance is the apparent lack of awareness by many physicians that hyperparathyroidism can occur during pregnancy. Serial calcium concentrations should be performed as part of all routine prenatal care. The diagnosis of maternal primary hyperparathyroidism can be made with virtual certainty when an elevated serum

Fig. 38-43. X-ray of the abdomen showing nephrocalcinosis. While this change sometimes occurs in hyperparathyroidism, it is not diagnostic of this condition.

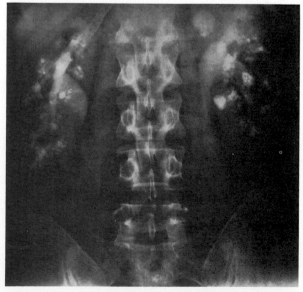

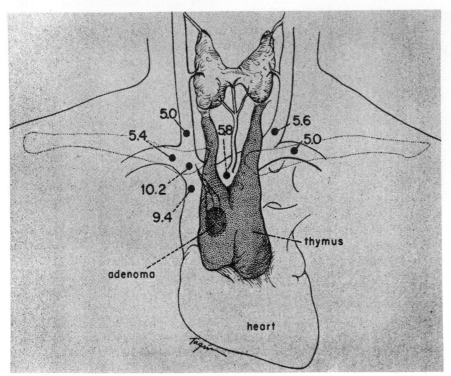

Fig. 38-44. Radioimmunoassay of blood samples obtained during venous catheterization of a patient with primary hyperparathyroidism. Localized increases in PTH values are demonstrated in the right innominate vein and the superior vena cava (10.2 and 9.4 mμg/ml). At operation a parathyroid adenoma was found in the thymus gland. Its venous drainage was to the right innominate vein and corresponded to the area of elevated PTH levels. (*From R. E. Reitz et al., N Engl J Med, 281:349, 1969.*)

Fig. 38-45. Plasma PTH concentrations in samples obtained at different points in the circulation. Veins are jugular (*J*), innominate (*I*), superior vena cava (*SVC*), superior thyroid veins (*STV*), and inferior thyroid veins (*ITV*). Samples also were obtained from the medial and lateral branches of the right inferior thyroid vein (*ITV—M* and *ITV—L*). Sites of sampling are indicated by • ; adjacent numbers indicate PTH concentration in mμg/ml. These data indicate an adenoma of the right lower parathyroid gland. Elevated PTH concentrations in samples from both sides of the neck indicate parathyroid hyperplasia. (*From J. T. Potts, Jr., et al., Am J Med, 50:639, 1971.*)

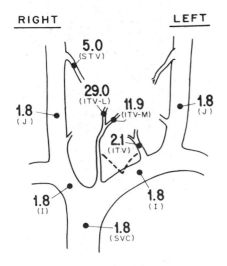

calcium concentration is accompanied at the same time by an elevated serum parathyroid hormone level, since ectopic hyperparathyroidism from occult malignancy is rare in these young women.

When maternal hyperparathyroidism is diagnosed during pregnancy, Kaplan feels that the proper therapy is parathyroidectomy. Optimally, the operation should be performed during the second trimester of pregnancy, since accidental abortion is lessened during this period. Furthermore, with correction of the hypercalcemic state at this early time, parathyroid development of the fetus can proceed normally.

The results in patients so managed are far better than those reported without operation. Only one instance of neonatal death and another of neonatal hypocalcemia occurred. Several recent studies clarify the pathophysiology of maternal hyperparathyroidism. It is known that both ionized and total calcium concentrations are somewhat higher in the fetal than in the maternal circulation. While calcium ion moves freely across the placenta, serum parathyroid hormone cannot cross from mother to fetus. In primary hyperparathyroidism the elevated serum calcium concentration of the mother results in an increased circulating serum calcium concentration in the fetus. Hypercalcemia, per se, may result in toxicity to the fetus. Also, it clearly causes suppression of fetal parathyroid function and possibly of parathyroid development. Following birth, hypocalcemia will occur in the newborn if its own parathyroid function is inadequate. Parathyroidectomy performed during early pregnancy permits restoration of the normal fetal calcium homeostasis and thus should eliminate this neonatal hypocalcemia.

Although there are other conditions which can cause neonatal tetany besides hyperparathyroidism in the mother, it is extremely important to obtain serum calcium and phosphorus values on mothers of children with neonatal tetany. This may be the best way that this cause for neonatal tetany can be definitely established, since the calcium level in neonates with tetany will be low whatever the cause of the tetany.

Multiple Endocrinopathies, Type 1 (M.E.A.-Type 1). The glands involved in the *endocrine polyglandular syndrome, Type 1,* are the parathyroid, the pancreatic islets, and the pituitary. The syndrome tends to fall into four main classifications: pancreatic beta cell tumor, hypercalcemia, Zollinger-Ellison syndrome, and acromegaly.

Pancreatic Beta Cell Tumor. In these patients the pancreatic beta cell tumor secretes insulin and produces symptoms of hypoglycemia. Rarely, there also may be parathyroid hyperfunction which gives rise to an elevated serum calcium level and renal stones in some patients. The pituitary tumors are usually asymptomatic. Peptic ulcers are sometimes present in these patients, but they are rarely intractable and usually respond to the resection of the parathyroid and pancreatic tumors. For those which do not respond, the usual ulcer treatment is effective. Total gastrectomy is not required.

Hypercalcemia. The second most frequent group is composed of patients in whom the pancreatic and pituitary tumors are nonfunctioning and who have symptoms of mild hyperparathyroidism. Peptic ulcers also occur in this group of patients and, again, respond readily to the usual therapy.

Zollinger-Ellison Syndrome. The third group of patients have pancreatic islet cell tumors of the non-beta cell type and are associated with severe enteritis or intractable ulceration. The parathyroid tumors are usually functionally hyperactive when present, and the patients may have hypercalcemia, whereas the pituitary tumors generally tend to be asymptomatic. Total gastrectomy is required for control of the severe ulcer diathesis.

Wilson (1973) has found that 27 percent of 677 patients with sufficient data for study in the Zollinger-Ellison Tumor Registry have one or more manifestations of multiple endocrine adenomatosis. Twenty percent have parathyroid disease documented either at neck operation or at autopsy. Our group has reported that some patients with the Zollinger-Ellison syndrome have elevated PTH levels despite normal or low serum calcium concentrations. We postulate that the parathyroid disease associated with Zollinger-Ellison syndrome may be due to secondary hyperparathyroidism (malabsorption) in some cases.

The pituitary tumors in the foregoing types of endocrine

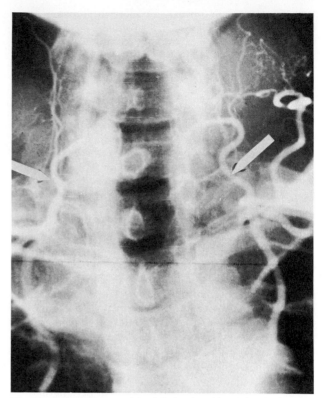

Fig. 38-46. Arteriogram of the inferior thyroid arteries, both sides being visualized simultaneously. The vessels are in their normal position. The patient was found to have hyperparathyroidism due to chief cell hyperplasia. Neither artery is larger than the other, and no displacement seems to have occurred. The arteries are indicated by the arrows. In some cases arteriograms result in a "tumor blush" because of the vascularity of the enlarged parathyroid glands.

polyglandular syndrome are generally made up of more than one cell type or else are chromaphobe adenomas and usually are nonfunctioning. The parathyroid glands show a variety of pathologic features and are characterized by having multiple gland involvement. Most cases of MEA-1 are found to have chief cell hyperplasia of the parathyroids when all glands are examined. Despite the elevated serum calcium levels which frequently accompany this disease the patients rarely show skeletal involvement, and renal complications are uncommon.

Acromegaly. There is a fourth type of multiple adenomas which consists of a pituitary tumor producing acromegaly with parathyroid and pancreatic islet cell tumors. Patients with this syndrome have died with perforated peptic ulcers, and there have been cases of acromegaly in which there was clinical hyperparathyroidism with impaired renal function. The early cases are well summarized by Underdahl et al.

General Considerations. The first account of chronic polyglandular syndrome, type 1, was given by Erdheim in 1903 and consists of a rather sketchy mention of a patient with acromegaly, eosinophilic adenoma of the pituitary, and four enlarged parathyroids. The first report of pituitary, parathyroid, and pancreatic islet cell tumors in combination was by Cushing and Davidoff in 1927, whereas the first report of acromegaly and clinical hyperparathyroidism was in 1948. Involvement of pituitary, parathyroids, and islet cells occurs in 34 percent, pituitary and parathyroids in 25 percent, pituitary and islet cells in 19 percent, parathyroids and islet cells in 22 percent. Twenty-five percent of the patients have peptic ulcer.

The syndromes of polyglandular disease are almost always associated with chief cell hyperplasia of the parathyroids but at times may consist of almost every conceivable combination of adenomas and hyperplasia. A dominant inheritance pattern seems to be characteristic of both chief cell hyperplasia and polyendocrine disease. Familial hyperparathyroidism is not uncommonly a part of the endocrine polyglandular syndrome, as evidenced by a large number of cases collected by Jackson and Boonstra.

Multiple Endocrinopathies, Type 2. Medullary carcinoma of the thyroid may be associated with all or part of a syndrome called *multiple endocrine neoplasia,* type 2, *familial medullary carcinoma syndrome,* or sometimes *Sipple's syndrome.* In its entirety it consists of pheochromocytomas (often bilateral), typical mucosal neuromas, and parathyroid gland abnormalities. Occasional individuals also have a Marfanoid habitus, coarse features, and ganglioneuromatous changes of the plexuses of Meissner and Auerbach.

The serum calcium level is almost always normal in these individuals but occasionally may be high or low. The parathyroid glands in this familial form of medullary carcinoma almost always demonstrate chief cell hyperplasia if they are abnormal. While it is attractive to think of the parathyroid gland abnormalities as compensatory for the calcitonin secreted by the medullary cancers, recent evidence suggests that they may be genetic in origin. Serum PTH is often elevated in cases of familial medullary carcinomas, but it is normal in sporadic cases of this same tumor despite similar high circulating levels of calcitonin. Renal stones have been noted occasionally in both normocalcemic and hypercalcemic individuals with this syndrome.

Hyperparathyroidism, Gout, Pseudogout, and Arthralgia. Gout has been observed from time to time in association with hyperparathyroidism. In most of the patients there has been some renal damage which might have interfered with the excretion of uric acid and thus produced the hyperuricemia. Uric acid calculi have been seen in hyperparathyroidism.

Other types of joint disease also occur in association with hyperparathyroidism. Sharp and Kelly have reported an acute monoarticular arthralgia occurring after the surgical correction of hyperparathyroidism. In each of their two cases the right knee was involved, and the patient had a leukocytosis, joint infusion, and low-grade fever. Sharp and Kelly felt that they had ruled out rheumatoid and infectious arthritis. This kind of arthralgia seems to occur when the serum phosphorous is at its highest, and it is associated with hyperuricemia, presumably because the tubular mechanisms for the excretion of phosphorus and uric acid are similar. Hyperuricemia can thus occur both

in hyperparathyroidism and in hypoparathyroidism. The arthritis described here is a transient one and disappears in a few days. It seems clear that some cases of hyperuricemia and gout in hyperparathyroidism are coincidental or due to renal failure and not related directly to the hyperparathyroidism. Some patients with hyperparathyroidism have symptoms of gout without hyperuricemia.

It has recently been noted that *pseudogout*—the intraarticular deposition of calcium pyrophosphate crystals—is seen in association with hyperparathyroidism. In three of six patients with pseudogout and hyperparathyroidism, pseudogout was the initial clinical manifestation of the hyperparathyroidism. This suggests that all patients with pseudogout should be carefully screened for hyperparathyroidism.

DIFFERENTIAL DIAGNOSIS. Some of the features of the differential diagnosis of hypercalcemia are shown in Table 38-7.

Parathyroid Disease versus Extraparathyroid PTH-producing Tumor. It may be very difficult to make the differential diagnosis between a parathyroid adenoma and an extraparathyroid PTH-producing tumor, since the effects on the patient are identical. The known presence of tumors which are likely to produce this syndrome—bronchogenic or small cell carcinomas of the lung, hypernephromas, hepatomas, epidermoid cancer, bladder, ovary, uterus, vulva, pancreas, liver, and lymphatic malignant tumors—should suggest this possibility. The history, physical findings, and appropriate x-ray studies may establish the diagnosis. As discussed earlier, ectopic production of PTH-like fragments may be diagnosed by radioimmunoassay by certain antisera which react with these substances. The ultimate diagnosis may require neck exploration and the demonstration of normal or atrophic parathyroid glands. In cases in which the differential diagnosis cannot be made with certainty it may be better, at times, to explore the neck than to miss the diagnosis of primary parathyroid overactivity.

Secondary Hyperparathyroidism. What usually distinguishes secondary hyperparathyroidism from the primary disease is that the serum calcium level is not elevated and the patient demonstrates an underlying condition which has caused the hyperparathyroidism, frequently chronic renal failure. In secondary hyperparathyroidism, the serum calcium is usually low, in fact. If this parameter becomes elevated, this is referred to as tertiary hyperparathyroidism (see further on). It may be extremely difficult or impossible to distinguish primary hyperparathyroidism with advanced renal failure from tertiary hyperparathyroidism, in which the renal failure was primary and led to secondary hyperparathyroidism and later to hypercalcemia. In both instances either chief cell hyperplasia alone or an adenoma and chief cell hyperplasia may be present.

When a patient with secondary hyperparathyroidism is operated upon and the parathyroids are removed, they invariably show chief cell hyperplasia, often with nests of oxyphil cells interspersed throughout the gland.

Vitamin D Poisoning. Vitamin D intoxication can be suspected when this vitamin has been administered in excess. The patients tend to have an increased, rather than de-

Table 38-7. THE DIFFERENTIAL DIAGNOSIS OF SOME DISEASES PRODUCING HYPERCALCEMIA, HYPERCALCINURIA, OR BONE CHANGES

Disease	Serum			Urine		Special tests and criteria	Parathyroid hormone
	Calcium	Phosphate	Alkaline phosphatase	Calcium	Phosphate		
Primary hyperparathyroidism	Increased	Decreased*	Normal or increased	Increased	Increased	TRP measurements	Increased
Secondary hyperparathyroidism (renal failure)	Decreased	Increased	Normal or increased	Decreased	Decreased	Chronic renal failure present	Increased
Vitamin D intoxication	Increased	Increased	Decreased	Increased	Increased	Ectopic calcification present	Decreased
Metastatic carcinoma	Increased	Normal	Normal or increased	Increased	Normal	X-rays showing metastases	Decreased†
Multiple myeloma	Increased	Normal	Normal	Normal or increased	Normal or decreased	X-rays showing lesions Bence-Jones protein present Increased plasma globulin	Decreased
Sarcoidosis	Increased	Normal or decreased	Normal or increased	Increased	Increased	Increased plasma globulin Hepatomegaly—biopsy Splenomegaly Kveim test positive	Decreased
Idiopathic hypercalcemia of infancy	Increased	Increased	Normal	Increased	Decreased	Presence of mental retardation Increased blood cholesterol Hypersensitivity to vitamin D	Decreased
Milk-alkali syndrome	Increased	Normal*	Normal	Normal or decreased	Normal or decreased	History of milk and alkali intake Renal insufficiency often present	Decreased
Paget's disease	Normal or increased	Normal	Increased	Increased	Normal	Bone changes on x-ray Serum calcium reduced by mobilization	Normal or decreased
Idiopathic hypercalcinuria	Normal	Decreased	Normal	Increased	Normal or increased	Renal calculi may be present	Normal

*Increased when renal failure supervenes.
†In ectopic hyperparathyroidism, PTH is also elevated.

creased, phosphate level in the serum. Metastatic calcification is much more common in vitamin D intoxication than in hyperparathyroidism (see Fig. 38-42). It is somewhat more apt to occur in the presence of renal failure. In vitamin D intoxication small yellowish deposits may be present underneath the fingernails, along the outer borders of the lips, in the skin, and in the corneal conjunctiva. Serum PTH level is low.

Metastatic Cancer. In metastatic cancer the phosphate level in the serum is usually not depressed. The cancer is usually of breast, kidney, lung, thyroid, or prostatic origin and may already have been established by previous procedures. Serum PTH is low unless the tumor secretes ectopic parathyroid hormone-like fragments. The bony involvement usually can be detected by x-ray. The plasma calcium level will usually fall in response to cortisone infusion. Sometimes the lesions in the bone may look quite similar to those seen with primary or secondary hyperparathyroidism as shown in Figs. 38-36 and 38-37.

Multiple Myeloma. This entity usually shows sharp, punched-out areas of destruction in the bone, generally well seen in the skull. At times rather similar lesions can be produced by hyperparathyroidism (see Fig. 38-36). The Bence-Jones protein is present in about 50 percent of the patients, and the plasma globulin level is high. Plasma cells are present in the bone marrow. The alkaline phosphatase level is usually not elevated. Serum PTH is low and the plasma calcium level is decreased with cortisol infusion.

Sarcoidosis. Hypercalcemia in sarcoidosis was first described by Harrell and Fisher. It occurs in about a third of the cases. Although bone destruction may be present in sarcoidosis, it is apparently not the basis for the hypercalcemia. There appears instead to be a hypersensitivity to vitamin D in some individuals with sarcoid, and exposure to sunlight or administration of vitamin D will produce hypercalcemia in the patients manifesting this phenomenon. Since band keratopathy of the eyes, bone cysts, renal calculi, nephrocalcinosis, and polyuria can occur, the incorrect diagnosis of hyperparathyroidism is sometimes made and neck exploration carried out.

The presence of an increased plasma globulin, hepatomegaly, and splenomegaly should suggest the correct diagnosis. In over 50 percent of the patients with sarcoidosis the Kveim reaction will be positive. This test consists of the intracutaneous injection of a heat-sterilized suspension of spleen or lymph node from patients with sarcoid. A positive test is indicated by the production of a papulonodular lesion with epithelioid tubercles demonstrated by biopsy 4 to 6 weeks after the initial injection. The administration of 150 mg of cortisone daily for 10 to 14 days reduces the serum calcium to normal (Dent test). A positive diagnosis may be established by biopsy of the liver, lymph nodes, or, when present, skin nodules. Serum PTH level is low.

Sarcoidosis and hyperparathyroidism may coexist in the same patient, the diagnosis being suspected when the serum calcium level fails to fall with cortisone administration.

Idiopathic Hypercalcemia of Infancy. This syndrome is believed to be due to a hypersensitivity to vitamin D, such as that seen in sarcoidosis. It occurs in infants who have mental retardation, an elevated serum cholesterol level, and hypercalcemia. The serum calcium level falls with the administration of cortisone.

The Milk-Alkali Syndrome. Burnett et al. described a syndrome in which hypercalcemia developed in patients ingesting large amounts of milk and absorbable alkali—such as sodium bicarbonate, usually for peptic ulcer. This is most apt to occur when there is some degree of renal insufficiency. The serum phosphate level is normal or elevated rather than low. Renal calculi and nephrocalcinosis may be present. Patients with primary hyperparathyroidism may develop renal failure, an elevated serum phosphate level, and peptic ulceration, at which point the picture may be difficult to distinguish from the milk-alkali syndrome. The history of ingestion of large amounts of milk and alkali, the improvement noted when these are stopped, and the absence of hypercalcinuria distinguish the latter condition. Serum PTH is low in this condition.

Paget's Disease (Osteitis Deformans). Paget's disease may occasionally be associated with an elevated serum calcium level. X-rays will show the characteristic lesion, usually in the pelvis, lower extremities, or skull. The blood calcium concentration may be normal, but hypercalcemia can develop, particularly if the patient is immobilized. Immobilization leads to disuse atrophy and osteoporosis with a diminished use of calcium for bone repair. Since the localized bone destruction which is the primary underlying feature of this disease continues, there is a net loss of calcium from the bone. The rate at which calcium enters the plasma may exceed the rate at which the kidney can excrete it, thus leading to hypercalcemia.

Paget's disease and primary hyperparathyroidism may coexist, making it difficult to establish the latter diagnosis. The measurement of PTH (not elevated in Paget's disease) and the failure of cortisone and mobilization to reduce the blood calcium should suggest the correct diagnosis.

Idiopathic Hypercalcinuria. This syndrome is characterized by hypercalcinuria, hypophosphatemia, and stone formation in the presence of a normal serum calcium value. It occurs almost exclusively in men. The bones are normal, and the alkaline phosphatase level is not elevated. The cause is unknown. However, hyperabsorption of calcium from the intestine may be responsible for some cases. If an elevated serum calcium level develops, studies for hyperparathyroidism should be carried out. This condition has been treated successfully by thiazide administration, which lowers the urinary calcium output.

Hyperthyroidism. Hypercalcemia occurs on rare occasions in association with hyperthyroidism. The serum calcium may return to normal when the hyperthyroidism is cured. Since hyperparathyroidism may coexist with hyperthyroidism, it is important to determine whether this may not be the cause of the hypercalcemia in any particular case.

Osteomalacia. In osteomalacia there is a failure to mineralize the skeletal matrix, leading to bone changes that might be confused with hyperparathyroidism. Since in osteomalacia the serum calcium level is not elevated and the urinary calcium and phosphate excretion is low rather than high, the conditions are fairly easily differentiated.

Thiazides. Hypercalcemia has been reported with increasing frequency in patients receiving benzothiadiazine diuretics. Hypercalcemia resulting solely from these diuretics is almost always mild. After cessation of the diuretic the serum calcium value usually returns to normal in less than 1 month. The thiazide diuretics can aggravate hypercalcemia in primary hyperparathyroidism. Thus when possible these diuretics should be stopped and the patient studied 1 to 2 months later. In patients with hypercalcemia greater than 12 mg/100 ml, this may not be practical, especially if the cause of the hypercalcemia is clear.

TREATMENT. Indications for Operation. Patients with primary hyperparathyroidism in whom the diagnosis has been established with relative certainty should definitely be subjected to parathyroid surgical treatment if they have either bony or renal manifestations of the disease, since these will almost inevitably become worse with time. The urgency is greater the higher the calcium level, the most impelling example being the patient with hypercalcemic crisis. Treatment is also indicated if peptic ulcer or pancreatitis is secondary to the hyperparathyroidism. Hypertension may or may not be benefited by parathyroidectomy, depending upon its relation to permanent renal damage which has been incurred by long-standing hypercalcemia.

As newer methods for establishing the diagnosis of hyperparathyroidism have developed, more and more cases are operated upon at an earlier stage. There is no question that it is advantageous to prevent the severe renal and bone changes which will eventuate if the patient is not operated upon. There may be an occasional case, however, in which the elevation of serum calcium level is so slight as to make a definitive diagnosis of the disease difficult. There is probably no harm in watching such cases for a few years until such time as the diagnosis can be established. The ability to measure PTH in the blood by immunoassay in an accurate and predictable fashion will facilitate early establishment of the diagnosis and will effect an improvement in the criteria for selection for operation. The mortality for this operation is so extremely low that unless the patient presents an unusually poor risk, operation should be undertaken when any of the indications listed above present themselves.

Some completely asymptomatic patients with minimal hypercalcemia (<11 mg/100 ml) are now being followed without surgery at the Mayo Clinic even though the diagnosis of primary hyperparathyroidism has been definitively made. At the end of a 5-year study period, 20 percent of these patients were operated upon because of complications attributable to the disease or a rise in serum calcium levels to above 11.0 mg/100 ml. Another 20 percent were dropped from the study because of lack of cooperation in the follow-up program. No criteria are evident that would permit identification of those patients who will ultimately require parathyroid operation. They have concluded that surgical treatment is correct in this asymptomatic group in most cases. We follow this same recommendation.

Treatment of Hypercalcemic Crisis. Hypercalcemia is a serious and potentially lethal complication of many diseases. The approach to therapy must be tempered by an appreciation of the underlying disease state and whether or not emergency reduction of serum calcium is required. Individual tolerance to hypercalcemia is variable and may reflect the rapidity with which the concentration of serum calcium rises. It is not uncommon, for example, to observe nearly asymptomatic patients with hyperparathyroidism with a serum calcium of 15 mg/100 ml yet virtually moribund patients with rapidly progressive cancer have a similar serum calcium. A very good review of this subject was written by Goldsmith.

General Support. Since patients with hypercalcemia often have had anorexia, nausea, and vomiting for some time prior to seeking medical assistance, severe dehydration and oliguria are common presenting features. Thus perhaps the most important treatment is restoration of the extracellular fluid volume with 0.9% sodium chloride. Hypokalemia is frequently present and may require replacement of large amounts of potassium for correction.

Calcium and digitalis are synergistic in effect on the myocardium and conducting system. Hence the fully digitalized patient may manifest digitalis toxicity if he becomes hypercalcemic. Thus it may be necessary to reduce or stop digitalis. Similarly, if digitalization is necessary in a hypercalcemic patient, a lower dose is generally required.

Treatment of the Underlying Disorder. An early assessment of the underlying disorder is essential so that specific therapy may be begun. Because of the increased hazard of general anesthesia in the ill, severely hypercalcemic patient it is unwise to rush into emergency surgery. Since specific medical therapy for hypercalcemia is generally adequate, it is no longer necessary to perform parathyroidectomy as an emergency procedure. Rather, dangerous levels of hypercalcemia should be controlled prior to surgery. Specific therapy after control of hypercalcemia would include surgical removal of neoplasms, radiation, cytotoxic drugs, corticosteroids, or withdrawal of milk and alkali, estrogens, thiazides, or vitamin D as appropriate.

Therapy of the Hypercalcemia Per Se (See Table 38-8). *Gastrointestinal Measures.* Attempts to lower intestinal absorption of calcium by use of a low-calcium diet are reasonably effective only for sarcoidosis or vitamin D intoxication. Cortisone appears to inhibit calcium absorption, which is related to vitamin D mechanisms.

Renal Excretion and Dialysis. In most instances, calcium excretion parallels sodium excretion. Hence mechanisms which increase sodium excretion are effective in lowering serum calcium levels. Isotonic saline solution is excellent in this regard but is limited by the cardiac and renal status of the patient. The use of furosemide or ethacrynic acid gives excellent results alone or with saline infusion. At present, furosemide with saline infusion is the treatment of choice for hypercalcemia. Fluid and electrolyte balance must be carefully monitored when these agents are used. Sodium sulfate does not seem to be better than sodium chloride and may be more dangerous. Therefore, it is rarely used.

EDTA chelates ionized calcium and also increases urinary excretion of calcium by forming soluble complexes. Its effects are difficult to monitor, and it produces pain at the site of infusion. It should be used only for emergency

Table 38-8. USUAL DOSES OF HYPOCALCEMIC AGENTS

Drug	Route	Dosage	Reported complications	Contraindications
Sodium chloride solution (isotonic)	Intravenous	1 liter every 3–4 hr	Pulmonary edema	Congestive heart failure, renal insufficiency, hypertension
Sodium sulfate solution (isotonic)	Intravenous	3 liters over 9 hr	Pulmonary edema, hypernatremia	Congestive heart failure, renal insufficiency, hypertension
Furosemide	Intravenous	100 mg/hr	Volume depletion, hypokalemia	Renal insufficiency
EDTA	Intravenous	50 mg/kg body weight over 4–6 hr	Renal failure, hypotension	Renal insufficiency
Cortisone	Oral or parenteral	150 mg/day	Hypercorticism	Emergency reduction of serum calcium required
Mithramycin	Intravenous	25 μg/kg body weight	Hemorrhage, thrombocytopenia, nausea, vomiting	Bleeding disorder, renal insufficiency, liver impairment
Phosphate	Intravenous	1 mM*/kg body weight over 6–8 hr	Extraskeletal calcification, hypocalcemia	Renal insufficiency, hyperphosphatemia
	Oral	1–2 mM*/kg body weight daily		
Calcitonin	Parenteral	1–5 MRC units/kg body weight/day	Nausea, vomiting	Thrombotic disorders

*1 mM of phosphate is equivalent to 31 mg of phosphorus.
SOURCE: Modified from W. N. Suki, J. J. Yium, M. Von Minden et al., Acute Treatment of Hypercalcemia with Furosemide, *N Engl J Med,* **283:**836–840, 1970.

reduction of life-threatening hypercalcemia, since doses in excess of 3 Gm have produced renal insufficiency.

If renal function is poor, temporary reduction of hypercalcemia may be obtained by peritoneal or hemodialysis.

Skeletal Factors—Reduction of Bone Resorption. Cortisone is especially useful in treatment of sarcoidosis, vitamin D intoxication, myeloma, and various leukemias or lymphomas. The effect is often slow; a lag period of 7 to 10 days is not exceptional. One of the major drawbacks to long-term therapy is the production of osteoporosis.

Phosphate given orally or intravenously has been demonstrated to be effective in lowering serum calcium levels. Intravenously administered phosphate may be risky;

when not used precisely as directed, death has resulted. Phosphate given orally is safe and efficacious but slower in effect. When given in excess, diarrhea will occur.

Calcitonin, by inhibiting bone resorption, should be the ideal emergency drug for treatment of hypercalcemia. Porcine calcitonin has proved far less effective than was predicted. Salmon calcitonin, which is available commercially, is more efficacious in human beings but has not been very useful in this regard.

Finally, mithramycin, a cytotoxic drug originally used

Fig. 38-47. Incision for parathyroidectomy. The dotted lines indicate the extension of the incision used for mediastinal exploration. The deep fascia is divided in the midline, and the strap muscles are divided.

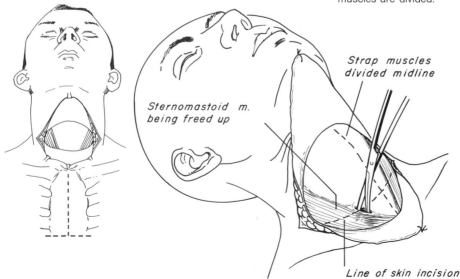

Strap muscles divided midline

Sternomastoid m. being freed up

Line of skin incision

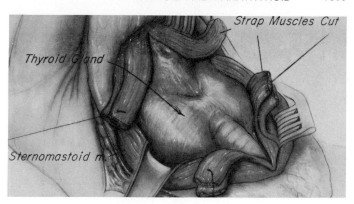

Fig. 38-48. Strap muscles are cut and retracted, and the gland is exposed. This may facilitate the exposure.

for therapy of testicular tumors, is very effective in reducing serum calcium concentrations but takes 12 to 24 hours to do so. Side effects are few when given as an infusion every 5 days at a dose of $25\mu g/kg$. In a recent study this schedule was shown to be effective in controlling the hypercalcemia of breast cancer. At present, we reserve this drug for cases of malignant tumor, although others have used it for benign disease.

Operative Technique. In general, parathyroid surgery requires an unrushed, meticulous dissection with a bloodless field. Intratracheal anesthesia with the neck somewhat hyperextended by means of a small pad between the shoulder blades is usually preferred for parathyroid exploration. The entire operating table may be tilted so that the head is somewhat elevated, thus diminishing bleeding.

The platysma muscle is elevated with the skin flap, and the superior flap is dissected to the hyoid superiorly and the upper border of the sternum inferiorly. The skin flaps may be held apart by a self-retaining retractor or by sutures, and the deep cervical fascia is divided longitudinally in the midline from the hyoid bone to the suprasternal notch. Others prefer to divide the sternohyoid and sternothyroid muscles routinely at the junction of the upper and middle third to facilitate exposure of the gland (Figs. 38-47 and 38-48); however, we usually do not find this necessary.

Locating the Parathyroid Glands. The thyroid gland is mobilized by dividing the middle thyroid veins and rolling the lobe of the thyroid anteriorly and mediad. The recurrent laryngeal nerve is then identified. The landmarks for this are the groove between the trachea and esophagus, and the inferior thyroid artery. The recurrent nerve may also be identified at the inferior cornu of the thyroid cartilage, as described by Wang. The areolar tissue is cleared from around the nerve, and the inferior thyroid artery is cleaned off and preserved at the same time. The best place to begin the search for a parathyroid adenoma is at the point where the recurrent laryngeal nerve crosses behind the inferior thyroid artery. The adenomas are very frequently tucked down under the lateral lobe of the thyroid in a little space alongside the esophagus lying just slightly posterior to the groove between the esophagus and the trachea or thyroid cartilage (Figs. 38-49 and 38-50). Tracing the branches of the inferior thyroid artery may sometimes be helpful in locating the hyperfunctioning parathyroid gland, since this vessel supplies the parathyroid adenoma with blood in

nearly 90 percent of the cases (Figs. 38-51 and 38-52). The adenoma can sometimes be located by tracing a branch of the inferior thyroid artery to its termination in the gland. After a preliminary search in this area the inferior parathyroid will usually be found just below the point at which the recurrent laryngeal nerve intersects the inferior thyroid artery. The superior parathyroid will often be found within 1 or 2 cm above this point, usually on a little prominence of the posterior surface of the thyroid.

An adenoma, particularly one of the lower gland, can be tucked well behind the thyroid or between the trachea and esophagus, so that it is not readily apparent until the thyroid has been rotated forward and the fatty tissue in this area has been gently teased away (Fig. 38-53). The adenoma is not usually bound down to the surrounding tissues, however, and usually can be popped out of its hiding place. It is generally red-brown, at times yellow-brown, smooth, and with a surface which is vascular and bleeds easily when rubbed or cut. On rare occasions, particularly when it lies beneath the capsule of the thyroid, it may look extremely similar to thyroid tissue itself.

Once the provisional location of the glands has been established, the procedure is repeated on the other side. We

Fig. 38-49. The middle thyroid veins are divided, and the lateral lobe of the thyroid is retracted anteriorly and mediad. The recurrent laryngeal nerve is exposed in the tracheoesophageal groove, and the inferior thyroid artery is dissected out and preserved. The inferior parathyroid is usually located just below the intersection of these two structures and is supplied by a branch of the inferior thyroid artery.

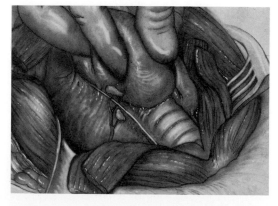

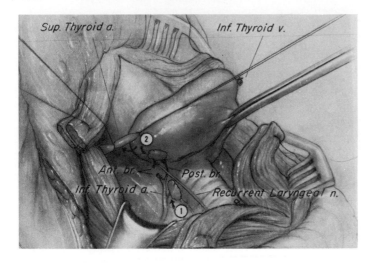

Fig. 38-50. It may be necessary to divide a branch of the inferior artery or to divide the superior thyroid artery to identify the upper parathyroid (2). The lower parathyroid gland (1) is not infrequently opposite the lower pole of the thyroid or below this and can sometimes be identified in the fatty tissue just behind the divided strap muscles.

make it a policy to identify by biopsy and frozen section all parathyroid glands which are questionable in appearance before removing any of them. This is to protect against circumstances which have been reported in which three enlarged parathyroid glands were resected as they were encountered, only to find that the patient had no fourth gland. When all the parathyroids cannot be found adjacent to the thyroid gland, further search is facilitated by dividing the superior pole vessels on the side on which the upper gland has not been identified and following the branch which joins the inferior artery to identify the blood supply of this gland. The lower parathyroid is not infrequently located below the lower pole of the thyroid, and it may be found by pulling the divided sternothyroid muscle superiorly and laterally and looking in the areolar tissue along the posterior surface of the muscle. The entire space leading down to the superior mediastinum should be carefully searched in order to find a missing inferior gland. The upper part of the thymus should also be removed if possible, since the lower parathyroid may be embedded in this tissue.

The upper gland may sometimes be found in unusual positions as well. It may be several centimeters above the upper pole of the thyroid gland. Furthermore, the retro-

Fig. 38-51. *A.* Blood supply of the parathyroids. *B.* The relation of the inferior thyroid artery to the recurrent laryngeal nerve.

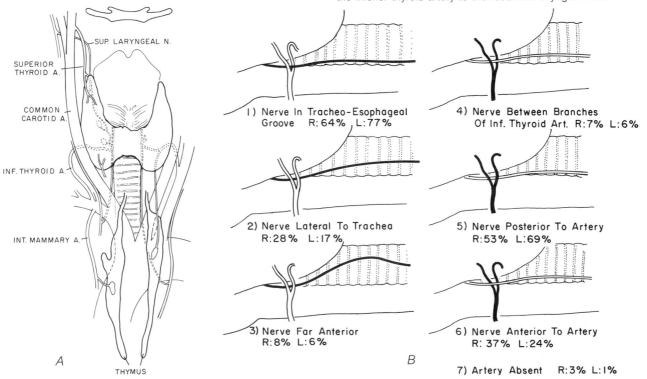

esophageal space of the lower neck and upper mediastinum should be explored, since adenomas of the superior parathyroid glands occasionally may be found in this location.

Most parathyroid glands can be found by utilizing a systematic, meticulous dissection. We have not found the injection of toluidine blue at operation to be helpful. This dye is said to selectively color the parathyroid glands blue or purple and thus to aid in their identification. Unfortunately, occasional cardiac arrhythmias and bone marrow depression have been reported. Furthermore, most experienced parathyroid surgeons have learned to recognize parathyroid glands, so that this technique does not add greatly to their efficiency.

Extent of Operation. Several different approaches regarding the extent of parathyroid resection for primary hyperparathyroidism have been proposed. Wang feels that a normal parathyroid gland in addition to an enlarged parathyroid gland is diagnostic of an adenoma and that the other side of the neck should not be explored. Paloyan, on the other hand, feels that the only way to prevent recurrent hyperparathyroidism is to perform a subtotal parathyroidectomy in each patient.

Our practice has been to take an intermediate approach—to try to identify all the parathyroid glands, to biopsy them at the time of operation, and then to decide which gland or glands should be removed. If only one gland is enlarged and the others are normal both in size and histologically on frozen section, only the enlarged gland is removed. If more than one gland is involved, a subtotal parathyroidectomy is performed, since we consider this to represent multiglandular disease. It is apparent that the surgeon must play a diagnostic as well as a therapeutic role at the time of exploration, regardless of which technique is chosen.

If hypoparathyroidism is to be prevented, a subtotal parathyroidectomy should be performed with the greatest of care. It is essential that the remnant of parathyroid tissue left behind have an intact blood supply. Generally, 40 to 60 mg of the smallest gland is left in place. It is first examined and seen to be viable before the other glands are removed. We mark it either with a metal clip or a suture to permit it to be found at a subsequent exploration, if necessary.

If three normal parathyroid glands have been found and the hyperfunctioning gland has not been identified, it is wise to resect the thyroid lobe on the side of the missing gland, since 3 percent of parathyroid adenomas have been reported by Goldman to be totally intrathyroidal.

If the possibility of *carcinoma of the parathyroid gland* is entertained at operation, the lesion should be completely removed with an adequate margin of surrounding tissue, including the thyroid lobe on that side. Great care should be exercised *not* to enter the lesion or to spill tumor cells, since recurrent disease in the neck is very common. With good surgical technique and an *en bloc* resection much of this local recurrence is avoidable.

Mediastinal Exploration. When a patient has been referred with an established diagnosis of hyperparathyroidism and neck exploration done elsewhere has failed to reveal a tumor, the neck operation should always be re-

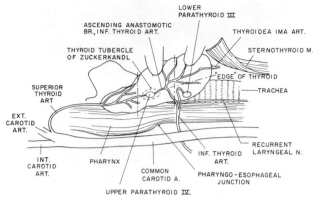

Fig. 38-52. Lateral view with the thyroid retracted anteriorly and mediad to show the surgical landmarks for locating the parathyroids.

peated, since in nearly every instance the tumor will be discovered there, rather than in the mediastinum. Increased difficulty with second or third operations is an added incentive to perform a satisfactory procedure the first time.

Since at least 95 to 98 percent of the parathyroid adenomas can be reached from the neck, mediastinal exploration is seldom necessary. We do not recommend a mediastinal exploration at the time of initial neck exploration, even if three normal glands have been found and the thyroid lobe on the side of the missing gland has been demonstrated to contain no parathyroid tissue. Even when four normal glands are found in the neck we do not recommend immediate exploration of the mediastinum, despite our realization that a fifth gland may be the culprit. Rather, we explore the superior mediastinum as carefully as possible from the neck, explore all other areas again, and then close.

Prior to reexploration and possible mediastinal exploration we feel that it is appropriate to reconfirm the diagnosis of primary hyperparathyroidism and then, if possible, to perform selective venous catheterization with PTH measurement to try to further localize the gland. This has been helpful in several instances.

If mediastinal exploration is necessary, the mediastinotomy may be done by splitting the sternum in the midline down to the level of the third interspace and making a short cut out into this interspace on each side. It is often easier to divide the entire sternum in the midline. The sternum is then held apart with a retractor, and the mediastinum is explored. If one is searching for the superior gland on that side, it may be located in the posterior part of the mediastinum, while if one is looking for the inferior parathyroid, it is generally located in the anterior mediastinum. It may be embedded in the thymus itself, or it may lie against the pericardium. One case of an intrapericardial parathyroid gland has been reported. In most instances it is in the upper portion of the mediastinum. The mediastinal exploration is usually carried out for a tumor which has arisen from a mediastinal parathyroid, rather than a tumor which has arisen from a parathyroid in the neck and descended during growth into the mediastinum—since these

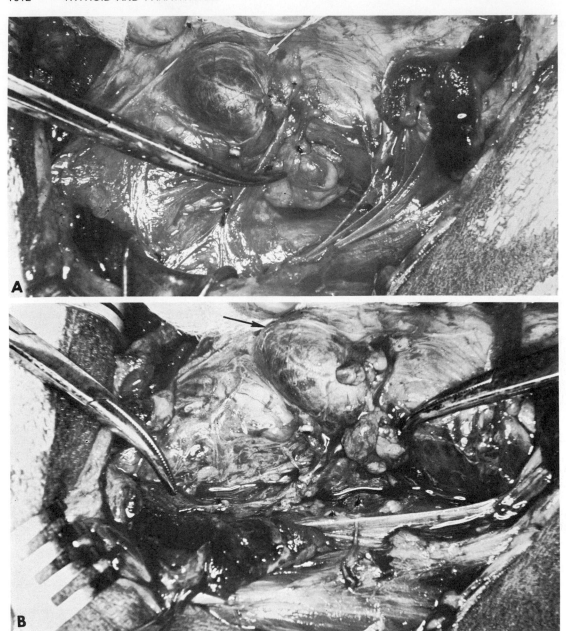

Fig. 38-53. Parathyroid exploration. *A.* The normal right lower parathyroid has been exposed and is identified by the end of the instrument. It is embedded in fat. It lies on top of the recurrent laryngeal nerve just below the inferior thyroid artery. An adenoma of the upper parathyroid gland is indicated by the arrow. *B.* Another adenoma is indicated by the arrow. The hemostat on the right side points to a normal-appearing parathyroid gland.

can usually be reached from the neck. The blood supply therefore will usually be from a mediastinal vessel (see Fig. 38-51).

In the Massachusetts General Hospital series only 19 of 400 parathyroid tumors (5 percent) required mediastinal exploration for removal. In the Mayo Clinic series, only 14 of 1,000 (1.4 percent) of patients with primary hyperparathyroidism were cured by a sternal splitting operation. Thus, a careful neck exploration is imperative at the initial operation.

Postoperative Complications. The postoperative complications consist of hypoparathyroidism, hemorrhage, recurrent laryngeal nerve damage, and persistent or recurrent disease.

Hypoparathyroidism can occur because of excision of all parathyroid tissue or because of permanent or temporary damage to the blood supply of the remaining parathyroid tissue. In thyroid and parathyroid operations, the inferior thyroid artery should *not* be ligated laterally, since this can devascularize the parathyroid glands. A temporary hypoparathyroidism often follows the excision of large parathyroid adenomas, and temporary calcium treatment may have to be instituted. This will usually correct itself in a week or two. The treatment of hypoparathyroidism is discussed in another section.

Hypocalcemia in the postoperative period is more apt to occur when a large adenoma has been removed, when there is impaired renal function, or when there is considerable bone disease. In the latter two cases the calcium level is depressed as a response to an elevated serum phosphorus level or by calcium deposition in calcium-starved bones. In this latter circumstance it may take many weeks for the calcium level to become normal. Examination of the serum phosphorus level is helpful postoperatively. If hypoparathyroidism is present, the phosphorus level is elevated; in "bone hunger" the phosphorus level may be low if renal function is not impaired.

It is our practice always to drain the wound after parathyroid exploration. The drain is brought out through one side of the incision and is usually removed in 24 hours. A loose dressing is applied so that if *hemorrhage* does occur, it will be less apt to compress the trachea and cause respiratory embarrassment. The wound is inspected frequently in the immediate postoperative period. A severe

hemorrhage will necessitate reopening the wound or re-exploration.

Damage to the recurrent nerve will rarely be a problem if the location of the nerve is determined as the first step in the surgical procedure as outlined above. Temporary malfunction of the nerve may occur if the nerve is stretched during the performance of the operation. The nerve will occasionally lie on top of the parathyroid adenoma. If the nerve is inadvertently divided, it should be resutured. Injury to the nerve is most apt to occur when there is a large adenoma located in the superior mediastinum pushing up into the neck, where it may displace the nerve anteriorly. If the recurrent laryngeal nerves are injured bilaterally, severe respiratory difficulty may occur, sometimes necessitating a tracheostomy.

Persistent disease means that hypercalcemia remains after operation. This occurs when the diagnosis of hyperparathyroidism is incorrect, or when the hyperfunctioning gland or glands have not been adequately removed. In the hands of experienced neck surgeons, this should occur only infrequently. *Recurrent disease* means that the calcium returns to normal postoperatively but that months to years later, hypercalcemia due to hyperparathyroidism returns. This condition is most commonly seen if primary chief cell hyperplasia is not recognized and one or two enlarged glands are removed because they are diagnosed as adenomas. When recurrent hyperparathyroidism does occur, the parathyroid disease should be treated as hyperplasia with subtotal parathyroidectomy. A lesser procedure, illustrated in Fig. 38-54, will be once more doomed to failure. Hyper-

Fig. 38-54. Recurrent hyperparathyroidism. In this patient, hypercalcemia and hypophosphatemia developed three separate times. On each occasion a single enlarged gland was removed. After removal of three glands, the patient has remained normocalcemic. While each of these glands was originally diagnosed as an adenoma, it is very likely that this process represents undiagnosed primary chief cell hyperplasia which was finally cured by the cumulative subtotal parathyroidectomy.

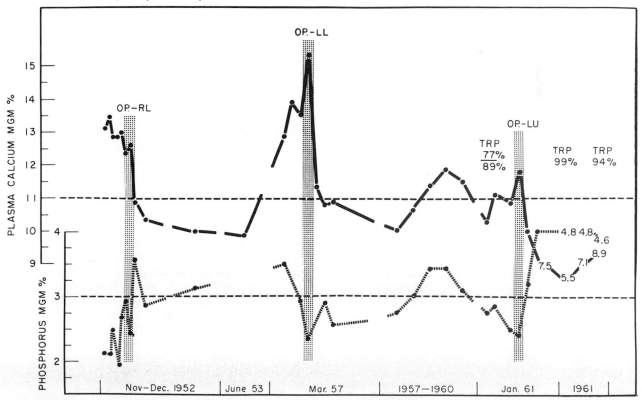

calcemia recurring several months after an apparently successful parathyroidectomy should alert the physician to the possibility of a parathyroid carcinoma, although inadequately treated hyperplasia is more likely. It is necessary to follow patients for many years following parathyroidectomy if the results of therapy are to be truly assessed.

Results of Therapy. In Table 38-9, the incidence of severe hypoparathyroidism and that of recurrent hyperparathyroidism are tabulated from some of the recent series of primary hyperparathyroidism. Note that although the recognition of multiglandular disease varied greatly from series to series, the incidence of recurrent hyperparathyroidism is low. Thus, when performed by an experienced surgeon, parathyroidectomy is generally successful. The series of Clark et al. points out clearly that those patients with multiple endocrine adenomatosis (MEA) or familial hyperparathyroidism (FHP) are most likely to get a recurrence. This may occasionally occur even following a subtotal parathyroidectomy. When these conditions were not present, recurrent disease occurred in only 0.4 percent of patients; when MEA or FHP was present, recurrent disease occurred in 33 percent of patients. Long-term follow-up studies are essential.

Severe hypoparathyroidism may occur more frequently following subtotal parathyroidectomy than after lesser operations if great care is not exercised in performing this operation. When done by experienced surgeons, however, the incidence of permanent hypoparathyroidism necessitating vitamin D therapy is quite low.

Secondary Hyperparathyroidism

In primary hyperparathyroidism there is an oversecretion of PTH which does not cease even in the presence of an elevated serum calcium level. In secondary hyperparathyroidism there is also an increased secretion of PTH but this is in response to a *lowered blood calcium* level which has been brought about by some factors, often renal disease or malabsorption syndromes. These diseases are associated with abnormalities in vitamin D metabolism [lack of production of $1,25-(OH)_2D_3$] and by poor calcium and vitamin D absorption from the intestines, respectively. The response of the parathyroids is thus a compensatory one, as the body attempts to raise the serum calcium level to the normal range. In secondary hyperparathyroidism there is a chief cell hyperplasia of the parathyroids, which is quite commonly accompanied by nests of oxyphil cells.

Other causes of secondary hyperparathyroidism include rickets and osteomalacia, where there is a deficient absorption of calcium from the intestine.

In secondary hyperparathyroidism the serum calcium level is usually low or low-normal. In rickets and osteomalacia the serum phosphate level is reduced, as it is in primary hyperparathyroidism, whereas in chronic renal failure it is usually elevated. The intestinal absorption of calcium is increased in primary hyperparathyroidism, and the fecal excretion is reduced, whereas the reverse is true in secondary hyperparathyroidism.

At times there may be some difficulty in differentiating between secondary and primary hyperparathyroidism be-

cause primary hyperparathyroidism can lead to renal failure through nephrocalcinosis and the effects of PTH and calcium on the kidney, thus producing an elevated serum phosphate level which may in turn lower the serum calcium level to some degree. The renal failure may lead to hyperplasia of the uninvolved parathyroid glands, thus leading to the coexistence of an adenoma and hyperplasia. This course of events is further discussed under Tertiary Hyperparathyroidism. The most significant differentiation between secondary (dependent) versus primary (autonomous) hyperparathyroidism depends upon the serum calcium level, which is seldom elevated in the former and almost always elevated in the latter. In parathyroid hypercalcemic crisis, in fact, there is usually a markedly elevated serum calcium level despite renal failure, azotemia, and an elevated serum phosphate level.

The skeletal changes of secondary hyperparathyroidism are identical to those of primary hyperparathyroidism except that ectopic calcification in the arteries, muscles, etc., is much more common in secondary hyperparathyroidism, especially if the patient has been given large doses of vitamin D (Fig. 38-42). Today severe bone disease associated with hyperparathyroidism is rare in primary hyperparathyroidism but is not infrequently seen in patients with chronic renal failure maintained on chronic hemodialysis.

The bone disease in chronic renal failure, commonly called *renal osteodystrophy,* is caused by at least several factors: Hyperphosphatemia results in a decreased serum calcium. Hypocalcemia results in secondary hyperparathyroidism. Impaired calcium absorption due to vitamin D insensitivity results in osteomalacia. Systemic acidosis may also contribute to bone resorption.

Recent advances in the treatment of renal osteodystrophy appear to be significant. By elevating the calcium in the dialysis bath, Arnaud and associates have demonstrated a decrease in serum PTH and a decreased incidence of bone disease in patients on chronic hemodialysis.

Patients with chronic renal failure may have an impaired ability to convert vitamin D_3 to its active metabolite $1,25-(OH)_2D_3$. This results in decreased calcium absorption from the intestine. In these patients, physiologic doses of vitamin D are usually ineffective, but improvement following administration of large pharmacologic doses of this vitamin may occur. The $1,25-(OH)_2D_3$ metabolite promises to be very effective. In a recent study it was given to uremic patients. Significant improvement in intestinal absorption of calcium and elevation of calcium concentrations were noted on a dose of only 100 units/day for 6 to 10 days. The same individuals were insensitive to 40,000 units of vitamin D_3. Thus administration of $1,25-(OH)_2D_3$ or other similar metabolites may be useful in the prevention and treatment of renal osteodystrophy. Medical therapy for the bone disease should be tried in all patients with secondary hyperparathyroidism before surgery is contemplated.

Stanbury et al. have advocated parathyroidectomy for patients in chronic renal failure with severe bone change who have developed intractable bone pain. The pain and severe itching, which is also sometimes present in patients on chronic dialysis, are often relieved in a dramatic fash-

Table 38-9. INCIDENCE OF RECURRENT HYPERPARATHYROIDISM AND SEVERE HYPOPARATHYROIDISM FOLLOWING OPERATION FOR PRIMARY HYPERPARATHYROIDISM

Author and year	Total no. of patients	Multiple gland involvement, %	Recurrent hyperparathyroidism, %	Severe hypoparathyroidism, %	Follow-up
Paloyan et al. (1969)	I 27	18	15	19	7 mo.–3 yr.
	II* 26	58	0	8	
Haff and Ballinger (1971)	38	50	3	5	18 mo. or longer
Bruining (1971)	I 267	45	0	1.2	3½ yr. (average)
	II* 11	...	0	27	
Clark and Taylor (1971)	99	15	1	2	
Johanssen et al. (1972)	203	18	0	3.8	
Paloyan et al. (1973)	98	65	1	2	
Romanus et al. (1973)	274	20	1	7	4 yr. average
Hines and Suker (1973)	51	10	0	...	To 15 yr.
Wang (1973)	256	...	0.8	...	10 mo.–15 yr.
Davies (1974)	350	10	3	5	mo.–38 yr.
Myers (1974)	82	13	1	...	1–6.5 yr.
Purnell et al. (1974)	475	13	0.6	0.2	
Block et al. (1974)	121	20	1	4	4½ yr. (average)
Muller et al. (1975)	352	50	1	...	
Palmer et al. (1975)	250	15	0.5	2	15 yr.
Farr (1976)	100	5	2	4	
Block (1976)	182	20	0	0	
Clark et al. (1976)	263	12	2.7	4	6 mo.–40 yr.
MEA or FHP‡	21	71	33	24†	
Without MEA or FHP	242	6	0.4	2.6	

*Subtotal parathyroidectomy.
†None permanent.
‡MEA, multiple endocrine adenomatosis; FHP, familial hyperparathyroidism.
SOURCE: Adapted from O. H. Clark, L. H. Wang, and T. K. Hunt, *Ann Surg,* **184:**391, 1976.

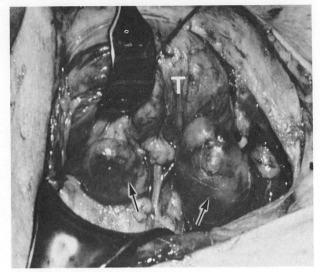

Fig. 38-55. Secondary hyperparathyroidism. Chief cell hyperplasia with four enlarged parathyroid glands was found in this patient with chronic renal failure and bone disease. Arrows point to two of the hyperplastic parathyroid glands. *T,* retracted thyroid lobe.

ion. Remineralization of the skeleton can be hastened by the administration of vitamin D postoperatively.

Patients with secondary hyperparathyroidism due to chronic renal failure are dialysed 1 day before surgery to reduce serum potassium. Before or during surgery washed frozen red cells may be administered. A subtotal parathy-

roidectomy is routinely performed leaving only 40 to 60 mg of vascularized parathyroid tissue behind (Fig. 38-55). Lesser operations may result in a reexacerbation of bone symptoms. Drains are always used. Postoperatively, the first dialysis is often accomplished with regional heparinization.

PARATHYROID TRANSPLANTATION. Following subtotal parathyroidectomy for secondary hyperparathyroidism, the remaining remnant of tissue is subjected to a continuing hypocalcemic stimulus. Thus, it is likely to hypertrophy and to cause symptoms again. To avoid reoperation in the neck, which is always more dangerous, Wells et al. have proposed that the parathyroid remnant be minced into small pieces and implanted into the muscles of the forearm. All other parathyroid tissues are removed. This technique has worked successfully in 29 patients with secondary hyperparathyroidism. Histologically viable parathyroid tissue has been biopsied in the arm, and the antecubital veins draining the grafted tissue have higher serum PTH

Fig. 38-56. The clinical course of a 19-year-old male who had undergone a total parathyroidectomy for severe bone pain in 1973 and then received a renal transplant 6 months later. Because of severe symptoms of hypocalcemia in the patient, two parathyroid glands were removed from his father (who had also contributed donor kidney) and implanted in the patient's forearm in November 1973. Thereafter serum calcium rose to normal values and calcium and vitamin D therapy was stopped. Serum PTH levels returned to normal and were higher in the antecubital veins on the side of the transplant. The patient remains on prednisone and cyclophosphamide (Cytoxan) therapy. (*From S. A. Wells, Jr., et al., Surgery, 78:34, 1975.*)

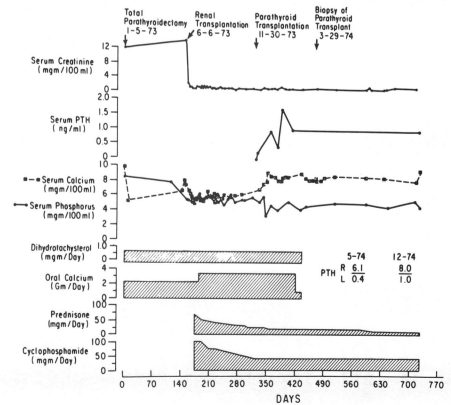

levels than do veins of the opposite, nongrafted arm. If hyperparathyroidism recurs, some of the tissue can be removed from the forearm using local anesthesia (a much safer procedure).

Parathyroid tissue which has been quick-frozen and stored at $-196°C$ for as long as 9 months has been successfully reimplanted in the arm. This could lead some day to a "parathyroid bank," in which some tissue is saved from each patient who undergoes a parathyroidectomy. In the event of hypoparathyroidism, some of his own parathyroid could be reimplanted.

Wells has suggested that patients with *primary* chief cell hyperplasia be treated by total parathyroidectomy and transplantation of tissue to the arm as well. We have not done this routinely but have successfully used this technique in one patient who developed recurrent hyperparathyroidism 3 years after a subtotal parathyroidectomy done elsewhere for hyperplasia.

Finally, one immunosuppressed, aparathyroid patient received a parathyroid allograft from a parent who previously had been his renal transplant donor (Fig. 38-56). This technique has only limited application, however, since most patients do well with vitamin D therapy.

Tertiary Hyperparathyroidism

Tertiary hyperparathyroidism is the term which has been employed to describe the situation in which secondary hyperparathyroidism with chief cell hyperplasia appears to have become "autonomous." The diagnosis is made when an elevated serum calcium level develops in the patient with chronic renal failure and secondary hyperparathyroidism or in a patient with known intestinal malabsorption who previously had hypocalcemia. Tertiary hyperparathyroidism may be present even when the blood calcium level is not grossly elevated but is simply in the upper normal range when it should have been low.

When renal transplantation is carried out in a patient with renal failure and secondary hyperparathyroidism, three patterns are characteristically seen: In the first the calcium level rises and the phosphorous level falls for a period of a week or two, after which they both return to normal levels. This is illustrated in Fig. 38-57. In the second pattern the elevated calcium and lowered phosphorus levels may persist for several weeks before gradually returning to normal (Fig. 38-58A). In the third pattern, hypercalcemia with hypophosphatemia persists for long periods of time. In the patient illustrated in Fig. 38-58B a staghorn calculus developed in the transplanted kidney within 6 months. Parathyroidectomy was carried out at this point, and the function of the kidney has remained excellent up to the present time, 5 years after transplantation.

Recent studies suggest that true parathyroid autonomy rarely occurs in patients with so-called tertiary hyperparathyroidism. It has been demonstrated that the hyperplastic glands found in chronic renal failure do suppress their secretion but cannot completely shut off their secretion of PTH despite the presence of hypercalcemia. Furthermore, because of their bulky size it may take a long time for them to involute. Johnson et al. have demonstrated that,

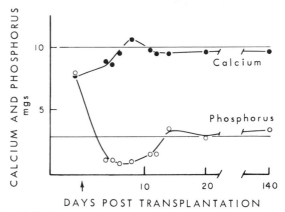

REVERSAL OF SECONDARY HYPERPARATHYROIDISM FOLLOWING RENAL HOMOTRANSPLANTATION

DAYS POST TRANSPLANTATION

Fig. 38-57. Serum calcium and phosphate values in a patient with secondary hyperparathyroidism who received a kidney transplant. Preoperatively the serum calcium level was low and the phosphate level high. After an initial rise in calcium level and fall in phosphate level to levels outside the normal range the values quickly returned to normal levels. No parathyroid exploration was carried out.

following renal transplantation, PTH concentrations in these patients slowly return toward normal within several months if renal function is good (see Fig. 38-59). Hypercalcemia posttransplantation may also be the result of increased end organ responsiveness, since abnormalities in vitamin D metabolism are corrected.

Some workers have a considerable fear that renal damage may occur very rapidly in the presence of hypercalcemia and advocate doing parathyroidectomy prior to renal transplantation in those patients suspected of having severe secondary or tertiary hyperparathyroidism. In view of the fact that in most of these cases normal serum calcium concentrations will return in a reasonable period after transplantation, it would seem a more appropriate policy to wait and watch the patient carefully posttransplantation for at least 6 months. Oral phosphate administration has been useful in restoring the elevated serum calcium level to normal if the serum phosphorus is low and should be tried. Only rarely will parathyroidectomy be necessary. Subtotal parathyroidectomy was only necessary in 3 of 111 patients following transplantation at the Mayo Clinic.

Hypoparathyroidism

ETIOLOGY. The most common cause of hypoparathyroidism is surgical removal of the parathyroids either during parathyroid surgical treatment or, more commonly, during operations on the thyroid. Postoperative tetany after thyroidectomy for goiter was first described by Reverdin and Kocher in 1882, although of course it was not recognized that this was due to parathyroid deficiency. Primary idiopathic hypoparathyroidism is extremely rare and is usually first noted in patients under the age of sixteen.

As mentioned earlier, transient hypoparathyroidism can

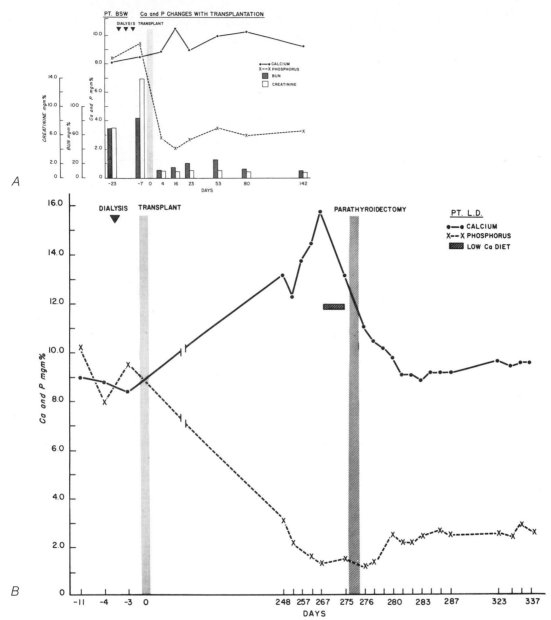

be noted after removal of a parathyroid adenoma or a resection of most of the tissue in parathyroid hyperplasia. This is made worse when the patient has some degree of renal disease which tends to lower the calcium level by itself or when the patient has serious bone disease, when the calcium tends to be deposited in the bone, thus producing hypocalcemia. In some instances the transient hypocalcemia is due to trauma to the remaining glands or to interference with the blood supply.

Idiopathic hypoparathyroidism is an uncommon disease of unknown cause. Recent evidence would suggest that in some cases it is due to the presence of antibodies against parathyroid tissue. The patients may also have antibodies against adrenal, thyroid, and gastric parietal cells. One hypothesis is that the parathyroid disease is part of a

Fig. 38-58. Serum calcium and phosphate values in patients with secondary hyperparathyroidism who received kidney transplants. *A.* Patient with secondary hyperparathyroidism whose serum phosphate level took somewhat longer to return to normal after renal homotransplantation. The calcium level remained in the high normal range for many days. *B.* Another patient with renal failure and secondary hyperparathyroidism. In this patient the preoperative serum calcium level was nearly in the normal range, whereas the phosphorus level was markedly elevated. After transplantation the serum calcium value steadily rose, while the phosphate value declined to abnormally low levels. No spontaneous return toward normal occurred, and it was apparent that tertiary hyperparathyrodism had developed. A parathyroidectomy was carried out on the 275th day after transplantation, and the patient was found to have chief cell hyperplasia with very large glands. By this time calcium deposits had developed in the walls of the calcyceal system of the transplanted kidney. After parathyroidectomy the serum calcium and phosphate values returned to normal. (*From D. M. Hume et al., Ann Surg, 164:352, 1966.*)

generalized autoimmune disease. Other diseases sometimes associated with this include monilial infection, Hashimoto's thyroiditis, and steatorrhea.

CLINICAL MANIFESTATIONS. Symptoms. The symptoms of hypoparathyroidism are those of hypocalcemia and are related to the greatly increased neuromuscular excitability brought about by a decrease in the plasma ionized calcium. The most striking manifestation is tetany. This may consist of carpopedal spasm in which the fingers at the metacarpal phalangeal joint and the wrist are flexed and the elbow, legs, and feet are extended. Tonic and clonic convulsions and laryngeal stridor may be present and may even prove fatal. In the milder forms paresthesias, muscle cramps, numbness, dysphagia, and dysarthria may be present. There may be some degree of anxiety. In chronic hypoparathyroidism cataracts and mental changes may occur.

Physical Signs. Chvostek's sign consists of a contraction of the facial muscles in response to a tap over the facial nerve in front of the ear. Occluding the circulation at the arm by inflation of a blood pressure cuff above the level of systolic pressure induces carpopedal spasm within 3 minutes. This is Trousseau's sign, a less reliable sign than Chvostek's sign.

The electrocardiogram shows a prolongation of the Q-T interval. The plasma calcium level is low, and the phosphate is increased.

Differential Diagnosis. Tetany can be caused by factors other than hypoparathyroidism. Alkalosis can produce tetany even in the presence of a normal blood total calcium level by lowering the ionized calcium level. Rickets in the child, osteomalacia in the adult, steatorrhea, and renal insufficiency all produce hypocalcemia. In rickets, osteomalacia, and steatorrhea there is a low plasma calcium level with a normal or low plasma phosphate level. This differentiates it from hypoparathyroidism, where the plasma phosphate level is generally elevated. Chronic renal insufficiency is associated with hypocalcemia with a markedly elevated plasma phosphate level—higher than that usually seen in hypoparathyroidism. This can further be distinguished from hypoparathyroidism by the elevated BUN level.

A low plasma magnesium level can also produce tetany. In some cases of tetany, hypomagnesemia and hypocalcemia are both present. The tetany often cannot be corrected until the circulating magnesium level is brought to normal. Renal tubular acidosis (the Fanconi syndrome) can also produce tetany. In these circumstances there is a failure of resorption of certain amino acids.

TREATMENT. Postoperative Hypocalcemia. When mild, no treatment is needed, but careful, watchful waiting should be employed. Serum calcium levels should be determined every 12 hours for the first few days and then daily thereafter. If the patient becomes symptomatic, 1 Gm calcium gluconate can be given intravenously, and then 1 to 2 Gm/8 hours of this preparation may be dripped continuously in an intravenous bottle to alleviate all symptoms. Within several days all calcium therapy can usually be stopped.

For more persistent hypocalcemia, oral calcium is also begun in a dose of 1.5 to 2.0 Gm calcium ion per day. It is

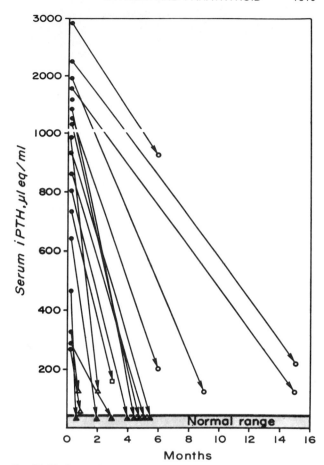

Fig. 38-59. Serum PTH concentrations before and after successful renal transplantation in patients with endogenous creatinine clearance of 60 ml/min/1.73 m² or greater. (*From W. J. Johnson et al., Med Clin North Am, 56:961, 1972.*)

important to note that to provide 1 Gm elemental calcium one must administer 5.5 Gm hydrated calcium chloride, 8 Gm calcium lactate, 11 Gm calcium gluconate, or 4 Gm calcium acetate. Calcium gluconate is palatable and therefore preferred. The patient may be sent home on oral calcium therapy when asymptomatic, and this can usually be discontinued after several weeks. It is preferable not to add vitamin D to this early regimen unless one strongly suspects that permanent hypoparathyroidism has occurred (or unless a parathyroid transplant has been performed).

If *permanent hypoparathyroidism* has occurred, in addition to the oral calcium therapy the patient is started on vitamin D_3, 50,000 to 100,000 units/day (1.25 to 2.5 mg/day). Others prefer to use dihydrotachysterol, 0.125 to 1.0 mg/day. In the future, metabolites of vitamin D_3 may prove more efficacious; however, they are not generally available at this time. The serum calcium concentration must be checked frequently, since some patients are insensitive to these preparations and need larger doses, whereas others develop vitamin D intoxication with severe hypercalcemia on relatively small dosages.

Serum PTH concentrations should be checked at intervals in patients being treated for permanent postoperative hypoparathyroidism. Several patients whom we have seen have been treated unnecessarily with vitamin D for many years because postoperative tetany had occurred. When serum PTH levels are detectable, vitamin D therapy should be slowly tapered and finally stopped if possible.

Other nonspecific factors may tend to influence the treatment of hypocalcemia. A diet high in phosphate or oxalate content should be avoided, since it may impair calcium absorption. Concomitant ingestion of anticonvulsants and tranquilizers may lower intestinal absorption of calcium both directly and by interfering with vitamin D metabolism. Estrogen and oral contraceptive therapy lower serum calcium level by suppressing bone resorption. Diuretics, such as furosemide, result in increased calcium excretion in the urine. Hypomagnesemia should be avoided since this leads to resistance to vitamin D therapy. Finally, the role of emotional stress in vitamin D resistance and hypocalcemia may be important.

Pseudohypoparathyroidism

Pseudohypoparathyroidism was first described by Albright et al. in 1942. This is a genetic disease in which the clinical and chemical features of hypoparathyroidism are present in association with the genetic stigmata of a round face, a short, thick body, and short, stubby fingers. There is a shortening of some of the metacarpal and metatarsal bones as a result of early epiphyseal closure, so that a dimple rather than a knuckle shows when the fist is clenched. Mental deficiency may be present, and there are sometimes areas of subcutaneous ossification. The manifestations are not due to lack of parathyroid secretion but to unresponsiveness of the end organ, the renal phosphaturic mechanism. The parathyroids are normal or hyperplastic, and serum PTH concentration is raised in these patients. There are hypocalcemia and hyperphosphatemia. Patients with this syndrome may show evidence of increased bone resorption and even osteitis fibrosa cystica, since PTH appears to act appropriately on bone but not on the kidney.

Pseudohypoparathyroidism can be distinguished from hypoparathyroidism not only by the characteristic physical picture of the patient but also because individuals with hypoparathyroidism respond to parathyroid extract while those with pseudohypoparathyroidism usually do not. The Ellsworth-Howard test has been designed to demonstrate this difference. The patient is slowly given 200 units of parathyroid extract intravenously, and the urinary phosphate excretion is determined for 3 hours before and 3 hours after the administration. The parathyroid extract produces a fivefold increase in urine phosphate excretion in normal persons, a tenfold increase in patients with hypoparathyroidism, and less than a twofold increase in patients with pseudohypoparathyroidism.

Recently it has been demonstrated that patients with pseudohypoparathyroidism have a deficient renal adenyl cyclase system. This offers a new diagnostic test for differentiating patients with idiopathic hypoparathyroidism from those with pseudohypoparathyroidism. In the former group, PTH administration results in increased urinary cyclic 3'5'-AMP, while in pseudohypoparathyroid patients PTH gives no change or only a slight increase in urinary cyclic AMP.

A high concentration of calcitonin has been found in the thyroid gland of some patients with this disease. This, however, appears to be the result of the hypocalcemia rather than its cause.

The treatment of pseudohypoparathyroidism is the same as that for hypoparathyroidism: low-phosphate diet, alumina gel, and vitamin D or its new metabolites.

Pseudopseudohypoparathyroidism

Pseudopseudohypoparathyroidism is also a genetic defect with the same physical features as pseudohypoparathyroidism. It differs from pseudohypoparathyroidism in that the plasma calcium and phosphate levels are normal and Chvostek's and Trousseau's signs are absent. The administration of PTH in one patient resulted in a normal rise in urinary cyclic AMP.

References

Thyroid: Anatomy

Durham, C. F., and Harrison, T. S.: The Surgical Anatomy of the Superior Laryngeal Nerve, *Surg Gynecol Obstet,* **118:**38, 1964.

Fish, J., and Moore, R. M.: Ectopic Thyroid Tissue and Ectopic Thyroid Carcinoma, *Ann Surg,* **157:**212, 1963.

Hung, W., Randolph, J. G., Sabatini, D., and Winship, T.: Lingual and Sublingual Thyroid Glands in Euthyroid Children, *Pediatrics,* **38:**647, 1966.

Hunt, P. S., Poole, M., and Reeve, T. S.: A Reappraisal of the Surgical Anatomy of the Thyroid and Parathyroid Glands, *Br J Surg,* **55:**63, 1968.

Riddell, V. H.: Injury to Recurrent Laryngeal Nerves during Thyroidectomy, *Lancet,* **2:**638, 1956.

Sloan, L. W.: Normal and Anomalous Development of the Thyroid, in S. C. Werner (ed.), "The Thyroid," chap. 19, Hoeber Medical Division, Harper & Row, Publishers, Incorporated, New York, 1955.

Ward, G. E., Cantrell, J. R., and Allan, W. B.: The Surgical Treatment of Lingual Thyroid, *Ann Surg,* **139:**536, 1954.

Thyroid: Physiology

Acland, J. D.: The Nature, Determination and Clinical Importance of Blood Iodine: A Review, *J Clin Pathol,* **2:**195, 1958.

Astwood, E. B., and Solomon, D. H.: Mechanisms of Action of Antithyroid Drugs, Iodides, and Other Thyroid Inhibitors, in S. C. Werner (ed.), "The Thyroid," chap. 6, Hoeber Medical Division, Harper & Row, Publishers, Incorporated, New York, 1955.

Burke, G.: Thyroid Stimulators and Thyroid Stimulation, *Acta Endocrinol (Kbh)* **66:**558, 1971.

DeGroot, L. J.: Current Views on the Formation of Thyroid Hormones, *N Engl J Med,* **272:**243, 1963.

——: Kinetic Analysis of Iodine Metabolism, *J Clin Endocrinol Metab,* **26:**149, 1966.

Greer, M. A.: Factors Regulating Triiodothyronine (T3) and Thyroxine (T4) in Blood, *Mayo Clin Proc,* **47:**944, 1972.

Hershman, J. M.: Hyperthyroidism Induced by Trophoblastic Thyrotropin, *Mayo Clin Proc,* **47:**913, 1972.

Hoch, F. L.: Biochemical Actions of Thyroid Hormones, *Physiol Rev,* **42:**605, 1962.

Ingbar, S. H.: Autoregulation of the Thyroid: Response to Iodide Excess and Depletion, *Mayo Clin Proc,* **47:**814, 1972.

———— and Woeber, K. A.: The Thyroid Gland, in R. H. Williams (ed.), "Textbook of Endocrinology," chap. 4, W. B. Saunders Company, Philadelphia, 1968.

Maloof, F., and Soodak, M.: Intermediary Metabolism of Thyroid Tissue and the Action of Drugs, *Physiol Rev,* **15:**43, 1963.

Means, J. H., DeGroot, L. J., and Stanbury, J. B.: "The Thyroid and Its Diseases," 3d ed., chaps. 2–4, McGraw-Hill Book Company, New York, 1963.

Reichlin, S.: Control of Thyrotropic Hormone Secretion, in L. Martini and W. F. Ganong (eds.), "Neuroendocrinology," Academic Press, Inc., New York, 1966.

Werner, S. C., and Ingbar, S. H.: "The Thyroid: A Fundamental and Clinical Text," 3d ed., Harper & Row, Publishers, Incorporated, New York, 1971.

Evaluation of Patients with Thyroid Disease

Alexander, W. D., Harden, R. McG., and Shimmins, J.: Thyroidal Suppression by Triiodothyronine as a Guide to Duration of Treatment of Thyrotoxicosis with Antithyroid Drugs, *Lancet,* **2:**1041, 1966.

Andrews, G. A., Sitterson, B. W., and Ross, D. A.: The Use of Scanning in Thyroid Cancer, in R. M. Kniseley, G. A. Andrews, and C. C. Harris (eds.), "Progress in Medical Radioisotope Scanning," chap. 15, Oak Ridge Institute of Nuclear Studies, Oak Ridge, Tenn., 1963.

Atkins, H. L., and Richards, P.: Assessment of Thyroid Function and Anatomy with Technetium-99m as Pertechnetate, *J Nucl Med,* **9:**7, 1968.

Becker, D. V., and Hurley, J. R.: The Impact of Technology on Clinical Practice in Graves' Disease, *Mayo Clin Proc,* **47:**835, 1972.

Boehme, E. J., Winship, T., Lindsay, S., and Kypridakis, G.: Evaluation of Needle Biopsy of Thyroid Gland, *Surg Gynecol Obstet,* **119:**831, 1964.

Gharib, H., Ryan, R. J., and Mayberry, W. E.: Triiodothyronine (T3) Radioimmunoassay: A Critical Evaluation, *Mayo Clin Proc,* **47:**934, 1972.

Mayberry, W. E., Gharib, H., Bilstad, J. M., and Sizemore, G. W.: Radioimmunoassay for Human Thyrotrophin: Clinical Value in Patients with Normal and Abnormal Thyroid Function, *Ann Intern Med,* **74:**471, 1971.

Meadows, P.: Thyroid Nodules, in R. M. Kniseley, G. A. Andrews, and C. C. Harris (eds.), "Progress in Medical Radioisotope Scanning," chap. 14, Oak Ridge Institute of Nuclear Studies, Oak Ridge, Tenn., 1963.

Means, J. H., DeGroot, L. J., and Stanbury, J. B.: "The Thyroid and Its Diseases," 3d ed., chap. 5, McGraw-Hill Book Company, New York, 1963.

Ormston, B. J., Garry, R., Cryer, R. J., Besser, G. M., and Hall, R.: Thyrotrophin-releasing Hormone as a Thyroid-Function Test, *Lancet,* **2:**10, 1971.

Riccabona, G.: "I^{125} in the Clinical Evaluation of Thyroid Disease," *N Engl J Med,* **273:**126, 1965.

Selenkow, H. A.: Tests for Circulating Thyroid Hormones, International Congress Series No. 227, Diagnosis and Treatment of Common Thyroid Diseases, in H. A. Selenkow and F. Hoffman (eds.), "Proceedings of a Symposium Held in San Francisco, California, U.S.A., March 6, 1970," Excerpta Medica Foundation, Amsterdam, 1971.

Solomon, D. H., Benotti, J., DeGroot, L. J., Greer, M. A., Pileggi, V. J., Pittman, J. A., Robbins, J., Selenkow, H. A., Sterling, K., and Volpe, R.: A Nomenclature for Tests of Thyroid Hormones in Serum: Report of a Committee of the American Thyroid Association, *J Clin Endocrinol Metab,* **34:**884, 1972.

Hyperthyroidism

Beahrs, O. H., Ryan, R. F., and White, R. A.: Complications of Thyroid Surgery, *J Clin Endocrinol Metab,* **16:**1456, 1956.

———— and Sakulsky, S. B.: Surgical Thyroidectomy in the Management of Exophthalmic Goiter, *Arch Surg,* **96:**512, 1968.

Bowers, R. F.: Hyperthyroidism: Comparative Results of Medical (I^{131}) and Surgical Therapy, *Ann Surg,* **162:**478, 1965.

Caswell, H. T., Robbins, R. R., and Rosemond, G. P.: Definitive Treatment of 536 Cases of Hyperthyroidism with I^{131} or Surgery, *Ann Surg,* **164:**593, 1966.

Goldsmith, R. E.: Radioisotope Therapy for Graves' Disease, *Mayo Clin Proc,* **47:**953, 1972.

Gould, E. A., Hirsch, E., and Brecher, I.: Complications Arising in the Course of Thyroidectomy, *Arch Surg,* **90:**81, 1965.

Green, M., and Wilson, G. M.: Thyrotoxicosis Treated by Surgery or Iodine 131 with Special Reference to Development of Hypothyroidism, *Br Med J,* **1:**1005, 1964.

Hales, I. B., and Rundle, F. F.: Ocular Changes in Graves' Disease: A Long-Term Follow-up Study, *Quart J Med,* **29:**113, 1960.

Hedley, A. J., Flemming, C. J., Chesters, M. I., Michie, W., and Crooks, J.: Surgical Treatment of Thyrotoxicosis, *Br Med J,* **1:**519, 1970.

Hollander, C. S., Nihei, N., Mitsuma, T., Scovill, C., and Gershengorn, M. C.: Elevated Serum Triiodothyronine in Association with Altered Available Iodide in Normal (NL) and Hyperthyroid Subjects, *Clin Res,* **19:**560, 1971.

Karlan, M. S., and Snyder, W. H.: Carcinoma of Thyroid following Treatment of Hyperthyroidism with I^{131}, *Calif Med,* **101:**196, 1964.

Michie, W., Pegg, C. A. S., and Bewsher, P. D.: Prediction of Hypothyroidism after Partial Thyroidectomy for Thyrotoxicosis, *Br Med J,* **1:**13, 1972.

Nofal, M. M., Beierwaltes, W. H., and Patno, M. E.: Treatment of Hyperthyroidism with Sodium Iodide I^{131}: A 16-year Experience, *JAMA,* **197:**695, 1966.

Ogura, J. H.: Transantral Orbital Decompression for Progressive Exophthalmos: A Follow-up of 54 Cases, *Med Clin North Am,* **52:**399, 1968.

Plested, W. G., III, and Pollock, W. F.: Radioactive Iodine, Antithyroid Drugs, and Surgery in Treatment of Hyperthyroidism, *Arch Surg,* **94:**517, 1967.

Riley, F. C.: Surgical Management of Ophthalmopathy in Graves' Disease: Transfrontal Orbital Decompression, *Mayo Clin Proc,* **47:**986, 1972.

Saenger, E. L., Thoma, G. E., and Tompkins, E. A.: Incidence of Leukemia following Treatment of Hyperthyroidism, *JAMA,* **205:**855, 1968.

Shapiro, S. J., Friedman, N. B., Perzik, S. L., and Catz, B.: Incidence of Thyroid Carcinoma in Graves' Disease, *Cancer,* **26:**1261, 1970.

Sheline, G. E., Lindsay, S., McCormack, K. R., and Galante, M.: Thyroid Nodules Occurring Late after Treatment of Thyrotoxicosis with Radioiodine, *J Clin Endocrinol Metab,* **22:**8, 1962.

Stanbury, J. B., and DeGroot, L. J.: Problems of Hypothyroidism after I[131] Therapy of Hyperthyroidism, *N Engl J Med,* **271:**195, 1964.

Trotter, W. R.: "Diseases of the Thyroid," Blackwell Scientific Publications, Ltd., Oxford, 1962.

Volpé, R., Edmonds, M., Lamki, L., Clarke, P. V., and Row, V. V.: The Pathogenesis of Graves' Disease: A Disorder of Delayed Hypersensitivity? *Mayo Clin Proc,* **47:**824, 1972.

Wahner, H. W.: T3 Hyperthyroidism, *Mayo Clin Proc,* **47:**938, 1972.

Hypothyroidism

Ingbar, S. H., and Woeber, K. A.: The Thyroid Gland, in R. H. Williams (ed.), "Textbook of Endocrinology," 4th ed., chap. 4, W. B. Saunders Company, Philadelphia, 1968.

Means, J. H., DeGroot, L. J., and Stanbury, J. B.: "The Thyroid and Its Diseases," 3d ed., McGraw-Hill Book Company, New York, 1963.

Van Welsum, M., Feltkamp, T. E. W., DeVries, M. J., Doctor, R., Van Zijl, J., and Hennemann, G.: Hypoparathyroidism after Thyroidectomy for Graves' Disease: Search for an Explanation, *Br Med J,* **4:**755, 1974.

Thyroiditis

Altemeier, W. A.: Acute Pyogenic Thyroiditis, *Arch Surg,* **61:**76, 1950.

Beahrs, O. H., Woolner, L. B., Engel, S., and McConahey, W. M.: Needle Biopsy of the Thyroid Gland and Management of Lymphocytic Thyroiditis, *Surg Gynecol Obstet,* **114:**636, 1962.

Block, M. A., Horn, R. C., Jr., and Miller, J. M.: Unilateral Thyroid Nodules with Lymphocytic Thyroiditis, *Arch Surg,* **87:**118, 1963.

Coons, A. H., and Kaplan, M. H.: Localization of Antigen in Tissue Cells: Improvements in Method for Detection of Antigen by Means of Fluorescent Antibody, *J Exp Med,* **91:**1, 1950.

Crile, G., Jr., and Hazard, J. B.: Incidence of Cancer in Struma Lymphomatosa, *Surg Gynecol Obstet,* **115:**101, 1962.

Greene, J. N.: Subacute Thyroiditis, *Am J Med,* **51:**97, 1971.

Hagan, A. D., Goffinet, J., and Davis, J. W.: Acute Streptococcal Thyroiditis, *JAMA,* **202:**842, 1967.

Hashimoto, H.: Zur Kenntriss der lymphomatösen Veränderung der Schilddrüse (Struma lymphomatosa), *Langenbecks Arch Klin Chir,* **97:**219, 1912.

Heimann, P.: Treatment of Thyroiditis, *Acta Med Scand,* **187:**323, 1970.

Hendrick, J. W.: Diagnosis and Treatment of Thyroiditis, *Ann Surg,* **144:**176, 1956.

Hirabayashi, R. N., and Lindsay, S.: The Relation of Thyroid

Carcinoma and Chronic Thyroiditis, *Surg Gynecol Obstet,* **121:**243, 1965.

Linden, M. C., Jr., and Clark, J. H.: Indications for Surgery in Thyroiditis, *Am J Surg,* **118:**829, 1969.

Mikal, S.: Hashimoto's Disease, *Surg Gynecol Obstet,* **121:**131, 1965.

Mulhern, L. M., Masi, A. T., and Shulman, L. E.: Hashimoto's Disease: A Search for Associated Disorders in 170 Clinically Detected Cases, *Lancet,* **2:**508, 1966.

Persson, P. S.: Cytodiagnosis of Thyroiditis: A Comparative Study of Cytological, Histological, Immunological, and Clinical Findings in Thyroiditis, Particularly in Diffuse Lymphoid Thyroiditis, *Acta Med Scand [Suppl]* 483, 1968.

Pollack, W. F., David, H., and Sprong, O. H., Jr.: The Rationale of Thyroidectomy for Hashimoto's Thyroiditis, *Western J Surg Obstet Gynecol,* **66:**17, 1958.

Quervain, F. de: Die akute, nicht eiterige Thyroiditis, *Mitt Grenzgeb Med Chir [Suppl],* **2:**1, 1904.

Roitt, I. M., Doniach, D., Campbell, P. N., and Hudson, R. V.: Auto-antibodies in Hashimoto's Disease, *Lancet,* **2:**820, 1956.

Rudman, I., Novota, O. J., and Keener, R. L.: Complications of Hashimoto Thyroiditis Surgery, *Arch Surg,* **83:**822, 1961.

Swann, N. H.: Acute Thyroiditis: A Clinical Report of Twelve Cases within a Four-Month Period, *Ann Intern Med,* **56:**68, 1962.

Volpé, R., Johnston, M. W., and Huber, N.: Thyroid Function in Subacute Thyroiditis, *J Clin Endocrinal Metab,* **18:**65, 1958.

Witebsky, E., Rose, N. R., Terplan, K., Paine, J. R., and Egan, R. W.: Chronic Thyroiditis and Autoimmunization, *JAMA,* **165:**1439, 1957.

Goiter

Astwood, E. B., Cassidy, C. E., and Aurbach, G. D.: Treatment of Goiter and Thyroid Nodules with Thyroid, *JAMA,* **174:**459, 1960.

Cole, W. H., Majarakis, J. D., and Slaughter, D. P.: Incidence of Carcinoma of the Thyroid in Nodular Goiter, *J Clin Endocrinol Metab,* **9:**1007, 1949.

Crile, G., Jr.: Treatment of Thyroid Cysts by Aspiration, *Surgery,* **59:**210, 1966.

Dobyns, B. M.: Goiter, *Curr Probl Surg,* January 1969.

Glassford, G. H., Fowler, E. F., and Cole, W. H.: The Treatment of Nontoxic Nodular Goiter with Dessicated Thyroid: Results and Evaluation, *Surgery,* **58:**621, 1965.

Ingbar, S. H., and Woeber, K. A.: The Thyroid Gland, in R. H. Williams (ed.), "Textbook of Endocrinology," W. B. Saunders Company, Philadelphia, 1968.

Jenny, H., Block, M. A., Horn, R. C., and Miller, J. M.: Recurrence following Surgery for Benign Thyroid Nodules, *Arch Surg,* **92:**525, 1966.

Liechty, R. D., Graham, M., and Freemeyer, P.: Benign Solitary Thyroid Nodules, *Surg Gynecol Obstet,* **121:**571, 1965.

Robinson, E., Horn, Y., and Hochmann, A.: Incidence of Cancer in Thyroid Nodules, *Surg Gynecol Obstet,* **123:**1024, 1966.

Shimaoka, K., Badillo, J., Sokal, J. E., and Marchetta, F. C.: Clinical Differentiation between Thyroid Cancer and Benign Goiter, *JAMA,* **181:**179, 1962.

Sokal, J. E.: The Incidence of Thyroid Cancer and the Problem of Malignancy in Nodular Goiter, in E. B. Astwood (ed.),

"Clinical Endocrinology," vol. I, Grune & Stratton, Inc., New York, 1960.

Benign Tumors

Ackerman, L. V.: "Surgical Pathology," The C. V. Mosby Company, St. Louis, 1964.

Means, J. H., DeGroot, L. J., and Stanbury, J. B.: "The Thyroid and Its Diseases," 3d ed., McGraw-Hill Book Company, New York, 1963.

Malignant Tumors

Beahrs, O. H., and Pasternak, B. M.: Cancer of the Thyroid Gland, *Curr Probl Surg,* December 1969.

Black, B. M., YaDeau, R. E., and Woolner, L. B.: Surgical Treatment of Thyroidal Carcinomas, *Arch Surg,* 88:610, 1964.

Block, M. A., Horn, R. C., Jr., Miller, J. M., Barrett, J. L., and Brush, B. E.: Familial Medullary Carcinoma of the Thyroid, *Ann Surg,* 166:403, 1967.

——, and ——: Medullary Carcinoma of the Thyroid: Surgical Implications, *Arch Surg,* 96:521, 1968.

——, and ——: Thyroid Carcinoma with Cervical Lymph Node Metastasis: Effectiveness of Total Thyroidectomy and Node Dissection, *Am J Surg,* 122:458, 1971.

——, Jackson, C. E., and Tashjian, A. H., Jr.: Medullary Thyroid Carcinoma Detected by Serum Calcitonin Assay, *Arch Surg,* 104:579, 1972.

Buckwalter, J. A., and Thomas, C. G., Jr.: Selection of Surgical Treatment for Well Differentiated Thyroid Carcinomas, *Ann Surg,* 176:565, 1972.

Crile, G., Jr.: The Fallacy of the Conventional Radical Neck Dissection for Papillary Carcinoma of the Thyroid, *Ann Surg,* 145:317, 1957.

——: Papillary Carcinoma of the Thyroid, in E. B. Astwood (ed.), "Clinical Endocrinology," vol. I., Grune & Stratton, Inc., New York, 1960.

——: Late Results of Treatment for Papillary Cancer of the Thyroid, *Ann Surg,* 160:178, 1964.

——: Lymphosarcoma and Reticulum Cell Sarcoma of the Thyroid, *Surg Gynecol Obstet,* 116:449, 1963.

——: Changing End Results in Patients with Papillary Carcinoma of the Thyroid, *Surg Gynecol Obstet,* 132:460, 1971.

——, Suhrer, J. G., Jr., and Hazard, J. B.: Results of Conservative Operations for Malignant Tumors of the Thyroid, *J Clin Endocrinol Metab,* 15:1422, 1955.

Doniach, I.: Aetiological Consideration of Thyroid Carcinoma, in D. Smithers (ed.), "Tumours of the Thyroid Gland," p. 55, E. & S. Livingstone, London, 1970.

Duffy, B. J.: Can Radiation Cause Thyroid Cancer? *J Clin Endocrinol Metab,* 17:1383, 1957.

Frazell, E. L., and Duffy, B. J.: Invasive Papillary Cancer of the Thyroid, *J Clin Endocrinol Metab,* 14:1362, 1954.

—— and Foote, F. W.: Papillary Cancer of the Thyroid: A Review of 25 Years of Experience, *Cancer,* 11:895, 1958.

Freund, H. R.: Surgical Treatment of Metastases to the Thyroid Gland from Other Primary Malignancies, *Ann Surg,* 162:285, 1965.

Glass, H. G., Waldron, G. W., Allen, H. C., Jr., and Brown, W. G.: A Rational Approach to the Thyroid Malignancy Problem, *Am Surg,* 26:81, 1960.

Gowing, N. F. C.: The Pathology and Natural History of Thyroid Tumours, in D. Smithers (ed.), "Tumours of the Thyroid Gland," p. 103, E. & S. Livingstone, London, 1970.

Harness, J. K., Thompson, N. W., Sisson, J. C., and Beierwaltes, W. H.: Differentiated Thyroid Carcinomas: Treatment of Distant Metastases, *Arch Surg,* 108:410, 1974.

Hill, C. S., Clark, R. L., and Wolf, M.: The Effect of Subsequent Pregnancy on Patients with Thyroid Carcinoma, *Surg Gynecol Obstet,* 122:1219, 1966.

Hirabayashi, R. N., and Lindsay, S.: Carcinoma of the Thyroid Gland: A Statistical Study of 390 Patients, *J Clin Endocrinol Metab,* 21:1596, 1961.

Kaplan, E. L., and Peskin, G. W.: Physiologic Implications of Medullary Carcinoma of the Thyroid Gland, *Surg Clin North Am,* 51:125, 1971.

Klopp, C. T., Rosvoll, R. V., and Winship, T.: Is Destructive Surgery Ever Necessary for Treatment of Thyroid Cancer in Children? *Ann Surg,* 165:745, 1967.

McDermott, W. V., Jr., Morgan, W. S., Hamlin, E., Jr., and Cope, O.: Cancer of the Thyroid, *J Clin Endocrinol Metab,* 14:1336, 1954.

Marchetta, F. C., and Sako, K.: Modified Neck Dissection for Carcinoma of the Thyroid Gland, *Surg Gynecol Obstet,* 119:551, 1964.

Medina, R. G., and Elliott, D. W.: Thyroid Carcinoma: An Analysis of 130 Cases, *Arch Surg,* 97:239, 1968.

Mikal, S.: Primary Lymphoma of the Thyroid Gland, *Surgery,* 55:233, 1964.

Sedgwick, C. E., and Konvolinka, C. W.: Management of Carcinoma of the Thyroid, *Surg Clin North Am,* 47:607, 1967.

Shapiro, S. J., Friedman, N. B., Perzik, S. L., and Catz, B.: Incidence of Thyroid Carcinoma in Graves' Disease, *Cancer,* 26:1261, 1970.

Silverberg, S. G., and Vidone, R. A.: Carcinoma of the Thyroid in Surgical and Postmortem Material: Analysis of 300 Cases at Autopsy and Literature Review, *Ann Surg,* 164:291, 1966.

Sipple, J. H.: The Association of Pheochromocytoma with Carcinoma of the Thyroid Gland, *Am J Med,* 31:163, 1961.

Smithers, D. W.: Malignant Lymphomas of the Thyroid Gland, in D. Smithers (ed.), "Tumours of the Thyroid Gland," p. 141, E. & S. Livingstone, London, 1970.

Tollefsen, H. R., and DeCosse, J. J.: Papillary Carcinoma of the Thyroid: Recurrence in the Thyroid Gland after Initial Surgical Treatment, *Am J Surg,* 106:728, 1963.

Wells, S. A., Jr., Ontjes, D. A., Cooper, C. W., Hennessy, J. F., Ellis, G. J., McPherson, H. T., and Sabiston, D. C., Jr.: Early Diagnosis of Medullary Carcinoma of the Thyroid Gland in Patients with Multiple Endocrine Neoplasia Type II, *Ann Surg,* 182:362, 1975.

Williams, E. D.: The Origin and Associations of Medullary Carcinoma of the Thyroid, in D. Smithers (ed.), "Tumours of the Thyroid Gland," p. 130, E. & S. Livingstone, London, 1970.

Wychulis, A. R., Beahrs, O. H., and Woolner, L. B.: Metastasis of Carcinoma to the Thyroid Gland, *Ann Surg,* 160:169, 1964.

——, ——, and ——: Papillary Carcinoma with Associated Anaplastic Carcinoma in the Thyroid Gland, *Surg Gynecol Obstet,* 120:28, 1965.

Surgery of the Thyroid

Adams, H. D.: Transthoracic Thyroidectomy, *J Thorac Cardiov Surg,* **19:**741, 1950.

Block, M. A., Jackson, C. E., and Tashjian, A. H.: Management of Parathyroid Glands in Surgery for Medullary Thyroid Carcinoma, *Arch Surg,* **110:**617, 1975.

Buckwalter, J. A., Soper, R. T., Davies, J., and Mason, E. E.: Postoperative Hypoparathyroidism, *Surg Gynecol Obstet,* **101:**657, 1955.

Chamberlin, J. A., Fries, J. G., and Allen, H. C., Jr.: Thyroid Carcinoma and the Problem of Postoperative Tetany, *Surgery,* **55:**787, 1964.

Colcock, B. P.: Surgery of Primary Hyperthyroidism, *Surg Clin North Am,* **40:**595, 1960.

———— and King, M. L.: The Mortality and Morbidity of Thyroid Surgery, *Surg Gynecol Obstet,* **114:**131, 1962.

Cope, O.: Surgery of the Thyroid, in J. H. Means, L. J. DeGroot, and J. B. Stanbury, "The Thyroid and Its Diseases," 3d ed., McGraw-Hill Book Company, New York, 1963.

Doyle, P. J., Everts, E. C., and Brummett, R. E.: Treatment of Recurrent Laryngeal Nerve Injury, *Arch Surg,* **96:**517, 1968.

Gould, E. A., Hirsch, E., and Brecher, I.: Complications Arising in the Course of Thyroidectomy, *Arch Surg,* **90:**81, 1965.

Halsted, W. S., and Evans, H. M.: The Parathyroid Glandules: Their Blood Supply and Preservation in Operations upon the Thyroid Gland, *Ann Surg,* **46:**489, 1907.

Hawe, P., and Lothian, K. R.: Recurrent Laryngeal Nerve Injury during Thyroidectomy, *Surg Gynecol Obstet,* **110:**488, 1960.

Holl-Allen, R. T. J.: Haemorrhage following Thyroidectomy for Thyrotoxicosis, *Br J Surg,* **54:**703, 1967.

Johnston, J. H., and Twente, G. E.: Surgical Approach to Intrathoracic (Mediastinal) Goiter, *Ann Surg,* **143:**572, 1956.

Lahey, F. H.: Routine Dissection and Demonstration of Recurrent Laryngeal Nerve in Subtotal Thyroidectomy, *Surg Gynecol Obstet,* **66:**775, 1938.

————: Intrathoracic Goiters, *Surg Clin North Am,* **25:**609, 1945.

———— and Hoover, W. B.: Tracheotomy after Thyroidectomy, *Ann Surg,* **133:**65, 1951.

Lee, T. C., Coffey, R. J., Mackin, J., Cobb, M., Routon, J., and Canary, J. J.: Use of Propranolol in Surgical Treatment of Thyrotoxic Patients, *Ann Surg,* **177:**643, 1973.

Perzik, S. L.: "Surgery in Thyroid Disease," Stratton Intercontinental Medical Book Corporation, New York, 1976.

Pimstone, B., and Joffe, B.: Use and Abuse of β-Adrenergic Blockade in Surgery of Hyperthyroidism, *S Afr Med J,* **44:**1059, 1970.

Smith, R. N., and Laljee, H. C. K.: Thyrocalcitonin Deficiency after Treatment of Thyroid Disorders by Surgery or Radioiodine, *Br Med J,* **4:**589, 1967.

Thompson, N. W., and Harness, J. K.: Complications of Total Thyroidectomy for Carcinoma, *Surg Gynecol Obstet,* **131:**861, 1970.

————, Olsen, W. R., and Hoffman, G. L.: The Continuing Development of the Technique of Thyroidectomy, *Surgery,* **73:**913, 1973.

Wade, J. S. H.: Three Major Complications of Thyroidectomy, *Br J Surg,* **52:**727, 1965.

Watkins, E., Jr., Bell, G. O., Snow, J. C., and Adams, H. D.: Incidence and Current Management of Post-thyroidectomy Hypoparathyroidism: Histologic Evidence of Rejection of Neonatal Aortic Pedicle Parathyroid Gland Homotransplants, *JAMA,* **182:**138, 1962.

Parathyroid: Embryology and Anatomy

Block, M. A., Miller, M., and Horn, R. C.: Minimizing Hypoparathyroidism after Extended Thyroid Operations, *Surg Gynecol Obstet,* **123:**501, 1966.

Durham, C. T., and Harrison, T. S.: The Surgical Anatomy of the Superior Laryngeal Nerve, *Surg Gynecol Obstet,* **118:**38, 1964.

Gilmour, J. R.: The Embryology of the Parathyroid Glands, the Thymus and Certain Associated Rudiments, *J Pathol,* **45:**507, 1937.

————: The Weight of the Parathyroid Glands, *J Pathol Bacteriol,* **44:**431, 1937.

————: The Gross Anatomy of the Parathyroid Glands, *J Pathol Bacteriol,* **46:**133, 1938.

Hunt, P. S., Poole, M., and Reeve, T. S.: A Reappraisal of the Surgical Anatomy of the Thyroid and Parathyroid Glands, *Br J Surg,* **55:**63, 1968.

State, D.: The Enlarged Inferior Thyroid Artery: A Valuable Guide in Surgery of Parathyroid Adenomas, *Surgery,* **56:**461, 1964.

Parathyroid Hormone: Chemistry

Brewer, H. B., Fairwell, T., Ronan, R., Sizemore, G. W., and Arnaud, C. D.: Human Parathyroid Hormone: Amino-Acid Sequence of the Amino-Terminal Residues 1–34, *Proc Nat Acad Sci USA,* **69:**3585, 1972.

————, and Ronan, R.: The Amino Acid Sequence of Bovine Parathyroid Hormone, *Proc Nat Acad Sci USA,* **67:**1862, 1970.

Habener, J. F., Potts, J. T., Jr., and Rich, A.: Pre-Proparathyroid Hormone. Evidence for an Early Biosynthetic Precursor of Proparathyroid Hormone, *J Biol Chem,* **251:**3893, 1976.

Kemper, B., Habener, J. F., Ernst, M. D., Potts, J. T., Jr., and Rich, A.: Pre-proparathyroid Hormone Analysis of Radioactive Tryptic Peptides and Amino Acid Sequence, *Biochemistry,* **15:**15, 1976.

Keutmann, H. T., Aurbach, G. D., Dawson, B. F., Niall, H. D., Deftos, L. J., and Potts, J. T., Jr.: Isolation and Characterization of Bovine Parathyroid Isohormones, *Biochemistry,* **10:**2779, 1971.

Niall, H. D., Keutmann, H. T., Sauer, R., Hogan, M. L., Dawson, B. F., Aurbach, G. D., and Potts, J. T., Jr.: The Amino Acid Sequence of Bovine Parathyroid Hormone I, *Hoppe-Seyler's Z, Physiol Chem,* **351:**1586, 1970.

Potts, J. T., Jr., Murray, T. M., Peacock, M., et al.: Parathyroid Hormone: Sequence, Synthesis, Immunoassay Studies, *Am J Med,* **50:**639, 1971.

————, Tregear, G. W., Keutmann, H. T., Niall, H. D., Sauer, R., Deftos, L. J., Dawson, B. F., Hogan, M. L., and Aurbach, G. D.: Synthesis of a Biologically Active *N*-terminal Tetra-triacontapeptide of Parathyroid Hormone, *Proc Nat Acad Sci USA,* **68:**63, 1971.

Parathyroid: Vitamin D

Brickman, A. S., Coburn, J. W., and Norman, A. W.: Action of 1,25-dihydroxycholecalciferol: A Potent, Kidney Produced

Metabolite of Vitamin D₃ in Uremic Man, *N Engl J Med,* **287:**891, 1972.

DeLuca, H. F.: Vitamin D: The Vitamin and the Hormone, *Fed Proc,* **33:**2211, 1974.

————: Vitamin D Endocrinology, *Ann Intern Med,* **85:**367, 1976.

Kodicek, E.: The Story of Vitamin D, from Vitamin to Hormone, *Lancet,* **1:**325, 1974.

Lawson, D. E. M., Fraser, D. M., Kodicek, E., et al.: Identification of 1,25-dihydroxycholecalciferol: A New Kidney Hormone Controlling Calcium Metabolism, *Nature (Lond),* **230:**228, 1971.

Teitelbaum, S. L., Bone, J. M., Stein, P. M., Gilden, J. J., Bates, M., Boisseau, V. C., and Avioli, L. V.: Calcifediol in Chronic Renal Insufficiency, *JAMA,* **235:**164, 1976.

Calcitonin and Medullary Carcinoma of the Thyroid

Aliapoulios, M. A., Goldhaber, P., and Munson, P. L.: Thyrocalcitonin Inhibition of Bone Resorption Induced by Parathyroid Hormone in Tissue Culture, *Science,* **151:**330, 1966.

Arnaud, C. D., Littledike, T., and Tsao, H. S.: Calcium Homeostasis and the Simultaneous Measurement of Calcitonin and Parathyroid Hormone in the Pig, in S. Taylor (ed.): "Calcitonin 1969: Proceedings of the Second International Symposium, London, 1970," pp. 95–101, William Heinemann Medical Books, Ltd., 1970.

————, ————, ————, and Kaplan, E. L.: Radioimmunoassay for Calcitonin: A Preliminary Report, *Proc Staff Meetings Mayo Clin,* **43:**496, 1968.

Beahrs, O. H., and Pasternak, B. M.: Cancer of the Thyroid Gland, *Curr Probl Surg,* December 1969.

Copp, D. H., Cameron, E. C., Cheney, B. A., Davidson, A. G. F., and Henze, K. G.: Evidence for Calcitonin: A New Hormone from the Parathyroid That Lowers Blood Calcium, *Endocrinology,* **70:**638, 1962.

————, Cockcroft, D. W., and Kueh, Y.: Calcitonin from Ultimobranchial Glands of Dogfish and Chickens, *Science,* **158:**924, 1967.

Deftos, L. J., Bury, A. E., Habener, J. F., Singer, F. R., and Potts, J. T., Jr.: Immunoassay for Human Calcitonin: II. Clinical Studies, *Metabolism,* **20:**1129, 1971.

Gonzalez-Licea, A., Hartmann, W. H., and Yardley, J. H.: Medullary Carcinoma of the Thyroid: Ultrastructural Evidence of Its Origin from the Parafollicular Cell and Its Possible Relation to Carcinoid Tumors, *J Clin Pathol,* **49:**512, 1968.

Hazard, J. B., Hawk, W. A., and Crile, G., Jr.: Medullary (Solid) Carcinoma of the Thyroid: Clinicopathological Entity, *J Clin Endocrinol Metab,* **19:**152, 1959.

Hennessy, J. F., Wells, S. A., Jr., Ontjes, D. A., and Cooper, C. W.: A Comparison of Pentagastrin Injection and Calcium Infusion as Provocative Test for the Detection of Medullary Carcinoma of the Thyroid, *J Clin Endocrinol Metab,* **39:**487, 1974.

Hirsch, P. F., Cauthier, G. F., and Munson, P. L.: Thyroid Hypocalcemic Principle and Recurrent Laryngeal Nerve Injury as Factors Affecting the Response to Parathyroidectomy in Rats, *Endocrinology,* **73:**244, 1963.

Kaplan, E. L.: Recent Advances in Calcium Metabolism: Application to Medullary Carcinoma of Thyroid and Hyperparathyroidism, *Surg Annu,* 1973.

————, and Peskin, G. W.: Physiologic Implications of Medullary

Carcinoma of the Thyroid Gland, *Surg Clin North Am,* **51:**125, 1971.

Ljungberg, O.: On Medullary Carcinoma of the Thyroid, *Acta Patholog Microbiol Scand [A] Suppl* 231, 1972.

Melvin, K. E. W., Tashjian, A. H., Jr., and Miller, H. H.: Studies in Familial (Medullary) Thyroid Carcinoma, *Recent Prog Horm Res,* **28:**399, 1972.

Pearse, A. G. E., and Polak, J. M.: Cytochemical Evidence for the Neural Crest Origin of Mammalian Ultimobranchial C cells, *Histochemie,* **27:**96, 1971.

Potts, J. T., Jr., Niall, H. D. Keutmann, H. T., and Lequin, R. M.: Chemistry of the Calcitonins: Species Variation plus Structure-Activity Relations, and Pharmacologic Implications, in R. V. Talmage and P. L. Munson (eds.), "Calcium, Parathyroid Hormone and the Calcitonins," pp. 121–127. Excerpta Medica, Amsterdam, 1972.

Queener, S. F., and Bell, N. H.: Calcitonin: A General Survey, *Metabolism,* **24:**555, 1975.

Tashjian, A. H., Jr., Howland, B. G., Melvin, K. E. W., and Hill, C. S., Jr.: Immunoassay for Human Calcitonin: Clinical Measurement, Relation to Serum Calcium and Studies in Patients with Medullary Carcinoma, *N Engl J Med,* **283:**890, 1970.

Wells, S. A., Jr., Ontjes, D. A., Cooper, C. W., Hennessy, J. F., Ellis, G. J., McPherson, H. T., and Sabiston, D. C., Jr.: The Early Diagnosis of Medullary Carcinoma of the Thyroid Gland in Patients with Multiple Endocrine Neoplasia, Type II, *Ann Surg,* **182:**362, 1975.

Wolfe, H. J., Melvin, K. E. W., Cervi-Skinner, S. J., Al Saadi, A. A., Juliar, J. F., Jackson, C. E., and Tashjian, A. H., Jr.: C-Cell Hyperplasia Preceding Medullary Thyroid Carcinoma, *N Engl J Med,* **289:**437, 1973.

Parathyroid: Pathology

Black, W. C., III.: Correlative Light and Electron Microscopy in Primary Hyperparathyroidism, *Arch Pathol,* **88:**225, 1969.

———— and Haff, R. C.: The Surgical Pathology of Parathyroid Chief Cell Hyperplasia, *Am J Clin Pathol,* **53:**565, 1970.

Castleman, B.: Tumors of the Parathyroid Glands, in "Atlas of Tumor Pathology," Fascicle 15, p. 1, Armed Forces Institute of Pathology, Washington, 1952.

Cope, O., Keynes, W. M., Roth, S. I., and Castleman, B.: Primary Chief-Cell Hyperplasia of the Parathyroid Glands: A New Entity in the Surgery of Hyperparathyroidism, *Ann Surg,* **148:**375, 1958.

Hall, E. M., and Chaffin, L.: Final Report of a Case of Malignant Adenoma of the Parathyroid Glands, *Western J Surg,* **48:**685, 1940.

Hellstrom, J., and Ivemark, B. I.: Primary Hyperparathyroidism: Clinical and Structural Findings in 138 Cases, *Acta Chir Scand [Suppl],* **294:**1, 1962.

Holmes, E. C., Morton, D. L., and Ketcham, A. S.: Parathyroid Carcinoma: A Collective Review, *Ann Surg,* **169:**631, 1969.

Holzmann, K., and Lange, R.: Zur Zytologie der Glandula parathyroeidea des Menschen: Weitere Untersuchungen an Epithelkörperadenomen, *Z. Zellforsch* **58:**759, 1963.

Roth, S. I.: Pathology of the Parathyroids in Hyperparathyroidism: Discussion of Recent Advances in the Anatomy and Pathology of the Parathyroid Glands, *Arch Path (Chicago)* **73:**495, 1962.

————: The Ultrastructure of Primary Water-clear Cell Hyperplasia of the Parathyroid Glands, *Amer J Path,* **61:**233, 1970.

————: Recent Advances in Parathyroid Gland Pathology, *Amer J Med,* **50:**612, 1971.

———— and Marshall, R. B.: Pathology and Ultrastructure of the Human Parathyroid Glands in Chronic Renal Failure, *Arch Intern Med, (Chicago)* **124:**397, 1969.

Schantz, A., and Castleman, B.: Parathyroid Carcinoma: A Study of 70 Cases, *Cancer,* **31:**600, 1973.

Steiner, A. L., Goodman, A. D., and Powers, S. R.: Study of a Kindred with Pheochromocytoma, Medullary Thyroid Carcinoma, Hyperparathyroidism and Cushing's Disease: Multiple Endocrine Neoplasia, Type 2, *Medicine (Balt)* **47:**371, 1968.

Utley, J. R., and Black, W. C.: Hyperparathyroidism: A Clinicopathologic Evaluation, *Amer J Surg,* **114:**788, 1967.

Wermer, P.: Endocrine Adenomatosis and Peptic Ulcer in a Large Kindred: Inherited Multiple Tumors and Mosaic Pleiotropism in Man, *Amer J Med,* **35:**205, 1963.

Primary Hyperparathyroidism

Arnaud, C. D., Goldsmith, R., Bischoff, J., Sizemore, G., Oldham, S., and Larsen, J.: Antibody Specificity, Immunochemical Heterogeneity and the Interpretation of Measurements of Plasma Parathyroid Hormone by Radioimmunoassay, *J Clin Invest,* **51:**5a, 1972.

————, Sizemore, G. W., Oldham, S. B., Fischer, J. A., Tsao, H. S., and Littledike, E. T.: Human Parathyroid Hormone: Glandular and Secreted Molecular Species, *Am J Med,* **50:**630, 1971.

————, Tsao, H. S., and Littledike, T.: Radioimmunoassay of Human Parathyroid Hormone in Serum, *J Clin Invest,* **50:**21, 1971.

Aurbach, G. D., and Chase, L. R.: Cyclic 3'5'-Adenylic Acid in Bone and the Mechanism of Action of Parathyroid Hormone, *Fed Proc,* **29:**1179, 1970.

Ballard, H. S., Frane, B., and Hartsock, R. J.: Familial Multiple Endocrine Adenoma-Peptic Ulcer Complex, *Medicine (Baltimore),* **43:**481, 1964.

Barreras, R. F., and Donaldson, R. M., Jr.: Role of Calcium in Gastric Hypersecretion, Parathyroid Adenoma and Peptic Ulcer, *N Engl J Med,* **276:**1122, 1967.

Barzel, U. S.: Parathyroid Hormone and the Buffering Function of Bone, *Hosp Practice,* **6:**131, 1971.

Bélanger, L. F., Robichon, J., Migicovsky, B. B., et al.: Resorption without Osteoclasts (Osteolysis), in R. F. Sognnaes, (ed.), "Mechanisms of Hard Tissue Destruction," p. 531, American Association for the Advancement of Science, Washington, 1963.

Bernstein, D. S.: Hypercalcemia Associated with Sarcoidosis, Hypernephroma, and Parathyroid Adenoma, *J Clin Endocrinol Metab,* **25:**1436, 1965.

Black, B. K.: Carcinoma of the Parathyroid, *Ann Surg,* **139:**355, 1954.

Black, W. C., III, and Utley, J. R.: The Differential Diagnosis of Parathyroid Adenoma and Chief Cell Hyperplasia, *Am J Clin Pathol,* **49:**761, 1968.

Block, M. A., Frame, B., Jackson, C. E., et al.: The Extent of Operation for Primary Hyperparathyroidism, *Arch Surg,* **109:**798, 1974.

————, ————, ————, et al.: Primary Diffuse Microscopical Hyperplasia of the Parathyroid Glands, *Arch Surg,* **111:**348, 1976.

Bruining, H. A.: "Surgical Treatment of Hyperparathyroidism," Assen, The Netherlands, Charles C Thomas, Publisher, Springfield, Ill., 1971.

Buckle, R. M., Smith, F. G., and Alexander, D. P.: Assessment of Parathyroid Glandular Activity in the Foetus, in R. V. Talmadge and P. L. Munson (eds.), "Calcium, Parathyroid Hormone and the Calcitonins," p. 127, Excerpta Medica, Amsterdam, 1972.

Cameron, J. R., and Sorenson, J.: Measurement of Bone Mineral In Vivo: An Improved Method, *Science,* **142:**230, 1963.

Canterbury, J. M., and Reiss, E.: Fractionation of Circulating Parathyroid Hormone (PTH) in Man, *J Lab Clin Med,* **78:**814, 1971.

Chase, L. R., and Aurbach, G. D.: Renal Adenyl Cyclase: Anatomically Separate Sites for Parathyroid Hormone and Vasopressin, *Science,* **159:**545, 1968.

Chaves-Carballo, E., and Hayles, A. B.: Parathyroid Adenoma in Children, *Am J Dis Child,* **112:**553, 1966.

Clark, O. H., and Taylor, S.: Persistent and Recurrent Hyperparathyroidism, *Br J Surg,* **59:**555, 1972.

————, Way, L. W., and Hunt, T. K.: Recurrent Hyperparathyroidism, *Ann Surg,* **184:**391, 1976.

Clunie, G. J. A., Gunn, A., and Robson, J. S.: Hyperparathyroid Crisis, *Br J Surg,* **54:**538, 1967.

Condon, R. E., Granville, G. E., Jordon, P. H., and Helgason, A. H.: Hypercalcemic Crisis and Intractable Gastrointestinal Ulceration in a Patient with Endocrine Polyglandular Syndrome, *Ann Surg,* **167:**185, 1968.

Cope, O.: The Study of Hyperparathyroidism at the Massachusetts General Hospital, *N Engl J Med,* **274:**1174, 1966.

Cushing, H., and Davidoff, L. M.: "The Pathological Findings in Four Autopsied Cases of Acromegaly with a Discussion of Their Significance," Monograph 22, The Rockefeller Institute for Medical Research, New York, 1927.

Cutler, R. E., Reiss, E., and Ackerman, L. V.: Familial Hyperparathyroidism: A Kindred Involving Eleven Cases with a Discussion of Primary Chief-Cell Hyperplasia, *N Engl J Med,* **270:**859, 1964.

Davies, D. R.: The Surgery of Primary Hyperparathyroidism, *Clin Endocrinol Metab,* **3:**253, 1974.

Delmonico, F., Neer, R. M., Cosimi, A. B., Barnes, A. B., and Russell, P. S.: Hyperparathyroidism during Pregnancy, *Am J Surg,* **131:**328, 1976.

Dent, C. E.: Cortisone Test for Hyperparathyroidism, *Br Med J,* **1:**120, 1956.

DiGiulio, W., and Beierwaltes, W. H.: Parathyroid Scanning with Selenium 75 Labeled Methionine, *J Nucl Med,* **5:**417, 1964.

Egdahl, R. H., Canterbury, J. M., and Reiss, E.: Measurement of Circulating Parathyroid Hormone Concentration Before and After Parathyroid Surgery for Adenoma or Hyperplasia, *Ann Surg,* **168:**714, 1968.

Farr, H. W.: Hyperparathyroidism and Cancer, *Cancer,* **26:**66, 1976.

Friderichsen, C.: Tetany in a Suckling, *Lancet,* **1:**85, 1939.

Gaeke, R. F., Kaplan, E. L., Lindheimer, M. D., Coe, F., and Shen, K-I.: Successful Treatment of Maternal Primary

Hyperparathyroidism of Pregnancy by Parathyroidectomy, *JAMA,* **238**(6):508, 1977.

Goldberg, M. F., Tashjian, A. H., Jr., Order, S. E., and Dammin, G. J.: Renal Adenocarcinoma Containing a Parathyroid Hormone-like Substance and Associated with Marked Hypercalcemia, *Am J Med,* **36:**805, 1964.

Graber, A. L., and Jacobs, K.: Familial Hyperparathyroidism, *JAMA,* **240:**542, 1968.

Haff, R. C., and Ballinger, W. F.: Causes of Recurrent Hypercalcemia after Parathyroidectomy for Primary Hyperparathyroidism, *Ann Surg,* **173:**884, 1971.

———, Black, W. C., and Ballinger, W. F., II: Primary Hyperparathyroidism: Changing Clinical, Surgical and Pathologic Aspects, *Ann Surg,* **171:**85, 1970.

Hartenstein, H., and Gardner, L. I.: Tetany of the Newborn Associated with Maternal Parathyroid Adenoma, *N Engl J Med,* **274:**266, 1966.

Hellstrom, J.: Hyperparathyroidism and Gastroduodenal Ulcer, *Acta Chir Scand,* **116:**207, 1959.

———, Birke, G., and Edvall, C. A.: Hypertension in Hyperparathyroidism, *Br J Urol,* **30:**13, 1958.

——— and Ivemark, B. I.: Primary Hyperparathyroidism: Clinical and Structural Findings in 138 Cases, *Acta Chir Scand [Suppl],* **294:**1, 1962.

Hillman, D. A., Scriver, C. R., Pedris, S., and Shragovitch, I.: Neonatal Familial Primary Hyperparathyroidism, *N Engl J Med,* **270:**483, 1964.

Hines, J. R., and Suker, J. R.: Some Unusual Manifestations of Parathyroid Disease, *Surg Clin North Am,* **53:**221, 1973.

Jackson, C. E.: Hereditary Hyperparathyroidism Associated with Recurrent Pancreatitis, *Ann Intern Med,* **49:**829, 1958.

———: The Association of Peptic Ulcer with Hereditary Hyperparathyroidism, *Gastroenterology,* **37:**35, 1959.

——— and Boonstra, C. E.: The Relationship of Hereditary Hyperparathyroidism to Endocrine Adenomatosis, *Am J Med,* **43:**727, 1967.

Jackson, W. P.: Gout Hyperparathyroidism: Report of a Case with Examination of the Synovial Fluid, *Br Med J,* **2:**211, 1965.

Johansson, H., Thoren, L., and Werner, I.: Hyperparathyroidism, *Upsala J Med Sci,* **77:**41, 1972.

Jowsey, J.: Quantitative Microradiography, *Am J Med,* **40:**485, 1966.

Lafferty, F. W.: Pseudohyperparathyroidism, *Medicine,* **45:**247, 1966.

Low, J. C., Schaaf, M., Earll, J. M., Piechocki, J. T., and Li, T. K.: The Value of Serum Ionized Calcium in the Diagnosis of Normocalcemic and Hypercalcemic Primary Hyperparathyroidism, *Clin Res,* **19:**375, 1971.

Ludwig, G. D.: Hyperparathyroidism in Relation to Pregnancy, *N Engl J Med,* **267:**637, 1962.

MacLeod, W. A. J., and Holloway, C. K.: Hyperparathyroid Crisis: A Collective Review, *Ann Surg,* **166:**1012, 1967.

Maurer, W. J., Johnston, J. R., and Mendenhall, J. T.: Mediastinal Parathyroid Adenoma, *J Thorac Cardiovasc Surg,* **49:**657, 1965.

Mintz, D. H., Canary, J. J., Carreon, G., and Kyle, L. H.: Hyperuricemia in Hyperparathyroidism, *N Engl J Med,* **265:**112, 1961.

Mixter, C. G., Jr., Keynes, W. M., and Cope, O.: Further Experi-

ence with Pancreatitis as a Diagnostic Clue to Hyperparathyroidism, *N Engl J Med,* **266:**265, 1962.

Muller, H.: True Recurrence of Hyperparathyroidism: Proposed Criteria of Recurrence, *Br J Surg,* **62:**556, 1975.

Myers, R. T.: Followup Study of Surgically-Treated Primary Hyperparathyroidism, *Ann Surg,* **179:**729, 1974.

Nathaniels, E. K., Nathaniels, A. M., and Wang, C.-A.: Mediastinal Parathyroid Tumors: A Clinical and Pathological Study of 84 Cases, *Ann Surg,* **171:**165, 1970.

Nolan, R. B., Hayles, A. B., and Woolner, L. B.: Adenoma of the Parathyroid Gland in Children: Report of Case and Brief Review of the Literature, *Am J Dis Child,* **99:**622, 1960.

Norris, E. H.: Collective Review: Parathyroid Adenoma; Study of 322 Cases, *Int Abstr Surg,* **84:**1, 1947.

Palmer, J. A., Brown, W. A., Kerr, W. H., Rosen, I. B., and Watters, N. A.: The Surgical Aspects of Hyperparathyroidism, *Arch Surg,* **110:**1004, 1975.

Paloyan, E., Lawrence, A. M., Baker, W. H., and Straus, F. H.: Near-Total Parathyroidectomy, *Surg Clin North Am,* **49**(1):43, 1969.

———, ———, and Straus, F. H.: "Hyperparathyroidism," Grune & Stratton, New York and London, 1973.

———, ———, Straus, F. H., II, Paloyan, D., Harper, P. V., and Cummings, D.: Alpha Cell Hyperplasia in Calcific Pancreatitis Associated with Hyperparathyroidism, *JAMA,* **200:**757, 1967.

———, Paloyan, D., and Pickleman, J. R.: Hyperparathyroidism Today, *Surg Clin North Am,* **53:**211, 1973.

Plimpton, C. H., and Gelhorn, A.: Hypercalcemia in Malignant Disease without Evidence of Bone Destruction, *Am J Med,* **21:**750, 1956.

Purnell, D. C., Scholz, D. A., Smith, L. H., Sizemore, G. W., Black, B. M., Goldsmith, R. S., and Arnaud, C. D.: Treatment of Primary Hyperparathyroidism, *Am J Med,* **56:**800, 1974.

———, Smith, L. H., Scholz, D. A., Elveback, L. R., and Arnaud, C. D.: Primary Hyperparathyroidism: A Prospective Clinical Study, *Am J Med,* **50:**670, 1971.

Pyrah, L. N., Hodgkinson, A., and Anderson, C. K.: Primary Hyperparathyroidism, *Br J Surg,* **53:**245, 1966.

Rapaport, A., Serp, A. H., and Brown, W. A.: Carcinoma of the Parathyroid Gland with Pulmonary Metastases and Cardiac Death, *Am J Med,* **28:**443, 1960.

Rasmussen, H.: Ionic and Hormonal Control of Calcium Homeostasis, *Am J Med,* **50:**567, 1971.

Reiss, E., and Canterbury, J. M.: Application of Radioimmunoassay to Differentiation of Adenoma and Hyperplasia and to Preoperative Localization of Hyperfunctioning Parathyroid Glands, *N Engl J Med,* **280:**1381, 1969.

——— and ———: Genesis of Hyperparathyroidism, *Am J Med,* **50:**679, 1971.

Riggs, B. L., Kelly, D. J., Jowsey, J., and Keating, F. R., Jr.: Skeletal Alterations in Hyperparathyroidism: Determination of Bone Formation, Resorption and Morphologic Changes by Microradiography, *J Clin Endocrinol Metab,* **25:**777, 1965.

Romanus, R., Heimann, O., and Hansson, G.: Surgical Treatment of Hyperparathyroidism, *Prog Surg,* **12:**22, 1973.

Roof, B. S., Carpenter, B., Fink, D. J., and Gordan, G. S.: Some Thoughts on the Nature of Ectopic Parathyroid Hormones, *Am J Med,* **50:**686, 1971.

Scholz, D. A., Purnell, D. C., Goldsmith, R. S., Smith, L. H.,

Riggs, B. L., and Arnaud, C. D.: Diagnostic Considerations in Hypercalcemic Syndromes, *Med Clin North Am,* **56:**941, 1972.

———, Purnell, D. C., Woolner, L. B., and Clagett, O. T.: Mediastinal Hyperfunctioning Parathyroid Tumors: Review of 14 Cases, *Ann Surg,* **178:**173, 1973.

Seldinger, S. I.: Localization of Parathyroid Adenomata by Arteriography, *Acta Radiol (Stockh),* **42:**353, 1954.

Selzman, H. M., and Fechner, R. E.: Oxyphil Adenoma and Primary Hyperparathyroidism, *JAMA,* **199:**359, 1967.

Sharp, W. V., and Kelly, T. R.: Acute Arthritis: A Complication of Surgically Induced Hypoparathyroidism, *Am J Surg,* **113:**829, 1967.

Sherwood, L. M., Lundberg, W. B., Targovnik, J. H., Rodman, J. S., Seyfer, A.: Synthesis and Secretion of Parathyroid Hormone In Vitro, *Am J Med,* **50:**658, 1971.

Smallwood, R. A.: Effect of Intravenous Calcium Administration on Gastric Secretion of Acid and Pepsin in Man, *Gut,* **8:**592, 1967.

State, D.: The Enlarged Inferior Thyroid Artery: A Valuable Guide in Surgery of Parathyroid Adenomas, *Surgery,* **56:**461, 1964.

Steiner, R. E., Fraser, R., and Aird, I.: Operative Parathyroid Arteriography for Location of Parathyroid Tumor, *Br Med J,* **2:**400, 1956.

Stevens, A. C., and Jackson, C. E.: Localization of Parathyroid Adenomas by Esophageal Cineroentgenography, *Am J Roentgenol Radium Ther Nucl Med,* **99:**233, 1967.

Stevens, L. E., Bloomer, A., and Castleton, K. B.: Familial Hyperparathyroidism, *Arch Surg,* **94:**524, 1967.

Underdahl, L. O., Woolner, L. B., and Black, B. M.: Multiple Endocrine Adenomas: Report of Eight Cases in Which the Parathyroids, Pituitary and Pancreatic Islets Were Involved, *J Clin Endocrinol Metab,* **13:**20, 1953.

Wang, C. A., Potts, J. T., Jr., and Neer, R. M.: Controversy of Parathyroid Surgery in Calcium Regulating Hormones, in R. V. Talmage (ed.), Excerpta Medica, p. 82, Amsterdam, 1975.

Wells, H., and Lloyd, W.: Hypercalcemic and Hypophosphatemic Effects of Dibutyryl Cyclic AMP in Rats after Parathyroidectomy, *Endocrinology,* **84:**861, 1969.

Wermer, P.: Genetic Aspects of Adenomatosis of Endocrine Glands, *Am J Med,* **16:**363, 1954.

———: Endocrine Adenomatosis and Peptic Ulcer in a Large Kindred, *Am J Med,* **35:**205, 1963.

Wills, M. R., and McGowan, G. K.: Plasma-chloride Levels in Hyperparathyroidism and Other Hypercalcemic States, *Br Med J,* **1:**1153, 1964.

Wilson, R. E., Bernhard, W. F., Polet, H., and Moore, R. D.: Hyperparathyroidism: The Problem of Acute Parathyroid Intoxication, *Ann Surg,* **159:**70, 1964.

Wilson, S. D.: Zollinger-Ellison Tumor Registry, University of Wisconsin at Milwaukee. (Personal communication.)

Hypercalcemia: Differential Diagnosis

Albright, F.: Cited in Case Records of the Massachusetts General Hospital: Case 27461, *N Engl J Med,* **225:**789, 1941.

Bachman, A. L., and Sproul, E. E.: Correlation of Radiographic and Autopsy Findings in Suspected Metastases in the Spine, *Bull NY Acad Med,* **31:**146, 1955.

Bekerman, C., Schulak, J., Shen, K.-L., and Kaplan, E. L.: Locali-

zation of a Parathyroid Adenoma by Gallium Scan, *J Nucl Med,* 1977. In press.

Berson, S. A., and Yalow, R. S.: Parathyroid Hormone in Plasma in Adenomatous Hyperparathyroidism, Uremia, and Bronchogenic Carcinoma, *Science,* **154:**907, 1966.

Boonstra, C. E., and Jackson, C. E.: Serum Calcium Survey for Hyperparathyroidism: Results in 50,000 Clinic Patients, *Am J Clin Pathol,* **55:**523, 1971.

Duarte, C. G., Winnacker, J. L., Becker, K. L., et al.: Thiazide-induced Hypercalcemia, *N Engl J Med,* **284:**828, 1971.

Genant, H. K., Heck, L. L., Lanzl, L. H., Rossmann, K., Vander Horst, J., and Paloyan, E.: Primary Hyperparathyroidism, *Radiology,* **109:**513, 1974.

Goldsmith, R. S., and Forland, M.: Rapid Calcium Infusion Test for Hyperparathyroidism: Further Experiences, *Arch Intern Med,* **113:**550, 1964.

Knill-Jones, R. P., Buckle, R. M., Parsons, V., et al.: Hypercalcemia and Increased Parathyroid-Hormone Activity in a Primary Hepatoma: Studies Before and After Hepatic Transplantation, *N Engl J Med,* **282:**704, 1970.

Koppel, M. H., Massry, S. G., Shinaberger, J. H., et al.: Thiazide-induced Rise in Serum Calcium and Magnesium in Patients on Maintenance Hemodialysis, *Ann Intern Med,* **72:**895, 1970.

Lafferty, F. W.: Pseudohyperparathyroidism, *Medicine (Baltimore),* **45:**247, 1966.

Monchik, J. M., Doppman, J. L., Earll, J. M., and Aurbach, G. D.: Localization of Hyperfunctioning Parathyroid Tissue. Radioimmunoassay of Parathyroid Hormone on Samples from the Large Veins of the Neck and Thorax and Selectively Catheterized Thyroid Veins, *Am J Surg,* **129:**413, 1975.

Moore, E. W.: Ionized Calcium in Normal Serum, Ultrafiltrates, and Whole Blood Determined by Ion-Exchange Electrodes, *J Clin Invest,* **49:**318, 1970.

O'Riordan, J. L. H., Kendall, B. E., and Woodhead, J. S.: Preoperative Localisation of Parathyroid Tumours, *Lancet,* **2:**1172, 1971.

Parfitt, A. M.: Chlorothiazide-induced Hypercalcemia in Juvenile Osteoporosis and Hyperparathyroidism, *N Engl J Med,* **281:**55, 1969.

Purnell, D. C., Smith, L. H., Scholz, D. A., et al.: Primary Hyperparathyroidism: A Prospective Clinical Study, *Am J Med,* **50:**670, 1971.

Reece, R. L.: An Analysis of 4000 Chemistry Graphs: Comments on Disease Patterns, *Minn Med,* **51:**351, 1968.

Reitz, R. E., Pollard, J. J., Wang, C-A., et al.: Localization of Parathyroid Adenomas by Selective Venous Catheterization and Radioimmunoassay, *N Engl J Med,* **281:**348, 1969.

Riggs, B. L., Arnaud, C. D., Reynolds, J. C., et al.: Immunologic Differentiation of Primary Hyperparathyroidism from Hyperparathyroidism Due to Nonparathyroid Cancer, *J Clin Invest,* **50:**2079, 1971.

Roof, B. S., Carpenter, B., Fink, D. J., et al.: Some Thoughts on the Nature of Ectopic Parathyroid Hormones, *Am J Med,* **50:**686, 1971.

Samuels, B. I.: The Present Status of Parathyroid Thermography, *JAMA,* **223:**907, 1975.

Seitz, H., and Jaworski, Z. F.: Effect of Hydrochlorothiazide on Serum and Urinary Calcium and Urinary Citrate, *Can Med Assoc J,* **90:**414, 1964.

Sherwood, L. M., O'Riordan, J. L. H., Aurbach, G. D., et al.:

Production of Parathyroid Hormone by Nonparathyroid Tumors, *J Clin Endocrinol Metab,* **27:**140, 1967.

Strott, C. A., and Nugent, C. A.: Laboratory Tests in the Diagnosis of Hyperparathyroidism in Hypercalcemic Patients, *Ann Intern Med,* **68:**188, 1968.

Yendt, E. R., and Gagne, R. J. A.: Detection of Primary Hyperparathyroidism, with Special Reference to Its Occurrence in Hypercalciuric Females with "Normal" or Borderline Serum Calcium, *Can Med Assoc J,* **98:**331, 1968.

Ectopic Hyperparathyroidism

Benson, R. C., Jr., Riggs, B. L., Pickard, B. M., and Arnaud, C. D.: Immunoreactive Forms of Circulating Parathyroid Hormone in Primary and Ectopic Hyperparathyroidism, *J Clin Invest,* **54:**175, 1973.

Drezner, M. K., Neelon, F. A., Curtis, H. B., and Lebovitz, H. E.: Renal Cyclic Adenosine Monophosphate: An Accurate Index of Parathyroid Function, *Metabolism,* **25:**1103, 1976.

Levine, R. J., and Metz, S. A.: A Classification of Ectopic Hormone-Producing Tumors, *Ann NY Acad Sci,* **230:**533, 1974.

Mundy, G. R., Luben, R. A., Raisz, L. G., Oppenheim, J. J., and Buell, D. N.: Bone-resorbing Activity in Supernatant from Lymphoid Cell Lines, *N Engl J Med,* **290:**867, 1974.

Samaan, N. A., Hickey, R. C., Hill, C. S., Jr., and Medellin, H.: Parathyroid Tumors: Their Preoperative Localization and Association with Other Tumors, Atlanta Endocrine Society (Abstr) A-298, 1974.

Seyberth, H. W., Segre, G. V., Morgan, J. L., Sweetman, B. J., Potts, J. T., Jr., and Oates, J. A.: Prostaglandins as Mediators of Hypercalcemia Associated with Certain Types of Cancer, *N Engl J Med,* **293:**1278, 1975.

Shaw, J. W., Oldham, S. B., Rosoff, L., Bethune, J. E., and Fichman, M. P.: Urinary Cyclic AMP Analyzed as a Function of the Serum Calcium and Parathyroid Hormone in the Differential Diagnosis of Hypercalcemia, *J Clin Invest,* **59:**14, 1977.

Treatment of Hypercalcemia

Albright, F., Bauer, W., Claflin, D., et al.: Studies in Parathyroid Physiology: III. The Effect of Phosphate Ingestion in Clinical Hyperparathyroidism, *J Clin Invest,* **11:**411, 1932.

Brewer, R. I., and LeBauer, J.: Caution in the Use of Phosphates in the Treatment of Severe Hypercalcemia, *J Clin Endocrinol Metab,* **27:**695, 1967.

Chakmakjian, Z. H., and Bethune, J. E.: Sodium Sulfate Treatment of Hypercalcemia, *N Engl J Med,* **275:**862, 1966.

Goldsmith, R. S.: Treatment of Hypercalcemia, *Med Clin North Am,* **56:**951, 1972.

——— and Ingbar, S. H.: Inorganic Phosphate Treatment of Hypercalcemia of Diverse Etiologies, *N Engl J Med,* **274:**1, 1966.

Henneman, P. H., Dempsey, E. F., Carroll, E. L., et al.: The Cause of Hypercalcuria in Sarcoid and Its Treatment with Cortisone and Sodium Phytate, *J Clin Invest,* **35:**1229, 1956.

Kennedy, B. J.: Metabolic and Toxic Effects of Mithramycin during Tumor Therapy, *Am J Med,* **49:**494, 1970.

Lazor, M. Z., and Rosenberg, L. E.: Mechanism of Adrenal-Steroid Reversal of Hypercalcemia in Multiple Myeloma, *N Engl J Med,* **270:**749, 1964.

Nolph, K. D., and Stoltz, M. L.: Treatment of Hypercalcemia with Calcium Free Peritoneal Dialysis (CFPD), *Clin Res,* **19:**481, 1971. (Abstract.)

Pak, C. Y. C., Wortsman, J., Bennett, J. E., et al.: Control of Hypercalcemia with Cellulose Phosphate, *J Clin Endocrinol Metab,* **28:**1829, 1968. (Letter to the Editor.)

Strauch, B. S., and Ball, M. F.: Hemodialysis in the Treatment of Severe Hypercalcemia, *JAMA,* **235:**1347, 1976.

Suki, W. N., Yium, J. J., VonMinden, M., et al.: Acute Treatment of Hypercalcemia with Furosemide, *N Engl J Med,* **283:**836, 1970.

West, T. E. T., Joffe, M., Sinclair, L., et al.: Treatment of Hypercalcemia with Calcitonin, *Lancet,* **1:**675, 1971.

Secondary and Tertiary Hyperparathyroidism

Bricker, N. S., Slatopolsky, E., Reiss, E., et al.: Calcium, Phosphorus and Bone in Renal Disease and Transplantation, *Arch Intern Med,* **123:**543, 1969.

Curtis, J. R., DeWardener, H. E., Gower, P. E., et al.: The Use of Calcium Carbonate and Calcium Phosphate without Vitamin D in Management of Renal Osteodystrophy, *Proc Eur Dialysis Transplant Assoc,* **7:**141, 1970.

Davies, D. R., Dent, C. E., and Watson, L.: Tertiary Hyperparathyroidism, *Br Med J,* **3:**395, 1968.

Easson, L. H., Faulds, J. S., and Hartley, J. N.: Van Recklinghausen's Disease of Bone Associated with Idiopathic Steatorrhoea, *J R Coll Surg Edinb,* **3:**193, 1958.

Fournier, A. E., Johnson, W. J., Taves, D. R., et al.: Etiology of Hyperparathyroidism and Bone Disease during Chronic Hemodialysis: I. Association of Bone Disease with Potentially Etiologic Factors, *J Clin Invest,* **50:**592, 1971.

Gittes, R. F., and Radde, I. C.: Experimental Model for Hyperparathyroidism: Effect of Excessive Numbers of Transplanted Isologous Parathyroid Glands, *J Urol,* **95:**595, 1966.

Glanville, H. J., and Bloom, R.: Case of Renal Tubular Osteomalacia (Dent Type 2) with Later Development of Autonomous Parathyroid Tumours, *Br Med J,* **2:**26, 1965.

Goldsmith, R. S., Furszyfer, J, Johnson, W. J., et al: Control of Secondary Hyperparathyroidism during Long-Term Hemodialysis, *Am J Med,* **50:**692, 1971.

Johnson, W. J., Goldsmith, R. S., and Arnaud, C. D.: Prevention and Treatment of Progressive Secondary Hyperparathyroidism in Advanced Renal Failure, *Med Clin North Am,* **56:**961, 1972.

———, ———, Beabut, J. W., Jowsey, J., Kelly, P. J., and Arnaud, C. D.: Prevention and Reversal of Progressive Secondary Hyperparathyroidism in Patients Maintained on Hemodialysis, *Am J Med,* **56:**827, 1974.

Jowsey, J., Johnson, W. J., Taves, D. R., et al.: Effects of Dialysate Calcium and Fluoride on Bone Disease during Regular Hemodialysis, *J Lab Clin Med,* **79:**204, 1972.

———, Massry, S. G., Coburn, J. W., et al.: Microradiographic Studies of Bone in Renal Osteodystrophy, *Arch Intern Med,* **124:**539, 1969.

Katz, A. I., Hampers, C. L., and Merrill, J. P.: Secondary Hyperparathyroidism and Renal Osteodystrophy in Chronic Renal Failure: Analysis of 195 Patients, with Observations on the Effects of Chronic Dialysis, Kidney Transplantation and Subtotal Parathyroidectomy, *Medicine (Baltimore),* **48:**333, 1969.

Kaye, M., Chatterjee, G., Cohen, G. F., et al.: Arrest of Hyperparathyroid Bone Disease with Dihydrotachysterol in Patients

Undergoing Chronic Hemodialysis, *Ann Intern Med,* **73:**225, 1970.

McPhaul, J. J., Jr., McIntosh, D. A., Hammond, W. S., and Park, O. K.: Autonomous Secondary (Renal) Parathyroid Hyperplasia, *N Engl J Med,* **271:**1342, 1964.

Mallick, N. P., and Berlyne, G. M.: Arterial Calcification after Vitamin-D Therapy in Hyperphosphatemic Renal Failure, *Lancet,* **2:**1316, 1968.

Messner, R. P., Smith, H. T., Shapiro, F. L., et al.: The Effect of Hemodialysis, Vitamin D, and Renal Homotransplantation on the Calcium Malabsorption of Chronic Renal Failure, *J Lab Clin Med,* **74:**472, 1969.

Ogg, C. S.: Total Parathyroidectomy in Treatment of Secondary (Renal) Hyperparathyroidism, *Br Med J,* **3:**31, 1967.

Oldham, S. B., Fischer, J. A., Capen, C. C., et al.: Dynamics of Parathyroid Hormone Secretion In Vitro, *Am J Med,* **50:**650, 1971.

Recker, R. R., and Saville, P.: Calcium Absorption in Renal Failure: Its Relationship to Blood Urea Nitrogen, Dietary Calcium Intake, Time on Dialysis, and Other Variables, *J Lab Clin Med,* **78:**380, 1971.

Reiss, E., and Canterbury, J. M.: Parathyroid Hormone in Renal Insufficiency, in Berglund, and B. Josephson (eds.), "Endocrinology: Metabolic Aspects (Proceedings of the Fourth International Congress of Nephrology, Stockholm, 1969)," vol. 2, pp. 164–174, S. Karger A. G., Basel, 1970.

Sherwood, L. M., Herrmann, I., and Bassett, C. A.: In Vitro Studies of Normal and Abnormal Parathyroid Tissue, *Arch Intern Med,* **124:**426, 1969.

Stanbury, S. W., Lumb, G. A., and Nicholson, W. F.: Elective Subtotal Parathyroidectomy for Renal Hyperparathyroidism, *Lancet,* **1:**793, 1960.

Hypoparathyroidism, Pseudohypoparathyroidism, and Parathyroid Transplants

Alvioli, L. V.: The Therapeutic Approach to Hypoparathyroidism, *Am J Med,* **57:**34, 1974.

Blizzard, R. M., Chee, D., and Davis, W.: The Incidence of Para-thyroid and Other Antibodies in the Sera of Patients with Idiopathic Hypoparathyroidism, *Clin Exp Immunol,* **1:**119, 1966.

Chase, L. R., Nelson, G. L., and Aurbach, G. D.: Metabolic Abnormality in Pseudohypoparathyroidism: Defective Renal Excretion of Cyclic 3'5'-AMP in Response to Parathyroid Hormone, *J Clin Invest,* **47:**18a, 1968.

Costello, J. M., and Dent, C. E.: Hypohyperparathyroidism, *Arch Dis Child,* **38:**397, 1963.

Dimich, A., Bedrossian, P. B., and Wallach, S.: Hypoparathyroidism: Clinical Observations in 34 Patients, *Arch Intern Med,* **120:**449, 1967.

Fisher, B., Fisher, E., Feduska, N., and Sakai, A.: Thyroid and Parathyroid Implantation: An Experimental Reevaluation, *Surgery,* **62:**1025, 1967.

Franz, A. G., and Lee, J. B.: Pseudohypoparathyroidism: Assays of Parathyroid Hormone and Thyrocalcitonin, *Proc Natl Acad Sci USA,* **56:**1138, 1966.

Jordan, G. L., Jr., Erickson, E., Gordon, W. B., Jr., and Rose, R. G.: The Treatment of Hypoparathyroidism by Parathyroid Transplantation, *Surgery,* **52:**134, 1962.

Kenney, F. M., and Holliday, M. A.: Hypoparathyroidism, Moniliasis and Hashimoto's Disease, *N Engl J Med,* **271:**708, 1964.

Kolb, F. O., and Steinberg, H. L.: Pseudohypoparathyroidism and Secondary Hyperparathyroidism and Osteitis Fibrosa, *J Clin Endocrinol Metab,* **22:**59, 1962.

Tashjian, A. H., Frantz, A. G., and Lee, J. B.: Pseudohypoparathyroidism: Assays of Parathyroid Hormone and Thyrocalcitonin, *Pathology,* **56:**1138, 1966.

Wells, S. A., Jr., Ellis, G. J., Gunnells, J. C., et al.: Parathyroid Autotransplantation in Primary Parathyroid Hyperplasia, *N Engl J Med,* **295:**57, 1976.

———, Gunnells, J. C., Shelburne, J. D., et al.: Transplantation of the Parathyroid Glands in Man: Clinical Indications and Results, *Surgery,* **78:**34, 1975.

Williams, E., and Wood, A. O. C.: The Syndrome of Hypoparathyroidism and Steatorrhea, *Arch Dis Child,* **34:**302, 1959.

Chapter 39

Pediatric Surgery

by R. Peter Altman, Judson G. Randolph, and Kathryn D. Anderson

GENERAL CONSIDERATIONS

The normal adaptive demands upon infants and young children are enormous. Add to these the compensatory requirements imposed by illness and by operation, and the role of the children's surgeon is brought into perspective. As the size of the patient is scaled down, the period of time in which a state of well-being turns to a surgical catastrophe becomes shorter. Thus, patients on a children's surgical unit must be guarded unceasingly against subtle changes in clinical signs.

In addition to the technical performance of an operation, pediatric surgery encompasses all phases of care, including the diagnosis, preoperative preparation, postoperative management, and long-term rehabilitation of the child.

This requires an appreciation of the unique physiologic and emotional requirements of infants, children, and adolescents. Most of all, pediatric surgery demands that the surgeon care about children, about their fears, about their expectations for themselves, and about the impact of surgical illness on the child and the family.

FLUID AND ELECTROLYTE BALANCE. In an infant or child the margin between dehydration and fluid overload is small. The infant is born with a surplus of body water, but within a few days this is excreted. At birth and for the first 10 days of life, fluid requirements are between 65 and 150 ml/kg (750 to 1,000 ml/m^2). Thereafter the maintenance fluid requirement approaches 1,500 to 2,000 ml/m^2/day. For infants and children with normal renal function, fluid calculations based on a rough guideline of 75 ml/kg generally fall within the limits of safe replacement. For short-term intravenous therapy, sodium 5 mEq/kg/day and potassium 2 mEq/kg/day will satisfy the daily need. Fluid and electrolyte losses secondary to protracted vomiting or diarrhea are corrected by modifying this formula according to the measured losses. An additional parameter for assessment of hydration is measurement of the serum and urine osmolarities. The normal serum osmolarity lies between 280 and 290 mOsm/liter. Because of the inability of the immature kidney to concentrate, it is not always possible to utilize the urine osmolarity as a guideline for fluid replacement in neonates. Even in a dehydrated infant the urine osmolarity rarely exceeds 400 mOsm/liter. No matter what formula is used to calculate the fluid replacement, there is no substitute for recording and analyzing all fluid losses, including the insensible depletion, then replacing the depleted constituents precisely.

ACID-BASE EQUILIBRIUM. The serum pH and P_{CO_2} reflect the respiratory and metabolic status of the patient. Their measurement permits estimation of the base excess and recognition of derangement in metabolic or respiratory status. These data are essential during the resuscitation of critically ill patients and constitute an integral part of the intraoperative and postoperative monitoring. Metabolic acidosis is usually corrected by the administration of sodium bicarbonate. In a fragile infant the risks of excessive sodium administration, hyperosmolarity, and cardiovascular overload are appreciable. Thus, for infants requiring extensive metabolic manipulation (such as those with congenital diaphragmatic hernia), all intravenous sodium solution should be as Na HCO$_3$. This maximizes the amount of buffer provided while restricting Na administered.

Fluid and electrolyte losses from the upper gastrointestinal tract in infants are generally equivalent to 0.45 N saline solution. Adjustments for ileostomy or biliary losses are made when these are significant by analyzing the individual drainage.

BLOOD VOLUME AND BLOOD REPLACEMENT. Replacement of volume with whole blood, blood components, plasma, and plasma substitutes is an integral part of pediatric surgical therapy. Because of the risks of immunologic sensitization, transfusion reactions, or hepatitis, blood or its fractions are administered only when absolutely indicated. Volume expansion with 5% or 25% albumin solutions is often chosen over the administration of blood. For transfusion in infants and children, whole blood can be subdivided into smaller packets of 125 ml. A useful guideline for blood replacement in the infant is to consider 10 ml/kg roughly equivalent to a 500-ml unit in the 70-kg adult. Replacement with packed red blood cells is calculated at 5 ml/kg.

Platelet transfusions are indicated in special circumstances, such as thrombocytopenia secondary to hypersplenism. Clotting is restored to normal when the platelet count is raised to 50,000 per milliliter. This is accomplished by transfusion of multiple platelet packs prepared from whole blood. The biologic half-life of platelets is limited, and therefore transfusion of platelets must be carried out promptly after their preparation.

In the child, as in the adult, coagulation deficiencies assume clinical significance after extensive blood transfusion. It is advisable to alternate whole blood transfusion with administration of fresh frozen plasma in order to replace the labile clotting factors, especially V and VIII.

HYPERALIMENTATION AND NUTRITION. The techniques of total parenteral nutrition have now been refined and are especially beneficial to infants, translating formerly hopeless clinical problems into situations where there is a good chance for survival.

When the gastrointestinal tract is not usable, because of mechanical, ischemic, or inflammatory disorders, several options for nutritional support are available. The original technique makes use of an indwelling central venous catheter for delivery of the nutritional substrate. The fundamental principle involves the provision of a source of calories (hypertonic glucose) in combination with a source of nitrogen (protein hydrolysate or amino acid solution). Since energy requirements are satisfied, the exogenous nitrogen is converted into body protein and an anabolic state is achieved. Essential fatty acid supplements, minerals, and vitamins are provided in the infusate, and long-term growth can be sustained even in the rapidly developing infant.

The risks, however, are not trivial. The concentration of infusate approaches 25 percent and therefore requires that administration be carried out through a major channel with rapid flow. Most often the superior vena cava is utilized. Sepsis, caval thrombosis, pneumothorax, hydrothorax, and hypertonic crises are constant threats. For these reasons, alternative techniques to central venous hyperalimentation have been developed. Peripheral alimentation, utilizing less concentrated but greater volume of solutions, has been used successfully to achieve positive nitrogen balance. Lipid emulsions prepared from soy extract (Intralipid) have largely eliminated the need for central alimentation techniques. The caloric yield from fat solution (11 kcal/Gm) reduces reliance upon hypertonic glucose. Positive nitrogen balance can thus be accomplished by the administration of isotonic solutions, which are provided through a peripheral vein. Advances in the techniques of parenteral nutrition have had a greater impact on survival for pediatric surgical patients than any other surgical development in the past decade.

THERMOREGULATION. Infants or children compromised by illness are exceedingly thermolabile. Premature infants are particularly susceptible to changes in environmental temperature. Unable to shiver, and lacking stores of fat, their potential for thermogenesis is severely impaired. Since these patients lack adaptive mechanisms to cope with the environment, the environment must itself be carefully regulated. This is true before, during, and after surgery. During transfer of an infant, attention to heat conservation is essential. The simple expedient of wrapping the infant in aluminum foil during transportation will diminish radiant heat loss. In the operating room the ambient temperature should approach thermal neutrality *for the patient.* This is 73°F. Supplementary heat is provided by means of direct warming lights during positioning and intubation when much of the body surface is exposed. Warm solutions are utilized for "prepping" the operative field. Excess preparatory solutions must be avoided to minimize evaporation with concomitant body surface cooling. Irrigation solutions employed during surgery should also be warmed. Intraoperative temperature is monitored by placement of a thermister probe in the axilla or esophagus.

After operation, a heated isolette should be immediately available to receive the baby. It has been demonstrated that infants have a better survival rate when temperatures are maintained above 95°F than when temperatures are permitted to fall below this level. Complications of hypothermia include increased blood viscosity, cardiorespiratory depression, and metabolic acidosis. Most of the currently available isolettes are provided with thermoregulatory devices which respond to constant recordings of the infant's temperature.

INTRAOPERATIVE MONITORING. The same physiologic parameters are monitored during a major surgical procedure in an infant or child as for an adult patient. The basic minimum requirements for conducting a safe pediatric surgical procedure include a temperature thermister, Doppler flow sensor, ECG, and a stethoscope placed either on the chest or in the esophagus. When necessary, ready access is obtained for central venous pressure monitoring, even in the neonate, by means of a catheter placed in the superior vena cava through the jugular vein or subclavian vein. Arterial access is available through radial or temporal artery cut-down or by percutaneous technique. Scrupulous attention to these detailed preparations is essential if the infant is to be guided safely through major operative procedures.

LESIONS OF THE NECK

Cystic Hygroma

ETIOLOGY AND PATHOLOGY. Cystic hygroma occurs as a result of imperfect formation of the lymphatic channels. The majority occur in the neck, posterior to the sternocleidomastoid muscle (Fig. 39-1). Other sites are the mediastinum, axilla, and groin. The term *hygroma* implies watery fluid contained within endothelial-lined spaces. The cyst may be unilocular, but more often there are multiple cysts which permeate the surrounding structures and distort the local anatomy. Supporting connective tissue shows extensive lymphocytic infiltration. Except in the case of single large cysts, no clear-cut cleavage plane is found between the hygroma and normal tissue. The lesion is usually apparent at birth. Occasionally, the mass occupies the entire submandibular region, distorting the subglottic tissues and compromising the airway. Local disfigurement may be severe. Not infrequently, an associated supraclavicular mass is seen which may become prominent with the Valsalva maneuver. This usually implies association with a mediastinal component.

CLINICAL MANIFESTATIONS. Symptoms are related to the location and size of the mass. Sudden enlargement of a hygroma generally indicates hemorrhage into a cyst. Infection in the mass may lead to dangerous regional cellulitis, but when the infection subsides, the resultant intracystic fibrosis and scar may significantly reduce the size of the mass.

TREATMENT. Surgical excision offers the best chance of cure. Total excision is often impractical because of the extent of the hygroma and its proximity to vital structures. Important nerves and vascular structures should not be sacrificed in an attempt to achieve total excision of this benign lesion; rather, repeated partial excisions of the residual hygroma are preferable. Some have favored repeated aspiration of the cysts with injections of sclerosing agents, but this approach has limited usefulness and is not recommended.

Thyroglossal Duct Remnants

PATHOLOGY AND CLINICAL MANIFESTATIONS. The thyroglossal duct originates as a diverticulum of the foregut, beginning at the base of the tongue in the foramen cecum and passing downward and forward through the hyoid bone to the normal anatomical position of the thyroid gland (Fig. 39-1). Persistence of a portion of the thyroglossal duct results in a midline cervical mass known as a *thyroglossal duct cyst.* These cysts can be troublesome because of repeated infection. The mass is usually discovered in the two- to four-year-old child when the baby fat subsides and irregularities in the neck are more readily apparent. The cyst is almost always found in the midline, but repeated infection and scarring may cause lateral displacement, which can lead to diagnostic confusion.

TREATMENT. Infected thyroglossal duct cysts should be treated with antibiotics; when an abscess is present, drainage is necessary. Removal of the cyst and thyroglossal duct tract, including the central portion of the hyoid bone, is carried out when infection subsides. The cyst occasionally presents in the mouth at the base of the tongue. A midline mass in the neck or at the base of the tongue which is thought to be a thyroglossal duct cyst may, in rare instances, be ectopic thyroid tissue. Therefore, if a normal thyroid cannot be palpated with certainty, a thyroid scan should be performed.

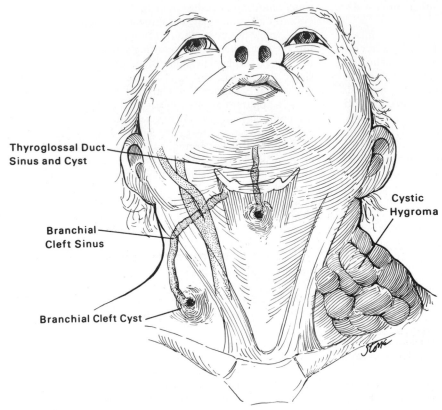

Thyroglossal Duct
Sinus and Cyst

Branchial
Cleft Sinus

Branchial Cleft Cyst

Cystic
Hygroma

Branchial Cleft Anomalies

Branchial clefts are those embryological grooves that ultimately evolve into the lower part of the face and neck. Persistence of various portions of the branchial apparatus

Fig. 39-1. Typical locations of lesions of the neck. Cystic hygroma—multilocular cysts in posterior triangle of neck. Thyroglossal duct cyst and sinus—usually a midline cyst with a sinus tract passing through the hyoid bone to the foramen cecum. Branchial cleft cyst and sinus. The sinus tract passes through the bifurcation of the carotid artery, ending in the pharynx.

leads to specific anomalies about the face and neck. A fistula or cyst orginating low in the anterior lateral region of the neck usually results from a malformation of the second branchial cleft. Typically the fistula extends from the skin of the lower part of the neck upward along the anterior border of the sternocleidomastoid muscle, then inward between the bifurcation of the carotid artery to enter the posterolateral pharynx just below the tonsillar fossa (Fig. 39-1). Cysts are typically found only in the lower end of the tract just above the clavicle. The presenting complaint is usually related to persistent or intermittent drainage onto the neck. Complete surgical extirpation is necessary for cure. Transverse "stair-step" incisions are preferred to a long incision encompassing the entire tract.

RESPIRATORY SYSTEM

Subglottic Stenosis

As more infants are being sustained with ventilatory support, acquired subglottic stenosis is assuming greater clinical importance (Fig. 39-2). Mild or moderate stenosis will usually respond to one or two tracheal dilatations. Severe tracheal stenosis may require tracheostomy, often

Fig. 39-2. Air tracheogram showing subglottic stenosis following protracted endotracheal intubation.

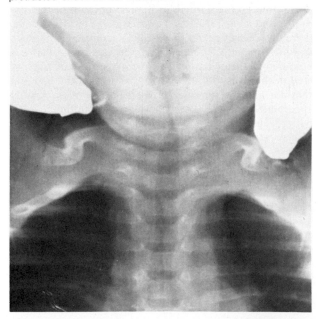

for a year or longer, with periodic dilatations. Tracheoplasty is reserved for the most severe stenoses, which do not respond to dilatation.

Subglottic Hemangioma

Hemangiomas in the subglottic area can compromise the airway and cause stridor. These tumors can often be demonstrated on a high-kilovolt neck film and confirmed by laryngoscopy and bronchoscopy. In some patients tracheostomy may be required, but the natural history of hemangioma is to increase in size during the first few months of life, after which there is a gradual involution and disappearance of the lesion. In critical circumstances involution of the hemangioma can be hastened by the systemic administration of steroids in combination with direct x-ray therapy (150 rads × three doses).

Diaphragmatic Hernia

PATHOLOGY. During formation of the diaphragm, the pleural and coelomic cavities remain in continuity via the pleuroperitoneal canal. Failure of this defect to close results in the congenital anomaly known as *Bochdalek hernia*. This anomaly has a predilection for the left side.

With incomplete closure of the posterior diaphragm, bowel fills the chest cavity during embryonic life. The abdominal cavity remains small and undeveloped. The presence of the intestinal loops in the chest interferes with the development of the lung, and prevents its expansion after birth. As the baby's bowel fills with air, further shift of the mediastinum occurs. Any newborn infant in respiratory distress who shows a scaphoid abdomen should be suspected of having a congenital diaphragmatic hernia (Fig. 39-3). Chest x-ray will confirm the diagnosis (Fig. 39-4).

TREATMENT. Diaphragmatic hernia is one of the most urgent surgical emergencies of the newborn infant. However, some severely compromised infants may benefit from a brief period of resuscitation with bicarbonate and 100 percent oxygen prior to surgical correction. Improved survival has been observed in infants in whom the pH can be partially corrected and the P_{CO_2} lowered toward normal.

Operative repair is best performed through a subcostal incision. There are advantages to the abdominal approach; withdrawing the bowel from the chest is technically simpler than pushing it from above, and a ventral hernia is usually necessary to accommodate the bowel which has lost its "right of domain" in the abdominal cavity. As a rule the anterior leaf of the diaphragm is well developed, since the defect is posterolateral. The posterior rim of the diaphragm is usually covered by a layer of peritoneum which is continuous with the parietal pleura. This must be incised and the diaphragm unrolled so that it can be sutured to the anterior diaphragmatic leaf. A single layer of nonabsorbable sutures is used to close the defect. A chest tube is positioned in the thoracic cavity and placed on gentle suction.

Fig. 39-3. Newborn with left congenital Bochdalek diaphragmatic hernia. Note scaphoid abdomen.

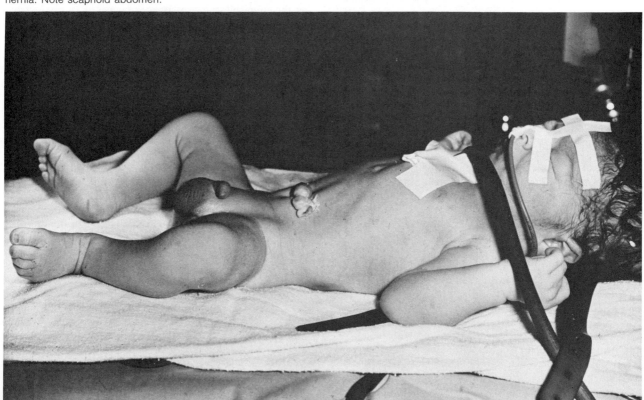

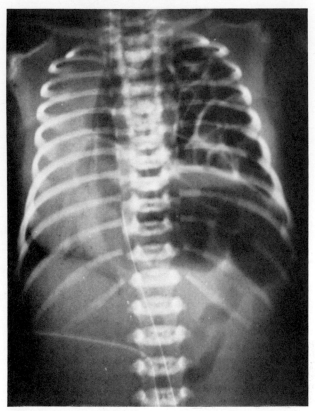

Fig. 39-4. X-ray showing left Bochdalek hernia. Intestine occupies the left side of the chest. Note the extreme mediastinal displacement.

A "prophylactic" chest tube is inserted on the opposite side, because pneumothorax, on the contralateral side, is a common life-threatening complication. Both chest tubes can be removed after the infant is weaned from the ventilator. The ventral hernia is repaired 10 days to 2 weeks after the abdominal cavity has expanded to accommodate the intestine. In spite of improvement in neonatal pulmonary support, diaphragmatic hernia is still associated with a 50 percent mortality. Perhaps technical developments in extracorporeal membrane oxygenation will be adapted to neonates and result in improved survival.

Congenital Lobar Emphysema

Hyperexpansion of a single lobe of the lung can produce a life-threatening respiratory crisis. Inspired air trapped in the affected lobe results in compression of the adjacent lung and displacement of the mediastinum. The right middle and left upper lobes are most frequently involved. In 10 percent of the cases the disease is bilateral. A chest x-ray which shows hyperaeration of the involved lobe and compression of adjacent lung parenchyma with mediastinal displacement to the contralateral side is diagnostic. In some patients, the lobar emphysema may pose a true surgical emergency and the affected lobe must be removed promptly. A bronchial abnormality is not usually identified in the resected specimen.

Pulmonary Sequestration

Accessory lung tissue may be present, either completely separate from adjacent lung parenchyma (extralobar sequestration) or invested within the visceral pleura of the adjoining normal lung tissue (intralobar sequestration). The former condition occurs most commonly in the left side of the chest, adjacent to the diaphragm. Typically there is no bronchial connection and the blood supply to the anomalous lobe emanates from the abdominal aorta. Symptoms are uncommon and this malformation is usually discovered on routine chest film. Arteriography is helpful in demonstrating the systemic arterial supply. Elective thoracotomy with excision is advisable.

Intralobar sequestration occurs in intimate association with normal lung parenchyma, usually in the lower lobes and more commonly in the left side of the chest. Unlike the asymptomatic extralobar sequestration, the intralobar sequestration may present with cough, hemoptysis, or pulmonary infection. The chest x-ray is usually diagnostic. There is no connection with the bronchus, but the sequestration may contain air which enters from adjacent alveoli. The sequestration may necessitate a lobectomy of the affected lobe, though segmental resection may be all that is required.

Bronchiectasis

Bronchiectasis is rare in children but can occur as a result of congenital cystic fibrosis. The condition also accompanies Kartagener's syndrome, with sinusitis drainage as the underlying cause. Bronchiectasis may result from infection secondary to a neglected bronchial foreign body.

Symptoms include chronic cough, which may be productive, and recurrent respiratory infection. Hemoptysis is not uncommon. The diagnosis is suggested on chest x-ray, and the saccular fusiform distortion of the peripheral bronchi can be confirmed by bronchography. Lobectomy or segmental resection is indicated if the disease is localized to a single lobe or portion of a lobe.

Foreign Bodies

Foreign objects aspirated into the larynx, trachea, and bronchi represent a major cause of respiratory difficulty in toddlers. Peanut aspiration is common, and severe lipid pneumonia secondary to the arachitic acid in the nut may result.

The history of choking while eating, often when the child is playing or laughing, should alert one to the possibility of foreign body aspiration. The coughing may then resolve and the only sign of the foreign body in the bronchus may be a unilateral wheeze. Fluoroscopy of the chest will often reveal air trapping and a swing of the mediastinum toward the side of the foreign body during expiration. Hyperaeration may involve a whole lung or be localized to a single lobe. In neglected cases where a foreign body is allowed to remain in the bronchus, atelectasis may ensue. Bronchiectasis is a late consequence of unrecognized bronchial foreign body.

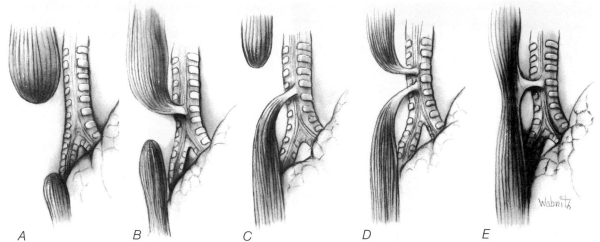

Fig. 39-5. Five major varieties of esophageal atresia and tra-cheoesophageal fistula. *A.* Esophageal atresia without associ-ated fistula. *B.* Esophageal atresia with tracheoesophageal fistula between proximal segment of esophagus and trachea. *C.* Esophageal atresia with tracheoesophageal fistula between distal esophagus and trachea. *D.* Esophageal atresia with fistula be-tween both proximal and distal ends of esophagus and trachea. *E.* Tracheoesophageal fistula without esophageal atresia (H-type fistula).

Endoscopic removal of the foreign body under general anesthesia is recommended, although some foreign bodies are expelled by treatment with vigorous pulmonary physi-otherapy.

Pneumothorax, Pneumomediastinum

The improved salvage of premature infants with respi-ratory distress syndrome has inevitably resulted in long-term maintenance on mechanic ventilation. Diminished compliance of lungs combined with positive-pressure ven-tilation has resulted in an increased incidence of pneumo-mediastinum and pneumothorax. The development of pulmonary interstitial emphysema (air surrounding the minor bronchi) precedes dissection of the air extrapleurally into the mediastinum or the pleural cavity. Pneumomedi-astinum is not usually clinically significant, but may con-tribute to respiratory distress and require needle aspiration. This can be safely accomplished by inserting a needle into the mediastinum beneath the xyphoid. Pneumothorax in neonates is almost always under tension and thus is life-threatening. Sudden deterioration of the infant's clinical status with a decrease in the arterial oxygen saturation and an increase in the P_{CO_2} may signal a pneumothorax. Chest x-rays are confirmatory, and the pneumothorax must be aspirated as an emergency. Even if immediate relief of the pneumothorax is obtained by needle aspiration, it is pru-dent to introduce a small chest tube for a few days. The tube is connected to suction of approximately 10 ml water since the infant is generally unable to generate the positive pressure necessary to evacuate the pneumothorax under unmodified water seal.

ESOPHAGUS

Tracheoesophageal Fistula and Esophageal Atresia

ESOPHAGEAL ATRESIA WITH LOWER-SEGMENT TRACHEOESOPHAGEAL FISTULA

PATHOLOGY. Esophageal atresia associated with distal tracheoesophageal fistulae (Vogt-Gross type C) (Fig. 39-5) accounts for 90 percent of the anomalies of the esophagus. The upper esophageal segment terminates as a blind pouch, and the proximal end of the lower segment of the esophagus joins the trachea, just above the carina. The fistula transmits inspired air to the stomach, and also al-lows acidic gastric secretions to reflux into the lungs. Asso-ciated anomalies are common. In nearly 20 percent of the infants born with esophageal atresia, some variant of con-genital heart disease occurs; imperforate anus is found in about 12 percent.

CLINICAL MANIFESTATIONS. The earliest and most ob-vious clinical sign of esophageal atresia is regurgitation of saliva at the first offered feeding. The aspiration of feed-ings is soon followed by pneumonia. The pulmonary prob-lem is magnified by refluxing gastric juice, and by the atelectasis which occurs consequent to aspiration secondary to gastric distension. When esophageal atresia is suspected, an attempt should be made to pass a catheter through the nose into the stomach (Fig. 39-6). Diagnosis of esophageal atresia is suggested if the catheter meets an obstruction and fails to advance. A lateral chest x-ray with 1 ml contrast media instilled in the upper pouch will outline the blind upper esophagus and confirm the diagnosis.

TREATMENT. Once the diagnosis of esophageal atresia with tracheoesophageal fistula has been established, use of the following is instituted: (1) infant warmer, in 30° head-up position; (2) sump catheter suction in the upper pouch (Repfogle tube); (3) parenteral antibiotics even if pneu-monia is not clinically manifest. Gastrostomy is a useful, often vital, adjunct in the management of these infants and can be performed before operative repair of the esophagus,

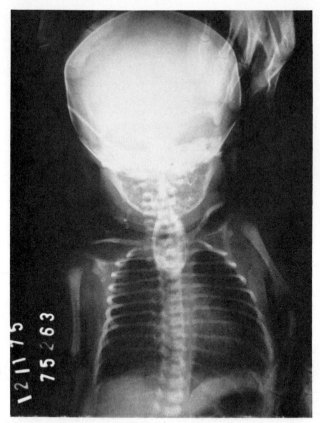

Fig. 39-6. Type C esophageal atresia with tracheoesophageal fistula. Catheter is coiled in upper pouch. Gas below diaphragm confirms the presence of a tracheoesophageal fistula.

if necessary. The gastrostomy accomplishes gastric decompression, improves ventilatory mechanics, and minimizes reflux of gastric contents through the fistula into the tracheobronchial passages (Fig. 39-7).

If the infant is full-term and has no pneumonia or other major congenital anomaly, then primary esophageal repair can be safely undertaken (Fig. 39-8). The approach is made through a right thoracotomy in the retropleural plane. The lower segment of the esophagus is detached from the trachea, and the tracheal fistula is meticulously sutured closed. The blind upper pouch is mobilized, and its end opened; a union between the two esophageal segments is then carried out. The classic repair described by Haight in 1941 continues to be popular. However, when utilizing a retropleural approach, a single-layer anastomosis using nonabsorbable sutures has also been successful.

If the patient has pneumonia, cardiac disease, or other serious anomaly, these clinical circumstances take precedence, and surgical correction is deferred. In this group of patients a gastrostomy is performed, often under local anesthesia. Up to a week is then spent employing upper-pouch suction, head-up position, antibiotics, intravenous feeding, and gastrostomy drainage. Thoracotomy with repair is carried out after the infant's condition has been stabilized, the heart assessed, and appropriate treatment instituted. With this approach, high-risk infants become

more satisfactory candidates for general anesthesia and definitive surgery.

For infants with overwhelming pneumonia, prematurity, or severe congenital heart disease, a staged approach may prove the wisest course. This involves temporary gastrostomy and fistula division, with complete repair of the esophagus weeks or months later.

The most frequent complication following surgical repair of esophageal atresia is stenosis at the site of the anastomosis. This may occur weeks after operation and is manifest by increasing difficulty in swallowing, followed by aspiration and pneumonia. Most patients with esophageal strictures can be managed by esophageal dilatation during the first year or two of life. In such instances, general anesthesia is preferred, and graduated tapered dilators can be guided down the esophagus with safety. When frequent repetitive dilations are needed, the gastrostomy should be maintained so that linked graduated rubber dilators (Tucker) can be pulled retrograde through the gastrostomy and up the esophagus to accomplish dilatation. In rare instances, when strictures are refractory to repeated dilations, resection may be advisable.

Overall survival for babies with esophageal atresia and tracheoesophageal fistula is approximately 80 percent in most reported series.

Fig. 39-7. Supportive measures for an infant with esophageal atresia and tracheoesophageal fistula include use of sump catheter in upper pouch, intravenous fluids and antibiotics, and gastrostomy for gastric decompression. (*From Randolph et al., J Thorac Cardiovasc Surg, 74:335, 1977, by permission.*)

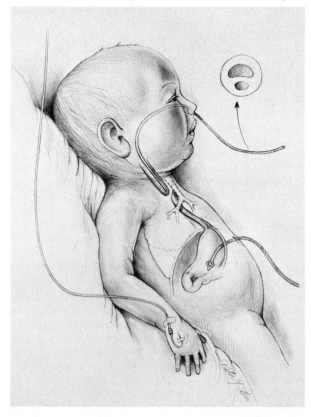

ISOLATED ESOPHAGEAL ATRESIA

Among those babies born with esophageal anomalies, 8 percent have isolated esophageal atresia. Characteristically, infants with isolated esophageal atresia present with a scaphoid abdomen, since the gastrointestinal tract is devoid of air. The x-ray finding of a blind upper pouch and the absence of air below the diaphragm is pathognomonic of isolated esophageal atresia without fistula.

Prompt esophagostomy with the upper esophageal pouch brought to the skin of the left side of the neck allows drainage of saliva and prevents aspiration. A gastrostomy is performed and serves for feeding in the early months of life. Esophageal replacement with colon or gastric tube is then recommended at a year of age. Some authors have shown that the esophageal ends can be dilated over a period of several months, allowing end-to-end union and avoiding esophageal replacement.

ISOLATED (H-TYPE) TRACHEOESOPHAGEAL FISTULA

In rare instances (3 percent), an isolated congenital fistula connecting the trachea to the esophagus may exist. In this anomaly both the trachea and the esophagus are otherwise normal, with no narrowing or obstruction. Infants with this condition seem to swallow normally. The clinical features are subtle; weeks or months may elapse before a correct diagnosis is made. The presence of an H-type tracheoesophageal fistula is suggested by the following triad of symptoms: (1) choking when feeding, (2) gaseous distension of the bowel, and (3) recurrent aspiration pneumonia. Diagnosis can usually be confirmed by cine contrast x-ray studies or by bronchoesophagoscopy using the recently available fiberoptic lens system. Definitive treatment consists of dividing the fistula. Surgical closure of the esophagus and trachea must be meticulous, and encroachment on the lumen of the trachea avoided. The fistula is usually accessible to surgical repair through an incision just above the clavicle.

Corrosive Injury of the Esophagus

Commercial cleaners stored in areas accessible to the toddler are commonly swallowed. These agents often contain a strong alkali which is hygroscopic and becomes firmly attached to the moist mucosal surface of the esophagus. The burn thus sustained coagulates protein and can involve the entire thickness of the esophagus. Children suspected of having swallowed corrosive materials should be admitted to the hospital and studied by esophagoscopy

Fig. 39-8. Primary repair of Type C tracheoesophageal fistula. *A.* Right thoracotomy incision. *B.* Azygos vein transected: proximal and distal esophagus demonstrated and fistula identified. *C.* Tracheoesophageal fistula transected and defect in trachea closed. *D.* End-to-end anastomosis between proximal and distal esophagus (posterior row). *E.* Anastomosis completed.

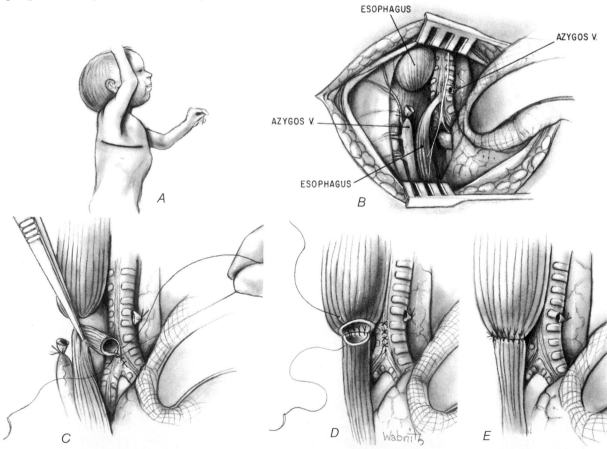

within 24 hours of injury. A burn will be seen as a whitish coagulum on the surface mucosa, surrounded by an area of hyperemia. If the esophageal injury is circumferential, it has been our practice to perform a gastrostomy for feeding, and to insert a string for subsequent dilatation.

Steroids seem to decrease the mucosal scarring and are therefore administered for 6 weeks. Antibiotics are used routinely for 3 weeks. After this interval, esophageal dilatation is begun. Dilatations are continued as often as twice weekly until either the stricture is resolved or it becomes apparent that esophageal substitution will be required. This latter decision is deferred for at least 6 to 12 months until healing is complete and the resulting esophageal injury can be fully assessed.

Esophageal Substitution

Esophageal substitution is required in children for two major conditions: severe esophageal strictures and isolated esophageal atresia. The colon has been the most widely used organ for esophageal substitution, reaching easily into the neck on the marginal artery of Drummond. It can be placed in a substernal tunnel or in the left side of the chest behind the lung root (Fig. 39-9). Since the colon acts as an aperistaltic conduit, antiperistaltic and isoperistaltic segments function equally well. An alternative method of esophageal substitution gaining popularity is the reversed gastric tube. This is fashioned from a flap cut from the greater curvature of the stomach, with a vascular pedicle based on the left gastroepiploic artery. The results of both

these methods of esophageal substitution are satisfactory. Children so treated are able to maintain normal growth and development, and the long-term complications are manageable.

Gastroesophageal Reflux

CLINICAL MANIFESTATIONS. Relentless vomiting in infants from pathologic gastroesophageal reflux is often caused by abnormal relaxation of the cardia ("chalasia"). Poor weight gain and recurrent aspiration pneumonia characterize the clinical course if esophageal reflux goes untreated.

Barium swallow is diagnostic for this condition. Recently, esophageal manometry has been adapted to young subjects. This has provided an important diagnostic adjunct in quantitating reflux. Esophagoscopy is helpful in those patients whose symptoms or x-ray studies suggest esophagitis.

TREATMENT. Upright propping of the infant in an infant seat and administration of small, frequent, thickened feedings constitute the conservative therapeutic approach. This is successful in relieving symptoms in the majority of patients. Many infants with gastroesophageal reflux recover function of the gastroesophageal junction spontaneously at about a year of age. Conservative measures fail in approximately 15 percent of infants and children, and

Fig. 39-9. Diagram showing coloesophagoplasty. Note that the colon can be placed in a substernal position or behind the root of the left lung. The vascular pedicle is supplied by the marginal artery of Drummond from the middle colic artery.

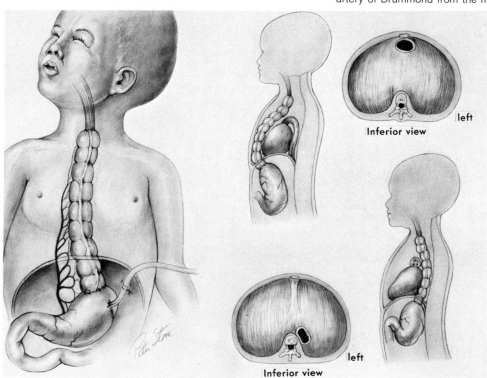

surgical correction is then necessary. The principal indications for surgery are (1) intractable vomiting despite conservative treatment, (2) failure to gain weight and grow normally, (3) recurrent aspiration pneumonia, (4) symptomatic esophagitis, (5) the formation of esophageal stricture. It is not necessary to demonstrate a hiatal hernia for the patient to be a candidate for surgical correction of esophageal reflux.

Both thoracic and abdominal approaches have been successful for surgical correction. Currently the most popular operation in infants and children is the Nissen fundoplication. Surgical correction is usually followed by gratifying clinical improvement and return toward normal growth and developmental parameters.

GASTROINTESTINAL TRACT

Pyloric Stenosis

CLINICAL MANIFESTATIONS. Hypertrophic pyloric stenosis affects male infants predominantly, often the firstborn. The typical history is one of projectile vomiting in an infant from three to ten weeks of age. The vomitus contains only ingested formula, never bile. The enlarged pyloric "olive" can usually be felt on abdominal examination but occasionally it may be necessary to confirm the diagnosis by upper gastrointestinal series. X-ray study shows a narrowed elongated pyloric channel with increased volume and peristaltic effort of the stomach.

TREATMENT. The extent of preoperative preparation depends upon the clinical status of the infant. If the diagnosis is recognized before electrolyte depletion has occurred, the infant may be operated on without elaborate preoperative preparation. Patients who have experienced days of vomiting, however, will show a metabolic alkalosis with a high serum pH and low chloride level. In this group of infants, there is a profound depletion of total body potassium. Correction is achieved by the administration of normal saline solution intravenously with added potassium, 2 to 4 mEq/kg, given over a 12- to 18-hour period. After resuscitation, surgical correction by the Fredet-Ramstedt pyloromyotomy is performed (Fig. 39-10). Postoperatively, cautious, small, frequent feedings are offered using dilute formula; feedings are gradually increased in strength and volume. In a few days a normal feeding schedule is resumed.

Pneumoperitoneum—Gastric Perforation

Pneumoperitoneum in the neonate usually constitutes a surgical emergency. Elevation of the diaphragm as a result of massive intraperitoneal accumulation of air can produce acute respiratory embarrassment. This air may be quickly and safely aspirated by abdominal-wall puncture, performed to the left or right of the midline. This simple maneuver can be lifesaving, as it improves respiratory dynamics until operative repair of the perforated viscus can be undertaken.

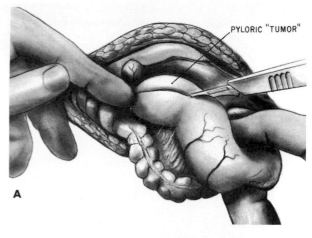

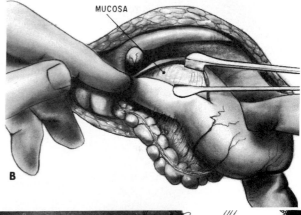

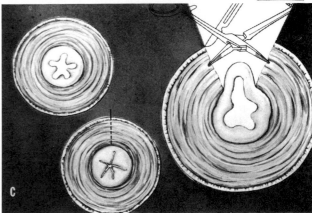

Fig. 39-10. Fredet-Ramstedt pyloromyotomy. *A.* Pylorus delivered into wound and seromuscular layer incised. *B.* Seromuscular layer separated down to submucosal base to permit herniation of mucosa through pyloric incision. *C.* Cross section demonstrating hypertrophied pylorus, depth of incision, and spreading of muscle to permit mucosa to herniate through incision.

Gastrostomy

A gastrostomy is a useful adjunctive procedure for neonates undergoing major abdominal surgery. It is preferred to an indwelling nasogastric tube, which has the potential for causing respiratory embarrassment and permitting gas-

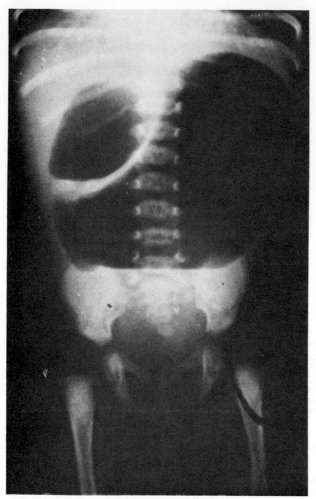

Fig. 39-11. Air-contrast study of an infant with congenital duodenal obstruction. Note size of stomach and distended duodenum, forming the "double bubble."

troesophageal reflux and aspiration. The gastrostomy is also useful to gain access to the gastrointestinal tract in infants who are too weak to take adequate calories by mouth or in infants with complicated oropharyngeal anomalies whose swallowing is impaired.

A Stamm gastrostomy is preferred, employing a Malecot catheter brought out through a separate stab wound in the abdominal wall. It can be removed without difficulty when it is no longer required, and the abdominal defect will usually close spontaneously.

Intestinal Obstruction in the Newborn

The hallmark of intestinal obstruction in the newborn is bilious vomiting. A mechanical obstruction in the intestine must be presumed before assigning this event to other causes such as sepsis or renal disease. Abdominal distension may not be a prominent feature if the obstruction is in the duodenum or the proximal jejunum. Flat and upright abdominal films will frequently indicate the level of the obstruction. A contrast enema will yield information about

intestinal rotation and the caliber of the colon. Contrast material given by mouth is avoided if possible. The upper part of the gastrointestinal tract can be well visualized by instilling air into the stomach.

DUODENAL MALFORMATIONS

Duodenal obstruction may be complete, as in duodenal atresia, or partial, as seen with duodenal stenosis, duodenal web, annular pancreas, and malrotation of the colon. Anomalous entry of the common bile duct and pancreatic duct may be associated with duodenal anomalies; thus, caution must be exercised in the surgical approach to the duodenum.

Duodenal atresia is characterized on x-ray by a "double bubble" (Fig. 39-11). Incomplete obstruction may show this double bubble as well as small amounts of air distally in the gastrointestinal tract. The surgical treatment of congenital duodenal obstruction varies according to the cause. Duodenal atresia is bypassed by either a duodenoduodenostomy or a duodenojejunostomy. An intraluminal web may be excised completely. Obstruction caused by annular pancreas is best treated by a bypass anastomosis, with the pancreas itself left undisturbed. Gastric decompression is accomplished by the insertion of a gastrostomy which should complement any of these procedures.

JEJUNO-ILEAL ATRESIA

Intestinal atresia probably results from intrauterine interruption of the vascular supply to a portion of the bowel. The defect can be reproduced experimentally in the laboratory by ligating branches of the mesenteric artery in the developing fetus. Atresias of the small intestine may be single or multiple. When there has been extensive vascular deficiency there is complete discontinuity of the bowel and a large mesenteric defect. These infants may be subject to the short-gut syndrome after surgical reconstruction.

The clinical presentation of newborn infants with atresia of the jejunum or ileum is similar to that found in other types of intestinal obstruction. Bilious vomiting is an early sign. Abdominal distension is progressive as crying and air swallowing result in dilatation of the bowel proximal to the atretic segment. An abdominal upright film then shows the characteristic stepladder picture of air and fluid in the distended loops. The number of obstructed loops and distribution of air-fluid levels on the x-ray offer some indication of the level of obstruction in the small bowel (Fig. 39-12). It is helpful to obtain a barium enema to determine the size of the colon and to demonstrate whether or not normal bowel rotation has occurred. The finding of a "microcolon" is indicative of distal small-bowel obstruction. The association of abdominal distension, bilious vomiting, and radiographic evidence of obstruction demands urgent surgical intervention unless there is a strong deterrent, such as overwhelming sepsis, severe dehydration, or cardiac failure. In the latter circumstance a limited period of resuscitation is warranted.

The technical problem in the surgical correction of intestinal atresia results from the enormous disparity in lumen size between the proximal distended bowel and the unused distal limb (Fig. 39-13). Anastomosis may be accomplished by (1) end-to-back technique, (2) tapering the proximal dilated limb preparatory to end-to-end union, (3) Bishop-Koop end-to-side anastomosis, (4) Mikulicz exteriorization (Fig. 39-14), or (5) simple temporary ileostomy and delayed anastomosis.

MECONIUM ILEUS

The bowel obstruction in meconium ileus results from impaction of tenacious meconium in the distal ileum. It is always associated with cystic fibrosis of the pancreas (mucoviscidosis). The abdomen of an infant with meconium ileus becomes progressively more distended, although bile vomiting is a relatively late feature. The failure to pass meconium is also a characteristic. The contrast enema will show the tiny caliber of the unused colon (Fig. 39-15). On the plain abdominal film there are dilated small-bowel loops and a "ground-glass" appearance in the right lower quadrant, representing small bubbles of gas trapped in the meconium. The air fluid levels typical of most mechanical obstructions are not seen, a feature which distinguishes meconium ileus. Until Noblett's report all infants with this condition required emergency surgical intervention. It is now standard practice to attempt a Gastrografin enema under fluoroscopic control. In a high percentage of cases this hygroscopic agent permeates the sticky meconium so that it can be evacuated through the rectum, thereby obviating surgery. Because of its powerful osmotic effect, Gastrografin instillation must be done under controlled conditions with an intravenous infusion running.

MALROTATION AND MIDGUT VOLVULUS

PATHOLOGY. During early fetal development, the diminutive abdominal cavity cannot accommodate the rapidly elongating intestine. The midgut, supplied by the

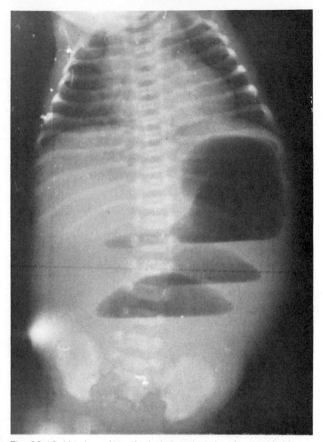

Fig. 39-12. Newborn intestinal obstruction showing several loops of distended bowel with air-fluid levels characteristic of jejunal atresia.

Fig. 39-13. Operative photograph of newborn with jejunal atresia. Note distended proximal portion; point of obstruction is seen just proximal of forceps.

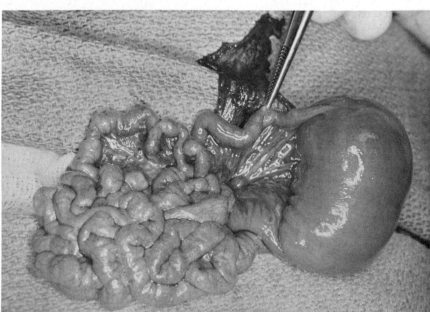

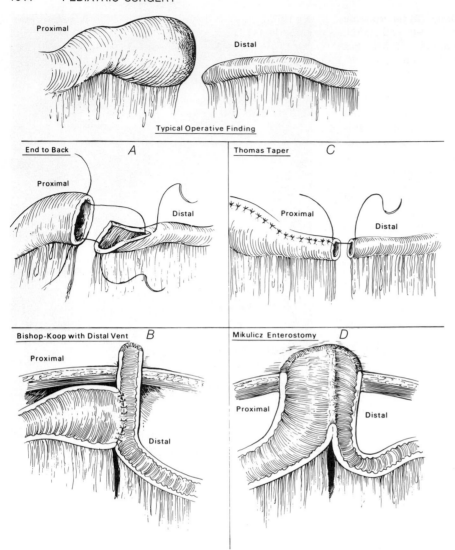

Fig. 39-14. Techniques of intestinal anastomosis for infants with small-bowel obstruction. (Typical operative findings: Proximal distension and discrepancy between ends of intestine to be anastomosed.) *A*. End-to-back distal limb has been incised, creating "fishmouth" to enlarge lumen. *B*. Bishop-Koop: Proximal distended limb joined to side of small distal bowel, which is vented by "chimney" to the abdominal wall. *C*. Tapering: Portion of antimesenteric wall of proximal bowel excised, with longitudinal closure to minimize disparity in the limbs. *D*. Mikulicz double-barreled enterostomy is constructed by suturing the two limbs together, then exteriorizing the double stoma. The common wall can be crushed with a special clamp to create one large stoma. The stoma can be closed in an extraperitoneal manner.

superior mesenteric artery, therefore prolapses into the umbilical cord. As the intestinal loops return to the abdominal cavity during the tenth week of fetal life, final rotation and fixation occur. The duodenum rotates to form a C loop, terminating in the left upper quadrant, and the cecum assumes its final position in the right lower quadrant. When the usual rotation process does not occur, bands extending from the abnormally positioned cecum to the right lateral abdominal wall may cause extrinsic duodenal obstruction. If the cecum remains in the epigastrium, the mesentery is foreshortened and the entire midgut may undergo torsion around the superior mesenteric artery, thereby severely compromising circulation to the bowel.

CLINICAL MANIFESTATIONS. Midgut volvulus may occur at any time during life but is common in the first postnatal week. Characteristically the infant vomits bile and later may begin to pass bloody stools. An abdominal film will often show a paucity of gas in the small bowel. The abnormally placed cecum is demonstrated definitively by barium enema.

TREATMENT. Immediate surgical intervention is mandatory. The intestine must be untwisted to relieve vascular obstruction to the midgut. The bands between the cecum and abdominal wall (Ladd's bands) are then divided. At the completion of this procedure the duodenum is positioned vertically on the right side of the abdomen and the cecum is placed in the left lower quadrant (Fig. 39-16). The appendix is removed. When the viability of the midgut is in doubt, then the volvulus is reduced and all compromised intestine returned to the abdomen. Twenty-four to thirty-six hours later a "second look" is carried out, and only then is a decision made to resect that portion of the bowel judged irretrievably necrotic. This approach will result in maximum salvage of intestine and avoid an irretrievable short-bowel syndrome.

NECROTIZING ENTEROCOLITIS (NEC)

CLINICAL MANIFESTATIONS. Advances in management of high-risk premature infants have introduced a population of neonates at risk from an ischemic bowel disease of uncertain cause. Necrotizing enterocolitis most frequently affects a premature infant with a compromised status. Those with respiratory distress syndrome requiring mechanical ventilation are at greatest risk. It has been observed that symptoms do not develop until feedings are offered.

NEC begins as an ischemic insult to the mucosa of the small and large bowel with invasion of the intestinal wall by gas-producing bacteria. The radiologic finding of air in the wall of the intestine is typical (Fig. 39-17). The ischemic process may progress to involve all layers of the bowel wall, and perforation is common (Fig. 39-18). The afflicted infant shows signs of generalized sepsis and disseminated intravascular coagulation. The abdomen is distended, tense, shiny, erythematous, and tender. Air in the portal vein is a late sign and associated with a grim prognosis.

TREATMENT. The indications for surgery in NEC include physical signs of peritonitis or the x-ray finding of free intraabdominal air. Resection of frankly gangrenous areas of bowel should be carried out and the viable margin ends of the bowel exteriorized. A decompressing gastrostomy should also be carried out.

For at least 2 weeks after surgery, the infant is maintained on total parenteral nutrition, following which oral alimentation is cautiously reintroduced. Although adequate length of the intestine may be preserved, there may be prolonged intestinal malfunction, with malabsorption and diarrhea. Parenteral nutrition may therefore be required for a prolonged period of time.

The formation of strictures in areas of intestine compromised but not frankly gangrenous is not unusual. Therefore, before closing intestinal ostomies a complete evaluation of the gastrointestinal tract by contrast x-ray is mandatory.

Intussusception

Intussusception is an important cause of intestinal obstruction in pediatric patients. The highest incidence is observed in infants eight to twelve months of age. Intussusception occurs when one segment of the bowel (intussusceptum) invaginates into the lumen of the intestine distal to it (intussuscipiens). The most frequent type of intussusception occurs as prolapse of the distal ileum into the cecum, or the ileocolic type. Less commonly, ileoileal and colocolic intussusceptions occur. In these instances a polyp or Meckel's diverticulum may act as a leading point. In many cases of intussusception, no specific lead point is identified.

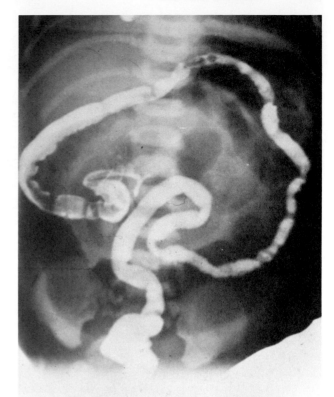

Fig. 39-15: Barium enema in an infant with meconium ileus. Microcolon is demonstrated. Colonic rotation is normal.

Frequently, intussusception is preceded by a viral syndrome characterized by abdominal pain, vomiting, and diarrhea. The symptoms merge into those of intussusception, thereby presenting a very difficult diagnostic dilemma for the physician. It was this association that led Zachary to the discovery that the adenovirus was frequently associated with intussusception. He reasoned that the intestinal inflammation caused enlargement of the ileal lymphoid tissue, or Peyer's patches, and that these tissues projected into the lumen of the ileum, forming the lead point of the intussusception.

Between paroxysms of intermittent crampy abdominal pain, the infant rests quietly, only to be awakened in 15 or 30 minutes with a recurrence of pain. Vomiting and the passage of bloody mucus per rectum (currant-jelly stool) are later signs. Unless the diagnosis is appreciated, and therapy instituted, serious vascular compromise of the bowel ensues, leading to infarction, peritonitis, and sepsis.

The pathognomonic physical finding in the infant with intussusception is an oblong mass in the right or midupper part of the abdomen and an absence of bowel in the right lower quadrant (Dance's sign). Bloody stool in the rectum is a late sign and indicates that venous compromise has already occurred.

The most important diagnostic procedure is the barium enema (Fig. 39-19). By this technique the intussusception is visualized as an obstructing filling defect preventing retrograde filling of the colon; typically, barium outlines the leading portion of the intussusceptum, giving an x-ray

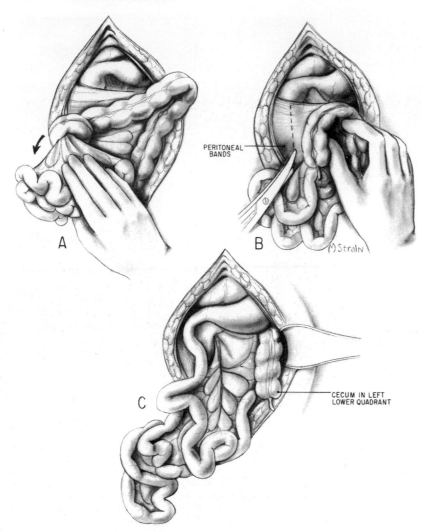

PERITONEAL BANDS

(M) Strain

CECUM IN LEFT LOWER QUADRANT

Fig. 39-16. Operative procedure for incomplete rotation of cecum and midgut volvulus. *A.* Unwinding of intestine to correct volvulus. *B.* Transection of peritoneal bands extending from cecum in right upper quadrant. *C.* Cecum relocated in left lower quadrant.

appearance of a coiled spring. The barium enema is diagnostic only for ileocolic intussusception; the results will be completely normal if the intussusception is confined to the ileum.

In the majority of patients hydrostatic reduction by barium enema will succeed. Reduction of the intussusception by this modality is not attempted if there are signs of peritonitis or peripheral collapse. Barium is instilled into the rectum under fluoroscopic control (from a height no more than 3 ft 6 in. above the table). Gradually the intussusception is pushed retrograde until the intussusceptum is reduced completely and contrast medium refluxes freely into the terminal ileum. Unless reflux into the ileum is observed unequivocally, the intussusception is regarded as unreduced and immediate surgery is advised.

When hydrostatic reduction fails, or is only partially successful, or when signs of systemic toxicity preclude reduction by this method, surgical exploration is mandatory. The operation is performed through a right lower quadrant transverse incision, through which the involved mass representing the intussusception is delivered. The intussusceptum is reduced by distal compression, pushing

the ileum from within the lumen of the colon until the prolapse is completely reduced. Unless the cecal wall is compromised, the appendix can be removed after reduction. It has recently been shown that the intravenous administration of the biologically active peptide, glucagon, will enhance the chances for successful hydrostatic reduction by its action on the smooth muscle in the intestinal wall. The recurrence rate is low whether the intussusception is reduced by hydrostatic or surgical means, and when the bowel is viable, the prognosis is excellent.

When serious circulatory compromise results in intestinal infarction, the intussusception will not reduce and ileocolic resection is required. Primary reconstruction is carried out, and the infant is given intravenous fluids and antibiotics for 5 to 7 days postoperatively.

Duplications and Mesenteric Cysts

DUPLICATIONS

Duplications can occur at any level in the gastrointestinal tract. They are most common in the small bowel and

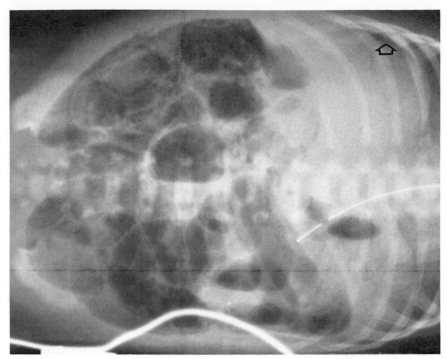

Fig. 39-17. X-ray study showing characteristic findings of necrotizing enterocolitis. There are distended, separated loops of bowel. Air is seen in the wall of the bowel (pneumotosis). The arrow depicts free air above the liver and below the diaphragm, signifying perforation.

affect primarily the ileum. These cystic masses are located on the mesenteric aspect of the intestine and lie within the leaves of the mesentery. They share a common wall with the contiguous small bowel. The duplications may be long and tubular, but more commonly are large, single cystic masses over which the normal intestinal tract is stretched. Duplications may cause obstruction by effacement of the adjacent small bowel; they may also undergo torsion, with gangrene and perforation. Bleeding into the lumen of the intestine occurs when ectopic gastric mucosa is present in the duplication. Although rare, these anomalies are troublesome and difficult to diagnose, since they are often mobile within the abdomen. Treatment consists of resection of the duplication and attached bowel. If extirpation is not possible, excision of a window from the septum between the cyst and intestine should be performed.

MESENTERIC CYSTS

Mesenteric cysts are similar to duplications in their location within the mesentery. However, they do not possess the muscular wall characteristic of duplications, and are not lined with mucosa. Chylous cyst is an unusual form of mesenteric cyst which develops secondary to congenital obstruction of the intestinal lymphatic drainage (Fig. 39-20). Mesenteric and chylous cysts can cause partial or complete intestinal obstruction, or may present as an abdominal mass. It is often necessary to resect a segment of involved intestine to circumscribe the mass surgically. Excision is curative, and there are no known malignant com-

ponents to these cysts. When these cystic structures involve a large portion of the intestinal mesentery they are best treated by partial surgical excision and marsupialization.

Hirschsprung's Disease

PATHOLOGY. The defect underlying this condition is congenital absence of ganglion cells in the rectum and rectosigmoid. Though the aganglionosis may involve the

Fig. 39-18. Operative photograph showing distended small bowel in an infant with necrotizing enterocolitis. Air is demonstrated beneath the serosa in the wall of the bowel.

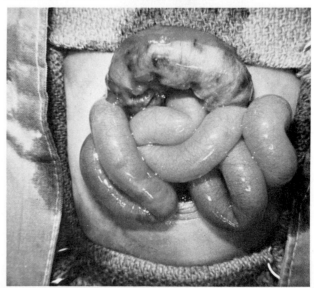

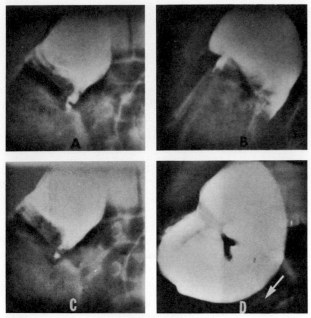

Fig. 39-19. Barium enema diagnosis and reduction of intussusception. *A* to *C.* Various stages of reduction. *D.* Reduction complete and radiopaque material noted in ileum.

entire colon, such extensive involvement is rare. Although this condition was originally described by Hirschsprung in 1888, appropriate surgical treatment was not devised until the classic work of Swenson in 1948. The absence of ganglion cells modifies the neuromuscular conduction. The area of aganglionosis in the bowel is inert and acts as an obstructing lesion. It is, however, the normally innervated proximal colon which dilates, distends, and undergoes muscular hypertrophy.

CLINICAL MANIFESTATIONS. The consequences of aganglionosis may be of such magnitude as to be life-threatening in the newborn period (Fig. 39-21). On the other hand the clinical presentation of Hirschsprung's disease may be subtle and in fact go unrecognized for months or years until the classic symptoms of constipation, abdominal distension, and secondary malnutrition become unmistakable. It is important to note, however, that the history of constipation almost always goes back to the early days of life in most patients with Hirschsprung's disease. Abdominal distension or debilitating enterocolitis brings the infant to the attention of the physician.

When an infant fails to pass meconium spontaneously in the first 24 hours of life, Hirschsprung's disease becomes a consideration. Though other forms of intestinal obstruction may be confused with Hirschsprung's disease, appropriate efforts will lead to a correct diagnosis.

In older children there are striking clinical findings. The abdomen is immense and out of proportion to the extremities, which are usually spindly. Children with long-standing megacolon are typically pale and cheerless. Growth and development are impeded. The major differential diagnosis in children with chronic constipation is Hirschsprung's disease or some form of habit constipation (psychogenic megacolon, chronic constipation, encopresis). The finding on physical examination of a dilated rectum, with stool well down against the anus, argues against the diagnosis of Hirschsprung's disease, since the aganglionic segment usually does not contain stool.

DIAGNOSTIC STUDIES. The barium enema in the newborn is not always a reliable study, since the characteristic disparity between the aganglionic distal segment and the

Fig. 39-20. Operative photograph depicting loops of ileum with a large chylous cyst in the mesentery. Note the relationship of the vascular supply to the bowel as it courses over the cyst. In most instances resection of the involved intestine is necessary.

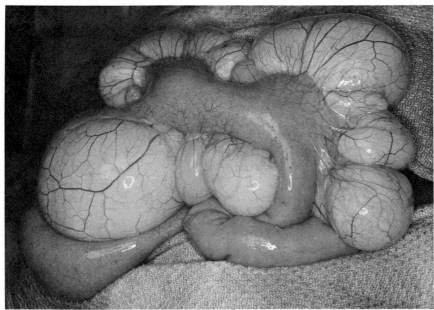

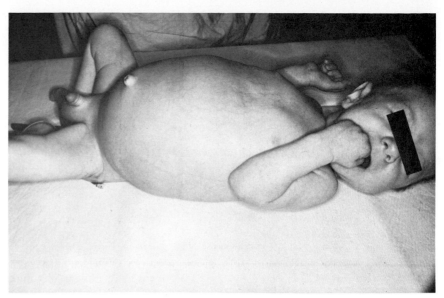

Fig. 39-21. Abdominal distension in a four-month-old infant with Hirschsprung's disease. The faint outline of an enlarged colon can be seen in the upper abdomen. Immediate decompressing colostomy is advised in such circumstances.

distended ganglionic segment proximal to it may not be seen early in life. In older children the barium enema is diagnostic. Typically there is a distal narrow segment, aganglionic bowel, with greatly distended colon proximal to this.

Rectal biopsy affords the definitive diagnosis in Hirschsprung's disease. There are several techniques of biopsy. The purpose of biopsy is to obtain a specimen of the rectal wall in which the ganglion cells can be evaluated. Experienced pathologists can interpret the more superficial biopsies which include only the submucosal tissue. The advantage of a partial-thickness rather than a full-thickness biopsy is that intramural scarring is minimized—a factor which is important to the subsequent performance of corrective surgical procedures. A suction biopsy technique is available and has particular application for infants. This bedside procedure usually provides adequate submucosal tissue for interpretation by an experienced pediatric pathologist.

TREATMENT. Treatment is surgical in all cases. Colostomy is appropriate for almost all children with the diagnosis of Hirschsprung's disease. After a period of months with adequate diet, the distended bowel returns to normal caliber. A definitive operation designed to eliminate the aganglionic segment is then possible. There are now three generally applied operations, based on the principal developed by Swenson, which are used for the definitive treatment of Hirschsprung's disease. The first is the original Swenson pull-through procedure. In this operation the rectosigmoid is carefully dissected in the pelvis and the distal anorectal junction is joined to the colon by an anastomosis carried out through a perineal approach (Fig. 39-22B). Variations of Swenson's technique have been devised by Duhamel and Soave (Fig. 39-22). In the former

procedure the ganglionic bowel is brought into the retrorectal space and anastomosed just above the anus posteriorly, with preservation of the anterior aganglionic rectal wall. In Soave's operation, the dissection is completely intramural, with removal of the mucosa of the rectum and anastomosis within the seromuscular sleeve of aganglionic rectum (Fig. 39-23). Following any of these repairs the outlook for most patients is for normal or near-normal bowel function.

TOTAL COLONIC AGANGLIONOSIS

An infrequent variant, total colonic aganglionosis presents special problems in diagnosis and management. The barium enema does not show the typical transition area characteristic of low-segment Hirschsprung's disease. Diagnosis is based upon a series of biopsies taken at the time of laparotomy which prove the entire colon to be aganglionic, back to and sometimes including the ileum. Surgical therapy is predicated upon transposing normally innervated distal ileum to the anus by end-to-side suture technique, or by low anterior resection with ileorectal anastomosis. The latter converts the patient's condition to a short-segment Hirschsprung's disease, which, with the low ileal anastomosis, can be compensated.

Imperforate Anus

Imperforate anus affects males and females with equal frequency and occurs in approximately one of every 20,000 live births. The anomaly results from a failure of differentiation of the urogenital sinus and cloaca. Imperforate anus is classified as high or low, depending upon the level to which the rectal pouch has descended. High imperforate anus in either sex implies that the rectal pouch is at or above the levator musculature. Low imperforate anus implies that the rectum has descended through this muscle complex and resides in a normal anatomical relationship to the levator sling and the puborectalis muscle. In an infant

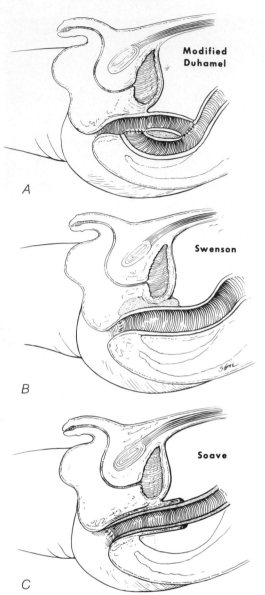

Fig. 39-22. The three basic operations for surgical correction of Hirschsprung's disease. A. The Duhamel procedure leaves the rectum in place and brings ganglionic bowel into the retrorectal space. The common wall, indicated by lines, is crushed to eliminate the septum. B. Classic Swenson operation (1948) is a resection with end-to-end anastomosis performed by exteriorizing bowel ends through the anus. C. The Soave operation is performed by endorectal dissection and removal of mucosa from the aganglionic distal segment and bringing the ganglionic bowel down to the anus within the seromuscular tunnel.

with low imperforate anus, the relationship of the rectum to the muscles of continence is normal, whereas patients with high imperforate anus will require a pull-through operation to establish the normal relationship between the levator muscles and the rectum.

Ninety percent of afflicted female infants will have imperforate anus of the low type. In these patients the rectum terminates by means of a fistula which presents anterior to

the normal location of the anus on the perineum, in the vaginal fourchette or low in the vagina. An emergency colostomy is not necessary in these infants, since satisfactory decompression can be accomplished through the fistula. Although it is technically feasible to perform an anoplasty in the newborn period, it is not necessary. In females with low imperforate anus and a vaginal fistula, dissection of the fistula and mobilization of the distal rectum from the vagina is optimally performed at three to six months of age. This dissection is performed entirely below the levator sling; thus continence should be assured. When the fistula is located high in the vagina, it is not accessible to dilation or surgical revision in the newborn period. For these infants, a colostomy is necessary. Definitive surgical therapy for high imperforate anus in the female is deferred until the baby weighs 15 to 20 lb.

In the male, the distribution of high and low imperforate anus is roughly equal. About half present with a fistula which opens on the perineum anterior to the normal location of the anus. In some the fistula terminates as far forward as the ventral surface of the penis. At birth, the opening of the fistula is not always apparent, and an interval of 12 to 24 hours may be required until meconium reaches the distal-most point in the gastrointestinal tract. For these infants, a perineal anoplasty supplemented by local dilatation will accomplish decompression of the bowel, and emergency colostomy is not needed.

When no fistula is visible on the perineum, the male infant must be presumed to have high imperforate anus with a fistulous connection to the posterior urethra. A colostomy is needed for decompression, and the definitive pull-through operation is generally deferred until the infant is about a year old. The colostomy should be placed high in the sigmoid colon. The definitive pull-through procedure can be performed through a sacroperineal or abdominosacroperineal approach, without taking down the colostomy. Urine refluxed through the urethral fistula is not exposed to excessive colonic surface and is not associated with reabsorption of urinary chloride and consequent acidosis. Even after the restoration of normal anatomic relationships the functional result may not be optimal. Analysis of long-term follow-up data has shown that in almost 50 percent of patients it is difficult to accomplish toilet training, and occasional soiling or minimal incontinence is not infrequent. In 50 percent continence is never achieved. Therefore, the families must be counseled truthfully, so that their expectations will be realistic.

JAUNDICE

General Considerations

PATHOLOGY. The primary surgical consideration in the evaluation of a jaundiced neonate is the differentiation between obstructive and nonobstructive causes. In addition to the physiologic jaundice of the newborn, other nonobstructive causes of hyperbilirubinemia include excessive red cell destruction from blood incompatibility, intrauterine infections such as toxoplasmosis, herpes, cytomegalic

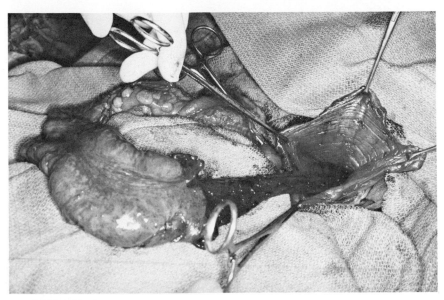

Fig. 39-23. Operative photograph of Soave procedure for Hirschsprung's disease. The seromuscular tunnel has been developed, and the circular muscle of the rectum is clearly seen. The mucosa has been stripped away from this tunnel and can be seen below the normally innervated sigmoid colon. The mucosal sleeve will be pulled through the rectum and the normal sigmoid colon drawn into the seromuscular tunnel for anastomosis at the anus.

inclusion disease, and syphilis; and genetically determined metabolic disorders such as alpha$_1$ antitrypsin deficiency. Additionally, there is a heterogeneous group of conditions labeled "neonatal hepatitis" which result in severe intrahepatic cholestasis. In addition to these medical causes of jaundice in the neonate, there are anatomic derangements which result in obstructive forms of jaundice. The most common of these is biliary atresia.

DIAGNOSTIC STUDIES. In the laboratory evaluation of an infant with hyperbilirubinemia, no single test is diagnostic. Laboratory studies should include measurement of prothrombin time, PTT, alkaline phosphatase, transaminases, and serologic evaluation to rule out intrauterine infection. The most useful evaluations are the rose Bengal scan and percutaneous needle biopsy. Although the isotope scan will not discriminate between intrahepatic cholestasis and extrahepatic obstruction, the presence of isotope in the gastrointestinal tract confirms patency of the extrahepatic bile ducts. Severe intrahepatic cholestasis may result in complete retention of the isotope within the liver. The percutaneous needle biopsy is diagnostic in about 85 percent of the cases. When the laboratory information is overlapping or unclear, it may be necessary to undertake surgical exploration, with biopsy of the liver and operative cholangiogram. Today, surgical exploration of the jaundiced neonate can be carried out in such a way as not to prejudice adversely the recovery of those infants who will be diagnosed as having a neonatal cholestatic syndrome with normal extrahepatic biliary structures. However, delay in the diagnosis of an infant with biliary atresia may eliminate any chance for surgical correction by the portoenterostomy procedure. This operative approach, pioneered by Kasai, should be performed before the twelfth week of life, after which, the microscopic biliary ductules seem to lose their patency. At the time of surgical exploration and operative cholangiography, if no gallbladder is present, it is justifiable to enlarge the incision and carry out formal exploration of the porta hepatis.

Extrahepatic Biliary Atresia

TREATMENT. In the vast majority of infants with extrahepatic biliary atresia, the entire extrahepatic biliary tree is affected. About 5 to 10 percent of these patients will have a patent hepatic or common hepatic duct with distal atresia; this is the so-called favorable type, which lends itself to reestablishment of biliary continuity in the gastrointestinal tract by means of Roux-en-Y choledochojejunostomy or choledochoduodenostomy. The portoenterostomy procedure now offers a chance of surgical relief of jaundice in some of those infants for whom there was formerly no hope (Fig. 39-24). Biliary atresia does not imply an absence of the extrahepatic biliary system; rather these structures are present as fibrous cords. Kasai's work demonstrates that the cords at the porta hepatis contain microscopically patent ductules.

It is to these channels that the jejunal conduit is anastomosed. When the operation is carried out before the twelfth week of life, bile drainage can be accomplished in many infants. It has been shown, however, that bile drainage is not tantamount to cure, for cirrhosis may continue even when bile drainage is achieved. However, a significant salvage rate has been accomplished in this group of infants, who formerly died usually by the end of the first year of life.

Biliary Hypoplasia

At the time of surgical exploration and operative cholangiography, the extrahepatic bile ducts may appear anatomically normal in distribution but have only a minute

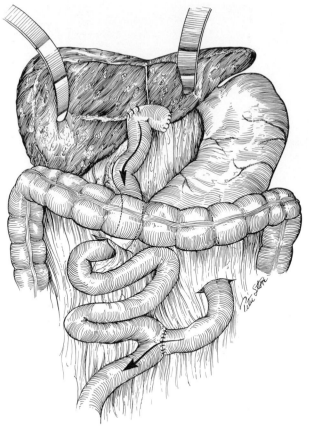

Fig. 39-24. Operative diagram of the Kasai portoenterostomy for biliary atresia. An isolated limb of jejunum has been brought to the porta hepatis and anastomosed to the transected ducts. The Roux-en-Y principle has been used to reconstitute intestinal continuity.

lumen. This has been termed *biliary hypoplasia* and is associated with a variety of hepatobiliary disorders resulting in intrahepatic cholestasis, including neonatal hepatitis and alpha$_1$ antitrypsin deficiency. Portoenterostomy is not applicable for this category of patients.

Choledochal Cyst

Extrahepatic biliary obstruction from choledochal cyst probably results from a localized obliterative process in the distal common duct. This disorder may be a more generalized alteration of the biliary drainage system, since many infants develop liver failure despite surgical relief of the obstructed bile flow. Diagnosis is often possible by palpation of the cyst. Barium studies of the upper gastrointestinal tract show displacement of the viscera by the cysts. Ultrasound echograms are also useful in defining cystic structures in the porta hepatis. The surgical options include drainage of the cyst to the duodenum or jejunum, or resection of the cyst with anastomosis of the bowel to the hepatic duct proximal to the origin of the choledochal cyst. The latter surgical approach is preferable, since malignant neoplasms may occur in the cyst wall and also the incidence of cholangitis is reduced.

ABNORMALITIES OF THE ABDOMINAL WALL
Umbilical Hernia

Most children with umbilical hernia heal spontaneously by about four years of age. Surgical repair is usually indicated if the hernia persists beyond this time. In younger patients, massive enlargement and distortion of the umbilicus dictate the need for earlier repair. Incarceration of umbilical hernia is extremely uncommon but has been seen in patients who have a small fascial defect associated with a large sac. A simple repair of the fascia is all that is required to correct this form of hernia. This can be done through a small curving infraumbilical incision which leaves an unobtrusive scar. Complicated fascial flap repairs are not necessary for children. The umbilicus is never excised.

Patent Urachus

During the development of the coelomic cavity, there is free communication between the urinary bladder and the abdominal wall through the urachus, which exits adjacent the omphalomesenteric duct. Persistence of this tract results in a communication between the bladder and the umbilicus (Fig. 39-25*B*). The first sign of a patent urachus is moisture or obvious urine emission from the umbilicus. Recurrent urinary tract infection may result. The urachus may be partly obliterated, with a remnant remaining beneath the umbilicus in the extraperitoneal position as an isolated cyst. Diagnosis of patent urachus is most reliably made by a cystogram in the lateral projection. Surgical correction is carried out via extraperitoneal exposure of the infraumbilical area. Identification and excision of the urachal tract with closure of the bladder is curative. Urachal cysts are also easily excised from this approach.

Patent Omphalomesenteric Duct

In fetal life, the omphalomesenteric duct is connected through the central wall of the coelomic cavity to the intestinal tract. Normally this duct involutes, but its persistence results in a tubular attachment between the ileum and the umbilicus (Fig. 39-25*A*). Liquid ileal content refluxes through the umbilical defect, soiling the abdominal wall. Diagnosis of a congenital fistula at the umbilicus is made by inspection, probing of the tract, and introduction of radiopaque material into the ostium. Proper surgical treatment consists of elective abdominal exploration with closure of the fistula on the antimesenteric border of the ileum and total excision of the fistulous tract, including its attachment to the undersurface of the umbilicus. Though not an emergency, this procedure should not be postponed, since there is a potential for intestinal volvulus to occur around this intraabdominal structure. Occasionally the peristaltic activity of the bowel will cause eversion of the intestine through this patent duct. The extruded intestine resembles a small ruptured omphalocele, and the lesion requires careful inspection at the neck of the defect to

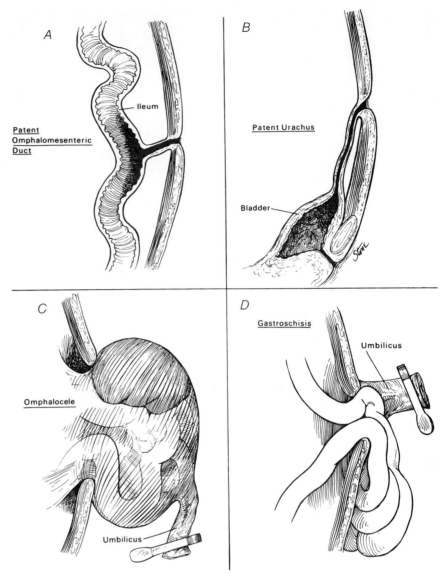

Fig. 39-25. Abnormalities at the umbilicus: *A.* Patent omphalomesenteric duct: persistent patent tract from ileum to abdominal wall, through which intestinal contents can be discharged or bowel can prolapse. *B.* Patent urachus: tract to umbilicus from bladder. Partial patency results in urachal cyst. *C.* Omphalocele: large abdominal wall defect with intestine and solid viscera within an intact sac. *D.* Gastroschisis: intestine prolapsing through small abdominal wall defect at the base of the umbilicus.

determine its true nature. In such cases the bowel has, in effect, turned inside out and prolapsed through the patent duct, forming an external intussusception. In this instance, immediate operation with reduction and correction is necessary.

Omphalocele

Interruption of normal formation of the abdominal wall can result in a central defect termed *omphalocele* (Fig 39-25*C*). In the newborn, the defect appears as a variable-sized mass of bowel and solid viscera in the center of the abdomen, covered by a translucent membrane. The size varies from 1 to 2 cm (Fig. 39-26) to a huge defect containing all the abdominal viscera. Usually the sac remains intact, but occasionally it is ruptured during delivery. The diagnosis of this anomaly is made by inspection, for it is readily apparent immediately after the birth. No pressure should be placed on the omphalocele sac in an effort to reduce it. This is not only hazardous to the integrity of the sac, but may interfere with abdominal venous return or impede the respiratory effort.

Small omphaloceles are usually amenable to complete one-stage reduction and anatomic surgical repair of the abdominal wall. For omphaloceles larger than 6 cm, a sheet of silastic with interwoven Marlex mesh is sewed around the edge of the defect to envelope the prolapsing viscera (Fig. 39-27). Continuous pressure on this prosthetic covering over a period of days brings about gradual reduc-

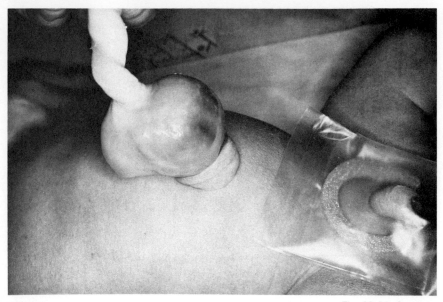

Fig. 39-26. Small omphalocele or hernia into the umbilical cord. Note that formation of the abdominal wall is nearly complete.

tion of the omphalocele, such that complete surgical closure of the abdominal wall can be accomplished as a staged procedure. The temporary use of a prosthetic covering allows gradual enlargement of the abdominal cavity, which then accommodates the extraneous viscera without compromising venous return or ventilatory dynamics. Intestinal atresia, congenital heart disease, and renal anomalies occur in approximately 30 percent of infants with omphalocele. The overall prognosis for these infants is affected by the existence and severity of associated anomalies.

Gastroschisis

Gastroschisis was originally thought to be a form of ruptured omphalocele, but now is recognized as a distinct embryologic phenomenon in which the abdominal wall has completed its development. There is no central defect, nor

is there any significant separation of the rectus muscles. There is a small defect at the base of the umbilicus through which part or all of the intestine herniates (Fig. 39-25D). The escape of intestine into the amniotic fluid can occur at different times in fetal life. Thus the bowel of some infants born with gastroschisis is glistening and normal-appearing, suggesting a recent onset, just prior to birth, while others show edematous and matted intestinal loops which appear to have been exposed to the amniotic fluid for many weeks or months (Fig. 39-28).

Immediately upon recognition of gastroschisis, the prolapsed intestine should be wrapped with a dressing soaked in warm sterile saline solution and an outer dry layer. Prompt surgical repair should be undertaken. In about half the cases, the viscera can be returned to the abdomen and secure closure obtained. It is usually necessary to enlarge the defect in order to accomplish this. When the bowel is matted and edematous it may take many weeks before recovery of intestinal function. In such instances, support by total parenteral nutrition is lifesaving. If the abdominal wall cannot be closed without undue tension, then an extra abdominal prosthetic compartment is fashioned from silastic-covered Marlex (Fig. 39-27). Once the prosthesis is in place, the capacity of the prosthetic envelope is gradually reduced over 7 to 10 days until complete surgical closure is obtained.

Fig. 39-27. Close-up of silastic prosthesis for temporary covering of gastroschisis. The remnant of the umbilicus is seen in the center of the photograph. A gastrostomy tube is seen.

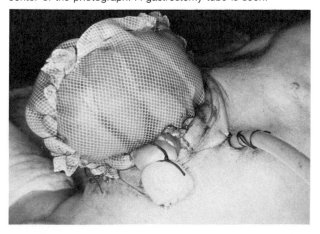

Exstrophy of the Cloaca (Vesicointestinal Fissure)

Exstrophy of the cloaca represents one of the severest forms of embryologic derangement. In infants with cloacal exstrophy, the normal ventral closure of the pelvis and the wall is imperfect. Major components of the cloacal exstrophy are (1) omphalocele, (2) exstrophy of the bladder, (3) external intestinal fistula through the bladder (ompha-

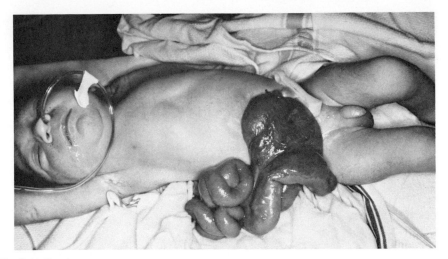

Fig. 39-28. Newborn with gastroschisis. The intestine has escaped through a defect just to the right of the umbilicus. The intestine is edematous and matted, indicating that these loops have been floating freely in the amnion for some period of time.

lomesenteric duct), (4) epispadias in the males, (5) imperforate anus, and (6) foreshortened colon (Fig. 39-29). In addition there is often an associated orthopedic deformity of the distal leg and foot. The summation of these physical defects is such that many of the newborns are not hardy enough to survive.

Early surgical intervention in these patients becomes necessary when extensive intestinal prolapse through the fistula causes intestinal obstruction. In such circumstances

Fig. 39-29. Close-up of baby with exstrophy of the cloaca. Note large omphalocele with clamp on the umbilical cord. Two halves of the exstrophied bladder are readily seen, with a prolapsed intestinal defect in the center. The imperforate anus is also shown. Pubic bones are widely separated.

an ileostomy is required. The colon is temporarily exteriorized as a mucous fistula. The omphalocele is closed primarily or treated with a topical agent which promotes epithelialization. There is no urgency about repairing the exstrophied bladder, and reconstruction of the urinary system need not be completed until the patient is two or three years of age. While most patients suffer a number of physical limitations, many have the potential for functional rehabilitation, which justifies aggressive surgical efforts on their behalf.

Congenital Deficiency of the Abdominal Musculature (Eagle-Barrett Syndrome; Prune-Belly Syndrome)

Congenital deficiency of the abdominal musculature is a rare anomaly occurring in males. In severely affected in-

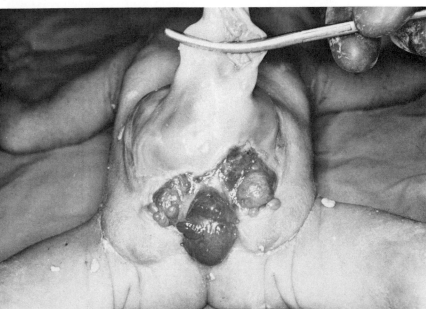

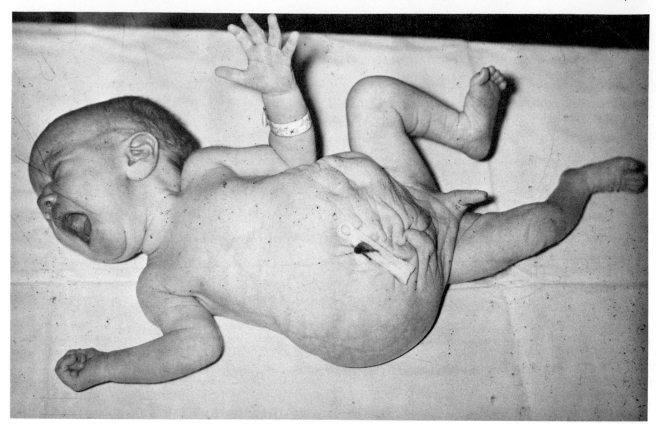

Fig. 39-30. Eagle-Barrett (prune-belly) syndrome. Baby with congenital absence of the abdominal musculature, showing lax, flaccid abdomen. This syndrome occurs in males and is associated with severe malformations of the urinary collecting system.

fants, there is marked wrinkling of the skin of the lower part of the abdomen and little or no muscular substance detectable beneath it (Fig. 39-30). In addition to the absent abdominal muscles, the bladder is large and the ureters are dilated and tortuous. The kidneys may be hypoplastic, but there is usually adequate renal parenchyma.

Advances in techniques of urinary reconstruction have improved the prognosis for this group. Temporary urinary diversion with subsequent stage reconstruction, by shortening, tapering, and reimplantation of the ureters, and reduction in the size of the bladder has been successful in rehabilitating the urinary tract. Various surgical procedures have been devised to tighten the lax abdominal musculature and reduce the redundancy of the abdominal wall, thereby providing adequate support. This approach has changed materially the dismal outlook that most of these children faced a decade age.

Inguinal Hernia

Inguinal hernia results from a failure of closure of the processus vaginalis, which is normally obliterated in males by two or three months of age. The processus is a fingerlike projection of the peritoneum which accompanies the testicle as it descends into the scrotum. Infants are at particular risk from incarceration of a hernia. The internal inguinal ring is narrow; therefore, intestine finding its way into the hernial sac in the inguinal canal can become trapped within the hernial sac. When there is diagnostic confusion between an incarcerated hernia and a hydrocele, a rectal examination with simultaneous abdominal palpation of the internal inguinal ring will delineate the structures passing through the internal ring into the inguinal canal. Using the vas deferens as a constant reference point, the presence of intestine adjacent to the vas between the examining fingers confirms the diagnosis of a hernia. Most often the hernia can be reduced. The infant is sedated, and moderate, bimanual pressure is applied by compressing the sac from below while a gentle counterforce downward is provided from the examiner's hand above the inguinal ring. Occasionally, these hernias will reduce spontaneously after sedation is given and the continuous struggling and crying are terminated. Surgery should be delayed 48 hours, until the local edema secondary to incarceration has resolved. If the hernia cannot be reduced, or, in cases of obvious intestinal obstruction, emergency operation, with reduction and repair, is necessary.

An inguinal hernia in the female usually is indicated by the appearance of a nontender groin mass. The mass represents an ovary herniated into the patent sac. Although the gonad can usually be reduced into the abdomen by gentle pressure, it often prolapses in and out until surgical repair is carried out. In some patients the ovary and fallopian tube constitute one wall of the hernial sac (sliding hernia), and in these cases the ovary can be effectively reduced only at the time of operation. Because of the frequency of bilaterality, contralateral exploration is recommended for all infants under one year of age except those in whom it is precluded by a coexisting medical condition or in whom the operation on the symptomatic side is unduly difficult.

Hydrocele is often associated with inguinal hernia. The hydrocele may communicate with the peritoneal cavity via the patent processus vaginalis and, therefore, wax and wane in size. Alternatively the hydrocele may be encysted and confined to the scrotum or to the inguinal canal. Usually a simple hydrocele does not require operation unless it is shown after 1 to 2 years of observation that it is not undergoing spontaneous regression.

GENITALIA

Undescended Testicle

One or both testicles may be absent from the scrotum of a newborn baby, or this finding may be noticed in the male child of any age. The empty scrotum can mean incomplete descent of the gonad or congenital absence. Confusion pervades the medical literature regarding the endocrinologic function and surgical treatment of the undescended testicle. The decision to operate is ideally made when the child is four to five years old. If the testicle can be drawn into the upper scrotum, then surgical therapy is delayed in favor of a period of observation, with the expectation that it will descend spontaneously. If the testicle cannot be brought into the scrotum by manual manipulation then it is unlikely that it will ever descend spontaneously. Operative repair cannot be delayed indefinitely, because spermatogenesis is reduced significantly when the testicle resides in the inguinal canal or within the abdomen where it is exposed to the normal body temperature. If the testicle cannot be palpated in the inguinal canal, it may occasionally be found in the perineum or medial thigh (ectopic testis). If an accompanying hernia is symptomatic, the surgical treatment of the undescended testicle and hernia should be performed as a combined procedure whenever the hernia manifests itself, even in infancy. Five specific reasons are generally advanced for operative replacement of an undescended testicle. These are (1) decreased or absent spermatogenesis; (2) embarrassment and concern to the boy with the empty scrotum, (3) increased incidence of malignancy, (4) increased incidence of torsion of the testicle, and (5) increased vulnerability to trauma (to the testicle which lies on the pubis).

Operative Technique. The operative approach to the undescended testicle is made through a groin incision exposing the retroperitoneum. The hernial sac is dissected from the cord and vascular pedicle. These structures are then freed of all connective tissue investments, which usually affords adequate length to allow the testicle to be placed in the scrotum. The testicle is brought through a new opening of the transversalis fascia immediately lateral to the pubic tubercle. In this way the internal ring is moved medially just behind the external ring. This shortens the distance that the cord and vessels must travel, thereby assuring adequate length. A scrotal pouch is dissected to accommodate the testicle outside the Dartos fascia. This maneuver ensures that the testicle remains in the scrotum without retraction into the inguinal canal.

In about 5 percent of patients an *abdominal testicle* will be found. In this group the artery and vein are short, precluding placement of the testicle in the scrotum even with a series of staged operations. In this circumstance it has been recommended that the artery and vein be divided and the testicle placed in the scrotum still attached to the vas deferens and its accompanying deferential artery. The deferential artery will supply enough blood to allow the testicle to remain viable. This approach is an attractive alternative to orchiectomy.

Intersexual Abnormalities (Ambiguous Genitalia; Hermaphrodite Syndromes)

The infant born with ambiguous external genitalia demands an urgent diagnostic workup (Fig. 39-31). Correct sex assignment must be made in the early days of life to avoid embarrassment and confusion on the part of the parents and the inevitable social stigma that results. Diagnostic procedures, including laparotomy when indicated, should be completed by the time the infant is a week old. However, hurried assignment of sex, without adequate understanding of the patient's anatomy, endocrine physiology, and chromosomes can lead to a mistaken diagnosis with tragic consequences.

Patients with ambiguous genitalia may be grouped into four categories:

1. True hermaphrodite (coexisting testicular and ovarian tissue)
2. Male pseudohermaphrodite (testicular gonads only) with hypospadias, one or both testes undescended, and persistent Müllerian duct remnants
3. Female pseudohermaphrodites (ovarian gonads only)
4. Absent or deficient gonads

Fig. 39-31. Ambiguous genitalia, manifest as enlarged clitoris and labioscrotal folds in a baby with the adrenogenital syndrome. This configuration can be confused with a normal penis and undescended testicles.

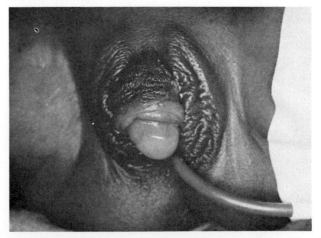

MOST COMMON SITES OF CANCER IN CHILDREN

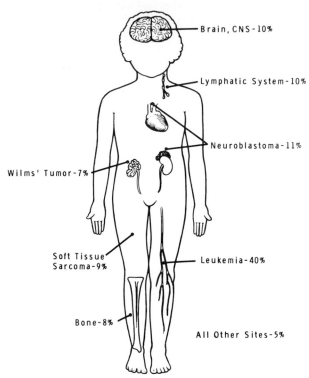

Brain, CNS - 10%

Lymphatic System - 10%

Neuroblastoma - 11%

Wilms' Tumor - 7%

Soft Tissue Sarcoma - 9%

Leukemia - 40%

Bone - 8%

All Other Sites - 5%

Fig. 39-32. Most common sites of cancer in children.

Securing a full family history, including details of the pregnancy with special attention to drug ingestion, is the first diagnostic step. Then the genitalia should be inspected and all orifices carefully defined. Rectal examination is helpful in detecting the uterus and cervix. Radiologic examination of the kidneys, urinary tract, and vagina discloses the presence and size of these structures. Chromosomal studies offer important information about genotypic sex, but this information alone should never constitute the basis for a final sex assignment without consideration of the anatomical and endocrine status of the patient. Elevated urinary excretion of pregnanetriol and 17 ketosteroids is diagnostic of congenital adrenal hyperplasia. When all other diagnostic maneuvers have been completed, a few patients will require laparotomy for identification of internal structures and biopsy of gonadal tissue. The laparotomy is for diagnosis only; excision of contradictory sexual structures is avoided at this stage until full disclosure of all the facts has been made before the family, and alternatives have been thoroughly discussed.

TREATMENT. Except for the diagnostic laparotomy, operative correction is usually begun at one or two years of age. Males require hypospadias repair and excision of remnants of the Müllerian ducts. In the case of true hermaphrodites, removal of the contradictory gonad is indicated. For many females, surgical revision of the enlarged clitoris may be necessary. A revision of the vaginal introitus may be needed in infancy to eliminate urinary

infection; a second surgical procedure may then be required in the premarital years. In some masculinized females, the distal vagina is congenitally absent and extensive reconstruction to unite the perineal skin and the proximal vagina is required.

Severe penile hypoplasia occurs in a small number of males. In these patients the testicles are histologically normal, albeit undescended; chromosome analysis reveals normal male genotype, but the phallus is a tiny clitoris-like structure. The phallus is inadequate for the male role, and there is presently no satisfactory medical or surgical treatment to alter the hypoplastic penis. Consequently, male patients in this small group are more successfully reared as females. The intersexual anomalies require effective teamwork between neonatologist, endocrinologist, geneticist, and surgeon to achieve the most satisfactory rehabilitation of these children.

MALIGNANT DISEASE

Approximately 12 percent of deaths in children is attributed to malignant disease. Of these, solid tumors account for 55 percent, while leukemia is responsible for death in the remaining children afflicted with cancer (Fig. 39-32).

Fig. 39-33. IVP from a patient with bilateral Wilms' tumor. Note bilateral distortion of calyceal systems.

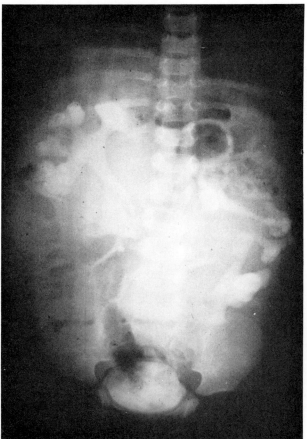

Wilms' Tumor (Nephroblastoma)

Approximately 500 new cases of Wilms' tumor are recorded in the United States each year. The discovery of an asymptomatic mass in the abdomen is the usual presentation of this malignant tumor. The incidence is greatest in the first 2 years of life. Males and females are affected equally. Intravenous pyelography is diagnostic in most cases. The collecting system typically shows a marked distortion, with the calyces appearing to be pulled apart (Fig. 39-33). Unless the tumor has invaded the renal pelvis obstructing the ureter, drainage appears normal. Renal function is generally unimpaired. Prompt nephrectomy with ipsilateral lymph node dissection is the preferred treatment. Some centers advocate preoperative radiation and/or chemotherapy to shrink the tumor, thus making subsequent resection technically easier. This necessarily reduces the amount of radiation that can be delivered to the tumor bed postoperatively. Chemotherapy with actinomycin D and vincristine has changed the outlook remarkably for patients with residual or recurrent disease. Actinomycin D has a synergistic effect when coupled with radiation therapy. Results obtained in the National Wilms' Tumor Study show 95 percent cure rate when the tumor is confined to the kidney or regional nodes (Stage I, II). Even when the tumor has spread to distant sites, the combination of radiation chemotherapy and, when appropriate, repeated excisional therapy has resulted in a cure rate of 80 percent of all children with Wilms' tumor.

Neuroblastoma

Following leukemia and tumors of the central nervous system, neuroblastoma is the third most frequent tumor of childhood, accounting for approximately 11 percent of all malignant disease. Neuroblastomas arise from the sympathetic nervous system, the typical sites being the adrenal glands and the posterior mediastinum. Some 50 percent of neuroblastomas occur in patients under a year of age, and 85 percent occur by age three. The younger children have a better prognosis. Patients seen before the age of one year have an overall survival rate of approximately 75 percent. This favorable survival is realized even when the bone marrow, liver, or adjacent lymph nodes are involved. Evidence is accumulating that immune mechanisms conferred by the mother are responsible for the extraordinary spontaneous regression rate seen when neuroblastoma appears in the early months of life.

Abdominal neuroblastoma is characteristically an irregular and hard mass which often crosses the midline. An intravenous pyelogram will show lateral or inferior displacement of the kidney but almost never calyceal distortion (Fig. 39-34), an important differentiation from Wilms' tumor. Thoracic tumors of neural origin are located in the posterior mediastinum, a distinguishing feature which is readily determined on the lateral chest film. Surgical excision is the treatment for neuroblastoma, regardless of the site of origin. In the abdomen and retroperitoneum this may be impossible because the tumor often invades adjacent organs surrounding the celiac axis and mesenteric artery. If it is feasible, the bulk of the tumor should be surgically excised. X-ray therapy offers only temporary control of this tumor's growth. Chemotherapy in the form of cytoxian, vincristine, and Carboximide has prolonged life, but these agents have not altered survival to the extent accomplished with other childhood tumors.

Teratoma

Teratomas are comprised of tissue from all three embryonic germ layers, although one cell type may predominate. Dermoids arising exclusively from ectodermal precursors are usually benign. Though teratomas may arise in any part of the body, a predilection for certain sites is well recognized. Those tumors arising in the chest are usually found in the anterior mediastinum and are generally benign. Teratoma arising in the retroperitoneum may present as a mass in the abdomen or flank. Such tumors may mimic other abdominal tumors in clinical presentation. The goal of therapy is complete surgical removal. If contiguous spread has not occurred, the cure rate for retroperitoneal teratoma is high.

SACROCOCCYGEAL TERATOMA

Sacrococcygeal teratoma usually appears as a mass originating from the buttocks and projecting forward to distort

Fig. 39-34. IVP from a patient with retroperitoneal neuroblastoma. Note that both kidneys are pushed aside and rotated by adjacent mass.

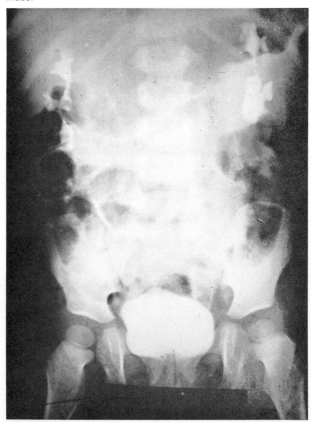

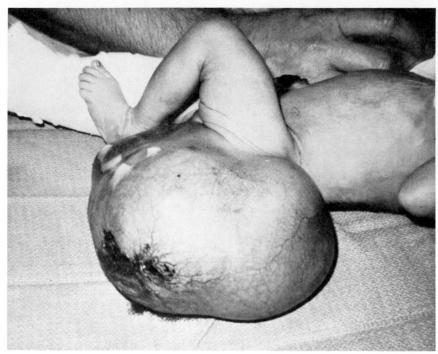

Fig. 39-35. Newborn with huge sacrococcygeal teratoma.

the perineum. The mass may vary in size from a few centimeters to a grapefruit-sized tumor (Fig. 39-35). Myelomeningocele, lipoma, and neural tumors with intraspinal extension should be considered in the differential diagnosis. The potential for malignant degeneration is high in these tumors, but this rarely occurs if operation is carried out in the early days of life. Complete excision is essential and usually can be accomplished without damaging the rectum or genital structures. If the tumor is completely excised the cure rate is excellent.

A form of sacrococcygeal teratoma exists which is not evident externally but projects inward into the retrorectal

Fig. 39-36. Operative photographs of hepatoblastoma in the right lobe of the liver in an eight-month-old child. Extended right hepatic lobectomy was curative.

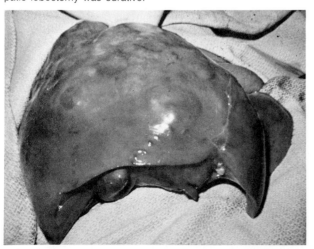

space and pelvis. Discovery of these tumors is often delayed until symptoms of rectal obstruction appear. The late discovery of this variant of sacrococcygeal teratoma allows malignant degeneration, and thus the cure rate is considerably decreased in this form.

Rhabdomyosarcoma

Once thought to originate only from striated muscle, rhabdomyosarcoma is now recognized as an embryonic tumor which can arise from a variety of mesenchymal tissues. The commonest sites of origin are the head and neck, the extremities, and the genitourinary system. This rapidly growing neoplasm invades surrounding structures. Metastases occur to regional nodes and the lungs. Wide local excision is now recognized as optimal surgical treatment for localized forms of rhabdomyosarcoma. Radical extirpation in the form of amputation does not improve survival. This latter change in concept has followed the extraordinary success of combined chemotherapy with actinomycin D, vincristine, and Adriamycin for this disease.

Hepatoma

Two main forms of liver disease occur in children, hepatoblastoma and hepatocellular carcinoma. Hepatoblastoma is slightly more frequent (Fig. 39-36), and its prognosis is considerably better than that of hepatic carcinoma. The child usually has an abdominal mass, often associated with anemia, low-grade fever, and anorexia. The patients are rarely jaundiced, and most tests of liver

Table 39-1. DEATHS IN CHILDREN AGED
1 TO 14 YEARS, UNITED STATES, 1974

Accidents	12,448
Cancer	2,961
Congenital anomalies	2,148
Pneumonia	1,277
Homicide	767
Heart disease	680
Cerebrovascular disease	375
Total all deaths	26,825

SOURCE: U. S. Bureau of Vital Statistics.

function are normal. Alpha fetoprotein, a protein usually not detectable in the serum after the first few weeks of life, is present in patients with hepatoblastoma and is a useful biologic marker. Prior to surgery complete radiologic evaluation, including selective hepatic angiography, is essential. Hepatic resection offers the only hope for cure, since no effective chemotherapy is known at present. The value of radiotherapy is limited, although some tumors have been reduced in size by x-ray therapy, making them surgically accessible. Extended radical hepatic surgery has increased the survival of children with primary liver tumors. For hepatoblastoma, approximately 60 percent of the children have a surgically accessible tumor, and of these patients, half are curable, for an overall survival of 30 percent. With respect to hepatocellular carcinoma, the outlook is much more dismal, with only 15 percent being cured by any surgical procedures.

TRAUMA

Accidents are the leading cause of death in children. Of the more than 26,000 deaths in 1974 in children from 1 to 14 years, almost one-half (12,448) were accidental (Table 39-1). Of the 12,448 deaths, 5,796 occurred as a direct result of motor vehicle accidents, 2,440 were drowning victims, and 1,218 children died of burns. Clearly the injured child needs immediate and expert management at the scene, prompt transport to a major pediatric trauma facility, and sophisticated surgical care in the hospital.

References

Fluid and Electrolyte Balance

Adamsons, K., Jr., and Towell, M. E.: Thermal Homeostasis in the Fetus and Newborn, *Anesthesiology,* **26**:531, 1965.

Altman, R. P., and Randolph, J. G.: The Applications and Hazards of Total Parenteral Nutrition in Infants, *Ann Surg,* **174**:85, 1971.

Asch, M. J., Shaw, K. N. F., and Hays, D. M.: Evaluation of Different Nitrogen Sources in High Calorie Parenteral Therapy, *J Pediatr Surg,* **7**:213, 1972.

Bill, A. H.: Immune Aspects of Neuroblastoma, *Am J Surg,* **122**:142, 1971.

Coran, A. G., and Nesbakken, R.: The Metabolism of Intrave-

nously Administered Fat in Adult and Newborn Dogs, *Surgery,* **66**:922, 1969.

————: The Long-Term Total Intravenous Feedings of Infants Using Peripheral Vein, *J Pediatr Surg,* **8**:801, 1973.

Filler, F. M., Eraklis, A. J., Rubin, V. G., et al.: Long-Term Parenteral Nutrition in Infants, *N Engl J Med,* **281**:589, 1969.

Goudsouzian, N. G., Morris, R. H., and Ryan, J. F.: The Effect of a Warming Blanket on the Maintenance of Body Temperature in Anesthetized Infants and Children, *Anesthesiology,* **39**:351, 1973.

Groff, D. B.: Complications of Intravenous Hyperalimentation in Newborns and Infants, *J Pediatr Surg,* **4**:460, 1969.

Ikeda, K., and Suita, S.: Total Parenteral Nutrition Using Peripheral Veins in Surgical Neonates, *Arch Surg,* **112**:1045, 1977.

Knutrud, O.: The Water and Electrolyte Metabolism in the Newborn Child after Major Surgery, Norwegian Monographs on Medical Science, Olso, Scandinavian University Books, Universitets Forlaget, 1965.

Roe, C. F., Santulli, T. V., and Blair, C. S.: Heat Loss in Infants during General Anesthesia and Operations, *J Pediatr Surg,* **1**:266, 1966.

Rowe, M. I.: The Role of Serial Serum Osmolality Measurements in the Management of the Neonatal Surgical Patient, *Surg Gynecol Obstet,* **133**:93, 1971.

————, Lankau, C., and Newmark, S.: Evaluation of Methods to Clinically Monitor Colloid Oncotic Pressure in the Pediatric Surgical Patient, *Surg Gynecol Obstet,* **139**:889, 1974.

Wilmore, D. W., and Dudrick, S. J.: Growth and Development of an Infant Receiving All Nutrients Exclusively by Vein, *JAMA,* **203**:860, 1968.

Lesions of Neck

Bill, A. H., Jr., and Sumner D. S.: Unified Concept of Lymphangioma and Cystic Hygroma, *Surg. Gynecol Obstet.,* **120**:79, 1965.

———— and Vadheim, J. L.: Cysts, Sinuses, and Fistulas of the Neck Arising from the First and Second Branchial Clefts, *Ann Surg,* **142**:904, 1955.

Brown, P. M., and Judd, E. S.: Thyroglossal Cysts and Sinuses: Results of Radical (Sistrunk) Operation, *Am J Surg* **102**:494, 1961.

Gross, R. E., and Connerly, M. L.: Thyroglossal Cysts and Sinuses, *N Engl J Med,* **223**:616, 1940.

Randolph, J. G.: On the Treatment of Lymphangioma in Children, *Surgery,* **49**:289, 1961.

Sistrunk, W. E.: The Surgical Treatment of Cysts of Thyroglossal Tract, *Ann Surg,* **71**:121, 1920.

Respiratory System

Aberdeen, E.: Tracheostomy and Tracheostomy Care in Infants, *Proc R Soc Med,* **58**:900, 1965.

Adelman, S., and Benson, C. D.: Bochdalek Hernias in Infancy: Factors Determining Mortality, *J Pediatr Surg,* **11**:569, 1976.

Anderson, K. D., and Chandra, R.: Pneumothorax as a Complication of Endotracheal Suction, *J Pediatr Surg,* **11**:687, 1976.

Boix-Ochoa, J., Peguero, G., Seijo, G., et al.: Acid-Base Balance and Blood Gases in Prognosis and Therapy of Congential Diaphragmatic Hernia, *J Pediatr Surg,* **9**:49, 1974.

Boles, E. T., Schiller, M. and Weinberger, M.: Improved Management of Neonates with Congenital Diaphragmatic Hernia, *Arch Surg,* **103:**344, 1971.

Gans, S. L., and Berci, G.: Advances in Endoscopy of Infants and Children, *J Pediatr Surg,* **6:**199, 1971.

Haller, J. A., Jr., and Talbert, J. L.: Clinical Evaluation of a New Silastic Tracheostomy Tube for Respiratory Support of Infants and Children, *Ann Surg,* **171:**915, 1970.

Hendren, W. H., and McKee, D. M.: Lobar Emphysema of Infancy, *J Pediatr Surg,* **1:**24, 1966.

Louhimo, I., Grahne, B., Pasila, M., et al.: Acquired Laryngotracheal Stenosis in Children, *J Pediatr Surg,* **6:**730, 1971.

McNamara, J. J., Eraklis, A. J., and Gross, R. E.: Congenital Posterolateral Diaphragmatic Hernia of the Newborn, *J Thorac Cardiovasc Surg,* **55:**55, 1968.

Mattila, M. A. K., Suutarinen, T., and Sulamaa, M.: Prolonged Endotracheal Intubation or Tracheostomy in Infants and Children, *J Pediatr Surg,* **4:**674, 1969.

Rowe, M. I., and Uribe, F.: Diaphragmatic Hernia in the Newborn Infant: Blood Gas and pH Considerations, *Surgery,* **70:**758, 1971.

Steele, R. W., Metz, J. R., Bass, J. W., et al.: Pneumothorax and Pneumomediastinum in the Newborn, *Radiology,* **98:**629, 1971.

White, J. J., Andrews, H. G., Risemberg, H., et al.: Prolonged Respiratory Support in Newborn Infants with a Membrane Oxygenator, *Surgery,* **70:**288, 1971.

Malformation of Esophagus

Anderson, K. D., and Randolph, J. G.: The Gastric Tube for Esophageal Replacement in Children, *J Thorac Cardiovasc Surg,* **66:**333, 1973.

Howard, R., and Myers, N. A.: Esophageal Atresia: A Technique for Elongating the Upper Pouch, *Surgery,* **58:**725, 1965.

Mahour, G. H., Woolley, M. M., and Gwinn, J. L.: Elongation of the Upper Pouch and Delayed Anatomic Reconstruction in Esophageal Atresia, *J Pediatr Surg,* **9:**373, 1974.

Mellins, R. B., and Blumenthal, S.: Cardiovascular Anomalies and Esophageal Atresia, *Am J Dis Child,* **107:**160, 1964.

Randolph, J. G., Lilly, J. R., and Tunell, W. P.: Gastric Division in the Critically Ill Infant with Esophageal Atresia and Tracheoesophageal Fistula, *Surgery,* **63:**496, 1968.

Waterston, D. J., Bonham, A., Carter, R. E., and Aberdeen, E.: Oesophageal Atresia: Tracheoesophageal Fistula. A Study of Survival in 218 Infants, *Lancet,* **1:**819, 1962.

Corrosive Injury of Esophagus

Anderson, K. D., and Randolph, J. G.: The Gastric Tube for Esophageal Replacement in Children, *J Thorac Cardiovasc Surg,* **66:**33, 1973.

Burrington, J. D., and Stephens, C. A.: Esophageal Replacement with a Gastric Tube in Infants and Children, *J Pediatr Surg,* **3:**246, 1968.

Ein, S. H., Shandling, B., Simpson M., et al.: A Further Look at the Gastric Tube as an Esophageal Replacement in Infants and Children, *J Pediatr Surg,* **6:**859, 1973.

German, J. C., and Waterston, D. J.: Colon Interposition for the Replacement of the Esophagus in Children, *J Pediatr Surg,* **11:**227, 1976.

Haller, J. A., Andrews, H. G., White, J. J., et al.: Pathophysiology and Management of Acute Corrosive Burns of the Esophagus:

Results of Treatment in 285 Children, *J Pediatr Surg,* **6:**578, 1971.

Sherman, C. D., Jr., and Waterston, D.: Oesophageal Reconstruction in Children Using Intrathoracic Colon, *Arch Dis Child,* **32:**11, 1957.

Webb, W. R., Koutras, P., Ecker, R. R., et al.: An Evaluation of Steroids and Antibiotics in Caustic Burns of the Esophagus, *Ann Thorac Surg,* **9:**95, 1970.

Weisskopf, A.: Effects of Cortisone on Experimental Lye Burn of the Esophagus, *Ann Otol Rhinol Laryngol,* **61:**681, 1952.

Gastroesophageal Reflux

Berenberg, W., and Neuhauser, E. B. D.: Cardioesophageal Relaxation (Chalasia) as a Cause of Vomiting in Infants, *Pediatrics,* **5:**414, 1950.

Cahill, J. L., Aberdeen, E., and Waterston, D. J.: Results of Surgical Treatment of Esophageal Hiatal Hernia in Infancy and Childhood, *Surgery,* **66:**597, 1969.

Carcassonne, M., Bansoussan, A., and Aubert, J.: The Management of Gastroesophageal Reflux in Infants, *J Pediatr Surg,* **8:**575, 1973.

Follette, D., Fonkalsrud, E. W., Euler, A., and Ament, M.: Gastroesophageal Fundoplication for Reflux in Infants and Children, *J Pediatr Surg,* **11:**757, 1976.

Johnson, D. G., Herbst, J. J., Oliveros, M. A., and Stewart, D. R.: Evaluation of Gastroesophageal Reflux Surgery in Children, *Pediatrics,* **59:**62, 1977.

Randolph, J. G., Lilly, J. R., and Anderson, K. D.: Surgical Treatment of Gastroesophageal Reflux in Infants, *J Thorac Cardiovasc Surg,* **55:**42, 1968.

Gastrointestinal Conditions

Bell, M. J., Kosloske, A. M., Martin, L. W., et al.: Neonatal Necrotizing Enterocolitis: Prevention of Perforation, *J Pediatr Surg,* **8:**601, 1973.

——, Ternberg, J. L., Askin, F. B., McAlister, W., and Shackelford, G.: Intestinal Stricture in Necrotizing Enterocolitis, *J Pediatr Surg,* **11:**319, 1976.

Clatworthy, H. W., Jr., Saleebe, R., and Lovingood, C.: Extensive Small Bowel Resection in Young Dogs: Its Effect on Growth and Development, *Surgery,* **32:**341, 1952.

deLorimier, A. A., Fonkalsrud, E. W., and Hayes, D. M.: Congenital Atresia of the Jejunum and Ileum in the Newborn, *Ann Surg,* **142:**478, 1955.

Ein, S.: Leading Points in Childhood Intussusception, *J Pediatr Surg,* **11:**209, 1976.

Gross, R. E., and Chisolm, T. C.: Annular Pancreas Producing Duodenal Obstruction, *Am Surg,* **119:**759, 1944.

Jackson, J. M.: Annular Pancreas and Duodenal Obstruction in the Neonate, a Review, *Arch Surg,* **87:**379, 1963.

Krasna, I. H., Becker, J. M., Schneider, K. M., et al.: Colonic Stenosis Following Necrotizing Enterocolitis of the Newborn, *J Pediatr Surg,* **5:**200, 1970.

Leonidas, J. C., Berdon, W. E., Baker, D. H., et al.: Meconium Ileus and Its Complications: A Reappraisal of Plain Film Roentgen Diagnostic Criteria, *Am J Roentgenol Radium Ther Nucl Med,* **108:**598, 1970.

Louw, J. H.: Jejunoileal Atresia and Stenosis, *J Pediatr Surg,* **1:**8, 1966.

Marks, R. M., Sieber, W. K., and Girdany, B. R.: Hydrostatic

Pressure in the Treatment of the Ileocolic Intussusception in Infants and Children, *J Pediatr Surg,* **1:**566, 1966.

Martin, L. W., and Zerella, J. T.: Jejunoilial Atresia: A Proposed Classification, *J Pediatr Surg,* **11:**399, 1976.

Nixon, H. H., and Tawes, R.: Etiology and Treatment of Small Intestinal Atresia: Analysis of a Series of 127 Jejunoileal Atresias and Comparison with 62 Duodenal Atresias, *Surgery,* **69:**41, 1971.

Noblett, H. R.: Treatment of Uncomplicated Meconium Ileus by Gastrografin Enema: A Preliminary Report, *J Pediatr Surg,* **4:**190, 1969.

Ravitch, M. M.: Intussusception, in W. T. Mustard, M. M. Ravitch, and W. H. Snyder, Jr., (eds.), "Pediatric Surgery," 2d ed., vol. 2, p. 914, Year Book Medical Publishers, Inc., Chicago, 1969.

Rowe, M. I., Furst, A. J., Altman, D. H., et al.: The Neonatal Response to Gastrografin Enema, *Pediatrics,* **48:**29, 1971.

Santulli, T. V., and Blanc, W. A.: Congenital Atresia of the Intestine: Pathogenesis and Treatment, *Ann Surg,* **154:**939, 1961.

Touloukian, R. J., Berdon, W. E., Amoury, R. A., et al.: Surgical Experience with Necrotizing Enterocolitis in the Infant, *J Pediatr Surg,* **2:**389, 1967.

———, Posch, J. N., and Spencer, R.: The Pathogenesis of Ischemic Gastroenterocolitis of the Neonate: Selective Gut Mucosal Ischemia in Asphyxiated Neonatal Piglets, *J Pediatr Surg,* **7:**194, 1972.

Intussusception

Hay, G. R., Boles, E. T., Jr., and Dunbar, D.: Use of Glucagon in the Diagnosis and Management of Ileocolic Intussusception, *J Pediatr Surg,* 1977. (In press.)

Ravitch, M. M., and McCune, R. M., Jr.: Reduction of Intussusception by Hydrostatic Pressure: An Experimental Study, *Bull Johns Hopkins Hosp,* **82:**550, 1948.

Zachary, R. B.: Acute Intussusception in Childhood, *Arch Dis Childhood,* **30:**32, 1955.

Hirschsprung's Disease

Asch, M. J., Weitzman, J. J., Hays, D. M., et al.: Total Colon Aganglionosis, *Arch Surg,* **105:**74, 1972.

Boley, S. J., Lafer, D. J., Kleinhaus, S., et al.: Endorectal Pull-Through Procedure for Hirschsprung's Disease with and without Primary Anastomosis, *J Pediatr Surg,* **3:**258, 1968.

Campbell, P. E., and Noblett, H. R.: Experience with Rectal Suction Biopsy in the Diagnosis of Hirschsprung's Disease, *J Pediatr Surg,* **4:**410, 1969.

Coran, A. G., Bjordal, R., Eek, S., et al.: The Surgical Management of Total Colonic and Partial Small Intestinal Aganglionosis, *J Pediatr Surg,* **4:**531, 1969.

Duhamel, B.: Retrorectal and Transanal Pull-Through Procedure for the Treatment of Hirschsprung's Disease, *Dis Colon Rectum,* **7:**455, 1964.

James, A. E., Jr., Greenfield, J. B., Pfister, R. C., et al.: The Roentgenologic Appearance of Postoperative Congenital Megacolon (Hirschsprung's Disease), *Am J Roentgenol Radium Ther Nucl Med,* **109:**351, 1970.

Martin, L. W.: Surgical Management of Hirschsprung's Disease Involving the Small Intestine, *Arch Surg,* **97:**183, 1968.

———: Surgical Management of Total Colonic Aganglionosis, *Ann Surg,* **176:**343, 1972.

Prevot, J., Bodart, N., Babut, J. M., et al.: Hirschsprung's Disease with Total Colonic Involvement: Therapeutic Problems, *Prog Pediatr Surg,* **4:**63, 1972.

Soave, F.: Hirschsprung's Disease: Technique and Results of Soave's Operation, *Br J Surg,* **53:**1023, 1966.

Soper, R. T., and Miller, F. E.: Modification of Duhamel Procedure: Elimination of Rectal Pouch and Colorectal Septum, *J Pediatr Surg,* **3:**376, 1968.

Swenson, O., and Bill, A. H., Jr.: Resection of Rectum and Rectosigmoid with Preservation of the Sphincter for Benign Spastic Lesions Producing Megacolon: An Experimental Study, *Surgery,* **24:**212, 1948.

———, Sherman, J. O., and Fisher, J. H.: Diagnosis of Congenital Megacolon: An Analysis of 501 Patients, *J Pediatr Surg,* **8:**587, 1973.

———, ———, ———, and Cohen, E.: Treatment and Postoperative Complications of Congenital Megacolon: A 25 Year Follow-up, *Ann Surg,* **182:**266, 1975.

Imperforate Anus

Kiesewetter, W. B.: Imperforate Anus. II. The Rationale and Technique of the Sacroabdominoperineal Operation, *J Pediatr Surg,* **2:**106, 1967.

Potts, W. J., Riker, W. L., and DeBoer, A.: Imperforate Anus with Recto-Vesical-Urethral-Vaginal and Perineal Fistula, *Ann Surg,* **140:**381, 1954.

Rehbein, F.: Imperforate Anus: Experiences with Abdomino-Perineal and Abdomino-Sacral-Perineal Pull-Through Procedures, *J Pediatr Surg,* **2:**99, 1967.

Santulli, T. V., Kiesewetter, W. B., and Bill, A. H., Jr.: Anorectal Anomalies: A Suggested International Classification, *J Pediatr Surg,* **5:**281, 1970.

Stephens, F. D.: "Congenital Malformations of the Rectum, Anus and Genitourinary Tract," E. and S. Livingstone, Edinburgh, 1963.

Wangersteen, D. H., and Rice, C. O.: Imperforate Anus: A Method of Determining the Surgical Approach, *Ann Surg,* **92:**77, 1930.

Jaundice

Adievre, M., Martin, J. P., Hadchouel, M., et al.: Alpha$_1$—Antitrypsin Deficiency and Liver Disease in Children: Phenotypes, Manifestations, and Prognosis, *Pediatrics,* **57:**226, 1976.

Altman, R. P., and Chandra, R.: Biliary Hypoplasia Consequent to Alpha$_1$ Antitrypsin Deficiency, *Surg Forum,* **37:**377, 1976.

——— and Lilly, J. R.: Technical Details or Surgical Correction of Extrahepatic Biliary Atresia, *Surg Gynecol Obstet,* **140:**952, 1975.

———, ———, and Chandra, R.: Ongoing Cirrhosis after Successful Porticoenterostomy in Infants with Biliary Atresia, *J Pediatr Surg,* **10:**685, 1975.

Clatworthy, H. W., Wall, T., and Watman, R. N.: A New Type of Porto-to-Systemic Venous Shunt for Portal Hypertension, *Arch Surg,* **71:**588, 1955.

Fonkalsrud, E. W.: Choledochal Cysts *Surg Clin North Am,* **53:**1275, 1973.

Kasai, M., Kimura, S., Asakura, Y., et al.: Surgical Treatment of Biliary Atresia, *J Pediatr Surg,* **3:**665, 1968.

Landing, B. H.: "Considerations of the Pathogenesis of Neonatal Hepatitis, Biliary Atresia, and Choledochal Cyst—the Concept of Infantile Obstructive Cholangiography," University Park Press, Baltimore, 1972.

Lilly, J. R.: The Surgery of Biliary Hypoplasia, *J Pediatr Surg,* **11**:815, 1976.

Suruga, K., Nagashima, K., Hirai, Y., et al.: A Clinical and Pathological Study of Congenital Biliary Atresia, *J Pediatr Surg,* **2**:558, 1967.

Portal Hypertension

Altman, R. P.: Portal Decompression by Interposition Mesocaval Shunt in Patients with Biliary Atresia, *J Pediatr Surg,* **11**:809, 1976.

Clatworthy, H. W., Jr., Wall, T., and Watman, R. M.: A New Type of Portal-to-Systemic Venous Shunt for Portal Hypertension, *Arch Surg,* **71**:588, 1955.

Drapanas, T.: Interposition Mesocaval Shunt for Treatment of Portal Hypertension, *Ann Surg,* **176**:435, 1972.

Marion, P.: Mesoenteric-Caval Anastomosis, *J Cardiovasc Surg,* **70**(Suppl):70, 1966.

Martin, L. W.: Changing Concepts of Management of Portal Hypertension in Children, *J Pediatr Surg,* **7**:559, 1972.

Tyson, K. R. T., Schuster, S. R., and Schwachman, H.: Portal Hypertension in Cystic Fibrosis, *J Pediatr Surg,* **3**:271, 1968.

Spleen

Eraklis, A. J., Kevy, S. V., Diamond, L. K., et al.: Hazard of Overwhelming Infection after Splenectomy in Childhood, *N Engl J Med,* **276**:1225, 1967.

Kiesewetter, W. B.: Pediatric Splenectomy: Indications, Technique, Complications and Mortality, *Surg Clin North Am,* **55**:449, 1975.

King, H., and Schumacker, H. B., Jr.: Splenic Studies: Susceptibility to Infection after Splenectomy Performed in Infancy, *Ann Surg,* **136**:239, 1952.

O'Mara, R. E., Hall, R. C., and Dombroski, D. L.: Scintiscanning in the Diagnosis of Rupture of the Spleen, *Surg Gynecol Obstet,* **131**:1077, 1970.

Pancreas

Cooney, D. R., and Grosfeld, J. L.: Operative Management of Pancreatic Pseudocysts in Infants and Children: A Review of 75 Cases, *Ann Surg,* **182**:590, 1975.

Filler, R. M., AvRuskin, T. W., Crigler, J. F., and Haryen, A. H.: The Role of "Total" Pancreatectomy in the Treatment of Unremitting Hypoglycemia of Infancy, *J Pediatr Surg,* **6**:284, 1971.

Hamilton, J. P., Baker, L., Kaye, R., and Koop, C. E.: Subtotal Pancreatectomy in the Management of Severe Idiopathic Hypoglycemia in Children, *Pediatrics,* **39**:49, 1967.

Miller, R. E.: Pancreatic Pseudocysts in Infants and Children, *Arch Surg,* **89**:517, 1964.

Otherson, H. B., Moore, F. T., and Boles, E. P.: Traumatic Pancreatitis and Pseudocyst in Children, *J Trauma,* **8**:535, 1968.

Abdominal Wall Abnormalities

Allen, R. G. and Wrenn, E. L., Jr.: Silon as a Sac in the Treatment of Omphalocele and Gastroschisis, *J Pediatr Surg,* **4**:3, 1969.

Gilbert, M. G., Mencia, L. F., Brown, W. T., et al.: Staged Surgical Repair of Large Omphaloceles and Gastroschisis, *J Pediatr Surg,* **3**:702, 1968.

Gross, R. E.: A New Method for Surgical Treatment of Large Omphaloceles, *Surgery,* **24**:277, 1948.

Mahour, G. H., Weitzman, J. J., and Rosencrantz, J. G.: Omphalocele and Gastroschisis, *Ann Surg,* **177**:478, 1973.

Raffensberger, J. G., and Jona, J. Z.: Gastroschisis, *Ann Surg,* **177**:478, 1973.

Schuster, S. R.: A New Method for the Staged Repair of Large Omphaloceles, *Surg Gynecol Obstet,* **125**:837, 1967.

Exstrophy

Marshall, V. F., and Muecke, E. C.: Variations in Exstrophy of the Bladder, *J Urol,* **88**:766, 1962.

Rosencrantz, J. G., Bailey, W. C., and Dumars, K. W., Jr.: Incomplete Exstrophy of the Cloaca, *J Urol,* **91**:549, 1964.

Williams, D. I., and Savage, J.: Reconstruction of the Exstrophied Bladder, *Br J Surg,* **53**:168, 1966.

Inguinal Hernia

Clatworthy, H. W., Jr., Gilbert, M., and Clement, A.: The Inguinal Hernia, Hydrocele and Undescended Testicle Problem in Infants and Children, *Postgrad Med,* **22**:122, 1957.

Gilbert, M., and Clatworthy, H. W., Jr.: Bilateral Operations for Inguinal Hernia and Hydrocele in Infancy and Childhood, *Am J Surg,* **97**:255, 1959.

Undescended Testicle

Gilbert, J. B., and Hamilton, J. B.: Studies in Malignant Testes Tumors: Incidence and Nature of Tumors in Ectopic Testes, *Surg Gynecol Obstet,* **71**:731, 1940.

Gross, R. E., and Jewett, T. C., Jr.: Surgical Experiences from 1,222 Operations for Undescended Testes, *JAMA,* **160**:634, 1956.

Koop, C. E.: Observations on Undescended Testes: I. Significance of Empty Scrotum, Indication for Orchiopexy, *Arch Surg,* **75**:801, 1957.

MacCollum, D. W.: Clinical Study of the Spermatogenesis of Undescended Testicles, *Arch Surg,* **31**:290, 1935.

Intersexual Abnormalities

Gross, R. E., Randolph, J. G., and Crigler, J. F.: Clitorectomy for Sexual Abnormalities: Indications and Techniques, *Surgery,* **54**:300, 1966.

Hendren, W. H., and Crawford, J. D.: Adrenogenital Syndrome: The Anatomy of the Anomaly and Its Repair: Some New Concepts, *J Pediatr Surg,* **4**:49, 1969.

Jones, H. W., Jr.: Clinical Significance of Anomalies of the Sex Chromosomes, *Am J Obstet Gynecol,* **93**:335, 1965.

Money, J., Hampson, J. G., and Hampson, J. L.: Hermaphroditism: Recommendations Concerning Assignment of Sex, Change of Sex and Psychologic Management, *Bull Johns Hopkins Hosp,* **97**:284, 1955.

Randolph, J. G., and Hung, W.: Reduction Clitoroplasty in Females with Hypertrophied Clitoris, *J Pediatr Surg,* **5**:224, 1970.

Rickman, P. P.: Vesico-intestinal Fissure, *Arch Dis Childhood,* **35**:97, 1960.

Wilkins, L.: The Diagnosis of Adrenogenital Syndrome and Its Treatment with Cortisone, *J Pediatr,* **41:**1952.

———: "The Diagnosis and Treatment of Endocrine Disorders in Childhood and Adolescence," 3d ed., Charles C Thomas, Publisher, Springfield, Ill., 1966.

Malignant Disease in Children

Altman, R. P., Randolph, J. G., and Lilly, J. R.: Surgical Treatment of Sacrococcygeal Teratoma, *J Pediatr Surg,* **9:**389, 1974.

Beckwith, J. B., and Martin, R. F.: Observations of the Histopathology of Neuroblastomas, *J Pediatr Surg,* **3:**106, 1968.

Bill, A. H., and Morgan, A.: Evidence for Immune Reactions to Neuroblastoma and Future Possibilities for Investigation, *J Pediatr Surg,* **5:**111, 1970.

Conference on the Biology of Neuroblastoma, *J Pediatr Surg,* **3:**101, 1968.

D'Angio, G. J.: Management of Children with Wilms's Tumor, *Cancer,* **30:**1528, 1972.

———, Evans, A. E., and Koop, C. E.: Special Pattern of Widespread Neuroblastoma with a Favorable Prognosis, *Lancet,* **1:**1046, 1971.

Evans, A. E.: Treatment of Neuroblastoma, *Cancer,* **30:**1595, 1972.

———, Heyn, R. M., Newton, W. A., et al.: Vincristine Sulfate and Cyclophosphamide for Children with Metastatic Neuroblastoma, *JAMA,* **207:**1325, 1969.

Farber, S.: Chemotherapy in the Treatment of Leukemia and Wilms's Tumor, *JAMA,* **198:**826, 1966.

Grosfeld, J. L., Smith, J. P., and Clatworthy, H. W., Jr.: Pelvic Rhabdomyosarcoma in Infants and Children, *J Urol,* **107:**673, 1972.

Hellstrom, I., Hellstrom, K. D., Bill, A. H., et al.: Studies on Cellular Immunity to Human Neuroblastoma Cell, *Int J Cancer,* **6:**172, 1970.

Holder, T. M., Stuber, J. L., and Templeton, A. W.: Sonography as a Diagnostic Aid in the Evaluation of Abdominal Masses in Infants and Children, *J Pediatr Surg,* **7:**532, 1972.

Koop, C. E.: Neuroblastoma: Two Year Survival and Treatment Correlations, *J Pediatr Surg,* **3:**178, 1968.

Towne, B. H., Mahour, G. A., Woolley, M. M., et al.: Ovarian Cyst and Tumors in Infancy and Childhood, *J Pediatr Surg,* **10:**311, 1975.

Trauma

Haller, A. J., Signer, R. D., Golladay, E. S., Shaker, I. J., and White, J. J.: Use of a Trauma Registry in the Management of Children with Life-Threatening Injuries, *J Pediatr Surg,* **11:**381, 1976.

Chapter 40

Urology

by Irwin N. Frank and Donald F. McDonald

ANATOMY

Knowledge of the anatomy of the genitourinary system and its anatomic relationships is a prerequisite to the accurate diagnosis and correct therapy of diseases involving these structures. Slight deviation of the axis of the kidney or the course of the ureter from normal may indicate a pathologic condition in adjacent organs. Disease within the genitourinary system may manifest itself in the form of gastrointestinal symptoms. Examples of this are the nausea and vomiting which so often occur with renal colic and ureteropelvic junction obstruction. Pathologic enlargement of structures situated in the pelvis commonly produces obstruction of the lower ureter and often leaves characteristic impressions on the bladder contour seen on a cystogram.

KIDNEY. The kidneys are paired retroperitoneal organs which weigh approximately 160 Gm each in the healthy adult. They are situated within the fascia of Gerota, and a variable amount of perinephric fat is present between the capsule of the kidney and this fascial envelope. Further protection of the kidneys is provided dorsally by their relationship to the lower ribs, the quadratus lumborum, and the psoas muscles. The ventral relationships of the kidney are illustrated in Fig. 40-1. They lie beneath the diaphragm, with the left kidney usually 1 to 2 cm. lower than the right kidney.

The renal arteries originate from the aorta at the upper level of the second lumbar vertebra, and the right artery is considerably longer than the left, since it crosses the midline behind the vena cava. About two-thirds of kidneys have a single renal artery, while multiple renal arteries are more prevalent in congenitally malformed or malpositioned kidneys. The main renal artery divides into five major branches, each of which represents an end artery. Partial occlusion of any branch produces ischemia, and complete occlusion produces infarction of the involved segment. However, the ureteral and capsular vessels can provide significant blood flow in the presence of marked renal artery occlusion. The renal veins are often multiple

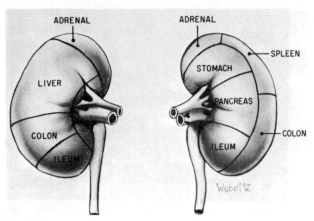

Fig. 40-1. Ventral relationships of the kidneys to adjacent organs.

and freely intercommunicate. The left renal vein crosses the midline ventral to the aorta after it has received blood from the left adrenal and gonadal veins. The renal lymphatics empty through a half-dozen hilar trunks in the region of the renal artery and vein. Capsular lymphatics travel through the perinephric fat to infradiaphragmatic periaortic nodes. The renal nerves, which receive contributions from T_4 to T_{12}, from the vagus nerve via the celiac axis, and from the splanchnics, contain vasomotor and pain fibers. Following total renal denervation, such as occurs with transplantation, no persistent abnormalities in renal function occur. The renal pelvis, which usually contains 5 ml of urine, lies dorsal to the renal vessels and has a transitional cell epithelium. The kidney's position with respect to the vertebral bodies and the axis of a line drawn through the upper and lower calyces offers a clue to focal diseases of the kidney and adjacent organs. The axis of the kidney often parallels that of the psoas muscle edge as noted on x-rays of the abdomen.

URETER. The ureters are muscular tubes which connect the renal pelvis to the bladder, traversing the retroperitoneal space in a linear course just lateral to the transverse processes of the lumbar vertebrae and crossing the common iliac arteries at their bifurcation. The lower ureter

Fig. 40-2. Posterior relationships of prostate, seminal vesicles, ureter, and bladder.

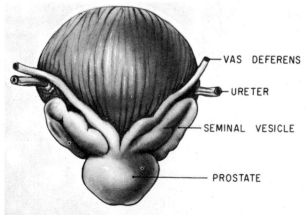

follows the contour of the pelvis and deviates laterally and then medially in a gentle curve to reach the trigone of the bladder above a line drawn between the spinous processes. The ureter is 28 to 30 cm long and about 5 mm in diameter. Its oblique course through the wall of the bladder measures 2 cm. The ureteral orifice is an oblique slit in the trigone. The function of the ureter is to transmit the urine from the renal pelvis to the bladder. Ordinarily urine is not modified in the ureter. However, during severe oliguria and dehydration the transitional epithelium acts as a semipermeable membrane which permits water and electrolyte changes in response to gradients. Normally, there are about four peristaltic waves per minute developing pressures of about 30 mm Hg. The ureteral blood supply originates from the renal, vesical, and lumbar arteries. Free intercommunication between these vessels permits extensive ureteral mobilization and transposition. Pain fibers refer stimuli to the T_{12} through L_2 segments, while the autonomic innervation is associated with intrinsic parasympathetic motor and sympathetic vasomotor ganglia. The lymphatic drainage is to segmental periaortic and caval nodes. The ureter may be drawn medially in retroperitoneal fibrosis and laterally as a result of enlargement of periaortic node involvement with tumor or an aortic aneurysm. It is essential to be aware of the course of the ureter during pelvic surgery and in difficult dissections of adjacent organs.

BLADDER. The urinary bladder is a muscular pelvic organ lined with transitional cell epithelium. It is related to the peritoneum superiorly, the sigmoid colon and rectum posteriorly in the male, and the uterus, cervix, and vagina in the female. In the male, the bladder is spherical, while in the female the uterus indents the dome. The smooth muscle (detrusor) is capable of stretching to a marked degree. The major blood supply originates from the superior, middle, and inferior branches of the hypogastric arteries. The lymphatics drain to the perivesical, hypogastric, and periaortic nodes. The autonomic nerve supply to the bladder is derived from the sacral cord and from the presacral and epigastric plexuses of nerves.

PROSTATE AND SEMINAL VESICLES. The chestnut-shaped prostate, which weighs approximately 25 Gm, surrounds the proximal male urethra. It is firmly attached to the bladder neck and symphysis pubis. Posteriorly, the fascia of Denonvilliers intervenes between the rectal ampulla and prostate (Fig. 40-2). Caudad, the prostate rests on the pelvic diaphragm, which contains the voluntary external sphincter. The blood supply derives from the inferior vesical and middle hemorrhoidal arteries, while the venous drainage communicates with an extensive pelvic plexus which empties into the hypogastric veins. This plexus also communicates with Batson's veins, thus explaining the common metastatic spread of prostatic carcinoma to the sacrum, ileum, and lumbar spine. The prostate receives secretory and motor (parasympathetic) innervation from S_3 and S_4 and vasomotor (sympathetic) fibers from the hypogastric plexus. The lymphatics drain into the external, internal, and common iliac nodes and then to the periaortic nodes. The seminal vesicles lie behind the bladder, lateral to the ampullae of the vasa deferentia. They are closely related to the ureters. Their secretions are rich in fructose, which may be of importance to survival of the spermatozoa.

PENIS AND URETHRA. The penis is composed of two lateral erectile bodies (corpora cavernosa) and a single ventral spongy erectile body (corpus spongiosum urethrae) through which the urethra passes. The latter terminates in the glans penis, which is also composed of erectile tissue. As the urethra emerges from the pelvic diaphragm, it enlarges to become the bulbous urethra which is invested by the bulbocavernosis muscle. The urethra continues as the pendulous urethra, which terminates in the fossa navicularis within the glans penis. The female urethra corresponds to the prostatic and membranous urethra in the male. It averages 4 cm in length and 32 mm in circumference. The principal blood supply to the penis and urethra originates from the internal pudendal arteries. Somatic sensory innervation of the penis is from S_3 and S_4 via the ilioinguinal and genitofemoral nerves. Sympathetic vasomotor innervation derives from the hypogastric plexus, while the parasympathetic innervation originates from S_2, S_3, and S_4 via the nervi erigentes. The lymphatic drainage is to the superficial and deep inguinal nodes and then to the external iliac and hypogastric nodes.

TESTIS AND EPIDIDYMIS. The testis is an ovoid firm scrotal organ which measures $4 \times 2.5 \times 2.5$ cm. The left testis commonly resides in the scrotum 2 to 4 cm lower than the right. The testis, which weighs approximately 20 Gm, is covered by a tough membrane, the tunica albuginea, except at its dorsal aspect where the epididymis and vascular pedicle are attached. The epididymis is a crescent-shaped body which curves around the dorsal portion of the testis. The vas deferens is a 4-mm thick-walled firm tubular structure which originates at the inferior pole of the epididymis and follows a cranial course with the spermatic vessels. The arterial blood supply to the testis and epididymis originates from the aorta just below the renal arteries. The left spermatic vein empties into the left renal vein, while the right spermatic vein empties directly into the inferior vena cava. The primary lymphatic drainage from the testis is to the periaortic nodes in the vicinity of the kidney. Crossover from these nodes to the opposite side is frequently observed.

DIAGNOSIS

SEQUENCE IN UROLOGIC DIAGNOSIS. Precision of diagnosis is a characteristic feature of the practice of urology. In order to maintain the achievable degree of accuracy, it is essential that a clinical problem be approached in a logical sequence. When so conducted, the diagnosis should be 95 percent accurate.

History

A variety of symptoms and signs are characteristic and often diagnostic of pathologic conditions involving the genitourinary system. The patient may spontaneously offer these clues, but in most instances it is necessary to ask them the proper questions to obtain this information. A brief

discussion of some of the more significant signs and symptoms follows, and suggestions for evaluating them are discussed.

GROSS HEMATURIA. The presence of gross blood in the urine is a significant sign which is quite alarming to the patient and warrants further evaluation. Even small amounts of blood in the urine occurring on one occasion may be the only indication of a malignant process in the urinary tract. Intermittent bleeding is common, and large tumors may manifest themselves with only a small amount of bleeding while small tumors may produce considerable loss of blood. The bleeding originates from lesions which cause erosion or disruption of blood vessels or from inflammatory changes which in turn lead to erosions and diapedesis of red cells.

In a series of 1,000 cases in all age groups, almost three-quarters of the patients were over forty, and two-thirds were male (Fig. 40-3). Gross hematuria was the sole complaint in only 18.8 percent, while associated symptoms in order of frequency were those due to bladder infections, 37 percent; renal colic, 27.3 percent; obstructive symptoms, 15.6 percent; urethral discharge, 5 percent; and urethral pain, 3 percent. The origin of bleeding and etiologic factors in this series are also represented in Fig. 40-3. Other factors implicated to a lesser extent include congenital abnormalities, medical causes, and idiopathic hematuria. Hemophilia, thrombocytopenic purpura, uremia, and drug-induced hypothrombinemia represented rare causes.

Infections, predominantly acute cystitis and urethritis,

Fig. 40-3. Gross hematuria: sex incidence, site of origin, and etiology.

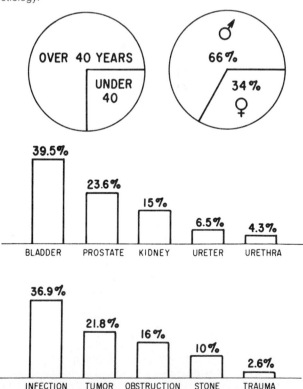

caused bleeding in 70 percent of male patients between the ages of eighteen and forty-one referred for a urologic consultation. Although 50 percent of the patients were referred with a diagnosis of glomerulonephritis none of them had it. Calculi were responsible for 4.9 percent; trauma, 6.1 percent; bladder tumors, 3.7 percent; medical, renal, and polycystic disease, 3 percent; and undiagnosed causes, 5.5 percent. In young individuals, gross hematuria is more likely to be the result of infection, while in older patients it is more likely to be related to tumors and prostatic disease. Three-quarters of patients with otherwise *asymptomatic* gross hematuria have bladder tumors.

It is important to determine whether hematuria appears at the beginning or end of voiding. Initial hematuria suggests lesions distal to the bladder neck, namely, the prostatic and membranous urethra. Predominantly terminal hematuria usually indicates involvement of the bladder neck and trigone. Uniform hematuria occurs with lesions of the ureter or kidney. The passage of blood clots suggests that the bleeding is quantitatively great, since urine inhibits coagulation of blood by the presence of citrate. Long, wormlike clots are apt to have been formed in the ureter. Reddish clots occur with recent bleeding, while brownish or grayish white clots indicate a time lapse between the bleeding episode and their passage.

ACUTE POSTRENAL RETENTION OF URINE. This term applies to an inability to empty a full bladder and is one of the most distressing symptoms. It should not be referred to as "anuria," since the latter indicates that urine is not being formed. The patient usually complains of lower abdominal distress, and the bladder is palpable as a tender suprapubic mass. A variety of afflictions may cause this condition.

Benign prostatic hypertrophy is the most common cause of acute retention in men. The vast majority have a long-standing history of increasing difficulty in voiding with gradually increasing nocturia. In contrast, *carcinoma of the prostate* is accompanied by a much shorter duration of symptoms. The history may be of months rather than years, and the urinary difficulties increase more rapidly. The patient with carcinoma of the prostate seldom presents with urinary retention when the lesion is early and amenable to surgical treatment. The presence of retention therefore suggests advanced disease, and symptoms of malignancy such as malaise, weight loss, anorexia, and sciatica are likely to be encountered. In young males, a *prostatic inflammation* is the most common cause of acute retention. This results from acute urethritis and prostatitis which have not been promptly or effectively treated. There is usually an antecedent history of frequent urination and dysuria progressing to acute retention. Fever, chills, and symptoms of systemic infection are common, and abscess formation occasionally occurs. Acute urinary retention may be the first manifestation of *urethral stricture* or may represent a recurrent problem related to the patient's unwillingness to undergo sufficiently frequent dilations. These patients usually give an antecedent history of gonorrhea, transurethral instrumentation, trauma, or radiation therapy. Many will have noted a gradual decrease in the force of the stream.

Neurogenic bladder dysfunction may lead to progressive increase in residual urine and eventual retention. This may be the first indication of spinal cord disease. In other patients, the retention may be preceded by difficulty in initiating voiding and overflow incontinence related to changes in abdominal pressure exerting force on a markedly distended bladder. Acute retention on a neurogenic basis may follow the administration of general anesthetics, spinal anesthesia, or the administration of certain drugs which influence the innervation of the bladder, bladder neck, proximal urethra, or external sphincter. Acute urinary retention in women is unusual and may be caused by neurogenic and psychogenic factors or urethral obstructions secondary to carcinoma, stricture, vaginal lesions, or cervical fibroids. A cystocele is seldom associated with acute retention.

INCONTINENCE. This is the situation in which a patient is unaware of the loss of urine until there is a sensation of wetness of the lower garments. The term is not a synonym for unintentional nocturnal bed wetting (enuresis) or urgency, where the patient knows he is going to wet himself but is unable to reach a suitable place to empty his bladder before the bladder empties itself. Patients with true incontinence have no residual urine. *True, or stress, incontinence* is the result of ineffective sphincter muscles which have been weakened by childbirth, stretched by an enlarged prostate, or traumatized by surgical procedures. A vesicovaginal or vesicoperineal fistula may also produce incontinence. Occasionally an ectopic ureter will open into the vagina, and this also will produce a constant leakage of urine. *Overflow, or paradoxical, incontinence* represents a second type, in which the bladder retains a large amount of residual urine. With each movement or breath the increased abdominal pressure causes overflow of a small amount of urine from a distended bladder. This condition may accompany neurogenic diseases of the spinal cord, or it may be the result of long-standing obstructive uropathy with detrusor decompensation. These patients may never really void, intermittently passing small quantities of urine without control. Incontinence of urine is a common manifestation of various neurologic diseases and spinal cord trauma.

URETERAL COLIC. This is related to a sudden increase in luminal pressure. Typically, there is sudden unilateral severe crescendo pain in the posterior subcostal region (lumbar triangle). The localization is frequently so precise that it can be defined by fingertip palpation. Obstruction at the ureteropelvic junction is associated with pain at the costovertebral angle, while obstruction lower in the ureter may have the added component of pain in the ipsilateral lower abdomen. With obstruction of the intramural ureter, pain, in addition to the above-mentioned sites, may be referred to the corresponding side of the scrotum or labia majora. Ureteral colic related to intramural obstruction is often associated with a sudden onset of urgency and frequency. Subsidence of these symptoms suggests that the stone has passed into the bladder and may be voided shortly. Narcotic addicts often simulate renal colic to procure drugs. Their deception may include fixing a radiopaque body to the skin in an appropriate area or placing blood from a finger prick in the urine sample.

FREQUENCY. This refers to the patient's voiding an excessive number of times. However, frequency of urination should not be confused with polyuria where the patient excretes large volumes of urine at more frequent intervals than normal. The correct term for frequency of urination with small volumes is pollakiuria. Most normal well-hydrated individuals void three to four times daily and do not arise from sleep to empty the bladder. Frequency may be related to reduction in bladder capacity associated with inflammation of the urinary passages or effective reduction in bladder capacity by increased residual urine, such as occurs with obstructive prostatic hypertrophy. Frequency is also a symptom of psychologic stress.

When patients complain of frequency, it is essential to question them carefully regarding fluid and caffeine intake. It is sometimes of value to have the patient record accurately the time and volume of the amounts of fluid ingested as well as the amount excreted in a 24-hour period. It is also essential to note the medications the patient is taking, since this may influence urinary frequency considerably. Further information regarding the relationship of urinary frequency to work, stress, weekend activity, and vacations is extremely helpful. Many patients have sought help from other physicians for this disturbing symptom, which may limit their activities because of the need to be close to a bathroom at all times. A careful history may lead to the information which will allow simple modification of habits, intake, and drug therapy to bring relief of this distressing and sometimes incapacitating problem.

NOCTURIA. Never normal, this condition may, however, be caused by consumption of an excessive amount of fluids prior to retiring, or it may be an expression of generalized restlessness. With cardiac decompensation, fluids which have accumulated in dependent portions of the body during the day are restored to the circulating blood when the patient maintains a horizontal position, thus causing nocturia. Patients with chronic renal disease who excrete large volumes because of an inability to concentrate the urine and patients on diuretics frequently experience nocturia. Prostatic hypertrophy and acute or chronic infection of the urinary tract cause nocturia by means of the same mechanisms described for frequency.

URGENCY. This is a symptom of vesical outlet inflammation and is most commonly due to prostatitis, urethritis, or cystitis. However, it may be a normal consequence of postponement of voiding for prolonged periods of time. The symptom may be so severe that the patient cannot restrain voiding.

DYSURIA. Difficult or painful urination is known as "dysuria." The sensation is commonly described as burning and may be referred to the glans penis or perineum. The symptom may be caused by urinary infection and the passage of clots, calculi, or crystals. However, it may also result from passage of highly concentrated urine. Pain at the termination of, or subsequent to, voiding is referred to as a "strangury" and may be associated with presence of a bladder calculus. Difficulty of urination is usually the result of an obstructive uropathy. "Hesitancy," indicating delayed voiding in response to mental command, is another symptom of chronic obstructive uropathy.

URINARY STREAM. The stream may lack force and have reduced projection in patients with obstructive uropathy. Stenosis of the meatus, which determines the caliber of the urinary stream, may be evidenced by a thin or duplicated stream.

IMPOTENCE AND EJACULATORY DYSFUNCTION. History taking in this area may prove to be quite difficult for the physician who has had little training in dealing with these problems. A careful history regarding medications is essential, since certain drugs will produce impotence and ejaculatory disturbances. However, in most situations, the underlying factor is situational or psychogenic, and this may become apparent during careful history taking. It is important to realize that in many instances patients wish to discuss their problems with a physician or have unsuccessfully attempted to do so before their present evaluation. In some instances, a physical or anatomic abnormality may be found to account for impotence.

Physical Examination

RENAL AREAS. The kidney regions may first be examined with the patient in the upright position. Observation may reveal obvious bulging or asymmetry of the costovertebral region. Scoliosis may be present from guarding in the presence of unilateral pain. Herpetic lesions occasionally may be encountered on the skin surface of this area and may be a clue to the etiology of pain in this area. Gentle palpation of the costovertebral angle areas may be followed by sharp percussion, disclosing an underlying obstructed or infected kidney. If the patient complains of pain in the flank region prior to examination, it is wise to start the evaluation on the contralateral side. Further examination of the kidney areas should be carried out with the patient supine, knees flexed, and arms at the side.

The examiner should stand on the side being examined. The posterior hand is placed parallel to the twelfth rib and below it. The anterior hand is placed 4 cm below the anterior rib cage and parallel to the posterior hand. Renal and retroperitoneal masses can be ballotted between the two hands. In slender individuals, the lower pole of the right kidney is often palpable. In others, the kidney may be palpable with deep inspiration. With unusually mobile kidneys (nephroptosis) the entire organ may be palpated. A solitary cyst may be distinguishable, while an irregular mass suggests a polycystic organ. Tenderness is usually related to obstruction or inflammation and is uncommon with uncomplicated tumors or cysts. The examiner again looks for evidence of asymmetry, rigidity of the costovertebral angle, tenderness, or bulging, which may suggest the presence of an underlying abscess, obstructed kidney, inflammation, or retroperitoneal extravasation of urine or blood.

URETERS. The deep retroperitoneal location of the ureters does not lend itself to palpation. It is unusual to be able to feel them when they are grossly dilated or to be able to localize a pathologic area within them.

BLADDER. The patient is examined in the supine position. The empty bladder is neither percussible nor palpable. In the markedly distended condition occurring with chronic obstruction, the bladder may be visible as a large abdominal mass rising out of the pelvis. However, under ordinary circumstances, the bladder is not percussible until it contains approximately 150 ml of urine. Persistence of a low abdominal mass following emptying of the bladder by catheterization documents the extravesical nature of the lesion.

PENIS. The penis may be examined with the patient in the upright position facing the examiner, who is sitting in a chair, or with the patient in a supine position on the examining table. If the patient is not circumcised, the foreskin should be retracted so that the underlying glans, urethral meatus, and inner aspect of the foreskin can be visualized. It is at this point in the examination that the patient may volunteer information regarding underlying fears, fantasies, or facts related to sexual dysfunction, erection, or impotence. If the patient does not do so, the examiner may utilize this opportunity to ask questions related to these topics. Further evaluation of the meatal caliber may be carried out with appropriate instrumentation, if indicated. A valid and recommended means of evaluating the presence of a meatal obstruction is observation of the patient voiding.

SCROTUM. Examination of the scrotum is carried out in conjunction with examination of the penis and with the patient in the positions noted above. Some patients are extremely sensitive to examination of this area, and the

Fig. 40-4. Differential diagnosis of scrotal lesions. *A.* Normal. *B.* Hydrocele. *C.* Spermatocele. *D.* Epididymitis. *E.* Tuberculous epididymitis and vasitis. *F.* Testis tumor. *G.* Hernia.

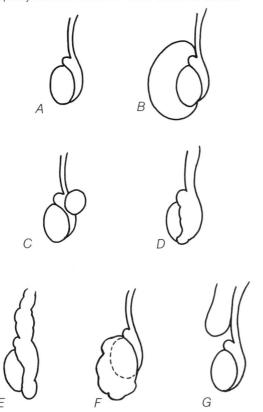

examiner may elicit a vasovagal response from the patient who is in the standing position. The examiner should be aware of this, since he may not appreciate that it is occurring while he is focusing his attention on the genital area. A knowledge of the normal scrotal contents and relationships is essential to the differential diagnosis of a variety of pathologic entities which occur in this area. Careful observation and palpation of this region and the use of a small flashlight to transilluminate lesions offer the only means of making an accurate diagnosis.

Scrotal Masses (Fig. 40-4)

As noted elsewhere in this text, an indirect *inguinal hernia* may present as a scrotal mass. The enlargement extends up into the inguinal region and may often be reduced with the patient in the supine position.

Epididymitis. Acute nonspecific pyogenic epididymitis is commonly a result of retrograde extension via the vas deferens from a focus of infection in the prostate or bladder. It may follow prostatic massage or instrumentation. The patient is frequently febrile and has a typical straddling gait to minimize contact with the inflamed scrotal contents. The scrotum is exquisitely tender and may contain a mass. The overlying skin is red and edematous. Nonspecific chronic epididymitis, which is a result of incompletely resolved acute epididymitis, presents with an indurated tender mass. Tuberculous epididymitis is characteristically nontender, stony hard, and may be associated with irregular indurated beadings of the vas deferens. It is the most common cause of scrotal fistulae. A sterile or chemical epididymitis may occur with the retrograde extravasation of fluid into the epididymis secondary to marked increase in intraabdominal pressure associated with heavy lifting while the bladder is distended. The urine is usually sterile in this situation, in contrast to the pyuria which is often present with epididymitis due to infection.

Varicocele. There is a predilection for the left side, because the left pampiniform plexus and spermatic vein drain into the left renal vein, which is usually 10 cm higher than the point at which the right spermatic vein enters the inferior vena cava. It is characteristically a lesion of puberty and becomes less obvious with age, usually disappearing after thirty-five. Acute onset of a left varicocele after the age of forty suggests left renal vein occlusion, commonly related to renal tumor. A varicocele on the right side may be secondary to vena caval obstruction or occlusion. This occasionally occurs with tumor thrombus from a hypernephroma invading and involving the lumen of the vena cava. The usual type of left varicocele is observed best with the patient in the standing position facing the examiner. The characteristic "bag of worms" appearance and feeling of the scrotum is noted. With the patient in the supine position, the varicocele collapses and usually cannot be palpated. Failure of drainage in the supine position is suggestive of left renal vein occlusion as noted above. The presence of a varicocele in a patient who is being examined for infertility may be a significant finding. This is especially true if the patient has a low sperm count with reduced motility of the sperm.

Hydrocele. Primary idiopathic hydrocele may be unilateral or bilateral and represents an increased collection of fluid between the tunica vaginalis and its contents. It is manifested as a large nontender mass which is translucent and obscures palpation of the testis and epididymis. It is ventral, superior, and inferior to the testis and frequently reaches the size of 25 cm in greatest dimension. Secondary hydroceles are the consequence of serous effusion in the vicinity of a disease process. Epididymitis, tuberculosis, trauma, and mumps are among the common causes. Twenty percent of acute hydroceles are secondary to testicular tumors. Aspiration of the hydrocele on the anterior ventral surface of the mass permits more precise palpation and differentiation from testicular tumors. A *communicating hydrocele* is a result of ascites in a patient with a patent processus vaginalis. In this situation, the scrotal mass fills and empties with varying positions.

Spermatocele. This is a cyst of an efferent ductule of the rete testis. It originates at the head of the epididymis and presents as a transilluminable cystic mass discrete from the testis. Spermatoceles are often bilateral and may be multiple. They are of no consequence except when they reach large proportions.

Testicular Tumor. A palpable nodule on or within the testis represents a potential malignant tumor until proved otherwise. The lesion is usually firm and nontender and is not transilluminable. It is often first noted by the patient or on a routine examination of this area. Prompt surgical exploration through an inguinal incision is indicated. One cannot stress enough the importance of being able to detect small lesions of the testis by careful palpation and the significance and urgency of proper management. The scrotal mass is usually hard, nontender, and irregular, and is not translucent. There is rarely associated pain, but the presentation of such a mass is regarded as surgical emergency requiring prompt inguinal exploration.

Mumps Orchitis. The lesion usually occurs in postpubertal males with acute parotitis. It commonly becomes apparent as the parotitis subsides, 7 to 10 days following the onset of the illness. Patients experience high fever, malaise, and marked testicular swelling which, unlike acute pyogenic epididymitis, is unaccompanied by scrotal edema.

Torsion of the Testis or Appendages. Torsion of the testis generally refers to torsion of the spermatic cord with a characteristic 540° rotation of the testis and an anterior presentation of the epididymis. The patient presents with sudden onset of pain accompanied by scrotal enlargement and edema. The testis, which appears to be elevated because the cord is shortened by twisting, is exquisitely tender. The differential diagnosis between acute epididymitis and torsion of the testis may be difficult. Since prompt treatment of the latter is important to save the testis from infarction, it may be necessary occasionally to explore patients with acute epididymitis to prevent loss of testis in patients with torsion. Four hours of torsion appears to be the limit after which the testis is irreversibly damaged. Because of the high incidence of bilateral anatomic predisposition to torsion, bilateral orchiopexy should be performed when surgical treatment for unilateral torsion is undertaken.

Torsion of the testis, per se, can occur only when there is a long mesorchium connecting it to the epididymis. In such a case, the testis, which is likened to a clapper in a bell, can twist inside the tunica vaginalis and undergo infarction. In this circumstance, the epididymis lies in its normal position, and the testis, which is enlarged, tender, and hard, is not drawn up high in the scrotum. A third condition of torsion involves the appendix testis. This normally present embryologic remnant lies at the upper pole of the testis. When it undergoes torsion, the patient presents with a painful lump on the surface of the testis. Transillumination before major swelling occurs may reveal a characteristic "black dot" sign, which is visualization of the infarcted appendage. Since testicular tumors are rarely tender, they are not likely to be confused with torsion of the appendix testis.

PROSTATE. The gland can best be evaluated after the patient has emptied his bladder, and it is preferable for the patient to be bending forward over the examining table or bed during the examination. If the patient is unable to stand, he should be examined while lying on his side with knees flexed and facing the standing examiner. If the examiner is right-handed, the patient should lie on his right side. Rectal examination should be carried out carefully, with very little pressure exerted while passing the finger through the anus and while the examining finger is on the prostate gland. It is seldom necessary to press hard on the prostate. Furthermore, exertion of pressure in this area may produce considerable discomfort and limit the examination. The normal prostate is two fingerbreadths wide with a 0.5 cm-deep sulcus between the two lobes. It is about 2.5 cm from apex to base. However, rectal examination is inadequate to define the precise size and must be combined with cystoscopy.

The consistency of both the normal prostate and the prostate with benign hypertrophy is similar to that of the thenar eminence. In contrast, carcinoma of the prostate feels stony hard, similar to the interphalangeal joint. Crepitations are related to multiple prostatic calculi. With benign hyperplasia, the gland can be delineated from surrounding tissues, and the contours are smooth. With carcinoma of the prostate, the surrounding tissues are frequently fixed to the gland, thus eliminating the usual discreteness of prostatic contour. Extension of the tumor may proceed into the seminal vesicle area superior and lateral to the prostate. Since 90 percent of carcinomas arise in the posterior portion of the gland, they are readily detectable on rectal examination as a single lump or a nodular mass. Acute suppuration of the prostate is accompanied by tenderness or fluctuation and dictates an atraumatic examination to avoid dissemination of the infection.

FEMALE URETHRA. Pelvic examination of the female patient in the lithotomy position is essential for evaluation of the lower urinary tract. Careful visualization and calibration of the urethral meatus can be carried out in this position. The presence of a cystocele or urethrocele can be determined with the patient bearing down. A urethral diverticulum may be detected by gentle pressure against the anterior vaginal wall, milking the urethra from the bladder to the meatus. Pressure in this region against the symphysis may result in release of purulent material or urine from a diverticulum of the urethra.

Urinalysis

A fresh two-glass specimen from the male or a catheterized specimen from the female provides optimal results. However, a carefully obtained, clean-voided midstream specimen from the female is useful. A midstream specimen from the circumcised male is usually satisfactory for culture and microscopic examination without any prior cleansing of the penis. The specimen should be examined while fresh, since refrigeration leads to sedimentation of phosphates and storage in a warm environment results in deterioration of formed elements and growth of bacteria.

A clear urine is usually normal. A cloudy urine may be normal if a few drops of dilute acetic acid render it clear, as in phosphaturia. The color may indicate disease, ingestion of certain foods, or administration of medications. Pyridium results in an orange-red color. Methylene blue incorporated in urinary medications leads to varying shades of green and blue. Pink urine may be due to food dyes or to medications like Serenium. Various degrees of bluish gray and brown may be associated with acute porphyria. The degree and timing of bleeding can often be best estimated by examination of the gross urine specimen.

The odor is often characteristic. A mousy odor which accompanies *Escherichia coli* infection is related to formation of ammonia. A pungent odor is characteristic of either necrotic bladder tumors or calculous pyonephrosis. Certain medications, such as ampicillin, have a characteristic and readily identifiable odor in the urine.

Chemical examination routinely includes tests for the presence of albumin, reducing sugars, acetone, and pH. Since there are no proteins in the secretions of the male

Fig. 40-5. Commonly used urologic instruments.

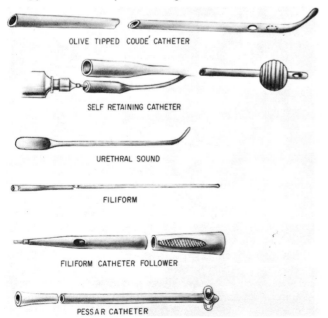

OLIVE TIPPED COUDE' CATHETER

SELF RETAINING CATHETER

URETHRAL SOUND

FILIFORM

FILIFORM CATHETER FOLLOWER

PESSAR CATHETER

genital organs, albuminuria cannot be ascribed to them. The various paper-dip tests are usually quite reliable but do have some limitation in the detection of hematuria.

Casts, crystals, and clumps of epithelial cells are identified under low-power *microscopic examination,* while the nature of cells, crystals, and bacteria are determined under higher powers. When the urine sediment is heavy, both the centrifuged and uncentrifuged specimens should be examined. Staining with methylene blue facilitates the diagnosis of bacteriuria. Exfoliative cytologic examination of urine may be helpful, but there is often a greater yield from study of the wet preparation, which may demonstrate clusters of cells with nucleocytoplasmic disparity characteristic of malignancy. The identification of bacteria in an unspun urine specimen is strongly suggestive of the presence of a urinary tract infection rather than contamination.

Genital Secretions

URETHRAL DISCHARGE. Collection is accomplished on a glass slide before the patient urinates. A heat-fixed and Gram-stained specimen identifies responsible organisms. Gonococcal urethritis is diagnosed by the presence of gram-negative diplococci within epithelial cells and leukocytes. In mimae infection, the cocci are quite similar. They are frequently polychromatic and are predominantly extracellular. Examination of the wet specimen is helpful in identifying the presence of trichomonads. Confirmation of the presence of infection is established by adequate culture of the urethral discharge.

PROSTATIC SECRETION. The specimen is obtained by gentle massage of the gland. Examination of the normally opalescent fluid reveals three to five white cells per high-power field and tiny refractile cephalin bodies. Epithelial cells are present in small numbers. Seminal vesicle secretion presents as a gelatinous and fibrinous tree-shaped cast of the seminal vesicle containing strands and granules. In the presence of prostatic infection, the secretions become granular, and large clumps of white cells are readily seen. An increased amount of prostatic secretion with the presence of very few white blood cells is suggestive of prostatic congestion.

SEMEN ANALYSIS. For purposes of standardization, the specimen should be obtained by masturbation and collected in a dry container after 5 days of sexual abstinence. Examination, performed less than 1 hour after ejaculation, normally notes a volume of 3 to 5 ml with liquefaction complete within 1 hour. There should be over 20 million spermatozoa per milliliter with at least 60 percent demonstrating motility and 80 percent appearing morphologically normal.

Instrumentation

The insertion of any foreign body or instrument into the urethra carries a risk of trauma, introduction of infection, sepsis, and the possibility of exacerbation of preexisting inflammatory or obstructive conditions. Figure 40-5 illustrates commonly used urologic instruments. Instruments are designated by the French numbering system relating to the circumference of the instrument in millimeters, i.e., a #24 French sound is 24 mm in circumference.

CYSTOURETHROSCOPY. This investigative procedure should be performed in most cases of gross or microscopic hematuria and in selected cases of patients with symptoms of lower urinary tract obstruction or infection. It can often be performed as an office procedure. Instillation of a local anesthetic agent into the male urethra makes the procedure tolerable. The smallest caliber instrument that will provide adequate visualization of the bladder and urethra is used. No anesthetic is usually required for female cystourethroscopy. The presence of very small lesions of the bladder measuring 1 or 2 mm in diameter can readily be detected, as well as small calculi, the configuration and location of the ureteral orifices, prostatic size, urethral strictures or valves, and other pathologic conditions which may be present in the bladder or the urethra.

THERAPEUTIC INSTRUMENTATION. An indwelling catheter affords temporary relief of the obstruction. However, since maintenance for over 3 days is almost always attended by ascending infection, an external collecting device, such as a sheath, is more appropriate to improve nursing care of the incontinent patient who has no obstruction. Relative contraindications to instrumentation include acute cystitis, urethritis, prostatitis, pyelonephritis, and epididymitis. In these instances, it is best to pretreat the patient for the organism present. An exception to the rule is that if obstruction is the predisposing cause of infection, i.e., prostatic hypertrophy with retention and acute cystopyelitis, immediate instrumentation is necessary. Temporary drainage during the acute infection stage may be carried out by suprapubic tap and the insertion of a small polyethylene or plastic tube connected to constant drainage. Therapeutic instrumentation may be applied in the endoscopic removal of calculi or foreign bodies, biopsy or excision of tumors, cysts, or other obstructive lesions, drainage of prostatic abscesses, and transurethral removal of the prostatic obstruction. Institution of transurethral drainage may represent the most important therapeutic factor in obstructions secondary to prostatic hypertrophy or impacted ureteral calculus associated with cystopyelitis or pyelonephritis.

Catheterization should be performed with aseptic technique and minimal trauma. For routine stat catheterization, a #16 or #18 olive-tip coudé rubber catheter is the easiest to pass and the least traumatic. For indwelling drainage in the absence of gross bleeding or clots, a #18 Foley catheter is usually satisfactory. If one plans to allow the catheter to remain for several days, it should not be a tight fit which leads to ischemic changes of the urethra and subsequent stricture. Closed system drainage should be instituted; periodic instillation of an antibacterial irrigating solution left in contact with the bladder mucosa may help prevent infection during this period of constant drainage.

The operator should wear sterile gloves or use a sterile clamp, and the patient should be prepped with germicidal soap and draped. For dilatation or instrumentation of the male urethra, a topical anesthetic is instilled. After the catheter, which has been lubricated with a water-soluble lubricant, is inserted into the urethra, the latter is drawn upward to straighten the curves and folds. Resistance of the sphincter is best overcome by gentle pressure. In the case of acute retention, complete bladder decompression should be effected. However, with chronic and prolonged distension, rapid decompression of the bladder may lead to distressing vesical spasm and hemorrhage. Therefore, gradual decompression over a period of 72 hours is indicated.

Special Diagnostic Studies

EXCRETORY UROGRAPHY. Certain intravenously administered organic substances are filtered and excreted by the kidney. When rendered opaque by iodinization, they opacify the renal parenchyma and collecting system. Hypaque (sodium orthoiodohippurate) and Conray (meglumine iothalamate) are two examples. These agents are potent osmotic diuretics and may lead to dehydration, especially in children. Therefore it is important to compensate for this effect by encouraging copious fluid intake following examination. Occasionally the study is followed by anuria and renal failure in elderly, dehydrated, debilitated patients who have evidence of renal dysfunction. Satisfactory hydration of these patients is essential to decrease the risk of this occurring.

If time permits, a 3-day low-residue diet and oral laxatives should be administered to eliminate fecal and gas shadows. Also, the patient should be dehydrated for 12 hours prior to the examination to concentrate the opacified urine. However, dehydration should not be carried out in the uremic patient, and in this situation the quantity of opaque can be doubled or tripled to improve the quality of films. Patients with reduced renal function and BUN (blood urea nitrogen) in the neighborhood of 60 mg/100 ml can excrete a sufficient concentration of opaque to give clinically useful information. Pyelograms with inadequate preparation may give useful information in emergencies. They may be adequate to determine the presence of obstruction, extravasation, or nonfunction.

Renal Size, Location and Axis. The adult male kidney averages 13 by 6.2 cm on pyelography. The left kidney is usually several millimeters longer and broader. The kidneys of females are 5 mm smaller in both dimensions. The upper pole of the left kidney lies at mid T_{12}, while the right kidney is a half vertebral body lower. In the upright position, the kidney descends one vertebral body. If lines are drawn through the uppermost and lowermost calyces of the two kidneys, they should converge at T_9 (Fig. 40-6). Any deviation from this axis is considered abnormal. The calyces should be adequate in number and delicately cupped. The infundibulae are straight and fine. The pelvis points medially and describes a smooth curve without redundancy or tortuosity. There may be several areas of incomplete ureteral visualization due to peristalsis. The diameter of the ureter usually does not exceed 4 mm. Late upright films should demonstrate emptying of the collecting system and visualization of the urinary bladder. On supine films the contrast may pool in the fundus of the bladder and lead to the erroneous interpretation of an outlet filling defect. A postvoiding film is helpful in reveal-

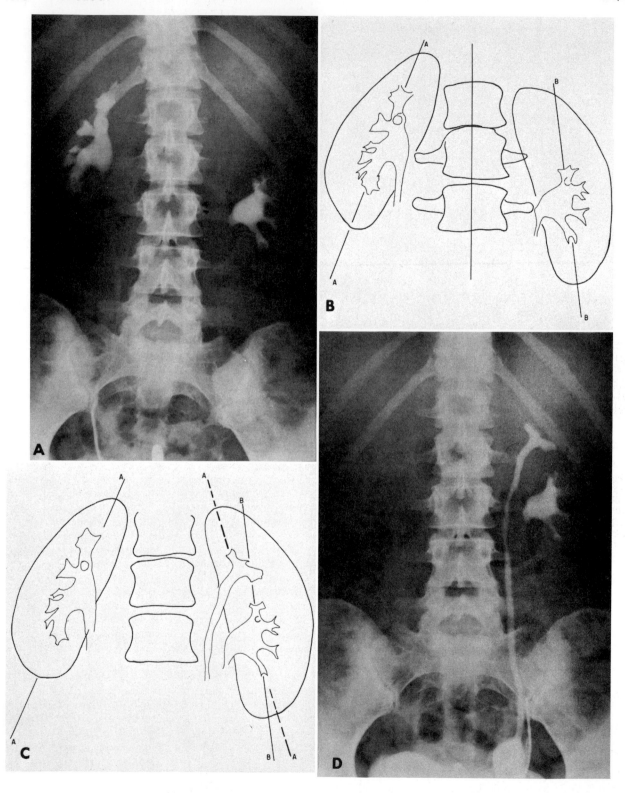

ing the lower ureter and indicating the amount of residual urine.

NEPHROTOMOGRAPHY. More detailed and accurate visualization of the kidney and pelvocalyceal system is available by this technique. Several "slices" of the kidneys are obtained beginning posteriorly and advancing anteriorly. This eliminates the overlying gas and fecal material in the bowel. Lucent areas such as fat and cysts are more readily identifiable. The poorly prepared patient may be evaluated more satisfactorily.

RETROGRADE PYELOURETEROGRAPHY. This study is indicated to further evaluate lesions of the pelvocalyceal system and ureter. "Filling defects" of these structures may not be evaluated adequately by excretory urography. Urine may be collected from the pelves for cytologic study and also to determine differential renal function. Instillation of contrast medium provides a more detailed visualization of these structures and is best done under fluoroscopic control. Improved techniques of excretory urography and nephrotomography have significantly decreased the need for retrograde pyeloureterography.

CYSTOURETHROGRAPHY. The patient's bladder and urethra may be evaluated by antegrade or retrograde studies. Fluoroscopic examination of the patient voiding may reveal the dynamics of micturition and evidence of obstruction or reflux of urine. Voiding cystourethrography is a useful diagnostic tool in the evaluation of children with voiding problems or recurrent urinary tract infections. Isotopic cystograms may be employed for the evaluation of reflux in children and offer decreased radiation exposure.

ANTEGRADE PYELOGRAPHY. Percutaneous insertion of a small catheter into the pelvocalyceal system may be a valuable diagnostic and therapeutic tool. The procedure is performed with local anesthesia and with fluoroscopic control. Once the small tube is placed properly within the drainage structures of the kidney, adequate drainage of an obstructed, infected pyohydronephrosis may be instituted and adequate x-ray visualization of the upper urinary tract may be obtained. Occasionally a ureter cannot be catheterized from below and may have to be visualized by this technique. It is an extremely valuable technique to use in the seriously ill, toxic patient. Adequate drainage may convert the situation from a surgical emergency to a relatively simple elective procedure in a nontoxic patient.

RENAL ARTERIOGRAPHY. Percutaneous, transfemoral renal arteriography is useful in the evaluation of possible renal vascular hypertension. The technique can demonstrate vascular lesions and thus direct the surgical approach. With congenital anomalies of the kidney arteriography is also helpful, since vascular anomalies frequently coexist and have an important bearing on surgical treat-

ment. Arteriography is also applied to the differential diagnosis of renal masses; a characteristic pooling of opaque is noted in tumor vessels within the parenchyma.

VENA CAVAGRAPHY. Percutaneous catheterization of the femoral vein with instillation of contrast material provides adequate visualization of the inferior vena cava. This study is particularly helpful in evaluating patients with carcinoma of the kidney and testicular neoplasms. Intrinsic involvement and obstruction of the vena cava and renal veins may be present with carcinoma of the kidney, and extrinsic compression of the vena cava may accompany enlargement of the periaortic nodes associated with metastatic testicular cancer. Preoperative evaluation with this study may help determine the most suitable type of surgical procedure for the patient.

LYMPHANGIOGRAPHY. Pedal lymphangiography may provide adequate visualization of the periaortic nodal drainage system as well as nodes of the pelvis. This study is usually employed in evaluation of patients with testicular, bladder, or prostatic carcinomas. A more adequate staging of the patient's disease may be possible with this technique.

RENOGRAPHY. The ^{131}I hippurate renogram provides an isotopic evaluation of the function of the individual kidneys. Dehydration, sodium depletion, and tubular blocking agents may alter the curves, and technical factors such as placement of detectors, dose of isotope, and paravenous injection may complicate interpretation. When properly performed, the renogram can be helpful in recognizing nonfunction or reduced function and delayed excretion, and in ureteral obstruction. It is also applied to differentiate between acute tubular necrosis and dehydration oliguria. Following renal arterial surgical procedures or homotransplantation, renography provides a simple and dependable method of evaluating the vascular status of the organ. Illustrative curves are shown in Figs. 40-7 to 40-10. The use of properly selected isotopes may provide further information regarding renal perfusion, drainage, and morphology.

ULTRASONOGRAPHY. This technique is useful in the differentiation of renal masses. Cystic lesions and hydronephrosis may be readily distinguished from solid masses of the kidney. Percutaneous needle aspiration of cystic masses may be carried out, providing drainage. The instillation of contrast material offers information as to the nature of the lesion. The noninvasive character of the

Fig. 40-6. *A* and *B*. Excretory urogram in complete left ureteral reduplication with ectopic ureteral orifice of nonvisualizing upper segment. Axis of the left kidney *BB* is abnormal. *C* and *D*. Left retrograde pyelogram demonstrating the upper segment. Note the correct axis of the right kidney *AA*. There is a ureterocele at the lower end of the ectopic ureter to the upper left renal segment.

Fig. 40-7. [131]I hippurate renograms. Both curves are normal.

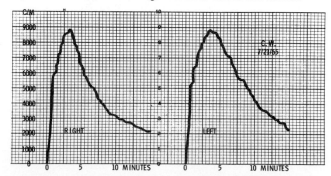

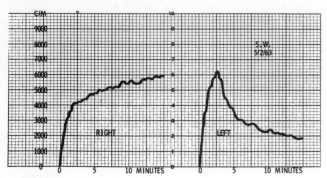

Fig. 40-8. ^{131}I hippurate renograms. Left renogram is normal. Delayed excretion on the right is due to obstructing ureteral calculus.

procedure and the lack of radiation exposure make it a useful screening, outpatient procedure, especially in children.

COMPUTED TOMOGRAPHY. The use of computed tomography for the evaluation of abdominal lesions is becoming a more common procedure. It is performed with and without contrast material. Lesions of the kidneys can be readily identified as to size, location, and consistency. Cystic lesions can be differentiated from solid lesions. The extent of tumor involvement with adjacent structures can be defined, allowing for improved staging of disease. As more experience is gained with this method, it will assume its proper place in the format of evaluation of patients with genitourinary disease.

CYSTOMETRICS, URETHRAL PRESSURE PROFILES, AND SPHINCTER ELECTROMYOGRAPHY. These studies are useful diagnostic tools for the evaluation of patients with micturition dysfunction, including problems which are due to obstruction, neurologic disease, functional disturbances, and dyssynergia.

PERCUTANEOUS RENAL CYST PUNCTURE. Under satisfactory local anesthesia and with fluoroscopic control, selected renal masses may be punctured. Fluid may be obtained for examination. Contrast material may be inserted into the cavity, and the differential diagnosis between cyst and tumor may be accurately determined.

Fig. 40-9. ^{131}I hippurate renograms. Right renogram is normal. Left kidney is surgically absent.

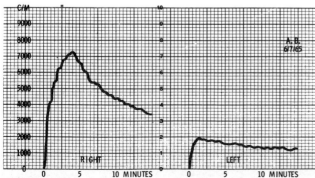

BLADDER FUNCTION

PHYSIOLOGY OF MICTURITION. As the empty bladder fills, the detrusor muscle stretches to accommodate the gradually increasing volume of urine. Normally, the pressure within the bladder is not significantly greater than intraabdominal pressure during the filling stage. When the volume of urine is sufficient, the pressure increases until it stimulates a spinal cord reflex which is under the control of cortical centers and leads to the contraction of the detrusor. This muscular contraction shortens the urethra and opens the bladder neck so that it resembles a funnel. Intravesical pressure at the initiation of voiding ranges between 15 and 30 cm of water. Voiding is resisted by the contraction of the striated muscles of the perineum and external sphincter, which overcome the tendency of the detrusor to effect urination.

In patients with obstructive uropathy, the pressure required to empty the bladder exceeds normal. This results in muscular hypertrophy of the detrusor and an increase in the pressure at the time of voiding so as to compensate for the obstruction. As long as the degree of the obstruction is counterbalanced by detrusor hypertrophy, the patient is able to empty the bladder with minimal amounts of residual urine. With overstretching of the detrusor muscle, the fibers lose their mechanical advantage and are unable to contract and empty the bladder effectively. Overdistension of the bladder occurs with obstruction, under the influence of certain drugs, and also in anesthetized patients with diuresis accompanying large amounts of intravenous therapy. This detrusor atonia is of short duration, disappearing rapidly following emptying of the bladder, while prolonged overdistension, such as occurs with chronic obstructive prostatic hypertrophy, may require several weeks of catheter drainage to effect complete recovery of function.

BLADDER INNERVATION. Sensations, including perception of heat and cold and pain of distension, are mediated by sensory fibers accompanying the sympathetic and parasympathetic nerves. They arise from T_9 to L_2 segments of the spinal cord. Motor pathways originate in the S_2 to S_4 segments and reach the bladder via the pelvic nerves. These parasympathetic nerves are responsible for the reflex contraction of the detrusor. The motor nerves of the external sphincter also originate in the S_2 to S_4 segments but travel via the pudendal nerves. The bladder is also richly supplied by sympathetic nerves which play a major role in detrusor function and outlet resistance.

Motor pathways may be evaluated by the bulbocavernosis reflex, which is elicited by gentle compression of the glans penis evoking contraction of the anal sphincter. *Cystometry* is the best method of evaluating motor function. This can be accomplished either by means of a recording gas or water cystometer or by an improvised system consisting of a reservoir with a drip chamber permitting regulation of fluid flow into the bladder. A Y tube connected to the indwelling urethral catheter and a graded column of fluid completes the system. The zero level of the column of fluid is positioned at the level of the symphysis, and warm saline solution is instilled into the bladder at the rate of 50 ml/minute. There is usually an increase of 10 to 15 cm of water pressure when flow is initiated. The normal cystometrogram shows a gradual increment in pressure during instillation of 400 ml of fluid, and at the end of this instillation the pressure rarely exceeds 20 cm. When bladder capacity is reached, there is a sudden increase in pressure as a result of detrusor response to the stretch reflex. Further information can be gained by combining cystometry with urethral pressure profile studies and a recording of sphincter electromyographic responses.

Neurogenic Bladder Dysfunction

Bladder dysfunction resulting from deficient innervation reflects the degree and type of nerve damage rather than the etiologic factor.

Uninhibited Neurogenic Bladder. Dysfunction is similar to that of the bladder of an infant in whom cortical integration is lacking. Etiology includes cerebral vascular accidents with cortical destruction, multiple sclerosis, and taboparesis. The condition presents as urgent voiding which is almost without voluntary control. A cystometrogram reveals many abrupt increases in pressure during filling, even at low volumes. Treatment with parasympatholytic drugs such as methantheline (Banthine), 50 mg four times daily, frequently produces a dramatic improvement in symptomatology by inhibiting the premature contractions.

Reflex (Automatic) Neurogenic Bladder. Dysfunction results from traumatic transection of the spinal cord. When the area between T_7 and C_7 is involved, a well-functioning reflex bladder usually results. In contrast, lesions above C_7 are often associated with extensive atrophy of the cord below the site of transection and may prevent the development of a reflex arc. The bladder with reflex function can frequently be rehabilitated to provide adequate emptying. This type of dysfunction is commonly associated with intense trabeculation of the bladder and, characteristically, produces a positive urecholine test result. Control pressure measurements are made through a urethral catheter with the bladder filled to 100 ml. Thirty minutes after the subcutaneous injection of 2.5 mg of urecholine, measurements are repeated. With upper motor neuron interruption, increased sensitivity of the neuromuscular junction and ganglionic synapses result in pressures which exceed 15 cm of water greater than control.

Centrally Denervated Neurogenic Bladder. Dysfunction is the result of traumatic, neoplastic, or congenital lesions of the sacral segments or cauda equina. Meningomyelocele or occult spina bifida are the most frequent lesions. The symptoms are overflow incontinence and recurring infections. Diagnosis is established by observing a large smooth-walled bladder containing a large amount of residual urine. Cystometry reveals large capacity associated with low pressures. Conservative management includes encouragement of the patient to strain and empty his bladder at frequent intervals, coupled with the administration of antibacterial agents to prevent the consequences of infection, namely, chronic pyelonephritis. Surgical treatment is directed at balancing the detrusor function

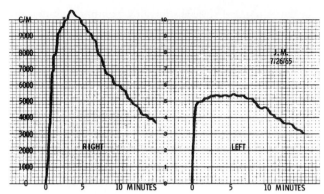

Fig. 40-10. ^{131}I hippurate renograms. Reduced left renal function with low urine volume is due to left renal artery stenosis with hypertension. Right renogram indicates functional hypertrophy.

with the resistance of the normal urethra by transurethral resection of the bladder neck or sphincterotomy. This results in improved emptying of the bladder and increased resistance to secondary infection. Long-term antibacterial therapy, however, is usually required. Intermittent self-catheterization may be required to maintain satisfactory emptying of the bladder at periodic intervals, which will decrease the incidence of infection and protect the upper urinary tract. Further balance between detrusor activity and peripheral resistance may be brought about by the proper use of drugs which will increase detrusor tone (cholinergic) and decrease bladder neck and proximal urethral resistance (sympatholytic).

Sensory Paralytic Bladder. Dysfunction results from the loss of sensory components of bladder innervation, such as in tabes dorsalis or combined cord degeneration. This leads to a huge bladder capacity and overflow incontinence. The patient is unaware of bladder filling. A cystometrogram shows a large capacity with lack of sensation and small response of pressure to volume change. Treatment is similar to that described above for the centrally denervated neurogenic bladder. The patient is then educated to void at regular intervals, since he never senses the need.

Motor Paralytic Bladder. Dysfunction may accompany poliomyelitis or infectious polyneuritis. Loss of motor activity is demonstrated on cystometry, and a large residual urine results. As the patient recovers from disease, bladder function returns to normal, but an indwelling catheter or intermittent catheterization may be required for a period of time.

MANAGEMENT OF POSTTRAUMATIC PARAPLEGIA WITH NEUROGENIC BLADDER DYSFUNCTION. A variety of methods have been utilized to establish bladder drainage in the initial paralytic, atonic phase. Multiple suprapubic aspirations, suprapubic cystostomy, and surgically constructed vesicocutaneous fistulae have been used. The indwelling urethral catheter is most commonly employed. A #16 or #18 indwelling balloon type is most practical and should be inserted in accordance with the previously proposed technique. The catheter should be attached to drainage in such a fashion that it can be irrigated by a closed system with a reservoir which is changed periodically. A

100-ml aliquot of sterile saline may be introduced into the bladder several times daily. Irrigations with $\frac{1}{4}$ percent acetic acid, mixtures of antibacterial drugs, and stone-dissolving agents have been proposed. It is seldom necessary to use irrigation to dissolve concretions, but if the situation arises, modified solution G (32.5 Gm of citric acid, 3.84 Gm of magnesium oxide, 8.84 Gm of sodium carbonate at a pH of 5) is useful.

Ascending infection around the catheter can be minimized by cleaning the meatus and surrounding tissue and by promoting the egress of urethral secretions. The latter can be accomplished by taping the penis parallel to the inguinal crease. The most important aspect of catheter care is the ingestion of sufficient fluids to produce an excess of 2 liters of urine daily. In addition to maintaining volume, the pH should be below 6, since an acid pH decreases the incidence of encrustation. The use of an acid-ash diet or ascorbic acid will result in an acid urine. Since paraplegic patients mobilize calcium from the bones and excrete it in the urine, multiple determinations of the 24-hour urinary calcium levels are indicated. If the urinary calcium excretion exceeds 300 mg/day, the patient should be placed on a low-calcium diet. Anabolic agents are also useful in reducing the urinary calcium excretion.

Periodic cultures of the urine and microscopic examination are directed at evaluating urinary infection. Methenamine mandelate is frequently useful to maintain an environment unfavorable for bacterial growth. High fever in a paraplegic is generally related to urinary tract infection. The specific complications of catheter drainage in these patients include acute cystitis and pyelonephritis, acute epididymitis, suppurative urethritis, periurethral abscess with fistula formation, and bladder or kidney stones.

A regimen of intermittent catheterization should be established as soon as possible in the early phase, so that the indwelling catheter can be removed. This can be carried out by self-catheterization, if the patient is able to learn this technique and has the necessary motor power in the upper extremities, or by trained personnel in the hospital ward or rehabilitation center.

Rehabilitation of Bladder. During the first 3 to 4 months of stabilizing a fracture, attention is directed at preventing infection and permanent damage to the urinary tract. Stabilization of the fracture permits the patient to assume an upright position and allows attempts at rehabilitation of the urinary tract. This should be initiated by cystometric and cystoscopic evaluation followed by a trial of catheter removal, if the patient has been on indwelling catheter drainage. In at least 70 percent of patients it is possible to reach a catheter-free state. Prior to and for several days subsequent to catheter removal, appropriate antibiotic therapy is directed at any organisms present. The patient's voiding habits and volume and character of urine should be noted. Success is anticipated when large volumes are voided at infrequent intervals. Frequent voiding of small volumes may precede total cessation of voiding, in which case the catheter is reinserted. A trial of urecholine is occasionally beneficial and may precede catheter reinsertion. If self-catheterization has not been instituted earlier and the patient is not able to empty the bladder satisfactorily, it can be taught at this time.

If necessary, a reinserted catheter should be left in place for an additional period of time during which reassessment of the anatomic status of the bladder by cystourethroscopy is performed. Over half the patients with upper motor neuron bladder dysfunction require resection of the bladder neck to relieve obstruction. Subsequent to surgical operations, such as sphincterotomy, the majority of patients void satisfactorily. The patients requiring prolonged or permanent catheter drainage are instructed in catheter care and the maintenance of a large urinary volume. Suppressive therapy with agents such as nitrofurantoin and methenamine mandelate is helpful in reducing the problem of chronic infection.

In females, incontinence may persist. If it is of the overflow type, self-catheterization may also be of value. In neglected patients with neurologic disturbance of bladder function, the resultant damage to the upper urinary tract requires a supravesical diversion. The cutaneous ureteroileostomy may resolve the problem, but attention must be given to watertight sealing of the collecting appliance.

ACUTE INFECTIONS

PATHOGENESIS. The most common portal of entry for urinary tract infection is the urethra. *Ascending infection* is potentiated by obstructive uropathy, foreign bodies, and also bladder tumor and papillary necrosis. The normal bladder possesses defense mechanisms which are capable of coping with introduced infection. In the obstructed, inflamed, or ulcerated organ, however, these mechanisms are rendered ineffective. In the presence of obstructive uropathy, the increased pressure required for evacuation frequently leads to retrograde infection by means of reflux of infected urine into the ureter and kidney. Voiding cystourethrograms document this occurrence. Ninety-six percent of pediatric urinary infections occur in the female, because of the shortness of the urethra. Many children who have recurrent urinary infections also have obstructive uropathy. In the adult, 65 percent of urinary infections are in females and are related to the trauma of sexual intercourse, childbirth, and gynecologic procedures. In older age groups, urinary tract infections increase in the male because of the incidence of obstructive uropathy secondary to prostatic hypertrophy.

Urinary tract infections also result from *hematogenous* spread, such as metastatic staphylococcal infection from cutaneous abscesses. This produces the entity known as staphylococcal kidney, or renal carbuncle. Severe hydronephrosis and renal calculi predispose to hematogenous infection. *Lymphatic transmission* of infection from the bowel and lower urinary tract via periureteral lymphatics is also proposed as a cause of pyelonephritis. Urinary tract infections are an infrequent result of spread from contiguous infections such as diverticulitis of the colon, regional enteritis, and appendiceal abscess.

BACTERIOLOGY. The most common organism causing

acute urinary tract infections is *E. coli,* which is responsible in 37 percent of the cases. Other commonly involved pathogens are *Proteus mirabilis, Klebsiella,* the enterococci, and *Pseudomonas.* Other organisms, encountered less frequently, include *Proteus vulgaris, morgagni* and *rettgeri* and the staphylococci. Most of these organisms are normal inhabitants of the fecal flora. With acute urinary tract infection, hundreds of thousands to millions of organisms per milliliter are present in the voided urine, and pure cultures are more prevalent in acute infections than in chronic infections.

TREATMENT. The ability to treat urinary tract infections with drugs is enhanced by the unique ability of normally functioning kidneys to concentrate a variety of antibacterial agents in the urine. Treatment involves proper selection of the right drug or drugs which can be adequately delivered to the urine, tissues, or blood. Drug selection is facilitated by culture and determination of sensitivities. However, these are usually not possible in the early stages of treatment. Further considerations include the age and general health of the patient, kidney function, history of allergy, previous drug therapy, relative cost of therapy, nature of the preparation, and possible complications of the drug to be administered.

Sulfonamides, which are rapidly excreted by the kidney in high concentration, are ideally suited to the treatment of urinary tract infections. Most acute urinary tract infections due to *E. coli* will respond to these drugs administered as 1 Gm four times daily for 7 to 10 days. In acute uncomplicated infections without upper tract involvement, this usually constitutes adequate therapy, but the urine should be reexamined microscopically and cultured at the end of 1 week. In the patient with manifestations of pyelonephritis, such as flank pain, chills, fever, malaise, nausea, vomiting, and leukocytosis, a more prolonged course of therapy is indicated. Other useful antibacterial agents are ampicillin, tetracycline, cephalexin, nitrofurantoin, nalidixic acid, and trimethoprim-sulfamethoxizole. The aminoglycosides, such as gentamicin, tobramycin, and amikacin, are particularly useful for the treatment of *Pseudomonas* infections. Antispasmodics and dye substances which relieve symptoms should be used only in conjunction with antibacterial agents.

The acute infection is sometimes secondary to an important factor which requires correction in order to prevent recurrence. Therefore, although it is justifiable to treat acutely ill patients before the diagnosis is made, complete investigation should be carried out as soon as possible. If the infection is related to defloration cystitis, vaginitis, diarrhea, or poor hygiene, simultaneous treatment of the two conditions will effect a cure. If the infection is secondary to obstruction, the obstruction must be eliminated.

Following subsidence of the acute episode, repeated urinalyses should be performed at 1-month intervals if the patient is asymptomatic and sooner if symptoms recur. Complete urologic evaluation should be performed in all patients who have had attacks of acute pyelonephritis or multiple attacks of cystitis. In the male, since the bladder is protected by a longer urethra, a single attack of cystitis

warrants investigation. If recurrent infections occur, long-term therapy for 3 to 12 months may succeed where short courses fail. Drugs useful for long-term therapy include nitrofurantoin, methenamine mandelate, methenamine hippurate, and trimethoprim-sulfamethoxizole. Patients receiving these medications should have periodic blood cell counts to detect granulocytopenia and anemia. Allergic and hypersensitive responses to these medicines are also relatively common.

GRAM-NEGATIVE BACTEREMIA. The syndrome is considered with urologic diseases, since in over half the patients with gram-negative bacteremia the urinary tract provides the portal of entry. Frequently the bacteremia follows instrumentation in the presence of preexisting urinary tract infection which has been ineffectively treated. The patients experience a shaking chill followed by high fever, peripheral vasodilatation, and hypotension. The organisms responsible are frequently resistant to the usual drugs and require large doses of parenterally administered antibacterial agents. Drugs which are bactericidal are preferable, in order to prevent liberation of additional quantities of the endotoxin by the multiplying bacteria. An aminoglycoside, such as gentamicin and ampicillin, or a similar drug used in combination has proved to be quite effective for the management of gram-negative bacteremia. Drug dosage is carefully regulated according to renal function and, when available, culture and sensitivities reports. The treatment of schock is discussed in Chap. 4.

Acute Staphylococcal Infections of the Kidney

Staphylococcal pyelonephritis or abscess is of hematogenous origin and usually the result of metastatic infection from furuncles. The symptoms include fever, flank pain, frequency, and dysuria. On examination, the patient is very ill, with marked tenderness over the kidney and leukocytosis. Urinalysis may reveal staphylococci on stain or culture. In the very acute phase, the urine may be negative, since the organisms are located in the cortex of the kidney and have not found their way into the urine. *Staphylococcus aureus* is the most common offending organism. Treatment consists of parenteral therapy with the appropriate antibacterial agent. Complications include renal carbuncle, which represents liquefaction necrosis, or perinephric abscess resulting from perforation of a renal carbuncle. *Renal carbuncle* usually occurs in patients who are ineffectively treated for the acute staphylococcal pyelonephritis. Clinical manifestations include flank pain and relapsing fever with enlargement and tenderness of the involved portion of the kidney. Treatment of the carbuncle with antibacterial agents is rarely effective, and surgical drainage is mandatory. Occasionally nephrectomy is necessary because of extensive involvement of the kidney with multiple abscesses.

PERINEPHRIC ABSCESS. This usually follows perforation of a renal abscess into the perinephric tissues. In some instances perinephric abscess may result from direct hematogenous spread or from a microabscess in the kidney which is not apparent. The patients present with an extremely high fever and boardlike rigidity of the abdominal wall. Roentgenograms reveal nonvisualization of the psoas shadow and concavity of the spine to the side of the lesion. If one takes a film during breathing, the involved kidney is fixed and does not blur. Nephrotomography, ultrasound, and percutaneous aspiration of the perinephric space may establish the diagnosis when conventional diagnostic procedures fail. Treatment requires prompt drainage and appropriate antibiotics.

Acute Papillary Necrosis

Necrosis of renal papillae occurs in patients with diabetes, sickle cell disease, tuberculosis, and excessive ingestion of phenacetin. In addition to the symptoms related to the associated acute infection of the kidney, renal colic may result from ureteral obstruction by the sloughed papillae. Diagnosis is made by demonstrating sloughed papillae or by characteristic appearance of the intravenous pyelogram showing loss of one or more of the papillae (Fig. 40-11). Loss of renal function may attend papillary necrosis, but recovery usually occurs, and initial measures are directed toward supporting the patient during the acute episode. Specific treatment for the involved organism is administered. If the patient remains febrile and there is ureteral obstruction, surgical intervention may be required to remove the obstructing soft tissue.

Acute Urethritis

Acute urethritis is usually ascending and venereal in origin. Included in the acute types of urethritis are those caused by gonorrhea, mycobacteria, *Chlamydia,* and *Trichomonas vaginalis.* Diagnosis is established by microscopy of the Gram-stained discharge and confirmed by adequate culture techniques. Reiter's syndrome, consisting of the

Fig. 40-11. Renal papillary necrosis. *A.* Retrograde pyelography in diabetic renal papillary necrosis. *B.* Necrotic papillae are indicated by arrows.

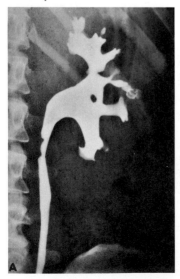
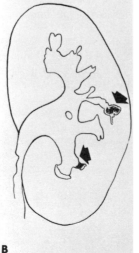

triad of arthritis, nongonococcal urethritis, and conjunctivitis, is considered by many to be of venereal origin and should be included in the differential diagnosis.

Gonorrhea is the most common venereal disease of man. The incubation period is 7 to 9 days, after which the symptoms of acute urethritis are manifest. Urethral stricture is a common sequela if the original infection is not adequately treated. Metastatic gonococcal infections include arthritis, tenosynovitis, bursitis, ophthalmitis, perihepatitis, and endocarditis. Gonococcal arthritis, which represents the only common manifestation of metastatic involvement, is polyarticular in 80 percent of the cases and accompanied by tenosynovitis in 50 percent of the cases. The diagnosis of gonococcal infection is established by demonstration of *Neisseria gonorrhoeae,* Gram-negative diplococci, intracellularly in a discharge. Since both syphilis and gonorrhea are contracted by the same exposure in about 3 percent of cases, the latter should be excluded by serologic tests at regular intervals for 6 months. Gonococcal urethral infections are best treated by adequate dosage of penicillin-type drugs. Oral tetracycline could be used for patients allergic to penicillin.

Penicillin therapy is also effective for mimae infection, while *Trichomonas* urethritis and prostatitis are best treated with metronidazole (Flagyl, 250 mg orally twice daily for men and three times daily for women for a period of 10 days). The tetracyclines are effective in the treatment of *Chlamydia* and mycobacteria.

Acute Infections of the Prostate

Acute prostatitis is commonly a complication of untreated or ineffectively treated acute urethritis. Acute prostatitis is particularly common in young or mature males in whom vigorous exertion or exposure may lead to spread of infection from the urethra. Retrograde instrumental trauma in the presence of urethral infection may cause prostatitis at any age. Formerly prostatitis was predominantly of gonococcal origin, but now it is more often associated with a mixed veneral flora including *Streptococcus fecalis, E. coli,* or *Corynebacterium hofmannii,* or exerosis. Acute prostatitis secondary to metastatic spread from furunculosis and caused by *Staphylococcus aureus* or *Staphylococcus albus* occurs less commonly.

Initial symptoms may be mild and consist of perineal discomfort with increasing frequency, initial hematuria, dysuria, and occasional retention. With progression, the perineal pain becomes continuous and severe and is attended by chills, high fever, malaise, and prostration. Leukocytosis is characteristic, and bacteremia is common. In extreme cases, the gram-negative bacteremia may be associated with endotoxin shock. Liquefaction necrosis of the local infection results in the formation of abscesses which may spontaneously or as a result of catheterization rupture into the urethra.

Culture of the urethral discharge should precede administration of antibacterial agents, but these should not be withheld until the culture reports are available. If necessary, the drug may be changed at a later date. Patients with retention should be catheterized gently with a small indwelling catheter. Rectal examination should be performed infrequently and with great care to avoid dissemination of the infection. Several days of treatment should result in symptomatic improvement and return of temperature to normal. Persistence of symptoms and fever suggests the presence of an abscess which will require drainage. The acutely ill patient should be at bed rest, hydrated, and treated with antibiotics until the acute phase of the process subsides. Warm sitz baths and prostatic massage are used to obviate the subacute and chronic phases. Prostatic abscesses occasionally occur with inadequate therapy and are treated by drainage performed either transurethrally with a resectoscope or perineally through a prostatectomy incision.

CHRONIC INFECTIONS

Chronic Prostatitis

"Chronic prostatitis" refers to a syndrome which causes genital discomfort, is associated with purulent prostatic secretion, and responds favorably to prostatic massage and antibacterial agents. It occurs most frequently in men over forty-five, and 35 to 50 percent in this age group are said to be affected. Thirty percent of normal asymptomatic males of military age have purulent prostatic secretions, and this is also present in some prepubertal males. An autopsy incidence of 6.3 percent has been reported by Moore. A variety of factors including gonorrhea, pyogenic urethritis, instrumentation, urethral stricture, prostatic hypertrophy, distant foci of infection, congestion, stasis, and postalcoholic changes have all been implicated as, but not proved to be, predisposing factors.

Chronic prostatitis is frequently caused by retrograde infection from the urethra. This is particularly true in those cases following acute urethritis and instrumentation. Hematogenous spread from distant foci has also been implicated as a cause, particularly in staphylococcal infection. The role of infection in chronic prostatitis has not been completely defined. Since the nonpathogenic bacterial flora of the urethra include staphylococci, streptococci, and diphtheroids, positive cultures from prostatic fluid collected at the urethral meatus are anticipated. In a series of patients with chronic prostatitis, 99 percent of prostatic fluid cultures demonstrated growth, but only 36 percent of the organisms were considered to be the pathogens. In contrast, prostatic secretions obtained through the urethroscope in patients with chronic prostatitis yield pathogens in only 4 percent of the specimens. The organisms include *E. coli, Streptococcus fecalis, A. aerogenes, P. aeruginosa, Staphylococcus aureus,* pleuropneumonia organisms, and *T. vaginalis.*

The pathologic changes in chronic prostatitis are minimal. Microscopically, the gland shows fibrosis and purulent secretions, interstitial fibroplasia, and lymphocytic infiltrations. Dilated acini and prostatic ducts are often filled with obstructing masses of cellular debris and leukocytes. The acini are frequently smaller than normal, and the epithelium may undergo metaplasia, becoming cuboidal or squamous. Associated seminal vesiculitis is seen infrequently, and therefore the term "prostatovesiculitis" is inappropriate.

Symptomatology includes discomfort in the lower abdomen or back and genitalia. In young men, the main complaint is a scanty mucoid urethral discharge. In middle-aged men the more common complaint is that of genital discomfort, while in older men symptoms suggesting obstruction such as nocturia, frequency, and dysuria are often elicited. On rectal examination, the prostate may be boggy or indurated but is of normal consistency in over half the patients.

Prostatic secretion for microscopic examination is obtained by prostatic massage. The normal secretion contains three to five white blood cells per high-powered field. Chronic prostatitis may be accompanied by an increase in number of white cells and a clumping of the leukocytes. However, in half the patients there is no abnormality in the number of white cells in the fluid. Also, no relationship has been demonstrated between changes in prostatic secretion during therapy and the remission or exacerbation of symptoms. The urine frequently contains shreds and leukocytes in the first portion of the voided specimen. Occasional red cells may be seen. The second glass of voided urine is usually normal, but 25 percent have pyuria. This finding is indicative of urinary tract infection, and the patient should be evaluated for obstructive uropathy and other urinary disease.

Treatment of chronic nonspecific prostatitis includes prostatic massage, warm baths, and antibacterial agents when indicated. The usual course includes increasingly vigorous massages at weekly intervals for 3 to 4 weeks, following which the intervals are extended, and finally the patient is advised to return only if recurrent symptoms do not respond to hot tubs. The prognosis for symptomatic improvement is excellent for a given episode, but there is a tendency toward recurrence. Antibacterial treatment is applicable in patients with urethritis or urinary tract infection. Hormones do not appear to be indicated. Instillations and irrigations have afforded symptomatic relief, and sedatives may be of benefit to the patient with psychogenic frequency of urination. Alcoholic beverages and highly seasoned foods are traditionally withheld. Normal frequency of sexual intercourse is not considered harmful, since it promotes emptying of the prostate.

The complications of chronic nonspecific prostatitis are also poorly defined. Acute cystitis, urethritis, epididymitis, and pyelonephritis have occurred during or following an episode of chronic nonspecific prostatitis. Benign prostatic hypertrophy and carcinoma of the prostate do not occur more frequently in the gland involved with chronic nonspecific prostatitis. Similarly, squamous metaplasia and squamous carcinoma have no increased incidence. A relationship between chronic prostatitis and associated arthritis or uveitis is questionable. Chronic prostatitis associated with prostatic calculi usually fails to respond to prostatic massage and may require operative removal of the calculi, with consideration of the fact that this operation interferes with potency.

Comparable infections of the urethra occur in the female. Treatment for acute urethritis of gonococcal origin is similar to that already outlined for the male. *Tricho-monas* infestation may require higher doses of the drugs used. Chronic urethritis in the female has been referred to as the "female urethral syndrome" and is probably the result of local inflammation or recurrent attacks of cystitis. The patients generally complain of frequency, nocturia, dysuria, and backache. Marked urgency and dyspareunia are also common symptoms. On examination, the urethra is enlarged, indurated, and tender; urethroscopy demonstrates injection, edema, and cystic changes. Injection and inflammation of the trigone may be an associated finding. A urine specimen obtained by catheterization rarely shows more than a few epithelial cells and occasional white cells. Progressive dilatation of the urethra to the size of #34 F may be helpful. Instillation of nitrofurazone (1:1,000) may prevent ascending cystitis. The prognosis for improvement is good, but, as in the male, the condition tends to recur. Complications include acute cystitis, pyelonephritis, and the development of a urethral caruncle.

Urinary Tuberculosis

Renal tuberculosis is the result of hematogenous spread from primary pulmonary or intestinal lesions. Although the involvement is probably bilateral and cortical in most individuals, some lesions progress to healing, while others assume clinical significance. Renal tuberculosis is generally undetected and asymptomatic until it ulcerates into the collecting system of the kidney. At that time the symptoms include gross hematuria, dysuria, frequency, and pyuria with an absence of bacteria on Gram stain. Many of the symptoms are a consequence of cystitis arising from organisms localizing in the bladder secondary to the renal involvement.

Special culture techniques will reveal the presence of *Mycobacterium tuberculosis*. Intravenous pyelography demonstrates calcification of caseous abscesses, ulceration of calyces, and failure of visualization of calyces filled with caseous debris (Fig. 40-12). Treatment consists of 1 to 2

Fig. 40-12. Renal tuberculosis. *A* and *B.* Left upper pole ulcerative renal tuberculosis. *C* and *D.* Chronic suppurative left pyelonephritis with atrophy.

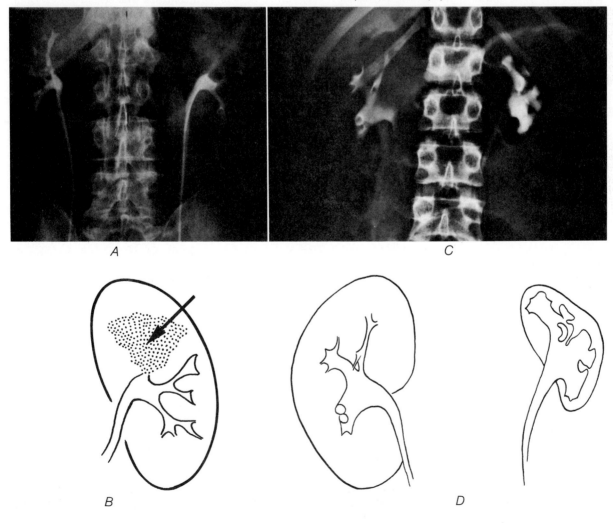

A

C

B

D

years of isoniazid (0.1 Gm three times daily), cycloserine (0.250 Gm twice daily), and sodium para-aminosalicylic acid (6 to 12 Gm daily). The patient is followed by repeated urine cultures and repeated pyelography, which should be performed at 3-month intervals during the first year.

Genital tuberculosis may accompany renal tuberculosis or may exist independently as a result of hematogenous spread. The epididymis is most frequently involved, and spread may take place from this source up the vas deferens to the prostate or through the scrotum in the form of a fistula. The vas deferens may become beaded with involvement. Epididymal tuberculosis may be successfully managed by chemotherapy, and epididymectomy is held in reserve.

URINARY CALCULI

The consequences of urinary calculi are responsible for 10 percent of the urologic hospital admissions in many parts of the world. An etiologic factor can be defined in only half the patients. Primary metabolic stones result from hyperexcretion of an offending substance. Cystine and uric acid stones form only in those individuals with excessive urinary excretion of these substances. In hyperparathyroidism, increased calcium and phosphorus excretion is responsible for the formation of the triple-phosphate stones. It is questionable whether the calcium oxalate stone is related to an excess excretion of oxalate.

Secondary stones arise as a result of foreign bodies, obstruction, or prolonged recumbency and consequent decalcification of bone with hyperexcretion of calcium salts in the urine. Infections with urea-splitting organisms result in ammonium-magnesium phosphate calculi, while chronic pyelonephritis and ulcerative processes lead to a suitable nidus for the deposition of encrustations and eventual stone formation.

COMPOSITION. Urinary calculi can often be identified by their external appearance. The calcium oxalate stones, which constitute 73 percent of calculi, are frequently small, under 50 mg, dark-colored, and have an external surface which is covered with sharp spicules. Ammonium-magnesium phosphate calculi account for 15.7 percent and are commonly found in infected urine. These stones are characteristically porous, soft, and either tan or white. Uric acid stones, which constitute 7.6 percent of all calculi, are commonly yellowish, orange, or pink. They are porous and easily broken. Cystine stones have been likened to maple sugar and represent only 1 percent of large series.

DIAGNOSIS. Calculi within the ureter usually present with typical renal colic. However, staghorn calculi and bladder stones associated with obstruction may be asymptomatic, except for a history of recurrent infection. Urinalysis may be negative during an attack of colic if the ureter is completely obstructed. As the colic subsides, the first voided urine may show copious quantities of red cells and crystals. The crystals are commonly similar to the constit-

uents of the calculi, and albuminuria, when present, is frequently proportionate to the number of red cells. Pyuria and bacteriuria are present in only 15 percent of the patients.

Ninety-five percent of urinary calculi are radiopaque. Most opaque stones contain calcium, but both ammonium-magnesium phosphate and cystine stones are sufficiently radiopaque to be detectable. Uric acid stones are usually nonopaque, and calculi, which are opaque, may be masked by overlying bony structures. Intravenous pyelograms may reveal the calculi, the point of obstruction, or delayed visualization of the obstructed side. When the latter obtains, delayed films taken up to 24 hours after injection may demonstrate the point of obstruction, since the opaque eventually mixes with the urine in the delayed collecting system (Fig. 40-13A to D). Roentgenographic examination, without adequate preparation, during acute renal colic may be less than satisfactory because of the gas in the colon secondary to reflex ileus. However, early x-ray examination in the differential diagnosis of flank pain is so important that the emergency pyelogram is indicated. Calculi which lie in the segment of ureter within the bony pelvis may be confused with phleboliths. Tomography may be helpful in this situation. However, the majority of calculi lie above a line drawn through the spinous processes of the ischium, and phloboliths have a characteristic spherical smooth configuration and, frequently, nonopaque centers. Occasionally, it is necessary to resort to retrograde ureteral catheterization to determine whether or not a given opacity lies within the ureter. In this circumstance, the combination of anteroposterior and oblique films, which demonstrate the opacity in contact with the catheter, is diagnostic of a calculus. Roentgenographic studies of the phalanges and lamina dura are useful in detecting the presence of bone changes associated with hyperparathyroidism.

MANAGEMENT. Symptomatic relief of the severe pain frequently must be initiated before the diagnosis is established. Narcotics are usually necessary to relieve severe renal colic, while moderate pain is improved by the application of heat. Roentgenographic determination of the size of the calculus and the nature of the urinary passages through which the calculus must pass is critical. The dilated ureter following pregnancy will permit passage of a larger stone than the normal ureter. Recognizable obstructive changes at the ureteropelvic junction may make passage of a small stone unlikely. Ninety-three percent of calculi less than 4 mm pass spontaneously, while only 20 percent of calculi greater than 6 mm in greatest dimension will pass. The patient who is followed expectantly should have renal function assessed at regular intervals, and the isotopic renogram has provided an excellent means for evaluating changes.

Indications for Removal. Although some surgeons feel that the presence of a stone indicates the need for surgical intervention, it seems unlikely that all calculi produce sufficient damage to warrant it. A small stone lodged in the calyx causes no marked loss of renal function, and there may be no alteration in size and no symptoms for

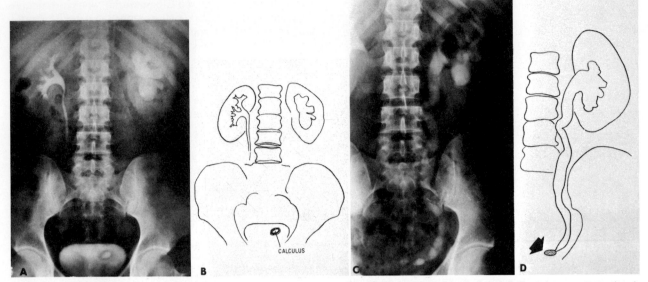

Fig. 40-13. Ureteral calculi. *A* and *B.* Excretory urogram showing left hydronephrosis with nonvisualization of left ureter on early films, calculus in region of left ureteral orifice. *C* and *D.* Excretory urogram, 2-hour delayed film, shows visualization of a dilated left ureter down to ureteral calculus in intravesical portion of ureter, thus establishing the diagnosis.

many years. The following are accepted indications for surgical treatment:

1. Nonfunction of the kidney on intravenous pyelogram or renogram, indicating severe obstruction. Loss of the kidney is inevitable if the obstruction persists.
2. Persistent hydronephrosis above an obstructing stone which fails to pass within a reasonable period of time. This may lead to pyelonephritis and irreparable renal damage.
3. Frequent episodes of incapacitating colic even in the presence of normal renal function.
4. An obstructing stone associated with infection, since the infection usually will not respond to medication.
5. Recurrent infections related to a calculus.

Following surgical or manipulative removal of stones, it is important to ensure that the passages are well flushed by a copious diuresis and that urinary infection is treated with appropriate antibacterial agents.

Surgery. Prior to surgical intervention, it is important to visualize the collecting system to determine if any abnormalities are present and require correction at the time of lithotomy. Calculi of small size may be removed from the lower ureter by means of transurethral instruments which snare the stone. These are referred to as "baskets" and consist of a special catheter with filaments attached so that when the catheter is passed beyond the stone and gradually withdrawn, the stone becomes entangled in the filaments. As peristalsis of the ureter expels the instrument, both the catheter and the stone are moved downward so that the stone passes into the urinary bladder, from which it can be removed easily. Bladder stones, especially soft magnesium-ammonium phosphate calculi, may be crushed and removed by the process of lithotripsy. Manipulative surgical treatment is usually not performed for calculi which lie in the ureter above the pelvic brim. Lithotomy may provide the least traumatic method for removing some stones. The high incidence of success is accompanied by an advantage over lithotripsy in that no fragments are left behind.

Urinary calculi sometimes can be dissolved by alkalinization or by irrigation through ureteral catheters. The latter technique is particularly applicable for some magnesium-ammonium phosphate and uric acid stones. The magnesium-ammonium phosphate stones may be dissolved in a modified solution G, while the uric acid stones are solubilized best by alkaline solutions such as 1% sodium bicarbonate. Although bladder stones may respond to modified solution G, litholapaxy is preferable, because these calculi are readily accessible.

Prevention of Recurrence. Even in the absence of obvious obstructive uropathy, stones tend to recur. In a series of patients presenting with renal colic due to calculi, 39 percent had previously passed stones.

Obstruction and infection must be treated, since stones in the kidney are associated with infection in half the cases. Treatment of infection and elimination of obstruction are particularly important in the stones of the magnesium-ammonium phosphate group and oxalate calculi. Ureteral calculi are associated with infection in only 8 percent of cases.

Hydration should be prescribed, since many patients with recurrent calculi are poor water drinkers and an adequate intake of fluids can prevent, or even result in the dissolution of, stones. The patient classified as a "chronic stone former" should imbibe 4,000 ml of fluid daily.

Urinary pH should be adjusted to favor solution of the components of the stone involved. This requires analysis of the calculus, since adjusting the pH of the urine in the wrong direction may be harmful. Uric acid and cystine stones form only in an acid urine. Changing the pH from 5 to 8 leads to a sixfold increase in the solubility of these substances in urine. This alkalinization may be accomplished by taking 1 tsp of sodium bicarbonate three to four times daily. Potassium citrate may also be used, and the alkalinity of the urine can be assessed by the patient with pH paper. Forty percent of uric acid stones dissolve when an alkaline urine is maintained. Calcium phosphate and magnesium-ammonium phosphate calculi are solubilized in an acid urine. Three to six grams daily of potassium acid phosphate are sufficient to acidify the urine, and the administration of the phosphate ion is also useful in binding calcium within the intestine and in reducing excretion in the urine. When urinary infection is present, the urea-splitting organisms may lead to the formation of ammonia and an intensely alkaline urine. This situation is difficult to handle with acid salts alone and requires active treatment of the infection. As the solubility of oxalate salts in the urine is not pH-dependent, manipulation of urinary pH is not useful for this variety.

Diet regulation is particularly pertinent for certain calculi. A low-protein diet plus anabolic agents is useful in decreasing the quantity of uric acid excreted in the urine. However, adjusting the urinary pH may be more successful and better tolerated. A diet which minimizes the amounts of amino acids containing sulfur may reduce the quantity of cystine excreted in the urine. The administration of penicillamine is also directed toward the cystine calculi, since it leads to the excretion of more soluble conjugates. Pyridoxine (vitamin B_6) has been prescribed to prevent an excess excretion of oxalate in the urine, but the evidence has not been convincing. Diets low in oxalate are available. However, oxalate stones are not necessarily associated with an excess excretion in the urine. For calcium-containing stones, a low-calcium diet which excludes dairy products can be combined with urinary acidifiers and chelating agents. Thiazides also decrease the urinary calcium excretion.

Treatment of acute gout with uricosuric agents may lead to uric acid calculi. Allopurinol, 0.1 Gm three times a day, reduces uric acid production, which lowers serum uric acid without dangers of urinary calculus.

HYPERPARATHYROIDISM. Eighty-four percent of patients with hyperparathyroidism (see Chap. 38) present with renal calculi or nephrocalcinosis, thus making the disease an important urologic consideration. The incidence of hyperparathyroidism among chronic stone formers varies considerably from one report to another. It may be as low as 1 percent and as high as 15 percent of the patients with recurrent renal calculi. The urinary symptoms include polydipsia, polyuria, recurrent renal colic due to calculi, and symptoms of hypertension. In patients with multiple recurrent urinary calculi the serum should be investigated for increased calcium ion and alkaline phosphatase and decreased phosphorus. Treatment consists of surgical removal of the hyperfunctioning parathyroid tissue followed by treatment of the urinary pathologic condition. In untreated patients, a renal death is common.

RENAL FAILURE

Renal failure is characterized by increased blood levels of certain products of metabolism normally excreted in the urine. These include urea, creatinine, potassium, phosphates, phenols, and aromatic oxyacids. The syndrome which accompanies this state has often been called "uremia," though properly this term refers only to an elevated level of blood urea. Since some of the metabolic end products are toxic in high concentrations, a series of symptoms develop. Mental confusion, restlessness, headache, fatigue, muscular twitching, convulsions, anorexia, nausea and vomiting, constipation changing to diarrhea, Kussmaul's breathing, pale dry yellowish skin, pruritis, anemia, anasarca, gastrointestinal bleeding, epistaxis, and heart failure may all be present in varying combinations. Although the specific factors responsible for some of these symptoms are known, the exact etiology of others remains in doubt.

Acute Failure

Acute renal failure is usually accompanied by an oliguria of less than 20 ml/hour or complete anuria. The blood metabolite level may become rapidly elevated, because acute renal failure often arises in association with several catabolic states. The acute changes in these metabolites are less well tolerated than the gradual changes which accompany chronic renal failure. One of the most common causes of oliguria and renal failure is decreased renal blood flow. Congestive heart failure, acute hypovolemia due to blood loss, severe dehydration, circulatory failure in association with overwhelming sepsis, marked fluid and electrolyte loss from the gastrointestinal tract associated with vomiting or diarrhea, tubular or cortical necrosis, nephritis, poisoning, and collagen diseases involving the kidney may all result in oliguria. Complete anuria usually indicates total ureteral or urethral obstruction or bilateral renal artery occlusion. Whenever anuria is present and the patient is not in clinical shock, obstruction should be suspected. The patients in clinical shock with a systolic blood pressure of less than 80 mm Hg cannot be expected to excrete much urine, and no further diagnostic studies are indicated until the hypovolemic shock is adequately treated. When a decreased renal blood flow is present, the urine proceeds through the renal tubule at a slow rate, so that reabsorption of electrolytes and water tends to produce a small volume with a high specific gravity and a low sodium concentration. Characteristically, the urine osmolarity exceeds that of plasma by a factor of two or three times. The urine sodium is usually less than 20 mEq/L.

In toxic nephropathies, the urine osmolarity is similar to that of plasma, and the urinary sodium exceeds 60 mEq/L. The differentiation of tubular necrosis from decreased renal blood flow and dehydration can also be elucidated by means of the PSP test with an indwelling catheter. The patient with marked oliguria and a urinary output of only 10 to 15 ml/hour will still excrete a significant amount of PSP if the oliguria is secondary to decreased renal blood flow but not if the primary lesion is acute tubular necrosis. Mannitol and water load (25 Gm of mannitol in 300 ml of fluid given intravenously over 30 minutes) will usually produce a diuresis if the patient has reduced renal blood flow or dehydration. In contrast, failure to respond to this infusion suggests acute tubular necrosis or toxic nephropathy.

LABORATORY FINDINGS. The serum generally shows an elevation of urea nitrogen, creatinine, phosphorus, and potassium levels, and a reduction in carbon dioxide, sodium chloride, and calcium. Prerenal azotemia is usually accompanied by an elevation of the serum urea nitrogen level combined with a normal serum creatinine level (Fig. 40-14). Dehydration, gastrointestinal bleeding, and catabolic processes associated with the administration of tetracycline, corticosteroids, and thiazide diuretics may produce prerenal azotemia.

With acute tubular necrosis, the urine specific gravity is usually fixed at 1.007 to 1.010. This is referred to as "isothenuria," which indicates that the specific gravity of urine is similar to that of plasma. In this situation, urine also often demonstrates red cell casts, albumin, and, occasionally, sugar in the presence of tubular necrosis.

Incipient or high-output renal failure is frequently undetected when estimations of renal function are based primarily on "adequate urinary volume." A simple method of detection is to perform a spot check of urinary and blood urea in milligrams per milliliter. A ratio of 20 : 1 or greater suggests extrarenal azotemia, while a ratio of 10 : 1 is borderline failure. A ratio as low as 5 : 1 or less, even in the presence of normal urinary volume, is indicative of incipient failure, usually on the basis of acute tubular necrosis.

TREATMENT. The treatment of acute renal failure consists of maintaining the patient in the best possible state until the function of the kidney returns. Therapeutic measures are directed along three main lines: (1) reducing toxic protein moieties in the blood, (2) correcting electrolyte imbalance including hyperkalemia, hyponatremia, and acidosis, and (3) preventing fluid overload. The first is accomplished by reducing or stopping protein intake, reducing catabolism by treating infection and/or draining an abscess, correcting other tissue injury, the use of anticatabolic agents, the administration of hypertonic intravenous glucose to spare protein breakdown, and the application of dialysis to decrease the blood and tissue levels. During this period, the patient's caloric requirements can be satisfied by carbohydrates and fats.

The electrolyte management requires frequent measurements of serum levels and serial electrocardiograms. Electrolyte replacement during oliguria or anuria is best managed conservatively. If there is significant loss from gastric aspiration, equivalent amounts of chloride should be administered. Hyperkalemia necessitates early correction to avoid cardiac asystole. Acute hyperkalemia with characteristic spiking T waves on the electrocardiogram may be treated with the intravenous administration of 25% glucose and 1 unit of regular insulin for each 2 Gm of glucose. Forty to eighty milliequivalents of sodium bicarbonate rapidly given intravenously may also temporarily avert an impending cardiac crisis due to hyperkalemia. The elimination of potassium intake, the administration of sodium exchange resins (Kayexalate) orally (30 to 90 Gm in 15 to 45 ml of sorbitol to reduce the constipating effect) or rectally (200 to 500 ml of a 10% solution two to three times daily) results in temporary reduction of the serum potassium level, but this can be effected more directly with dialysis. Hypocalcemia in patients with oliguria may lead to tetany, especially when efforts are directed toward correction of acidosis. Therefore, calcium gluconate (0.5 to 1 Gm daily) should be administered intravenously with alkalinizing agents. In the digitalized patient, the administration of calcium gluconate may be dangerous, since the calcium ion potentiates the effect of digitalis on the myocardium.

Perhaps the foremost therapeutic measure in patients with acute renal failure is fluid restriction. Death from pulmonary edema and congestive failure is not an unusual circumstance. The daily fluid intake should be limited to 400 ml (600 ml insensible loss minus 200 ml of water gained through oxidation) plus replacement of any fluid loss from urine or gastrointestinal tract. If the patient is febrile or if the air temperature and humidity are high, replacement of fluids should be increased slightly. The most valuable single means for estimating fluid requirements is an accurate daily weight. The anticipated weight loss by the starving patient is $\frac{1}{2}$ to 1 lb/day.

Frequent dialysis during the period of renal shutdown represents the most effective treatment, especially when catabolism is marked. In reversible acute renal failure, the salvage rate with extracorporeal hemodialysis should exceed 50 percent.

When patients have been successfully sustained through the acute oliguric failure, a period of polyuria may ensue. Electrolyte losses during this stage may be dangerously high, since the kidney is temporarily incapable of reabsorbing sodium and potassium. Replacement of these anions is indicated. If the patient has been digitalized during acute renal failure, digitalis intoxication may result

Fig. 40-14. Prerenal azotemia due to gastrointestinal hemorrhage.

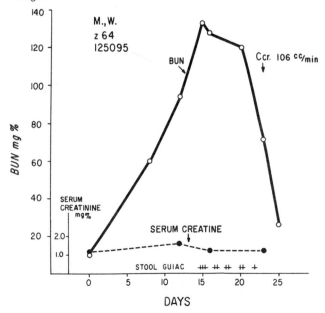

when serum potassium is reduced either during the polyuric phase or by dialysis. Digitalis intoxication should be prevented by using half the usual dose, removing potassium slowly, and replacing potassium losses during the polyuria.

Chronic Failure

Although complete recovery or death frequently occurs, acute renal failure may progress to chronic failure. Chronic failure may also be the end result of a variety of renal diseases including glomerulonephritis, pyelonephritis, nephrosclerosis, congenital polycystic disease, obstructive uropathy, primary hyperparathyroidism, vitamin D poisoning, gout, collagen diseases, vascular diseases, diabetic nephropathy, medullary necrosis, and various nephrotoxic poisons including phenacetin.

Diagnosis is suspected on the basis of clinical signs and symptoms and confirmed by laboratory evaluation. Since progressive uremia is often well tolerated, the urea level may be higher than the patient's condition indicates. The presence of anemia and acidosis is reflected clinically in a patient's ease of fatigability. Hyponatremia, which leads to further reduction in the glomerular filtration rate, may result from the inability of the kidney to preserve sodium because of tubular damage. The diagnosis of salt depletion is based on examination of intake and sodium loss in urine rather than the serum sodium levels.

Treatment of chronic renal failure includes the same modalities mentioned above for acute failure. Urinary infections must be eradicated and intercurrent infections promptly recognized and treated. Drugs which are excreted by the kidney should be administered in reduced doses, but penicillin may be given in usual doses to patients with oliguria and in half doses when complete anuria is present. Tetracycline and streptomycin, which are excreted predominantly by the kidney, should be given in usual doses at intervals of 2 to 4 days rather than daily. Chloramphenicol, which is detoxified by the liver, may be administered in usual doses over short periods of time. Kanamycin is given in half the usual dose with oliguria, and if anuria is present, this should be administered every 3 days rather than daily. Colistin can be given at the rate of half the usual dose every 2 days in oliguria and every 5 days in anuria. Aminoglycosides must also be given in altered dosage in the presence of renal failure.

Correction of acidosis by oral sodium bicarbonate or citrate therapy often gives marked symptomatic relief. However, increasing the serum pH decreases the ionizable calcium and may result in hypocalcemic tetany. In this circumstance, parenteral calcium gluconate or oral calcium lactate can be used, while calcium chloride is contraindicated.

A high-carbohydrate, low-protein ($\frac{1}{2}$ Gm/kg of body weight daily), low-potassium (less than 15 mEq/L), low-sodium (200 to 500 mg) diet is applicable to prevent tissue catabolism and electrolyte imbalance. Norethandrolone (50 mg three times daily), an anabolic agent, may also have a protein-sparing effect.

Accurate daily weights are valuable for determining the optimal amount of water to be taken daily. A gain of weight denotes an excess intake and may presage pulmonary edema. Optimal urinary volume may be ascertained by gradually increasing fluid intake in these patients. Sodium intake must be reduced to control water metabolism unless the patient has a salt-losing nephropathy with normal or increased volumes of urine. Under these circumstances, large amounts of sodium bicarbonate may be required.

Chronic dialysis and renal homotransplantation are therapeutic modalities available at certain medical centers. They are discussed in Chap. 10. Increasing experience with these methods establishes their merit for relatively stable uremic patients. Periodic dialysis may support the patient through episodes of intercurrent infection associated with diarrhea and vomiting which cause a temporary exacerbation of the uremic state. Peritoneal dialysis or extracorporeal dialysis may reverse the course in such patients for a period of time. Dialysis also may be helpful in preparing the patient with obstructive uropathy for supravesical diversionary surgical treatment.

PEDIATRIC UROLOGY

Both congenital abnormalities of the urinary tract and tumors in children demand prompt and thorough investigation because of their significant incidence and consequences. The genitourinary system should be evaluated in all instances of "failure to thrive" syndrome, undiagnosed febrile illnesses, externally apparent congenital anomalies, and abdominal masses. Sixty-seven percent of surgically correctable abdominal masses in children involve the adrenals or kidneys. Wilms' tumor of the kidney and neuroblastoma of the adrenal are the most common solid tumors in children and are of equal prevalence. Hydronephrosis constitutes 40 percent of renal masses.

Wilms' Tumor (Adenomyosarcoma)

Neoplastic degeneration of embryonal rests has been implicated in the evolution of this tumor. The lesion is often present at birth and frequently becomes clinically recognizable when the patient is under the age of two. The patients most commonly present with a unilateral flank mass recognized by the parent. Hematuria, weight loss, and pain are unusual manifestations and occur late in the course of the disease. On examination, the flank mass is firm and nontender. The blood pressure may be elevated because of renal artery compression, and the urine is usually negative.

Abdominal radiograms show displacement of the intestinal gas shadows and obliteration of the psoas shadow on the side of the lesion. Chest films may demonstrate spherical densities of metastases. Excretory urography is frequently difficult to interpret because of the small rim of displaced functioning renal tissue, which visualizes poorly. In general, since the renal tumor is focal and protrudes from the kidney, some portion of normal kidney is usually visualized (Fig. 40-15). When the tumor invades the renal

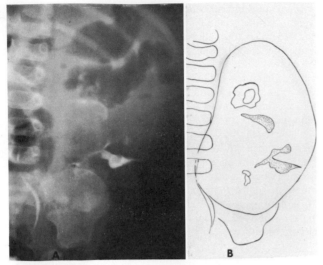

Fig. 40-15. Wilms' tumor of the left kidney in a one-year-old male deforming calyces of the left kidney and displacing left abdominal gas shadows.

vein causing occlusion, the kidney on the side of the lesion may not be visualized by intravenous pyelogram. In this circumstance, a retrograde pyelogram should establish the diagnosis. Five percent of Wilms' tumors are bilateral, and it is important preoperatively to estimate the function of the apparently uninvolved kidney.

Differential diagnosis includes adrenal neuroblastoma, hydronephrosis, and renal cystic disease. Neuroblastoma is usually more medial in location. It frequently displaces but does not deform the adjacent kidney, and interstitial calcification may be noted on x-ray. Hydronephrosis with nonvisualization on the excretory pyelogram may be differentiated by retrograde pyelography. Renal cystic disease can be recognized on nephrotomograms or renal arteriograms, but these techniques are not usually required.

The treatment of Wilms' tumor usually consists of immediate transperitoneal surgical excision. This may be followed by postoperative radiation therapy or chemotherapy, or both. Postoperative chemotherapy consists of intravenous actinomycin D (15 μg/kg daily for 5 days). Radiation to the tumor bed (3000 r) is usually adequate when administered in conjunction with actinomycin. There is indication that cyclic courses of actinomycin may double the survival rate. Vincristine, used alone or in combination with actinomycin, has also proved to be a valuable chemotherapeutic adjunct.

The prognosis of Wilms' tumor is related to the patient's age. When the lesions are removed from children under the age of two, the survival rate is 73 percent, whereas over the age of two it is 18 percent according to Lattimer et al. The presence of metastases in lungs, bones, or at the site of surgical treatment is associated with an unfavorable prognosis, and both chemotherapy and radiation therapy are less effective in this situation. However, chemotherapy has been demonstrated to be of significant value in lengthening the survival of patients with proved metastatic Wilms' tumor.

Congenital Anomalies

PHIMOSIS (REDUNDANT PREPUCE) This condition predisposes to difficulty secondary to poor hygiene, infection, and carcinoma of the glans penis. Circumcision is usually performed during the neonatal period. If it is not performed at this time, it can be done when medically indicated or when requested electively by the patient or his family. Risk of anesthesia and psychologic implications should be considered in the selection of cases and timing of the operation.

MEATAL OR DISTAL URETHRAL STENOSIS. This is the most common cause of impaired voiding in children, occurring more frequently in girls. Boys may present with recognizable impairment of the urinary stream or distress during voiding. However, since the longer male urethra offers protection against secondary urinary infection, obstructive changes, such as enlargement of the bladder and ureteral dilatation, may result before the condition is suspected. In girls, urinary infection is a more frequent accompaniment of stenosis and leads to earlier appreciation of the pathologic condition. Girls commonly present with high fever related to pyelonephritis. Other symptoms include enuresis, urgency, diurnal incontinence, and urethral distress. Anorexia and weight loss may accompany chronic or recurrent infections.

The diagnosis is established with acorn-tipped bougies à boule under anesthesia. Insertion and, more particularly, withdrawal of the bougie is accompanied by a sensation of passage through a constriction. With a stenosis in the distal urethra or at the meatus the constricting fibromuscular ring can be visualized as the bougie is withdrawn. Urethral stenosis may also be recognized by a "hang." In the first two years of life a #14 French bougie should pass easily. Between the ages of two and six the normal female urethra should accept a #18, while from six to thirteen years of age a #22 French can be passed. Over the age of thirteen a #26 French should pass easily.

Cystourethroscopy may be indicated to disclose secondary consequences of urethral obstruction such as bladder trabeculation, diverticula, calculi, vesicoureteral incompetence (reflux), and any ureteral obstruction. Radiologic examination, such as voiding cystourethrograms and excretory urograms, are also helpful in establishing the degree of urethral obstruction and the presence of sequelae (Fig. 40-16). Voiding studies have definite limitations.

Treatment of urethral meatal stenosis is dependent upon the extent of secondary involvement. Uncomplicated cases will be satisfactorily treated by meatotomy or dilatations. Most patients with accompanying infection require continuation of antimicrobial treatment followed by suppressive therapy with sulfonamides or nitrofurantoin for 3 or more months. Growth and development are allies in the rehabilitation of pediatric urologic patients. Where morphologic abnormalities are recognized on initial evaluation, follow-up examinations are necessary to determine the course.

About 10 percent of girls with urethral obstruction either fail to respond to conservative therapy or have advanced secondary upper tract damage at the time the condition is recognized. In these cases, corrective procedures are necessary to prevent progressive damage to the kidneys. These are directed at reducing resistance to voiding, preventing reflux of urine (ureteral reimplantation), and diversion of the urine from poorly functioning excretory passages (nephrostomy, ureterostomy, or cutaneous ureteroileostomy). These are to be considered as lifesaving procedures, since they are associated with difficulties. In the female who has had surgical enlargement of the bladder neck (Y–V-plasty), urinary incontinence may develop following pregnancy. The male who has had bladder neck surgical treatment may experience infertility due to retrograde ejaculation. The patient who undergoes a ureterostomy or cutaneous ureteroileostomy requires a permanent appliance.

URETHRAL VALVES. Unlike distal urethral and meatal stenosis, these are more commonly seen in boys. The length of the male urethra serves as protection from secondary infection. The symptoms leading to diagnosis of membranous posterior urethral valves are related to uremia and hypertension. Diagnosis is made by voiding cystourethrography, which clearly depicts the site of obstruction. Dilatation of the proximal urethra and bladder is commonly noted, and marked hydroureteronephrosis is frequent. This advanced degree of secondary dilatation of the bladder, ureter, and calyces necessitates diversion of the urine. Operative excision of the urethral valves may not afford adequate treatment. Cutaneous pyeloileostomy, nephrostomy, or loop cutaneous ureterostomies may be required to bypass the tortuous dilated atonic ureters. Nephrostomy has the disadvantage of periodic need for tube changes and the constant threat of ascending infection. The prognosis for restoration of normal urinary function is dependent upon the degree of secondary changes in the proximal collecting system and the renal function at the time of diagnosis. Since males usually present with more advanced renal deterioration, their prognosis is usually less favorable.

NEUROGENIC BLADDER. This is usually due to autonomic dysfunction accompanying meningomyelocele. Impaired sensation of filling leads to a large residual urine with overflow incontinence. The patient may present with symptoms of infection, diurnal incontinence, or impaired voiding. Diagnosis is established by excretory urography, voiding cystourethrogram, and cystometry. The latter study reveals a large residual urine with low-pressure high-volume tracing and lack of sensation of filling until large volumes have been instilled. Treatment for mild dysfunction may be manual assistance in voiding, coupled with therapy for infection. With moderately severe involvement, treatment is directed at eliminating the residual urine. This may be accomplished by transurethral resection of the bladder neck. If the children are reminded to void at intervals of 2 hours, many become continent. Children may be taught intermittent catheterization when they reach six to eight years of age. For severely compromised urinary tracts with marked loss of renal function, urinary diversion may be indicated.

URETEROCELE. This is a consequence of a stenotic ureteral orifice. As the intravesical ureter dilates, it forms a cystic intravesical mass which may become sufficiently

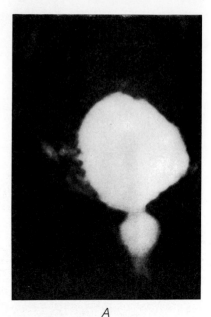

A

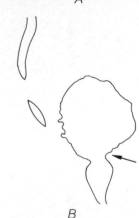

B

Fig. 40-16. Urethral stenosis. Voiding cystourethrogram in distal urethral stenosis. Proximal urethra is markedly dilated. The bladder is irregularly trabeculated. Reflux of contrast is seen in the markedly dilated right ureter. Arrow in *B* indicates the bladder neck.

large to obstruct the bladder neck during voiding. Occasionally, the ureterocele prolapses through the urethra. Diagnosis is established by means of delayed films during intravenous pyelography (Fig. 40-17). The opaque-filled intravesical mass has a thin, nonopaque rim (the ureterocele wall) which contrasts with the opacity of the bladder content, giving the appearance of "cobra head deformity." Many ureteroceles cause sufficient ureteral obstruction to warrant surgical treatment. Small lesions may be removed by endoscopic incision or excision. Prolapsing ureteroceles with urethral obstruction require transvesical excision. In children, ureterocele is often associated with ureteral duplication.

HYDRONEPHROSIS. This is often the result of a congenital stenosis at the ureteropelvic junction. Although narrowing may not be severe, impaired passage of urine through this area leads to dilatation of the renal pelvis and

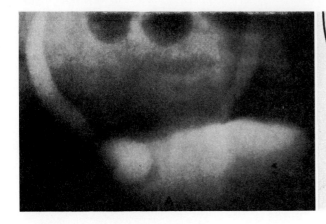

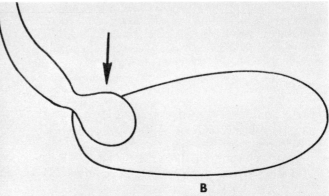

Fig. 40-17. Ureterocele. *A.* Excretory urogram of right ureterocele bulging into bladder. Ureter is obstructed and dilated. *B.* Ureterocele is indicated by arrow.

calyces (Fig. 40-18). Pressure atrophy results in severe loss of renal function. Patients most frequently complain of pain which, on occasion, may mimic the pain of appendicitis. Gastrointestinal symptoms such as nausea and vomiting are common. Abdominal mass represents another presenting finding. A familial history may be present. Diagnosis is established by means of excretory pyelography with delayed films demonstrating an impairment in renal excretion of contrast material. Pyeloplasty should be attempted whenever renal function is not too seriously compromised. With contralateral compensatory hypertrophy noted on the pyelogram, the pyeloplasty may not improve kidney function. Since there is a distinct tendency for hydronephrosis to be manifest on one side and incipient on the other, the patients should be followed with repeated pyelograms until they reach their maximal longitudinal growth in order to determine the presence of progression in the less involved kidney.

CONGENITAL NONOBSTRUCTIVE RENAL DISEASE. The disease may be suspected when kidneys fail to be visualized on intravenous pyelography and the BUN is normal. Congenital or neonatal glomerular disease, which represents a histologic diagnosis, is usually fatal. Cystic disease

Fig. 40-18. Hydronephrosis. This was due to intrinsic ureteral stenosis indicated by arrow in *B.*

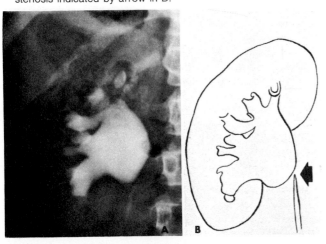

of the kidney has a broad spectrum. The collecting ducts may be ectatic, as in *medullary cystic disease.* There may be failure of communication between tubules and glomeruli, as in *polycystic disease.* Failure of development of the metanephric blastema accounts for *nonfunctioning multicystic renal disease.* Clinically recognizable *simple renal cysts* are infrequently seen in children. Failure to visualize the kidneys on intravenous pyelography in any of these disease states is indication for retrograde pyelography to assess long-term prognosis.

CRYPTORCHIDISM (UNDESCENDED TESTIS). This is the result of a congenital arrest of testicular descent. About 4 percent of full-term infant males have undescended testes at birth. Twenty-one percent of premature males have undescended testes. If the testis fails to reach a scrotal position within 6 weeks (3 months for the premature), it rarely descends in later life. When the testis lies in a position other than the normal scrotal location, it is subjected to a 2.5° increase in temperature, which is injurious to the seminiferous tubules. The normal testis may begin to show active differentiation of the spermatocytic series when the patient is five years old. This does not occur in the cryptorchid. With bilateral cryptorchidism, which is present in 24 percent of the cases, spermatogenesis never develops, and the individual is infertile. After the age of fourteen, the undescended testis may be damaged beyond recovery. Testicular tumors are more common in undescended testes. These tumors occur fifty times more frequently in the abdominal testis and eleven times more often in the inguinal testis than in the normally located organs. Following orchiopexy the tendency to neoplasm is not altered, but examination is more feasible. Orchiopexy should be performed prior to puberty, and it is an advantage to operate before the patient is of school age. Ninety percent of undescended testes are associated with indirect inguinal hernia, and simultaneous repair of the defect should be performed. Nonsurgical treatment with chorionic gonadotropin is occasionally effective but does nothing for the associated hernia.

HYPOSPADIAS. This is the most frequent fusion defect of the urethra. It occurs in approximately 1 of 900 pediatric hospital admissions. The abnormality consists of a dorsal hood (absent ventral foreskin), chordee (ventral curvature of the glans penis on the shaft), and proximal location of the urethral meatus. The urethral meatus may be located anywhere from the coronary sulcus to the perineum but is more frequently distal. Multiple urethral orifices may be present, but only one communicates with the urethra per se.

Hypospadias results in an abnormal urinary stream. The downward deformity of the glans penis causes the urine issuing from the urethral meatus to be deflected. Infertility is frequently associated with a scrotal or perineal meatus. Hypospadias with urethral meatus in the scrotal area is often accompanied by bilateral undescended testes and must be differentiated from adrenogenital syndrome and pseudohermaphroditism. Before performing urethroplasty on such a patient, determination of the genetic sex by karyotyping and adrenal function by determination of 17-oxysteroids and 17-ketosteroids is indicated. Visualization of the lower urinary tract by means of retrograde opaque studies may disclose the presence of a vagina and abdominal exploration may reveal that the child's sex organs are more female than male, in which case excision of the hypertrophied clitoris should be performed.

Treatment of hypospadias may be by staged operations. First the chordee is corrected, and then the urethra is reconstructed. In some cases, stenosis of the original urethral meatus may require meatotomy before the definitive operations are undertaken. One-stage hypospadias repairs are also performed, with simultaneous chordee repair and urethroplasty. Postoperative urethral fistula formation may require further surgical correction. A minimum period of 6 months should be allowed for adequate healing between stages or before a fistula is excised. (See Chap. 51.)

EPISPADIAS. A dorsally cleft urethra is only one-fifth as common as hypospadias. It is the consequence of failure of dorsal fusion and in its most marked form involves the urethral sphincter and may be associated with urinary incontinence. Surgical repair is indicated.

EXSTROPHY OF THE BLADDER. This represents an extremely rare advanced stage of epispadias. Although techniques have been devised to reconstruct the bladder, function is seldom normal. Therefore, a supravesical diversion of urine by cutaneous ureteroileostomy or ureterosigmoidostomy and cystectomy is advisable. The urethra can be reconstructed in the male to permit siring of offspring.

ECTOPIC URETERAL ORIFICE. The ectopic ureteral orifice usually drains the upper part of a double kidney, with complete duplication of the ureters. The condition is four times more prevalent in females. In order to be manifest symptomatically, the ectopic ureteral orifice must empty outside the urethral sphincter in the urethra or vagina. The characteristic complaint is of urinary incontinence despite normal voiding habits. The ureteral segment drained by the ectopic ureter is frequently severely hydroephrotic and may not be visualized on the excretory pyelogram (Fig. 40-6). Treatment is excision of the upper renal segment and ureter in most instances, but at times it is possible to reimplant the ureter into the bladder.

ENURESIS. Nocturnal loss of urine is normal until the age of three. After that age a normal child may occasionally wet the bed. Habitual bed wetting after the age of three may be associated with organic lesions of the bladder or urethra; the presence of additional urinary symptoms suggests such a lesion, and investigation is indicated before ascribing the enuresis to psychogenic factors.

NEOPLASMS

Renal Tumors

INCIDENCE AND ETIOLOGY. Renal tumors account for approximately 3 percent of cancer deaths. The frequency in males is twice that in females. The histologic origin of most carcinomas in males is probably from the renal tubular cell. Experimentally, renal tumors occur in male hamsters treated with estrogens. A virus has been implicated as the cause of the Lücke renal adenocarcinoma in frogs. The intrarenal injection of zinc chloride or Thorotrast has also been observed to produce renal tumors in animals. None of these factors has been implicated in the formation of human renal tumors, and the cause remains unknown.

PATHOLOGY. There are three major types of malignant tumors of the renal parenchyma. The foamy or granular cell carcinoma and tubular adenocarcinomas constitute 60 percent. Wilms' tumor (adenomyosarcoma), which characteristically occurs in children, accounts for 14 percent. Renal sarcoma, originating from the interstitial renal tissue, the renal capsule, and blood vessels, is defined in 6 percent while tumors of the collecting system constitute 14 percent of the total. Benign renal tumors (adenomas) are frequent postmortem findings but are not commonly associated with clinical manifestations.

CLINICAL MANIFESTATIONS. The classic triad of pain, mass, and hematuria occurs late and is seen in its entirety in less than half the patients. Marked variations in the prevalence of these symptoms have been noted in reported series: gross hematuria, 31 to 76 percent; pain, 24 to 75 percent; mass, 6 to 50 percent; fever, 16 percent; metastatic pain, 6 percent. Hematuria is a late manifestation which represents erosion of the tumor into the collecting system. A palpable mass is more frequently present if the tumor involves the lower pole of the right kidney. Pain has been related to the stretching of the renal capsule, in which instance it is usually mild but persistent. Sudden severe flank pain may accompany bleeding into the tumor. The passage of blood clots mimics colic from a ureteral stone. Fever is probably caused by necrosis of a tumor. Although adult parenchymal tumors are usually not associated with hypertension, this is a frequent accompaniment of Wilms' tumor. Hypertension has been related to compression of the renal artery with resultant renal ischemia.

Utz described an interesting group of 27 patients with hepatosplenomegaly and renal tumors. They presented with fatigue, anemia, and fever but had no pain, mass, or hematuria. The sedimentation rate exceeded 100 mm/hour, and the prothrombin time, α-2-globulin, alkaline phosphatase, and Bromsulphalein retention were all increased. Both the hepatosplenomegaly and laboratory

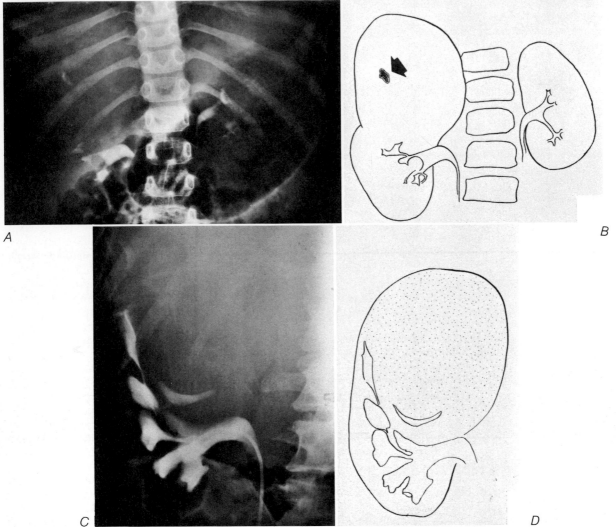

Fig. 40-19. Renal tumor. *A* and *B*. Right upper pole renal cell carcinoma (hypernephroma) deforms calyces on excretory urogram. Calcification is indicated by the arrow on *B*. *C* and *D*. Retrograde pyelogram of a large renal tumor (stippled on *D*) deforming upper calyces.

abnormalities reverted to normal when the tumor was curatively excised. It is thought that the syndrome is caused by a glycoprotein present in the tumor. Erythrocytemia is present in 2 percent of cases with hypernephroma, which accounts for 7 percent of patients evaluated for polycythemia. Erythropoietin has been extracted from these renal tumors.

Despite the nature of the symptoms, the delay between onset and medical consultation has been long, averaging 23 months from the onset of hematuria and 14 months from the onset of pain in one series. Metastases were demonstrated in 37 percent of patients at the time of diagnosis and included involvement of the hip, shoulder, back, and lungs. Skull metastases simulating sebaceous cyst are not uncommon.

DIAGNOSIS. Excretory pyelography is frequently diagnostic. Since the renal tumor is focal, the uninvolved portion of the kidney is usually visualized. The exception to this rule is the presence of renal vein occlusion. Charac-

teristically, there is enlargement of the renal silhouette with deformity of the calyces in the area of the mass (Fig. 40-19). On early films, the renal neoplasm opacifies because of vascularity of the tumor. This may distinguish an opacifying tumor from a nonopacifying cyst (Fig. 40-20). Approximately 30 percent of renal lesions are neoplasms, while 58 percent are cysts and 12 percent represent polycystic disease (Fig. 40-21). Nephrotomography is helpful in differentiating cyst from tumor. While tumors usually opacify, with hemorrhage or necrosis the opacification may be impaired and a false diagnosis of cyst made. The presence of calcium at the edge of the mass is more suggestive of tumor than cyst, with the exception of the echinococcal renal cyst. Ultrasonography is helpful in the differentiation between cystic and solid tumors. Percutaneous cyst aspira-

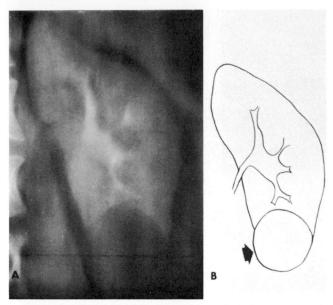

Fig. 40-20. Renal cyst. Nephrotomogram disclosing a nonopacifying lower pole cyst indicated by arrow on *B*.

rate for renal tumors without metastases is about 50 percent for 5 years and 33 percent for 10 years.

CARCINOMA OF THE RENAL PELVIS

Tumors of the renal pelvis constitute 14 percent of kidney tumors. Half of these are epidermoid and have been associated with infection or calculus-induced metaplasia of the transitional epithelium of the pelvis. The associated infection or calculus frequently masks the tumor. The patients characteristically have no gross hematuria, flank pain, or mass and frequently present with a resistant urinary infection and markedly reduced function noted on

Fig. 40-21. Polycystic disease. Excretory urogram of a nineteen-year-old girl with congenital polycystic renal disease. Huge left kidney shows classic deformity of calyces and elongation of infundibula by multiple cysts.

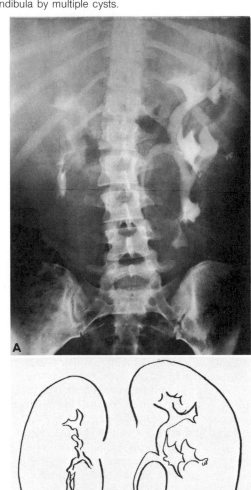

tion with analysis of the fluid extracted and instillation of contrast material may offer a definitive diagnosis. Renal arteriography (Fig. 40-22) is indicated for solid lesions, followed by vena cavagraphy (Fig. 40-23) for evaluation of venous involvement. Computed tomography may prove valuable in determining the nature and extent of a kidney lesion (Fig. 40-24). Metastatic series, including chest films and isotopic scans, should be routine for the evaluation of patients with suspected malignant disease (Figs. 40-25 and 40-26).

Abnormalities in serum electrolytes or proteins are rarely noted. If the total renal function is compromised, preoperative evaluation of the uninvolved kidney's function is imperative. The individual renal creatinine clearances and isotopic perfusion studies will aid in the assessment of the situation prior to therapy.

TREATMENT. In some instances it is necessary to explore the renal fossa. The operative approach to renal tumor may be through the flank, chest, or abdomen. Removal of the perinephric fat with the kidney provides the best margin. Early ligation of the renal vessels minimizes venous tumor spread and blood loss. Preoperative radiation therapy and chemotherapy are rarely prescribed, but postoperative radiation may be of some benefit when adequate local resection is compromised. Removal of primary renal tumor has been observed to be followed by regression of metastases in lung and bone. Also, in a few cases, resection of metastatic lesions in the lung or extremities has been associated with prolonged survival.

PROGNOSIS. This depends on the histologic type, the presence of local extension into the renal vein, perinephric tissues, or lymph nodes, and distant metastases. For patients with low-grade local lesions, the survival rate equals the actuarial life expectancy. The overall survival

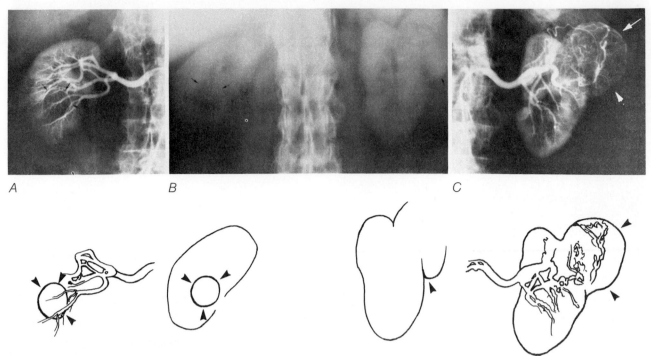

Fig. 40-22. Renal neoplasm and renal cyst. *A.* Selective right renal arteriogram showing avascular lesion which, on needle aspiration, proved to be cyst. *B.* Nephrotomogram showing right renal cyst and left upper pole renal carcinoma. *C.* Selective left renal arteriogram demonstrating vascular renal neoplasm. Diagrams below demonstrate the pathology.

intravenous pyelography. Ureteral urinary cytology may demonstrate epithelial pearls. The treatment for squamous carcinoma is surgical excision, but the prognosis is exceedingly poor because of late diagnosis. Adjuvant radiation therapy and chemotherapy are ineffective.

Transitional cell tumors of the renal pelvis and ureter are histologically similar to the vesical counterparts. They occur more frequently in the male and are seldom seen in patients under the age of fifty. Gross hematuria and renal colic due to the passage of blood clots are common presenting symptoms. Lesions usually become manifest before a tumor is palpable. Intravenous pyelography frequently establishes the diagnosis, showing a filling defect in the portion of the pelvis or ureter (Fig. 40-27). Differential diagnosis of the filling defects include blood clot and nonopaque (uric acid) calculi. Urine obtained by ureteral catheter lavage or brushing may demonstrate clusters of transitional cells. Transitional cell tumors of the pelvis tend to be multiple, and frequently there are ureteral implants involving the distal ureter or the bladder. Treatment therefore consists of removing the kidney, the ureter, and a margin of the bladder around the ureteral orifice. The prognosis for survival is markedly reduced when the tumor infiltrates the adjacent parenchyma. Postoperative radiation therapy and chemotherapy have not been demonstrated to be of value in improving the statistics.

Tumors of the Urinary Bladder

INCIDENCE AND ETIOLOGY. Although tumors of the bladder cause only 3 percent of all cancer deaths, the estimated incidence in the general population is 0.02 percent. The peak age incidence is fifty to seventy years of age.

In 1978, the estimated number of deaths from cancer of the bladder was reported as 6,900 for men and 3,000 for women.

Papillary bladder tumors have been related to the inadvertent ingestion of chemicals which are excreted in the urine as conjugated orthoaminophenols. These include beta-naphthylamine and para-aminobiphenyl. Prolonged periods of exposure are apparently necessary. Certain carcinogenic tryptophan metabolites are present in higher concentrations in the urine of patients with recurring bladder tumors. Tobacco tar applied to the oral mucosa in mice produces vesical papillomas, and there appears to be a prevalence of heavy cigarette smokers among the group with bladder tumors. Chronic infection with schistosomiasis and mechanical trauma due to calculus may cause metaplasia and neoplasia of the bladder epithelium.

CLINICAL MANIFESTATIONS. The patients usually present with gross painless hematuria secondary to partial infarction of a tumor. Hematuria is the initial symptom in 75 percent of cases and is present in 95 percent of cases at the time of diagnosis. Frequency and painful urination are late symptoms which result from sloughing of the tumor and secondary infection.

The physical findings in early cases are minimal, since the tumor remains within the confines of the bladder. Metastases and local extension occur quite late in the course of disease; in one series at the time of death 80 percent of the tumors were confined to the bladder. In

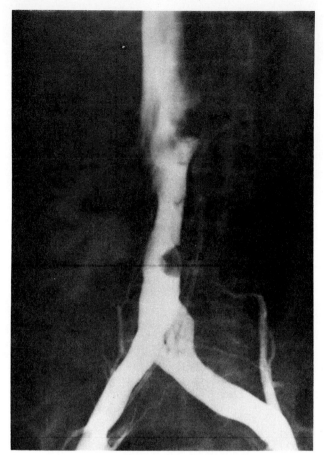

Fig. 40-23. Tumor involvement of vena cava. *A.* Renal vein tumor extending into lumen of vena cava. *B.* Direct extension of renal tumor into vena cava.

untreated cases, the neoplasm may occlude the ureter and lead to uremia. Local extension of the tumor may result in a stony nodular induration at the base of the bladder with fixation to the wall of the pelvis. Lymphatic spread may involve the pelvic and periaortic nodes. Osseous lesions are usually osteolytic and may cause nerve root pain.

Laboratory studies may be normal in early cases but may reveal anemia and uremia in late cases. Urinalysis usually demonstrates red blood cells. White blood cells are seen at times if there is associated infection and necrosis, and clusters of abnormal transitional cells may occasionally be identified. Tumor biopsies provide tissue for histologic diagnosis, and deeper biopsies offer information regarding depth of penetration (staging).

TREATMENT AND PROGNOSIS. Endoscopic resection and electrodesiccation are suitable for superficial small tumors. Many patients have survived for prolonged periods of time with recurring superficial bladder tumors requiring periodic endoscopic treatment. Others demonstrate more rapid recurrences with change toward anaplastic and invasive characteristics. The most satisfactory treatment for locally invasive, resectable carcinoma of the bladder is preoperative radiation therapy followed by cystectomy,

with supravesical diversion of the urine by means of the cutaneous ureteroileostomy (ileal loop) or cutaneous ureterocolostomy (colon loop). Experience with combinations of chemotherapeutic agents and radiation therapy followed by cystectomy has not demonstrated improved survival.

For patients with nonresectable disease, urinary diversion may relieve frequency and reduce hemorrhage. Palliative radiation therapy may also reduce the bleeding. No systemic chemotherapeutic agent warrants enthusiastic recommendation. Thiotepa instilled at weekly intervals for a month has destroyed superficial tumors. The prognosis of bladder tumor depends on the nature and extent of the tumor. When there is no invasion of muscle, the 5-year survival is 77 percent. With deep invasion of the muscle, 5-year survival is less than 10 percent.

Fig. 42-24. *A.* Computed tomography demonstrating cyst of the left renal pelvis. *B.* Diagram for orientation.

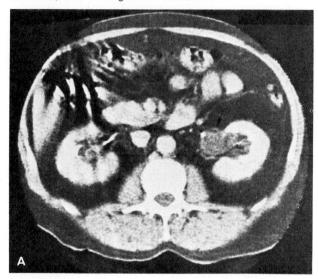

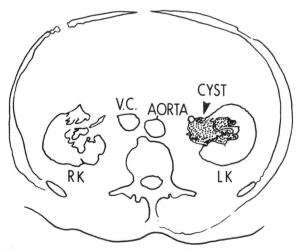

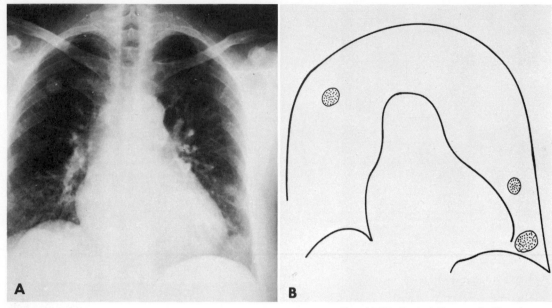

Fig. 40-25. Typical "cannonball" pulmonary metastases from renal carcinoma.

Prostatic Tumors

BENIGN PROSTATIC HYPERTROPHY

INCIDENCE AND ETIOLOGY. Benign prostatic hypertrophy is a benign tumor, adenoleiomyofibromatosis, which originates from the periurethral tissues. The lesion is rare before the age of forty and does not occur in eunuchs. After the age of forty, 55 percent of males manifest typical lesions histologically, and after the age of eighty, 75 percent of males are so affected. However, Chinese males living in their native land have an incidence of only 6 percent after the age of forty.

CLINICAL MANIFESTATIONS. The symptoms are related to mechanical obstruction. Although the initial symptoms consisting of diminished forcefulness and projection of the stream may be apparent, the onset of obstruction is usually so insidious that most patients are unaware of difficulty until it becomes more pronounced. Nocturia is a frequent symptom and is usually due to residual urine, but in the early stages the bladder capacity may be functionally reduced because of compensatory detrusor hypertrophy. Hematuria may result from straining to void. However,

Fig. 40-26. Typical osteolytic metastasis to the calvarium from clear cell renal carcinoma (hypernephroma).

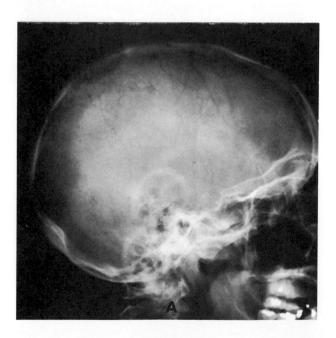

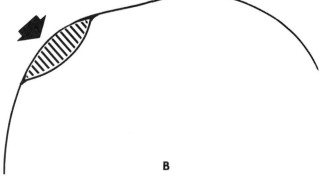

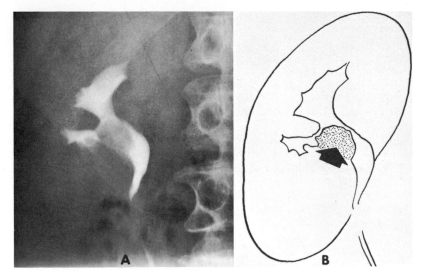

Fig. 40-27. Carcinoma of renal pelvis. *A.* Excretory urogram pyelogram showing a filling defect in the renal pelvis due to papillary carcinoma. *B.* Tumor is indicated by arrow.

other causes of hematuria such as bladder tumor and vesical calculus should be excluded cystoscopically before a prostatic cause is accepted. Acute retention of urine is the ultimate consequence of detrusor decompensation and frequently is the symptom for which the patient first seeks medical assistance.

On examination, 90 percent of patients demonstrate a smooth symmetrical enlargement of the prostate which has the consistency of the thenar eminence. Ten percent of the patients with intravesical enlargement or median bar prostatic hypertrophy have a normal gland on rectal examination. A palpable percussible bladder is indicative of retention of urine. Presence of bilateral direct inguinal hernia and/or external hemorrhoids of recent origin is often an indication of the degree of straining that the patient has experienced to pass his urine. Observation of the urinary stream will evaluate the degree of difficulty. A self-activating flowmeter may be used to estimate the degree of obstruction. Normally, when more than 200 ml is voided, the flow rate will be 20 ml/second. In patients with prostatic obstruction, rates of less than 5 ml/second are common. Cytoscopic and roentgenographic evidences of benign prostatic hypertrophy include trabeculation and thickening of the bladder wall, formation of pulsion diverticula (Fig. 40-28), vesical calculi, ureteral dilatation, hydronephrosis, and a smooth filling defect (the prostate) at the base of the bladder on films made with the patient upright.

RESIDUAL URINE. The amount of residual urine may be determined directly by catheterization or by indirect methods. Following voiding, the bladder is normally empty except for a few drops of urine. A postvoiding film after an intravenous pyelogram may also determine the presence of residual urine.

The mechanism of prostatic obstruction includes functional reduction in the cross-sectional area of the prostatic urethra, attenuation of the muscle fibers which normally open the vesical neck, decreased mechanical advantage of these muscles by virtue of a longer course overlying the adenoma, and increased tissue resistance to opening of the vesical outlet.

Residual urine is the result of stretching of the detrusor muscle when the ability of the bladder to compensate and expel urine against an increased resistance is exceeded. As the degree of obstruction reduces the flow rate with maximal bladder pressures, the percent of bladder volume emptied with each voiding decreases. Thus, the residual urine volume increases. The formation of vesical diverticula and vesicoureteral reflux, which are consequences of the obstructive uropathy, also increase the amount of residual urine. The functionally reduced bladder capacity becomes manifest by the need for multiple voiding, particularly early in the morning. The patient soon learns that it is wiser to void when the need first becomes apparent, since procrastination compounds the difficulty. The patient

Fig. 40-28. Vesical diverticulum. Cystogram showing a large vesical diverticulum (arrow), an important cause of residual urine and persistent infection associated with prostatic hypertrophy.

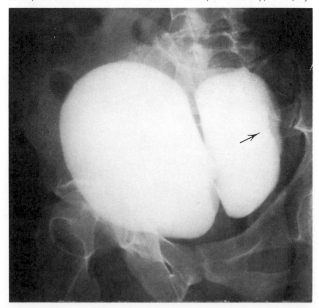

with residual urine secondary to benign prostatic hypertrophy is always in danger of acute retention if he defers urination until the bladder is so distended that a detrusor contraction cannot be initiated. The diuretic and analgesic responses to alcohol and the effects of anesthesia and of anticholinergic and sympathomimetic drugs also increase the likelihood of acute retention.

The presence of residual urine favors formation of vesical calculi (Fig. 40-29). These may be associated with sharp twinges of pain, the "curbstone" symptom, when the patient descends a stairway or steps down from the curb. This is related to the calculi bouncing on the trigone. Following voiding, the patient may have severe strangury and terminal gross hematuria. Residual urine also predisposes to infection. The normally functioning bladder is capable of eliminating a heavy inoculum of bacteria, while the obstructed bladder remains infected.

TREATMENT. The patient who is a good operative risk with a reasonable life expectancy is best treated by prostatectomy. However, circumstances may dictate a nonsurgical or an altered surgical management. Patients with significant residual urine but without compromised renal function can often be managed without an indwelling catheter. Specific treatment of infection followed by long-term suppressive therapy with mandelic acid or nitrofurantoin is indicated. The patient should be instructed to avoid overdistension of the bladder and to void at the first indication of need. Caution against long automobile trips and ingestion of alcoholic beverages, anticholinergic medications, and diuretics is indicated. Hot tub baths and prostatic massages effect symptomatic relief.

Fig. 40-29. Vesical calculus secondary to long-standing benign prostatic hypertrophy. Note intravesical intrusion of huge middle lobe.

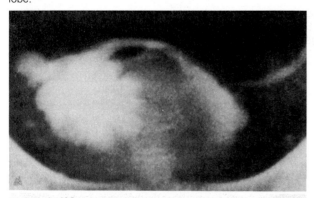

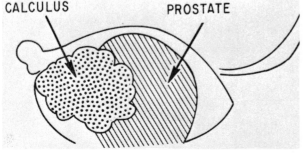

CALCULUS   PROSTATE

The patient with compromised renal function can be managed with an indwelling retention catheter, but if prolonged treatment is anticipated, bilateral partial vasectomy to prevent descending epididymitis should be performed. Patients who fail to tolerate the urethral catheter may be more comfortable with a suprapubic cystostomy performed under local or regional anesthesia. In either situation, the catheter care outlined previously should be adhered to. A leg bag for collection is convenient while the patient ambulates, whereas a floor bottle is preferred for night collection.

The indications for surgical intervention include significant residual urine, difficulty in voiding, and annoying frequency and nocturia, as well as the secondary effects of obstruction such as vesical diverticula, calculi, hydroureteronephrosis, and persistent infection. Presence of benign prostatic hypertrophy per se and symptoms of prostatitis do not constitute indications. As the size of the adenomatous mass increases, the normal prostate is compressed into a 0.5-cm-thick surgical capsule. This portion remains after simple prostatectomy for benign prostatic hypertrophy. Although it is appreciated that carcinoma of the prostate may subsequently arise in the remaining gland, simple prostatectomy is most appropriate, since it is attended by a low morbidity and mortality, and secondary recurrences and neoplasms are infrequent.

Transurethral Prostatectomy. This is performed by application of a high-frequency current to a tungsten wire loop. Multiple fragments of the obstructive tissue are removed by successive cuts under direct endoscopic vision. Hemostasis is effected by sealing the vessels with the coagulating current. Because of low mortality and morbidity, transurethral resection is favored in the elderly patient. It represents an excellent operation for the young patient who values sexual potency. Transurethral resection is particularly adaptable to a median bar prostatic hypertrophy and the removal of small or inflamed glands which do not enucleate easily by the open route. The procedure can be combined with lithotripsy (crushing and removal of a vesical calculus). The technique is also applicable for the relief of urinary obstruction due to surgically incurable carcinoma of the prostate. Transurethral prostatectomy may be precluded by hip disease which interferes with the lithotomy position.

Open Prostatectomy. Whether performed through a suprapubic bladder incision, retropubically, or perineally, it employs similar techniques. Cleavage is developed with fingers or instruments so that the adenomas and attached prostatic urethra are removed. This leaves the entire prostatic cavity to reepithelialize from the bladder neck and urethral epithelium and from ducts of the acinar glands in the remaining surgical capsule. The transvesical suprapubic approach is particularly applicable to the removal of large vesical diverticula and calculi. The retropubic approach is ideal for coping with inguinal hernia at the time of suprapubic prostatectomy.

Open prostatectomy is associated with a four times greater mortality rate than transurethral resection. This is related to the increased bleeding problems, wound healing, and urinary fistulae. The catheter drainage for open prostatectomy usually extends over 5 days, as compared with 2 to 3 days for transurethral prostatectomy. The attendant increase in the risk of ascending epididymitis makes bilateral prophylactic vasectomy at the time of open prostatectomy advisable. The postoperative stay with transurethral resection is usually 5 days in contrast to approximately 9 days for open prostatectomy.

With either approach, adequate drainage of the catheter and appropriate antibacterial agents are indicated. Early ambulation should be encouraged and constipation prevented by oral laxatives. Enemas are usually best avoided, since they may initiate bleeding. Upon discharge, the patient should be cautioned that long, bumpy automobile trips, heavy lifting, straining during defecation, and inadequate hydration may lead to bleeding. Oral antibacterial agents are continued when urine cultures are positive. The patient is seen at intervals to evaluate the character and frequency of voiding. A thin stream may be due to metal stricture resulting from the indwelling catheter, a situation which can be corrected by dilation. The majority of patients who do office work may return to their work at 4 weeks. Laborers should not resume work for 2 to 3 months.

PROGNOSIS. Ninety percent of patients have improvement or relief of symptoms. Ten percent develop urethral stricture which must be treated. Many patients have persisting low-grade pyuria which is difficult to eradicate and require continued suppressive therapy until reepithelization is complete. Five-year results indicate that recurrent obstruction requiring additional surgical treatment develops in about 10 to 25 percent. It is important to appreciate the fact that carcinoma may develop in the remaining tissue.

CARCINOMA OF THE PROSTATE

INCIDENCE AND ETIOLOGY. Although the cause of prostatic carcinoma is unknown, it seems to be related to long-standing androgen stimulation. It does not occur in eunuchs and is rare below the age of thirty. However, administration of testosterone to the elderly does not appear to significantly increase the incidence. The new case rate is estimated at 57,000 per year, with approximately 20,600 deaths per year. It is further estimated that approximately 5 million men are living with histologic cancer of the prostate. Although the autopsy rate has doubled recently, the tumor accounts for only 3.5 percent of deaths in males. For each decade over fifty years, the death per 100,000 doubles, reaching 400 at age eighty (Fig. 40-30). Carcinoma of the prostate represents the most frequent malignant tumor in males over the age of sixty-five, but many men die *with* carcinoma of the prostate and not *of* it.

EARLY CARCINOMA. This represents the stage in which prostatic carcinoma is potentially curable. In most series, less than 10 percent of patients present as early cases, and a vast majority are completely asymptomatic with the tumors detected on routine physical examination. Over 50 percent of prostatic nodules palpated on rectal examination are positive for carcinoma on biopsy. Following a positive biopsy, the patient should be evaluated for total prostatoseminal vesiculectomy. This operation is more demanding on the patient's general condition than the simple prosta-

tectomy. During the radical operation, the bladder neck is sutured to the urethra, and the postoperative course is frequently less eventful than that following simple prostatectomy. An indwelling urethral catheter is necessary for 10 days, and constipation should be avoided to prevent straining and bleeding. An adequate operation abolishes sexual function.

An alternative method of treatment for the patient with early carcinoma is radiation therapy. If the patient is not a candidate for either radical surgery or radiation therapy, he may be treated with estrogen therapy or orchiectomy, or in some instances followed without any specific therapy. However, only surgical excision or radical radiation therapy can offer a cure for this disease, and the 5- and 10-year rates associated with these forms of treatment are fairly similar in several series of cases. One can hope to achieve better than a 50 percent 5-year cure in selected cases.

ADVANCED CARCINOMA. The average age of the symptomatic patient who presents with advanced prostatic cancer is seventy-two. Typically, the symptoms are of a few months' duration with rapid progression of frequency and nocturia leading to acute retention in 28 percent. Weight loss is common, severe back pain occurs in 14 percent, and sciatica in 56 percent. Gross hematuria occurs in only 8 percent of patients, and lymphedema secondary to lymphatic obstruction is present in 4 percent.

Rectal examination characteristically demonstrates a fixed, enlarged, nodular, stony hard prostate. Virchow's node and axillary and inguinal nodes may be palpable. The serum acid and alkaline phosphatase levels are elevated in 72 percent of the patients. Combined osteoblastic and osteolytic bony metastases are present in 60 percent, while isolated osteolytic metastases are rare. Pulmonary metastases occur in 1 percent of patients and are usually miliary in appearance.

The diagnosis is established by transperineal or transrectal needle biopsy. Indurations of the prostate also are observed in tuberculosis, prostatitis, calculus, benign prostatic hypertrophy, and carcinoma of the bladder and rec-

Fig. 40-30. Prostatic cancer death rate versus age.

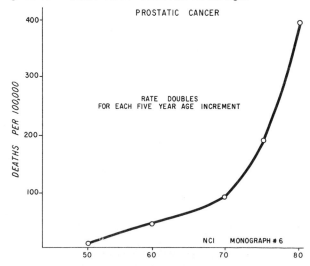

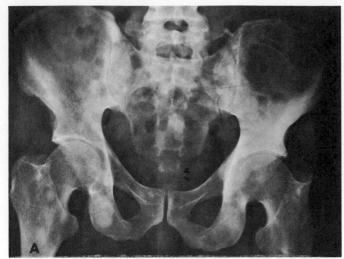

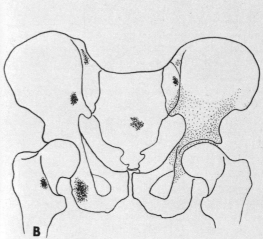

Fig. 40-31. Multiple focal osteoblastic metastatic prostatic carcinoma lesions in the pelvis.

tum with prostatic extension. The differential diagnosis of the osseous lesions (Fig. 40-31) is primarily concerned with Paget's disease. The latter is more diffuse, while the bony lesions of carcinoma of the prostate are usually focal and multiple. The wavy, coarsened, trabecular pattern associated with cystic lesions is characteristic of Paget's disease. Elevation of the serum acid phosphatase level is also associated with myeloma and other bony tumors. Hemolysis of the blood and the drawing of blood within 24 hours subsequent to vigorous rectal examination may also raise this level. The alkaline phosphatase level is also elevated in other bone diseases such as Paget's, multiple myeloma, osteogenic sarcoma, and metastatic tumor. Obstructive lesions of the common bile duct also cause an increase in the serum alkaline phosphatase.

Histopathologically, prostatic malignant tumors are adenocarcinomas, and the majority are highly differentiated. Local extension of the tumor into perineural spaces is present in 92 percent of the cases. The prognosis is particularly dependent upon the extent of differentiation of the tumor; with highly differentiated tumors, the life expectancy approaches actuarial levels. Five- and ten-year survival rates also depend on the stage of the disease. If metastatic carcinoma is present, the figures are 20 and 10 percent, respectively. If the prostatic cancer is localized without evident metastases, 5- and 10-year survival rates are 56 and 26 percent.

Fig. 40-32. Age incidence of testicular tumors.

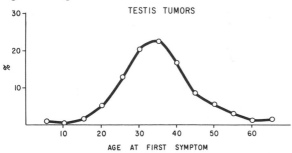

Treatment of advanced carcinoma consists of estrogen therapy and/or orchiectomy. This treatment rapidly improves pain and anorexia and gradually relieves the obstructive urinary symptoms. If a large residual urine persists, transurethral prostatic resection may be indicated. The endocrine therapy is accompanied by palliation in about 90 percent of patients. Diethylstilbestrol (1 mg daily) is generally adequate for long-term therapy and is not associated with significant thromboembolic complications. Increased dosage of stilbestrol may be necessary in the patient who has not had an orchiectomy. Recurrence of symptoms is attended by a poor prognosis. Symptomatic relief may be achieved by large doses of diethylstilbestrol diphosphate administered intravenously. X-ray therapy to isolated metastatic lesions is also palliative. ^{32}P, which localizes in prostatic cancer cells, may relieve metastatic bone pain but is associated with adverse effects on the hemopoietic tissues. Antiandrogen therapy and treatment with compounds such as estramurine phosphate (Estracyt) have proved to be of some value in treatment. The latter drug has been shown to be effective in some patients who are no longer estrogen-responsive. Corticosteroids in large doses are symptomatically beneficial but have no direct effect on the tumor. Hypophysectomy may offer dramatic relief to 10 percent of patients. Five- and ten-year survival rates depend on the stage of disease at the time of institution of therapy. With metastatic carcinoma present, the figures are 20 and 10 percent, respectively.

Testicular Tumors

INCIDENCE AND ETIOLOGY. Testicular tumors account for 2 percent of cancers in the male, and the average age at diagnosis is thirty-two years (Fig. 40-32). The cause of human testicular tumors is unknown, but they occur eleven times more frequently in undescended testes and fifty times more often in abdominal undescended testes. Therefore, they may be related to imperfect embryogenesis. Experimentally, intratesticular injections of zinc chloride result in teratomas, and systemic administration of estrogen produces Leydig cell tumors.

CLINICAL MANIFESTATIONS. Patients usually present with a nonpainful "lump" in the testis. On examination, the lesion is hard, nontender, and solid, and does not transilluminate. About 20 percent of tumors are misdiagnosed as simple hydroceles because of the formation of a secondary hydrocele. The diagnosis of epididymitis may be made erroneously in some situations and delay the appropriate diagnostic surgical intervention. In the patient with a testicular tumor a large scrotal mass may also develop as a result of laceration of the tumor with formation of a hematocele. Late symptoms of metastatic disease include weight loss, fatigue, hemoptysis, and enlargement of the regional lymph nodes.

DIAGNOSIS AND TREATMENT. If a testicular tumor is suspected, surgical exploration is indicated. Measurement of urinary gonadotropins, radioimmunoassay of HCG and AFP markers, may be useful, but surgical treatment should not be delayed. If the lesion is confined to the testis on physical examination, an inguinal surgical approach is preferred. The spermatic vessels are occluded before the testis is exteriorized for inspection, in order to prevent the spread of tumor. Palpation of induration in the testis is indication for orchiectomy, and there is essentially no place for biopsy, since over 90 percent of solid lesions of the testis in this age group are malignant. In patients with apparent lymphatic or pulmonary spread, the primary tumor should be resected for pathologic evaluation. About one-third of the tumors are seminoma, and another third are embryonal cell tumors. The remainder are made up of teratocarcinoma, with 4 percent choriocarcinoma, 5 percent teratoma, and 1 percent interstitial tumors.

Subsequent therapy is dependent upon the histologic diagnosis. Additional surgical treatment is of little use with choriocarcinoma, since this tumor is associated with pulmonary metastases in 81 percent of cases. Pulmonary lesions are present in only 19 percent of cases with seminoma, but bilateral retroperitoneal lymph node resection appears unnecessary for this lesion, since it is extremely radiosensitive. As little as 100 r may sterilize seminomatous lymph node metastases. Lymph node resection is not indicated for benign teratomas but usually is performed for embryonal carcinoma and teratocarcinoma without supradiaphragmatic spread. Lymphadenectomy in such patients increases the 5-year survival significantly.

The use of such chemotherapeutic agents as vinblastine, actinomycin, bleomycin, cisplatinum, and other drugs in combinations has markedly increased the survival of patients with advanced metastatic testicular tumors. These agents may cause severe hemopoietic changes, especially when combined with x-ray therapy. The overall 5-year survival depends on the cell type and stage of disease at the time of diagnosis.

Carcinoma of the Penis

Carcinoma of the penis develops in the squamous epithelium of the glans and foreskin. The risk of squamous carcinoma of the penis is prevented by circumcision in infancy, but the incidence is not altered when the procedure is carried out in adulthood. The lesion is uncommon in the United States, and the average age of onset is over sixty. Patients characteristically present with a sore that does not heal or a palpable nodule under the nonretractable foreskin (phimosis). Because of poor hygiene and associated infection the diagnosis may be difficult. Biopsy provides a definitive diagnosis. Squamous carcinoma of the glans is slow-growing, and local excision or x-ray therapy is associated with a 90 percent 5-year cure rate when no distant spread is present. With nodes involved by tumor, the 5-year survival is reduced to 32 percent, and excision of both inguinal and femoral nodes is attended by improved survival.

GENITOURINARY TRACT INJURIES

Renal Injury

A direct blow or crushing injury to the renal area represents the most frequent type of trauma. Knife and bullet wounds are less common. Change in momentum, such as accompanies a fall from a height, may result in a tear of the renal vessels. The patient frequently indicates pain in the renal area. Physical findings include local cutaneous ecchymoses, guarding, mass, and tenderness. Gross hematuria or microhematuria indicates a need for urologic evaluation; if either occurs without local findings or after trivial hematuria, a predisposing renal lesion should be suspected. In children, 21 percent of renal injuries occur in abnormal kidneys involved with hydronephrosis or tumors and enlarged to the extent that they are not protected by the rib cage.

Diagnosis of renal injury is confirmed by excretory pyelography. The preinjection film may show obliteration of the psoas shadow, scoliosis with the concavity to the side of the injury, and displacement of intestinal gas. Postinjection films may demonstrate delayed, absent, or partial visualization of the injured kidney or extravasation of the opaque medium. The uninjured kidney should be evaluated particularly if nephrectomy is entertained. Arteriography and retrograde pyelography may be applicable and are of definite value if the kidney is not visualized.

Patients with renal contusions and lacerations which do not result in extravasation of urine may be treated by bed rest for 10 days and avoidance of strenuous activity for 3 weeks. When significant segments of the kidney fail to visualize on pyelography and arteriography or when there is extravasation, surgical treatment is considered. Preoperative evaluation of multiplicity of injuries is important. At the time of surgical treatment, perinephric hematoma and necrotic renal parenchyma should be removed. The kidney can be reconstructed by suturing its torn capsule, and the perinephric tissues should be well drained. The transperitoneal approach facilitates exploration and early pedicle control. With massive trauma to the kidney, nephrectomy may be indicated to control the immediate situation and because hypertension due to perinephric scarring may result. Delayed bleeding, urinary extravasation, abscesses, and calculus may require surgical attention.

Bladder Injury

The full bladder is vulnerable to trauma. This situation often prevails in the patient who has recently had an excessive alcohol intake. Direct blows, penetrating injury by spicules of bone associated with pelvic fractures, stab wounds, and gunshot wounds may all result in rupture of the bladder. Direct blows without bony fracture usually cause intraperitoneal rupture, while pelvic fractures are more often associated with an extraperitoneal rupture. The patient may be unable to void, and either a low abdominal or anterior rectal mass may be palpable. The urine obtained by voiding or catheterization is grossly or microscopically bloody. If catheterization is not possible, this suggests that the urethra may have been avulsed from the bladder. Cystography with postevacuation films define the site of extravasation.

Treatment usually consists of surgical repair of the bladder and cystostomy drainage, which should be maintained for a minimum of 10 days. Occasionally, conservative management without an operation may prove satisfactory. This is especially true in the extraperitoneal rupture of the bladder, where catheter drainage may be all that is required in certain circumstances. If the urethra is avulsed, a splinting urethral catheter is also inserted. Perivesical and perineal hematomas should be drained. When trauma is extensive and the patient's condition poor, cystostomy under local anesthesia may be adequate to allow the sites of rupture to heal themselves. Differences of opinion exist regarding the surgical management. Some authors advocate simple suprapubic cystostomy drainage, while others suggest more extensive primary repair of the ruptured urethra.

Ureteral Trauma

Injuries to the ureter occur mainly as the result of trauma during operation. If the injury is recognized at the time of the operation, a direct repair over an indwelling catheter should be performed. If the condition is not recognized at operation, it may become manifest by anuria in the case of bilateral ligation or, more frequently, a urinary tract fistula or an expanding urinoma. Excretory pyelography frequently demonstrates obstructive changes in the site of the ureteral fistula or urinoma. Treatment of the sequelae of ureteral trauma consists of surgical repair. The ureter occasionally may be injured by penetrating objects such as bullets and knives. This situation must be suspected when the patient who has sustained such an injury has microhematuria. There is a definite strong indication for an excretory urogram on a patient who sustains a penetrating injury of the abdomen.

OPERATIONS ON GENITOURINARY ORGANS

Lumbar Nephrectomy

The retroperitoneal approach to the kidney is the traditional route, since in the preantibiotic era a major proportion of renal operations were performed for pyogenic disease and the avoidance of contamination of the peritoneum with urine was considered advantageous. Today, the lumbar renal approach (Fig. 40-33) remains popular but is supplanted on many occasions by the transabdominal route when early access to the renal vessels is required, as in renal tumor, trauma, or renal vascular disease.

Indications for the lumbar approach include inflammatory renal disease, calculi, tumor (especially of the upper pole), pyelonephritis, hydronephrosis, renal trauma, and renal cystic disease. Since it offers a most expeditious exposure, it is frequently used in poor-risk patients or for secondary nephrectomy. The disadvantages are a limited exposure for abdominal exploration, the fact that it may be poorly tolerated by the patient, and that it precludes bilateral renal or adrenal exploration. In addition, the lumbar approach makes early control of the renal pedicle without manipulation of the kidney difficult and therefore should not be applied for certain renal tumors.

The procedure is carried out with the patient in the lateral flexed position, with the involved side on stretch. The incision extends from the lumbar triangle (just below the twelfth rib) to a point 4 cm above the anterior superior

Fig. 40-33. Lumbar nephrectomy. (See text.)

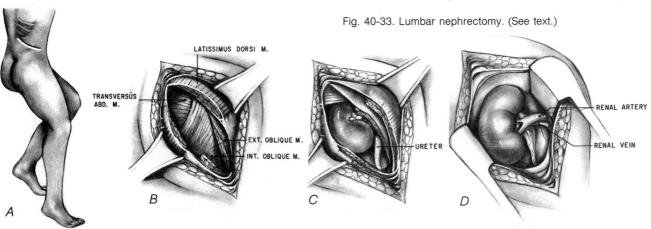

LATISSIMUS DORSI M.

TRANSVERSUS ABD. M.

EXT. OBLIQUE M.
INT. OBLIQUE M.

URETER

RENAL ARTERY
RENAL VEIN

A   *B*   *C*   *D*

spine of the ileum. The latissimus dorsi and the external and internal oblique muscles are divided in the line of the incision. The transversus muscle is separated, and the aponeurosis of the transversus and the costovertebral ligament to the twelfth rib are divided. At the level of the internal oblique muscle, the large ilioinguinal nerve is encountered. After separating the transversus abdominis muscle in the line of its fibers, the retroperitoneum is exposed, and the peritoneum is displaced toward the midline. The fascia of Gerota is opened, thus exposing the kidney and the perinephric fatty tissue. The important structures within the renal pedicle are located anteriorly (ventrally). During mobilization of the kidney, particular care is necessary in the region of the upper pole because of the adrenal vessels and in the region of the lower pole because of aberrant arteries. Usually the renal artery and vein can be dissected free of fatty areolar tissue, so that individual ligation may be applied. Under adverse circumstances, a renal pedicle clamp can be used to control bleeding and permit transection of the hilus. Suture ligature of the renal pedicle en masse may fail to control the bleeding and can lead to arteriovenous fistula. Absorbable sutures are often used when wound infection is present. Whenever the urinary conductive passages are opened, it is advisable to institute drainage, and a latex tissue drain has been effective. The incision is closed in layers with chromic catgut with the exception of the skin, which is closed with nonabsorbable suture. Nonabsorbable sutures with increased tensile strength, such as Prolene, may be used in the fascia to increase the strength of closure in debilitated patients or those in whom poor wound healing is expected. The drain may be conveniently advanced so that it is removed on the fifth postoperative day.

Cutaneous Ureteroileostomy (Ileal Conduit)

Currently, the most popular method of supravesical urinary diversion for pelvic malignant tumors, neurogenic bladder dysfunction, and chronic lower urinary tract obstruction or infection with deterioration of renal function is cutaneous ureteroileostomy (Fig. 40-34). The major indications for this form of diversion are (1) required removal of the bladder and (2) poor urinary conduction from the kidney with accompanying reduced renal function. The disadvantages of the procedure are the extent of the operation and an increased incidence of postoperative complications compared to cutaneous ureterostomy or nephrostomy. Additional minor disadvantages include reabsorption of urea by the ileum and the requirement of a meticulously applied collection device. These disadvantages are counteracted by the advantages of the ileal conduit in providing a continuous unobstructed drainage of urine and its versatility in coping with varying requirements. The use of colon instead of ileum offers some advantages and is being utilized with increasing frequency (colon conduit).

Preoperative preparation is an integral part of the procedure and the blood volume, cardiac, pulmonary, and renal status should be optimal. Treatment of preexisting

infections or metabolic disturbances should be instituted at this time. Antibacterial preparation of the intestinal tract is not necessary, but adequate deflation should be accomplished by a low-residue diet for 3 to 4 days. The urinary appliance should be worn by the patient preoperatively in order to determine his tolerance to adhesive and identify the optimal location of the stoma.

This procedure is best performed through a midline abdominal incision. Prior to making this incision, it is preferable to create the abdominal wall defect for the ileostomy. This results in the creation of a tract through muscles which have not been distorted by the major incision and avoids the problem of mechanical obstruction of the ileostomy. The abdomen is then entered. Appendectomy is performed. A segment of the ileum approximately 20 cm in length is selected for the formation of the conduit. A segment supplied by two arteries is preferred. The ileum is divided at the selected sites, and the isolated segment is irrigated with saline solution. The continuity of the ileum is restored, and the isolated ileal segment is positioned posterior to the ileoileal anastomosis. The proximal end of the ileal segment to be utilized for the conduit is closed with a continuous inverting chromic catgut suture. The left ureter is brought through the sigmoid mesentery and mobilized to provide length and eliminate the possibility of kinking or obstruction. The full thickness of ureter is sutured to the ileal mucosa. If the left ureter is markedly dilated, an end-to-end ureteroileostomy is performed. Calibrated catheters may be used to splint the anastomosis for a few days and to encourage good position of the ureters. The right ureter is anastomosed in a similar fashion over a catheter stent. The isolated segment of ileum and its mesentery are sutured to the posterior peritoneum to prevent an internal hernia. The distal end of the ileal conduit is brought to the previously prepared abdominal opening. The peritoneum or fascia is secured to the serosa of the ileum to prevent hernia. The ileostomy is everted and sutured to the skin and itself. A 1-cm protuberant cuff under no tension is considered optimal. Stay sutures may be used to reduce the tension on the wound, which is closed with catgut for the fascial layers and silk for the skin. A nasogastric tube is necessary postoperatively for 3 to 5 days. Another variation of the procedure involves the joining of both ureters together with one large stoma, which is then anastomosed to the proximal end of the ileal loop as a "cap." This may provide a larger anastomotic opening between the ureters and the segment of ileum and decrease the incidence of the complication of stricture at this vital site.

Cystostomy, Cystolithotomy

Surgical treatment of the bladder (Fig. 40-35) is facilitated by filling the organ, since this elevates the peritoneum out of the line of the incision. A low transverse abdominal incision 4 cm above the pubis is carried through the skin, subcutaneous tissue, and rectus abdominis fascia. The recti are mobilized from their midline attachments and separated. The bladder is easily recognized by its characteristic muscular and vascular pattern. The bladder

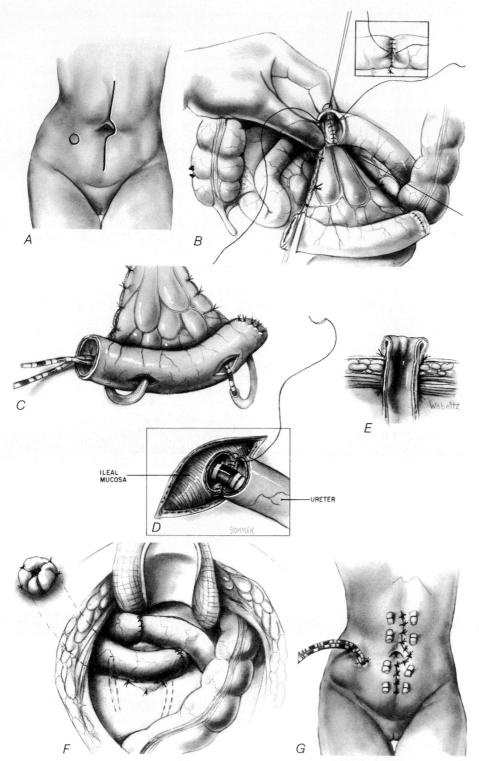

ILEAL
MUCOSA

URETER

Fig. 40-34. Cutaneous ureteroileostomy (ileal conduit).

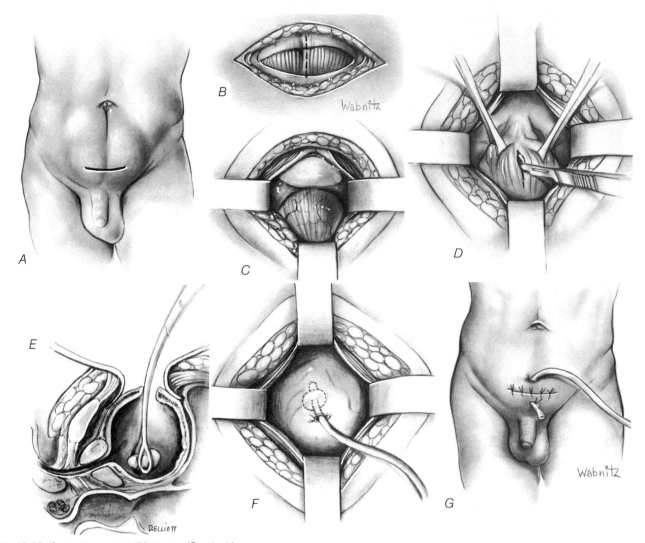

Fig. 40-35. Cystostomy, cystolithotomy. (See text.)

is entered longitudinally, and if calculi are present, they can be removed digitally or with stone forceps. Thorough digital and visual exploration is indicated. Drainage is best provided by a de Pezzer or Malecot cystostomy catheter brought out through a stab wound above the incision. A prevesical tissue drain should be used and brought out through a separate stab wound below the incision. The bladder is closed with a one-layer continuous zero chromic catgut suture which incorporates the seromuscular wall of the bladder. The rectus fascia is approximated with interrupted zero chromic catgut sutures. The subcutaneous fat may be approximated with 3-0 interrupted plain catgut sutures and the skin edges with nonabsorbable suture material, such as 4-0 silk or nylon.

Prostatectomy (Fig. 40-36)

TRANSURETHRAL PROSTATECTOMY. The most commonly employed operation for removal of prostatic obstruction is the endoscopic approach. Following adequate dilatation of the urethra, the resectoscope sheath is inserted. Excellent visualization through the resectoscope allows for identification of the ureteral orifices, verumontanum, and external sphincter. With a cutting loop, the prostatic tissue is resected and hemostasis is secured with electrocoagulation. A catheter is inserted at the end of the procedure, and further hemostasis may be obtained by pulling the catheter bag against the bladder neck and prostatic fossa. This procedure is well tolerated by the patient, with minimal postoperative discomfort and early removal of the catheter. Contraindications to the transurethral resection are an excessively enlarged prostate gland and the presence of other intravesical pathologic conditions which warrant open exploration. The skilled operator is able to avoid the complications of excessive bleeding, ureteral orifice injury, perforation, and injury to the external sphincter. The results of this procedure are gratifying, and it can be performed on elderly, debilitated patients with minimal morbidity and mortality.

SUPRAPUBIC PROSTATECTOMY (Fig. 40-36C and D). This is performed through the cystostomy approach previously described. The compressed normal prostate represents the surgical capsule from which adenomatous tissue is mobilized by finger dissection. The prostatic urethra and adenomas are removed together. The distal urethral attachment is transected, and the prostatic fossa is packed while the prostatic arteries which are located on either side of the posterior bladder neck are suture ligated. Redundant mucosal fragments or small adenomas may be removed by sharp dissection. After the pack is removed, a #22, 30-cc urethral retention catheter is inserted. If oozing from the bladder neck or prostatic fossa occurs, gentle traction on the urethral catheter may effect hemostasis. A de Pezzer or Malecot catheter and tissue drain are employed in a similar fashion to that described for suprapubic cystostomy.

RETROPUBIC PROSTATECTOMY. This is also accomplished through the incision described for cystostomy. After the bladder wall is identified, the bladder is decompressed, and a 5-cm transverse incision is made 1.5 cm distal to the bladder neck. An alternative approach, known as a vesicocapsular prostatectomy, employs a vertical incision in line with the urethra and into the bladder and has the advantages of easier closure and avoidance of the anterior prostatic venous plexus. After the prostatic capsule is incised, the adenomas are mobilized by finger dissection. The distal urethra and bladder neck attachments are transected, and hemostasis is effected by suture ligature. The prostatic capsule is closed with interrupted catgut sutures, and a watertight closure is desirable. The bladder is drained by a retention catheter. Traction on the catheter following retropubic prostatectomy is not as effective for hemostasis as it is following transvesical prostatectomy and

may interfere with closure of the capsule. If additional security against catheter obstruction is desired, a suprapubic cystostomy can be performed.

PERINEAL PROSTATECTOMY (Fig. 40-36B). A curvilinear perineal incision extending from the two ischiorectal fossae is employed. The prostate is approached by dissecting along the anterior wall of the rectal ampulla. The central tendon is divided, and the portion of the levator ani which is attached to the membranous urethra is separated and reflected posteriorly. During this dissection, it is helpful to insert a urethral sound in order to identify the urethra. When the prostatic capsule is identified, a Young prostatic tractor is used to present the prostate into the perineal incision. After the apex has been carefully identified, two incisions extending laterally and superiorly in the shape of an inverted V prepare for the enucleation of the adenomas. Downward traction with a short Lowsley tractor which replaces the urethral tractor facilitates enucleation of the adenomas. Hemostasis is effected by suture of the bladder neck. A #22, 30-cc urethral retention catheter is inserted, and the prostatic capsule is closed with interrupted 2-0 chromic catgut sutures. A space between the prostate and the rectal ampulla is left open, and the levator ani muscles are brought together in the midline with interrupted chromic catgut. Subcutaneous tissues are closed with plain catgut, and a latex tissue drain is brought out through one corner of the incision. The skin is closed with nonabsorbable sutures.

Fig. 40-36. A. Types of open prostatectomy. B. Perineal prostatectomy. C and D. Suprapubic prostatectomy.

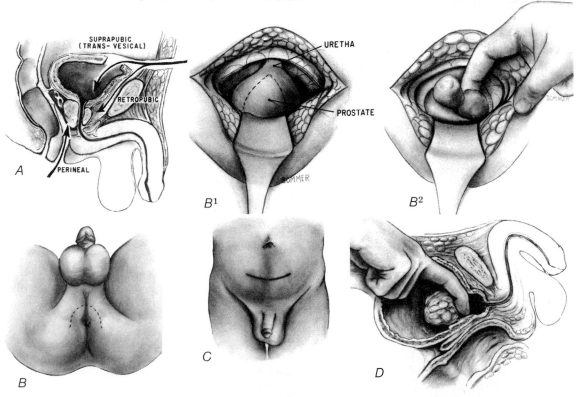

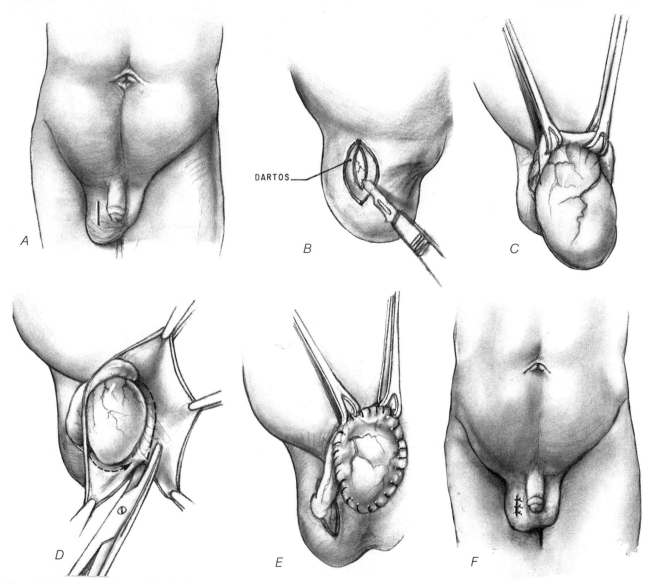

DARTOS

A *B* *C*

D *E* *F*

Fig. 40-37. Hydrocelectomy. (See text.)

Postoperative patency of the catheter is maintained by induction of osmotic diuresis. The suprapubic cystostomy catheter is usually removed in 24 to 48 hours, while the urethral catheter is usually not necessary after the fifth day.

POSTOPERATIVE MANAGEMENT. Postoperative patency of the catheter or catheters is maintained by irrigation. This may be carried out manually or by continuous drip irrigation. Continuous irrigation may be performed through a three-way catheter if there is no suprapubic tube present. If a suprapubic tube is present, the continuous irrigation flows from the urethral catheter through the bladder and out the suprapubic tube. The suprapubic cystostomy catheter is usually removed in 24 to 48 hours if good hemostasis is present. The urethral catheter is usually removed by the seventh postoperative day, and sooner if the retropubic or perineal approach has been used.

Hydrocelectomy (Fig. 40-37)

A vertical scrotal incision is usually employed. It is carried through the skin, dartos fascia, and overlying coverings of the hydrocele sac. It is desirable to avoid opening the hydrocele until the sac is totally mobilized. The tunica vaginalis is then opened and the excess tunica excised. Hemostasis is secured with multiple ligatures or electrocoagulation of the small bleeders in the cut edge. The edges of the tunica may be sutured together behind the testis with a continuous 3-0 chromic suture. If hemostasis is satisfactory, this may not be necessary. A drain may be brought out through a stab wound in a dependent portion of the scrotum if the hydrocele is excessively large, but in most instances a drain is not required. The incision is then closed in layers. A scrotal suspensory provides an excellent dressing in the postoperative period, and the use of an ice bag decreases the swelling. Hydrocelectomy in children is car-

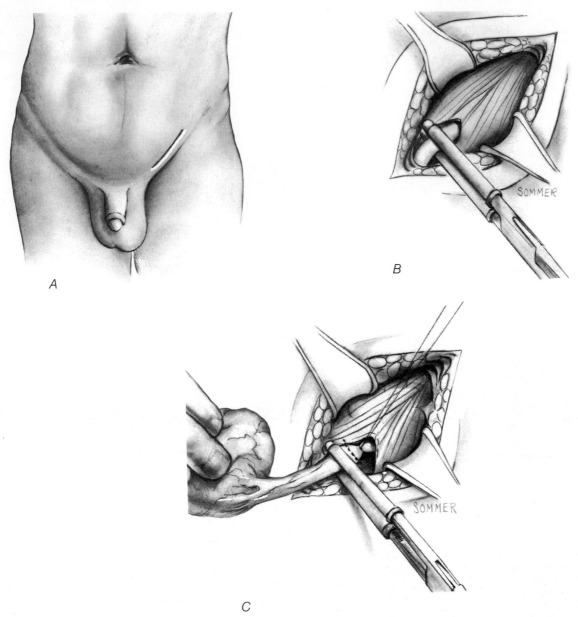

A

B

C

Fig. 40-38. Inguinal orchiectomy. (See text.)

ried out through an inguinal incision so that an associated hernia can be repaired at the same time.

Inguinal Orchiectomy (Fig. 40-38)

This approach is utilized when a testicular tumor is suspected. It provides access to the spermatic vessels prior to manipulation of the testis. The incision is identical to that performed for repair of a hernia, and the spermatic cord is identified at the external inguinal ring. After a rubber-shod or bulldog clamp has been applied to the cord at this level, the testis is mobilized from its scrotal attachments and exteriorized through the inguinal incision. The tunica vaginalis is opened to permit examination of the testis, and if the lesion looks neoplastic, the cord is ligated and transected. Any solid lesion within the testis is considered potentially malignant, and biopsy is seldom performed. A metal clip is placed in the end of the remaining cord as a marker for future surgery or radiation therapy localization. After the testis has been removed, the inguinal incision is closed. The incision is *not* drained.

Transseptal Orchiopexy
(Fig. 40-39)

This has largely replaced the Thorek and Bevan procedures. The testis is identified through an inguinal incision which permits mobilization of the spermatic cord and correction of an indirect hernia which usually accompanies the undescended testis. After sufficient cord structures have been mobilized to permit placement of the testis in the scrotum, a small incision is made in the contralateral scrotum and a subdartos pouch is prepared to receive the cryptorchid testis. The scrotal septum is incised over a clamp, and traction is applied to the gubernaculum so that the testis is brought down through the scrotal septum into the contralateral scrotum. The septal defect may require a partial closure to prevent the testis from pulling back but should not be closed too tightly, since strangulation of the cord could occur. The scrotal and inguinal incisions are closed, and the patient is usually able to leave the hospital in 24 to 48 hours.

Bilateral Vasectomy (Fig. 40-40)

This male sterilization procedure usually is carried out under local anesthesia in an outpatient setting. Previous consultation with the patient and his wife has allowed for careful selection, instructions to the patient, and the signing of the required papers for sterilization and informed consent. The patient or his wife has been instructed to shave the scrotum on the night before the procedure, and the patient brings a scrotal suspensory with him to the office. The procedure is carried out with the patient in the lithotomy or supine position. The vas on one side is isolated between the thumb and index finger of the operator, and the overlying skin is infiltrated with 1% lidocaine or a similar local anesthetic agent. The underlying cord is also infiltrated. A towel clip is then used to isolate the vas. A small incision is made over the vas and it is delivered into the incision. An Allis clamp is then used to pick up the vas and separate it from the surrounding cord structures. The vas is then mobilized for approximately 3 cm. A segment measuring approximately 1 to 2 cm is excised between clamps. The edges of the vas are then transfixed with sutures. Another suture is placed approximately 1 cm below the previous suture and tied. The end of that suture is then passed through the end of the vas and tied, produc-

Fig. 40-39. Transseptal orchiopexy. (See text.)

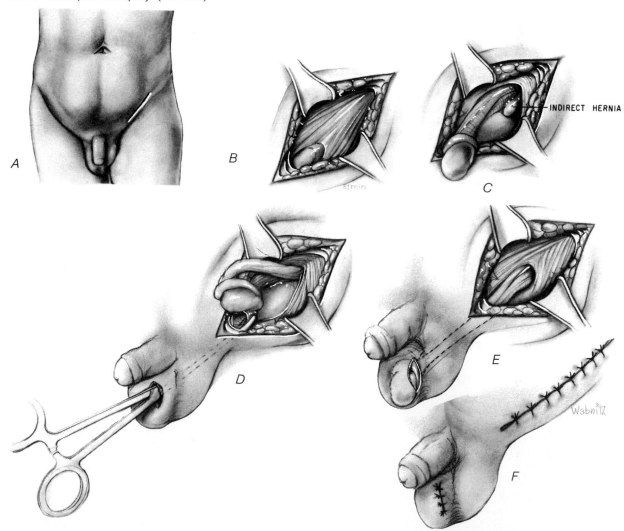

A

B

C
INDIRECT HERNIA

D

E

F

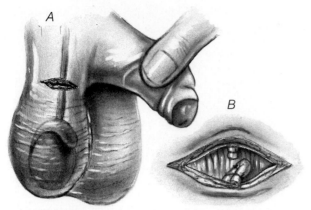

Fig. 40-40. Vasectomy. *A.* Scrotal incision. *B.* Double ligation of vasa.

ing a means of bending the vas back on itself so that the ends are no longer in close proximity. One of the ends can also be buried in the adjacent tissues to prevent recanalization. An alternative technique involving electrocoagulation of the lumen of each end is commonly employed. After satisfactory hemostasis has been secured, the ends of the vas are dropped back into the incision. The edges of the skin and underlying dartos are then approximated. A similar procedure is then carried out on the other side. Incorporating the underlying dartos in the skin closure provides excellent hemostasis. A collodion dressing is then applied, and the patient uses the scrotal suspensory over a small gauze dressing. He is instructed to use an ice bag on that area for the remainder of the day and returns to work wearing the scrotal suspensory the following day. He is advised to expect a minimal amount of discomfort, swelling, and ecchymosis. When he resumes intercourse, he

continues contraception until an examination of his semen reveals no sperm. This usually requires a period of 6 weeks or at least 10 ejaculations to evacuate the remaining sperm which are distal to the anastomotic sites.

Vasovasostomy (Fig. 40-41)

This procedure is usually carried out on an in-hospital basis and with the patient under general anesthesia. An incision is made in the scrotum, and the underlying cord structures are delivered into view. The previous site of vasectomy is usually palpable unless a large segment of the vas has been excised. Magnifying lenses, or the use of the operating microscope, facilitate the operation and improve the results. Once the ends of the vas have been isolated, they are excised back to a normal-appearing vas deferens. The ends are then carefully approximated and sutured with 6-0 Prolene sutures. Finer suture material may be utilized when the operating microscope is employed. The lumen is usually reestablished by passage of some of the sutures through it. Care must be taken to prevent excessive tension on the completed anastomosis. Bleeding is minimal, and the reconstituted vas is then dropped back into the scrotum and the skin and dartos approximated. A similar procedure is then carried out on the other side. The patient is often able to leave the hospital the following day. Sperm may begin to appear in the ejaculate as early as 1 month following the procedure, but most often this does not occur until 2 or 3 months following the procedure, at which time the edema may subside enough to allow for passage of sperm through the small lumen of the vas deferens. Satisfactory reconstitution with sperm in the ejaculate occurs in

Fig. 40-41. Vasovasostomy. *A.* Scrotal incision. *B.* Excision of ligated (scarred) ends. *C.* Reanastomosis of ends, restoring continuity.

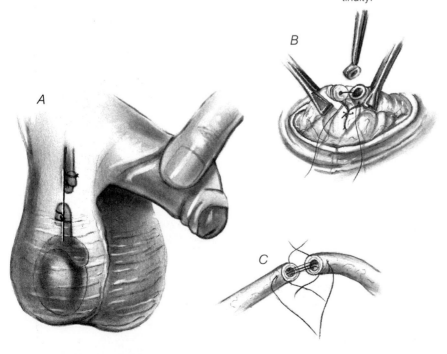

approximately 50 percent of cases. A higher percentage of success is reported when microsurgery is used. A satisfactory surgical result does not ensure that a pregnancy will result; other factors such as sperm quality and antisperm antibodies may play a role in persistent infertility.

References

Bagshaw, M. A., Ray, G. R., Pistenma, D. A., Castelino, R. A., and Meares, E. M., Jr.: External Beam Radiation Therapy of Primary Carcinoma of the Prostate, *Cancer,* **36:**723, 1975.

Bars, E., and Comarr, A. E.: "Neurological Urology," University Park Press, Baltimore, 1971.

Byar, D. R.: The Veterans Administration Cooperative Urological Research Group's Studies of Cancer of the Prostate, *Cancer,* **32:**1126, 1973.

Campbell, M. F., and Harrison, J. H. (eds.): "Urology," 3d ed., W. B. Saunders Company, Philadelphia, 1970.

Creevy, C. D.: The Correction of Hypospadias: A Review, *Urol Surv,* **8:**2, 1958.

D'Angio, G. J., Evans, A., et al.: Treatment of Wilms' Tumor: Results of the National Wilms' Tumor Study, *Cancer,* **38:**633, 1976.

Einhorn, L. H., and Donahue, J.: Cis-diaminodichloroplatinum, Vinblastine, and Bleomycin Combination Chemotherapy in Disseminated Testicular Cancer, *Ann Int Med,* **87:**293, 1977.

Farber, S.: Chemotherapy in Leukemia and Wilms' Tumor, *JAMA,* **198:**826, 1966.

Flocks, R. H.: Clinical Cancer of the Prostate: A Study of 4,000 Cases, *JAMA,* **193:**559, 1965.

Gartman, E.: The Significance of Hematuria in Young Men, *J Urol,* **75:**135, 1956.

Glenn, J. F. (ed.): "Urologic Surgery," 2d ed., Harper & Row, Hagerstown, 1975.

Herring, L. C.: Analysis of Ten Thousand Urinary Calculi, *J Urol,* **88:**545, 1962.

Hinman, F., Jr.: Vesical Defense against Infection, *Postgrad Med,* **37:**397, 1965.

Horton, C. E., and Devine, C. J.: Hypospadias and Epispadias, *Ciba Found Clin Symp,* vol. 24, no. 3, 1972.

Javadpour, N., and Scardino, P. T.: Recent Advances in Immunobiology of Genito-urinary Cancer, *Urology,* **9:**377, 1977.

Jewett, H. J., et al.: The Palpable Nodule of Prostatic Cancer: Results 15 Years after Radical Excision, *JAMA,* **203:**403, 1968.

Kelalis, P. P., King, L. R., and Belman, A. B. (eds.): "Clinical Pediatric Urology," W. B. Saunders Company, Philadelphia, 1976.

Lindberg, B.: Treatment of Rapidly Progressing Prostatic Carcinoma with Estracyt, *J Urol,* **108:**303, 1972.

Melicow, M., and Uson, A. C.: Palpable Masses in Infants and Children: A Report Based on a Review of 653 Cases, *J Urol,* **81:**705, 1959.

Symposium on Renal Lithiasis, William H. Boyce (guest editor), *Urol Clin North Am,* Vol 1(2) June, 1974.

Robson, C. J., Churchill, B. M., and Anderson, W.: Results of Radical Nephrectomy for Renal Cell Carcinoma, *Trans Am Assoc Genitourin Surg,* **60:**122, 1968.

Rubin, P. (ed.): "Current Concepts in Cancer," pts. IX–XX: Cancer of the Urogenital Tract, p. 117, American Medical Association, Chicago, 1974.

Skinner, D. G.: Non-seminomatous Testis Tumors: A Plan of Management Based on 96 Patients to Improve Survival in All Stages by Combined Therapeutic Modalities, *J Urol,* **115:**65, 1976.

Symposium on Urinary Calculi, *Am J Med,* vol. 45, November, 1968.

Van der Werf-Messing, B.: Carcinoma of the Bladder Treated by Preoperative Irradiation Followed by Cystectomy: Second Report, *Cancer,* **32:**1084, 1973.

Wax, S. H., and Frank, I. N.: A Retrospective Study of Upper Urinary Tract Calculi, *J Urol,* **94:**28, 1965.

Whitmore, W. F., Jr., et al.: Preoperative Irradiation with Cystectomy in the Management of Bladder Cancer, *Am J Roentgenol,* **102:**570, 1962.

Yendt, E. R., Gagne, R. J. A., and Cohanim, M.: The Effects of Thiazides in Idiopathic Hypercalcuria, *Am J Med Sci,* **251:**449, 1966.

Chapter 41

Gynecology

by Arthur L. Herbst, Howard Ulfelder and Donald R. Tredway

FEMALE REPRODUCTIVE TRACT

Embryologic Development

Fertilization of the ovum by a sperm carrying the X chromosome initiates the development of a feminine individual, but it is not before the eighth week that the structures specific for this sex attain noticeable dominance. These are the primordial ovaries and the Müllerian ducts. The latter drift medially and become fused throughout their lower two-thirds before the eleventh week of gestation; from this evolves the adult internal genital apparatus (Fig. 41-1). At the lower end it establishes communication with an entodermal derivative, the urogenital sinus, which, when fully differentiated, provides distinct and separate orifices for the urethra and vagina. The distal colon and anus lie well posterior.

The external genitalia begin as folds of ectoderm from the genital tubercle (clitoris), passing back on either side of the orifices and eventually forming the vulva with its major and minor labia (Fig. 41-2). The hymenal membrane partially occludes the vaginal canal at the level of the urogenital diaphragm, below the point of juncture between the urogenital sinus and the Müllerian ducts. Although the male structures (Wolffian ducts) normally regress, remnants can often be seen as small cystic swellings near the ovaries (parovarian cysts), as histologically recognizable rests in the broad ligaments or cervix, or as cystic tumors of the vagina (Gärtner's duct cysts).

A variety of anomalies of the tubes, uterus, cervix, and vagina have been described (Fig. 41-3). All are easily

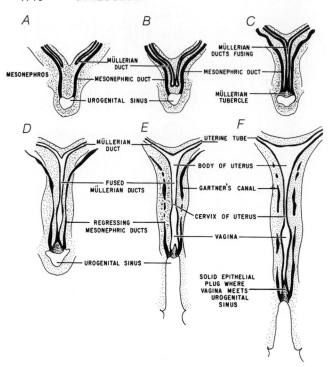

Fig. 41-1. Fusion of the Müllerian ducts to form the uterus and vagina. (*Redrawn after Koff, Carnegie Contributions to Embryology, vol. 24, 1933.*) *A.* 23 mm. *B.* 25 mm. *C.* 32.9 mm. *D.* 48 mm. *E.* 63 mm. *F.* 69 mm.

Fig. 41-2. Schematic diagram showing plan of developing female reproductive system. (*After B. M. Patton, "Human Embryology," 2d ed., McGraw-Hill Book Company, New York, 1953.*)

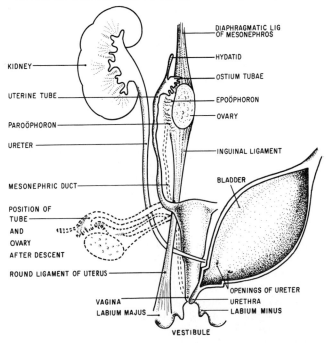

explained as improper Müllerian duct development, by partial or complete failure to fuse, by asymmetrical growth, or by unilateral or bilateral failure to develop at all. These Müllerian anomalies are frequently accompanied by renal (Wolffian) abnormalities, including absent or malformed kidneys; therefore an intravenous pyelogram (IVP) should be performed in individuals with these congenital uterine abnormalities. Abnormal development of the external genital structures usually takes the form of some degree of masculinization. There is enlargement of the clitoris and occasionally fusion of the labial folds caused by excessive androgen stimulation of the fetus in utero. When the hymen is imperforate, there is complete mechanical obstruction of the outlet of the vagina, usually resulting in a blood-filled pelvic mass, a "hematocolpos," first noted months or years after menstruation should have started. Transverse fibrous ridges of the vagina and cervix, as well as distortions of the cavity of the uterus, have been described in association with intrauterine exposure to diethylstilbestrol (DES) and similar compounds. These presumably result from a disturbance in the development of the Müllerian ducts; in the case of vaginal ridges, the urogenital sinus development may have been affected.

Morphologic Anatomy

EXTERNAL GENITALIA. The external genitalia are shown in Fig. 41-4. The entrance to the vagina (introitus) is bounded laterally by two folds of skin, the external labia majora and the internal labia minora. The labia majora form the lateral boundary of the vulva. They meet anteriorly toward the lower abdomen and fuse in an area over the pubis known as the "mons veneris." The posterior extensions of the labia meet in an area known as the "posterior commissure." Just above the posterior commissure is the caudal part of the vaginal opening known as the "posterior fourchette." The "vestibule" consists of that area into which the vagina and the urethra open and which is bounded laterally by the labia. The vulva includes both labia, the vestibular structures, and the clitoris. The clitoris lies immediately above the urethral meatus and is the analog of the male phallus. The "perineum" refers to the area between the rectum and the vagina, and it is through the tissues of this area that obstetric episiotomies are made.

Two types of glands can be considered with the external genitalia of the female. Skene's glands are located about the urethra and are important as a site of infection in cases of gonorrhea. Bartholin's glands supply lubrication to the vagina during times of sexual excitation and are located immediately deep to the labia majora. These glands can be invaded by bacterial organisms resulting in acute bartholinitis and Bartholin's abscesses.

INTERNAL GENITALIA. The internal genitalia and surrounding structures are demonstrated in Fig. 41-5. The uterus is divided into its main body (fundus) and lower portion (cervix). The fallopian tubes open into either side of the endometrial cavity of the uterus, traversing the wall of the uterus at the interstitial, or cornual, end of the tube. The tube widens throughout its course laterally to its ampullary, or infundibular, end. The ovaries are suspended

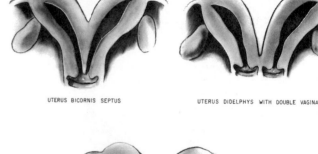

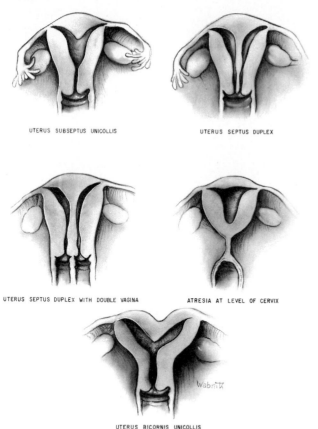

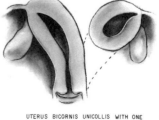

UTERUS SUBSEPTUS UNICOLLIS   UTERUS SEPTUS DUPLEX   UTERUS BICORNIS SEPTUS   UTERUS DIDELPHYS WITH DOUBLE VAGINA

UTERUS SEPTUS DUPLEX WITH DOUBLE VAGINA   ATRESIA AT LEVEL OF CERVIX   UTERUS BICORNIS UNICOLLIS WITH ONE UNCONNECTED RUDIMENTARY HORN

UTERUS BICORNIS UNICOLLIS

Fig. 41-3. Schematic diagram of various types of abnormal uteri.

immediately posterior to the tubes by a mesentery (meso-varium). The round ligaments run laterally from the uterus through the inguinal ring in the anterior abdominal wall and end in the labia majora. They lie anteriorly to the fallopian tubes, a fact that is useful in orienting surgical specimens. The round ligament forms the apex for the folds of peritoneum that contain the uterine blood supply (broad ligament). At the base of the broad ligament, running from the cervix to the lateral pelvic wall, are important supporting structures known as the "cardinal" (Mackenrodt) ligaments. Posterior to these and running from the cervix to the sacrum are the uterosacral ligaments. These ligaments and the relationship of the cervix to the bladder and the rectum with the spaces surrounding these structures are shown in Fig. 41-6.

The blood supply to the female pelvis is illustrated in Fig. 41-7, which shows the distribution of the common iliac, external iliac, and internal iliac arteries (hypogastric arteries). It should be noted that the posterior division of the internal iliac artery gives off its superior gluteal branch and then continues further to split into its varying visceral branches. The remainder of the hypogastric artery continues inferiorly into the pelvis and gives off the obturator artery and the obliterated internal iliac artery distal to the superior vesical branch, which runs to the bladder; other branches, including the uterine artery, run to the central pelvic organs. Each ureter enters the pelvis near the bifurcation of a common iliac artery. It passes medial to the

internal iliac artery and runs immediately beneath the uterine artery, an important landmark in the anatomy of pelvic dissection (Fig. 41-32). The ureter then passes forward over the lateral aspect of the cervix and vagina to reach the bladder.

THE PELVIC ENVIRONMENT. Between the uterosacral ligaments anterior to the rectum and posterior to the cervix is a space known as the cul-de-sac, or pouch of Douglas, the most dependent extension of the free peritoneal cavity. This important area can be used for diagnostic exploration of the pelvis via the vagina. The uterosacral and cardinal ligaments form important stays for preventing prolapse of the uterus by helping to fix the position of the cervix back toward the hollow of the sacrum. Their effects can be

Fig. 41-4. External genitalia of the female.

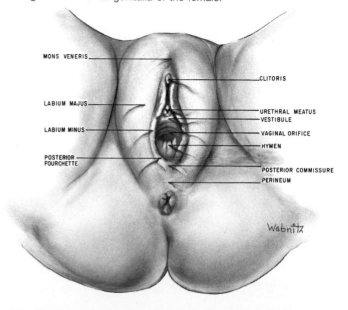

MONS VENERIS

LABIUM MAJUS

LABIUM MINUS

POSTERIOR FOURCHETTE

CLITORIS

URETHRAL MEATUS
VESTIBULE

VAGINAL ORIFICE

HYMEN

POSTERIOR COMMISSURE

PERINEUM

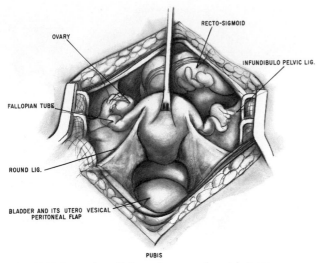

Fig. 41-5. Internal genitalia and surrounding structures.

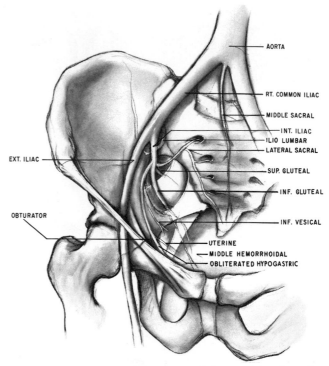

Fig. 41-7. Anterior and superior view of the arterial system of the pelvis showing the named primary arteries and their relationships to the bony and ligamentous structures.

demonstrated at the operating table by the great increase in mobility of the uterus and cervix after these ligaments are cut. The round ligament, though a firm structure, does not prevent descensus, i.e., downward motion of the uterus and cervix in the plane of the vagina. Changes in the length of the round ligaments do appear to accompany changes in the anterior or posterior orientation of the uterus and cervix. Posterior displacement of the fundus is termed "retroversion," a common finding in females during their reproductive years, especially following pregnancy. It is, in fact, so common that one should be extremely cautious before ascribing any pain or pelvic complaint to the existence of a retroverted uterus.

In addition to the ligamentous supports noted above, a firm and strong supportive shelf is provided by the levator ani muscles, as shown in Fig. 41-8. In the female this muscular complex is pierced by the urethra, vagina, and

rectum, and these orifices provide a structural weakness for the start of herniation that may be seen in adult life. A second layer of reinforcement beyond the shelf of the levator ani muscles is provided by the muscles of the urogenital diaphragm, which is located between the ischial tuberosities and the pubis, as shown in Fig. 41-9. This secondary layer provides muscular support anteriorly to the main mass of the levator ani muscle. Thus it can be

Fig. 41-6. Diagrammatic cross section of the pelvis to show the concentration of connective tissue forming ligamentous bands, the junction with the cardinal ligament (Mackenrodt's ligament), and the spaces and tissue planes. (*From Peham and Amreich.*)

Fig. 41-8. Components of the levator muscles viewed from below.

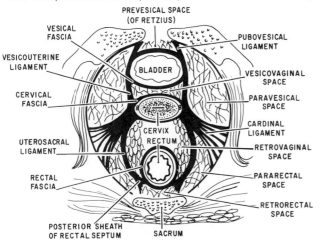

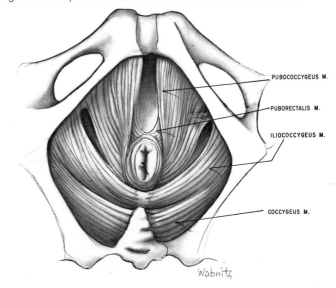

seen that in addition to the bony pelvis, the main support to the pelvic organs in the erect human female is provided by striated muscle, mainly of the levator ani complex, and partially by the urogenital diaphragm. The firm ligamentous attachments at the base of the cervix (the cardinal and uterosacral ligaments) stabilize the uterus at the apex of the vagina.

Weaknesses which give rise to various forms of herniation can occur in this area. Protrusion of the anterior vaginal wall, which includes the bladder, is referred to as a "cystocele," while protrusion of the posterior vaginal wall, which includes the rectum, is referred to as a "rectocele." The latter will occur especially after separation of the levator muscles following childbirth. If weakness develops in the area of the cul-de-sac, then this portion of the vaginal wall descends, occasionally accompanied by the small bowel, resulting in an "enterocele." A weakness can occur in the distal anterior vaginal wall with a bulging of the urethra. This occurs after destruction of the fascial support of the urethra and the bladder neck, and usually urinary incontinence accompanies the hernia in these patients. Weakness can develop in the ligamentous support of the uterus as well as in the muscular support, and this results in varying degrees of uterine and cervical prolapse, as illustrated in Fig. 41-10.

ENDOCRINOLOGY

Hypothalamic Releasing Factors and Gonadotropic Hormones

Releasing factors are polypeptides that originate from the base of the brain (hypothalamus) near the pituitary gland and affect secretion of all the various pituitary hormones. A decapeptide, luteinizing hormone releasing factor (LRF), has been identified and seems to control gonadotropin synthesis and release.

Gonadotropins, polypeptide hormones associated with carbohydrates (glycoproteins), stimulate the gonads. The gonadotropins of pituitary origin are follicle-stimulating hormone (FSH) and luteinizing hormone (LH). The development of sensitive radioimmunoassays for these hormones permits their measurement in human serum, allowing new and more precise investigation of their circulating levels in various physiologic as well as pathologic conditions.

FOLLICLE-STIMULATING HORMONE (FSH). In the female, in the presence of small amounts of LH, this hormone stimulates the immature ovarian follicle to antral formation (Fig. 41-11). In the male, FSH stimulates the cells of the seminiferous tubules and increases spermatogenesis.

LUTEINIZING HORMONE (LH, ICSH). This is the ovulatory hormone. Ovulation occurs after the midcycle LH surge (Fig. 41-11), and luteinization of the ovarian theca cells occurs following the rupture of the graafian follicle. Although another stimulant, luteotropic hormone (LTH), maintains corpus luteum function in rats, only LH appears to have any relation to corpus luteum activity in man. In

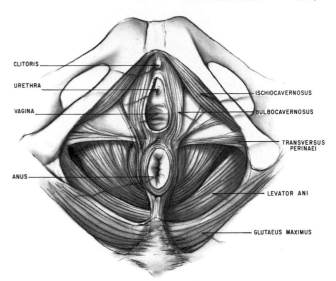

Fig. 41-9. Superficial layer of the urogenital diaphragm in the female.

the male LH stimulates the Leydig cells (interstitial cells), causing androgen secretion. Administration of ovulatory-suppressing oral contraceptives abolishes this peak.

HUMAN CHORIONIC GONADOTROPIN (HCG). This hormone is normally secreted in the human being by the placenta during pregnancy. It is occasionally elaborated by testicular or ovarian tumors. In the pregnant female, it can be detected in the second week of pregnancy or at about the time of the missed period, when it appears in the urine as well as other body fluids. This hormone is secreted maximally in about the third month of pregnancy and then decreases. It rapidly disappears approximately 2 weeks after delivery. Excessive quantities of HCG are secreted by patients with trophoblastic disease (hydatidiform mole and choriocarcinoma). The hormone has primarily a luteinizing effect, although it is not chemically identical with LH from the anterior pituitary. Its biologic action in various animals has formed the basis of many pregnancy tests. HCG causes hemorrhagic follicles and corpora lutea formation in immature mice (Aschheim-Zondek test) and in mature female rabbits (Friedman test).

Fig. 41-10. Diagrammatic representation of first- and second-degree prolapses of the uterus.

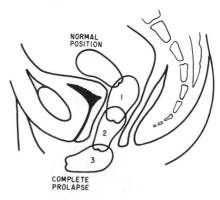

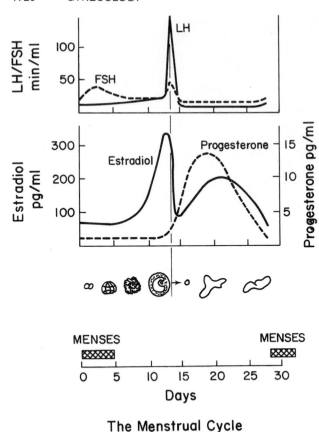

The Menstrual Cycle

Fig. 41-11. Hormonal changes during the menstrual cycle.

It also causes spermiation in the toad and frog, making possible the highly sensitive biologic *Rana pipiens* test. Although chorionic gonadotropin is secreted and is detectable by the time of the first missed period, most of these biologic tests do not become positive until 1 or 2 weeks after the first missed period and occasionally even later. The biologic tests now are rarely used clinically. They have been replaced by immunologic assays which are usually based on agglutination of sensitized red cells or latex particles. These immunologic assays are sensitive and clinically useful tools, although false-positive and false-negative reactions can result with these as well as with biologic assays. Radioimmunoassays permit precise and sensitive measurement of HCG and β-HCG in serum and urine and are useful for monitoring patients who have been treated for trophoblastic disease.

Clinical Gonadotropic Estimation. Many clinical studies dealing with problems of reproduction have noted altered gonadotropic activities in terms of the bioassays and radioimmunoassays. Low levels suggest lack of gonadotropic secretion from the anterior pituitary. Very high levels are detected during the menopause and in cases of premature ovarian failure due to excessive gonadotropin production from the pituitary. The urine bioassays are much less accurate than serum assays, which permit measurement of FSH and LH.

Steroid Hormones

A schema of steroid metabolism, starting with cholesterol and ending with estrogen, is shown in Fig. 41-12. However, for simplicity alternative pathways and many steps are omitted.

ESTROGENS

These are female sex hormones secreted primarily from the ovary with a small contribution from the adrenal. In the pregnant female the placenta is a major source of both estrogen and progesterone. Estrogens occur in many chemical forms but in the urine they are usually measured as estrone, estradiol, and estriol. Recent development of sensitive competitive binding assays has allowed their measurement in serum. They are secreted throughout the menstrual cycle, with greater quantities detected after ovulation (Fig. 41-11). These hormones cause an increase in the size of genital tissues, i.e., of the uterus, fallopian tubes, and breasts. Under their stimulation, there is increased mitotic activity in both the myometrium and endometrium. The vaginal mucosa thickens with proliferation of vaginal epithelium and cornification of surface cells. With increased glycogen deposition in the vaginal cells and under the action of the Döderlein bacilli, lactic acid is formed, decreasing the pH of the vagina and providing some protection against vaginal infection.

In addition to the effect on the myometrium, estrogens may cause a growth in the size of fibroids (leiomyomas), a fact that should be remembered when giving patients estrogen-containing oral contraceptives.

PROGESTERONE

This hormone is secreted throughout the cycle but is released in significant quantities mainly from the corpus luteum after the rupture of the graafian follicle (Fig. 41-11). Therefore, changes induced by this increase in progesterone are taken to be reasonable circumstantial evidence for the occurrence of ovulation. However, the only proof of ovulation in the human being is pregnancy, since progesterone can be secreted from an ovary which has undergone theca luteinization without corpus luteum formation.

Progesterone is thermogenic and, as a result, causes a rise of $\frac{1}{2}$ to 1°F in body temperature. This is the basis of the use of a monthly basal body temperature chart as an indirect indication of ovulation. Progesterone can be measured chemically in serum by competitive binding radioimmunoassays available in research laboratories and more recently in commercial laboratories. It can be indirectly measured in the urine in the form of its metabolite, pregnanediol, and 5 to 10 mg/24 hours are usually excreted during the secretory phase of the menstrual cycle.

ANDROGENS

The normal ovary secretes a small amount of androgens during the normal cycle, with a small midcycle peak. As one follicle develops, the other follicles become atretic and stromal cells are formed. These stromal cells secrete prin-

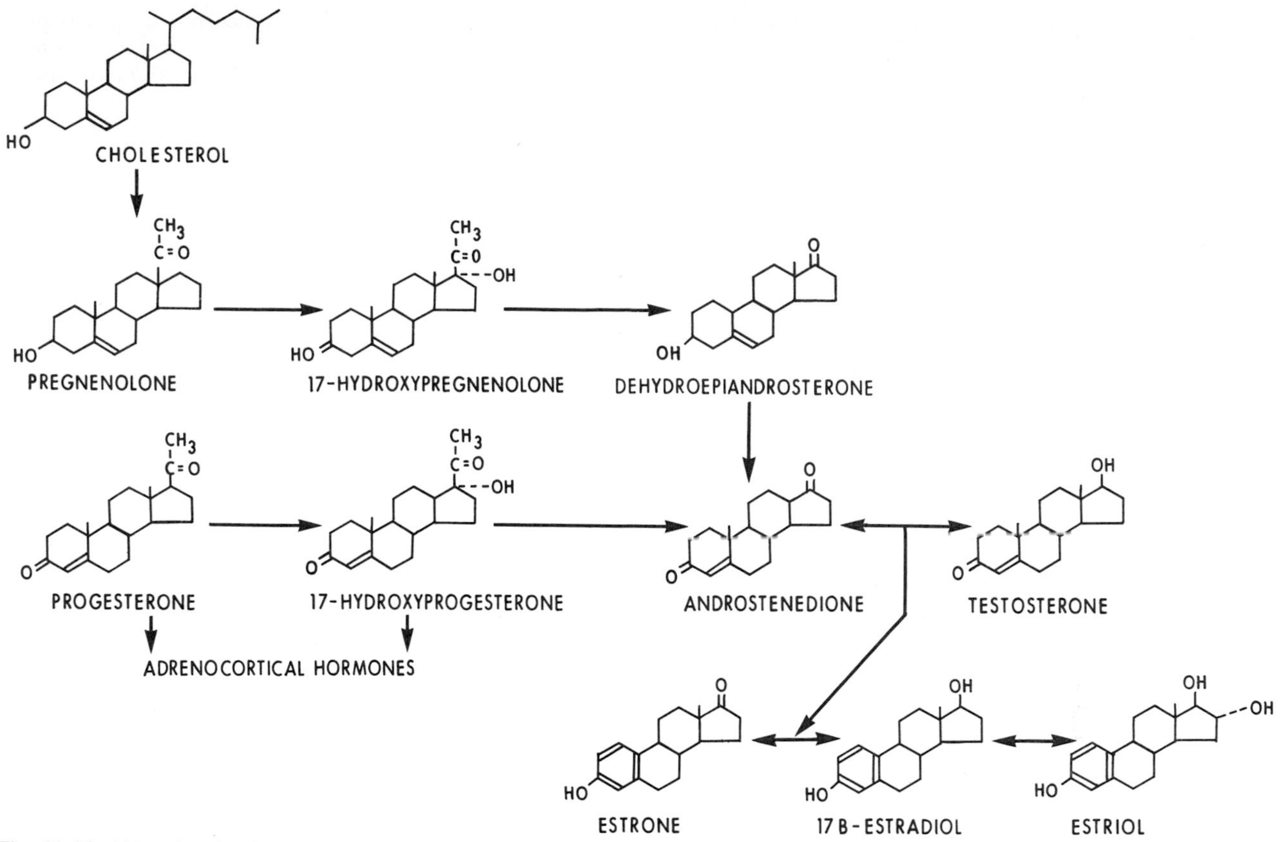

Fig. 41-12. Abbreviated schema of steroid metabolism.

cipally the 17 β-hydroxysteroids (androstenedione, testosterone, etc.).

17-Ketosteroid determinations have been used as an assessment of androgen function. These metabolic products of adrenal and testicular secretion are measurable in the urine. There is only a small contribution from the ovary in the female. Although 17-ketosteroid output may be elevated in certain masculinizing conditions, it is not necessarily a good guide to androgenic function in the female. For example, doubled secretion of testosterone, a potent androgenic hormone, from the adrenal or the ovary would cause very noticeable masculinizing effects. However, because of the small amount of this hormone that would be chemically present, there would not be any detectable change in the 17-ketosteroid output. The recent availability of sensitive radioimmunoassays to measure serum testosterone and other androgens permits more precise investigation of masculinizing conditions.

Hormonal Events in the Menstrual Cycle

At this point it is important to note the dynamic relationship of these hormones during the menstrual cycle. The menstrual cycle can be described in three phases: the follicular, ovulatory, and luteal phases. These phases are determined by the steroid, gonadotropin, and hypothalamic feedback mechanisms.

During the reproductive life of the female, a certain number of follicles begin to grow. The mechanisms that determine which follicles or how many will grow per cycle are undetermined. This selection is probably a matter of timing and morphologic characteristic. Shortly before menses, a rise in FSH (Fig. 41-11) results in stimulation of a follicle or follicles. This rise in FSH probably represents an escape from the negative feedback of estradiol during the previous luteal phase. However, the estradiol level never becomes low enough in the normal menstrual cycle to allow a negative feedback escape for LH. Consequently LH is probably not essential in initiation of the menstrual cycle.

As the follicle grows there is a concomitant rise in estradiol level. The source of estradiol seems to be predominantly the thecal cells surrounding the follicle. With a rise in level of estradiol the negative feedback of FSH occurs and FSH levels begin to drop. The little amount of FSH that remains probably is selectively bound in the developing follicle as a result of the high follicular levels of estradiol. Thus the follicle continues to develop, and this mechanism ensures that only one follicle will reach ovulation. As midcycle approaches, the lesser follicles begin to undergo atresia.

At midcycle a surge of estradiol triggers a midcycle surge of LH and also a small surge of FSH. The actual release of the egg occurs approximately 24 hours after this LH peak. The LH surge also results in the beginning luteinization of the follicle. Consequently, at midcycle the progesterone level begins to rise and remains elevated during the luteal phase.

During the luteal phase, progesterone has a negative effect on LH, especially in the presence of estradiol. FSH is also suppressed because of the high estradiol levels. Although suppressed, small amounts of gonadotropins, especially LH, are necessary for normal corpus luteum function. Also for the first few days after ovulation the granulosa cells enlarge and capillaries penetrate into the granulosa layer, often filling the central cavity with blood. The peak of vascularization occurs by day 8 or 9 after ovulation and is usually associated with the peak serum levels of progesterone and estradiol. After this the corpus luteum enters a period of regression, as noted by decreasing progesterone levels. This life-span for the corpus luteum is consistently 14 days. At the end of this time the steroid levels fall and the whole cycle begins again with menses.

Fig. 41-13. *A.* Proliferative endometrium. *B.* Secretory endometrium.

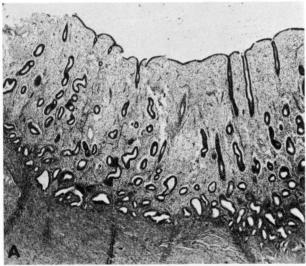

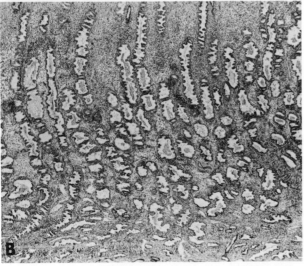

With pregnancy, survival of the corpus luteum is prolonged by the trophoblastic production of HCG. This new stimulus first appears at the peak of corpus luteum development, just in time to prevent luteal regression. HCG then maintains the corpus luteum until 8 to 10 weeks of gestation, by which time placental steroidogenesis is established.

The gonadotropins are under the control of hypothlamic releasing factors. LRF seems to control both FSH and LH functions. The control of the reproductive cycle seems to depend upon the level of LRF at any given moment. This function, in turn, seems to depend upon complex and coordinated interrelationships among the releasing factor(s), other neurohormones, pituitary gonadotropins, and gonadal steroids. These relationships are governed by feedback mechanisms of both stimulatory and inhibitory nature.

CHRONOLOGIC DEVELOPMENTAL FEMALE PHYSIOLOGY

The normal female infant is born with a small uterus, most of which consists of cervix. The ovaries and fallopian tubes are present but much smaller than in the adult. A small vagina opens to the exterior through the folds of the hymenal ring. Except for the effects of maternal hormones that may be present immediately after birth, the female infant has little, if any, gonadotropin or ovarian hormone present.

Normally puberty will begin between the ages of nine and seventeen (average at twelve and one-half) years of age. If menstruation occurs prior to age nine, precocious puberty is diagnosed, while menstruation after age seventeen warrants the diagnosis of delayed puberty. It appears that menstrual function begins earlier in Western populations, possibly as the result of improved hygiene and nutrition.

The first anatomic evidence of puberty is development of breast budding and then of pubic hair at about the age of ten or eleven. In addition there is an increase in the size of the internal and external genitalia. The uterine fundus increases in volume at a greater rate than the cervix, and in the adult the uterine fundus is approximately twice the size of the cervix. Axillary hair also develops during puberty, but this usually does not take place until after breast and pubic hair development. The adolescent growth spurt is also occurring at this time.

Menstrual bleeding usually follows the development of the secondary sexual characteristics already described. Initial bleeding is usually anovulatory and irregular. Ovulatory cycles, which may occur at 4- to 6-week intervals, begin in about 1 year. Their onset is often heralded by pelvic pain occurring at the time of menses. The characteristic hormonal changes which occur during the menstrual cycle are illustrated in Fig. 41-11. By definition the first day of menstrual bleeding is considered to be day 1 of the cycle. The average volume of blood loss during a normal menstrual cycle is estimated to be from 35 to 150 ml, and it will usually last from 3 to 6 days, with much individual variation. An interval between menses of 6 to 8 weeks is not uncommon.

During menstruation the superficial layers of endometrium are cast off, leaving the stratum basalis and much of the stratum spongiosum, which lies superficial to the basalis, in situ and ready to begin regeneration during the cycle. Estrogen stimulation during the first part of the menstrual cycle causes mitoses in the endometrial glands and stroma, resulting in a proliferative endometrial pattern (Fig. 41-13A). During this proliferative phase of the cycle the endometrium increases in thickness. As the middle of the cycle approaches, estrogen output from the ovary increases (Fig. 41-11). Ovulation occurs, and corpus luteum formation resulting in progesterone secretion follows. Progesterone stimulates coiling of the glands of the endometrium, which become filled with fluid, resulting in a secretory pattern (Fig. 41-13B).

The cervical mucus and vaginal cytologic features are also altered during the menstrual cycle. In the proliferative phase the cervical mucus forms a fernlike pattern when it is allowed to dry. At ovulation the volume of cervical mucus greatly increases. It becomes tenacious and can be drawn into a long thread (*Spinn barkheit* phenomenon). At this time the mucus is maximally receptive to sperm and thus ideally suited to fertilization of the recently released ovum. The cervical mucus then decreases in volume, and because of the influence of progesterone, loses its ability to fern. Serial examination of the vaginal smear during the proliferative phase of the cycle shows a gradual increase in the number of superficial cornified cells. After ovulation these cells are less prevalent because of the influence of progesterone. Thus, a rough estimate of hormonal status can be gained by examining the cervical mucus and vaginal smear during the menstrual cycle.

As menopause approaches, anovulatory periods begin to occur with increased frequency. Occasionally a period will be missed or will come later than expected. Menopausal bleeding is characterized by skips and delays. If menses are absent for more than 6 months, any subsequent vaginal bleeding should be considered abnormal and deserves further investigation. With the decrease in hormonal function and drop in estrogen output, there is a concomitant rise in gonadotropin secretion. The vaginal pH becomes more alkaline, because of decrease in glycogenation of the vaginal epithelium and decreased action of the Döderlein bacillus. The vaginal mucosa becomes thinner and is more prone to secondary infection. The patient may complain of sudden and sharp feelings of heat (hot flashes), which can usually be controlled by small doses of oral estrogen.

GYNECOLOGIC EXAMINATION

The gynecologic history includes careful attention to all the details of menstrual and reproductive function such as onset and frequency of menstruation, length and amount of menstrual bleeding, and the dates of the two most recent menstrual periods. If pain is a problem, when does it occur? Is it related to the menstrual cycle? Where

is it? How severe is it? Does it radiate? What relieves it, and what, if anything, makes it worse? Are there any urinary or gastrointestinal symptoms? Physical examination includes pelvic examination, which is most comfortably done with the patient in the lithotomy position, suitably draped and always accompanied by a nurse chaperone. The external genitalia are first visualized, special note being made of hair distribution, the size of the clitoris, the patency of the hymen, and any enlargements or inflammations, such as may be associated with Bartholin's glands. Skin lesions, such as may be seen with venereal infection, and vaginal discharges are also noted. The cervix is exposed with a water-lubricated speculum. Surgical jelly is not used because it will interfere with cytologic sampling (PAP smear). After cytologic sampling is complete, a bimanual examination is carried out and palpation performed, as illustrated in Fig. 41-14. First the fundus is felt; its position, its size, and the contour of the surface are noted. Leiomyomas (fibroids) cause smooth irregularities in the uterine surface which may vary in size from a few millimeters to several centimeters. A smooth indentation at the apex of the fundus may suggest a bicornuate or arcuate uterus. The left and right adnexal regions are then carefully palpated bimanually. The patient is asked to cough, and the support of the pelvis is carefully noted. If there is a weakness in the anterior wall (cystocele), the support of the urethra is carefully examined, and the patient is evaluated for stress incontinence. Separation of the levators will develop a weakness and herniation of the posterior vaginal wall (rectocele), and occasionally these may become sufficiently severe to cause constipation. Herniation near the apex of the vagina between the uterosacral ligaments usually contains small bowel (enterocele) and frequently is seen in patients with pelvic relaxation. If the ligamentous attachment and levator supports of the uterus and cervix should become weakened, descensus will be noted, and occasionally the cervix may even be seen to protrude through the introitus. Finally a rectal examination is performed, both to confirm the findings of the vaginal examination and also to palpate carefully the uterosacral ligaments, the back of the cervix and uterus, and the contents

Fig. 41-14. *A.* Bimanual abdominovaginal palpation of the uterus. *B.* Bimanual abdominovaginal palpation of the adnexa.

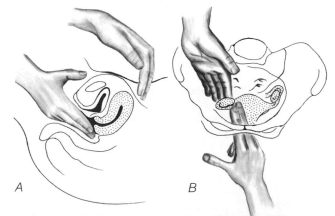

of the cul-de-sac (pouch of Douglas). These areas are often sites of nodularity and tenderness in cases of endometriosis and are important areas to be checked for spread in cases of cervical carcinoma.

SYMPTOMS

Pain

Cyclic pain associated with the menstrual cycle is known as *"dysmenorrhea."* When no demonstrable pathologic condition is present, the diagnosis is "primary, or idiopathic, dysmenorrhea." This is thought to occur only at the end of the ovulatory cycle. It would appear that some of the pain associated with menstrual bleeding is caused by the dilatation of the cervix due to mechanical stretching of the endocervical canal that accompanies the passage of blood and clot. This pain sensation is believed to be transmitted to the cervicouterine ganglion (Frankenhäuser's plexus) which is located on the posterior wall of the uterus near the uterosacral ligaments. Pain is then transmitted via the hypogastric presacral plexus to the spinal cord, to enter at the level of approximately T_{11} and T_{12}. The pain is usually sharp and may occasionally be colicky. It is usually confined to the lower abdomen and can radiate to the back and sides. The patient often complains of a dull, heavy ache and may also have nausea and a feeling of bloating. In severe cases there may even be vomiting.

The pain may begin prior to, or just with, the onset of menstruation, but as a rule the worst pain occurs early during the menstrual flow. It may be that some of the menstrual pain is due to hyperirritability and irregular contractions of the uterine musculature in addition to the dilatation of the cervix. Constriction of the spiral arterioles in the uterine musculature may result in ischemic pain, which could contribute to the discomfort noted at the time of the menstrual flow.

In dealing with primary dysmenorrhea and premenstrual tension, conservative measures are usually the best. Simple analgesics, such as aspirin and occasionally codeine, are helpful. Sympathomimetic drugs are helpful for menstrual cramps. For those patients who complain of premenstrual tension and the feeling of bloating prior to the onset of menses, salt restriction and even diuretics for approximately a week prior to the onset of menses and for the first few days of the cycle may give symptomatic relief. Since these symptoms are noted with ovulatory cycles, a severe case can be treated by the administration of cyclic oral contraceptives. If all these measures fail and the patient is either incapacitated by pain or requires long-term narcotics for its control, then surgical therapy can be tried. In such cases, removal of the hypogastric plexus, i.e., a presacral neurectomy, is indicated. Care should be taken to remove all the nerve tissue located anterior to the sacrum, which means a complete dissection between the hypogastric vessels and identification of both ureters. It is almost never necessary to undertake this procedure for primary dysmenorrhea.

In cases where there is demonstrable pathology, the term "secondary dysmenorrhea" is applied to the menstrual pain. It is treated by attempts to correct the specific cause. One of the most common causes is endometriosis. The patients complain of severe and increasing menstrual discomfort that progressively becomes worse. A few patients have an extremely tight cervical os, either on a congenital basis or as the result of extensive cauterization or cryosurgical treatment, and nulliparous females are especially prone to stenosis. In such cases, dilation of the stenosed cervix may occasionally help. Some patients will have acute pain and some fever, with diffuse abdominal symptoms at the time of menses. These patients are often previous victims of pelvic inflammation, and their pain during menstruation is believed to be associated with the residual effects of chronic pelvic inflammatory disease (PID). Occasionally, pain is related to an endometrial polyp or an intraluminal fibroid (leiomyoma) which is being extruded from the uterine cavity.

Lower abdominal pain may occur at times other than during menstruation. Chronic pelvic inflammation and adhesions can cause diffuse nonmenstrual abdominal pain. These patients have vague and continuous symptoms of pelvic pain. Pain coming in the middle of the cycle at about the tenth or fourteenth day of the period should suggest ovulation pain (mittelschmerz) or a ruptured ovarian cyst. Ectopic pregnancy should be considered in patients with midcycle pain, especially if the previous period is scanty or of an irregular nature.

Both the gastrointestinal and genitourinary tract can cause pelvic symptoms, and it is important to consider the kidney, ureters, the appendix, and the lower bowel in any evaluation of pelvic pain.

GYNECOLOGIC EVALUATION OF ACUTE ABDOMINAL PAIN. An assessment of the female patient with acute lower abdominal pain necessitates separation of those problems which require operative intervention from cases in which surgical treatment is unnecessary or even undesirable. Ectopic pregnancy, twisted ovarian cyst, ruptured tuboovarian abscess, and appendicitis all require surgical intervention, while a ruptured corpus luteum cyst usually requires no therapy and acute pelvic inflammation is preferably treated without surgical intervention. The character and location of the pain combined with the patient's history and physical findings usually provide sufficient clues to lead to a reasonable therapeutic course.

Pregnancy symptoms combined with an adnexal mass suggest ectopic pregnancy. Pain, when present, is often unilateral. Bilateral lower abdominal pain intensified by cervical motion and accompanied by fever is usually seen in patients with acute pelvic inflammatory disease. A tender adnexal mass may be an ovarian cyst, an ectopic pregnancy, or an inflammatory mass. An accompanying high fever and high white blood cell count suggest tuboovarian abscess or pyosalpinx. Further details to be considered in the differential diagnosis of lower abdominal pain in the female patient are discussed in the sections on pelvic inflammatory disease and ectopic pregnancy.

When a pathologic condition of the tube or ovary is suspected (ectopic pregnancy, ruptured ovarian cyst), direct visualization of the internal genitalia through the laparoscope (Fig. 41-15) can provide an accurate diagnosis. The procedure is carried out in the operating room under general and occasionally local anesthesia. The laparoscope is usually introduced through a small subumbilical incision after carbon dioxide has been introduced to distend the peritoneal cavity. The laparoscope provides an excellent view of the pelvis and intraabdominal contents. Laparoscopy is usually performed with the patient in the Trendelenburg position. A second small probe introduced a few centimeters above the symphysis aids in manipulation and helps to provide a complete evaluation of the internal genitalia.

Disorders of Support—Pelvic Hernias and Urinary Incontinence

The involuntary loss of urine is termed "incontinence." If this follows coughing, sneezing, or straining, the term "stress incontinence" applies. Stress incontinence is secondary to inadequate pelvic support and must be differentiated from other causes of incontinence. "Urgency incontinence" is characterized by an involuntary loss of urine accompanied by a frequent urge to urinate. This suggests

Fig. 41-15. *A.* Method of transparietal laparoscopy. (*After Steptoes.*) *B.* View of laparoscopy of normal uterus and adnexa with minimal endometriosis. (*After M. R. Cohen.*) Figure reprinted from Gynecological Laparoscopy, Symposia Specialists, P.O. Box 610397, Miami, Fl. 33161.

a urinary tract infection, nonspecific inflammation at the base of the bladder (trigonitis), or occasionally bladder sphincteric spasm. "Overflow incontinence" is due to persistently large, retained urinary volumes which occur in neurogenic atonic bladders of diabetics and are associated with large cystoceles. The involuntary loss of urine unassociated with stress is a characteristic of neurologic disease, such as multiple sclerosis. Involuntary loss of urine occurs with vesicovaginal or urethrovaginal fistulas.

Once it has been established that the patient has stress incontinence requiring correction, further evaluation should include urine culture to rule out urinary tract infection, cystoscopy to rule out trigonitis, a demonstration of stress incontinence at the time of pelvic examination and correction of this when the examiner elevates the bladder neck in such a way as to restore the posterior urethrovesical angle to prevent the loss of urine (Marshall test). Finally, a cystometrogram and measurement of postvoiding residual urine are important to rule out neurogenic causes of urinary complaints. Some investigators find x-ray definition of the posterior urethrovesical angle helpful in evaluating the extent of anatomic derangement.

CONSIDERATIONS IN THE THERAPY OF PELVIC RELAXATION AND URINARY STRESS INCONTINENCE. In certain cases, the amount of stress incontinence is mild. The patient can be helped by practicing starting and stopping her urinary stream during the course of voiding (Kegel exercises). If the patient is found to have urinary frequency and urgency, then conservative therapy of antispasmodics is occasionally helpful. Dilation of the vesical sphincter may give symptomatic relief, especially in elderly patients

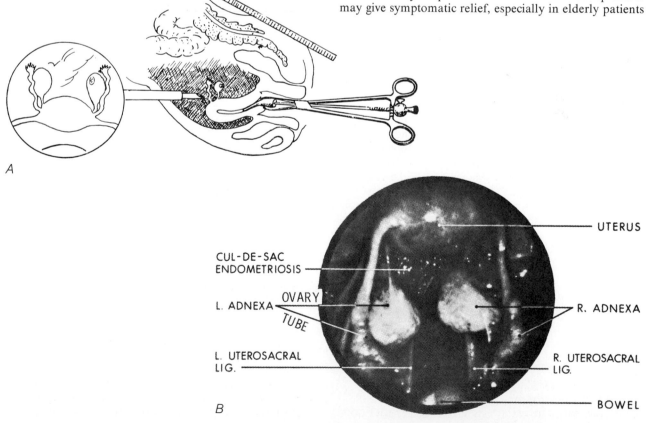

A

CUL-DE-SAC
ENDOMETRIOSIS

L. ADNEXA

OVARY

TUBE

L. UTEROSACRAL
LIG.

UTERUS

R. ADNEXA

R. UTEROSACRAL
LIG.

BOWEL

B

troubled with nocturia. Surgical intervention is indicated for those patients who are wet much of the time and suffer social embarrassment or limitation as a result of urinary stress incontinence. If there is simple loss of the posterior urethrovesical angle without a change in the angle of the urethra with respect to the horizontal axis when the patient strains, then the patient is said to have Type I stress incontinence. If, in addition to the loss of the posterior urethrovesical angle, there is rotational descent of the urethra with respect to the horizontal axis, then Type II stress incontinence exists.

If a patient complains of stress incontinence and is noted to have a cystocele and rectocele without descent of the uterus and cervix, then an anterior and posterior colporrhaphy should usually provide a good repair. In deciding whether or not to repair a cystocele, not only is the size of the hernia important but also the degree to which the patient is bothered by it, including prior urinary symptoms. If she has not had stress incontinence but appears to have had recurrent urinary tract infection or overflow incontinence due to a persistently large residual urine as a result of the cystocele, then a repair is also indicated. However, surgical repair is not indicated if the cystocele is asymptomatic and there have been no prior related complaints.

During the repair, the posterior urethrovesical angle is supported, and a sharp angulation of approximately 90° is reconstructed in this area. This is necessary not only to repair the causes of stress incontinence but also to avoid a flattening of the angle at the time of routine cystocele repair, which can lead to post-cystocele-repair stress incontinence. Support of the posterior vaginal wall must be achieved at the time of perineal repair by approximating the pubococcygeus muscle, which reconstitutes the muscular support of the pelvic floor. It is probably wise to avoid repairs in patients wishing to have more children.

If in addition to the above complaints, the patient has descensus of the uterus, then a vaginal hysterectomy may be combined with the repair. When a vaginal hysterectomy is done, the uterosacral ligaments should be used for apical vaginal supports, both to support the vagina and to prevent future enterocele. In certain cases, there is elongation of the cervix with moderately good support of the fundus, in which case a cervicectomy (Manchester-Fothergill operation) can be performed. This operation is also used in cases where there is a severe symptomatic pelvic hernia in patients who wish to preserve childbearing function. Although vaginal hysterectomy can usually be accomplished at the time of most repairs, there are certain relative contraindications:

1. A greatly enlarged uterus, since it is unwise to attempt vaginal hysterectomy if the uterus is much larger than 10 or 12 cm. In many cases an enlarged descended uterus may be removed by splitting it into many small pieces during dissection (morcellation).
2. Extensive pelvic adhesions from previous infection or surgical treatment.
3. A previous abdominal uterine suspension, since the fundus is firmly adherent to the anterior abdominal wall.

If severe stress incontinence exists, especially without uterine descensus, it is less likely that a good repair can be obtained by the vaginal approach. However, in certain obese patients, this approach still can be used with hope of success. In most cases, a Marshall-Marchetti procedure is accomplished by a dissection of the retropubic space of Retzius. The urethra and bladder neck are supported anteriorly toward the symphysis by paraurethral sutures which restore the posterior urethrovesical angle. This operation is also used to treat recurrent stress incontinence previously treated by vaginal repair. If there is failure following Marshall-Marchetti repair, then a second Marshall-Marchetti procedure is occasionally attempted or a sling procedure may be carried out. The latter consists of a repeat dissection of the space of Retzius and also the urethra. A strip of anterior rectus abdominis fascia is passed under the urethra and tied to the opposite rectus abdominis fascia in order to suspend the posterior urethrovesical angle.

Prolapse of the vagina following hysterectomy may be corrected through an abdominal or vaginal approach, depending upon the patient's health as well as upon her desire to keep a functioning vagina. In elderly patients, a complete obliteration of the vagina can be carried out to eliminate space for future potential hernias. In patients who desire to keep a functioning vagina, the abdominal route can be used to fix the vaginal apex to the periosteum of the presacral area, thus providing the vagina with permanent support.

The use of a vaginal pessary should be considered, especially in the elderly patient who is not a good surgical candidate. This is particularly useful when the posterior vaginal wall is adequate to support the pessary. Three commonly used pessaries are shown in Fig. 41-16. The pessary used will depend upon the size of the vaginal opening and the comfort of the patient. The Smith-Hodge pessary is useful in younger patients where retroversion exists and where trial replacement of the uterus in an anterior position is desired.

Disorders of Bleeding

In the neonatal period, bleeding can occur secondary to withdrawal of maternal hormone stimulation. Bleeding in the infant and child is exceedingly rare and is usually a sign of vaginal foreign body, a hormonally functional tumor, or a genital tract tumor. Heavy vaginal bleeding may appear in the female with the onset of puberty. During this time, ovulation is not occurring, and partial development of ovarian follicles may result in low estrogen production. The endometrium fails to proliferate and may be atrophic. Surface necrosis appears to occur, and instead of the sharp disintegration that accompanies menstruation, there is a slow and prolonged surface oozing. The resulting bleeding can vary from a slight stain to a severe hemorrhage, and it can be sufficiently severe to require blood transfusion. Since estrogen lack is the cause, high doses of intravenous estrogen can be excellent therapy. Occasionally, prolonged estrogen stimulation without progesterone interaction leads to endometrial hyperplasia and menorrhagia. The bleeding and clotting factors should also be checked, since blood dyscrasia (idiopathic thrombocytopenia) can also be the cause of heavy vaginal bleeding

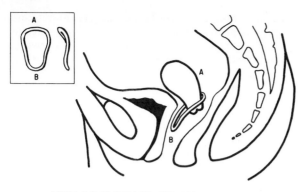
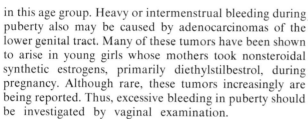
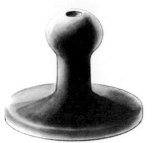
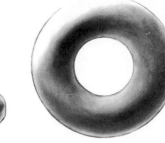

SMITH-HODGE PESSARY FOR RETROVERSION OF UTERUS

GELLHORN PESSARY   SIMPLE RING PESSARY

Fig. 41-16. Types of vaginal pessaries.

in this age group. Heavy or intermenstrual bleeding during puberty also may be caused by adenocarcinomas of the lower genital tract. Many of these tumors have been shown to arise in young girls whose mothers took nonsteroidal synthetic estrogens, primarily diethylstilbestrol, during pregnancy. Although rare, these tumors increasingly are being reported. Thus, excessive bleeding in puberty should be investigated by vaginal examination.

During the reproductive years, there can be great variation in the menstrual pattern. It is not unusual for a normal, healthy female to have two menstrual periods in a month or to miss a menstrual period without any underlying pathologic condition. Cyclic bleeding at midcycle, corresponding to the time of ovulation, is frequently seen. Changes in the menstrual pattern for which no pathologic explanation is readily available are referred to as "dysfunctional" bleeding. When this is diagnosed, simple observation for a few months is often sufficient.

During the reproductive years, ovulation probably does not occur every month, so that even in the normal individual there may be a few cycles during the year which are anovulatory. These cycles provide the variations in length of flow or intervals between flow that many healthy women occasionally notice. In addition, emotional stimuli can result in anovulation, delaying or changing the menstrual pattern. The bleeding can become extremely heavy and cause anemia. Anovulatory bleeding may be a consequence of old pelvic inflammation. Ovaries encased in adhesions have fewer ovulations as judged by histologic criteria.

Submucous fibroids may cause prolonged and heavy bleeding at the time of menstruation. A similar menstrual pattern is often seen in association with an enlarged uterus in which the myometrium is greatly thickened. The cause of such heavy bleeding may be the large surface of endometrium which is shed at the time of menstruation. Adenomyosis, referring to the condition in which glands of the endometrium grow into the myometrium, may, on rare occasions, be responsible for heavy bleeding. Blood dyscrasias and endocrine imbalance such as hypothyroidism are also very rare causes of heavy menstrual bleeding. Heavy menstrual bleeding may be associated with or produce iron deficiency anemia, which is corrected by oral iron therapy.

Postmenstrual staining is commonly due to endometrial or endocervical polyps, which are usually benign polypoid masses. A severe vaginitis or cervicitis may also be found to be the cause of this symptom. In addition, postmenstrual staining is seen with abnormalities of the secretory phase of the cycle. The syndrome, known as "irregular shedding of endometrium," appears to be caused by a slow shedding of the secretory endometrium, associated with prolonged progesterone secretion extending into the subsequent cycle. The diagnosis is made by performing an endometrial biopsy or a dilation and curettage on the fifth or sixth day of the cycle.

Intermenstrual bleeding can occur at the time of ovulation. Premenstrual staining may result when there is an inadequate luteal phase with a premature drop in progesterone output.

Bleeding unrelated to the menstrual cycle may be due to carcinoma of the cervix, which is the most common malignant condition in women in the reproductive years. The bleeding associated with this lesion is characteristically irregular, consists of postmenstrual staining, and often is accompanied by intermenstrual bleeding and staining. There may be postcoital staining or bleeding. Carcinoma of the ovary does not usually cause nonmenstrual bleeding unless hormonally functional tumors are present.

Tumors of the fallopian tubes rarely cause intermenstrual bleeding. There may be an intermittent mucous or serous discharge with the bleeding or staining, "hydrops tubae profluens." This occurs presumably as a result of blockage of the tube by a tumor. The tumor can occur at any age but is usually seen in older women and often occurs postmenopausally. Similarly, carcinoma of the endometrium is primarily a disease of postmenopausal women but may cause nonmenstrual bleeding in a younger woman.

Brisk bleeding can occur in early pregnancy. It may accompany implantation of the blastocyst a few days after fertilization. It is not unusual to have a small amount of bleeding or staining during the first few weeks of pregnancy. If the patient has bleeding during early pregnancy, then the diagnosis is "threatened abortion." If, however, tissue is passed, then abortion is considered to have taken place. Ectopic pregnancy can cause irregular bleeding early in pregnancy. *Although there is no characteristic history obtained with an ectopic pregnancy,* many patients will complain of a delay in menses followed by scanty bleeding or staining, often in association with pelvic pain. There may or may not be symptoms of pregnancy. Finally, irregular bleeding early in pregnancy, especially if the uterus is larger than anticipated by the menstrual history, suggests trophoblastic disease.

Postmenopausal bleeding frequently is caused by an endometrial or endocervical polyp or atrophic vaginitis. Carcinoma of any part of the reproductive tract or premalignant change in the endometrium may exist in the postmenopausal female. In all cases of vaginal bleeding, the bladder and rectum must be ruled out as origins of the blood.

AMENORRHEA

Primary amenorrhea is the failure to initiate menstruation prior to age eighteen. Secondary amenorrhea is diagnosed in a patient who has menstruated monthly but then fails to bleed for at least 6 months. Primary amenorrhea can result from anatomic abnormalities such as imperforate hymen, atresia of the vagina, and other congenital defects. However, there are numerous nonanatomic conditions which occur with either primary or secondary amenorrhea. In a few patients with recent weight gain and marked obesity, infrequent periods and finally amenorrhea may develop. Often simple diet and weight control will result in a resumption of menstruation. Emotional stimuli also serve as an important cause of amenorrhea.

Although emotional factors certainly must be considered in evaluating any patient, this is a diagnosis of exclusion since there are many endocrine causes of amenorrhea. Pituitary tumors, such as chromophobe adenoma or, in the young person, craniopharyngioma, can cause amenorrhea. In such cases, there may often be signs of failure of other endocrine systems due to the loss of pituitary function. Severe thyroid disturbance may be responsible for amenorrhea, and hyperthyroidism can be involved in varieties of menstrual dysfunction. Overactivity of the adrenal gland, as with adrenocortical hyperplasia or adrenal tumor with excessive hormone production, can result in disorders of ovulatory function and amenorrhea, and occasionally masculinization.

The ovary, itself, rarely can be the hormonal source causing amenorrhea. Functioning ovarian tumors can produce large amounts of estrogen or androgen. On occasion the ovary fails to function even in the early twenties, and the diagnosis of primary ovarian failure or premature menopause can be made in these cases by noting the abnormally high gonadotropin level. Oligomenorrhea or amenorrhea in the presence of polycystic ovaries with thickened capsules represent the Stein-Leventhal syndrome. Such patients may have increased production of ovarian androgens, and in some cases hirsutism and obesity are noted.

Pregnancy per se is the most common cause of amenorrhea in the reproductive age group. The sequelae of pregnancy are often pathologic causes of amenorrhea. Usually menstruation will recur within a month or two following pregnancy, with menses occurring later in patients who breast-feed. However, occasionally patients who undergo severe hemorrhage or shock during delivery do not have recovery of menstrual function and are unable to lactate. This is caused by pituitary insufficiency and is known as "Sheehan's syndrome." In this group of patients the tropic hormones associated with thyroid and adrenal function may or may not be impaired, while gonadotropic hormone is lost.

After delivery, persistent amenorrhea and milk production for a period of at least 6 months suggests the "Chiari-Frommel syndrome." Amenorrhea and galactorrhea not associated with pregnancy is known as "Del Castillo syndrome." In all patients with amenorrhea and persistent lactation, a pituitary tumor must be ruled out.

Occasionally, a patient bleeds following delivery due to retained products of conception and requires a dilatation and curettage. In a few instances, especially with repeated curettage, the lining of the endometrial cavity is so extensively removed that intrauterine synechiae result. This will cause a mechanical and persistent amenorrhea known as "Asherman's syndrome."

Anatomic defects, such as an imperforate hymen or absence of the uterus, are often apparent on physical examination. Evaluation of the pituitary-gonadal axis can be initiated by testing the amenorrheic person with an injection of progesterone. If there is estrogen priming of the endometrium, withdrawal flow will ensue. Similarly, one can examine the cervical mucus; ferning suggests adequate ovarian estrogen secretion and an intact pituitary with gonadotropin function capable of stimulating the ovary.

Thyroid function can be evaluated by one of the serum tests (protein-bound iodine concentration [PBI], resin-T3 uptake, serum thyroxine level). Any recent injections of iodine (uterotubogram, intravenous pyelogram) can alter the PBI. In addition, estrogen administration and oral contraceptives alter the protein binding of thyroid hormones and the results of serum thyroid tests. However, free thyroxine concentration (Free-T4), or T3, can be a useful determination since this substance is not bound to plasma proteins, and the concentration will remain unchanged in euthyroid patients receiving exogenous estrogen.

Adrenal function can be estimated by 24-hour urinary determination of 17-ketosteroid or 17-hydrocorticosteroid concentrations. Radioimmunoassays have become available to measure the plasma testosterone level as well as levels of other androgens such as dehydroepiandrosterone sulfate and androstenedione. Plasma cortisol (hydrocortisone) concentration also can be measured by these techniques.

If the 17-ketosteroid or 17-hydroxycorticosteroid levels are elevated, suppression can be attempted by administering one of the adrenocortical hormones or their analogs. Dexamethasone, 0.5 mg given four times a day, will cause suppression in cases of adrenocortical hyperplasia but not in cases of adrenal tumor. Low urinary steroid levels suggest adrenocortical or pituitary insufficiency. These can usually be differentiated by an ACTH stimulation test and a metyrapone (SU-4885) test. The patient is hospitalized, and 40 I.U. of ACTH is given intravenously over an 8-hour period on two successive days; serial 24-hour urine specimens are collected. A patient with normal adrenocortical function will at least double base-line 17-ketosteroid and 17-hydroxycorticosteroid outputs on the day following ACTH infusion.

If there is adrenocortical insufficiency, a low urinary steroid level will be followed by a small increase in response to ACTH infusion. Since metyrapone blocks 11-β-hydroxylation, its administration inhibits the conversion of progesterone to hydrocortisone. Thus, the normal inhibition of ACTH secretion from the pituitary by hydrocortisone is prevented when metyrapone is given. This results in an outpouring of pituitary ACTH and a concomitant increase in adrenocortical secretion. In patients with normal pituitary reserve, a doubling or tripling of 17-hydroxycorticosteroids follows metyrapone administration. With pituitary insufficiency, the decrease in hydrocortisone formation is unable to evoke an increase in ACTH secretion, and the rise in adrenocortical output and 17-hydroxycorticosteroids does not occur.

Hormonally active tumors should be removed. In cases of adrenal hyperfunction, therapy with 30 to 40 mg/day of cortisone can be tried. Hirsute patients may note a decrease in hair with this therapy. Some amenorrheic patients have been helped by clomiphene citrate (Clomid), which is a potent agent for the induction of ovulation. The drug has been particularly helpful in patients with intact pituitary function as indicated by normal gonadotropin excretion. Patients with the Stein-Leventhal syndrome have been successfully treated with this drug. For an occasional patient who truly fits the category of the Stein-Leventhal syndrome and cannot be treated successfully with clomiphene bilateral wedge resection of the ovary has also proved successful. Finally, there is a group of patients who will not respond to any of the above measures. For them, human menopausal gonadotropin has been useful, especially in cases with pituitary failure or removal due to tumor. These gonadotropins are potent and frequently may cause multiple pregnancies and large ovarian cysts.

A small number of twenty- to thirty-year-old patients are amenorrheic with high gonadotropin values. These patients have premature menopause or primary ovarian failure. Their menopausal symptoms can be controlled by small doses of cyclic estrogen therapy.

If a patient has Asherman's syndrome, attempts can be made surgically to break up the synechiae, which may re-form. In general, therapy of this condition has been disappointing, probably partly because of the necessary retention of residual endometrial tissue, which is capable of regenerating, in order to achieve an effective, new endometrial cavity.

Hirsutism and Masculinization

The amount of hair will vary with the individual's coloring and the family patterns. The amount to be expected on a young female may be estimated by examining the patient's parents. There is an increase in hair over the body, including the trunk, legs, and face, through menarche. Any significant increase in the amount or distribution of hair after the age of twenty-five is unusual.

Although hirsutism may be an early sign of virilization, in most cases it is usually a variant for the individual and not amenable to therapy. Excessive hairiness due to the virilization syndrome may be due to overactivity of the adrenal cortex such as is seen in Cushing's disease, a tumor of the adrenal, or masculinizing tumor of the ovary. Hirsutism is also seen with the Stein-Leventhal syndrome. Adrenal hyperactivity may be diagnosed by tests outlined in the previous section. Cortisone administration suppresses elevated 17-ketosteroid levels in cases of excessive adrenal activity. However, unlike cases of adrenal hyperplasia, functioning tumors will not respond to exogenous hormonal stimulation. Direct visualization of the ovary via the laparoscope (Fig. 41-15) permits diagnosis of the ovarian tumor of Stein-Leventhal syndrome.

Inherited Reproductive Defects

Genetic material is transmitted via the chromosomes, of which the normal human complement is 46, i.e., 23 pairs. These can be studied morphologically and arranged according to size in a karyotype. There are 22 autosomes and two sex chromosomes designated X and Y. The presence of two or more chromosome complements in an individual is termed a "mosaic." In the female there are normally two X chromosomes, and one of these chromosomes is believed to be the basis of a discrete bit of chromatin material in the nucleus of many female cells. This is referred to as the "Barr body" (Fig. 41-17). In general, the number of X chromosomes is one greater than the number of Barr bodies seen. Thus, if there are three X chromosomes, there would be two Barr bodies present in most cells examined. In the normal male (X-Y), no Barr bodies are present. Some of the common chromosomal abnormalities are as follows:

GONADAL DYSGENESIS (TURNER'S SYNDROME). These patients are characteristically short and have primary amenorrhea with high urinary gonadotropins and low estrogen. They are usually of the X-O chromosomal type and thus are negative for Barr bodies. The ovaries are absent or of the so-called streak variety.

MALE PSEUDOHERMAPHRODITISM. A pseudohermaphrodite is defined by the sex which is the true genetic pattern; i.e., the presence of a testicle would result in a male classification, but the patient would be phenotypically female. Thus, a patient with the syndrome of testicular feminization is a male pseudohermaphrodite. These patients are always chromosomally X-Y. The abnormal testis secretes androgen, but there appears to be "target insensitivity," and the patients have breast development with sparse axillary and pubic hair. The testes should be surgically removed, usually in the late teens, because of the high danger of malignancy. This should be followed by female sex hormone replacement, since the patients are psychologically adjusted to female life.

FEMALE PSEUDOHERMAPHRODITISM. In this condition a female patient with an ovary and X-X chromosomal complement develops male external characteristics. Many of these patients present as newborn females who were masculinized in utero from androgens or progestational

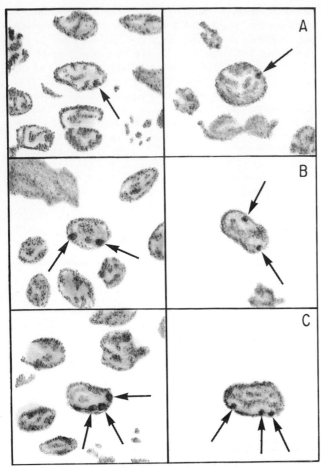

Fig. 41-17. Sex chromatin masses in cells of human skin (left) and vaginal mucosa (right). *A.* Normal female: XX. *B.* Klinefelter's syndrome with mental deficiency: XXXY. *C.* Eunuch with microorchism and mental deficiency: XXXXY. The finding of duplicate Barr bodies suggests the presence of a mosaic of an undetected third stem line, such as XXX or XXXY. (*After A. R. Sohval, Am J Med, 31:397, 1961, and M. L. Barr and D. H. Carr, Canad Med Assoc J, 83:979, 1960.*)

hormones administered to the mother during pregnancy. This syndrome can also develop from overactivity of the female adrenal cortex, which produces androgen and thus masculinization, such as in congenital adrenal hyperplasia and the adrenogenital syndrome.

THE POLY-X SYNDROME. This is a syndrome in which females have more than two X chromosomes, such as 47-XXX or 48-XXXX. These are referred to as "super-females." They are usually mentally deficient with underdeveloped female secondary sex characteristics.

TRUE HERMAPHRODITES. This is rare in the human being, although patients have been reported with both testicular and ovarian tissue. It is important to determine early how the patient would function best as an adult. As a rule, it is simpler to create a functioning vagina than to reconstruct the phallus.

FAULTY DEVELOPMENT OF GENITALIA. Patients are

encountered with faulty development of the external genitalia. The two most commonly encountered situations are the imperforate hymen and complete absence of the vagina. In the case of the imperforate hymen, a pelvic mass is usually noted in either the pubertal or newborn female. In the newborn infant such a tumor may be produced by secretions trapped behind the hymen. The infant should be catheterized to rule out bladder distension. Before any newborn female is explored abdominally for a pelvic mass, an imperforate hymen or transverse vaginal septum should be ruled out, for these conditions can be treated quite simply by a hymenotomy or incision of the septum with release of the trapped fluid. Abdominal exploration can result in destruction of the small female pelvic organs with lifelong consequences.

If no vagina exists, one can be constructed. After an adequate space is created, split-thickness skin grafts are placed and held with a vaginal mold. This is usually carried out in the patient's late teens or early twenties when she has sufficient psychosexual maturity and also is able to keep the mold in situ and change it by herself. The mold must be used unless the patient is having frequent intercourse. Delaying this procedure until the patient is ready to marry can result in severe emotional problems for her and her fiancé.

Disorders of Reproductive Capacity

A couple is not usually evaluated for infertility unless there has been 1 year of deliberate effort to conceive. The diagnostic scheme can be divided into four parts as follows (Fig. 41-18).

PROOF OF OVULATION. Since there is no proof except pregnancy, circumstantial evidence is used. A biphasic basal body temperature, an elevated serum progesterone level, and a secretory endometrial biopsy obtained in the luteal phase of the cycle, can be considered as a reasonable indication of ovulation.

THE TUBAL FACTOR. The patency of the tubes must be established. The passage of CO_2 through the tubes (Rubin's test) is recorded by alterations in CO_2 pressure during the test. Confirmation of passage of CO_2 is noted by shoulder pain in the erect patient a few minutes after the completion of the procedure. Since the test does not permit visualization of the tubes, it is possible that only one tube could be open. Direct visualization of the tubes can be obtained radiologically by a uterotubogram (hysterosalpingogram). In such cases the endometrial cavity is outlined, and tubal patency is established. Laparoscopy (Fig. 41-15) is an essential step in the evaluation. When laparoscopy is performed, the tubes can be lavaged with a dye, such as indigo carmine, at the time of the surgical procedure; efflux of the dye through the fimbriate ends of both tubes proves patency. At the same time the pelvic organs are inspected for other pathologic changes, including peritubal adhesions, endometriosis, etc.

PROBLEM OF IMPLANTATION. This includes an evaluation of the adequacy of the size and shape of the uterus, particularly in patients who have repeated first trimester

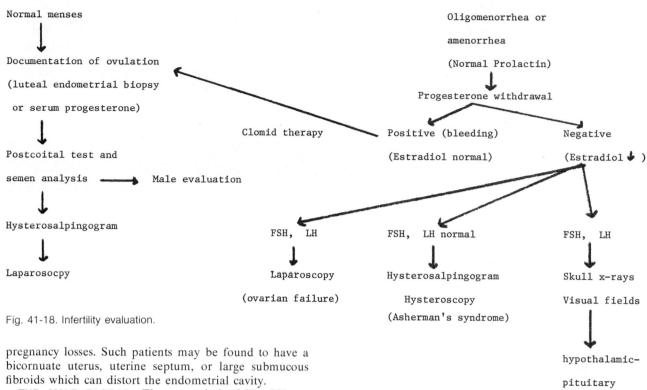

Fig. 41-18. Infertility evaluation.

pregnancy losses. Such patients may be found to have a bicornuate uterus, uterine septum, or large submucous fibroids which can distort the endometrial cavity.

THE MALE FACTOR. The postcoital (PCT, PK, or Huhner's) test evaluates this factor. The patient is instructed to have coitus with her husband about the time of midcycle, because it is at this time that the cervical mucus is most plentiful and most receptive to sperm. The mucus is then examined, optimally within 2 hours after coitus, at which time there should be numerous motile active sperm in a high-powered field (hpf). The number will vary depending upon the time the test is done and the amount of cervical mucus present. Usually 15 or more active sperm per hpf are seen. When the PCT contains this many sperm per hpf, the semen analysis will usually be at least 30 million sperm per cubic milliliter. When the PCT is less than that, repeated semen analyses should be done. The minimum accepted value is 20 million sperm per cubic milliliter, and a normal range is 40 million to 100 million sperm per cubic milliliter. A few pregnancies have been conceived by patients with counts as low as 10 million sperm per cubic millimeter. If a period of continence is followed by frequent intercourse, a gradual lowering of the sperm count can result.

Therapy of the infertile couple depends on the causative factor. If anovulation is the problem, then this should be treated according to the previously mentioned outline. In cases of uterine distortion, a myomectomy, reunification of a bicornuate uterus (Strassmann procedure), or removal of the uterine septum is usually necessary to achieve term pregnancy. If pelvic adhesions are present, chances for pregnancy can be improved if they are lysed, providing ovulatory and sperm functions are normal. Areas of endometriosis should be resected. Although the value of a ventral suspension is unproved, it is usually performed to improve theoretically the cervical exposure to the vaginal pool of semen. Tuboplastic procedures are performed to correct occlusion of the tube. Such surgical procedures should be avoided in cases of severe tubal destruction and are contraindicated in the cases of tuberculosis. A few pregnancies will result from tuboplasty procedures, but in most cases the results have been disappointing.

Pregnancy and Its Disorders

Amenorrhea in the reproductive years is most frequently caused by pregnancy. During the first weeks of normal pregnancy, the cervix becomes blue and soft. The cervicouterine junction softens, and the fundus of the uterus becomes boggy, especially near implantation site. The cervical vessels enlarge and are easy to palpate. Enlargement of the uterus may be noted as early as 2 to 3 weeks after the first missed menstrual period. Uterine enlargement continues, and by the tenth week the fundus can be felt just above the symphysis. Usually the patient will notice fetal movement (quickening) by the sixteenth to eighteenth week of gestation. The examiner may hear the fetal heart as early as the seventeenth to twentieth week of gestation, depending upon the size of the patient. The fundus reaches the umbilicus by about the twentieth week of gestation and extends to the xiphoid of the sternum by the thirty-sixth week.

A small amount of staining early in the first trimester of pregnancy is not uncommon. However, if bleeding is severe and is unaccompanied by the passage of tissue or dilatation of the os, then the diagnosis of *threatened abortion* is made. The uterine size is usually consistent with the dates of gestation. The urinary test for chorionic gonadotropin remains positive. If tissue has been passed through a dilated cervical os, then usually some products of conception remain in the uterus. Under such circumstances, the diagnosis of *incomplete abortion* is made, and a curettage, usually performed with a suction apparatus, is indicated to prevent further hemorrhage and also to prevent infection from the retained products of conception. Occasionally, in the first trimester of pregnancy, the entire products of conception are passed, and the complete sac of the total pregnancy can be identified. These complete abortions do not require further surgical therapy.

Induced (therapeutic) abortions are frequently performed for a variety of indications, including the preference of the patient. Usually, under local anesthesia, the products of conception are removed by suction curettage after the cervix has been dilated. It is preferable to perform the procedure prior to the twelfth week of pregnancy.

Some first trimester pregnancy losses are complicated by infection. These are almost invariably due to instrumentation to induce abortion. The patient usually presents with lower abdominal pain, fever, and occasionally cervical discharge. The uterus is tender, and there is pain on cervical motion. The white cell count is elevated. In severe cases, septicemia and septic shock may ensue. The patient becomes moribund and is unable to maintain her blood pressure. There is then decreased or absent urinary output.

Therapy of septic abortion is initiated by high doses of intravenous antibiotics. Hyperbaric oxygen has been used for clostridial infections. The treatment of septic shock is discussed in Chap. 4. Once the infection appears controlled and the patient stabilized, gentle evacuation of the uterus is carried out. A vigorous curettage should not be done, as bacteremia and septic shock can result from excessive surgical manipulation. If the patient does not respond to gentle evacuation of the uterus, or if there is persistent shock and decreased urinary output, or if there is a history of the intrauterine injection of a powerful chemical toxin such as soap, detergent, or lysol, then a hysterectomy may be required as a lifesaving procedure. In such cases it is important to remove both the tubes and ovaries, since these are often areas of microabscesses and toxic products which have accumulated as a result of sepsis.

A diagnosis of *missed abortion* is applied if the fetus does not remain viable and there is no sign of external bleeding or loss of the pregnancy. The uterus shrinks in size, and there is necrosis of the fetus and placenta. The chorionic gonadotropin test becomes negative. If the uterus is smaller than a 12-week size, it can usually be safely evacuated by a curettage. In very rare cases, a hysterotomy is necessary.

ECTOPIC PREGNANCY. Implantation of the fertilized ovum outside the endometrial cavity, usually in the tube or, occasionally, on the surface of the ovary or in the abdomen, results in an ectopic pregnancy. It occurs in less than 1 percent of pregnancies. Tubal ectopic pregnancy is believed to result from the improper transport of the fertilized ovum through the tube, either because of a congenital

defect in the tube or as the sequela of infection. It has been noted in many cases of ectopic pregnancies that the corpus luteum of pregnancy will exist in one ovary while the ectopic pregnancy is found to exist in the tube on the opposite side. Thus, there may have been transmigration of the fertilized ovum from one ovary to the contralateral tube; the time involved in this passage resulted in abnormal implantation into the tube rather than into the endometrial cavity. Patients who have had an ectopic pregnancy on one side are predisposed to the same problem in the opposite tube.

This is a disease of diagnostic surprises. There may be symptoms associated with early pregnancy such as breast tenderness, nausea, vomiting, and a delay in menses. There may be some bleeding or staining which follows a previously scanty period. The uterus often grows, but if an increase in size is noted, it will usually be less than expected for pregnancy, the duration of which is estimated from the menstrual history. Pain and cramps are often present. On physical examination, in addition to change in uterine size, an adnexal mass is occasionally palpable but may not be felt. Pain on cervical motion does occur and is usually localized to the side of the ectopic pregnancy. The pregnancy test may be positive or negative and often is not useful.

Occasionally, a patient will present with the pregnancy ruptured from the tube or extruded from the tip of the tube into the peritoneal cavity. The symptoms will then be of local peritoneal irritation due to the presence of blood. Characteristically, the patient complains of pain in the shoulder due to diaphragmatic irritation. In advanced cases, shock occurs because of heavy blood loss. Most ectopic pregnancies should be diagnosed before a vascular emergency occurs, but shock is seen in approximately 10 percent.

Ruptured ovarian cysts and pelvic inflammatory disease present with similar findings. Culdocentesis may aid in establishing the correct diagnosis. In most cases, the diagnosis can be made by laparoscopy. If this procedure is not feasible, an abdominal exploration is indicated.

The treatment of ectopic pregnancy consists of removal of the products of conception at the time of laparotomy. In certain cases, this measure can be followed by a tuboplastic procedure, which can preserve tubal patency. However, the tube is usually destroyed, and in such cases a salpingectomy must be performed. It is important to resect the cornual end of the tube to prevent the development of a future ectopic pregnancy in this site. Some authors recommend the removal of the ovary on the same side as the ectopic pregnancy in order to prevent future transmigration into the opposite tube, but such therapy should be reserved for patients in their later reproductive years.

ABNORMAL PREGNANCY GROWTH

Occasionally the products of conception will undergo abnormal growth and even malignant degeneration.

Trophoblastic Disease

Most cases of trophoblastic disease are benign *hydatidiform moles* which can be removed by curettage or hysterotomy. Locally invasive trophoblastic disease is usually referred to as "chorioadenoma destruens"; a truly malignant tumor is referred to as "choriocarcinoma." One cannot accurately predict the malignancy of trophoblastic disease from histologic appearance, but Hertig has devised a useful diagnostic categorization which divides trophoblastic disease into six groups: group I, benign; group VI, malignant; and the intervening groups ranging from the obviously benign to the obviously malignant. The disease occurs rarely and in the United States appears in approximately 1 out of every 2,000 pregnancies. There is a higher incidence in Asia, where there is approximately 1 case per 200 to 250 deliveries. The clinical picture is one of persistent bleeding and staining in early pregnancy with a uterus that is much larger than indicated by the menstrual history. Multiple pregnancies can be confused with this disease. Chorionic gonadotropin determinations often reveal levels higher than seen in normal pregnancy, while human placental lactogen (HPL) titers are lower. These can be measured in the patient's serum by radioimmunoassay. The use of ultrasonography aids in establishing the diagnosis of a normal or an abnormal pregnancy.

Placental polyp is not a true polyp but a focally retained part of the placenta. There is necrosis, inflammation, and occasional bleeding. Hertig classifies a placental polyp as being potentially malignant. It may have neoplastic trophoblast at its base. On the other hand, *syncytial endometritis*, which histologically can be confused with choriocarcinoma, is probably a benign lesion from the placental site that contains many inflammatory cells.

Trophoblastic disease can metastasize, and the most common sites of metastases are the lungs, vagina, brain, and liver, in decreasing order of occurrence. Antitumor agents provide excellent treatment. Methotrexate, actinomycin D, and Velban have been the most commonly used chemotherapeutic agents. It has been estimated that there is complete remission in approximately 50 percent of cases following the use of methotrexate or actinomycin D in the treatment of trophoblastic disease. In certain cases, surgical intervention is necessary, either to control hemorrhage or infection or to irradicate a solitary site which has been refractive to chemotherapy. However, primary surgical treatment of malignant trophoblastic disease does not appear to offer the patient as much benefit as chemotherapeutic agents.

SPECIFIC GYNECOLOGIC DISEASES

Infections and Discharges

During childhood, a whitish discharge, leukorrhea, may develop. At birth this increased vaginal secretion is usually due to maternal hormones and is entirely physiologic. A similar discharge may be seen in the pubertal female with the onset of estrogen stimulation. Severe leukorrhea during childhood is usually the result of infection caused by a foreign body in the vagina. The majority of vaginal discharges of children are caused by coliform organisms. Occasionally pinworm infection is the cause. The correct diagnosis can be established by direct visualization of the foreign body and culturing for pathologic organisms, or by doing a Scotch tape test for pinworms (*Enterobius vermicularis*). With the onset of menarche, various organisms can be implicated as the cause of a discharge.

The most common of these conditions caused by organisms follow.

TRICHOMONAS VAGINALIS INFECTION. This discharge is caused by a parasite. The trichomonad can be identified by its very active flagella, which can be seen beating, when the vaginal discharge mixed with a drop of saline solution is examined microscopically. The parasite flourishes in an alkaline pH. It often causes a strawberry red inflammatory reaction of the cervix and is usually accompanied by a green and extremely odorous discharge that is often worse at the time of menstruation, because of the alkalinity of the menstrual discharge. Treatment is carried out with a trichomonacidal drug, metronidazole (Flagyl) Vinegar douches are occasionally of symptomatic help. The male carries the infection asymptomatically and occasionally must be treated when there is recurrent infection in the female.

MONILIA VAGINITIS (*CANDIDA ALBICANS*). This fungus infection can occur at any time but is often seen during pregnancy, after the use of antibiotics, and frequently in diabetics. It flourishes in an acid environment. The fungus can be cultured on Nickerson's medium. Mycelial budding can be seen on direct examination of the vaginal secretion which has previously been treated with 10 percent potassium hydroxide to lyse epithelial cells. Grossly, the discharge looks like a thick white cottage cheese. It is extremely irritating, and the patients usually complain of marked itching. Local antifungal agents are effective, and it is usually wise to treat the gastrointestinal tract at the same time to eradicate the fungus. Alkaline douches occasionally help, and gentian violet staining of the vagina may also provide relief. Anti-inflammatory agents such as cortisone can be used for the irritated vulva.

NONSPECIFIC VAGINITIS. This discharge is due to bacteria, generally *H. vaginalis*, and is not associated with either *Trichomonas* or *Candida* infections. A purulent discharge is present, and polymorphonuclear cells as well as many bacteria can be seen on examination of the vaginal secretion. Specific bacterial cultures occasionally are done, but usually a gram-negative organism is the offender. There is often secondary infection of a chronically eroded cervix. Triplesulfa creams are effective, and if chronic cervicitis exists, improvement can often be obtained by cauterization of the erosion.

ATROPHIC VAGINITIS. This occurs in the elderly female or in the young patient after removal of the ovaries. The vaginitis is usually of a bacterial origin and results from secondary invasion of the atrophic vaginal tissues which have lost their thickness as well as acid protection. Vinegar douches are occasionally helpful, and small doses of estrogen either locally or orally can restore the integrity of the vaginal mucosa.

BARTHOLINITIS. Infection of Bartholin's duct may lead to obstruction and eventual dilatation, with the formation of a Bartholin's cyst. Occasionally these are asymptomatic and require no treatment. If the cyst is acutely inflamed, drainage by marsupialization is usually successful; in cases of recurrent infection, removal of the cyst and gland may become necessary.

VENEREAL INFECTIONS AND PELVIC INFLAMMATORY DISEASE

SYPHILIS. This disease should be suspected in any genital lesion. Serologic screening (VDRL) tests can be done. Definitive diagnosis is made by dark-field examination of scrapings of ulcers to demonstrate the spirochetes or fluorescent treponema antibody absorption (FTA-ABS) blood tests. The diagnosis may be made by examination of the spinal fluid in more advanced cases. Treatment is with penicillin.

CHANCROID. This is a painful ulcer of the vulva caused by the organism *Hemophilus ducreyi,* which can be cultured from the ulcer and responds to sulfonamide or streptomycin therapy.

GRANULOMA INGUINALE. This is a chronic inflammatory disease. The offending *Klebsiella* bacteria cause inclusion bodies to occur in the cells obtained from the ulcerating area (Donovan bodies). There are usually nontender ulcers, and streptomycin therapy is usually effective.

LYMPHOPATHIA VENEREUM. This is a viral disease which infiltrates the lymphatics and spreads to regional nodes, causing a severe adenitis. The groins, perineum, and lower gastrointestinal tract can be involved. The diagnosis is made by a skin test (Frei test), and therapy is effective with chloramphenicol or sulfonamide. Scarring in the region of the anorectum can become so severe that colostomy may be necessary.

CONDYLOMA ACCUMINATUM. These venereal warts are not truly venereal but often occur secondarily to vaginal discharges. Viruses have been implicated. If the primary cause can be found and the discharge corrected, the condylomas may disappear. They may be removed by hot cautery or chemically with podophyllin, but they frequently recur.

GONORRHEA. This common disease is caused by bacteria of the genus *Neisseria gonococcus.* The diagnosis can be established by examining the purulent discharge from the cervix, urethra, or Skene's glands. Polymorphonuclear leukocytes are present, containing gram-negative intracellular diplococci. The organisms can be cultured from the secretions, but the culture must be done immediately, since the organisms die soon after exposure to air, and a false-negative culture can result. There has been a recent sharp increase in the number of cases treated, and changes in sexual behavior patterns are resulting in continuing spread of the disease to individuals in all socioeconomic categories. Penicillin is the primary mode of therapy, but resistant strains of the organism are being detected. For the female, 4.8 million units of aqueous procaine penicillin plus 1 Gm of probenecid usually are given, and the dosage is repeated if the culture remains positive. For patients allergic to penicillin, tetracycline can be used, although it is usually less effective than penicillin. Tetracycline can be given orally; after a loading dose of 1.5 Gm, 0.5 Gm is given four times daily for 4 additional days. Ampicillin, 3.5 Gm given orally as one dose, or spectinomycin, 4 Gm intramuscularly, may be used.

PELVIC INFLAMMATORY DISEASE. Neisserian infection is frequently the initial cause of pelvic inflammatory disease in many patients. However, nongonoccal infection of the adnexa and pelvic tissue can follow abortion or pregnancy and has been reported with the use of intrauterine devices (IUD). The patients characteristically present with acute diffuse lower abdominal pain and a high fever, which may reach 103 to 104°F. There is severe pain on even slight motion of the cervix. The vagina is hyperemic and extremely warm. The tenderness noted on pelvic examination usually is bilateral because of the presence of a diffuse cellulitis. There may be some minor gastrointestinal complaints, but normal bowel sounds are usually present. The white blood cell count is elevated out of proportion to the degree of morbidity. In many cases, it is not possible to culture the pathogenic organism, but certainly an attempt should be made to rule out gonorrhea. Acute lower abdominal pain may also suggest appendicitis, ectopic pregnancy, twisted or ruptured ovarian cyst, or occasionally involvement of the urinary tract or the lower gastrointestinal tract.

Therapy. Treatment consists of antibiotics and bed rest. The response is usually rapid. If an IUD is present, it should be removed. There is danger that a focus of chronic infection will exist in the pelvis and that repeated attacks will predispose to infertility. Therefore, complete and adequate therapy, which in many cases may require hospitalization, is necessary. Occasionally, acute attacks are followed by scarring in the pelvis. This may then result in chronic pain and menstrual irregularity. In such patients blocked tubes, sterility, and adnexal adhesions may then develop. In certain cases, the secretions from the lining of the tube are trapped in the tube, and hydrosalpinx develops. In more advanced cases, an abscess develops between the tube and the ovary. These tuboovarian abscesses are best treated by surgical removal. If the abscess has leaked or ruptured, there will be signs of generalized peritonitis. If prompt surgical therapy is not instituted, a significant percentage of these patients will be lost. Total hysterectomy with bilateral salpingo-oophorectomy is the treatment of choice for ruptured tuboovarian abscesses. Occasionally, massive doses of antibiotics and supportive therapy with blood replacement and plasma must precede surgical procedures in order to bring the patient into optimal preoperative condition.

TUBERCULOUS PELVIC INFECTION

Tuberculosis is an uncommon cause of chronic pelvic inflammatory disease in the United States. It is generally associated with irreversible infertility. Tuberculosis is usually not a primary infection of the genital tract and is either of pulmonary or gastrointestinal origin. The diagnosis is made by curettings obtained at the time of menstruation and stained, cultured, and inoculated into guinea pigs. Chemotherapy with antituberculous drugs is the preferred treatment. Attempts to restore fertility by corrective surgical procedures in these cases have uniformly met with poor results.

Endometriosis

The growth of endometrial glands and stroma in areas outside the uterus is known as endometriosis. Such areas may undergo cyclic changes during the menstrual cycle, although histologically the changes do not necessarily mimic that of the endometrium. The sites of occurrence are wide and varied, and may be anywhere in the pelvis. The uterosacral ligaments are typical locations for this disease, and tender nodularity felt along these ligaments is diagnostic. Endometriosis may also be found on the ovaries, where it exists as large chocolate cysts, or endometriomas. Posterior cul-de-sac peritoneal implants are very common, and multiple 2- to 3-mm nodules are often seen in this area. Endometriosis may be on the vulva or vagina and may undergo cyclic changes during the menstrual cycle which can be directly observed. Endometrial implants on the bowel can be the cause of cyclic lower gastrointestinal tract bleeding, and cases of cyclic hemoptysis have been reported from lesions in the lung.

Many theories have been proposed to explain the origin of endometriosis. None has been proved. One widely held theory postulates that implantation of endometrium occurs at the time of menstruation as a result of reflux of endometrial tissue into the peritoneal cavity through the fallopian tubes. The reflux theory is given some support by the fact that implantation of endometrial tissue can occur in cesarean section scars. Embryologic changes have also been suggested as a cause for endometriosis. It has been postulated that a change occurs in the coelomic epithelium, which gives rise to endometrial cell nests. This assumes that the cells with the potential of undergoing change to endometriosis are present at birth and transform during the reproductive years. Such a theory is given strength by endometrial implants found, not only on the bowel, but also in the lung and in other places in the body at a distance from the pelvis. Other theories have been advanced, but none can claim any greater acceptability.

A patient with endometriosis may have no symptoms or may complain of severe dysmenorrhea that becomes increasingly debilitating with the passage of time. Severe dysmenorrhea is usually seen in a patient in her late twenties who has never been pregnant, although endometriosis can occur in an older patient who has not been pregnant for years. The origin of the pain is uncertain but is probably due, in part, to cyclic bleeding into the sites of endometriosis at the time of menstruation. Large endometrial implants are often asymptomatic, while millimeter-size nodules are often associated with severe pain. Although it cannot be stated that endometriosis per se will cause infertility, it is generally accepted that patients with endometriosis will have a smaller chance of becoming pregnant than the general population.

Clinically, the diagnosis can be confirmed by direct visualization of the endometriosis either at laparotomy, laparoscopy, or culdoscopy. However, endometriosis often causes obliteration of the cul-de-sac, and culdoscopy can lead to rectal perforation. Therefore, it should not be attempted in those cases where marked uterosacral or cul-de-sac scarring exists. In order to make a microscopic diagnosis of endometriosis, endometrial glands, endometrial stroma, or blood should be demonstrated. The blood may appear in the form of hemosiderin. If two of these three diagnostic criteria are present, then the histologic diagnosis of endometriosis is justified.

Many patients with endometriosis have no symptoms and require no special therapy. Since there is an increased incidence of infertility in these patients, pregnancy preferably should not be delayed. If this is not possible, hormonal treatment with progestational agents accompanied by estrogen (pseudopregnancy) has been suggested to induce long periods of amenorrhea. This may decrease the size of endometrial nodules, but endometriosis may recur following such long-term therapy. Danocrine, a new but expensive hormonal treatment, has been reported to be very successful. However, primate studies have suggested that artificially induced endometriosis lesions do not disappear following hormonal therapy but remain functional. Small doses of methyltestosterone can be given on a cyclic basis for a short period of time for relief of pain. It should be avoided in dark-skinned or hirsute people, since they can become masculinized by androgen therapy.

In certain cases, surgical treatment must be performed. Conservative surgical measures consist of complete removal of as much of the endometriosis as possible, taking care to preserve normal anatomic structures, especially in the areas of the tubes and ovaries. A presacral neurectomy, as outlined in the section on pelvic pain, is also usually performed. In cases where the endometriosis can be completely excised, excellent results are obtained, and the patients usually remain pain-free. If symptomatic endometriosis exists in an older patient who no longer desires to have children, then a total hysterectomy with bilateral salpingo-oophorectomy can be considered. By surgical castration, the endogenous hormonal support of the endometriosis is removed, and the disease is cured.

Intrauterine (DES) Exposure

Clear-cell adenocarcinomas of the vagina and cervix have been observed in young women whose mothers were treated with DES and similar compounds during pregnancy. Fortunately these cancers are rare among the exposed. They have been noted to occur primarily after puberty, with a peak incidence at age nineteen. Through age twenty-four the risk of cancer is estimated to be 1:1,000 or less. Since most of the exposed population is under thirty years of age, it is not known what effect, if any, the exposure may have on these women as they age.

In spite of the low risk of malignancy, DES-exposed females should have a complete gynecologic evaluation once they begin to menstruate or reach the age of fourteen, in order to rule out the presence of malignancy as well as to detect the common nonneoplastic changes that have been found in their vaginas and cervixes. These changes include vaginal adenosis, the presence of columnar tissue or its mucinous products in the vagina; cervical eversion (or ectropion), the presence of columnar epithelium or its mucinous products on the cervix; and transverse vaginal and cervical fibrous ridges. The ridges are found in about

20 percent of the exposed; while vaginal adenosis occurs in about one-half (depending upon the time in pregnancy when DES was started), and cervical eversion occurs commonly among the unexposed population, vaginal adenosis and transverse ridges are rare in the absence of intrauterine DES exposure.

Adenosis appears to be a benign lesion that is usually found near the vaginal clear-cell adenocarcinoma. Current evidence suggests that adenosis does not require therapy. The columnar epithelium of vaginal adenosis and cervical eversion is usually physiologically replaced by squamous epithelium (metaplasia). Occasionally neoplastic, squamous epithelium develops (dysplasia, carcinoma in situ), as is discussed in the section on the cervix. The degree to which squamous malignancies may be a problem in the DES-exposed female is unknown at present.

The complete evaluation consists of careful palpation, direct visualization, and cytologic sampling of the vagina and cervix. This is usually followed by colposcopy to study transformation areas of metaplasia, followed by an iodine stain to delineate the extent of the nonglycogenated epithelium. Biopsies are taken from the areas which are markedly abnormal on colposcopic examination or from nodules that are suggestive of malignancy.

Fig. 41-19. Uterine fibroids. *A.* Types. *B.* Various locations.

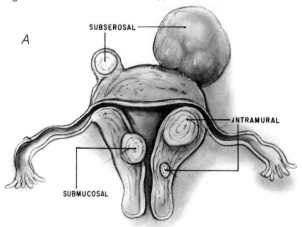

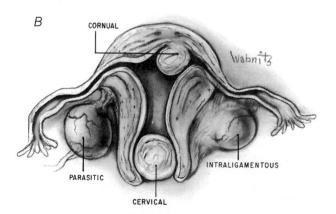

Benign Disorders of the Uterus

FUNDUS

Fibroids

Fibroids (leiomyoma) are extremely common, occurring in perhaps 50 percent of women. They are collections of whorls of interlacing, smooth muscle fibers. Fibroids vary tremendously in size, being as small as a few millimeters or growing sufficiently large to fill the entire pelvis. They are usually named by their location, as shown in Fig. 41-19, where subserosal, intramural, and submucous fibroids are illustrated. Occasionally, a subserosal fibroid develops with a large stalk attached to the fundus of the uterus, in which case it is referred to as a "pedunculated fibroid." This is easily confused on physical examination with an adnexal mass or ovarian tumor. The origin of these benign tumors is unknown, but there appears to be a definite hormonal influence, as the tumors are rarely seen prior to the age of twenty and are known to involute after the menopause. In addition, leiomyomas can be stimulated to grow by administering estrogens. Therefore estrogen-containing medication, such as oral contraceptives, must be used judiciously in the presence of these tumors.

Their presence is not in itself an indication for any therapy. The therapy of leiomyomas is dependent upon the symptoms and problems which are associated with them. Fibroids are associated with four major problems. These are bleeding, pain, increase in size, and infertility.

Bleeding. An increase in menstrual flow or prolongation of the menstrual period sufficient to cause anemia can be associated with submucous fibroids. The endometrial cavity is markedly enlarged and distorted, and there is incomplete endometrial regeneration over the surface of the fibroid, leading to continuous oozing or bleeding and sometimes hemorrhage.

Pain. This is not a common symptom. It occurs primarily when there is degeneration, which usually results when one of these large tumors outgrows its blood supply. It may also occur when a pedunculated fibroid twists and becomes infarcted. Rarely pain is associated with a large leiomyoma that has impinged or caused pressure on local adjacent viscera, and the discomfort would be referred to the involved organ.

Growth. Fibroids do grow during the reproductive years. Usually the growth is at a slow rate, unless there is excessive hormonal stimulation as a result of medication or in association with pregnancy. Since malignancy occurring in a fibroid is an exceedingly rare event, malignant change need only be considered if the growth of the fibroid is extremely rapid, especially during the menopausal years.

Infertility. Many patients who present with problems in conception and infertility are found to have fibroids. Usually fibroids interfering with conception cause distortion of the endometrial cavity and can interfere with implantation. They also can distort the fallopian tube and by their size interfere with the transport of the ovum. Small subserosal fibroids, which do not distort the endometrial cavity and are not in a position to interfere with tubal transport, probably are not related to a patient's infertility problem.

A submucous fibroid will occasionally extrude through the cervix and present as a bleeding and infected mass attached by a stalk to the endometrial cavity. These fibroids are safely treated by removing the stalk, followed by a few weeks' rest period to allow infection to clear from the pelvic lymphatics prior to undertaking further surgical treatment. Attempts at surgical procedures without this waiting period usually result in a high incidence of postoperative complications and wound sepsis. In general, the surgical therapy of fibroids consists of either hysterectomy or myomectomy.

Adenomyosis

Adenomyosis is a growth of endometrial tissue in the myometrium of the uterus and is sometimes referred to as "endometriosis of the uterine corpus." The condition occurs primarily during the reproductive years and leads to a thickening of the myometrial wall with subsequent uterine enlargement. Adenomyosis usually occurs in women who have had a number of pregnancies. Occasionally patients with adenomyosis will complain of dysmenorrhea, and some present with increased uterine bleeding and heavy menstrual flow. However, a number of patients with adenomyosis in hysterectomy specimens have been asymptomatic. Therefore, the association of adenomyosis with heavy menstrual bleeding and dysmenorrhea is questionable.

Polyps

Endometrial polyps can occur at any time after puberty. A polyp is a local hyperplastic growth of endometrial tissue which usually causes postmenstrual or postmenopausal bleeding or staining. The polyps are usually benign, but rare cases of malignant tumor of the endometrium arising in a polyp have been reported. Removal of polyps at the time of curettage is generally curative, although they can recur.

Endometritis

Occasionally patients with menstrual irregularity and postmenstrual staining are found to have endometritis. Histologically, the lesion demonstrates massive inflammatory cell infiltration of the stroma of the endometrium. The infiltration is greater than that normally seen at the time of menstruation and is usually accompanied by plasma cells. Antibiotics and curettage usually are sufficient treatment. Instrumentation or procedure such as obtaining a tubogram should not be performed in the presence of endometritis, since a severe exacerbation of diffuse pelvic inflammation could result.

CERVIX

Common benign conditions of the uterine cervix include inflammation, Nabothian cysts, and polyps. *Cervical polyps* cause the same symptoms as endometrial polyps. Since they are often quite small and are visible at the external os, they often can be removed as an outpatient procedure followed by cauterization of the base of the polyp. *Nabothian cysts* are mucous inclusion cysts of the cervix. They are occasionally associated with chronic inflammation and can easily be removed with a cautery. However, they are harmless, usually asymptomatic, and generally do not require therapy.

During reproductive years the portio of the cervix is covered primarily with glycogenated squamous epithelium, and columnar epithelium is normally found centrally near the external os in most women. This exposed columnar epithelium is termed *ectropion* or *eversion* and usually is bright red. Unless accompanied by inflammation and a purulent discharge (cervicitis), it requires no treatment. During adult life, the columnar epithelium is usually replaced by squamous metaplasia, and this physiologic process occurs in the transformation zone at the interface of squamous and columnar epithelium. After menopause the squamous columnar junction is usually in the endocervical canal.

Malignant Disease of the Uterus

CARCINOMA OF THE CERVIX

Carcinoma of the cervix is the most common malignant tumor of the female reproductive tract, although recently carcinoma of the endometrium appears to have become almost as common. Carcinoma of the cervix comprises 40 to 50 percent of genital tract cancers. Most of the tumors are epithelial cell or squamous cell carcinomas, while approximately 5 percent are adenocarcinomas. The tumor occurs more frequently in women who have started to bear children at an early age. The malignant change develops at the squamocolumnar junction, and this area is also involved with inflammatory changes following pregnancy. These tumors are not often seen in the virgin female. There is a possibility that a male factor may be etiologically related, and it has been suggested that the disease is less common in women married to circumcised males.

SYMPTOMS. Carcinoma of the cervix may be discovered in a patient who has no symptoms or complaints. She may have intermenstrual bleeding or staining and may complain of bleeding which occurs following douching or intercourse. Any bleeding of an irregular nature which is not associated with menstruation is a danger signal in the female of reproductive years. Postmenopausal bleeding also may be caused by cervical carcinoma, but it occurs more commonly with endometrial malignancy. Pain is a late manifestation of this disease, as is general malaise.

DETECTION AND DIAGNOSIS. The advent of the Papanicolaou smear has offered the possibility of screening large segments of the population for cervical tumor by methods that are approximately 95 percent accurate. The smear may be taken as a vaginal aspiration or by direct aspiration or scraping from the cervix. The stained smear can then be categorized as showing normal, suspicious, or malignant changes. Although malignancy can be suggested by the Papanicolaou smear, the diagnosis of cervical carcinoma can be made *only* on biopsy. Even in the presence of malignant disease, a benign smear may be obtained, especially where there is a great deal of secondary infection accompanying the tumor. Therefore, a malignant tumor of the cervix is not definitely ruled out by a benign Papanicolaou smear, and grossly suspicious areas should be biopsied. A suspicious Papanicolaou smear or report of malignant cells in the smear also require further investigation by biopsy.

By helping the examiner identify abnormal epithelial and vascular patterns in the transformation zone, the col-

Fig. 41-20. *A.* Cervical dysplasia. *B.* Carcinoma in situ of cervix. *C.* Invasive squamous cell carcinoma of cervix.

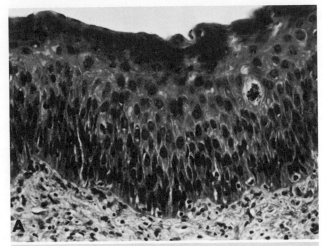

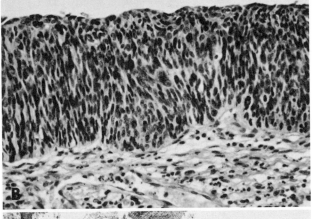

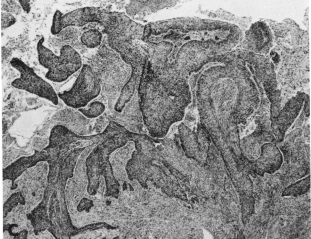

poscope aids in directed biopsy of the most suggestive areas. It is important that the entire transformation zone be visible on the portio of the cervix for a satisfactory colposcopy to be performed. If colposcopy is unsatisfactory, a diagnostic conization of the cervix will usually be necessary to rule out the presence of invasive carcinoma. Schiller's or Lugol's iodine stain can also be used as a nonspecific guide for biopsy. Nonglycogenated epithelium will usually appear grossly normal but does not stain with iodine. These suggestive areas are then biopsied, although such areas may contain only nonneoplastic or inflammatory changes.

The Papanicolaou smear is particularly important in that it not only can detect the cells of a frankly malignant condition but also can detect changes in the cervical epithelium which are potentially malignant. These changes are termed "anaplasia" (dysplasia) and "carcinoma in situ," depending upon the severity of the alterations in the cervical epithelium.

Colposcopy, which consists of the examination of the cervix with a low-power microscope and built-in light source, has recently gained popularity. It is a technique which aids in differentiating pathologic processes and other atypical lesions.

Dysplasia. Figure 41-20*A* shows an area of dysplasia of the cervix in which the architecture of the squamous epithelium has been disturbed and there is progressive loss of differentiation of the squamous epithelial cells. Dysplasia is in itself not a malignant change and can be treated successfully by cauterization. However, patients with dysplasia must be thoroughly investigated and followed to make sure that a more serious cervical change does not exist or develop in the future.

Carcinoma In Situ. The lesion consists of malignant epithelium that is confined to the surface of the cervix (Fig. 41-20*B*). There is no invasion of the deep layers of the cervix by malignant cells. In spite of its malignant potential, the lesion is benign. Carcinoma in situ is considered a precursor of invasive carcinoma for the following reasons:

1. The peak rate of occurrence of carcinoma in situ precedes by approximately 10 years in age distribution the peak occurrence of invasive carcinoma of the cervix. In situ lesions are seen at about the age of thirty-eight, while invasive carcinoma occurs most frequently at age forty-eight, and both diseases occur at approximately the same rate with the 10-year span separating them.
2. There is a similar racial and ethnic distribution. The disease is uncommon in Jewish women when compared to non-Jewish women and is more frequently seen in Negroes than in whites.
3. It is common in cases of carcinoma of the cervix to note microscopically coexisting, adjacent areas of carcinoma in situ.
4. A few patients with carcinoma in situ have been known to develop invasive carcinoma later.

Once the question of malignancy of the cervix has been raised, either by Papanicolaou smear or by biopsy, carcinoma in situ must be differentiated from invasive carcinoma of the cervix, since these lesions can coexist. Colposcopy is used to identify the most abnormal areas, but iodine stain with multiple biopsies and an endocervical curettage can be effectively used by competent examiners. It is vital to rule out invasive cancer, and hospitalization for diagnostic conization of the cervix is occasionally required.

THERAPY. Treatment is determined by the nature of the lesion and most particularly by the extent of involvement.

Carcinoma In Situ. If the diagnosis of carcinoma in situ without invasion can be made, adequate therapy consists of a total abdominal hysterectomy with removal of at least 1 cm of vaginal cuff. The cervix and vagina may be stained with Schiller's solution prior to surgical treatment to detect any parts which do not take Schiller's stain, and these parts are included with the specimen.

All patients treated for carcinoma in situ should be followed by yearly vaginal smears, since the remaining squamous epithelium of the vagina can undergo malignant changes in future years. Patients with carcinoma in situ in whom preservation of reproductive function is desired can be treated by a therapeutic conization of the cervix. Some investigators have utilized locally destructive procedures such as cryosurgery or cauterization to treat carcinoma in situ, with apparently good results, but such treatment is generally performed for dysplasia of the cervix. The follow-up of these patients is particularly important, since future epithelial change can occur in both the vagina and retained cervix.

Invasive Carcinoma. Carcinoma of the cervix is a slow-growing tumor (Fig. 41-20C). It spreads over the surface of the adjacent epithelium of the cervix and may invade the underlying muscular walls and disseminate via lymph channels. Parametrial areas and paracervical areas are prime sites for the spread of the disease. The first metastases are usually found in the lymph nodes of the pelvis and often in the parametrium and paracervical tissues. The tumor spreads to the pelvic wall along the hypogastric vessels and then to the areas of the external and common iliac arteries. The tumor will extend outside the true pelvis as a late manifestation. In untreated cases, death can result from hemorrhage due to major vessel erosion or from urinary tract obstruction which leads to subsequent uremia while the disease may be confined to the pelvic cavity.

STAGING. In order to determine the proper therapy of carcinoma of the cervix, the precise extent of the disease must be defined. This is accomplished by diagnostic x-rays, sigmoidoscopy, cystoscopy, and pelvic examination under general anesthesia. The tumor spread is classified according to international agreement which divides the various categories into the stages depicted in Fig. 41-21.

Stage I refers to invasive carcinoma which is confined to the cervix. If invasive tumor is not clinically evident and a small focus is discovered microscopically, microinvasion or preclinical carcinoma is diagnosed and assigned to Stage I-A. The diagnosis of microinvasive carcinoma is made if invasion is 3 mm or less and vascular or lymphatic involvement is absent. All other Stage I carcinomas then are assigned to Stage I-B. *Stage II* refers to carcinoma that extends beyond the cervix but has not yet reached the pelvic wall and is confined to the upper two-thirds of the vagina. The stage is subdivided by most clinics into Stage II-A, which indicates involvement only of the vagina, and Stage II-B, which indicates involvement beyond the vagina, into the parametrial and paracervical areas. *Stage III* refers to involvement of either the lower third of the vagina or the extension of tumor to the pelvic wall. If tumor has caused hydronephrosis or a nonfunctioning kidney as determined by intravenous pyelogram, the tumor is assigned to Stage III. *Stage IV* represents either spread of tumor outside the pelvis or invasion of the mucosa of the bladder or rectum by malignant disease.

CHOICE OF THERAPY. Radical surgical procedures and radiation therapy both provide effective treatment for carcinoma of the cervix. The modality of therapy will depend upon the extent of the tumor, the condition of the patient, and the capabilities of the clinic. There are a large number of cases that can be treated successfully by either method with similar likelihood of cure. Although attempts have been made to measure the patient's responsiveness to radiation by studying the histology of cervical tumor following external radiation and by examining the cellular components of the smear, there is no available test which permits one to separate those cases that will best respond to surgical treatment from those that will do better with radiation.

Stage I and II-A. Most young patients with Stage I carcinoma of the cervix or early Stage II-A lesions can be treated equally satisfactorily by either radical surgery or radiation. If radical surgery is performed, ovarian function occasionally can be preserved. Patients with local inflammation or pelvic infection should be treated surgically, since massive sepsis can result if radiotherapy is undertaken. The development of a wide en bloc dissection is an integral part of adequate surgical therapy for this disease, and the extent to which an adequate dissection can be done is illustrated in Fig. 41-22. It can be seen that wide areas of the parametrial and paracervical tissues can be removed. Many investigators feel that microinvasive carcinoma can be effectively treated with total (extrafascial) hysterectomy.

RADIATION CONSIDERATIONS. Adequate radiation therapy requires the delivery of tumoricidal doses of radiation to all areas that either are or can be affected by tumor. The dose of radiation delivered is inversely proportional to the distance between the source and the point being treated. In addition, the tissue absorption of radiation is inversely proportional to the wavelength of the administered dose. Thus, by lowering the wavelength, one increases penetration of the radiation. This can be done by raising the therapeutic voltage, as for example, with the million-electron-volt machines, or it can be accomplished by using filters to eliminate the longer wavelengths. Time and volume factors are important. When a given dose is administered over a long period of time, the tissue reaction is less than if it is given in a short interval. Similarly, a dose which is distributed throughout a large volume causes greater tissue damage than one which is confined to a small volume. The unit of exposure in radiation is usually expressed as the rad, which is equivalent to the transfer of 100 ergs of energy/Gm of tissue. For practical purposes, this is equivalent to 1 r. Thus, 10,000 r given to the cervix is a dose that can be tolerated, while the same dose given to the entire pelvis would cause necrosis of normal tissue. Occasionally, radium doses are expressed in terms of milligram-hours, a quantity determined by multiplying the milligrams of radium used by the number

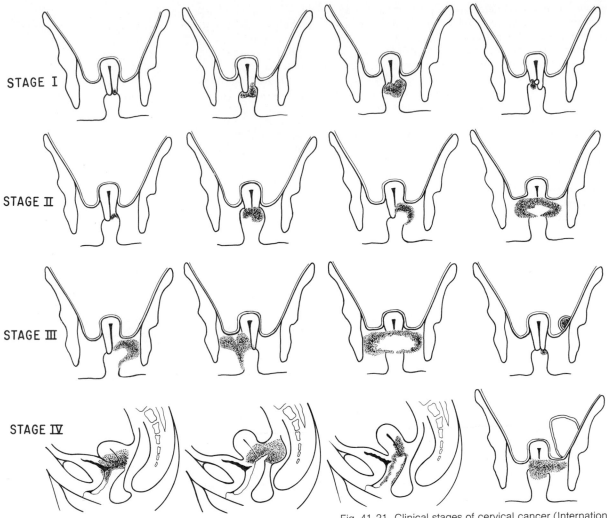

STAGE I

STAGE II

STAGE III

STAGE IV

Fig. 41-21. Clinical stages of cervical cancer (International Classification).

of hours it is in place. However, this gives no indication of the overall effect or distribution of the dose in relation to surrounding tissue. For convenience, two standard reference points, identified as A and B, are used to specify the dose of radiation given. Point A is 2 cm superior to

Fig. 41-22. Radical hysterectomy section.

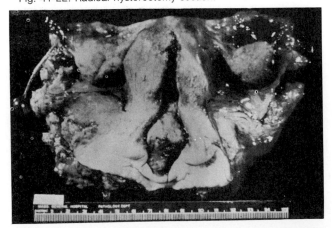

the fornix and 2 cm lateral to the uterine canal. Point B lies in the same plane but is located 5 cm laterally.

The radiosensitivity of a tissue is proportional to its reproductive capacity and degree of differentiation. Since neoplastic tissues are generally poorly differentiated and have increased mitotic activity, they are, as a rule, more sensitive to radiation than normal tissue. The radiosensitivity of a tumor is an expression of its ability to respond to radiation, and this is not necessarily the same as its ability to be cured by radiation. The radiocurability of a tumor depends upon the ability to deliver sufficient radiation to destroy the tumor completely and eliminate it from the host. The presence in the pelvis of vital structures immediately adjacent to the anatomic distribution of the tumor limits the amount and dose of radiation that can be given, just as it limits surgical treatment.

A useful method of applying radium consists of a stem and box (Stockholm), as demonstrated in Fig. 41-23, where various types of applications are shown. The stem and box are usually applied in two applications, separated by a 3-week interval. By dividing the application, the tumor is given a chance to shrink following the first local application, and a better radium application can be accomplished the second time. The radium treatments are then supplemented with external therapy to the entire pelvis, usually with shielding of the midline. As a rule, 6000 to 8000 r are delivered to Point A and approximately 5000 r to Point B. Afterloading devices, utilizing a central stem and side ovoids (Fletcher-Suit applicator), permit the appliance without radiation exposure to medical personnel. An x-ray film of the application is taken and dosemetry calculated on a computer, depending upon the arrangement of stem and ovoids.

Stages II-B, III, and IV. In cases of extensive Stage II-B carcinomas of the cervix or in Stage III or IV lesions, external radiation is usually initially employed. Since radium is effective only for local cervical disease, external therapy permits treatment of the entire bulk of the tumor before concentrating on the small central part. Following preliminary external radiotherapy, radium application usually can be more effectively completed. If Stage IV lesions involve the bladder or rectum but not the pelvic wall, then a radical surgical procedure removing the bladder (anterior exenteration) or rectum (posterior exenteration) is used, since radiation cure of these lesions is usually less than 5 percent and fistulas can result from radiation treatment. However, preliminary external radiotherapy can be useful to reduce the size of the tumor as well as secondary infection. Smaller doses of radiotherapy are used when future surgical therapy is planned.

PROBLEMS OF SURGERY AND RADIATION. The immediate problems concerned with radiation therapy relate to discomfort of the patient as a result of gastrointestinal upset. Nausea, vomiting, or diarrhea are frequently encountered. However, long-term complications can also occur, and these usually relate to bleeding or inflammation of the lower bowel or chronic irritation of the bladder. Radiation proctitis or cystitis can occasionally become extremely debilitating. Fistulas may result either between the bowel and the vagina or between the bladder and the vagina, especially where extremely heavy doses of radiation have to be used. With recent refinements in radiation techniques, these complications are occurring less frequently.

Surgical complications usually occur early and relate to damage of either the genitourinary tract or the bowel. Urinary fistula is the most common complication and occurs in approximately 1 to 2 percent of cases treated by radical hysterectomy. Many of these close spontaneously, but a few require further surgical treatment, such as repair of a damaged ureter or removal of the affected kidney.

RESULTS OF THERAPY. The curability of carcinoma of the cervix is directly related to the extent of the disease at the time therapy is initiated. Comparable results have been obtained following the effective use of surgical and radiation therapy. Average approximate 5-year survival rates for the various stages are as follows: Stage I, 75 percent; Stage II, 50 percent; Stage III, 25 percent; Stage IV, 10 percent. In Stage I lesions with negative nodes, the 5-year survival approaches 90 percent. When the nodes are positive, the rates drop to 45 percent. In Stage II lesions

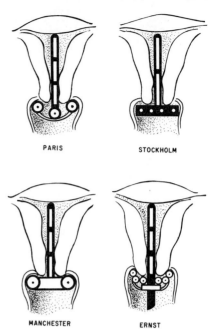

Fig. 41-23. Various types of radium applicators employed in radiation therapy of cervical cancer.

the comparable figures for negative and positive nodes are approximately 75 and 20 percent, respectively.

Recurrent Cervical Carcinoma. Carcinoma of the cervix can metastasize to any part of the body, but most recurrences are found in the pelvis. If the patient has pelvic recurrence after primary surgical therapy, then radiation can be tried to treat local disease. If recurrence occurs after primary therapy with radiation, then only by radical removal of the contents of the pelvis is there hope of curing the patient. This usually requires removal of both the lower bowel and bladder (total exenteration), and this procedure is reserved only for those cases where there is some hope of cure. It is occasionally done for palliation. In properly selected cases, a 20 to 30 percent 5-year survival can be obtained by using exenteration for therapy of recurrent carcinoma of the cervix.

Carcinoma of the Cervix in Pregnancy. In general, the therapy of carcinoma of the cervix which occurs during a pregnancy follows the same principles that would pertain if the patient were not pregnant. Consideration for the viability of the fetus is important only in the latter stages of pregnancy and should not be allowed to change treatment in a way that will diminish the chances of curing the mother. In the first trimester of pregnancy, therapy for early Stage I lesions can be accomplished either by radical hysterectomy or by radiation therapy. The latter is followed by spontaneous delivery of the products of conception about 2 weeks after radium therapy. In the second and third trimesters the fetus has become sufficiently large that the size of the uterus becomes a technical problem. It is usually necessary to empty the uterus by hysterotomy before proceeding with either surgical or radiation therapy, but once hysterotomy has been performed, a radical hysterectomy can usually be accomplished at the same time.

Frequently it is advisable to precede surgical exploration with a course of 2000 r external therapy prior to abdominal exploration. Then either radical hysterectomy or further radiation therapy can be accomplished, depending upon the extent of the lesion. For the advanced Stage II and III cases, radiation therapy remains the treatment of

Fig. 41-24. *A.* Endometrial hyperplasia (cystic and adenomatous). *B.* Carcinoma in situ. *C.* Adenocarcinoma of endometrium.

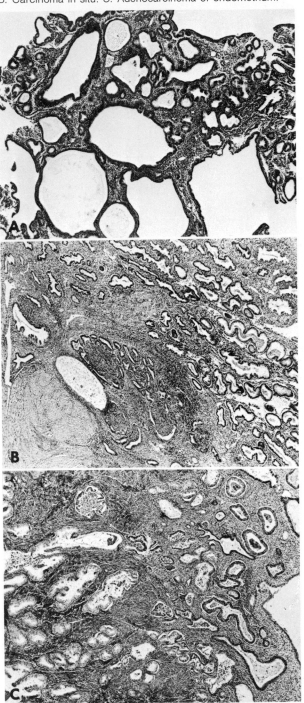

choice. Results of therapy indicate that for each stage the survival following treatment for carcinoma of the cervix in pregnancy is much the same as it is in the nonpregnant patient.

TUMORS OF THE FUNDUS OF THE UTERUS

Endometrial Carcinoma

Most malignant tumors of the fundus of the uterus arise in the glands of the endometrium. Adenocarcinoma (Fig. 41-24*C*) is the most frequently found tumor, although a few adenocarcinomas with squamous tissue elements (adenoacanthoma) are seen. These tumors are histologically different but appear to have a similar clinical behavior.

Carcinomas of the endometrium are less common than malignant tumors in the cervix. They constitute approximately 20 percent of the tumors seen in the female reproductive tract. Most cases occur in the sixth decade of life and are associated with nulliparity or late childbirth. There is also an increased incidence of endometrial carcinoma in patients who are obese, diabetic, and hypertensive. Thus, these patients will generally present a markedly different social history, reproductive history, and somatic appearance than patients with carcinoma of the cervix.

The endometrium is exquisitely sensitive to hormonal stimulation, and it appears that abnormal stimulation of the endometrium could play a part in the development of certain endometrial carcinomas. It has been observed that there is an increased incidence of endometrial carcinomas in cases of prolonged and excessive estrogen stimulation, such as with estrogen-secreting tumors.

A scheme of development of malignancy has been suggested which begins with a local hyperplastic growth of endometrial glands in the form of an endometrial polyp; then cystic hyperplasia develops, followed by both cystic and adenomatous hyperplasia (Fig. 41-24*A*) and finally carcinoma in situ (Fig. 41-24*B*) of the endometrium. This sequence of changes might occur in a fashion similar to that already described for carcinoma of the cervix, although the stimuli are evidently quite different. Patients who have had prolonged anovulatory cycles and continuous estrogen stimulation without progesterone appear to be prime candidates for the development of hyperplastic changes and endometrial carcinoma.

Corpus carcinoma can be staged as follows:

Stage I—the carcinoma is confined to the corpus.
      I*a*—the uterus sounds to 8 cm or less.
Stage II—the carcinoma involves the corpus and cervix.
      I*b*—the uterus sounds to more than 8 cm.
Stage III—the carcinoma extends outside the uterus but is confined to the true pelvis.
Stage IV—the carcinoma extends outside the true pelvis or involves the mucosa of the bladder or rectum.

The grade of endometrial carcinoma is also important. Three grades (G1, G2, G3) are usually assigned, with the latter identifying the least differentiated lesion.

Initially, carcinoma of the endometrium invades the myometrium and then the lymphatics. When the tumor is low in the uterus and involves the cervix, the paths of spread are the same as those for cervical carcinoma. In contrast, spread of tumor from the upper part of the fundus goes directly to the aortic or inguinal nodes, which are sites outside the limits of radical pelvic surgical therapy.

THERAPY. The primary method for carcinoma of the endometrium is surgical therapy. This consists of a simple total hysterectomy when the carcinoma is well differentiated and confined to the fundus. To reduce the incidence of vaginal recurrence, a postoperative vaginal radium application is usually done in 4 to 6 weeks. In those cases where the cervix also is involved, therapy is best carried out in accordance with the principles outlined under the discussion of carcinoma of the cervix. External radiation therapy is employed preoperatively in cases where there is a large uterus filled with tumor or if the tumor is poorly differentiated on microscopic examination. Radiotherapy alone is used for patients who are unable to tolerate surgical therapy. These patients are then given additional radium therapy.

RESULTS OF THERAPY. The results of therapy in cases of carcinoma of the endometrium will vary with the extent of the lesion originally treated. For tumors confined to the fundus and treatable by surgical methods, approximately 70 to 80 percent will be alive and free of disease 5 years following treatment. For those who are not, because of medical reasons or spread of tumor, able to be treated by primary surgical procedures, the 5-year survival is markedly reduced. The overall salvage is approximately 50 to 60 percent.

PROBLEMS OF RECURRENCES. Recurrences of carcinoma of the endometrium are most frequently seen in the vagina, especially in the suburethral area or at the vaginal apex. They occasionally occur in the pelvis. Distant metastases are most commonly found in the lung and in the liver. Occasionally, there are intraperitoneal, nonpelvic sites of metastatic disease, but these are less common. Therapy for recurrence of endometrial carcinoma depends upon its location and extent of tumor. In cases where there is a local recurrence in the pelvis, either in the vagina or intraperitoneally, radiation is the treatment of choice. Occasionally, local vaginal radium applications are possible. If there is a large recurrence located centrally within the pelvis and especially if there has been prior radiation therapy, then radical pelvic surgical therapy should be considered. However, as in the case of carcinoma of the cervix, exenteration is generally considered for cure of a patient who is in good medical condition. Distant metastases of carcinoma of the endometrium have been successfully treated by high doses of progestational agents. Delalutin (17-hydroxyprogesterone caproate), Depo-Provera (medroxyprogesterone), and Megace (megestrol acetate) have been employed and in some cases have resulted in regression of metastatic nodules particularly in the lung. Well-differentiated tumors respond most favorably, while highly undifferentiated tumors or those which have been previously irradiated have a less satisfactory response. A response rate of about 25 percent has been obtained.

Sarcomas

These are rare tumors, comprising less than 5 percent of uterine malignant disease. They primarily occur in the postmenopausal female. The following types are those most frequently encountered.

Carcinosarcoma. This is a mixed tumor, probably of endometrial origin, which contains carcinomatous elements which probably arise from Müllerian structures and also have a sarcomatous stroma.

Endolymphatic Stromal Myosis. This refers to an endometrial tissue infiltration into the myometrium. It is a form of low-grade stromal sarcoma. The more mitoses noted in these tumors, the more malignant is the behavior.

Leiomyosarcoma. This category is the most common variety of sarcoma. These tumors generally arise from the myometrium and may be either smooth muscle leiomyosarcomas or may contain more fibrous tissues in the form of fibrosarcoma. Occasionally, one encounters malignant degeneration in a fibroid, but this is a rare occurrence. The prognosis is believed to be better if the sarcomatous change is confined to a leiomyoma.

Stromal Sarcoma. This is a sarcoma which arises from a stromal cell of the endometrium, which then invades the myometrium. It is the more malignant expression of endolymphatic stromal myosis. There are pleomorphic endometrial cells with occasional giant cell formation present inside the tumor. Many of these tumors appear to arise in patients who have had previous radiation. These tumors are usually found in the older age group and are seen primarily in the postmenopausal female. Many of them are associated with pyometrium, since the endocervix becomes closed and there is some accumulated secretion and infection behind it developing into purulent contents contained within the endometrial cavity. It has been estimated that approximately 2 to 4 percent of all patients with uterine cancer, regardless of the histologic features, may be found to have pyometrium.

THERAPY. The primary therapy of sarcoma of the fundus is surgery, consisting of total simple hysterectomy. In general, the prognosis for all these tumors is poor unless they are detected early and confined to the uterus. Radical surgical treatment generally has not been successful. Although some sarcomas have been found to be radiosensitive, they have not, as a rule, been radiocurative. Some additional palliation has been obtained by the use of chemotherapeutic agents.

Disorders of the Vulva

BENIGN AND PREMALIGNANT CHANGES

The vulva is an area which is readily accessible to examination and treatment. Therefore, much attention has been focused on the local changes which precede the development of malignancy. Whitish areas have been noted to coexist with vulvar malignancy, and in many cases these white areas have existed prior to tumor development. Such areas have been termed "leukoplakia" (white patch). However, confusion has arisen, since many white areas of

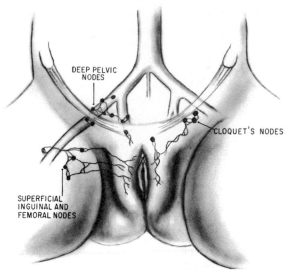

Fig. 41-25. Routes of lymphatic spread in carcinoma of the vulva.

Fig. 41-26. Radical surgical treatment for carcinoma of the vulva. *A.* Incision for a one-stage approach to radical vulvectomy in continuity with bilateral groin and deep pelvic lymph node dissections. *B.* Final operative specimen.

A

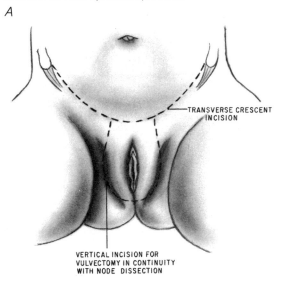

B

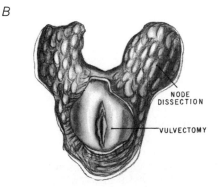

the vulva are associated with pruritic irritations that bear no relationship to malignancy and are without malignant potential. The correct diagnosis of a white vulvar lesion can be made only by biopsy, and this examination should be performed for lesions which are not temporary irritations.

Although the term leukoplakia is often used for any white patch of the vulva, it is properly reserved for areas which show histologically atypical epithelial activity. These alterations may precede the development of malignant changes. In many instances, chronically irritated and itchy white areas of the vulva will show sclerosing atrophy of the skin (lichen sclerosus et atrophicus). The term "kraurosis" is applied when hyperkeratinization becomes part of the sclerosing picture. Lichen sclerosus et atrophicans and kraurosis are pruritic lesions which do not appear to be premalignant. They are chronic problems for which transient relief can occasionally be obtained by the local application of cortisone or some other anti-inflammatory agent. Rarely, however, in severe cases, simple vulvectomy has been used to provide relief.

Noninvasive malignant change of the surface squamous epithelium of the vulva occurs in the same way that has been described for the cervix. Carcinoma in situ of the vulva, both histologically and clinically, behaves like carcinoma in situ of the cervix. The changes are confined to the squamous elements of the vulva, and the condition is sometimes referred to as "Bowen's disease." In certain instances, the apocrine glandular elements of the vulva are involved in association with an intensely pruritic area. Histologically, large, foamy Paget's cells are seen, similar to those noted in the breast, although invasive carcinoma occasionally can accompany Paget cells. Both Bowen's disease and usually Paget's disease are considered part of the carcinoma in situ complex of the vulva and are adequately treated by wide local surgical excision which consists of a simple vulvectomy.

VULVAR MALIGNANCY

Most malignant tumors of the vulva are of the squamous cell variety. These tumors comprise approximately 5 percent of all gynecologic malignant tumors and occur primarily in elderly patients. The average age of a patient treated for this disease is about sixty-one years, and the incidence of vulvar carcinoma increases in each decade. As with carcinoma of the endometrium, vulvar carcinoma tends to occur in obese patients and in nulliparous patients, and the incidence of diabetes is increased in those with this disease. In addition, as many as 10 percent of these patients may have malignant tumors at other sites.

As a rule, the carcinoma arises unilaterally and may be present on any part of the vulva. It may be multicentric in origin. The disease spreads via the lymphatics and in spite of the unilaterality of the primary lesion the lymphatics carry the tumor to both sides. Initially, metastases occur from the vulva to the superficial inguinal and femoral nodes. Then spread progresses to the deep pelvic nodes of the external iliac group (Fig. 41-25). Vulvar carcinomas tend to be slow-growing, locally spreading tumors with distant metastases occurring as late manifestations of the disease.

The rate of cure of this tumor formerly was poor because of attempts at treatment by simple local excision. The recent advent of a wide surgical en bloc resection (Fig. 41-26) has markedly improved the survival rate of these patients. Adequate therapy consists of a radical vulvectomy combined with bilateral superficial and deep groin node dissection (Fig. 41-26B). Dissection includes both groins, even though the tumor is confined to one side of the vulva, because of the high incidence of bilateral spread through the rich supply of anastomosing vulvar lymphatics. In certain cases where the patient is considered not to be an optimal surgical risk and where the upper femoral node (Cloquet's node) is found to be free of tumor, the deep iliac node dissection is omitted.

Approximately half the patients treated in this fashion are cured of the carcinoma. If the lymph nodes are un-involved with tumor, the cure rate rises to 80 or 90 percent. Even if the lymph nodes are involved, almost half the patients treated by radical vulvectomy and bilateral node dissection can be salvaged. Involvement of the deep nodes markedly diminishes the prognosis. Radiotherapy has not proved to be as satisfactory a method as surgical therapy, especially since the vulvar skin becomes chronically irritated and pruritic after treatment.

Tumors other than epithelial carcinomas can occur in the vulva. Basal cell carcinomas are treated by simple excision. The vulva is a common site for malignant melanoma, and approximately 8 percent of melanomas that occur in females are noted in this region. However, they constitute only about 2 percent of all vulvar malignant tumors. Melanomas occur at any time but are usually noted in later years. Vulvar melanoma is treated similarly to epithelial cell carcinoma by radical vulvectomy and bilateral superficial and deep node dissection.

Carcinomas of Bartholin's glands have been reported, but these are exceedingly rare. Since the tumors are often diagnosed late in the course of the disease, they have generally disseminated through lymphatics. The results of therapy have been poor, although a wide local resection with node dissection would appear to offer the best opportunity for eradication.

Finally, tumors of sweat gland origin are seen in the vulva. These are referred to as "hidradenomas." There is some disagreement as to whether or not these tumors can occur as carcinomas. However, they are locally invasive, and therefore minimum adequate therapy consists of wide local excision.

Malignant Tumors of the Vagina

Although the vagina is frequently a site of extension from vulvar, cervical, or endometrial tumors, it is the rarest site for the origin of a malignant tumor in the female genital tract, with the exception of the fallopian tube. Usually vaginal malignant tumors occur in postmenopausal females around the age of sixty. One exception to this is the sarcoma botryoides, which is a tumor of young children. This malignant sarcoma usually presents as a mass in young infants. It is a bulky, polypoid tumor which is radiation-resistant, and the only hope of cure lies with radical surgical therapy.

Most primary cancers of the vagina are squamous cell carcinomas. Their clinical behavior depends upon the location in the vagina. Those that occur in the upper vagina usually behave as cervical tumors and therefore are treated by the same criteria used in therapy of carcinoma of the cervix. If a squamous cell carcinoma appears to be primarily occupying the vagina but is also on the cervix, it must be classified as a primary cervical tumor. For tumors located in the anterior vagina, either radiotherapy or an anterior exenteration will provide adequate therapy. For those lying in the posterior or upper vagina, either a posterior exenteration or radiotherapy must be considered. The tumors involving the lower vagina are treated as vulvar tumors, since the lymphatic spread in these instances is similar to that noted for vulvar carcinoma.

Recently, adenocarcinomas of the vagina and cervix have been noted in young girls in their late teens and early twenties, many of whose mothers took diethylstilbestrol and similar hormones during pregnancy (see section on disorders of bleeding). Histologically, the tumors consist of clear cells containing glycogen and so-called "hobnail cells." Therefore, they are called "clear cell carcinomas," although they also have been called "mesonephromas." Benign glandular infiltration of the vagina (vaginal adenosis) often accompanies these tumors, and transverse vaginal septa occasionally are seen, presumably resulting from in utero exposure to diethylstilbestrol. Diagnosis is made by vaginal examination. Although vaginal cytology occasionally can detect the tumor, the smear sometimes is negative with tumor present. Thus a complete pelvic examination including inspection of the walls of the vagina is necessary to rule out this malignancy. Therapy is accomplished by the usual considerations governing the treatment of malignancy in this area. Both operative resection and irradiation have been effective in eradicating these tumors. The operative approach is favored for young patients with early resectable lesions. When recurrences occur, they are most frequently noted locally, in the lungs, and in supraclavicular nodes. The results with chemotherapy have been disappointing.

Ovarian Tumors

DIAGNOSIS. Many types of ovarian tumors can occur in both benign and malignant forms, and a few tumors cannot be classified until their clinical behavior has been clarified by following the patient for a number of years. This multipotential behavior of ovarian tumors necessitates the consideration of benign and malignant lesions together. Ovarian malignant tumors occur less frequently than those from either the cervix or the endometrium. In general, there is an increased incidence of malignancy in ovarian tumors with advancing age.

In an infant or child, ovarian tumors may present as large pelvic masses. Adequate evaluation requires an intravenous pyelogram to rule out the urinary tract as the cause of the mass (Wilms' tumor). Patency of the hymen and vagina should be checked to rule out hydrocolpos, and the patient should be catheterized to be sure the mass is not a urine-filled bladder. An ovarian tumor in these young patients is most likely to be a teratoma, usually of the cystic variety (dermoid), or a follicle cyst. Ovarian malignant tumors do occur in the young age group, but they are rare.

During puberty and the reproductive years, ovarian tumors become more common. There is little need for concern about an enlargement unless it has become 5 cm or larger. Most 5-cm tumors in this age group are benign follicle cysts and may be followed through two menstrual periods. If the lesion persists for this length of time or appears to be enlarging, then diagnosis through direct visualization is indicated. Depending upon the size and location of the mass and the age of the patient, this may be accomplished by laparoscopy or abdominal exploration. For patients who are over age forty or in the menopausal years, the ovarian masses estimated to be 5 cm or larger should be explored.

Since ovarian enlargements are often asymptomatic, there can be significant spread of an ovarian tumor before the diagnosis is made. Common subjective symptoms consist of lower abdominal discomfort occasionally accompanied by the feeling of distension. Pain is rare unless there is advanced disease. In about one-third of the cases, the patient may complain of abnormal vaginal bleeding, and in a few cases urinary or intestinal complaints may be elicited.

NONNEOPLASTIC CYSTS

By definition a cystic enlargement of the ovary should be at least 2.5 cm in diameter to be termed a cyst. Some of the more common cysts are as follows.

FOLLICULAR CYSTS. These are unruptured, enlarged graafian follicles. They may grossly resemble true cystomas which are described in the following section. They can rupture, causing acute peritoneal irritation, but more commonly they are associated with torsion and infarction of the ovary or infarction of the tube and ovary.

CORPUS LUTEUM CYSTS. At times these cysts may become as large as 10 to 11 cm. They can rupture and lead to severe hemorrhage and occasionally vascular collapse from blood loss. The symptoms and physical findings of these cysts may mimic those of ectopic pregnancy, and they are thought by some to be associated with delayed menses and spotting.

ENDOMETRIOMAS. These account for most "chocolate cysts" and are simply cystic forms of endometriosis of the ovary.

WOLFFIAN DUCT REMNANTS. These are not ovarian cysts but often cannot be distinguished clinically from tumors of the ovary. They are small unilocular cysts. Occasionally, they enlarge and may twist and infarct. In most instances, they are incidental findings at laparotomy and cause no difficulties or symptoms.

MÜLLERIAN DUCT REMNANTS. These can appear as paraovarian cysts or as small cystic swellings at the fimbriated end of the fallopian tube (hydatids of Morgagni).

NONFUNCTIONING TUMORS

Cystadenomas

Many of the common, benign, cystic tumors of the ovary are believed to arise from the surface germinal epithelium. Some of these tumors, referred to as "serous cystadenomas," appear as cysts with thin, translucent walls containing clear fluid and lined by simple ciliated epithelium. They frequently are on a pedicle and may undergo torsion leading to pain and infarction. When encountered surgically, they are adequately treated by simple excision. Many serum-containing cystic tumors of the ovary are also accompanied by papillary projections and are known as papillary serous cystadenomas. Because of epithelial variation in these tumors, it is often difficult to be sure where they fit in the spectrum of benign to malignant disease. A similar problem of malignant potential exists for the mucinous cystadenoma, which is a cystic tumor containing sticky, gelatinous material. These mucinous tumors are less likely to be malignant than the serous cystadenomas. About 20 percent of the serous tumors and 5 percent of the mucinous tumors are bilateral.

It is not always possible to be sure by gross inspection whether cystic tumors with solid components are benign or malignant. It is usually necessary to excise the involved ovary completely, even though there is no definite evidence of malignancy. The malignant potential of the cystoma is then determined by histologic examination. Frozen-section examination of the tumor at the time of surgical intervention is necessary to determine the proper course of therapy for patients in the reproductive age group. The opposite ovary should be examined for a lesion and may be bivalved.

Occasionally, a condition is encountered known as "pseudomyxoma peritonei," which is a locally infiltrating tumor composed of multiple cysts containing thick mucin. These tumors arise either from ovarian mucinous cystadenomas or from mucoceles of the appendix, both of which commonly coexist. Histologically, they are benign, but by local spread and infiltration they compromise surrounding vital structures. Localized tumors should be completely excised, if possible. Both ovaries and the appendix are removed even though they grossly appear to be normal.

Primary Carcinomas

Primary carcinomas of the ovary most commonly are serous, mucinous, or endometroid cystadenocarcinomas. These are malignant variations of the previously discussed cystadenomas and of endometriosis. A useful method of staging these tumors is as follows:

Stage I—tumor confined to the ovaries
Stage II—tumor confined to the true pelvis
Stage III—tumor extends to peritoneum outside pelvis
Stage IV—spread beyond the abdominal cavity or intrahepatic metastases.

The Stage III and IV tumors have a markedly poorer prognosis than in those cases with malignancy confined to the ovary.

Malignant tumors of the ovary usually spread locally,

and it is common to see seedings on both peritoneum and serosal surfaces of bowel. Giant masses can develop and slowly spread to fill the entire peritoneal cavity encasing the bowel but rarely invading the lumen. Fluid retention occurs, and both ascites and hydrothorax may be present. Lower leg edema may be seen secondary to abdominal lymphatic obstruction. The patient may experience an increase in abdominal girth and, possibly, weight gain accompanied by wasting of the extremities, loss of appetite, and reduction in muscle mass. Increase in fluid retention and in the size of the abdomen continues with the growth of the intraabdominal tumor.

Surgical intervention is the primary therapy for ovarian malignancy and consists of hysterectomy and bilateral salpingo-oophorectomy. If ascites is present, ascitic fluid is examined cytologically for malignant cells. If there is no obvious extension of tumor outside the ovaries, peritoneal saline washings are examined for malignant cells. The omentum is also sampled or excised. An attempt should be made to remove all sites of the tumor, including local peritoneal metastases. However, in widespread cases radical pelvic surgical treatment with removal of the bladder or the rectum has generally not proved to be helpful. Therefore, if a few discrete peritoneal metastases exist, it is wise to remove them and it is generally accepted that maximum tumor reduction surgery is beneficial if it does not seriously expose the patient to the risk of life-threatening complications. Reduction of tumor mass appears to be helpful in improving the response to chemotherapy or irradiation.

When complete surgical removal cannot be accomplished, it has been customary to treat the residual tumor with radiotherapy. Usually there is sufficient response to produce an interval without symptoms during which the patient is comfortable and active. Rarely this is of long duration, but cure is so unlikely that most clinics now prefer to treat patients with known or suspected residual cancer of the ovary with one or another program of systemic chemotherapy.

Chemotherapy has also been effective in treatment of metastatic tumors and has been used with increasing frequency. The alkylating agents Cytoxan, chlorambucil, and phenylalanine mustard have been the most effective drugs. They have radiomimetic effects. These potent agents interfere with rapidly growing cells and thus particularly affect the bone marrow and gastrointestinal tract as well as the tumor. Nausea, vomiting, diarrhea, and loss of hair can accompany their use. Blood indices must be carefully observed since leukopenia and thrombocytopenia may occur, especially in patients who have received radiotherapy. Cytoxan, chlorambucil, and phenylalanine mustard can be taken orally; the dosage is adjusted to maintain a slight leukocyte depression with the white blood cell count kept in the range of 3,500 to 5,000 cells per cubic millimeter. The antimetabolite 5-fluorouracil (5-FU) also is used but is less effective than the alkylating agents. Efforts have been made to improve results by administration of a number of agents at reduced dosages simultaneously.

In addition, another alkylating agent, thiotepa, can be instilled into the peritoneal cavity to help to control the growth of the tumor and ascites formation. Radioactive gold has been used in a similar fashion. One must be careful in using intraperitoneal instillations, since there is often loculation of fluid between areas of tumor and bowel which can cause a high local concentration of the chemotherapeutic agent or the radioactive gold. Bowel perforation can result.

Radiation therapy is useful in situations in which regression can be assessed. It is offered for the relief of ascites when all other modalities have failed. It is also used as adjuvant therapy when the pelvis is contaminated with tumor cells or when there are external papillary projections or cytologically positive peritoneal fluid. In the latter situation, alkylating agents are frequently used.

The ovary is a site for metastases from tumors originating elsewhere in the body. Solid ovarian tumors containing malignant disease which is usually metastatic from the stomach are known as "Krukenberg tumors," identified histologically by the presence of signet cells. However, ovarian metastases from other intestinal malignant tumors are more common. In cases where a Krukenberg tumor can be diagnosed, it is felt by some that oophorectomy may offer a palliation to the patient, even though the primary malignant tumor cannot be found. The ovary is also a common site for metastases from breast carcinoma.

Dysgerminoma

This rare tumor is most often seen in females in the age group of ten to thirty. It often occurs in pseudohermaphrodites. Dysgerminomas are often found during pregnancy, perhaps because they occur most frequently during the reproductive years. Histologically (Fig. 41-27C), the tumors contain masses of germ cells infiltrated with lymphocytes. If the tumor is unilateral and has not broken through its capsule, then a simple oophorectomy is usually sufficient therapy. If it has broken through its capsule but has not spread beyond the ovary and the contralateral ovary is normal, then preservation of the contralateral ovary with radiation to the side of the surgically removed specimen may be considered. If the tumor has spread or metastasized locally in the pelvis, then the prognosis is poorer. The tumor is sensitive to radiation, resembling the seminoma of the male, but is frequently not radiocurable.

Teratoma

These tumors are thought to arise from the totipotential germ cells of the ovary. The tumors often contain calcified masses, and occasionally either teeth or pieces of bone can be seen on abdominal x-rays. Teratomas occur at any age but are more frequent in patients between twenty and forty years. They are usually benign dermoid cysts but occasionally are solid and then are usually malignant (solid malignant teratomas; teratocarcinomas). The embryonal carcinoma is thought to be an undifferentiated form of teratocarcinoma, and the prognosis associated with these tumors is exceedingly poor even if there is complete excision with no apparent tumor extension at the time of surgical treatment.

If a cystic teratoma (dermoid) is encountered in a young woman, it is preferable to shell it out from the ovarian stroma, preserving functioning tissue in the affected ovary.

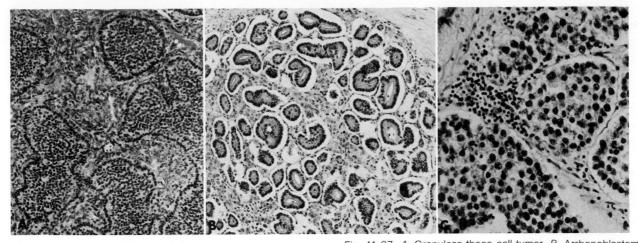

Fig. 41-27. A. Granulosa-theca cell tumor. B. Arrhenoblastoma. C. Dysgerminoma.

Usually these cysts contain ectodermal, mesodermal, and entodermal tissues, in addition to a thick, greasy, fatty material. If this material is spilled during surgery, a chemical peritonitis may result, and, therefore, it is important to remove these tumors intact. The opposite ovary should be inspected and bivalved at the time of removal of cystic teratomas, because in approximately 12 percent of the cases these tumors are bilateral. Malignant teratomas are treated as a carcinoma of the ovary by hysterectomy and bilateral salpingo-oophorectomy.

Brenner Tumor

These are fibroepithelial tumors which are rare and usually do not secrete hormones. Histologically, the epithelial elements are similar to Walthard rests and are believed to arise from these. These tumors occur primarily in later life and have a small malignant potential. Simple oophorectomy is usually sufficient therapy, and the prognosis is excellent.

Clear Cell Carcinomas

These account for as many as 5 percent of primary carcinomas of the ovary. Histologically they consist of clear cells containing glycogen and "hobnail" cells. In most cases the ovaries and uterus are removed since the tumors predominantly occur in older women.

Meigs' Syndrome

This pertains to ascites with hydrothorax, seen in association with benign ovarian tumors with fibrous elements, usually fibromas. It is more common to see fluid accumulation with ovarian fibromas that are more than 6 cm in size. The cause of the condition is unknown, but the ascitic fluid may originate from the tumor, as a result of lymphatic obstruction of the ovary. Frequently, this clinical picture is encountered with other ovarian tumors, especially ovarian malignancy, which can produce a cytologically benign plural effusion; in such cases it is termed a "pseudo-Meigs" syndrome. Meigs' syndrome can be cured by excising the fibroma.

FUNCTIONING TUMORS

Granulosa-Theca Cell Tumor

Pure theca cell tumors (thecomas) are benign, but those with granulosa cell elements may be malignant. It is often impossible to predict their behavior from the histologic features (Fig. 41-27A), and prolonged followup is necessary in order to judge the nature. Usually, granulosa cell tumors elaborate estrogen, but some of these tumors have no hormone production. In the young girl they are characteristically manifested by precocious puberty, and in the elderly female they are sometimes associated with endometrial carcinoma. The tumor can occur at all ages from childhood to the postmenopausal period but are most common in later life, with maximal occurrence between the ages of forty and sixty. If the tumor is discovered in the reproductive years and confined to one ovary without signs of surface spread or dissemination, a simple oophorectomy may be sufficient therapy. If it is discovered in later life, then removal of both ovaries with the uterus is indicated.

Sertoli-Leydig Cell Tumors (Arrhenoblastomas)

These are rare but potentially malignant tumors which are associated with androgen output and masculinization. Rarely, they elaborate estrogen. They usually occur in the reproductive age group and appear to contain tubular structures as well as Leydig-type cells (Fig. 41-27B). In young patients with a singly involved ovary, unilateral oophorectomy is adequate therapy, provided there is no extension of the tumor. For older patients or for those with bilateral involvement, total hysterectomy and bilateral salpingo-oophorectomy are performed.

Hilus Cell Tumors

These are also rare tumors and consist of nests of cells resembling the hilus cells of the ovary. They are characteristically associated with masculinization. They occur primarily in the later years of life and often in the menopausal female. None of the reported cases was malignant.

Struma Ovarii

This term refers to the presence of grossly detectable thyroid tissue in the ovary, usually as the predominant element in dermoid cysts. This tissue occasionally may produce the clinical picture of hyperthyroidism.

Choriocarcinoma

These very rare primary tumors of the ovary elaborate chorionic gonadotropin, and the therapy follows similar considerations already outlined for trophoblastic disease, but the therapeutic results for the ovarian tumors have been disappointing.

Adrenal Rest Tumors

These are also very rare tumors of the ovary which may occur at any age and are not always associated with hormonal activity. Those with adrenal tissue usually show masculinization and are, as a rule, benign. Although most of the signs of masculinization regress after surgical therapy, some of the effects, such as enlarged clitoris, may remain.

Tumors of the Fallopian Tube

BENIGN TUMORS

Tumors of the fallopian tube are rare. Occasionally one sees a tube with thick nodularities at its proximal end. This benign condition is referred to as "salpingitis isthmica nodosa," and although its origin is not definitely known, it is thought to be a sequela of tubal inflammation. It is associated with infertility due to blockage of the tubes. In cases of infertility, a tuboplastic procedure can be attempted in the hope of restoring tubal patency, but the prognosis is poor.

Another type of benign lesion is referred to as "adenomatoid tumor." These are small gland-containing enlargements of the tube which are usually located in the tubal muscularis and are often incidental findings at the time of surgical intervention. Other enlargements of the tube secondary to inflammation or associated with pregnancy are discussed in previous sections of the chapter.

MALIGNANT TUMORS

Primary malignant tumors of the tube are the least frequently seen cancers of the female genital tract. There may be an association between previous tubal inflammation and subsequent development of carcinoma in the tube. Usually these tumors are papillary adenocarcinomas. They may present as a pelvic mass. Occasionally, the tumors block the distal end of the fallopian tube and cause a bloody, mucous vaginal discharge. These tumors are occasionally seen during the reproductive years but occur more often in the postmenopausal age group. Because of the paucity of symptoms and physical findings associated with them, tumors of the fallopian tube are difficult to diagnose early. They may metastasize locally and occa-

sionally spread to the inguinal nodes. Primary therapy is by surgical excision, preferably removal of the tumor and of the uterus and opposite tube and ovary as well. In cases where there appears to be some lymphatic spread of the tumor in the area of the cervix, a radical hysterectomy may effect a cure. The 5-year survival ranges between 10 and 40 percent. Radiotherapy may be tried as palliation or as adjunctive therapy.

TECHNICAL CONSIDERATIONS OF GYNECOLOGIC OPERATIONS

Dilatation and Curettage

Dilatation and curettage (D and C) are frequently indicated in a variety of clinical problems. In patients of reproductive age it is often advisable to perform a curettage after a first-trimester pregnancy loss. In such circumstances, as has been noted in this chapter, an incomplete abortion may have occurred, and curettage is advisable both to prevent further blood loss and to reduce the incidence of postabortal infection. These considerations apply only to cases of spontaneous noninfected abortion. In those cases where instrumentation or sepsis have supervened, a curettage should not be carried out until the patient is adequately treated with antibiotics. Any manipulation of a pregnant uterus should be carried out with extreme care because of the high risk of uterine perforation. In addition, only the major products of conception need be removed. Excessively vigorous curettage at this time can denude the uterine cavity of regenerative tissue, which may result in postcurettage intrauterine synechiae (Asherman's syndrome).

A curettage may also be indicated during reproductive years for excessive bleeding and hemorrhage not associated with pregnancy. In such instances, it is important to carry out a meticulous exploration of the endometrial cavity to be sure that neither endometrial polyps nor submucous fibroids are present. During the menopause, excessive bleeding may necessitate a curettage for diagnostic as well as therapeutic reasons. In these circumstances, a thorough curettage of the endometrial cavity is mandatory, not only to remove all foci that might harbor malignancy, but also to denude the cavity of excess endometrial tissue which may be the cause of the bleeding. A thorough curettage is also required in cases of postmenopausal bleeding. In such cases, a "fractional" curettage is accomplished by first curetting the cervix and then dilating the cervix and curetting the uterine fundus. In this way separate endocervical and endometrial specimens are submitted for pathologic examination. If endometrial carcinoma is discovered, the presence or absence of endocervical involvement is immediately determined, and therapy is planned accordingly (see section on therapy of endometrial carcinoma). In all cases a thorough pelvic examination should be performed, since the anesthetized patients provide the physician with an excellent opportunity to find previously unsuspected intrapelvic pathologic conditions.

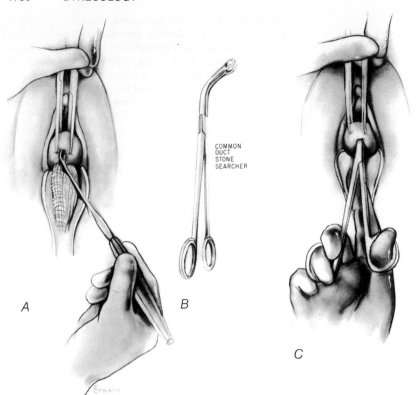

COMMON
DUCT
STONE
SEARCHER

A   *B*

C

Fig. 41-28. Dilatation and curettage. (See description in text.)

TECHNIQUE (Fig. 41-28). The cervix is grasped with a tenaculum. Dilatation of the cervix following abortion is not necessary, and in other cases a dilatation is carried out with graduated dilators of increasing diameter. The Goodell dilator, which can cause great pressure on the endocervix, should not be used as it can split the cervix. A blunt curet is gently introduced into the cervix and endometrial cavity using only minimal force. Extra pressure on the curet is avoided during this time. The curet is then withdrawn, scraping sharply against the sidewalls of the uterus. Firm pressure on the curet is applied during the withdrawal stroke. The cavity is further explored with a common duct stone searcher in order to remove any large masses of tissue. A sharp curet is often unnecessary in cases associated with pregnancy but is used routinely when a diagnostic or therapeutic curettage is being performed in the nonpregnant uterus.

There are numerous surgical procedures that can be performed vaginally. The uterus can be removed by this route in cases of pelvic relaxation, and many disorders of pelvic support can be corrected by a vaginal operation. A few general guidelines are worth considering: exposure at all times should be adequate, small bites of tissue should be taken under direct vision, and a meticulous dissection should be carried out. An enlarged uterus or adnexal mass may preclude a safe vaginal dissection; under these circumstances the abdominal route is used. The excess blood loss that all too frequently accompanies vaginal surgical procedures must be avoided. Damage to surrounding structures, including bladder, ureter, and rectum, can be prevented by adhering to these principles.

Abdominal Gynecologic Procedures

Incisions

The lower abdomen may be conveniently entered through a transverse or vertical incision. For most gynecologic procedures, either a midline or paramedian incision will provide good exposure. The right paramedian incision is frequently used when there is a pathologic condition in the right lower quadrant, especially in cases where the appendix or right adnexal structures could be involved. If a paramedian incision is used, the rectus abdominis muscle is retracted laterally away from the midline. If a midline approach is used, both the right and left rectus sheaths are opened and then resutured at the close of the procedure, since approximation prevents postoperative diastasis and adds to the long-term strength of the wound. Permanent suture material or heavy absorbable suture material can be used to reapproximate the anterior rectus fascia, since this is the layer that provides the main strength of the wound closure.

In certain instances, where surgical treatment is performed on young patients, a Pfannenstiel incision may be used. This incision provides a better cosmetic result, and although there may be slight decrease in exposure, this usually poses no problem. The incision can provide adequate exposure for operations confined to the uterus or to the adnexa. The risk of hematoma formation and subsequent sepsis is somewhat higher in a Pfannenstiel incision. The incision is placed transversely just above the pubic hairline and extends beyond the border of both rectus abdominis muscles (Fig. 41-29*A*). The subcutaneous tissue is divided, and the rectus fascia is split transversely (Fig. 41-29*B*). With traction placed on the lower rectus fascia it is separated from the rectus muscle, and the pyramidalis muscle is preserved on its fascial attachment. After the inferior border of the incision has been delineated, the upper segment of the incision of the anterior rectus fascia is also freed from the underlying muscles (Fig. 41-29*C*). The rectus abdominis muscles are separated in the midline, and the peritoneum is entered in a vertical fashion (Fig. 41-29*D*). After the conclusion of the procedure, the peritoneum is reapproximated in the midline. The muscles are then reapproximated with loose interrupted sutures, and then the rectus sheath is reapproximated in a transverse direction. The skin and subcutaneous tissues are closed in routine fashion.

OPERATION FOR ECTOPIC PREGNANCY

Death from intraperitoneal hemorrhage can occur, and rapid entry into the abdomen through a vertical incision may be necessary. In most cases, the architecture of the tube is destroyed. In rare circumstances the tube may be left in situ. Unfortunately a second ectopic pregnancy is a significant risk in these patients, and thus the tube usually is removed.

Fig. 41-29. Pfannenstiel incision. (See description in text.)

The question of prophylactic removal of the ipsilateral ovary with the tube in cases of ectopic pregnancy has received a great deal of attention due to the introduction of the theory of transmigration, discussed previously in this chapter. Therefore, it has been suggested that the removal of both the tube and the ovary on the same side may prevent a future ectopic pregnancy in the remaining opposite tube. However, this practice is not routinely adopted in younger patients whose reproductive life is just beginning and who do run the risk of a pathologic condition developing in the opposite ovary. This is consistent with the general concept of retaining normal tissue in conservative operations on the reproductive tract.

TECHNIQUE. A traction suture is placed on the uterus, which is retracted to the side opposite the tube. The tube is brought up into view, and the mesentery of the tube is divided (Fig. 41-30*A*). After the tube has been freed from its mesentery, it is placed on traction, elevated and dissected free at its base, in order to be sure that the cornual end of the tube is removed (Fig. 41-30*B*). This prevents the occurrence of future cornual pregnancy. A mattress suture placed in the cornual end of the tube prior to cornual resection helps control hemorrhage. The uterus is repaired, and the mesentery of the ovary is brought to the posterior edge of the broad ligament in order to cover any remaining raw surface (Fig. 41-30*C*).

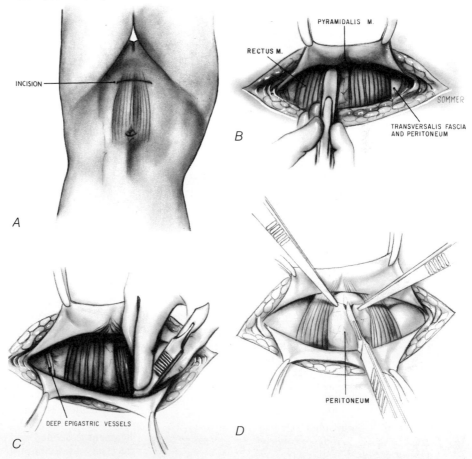

A

B

C

D

INCISION

PYRAMIDALIS M.

RECTUS M.

TRANSVERSALIS FASCIA AND PERITONEUM

SOMMER

DEEP EPIGASTRIC VESSELS

PERITONEUM

SALPINGO-OOPHORECTOMY

In cases of large ovarian tumors or with torsion of the adnexa, the architecture of the tube and ovary may be destroyed. In this instance, unilateral removal of both is performed. First the infundibulopelvic ligament is divided after the ovarian vessels are sutured (Fig. 41-31*A*). The

Fig. 41-30. Salpingectomy. (See description in text.)

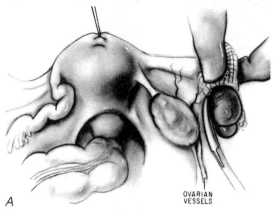

A

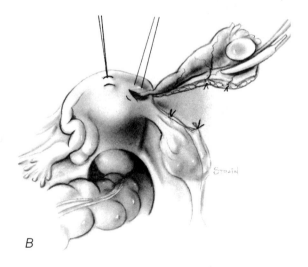

B

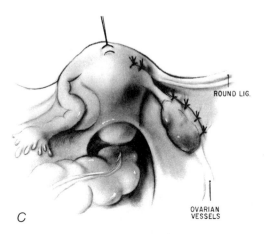

C

broad ligament is divided and dissection carried to the insertion of the tube into the uterus near the origin of the round ligament (Fig. 41-31*B*). The ovarian branch of the uterine artery is ligated (Fig. 41-31*C*). The cornual end of the tube is excised (as in Fig. 41-30*B*), and the defect in the peritoneum is closed (Fig. 41-31*D*).

ABDOMINAL HYSTERECTOMY

In cases of ovarian or endometrial malignancy, the ovaries and tubes are removed with the hysterectomy specimen. In younger patients who are undergoing surgical treatment for other diseases, ovarian conservation may be practiced. The ureter, bladder, and adjacent intestine can be injured during the course of hysterectomy unless careful surgical technique and adequate exposure are maintained (Fig. 41-32). The ureters are particularly prone to injury in the areas of uterosacral ligaments and the uterine artery, since they pass close to these structures. In cases where there is any doubt, the ureter should be visually identified.

TECHNIQUE. The uterus is placed on tension by a tenaculum in the fundus. The anterior leaf of the broad ligament is opened (Fig. 41-33*A*), and the peritoneum above the bladder is separated away from the anterior portion of the uterus (Fig. 41-33*B*). The bladder is then advanced off the uterus and cervix (Fig. 41-33*C*), with the peritoneal sheath kept on tension during the course of this dissection in order not to injure the dome of the bladder.

If the ovaries are to be preserved, the ovarian vessels with the fallopian tube are ligated approximately 1 in. lateral to the uterus (Fig. 41-33*D*). If the ovaries are to be removed, the technique is similar to that shown in Fig. 41-31. The round ligament is then divided, and the anterior and posterior leaves of the broad ligaments are separated. The uterine vessels lie at the base of the broad ligament, and the ureter can be palpated as it passes beneath the uterine vessels (Fig. 41-33*E*). The uterosacral ligaments are next divided, and once again careful attention should be paid to the location of the ureter (Fig. 41-33*F*). After both uterosacral ligaments have been divided, the posterior peritoneum is separated from the back of the specimen, and care is taken to ensure that the rectosigmoid is separated from the posterior part of the dissection. In this fashion, the posterior wall of the vagina is exposed, and the uterus is separated from its peritoneal attachment.

The uterine vessels are then secured. Clamps should be applied under direct vision (Fig. 41-33*G*). The branches of the uterine artery and vein run close to the cervix and cervicouterine junction, and hemostasis must be obtained at the lateral edge of the cervix and lower portion of the uterus. Traction is placed on the fundus, and the uterine vessels are clamped. A second clamp is added to protect against back-bleeding. The vessels are divided, and an additional clamp is placed to ensure against loss of control of the uterine vessel pedicle. The vessels are ligated, removing the lateral clamp first, following which a second suture is placed.

The bladder is mobilized anteriorly to free it completely from the vagina in the area of the cervix. The cardinal ligament is divided and sutured (Fig. 41-33*H*). It may be necessary to accomplish this step in a number of small bites. The vagina is then entered. This can be accomplished by elevating the uterus and placing clamps at the lateral corners of the vagina. The tissue above the clamps is then divided (Fig. 41-33*I*). The specimen is removed by dividing the vaginal tissue under direct vision. Sutures are placed at each angle of the vagina to ensure hemostasis, and the vaginal tissue is then repaired by a running atraumatic chromic catgut suture placed around the apex, which is then left open for improved drainage (Fig. 41-33*J*).

The pelvis is reconstructed by suturing the uterosacral ligaments to the posterior vaginal wall (Fig. 41-33*K*). This provides important support to the vagina. The round ligaments are then brought to the corners of the vagina (Fig. 41-33*L*). Although this maneuver does not add to the permanent support of the vagina, it does aid in reperito-

nealization of the pelvis. The procedure is completed by bringing together the edges of the remaining peritoneum in order to leave a smooth operative field (Fig. 41-33*L*).

Wertheim Hysterectomy with Pelvic Lymphadenectomy

This operation is performed primarily for cancer of the cervix when the disease appears to be confined to the cervix itself or the immediately adjacent vaginal wall. It has also been performed for treatment of cancer of the endometrium. The operation removes the contents of the pelvis from one obturator fossa to the other, including the lymph nodes in the common iliac, hypogastric, external iliac, and obturator artery areas. The ureters are identified through their entire course from bifurcation of the aorta to entrance into the bladder. Complete mobilization of the bladder and ureters from the vagina permits removal of all the tissue extending from the side wall of the pelvis

Fig. 41-31. Salpingo-oophorectomy. (See description in text.)

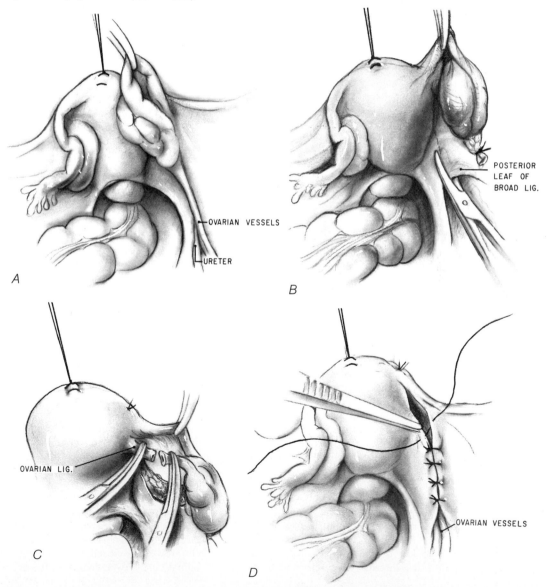

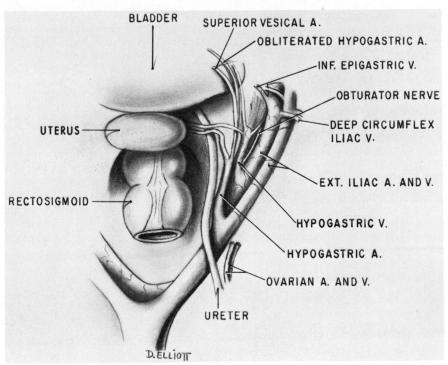

BLADDER   SUPERIOR VESICAL A.
OBLITERATED HYPOGASTRIC A.
INF. EPIGASTRIC V.
OBTURATOR NERVE
DEEP CIRCUMFLEX ILIAC V.
EXT. ILIAC A. AND V.
HYPOGASTRIC V.
HYPOGASTRIC A.
OVARIAN A. AND V.
UTERUS
RECTOSIGMOID
URETER
D. ELLIOTT

Fig. 41-32. Surgical anatomy of pelvis.

to the paracervical and paravaginal area. The entire uterus, the adnexa, and a wide block of lymphatic tissue are removed in one piece, together with a large segment of vagina.

TECHNIQUE. The operation is performed through a low abdominal vertical incision. Most of the points of technique enumerated for hysterectomy apply; those specifically applicable to the Wertheim hysterectomy are outlined in this discussion. The ureter is initially identified at a point where it crosses the common iliac artery (Fig. 41-34A); the ovarian arteries are dissected free of the ureter and underlying common iliac artery. The ovarian vessels are then divided. The bladder flap is then developed as in the technique of total hysterectomy. The round ligament and broad ligament are transected. The uterus is then retracted medially to permit exposure of the areolar tissue overlying the external and internal iliac arteries. Dissection begins lateral to the artery on the psoas muscle and continues down along its medial surface to enter the upper portion of the obturator space. The genitofemoral nerve lies on the psoas and should be preserved. This dissection exposes the lateral and inferior surface of the external iliac vein and mobilizes all areolar tissue toward the midline (Fig. 41-34B). The common iliac lymph nodes and the external iliac lymph nodes are freed. Dissection of this areolar tissue mass permits exposure of the pubic ramus. The obturator and internal iliac nodes are also dissected free. In the course of this dissection, the obturator nerve is identified and spared. The uterine vein is identified at a point where it enters the internal iliac vein and is tran-

sected (Fig. 41-34C). The same dissection is carried out on the opposite side up to this point.

Attention is next directed to the original side, and freeing of the ureter continues. The ureter is dissected down to its entrance into the bladder. The ureter must be cleared from its tunnel along the anterior vaginal wall to permit excision of the paracervical and paravaginal lymphatics. A plexus of vaginal veins lies above and below it, and these must be transected (Fig. 41-34D). The ureter is now completely free from its bed, and the junction with the bladder can be identified. This permits dissection of an adequate length of vagina and paravaginal tissue.

The rectum is then separated from the posterior vaginal wall. All posterior attachments of the uterus are transected, and attention is directed to the anterolateral attachments. The uterus is drawn sharply back toward the promontory of the sacrum, and the bladder and ureters are carefully elevated so that dissection can begin beneath the bladder, freeing it laterally first on one side and then on the other. This represents the most important area of dissection; in order to avoid risk of recurrence, it is imperative that a wide block of tissue containing the paravaginal lymphatics be removed (Fig. 41-34E). This maneuver permits demonstration of the vaginal wall and allows transection and removal of one-half of the vagina. Complete dissection clears both iliac areas and the obturator fossa of all intervening lymphatic tissue. The bladder and ureters lie mobile above the closed vaginal stump (Fig. 41-34F). The vaginal cuff is oversewn, and the area is reperitonealized.

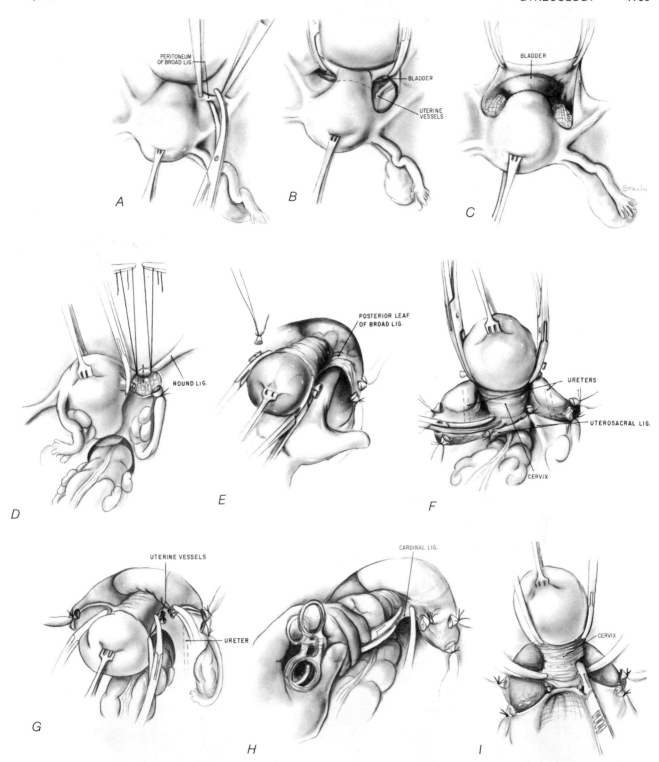

Fig. 41-33. Hysterectomy. (See description in text.)

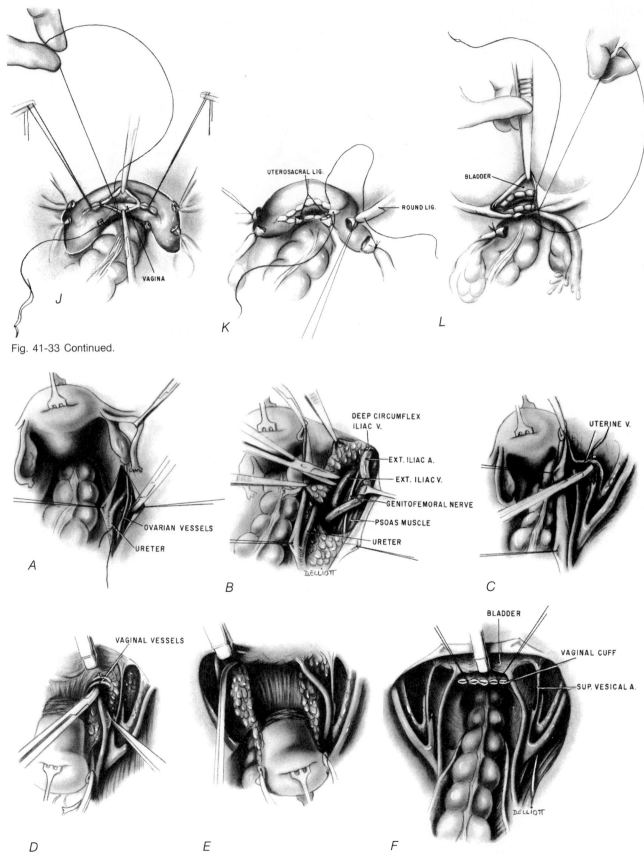

Fig. 41-33 Continued.

J

K

UTEROSACRAL LIG.

ROUND LIG.

VAGINA

L

BLADDER

A

OVARIAN VESSELS

URETER

B

DEEP CIRCUMFLEX
ILIAC V.

EXT. ILIAC A.

EXT. ILIAC V.

GENITOFEMORAL NERVE

PSOAS MUSCLE

URETER

DELLIOTT

C

UTERINE V.

D

VAGINAL VESSELS

E

F

BLADDER

VAGINAL CUFF

SUP. VESICAL A.

DELLIOTT

Fig. 41-34. Wertheim hysterectomy with pelvic lymphadenectomy. (See description in text.)

References

General

Glass, R.: "Office Gynecology," Williams & Wilkins Company, Baltimore, 1976.

Green, T. H., Jr.: "Gynecology: Essentials of Clinical Practice," 3d ed., Little, Brown and Company, Boston, 1977.

Herbst, A. L. (ed.): "Intrauterine Exposure to Diethylstilbestrol in the Human," American College of Obstetrics and Gynecology, 1978.

Kistner, R. W.: "Gynecology: Principles and Practice," 2d ed., Year Book Medical Publishers, Inc., Chicago, 1971.

Novak, E. R., Jones, G. S., and Jones, H. W., Jr.: "Textbook of Gynecology," 9th ed., The Williams & Wilkins Company, Baltimore, 1975.

Parsons, L., and Sommers, S. C.: "Gynecology," W. B. Saunders Company, Philadelphia, 1977.

Taynor, M. L., and Green, T. H.: "Progress in Gynecology," vol. VI, Grune & Stratton, Inc., New York, 1975.

Wynn, R.: "Obstetrics and Gynecology: The Clinical Care," Lea & Febiger, Philadelphia, 1974.

Gynecologic Procedures and Techniques

Coppleson, M., Pixley, E., and Reid, B.: Colposcopy: A Scientific and Practical Approach to the Cervix in Health and Disease, in "American Lectures in Gynecology and Obstetrics," American Lecture Series, no. 799, Charles C Thomas, Publishers, Springfield, Ill., 1971.

Kolstad, P. and Stafl, A.: "Atlas of Colposcopy," Scandinavian University Books, Oslo, 1972.

Mattingly, R. F.: "TeLinde's Operative Gynecology," 5th ed., J. B. Lippincott Company, Philadelphia, 1977.

Parsons, L., and Ulfelder, H.: "An Atlas of Pelvic Operations," 2d ed., W. B. Saunders Company, Philadelphia, 1968.

Related Texts of Special Interest

Behrman, S. J., and Kistner, R. W.: "Progress in Infertility," 2d ed., Little, Brown and Company, Boston, 1975.

Gold, J. J.: "Gynecologic Endocrinology," 2d ed., Harper & Row, Publishers, Incorporated, New York, 1975.

Jones, H. W., Jr., and Scott, W.: "Hermaphroditism; Genital Anomalies and Related Endocrine Disorders," 3d ed., The Williams & Wilkins Company, Baltimore, 1971.

Moore, K. L.: "The Developing Human: Clinically Oriented Embryology," W. B. Saunders Company, Philadelphia, 1973.

Morris, J. M., and Scully, R. E.: "Endocrine Pathology of the Ovary," The C. V. Mosby Company, St. Louis, 1958.

Reid, E. D., Ryan, K. J., and Berdirschke, K.: "Principles and Management of Human Reproduction," W. B. Saunders Company, Philadelphia, 1972.

Speroff, L., Glass, R. H., and Kage, N. G.: "Clinical Gynecologic Endocrinology and Infertility," The Williams & Wilkins Company, Baltimore, 1973.

Chapter 42

Neurologic Surgery

by **William F. Collins, Jr., Joan L. Venes, Franklin C. Wagner, Jr., and Dennis D. Spencer**

GENERAL CONSIDERATIONS

Neurologic surgery includes the surgical treatment of diseases of the nervous system, correction of malformations of the nervous system, the care and repair of traumatic lesions of the nervous system, and the surgical palliation of pain and abnormal motor movements. Anatomy and physiology of the nervous system, the pathophysiology of neurologic disease, and surgery in the broadest sense constitute the foundations of neurologic surgery. The goal is to preserve or restore the maximal degree of neurologic function possible within the disease state. This section will discuss a few salient concepts that provide insight into the surgical therapy of nervous system disease.

Consciousness is a prime sign of the working brain, and loss of consciousness can result from many conditions, for the function of the brain not only is dependent upon controlled excitability in many interrelated and interconnected neurons and the integrity of their supporting glia but also upon adequate function in the rest of the organism. Normal central nervous system function presupposes adequate cardiac output of oxygenated blood with normal ionic and molecular constituents and intact vascular channels for perfusion. Loss of consciousness as a presenting symptom requires not only consideration of central nervous system pathology but evaluations of cardiac output, competence of blood vessels, causes of aberrant serum chemistries, possible circulating toxic substances alterations in body temperature, and the myriad causes of each.

One of the important insights into the physiology of the

brain in recent years has been the definition of the relationship of the reticular formation of the brainstem to overall function of the nervous system. Small lesions placed in the mesencephalic reticular formation of experimental animals produce a state of coma. Sudden isolation of the spinal cord from descending influences of the reticular core of the brainstem by transsection at the cervical medullary junction or more caudad in the spinal cord produces areflexic paralysis or spinal shock distal to the section, followed by mass withdrawal reflexes when spinal shock ceases. Isolation of the brainstem reticular formation from descending hemispheric impulses by a section at the upper midbrain produces facilitation of antigravity musculature, or the state known as *decerebrate rigidity*. Removal of the cerebellum in the midbrain-sectioned animal decreases the extensor tone, while sensory stimuli of any sort enhance it.

Electrophysiologic studies have shown that the reticular core is activated by all sensory stimuli and, conversely, that with total sensory deprivation, that is, section of all sensory nerves, a sleep record is obtained from the electroencephalogram that is altered or "activated" by stimulation within the reticular core. For this reason the ascending cortical influences of the reticular core of the brainstem have been called the *reticular activating system*. The reticular core is more than this. Its reticulum, or network of neurons, influences cortical and subcortical function in the broadest sense in that consciousness and gnosis (recognition of sensation), and motor function are all dependent upon its integrity. For these reasons small lesions in the reticular core of the brainstem can cause loss of consciousness, as seen with contusions of the brainstem or infarcts following thrombosis of perforating branches of the basilar artery. These lesions also can alter motor function and motor tone and muscle tone from areflexic paralysis to decerebrate rigidity.

Surgical diseases of the nervous system are manifestations of space-occupying lesions, be they tumor, hemorrhage, abscess, edema, spinal fluid, or foreign body. The technique of their removal or the control of their effects, as well as an understanding of the mechanisms involved in their producing malfunction in the nervous system, makes neurologic surgery a specialty. The fact that the intracranial space and the spinal canal are nearly closed boxes determines a set of mechanical conditions basic to many considerations of the effect of mass lesions on the nervous system. The intracranial space, compartmentalized by the falx and tentorium cerebri, has communication to the spinal space through the incisura of the tentorium and the foramen magnum of the skull. This represents its only major extracranial communication. The brainstem passes through these areas of communication, i.e., from the incisura of the tentorium through the posterior fossa to the foramen magnum. Rostrally it is continuous with the diencephalon and the internal capsule of each hemisphere, where the medial portion of the temporal lobes have immediate lateral relation to the upper brainstem, with a portion of the circle of Willis, the subarachnoid space, and the oculomotor, or third cranial, nerve between them. Caudad it is continuous with the cervical spinal cord,

where at the foramen magnum it lies immediately anterior to the inferior portion of the ansiform lobes of the cerebellum, more commonly known as the *cerebellar tonsils*.

Central nervous system tissue has many of the properties of a fluid; that is, it is deformable but not compressible, and when deformed it flows in the course of least resistance. Deformation over months or years causes "internal" flows, or loss of substance, mainly of myelin, but rapid deformation varying with the imposed pressure causes flow toward sites of decompression, the incisura of the tentorium and the foramen magnum. While the tissue is not compressible, the lumen of its blood supply is, and obstruction of veins, capillaries, and arteries occurs with deformation. The lethal factors of the flow toward decompression areas are in part the limitation of the accommodation allowed by the semirigid infolded meningeal structures of the falx and the tentorium and the sheer stress at their edges, and the unyielding character of the bony rim of the foramen magnum. In addition, the axial as well as lateral shift of the brainstem is functionally limited by the mobility of the circle of Willis, fixed by the carotid arteries where they pierce the dura. The circle of Willis plus the basilar arteries (Fig. 42-1) supply blood to the brainstem by vessels that enter perpendicular to its surface. With progressive axial shift the normally lax vessels become straightened and eventually tether the brain. With continuing shift there is collapse of the vessels with infarction and rupture of the smaller vessels with hemorrhage. At the foramen magnum compression of the medulla by the decompressing (herniating) cerebellar tonsils causes the same phenomena, but failure of perfusion of this area more commonly causes death before gross visible changes occur.

The situation of a noncompressible tissue nurtured by vessels whose lumens are compressible allows the compressing force to set in motion a cycle that includes production of further mass by edema with consequent increase of the size and compressing force of the original mass. The incisural syndrome of altered consciousness followed by loss of function of the oculomotor nerve, decerebrate rigidity, and death reflects the cycle in supratentorial mass lesions. At the foramen magnum, altered consciousness, followed by depression of respiration requiring the stimulus of increased blood CO_2, or Cheyne-Stokes respiration, depression of reflexes, cessation of respiration, and death represent progression of the cycle. The early recognition of any portion of these patterns is necessary if the lethal effects of intracranial masses are to be reversed. Their recognition and treatment is a sine qua non of neurologic surgery.

It is beyond the scope of this section to review all the neurodiagnostic techniques (and their indications) that can or should be used to investigate neurological diseases requiring neurosurgical intervention. With the recognition that the central nervous system requires a degree of homeostasis in the patient in order to function normally, it becomes obvious that a complete history, physical examination, neurological examination, and basic laboratory studies are requisites for any evaluation of neurological disease. The history should be carefully done, since there is a high probability of its indicating the cause of the condition being studied. In contrast, neurological examination indicates the area or areas of the central nervous system involved and when combined with the history will define questions that can be answered by special diagnostic studies.

DIAGNOSTIC STUDIES. These studies may be benign, that is, of no significant risk to the patient, as with skull x-rays or electroencephalogram, or they can be dangerous enough to require the immediate availability of an operating room, as with pneumoencephalography. The accuracy of the special studies depends not only on the technical skill with which they are performed but also on knowing what question is being asked of the test and what answers can be gained. This latter aspect, as well as knowing what the risks of the test are, is why as much knowledge of the patient as a whole should be gained before using the tests and why their use in neurological evaluation is restricted to physicians knowledgeable in nervous system disease.

X-rays of the skull can be helpful in the diagnosis of neurological disorders, for increased intracranial pressure may be reflected in springing of the sutures in the infant or decalcification of the sella turcica in the adult. A calcified pineal gland that defines the posterior position of the third ventricle may be shifted from its usual midline position by a supratentorial mass. Many tumors contain radiopaque calcification which may be visible in skull x-rays. Meningiomas may contain calcification but usually are recognized, because they evoke hyperostosis in the adjacent bones of the skull. Other stigmata of brain tumor in skull x-rays are erosions of the internal auditory meatus with an eighth nerve tumor or erosion of the optic foramen or anterior clinoid with an optic nerve tumor.

Special diagnostic studies can indicate the position, the size, and the blood supply of the tumor, and also may give information as to the amount of brain shift. The studies that involve no risk to the patient are electroencephalography, echo encephalography, brain scan, and computerized axial tomography (CT scan).

Electroencephalography. The electroencephalogram, or EEG, is the recording of electrical activity of the brain from amplification of the cerebral potentials recorded from the scalp. Alterations in cortical cellular excitability are reflected in the electroencephalogram. The most common abnormalities seen with mass lesions are focal slowing or focal paroxysmal activity. Since this is a record of the surface activity of the cerebral hemispheres, lesions not affecting cortical function directly by metabolic changes, by interrupting subcortical projection, or by pressure will not cause alteration in the electroencephalogram.

Echo Encephalography. The echo encephalogram uses the reflection of ultrasonic waves from intracranial structures to locate them within the skull. The third ventricle has a fairly constant ultrasonic echo, and therefore its position can often be determined. As with the pineal gland, shift of this structure by a supratentorial mass is not uncommon. An echo also occurs at any tissue density interphase, and with special equipment solid tumors as well as the lateral ventricles of the hemispheres at times can be located.

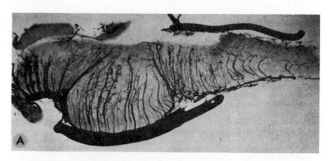

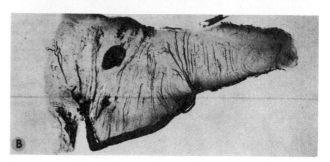

Fig. 42-1. Angiograms of thick longitudinal sections of the midline brainstem. *A.* Normal specimen with demonstration of the basilar artery and its paramedian branches. *B.* Specimen from a case with an expanding supratentorial mass. Caudal displacement of the brainstem has occurred with longitudinal shortening of the brainstem and an increase in the anteroposterior dimension. There are several paramedian arteries which have been ruptured with the demonstration of parenchymal hemorrhages. (*From O. Hassler, Neurology, 17:368, 1967.*)

Radioactive Brain Scan. The brain scan uses radioactive materials such as mercury 203 or technetium 99 that will not cross the intact blood-brain barrier. Since most brain tumors are not included within the barrier, an abnormal amount of radioactive material will be present in the area of the tumor and can be localized by counting this radioactive material with a scintillation counter. This counter localizes the abnormal activity through the intact skull, producing a graphic display. Since there are many causes for breakdown of the blood-brain barrier, positive brain scans can be found in conditions which are not caused by tumors, such as in vascular occlusion, infection, or trauma. The problem of false-negative studies of lesions contained within the blood-brain barrier further limits the value of the study.

Computerized Axial Tomography. Computerized axial tomography (Fig. 42-2) is a major advance in radiological diagnosis whose unique attributes are particularly advantageous for diagnosis of intracranial disease. Conventional x-rays use photographic film to measure the relative amount of x-ray absorbed by the structures through which the beam has passed. Limitations of conventional x-ray include the fact that with photographic film, quantitative definition of the amount of x-ray absorbed is poor and slanted towards high-absorption matter such as bone, and the resulting image is only two-dimensional. In the early 1970s, Geoffrey Houndsfield, a British engineer, developed

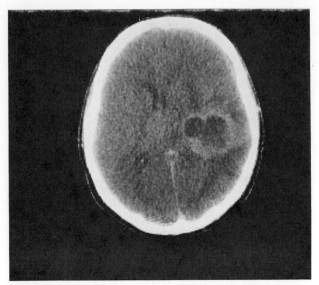

Fig. 42-2. Computerized axial tomography of a right temporal parietal tumor. The breakdown in the blood-brain barrier is enhanced by use of radiopaque intravenous material (Renografin). Note central area of decreased density (necrosis), surrounded by area of no blood-brain barrier, surrounded by edema (lower density). The mass has also shifted the ventricles. The tumor was a glioblastoma.

a technique of a carefully controlled small beam of x-ray, a focused crystal scintillation counter, to measure accurately the amount of x-ray remaining after the beam passed through an object, and computer technology along with matrix mathematics and pattern storage techniques to produce a three-dimensional array in a computer of the object being studied, which he called *computerized axial tomography.* The small x-ray beam is passed through the object being studied through multiple directions, and the matrix is formed in the computer so that by simultaneously solving a number of equations, the amount of x-ray absorbed in each portion of the matrix is determined. The size of the area in each point is determined by the size of the matrix; with recent scanners, the image resolution is approximately 1 mm in diameter. Since brain, cerebrospinal fluid, and bone have different x-ray absorption coefficients, with the technique of computerized axial tomography, the amount and position of each of these structures can be determined, and with the use of radiopaque compounds, areas of abnormal vascularity or breakdown in the blood-brain barrier can be accurately determined. The ability to show enlarged ventricles, altered cortical surfaces, tumors, and abscesses has allowed accurate diagnosis of many neurological conditions without any significant risk to the patient. By 1974, Ambrose at the Atkinson Morley Hospital in England had demonstrated both the value and the accuracy of the technique. In the past few years, it has become a standard neuroradiological diagnostic technique.

Pneumoencephalography. Pneumoencephalography, or the x-ray study of the brain with air, utilizes the difference in the absorption of x-rays between air, brain, and fluid. Air studies are done in one of two ways and in general outline the ventricles, the basal cisterns, and a portion of the subarachnoid spaces around the cerebral hemispheres. A patient who is suspected of a major shift of the cerebral hemispheres or who has significant symptoms from intracranial pressure is not a candidate for a lumbar puncture, and therefore the air study is usually done by a technique known as ventriculography. This consists of making openings in the skull, usually in the posterior parietal bone, tapping the lateral ventricles directly, and replacing fluid in the ventricle with air. A series of x-ray films is then taken with the head manipulated to move the air around to show the different portions of the ventricle and to fill the basal cisterns and subarachnoid spaces.

Pneumoencephalography also may be performed with the patient in the upright position. In this position a lumbar puncture is performed, and small increments of air are placed in the lumbar subarachnoid space. The head is positioned so that the ascending air will fill the different portions of the subarachnoid space. Since both studies alter the cerebrospinal fluid circulation and may precipitate sudden shifting of the intracranial contents with possible sudden loss of brainstem function, it is always best to have an operating room and neurosurgeon available at the start of such studies; rapid decompression of the intracranial pressure and/or removal of a tumor or mass can be accomplished if the patient's condition starts to deteriorate. Computerized axial tomography has decreased the need for pneumoencephalography in many conditions, but one of the problems with computerized axial tomography is the difficulty of separating lesions which are close to the bone, so that pneumoencephalography remains an important diagnostic tool for conditions along the base of the skull, particularly pituitary tumors, useful in determining if the tumor has extended past the confines of the sella.

Cerebral Angiography. Cerebral angiography, or what is more commonly called carotid or vertebral arteriography, is the x-ray study of the intracranial circulation as demonstrated by the injection of contrast material. These studies can define the position of the arteries and the presence or absence of abnormal vasculature, and thereby often define not only the presence of a brain tumor but also its blood supply and how it has affected the adjacent structures. Angiography is the main method of demonstrating vascular lesions such as arteriovenous malformations, aneurysms, and vascular occlusive disease. These studies are usually done by injecting the contrast material into the common carotid artery, the subclavian artery, or the arch of the aorta, so that the material is carried into the intracranial vessels; films to demonstrate the arterial or capillary and venous spaces can then be taken.

HEAD INJURY

Included within the term "head injury" are injuries of the scalp, skull, and brain. The immediate care of patients with head injury is no different from that of any injured patient. Primary consideration must be given to the establishment of adequate respiratory exchange, control of hemorrhage, and maintenance of peripheral vascular circulation. Physicians caring for the patient with traumatic injury to the nervous system too often forget these cardinal necessities or blame apparent respiratory difficulty or peripheral vascular collapse on central nervous system factors that they feel unable to alter. During the initial period of treatment of a patient with head injury, as measures are instituted for the control of the vital functions, a preliminary evaluation of the nervous system function is essential and should be followed as soon as possible by careful repetitive neurologic examinations. The reason for repetitive neurologic examinations will become clear as complications of head-injured patients are discussed, but it suffices to state that the care of patients with traumatic lesions of the nervous system is mainly based on the detection of deterioration or improvement in neurologic function.

Scalp

Although the scalp consists of five layers, from a surgical point of view its two important layers are the dermis and the galea. The principles in the care of scalp lacerations are the same as in the care of any laceration, that is, to change a contaminated open wound into a closed clean wound, but some unique problems arise because of the structure of the scalp and its anatomic relationships. The unyielding character of the scalp with its major blood supply lying between the galea and the dermis has a tendency to hold blood vessels open following laceration with the possibility of considerable loss of blood. Hemostasis of the scalp is easily obtained, if the skull is intact, by compression of the scalp against the skull either in a circumferential fashion at the base of the scalp or by direct pressure on the wound edges. When the skull is not intact, traction on the galea by a clamp which grasps the galea, pulling it back over the dermis, will usually control the hemorrhage. The minor hemorrhage of contusions lying between the galea and the skin rarely causes any significant difficulty, but hematomas of the scalp which lie beneath the galea can attain considerable size, causing elevation of a major portion of the scalp from the skull. Early control of such hemorrhage sometimes can be accomplished by pressure and a firm dressing. Such subgaleal hematomas may take weeks to absorb, but with intact skin over them they are best treated by allowing natural absorption to occur. However, if the hematoma is of significant size to embarrass circulation of the scalp or if there is a question of infection as manifested by heat, swelling, and fever, evacuation of the hematoma is indicated. This should be done under sterile conditions, the hematoma totally evacuated, and any dead space obliterated by a compression dressing.

The approximation of the scalp to the skull not only allows lacerations to occur with blunt injury but also causes increased morbidity with infections of the scalp. Infections of the scalp may spread into the intracranial epidural space through the connecting emissary veins in the diploic spaces of the skull and into the veins on the surface of the brain. With these channels for spread of infection, epidural abscess, subdural abscess, cerebral thrombophlebitis, cerebritis, or brain abscess can occur.

Finally the galea is not only a strong fascial layer that is firmly attached to the skin by numerous fascial bands but is also the attachment of the occipitalis and frontalis muscles. These muscles tend by their contraction to separate any weak area of the galea. The problem of such contraction is that any laceration of more than a few centimeters in size will have a tendency to pull open unless the galea is closed at the time that the dermis is closed; any large laceration of the scalp which is allowed to remain open for more than 5 to 6 days may show a significant amount of contraction with fibrosis, so that it cannot be closed without special plastic techniques.

Thus, the toilet of a scalp wound must be thorough and include shaving of hair in the immediate vicinity, debridement of all the devitalized tissue, and removal of any foreign body. The wound closure must include closure of the galea, either as a separate layer or as a layer included within the dermis. If the laceration is of a large size with separation of a major portion of the galea from the subgaleal tissue, a compression dressing will make the patient more comfortable and decrease the chances of a subgaleal hematoma and infection.

Skull

ANATOMY. The skull is divided into the cranium, which contains and protects the brain, and the facial bones. The cranium consists of eight bones: two parietal and temporal bones and one frontal, occipital, ethmoid, and sphenoid bone. The superior, or rounded, portion of the skull is called the *vault,* and its bones are formed as membranous bone. In the adult the bone consists of firm inner and outer tables with cancellous bone, or diploë, lying between them. The skull contains within the frontal, ethmoid, and sphenoid bones mucous membrane-lined sinuses which connect to the nasal cavities. The basilar, or petrous, portion of the temporal bones contains the middle ear and mastoid air cells, which also connect to the nasopharynx via the eustachian tube.

CLASSIFICATION OF SKULL FRACTURE

The clinical term "skull fracture" is used for fractures of the cranium. Such fractures are described by using a term describing the pattern of the fracture (linear, stellate, comminuted), by using the term "depressed" to denote an inward displacement of a portion of the vault, by naming the bone involved, by including the term "basilar" for fractures traversing the base of the skull, and by describing a break in the scalp or mucous membrane over such a fracture with the term "compound fracture." Thus, a compound comminuted depressed fracture of the left parietal bone states that there is a scalp laceration over a fracture of the parietal bone on the left that consists of multiple fragments of bone driven beneath the surface of the cranial vault.

Fractures of the skull may occur in any area of the skull and have a tendency to radiate from the point of contact into the weaker areas of the skull, e.g., basilar or temporal areas. Most skull fractures require no treatment in themselves, but compound and depressed fractures must be treated. A compound fracture of the cranial vault should be cleansed and debrided, and the wound closed. Replacement of large skull fragments in the area of a compound fracture requires surgical judgment and depends upon the degree of contamination, intactness of the dura, the area of the skull involved, and the ability to watch the patient closely after injury. If the surgeon is in doubt in any of these respects, it is always wisest to remove all fragments of a compound fracture.

With depressed fractures the rule is to elevate all of them, but again this should be based on surgical judgment of the size of the depressed segment, the depth to which it is depressed, and the area of the skull depressed, and the ability to be certain that the dura has not been torn. Any fragment which has been depressed more than a centimeter, a fragment which is over the motor strip, and most small fragments that appear sharp on x-ray usually should be elevated, since they may tear the dura and cause damage to the brain. The combination of a depressed and compound fracture will always require elevation to be certain that contamination has not been driven through the dura into the subarachnoid space or the brain.

Another type of compound skull injury, one that is not as obvious as a penetrating injury, is the injury in which a fracture of the skull traverses one or more of the paranasal sinuses, the mastoid air cells, or the middle ear. The indication that this type of open head injury has occurred is the presence of cerebrospinal fluid drainage from the nose or ear. It signifies a rupture of the protective meningeal coverings of the brain and requires observation and prophylactic antibiotics to be certain that infection of the subarachnoid space or brain does not occur. The posttraumatic cerebrospinal fluid fistula of the ear almost always heals within a few days, but healing of rhinorrhea may be more difficult. It is important in both injuries that the patient remain under medical supervision until such drainage ceases, and usually if either otorrhea or rhinorrhea continues for more than 10 to 14 days, surgical repair of the dural tear is necessary.

Brain

MECHANISMS OF INJURY

The most critical aspect of head trauma is what happens to the brain. The immediate brain damage that results from head trauma is dependent upon the force applied to the head, the area of its application, and whether the head is fixed or freely movable. The damage can be caused by the injuring object or a portion of the skull lacerating the brain, the effects of force transmitted to the brain, and the effects of acceleration and deceleration of the head on the brain confined by the semirigid dura and rigid skull. Delayed brain damage is mainly caused by the reactions of the tissues within the skull. When viable tissue receives an application of force strong enough to be injurious, it responds by alteration in intracellular and extracellular fluid content, by extravasation of blood, by increasing blood supply to the local area, and by mobilization of cells capable of removing cellular debris and repairing any disruption. The same mechanisms occur in injuries of the brain, and these mechanisms, as well as alteration of vasomotor control or autoregulation of cerebral circulation, may have secondary deleterious effects on the brain because of the unique anatomic position of the brain within the skull and the brain's unique dependency on a constant supply of oxygen and glucose.

It is simplest and easiest to consider the initial brain injury of head trauma as being caused in one of two ways: by the application of a focal, or local, force to the skull or by the application of a generalized, or diffuse, force to the skull. There is considerable overlap between the two, since a patient may have both types of injuries at the same time, but the mechanisms and results of the two types of injury are different. In focal injury, a sharp object of low velocity strikes the head and may cause disruption of the scalp, fracture of the skull, and laceration of the brain, either directly or by driving fragments of the skull through the dura mater. The resulting neurologic dysfunction relates to the area of the brain involved, since no significant force is transmitted to the skull or brain generally. There is usually brief loss or no loss of consciousness, and the main problem is the care of the local wound.

Following the application of a more generalized force to the skull, there are three other mechanisms that may cause brain injury and complicate or amplify any focal injury that has occurred. Such an application of force may occur following high-velocity missile injuries, such as a gunshot wound, but is most commonly seen in blunt head injuries or injuries in which the freely movable head is struck by a heavy object or when the head is propelled against a solid structure as seen in a high-speed vehicle accident. These mechanisms of brain injury in the more generalized application of force to the skull are injury caused by the direct transmission of energy to the brain, injury caused by the inertia and momentum of the brain when the head is accelerated and decelerated causing the brain to strike against the skull and edges of the dura, injury caused by the torque or compressive force applied to the relatively fixed upper brainstem with the rotation of the cerebral hemispheres during such acceleration and deceleration, and the stretching effect of this movement on the various tissues of the intracranial content.

The effects of transmitted energy to the brain relate to the amount of force applied minus the amount of energy dissipated by disruption of the scalp or skull. The force dissipated in fracturing the skull can be considerable and in part accounts for the paradoxic situation in which brain injury appears inversely related to the skull injury. The remaining energy after disruption of scalp and skull can either be transmitted through the skull or be directly applied to the brain, if the injuring object penetrates the skull. The energy spreads concentrically from the point of application with maximal transmission in the primary direction in which the force was applied. As this energy passes through the tissues of the brain, and particularly through the interphases of the vascular channels and cerebral spinal fluid spaces, a change in direction of the force occurs and may cause disruption or damage to the tissue.

This type of damage will usually be most marked at cortical and ventricular surfaces and adjacent to blood vessels within the hemispheres, since these are areas of major changes in tissue density and tensile strength.

The other mechanisms of brain injury following head trauma are more commonly the cause of severe brain damage and neurologic dysfunction in the head-injury patient and therefore are more frequently the cause for major difficulty in the care of these patients. The mechanisms relate to induced acceleration and deceleration of the head, the inertia of the brain at the moment of acceleration, and the momentum of the brain at the time of deceleration. These forces cause motion of the head and its contents, forcing the brain against the inner surface of the skull where the force has been applied, as well as against the opposite inner surface of the skull (contrecoup injury). Such contact may cause damage to any surface of the brain but is usually most severe when it involves a motion which throws the brain against the sphenoid ridges and/or the free edges of the tentorium cerebelli. This latter action is most likely to occur when the head is struck in such a way as to produce rotation of the skull. The areas of the brain most likely to receive severe damage are the anterior portions of the frontal and temporal lobes, the posterior portions of the occipital lobes, and the upper portions of the midbrain. The intrinsic movement of the brain tissue with the varying degrees of resistance to such movement of blood vessel, fiber tracts, glia, and neurons results in stretching and rupture of the tissue, with maximum effect on the perivascular tissue and the white matter of the hemispheres and brainstem. The torque effect on the upper brainstem is also most easily obtained in the freely movable head that is struck in a manner to cause marked rotation. The effects of such torque applied to the upper brainstem cause almost instant alteration in neuronal function with resulting change in consciousness. This loss of function is probably the cause of the immediate loss of consciousness seen with "concussion." The leverage of a blow applied to the point of the jaw easily gives this rotational effect to the skull and may explain the "knockout" effect of the uppercut in boxing.

In summary, a force applied to the skull may have a local effect of laceration of the scalp, fracture of the skull, and laceration and contusion of the brain, or it may have a more generalized effect caused by the effect of energy transmitted through a semisolid substance, a contusing and lacerating effect when the brain is driven against the inner portion of the skull and edges of the dura, the stretching and tearing effect of the resulting internal movement of tissue, and the loss of function by the compressive effect of the torque or stress applied to the upper portion of the midbrain with rotational movement of the brain. These mechanisms result in the clinical conditions of cerebral concussion, cerebral contusion, and cerebral laceration. They, plus the effect of alteration in total function of the nervous system, the alterations in cerebral circulation, the changes in respiration and vasomotor control, and the reaction of the nervous system tissue to injury, are the main reasons for the clinical syndromes seen in the head-injured patient.

Care of the Head-injured Patient

The care of the head-injured patient can be divided into temporally sequential aspects. These are first aid; evaluation; protection from the loss of nervous system function; protection from the response of injured nervous system tissue; prevention, recognition, and treatment of complications; and rehabilitation. The eventual morbidity and mortality of the head-injured patient can be markedly improved by knowledgeable and effective care throughout the course of the illness. In general, hospitals with specialized centers for neurosurgical patients and for rehabilitation for neurologically disabled patients should be utilized as soon as it is feasible to move the patient. As a rule the patient is best transferred to such an area for definitive care as early as possible, since with few exceptions the patient is most capable of transport immediately after first aid and evaluation have been completed.

FIRST AID. The basic principles for first aid of the head-injured patient have already been discussed in the opening paragraphs of this section on head trauma. They consist of maintenance of respiration, control of hemorrhage, and maintenance of peripheral vascular circulation. The importance of such measures cannot be stressed too much, since any failure of these vital functions not only is a significant factor in the mortality of head injury but can be significant in increasing eventual morbidity. The addition of anoxia or loss of circulation, either from respiratory obstruction or peripheral vascular collapse, can cause a marked increase in neuronal damage and may contribute to the degree of reaction the brain has to the original injury.

Another aspect of first aid is the transport of the patient, either from the scene of the accident or to a hospital for definitive therapy. The unconscious head-injured patient should always be accompanied by an attendant who can clear the nasopharynx and assist respiration. The patient is most safely transported in a two-thirds prone position with his head slightly elevated by a firm roll or his arm above a firm surface. This allows secretions from the nasopharynx and vomitus to drain onto the stretcher rather than be aspirated into the trachea.

EVALUATION. Evaluation of a head-injured patient includes careful examination for other injuries. Visible lacerations and obvious deformities of the extremities signify lesions which must be treated, but internal injury to the thorax, abdomen, or pelvis may be difficult to diagnose in the unconscious patient. Continued hypotension and tachycardia are the most consistent signs of such injuries and should always indicate further investigation, since peripheral vascular collapse from central nervous system damage is seen only as a terminal event. Injury to the cervical spine may occur in head injury, and x-rays of the cervical spine may be necessary to rule out such injuries.

A complete neurologic examination should be recorded as soon as possible, and this must include an accurate evaluation of the state of consciousness. The most common neurologic deficit that occurs with head injury is altered consciousness. Accurate evaluation of the state of consciousness and comparison of the initial examination with subsequent examinations are the most reliable means for evaluating the progress of the head-injured patient. Terms such as "comatose," "semicomatose," and "stuporous" that are commonly used to describe states of consciousness have little meaning and are best used, if used at all, as a means of introducing descriptions that have objective findings as their method of evaluation. The evaluation of the state of consciousness is done by utilizing the response of the patient to various stimuli. If the stimulus and the response are described, the evaluation can be repeated and compared later by the same examiner or others. Table 42-1 offers a general description of the levels of consciousness to be determined by this method. Levels between those described can be easily devised when required.

By utilizing objective responses to stimuli it is not difficult to recognize progressive neurologic deficit. The difference in neurologic function between the confused patient who follows commands and the patient who responds to painful stimuli with nonpurposeful movements is obvious, and the time it takes for such neurologic deficit to develop indicates how rapidly definitive treatment must be started. Decerebrate posturing as a description of a level of consciousness is the posture assumed by a patient with physiologic or anatomic section of the upper brainstem. It is basically the posture assumed when there is facilitation of all antigravity musculature. The patient therefore extends and internally rotates his extremities, extends his neck, and arches his back. Fragments of decerebrated posturing usually appear first with thrusting of the lower extremities. Since it signifies failure of function of the upper brainstem, it is an ominous sign that requires immediate definitive therapy. It is seen with shift of the brain by a supratentorial mass and therefore is often the preterminal event in the patient with untreated posttraumatic intracranial hemorrhage.

Jennett and coworkers over the past decade have utilized a simple scale to assess the level of severe head injuries in order to study and compare various forms of therapy. Though the outcome of the study comparing various forms of therapy is not complete, the reliability of the "Glasgow Coma Scale" in predicting the outcome of severely traumatized patients who have received good neurosurgical treatment in various clinics and countries has been demonstrated. The scale (Table 42-2) is applied to a patient who has been unconscious for more than 6 hours, thus eliminating relatively minor head trauma. The score is the sum of the highest numbers obtained in each section of the scale, i.e., motor response, verbal response, and eye opening. Jennett has demonstrated that patients with less than 5 on the scale have an overall mortality rate of over 50 percent. The scale basically shows that the levels of consciousness and brainstem function closely parallel the severity of the injury and thus the mortality rate. It further points out how evaluation of general function of the brain, i.e., consciousness and a portion of the brain that responds to shift and flow of intracranial contents, the midbrain, can give a fairly accurate picture of the amount or progression in amount of injury to the central nervous system.

OBSERVATION AND DIAGNOSTIC STUDIES. Therapy is dependent upon the evaluation of the initial and repeated neurologic examinations. Most patients can be observed over a short period of time, 30 minutes to a few hours, while first aid is given and other areas of the body evaluated; following observation a more accurate decision can be made as to what is necessary for treatment. Studies other than observation and neurologic examination are helpful but are never indicated if they remove a seriously ill patient from medical and nursing observation.

Roentgenograms of the skull can be helpful especially if the pineal gland is calcified, since shift of its midline position in the anteroposterior view will signify a mass lesion. The skull roentgenograms may show depressed fractures or fractures that traverse arterial vessel grooves in the skull (middle meningeal artery), indicating a possible source for bleeding (epidural hematoma). They may demonstrate air within the skull, indicating a tear in the coverings of the brain, or they may show a foreign body. Computerized axial tomography has altered the evaluation of acute head problems since it can demonstrate recent

Table 42-1. LEVELS OF CONSCIOUSNESS

Responds to spoken word, is alert, cooperative, and oriented.
Responds to spoken word, is confused, and obeys simple commands.
Responds to spoken word only after receiving painful stimuli of supraorbital pressure; obeys commands only while receiving painful stimuli.
Does not respond to auditory stimuli before or while receiving painful stimuli but has purposeful, effective motor response to painful supraorbital and sternal pressure.
Responds to painful supraorbital and sternal pressure with purposeful but noneffective motor movements.
Responds to painful supraorbital and sternal pressure with nonpurposeful movement.
Responds to painful stimuli only with alteration in pulse and respiratory rate or with decerebrate posturing.
No response to painful stimuli, but cough and gag reflexes are present.
No response to stimuli.
Lowest level is unconsciousness; the only step below this is death.

Table 42-2. GLASGOW COMA SCALE

Best motor response	Obeys	M6
	Localizes	5
	Withdraws	4
	Abnormal flexion	3
	Extensor response	2
	Nil	1
Verbal response	Oriented	V5
	Confused conversation	4
	Inappropriate words	3
	Incomprehensible sounds	2
	Nil	1
Eye opening	Spontaneous	E4
	To speech	3
	To pain	2
	Nil	1

NOTE: The coma scale score is the sum of the sectional scores. See text for details.

intracranial hemorrhage quite accurately and indicate both its size and location. The scanner can also define shift of intracranial contents, as well as areas of localized edema. No diagnostic procedure should displace clinical observation, but in the critically ill, head-injured patient, the accurate knowledge that intracranial hemorrhage or mass exists or does not exist allows more accurate control of intracranial pressure and cerebrovascular perfusion pressure without invasive x-ray procedures such as angiography and ventriculography, and quickly defines the need or lack of need for surgical excision of intracranial masses from the injury. If a scanner is not available, further studies such as carotid arteriography or exploratory perforator openings of the skull are indicated only when the patient's condition precludes serial evaluations or a course of progressive neurologic deficit has been established.

During and following the period of initial evaluation frequent recording of the blood pressure, pulse rate, and respiratory rate is indicated, since elevation of blood pressure and decrease in pulse and respiratory rate are seen with increasing intracranial pressure and may indicate impending medullary failure. As these changes in vital signs are less sensitive and usually occur later than alteration in levels of consciousness, they are helpful but not as accurate in defining the need for active intervention.

Lumbar puncture has little place in the early evaluation of head trauma. The risk involved in altering spinal fluid pressure when the possibility exists of mass lesion in the calvarium far outweighs any information gained. The presence or absence of blood in the spinal fluid or the presence or absence of increased spinal fluid pressure do not signify the need for, or the contraindication for, any form of therapy. Lumbar puncture can at times be helpful in deciding that an unconscious patient without history has had a subarchnoid hemorrhage or meningeal infection before, or instead of, head trauma.

SUPPORTIVE THERAPY. During the entire period of treatment of the head-injured patient measures must be instituted to provide substitutes for the protective nervous system reflexes that may have been lost. Any obstruction to the airway or any difficulty with keeping clear the pharynx, larynx, or trachea should be handled by tracheostomy. This is usually best done as an elective procedure within 24 hours after intubation with a cuffed endotracheal tube. At times with facial or cervical spine injuries an emergency tracheostomy may have to be done. Gastric suction through a nasogastric tube is helpful not only in preventing gastric dilatation and the resulting respiratory difficulty but also in preventing the regurgitation of gastric contents into the nasopharynx and trachea. A Foley catheter for bladder drainage allows accurate measuring of urinary output and prevents overdistension of the urinary bladder.

Control of water balance may be altered so that diabetes insipidus or lack of antidiuretic hormone release may occur. Accurate recording of urinary output, the replacement of fluid, and the use of Pitressin tannate in oil can control this. The opposite effect or the inappropriate secretion of antidiuretic hormone is more common and may cause water retention despite decreasing serum osmolarity.

Water restriction is necessary to avert the complications of water intoxication that will ensue.

Temperature regulation may be deficient with head trauma; most commonly the deficiency is in the heat-loss mechanism, that is loss of superficial vasodilation and sweating. The resulting hyperthermia can contribute to the central nervous system damage and to central nervous system response to damage. Frequent rectal or esophageal temperature should be taken. If fever ensues, exposure of major portions of the body, tepid-water sponging, and water-cooled mattresses should be used to control the fever.

PREVENTION AND TREATMENT OF CEREBRAL EDEMA. The nervous system tissue, like other tissue, responds to injury by formation of edema. Since the brain is encased within the skull and dura, the formation of edema causes increased intracranial pressure which may become of such magnitude that it equals systemic arterial pressure. At that point circulation through the brain ceases, and death of tissue ensues. When this happens, the situation is usually irreversible, because relief of pressure must be accomplished within 4 to 5 minutes in order to avert neuronal death. Since the formation of edema is gradual, starting a few hours after injury and reaching its maximum in 36 to 48 hours, protective measures instituted promptly can have considerable value.

Intracranial pressure in the head-injured patient is dependent upon a number of factors. One of the main ones is the volume of fluid in each of the intracranial compartments, i.e., cerebrospinal fluid and fluid in vascular, intracellular, and extracellular spaces. The extracellular space is small, and its contribution to brain swelling is open to argument; the increase in intracranial pressure appears to relate to alteration in volume of the vascular bed, intracellular space, and the cerebrospinal fluid space. Modification in the reaction of the brain to injury is dependent upon modifying the volume responses of these spaces.

The vascular bed volume is dependent upon venous pressure, CO_2 content of the circulating blood, and arterial pressure. It is generally unwise to alter arterial pressure except to raise it toward normal. The blood CO_2 level and venous pressure can be reduced by making certain there is no obstruction to the airway, by assisting respiration with a short positive and longer negative cycle respirator, and by elevating the head of the bed 15 to 20°. The intracellular response depends on breakdown of the blood-brain barrier, the metabolism of the cells, the osmolarity of the blood, and the availability of free water. Keeping the head-injured patient at normothermic or slightly hypothermic temperature (34 to 37°C) decreases metabolism and protects cells that may have regionally poor perfusion.

Removal of fluid in the hydrated or overhydrated patient with solute diuretics such as mannitol or urea, plus limitation of fluid intake to insensible water loss and urinary output, are helpful for the control of intracellular edema. The fluid intake to accomplish this usually is 1,800 to 2,000 ml/24 hours and should include at least 150 mEq of sodium chloride. One-half normal saline solution and $2\frac{1}{2}$% glucose approximates these requirements for intravenous fluids. The inflammatory response may be decreased and the blood-brain barrier protected by the use of glucocorticosteroid compounds. Dexamethasone is commonly used in intravenous doses of 10 mg shortly after injury and 4 mg every 6 hours for the first 36 to 72 hours. The dose is later tapered at a rate dependent upon the course of the patient. Fluid restriction also helps control the volume of the cerebrospinal fluid compartment.

Lumbar puncture would appear to be of help, but since the possibility of a mass lesion (hemorrhage) always exists and since asymmetric contusion and swelling frequently exists in the head-injured patient, drainage of spinal fluid via the lumbar route is too dangerous. Such drainage may cause herniation of the temporal lobe into the incisura of the tentorium and compression of the upper brainstem or herniation of the cerebellum through the foramen magnum and compression of the lower brainstem.

Recent studies have shown that although posttraumatic edema of the brain can cause such raised intracranial pressure that cerebral perfusion ceases, it is rare, and that most cases of "malignant" posttraumatic edema after head trauma are caused by repetitive episodes of inadequate cerebral perfusion that relate to transient waves of intracranial pressure. These "plateau waves," first described by Lundberg and coworkers, have been shown to relate to dilatation and later constriction of the cerebrovascular resistant vessels. In the injured brain, such changes in cerebrovascular resistance cause changes in blood flow and blood volume, and since the brain has lost its compliance or ability to tolerate small changes in volume without major changes in pressure, these waves of pressure are seen if intraventricular recording of pressure is done. Since cerebral blood flow relates directly to systemic arterial pressure minus intracranial pressure and inversely to the cerebrovascular resistance $\left[CBF = \dfrac{K(SAP - ICP)}{VR} \right]$, during episodes of plateau waves, effective cerebral perfusion is impaired and repetitive inadequate perfusion of the brain occurs. With each occurrence, further damage to the blood-brain barrier, neurons, and glia occurs. When these episodes have caused enough damage or when there is vasomotor paralysis from injury, the increased intracranial pressure causes bradycardia and hypertension systemically or the Cushing effect, which then causes further increase in intracranial pressure from the effect of increased blood volume and pressure intracranially. As mentioned above, this is often a late sign and in the head-injured patient may be the initial sign of impending respiratory arrest and total loss of effective intracranial vascular perfusion.

Since it has been demonstrated that effective cerebral perfusion pressure requires that systemic arterial pressure be at least 50 mmHg greater than intracranial pressure, in the severely injured patient, direct measure of intracranial pressure by placing a catheter in the frontal horn of the lateral ventricle makes it possible, when systemic arterial pressure is also monitored, not only to recognize the presence of plateau waves and inadequate cerebral perfusion pressure but also to undertake treatment to control the pressure and thus avert these transient episodes. The measures described above to control respirations and thus levels of CO_2, the use of solute diuretics such as mannitol or urea, and, since there is a catheter in the ventricle, drainage of spinal fluid can markedly protect the brain against this secondary injury. Many neurosurgical services routinely monitor intracranial pressure in all patients in whom there is major impairment of levels of consciousness for more than 6 to 10 hours and in all patients whose function on the Glasgow Coma Scale is 6 or less. With these techniques, malignant cerebral edema following trauma is rare and protection of the brain against secondary injury from inadequate cerebral perfusion allows a better functional result, although the mortality rate of severely head-injured patients has not been significantly altered.

INTRACRANIAL HEMORRHAGE

Progressive neurologic deficit, the most common being progressive loss of consciousness, following head trauma should always be assumed to be due to intracranial hemorrhage until proved otherwise. The patterns of neurologic change vary with the type of hemorrhage, but all have as a major component the neurologic deficit of progressive loss of consciousness.

The most common intracranial hemorrhage following head trauma is subarachnoid hemorrhage. It has little surgical significance and usually causes signs of meningismus or stiff neck and headache. It may, in the young male, produce maniacal behavior. It has little significance surgically, because the blood is rapidly diluted by the cerebrospinal fluid and flows throughout the subarachnoid space, so that no significant localized mass effect occurs. It may have significance as a late complication of head injury, namely, progressive communicating hydrocephalus. This complication is rare, occurring weeks or months after injury, and presents as a progressive dementia with motor apraxia, usually most marked as a gait disturbance. The mechanism is thought to be obstruction of the arachnoid villi and/or basal cisterns so that the absorption of cerebrospinal fluid is altered. The treatment is the same as for infantile hydrocephalus with the construction of an artificial path for the absorption of cerebrospinal fluid. Most commonly this is done with a shunt from the lateral ventricle to the superior vena cava, using a Holter or Pudenz valve to prevent blood reflux and to stabilize the pressure in the ventricle at 50 to 70 mm of water.

Surgically significant intracranial hemorrhages are best classified by their anatomic positions, i.e., subdural hematoma, epidural hematoma, and intracerebral hematoma. While they are relatively rare, unrecognized and untreated posttraumatic intracranial hematomas have almost a 100 percent mortality rate. Since most of this mortality can be averted by surgical treatment, early and accurate diagnosis is important.

SUBDURAL HEMATOMA

One of the most common types of posttraumatic intracranial hemorrhage is subdural hematoma. It is caused by either rupture of the veins traversing the subdural space from the brain to the dural sinuses or by a laceration of the brain that has torn the overlying piarachnoid. The symptoms may appear as early as within the first few minutes or as late as 6 to 8 weeks after injury. The pattern of symptoms, the findings, the treatment, and the prognosis vary with the rapidity of formation of the hematoma, so that it is logical to consider the syndrome of subdural hematoma as three different types: acute subdural, subacute subdural, and chronic subdural. Subdural hematomas plus epidural and intracerebral hematomas are the common surgically important intracranial hemorrhagic complications of trauma. Although each has a different symptom pattern, all have somewhere in their history the finding of decreased level of consciousness out of proportion to focal neurologic deficit. Portions of the basic patterns are usually present in all patients with subdural hematoma, but at times discovering them can tax the most astute clinician. The following descriptions are to be taken as outlines of patterns commonly presented by the patient with the different types of intracranial hematoma, but the reader should always keep in mind the protean signs and symptoms possible in a patient with intracranial hematoma.

Acute Subdural Hematoma

Acute subdural hematomas are defined as hematomas that cause significant progressive neurologic deficit within 48 hours of injury. They almost always occur following severe head trauma, and since they may have both arterial and venous sources for bleeding, the progression of the neurologic deficit can be rapid, often in terms of minutes or hours. The source of the arterial bleeding is frequently a laceration of the brain, and therefore focal neurologic deficit such as a hemiparesis is common.

Clinical Manifestations. When first seen the patient is usually unresponsive with a focal neurologic deficit. Progressive decrease in sensorium with or without progressive focal neurologic deficit is the warning of increasing intracranial mass. Without treatment the brainstem will be compressed by hemorrhage, edema, and herniation until death results. Death may occur within hours, with cessation of respiration, maintenance of pulse and blood pressure for a short time, and then peripheral vascular collapse as the medulla fails. Diagnosis is made by always considering the possibility of acute subdural hematoma in the severely head-injured patient who shows any deterioration in neurologic status. Aid in the diagnosis and in determining the side of major hemorrhage can be gained by the localization of any focal neurologic deficit, the presence of a lateral shift of a calcified pineal gland, and shift of the midline in the echo encephalogram. As mentioned above, computerized axial tomography is accurate in defining the position and size of recent intracranial hemorrhage and therefore, is the best method, if there is time, of diagnosing acute subdural hematomas. It also can define adjacent intracerebral hematomas, a common concomitant of acute subdural hematomas, making surgical approach to the hemorrhage more accurate and effective. More than half of acute subdural hematomas are bilateral, so that evaluation by either perforator openings or arteriograms of both subdural spaces is indicated.

Treatment. Treatment consists of removal of the hematoma through a large craniotomy with control of bleeding

areas, decompression by excision of large areas of the skull and relaxation of the compressing dura, and, when necessary, internal decompression by excision of portions of the frontal or temporal lobes. The methods for controlling edema and secondary injury from loss of effective cerebral perfusion pressure, as outlined in a preceding section, have decreased the necessity for excising large areas of the skull and, therefore, decreased both the problem of shift of the brain and the damage that can occur as an area of brain protrudes through a decompression site, as well as the later need for repair of surgical defect in the skull. Drainage of the hematoma through perforator openings is never satisfactory, since the major portion of the hematoma is solid clot and the problem is a combination of mass from clot and reaction of the brain to severe trauma. Without prompt surgical care mortality is 100 percent, and even with the best care it can be as high as 80 to 90 percent.

Subacute Subdural Hematoma

Subacute subdural hematomas are complications of head trauma that cause significant neurologic deficit more than 48 hours but less than 2 weeks after injury. They are usually caused by venous bleeding into the subdural space.

Clinical Manifestations. The basic pattern of symptoms and signs is a history of head trauma with unconsciousness, gradual improvement in the first few days followed by lack of improvement, fluctuation in levels of consciousness, and then decompensation with progressive loss of consciousness and often partial loss of hemispheric function. The patients are usually not as severely injured as are the patients with acute subdural hematomas. The phase of fluctuation in level of consciousness often heralds that significant shift of the intracranial contents has occurred, and the patient may change from relatively alert to difficult to arouse even with painful stimuli and back to his alert status within a few hours. Herniation of the medial temporal lobe through the incisura of the tentorium and compensation of the midbrain to the pressure of such herniation is a possible mechanism of such fluctuation in levels of consciousness. The presence of a third nerve paresis with dilatation of the pupil is often a warning that midbrain decompensation is imminent. The computerized scanner may not identify subacute subdural hematomas, since they can become isodense within the first 10 to 12 days after injury (i.e., the x-ray absorbed is approximately the same as brain). If the hematoma is unilateral or asymmetrical, the shift of the ventricular system as seen on computerized scanning will suggest the location of the hematoma. If the clinical history and signs suggest subdural hematoma, the diagnosis is better made by multiple perforator openings or by angiography.

Treatment. Treatment is dependent upon how critical the patient's condition is, how much liquid clot there is, and whether significant temporal lobe herniation has occurred. The patient with solid clot, unresponsive from uncal herniation, requires craniotomy, removal of the clot, and elevation of the temporal lobe herniation with or without incision of the tentorial edge. In the less critically ill patient and in the patient with considerable liquefaction of the hematoma the removal of a major portion of the clot through a small craniectomy and multiple perforator openings followed by external drainage of the subdural space may be all that is required. As with acute subdural hematomas, these hematomas are commonly bilateral, and exploration of both subdural spaces is always indicated unless bilateral angiograms have ruled out the presence of bilateral hematomas.

Chronic Subdural Hematoma

Although the initial cause of the chronic subdural hematoma is usually rupture by head trauma of one of the veins traversing the subdural space, the symptoms are caused by the increasing mass effect of the hematoma surrounded by a semipermeable membrane. Within 7 to 10 days after bleeding has occurred in the subdural space the blood is surrounded by a fibrous membrane. As the blood cells within the membrane break down, fluid is osmotically pulled into the hematoma, causing an increase in its volume. This may cause further bleeding from tears in the membrane or by rupturing other traversing veins with the reestablishment of the same process and an increasing size of the semiliquid-filled membrane.

Clinical Manifestations. Chronic subdural hematomas may occur at any age but are most frequent in the infant or the elderly. The causative trauma, particularly in the elderly, may be so slight that the patient does not remember it and gives no history of trauma. The symptoms and signs are best classified as a progressive alteration in mentation and level of consciousness of 4 to 6 weeks' duration out of proportion to the focal neurologic deficit. Therefore, any patient presenting with a progressive change in mental faculties and fluctuation or decreasing level of consciousness should be considered a subdural hematoma suspect.

Treatment. Since the hematoma is liquid, drainage through perforator openings is usually all that is required. In the past many neurosurgeons have felt that removal of the membranes is required, since they may be quite thick. However, experience has shown that there is increased mortality and morbidity from craniotomy removal of membranes and no improvement in the long-term results over those achieved by simple drainage of chronic subdural hematomas.

Subdural Hygroma

Although subdural hygromas are not a part of intracranial hemorrhage, they can produce similar symptoms. Subdural hygroma is usually caused by a tear in the piarachnoid that acts as a one-way valve with leakage of cerebrospinal fluid into the subdural space. The hygroma can increase in size quite rapidly and therefore can mimic an acute or subacute subdural hematoma. Perforator openings of the skull with external drainage is the treatment of choice, but at times formation of an artificial fistula between the subarachnoid space and the subdural space must be made in order to control continued formation of the hygroma.

EPIDURAL HEMATOMA

Epidural hematomas may be caused by either venous or arterial bleeding. They lie between the skull and the dura. The most common cause is venous bleeding, but the surgically important epidural hematomas most frequently are formed by arterial bleeding. Occasionally the patient with a skull fracture may have a significant venous epidural, the removal of which allows decrease in intracranial pressure or release of focal compression of the brain, but generally venous epidural hematomas are limited by the firm adherence of the dura to the inner surface of the skull. The central point of the venous epidural is almost always at the site of a fracture.

The epidural hematoma from arterial bleeding commonly occurs from rupture of the middle meningeal artery. This may be caused by a fracture of the temporal bone where the artery is in close proximity to the bone or by a tear of the middle meningeal artery when a blow causes angular acceleration of the head or sudden decrease or increase in any diameter of the skull. The tear may occur at the foramen spinosum, where the artery enters the skull, or anywhere along its branches.

CLINICAL MANIFESTATIONS. The basic historical pattern of the epidural hematoma is a young adult who has received a relatively minor blow causing momentary alteration in consciousness, followed by a lucid interval extending from a few minutes to a few hours. This interval terminates by rapid progressive loss of consciousness, dilatation of the pupil on the side of the epidural hematoma, evidence of compression of the upper midbrain, either by the production of a hemiparesis or decerebrate rigidity, and then evidence of compromise of the entire brainstem and death. The frequency of the hematoma being over the temporal area, the direct pressure onto the temporal lobe and therefore the maximal chance of herniation of the medial temporal lobe through the incisura, plus the arterial pressure as a source of bleeding are the main reasons for the rapidity with which the entire syndrome can be completed.

TREATMENT. Treatment consists of early recognition, a temporal craniectomy, evacuation of the hemorrhage, and control of the bleeding artery either at the foramen spinosum or at the point of tear in the dura. The mortality from epidural hematoma remains approximately 50 percent, partly because of the difficulty in recognizing the syndrome and partly because even upon recognition rapid control of the hemorrhage is necessary to avert a fatal outcome.

INTRACEREBRAL HEMATOMA

Posttraumatic intracerebral hematomas are most often seen in patients with severe head trauma, often mimic the symptom patterns of an acute or subacute subdural hematoma, and frequently are found in conjunction with them. In some series of posttraumatic intracranial hemorrhage intracerebral hematomas are as frequent as subdural hematomas, especially if the series includes many patients injured in high-speed vehicle accidents. The hematoma usually presents either beneath a cortical laceration or as a confluence of small hemorrhages in a contused area of the brain. Intracerebral hematomas are most commonly found in the anterior third of the temporal lobe where the temporal lobe may strike the sphenoid bone, and less frequently in the tips of the frontal or occipital lobes. They can be seen in any area of the cerebrum. The symptoms of clinically significant posttraumatic intracerebral hematomas are similar to the symptoms of an acute or subacute subdural hematoma. There are many intracerebral hematomas that do not alter the clinical course of a patient, are not diagnosed, and resolve by liquefaction, phagocytosis, and gliosis. The surgically significant intracerebral hematomas present with progressive decrease in consciousness and/or progressive focal neurologic deficit. Most frequently, focal deficits are third nerve palsy and hemiparesis. These symptoms may develop within a few hours or a few days of the injury. An important concept is the fact that these hematomas can cause significant neurologic deficit and, therefore, may explain progressive neurologic deficits in the head-injured patient in whom exploratory trephines have failed to reveal subdural hematoma. As with acute subdural hematomas, computerized axial tomography accurately diagnoses, localizes, and determines the extent of intracerebral hematomas. If a scanner is not available, arteriography is usually the best method to localize the hematoma, and ventriculography the next best. Occasionally an intracerebral hematoma is an incidental finding in surgery for acute subdural hematoma or is diagnosed by exploring the areas where occurrence is anticipated.

TREATMENT. The only effective treatment of surgically significant posttraumatic intracerebral hematomas is craniotomy or craniectomy with incision of the hemisphere at the most superficial area of the hematoma and evacuation of the clot. Simple aspiration of the lesion is not adequate since the majority of the hemorrhage is usually solid clot. The evacuation often must include excision of part of the lobe involved in order to remove devitalized brain and to obtain effective decompression of the injured cerebrum.

REHABILITATION. Rehabilitation of the head-injured patient starts with his initial care and finishes when his function is stabilized at its highest possible level. The rehabilitation of the brain-injured patient is a specialty in itself, but fortunately few patients require retraining or reconstructive surgical procedures to overcome their neurologic deficits. A majority of head-injured patients require only the support and care of a knowledgeable physician. Special problems of the head-injured patient during convalescence fall within three categories: psychologic problems, convulsions, and problems with cerebrospinal fluid circulation.

Psychologic Problems. Changes in personality and mood during the period of convalescence are one of the most common and often one of the most difficult symptoms for both patient and physician. The symptoms usually fall into the broad psychiatric category of a reactive depression with an overlay of anxiety. Complaints of headache, fatigue, loss of memory, excessive difficulty with performing tasks, transient despondency, and overreaction to emotional stimuli demonstrate a mixture of possible organic and psychologic bases for the symptoms. On the organic side is the suggestion of temporal and frontal lobe malfunction, while on the psychologic side is the reaction to physical and mental fatigue with a superimposed anxiety from the fear that the change may be permanent.

Gradually increasing physical activity in a planned fashion with limited goals that can be reached in reasonable periods of time and a planned return to increasingly difficult mental tasks is usually the best method for overcoming the problem. The settlement of any pending litigation is important when psychologic problems become paramount, for unnecessary delay can make a psychologic cripple of the patient. The physician should not abandon these patients or allow them to become dependent but rather insist that they get psychiatric help when necessary and that they work toward any physical and mental goals that seem possible. The best method of giving such support is for the physician to see the patient at planned intervals and during the visits to evaluate the neurologic progress of the patient to be certain that a portion of the problem is not coming from seizures or altered cerebrospinal fluid circulation.

Convulsions. Approximately 30 to 45 percent of patients with a compound injury that involves a laceration of the brain will have seizures if they are not on anticonvulsive medication. In contrast, the incidence of convulsions in the closed-head-injury patient is much lower. It is difficult to obtain any significant figures on the incidence of convulsion in the closed-head-injury patient, for in large series it varies from 0.5 percent to as high as 10 percent. In general it is safe to assume that a patient who has had less than 4 hours of either markedly altered consciousness or focal neurologic deficit will have no significant chance of convulsions' developing late in the convalescence that relate to the head injury. In the group with more serious head injuries there remains a small but persistent percentage in whom convulsions will develop that appear to relate to the head injury. The period in which convulsions may develop extends over many years. It is often difficult to recognize that focal or partial seizures are occurring, but they always should be considered when any paroxysmal symptoms occur, that is, symptoms of relatively brief duration that end with excessive fatigue. Electroencephalograms may be of help in diagnosing the cause of such symptoms as seizures, but at times trials of anticonvulsants are necessary to rule them out. Control of posttraumatic seizures with Dilantin and phenobarbital is usually sufficient, but occasionally resection of the damaged area is necessary for control with anticonvulsant drugs.

Problems of Cerebrospinal Fluid. Alteration in cerebrospinal fluid circulation is probably common in the early convalescence after head injury and may account for some of the complaints of headache, postural vertigo, and feelings of lightheadedness. These symptoms usually require no therapy other than the passage of time. Occasionally mild elevation of cerebrospinal fluid pressure continues and requires investigation by arteriography or air study. If no mass lesion is found to explain the increased pressure, intermittent lumbar spinal drainage over a few days will often control this. Prolonged elevation of cerebrospinal fluid pressure with enlargement of ventricles is a rare but serious complication. Its cause is probably obstruction of the arachnoid villi or basal cisterns by blood. It usually presents weeks or months after the injury with a gradual dementia and motor apraxia or loss of complex coordinated motor movements. The treatment is to shunt the cerebrospinal fluid from the lateral ventricles to the superior vena cava via a Holter or Pudenz valve to maintain the cerebrospinal pressure at 50 to 70 mm of water.

In general, with patience, support, and guidance the head-injured patient will recover and return to useful existence. This may take many months and requires that both the physician and the patient not become discouraged. The degree of recovery of even the very seriously injured patients will justify for the physician the amount of effort and time that he must give to this group of patients.

SPINAL CORD INJURIES

In the treatment of spinal cord injuries the prime objectives are the preservation of neural function and, when possible, restoration of neural function, followed by the reestablishment of the integrity of the vertebral column and the rehabilitation of the patient.

MECHANISMS OF INJURY. In contrast to skull injuries, in which fracture and brain damage may have an inverse relationship, bony vertebral damage and spinal cord injury have a high correlation, for the bony vertebrae and their attached soft tissue are usually the agents directly causing the spinal cord injury. The construction of the vertebral column with its circumferential bony ring provides ideal protection for low-velocity penetrating injuries or concussive blows, but the intervertebral articulations are weak points for flexion, extension, or rotary stresses. Dislocation and fractures that do not break the vertebral ring allow the vertebrae above and below the area of injury to act as a fulcrum for another vertebra and its attached soft tissue to concuss, stretch, contuse, or disrupt the spinal cord. The rarer fracture-dislocation that separates the posterior arch from the vertebral body demonstrates how much dislocation of the body can occur without permanent spinal cord damage and suggests methods of protecting the damaged cord, namely, laminectomy or removal of the posterior segments of the vertebrae. The stress of flexion, extension, and rotation and the relative weakness of the articulations of the vertebrae operate to make fractures and dislocations most common at points of junction between mobile and relatively fixed segments of the spinal column. These are the lower cervical region (Fig. 42-3) and the upper lumbar region related to the thoracic spine, that is relatively fixed by the ribs.

Most of the spinal cord damage occurs at the time of injury. However, recent studies of experimental spinal cord trauma in animals suggest a progressive hemorrhagic destruction of the central gray matter followed by edema in the white matter. Progressive damage to the white matter may occur during the first 4 to 6 hours after injury and plays a role in eventual spinal cord dysfunction. The mechanism of the pathophysiology is not clear, but in the experimental animal cooling of the injured segment, steroids, and myelotomy have protective value and alter this progressive posttraumatic process. This suggests possible therapeutic approaches to the problem of spinal cord injury, and clinical studies are in progress. Secondary spinal cord damage can occur from further movement of the unstable vertebral column, the movement of the spinal cord against sharp fragments of bone in the canal, and continued compression of the spinal cord. Therapy to prevent any secondary damage to the spinal cord requires stabilization of the vertebral column, removal of any foreign body or fragments of bone from the spinal canal, and decompression of the spinal cord when necessary.

REDUCTION AND STABILIZATION OF VERTEBRAL COLUMN. In the cervical region stabilization of the vertebral column is most effectively obtained by skeletal traction, using skull tongs (Barton, Vinke, or Crutchfield tongs). Stabilization is achieved by anatomic reduction and by tension of the spinal ligaments and soft tissue of the cervical region. Slight extension of the neck will give tension to the anterior spinal ligament, the strongest of the spinal ligaments, and therefore is preferred unless there is evi-

Fig. 42-3. Fracture-dislocation with anterior displacement of C_5 on C_6 and unilateral locking of the left facets in a twenty-year-old man who, following a fall from a horse, presented with signs of weakness and sensory loss in his arms and legs. Radicular (local) signs were weakness of the muscles innervated by the C_6 root, i.e., biceps and brachioradialis muscles. Tract signs were weakness of both lower extremities, the left more than the right, with bilateral plantar extensor responses. Following reduction his neurologic recovery was complete except for residual weakness of the left biceps.

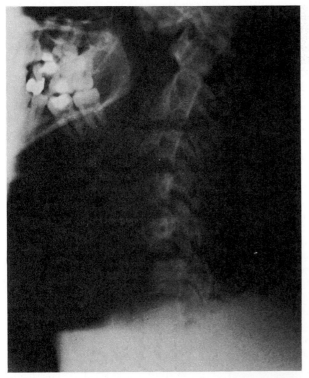

dence of rupture of the ligament. This is usually apparent from an x-ray that shows avulsion of the anterior lip of a vertebral body, the site of insertion of the ligament. Stabilization is promoted by placing the patient on a firm surface. A Stryker or Foster frame bed makes an excellent support, since the patient can be turned from the prone to supine position without changing the relative position of the spinal column.

Reduction of fracture-dislocations of the thoracic or lumbar spine should not be done unless the spinal cord or cauda equina is exposed by laminectomy before the reduction, since the force necessary for such closed reduction carries too high a risk of further damage to the spinal cord or cauda equina. Simple compression fractures of the body of the vertebra, with flexion angulation of the spine but without spinal cord deficit, may be gently extended by positioning in a Foster frame, utilizing extension to stretch the anterior spinal ligament and expand the vertebral body. A foreign body or bone fragment in the canal is a contraindication for any manipulative maneuver, since it may act as a disrupting agent during such maneuvers. The presence of foreign bodies adjacent to or in the spinal cord also allows possible continuing damage from any body movement or from the natural movements of the spinal cord with respirations and pulse. If any continuity of spinal cord function remains across such an area, laminectomy and removal of the fragments is indicated.

DECOMPRESSION OF SPINAL CORD. The most difficult judgment in the early care of spinal cord injury is the decision to decompress the spinal cord. Some surgeons have solved this problem by always doing a laminectomy in any severe spinal cord injury, while others are firmly convinced that it is of value in only the rare case with later progression of neurologic deficit. The first group base their judgment on the concept that there is always edema and swelling of the spinal cord and surrounding tissue and therefore laminectomy with decompression is always of some potential value. Complications of such therapy have to be considered, and in unskilled hands they may be considerable. An argument used by the latter group is that severe injury of the spinal cord rarely can be reversed, since neuronal loss is complete within a short time of the injury and the life of the patient is placed in jeopardy by surgical therapy with little chance of helping spinal cord function.

Experimental evidence in animals demonstrates that the tracts of the spinal cord can tolerate many hours of anoxic compression and recover, even though the neurons within the anoxic area cannot. Since the total functional result is mainly dependent upon the tracts traversing the segment, preservation of viability in these tracts is worthwhile. Evidence that there is compression consists of any progression in neurologic deficit, or a block of cerebrospinal fluid circulation. The Queckenstedt test consists of a measurement of lumbar cerebrospinal fluid pressure before and after compression of the jugular veins of the neck by a blood pressure cuff. If rapid rise and fall in the lumbar pressure does not occur with the compression and release of the neck veins, the test shows evidence of a block in the cerebrospinal fluid circulation between the foramen mag-

num and the lumbar puncture needle. The Queckenstedt test is both inaccurate and dangerous, since an opening at the site of compression just larger than a spinal needle may give a negative test (no evidence of block) despite considerable compression, and increasing cerebrospinal fluid pressure above a block of the spinal canal can cause further spinal cord damage. For these reasons, when a compressive block is suspected, contrast myelography with air or Pantopaque, usually placed in the spinal canal through a lateral C_1-C_2 spinal puncture, is indicated. With such evidence of block in cerebrospinal fluid circulation, laminectomy with opening of the dura is indicated unless rapid improvement in neurologic function is occurring. With trained neurosurgeons the morbidity and mortality of the procedure is far below the risk of allowing progressive spinal cord damage from further compression of the cord.

COMPOUND INJURIES. Trauma to the spinal cord may also result in open or compound injuries. The principles for the care of both closed and open injuries are not substantially different except that compound injuries require debridement and closure of the wound and they rarely have vertebral instability. Compound wounds of the spinal cord may occur from sharp penetrating objects but are most commonly from gunshot wounds. The concussive force of the bullet causes widespread damage and therefore more widespread reactive edema. If there is any possibility of cord continuity, early exploration, wide decompression, and removal of devitalized tissues both within and around the spinal cord are indicated in order to give the patient any significant chance of recovery. Without such surgical measures secondary compressive anoxia of the tracts is certain to occur.

BONY UNION. Reestablishment of vertebral integrity requires time for bony union. If instability is marked, fusion is usually indicated. Marked instability occurs when the articulating facets and ligaments are disrupted or when there is some combination of injury to the vertebral body, pedicles, and facets. If open fusion is indicated, it is best to allow 2 to 3 weeks for reaction of injury within the cord to subside before performing a spinal fusion, since further reaction within the surrounding tissue occurs with such a procedure. Total immobilization of at least 6 weeks is indicated in most cervical injuries, with 6 to 8 weeks of support following this to ensure firm union. In other areas of the spinal column where weight-bearing stresses are greater, the time for sufficient union varies with the area and the type of bony injury but in general is longer than in the cervical area.

REHABILITATION. Rehabilitation of the patient with a spinal cord injury is a specialty by itself. The early care of the skin and bladder, however, can be as important for the time required for rehabilitation as any factor other than neurologic deficit. Following cord injury, spinal shock of varying degree occurs, and protective skin and bladder reflexes are lost. Support of the body is necessary so that the pressure points, such as the sacrum and the heels, take as little weight as possible. A dry smooth covering against any weight-bearing skin, good nutrition, cleanliness, and, most important, turning the patient at least every 2 hours are the necessary nursing measures to protect the skin of the cord-injured patient. Initial constant catheter drainage of the bladder should be followed by intermittent catheter drainage plus high fluid intake to protect the urinary tract from distension and infection.

Illustrative Case

Perhaps the easiest way to summarize the acute neurosurgical care of the cord-injured patient is to review the care of a patient who, immediately following an automobile accident, entered the hospital with weakness and sensory loss from the arms down. Initial examination revealed normal movement of the deltoid and biceps muscles, weakness of both triceps muscles, and only slight movement of the fingers, legs, and toes. Sensory examination showed preservation of deep pain and some touch sensation in both lower extremities but marked hypesthesia and hypalgesia from the ulnar side of the hands and arms caudad bilaterally. There were absent deep tendon and superficial reflexes except for the biceps reflexes. X-rays of the cervical spine were reported as negative.

The history and the examination indicated a C_6-C_7 or C_7-T_1 vertebral column injury, and with this knowledge the x-rays were found to be not negative but inadequate, since they showed only the upper portion of C_6 and more cephalad vertebrae. Further x-rays showed a fracture dislocation with the C_6 vertebra anteriorly displaced on the C_7 vertebra. The patient was placed on a Stryker frame; the bladder was catheterized and connected to constant drainage. Barton tongs were applied to the skull, slightly anterior to the coronal plane traversing the mastoid tips, and 15 lb of weight was applied. Neurologic examination showed no change in function. X-rays showed no evidence of reduction. Five more pounds of weight was applied. Neurologic examination remained unchanged, and x-rays showed slight reduction of the dislocation. Five more pounds, or a total of twenty-five pounds, was applied, and neurologic examination remained unchanged, but x-rays showed reduction of the dislocation. Because of the lack of improvement, a myelogram was done and showed posterior and anterior compression of the spinal cord at approximately the C_6 level. The patient was taken to the operating room for laminectomy, and at operation the laminae and facets of C_6 and C_7 were found to be fractured. The laminae and spinous processes of C_5, C_6, and C_7 were removed, and the dura was opened. The spinal cord appeared posteriorly displaced and swollen. Because closure of the dura appeared to cause constriction of the spinal cord, a fascial graft was placed for dural relaxation, and the dura, muscles, fascia, and skin were sutured with interrupted silk sutures.

The patient showed gradual improvement for approximately 1 week, at which time over a 2-day period the strength of his finger flexors gradually decreased. The Pantopaque that had been left in the canal at the previous myelogram was repositioned into the cervical canal under fluoroscopy, and an anterior filling defect was demonstrated at the C_6-C_7 interspace. The patient was returned to the operating room, and the C_6-C_7 interspace was approached anteriorly. The interspace was exposed and the remains of damaged nucleus pulposus were removed along with the cartilaginous end plates. A fragment of nucleus pulposus was found free in the anterior part of the spinal canal and removed. A piece of bone taken from the ileum was wedged into the hole for stability and future bony fusion. The patient made a gradual recovery over the next 6 months.

The points illustrated are the same as those discussed in the initial portion of this section. It is important that the area of damage be identified from the neurologic examination, so that the examiner is certain that x-rays of the spinal column include the area. When any manipulation is done, both the x-rays and the neurologic function should be checked. If despite reduction there remains evidence of cerebrospinal fluid circulation obstruction and there is no sign of neurologic improvement, decompressive laminectomy is indicated at that time, and the decompression should be complete, so that not even the dura binds the spinal cord. In the case reviewed above, even though there was a question of something displacing the spinal cord when it was seen at laminectomy, it was felt that further manipulation of the cord in order to expose the anterior surface was not indicated, since the spinal cord had already sustained significant trauma. The signs of progressive neurologic deficit even in the late postoperative period indicated either further compression of the spinal cord or instability of the vertebral column despite the traction. When a myelogram demonstrated a filling defect in the anterior portion of the spinal canal, both problems were definitively treated by ventral exposure of the damaged intervertebral space, removal of the free fragment of nucleus pulposus, and placement of an interbody bone graft to allow fusion.

PERIPHERAL NERVE INJURIES

The common types of peripheral nerve injuries are laceration, contusion, and stretch or compression, with or without disruption. The agents causing such injuries are numerous but from a therapeutic view can be divided into those causing a focal injury, such as a knife or a piece of glass; those causing relatively localized injury but imparting force to adjacent areas, such as a gunshot wound; and those causing damage to long segments of the nerve, as with stretch following a dislocation of extremity or compression from swelling under a rigid cast or dressing. Evaluation of nerve injuries includes accurate knowledge of the anatomy and function of the nerve suspected of injury, identification of the agent causing the injury, and recognition of the type of injury resulting. Treatment is based on the evaluation as well as knowledge of the factors influencing the comparative prognosis of the different forms of therapy available and the skill of the surgeon, not only to repair the nerve involved and the adjacent tissues, but also to utilize all reconstructive measures available.

EVALUATION. The evaluation of peripheral nerve injuries is in part similar to the evaluation of central nervous system injuries, for comparison of serial observations and recognition of progressive neurologic deficit or improvement often determine the type of therapy required. The treatment differs from that for central nervous system injuries in that regeneration and reinnervation can occur and therefore the treatment of peripheral nerve injury includes neurorrhaphy, or the surgical repair of the nerve. Since comparison of later examinations with the initial one is important in therapy, it is essential to have an accurate examination that includes the sensory and motor function of all nerves thought to be injured. Peripheral nerve injuries often occur as part of more extensive injuries, and since an accurate examination can be done only on a cooperative patient, all patients suspected of nerve injury should be reexamined when well enough to cooperate.

Accurate knowledge of the anatomy and function of the nerve suspected of injury is a minimal requirement for a competent examination and evaluation. Nerve injuries are a relatively rare experience for the average physician; since the accuracy of even an experienced neurosurgeon can be enhanced by reviewing the anatomy and functions of nerves suspected of injury, the physician making the initial examination or treating the patient at any time should not hesitate to consult an anatomy book and review the anatomic relations and the motor and sensory function of the nerves involved. With this help accurate localization and accurate definition of the neurologic deficit can usually be made.

TREATMENT. The problem after diagnosis is what to do and when to do it. There are only a few alternatives for treatment of peripheral nerve injury: suture of the nerve, resection of damaged areas and resuture, or no treatment of the nerve but reestablishment of function of the part by utilizing other muscles and internal or external support.

A few axioms should be kept in mind. Complete functional loss in a nerve can occur without anatomic disruption, and functional return can occur within 60 to 90 days. This segmental loss of conduction in the nerve following trauma is caused by alteration in the ability of the axons to reestablish their membrane potential and is called *neuronapraxis*. The mechanism of recovery is not known, but the nerve recovers its function in all segments distal to the injury at approximately the same time, and therefore the recovery cannot be secondary to regrowth of the axons.

Although immediate repair gives the best functional results, little is lost by a delay of 3 to 5 weeks. After disruption and reapproximation of a nerve the axons require about 3 weeks to grow across the suture line and then grow at about 2 cm/month. In general, counting the delay across the suture line and the time for reinnervation of the muscle end plates or peripheral end organs, an estimated functional growth of 1 in./month is usually accurate. Following denervation, muscle end plates atrophy and muscle fibers progressively degenerate, so that within 20 to 24 months no significant muscle contraction can be expected from reinnervation. While muscle tone reappears and some movement will occur up to that time, significant strength in a muscle rarely can be regained past 15 months. Since functional nerve regeneration proceeds at approximately 1 in./month, a nerve suture that is more than 15 in. from the denervated muscle cannot be expected

to give significant motor return, and tendon transplants, joint fixation, or bracing should be considered as the treatment for the motor loss. Tone in facial muscles will return up to 24 months past denervation, but as the end of the 24-month period approaches, no movement of expression can be expected.

All nerve injuries are painful, and the pain will continue with varying intensity for many months. Narcotics have no place in the treatment of chronic pain and therefore should not be used after the immediate wound pain has ceased. Functional use of the extremity is the best therapy for the pain and is an important reason for using passive and active motion and functional bracing as soon as possible. It is also a major reason for not waiting for an improbable result, such as reinnervation of a muscle too distant from the point of suture, before using other reconstructive methods.

In contrast to the time limits on return of motor function, sensory function of a significant degree can return whenever reinnervation of the part occurs and often is of help in relieving the discomfort as well as in providing protection of an extremity. This is especially true of the protection offered by sensory reinnervation of the foot.

In general, nerve grafts have not been successful as a method of bridging areas of nerve loss in order to restore function. The delay in crossing two suture lines, the loss and mixing of fibers at each suture line, and the associated tissue damage that usually occurs when grafts have been required have been suggested as the main reasons for functional failures. In almost all nerves, gaps of 8 to 10 cm can be bridged by proximal and distal dissection to release the nerve from surrounding tissue and by positioning of the nerve or the extremity to minimize the distance across joints. This may require wide dissection and positioning of more than one joint of the extremity. When neurorrhaphy is planned, skin preparation and draping should allow for such maneuvers. The problems with these maneuvers are that they may not allow closure of the ends of the nerve without tension, or may, after initial healing of the neurorrhaphy, allow tension and interference with blood supply of the regenerating nerve as the joints are extended. A recent microsurgical technique of perineural suture, i.e., approximation of the perifascicular tissue of the nerve rather than closure of the epineural tissue, suggests improved distal growth both in number and rate of regenerating axons. The technique allows no tension at the site of closure, since very fine suture and low-tensile-strength tissue are used in the approximation. Interfascicular grafts, composed of homologous nerve, usually the sural nerve of the patient, interposed in a defect and sutured by these techniques, are reported to give better results than end-to-end epineural neurorrhaphy under tension. These grafts, by averting the mixture of interfascicular fibers and altered blood supply of a nerve under tension, appear to be an advance in nerve repair and have improved the expected results from some neurorrhaphies that had been done under tension and from some nerve grafts that had been required because of a long area of deficit. Interfascicular (perineural) neurorrhaphy allows better approximation and has reactivated interest in homologous nerve grafts.

EVALUATION OF FUNCTIONAL RECOVERY. In the evaluation of the injured nerve, evidence for functional recovery of the nerve is important, for it determines the success or failure of the therapy. Evidence that the nerve functions is not the same as functional recovery, for nerve function means only that some portion of the nerve has anatomic continuity. Definite evidence of functional recovery consists of:

1. Voluntary motor function of a muscle innervated by the nerve distal to the injury. This means that a major number of the motor fibers have reinnervated the muscle and that with time increase in strength will occur, either through increased strength of the individual reinnervated muscle fibers or by further innervation.
2. Muscle contraction on electrical stimulation of the nerve distal to the point of injury when performed more than 7 days after injury. Since the distal segment of a divided nerve will conduct impulses for only 5 to 6 days, evidence of ability to conduct later than 7 days after injury indicates functional continuity or regeneration. Muscle contraction following the stimulation means a major portion of the motor fibers are conducting. Direct electrical stimulation of the muscle does not give evidence of functional recovery, since contraction with this type of stimulation will occur until atrophy of the muscle is complete.
3. Recovery of sensation in an autogenous area of innervation. There are few such areas for individual nerves. The distal phalanx of the index finger for the median nerve and the distal phalanx of the little finger for the ulnar nerve are the only two in the upper extremity. The distal phalanges of the middle three toes of the foot are autogenous for the sciatic nerve but only if both peroneal and tibial divisions are involved.

Evidence of anatomic continuity but not of prognostic significance for functional recovery consists of:

1. Tinel's sign distal to the site of injury. Tinel's sign is elicited by percussing the nerve and obtaining paresthesias referred to the superficial area of skin innervation. It requires activation of only a small percentage of the fibers, far less than is required for functional recovery.
2. Alteration in electromyographic activity with attempted voluntary motion or nerve stimulation. As with Tinel's sign, the activation of far fewer fibers than is necessary for functional return of a muscle is required to elicit alteration in the recorded electromyographic activity.

Evidence that indicates neither anatomic nor functional continuity of an injured nerve consists of:

1. Shrinkage of the area of sensory loss. The marked overlap of sensory innervation in all areas of the body has been alluded to with the description of the very few autogenous zones of peripheral nerve innervation. Decrease in an area of sensory loss after nerve injury can occur from recovery of the nerve function, but even without reinnervation adjacent nerves reestablish sensation in the area. The mechanism appears to be both utilization of fibers which function with the damaged nerve but which without the spatial summation of the damaged nerve activity do not reach consciousness, and branching of the superficial nerve fibers of the remaining nerves with growth into the denervated area.
2. Improved use of the extremity. The adaptability of the child to use any remaining function to accomplish coordinated tasks is a major example, but use of gravity, momentum, and muscles with remaining function to simulate the lost function must not be confused with reinnervation.

Illustrative Cases

The application of these concepts is most easily understood in relation to examples of the three major groups of peripheral nerve injury, laceration, or focal sharp injury, focal contusion, and compression or stretch injury.

Focal Laceration. An example of focal sharp injury is a knife wound of the upper extremity at approximately the midhumeral level, resulting in loss of median nerve function. Motor loss would consist of paralysis of all flexors of the wrist and fingers except the flexor carpi ulnaris and the ulnar portion of the flexor digitorum profundus. These latter two muscles would give wrist flexion with ulnar deviation and flexion of the ring and little fingers. Sensory loss would consist of loss of superficial sensation of the palmar surface of the hand extending to the thumb and first two fingers and the radial half of the ring finger. Deep as well as superficial sensation would be lost in the distal phalanx of the index finger.

Immediate repair is indicated *except* when any of the following apply: (1) The nerve appears contused for more than a few millimeters on either side of the injury. (2) There is blood loss from arterial injury that would jeopardize the life of the patient in undergoing a long (2- to 3-hour) operation for repair of the artery and nerve. (3) The wound is older than 5 to 6 hours, and dissection might spread contamination. (4) The surgeon is not certain of his ability to perform adequate neurorrhaphy.

If inadequate repair is done so that regeneration does not occur (no matter what the reason), it will take approximately 6 months, or the time it takes the nerve to grow 6 in. to the flexor muscles of the forearm, before the inadequacy of the repair is recognized. Since the opponens of the thumb is beyond the distance where significant strength can be expected to be regained, as soon as the flexor muscles of the forearm are reinnervated, tendon transplant of one of the flexors to strengthen the apposition of the thumb is indicated.

Focal Contusion. The most common focal contusion of nerve is that secondary to a gunshot wound, and the treatment of a gunshot wound of the midthigh resulting in loss of sciatic nerve function is an example of such an injury. Immediate repair of the nerve is not indicated, since the damage extending up and down the nerve cannot be determined by inspection and after a high-velocity-missile injury it is always present in varying degrees.

The wound is treated to prevent infection, and the patient is fitted with a short leg brace for stabilization of the ankle. Stabilization is necessary, since motor function in all flexors, extensors, evertors, and invertors of the foot, as well as in the intrinsic muscles of the foot, will be lost. The patient is ambulated with a brace as soon as possible and taught to inspect the skin of the foot three or four times a day in order to protect it from unrecognized injury in the anesthetic area. Four to five weeks later, if no function has returned or if only minimal function in one portion of the sciatic nerve has returned, exploration is indicated. By this time fibrosis or neuroma formation will define the area of injury. Resection and resuture may be indicated. Three weeks after repair, when the anastomosis is secure, active use of the leg with the same precautions that were observed preoperatively should be started. Fifteen months later the stability of the ankle should be evaluated, and internal stabilization or arthrodesis may be indicated because of failure of adequate reinnervation.

Stretch or Compression Injury. The problem of the nerve with stretch or compression injury is more difficult. The segment of injury is often longer than can be bridged by any technique, and the loss is usually incomplete, so that even if the area might be bridged by surgical technique, comparison of the deficit from the injury with what might be obtained by resection and suture is essential in the decision for treatment. A common area of stretch injury is the brachial plexus, as might be seen following a shoulder injury. Careful recording of all sensory and motor loss is necessary, and if the pattern of loss suggests a radicular pattern, that is, loss of root function such as at C_5 and C_6, myelography or the fluoroscopic study of the spinal arachnoid space with radiopaque substance is indicated. Rupture of the arachnoid root sleeve with formation of a traumatic meningocele or pouching of the arachnoid through the intervertebral foramen may be demonstrated, indicating avulsion of the roots from the cord. Root avulsions are not repairable, and reconstructive measures such as fusion of the shoulder and triceps transplantation for elbow flexion are indicated rather than surgical exploration of the area of injury.

The possibility of surgical repair of compression or stretch injury is slight, since the area of injury is so long, and 2 to 3 months of evaluation are indicated to determine that the loss is not due to neuronapraxis, with spontaneous recovery occurring. In the brachial plexus injury loss of motion in the forearm would not be significantly improved by resection and suture, and loss of intrinsic muscles in the hands is not an indication for surgical intervention, since return of function cannot be expected. The usual early treatment indicated is protection of the denervated muscles from overstretching by a supporting brace, while later functional bracing, fusion of joints, and transplantation of remaining functioning muscles are the appropriate means of gaining maximum possible function.

BRAIN TUMORS

Although uncommon in the experience of the average physician, brain tumors are not rare. As a clinical entity they are best brought into perspective by realizing that brain tumors constitute almost 10 percent of all benign and malignant tumors requiring hospitalization for surgical removal and that just under 1 percent of all deaths are caused by primary intracranial neoplasm. One reason that brain tumors seem to be uncommon in the experience of physicians is that they are not suspected as the cause of the patient's complaints, for the presenting symptoms are diverse and confusing, and their recognition can be difficult.

CLASSIFICATION AND CHARACTERISTICS. The classifications of brain tumors are at best confusing, partly because the naming of tumors has usually been on the basis of cellular characteristics. The difficulties of such classifications arise not only from the many different names that can be applied to the same tumor in different situations but also from the difficulty of describing the different characteristics of even the same cell type within a tumor. Clinically a useful classification of brain tumors is the one proposed by Kernohan and Sayre based on naming the tumors for the cells present in the adult nervous system, vascular tissue, and developmental defects, combined with a grading of the malignancy of the tumor from grade I to grade IV, with IV the most malignant (Table 42-3).

Certain types of tumors are more frequent at certain ages and occur with greater frequency in those ages in different areas of the brain. For example, 70 percent of adult tumors are supratentorial, that is, in the middle or anterior fossa, while 75 percent of childhood tumors occur in the posterior fossa. The most common primary tumor of the brain in the middle-aged and elderly is a grade III or grade IV astrocytoma (glioblastoma multiforme), while the most common tumor of childhood is the grade I and II astrocytoma of the cerebellum. Malignant astrocytomas are by far the most common primary brain tumor in adults, followed by meningiomas, pituitary tumors, and neurilemomas, while in childhood the most common tumors are the relatively benign astrocytomas of the posterior fossa, followed very closely by the highly malignant medulloblastomas, and then by ependymomas and craniopharyngiomas. Tumors of childhood occur characteristically near the midline of the brain, as with the tumors of developmental defects, the medulloblastomas, and the astrocytomas of the brainstem and cerebellum. Gliomas in adults occur at a frequency that is related to the volume of the brain itself and therefore are more common in the cerebral hemispheres. Meningiomas have a predilection for areas of arachnoid villi and arachnoid invaginations that contain cells similar to those seen in the meningioma. These areas of predilection are along the sagittal sinus, the sella, the olfactory groove, the tentorium, and the petrous ridges.

Table 42-3. BRAIN TUMORS

	Percent
Gliomas	40–50
Astrocytoma, grade I	5–10
Astrocytoma, grade II	2–5
Astrocytoma, grades III and IV	
(glioblastoma multiforme)	20–30
Medulloblastoma	3–5
Oligodendroglioma	1–4
Ependymoma, grades I–IV	1–3
Meningioma	12–20
Pituitary tumors	5–15
Neurolemmomas (mainly eighth nerve)	3–10
Metastatic tumors	5–10
Blood vessel tumors	
Arteriovenous malformations	
Hemangioblastomas	
Endotheliomas	0.5–1
Tumors of developmental defects	2–3
Dermoids, epidermoids, teratomas	
Chordomas, paraphyseal cysts	
Craniopharyngiomas	3–8
Pinealomas	0.5–0.8
Miscellaneous	
Sarcomas, papillomas of the choroid plexus, lipomas,	
unclassified, etc	1–3

PATHOPHYSIOLOGY. This difficulty is minimized if the physician has a concept of the basic pathophysiology of brain tumors. The basic pattern is one of progressive neurologic deficit. This deficit can be a progressive focal deficit or a progression in the neurologic dysfunction that occurs secondary to increased intracranial pressure. Since these clinical patterns are a continuum, the historical examination of the patient must include the factor of time and its relationship to the development of the symptoms and signs. Their development may vary within the basic patterns because of the different mechanisms by which tumors disturb normal function, the different positions the tumor may occupy within the skull, and the diverse growth potentials of the different tumor types. These variables, when combined with the concepts discussed in the opening portion of this chapter, namely, the anatomic confinement within compartments of the skull of a deformable but relatively noncompressible brain and the changes in neural function that occur from compression of the brainstem passing through the incisura of the tentorium and the foramen magnum, explain in part the diversity of the presenting symptoms produced by brain tumors. With so many combinations of variables possible, learning the symptoms for the different types of tumors in their different clinical stages is almost an endless task unless it is related to functional anatomy of the brain, the mechanisms used by tumors in producing signs and symptoms, and a classification of the tumors by frequency of occurrence and growth potential.

Tumors of the central nervous system manifest themselves most frequently by effects caused by one or more of the following mechanisms:

1. Compression of neural tissue, either direct or secondary to displacement of the brain
2. Infiltration or direct invasion with destruction of neural tissue
3. Alteration in the blood supply to neurons
4. Alteration in neuronal excitability
5. Increase in mass within the skull
6. Alteration in cerebrospinal fluid circulation

CLINICAL MANIFESTATIONS. Direct compression of neural tissue produces a progressive focal neurologic deficit which is the most easily recognized sign of brain tumor. The deficit will vary depending upon the area of the brain involved and is usually partial rather than complete. Thus, hemiparesis rather than hemiplegia is more frequently seen, and sensory loss is more commonly a partial rather than a total deficit.

Progressive focal neurologic deficit can be produced by other mechanisms, such as direct destruction of neural tissue by malignant cells and loss of neural function by alteration in local blood supply. Direct destruction of neural tissue by involvement of malignant cells is uncommon, but alteration in local blood supply does occur and particularly may be seen in the older patient with a highly malignant glioma. Interference with arterial blood supply by tumor usually manifests itself as an acute loss of function, suggesting primary vascular disease, and only the later focal progression from increasing mass effects, or further involvement of local blood supply, completes the pattern of progressive focal neurologic deficit, indicating the diagnosis of brain tumor.

Compression, invasion, and altered blood supply may also cause altered neuronal excitability which is manifested by convulsions. Convulsions are paroxysmal episodes of uncontrolled neural activity, and since the neurons of the cerebral cortex have the lowest threshold for such paroxysmal activity, seizures caused by tumors are most commonly seen in lesions adjacent to or within the cerebral cortex. A focal or a Jacksonian seizure and especially a postictal neurologic loss (Todd's paralysis) indicate the localization of the lesion, and progression in either frequency or severity of the seizures or in the postictal neurologic deficit is strongly suggestive of a brain tumor.

The signs and symptoms of generalized increase in pressure are cloudy mentation and consciousness, headache, papilledema, vomiting, bradycardia, and systolic hypertension. It is rare to have all these findings except as terminal events. Increased pressure can also produce abducens, or sixth cranial nerve palsy, which may have no localizing value, for the abducens nerve is particularly prone to loss of function secondary to increased intracranial pressure. Increased intracranial pressure from brain tumors can result from mass, impaired cerebrospinal fluid circulation, or a combination of these.

The increase in mass may result from a number of factors. There is the neoplastic growth itself and edema formation. Malignant tumors especially produce edema in the adjacent brain. The cause of this edema is not understood, but it can result in massive swelling at considerable distances from the tumor. Some tumors form cysts that have osmotic gradients that cause an enlargement of the cyst by absorption of fluid. Infrequently rapid enlargement may result from hemorrhage within a tumor. Changes may occur in the surrounding nervous tissue, such as edema from venous obstruction or edema from breakdown of the integrity of the blood-brain barrier, secondary to either arterial or venous insufficiency.

The increased intracranial pressure caused by alteration in cerebrospinal fluid circulation usually occurs from obstruction of the passage of cerebrospinal fluid from the lateral ventricles to the subarachnoid space. This can occur when tumors arise within the ventricular system. Obstruction in the flow of cerebrospinal fluid may also occur when there is a shift of the brainstem so that the aqueduct of Sylvius is compressed or the outlets of the fourth ventricle are blocked. Tumors in the basal cisterns may also obstruct cerebrospinal fluid flow.

There are compensatory intracranial mechanisms for altering the effects of increased mass and pressure. Most of them require days or months to be effective and therefore are best utilized in controlling pressure from a slowly growing, benign tumor. These mechanisms include decreases in intracranial blood volume, cerebrospinal fluid volume, intracellular fluid contents, and parenchymal cell numbers.

EVALUATION. The primary necessity in the diagnosis of brain tumor is the suspicion which should be initiated by the patient's history of a progressive neurologic deficit. The more knowledgeable the physician is of the functional anatomy of the brain, the more accurately he will recognize progressive neurologic deficit. While hemiparesis and hemisensory loss or lack of motor function in a cranial nerve are easily recognizable, slow progressive dementia, decrease in pituitary function, or progression in the severity of seizures are more difficult neurologic deficits to recognize as indicating brain tumor.

It is beyond the scope of this section to review the diagnostic investigation that should be completed in evaluating a patient suspected of having a brain tumor, but complete physical and neurologic examinations are the minimal requisites to the use of special diagnostic tests that have been described in the opening section of this chapter. The dangers of alteration in intracranial pressure by some of the studies, such as pneumoencephalography, and the dangers inherent in angiography must be weighed against the benefit of obtaining information needed for treatment, realizing that these special diagnostic studies such as brain scan, computerized axial tomography, echo encephalogram, air study, and arteriography have a high degree of accuracy and aid considerably in the final judgment as to what should be done with a brain tumor.

TREATMENT. The primary goal of tumor therapy is cure, and surgical excision is the method most likely to accomplish a cure. Unfortunately, in the case of brain tumor surgical removal is not always possible or even desirable, since the resulting neurologic deficit may leave the patient so impaired that saving his life is of no significance. The treatment of brain tumors therefore is not just their surgical removal, and it requires experience and knowledge combined with surgical skill in order to obtain the maximal functional result. At times the repetitive use of these special diagnostic tests and evaluation over a period of time are necessary to be certain of what would be the optimal therapy. As often as possible total removal is attempted, but when this is deemed impossible, palliation by partial removal of the tumor for internal decompression, relief of intracranial pressure by shunting of blocked spinal fluid, or treatment of the tumor by x-ray therapy and/or chemotherapy may control the tumor or give significant relief and allow the patient extended periods of normal existence. Combinations of these palliative and curative techniques allow a large percentage of patients to obtain significant relief of symptoms or cure of the brain tumor.

SUMMATION. In summary, it is the evidence of a progressive neurologic deficit that should raise the suspicion of diagnosis of a brain tumor, for progressive neurologic deficit is the most common presenting symptom of brain tumor. This deficit may be of a focal nature which varies according to the area of the brain involved or may be a more generalized type secondary to increased intracranial pressure. The focal neurologic deficit may be a loss of function or can be altered excitability. Loss of neural function secondary to brain tumor is most frequently incomplete, and altered excitability usually presents as a convulsion. The effects of generalized increased intracranial pressure can be secondary to increased mass, alteration in cerebrospinal fluid circulation, or a combination

of these. The deficits seen in brain tumor have a common denominator, that is, evidence of progression in symptomatology and signs over a period of time. A knowledge of the functional anatomy of the brain, classification of brain tumors, their frequency of occurrence and growth potential, and the mechanisms by which tumors manifest themselves will facilitate a high degree of accuracy in suspecting brain tumors, thereby allowing the physician to have the aid of the specialist in diagnosing and treating the tumor.

SPINAL CORD TUMORS

The term *spinal tumors* includes all tumors encroaching on the spinal cord. Primary tumors of the spine are approximately one-sixth as common as intracranial tumors but have a much better prognosis, since almost 60 percent are benign and a high percentage of the remainder respond to therapy, so that prolonged functional palliation can be expected. Metastatic spinal tumors are reported to present as often as primary spinal tumors. Any malignant tumor may metastasize to the bones of the spinal column or to the spinal epidural space, but the most common are from lung, breast, lymphoid tissue, prostate, kidney, and thyroid. Metastatic spinal tumors usually cause pain, followed by neurologic deficit. Since these tumors rarely cause death, palliation by surgical and radiation therapy is indicated in order to preserve neurologic function and decrease suffering during a terminal illness.

CLASSIFICATION AND CHARACTERISTICS. The symptoms, the type of tumor, and the prognosis correlate with where the tumor is in relation to the dura and spinal cord. Therefore, the classification of tumors into extradural and intradural groups and the subdivision of the intradural group into extramedullary and intramedullary has significance from both a clinical and pathologic point of view. Ninety percent of extradural tumors are malignant, while sixty percent of intradural tumors are benign. Seventy-five to eighty percent of extradural tumors are metastatic, while ninety-eight percent of intradural tumors are primary tumors. The common clinical course of extradural tumors is one of rapid compression of the spinal cord, either by the tumor itself or from collapse of involved vertebrae. The patient may present with rapidly progressing flaccid paraparesis and sensory loss that requires rapid recognition and surgical decompression in order to have significant palliative effect. The common clinical course of the intradural tumor is usually much slower and may extend over months or years with the patient presenting with spastic paraparesis and partial sensory loss.

Knowledge of the types of tumors, their potential for growth, and their mechanisms of production of symptoms is the means by which the finer aspects of diagnosis of spinal cord tumor are best attained, but the clinician should always consider the diagnosis of spinal cord tumor when any bilateral progressive neurologic loss occurs below any transverse level of the body. The value of such constant suspicion is the high degree of functional return and the high percentage of cure or palliation of symptoms resulting from the early surgical treatment.

EVALUATION. A suspected spinal cord tumor is localized by utilizing the findings of the neurologic examination, the bony changes in spinal x-rays, and the results of spinal contrast studies, or myelography.

CLINICAL MANIFESTATIONS. The diagnostic neurologic examination findings are of two types, local signs and tract signs. The local signs are segmental changes and localize the lesion along the rostral-caudal axis. The local motor signs are weakness and loss of reflexes with normal above and normal or hyperactive reflexes below the level, fasciculations over a segmental distribution, and atrophy in a myotome pattern. These indicate involvement of the anterior motor horn cells or the anterior spinal roots. Local sensory signs are localized pain and spinal tenderness, radicular or radiating pain, and loss of sensation over a dermatome pattern, indicating involvement of the dorsal root or dorsal root entry zone. Segmental loss of pain and temperature with preservation of touch (sensory dissociation) is also a local sign and indicates involvement of the crossing fibers in the anterior commissure of the spinal cord from a central lesion of the cord.

Tract signs only indicate that the lesion must be cephalad to the highest point of involvement, and the motor changes may vary from increased tone and reflexes to flaccidity with absent reflexes. The difference usually relates to the rapidness of onset, since with rapid loss of spinal cord function spinal shock with flaccid, areflexic paralysis may result whereas spastic paraparesis is more common with the slow, progressive loss of motor function. The other tract signs may relate to involvement of any portion of the spinal cord and thus can consist of loss of pain and temperature (anterolateral fasciculus); loss of position and vibratory sense (dorsal column); weakness, spasticity, hyperreflexia, and Babinski signs (posterolateral fasciculus).

DIAGNOSTIC STUDIES. Roentgenograms are of diagnostic aid if they are taken of the correct area. When doubt exists or when there is a question of multiple levels, the entire spinal column should be visualized. Diagnostic findings in the roentgenograms relate to the type of tumor present. With malignant tumors areas of invasion and destruction, particularly of the vertebral body and pedicles, may give localization. With benign or slowly growing tumors widening of the interpedicular and anteroposterior diameter of the neural canal, erosion of a pedicle or of a body, and enlargement of the intervertebral foramina are diagnostic.

Definitive localization, however, is done by myelography. It is usually best to do the lumbar puncture and obtain fluid, at the time that myelography is done. Prompt surgical intervention may be required with lumbar puncture or myelography, since increase in deficit may follow removal of spinal fluid below the level of the lesion. For this reason none of these should be done unless the patient is in an area where definitive neurosurgical care is available and the patient is under the observation or care of a neurosurgeon.

Extradural Tumors

The different types of patterns of symptoms and the local and tract signs are best remembered in relation to the different types of spinal cord tumors, namely, extradural, intradural-extramedullary, and intradural-intramedullary.

Aside from a rare extradural meningioma, neurofibroma, and benign osteoma of the vertebra, extradural tumors are malignant with rapid growth and a tendency to destroy the spinal column. The symptom pattern of the extradural tumor is one of pain, both localized to the area of involvement and radiating over the dermatome level of the adjacent spinal roots (local sign). This is followed by rapidly progressive transverse loss of spinal cord function (tract sign). The local pain is frequently more severe at night and at rest, while the radicular pain relates to movement, coughing, and straining. Both types of pain may be present for weeks or months before spinal cord involvement. The progressive transverse loss of spinal cord function can be as rapid as a few hours or as slow as a few days, and effective palliation is possible only if surgical decompression is done before total loss of spinal cord function has occurred.

Since these tumors frequently involve the adjacent vertebrae, x-rays of the spine with particular attention to the integrity of the vertebral body and pedicles will often suggest the diagnosis before as well as after the onset of progressive neurologic deficit in the spinal cord. Decompression by removing the posterior neural arch or laminectomy followed by x-ray therapy gives the best palliative result in this malignant group of tumors, and laminectomy with excision of the lesion is the treatment of choice for the few benign tumors.

Intradural-Extramedullary Tumors

Approximately 65 percent of all intradural tumors are extramedullary, and 90 percent are either neurofibromas or meningiomas. Neurofibromas are slightly more common and often are multiple. They have no sex predilection and are more common in the cervical and thoracic areas, while meningiomas are more frequent in females and more common in the thoracic region. It has been stated that the frequency of occurrence of both these tumors in the thoracic areas is in the same ratio as the length of the thoracic spine to the length of the spinal column.

Angiomas are also common in the thoracic area. They are arteriovenous malformations and not true tumors but may at times present like an extramedullary tumor. This is particularly true during the last trimester of pregnancy. Other tumors that occur in the extramedullary-intradural area are epidermoids, dermoids, and lipomas. The basic pattern of symptoms of the extramedullary-intradural tumor is similar to the extradural tumors, namely, local pain and radicular pain (local sign), followed by progressive spinal cord malfunction (tract sign). The course is slower, and the development of the spinal cord deficit is often prolonged so that partial patterns of loss are seen. A common partial pattern is the modified Brown-Séquard pattern in which loss to temperature and pinprick is more marked on one side below the level of the lesion and weakness and spasticity are more marked on the opposite side (tract signs).

Intramedullary Tumors

Over 95 percent of intramedullary tumors are gliomas. In contrast to intracranial gliomas they tend to be more benign histologically and to have a more benign course. This is in part because of the low grade of their malignancy and in part because of their frequently nonlethal position in the spinal cord. Except for the preponderance of ependymomas occurring in the conus medullaris and the filum terminale, they occur equally frequently in all areas of the spinal cord. Approximately one-half of intramedullary tumors are ependymomas, and 45 percent are astrocytomas, with a few oligodendrogliomas, hemangioblastomas, and ganglioneuromas making up the remainder. Arterial venous malformations and syringomyelia may present as intramedullary spinal cord tumors but are developmental abnormalities and not neoplasms.

The basic pattern of symptoms for the intramedullary tumor is different from the extradural and extramedullary tumor in that radicular or radiating pain is rare and the complaint of local pain is uncommon. These tumors tend to grow into the central part of the spinal cord and to destroy crossing fibers and neurons of the gray matter. The destruction of crossing fibers causes segmental loss of pain and temperature sensation with preservation of touch (sensory dissociation), resulting in damage to peripheral skin areas because of lack of protection of pain and temperature sensation (local sign). Trophic changes with alteration in vasomotor control and sweating may cause symptoms that resemble Raynaud's phenomenon or erythromelalgia. Alteration in the function of descending motor pathways or ascending sensory pathways is usually late in appearance, but alteration in sexual function and bladder function may occur early (tract sign). Segmental lower motor neuron destruction is common, and the signs of such destruction, namely, weakness, atrophy, loss of reflex, and fasciculations, should always be searched for in these patients, since they have localizing value (local sign).

Summation

In summary, spinal cord tumors have a good prognosis if treated early. It is important to keep in mind that a progressive decrease in spinal cord function must always be considered to indicate a spinal cord tumor until proved otherwise. Early diagnosis, accurate localization, and surgical therapy can be expected to give a large percentage of cures with good functional result and in the remainder to give considerable and prolonged palliation of symptoms.

MALFORMATIONS OF THE NERVOUS SYSTEM

More than one-half of all congenital defects involve the central nervous system or its coverings. Some anomalies such as anencephaly are lethal; many, such as mongolism and micrencephaly, preclude development of normal intellectual function, while others, such as spina bifida occulta, cause no disturbance of neurologic function. Within the diverse group of prenatal malformations affecting the nervous system directly or indirectly there exist some which necessitate surgical treatment for several reasons: they may provide an actual or potential communication to the body surface, produce compression of neural structures, impede normal circulation of cerebrospinal fluid, restrict normal growth of the nervous system, or act as a source of bleeding or seizures. The more common malformations in this category include the overt forms of cranium and spina bifida, dermal sinus tracts, congenital forms of hydrocephalus, craniosynostosis, congenital tumors, and vascular malformations. Some anomalies such as the leaking myelomeningocele have to be dealt with within hours after birth; others, as for example, vascular malformations of the brain and spinal cord, may not become symptomatic until late in life; most, however, require attention during infancy or early childhood.

Many prenatal defects affecting the nervous system produce or are associated with external evidence of their presence, and a diagnosis often can be made on inspection. Once seen, one is unlikely to forget the enlarged head, bulging fontanel, and prominent scalp veins of the infant with hydrocephalus, the misshapen head of the child with craniosynostosis, or the midline hair-containing dimple in the lumbar or occipital region indicating a dermal sinus tract. By the simple maneuver of transillumination with a strong flashlight in a dark room it is frequently possible in young infants to diagnose abnormal cystic cavities within the cranium and to make the important clinical distinction between a meningocele containing only cerebrospinal fluid and a myelomeningocele or encephalocele which contains nervous tissue as well.

Because of frequently associated bony anomalies, typical locations of certain lesions, and ease of deformation of the growing skull and spine, plain x-rays are fruitful in the diagnosis of congenital abnormalities. Contrast x-ray studies such as ventriculography, angiography, and myelography are, however, often necessary for diagnosis of the occult lesion as well as for better definition of the extent of those that are more obvious.

It is not possible surgically to repair damaged or abnormally constituted portions of the brain or spinal cord. One can only restore the integrity of the protective coverings; relieve pressure caused by space-occupying lesions, compressing bone, or impaired cerebrospinal fluid circulation; repair or occlude abnormalities of the vessels; or destroy malfunctioning nervous tissue when it interferes with normal neurophysiologic processes. In many instances, operations for congenital defects should be carried out early in life to allow unimpeded development of the growing nervous system. Thus, the dermal sinus tract should be recognized and excised before the first attack of meningitis and the fused coronal suture opened before the onset of increased intracranial pressure. The results of such prophylactic surgical measures are often undramatic but are obviously more valuable than if done after the nervous system is compromised.

EMBRYOLOGY. Malformations of the nervous system may result from failure of initial development, from incomplete or aberrant development, or from destruction of already formed tissues by intrauterine infection or infarction. Teratologic studies in animals have revealed that dissimilar insults to the embryo, if delivered at the same stage of development, may produce the same malformation, making it extremely difficult to classify most central nervous system malformations on the basis of etiology.

A better understanding of a number of surgically important prenatal defects can be obtained from a knowledge of the basic details of embryology of the nervous system. The neurons and supporting glia of the brain, spinal cord, and peripheral ganglia are derivatives of the ectoderm. The nervous system begins as a proliferation of ectodermal cells in the craniocaudal axis of the embryo dorsal to the notochord. Growth proceeds in the neural plate so that a longitudinally oriented groove, flanked on either side by a crest, is formed on its dorsal aspect. This process of invagination continues until the dorsal lips of the groove meet and fuse to form a hollow tube extending the length of the embryo. Normally the neural tube which represents the primitive brain and spinal cord completely separates from the cutaneous ectoderm which comes to overlie it, from the underlying notochord around which the vertebral bodies are formed, and from the entodermal structures beneath the notochord. The spinal and peripheral ganglia are formed from cells of the neural crest. Local concentrations of mesoderm give rise to the vascular structures of the nervous system and to its coverings, both meningeal and bony.

Closure of the dorsad situated neural groove and separation of the neural elements from the cutaneous ectoderm commences in its midportion and progresses craniad and caudad. This process occurs during the third and fourth weeks of gestation and if not completed, either because of an insult to the embryo during this period or because of a genetic abnormality, results in a group of malformations characterized by a local defect in any of or all the coverings of the central nervous system. Such defects can occur anywhere in the dorsal midline along the neuroaxis but are most common at its extremes, namely, the lumbosacral and occipital regions.

Spina Bifida and Cranium Bifida

The common denominator in these lesions is a midline bony defect; hence the general terms *spina bifida* (cleft spine) and *cranium bifida* are useful. The spectrum encountered ranges from (1) spina bifida occulta, or incomplete fusion of the two halves of the neural arch of one or two lumbar or sacral vertebrae with intact skin and meninges, present in about 20 percent of the population,

through (2) the meningoceles, in which there is protrusion of the meninges through a defect in the skull or spine to form a sac filled with cerebrospinal fluid, and (3) the myelomeningoceles and their cranial counterparts, the encephaloceles, in which nervous tissue, usually malformed, is present within the sac, to (4) the unclosed neural plate bare of coverings. Closure defects of the spine far outnumber those of the cranium, and myelomeningoceles are many times more common than spinal meningoceles. Rarely herniation of the meninges and sometimes nervous tissue as well occur through ventral bony defects to present in the nasal cavity, thorax, abdomen, or pelvis.

SPINA BIFIDA OCCULTA

Spina bifida occulta most commonly is hidden (occulta) or unable to be diagnosed from examination of the surface over the spine. It is most commonly picked up in adults from an x-ray examination. These lesser degrees of spinal closure defects, however, often have associated cutaneous stigmata, e.g., midline skin angioma, or pigmentation, or tufts of hair. The presence of these superficial lesions should alert one to the possibility of a closure defect of the spine beneath them. Although the closure defect of spina bifida occulta is usually asymptomatic, its presence in a child suspected of neurologic dysfunction or with enuresis should lead one to suspect an underlying lesion of the neural tube. Not uncommonly, in these circumstances, one may find a hamartoma, frequently lipomatous, or a "tethered" filum terminale. Both these lesions may lend themselves to surgical correction with gratifying results. Every child with enuresis in whom the diagnosis of neurogenic bladder is suspected should have careful neurologic examination, plain films of the spine, and positive contrast myelography when indicated. Many of these children have subtle neurologic deficits that can be elicited only by thorough and repeated examinations.

Diastematomyelia (separation of the cord) is often associated with similar midline skin stigmata. In this anomaly, the cord is divided into two halves, each of which undergoes normal maturation. The two parallel spinal cords are often separated from one another by a bony projection or fibrous band arising from the dorsal surface of the body of the vertebra dividing the intradural space into two separate compartments. Because of the high incidence of vertebral abnormality, diagnosis often can be made from the spinal column x-rays. These children usually present with sphincter dysfunction, difficulty in walking, and/or deformities of the feet. When the diagnosis is made in infancy, removal of the bony or fibrous spur is indicated, since with growth there is often traction on the spinal cord and insidious loss of bladder and bowel function may go unsuspected. In the older child, removal is indicated when progressive neurologic deficit ensues.

Dermal Sinus Tracts

This closure defect apparently results from incomplete separation of the neural ectoderm from either the cutaneous ectoderm or the entoderm. These epithelial-lined tracts may provide a direct communication between the skin surface and the subarachnoid space. The opening at the skin, which consists of a small midline pore located in the lumbar or occipital region, is usually inconspicuous and may be completely hidden by surrounding hair. In the occipital region the tract penetrates the skull through a small midline opening that may or may not be apparent on x-rays and is directed caudad toward the posterior fossa. In the lumbar region, the tract may begin as low as the gluteal cleft but always extends in a cephalic direction toward the conus medullaris. In either location the tract may extend for varying distances. It may end at or above the dura, or it may continue through the subarachnoid space to end in the pia or even penetrate nervous tissue. The tract may expand at any point along its course into a dermoid cyst. This lesion therefore not only may be responsible for meningitis but also may cause dysfunction by compression of nervous tissue. In any case of meningitis due to *Escherichia coli,* caused by a mixture of skin organisms, or in infants with recurrent meningitis, a sinus tract should be sought. This includes shaving the occiput and taking x-rays of the skull and spine. It is advised that all sinus tracts be excised before the infant is six weeks of age. This is best done by a neurosurgeon, since, on occasion, laminectomy and intradural exploration are indicated.

Neurenteric cysts are extremely rare lesions that present as a spinal cord tumor. They represent incomplete separation of the neural tube and the underlying entoderm. They usually occur in the upper thoracic region and may be suspected if x-rays reveal vertebral anomalies. The lesion consists of a cyst or solid tumor adherent to the anterior surface of the spinal cord and is lined with, or composed of, entodermal derivatives. A stalk may traverse the opening in the vertebra and connect with a similar mass in the thorax.

MENINGOCELES

Meningoceles are often completely covered by skin at birth, and the communication with the subarachnoid space at the neck of the sac is frequently quite small. Treatment consists of excision of the sac and closure of the dura, fascia, and skin. Surgical intervention should be considered urgent if the sac is extremely thin, is ulcerated, or is leaking cerebrospinal fluid. Patients with meningoceles alone do not have neurologic dysfunction and do not usually develop hydrocephalus. They are at risk for the later development of neurological dysfunction as a result of other anomalies, e.g., tethered filum terminale are often found in association with an initially asymptomatic meningocele.

ENCEPHALOCELES

The majority of encephaloceles occur in the occipital region and are often associated with malformation of the occipital lobes or cerebellum, and either portion of the brain may be present within the sac. These lesions can be huge, often approaching the size of the baby's head. However, size of the encephalocele is not correlated with the degree of neural dysgenesis. Arteriography is of value in

differentiating meningocele from encephalocele and in determining the position of the venous sinuses in preparation for surgical repair. Ideal treatment consists of replacing the herniated brain within the cranium, removing the sac, and effecting a tight closure of dura and skin. Unfortunately, amputation of the herniated nervous tissue often must be carried out, because it is grossly malformed or infarcted or because the cranium is too small to allow its return. Hydrocephalus occurs commonly in infants with encephalocele, including those patients with only a meningocele. It most commonly results from adhesions in the posterior fossa but may include all the causes of hydrocephalus. The hydrocephalus may not become apparent until some weeks following surgical repair. The prognosis in many of these children is quite good, although there is an increased incidence of learning disability and mental retardation. The presence of neural tissue in the sac is associated with a poor prognosis, and the greater the amount of tissue, the poorer the prognosis.

MYELOMENINGOCELES

Myelomeningoceles are the most common of the closure defects. The incidence in United States is about 2.5 per 1,000 live births. All these children have neurologic deficit, the vast majority have hydrocephalus, and many have associated congenital anomalies of other systems, mainly skeletal and urinary. Most myelomeningoceles occur in the lumbosacral region. The bony defect, best seen on x-ray, usually extends over three or more segments, and the spinal canal is often widened. Although the sac is occasionally covered by skin, its dorsum is usually formed of arachnoid. The dysplastic cord can often be seen through this membrane attached to its undersurface. Frequently an unclosed neural plate with both posterior and anterior roots emerging from its ventral surface lies at, or just below, the surface at the cephalic end of the sac. The central canal of the spinal cord may be dilated and may open directly into the sac. If spinal cord is present below the lesion, it too is usually grossly malformed. Duplication of the cord (diplomyelia) extending for various distances proximally is commonly seen with large lesions. The dorsal nerve roots and peripheral nerves are well formed but may not be in continuity with the affected portions of the spinal cord.

Neurologic deficit attributable to the spinal cord lesion is both motor and sensory; its degree depends upon the site and severity of the malformation as well as secondary factors such as infection and infarction of the exposed cord. Most patients have a flaccid paraparesis, the sensory level usually being somewhat lower than the motor level. Virtually all patients have urinary incontinence. Occasionally because of partial lesions of the spinal cord, there is a mixed upper and lower motor neuron deficit in the lower extremities.

Malformations of the nervous system in patients with myelomeningocele are not confined to the spinal cord but are frequently present in the hindbrain, midbrain, and forebrain. The almost constant presence of the Chiari II malformation and frequent occurrence of aqueductal malformation lead to the almost uniform presence of hydrocephalus. The Chiari II malformation consists of an elongation of the medulla and cerebellar tonsils and vermis with displacement of these structures including the fourth ventricle through the foramen magnum into the upper cervical spine canal. Careful pathologic studies have demonstrated that these patients also often have malformations of the cerebrum including an enlarged massa intermedia, heterotropias, and agenesis of the corpus callosum.

In addition to spina bifida, other anomalies of the spine, such as hemivertebrae, are often present. Other structural abnormalities due to muscular hypotonicity and imbalance, including scoliosis, kyphosis, dislocation of the hips, and clubfoot, are common. Disorders of the urinary tract are mainly secondary to neurogenic vesicular dysfunction. No definite correlation has been made between these lesions and intellectual performance, although many of these children have visuomotor perceptual difficulties. There is also an increased incidence of mental retardation within the group as a whole.

TREATMENT. Treatment of patients with myelomeningoceles can be divided into acute and chronic phases. The immediate problems relate to the myelomeningocele and altered cerebrospinal fluid circulation. Long-term problems are the continuing treatment of hydrocephalus, the musculoskeletal abnormalities, and problems associated with bladder dysfunction, including hydronephrosis and infection. Whenever possible an excision of the membranous sac, replacement of the herniated spinal cord within the spinal canal, and closure of the dura, fascia, and skin should be carried out. There is now good evidence to suggest that this operation should be done within the first few hours of life. At this time the sac is smaller and the skin more pliable; there are fewer adhesions between the nervous tissue and the sac; and the risk of infection is lower, because the skin flora have not yet become established. The major advantage in early closure is that neurologic deficit can be reduced to a minimum by surgical intervention before the spinal cord is exposed to infection.

Although the head circumference measurement at birth may be normal, the ventricular system is usually enlarged, and overt evidence of hydrocephalus frequently occurs within the first few weeks of life. Occasionally the hydrocephalus is arrested spontaneously, but all patients should be closely followed by serial head measurements and cerebrospinal fluid shunting procedures carried out if there is progressive ventricular enlargement.

X-rays of the skull, entire spine, and hips, intravenous pyelogram, urinalysis and urine cultures, as well as urologic and orthopedic consultations should be obtained as a base line before discharge and repeated as necessary during follow-up. Long-term care involves multiple disciplines, including neurosurgery, orthopedic surgery, urology, and physical therapy.

Infantile Hydrocephalus

The central canal in that portion of the neural tube which becomes the spinal cord progressively decreases in size and in the adult is seldom patent, its position usually marked only by a collection of ependymal cells. The central canal at the cephalic end of the neural tube, however, ultimately forms the interconnecting ventricular system. Although a small amount of cerebrospinal fluid, considered to be identical with the extracellular fluid of the brain, is formed outside the ventricles as well as within them, there is apparently a net production of fluid secreted by the choroid plexuses. This excess fluid must exit through the openings in the fourth ventricle and through the foramina of Luschka and Magendie, and pass into the subarachnoid cisterns surrounding the brainstem which communicate through the tentorial notch with the subarachnoid space over the cerebral hemispheres. The fluid is finally absorbed by passing into the lumen of the venous sinuses via the arachnoid villi. Major obstruction to this flow at any point in the pathway results in progressive enlargement of the ventricles proximal to the obstruction. With the possible exception of one rare tumor (papilloma of the choroid plexus), in which the production of cerebrospinal fluid may exceed the resorptive capacity of the system, all hydrocephalus can be considered as an obstructive phenomenon, having, however, a diversity of causes including congenital or acquired, neoplastic, and inflammatory.

Confusion frequently exists in regard to the term "communicating hydrocephalus." This means only that there is communication between the lateral ventricles and the lumbar subarachnoid space, tested traditionally by inserting a dye in one of these two compartments and recovering it in the other. The obstruction in communicating hydrocephalus is usually in the subarachnoid cisterns in the posterior fossa or at the base of the cerebrum. Known causes are adhesions following meningitis or subarachnoid bleeding. Hydrocephalus from basal arachnoiditis is quite common in infancy and, although the cause can rarely be determined, is presumably secondary to subarachnoid bleeding from birth trauma or intrauterine or neonatal subclinical meningitis. The prognosis for normal mental development is poor in those instances where hydrocephalus is associated with anoxia, meningitis, or brain trauma, i.e., concomitant with brain injury.

There are several congenital malformations that result in hydrocephalus. Two congenital defects, the Chiari II malformation and malformations of the aqueduct, are common causes of hydrocephalus in infancy. Both are frequently associated with myelomeningocele, but aqueductal malformations are also a common cause of an isolated hydrocephalus in early life. With the Chiari malformation, passage of cerebrospinal fluid around the dislocated brainstem is impeded by the abnormal mass of tissue in the foramen magnum and by surrounding adhesions. The pathology in congenital aqueductal obstruction is more varied; obstruction usually occurs in the upper portion of the aqueduct. The commonest abnormality causing obstruction of the aqueduct in this upper portion is forking or lack of development of a single tube. Although the term "stenosis" is used, it is misleading since it implies constriction rather than the more common failure of development. A glial septum may occlude the lumen at its junction with the fourth ventricle. Progressive gliosis (scarring) of the aqueduct of unknown cause may be responsible for hydrocephalus arising at a later age; it may become symptomatic as late as the second or third decade.

Other malformations are also occasionally responsible for hydrocephalus. Failure of development of the foramina of the fourth ventricle (Dandy-Walker syndrome) results in massive cystic dilatation of the fourth ventricle. The posterior fossa is markedly enlarged, and the cerebellum is reduced to small atrophic remnants on either side of the cyst. The vermis is usually completely atrophied. Congenital cysts within the arachnoid of the posterior fossa may result in a similar picture.

Tumors are a rare but possible cause of hydrocephalus in the infant. These include intraventricular tumors such as ependymomas, medulloblastomas occurring in the fourth ventricle, and tumors adjacent to the ventricular system such as cerebellar astrocytomas, craniopharyngiomas, meningiomas, or pinealomas. Most of these tumors cause hydrocephalus by blocking the cerebrospinal fluid pathways or by compressing the aqueduct.

EVALUATION. The diagnosis of hydrocephalus is to a large extent clinical. Accurate measurement of head circumference and plotting on a chart of normal distribution of head size and palpation of the fontanel should be a routine part of the examination during the first few years of life. Any child with a head circumference outside the normal range should be evaluated by a neurosurgeon.

For years the only adequate means of visualizing the ventricular system was by air encephalography. The advent of computerized axial tomography has replaced ventriculography as the diagnostic procedure of choice in those institutions in which it is available. The advantages of this method are that it is noninvasive, does not alter cerebrospinal fluid dynamics, and may identify associated tumors and/or hematoma. The major disadvantage is that is does not give any information concerning communication between the various cerebrospinal fluid compartments. For this reason, a limited or "bubble" ventriculogram is performed. In infants this is best carried out by introducing a spinal needle into the ventricular system through the coronal suture. Preliminary bilateral subdural taps are carried out to rule out the other most common cause of an enlarged head in infancy, namely, subdural hematoma. The primary aim of the ventriculogram is to demonstrate the site and cause of the block in the cerebrospinal fluid pathways and to determine if the hydrocephalus is communicating or noncommunicating. Communication is verified by the demonstration of air passing into the subarachnoid space. Cerebrospinal fluid is also obtained for aerobic and anaerobic cultures, protein and glucose determination, and cell count. Indolent meningitis or ventriculitis may be the cause of hydrocephalus in infants even in the absence of fever or other clinical signs and symptoms.

More recently, angiography has been used for diagnosing hydrocephalus. It also appears to have value in prognosis, since the presence of normal vasculature, allowing for the distortion from the hydrocephalus, has been associated with a better prognosis than when arteriography shows absence of major arterial branches. This latter may indicate atrophy or lack of development of areas of the brain.

TREATMENT. The treatment of infantile hydrocephalus depends on etiology. There is a small but important group of patients who may be cured by a single operation. These include those in whom hydrocephalus is caused by choroid plexus papillomas, benign tumors obstructing the cerebrospinal fluid pathways, posterior fossa cysts, and occlusion of the aqueduct by thin glial septa. The remainder of the patients require procedures which shunt the cerebrospinal fluid around the obstruction within the cranium, into another body cavity, or into the bloodstream.

The procedure for shunting spinal fluid around an obstruction of the posterior third ventricle or the aqueduct is known as the Torkildsen procedure. It consists of placing a tube from the lateral ventricle to the cisterna magna or cervical subarachnoid space. Although it is an effective method of therapy in many cases of hydrocephalus, it is dependent upon patent subarachnoid spaces with normal absorptive mechanisms. In the infant, these conditions are frequently absent, and in ventricular or midbrain tumors the subarachnoid spaces may be blocked at the incisura of the tentorium. With the development of pliable, nonreactive materials, such as silastic, it has become possible to utilize shunts between the ventricles or the subarachnoid space and the pleural and peritoneal cavities for absorption of spinal fluid. These can be maintained for prolonged periods. Although reactive scarring may occur and, at times, significant effusion develops in some patients following immunization or mild viral illnesses, these shunts have an advantage over the vascular shunting in that there is no foreign body in the venous system, and they are simpler and require less frequent revision for growth in the young infant.

By far the most successful treatment of hydrocephalus has been the ventriculoatrial shunt. A catheter is placed in one lateral ventricle, and a second via the internal jugular vein into the right cardiac atrium. A one-way valve is incorporated between the two catheters so that cerebrospinal fluid at normal pressures can pass into the vascular system but blood cannot reflux. There are three major problems with the ventriculoatrial shunt: The first is the chronic presence of a foreign body within the vascular system that may act as a nidus for infection, especially if the cardiac catheter impinges on the tricuspid valve. The most common organism causing the septicemia is *Staphylococcus albus*. The infection can develop at any time after the shunt has been inserted and should be suspected if there is intermittent or persistent unexplained fever, anemia, and/or splenomegaly. If infection is proved by blood culture, removal of the shunt and antibiotic treatment are indicated. Treatment with antibiotics alone almost invariably fails. The second problem results from progressive upward displacement of the atrial catheter with growth. Once the tip of the catheter reaches the upper superior vena cava, it often becomes obstructed. Periodic chest x-rays are necessary to determine the position of the radiopaque catheter, so that elective lengthening can be done before the shunt obstructs. The third problem, common to all shunts, is obstruction of the ventricular catheter by inspissated protein, brain, or choroid plexus.

Children with hydrocephalus require close and knowledgeable follow-up, and parents should be taught to recognize signs of increased intracranial pressure. Increasing head circumference is a useful guide in evaluating hydrocephalus in the infant, but a gradual fall in psychometric level or school performance may be the only sign of progressive hydrocephalus in an older child. Although hydrocephalus presents a difficult and often frustrating problem, an increasing number of patients with hydrocephalus beginning in infancy are growing up to be useful individuals. It is apparent that many of these patients if adequately treated can develop intellectual capacity to superior levels.

Craniosynostosis

The normal stimulus for growth of the skull is provided by expansion of the growing brain. This fact is easily demonstrable in cases of micrencephaly, in which there is a head size comparable to the size of the brain, and in hemiatrophy of the cerebrum of infancy, in which the hemicranium on the affected side is smaller than on the side with the normal hemisphere. To a large extent, increase in the size of the cranial bones proceeds by incremental growth at the sutural margin. Fifty percent of the brain growth occurs in the first six months and 85 percent by the first year. The major sutures remain open until the growing brain has achieved its maximal volume in the middle of the second decade. Premature closure of a suture (craniosynostosis) therefore results in skull deformities and may also restrict the capacity of the cranium to such an extent that there is compression of the growing brain and a generalized increase in intracranial pressure.

INCIDENCE. The cause of craniosynostosis is unknown. Some cases are clearly familial, but many are sporadic. There is a sexual predilection in some types of craniosynostosis. Isolated closure of the sagittal suture occurs predominantly in males in a ratio of about 4:1, but isolated coronal synostosis is more common in females. In the majority of patients with premature closure of a single suture, no other abnormalities exist. In isolated coronal suture synostosis, an increased incidence of congenital anomalies of the brain, such as agenesis of the corpus callosum, has been reported. In the familial, multiple, or even complete synostosis, such as Apert's syndrome, there is the coexistence of the synostosis, syndactyly, and craniofacial dysostosis; in Crouzon's disease, along with the cranial synostosis, there is facial bone dysostosis with maxillary hypoplasia. In both these conditions, early operative opening of the cranial sutures and decompression of the orbit are indicated to preserve mental functions and vision. Later, cosmetic surgery for the face is often indicated.

The incidence of the different sutures involved in craniosynostosis varies. Isolated sagittal synostosis is the most common, followed in order by premature closure of the coronal sutures, closure of three or more cranial sutures, the metopic suture alone, and finally various combinations of sagittal, coronal, and lambdoid sutures. Closure of the coronal and lambdoid sutures may be unilateral or bilateral.

CLINICAL MANIFESTATIONS. The resulting shape of the head depends on the suture involved and at what age it closes. Deficiency in skull growth with synostosis occurs in a direction perpendicular to the involved suture. Premature closure of the sagittal suture results in a long, narrow head and that of the coronal in a wide, short skull. Total synostosis produces a high vertex with an abnormally small circumference. This entity must be distinguished from micrencephaly, in which the sutures are fused early because there is little or no brain growth. Unilateral synostosis of the coronal suture produces a flat forehead on the involved side. The metopic suture, normally closed at birth, may be involved, giving a characteristic prow-shaped deformity of the forehead, indicating craniosynostosis in utero. Most of these deformities are obvious within a few weeks following birth. Any child with an abnormally shaped head after the effects of molding have subsided should have skull x-rays. Even though accurate diagnosis by x-ray is difficult, it is important to have a base-line determination of the sutures involved. The diagnosis is usually apparent from head shape alone and verified by palpation of a ridge along the involved suture.

TREATMENT. Treatment of craniosynostosis consists of creating an artificial suture at the site of, or parallel to, the natural suture by cutting out a strip of skull. To retard fusion, the periosteum is widely removed from the exposed bone, and strips of plastic, e.g., polyethylene film, are fastened to the margins of the craniectomy. There is little evidence to suggest that brain growth is compromised in metopic, sagittal, and lambdoid or unilateral coronal synostosis. The very significant deformity and negligible operative risk nevertheless justify surgical intervention for cosmetic reasons alone in these types of synostosis. In these conditions, early surgical intervention is indicated to achieve a good cosmetic result.

Surgical treatment for total synostosis and bilateral coronal synostosis must be carried out early to prevent brain damage and visual dysfunction. In these conditions, reoperation at periodic intervals into the early teens may be necessary to keep the artificial sutures patent. In operations of this type, both cosmetic and therapeutic results are better the earlier the operations are done. The optimal time for surgical repair of total and bicoronal synostosis is in the neonatal period. Cosmetic results of any synostectomy are better before four months of age, since the growing brain molds the skull. There is little likelihood that significant change in appearance can be achieved after one year of age. Surgical treatment after the age of eighteen to twenty-four months should be restricted to those patients with symptomatic varieties of synostosis.

VASCULAR DISEASES OF THE NERVOUS SYSTEM

ETIOLOGY. Vascular disease constitutes a set of major causes of neurologic morbidity and mortality spanning several pathologic categories. Congenital lesions are represented by saccular aneurysms which appear and enlarge consequent to defective muscular and elastic layers at vessel bifurcations, and by arteriovenous malformations that result from failure of formation of a capillary bed between segments of the arterial and venous circulations. Infectious and inflammatory conditions of the vessels of the central nervous system occur. These include arteritis and phlebitis accompanying chronic meningitis, thrombophlebitis or dural venous sinus thrombosis accompanying subdural and epidural infections, mycotic aneurysms secondary to septic emboli, and the less specific arteritis as exemplified by temporal arteritis. The degenerative or metabolic disease complex subsumed by the term "atherosclerosis" constitutes one of the characteristic afflictions of the twentieth-century man. Brain ischemia or infarction due to thrombosis of involved vessels or their occlusion by emboli from vessels more proximal with diseased endothelium constitutes a frequent form of this disease. A less frequent but even more catastrophic form of the disease is the intracerebral hemorrhage that can occur with the same basic set of conditions upon which has been superimposed an elevation in blood pressure.

ANATOMY. The major arterial supply to the brain consists of paired internal carotid and vertebral arteries. The internal carotid arteries begin in the neck at the division of the common carotid artery into the external and internal carotid arteries. The internal carotid arteries can be divided into cervical, petrous, cavernous, and intradural portions. The cervical portion has no branches, but the remaining portions have branches that can be significant in collateral blood supply to the brain following obstruction in the internal or common carotid artery. Branches of the petrous portion that anastomose with the internal maxillary artery are the caroticotympanic and pterygoid canal arteries. These are relatively small branches and rarely have significant anastomotic capacity. In the cavernous portion are branches to the cavernous sinus, the hypophysis, semilunar ganglion, meninges, and orbit. The semilunar and meningeal arteries can have significant anastomosis with the meningeal branches of the internal maxillary artery, and the ophthalmic artery is commonly a significant anastomotic channel with the terminal branches of the external maxillary artery. The cavernous sinus branches may be a source of communication between the carotid artery and the cavernous sinus, a carotid cavernous fistula, when they are ruptured by trauma or disease. The intradural branches of the internal carotid artery are the anterior cerebral, the middle cerebral, the posterior communicating, and the choroid arteries. The posterior communicating artery forms an anastomosis with the posterior cerebral artery, and the anterior cerebral artery with the anterior communicating and the opposite anterior cerebral artery to complete the anterior portion of the circle of Willis. The vertebral arteries in their cervical or extradural portion have anastomotic branches with the thyrocervical trunk of the subclavian artery and with the posterior branches of the external carotid. After traversing the dura, they join to form the basilar artery giving branches to the brainstem. The division of the basilar artery into the posterior cerebral arteries completes the posterior portion of the circle of Willis.

There are, therefore, extensive anastomoses between the vertebral basilar system and the carotid system. The collateral circulation can be divided into the extracranial, extracranial-intracranial, and intracranial. The extracranial anastomoses have been described in the paragraph above but, in general, consist of posterior branches of the external carotid and the vertebral and the thyrocervical trunk of the subclavian, the internal maxillary branch of the carotid through the meningeal branches of the internal carotid, and between terminal branches of both external carotid arteries. Most of these anastomoses are normally small but have the capacity to enlarge following proximal or distal occlusion of a carotid or vertebral artery. For example, after obstruction of the cervical common carotid artery below the bifurcation, anastomosis through the external carotid arteries can result in retrograde flow in the ipsilateral external carotid artery to its origin and consequent forward flow in the external carotid artery to the brain, bypassing the obstruction. Extracranial-intracranial collaterals are principally by anastomosis of the external carotid artery to the intracranial circulation by the ophthalmic artery and by collaterals developed between meningeal vessels and the intracranial arteries of the pia on the convexity of the cerebral hemispheres. The major intracranial anastomosis is the circle of Willis described above. In only 18 percent of brains is the circle of Willis fully developed, there being various degrees of hypoplasia in one or more vessels in the majority of cases. Extensive end-to-end anastomoses of arterial branches of the anterior, middle, and posterior cervical arteries have been demonstrated by arteriography following occlusion of major intracerebral vessels. Although these anastomoses are, in general, not present in the normal state, they develop rapidly following vascular compromise and may be, in part, the reason for neurologic recovery following cerebrovascular accidents secondary to occlusion of a major vessel. All the anastomoses, but particularly the larger extracranial-intracranial and intracranial anastomoses, play a significant role in the protection of the brain against neurologic dysfunction in vascular disease and major occlusion.

PHYSIOLOGY. Intracranial circulation is dependent upon many factors, but the main determinants are arterial and venous pressure at the level of the brain, intracranial pressure, blood viscosity, and the state of the vascular bed and its resultant resistance. The brain is one of the most metabolically active organs in the body, requiring a constant supply of oxygen and glucose and, therefore, constant blood flow containing these substances. Intracerebral blood flow has been calculated by several techniques with variations between 44 and 80 ml/100 Gm of brain/minute, but the generally accepted value in the adult normal brain is approximately 50 to 55 ml/100 Gm of brain/minute, or approximately 750 ml of blood/minute in the adult. Thus, the brain, representing only 2 percent of the body weight, ordinarily receives between 17 to 18 percent of the heart's output and consumes nearly 20 percent of the oxygen supply of the body. Gray matter blood flow has been measured at 80 ml/100 Gm of brain/minute, while that of the white matter is 20 ml/100 Gm of brain/minute or roughly one-fourth of the gray matter, indicating further the metabolic activity of the two areas.

There are several intrinsic factors regulating the cerebral blood flow which are unique to the cerebral vasculature, and extrinsic factors which relate to blood flow and its constituents, both of which tend to keep cerebral blood flow and availability of oxygen and glucose constant despite wide variation in systemic flow to other areas of the body. The intrinsic factors are referred to by the term *autoregulation.* In experimental animals with normal autoregulation of the cerebral vessels if the parameters of P_{CO_2}, P_{O_2}, and body temperature are kept constant, cerebral blood flow remains constant between systolic pressures of 80 to 180 mm Hg. Not all the factors affecting autoregulation are clear, but two are well substantiated and a third has been suggested by recent experimental work. Evidence of a local myogenic factor is based on the demonstration that the intrinsic smooth muscle cells of intracranial arteries and arterioles respond to change in intraluminal pressure by contracting with increasing pressure and dilating with decreasing pressure. It has also been demonstrated that intracranial arteries constrict in response to increased levels of oxygen and to decreased levels of P_{CO_2} and expand to the opposite changes in these gases. Alteration in pH cause similar changes to P_{CO_2} alteration, i.e., vasodilation with increase and vasoconstriction with decrease in level of pH. A neurogenic basis for intrinsic control of the intracerebral arteries has been proposed based on physiologic experiments demonstrating areas of the brainstem, whose stimulation or ablation affects the autoregulation of the arteries and larger arterioles of the cerebral circulation.

Loss of autoregulation is seen in toxic states, following injury, and after hypoxia or hypotension; if autoregulation is lost, hypertension or hypotension can in itself be a factor for further brain injury. Methods for determining the intactness of autoregulation are available in the experimental animal and may be estimated in the clinical situation when intracranial pressure (ICP) is being monitored. It has been demonstrated that ICP will passively follow a change in mean arterial blood pressure (MABP) in animals and humans who have lost cerebral autoregulation. Thus, one may observe simultaneously recorded ICP and MABP during physiological fluctuations, or the physician may artificially lower or raise the MABP, noting the effect on ICP. The importance of these measurements is rapidly becoming more apparent in clinical problems such as head trauma or vascular disease.

Extrinsic factors for control of cerebral circulation are intracranial pressure, and vasomotor and cardiac reflexes from special receptors in the carotid artery, the aortic arch, pulmonary arch, vena cava, and splenic artery, via brainstem nuclei to raise or lower systemic pressure toward adequate cerebral perfusion. Elevated P_{CO_2} levels or reduction in oxygen tension via these receptors tend to raise systemic blood pressure. Hypoxia or decrease in blood flow in the hindbrain by direct effect on the muscle causes slowing of the heart, peripheral constriction, and, therefore, relative increase in available circulation to the brain.

In the past, knowledge of the action of autoregulation and reflex activity have been used for diagnosis and prognosis of disease states. More accurate methods of determining their intactness and functions and pharmacologic agents now have therapeutic possibilities.

CLINICAL MANIFESTATIONS. The history of neurologic dysfunction in the patient with vascular disease is one whose course in time is characterized by an abrupt change in neurological function. There may be sudden deterioration, followed by relatively immediate or full recovery, called *transient ischemic attacks* (TIA). The term *stroke* denotes sudden loss of perfusion to a portion of the brain, which may be followed by a prolonged return to the premorbid state (reversible ischemic neurological deficit) or leave the patient with residual deficit (completed stroke). The vascular accident of intracerebral hematoma often results in progressive neurological dysfunction and a decreasing level of consciousness as the mass expands. This same abrupt onset is seen with the subarachnoid hemorrhage as sudden headache, alteration in consciousness, and changes in neurologic function occurring in a very few moments. The symptomatology resulting from vascular disease infrequently can be quite nonspecific, but more commonly the gradual loss of function in the cerebral hemisphere thought to be caused by "little strokes" is found at postmortem not to be vascular but to be a neuronal degeneration. Changes in function of the spinal cord considered to be vascular are rarely proved to be so unless the vascular compromise is secondary to mechanical factors involving the blood supply passing through the intervertebral foramen or mechanical factors in the canal, such as hypertrophic osteoarthritic spurs at the intervertebral spaces causing both vascular and nervous system tissue compression.

Occasionally the patient with a history typical of cerebrovascular disease, on more complete work-up, proves to have a tumor. Conversely, the progressive neurologic deficit which has caused a patient to be suspected of having a tumor turns out to be recurrent transient ischemic attacks, secondary to extracranial vascular disease.

Surgically significant lesions of the cranial vasculature, that is, lesions in which surgical therapy can improve the prognosis for life or can decrease morbidity, are relatively rare compared with the common occurrence of cerebrovascular accidents or strokes. However, since surgery may decrease the morbidity and mortality of cerebrovascular disease and since there is relatively little other than supportive therapy, it is important to keep in mind the possibility of surgical intervention whenever cerebrovascular disease cases are seen. Surgical lesions fall into four groups of conditions with overlapping categories, such as infarction from congenital lesions and hematomas with infarcts. The groups are:

Transient ischemic attacks
Cerebral infarctions
Cerebral and cerebellar hematomas
Congenital lesions
    Aneurysms
    Arteriovenous malformations

Cerebral Ischemia and Infarction

Cerebral ischemia is a multifaceted problem which may originate with progressive atherosclerosis and which encompasses cerebral thrombosis, embolism, altered metabolic substrates, and hypoxia. Its ultimate pathological end point, a stroke, is the third leading cause of death and disability in the United States and accounts for the disability of some 2 million persons today. The logic of surgical intervention in this disease is predicated upon the reversibility of the process and demonstration of statistically significant prophylaxis.

The sites of atherosclerosis are generally bifurcations of major vessels. In decreasing order they are the carotid bifurcation in the neck; the vertebral basilar junction; the middle cerebral (MCA), posterior cerebral (PCA), and anterior cerebral (ACA) arteries; and the major ascending vessels from the aorta. Hypertension increases the predilection for atherosclerosis at each of these sites. Embolic phenomena are generally fibrin-platelet aggregates, and most of them arise in the heart, but many originate from one of the "local" vessels mentioned above. Embolic episodes usually affect the more distant vessels of the intracranial circulation, such as MCA and PCA, while the internal carotid artery (ICA) and vertebral are more subject to thrombosis.

The diagnosis of an occluded artery based on focal neurologic deficit was accepted for a long time, though it rarely was proved to be accurate at postmortem. Since arteriography, the assignment of the site of vascular disease on the basis of neurologic dysfunction has become even more insecure. A wide range of capability for adequate perfusion of the brain is maintained by the anastomoses described above, and these can alter the resulting neurologic dysfunction following occlusion of any of the major vessels.

The syndrome of "middle cerebral artery occlusion," described as a hemiparesis most severe in the arm with cortical sensory dysfunction, a partial visual field defect, and, if the hemisphere involved is the dominant hemisphere, dysphasia, does not necessarily require occlusion of the middle cerebral artery. It may result from narrowing of proximal vessels, the common sites being in the internal carotid artery at its origin in the neck or intracranially in its cavernous portion. In contrast, an individual may have a clinically silent carotid occlusion with maintenance of normal cerebral function distal to it because of adequate perfusion of the vessels by segments of the circle of Willis. Such a patient may eventually present with a "middle cerebral artery" syndrome when his opposite internal carotid has become sufficiently narrowed by atheromas to impair the adequacy of collateral flow. Thus, the effects of ischemia may be first apparent in the most distant reaches of the circulation on the side of the originally silent carotid occlusion. Anomalies and imperfections of the circle of Willis may remove its safety factor for some and make them early victims of arteriosclerosis, for they are less likely to have been protected from the effects of the loss of individual vessels.

The premorbid recognition of cerebrovascular disease often begins with an awareness of marginal cerebral blood flow presenting as transient ischemic attacks (TIAs), defined as focal neurological signs or symptoms of less than 24 hours in duration which have a tendency to recur. In the region of carotid perfusion, they are associated with local embolic phenomenon and herald a completed stroke in one-third of patients within 5 years. Some patients progress to stroke after only one or two warning TIAs. Symptoms include hemiparesis, hemisensory disturbance, and, commonly, decrease or loss of vision in the eye of the involved side (amaurosis fugax). Vertebrobasilar TIAs less frequently progress to stroke with statistical predictability; symptoms include vertigo, dysarthria, facial paresthesia, diplopia, sometimes paresis, and drop attacks. Immediate mortality rates from intracerebral hemorrhage, embolism, and thrombosis are approximately 93 percent, 60 percent, and 37 percent respectively. For those that survive, death rates from 16 to 18 percent per annum should be expected. A portion of this group with TIAs and more major infarctions may have a focal problem amenable to surgical treatment.

Identification of this group which may be helped by surgery is difficult, but a few guidelines are apparent. The workup of patients with TIAs should begin with a physical examination, including auscultation for a focal bruit over the suspected vessel—the carotid in hemispheric lesions, the subclavian or vertebral in brainstem disease. Next, regional cerebral blood flow is ascertained either with conventional nuclear brain scans or with more accurate xenon washout techniques that quantitate cerebral blood flow in milliliters per minute per 100 Gm cerebral tissue. Numerous Doppler systems now available are also able to pinpoint stenotic extracranial vessel disease and determine flow direction. Arch and cerebral angiography, however, must be performed to delineate accurately all the vascular pathologic change. There is a 5 to 7 percent morbidity from angiography in most series. It is important, therefore, to choose those patients in whom the chance of finding a remedial lesion is high enough to warrant this risk. If a stenotic or ulcerative lesion is localized, surgery may be appropriate. Treatment involves excision of the ulcerative or stenotic plaque, with or without vascular reconstruction or bypass around the obstruction. The most ideal patient for extracranial vascular surgery has TIAs, an isolated lesion, and no neurological deficit. In Ojemann's endarterectomy series, 104 patients with TIAs had a 1/104 mortality, 2/104 had neurological morbidity, and 101/104 resumed normal function. Fifty patients with persistent neurological deficit before surgery showed a 45/50 recovery, 2/45 mortality, and 5/45 neurological morbidity. A low surgical morbidity and mortality are dependent upon preoperative blood flow studies to identify the patient with borderline cerebral ischemia. At Yale, intraoperative distal internal carotid artery pressures are obtained and correlated with EEG and evoked cortical response recordings. Temporary bypass shunts are placed when the EEG or cortical evoked responses indicate inadequate perfusion.

Extracranial focal vascular lesions are accessible to direct intervention; however, a joint study of extracranial arterial occlusion concluded that about 33 percent of patients suffered from a surgically inaccessible lesion such as intracranial ICA stenosis, MCA occlusion, or complete ICA occlusion. In 1967, Donaghy and Yasargil successfully anastomosed the superficial temporal artery to a cortical branch of the MCA in two patients with inaccessible vascular disease. Since then, this operation has been performed in hundreds of patients, with low morbidity and mortality rates but without long-enough follow-up for statistical analysis of results. Recently, not only has the STA-MCA bypass been utilized but also occipital to posterior inferior cerebellar artery anastomoses have appeared in the treatment of vertebral basilar disease. At this time, indications for bypass procedures may include low-perfusion syndromes which are accompanied by ICA occlusion, carotid siphon stenosis, and MCA stenosis or occlusion. It has also been successfully employed as an additional source of flow to cerebral regions perfused by major intracranial vessels which may require occlusion during the treatment of another primary disease such as aneurysm, carotid cavernous fistulas, or neoplasms.

The other indication for surgical therapy for patients with cerebrovascular occlusion is in those patients with completed infarcts in whom symptoms of progressive focal neurologic deficit and brainstem involvement occur. The progression most commonly occurs from 12 to 36 hours after the stroke; it consists of increase in the initial focal deficit, such as hemiparesis to hemiplegia; decreasing levels of consciousness; and signs of third nerve paresis (dilated pupil) and midbrain dysfunction. This progression occurs since occasionally a major infarct constitutes a mass because of the volume of swollen edematous and, at times, hemorrhagic brain. In such circumstances, it behaves like other cerebral tumors in producing clinical signs and symptoms of progressive focal neurologic deficit and progressive brainstem involvement. The condition may be amenable to surgical removal or internal decompression of the swollen brain by craniotomy for relief of the pressure.

Cerebral and Cerebellar Hemorrhage

Although intracranial hemorrhage may result from any structural cause of an abnormality in the blood vessels or circulating blood, the most common cause of intracranial hematoma is hypertensive arteriosclerotic vascular disease. In patients succumbing to hypertensive intracranial hemorrhage, the larger arteries show hypertrophic and degenerative changes in their media and intima; the arterioles demonstrate thickness of the vessel walls and reduction in lumen caliber secondary to hypertrophy of the intimal lining; and only minor structural changes are present in the capillaries. The pathogenesis of hypertensive hemorrhage is unclear and thought to involve many factors. The blood pressure fluctuates in hypertension and, during periods of decreased systolic pressure, ischemia of tissue supplied by these diseased vessels and/or the arteries themselves may occur. The lack of arterial support from surrounding tissue (evidenced by "état lacunaire") and weakness in the vessel wall result in hemorrhage when the increased intraluminal pressure returns to the damaged segment. Arterial spasm with distal ischemia and decreased tonus may be significant mechanisms with hemorrhage resulting at the devitalized or necrotic channel after relaxation of the spasm.

The commonest sites of hypertensive hemorrhages are in the regions of the lentiform nucleus, deep white matter or cerebellar hemispheres, pons, and midbrain. Hemorrhage into the basal ganglion can be divided into lateral and medial involvement. The latter arises medial to the putamen and destroys the hypothalamus, usually resulting in death; however, the lateral group are in the putamen, external capsule, and claustrum and often are compatible with survival. In contrast to hemorrhagic infarction in which all tissue in the area is destroyed, hemorrhage has a tendency to track along tissue planes, separating rather than destroying the nervous tissue. This phenomenon is especially true when the hematoma has its origin in white matter and may result in relatively minor permanent neurologic deficit.

CLINICAL MANIFESTATIONS. Initial symptoms of intracranial hemorrhage may be nonspecific and include headache, dizziness, paresthesias, or mild speech disturbances. These symptoms are followed by a sudden "strokelike" syndrome of paresis, severe headache, severe speech disturbances, vomiting and/or loss of consciousness. The space-occupying hemorrhage may continue to enlarge and result in herniation of brain, secondary brainstem hemorrhage, and death. In instances where hemorrhage is situated in the medial basal ganglia, hypothalamus, brainstem, and dominant hemisphere temporal parietal speech areas in patients over fifty-five years of age, surgical intervention is probably not indicated because of the severe mortality and morbidity. However, intracranial hemorrhage at other sites may be surgically evacuated, frequently with little or no neurologic residual.

Approximate localization of the surgically accessible hematomas in the cerebral hemispheres is not difficult, since the patients present with neurologic dysfunction of the area involved. Usually carotid angiography is necessary to accurately localize the lesion in order to minimize surgical trauma. Hematomas of the cerebellar hemisphere are more difficult to recognize. A history suggestive of acute cerebellar dysfunction is most helpful but frequently not obtained, since initial loss of consciousness in patients with cerebellar hemorrhage is not uncommon. Cerebellar dysfunction with altered consciousness followed by progressive lower brainstem dysfunction, but without the pupillary signs and deep unconsciousness seen with pontine hemorrhages, should raise the suspicion of cerebellar hematoma. The brainstem signs most frequently seen in these conditions are slow respiratory rate, often with Cheyne-Stokes characteristics, slow pulse, hiccups, and difficulty with swallowing secretions. Early recognition of a cerebellar hematoma before major compromise of the lower brainstem occurs is necessary if a favorable outcome is to be achieved with surgical intervention.

Congenital Lesions

The vascular diseases most amenable to surgical intervention are those due to congenital lesions, namely, the saccular, or berry, aneurysm and the arteriovenous malformation.

ANEURYSMS

Most cerebral aneurysms are silent lesions that do not cause clinical disease and are often therefore incidental findings at autopsy. However, rupture of an aneurysm initiates a distinctly morbid train of events. The natural history of patients with ruptured aneurysms is still the subject of brisk controversy, since the reported mortality during the initial hemorrhage and during subsequent therapy varies from 20 to 75 percent. It is fair to state that there is a high initial mortality and that some of the lower figures do not take into account patients who never arrived at a surgical service. Although the prognosis is directly related to the degree of neurologic deficit following subarachnoid hemorrhage, approximately 27 percent of patients will die in the first week subsequent to ruptured aneurysm, the percentage declining thereafter. A second hemorrhage has a mortality of 42 percent, the incidence having its peak between 7 and 12 days following the initial hemorrhage. The likelihood of rebleeding then decreases through the ensuing 4 weeks to drop off sharply after 6 weeks; however, 10 percent of patients will re-hemorrhage after 1 year. From the onset of the rupture to the second or third month after the rupture there appears to be a mortality between 30 and 40 percent.

The majority of intracranial aneurysms arise from the larger intracranial arteries of the circle of Willis and at the origin of large vessels from the vertebrobasilar system. Intracranial arteries have a thin, poorly developed, adventitial layer, a media which is partially or completely devoid of elastic fibers, and an intima consisting of an elastic lamella and thin collagenous tissue covered by an endothelial lining. Aneurysms develop at the arterial bifurcation and are probably caused by the effect of hemodynamic factors on defects in the medial musculature and elastic layers of the artery.

The most common sites of intracranial aneurysms are the internal carotid artery (42 percent), anterior cerebral artery (43 percent), and middle cerebral arteries (20 percent), with 6 percent of aneurysms arising from the vertebrobasilar system in the posterior fossae. The majority of aneurysms are single; however, there is a 20 percent incidence of multiple aneurysms. When two aneurysms are present, they have a proclivity either for being symmetric in location or for arising from the same parent vessel.

The immediate cause of rupture of aneurysms usually cannot be determined, but the coincidence of hypertension and a congenital aneurysm appears to increase the possibility of rupture no matter what the cause of hypertension. Thus, in young patients with coarctation of the aorta with hypertension in the cerebral circulation ruptured aneurysms are common. There also seems to be a correlation between systolic hypertension and rupture of the aneurysm. Silent aneurysms are seen with approximately the same incidence in patients with or without hypertension, while rupture is more frequent in patients with hypertension.

CLINICAL MANIFESTATIONS. The syndrome of nontraumatic subarachnoid hemorrhage is one of sudden onset of headache followed by altered consciousness. Focal neurologic deficit may occur, but, in contrast to the occlusion of a major intracranial vessel, headache, meningeal signs, and altered consciousness are usually much more prominent and the focal neurologic deficit less prominent. The most common cause of this syndrome is a ruptured berry aneurysm. Other possible causes are hypertensive hemorrhage and a bleeding arteriovenous malformation.

The most benign syndrome of subarachnoid hemorrhage occurring from aneurysm is a sudden headache; maintenance of, or perhaps only transient loss of, consciousness; and the absence of any objective neurologic signs. The presence of the stiff neck and perhaps photophobia, reflecting the presence of blood in the cerebrospinal fluid, are the only signs that a major pathologic vascular syndrome has occurred. A patient with this syndrome is considered to be grade I in each of several schemas for evaluating patients with subarachnoid hemorrhage and presents an excellent opportunity for surgical intervention to alter the natural course of the disease. On the other end of the spectrum of subarachnoid hemorrhage, when a large amount of bleeding occurs in a short period of time, the basal cisterns may be filled with clotted blood, or dissection of the hematoma into the hemispheres may occur. At this time the patient is unconscious, and therapeutic manipulation or angiography has a high probability of increasing morbidity or mortality.

TREATMENT. A major factor in the mortality and morbidity of subarachnoid hemorrhage is vasospasm of the branches of the circle of Willis due to an irritating effect of the blood on the vessels. This may produce neurologic deficit without the presence of mass and has been considered by most surgeons to be a contraindication to early surgical treatment, since it is associated with a high operative mortality. The goal of the treatment is to remove the aneurysm from the force of systolic blood pressure; since recent evidence suggests that the probability of a second hemorrhage increases in a linear manner with time, the earliest possible accomplishment of this is indicated. The most favorable lesion is one in which the aneurysm has a narrow neck which can be occluded without interference of the parent vessel circulation. Not all aneurysms can be so treated; some may be coated with synthetic plastics to reinforce their walls, and others may be treated by occlusion of parent vessels, such as the common or internal carotid artery in the neck, to decrease the pulse pressure applied to an aneurysm of the internal carotid artery intracranially.

ARTERIOVENOUS MALFORMATIONS

A second major type of congenital vascular disease is arteriovenous malformation, which results from replacement of the capillary bed by clusters of abnormal vessels interposed between arterial and venous systems in a segment of the circulation. Such malformations tend to enlarge with time and may present in a variety of ways. Because the contiguous cerebral tissue may be chronically ischemic, neurologic symptoms and signs will include focal loss of neurologic function and altered excitability. For this reason focal neurologic deficits of a minor or major nature and seizures are frequently seen in these patients. Arteriovenous malformations also are causes of subarachnoid hemorrhage and intracerebral hematoma.

Subarachnoid hemorrhage due to arteriovenous malformation occurs generally at a younger age than that due to aneurysm. The majority of cases occur between twenty and forty-nine years of age without a peak incidence, whereas with aneurysm the majority occur between forty and sixty-four years of age with a peak incidence between fifty and fifty-four years.

Intracerebral hematoma resulting from "cryptic" vascular malformations is probably more common than generally appreciated and is frequently mistaken for hypertensive hemorrhage. These small arteriovenous malformations, measuring less than 3 cm maximum size, are usually clinically silent and may be more common than the classic arteriovenous anomaly. The cryptic anomaly may be destroyed by the hematoma and its pathogenesis impossible to determine. In contrast to hypertensive hemorrhage, hematoma secondary to arteriovenous anomalies tend to occur outside the basal ganglion in the cerebral hemisphere white matter and may be present in the cerebellum, spinal cord, and brainstem.

TREATMENT. Because of the possibility of increase in size of the malformation with increased shunting of blood to impair further the oxygenation of surrounding tissue, the continued problem of seizures, and the constant possibility of hemorrhage, surgical excision of the malformation is indicated whenever it is feasible. Feasibility of resection relates to size, position, and source of arterial supply. Arteriovenous malformations that are deep in the hemisphere are in general nonresectable, since according to their natural history they would have a lower morbidity than would be expected from surgical treatment. Excision of arteriovenous malformations in the tip of the occipital, frontal, or temporal lobe not only may be lifesaving in the face of hemorrhage but may control seizures and improve circulation in the involved hemisphere.

THE SURGERY OF EPILEPSY

Epilepsy is perhaps the oldest recorded neurological disorder. Its history traces a fascinating path from mysticism to accurate descriptions of cortical physiology and pathology. Although its study has provided insight into cerebral pathways and cortical functional localization, the cure or control of this disorder continues to frustrate the physician devoted to caring for seizure victims. There is controversy surrounding the incidence of convulsive disorders because of the lack of a universally accepted classification. Most studies place the incidence of epilepsy between 3.7 and 6.2 per 1,000 population. Two-thirds of patients with seizures have their initial seizure before the age of twenty. The older the patient, however, at the onset of epilepsy, the more likely a focal etiological cause will be found. In patients presenting with their first seizure after age twenty, between 10 and 25 percent will have a focal lesion (such as a tumor or arteriovenous malformation) demonstrated on a complete neurological workup.

The cornerstone of seizure control is medical therapy for those patients without obvious cerebral pathologic change. Anticonvulsant drugs will control seizures in more than half of the patients with epilepsy and achieve partial to almost complete control in another 25 percent. Surgical therapy is reserved for patients whose seizures are not well controlled with medication and whose history, description of the seizures, neurological examination, or electroencephalogram suggests a focal cerebral origin. Success of surgical treatment correlates best with accurate identification of these patients with focal seizures, precise localization of the point of origin, and careful surgical excision of the area. Accurate localization of the area and identification of any motor, sensory, or intellectual deficit that may be caused by excision of the focus require a team approach, utilizing the neurosurgeon, neurologist, electroencephalographer, neuroradiologist, and neuropsychologist, as well as the proper electrophysiological equipment and techniques.

The preliminary workup for a patient being considered for surgery includes a careful general physical and neurological examination, with evaluation of past medication and dosages and an additional medical trial if medication has not been used adequately. If the decision is to continue the presurgical workup, continuous electroencephalographic monitoring with scalp electrodes is begun, since the most accurate method of identifying the area of seizure onset is to record the electrical activity of spontaneously occurring seizures. To enhance the opportunity of recording spontaneous seizures, the anticonvulsant medication of the patient is often stopped or markedly decreased. This in itself can be dangerous because it may precipitate a series of seizures or even status epilepticus; therefore, constant observation by specially trained nursing and medical personnel is required. If the candidate's electroencephalogram is not so diffusely abnormal as to obviate further consideration, his workup continues. In search of a focal lesion, x-rays of the skull and computerized axial tomography are usually the first of the special tests. Additional neuroradiographic tests, such as pneumoencephalogram and arteriogram, are usually necessary. At the time of arteriography, with EEG surveillance, a short-acting barbiturate is injected selectively into each internal carotid artery and behavioral testing is carried out to determine speech dominance and the memory capacity of each temporal lobe (Wada test). Extensive neuropsychological testing is always indicated but is often difficult to evaluate because of the sedative effect of the anticonvulsant medication. If the scalp electrode electroencephalography and the special neuroradiological procedures have not identified an epileptic focus but suggest focality in one hemisphere or portion of a hemisphere, depth electrodes are implanted, especially in the deep medial frontal temporal regions where the majority of focal resectable lesions are located. With depth electrodes in place, the patient's condition is again monitored in a special nursing unit and medication again withdrawn if necessary to precipitate typical clinical and subclinical seizures.

A review of cerebral focal pathologic change in patients with intractable seizures was undertaken at the Montreal Neurological Institute. Among patients with intractable seizures, focal resectable lesions were found in the following distribution: temporal lobe, 60 percent; frontal lobe, 9 percent; combined frontal and temporal, 10 percent; parietal, 3 percent; central, 7 percent; occipital, 1 percent; and multilobular, 10 percent. This series does not imply that the majority of intractable seizures arise in the temporal lobe, although it has been well recognized for years that temporal lobe seizures are difficult to control medically and may respond to surgical excision of lesions. The series implies that a majority of potentially resectable lesions will lie in the temporal lobe. The Montreal Neurological Institute's most common findings were medial temporal sclerosis or the scarring secondary to injury of the medial temporal lobe, low-grade gliomas, and a few focal lesions including meningocerebral cicatrix, granulomatous disease, parasitic disease, tuberous sclerosis, vascular abnormalities, and scarring from an infarct. The follow-up of 1,145 patients surgically treated at the Montreal Neurological Institute for intractable epilepsy revealed at the end of 10 years that 36 percent remained seizure-free and 28 percent had rare attacks or reduction to less than 1 percent of their preoperative frequency. However, almost all patients required continuation of their anticonvulsive medication. Thus, 64 percent have almost complete control of their seizures while 36 percent continue to have seizures at variably reduced rates. These results certainly indicate the efficacy of surgical treatment in selected patients with intractable epilepsy. They point out, however, that despite careful evaluation, multiple areas of epileptogenic activity occur in almost one-third of the patients who appear to have a focal seizure disorder, and suggest either the failure of the evaluation techniques or generalized altered neuronal excitability in patients with intractable seizures.

Electrophysiological studies in animals have indicated that subcortical structures alter the excitability of the cortex. Much work has been done in an attempt to utilize this information clinically. As yet, such therapeutic trials are experimental and require further evaluation. The technique which appears most likely to be of value is stimulation of the cerebellum, and surgical and electronic techniques for doing this are well developed. The results are controversial, but the concepts offer the possibility that in the future some patients with diffuse or multicentric origin of seizures may be returned to a more normal existence.

INTRACRANIAL INFECTIONS

Infections of the central nervous system and its coverings have surgical significance if they produce a mass, hydrocephalus, or osteomyelitis, or are the result of a break in, or absence of, continuity of the nervous system coverings.

A mass can be caused by pus, as in abscess or empyema, by the edema of the reaction of the nervous system to infection, by the edema of venous occlusion, or by an effusion in the subdural space. Hydrocephalus may be caused by the interruption of cerebrospinal fluid flow by blockage at the villi or basal cisterns, or within the ventricular system. Osteomyelitis of the skull and spine has surgical significance because of the propensity for the

infected bone to become necrotic and sequester, forming the nidus for chronic inflammation, abscess, and progressive infection of adjacent bone and intracranial contents.

Surgical therapy of infections of the nervous system falls into one or more of the following categories: excision of infected bone, drainage or excision of abscess or empyema, decompression to relieve the effects of edema, shunting to relieve obstruction of cerebrospinal fluid circulation, and the repair or establishment of anatomic barriers to infection. This last category may involve surgical procedures as diverse as repair of a congenital heart lesion, eradication of a chronic middle ear infection, or removal of a pituitary tumor that has eroded into the sphenoid sinus.

Osteomyelitis of the Skull

Infections of the skull are relatively rare. The pathogenesis of osteomyelitis of the skull includes three major avenues of origin: (1) direct extension of preexisting infection in a paranasal sinus, middle ear, or mastoid air cells; (2) infection from a wound of the scalp that extends into or below the subgaleal space; and (3) hematogenous spread from elsewhere in the body. Any organism can be the causative agent, but by far the most common are *S. aureus* and the gram-negative contaminants of ear infection, such as *Bacillus proteus* and *B. pyocyaneus*. Once the infection is established, it usually spreads through the diploic spaces and the epidural space. Although spread under the outer periosteal layer or pericranium does occur, the pericranium is so firmly attached to the skull that it limits this as an important avenue of spread. This same attachment of the pericranium sometimes gives a false impression of the extent of the skull infection. Part of the mechanism of spread of the infection includes damage to the blood supply of the skull, and therefore necrosis and sequestration of the bone is common.

CLINICAL MANIFESTATIONS. The signs and symptoms of pyogenic infection of the skull are those of generalized infection, that is, fever, malaise, and leukocytosis, with focal tenderness and swelling. At times the infection can be indolent and manifest itself first by drainage through an area of the scalp, but more often it is highly virulent with spread into the intracranial structures, resulting in irritation and inflammation of the brain.

TREATMENT. The only effective treatment is excision of the involved bone and drainage of the area. Care must be taken to be certain that no infection remains in the epidural space to strip away the dura or in the diploic spaces to further necrose and infect adjacent bone. Appropriate antibiotics are helpful in protecting the bone edges and epidural space from further spread of the infection but are of little help without surgical excision of infected necrotic bone.

Epidural Abscess

Intracranial epidural abscesses are most commonly seen adjacent to infections of the skull and therefore are common near the middle ear, mastoid air cells, and nasal sinuses. Although the dura is a good protective barrier against inward spread of infection and although many epidural abscesses are discovered as incidental findings of surgical treatment for mastoid and sinus infection, they should not be considered benign processes. The infection can and often does break through the dural barrier, meningitis being the most common result and brain abscess the next most common. As already mentioned, the epidural space is an avenue for progression of osteomyelitis of the skull.

CLINICAL MANIFESTATIONS. The symptoms of epidural abscess are quite similar to skull infections, except that seizures and focal neurologic deficits are more common. These are commonly secondary to thrombophlebitis of superficial cortical veins.

TREATMENT. Treatment of epidural abscess is trephination, drainage, excision of infected bone, and the use of appropriate antibiotics. The excision of any infected bone and the drainage of any infected sinus or mastoid air cells are mandatory if the infection is not to recur.

Subdural Empyema

Although intracranial spread of paranasal sinus, ear, and mastoid infections to the epidural and subarachnoid spaces is more common, the high rate of morbidity and mortality seen with delayed or inadequate treatment with spread to the subdural space requires that this possibility always be kept in mind. Infections of the paranasal sinuses are the most common source of subdural empyema, and the spread of the infection to the subdural space is felt to include direct extension along emissary veins and via dural sinuses.

CLINICAL MANIFESTATIONS. The symptom complex of subdural empyema is related to five factors: First is the pathogenicity of the organism. Although staphylococci, *B. proteus,* and *B. pyocyaneus* are common chronic infecting agents of the sinus, ear, and mastoid areas and may cause subdural empyema, the infection is more often caused by staphylococci or streptococci that are acutely superimposed on a chronic infection. With these highly pathogenic organisms the course of subdural empyema may proceed to serious neurologic deficit in hours and to death within days. Second, there is no natural barrier to spread of the infection within the subdural space. Because of this the surface of an entire hemisphere may be involved within a very short period of time, and progression beneath the falx to the opposite hemisphere may occur as soon as significant pus has accumulated. Third, the veins traversing the subdural space from cortex to the dural sinuses are particularly vulnerable to inflammatory response from the infection, with progressive thrombosis of the cortical veins and dural sinuses resulting. Fourth, the reaction in the subarachnoid space and surface of the hemisphere through the thin piarachnoid causes a sterile meningitis and an acute encephalitis. Finally, there is the mass effect, mainly secondary to the inflammatory reaction and the occlusion in venous drainage but also in part secondary to the volume of pus.

The first factors relate to rapidity of onset and the in-

volvement of the entire hemisphere within a short period of time, while the last three explain in part the high incidence of seizures, signs of meningitis, neurologic deficit, and massive edema. Thus the symptom pattern of a patient with subdural empyema may vary but is best characterized as follows: A patient with a history of chronic sinusitis or chronic ear infection has an acute upper respiratory tract infection. Two or three days later when he should be making an uneventful recovery, he has a sudden secondary rise in temperature, shaking chills, and a convulsion. On regaining consciousness he complains of severe lateralized headache and of mild weakness or numbness on the opposite side of the body. Within a short period of time, a few moments to a few hours, he has another convulsion and then progressive decrease in his sensorium. At this point he is frequently either brought to a hospital or seen by a physician. Initial examination reveals an acutely ill patient with signs of meningitis. Lumbar puncture shows increased cellular response, but the spinal fluid sugar is within normal limits, and the microscopic smears fail to reveal any evidence of bacteria.

Within a few hours the patient can be in severe difficulty, often with total loss of function in the involved hemisphere, evidence of herniation of the temporal lobe with a dilated pupil on the side involved, and the beginning of decerebration.

TREATMENT. Treatment varies with the severity of the symptoms at the time that the patient is seen and the rapidity with which they have progressed. However, early trephination and drainage alone would be a satisfactory treatment only if the patient shows no signs of increased intracranial pressure, major alteration of conscious level, or shift of the midline structures. If the patient already shows any of these signs, drainage of the subdural space, external decompression by removal of a major portion of the skull on the side involved, and opening of the dura to allow expansion of the hemisphere are mandatory if the patient is to survive with good neurologic function. Although this appears to be a rather heroic treatment, the fact that the major deficit is secondary to inflammation and venous occlusion allows a degree of recovery to occur that is most gratifying, provided the treatment is started before the upper brainstem becomes irreversibly damaged.

Brain Abscess

Intracerebral pyogenic infection can be categorized as acute, subacute, or chronic. The symptoms and signs of suppuration within the brain encompass a range that extends from rapidly progressive focal neurologic deficit with a systemic response indicative of severe infection to evidence of an expanding intracranial mass with no suggestion of infection. In the former, the symptoms usually relate to a focal pyogenic encephalitis with little or no frank pus that will either resolve into an abscess or cause death if it continues to spread unchecked, while in the latter the abscess has a well-formed capsule of fibrous tissue and glial reaction.

The brain is resistant to infection by bacteria. Experimentally it is difficult to produce an abscess or focal en-

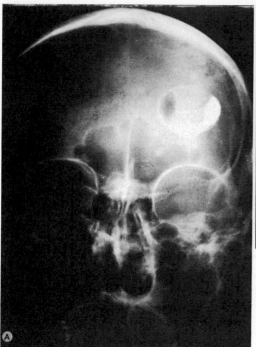

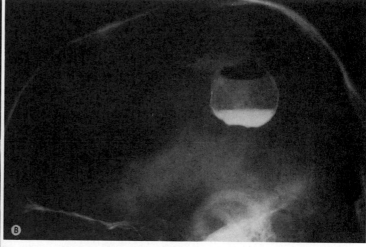

Fig. 42-4. Roentgenograms of brain abscess. A middle-aged man with a neurologic syndrome compatible with an expanding parenchymal mass in the dominant hemisphere. Diagnosis of brain abscess was established by carotid arteriography and ventriculography. The abscess cavity was tapped, producing 30 ml of pus. One milliliter of microbarium sulfate and several milliliters of air were injected into the cavity to mark the lesion before these x-rays were taken.

cephalitis within the brain unless the area in which bacteria are placed is damaged beforehand, as by trauma, hemorrhage, or anoxia. Although the brain initially responds to infection in the same fashion as any tissue, its ability to wall off the infection by granulation and glial tissue is so effective that it often isolates the infection not only from the brain but even from significant contact with the systemic blood supply. For this reason the contents of a localized brain abscess usually cannot be sterilized by systemic antibiotics.

The pathogenesis of brain abscess includes, in the order of frequency of occurrence, three main routes of entry of the infecting organism: by direct extension from middle ear, mastoid, and paranasal sinus infections; through the blood supply to the central nervous system; and by direct traumatic penetration. Posttraumatic brain abscess is now rare, since adequate surgical care of the wound and antibiotic protection are excellent preventives. The ear is three or four times more common as a source of the infection for brain abscess than are the sinuses, and the temporal lobe and cerebellar hemispheres are the more common sites for abscesses secondary to these infections. Hematogenous abscesses can occur following any bacteremia but are more commonly seen with lung abscess, infected bronchiectasis, and cyanotic heart disease. In the patient with cyanotic heart disease the presence of a right-to-left heart

shunt with the loss of the lung as a filter to remove bloodborne bacteria is felt to be the mechanism responsible for the high frequency of occurrence of brain abscess. The organisms commonly seen in brain abscess are streptococci, pneumococci, and staphylococci. The most common streptococci are the anaerobic strains.

CLINICAL MANIFESTATIONS. The symptom complex of brain abscess will vary according to whether the infection is acute, subacute, or chronic. As was noted earlier, in the chronic walled-off brain abscess there may be no signs of systemic reaction to infection, that is, no fever or leukocytosis. Brain abscess should be considered as a possible diagnosis in any patient with progressive focal neurologic deficit and increasing mass with a short, that is a 2- to 3-week, history. Often with questioning a source of possible brain abscess or an episode suggestive of bacteremia can be found in the recent past. Acute pyogenic encephalitis has a course quite similar to a subdural abscess, from which it is often difficult to differentiate.

The subacute abscess varies between these two extremes, so that the combination of signs of inflammation, progressive focal neurologic deficit, and increasing mass effect not only suggests the presence of a brain abscess but also frequently from the neurologic signs localizes it. Further studies that help in localizing the brain abscess are skull films (Fig. 42-4), which may show shift of the pineal; electroencephalogram, which characteristically has a very high incidence of marked slow-wave activity over the area of abscess; brain scan; and computerized axial tomography. The fibrous tissue and breakdown of the blood-brain barrier around an abscess cause a high uptake of the radioactive material with good localization in the brain scan, but CT scan has become the best method of identifying the presence of one or more brain abscesses, accurately localizing them and demonstrating the presence or absence of a capsule.

TREATMENT. Although in the past it was taught that suppurative intracranial encephalitis could not be treated surgically, decompression, removal of portions of the infected brain, and the use of antibiotics may be lifesaving and function-saving when applied to the critically ill patient in the acute stage. Usually the patient can be carried through the acute stage by the use of antibiotics and anti-inflammatory agents, such as steroids, and by careful control of fluids. Within 10 to 12 days the abscess usually is walled off and can be localized by combining the findings on neurologic examination, electroencephalography, radioactive brain scan, and arteriography. Occasionally ventriculography is necessary.

Once localization has been accomplished, drainage of the abscess by intermittent tapping through a perforator opening, by constant drainage, or by excision of the abscess will give a high percentage of cures. In hematogenous abscesses more than half will be multiple, and care must be taken to be certain that an abscess is not missed. The major dangers to the patient with abscess of the brain are (1) the early acute edematous response the brain has to pyogenic infection, (2) the continued problem of a mass lesion from both the edema and the suppuration itself, and (3) the continued possibility of rupture of the abscess into the ventricular system. This latter complication can be rapidly fatal. With the advent of antibiotics and anti-inflammatory agents such as steroids, brain abscess should have low mortality and, depending upon its location, low morbidity rates. However, failure to diagnose its presence until late in its course, failure to realize the dangers of mass effects from the abscess, the surrounding reaction of the brain, and the concurrence of cardiac disease and systemic infection have kept the mortality rate in most reported series between 35 and 45 percent.

PAIN

Pain, the symptom that most commonly brings a patient to a physician, can be simultaneously the protector and the debilitator. As a protector it calls for diagnostic inquiry, but when it no longer has protective value, it can be a disease in itself. The best treatment of pain is the removal of its cause. When this is not possible or must be delayed, drugs, and particularly opiates and their derivatives, can be used for relief. All potent analgesics, however, have addicting qualities and therefore decreasing effectiveness with continued use, so that if more than a few months of pain relief is required, drugs not only are ineffective but also can contribute to physical deterioration and mental depression. The need for prolonged effective control has been the impetus for surgeons to devise surgical means for relieving pain. Horsley's resection of the gasserian ganglion (1891), section of dorsal roots by Bennett and Abbe (1889), and Martin's incision into the anterolateral portion of the spinal cord (1911) were milestones in this quest, but further success has been limited by the same lack of information that has limited the control of pain by any method. This lack of knowledge exists not only in the spheres of anatomy and physiology but even in defining pain. Is pain a sensory modality with its own anatomic and physiologic correlates, or is it a learned response to environmental alteration which threatens the organism? Is pain an emotional reaction evoked with or without stimuli, or is it the recognition that a central nervous system pathway or area has been activated, indicating that a portion of the organism has reached or exceeded its functional limits? There is justification for the concept that pain contains some or all of these attributes.

ANATOMY AND PHYSIOLOGY. There are many theories concerning the anatomy and physiology of pain, but they usually fall within two extremes: on the one hand pain is considered a sensory modality with specific end organs, peripheral nerve fibers, and central nervous system pathways, while on the other hand pain is regarded as a learned response to patterns of nervous system activity that denotes damage or threatened damage to the body. There is evidence in support of both theories, and there are phenomena that cannot be explained by either. It has been shown that the smaller peripheral nerve fibers and their free endings must be activated to recognize a stimulus as painful, but these fibers and endings have also been shown to be activated by nonpainful stimuli, and with such activation touch, hot, and cold can be recognized. A lesion of the anterolateral spinal cord causes loss of pain and temperature sensation on the opposite side of the body, but return of pain perception in the area occurs over many months or years without evidence of regeneration. Section of several adjacent dorsal roots causes loss of all sensation, including recognition of noxious stimuli over their peripheral distribution, but often is associated with paresthesias that are described as "unbearable" pain in the anesthetic area. Although the expression of pain contains many attributes of learned processes, the person with congenitally absent pain sensation learns to protect his body only from the effects of visible damage, and the newborn infant without significant periods of learning responds to painful stimuli with effective movement and characteristic vocalization.

The diversity of these theories not only reflects the incompleteness of basic knowledge but foretells the difficulties of ablative control of pain. According to theories at the first extreme a correctly placed surgical lesion should always relieve pain, while it would follow from theories at the opposite extreme that a procedure should rarely relieve pain. Neither is the case, nor do the theories at either extreme explain the problems encountered in the surgical relief of pain.

The analogies of the physiology of pain comparing experimental findings in animals and human beings with observations in human beings can be a basis for understanding pain in patients, but the concept must include suffering and its treatment. In the patient pain causes suffering, but suffering alone can be expressed as pain. In the former the removal of the cause of the pain or a lesion to block the conduction of pain from the area will relieve the suffering, but in the latter, since pain is not caused by physical stimuli but is the expression of an emotional problem, alteration in pain perception may increase the suffering and therefore the expressed pain. Differentiating the part each plays in the clinical situation is difficult and at times impossible, but failure to recognize that both exist is probably the most common reason for failure to relieve pain by surgical means.

Studies of the anatomy and physiology of pain encompass many techniques and have engendered much controversy, but despite the lack of a solution as to what is pain, they have indicated directions for conceptualization of pain. Classically, or at least since Edinger's description of the crossed afferent pathway, the spinothalamic tract has been considered to be the pain pathway. Its anatomy consists of a primary neuron in the dorsal root ganglion with its central axon entering the spinal cord in the lateral portion of the dorsal root synapsing on cells of the dorsal root entry zone. The axons of these cells ascend three to four segments and then cross in the anterior commissure of the cord. Its cephalad course continues through the anterior and lateral funiculi of the cord into the lateral portion of the reticular formation of the medulla, through the pons just lateral to the medial lemniscus and ventral to the lateral lemniscus, continuing adjacent to the lateral side of the medial lemniscus in the midbrain, and ending in the nucleus ventralis posterolateralis of the thalamus.

The pathway was defined by staining the altered myelin of wallerian degeneration after section of the dorsal roots and after lesions in the dorsal root entry zone and anterolateral quadrant of the spinal cord. Its function was suggested from the animal experimentation of Schiff, Voroschilov, and Sherrington, and the clinical observations of Gowers, Brown-Séquard, and Spiller. These suggestions were confirmed by the operative section of the anterolateral portion of the spinal cord by Martin and Frazier. The first central ablative procedure for pain, anterolateral chordotomy, has continued to the present to be one of the most effective methods of relieving pain in the lower portions of the body.

Is the spinothalamic tract the pain pathway? As was mentioned above, activation of smaller fibers (less than 6 μ diameter) of peripheral nerve appears necessary for the appreciation of noxious stimuli, and these smaller fibers have been shown to project to central pathways composed of similar or smaller-sized fibers. The Marchi stain, used for staining degenerating myelin in the central nervous system, only stains fibers 6 μ or larger, and a pathway defined by this technique would only coincidentally define a pain pathway. Of the thousands of fibers lying in the anterior and lateral funiculi of the spinal cord only a small percentage can be traced to the posterior ventral nucleus of the thalamus in human beings, and in subprimates none can. Lesions placed in the spinothalamic tract as outlined by the Marchi degeneration at the midbrain level often cause burning dysesthesias rather than relief of pain, and lesions placed anywhere in the tract not only do not give permanent loss of pain but cause only a relative even though marked analgesia.

The Nauta-Glees method of staining degenerating axons also has been used to trace degeneration following a lesion in the anterolateral funiculi of the spinal cord. This method not only allows the smaller fibers to be followed but shows terminal degeneration, i.e., degeneration at synaptic junctions. The technique has shown that in human beings there is little evidence of synaptic transfer as the axons ascend to the cervical medullary junction. It is a lesion of this portion of the central nervous system, that is, the anterolateral quadrant of the spinal cord, that produces marked analgesia. In subprimates there is considerable loss of stainable fibers as each segment of the spinal cord is passed, and there is also degeneration signifying synapses in the gray matter of the cord. This agrees in part with the impression of Brown-Séquard that pain may travel in the central gray matter of the cord. In primates the loss of fibers is less until the medulla is reached, but even these few fibers may explain the gradual decrease in analgesia seen after chordotomy. In both primates and subprimates a major synaptic area is seen at the lower end of the brainstem in the medial portion of the reticular core with many fibers turning into, and projecting to, this area.

Comparison of the findings of the Nauta-Glees technique with the Marchi technique shows major differences. With the Nauta-Glees technique the fibers are more widely disseminated at each level of observation within the central nervous system, and major areas of synapse are seen at the cervical medullary junction, in the midpontine level at the oral pole of the nucleus gigantocellularis, and in the tegmentum. The fibers appear to be more dorsally placed at the level of the colliculus, and in the thalamus only a very few fibers go to the posterior ventral nucleus, more being seen medially approaching the centramedian and parafascicularis nuclei.

The concept that there are specific peripheral nerve fibers and central nervous system neurons responsive only to pain has recently been reexamined; evidence for peripheral receptor units uniquely responsive to noxious stimuli have been demonstrated by Perl and his coworkers, and neurons uniquely responsive to strong mechanical stimuli in the dorsal root entry zone and trigeminal system also have been identified. The fibers have been small myelinated or unmyelinated fibers, and the anatomic characteristics of the receptors are not known. Although this recent evidence further dilutes a basis for the pattern theory of pain, that an isolated receptor or fiber can be stimulated and produce pain has not been demonstrated. The demonstration of such structures uniquely responsive to noxious stimuli still does not explain some of the pain syndromes seen clinically, e.g., causalgia, postherpetic neuralgia, and thalamic pain. These all have the common finding that usually nonpainful stimuli, such as light touch, are painful and that the pain continues after the stimulus and spreads to contiguous areas. This indicates an altered excitability has occurred with a peripheral nerve lesion in the first condition, a peripheral nerve and dorsal root ganglion lesion in the second, and a central nervous system lesion in the third. Little is known concerning the control of excitability of afferent pathways and even less concerning pain. Melzack and Wall, elaborating on experimental studies in animals, suggested that activity in larger peripheral nerve fibers alters excitabilities of the cells upon which the smaller fibers synapse. This suggests an inhibitory influence of the large fibers on pain conduction. Since the peripheral nerve lesion in causalgia and herpetic neuralgia is mainly damage to large fibers, Melzack and Wall offered both pain syndromes as examples of loss of peripheral control. They further postulated that descending influences from upper centers impose control at each synaptic junction.

Anatomical and physiological studies have demonstrated significant evidence for direct and indirect descending cortical, subcortical, and brainstem control of afferent input at various levels of the neuro axis from the dorsal root entry zone to the midbrain. Although this evidence might a priori be assumed to apply to modulation of the afferent input of noxious stimuli, more specific information concerning modulation of the input from noxious stimuli has been gathered from diverse experimental approaches, a portion of which has included activation of spinal descending pathways. The evidence includes a demonstration of effective analgesia in rats from electrical stimulation in the brainstem, the presence of opiate receptors in the paraventricular and brainstem gray matter in vertebrates, and the isolation of endogenous polypeptides from the brain and pituitary gland with opiate properties. Other studies have shown that minute amounts of opiates injected into areas with opiate receptors produce analgesic effects without significant systemic levels of the opiate compound, and that opiate antagonists such as naloxone can reverse the opiate effects of brainstem stimulation in areas of opiate receptors, the opiate effect of focally injected opiates, and some of the analgesic effects of paraventricular stimulation in humans. In rats, analgesic effects from systemic opiates, from brainstem injection of opiates, and from stimulation of the brainstem have been shown to be markedly reduced below lesions sectioning the dorsolateral funiculus of the spinal cord. This information has not only altered some concepts of analgesic actions of opiates but, because of the correlation of many of the sites of opiate receptors and brainstem analgesic responses with what has been designated as a limbic system and its input, has also brought forth hypotheses for unifying some pain states and affective disorders. The combination of the demonstration of specific opiate receptors and peptide ligands that interact with these receptors to produce opiate effects has further melded the anatomy and pharmacology of pain and opened significant new avenues for its study.

Surgical Relief of Pain

Despite the paucity of knowledge concerning pain, empiric observations combined with physiologic studies have given neurosurgeons effective methods for surgically relieving pain. They fall into one of five different categories:

1. Section of the peripheral nerve pathway: neurectomy, sphlanchnicectomy, dorsal rhizotomy
2. Section of central nervous system pathways: anterior lateral chordotomy, and trigeminal tractotomy
3. Procedures to alter affective response to pain: thalamotomy, lobotomy, cingulumotomy
4. Section of the efferent arc of the vasomotor reflex: sympathectomy
5. Suppression by stimulation

Despite many variations in technique and many claims for various procedures, clinical experience has demonstrated that all the procedures for relief of pain from lesions of the nervous system fall into one of the first four categories and that each category has its area of application, its inherent rate of success, and its complications. Experience with suppression of pain by stimulation, if related to acupuncture, has accumulated for centuries. However, there is still too little objective evidence to determine the extent of its usefulness and its long-term effectiveness. Application of the correct procedure at the correct time to a suitable patient is the most difficult aspect of the surgery for pain.

SECTION OF THE PERIPHERAL PATHWAY

Section of the peripheral pathway for pain causes loss of all sensation distal to the area of section. Permanent loss occurs only when the pathway is sectioned proximal to the sensory ganglion, that is, section of the dorsal roots, termed *rhizotomy*. Any procedure that damages primary sensory neurons gives subjective sensory loss, which has as a complication painful paresthesias or spontaneous pain in the anesthetic area in 5 to 8 percent of cases. The explanation for this pain may be altered excitability of the dorsal root entry zone neurons. However, since further pain pathway interruption usually intensifies the pain, a more logical explanation appears to be that in this group of patients the subjective sensation of sensory loss signifies something wrong with the area and is painful. Any further alteration in sensation increases the pain. The psychologic basis of this may be that anything painful is abnormal, and therefore anything abnormal is painful. Stressing the lack of significance of such feelings at times helps, but alteration in affective response either by psychotherapeutic drugs or surgical intervention sometimes is the only recourse when the paresthesias become unbearable.

Section of multiple dorsal roots is seldom considered for relief of pain in a functioning limb, since loss of position sense, gamma afferents, and sense of touch leave the limb useless. It is of value in the thoracic area or where only one root is directly involved. In the former, touch and position senses are not of functional significance, and in the latter, sensory overlap of adjacent roots makes the peripheral sensory loss minimal. This sensory overlap of adjacent roots makes section of at least two and usually three roots necessary for significant deafferentation of any peripheral area.

Rhizotomy of the trigeminal nerve is used to control pain of malignant tumors of the face and trigeminal neuralgia. Trigeminal neuralgia, or tic douloureux, is a painful condition of the trigeminal nerve of unknown cause, characterized by paroxysms of pain over one or two adjacent divisions of the fifth cranial nerve. The paroxysms are often initiated by any stimulus in localized areas of the division involved, known as "trigger zones." Section of the preganglionic fibers of the trigeminal nerve or of the descending trigeminal tract in the brainstem permanently controls the pain, but as with other peripheral nerve section painful paresthesias may arise.

An observation by Jennett that patients with trigeminal neuralgia frequently have vascular compression of the trigeminal rootlets as they exit from the pons suggests altered conduction and excitability at the root entry zone of the brainstem as the cause of the syndrome of trigeminal neuralgia. Jennett also has suggested that other paroxysmal disorders of cranial nerves, such as glossopharyngeal neuralgia and facial tic, have the same cause. Compression of the trigeminal nerve more distally does not correlate with the syndrome, and decompression of the compressing vessels from the trigeminal rootlets has achieved a high percentage of relief without significant sensory loss.

Peripheral pathway section was the first procedure used for relief of pain, but because of the annoyance of the feeling of numbness, the incidence of paresthesias, nerve regeneration, and the availability of other procedures, it is now rarely used except for denervating trigger areas in the control of trigeminal pain by avulsion of either the supraorbital or infraorbital nerve.

Sphlanchnicectomy effectively denervates the upper abdominal viscera and is used for relief of intractable pain of the upper abdomen. Although the sphlanchnic nerves are part of the sympathetic nervous system, it is the interruption of the visceral afferent fibers coursing within the sympathetic nerves that gives the relief of pain. Their cells of origin are in the dorsal root ganglion, as are the cells of all peripheral sensory nerves, but since they have no surface innervation and paresthesias of denervation are always referred to the surface, painful paresthesias are not seen following their interruption. Since at times with malignant disease of the upper abdomen somatic sensory fibers in the intercostal nerves are involved, dorsal root section or chordotomy may be more effective than sphlanchnicectomy.

SECTION OF CENTRAL NERVOUS SYSTEM PATHWAYS

When Martin in 1911 made an incision in the anterolateral quadrant of a patient's spinal cord, the era of surgical control of intractable pain commenced. Anterolateral chordotomy has remained an effective means of controlling intractable pain, and many surgeons have contributed their skill and knowledge to modify Martin's original procedure so that it is a simple and reliable method for production of analgesia. Section of the tract in the spinal cord causes no subjective sensory loss and therefore rarely causes dysesthesias or paresthesias, but it has limitations. Since the fibers projecting to the anterolateral quadrant of the spinal cord ascend three to four segments before crossing in the spinal cord, incision of the quadrant gives loss of pain and temperature sensation on the opposite side of the body three or more segments below the level of the chordotomy. Thus, even a perfectly performed high cervical chordotomy fails to block pain in the upper arm, shoulder, or neck; therefore the procedure is best used for control of pain below the upper thoracic level. The loss of pain, although marked, can be demonstrated to be incomplete, and with time islands of pain perception appear, and with them the original pain usually returns. This may take a year or more to occur and limits in part the usefulness of the procedure for pain from benign conditions.

Lesions further cephalad in the spinothalamic tract, that is, at the midbrain, although causing loss of pain without subjective sensory loss, may also cause dysesthesias or the sensation of pain from nonpainful stimuli. The cause of this dysesthesia is unknown.

Section of the descending, or spinal, tract of the trigeminal nerve in the medulla causes loss of pain and temperature sensation in the ipsilateral face. It is used to control pain in the face, but since the operation has a higher morbidity and mortality than preganglionic section of the trigeminal nerve in the middle fossa, it is usually used only when it is feared a patient would not tolerate anesthesia of the face or when paralysis of the motor portion of the trigeminal on the opposite side is already present. In this latter condition the danger of bilateral paralysis of the muscles of mastication by approaching the nerve distad is higher than the morbidity of medullary tractotomy.

Stereotaxic lesions have been placed in the posterior medial thalamus in the area of the centramedian and nucleus parafascicularis, structures suggested by electrophysiologic and axonal degeneration studies as projections of the medial spinal reticular tracts. These procedures have been reported to relieve pain without any loss of pinprick or temperature sensation in the periphery, but their effectiveness is short-lived. It can be hoped, however, that with more basic information lesions for control will be devised that either interrupt major projections of the impulses defining a stimulus as noxious or increase the blockade of such impulses as they attempt to pass each controlled synaptic junction.

PROCEDURES TO ALTER AFFECTIVE RESPONSE TO PAIN

On a basis of the work in primates of Fulton and Jacobson, Egas Moniz in 1935 persuaded his neurosurgical colleague Lima to perform a prefrontal lobotomy on a psychiatric patient with marked anxiety as part of the basis for the psychiatric problem. The success of the procedure prompted many other surgeons to try prefrontal lobotomy for psychiatric illness. Altered affect, particularly in response to peripheral stimuli, and relief of anxiety was seen in the patients as it had been seen in the animals, and it seemed probable that the reaction of the patients to pain might be similarly altered. Van Wagenen in 1942 performed bilateral prefrontal lobotomies on a mentally ill patient who had phantom limb pain, and his success in altering the patient's complaint prompted other surgeons to use the same procedure in patients with intractable pain. Experience with the procedure of prefrontal lobotomy has shown that the lobotomy patient is unconcerned with the pain but when questioned still reports the pain as present. This lack of concern is no different for pain than it is for other stimuli, and therefore the procedure alters not only the response to pain but the entire affect of the patient. Lesions of the nonspecific nuclei of the thalamus, as in the dorsal median nucleus, lesions of the limbic system, such as cingulumotomy, or excisions of gyri in the prefrontal cortex all produce the same response with varying degrees of affective change.

The major limitation of these procedures is this change in personality. The same effect can be obtained with psychotherapeutic drugs, such as chlorpromazine, but with drugs it can be reversed. For this reason, the procedures for altering affective response to pain are rarely used but still should remain a part of the physician's armamentarium for care of the terminally ill patient whose fears make the situation and the pain unbearable for the patient and the family alike, and for the occasional patient where relief of anxiety will make it possible to resume a more normal life.

SECTION OF THE EFFERENT ARC OF THE VASOMOTOR REFLEX

Pain that occurs in diseases which cause alteration in blood flow of an extremity, such as Raynaud's syndrome or erythromelalgia, or conditions which cause marked vasospasm, such as causalgia following nerve injury, and the pain of obstruction of the major vessels in an extremity where circulation can be reestablished by dilatation of collateral vessels will respond to sympathectomy. Much has been written about possible sensory function in the sympathetic nervous system; however, aside from the visceral afferent fibers in the sphlanchnic nerves, no evidence of sensory function has been demonstrated. The clinical experience that sympathectomy does not relieve pain unless evidence of altered blood flow is present before sympathectomy bears this out. The occasional exception experienced by surgeons is more likely related to the placebo effect of any form of therapy rather than to alteration in peripheral afferent pathways.

Surgical treatment for pain is a useful adjunct to the care of patients and can be effective in prolonging useful life in many situations. An understanding of what it can and cannot do and an awareness of its limitations is an important aspect of its use. The striking relief afforded a patient with intractable pain of malignant pelvic tumor and the return of such a patient to normal interpersonal relationships is an experience that can demonstrate to any physician the effectiveness of chordotomy. The failure of ablative surgical procedures for pain in the patient using pain as a means of removing himself from an intolerable situation should demonstrate just as strikingly to the physician that no therapy should be applied just because a symptom is present.

SUPPRESSION OF PAIN BY STIMULATION

Counterstimulation based on theories foreign to most Western neurophysiologic concepts has been used for centuries. Unfortunately, scientific evaluation of the results is not available, and allegorical reports not recognizing placebo effects, emotional factors, and the striking immediate effect of one pain to suppress a less severe pain are the only evidence available for evaluation. More recently, electrical stimulation applied to peripheral nerves, dorsal columns of the spinal cord, and various subcortical cerebral structures have been used for a variety of intractably painful states with varying clinical results.

Although the initial rationale for using these techniques was based on physiologic concepts, the development of the techniques appears to be more empirically than theoretically based. Stimulation of peripheral nerves is done for painful dysesthesias limited to an area innervated by a single nerve. The technique is based on electrophysiologic evidence mentioned in the introduction of this section that the larger nonpainful fibers of peripheral nerves inhibit the subsequent spinal cord activity secondary to smaller fibers, the latter being essential for pain conduction. Stimulation of nonpainful myelinated fibers by implanted cuff electrodes on peripheral nerve has had limited success in alleviation of pain, and the method is limited to painful entities in a single nerve distribution. It has been more effective in the upper extremity than in the lower extremity.

Electrical stimulation of the spinal cord dorsal column by implanted electrodes has been used for more diffuse intractable pain, particularly of the lower extremities. A theoretic basis for this type of stimulation includes increasing descending inhibition in the dorsal root entry zone, and experimental evidence that such stimulation inhibits the central conduction of smaller fiber activity has been demonstrated. Using nonpainful paresthesias to determine the threshold, implanted dorsal column stimulators have had effective short-term results for relief of intractable pain in many patients.

Electrical stimulation of the thalamus, amygdaloid body, caudate nucleus, and hypothalamus, regions in which lesions have been placed for controlled affective states, has been shown to have varying beneficial effects on some painful syndromes. Although none of these techniques have been universally effective for the control of pain, with further understanding of its etiology by experimental patient and clinical investigation, perhaps newer knowledge in the treatment of pain will be forthcoming.

STRUCTURAL ABNORMALITIES OF AXIAL SKELETON

General Considerations

ANATOMY. The vertebral column with its ligaments and musculature serves two functions: the support of body weight and protection of the neuraxis. The same dual role is played by the basiocciput, which may be considered from an embryologic and functional standpoint as an extension of the spine. In health, the spine is a sturdy yet flexible weight-bearing structure. Most of its weight-bearing property is provided by the vertebral bodies and intervertebral discs. The neural arch formed by the pedicles and laminae complete a bony ring at each vertebral level defining the vertebral canal, while the articular processes and attached facets bridge the intervertebral spaces posterolaterally, providing further support and protection. The spinous and transverse processes of the neural arch serve as attachments for the spinal musculature. The ligamentum flavum and the posterior atlantooccipital ligament, both thick elastic structures, complete the bony and ligamentous tube which extends from the foramen magnum to the lowest part of the sacrum. In the normal skeleton there is ample room within the foramen magnum and the vertebral canal for the contained neural and vascular elements, and the intervertebral foramina provide unrestricted passage of the nerve roots and blood vessels.

There is a considerable discrepancy between the cross-sectional area of the vertebral canal and that of the spinal cord at all levels, the additional space being occupied by the cerebrospinal fluid-filled subarachnoid space and the fat-filled epidural space. The fluid and fat suspend and cushion the neuraxis and, because they are displaceable, provide room for lateral and anteroposterior movement of the neuraxis that must take place with normal motion of the axial skeleton. Radiologic and postmortem studies have shown that the spinal cord and nerve roots also undergo grossly perceptible axial movement when the spine is flexed or extended. The spinal cord and roots must, therefore, be free to move up and down the vertebral canal, and the stress applied to the nerve roots through the movement of the peripheral nerves must be relieved by movement within the intervertebral foramina.

PATHOPHYSIOLOGY. Structural abnormalities which markedly decrease the dimensions of the foramen magnum, the vertebral canal, or the intervertebral foramina may result in damage to the nervous system. The mechanism of injury is primarily that of direct compression of nervous tissue, although in some instances concomitant interference with blood supply may be a factor. Injury to the nervous system may be caused by acute angulation of the vertebral axis, subluxation of one part of the axial skeleton upon another, or encroachment of a mass upon the vertebral canal or intervertebral foramina. Not only the degree but the rate of compression is important. Angulation of the spine, for example, in idiopathic scoliosis may be extremely severe but rarely causes neurologic deficit because of the ability of the cord and roots to accommodate to their distorted position. In contrast, less pronounced angulation from an acute process such as collapse of vertebra in an osteoporotic spine may result in complete destruction of the spinal cord.

The causes of structural abnormalities of the spine which affect the nervous system are extremely diverse. The bones, joints, and associated muscles of the axial skeleton are subject to the same diseases as they are elsewhere in the body. They may be congenital or acquired, local or diffuse. Symptomatic abnormalities often result from a combination of these factors. As an example, the foramen magnum and the vertebral canal in achondroplasia is malformed and disproportionately small as compared with the normal size of the spinal cord. A relatively minor degree of disc protrusion or scoliosis in these patients often causes severe neurologic deficit. It is becoming increasingly apparent as careful measurement of the spinal canal becomes more prevalent that individual differences in response to structural disease in the general population can, at least in part, be accounted for by differences in the size of the vertebral canal. Those persons with congenitally small but undistorted vertebral canals are much more liable to major neurologic deficit in response to degenerative disc disease or relatively minor spine trauma.

It is not the intention of this section to discuss all the etiologic agents that may result in structural abnormalities of the spine. What will be emphasized are the often misunderstood structural lesions occurring at the craniovertebral border and the common lesions resulting from disease of the intervertebral discs.

Abnormalities of the Craniovertebral Border

Structural abnormalities involving the basiocciput and the cephalic portion of the cervical spine are uncommon as compared to those of the remainder of the axial skeleton. Their importance lies in the fact that they may produce profound neurologic dysfunction, which is not infrequently misinterpreted as the result of other causes. Craniovertebral abnormalities are usually congenital but may be acquired. Anatomically these lesions divide into two basic categories, those which affect the basiocciput and those which primarily involve the first and second cervical vertebrae. Both limit the space available for the cervicomedullary junction and can produce similar neurologic dysfunction.

PATHOLOGY. Maldevelopment of the occipital bone resulting in an abnormally small and irregularly shaped foramen magnum occurs in achondroplasia and occasionally in craniosynostosis. More common deformities of the basiocciput are those termed *platybasia* (*platys,* flat) and *basilar impression.* To accommodate the cerebellum and the brainstem, which lie in approximately the same axis as the spinal cord, the level of the floor of the posterior fossa is normally well below that of the anterior and middle fossae. In platybasia, the entire floor of the posterior fossa appears elevated. As seen in a lateral x-ray of the skull, the angle formed by the floor of the anterior fossa and the posterior border of the clivus approaches 180°, and the posterior fossa is therefore extremely shallow. In basilar impression the margins of the foramen magnum are indented as if the weight of the head had caused it to sink toward the vertebral column. This may be the case in acquired basilar impression associated with rickets and Paget's disease. In both platybasia and basilar impression the capacity of the posterior fossa is reduced, and the dimensions of the foramen magnum, especially the anteroposterior diameter, are decreased. In accommodating to the small and abnormally shaped posterior fossa, the hindbrain may be distorted with resulting pressure applied, especially to its ventral surface. Thus the lower cranial nerves and the cervicomedullary junction may be compressed directly or stretched, and hydrocephalus can result from local obstruction to cerebrospinal fluid pathways.

The most significant structural abnormality of the upper cervical spine is atlantoaxial dislocation. This can occur for a variety of reasons. As with dislocations at other levels, it may be the result of trauma, infection, or degenerative bone disease. It most commonly, however, occurs in association with maldevelopment of the atlas. The atlas may be fused to the base of the occiput, and the odontoid, which represents the body of the atlas, may be maldeveloped. Failure of fusion of the odontoid process to the body of the axis may occur without other abnormalities. In occipitalization of the atlas, the head can no longer nod at the atlantooccipital joint, and the added stress on the ligaments holding the odontoid process in place may eventually produce a dislocation. The same ventral dislocation of the atlas on the axis may occur if the odontoid process is rudimentary or ununited to the atlas. With atlantoaxial dislocation the upper cervical spinal cord may be compressed between the odontoid process and the posterior arch of the atlas. The lower medulla may become compromised as well, presumably by resulting angulation at its junction with the posteriorly displaced spinal cord.

CLINICAL MANIFESTATIONS. Structural abnormalities of the craniovertebral border frequently remain asymptomatic until adult life and then frequently are in response to relatively minor trauma. Cranial nerve signs include disassociated sensory loss over the face (descending trigeminal tract) and palatal and vocal cord weakness. Nystagmus and spastic weakness of the extremities are common, and the patient may have loss of position sense, ataxia, bladder dysfunction, and atrophy of the shoulder musculature and small muscles of the hand. Although examination may reveal a short neck and restriction of head movement, diagnosis is confirmed by x-ray studies. Myelography in questionable cases usually reveals a partial or complete obstruction of passage of the contrast agent.

TREATMENT. Immobilization of the neck is indicated for patients with minor degrees of impairment. If the dysfunction is progressive or is already severe, decompression of the craniovertebral border is indicated. The mechanisms of continued compression, however, must be demonstrated. Most frequently, the mechanism is occlusion of the outlet of the cerebrospinal fluid from the fourth ventricle, causing hydrocephalus and increased intracranial pressure. A shunt from the ventricle to the venous system, as described earlier under Infantile Hydrocephalus, will often reverse this process and allow a return toward normal neurological function. If hydrocephalus is not found, air myelography or Pantopaque myelography will demonstrate, in most cases, the direction of the compression of the cervical medullary junction and thus indicate either anterior or posterior decompression of the area. In atlantoaxial dislocation, surgical procedures should be done with the patient in skeletal traction and stabilization obtained by bony fusion.

Degenerative Disease of the Intervertebral Disc

Degenerative disease of the intervertebral disc is one of the most common, yet one of the least understood and often one of the most mistreated, disorders of the spine (see Chap. 43). Although many patients have benefited from removal of herniated portions of an intervertebral disc compressing neural tissue, too many have been crippled by ill-advised operation for symptoms mistakenly interpreted as being due to this same cause. Just as not all right lower quadrant abdominal pain is caused by appendicitis, not all neck and low back pain is caused by surgical disease of the intervertebral disc.

ANATOMY. The intervertebral disc is well suited for its task of supporting considerable weight while still allowing mobility of the spine. It is classically and practically described as consisting of two parts: a tough yet slightly flexible outer ring, the annulus fibrosis, which joins the periphery of adjacent vertebral bodies to one another, and a semisolid plastic center, the nucleus pulposus, interposed between the hyaline cartilage faces of the vertebral bodies.

The joint is further reinforced by the anterior and posterior longitudinal ligaments, which extend the length of the spine. Actually, the intervertebral disc is a composite structure in which three zones grading into one another may be recognized. The outer zone, which may be regarded as the joint capsule, is composed of lamellae of interlacing bundles of fibrous tissue that blend with the longitudinal ligaments. Beneath this fibrous capsule and intimately adherent to it lies a thick envelope of fibrocartilage that in turn surrounds and attaches to the less dense nucleus pulposus. This latter substance is composed primarily of collagenous fibrils and cartilage cells suspended in a fluid matrix. In younger persons remnants of the notochord may be found here as well. Motion between vertebral bodies is allowed by the flexibility of the outer layers, the more fluid center responding to variations in weight distribution by flowing into areas of least pressure within the confines of the annulus.

ETIOLOGY AND PATHOLOGY. Although the intervertebral disc may be damaged by infection, collagen disease, and severe trauma, it is, in comparison with other weight-bearing structures, particularly liable to early degenerative changes. Knowledge of the basic cause of this deterioration, which secondarily involves surrounding bone as well, is uncertain, but it is at least presumably in part a response to the trauma of daily normal activity. It is more prevalent in men than in women and in laborers than in sedentary workers. Degenerative changes occur most frequently in portions of the spine where there is a transition between a relatively mobile segment and a less mobile one, namely, in the lower cervical and lower lumbar region. This distribution again implicates trauma as a causative factor, since there is relatively more motion and therefore more stress at these levels.

Pathologically there is thinning of the fibrous layers of the annulus, destruction of fibrocartilage, and dehydration of the nucleus pulposus. The interspace becomes narrowed and, presumably because of loss of normal joint function, there is frequently new bone formation (osteoarthritis) at the margins of the interspace. These changes are often relatively asymptomatic, producing only transient local pain and the progressive loss of spine mobility usually taken as a matter of course with advancing age. Under certain circumstances, however, essentially the same degenerative processes may have more serious consequences. The nucleus pulposus may herniate through the weakened annulus, and/or large bony spurs may develop to project into the vertebral canal or intervertebral foramina. Of the two processes, herniation of the nucleus pulposus is a much more common cause of neurologic dysfunction and occurs at an earlier age. Approximately three-quarters of symptomatic herniations of the nucleus pulposus occur between the ages of thirty and fifty years. Neurologic disability resulting from osteoarthritis occurs predominantly in the individuals fifty years of age or older.

The effects of herniation of the nucleus pulposus depend on its location, both in respect to the transverse plane and the disc involved, its size, rate of development, and individual differences in surrounding structures. The most common type of herniation of the nucleus pulposus is not through the annulus but rather into the cancellous portion of the vertebral bodies, the so-called "Schmorl's nodules." Such herniation produces no neurologic deficit but by impairing joint function often results in reactive bone formation at the disc margins. Herniation of the nucleus pulposus through the annulus may likewise be asymptomatic. It most commonly occurs at its weakest portion just lateral to the posterior longitudinal ligament near the intervertebral foramen. Herniation into the center of the vertebral canal is relatively uncommon. When it does occur, however, it may result in compression of the spinal cord or of multiple nerve roots if it is below the conus medullaris. The size of the herniated mass varies considerably; it ranges from a protrusion still covered by thinned-out annulus to complete extrusion of the nucleus pulposus as well as the fibrocartilage layers of the annulus into the vertebral canal. The largest intervertebral discs are those in the lumbar region, and, as might be expected, the largest herniated masses occur there. Herniations of the same size are better tolerated in the lumbar area than in other regions, since the spinal cord ends at the thoracolumbar junction, and the lumbar vertebral canal and the intervertebral foramina are larger.

Occasionally in response to severe trauma, especially flexion injuries, an acute rupture of the annulus occurs with massive herniation of the nucleus pulposus and immediate onset of severe neurologic deficit. In the vast majority of patients, however, signs and symptoms resulting from herniation of the nucleus pulposus are more chronic. Although patients often relate their disability to a recent event, such as bending, turning, or lifting, they almost invariably also give a history of past neck or back pain with or without symptoms of nerve root compression. Herniation of the nucleus pulposus is therefore usually a gradual and intermittent process. Signs and symptoms appear when surrounding pain-sensitive structures, such as the annulus, longitudinal ligaments, and dura, are stimulated or nervous tissue, usually roots, is compressed. Anatomic and pathologic adjustments then often occur, and the symptoms regress, perhaps to reappear when the mass enlarges or anatomic relationships change.

CLINICAL MANIFESTATIONS. The clinical picture produced by the common posterolateral disc herniation is characteristic. Diagnosis often can be made by history alone. Signs and symptoms are primarily those of extradural mass: pain over the distribution of the nerve root involved and evidence of lower motor neuron functional loss. Complaints of sensory disturbance over the peripheral distribution of the nerve root involved is commonly of a "pins and needles" type or just a slightly numb feeling. While weakness may be a symptom, it is much less common. The other root signs are loss or decrease in the deep tendon reflex and weakness and atrophy. Examination of the involved area of the spine reveals muscle spasm that may cause loss of normal lumbar or cervical lordosis. In lumbar lesions scoliosis is frequently present, the convexity usually occurring on the side of the lesion. Motion in the affected portion of the spine is limited and painful, especially on lateral flexion toward the lesion. Palpation over the corresponding spinous process and along the major

nerve trunks produces pain. Maneuvers such as straight-leg raising which increase the tension of the nerve roots are painful.

DIAGNOSTIC FINDINGS. Plain x-rays may be normal or reveal distortion of alignment of the spine produced by muscle spasm. They may, however, show narrowing of the interspace, lipping of the margins of the vertebral bodies bordering on the disc, and osteoarthritic spurs. X-rays also serve to rule out bone erosion that may be present with spinal neoplasms and congenital bony anomalies such as spondylolisthesis. Computerized axial tomography has recently been used as an adjunct to plain x-ray when stenosis of the spinal canal is suspected. Most commonly caused by hypertrophy of the articular facets, impingement of the neural canal is readily identified by this method. Myelography is often used as final verification of a herniated disc, especially in the cervical and thoracic region. This procedure is best carried out after making the decision to operate based on the course of the disease and the findings on examination.

HERNIATED LUMBAR DISC

The highest incidence of symptomatic herniation of the intervertebral disc is in the lumbar region. Ninety-five percent of lumbar herniations occur at the last two interspaces. The relative frequencies of herniations at these two interspaces are approximately equal. Most of the remainder of the herniated lumbar intervertebral discs occur at the third lumbar interspace. The vast majority of herniations in the lumbar as well as in other locations are unilateral. The disposition of the nerve roots in the lumbar space is such that posterolateral herniation does not compress the nerve exiting at the corresponding intervertebral foramen but rather impinges on the set of anterior and posterior nerve roots, contained in a single dural sleeve, which cross the disc in their course to the foramen immediately caudad.

CLINICAL MANIFESTATIONS. Herniation at the interspace between the fourth and fifth lumbar vertebral bodies usually compresses the fifth lumbar roots, and herniation at the disc located at the lumbosacral junction produces signs and symptoms referable to the first sacral roots. The fifth lumbar anterior root serves as a major supply to the anterior crural muscles, which dorsiflex the foot, and the peroneal muscles, which evert and plantar-flex the foot. The dermatome served by the fifth lumbar posterior root includes the anterolateral aspect of the leg and crosses anteriorly at the ankle to supply the medial aspect of the foot including its dorsum. Compression of the fifth nerve root by a herniated nucleus pulposus occasionally produces a foot drop. The motor deficit, however, is usually less severe; the most common finding is weakness of dorsiflexion of the great toe. Hypesthesia and hypalgesia are usually most evident on the dorsum of the foot between the great and second toes. The motor root of the first sacral nerve supplies some innervation to the gluteal and hamstring muscles but gives a larger supply to the muscles of the calf and the small muscles of the foot. Its sensory distribution covers a narrow strip on the posterior aspect of the leg and the lateral aspect of the foot. The most common motor deficit in patients with herniation at the lumbosacral interspace is weakness of plantar flexion. Minor degrees of weakness may be brought out by having the patient attempt to walk on his toes. In addition, the ankle reflex is diminished or absent, and sensory deficit is found on the lateral aspect of the foot.

TREATMENT. For the majority of patients with herniated lumbar intervertebral discs the appropriate treatment includes a regimen of strict bed rest on a firm mattress, local heat, and analgesics. Pain usually subsides in 1 to 2 weeks, and the patient may then be started on a graded program of exercises designed to strengthen the back musculature. The patient should be instructed to refrain from heavy lifting and from activities that involve sudden bending or twisting of the lumbar spine. Early operation is reserved for those patients who have evidence of major neurologic dysfunction such as a foot drop or bowel and bladder disturbances which indicate a massive disc protrusion. If the patient has not responded to conservative management in a few weeks or is losing considerable time from work each year from repetitive episodes, operation should probably be carried out. Back pain alone is not an indication for operation. The aim of the operation, done through a limited hemilaminectomy, is to relieve nerve root compression by excision of the mass of herniated nucleus pulposus. Relief of signs and symptoms referable to such compression is usual, but many of the patients have residual low back pain. In our experience fusion of the vertebrae does not often solve this latter problem.

HERNIATED CERVICAL DISC

The lower cervical region is the next most common site of herniated discs. Approximately 90 percent of the herniations in this region occur at the interspaces between C_5 and C_6 and between C_6 and C_7 with the lower level predominating. In contrast with the lower lumbar region, cervical nerve roots are short and almost horizontal.

CLINICAL MANIFESTATIONS. Relatively small herniations are often symptomatic, usually lying just beneath the corresponding roots as they enter the intervertebral foramen. It is fortunate that large or medially placed herniations are rare, for when they do occur, they often result in quadriparesis.

With lateral herniations at the lower cervical levels, patients complain of neck pain radiating into the corresponding shoulder and arm. Referred interscapular pain is also common. Localization of the compressed roots by physical signs is somewhat less precise than in the lumbar area. Compression of the sixth cervical roots by posterolateral herniation at the C_5–C_6 interspace usually results in clinically evident weakness of the biceps muscle, depression or absence of the biceps tendon reflex, and sensory loss on the dorsal and lateral aspect of the thumb and radial aspect of the hand often including the index finger. The syndrome of the seventh cervical roots includes weakness of the triceps muscle, decrease or absence of the triceps reflex, and sensory deficit of the distal portions of the corresponding dermatome, which is medial to that of the sixth cervical dermatome. It usually includes both the dorsal and palmar aspects of the index and middle fingers.

TREATMENT. The rationale of treatment of cervical disc herniation is similar to that in the lumbar region. Signs and symptoms in the majority of patients will regress with conservative management. Neck traction is especially useful. Operation is indicated only in patients with evidence of spinal cord compression and those not responding to conservative measures. Central herniations are best removed through the interspace from the anterior aspect of the spine. The common lateral herniations can be removed effectively either from the same anterior approach or by hemilaminectomy.

HERNIATED THORACIC DISC

Disc herniation in the thoracic region is rare. When it does occur, it is usually in the lower thoracic spine and is apt to produce major neurologic deficit, often with little associated pain. This lesion may be suspected on the basis of a past history of trauma to the thoracic spine, but it is usually clinically indistinguishable from the more common neoplasms occurring in this region. Diagnosis is made by x-ray studies. There may be narrowing of an interspace and, in contrast to disc disease in other regions, calcification in the interspace. Myelography is essential for diagnosis. Results of operation by the classic approach, i.e., laminectomy, are in general poor with no improvement or with increased deficit in about one-half of the patients reported in larger series. The reasons for these poor results include the fact that most of these lesions are anterior to the cord and are firm and partially calcified. Their removal with a posterior exposure therefore often necessitates major retraction of an already compressed spinal cord. Removal of the herniated disc by approach through the interspace, either by removing the adjacent ribs and transverse processes or by going through the chest cavity, has been more effective in relieving the myelopathy without causing further neurological deficit.

SPONDYLOSIS

Hypertrophic bone changes are not infrequently associated with disc herniation even in younger individuals. They are especially prevalent in cervical herniations in which spurs of bone projecting into the intervertebral foramina are often a contributing cause of nerve root compression. In relation to its almost uniform presence in the elderly, hypertrophic bony change alone as a cause of significant neurologic dysfunction is uncommon. However, in some patients with advanced hypertrophic bone disease of the cervical spine, often termed *spondylosis,* major spinal cord and nerve root dysfunction develop. This entity, which usually affects two or more lower cervical interspaces, is characterized by narrowing of the interspaces and extensive bony proliferation on the lips of the vertebral bodies adjacent to the discs, producing transverse ridges which project into the vertebral canal. The corresponding intervertebral foramina are narrowed, and in advanced disease minor degrees of subluxation of one vertebra on another may exist.

Why many persons tolerate advanced cervical spondylosis without significant disability while in others a severe spastic quadriparesis may develop is largely unknown. It has been demonstrated that a greater number of patients with symptomatic spondylosis have congenitally narrow cervical vertebral canals than those without spinal cord signs. A simple compressive mechanism, however, does not entirely suffice to explain the problem, since return of function often does not follow seemingly adequate decompression which includes extensive laminectomy combined with removal of bony spurs and fusion from the anterior approach. Chronic vascular insufficiency resulting from a combination of such factors as arteriosclerosis, compression of a long segment of spinal cord, and compression of the arterial supply entering through the intervertebral foramina may explain the difference in the results of surgical therapy for cervical spondylosis as compared with more localized mass lesions in the same region.

CLINICAL MANIFESTATIONS. The clinical picture of symptomatic cervical spondylosis varies considerably. Neck pain radiating bilaterally into the shoulders is frequently but not invariably present. Examination reveals evidence of compression of multiple cervical nerve roots and signs of cervical spinal cord compression. The course of the disease is also variable. Occasionally there is rapid progression which may lead to a severe spastic quadriparesis within a year or less. More often the onset of signs is insidious, and progression is slow. Spontaneous regression of neurologic deficit is rare, but on the other hand progression of deficit may halt at any point.

TREATMENT. The variability of the course makes it difficult to evaluate the effectiveness of operative procedures. In the early stages of the disease immobilization of the cervical spine by a well-fitted collar brace may be of benefit. Traction occasionally may reduce root pain but often is not successful. Operation early in the course of the disease should probably be reserved for those patients with involvement of only one or two interspaces and those with obviously small vertebral canals. With severe and seemingly unrelenting progression of neurologic deficit associated with widespread bony changes, the patient should be informed that a halt in progression may be all that can be hoped for from operation.

References

General Considerations

Jefferson, G.: "Selected Papers," Pitman Medical Publications, London, 1960.

Mullan, S.: "Essentials of Neurosurgery," Springer Publishing Co., Inc., New York, 1961.

Plum, F., and Posner, J.: "The Diagnosis of Stupor and Coma," F. A. Davis Company, Philadelphia, 1972.

Head Injury, Mechanisms of Injury, Care of Head-injured Patient

Adams, J. H.: "The Neuropathology of Head Trauma: Handbook of Clinical Neurology," pp. 35–65, North-Holland Publishing Company, Amsterdam, 1975.

Browder, E. J., and Cook, A. W.: Indications for Surgical Intervention in Head Injuries, *Surg Clin North Am,* **35:**577, 1955.

Ingraham, F., and Matson, D.: "Neurosurgery of Infancy and Childhood," pt. III, chap. 5, Charles C Thomas, Publisher, Springfield, Ill., 1954.

Jennett, B., Teasdale, G., Galbraith, S., Pickard, J., Grant, H., Braakman, R., Avezaat, C., Maas, A., Minderhound, J., Vecht, C. J., Herden, J., Small, R., Caton, W., and Kurze, T.: Severe Head Injuries in Three Countries, *J Neurol Neurosurg Psychiatry,* **40:**291, 1977.

Johnson, R. T., and Yates, P. O.: Brain Stem Haemorrhages in Expanding Supratentorial Conditions, *Acta Radiol (Stockh),* **46:**250, 1956.

Lewin, W.: Factors in the Mortality of Closed Head Injuries, *Br Med J,* **1:**1239, 1953.

Lindenberg, R.: Compression of Brain Arteries as a Pathogenetic Factor for Tissue Necroses and Their Areas of Predilection, *J Neuropathol Exp Neurol,* **14:**223, 1955.

Schneider, R. C., and Tytus, J. S.: Extradural Hemorrhage: Factors Responsible for the High Mortality Rate, *Ann Surg,* **142:**938, 1955.

Walker, A. E.: Practical Considerations in the Treatment of Head Injuries, *Neurology,* **1:**75, 1951.

Ward, A. A.: Physiological Basis of Concussion, *J Neurosurg,* **15:**129, 1958.

Spinal Cord Injuries

Holdsworth, F.: Review Article. Fractures, Dislocations, and Fracture-Dislocations of the Spine, *J Bone Joint Surg,* **52-A:**1534, 1970.

Schneider, R. C., Crosby, E. C., Russo, R. H., and Gosch, H. H.: Traumatic Spinal Cord Syndromes and Their Management, *Clin Neurosurg,* **20:**424, 1973.

Symonds, C. P.: The Interrelation of Trauma and Cervical Spondylosis in Compression of the Cervical Cord, *Lancet,* **1:**451, 1953.

Tarlov, I. M.: Spinal Cord Compression Studies: III, *Arch Neurol Psychiatry,* **71:**588, 1954.

——— and Herz, E.: Spinal Cord Compression Studies: IV, *Arch Neurol Psychiatry,* **72:**43, 1954.

Wagner, F. C.: Management of Acute Spinal Cord Injury, *Surg Neurol,* **7:**346, 1977.

Peripheral Nerve Injuries

Lyons, W. R., and Woodhall, B.: "Atlas of Peripheral Nerve Injuries," W. B. Saunders Company, Philadelphia, 1949.

Millese, H., Meissl, G., and Berger, A.: Further Experiences with Interfascicular Grafting of the Median, Ulnar and Radial Nerves, *J Bone Joint Surg,* **58-A:**209, 1976.

Smith, J. W.: Microsurgery of Peripheral Nerves, *Plast Reconstr Surg,* **33:**317, 1964.

Woodhall, B.: Surgical Repair of Acute Peripheral Nerve Injury, *Surg Clin North Am,* **30:**1369, 1951.

Young, J. Z.: The Functional Repair of Nervous Tissue, *Physiol Rev,* **22:**318, 1942.

Brain Tumors

Bailey, P.: "Intracranial Tumors," Charles C Thomas, Publisher, Springfield, Ill., 1948.

Kernohan, J. W., and Sayre, G. P.: "Tumors of the Central Nervous System," sec. X, fasicles 35, 37, Armed Forces Institute of Pathology, Washington, 1952.

Russell, D., and Rubenstein, L.: "Pathology of Tumors of the Nervous System," The Williams & Wilkins Company, Baltimore, 1963.

Spinal Tumors

Dodge, H. W., Jr., Keith, H. M., and Campagna, M. J.: Intraspinal Tumors in Infants and Children, *J Int Coll Surg,* **26:**199, 1957.

Kennady, J. C., and Stern, W. E.: Metastatic Neoplasms of the Vertebral Column Producing Compression of the Spinal Cord, *Am J Surg,* **104:**155, 1962.

Woltman, H. W., Kernohan, J. W., Adson, A. W., and Craig, W. M.: Intramedullary Tumors of Spinal Cord and Gliomas of Intradural Portion of Filum Terminale, *Arch Neurol Psychiatry,* **65:**378, 1951.

Congenital Malformations of the Nervous System

Bunch, W. H., Cass, A. S., Bensman, A. S., and Long, D. M.: "Modern Management of Myelomeningocele," Warren H. Green, Publisher, St. Louis, 1972.

Forrest, D. M., Hale, R., and Wynne, J. M.: Treatment of Infantile Hydrocephalus Using Holter Valve: An Analysis of 152 Consecutive Cases. *Dev Med Child Neurol Suppl,* **11:**27, 1966.

Lorber, J., and De, N. C.: Family History of Congenital Hydrocephalus, *Dev Med Child Neurol Suppl,* **22:**94, 1969.

Matson, D. D.: "Neurosurgery of Infancy and Childhood," chaps. 1–14, Charles C Thomas, Publisher, Springfield, Ill., 1969.

Mealey, J., Dzenitus, A. J., and Hockey, A. A.: The Prognosis of Encephaloceles, *J Neurosurg,* **32:**209, 1970.

Norman, R. M.: Malformation of the Nervous System, in W. Blackwood et al. (eds.), "Greenfield's Neuropathology," chap. 6, The Williams & Wilkins Company, Baltimore, 1967.

Raimondi, A.: Angiographic Diagnosis of Hydrocephalus in the Newborn, *J Neurosurg,* **31:**550, 1969.

Russell, D. S.: Observations on the Pathology of Hydrocephalus, Her Majesty's Stationery Office, London, 1949.

Scarff, J. E.: Treatment of Hydrocephalus: An Historical and Critical Review of Methods and Results, *J Neurol Neurosurg Psychiatry,* **26:**1, 1963.

Shilleto, J.: Craniosynostosis: Review of 519 Cases, *Pediatrics,* **41:**829, 1968.

Surgical Aspects of Central Nervous System Infections

Evans, W.: The Pathology and Aetiology of Brain Abscess, *Lancet,* **1:**1231, 1931.

Irsigler, F. J.: "The Neurosurgical Approach to Intracranial Infections," Springer-Verlag OHG, Berlin, 1961.

Kerr, F. W. L., King, R. B., and Meagher, J. N.: Brain Abscess, *JAMA,* **168:**868, 1958.

Lewin, W.: Cerebrospinal Fluid Rhinorrhea in Closed Head Injuries, *Br J Surg,* **62:**1, 1954.

Matson, D. D., and Salvin, M.: Brain Abscess in Congenital Heart Disease, *Pediatrics,* **27:**772, 1961.

Vascular Disease of the Nervous System

Blackwood, W., et al. (eds.): "Greenfield's Neuropathology," chap. 2, The Williams & Wilkins Company, Baltimore, 1963.

Crawford, T.: Some Observations on the Pathogenesis and Natural History of Intracranial Aneurysms, *J Neurol Neurosurg Psychiatry,* **22:**259, 1959.

Hamby, W. B.: "Intracranial Aneurysms," Charles C Thomas, Publisher, Springfield, Ill., 1952.

Jefferson, G.: Subarachnoid Hemorrhage from Angiomas and Aneurysms in the Young, *Rev Neurol (Paris),* **80:**413, 1948.

Report on the Cooperative Study of Intracranial Aneurysms, *J Neurosurg,* 24:782, 24:789, 24:792, 24:807, 24:922, 24:1034, 25:98, 25:219, 25:321, 25:467, 25:574, 25:593, 25:660, 25:683, 1966.

Russell, D. S.: The Pathology of Spontaneous Intracranial Hemorrhage, *Proc R Soc Med,* **47:**689, 1954.

Yasargil, M. D.: "Microneurosurgery Applied to Neurosurgery," Academic Press, Inc., New York, 1969.

The Surgery of Epilepsy

Blaisdell, W. F., Clauss, R. H., Galbraith, J. G., et al.: Joint Study of Extracranial Arterial Occlusions: IV. A Review of Surgical Considerations, *JAMA,* **209:**12, 1969.

Earle, K. M., Baldwin, M., and Penfield, W.: Incisural Sclerosis and Temporal Lobe Seizures Produced by Hippocampal Herniation at Birth, *Arch Neurol Psychiatry,* **69:**27, 1953.

Hassler, O.: Arterial Pattern of Human Brain Stem, *Neurology,* **17:**368, 1967.

Marshall, J.: The Natural History of Cerebrovascular Diseases, in "Modern Concepts of Cerebrovascular Disease," Spectrum Publications, Inc., New York, 1975.

Ojemann, R. G., Crowell, R. M., Roberson, G. H., and Fisher, C. M.: Surgical Treatment of Extracranial Carotid Occlusive Disease, in "Clinical Neurosurgery," vol. 21, 1976.

Penfield, W., and Jasper, H.: "Epilepsy and the Functional Anatomy of the Human Brain," Little, Brown and Company, Boston, 1954.

Pond, D. A., Bidwell, B. H., and Stein, L.: A Survey of Epilepsy in 14 General Practices: I. Demographic and Medical Data, *Psychiatr Neurol Neurochir,* **63:**217, 1960.

Purpura, D. P., Perry, J. K., and Walter, R. D.: Neurosurgical Management of the Epilepsies, p. 44 in "Advances in Neurology," vol. 8, Raven Press Publishers, New York, 1975.

Yasargil, M. G.: "Experimental Small Vessel Surgery in the Dog Including Patching and Grafting of Cerebral Vessels and the Formation of Functional Extra-intracranial Shunts," The C. V. Mosby Company, St. Louis, 1967.

Pain

Bessou, P., and Perl, E. R.: Response of Cutaneous Sensory Units with Unmyelinated Fibers to Noxious Stimuli, *J Neurophysiol,* **32:**1025, 1969.

Bowsher, D.: Termination of the Central Pain Pathway in Man: The Conscious Appreciation of Pain, *Brain,* **80:**606, 1957.

Keele, K. D.: "Anatomies of Pain," Blackwell Scientific Publications, Ltd., Oxford, 1957.

Knighton, R. S., and Dumke, P. R.: "Pain," Little, Brown and Company, Boston, 1966.

Melzack, R., and Wall, P.: Pain Mechanisms in a New Theory, *Science,* **150:**971, 1965.

Stookey, B., and Ransohoff, J.: "Trigeminal Neuralgia: Its History and Treatment," Charles C Thomas, Publisher, Springfield, Ill., 1959.

White, J. C., and Sweet, W. H.: "Pain: Its Mechanisms and Neurosurgical Control," Charles C Thomas, Publisher, Springfield, Ill., 1955.

Structural Abnormalities of Axial Skeleton

Hinck, V. C., and Sachdev, N. S.: Developmental Stenosis of the Cervical Spinal Canal, *Brain,* **89:**27, 1966.

List, C. F.: Clinical Syndromes of Craniovertebral Anomalies, *Arch Neurol Psychiatry,* **45:**577, 1941.

Spurling, R. G.: "Lesions of the Lumbar Intervertebral Disc," Charles C Thomas, Publisher, Springfield, Ill., 1953.

———: "Lesions of the Cervical Intervertebral Disc," Charles C Thomas, Publisher, Springfield, Ill., 1956.

Wilkinson, M.: The Morbid Anatomy of Cervical Spondylosis and Myelopathy, *Brain,* **83:**589, 1960.

Chapter 43

Manifestations of Musculoskeletal Disorders

by **Robert B. Duthie and Franklin T. Hoaglund**

PAIN

Since pain is the major manifestation of many orthopedic disorders, careful evaluation of its character and properties is essential in the diagnosis, treatment, and understanding of such conditions.

Pain, defined by Sherrington as "the physical adjunct of an imperative protective reflex," is a sensation one feels when injured. Because it appears to vary in quality with each individual, its precise definition is very difficult.

The afferent nociceptive impulses produced by injurious agents stream into the central nervous system, where they are given meaning by the emotional state of the individual based upon the past and present experience. Pain is, therefore, an *experience* rather than a sensory modality in a strict neurologic sense, and psychologic events play an essential role in determining the quality and quantity of its ultimate perception.

Anatomy and Physiology

PAINFUL STIMULUS. The old theory which postulated that pain was the result of stimuli exceeding the intensity threshold for sensory nerve endings can no longer be accepted in the light of modern anatomic and physiologic studies. Weddell has suggested that stimulation of peripheral receptors by noxious agents produces a spatiotemporal pattern of nervous impulses which is interpreted as pain within the higher cerebral centers. Such patterns of nervous activity may be produced by many physical phenomena such as pressure, puncturing, squeezing, and tension;

by alteration in temperature; or by chemical effects, such as the alteration in pH or the concentration of histamine-like substances, serotonin, bradykinin, and other polypeptide compounds. Tissue changes in inflammation are accompanied by a local acidosis. Pus formation, and fibrosis, by virtue of pH changes or internal pressure effects, may convert normal stimuli into stimuli with certain patterns of nervous activity which will be interpreted as pain.

SENSORY END ORGANS. Specialized end organs for pressure and stress do occur in skin and tendons, respectively. However, the old concept of absolute *specificity* of end organs for pressure (Pacini), cold (Krause), and traction (Meissner and Ruffini) requires revision. Weddell and others have demonstrated that most cutaneous sensory nerve endings are unmyelinated fibers forming a dense dermal network. These, when stimulated, may produce sensations of pressure, touch, or pain, depending upon the impulse pattern invoked, rather than the excitation of specific fibers beyond their normal threshold. Similar networks of unmyelinated nerve fibers are found in the walls of blood vessels, particularly arteries, in periosteum, in bone, in synovium, and in joint capsule. In muscles, a similar role is conducted by small myelinated fibers. Cartilage has no sensory end organs.

Specialized end organs, i.e., Pacinian for pressure, can be seen occasionally within the dermis. End organs of Golgi can be identified in ligaments and tendons, where they act as stretch receptors, for muscle control, and perhaps for pain. Bone and periosteum respond to pressure, percussion, or tension. Capsule responds to both tension and traction and is certainly the most sensitive of all joint structures. Although synovium contains scattered free nerve endings, it is difficult to elicit their function experimentally because of the proximity of synovium to capsule.

SENSORY PATHWAYS. The conduction velocity and frequency of impulses in afferent nerve fibers is dependent upon fiber diameter (Table 43-1). The afferent fibers are carried within the peripheral nerves to spinal root ganglia and then to the cord, where they synapse within one or two segments of the dorsal column before crossing the midline to form the contralateral lateral spinothalamic tract. At the site of dorsal column synapse, the pathway

Table 43-1.

Type	Velocity	Fiber diameter	Fiber function
A	120 m/sec	15–25 μ	Proprioceptive afferents from the skin and joints
B		Less than 2 μ	Unmyelinated pain afferents accompanying sympathetic fibers from muscle and bone
C	10 m/sec	5–15 μ	Afferents from muscle and tendon
D			Myelinated fibers in association with visceral nerves

of pain fibers is regulated by fibers descending in the ipsilateral corticospinal tract. There is a controlling mechanism acting at every junction at which nerve impulses are relayed from one neuron to the next on their cerebral ascent. Melzack described this as the mechanism by which psychologic or emotional events determine the quality and quantity of ultimate perception of pain. There are five links in the path by which pain reaches the cerebrum (Fig. 43-1):

1. The spinothalamic tract, excitatory in function and carrying the majority of pain impulses.
2. The central tegmental tract, inhibitory in function. Division increases pain sensitivity.
3. The central gray pathway. Division decreases pain sensitivity.
4. The ascending reticular system, which alerts the entire brain.
5. The medial lemniscal tract, for proprioception and light touch.

The first three of these pathways are depressed by analgesic agents, while the fifth maintains the function of spatial awareness.

Livingston explained the *phantom limb syndrome* in amputees as a disturbance of neural activity in the posterior horn internuncial pool, which produces reverberatory patterns of neural activity. These may be aggravated by minor cutaneous irritations, stimulations of nerve stumps, and emotional upset.

Characteristics

Pain may be expressed in many ways. A deep boring ache is characteristic of tension, whereas a "burning" pain with paresthesias, especially if accompanied by vasomotor phenomena (sweating or redness), indicates a sympathetic as well as a somatic sensory involvement.

Sites

Pain may be described as localized, diffuse, radicular, or referred.

Local pain. Local pain is felt at the site of pathologic processes in superficial structures and is usually associated with local tenderness on palpation or percussion.

Diffuse pain. Diffuse pain appears to be more characteristic of deep-lying tissues and has a more or less segmental distribution.

Radicular pain. Radicular pain, as seen in sciatica and brachalgia, is characterized by its radiation from the center to the periphery in a strict anatomic sense. It is often associated with paresthesia and tenderness along the nerve root. Clinical examination frequently reveals neurologic deficits such as sensory loss, reflex depression, and muscle paresis or paralysis.

Referred pain. Referred pain occurs with injury to, or disease affecting, deep structures such as the spine or the viscera and is a result of misplaced pain projection caused by cortical misrepresentation. For this to occur, sensory pathways must converge on a single cell within the cord or higher centers. Gaze and Gordon and McLeod demonstrated confluence of visceral and cutaneous impulses in the thalamus of the cat. Whitty and Hockaday indicate that there is possible influence upon such convergence points of stored "pain experience," from cells within the brain, rather than only at the spinal cord level.

The experiments of Kellgren and Samuel have helped to define some characteristics of referred pain in different body tissues (Fig. 43-2). Pain resulting from the injection of 6% saline solution into muscle was diffuse and referred into the spinal segments from which the muscle receives its motor innervation, and it varied with the individual. Pain resulting from injection into deep fascia, periosteum, ligament, or tendon was more accurately localized when these tissues were close to the body surface (Fig. 43-3). When the structures were deeper, the pain was more diffuse and had minimal segmental distribution.

Feinstein et al. demonstrated that similar injection of muscle and intervertebral articulations produced gripping, boring, and cramplike pain, often accompanied by muscle spasm and autonomic effects such as hypotension, nausea, and bradycardia. There was less segmental distribution of pain because of extensive arborization of nerve endings and excitation within the internuncial pools, which resulted in extensive overflow into neighboring segments.

Tissue Patterns

BONE PAIN. Pain originating in bone is carried by small myelinated and unmyelinated fibers from the periosteum and small blood vessels. It has a characteristic deep, boring quality usually attributable to the stimulus of internal tension. Such pain is characteristic of osteomyelitis, tumors, and vascular lesions of bone such as those of Paget's disease.

The deep, boring night pain of osteoarthritis is probably of vascular origin. However, this type of pain in osteoarthritis must be differentiated from that due to capsular fibrosis and muscle spasm often aggravated by unguarded movements. Pain of a similar boring nature but of a somewhat diffuse character occurs in generalized osseous diseases such as osteomalacia, osteoporosis, and hyperparathyroidism or metastatic lesions (myelomatosis, carcinomatosis) of the vertebral column, ribs, and pelvic and shoulder girdles. These conditions may have more severe acute pain superimposed as a result of pathologic fractures.

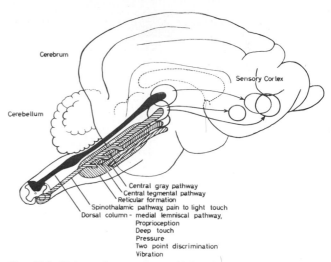

Fig. 43-1. Major pathways along which pain reaches the brain. (*After Melzack, 1961. Taken with permission from Scientific American, 1961.*)

Bone pain associated with fracture has quite a different character. It is often described as sharp or piercing and is characteristically relieved by rest. Pain which is unrelieved by rest is ominous and points toward serious disease processes.

MUSCLE AND TENDON PAIN. Muscle contains many unmyelinated nerve fibers, especially related to its rich blood supply. Many efferent motor fibers to the muscle end plate may subserve a sensory function by virtue of their control over muscle contraction, which, when abnormal, is experienced as pain.

Muscle pain may be the result of direct injury or the effect of chemical irritants such as lactic acid and other products of tissue anoxia. That due to direct injury is usually described as "tearing" and is followed by a soreness aggravated by movement, whereas that consequent upon anoxia is described as a "cramplike" pain. Such a cramplike pain is characteristic of intermittent claudication secondary to atherosclerosis, Volkmann's ischemia, and the anterior tibial syndrome. The pain is aggravated by muscle movement, either passive or active. It is the result of edema secondary to tissue necrosis and the release of chemical irritants which in turn alter the circulation.

Muscle spasm refers to sustained muscular contraction

Fig. 43-2. *A.* Characteristics of muscle pain when stimulated by injected saline solution. *B.* Characteristics of ligament pain when stimulated. (*After Kellgren, 1943. Taken with permission from Mercer and Duthie [eds.], "Orthopaedic Surgery," Edward Arnold [Publishers] Ltd., London, 1972.*)

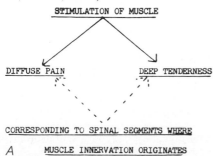

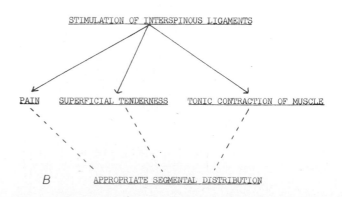

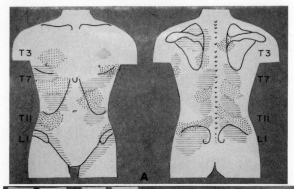

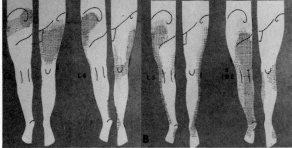

Fig. 43-3. Distribution of pain in the trunk when the interspinous ligaments between various vertebrae were stimulated. *B*. Distribution of pain in the lower extremities when interspinous ligaments were stimulated. (*After Kellgren, 1943. Taken with permission from Mercer and Duthie [eds.], "Orthopaedic Surgery," Edward Arnold [Publishers] Ltd., London, 1972.*)

and is felt as deep, diffuse, persistent pain often described as "like a toothache." Characteristically, in sciatica it produces a scoliosis and in brachialgia a torticollis due to lumbar and cervical nerve root irritation. It is accompanied by local tenderness and a feeling of hardness of the muscles.

The mode of production of painful symptoms by root compression has been clarified by Frykholm, who stimulated nerve roots in patients under local anesthesia. He found that compression of the motor root produced deep, boring ache which could be abolished by blocking the related sensory root. Then stimulation of the motor root continued to produce contraction but did not produce pain. Stimulation of the sensory root, on the other hand, produced sharp, shocklike pain radiating in a peripheral fashion into the appropriate dermatome. Referred pain also may occur when muscle spasm is associated with visceral disorder, e.g., peptic ulceration, appendicitis, and peritonitis.

Paroxysmal cramplike pain accompanied by rigidity or excessive muscle spasm is seen in tetany, which is due to increased sensitivity of the neuromuscular unit consequent upon hypocalcemia or alkalosis. Muscle cramps are also noted with sodium depletion due to hypermotility of muscle cells, a condition rapidly reversed by restoration of the electrolyte balance. Peripheral neuritis may also present cramping of muscle masses as well as paresthesias. The pain and accompanying tenderness of fibrositis is related

to a specific muscle group, but its pathology is not understood.

JOINT PAIN. It is difficult to define joint pain because of the complexity and number of tissues involved in its structure.

The synovium contains two plexuses of nerve fibers, a superficial plexus lying in close proximity to the capsule and a deeper one in the synovial villi. This plexus is intimately related to blood vessels which carry within their tunica media many unmyelinated sensory fibers.

The capsule has a rich supply of somatic sensory fibers and proprioceptive fibers in the form of specialized Golgi apparatus, Vater-Pacini corpuscles, and Ruffini-like endings. Its connection with joint pain appreciation was demonstrated by Leriche, who showed that local anesthetic injected into the capsule was more effective than a simple intraarticular injection.

Coomes produced patterns of pain around the hip, depending upon the aspect of the capsule stimulated. Stimulation of the anterior capsule produced pain in the groin, buttock, anterior thigh, and knee, whereas posterior capsule stimulation produced pain in the buttock, posterior aspect of the thigh, and heel.

Cartilage is avascular and aneural and, therefore, insensitive to stimuli.

There are many sensory endings in the periosteum and accompanying the blood vessels in bone. Bone pain appears to be commonly associated with increased internal tension.

Thus, pain in joints may be attributable to a number of factors:

1. Hyperemia, both of the synovium and bone
2. Joint effusion, producing capsular distension and ligamentous laxity
3. Joint instability, producing traction on capsular structures
4. Asymmetry of the joint surfaces, particularly in the presence of exposed subchondral bone or cyst formation with tension
5. Muscle spasm

PERIPHERAL NERVE PAIN. Peripheral nerve fibers may be subject to:

1. External pressure—neuralgia
2. Ischemia
3. Infection—herpes zoster
4. Metabolic disturbance—avitaminosis⎫ neuritis
5. Toxins—lead or arsenic ⎭

The pain of neuralgia is usually paroxysmal and radicular in type. Paresthesia is common, and examination frequently reveals changes in reflexes, loss of sensation, muscle atrophy, etc. The pain of neuritis, however, tends to be continuous until relief of the disease process or total destruction of neural tissue ensues. The special pain of herpes zoster or Guillain-Barré syndrome due to viral involvement of the internuncial element is accompanied by hyperesthesias, with or without sympathetic vasomotor changes.

PAIN ARISING FROM THE VERTEBRAL COLUMN AND/OR ITS CONTENTS. Lesions of the Cord. *Intraspinal Tumors.* To differentiate between vertebral tumors proper and intraspinal soft tissue tumors with their common symptoms of backache and root pain and occasional signs of spinal block is not always possible. However, intraspinal lesions tend to be progressive without periods of remission. The pain is not relieved by rest, and any progression of the intramedullary compression will produce a rapid loss of motor power in the extremities and loss of sphincter control.

Benign nerve sheath tumors and meningiomas are much more common than tumors of the spinal cord itself, i.e., metastatic carcinoma, glial and ependymal tumors, and more rarely connective tissue tumors.

Infection. Infections involving the spinal cord such as poliomyelitis, meningitis, and the Guillain-Barré syndrome tend to produce lancinating peripheral pain due to the involvement of the internuncial pool cells by the virus. In Guillain-Barré disease the peripheral sensory neurons outside the spinal cord are primarily involved rather than those within the spinal ganglia.

Ischemic and Degenerative Lesions. The conditions of amyotrophic lateral sclerosis, multiple sclerosis, subacute combined degeneration of the cord, and tabes dorsalis will all present with lancinating pain radiating to the extremities. Loss of reflexes are commonly found. Syringomyelia can usually be diagnosed by the loss of both pain and temperature sensations.

Lesions of the Vertebrae and/or Joints. Primary and secondary neoplasms, osteoporosis with pathologic fractures, and tuberculous and pyogenic infections affecting bones of the spine will produce severe local pain with local tenderness on palpation and percussion. Radicular pain does not occur unless the peripheral nerves are involved by the lesion. Carcinoma metastases to the skeletal structures from the prostate, breast, kidney, gastrointestinal tract, female genital organs, thyroid, or lung may produce significant symptoms before there are visible radiographic changes. Determination of the acid and alkaline phosphatase levels are indicated. Sternal puncture may demonstrate myeloma cells, and biopsy of the involved area may reveal the lesion.

Coccygodynia is deep, throbbing pain in the vicinity of the lower end of the sacrum and coccyx aggravated by sitting. It tends to be progressive and to last several months, but without any radicular expression or involvement of sphincteric function. It can be traumatic in origin, from arthritis involving the sacrococcygeal joint or from a disc protrusion at the lumbosacral junction. Localized tenderness on rectal examination is present, and radiographic changes of the joint may be noted. Treatment is usually conservative and consists of application of local heat and cushioned sitting. Rarely does the patient require excision of the coccyx.

Lesions Involving Peripheral Nerves. Peripheral nerves may be compressed in the intervertebral foramina by such conditions as neurofibromas, trauma, osteophyte formation associated with osteoarthrosis, and intervertebral disc protrusions. The pain is usually radicular over the area supplied by the nerve roots involved. Pain also may be referred to the back and limbs from visceral involvement as seen in mediastinitis, esophagitis, and diseases of the kidney, stomach, or gonads.

Pain in the Upper Limbs

The diagnosis of the cause of pain in the neck, head, shoulder, and upper limb requires understanding of anatomic, mechanical, and pathologic factors. In the cervical spine, the thoracic outlet region, and the upper extremities there are numerous soft tissues, e.g., muscles ligaments, and capsules around joints, all of which are plentifully supplied with pain nerve endings. Moreover, all these tissues are compressed into small areas and subjected to numerous stresses and strains in relation to movement. Any decrease in the dimensions of these spaces can result in pain and possible loss of function. Pain is more likely to occur if the pressure is acute and transient, whereas loss in function is more likely if pressure is prolonged and continuous.

DIFFERENTIAL DIAGNOSIS OF PAIN IN THE UPPER LIMB, BASED UPON ANATOMIC REGIONS. Pain in the Shoulder-Scapular Area. This will arise from cervical disc protrusion, diseases of the cervical vertebrae, and affections of the shoulder joint, e.g., supraspinatus tendinitis and subacromial bursitis, or it may be referred visceral pain arising from disease of the heart, lungs, or pleura.

Pain in the Vicinity of the Elbow. This may result from local conditions such as arthritis of the radiohumeral articulations or lateral epicondylitis ("tennis elbow"), or it may be referred pain with involvement of the fifth, sixth, or seventh cervical vertebrae or associated discs.

Pain in the Wrist and Hand. This may be the result of local lesions such as tendon sheath disease, e.g., Quervain's disease, radiocarpal arthritis, neoplastic or infective diseases of the bones, or compression of the median nerve within the carpal tunnel. Radicular pain may be due to compression of the ulnar nerve at the elbow or of the brachial plexus at any point from the roots at the intervertebral foramina or in the thoracic outlet; these conditions will be accompanied by other signs of neurologic deficit such as paresthesias, muscle atrophy, reflex changes, and overlying skin changes. Associated vasomotor trophic changes suggest Sudeck's atrophy or the shoulder-hand syndrome.

BRACHIALGIA (BRACHIAL NEURALGIA)

This pain involves the neck, shoulder, or upper extremity; i.e., it is distributed within the brachial plexus dermatome and sclerotome. It may be characterized by:

Upper extremity pain, either unilateral or bilateral
Paresthesias, in a dermatome with altered sensation
Deep tendon reflex changes in the jaw and/or in the upper extremity
Muscle weakness, with atrophy and possibly fibrillation
Vertebral artery or sympathetic plexus disturbance with giddiness or tinnitus or visual disturbance

The disease process may involve the motor neuron, the pyramidal tract, the root, or the surrounding vertebrae. Muscle pain which can be temporarily relieved by physical therapy is unlikely to be due to true nerve root involvement. These features, which are found in the upper extremity, may also involve the lower. Therefore, examination should be made of the reflexes, vibratory sense, and proprioceptive sense in the lower extremities as well as in the abdominal wall.

Radiography (AP and lateral, as well as oblique views), lumbar puncture to show the presence of some degree of block on jugular compression, examination of cerebrospinal fluid for changes in protein and other chemical constituents, and a cell count should be carried out. The differential diagnosis of brachialgia includes:

1. Tumors of the cord and its membranes or of the vertebral column, e.g., ependymoma, neurofibroma, or neurolemmoma
2. Infections, such as acute tuberculosis, osteomyelitis, actinomycosis
3. Prolapsing intervertebral disc, or degenerative disc with arthritis
4. Pancoast's tumor of the apex of lung
5. Congenital anomalies of the cord, e.g., syringomyelia
6. Atlantoaxial dislocation

CERVICAL COMPRESSION SYNDROME (CERVICAL DISC DISEASE)

Maximal movement of flexion or extension and static curvature occur at the level of C_4 to C_6. Maximal stress is to be expected at this level, and this is the most common site for herniations of the cervical intervertebral discs (Fig. 43-4). In addition, the cervical spinal canal contains a relatively immobile and thick spinal cord anchored

Fig. 43-4. Lateral radiograph of the cervical spine to show narrowing of disc spaces between C_4–C_5 and C_5–C_6 with osteophyte formation.

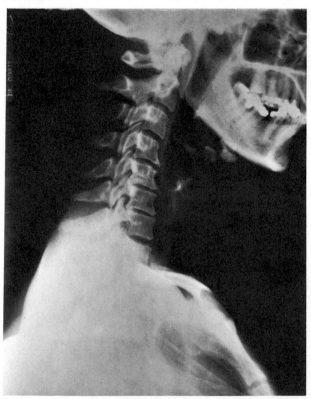

through the meninges by the denticular ligament and by the short, almost transversely directed nerve roots. These nerve roots continue their short horizontal course outside the thecal sac, remaining intradural, to the region of the intervertebral foramina, where they lie close to the intervertebral bodies opposite the intervertebral discs.

The precise situation of the disc protrusion or the osteophytic compression is important, because it determines whether the spinal cord and/or the nerve root will be affected. A prominence in the midline will compress the whole spinal cord and the anterior nerve roots which emerge at this level, but a bulge to one side of the midline will cause unilateral cord compression with a Brown-Séquard type of syndrome. The most common variety of protrusion, however, is that arising from the lateral portion of the disc in relation to the nerve root and is either dorsolateral or intraforaminal in location. An intraforaminal lesion may also be the result of narrowing of an already small intervertebral foramen by osteophytic lipping of the margins of the neurocentral joints of Luschka. These "neurocentral" joints are set at the lateral margins of the vertebrae facing into the intervertebral foramina and lie anteromedial to the nerve roots but posteromedial to the vertebral arteries and veins.

Protrusion of a cervical intervertebral disc can produce:

1. Nerve root compression alone, with pain down the arm
2. Compression of the spinal cord structures
3. A combination of both
4. Local and referred pain in the absence of nerve root compression

When there is nerve root compression, there are additional local symptoms in and about the neck resulting from local disease process in the cervical spine.

CLINICAL MANIFESTATIONS. Symptoms of nerve root compression, when present, usually constitute the chief complaint. However, the majority of patients have only symptoms of local and referred pain as a consequence of the disc degeneration. Occasionally, there is a history of trauma, but usually it is minor in nature. A form of precipitating injury may be an unexpected and abrupt forward jerk of the head as with sudden acceleration or deceleration of an automobile when hit from behind or in a head-on collision. The patient may sometimes notice restriction of neck movement.

The predominant feature of nerve root compression from a laterally placed protrusion is pain distributed according to the level of the disc lesion and the nerve root involved. There are eight cervical nerve roots, the first leaving the canal between the occiput and the atlas, where there is no disc. Therefore, a disc herniation at a particular level will compress the nerve root immediately below it; e.g., a sixth cervical disc will compress a seventh cervical nerve root. Lesions of the sixth cervical nerve produce pain and paresthesia over the radial aspect of the forearm, thumb, and index finger. There is wasting, weakness, and loss of biceps reflex. Involvement of the seventh cervical nerve root will produce pain and paresthesia referred to the dorsal aspect of the forearm and wrist and to one or all of the three middle fingers. On the left side, involvement of the seventh cervical nerve root frequently produces chest pain, which may be misdiagnosed as a coronary thrombosis.

The pain has the usual persistent aching quality associated with nerve root compression, lasting from weeks to months. Attacks tend to recur, and the intervals of relief become shortened until the pain in the upper limb becomes intractable. However, in general, the root symptoms are of a subacute or chronic nature, permitting the patient to carry on with mild restricted activity in spite of some persistent paresthesia of the fingers.

The mode of production of symptoms by nerve compression, as described by Frykholm, has been referred to. Nerve root compression results in pain in the myotome, sclerotome, and dermatome with a wide and diffuse distribution proximally but a more narrow and more localized radiation distally.

There is usually a reduction of mobility in the cervical spine in both lateral and anteroposterior flexion, but any limitation in extension tends to be obscured by free movement of the head at the atlantoaxooccipital articulations. However, even in the presence of marked neurologic signs, cervical movements may sometimes be quite unrestricted.

The compression test of steady downward pressure on the vertex of the skull or forehead from behind with flexion and extension toward the affected side will often produce severe radicular pain, whereas suspension of the head may relieve the pain. Localized tenderness in muscle at the affected level is common, as is tenderness in areas of the shoulder girdle and the upper limb secondary to localized muscle spasm caused by anterior rami irritation.

Neurologic signs such as selective wasting of muscles, reduction or abolition of deep tendon reflexes, e.g., the biceps, triceps, or brachioradialis, and sensory changes in an area of dermatome distribution may be present.

Radiologic examination will reveal absence of the normal cervical lordosis and narrowing of the involved intervertebral space. Oblique views of the cervical spine may reveal narrowing of the anteroposterior diameter of the intervertebral foramina by osteophytes or by osteoarthritic changes of the lateral articulations.

In uncomplicated nerve root compression, examination of the cerebrospinal fluid and/or myelography are usually unnecessary. However, myelography may show a partial block, and the protein content of the cerebrospinal fluid may be increased.

Cervical Myelopathy

This condition will present as weakness and spasticity in one or both legs, with associated exaggerated reflexes and an extensor plantar response. Sensory changes in the legs and trunk are less common and usually are paresthesias, patchy in distribution and rarely with a sharp upper level. In the upper limbs a more complex picture may result from the relative balance of spinal cord versus peripheral nerve root involvement. There may be weakness and wasting, which may be limited to a single root distribution or confined to the small muscles of the hand on one side or both or may be generalized throughout the arm with fasciculation.

Sphincter disturbances occur in about a third of the patients but are not severe and consist mainly of hesitancy or urgency of micturition. Incontinence is unusual.

ETIOLOGY. Simple compression of the spinal cord and its fibers is not the only mechanism responsible for neurologic signs in cervical myelopathy. A purely mechanical cause in the nature of a tethering effect of the dentate ligament which, in preventing backward displacement of the cord, compresses the pyramidal fibers lying beneath its attachments against the osteophyte has been suggested. O'Connell believed that the myelopathy did not result from any sustained compression of the nerve tissues but rather from compression by the discs of the anterior spinal arteries during movement, particularly between C_5–C_6, and C_6–C_7. Changes in the vascular supply also have been implicated, since demyelination is greatest in the territory of supply of the anterior spinal artery and its branches.

Most probably the cause of cord damage is interference with the blood flow in the anterior spinal artery and branches brought about either by intermittent compression or by frictional injuries of the vessel during neck movement.

DIFFERENTIAL DIAGNOSIS OF CERVICAL COMPRESSION OR IRRITATIVE LESIONS. Spinal Cord Tumors and Syringomyelia. In the former, absence of trauma in the history, a slow progressive course, negative clinical tests and radiographs for protrusion, and finally a positive myelogram will aid diagnosis.

In syringomyelia, there is segmental sensory loss over the neck, shoulders, and arms, amyotrophy, and thoracic scoliosis. Symptoms usually begin in late childhood, adolescence, or adult life and progress irregularly, being arrested for long periods of time.

Osteoarthritis of the Cervical Spine. This occurs in middle age groups and affects the spine over more than one segment. It has a slow, episodic, chronic course, with stiffness and sometimes diffuse tenderness on palpation of the cervical spine. Irritative symptoms are sometimes present, but objective neurologic signs from root compression as a rule are absent. X-rays, apart from the usual features of osteoarthritis, may show osteophytes adjacent to the vertebral foramina giving rise to radicular pain and paresthesias.

Direct Injury Producing Laminar Fractures. There is a history of trauma. At times only exploration will establish the diagnosis if the radiographs are negative.

Thoracic Inlet Syndrome. *Cervical Rib.* The rudimentary rib, although usually symptomless, may affect the lowest trunk of the plexus composed of C_8 and T_1 nerve roots. The course is gradual, without remissions or exacerbations. Motor signs usually involve the median or ulnar nerves, and sensory findings are within the C_8 dermatome. Vasomotor symptoms may be present.

Scalenus Anticus Syndrome. This is due to an abnormal insertion and can simulate the above findings.

Pancoast Tumor (Superior Pulmonary Sulcus Tumor). This is an unusual involvement of the apex of the lung parenchyma in the supraclavicular area by a pleomorphic adenocarcinoma. Radicular pain into one of the extremities, paresthesias, and sensory loss involving the dermatomes of C_5 and C_6 in the forearm and hand or of the C_8 and

T_1 roots are seen. Horner's syndrome of the eye with ptosis and constriction of the pupil may be produced by involvement of the sympathetic inferior cervical ganglion. On radiography, the tumor may be seen as an opacity in the apical area with or without destruction of the ribs, particularly the second thoracic rib, or of the vertebral column itself.

TREATMENT OF THE CERVICAL COMPRESSION SYNDROME. In the most acute case, particularly if the pain persists for more than a few weeks, strict recumbency and immobilization of the neck in cervical traction are indicated with adequate sedation and physiotherapy. Once the pain has subsided and in less severe attacks, the patient may be placed in a cervical collar during the period of the spasm.

Active resistance exercises should be carried out to elongate the soft tissues within their normal range and reduce periarticular fibrous contracture. The accompanying increased circulation to the deep neck tissues improves flexibility, muscle tone, and neck posture.

If there is progression of the neurologic deficit or cord structure compression, surgical intervention is indicated.

Occasionally it may be found that a lateral protrusion produces symptoms of cord compression due to interference with the vascular supply of a segment of the cord. In cases with a more centrally situated lesion, laminectomy is necessary, and, to facilitate the safe retraction of the cord in its coverings, mobilization of the cord by division of several slips of denticulate ligament is advisable prior to removal of the herniation.

Fusion of the spine may be required, particularly if an extensive laminectomy has been necessary. Smith and Robinson have noted that when symptoms are bilateral, disc removal and fusion of the cervical spine by the anterior approach are indicated. This procedure produces less morbidity and less disturbance of the spinal cord than the posterior exposure.

However, Campbell and Phillips, as a result of experience with 60 cases of myelopathy of the spinal cord or radiculitis due to cervical intervertebral disc lesions and spondylosis, believe that brachial neuritis and true disc prolapse with cord compression have a good prognosis. They recommend the use of a light Minerva plastic jacket with both chest and back pieces extending up to form a head halter.

Low Back Pain

Low back pain has a multiplicity of causes, and although few of them result in mortality, this complaint is associated with high morbidity, great inconvenience, and severe economic burden. "Low back syndrome" refers to a disease or injury of the lumbosacral spine with or without an underlying predisposing condition. The condition may be acute, producing a temporary or permanent change in the physical state of the individual, or may be a chronic condition exhibiting variable degrees of frequency, duration of symptoms, and degrees of physical deterioration.

Rowe described the varying conditions which can produce the low back syndrome. These are presented in Table

Table 43-2. CAUSES OF LOW BACK PAIN

A. Structural defects
  1. Segmentation defects
    a. Six lumbar vertebrae
    b. Four lumbar vertebrae
    c. Transitional lumbosacral junction
  2. Ossification defects
    a. Spina bifida
    b. Spondylolysis
    c. Spondylolisthesis
  3. Facet abnormalities
    a. Asymmetry (tropism)
    b. Anteroposterior lumbosacral facets
  4. Increased lumbosacral angle
B. Functional defects
  1. Lateral imbalance (leg-length discrepancy, scoliosis, work or postural attitudes, etc.)
  2. Anteroposterior imbalance (pregnancy, potbelly, flexion contracture of hips and knees, etc.)
C. Infections
  1. Bone and joint
    a. Arthritis
    b. Tuberculosis
    c. Brucellosis
    d. Osteomyelitis
  2. Soft tissue
    a. "Myositis"
    b. "Fibrositis"
D. Degenerative processes
  1. Osteoarthritis
  2. Senile osteoporosis
  3. Degenerative disc disease
E. Neoplastic processes
  1. Primary
    a. Multiple myeloma
    b. Hemangioma
    c. Giant cell tumor, eosinophilic granuloma, osteogenic sarcoma
  2. Metastatic
    a. Prostate and breast
    b. Lung, kidney, thyroid, gastrointestinal tract
F. Traumatic
  1. Compression fracture
  2. Vertebral process fracture (facet, transverse, and spinous process)
  3. Sprain and strain
  4. Ruptured disc

SOURCE: From M. L. Rowe, *J Occup Med,* 2:219, 1960.

43-2, which does not include lumbosacral pain consequent to visceral disease or psychosomatic disorder.

The low back syndrome usually occurs in the third, fourth, or fifth decades of life as an acute low back pain associated with muscle spasm. The pain may be aggravated by coughing, sneezing, defecation, or any other maneuver which raises the intrathecal pressure, but it is rarely of true radicular nature and is usually relieved by lying down with the knees flexed.

On examination, there may be tenderness in the lumbosacral angle or of the spinous processes and interspinous ligaments. There is frequently limitation of vertebral movement with or without spasm of the paravertebral muscles, and very occasionally nerve root involvement may be found. Radiologic examination may show narrowing of the L_4, L_5, or S_1 disc spaces with some associated lumbar spondylosis or posterior facet joint subluxation (Fig. 43-5). However, radiographic evidence of such underlying lesions should not be taken as necessarily indicative of the causative pathologic condition. Rumbold noted that routine preemployment x-rays of the lumbar spine of 1,000 consecutive applicants for work revealed specific conditions such as narrowing of the intervertebral disc or acute lumbosacral angles in 660 of the individuals. Similarly, Splithoff compared the radiographs of the lumbosacral spines of 100 so-called "normal" people with 100 patients complaining of "backache." He found that such conditions as spina bifida, spondylosis, and osteoarthritis occurred just as frequently in the "normal" as in the "backache" group.

ETIOLOGIC FACTORS. Rowe has emphasized the concept of degenerative disc disease as an etiologic factor in the low back syndrome. During the normal aging process, the mechanical stresses in the lumbar spine fall primarily on the posterior aspect of the annulus fibrosus, particularly at L_4 and L_5, so that multiple, though minor, traumas produce gradual loss of disc material. This may result in irritation of the adjacent nerve roots to give the clinical manifestations of a "lumbosacral strain," "lumbago," "myositis," or "sacroiliac strain." Narrowing of the intervertebral space may progress so that the intervertebral foramen becomes smaller and distorted, and spondylosis or even a reverse spondylolisthesis may occur with further narrowing of this intervertebral foramen. Involvement of the nerve root results in a pain-spasm reflex, which may produce some degree of ischemia of muscle tissue and further pain.

Another condition contributing to the low back syndrome was described by Morgan and King, namely, instability in the anteroposterior plane of the adjacent vertebrae, during flexion and extension, presumably due to incomplete tears of the posterior aspects of the annulus fibrosus. This may produce severe low back pain with pain radiating down the thighs, but not of a truly radicular nature. Morgan and King believe that this condition of an "unstable back" makes up nearly 30 percent of all cases of low back pain in the middle age range. They advise educating the patient to avoid forward flexion and lifting strains, and exclusion of other pathologic causes.

CLINICAL HISTORY. In evaluating the clinical history of low back pain, it is important to assess the type of pain, its site, whether it is referred, its duration, its mode of onset, its relationship to activity and to rest, and its association with symptoms relevant to other systems such as the genitourinary, gynecologic, and alimentary organs.

In disease processes such as neoplasm, tuberculosis, and various types of osteomyelitis of the spine, the pain is usually severe, localized, and not relieved by rest. In mechanical lesions, rest usually relieves the pain, except in the presence of severe root irritation. Diurnal variation of the pain and associated stiffness are important. Ankylosing spondylitis is characterized by early morning pain, relieved as activity increases. Pain due to intervertebral disc lesions or lumbar spondylosis is usually relieved by bed rest and aggravated by activity.

CLINICAL EXAMINATION. First, the patient is examined standing; posture, weight, muscular development, the state

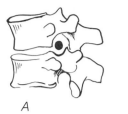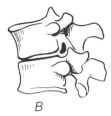

Fig. 43-5. Narrowing of lumbar disc space with a reversed spondylosis and deformation of the peripheral nerve. (*After Rowe, 1960. Taken with permission from Mercer and Duthie [eds.], "Orthopaedic Surgery," Edward Arnold [Publishers] Ltd., London, 1972.*)

of lumbar lordotic curve, and the presence of any structural or "discogenic" scoliosis are noted (Fig. 43-6). Ranges of flexion, extension, and lateral flexion of the lumbar spine are determined, especially if there is restriction because of spasm or pain.

The patient is then examined supine. The abdomen is palpated for any mass or tenderness. Particular attention is paid to the presence or absence of peripheral pulses. Joints of the lower limbs are put through the range of movement, and then the straight-leg-raising test is carried out. In this test the patient's straight leg is flexed at the hip and can, under normal circumstances, be lifted to almost 90° depending on the tightness of the hamstrings. Limitation of this movement is usually present in low back pain and sciatica. When dorsiflexion of the foot (Bragard's test) is superimposed upon straight-leg raising, the pull on

Fig. 43-6. Exaggeration of a "discogenic" scoliosis (left) by forward flexion (right) which is restricted in range. (*Taken with permission from Mercer and Duthie [eds.], "Orthopaedic Surgery," Edward Arnold [Publishers] Ltd., London, 1972.*)

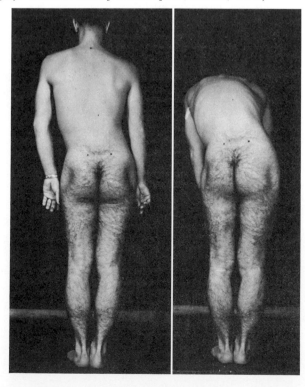

the sciatic produces sciatic pain. With straight-leg raising, there is a 4-mm excursion of the L_4, L_5, S_1, and S_2 nerve roots within the intervertebral foramen. This is restricted by adhesion formation, by tumor, or by prolapse of an intervertebral disc.

Finally, a comprehensive neurologic examination is carried out, with assessment of the reflexes, the presence of sensation, and motor power.

A rectal and prostatic examination of the male and a gynecologic examination of the female are essential.

ANCILLARY TESTS. Anteroposterior, lateral, and oblique views of the lumbosacral spine including cone views of the lumbosacral junction are necessary in a patient complaining of back pain. In certain circumstances, it is necessary to carry out detailed examinations of the urine, the blood, and cerebrospinal fluid, and a Wassermann test.

TREATMENT OF LOW BACK SYNDROME. The treatment of low back syndrome should be essentially conservative, with adequate bed rest in a low Fowler position, sedation, and some type of superficial heat to relieve the muscle spasm. Some authorities believe that when the pain improves, knee-to-chest flexion exercises or lumbar flexion and hanging exercises and, in some cases, the restriction of back movements by the use of a corset or brace will help both to relieve symptoms and to prevent recurrence.

SPONDYLOLISTHESIS AND SPONDYLOLYSIS

The term "spondylolisthesis" was first used by Kilian in 1853 and is derived from the Greek word *olisthesis,* meaning a "slipping" or a "falling," and is used to describe the condition of forward subluxation of one vertebral body upon another. The condition is not limited to any specific segment of the vertebral column, but most commonly the term refers to displacement of the fifth lumbar vertebra on the body of the first sacral vertebra. The term "spondylolysis" is used to describe a bony defect of the neural arch, a condition which is felt to be one of the predisposing factors in the production of spondylolisthesis.

There is some evidence that this condition is genetically inherited with an increased penetrance caused by inbreed-

Fig. 43-7. *A.* Normal lumbosacral vertebrae. *B.* Defect at the pars interarticularis with forward slip of the body of the fifth lumbar vertebra upon the sacrum. This is particularly seen on aligning the posterior surface of the bodies of the fifth lumbar and first sacral vertebrae.

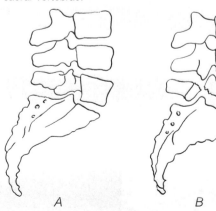

A   *B*

ing. Baker and McHolick examined the x-rays of the lumbosacral region of 400 school children between the ages of six and seven and found an incidence of arch defect in 4.5 percent. Upon examination of the parents of these children it was found that the incidences of arch defect was 27.6 percent, which is more than five times greater than the incidence in the general population.

The incidence obviously varies throughout the world and is higher in certain races or occupations. Roche and Rowe, in an extensive study of 4,000 skeletons, found that white and Negro incidences varied as follows:

White   male : female :: 6.4 : 2.3 percent
Negro   male : female :: 2.8 : 2.3 percent

Stewart described an incidence of 50 percent in the Alaskan Eskimos, a finding which may result from inbreeding.

PATHOLOGY. Spondylolisthesis usually results from a structural defect in the fifth lumbar vertebra, the defective vertebra being divided into two separate parts by a deep bilateral defect in the pars interarticularis of the neural arch. The anterior segment of the vertebra is composed of the body, pedicles, transverse processes, and superior articular facets, while the posterior fragment includes the spinous process, the laminae, and the inferior articular facets (Fig. 43-7).

There is no certainty as to the manner by which the defect develops, although it does not appear to be congenital. None of the series of examinations carried out upon the spines of the newborn has yet yielded a single example of spondylolisthesis or any defect in normal ossification. There are three primary centers of ossification for a vertebra, i.e., one for the body and one for each half of the neural arch from the point where the base of the pedicle is attached to the vertebral body to the tip of the spinous process. Each lateral center forms a pedicle, superior articular facets, pars interarticularis, inferior articular facets, laminae, and half the spinous process.

Wiltse described the etiology of spondylolisthesis as resulting from a defect in the pars interarticularis due to:

1. An inherited dysplasia in the cartilaginous arch of the affected vertebra.
2. The physical forces resulting from the erect position and the curvature of the lumbar spine acting on a weakened pars interarticularis. He believes that bone reabsorption results rather than any new bone formation defect. In his series, the condition was never present at birth and seldom present below the age of four, and the greatest incidence of slipping was seen between the ages of ten and fifteen years.

Spondylolysis, however, is not the only cause of spondylolisthesis, which can occur in the absence of any defect of the neural arch. Newman has described the following types of spondylolisthesis:

1. Infantile spondylolisthesis
   a. Facet deficiency or subluxation
   b. Attenuation of the pars interarticularis
   c. Loss of continuity of the pars interarticularis (spondylolysis)
2. Adult spondylolisthesis
   a. Stress fracture in mature bone
   b. Facet deficiency due to degenerative joint disease

CLINICAL MANIFESTATIONS. In children the condition is usually painless, although the parents may notice an unduly prominent abdomen and buttock. In adolescents and adults, backache may be the presenting symptom. It is usually intermittent, coming on after exercise or strain, and in some cases there may be sciatica as a consequence of root pressure. There are two mechanisms for this root pressure: the first occurs when the displacement of the intervertebral body is marked, producing distortion and narrowing of the intervertebral foramina with root pressure; the second mechanism, producing first sacral root pressure, is the result of a protrusion of the disc or pressure by an irregular osteophytic margin about the defect in the neural arch. Probably the most commonly experienced pain is that which arises in the disc adjacent to the unstable vertebrae as a consequence of altered spine mechanics and increased forces on the disc.

Spondylolisthesis can be completely asymptomatic and may be found during examination for other complaints. It would be difficult otherwise to explain the discrepancy between the 5 percent incidence of the defect in adult skeletons in anatomic museums and the much smaller numbers of the general population who present for treatment. Many patients first appear for treatment in the middle or late decades of life, but they have probably had the defect since early childhood.

Spondylolisthesis may be seen as a characteristic deformity which is the result of forward displacement of the involved vertebra and the vertebrae above. The spinous process above forms a "step" kyphosis in contrast to the "angular" kyphosis of tuberculous disease.

The pelvis is rotated about a transverse axis passing through the hip joints so that the anterosuperior iliac spines are raised to the same level as the posterosuperior iliac spines. This rotation may be so great that the thighs are not in a straight line with the trunk even when they are fully extended. Consequently the patient must stand with his trunk thrust forward if the legs are vertical or with the hips and knees flexed if the trunk is held erect. As the trunk is shortened by the downward displacement accompanying the forward slip, the ribs overlap or approach the iliac crest, and transverse creases appear above the waist.

RADIOLOGIC DIAGNOSIS. In the early stages of disease, especially in cases of simple spondylolysis, a simple translucency may be seen in the pars interarticularis. The lateral radiograph will show the presence of any spondylolisthesis (Fig. 43-8), but doubtful cases are best shown by an oblique view of the pars interarticularis. Under normal circumstances the pars interarticularis and the superior articular facet forms the outline of a "Scottish terrier." In the condition of spondylolysis without slip, the terrier is seen to wear a collar of translucency as compared with the rest of the bone, whereas in spondylolisthesis, when there has been movement forward of the superior articular facet, the terrier is seen to be decapitated.

TREATMENT. The surgical treatment of spondylolisthesis consists of fixing the involved segment by bony fusion, but this is a major undertaking. Therefore, consideration must be given to the age, sex of the patient, severity of the

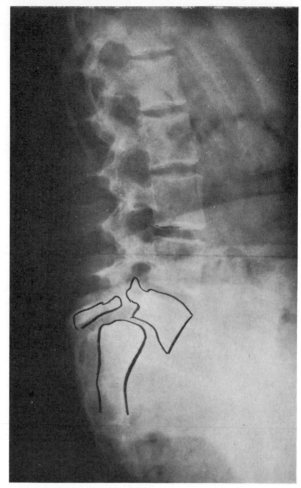

Fig. 43-8. Radiograph showing a spondylolisthesis of the fifth lumbar upon the first sacral vertebra, with an obvious defect in the pars interarticularis.

deformity, and physical occupation of the individual as well as the severity of his symptoms.

Younger patients are best treated by lumbosacral fusion, but in older people this approach is open to question. A successful fusion will relieve them of all their symptoms, but because the operation is a major one, these patients are probably best treated by the use of spinal brace or corset, combined with sleeping on a firm mattress.

The actual method of lumbosacral fusion is still controversial. Ideally the fusion should be a posterior or posterolateral one uniting the spinous processes, laminas, and transverse processes of the involved vertebrae to the normal vertebrae above and below. Other types of fusion such as anterior, transperitoneal, extraperitoneal, and posterior interbody fusions have been used, but these operations have limited application.

SCIATICA

Sciatica is a symptom and not a disease. It is a term used to describe pain of a radicular nature occurring in one or both lower limbs consequent to inflammation or pressure on one or more nerve roots involved in the formation of the lumbosacral plexus.

Causes of Sciatica

A. Nerve root compression
   1. Intraspinal compression. This may be due to a prolapsed intervertebral disc, an intraspinal tumor, or an intraspinal abscess.
   2. Compression within the intervertebral foramen. This may arise through a tumor of the nerve roots, such as neurofibroma, or a narrowing of the foramen due to a spondylolisthesis, spondylosis, or osteoarthritis of the posterior apophyseal joints.
   3. Compression within the pelvis or buttock. This may arise as a result of intrapelvic or gluteal abscess, or a tumor in one or the other of these sites.
B. Inflammation of nerve and nerve roots
   1. Toxic
      a. Alcoholism
      b. Diabetic neuritis
      c. Arsenical poisoning
      d. Lead poisoning
   2. "Infective"
      a. Focal sepsis
      b. Rheumatism
      c. Syphilis

Of all the causes of sciatica listed above intervertebral disc protrusion is by far the most common.

LUMBAR AND INTERVERTEBRAL DISC PROTRUSION

ANATOMY. Intervertebral discs, which unite the bodies of successive vertebras from the second cervical vertebra to the sacrum, form a series of amphiarthrotic, or slightly movable, joints with no synovial cavity. Structurally, intervertebral discs consist of three parts: the cartilage end plate, the annulus fibrosus, and the nucleus pulposus.

The cartilaginous end plate is a thin layer of hyaline cartilage adherent to the trabeculae of cancellous bone comprising the major portion of the vertebral body.

Nucleus Pulposus. The nucleus pulposus comprises the central portion of the intervertebral disc; it is a soft, semifluid mass containing over 80 percent water by weight, the water being bound to mucopolysaccharides as in myxoid tissue. Because it contains so much water, the nucleus is virtually incompressible and inelastic, although subject to a great range of changing pressures.

Annulus Fibrosus. Surrounding the nucleus pulposus is the annulus fibrosus, comprised of laminas, fibrocartilage, and fibrous tissue, and containing more cells, a greater abundance of collagen, and a lesser amount of mucopolysaccharide ground substance than the nucleus. The annulus is somewhat elastic; it bends with the overlying spinal ligaments, its fibers running obliquely from vertebra to vertebra, continuous with the fibrils in the cartilaginous end plates and ossified epiphyseal rings in the vertebral bodies. The function of the annulus fibrosus would appear to be twofold: to restrict and regulate movements of the vertebral column and to enclose and retain the nucleus pulposus.

The two components of the intervertebral discs, the annulus fibrosus and the nucleus pulposus, are avascular except for the most peripheral fibers of the annulus, which receive a small blood supply from adjacent vessels. The nutrition of the intervertebral disc therefore would appear to be dependent on the diffusion of fluid into it from the vertebral bodies and the vessels of the peripheral portion of the annulus.

With respect to nerve supply, fine unmyelinated nerve fibers have been found in the posterior longitudinal ligament and a lesser number in the annulus fibrosus. None are in the nucleus pulposus. The ligamentous and articular structures of the vertebral column have a considerable sensory innervation from the nervus sinuvertebralis of Luschka.

MECHANISM OF HERNIATIONS AND PROTRUSIONS OF THE INTERVERTEBRAL DISC. With aging, the collagen increases and becomes coarser. The mucopolysaccharides decrease, with the ratio of karatan sulfate to chondroitin sulfate increasing. The proteoglycans become smaller in molecular size and more firmly adherent to the collagen fibrils. The elasticity, viscosity, and water-binding capacity of the ground substance decrease. The proportion of water decreases from 90 percent in childhood to less than 70 percent in old age.

The nucleus is constantly under compression, and the turgid nucleus of a living person, bounded laterally by the strong elastic laminas of the annulus and vertically by the cartilaginous end plate, may burst through either one of these barriers. Spontaneous herniation of an intervertebral disc may take place either vertically into the spongiosa of the vertebral body or horizontally. Prolapse of nuclear substance can take place only when the nucleus retains its turgescence. This cannot occur in older people whose nuclei pulposi have undergone desiccation.

Vertical prolapse of an intervertebral disc into the vertebral bodies produces the phenomenon known as "Schmorl's nodes." It cannot be detected radiologically until it becomes outlined by a shell of reactive bone. It is of no clinical importance.

On the other hand, horizontal prolapse is of considerable clinical importance. Two forms of horizontal prolapse may occur, namely, nuclear herniation and annular protrusion (Fig. 43-9). In nuclear herniation the nucleus usually displaces posteriorly, but in annular prolapse there is convex bulging of the relaxed annulus fibers in all directions.

Posterior herniation of the nucleus pulposus is seldom accompanied by any gross breach of the annulus, and the semifluid material seems to escape by dissecting its way through the annulus. Most of these posterior herniations lie to one side of the midline, because the posterior longitudinal ligament prevents direct posterior herniation. Consequently, neurologic symptoms caused by direct pressure on the neural tissues tend to be unilateral.

Annular protrusions follow the narrowing of the disc space resulting from desiccation or vertebral prolapse of the nucleus, and the relaxed annulus fibers are squeezed outward. It is these anterolateral protrusions of the fibers of the annulus that account for the common and well-known form of osteophytosis or spondylosis of the vertebral column.

PATHOLOGY OF NUCLEAR PROTRUSIONS. As stated

above, the most common site for posterior herniation of nuclear material is posterolateral. This herniation may enlarge and may impinge on neighboring nerve roots, producing symptoms and signs similar to any other space-occupying lesion in the intraspinal canal. There may be irritation of the nerve root by compression, by stretching, or by friction, an occlusion of its vasa nervorum, or a combination of all these factors. The compressed nerve root becomes edematous, enlarged, and later adherent to the protrusion.

A nerve root may be stretched tautly over a nuclear protrusion in close proximity to the ligamentum flavum. On straight-leg raising there is an excursion of 4 mm of spinal roots at L_4–L_5 and S_1–S_2. Therefore any pressure from a nuclear protrusion on such a nerve root will interfere with its range of movement. This is the basis of the restricted straight-leg raising test. Of course, if the pressure is severe and prolonged, impairment of axonal conductivity will occur in the nerve root, producing symptoms and signs of motor and sensory loss in the lower limb.

CLINICAL MANIFESTATIONS. Fifty percent of cases of intervertebral disc protrusion present initially as low backache followed later by radicular sciatic pain, whereas about one-third of patients may give a history of sciatica preceding the backache and in the remainder sciatica and backache commence simultaneously.

The onset may be acute following a minor degree of trauma such as a fall in the sitting position or the lifting of a heavy weight in the stooping position, but in many cases there is absolutely no evidence of any traumatic incident. In some cases the first attack may be the most severe one, followed by a series of perhaps minor but annoying exacerbations, but in others the reverse sequence of presentation may be the case. The reason for spontaneous remissions in this condition is not clearly understood, but they may occur by degeneration of compressed nerve fibers and the adjustment of the nerve root to its displaced position. Again, there may be diminution of the swelling associated with the herniation and reduction of edema of the nerve root.

Characteristically the pain of sciatica is usually described as a "dull ache," "like a toothache," a "dragging" pain, or a "shooting" pain radiating from the lower lumbar region to the buttock and farther distally into the lower limb. It is important to assess the actual distribution of pain, since it is referred to the dermatome of the involved nerve root and is a valuable method of localizing the site of the occlusion.

It is most important also to ask the patient whether there is any loss of sensation or motor power. It is quite common to find that there is subjective loss of motor power when no such loss is detectable on clinical examination. Inquiry as to urgency or frequency of micturition is most important, since this is an early sign of the rare but serious condition of central protrusion which embarrasses the cauda equina.

The patient is usually an adult male found to be in relatively good health, and in the majority of cases urine examination and rectal examination will be completely normal. It is essential never to omit a general examination

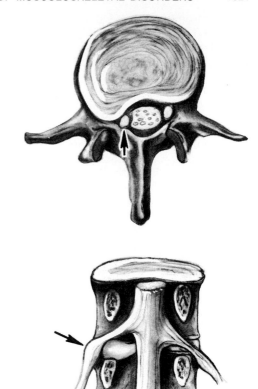

Fig. 43-9. Posterolateral herniation, or prolapse, with deformation of the peripheral nerve. (*Taken with permission from Mercer and Duthie [eds.], "Orthopaedic Surgery," Edward Arnold [Publishers] Ltd., London, 1972.*)

of the patient, however, because back pain and sciatica can have sinister significance.

Examination of the patient is first carried out with the patient standing and undressed. Special note is taken of the presence of any alterations of the spinal curvature with respect to both lumbar lordosis and the presence of any discogenic scoliosis, and then movements of flexion, extension, and lateral flexion to either side are assessed. Where these initially appear to be normal, attention should be paid to the rhythm of flexion and extension of the lumbar spine. It is also important to make sure that what appears to be relatively normal lateral flexion on one side or the other is actually being carried out at the lumbar spine and not at the thoracolumbar junction.

The patient is then asked to assume the supine position, and attention paid to the degree of difficulty he has in mounting the couch. With the patient in the supine position the abdomen can be palpated and the range of movement of the hips and knees examined.

The effects of straight-leg raising or the possible presence of a positive Lasègue sign is then assessed. In the presence of a protrusion, the straight-leg-raising test will aggravate the pain and may actually aggravate the radiation to the extremity. The greater the restriction of straight-leg raising, the larger the protrusion. Such symptoms are aggravated in the straight-leg-raising position by forced dorsiflexion of the foot and then are known as Lasègue's sign.

Finally, a neurologic assessment with respect to reflexes, motor power, and sensation is carried out on the lower limbs. Impairment of sensation may be found along the dermatome of the nerve root involved, especially along the outer thigh, the calf, and the foot. Examination for motor power may reveal weakness of the long extensor or flexor of the great toe and occasionally of the gluteal muscles, where of course the symptom must be assessed with the patient in the prone position. In the presence of a severe protrusion at the L_5–S_1 disc space the ankle jerk may well be diminished. The absence of a knee jerk indicates a higher prolapse than usual.

SPECIAL EXAMINATIONS. Radiography. Anteroposterior and lateral views of the lumbosacral spine and similar cone views of the lumbosacral junction are taken routinely. The major purpose of these x-rays is to exclude diseases of a more sinister nature. They also help to assess the possible presence of discogenic scoliosis and the state of the intervertebral discs (Fig. 43-10). The lumbar disc spaces normally show progressive widening in a caudal direction, the space between L_2 and L_3 being wider than the one above. The lateral view may show diminished disc spaces, but a normal space does not always exclude a small disc protrusion at this level.

Myelography. Myelography is a valuable additional radiologic investigation to exclude other conditions and to help

Fig. 43-10. Lateral radiograph of lumbar spine to show narrowing of the disc space between L_4 and L_5 due to a disc prolapse.

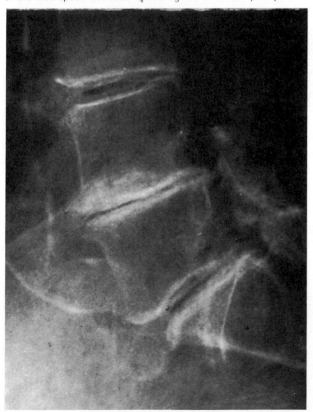

localize the site of the intervertebral disc protrusion (Fig. 43-11). It is especially valuable where the diagnosis is in doubt, as in the presence of an intraspinal tumor. But it is not always necessary as a preliminary to operative removal of the disc protrusion, because neurologic assessment of the level of the herniation, even without myelography, is highly reliable.

Three methods of myelography are available, namely, gas, water-soluble medium, and oily contrast medium.

Since the process of myelography involves lumbar puncture, the opportunity should be taken to test the dynamics of the cerebrospinal fluid as well as to obtain a specimen for biochemical assessment.

DIFFERENTIAL DIAGNOSIS. Although most cases of backache and sciatica are a result of a prolapsed intervertebral disc, it is most important in all cases to exclude the possibility of tuberculosis or tumors of the vertebral column, meninges, or nerve roots, and especially secondary deposits.

In a prolapsed intervertebral disc the complaint is usually episodic, whereas in most other conditions of tumor or infection the symptoms and signs tend to be constant and progressive. When a case of herniated intervertebral disc is examined, the patient is obviously well, whereas in more serious conditions he may be obviously ill or cachectic and the limitation of back movement is usually far more restricted than in an intervertebral disc lesion.

On radiologic examination tuberculous foci and primary or secondary deposits in the vertebral bodies are easily detectable, and other conditions such as spondylolisthesis, spondylosis, or old fractures are also clearly seen. In cases of doubt, myelography should be performed as indicated above.

TREATMENT. Conservative Treatment. With few exceptions conservative treatment is recommended initially in all cases of prolapsed intervertebral discs; in about 80 percent of cases this may effect complete and permanent relief.

The ideal method of instituting conservative treatment is to advise strict recumbency for a period of at least 3 weeks, and if the attack is severe, up to 6 weeks. This forced bed rest should be accompanied by adequate sedation, simple analgesics, and the use of heat. When the symptoms have subsided to some degree, and in some cases as a primary method of treatment, immobilization of the lumbar spine in a plaster jacket which permits the patient to remain mobile is useful. Recurrence of the intervertebral disc protrusion may be prevented by instructing the patient to avoid stooping and lifting as far as possible. A Knight back brace or a lumbosacral corset is of value in limiting motion of the lumbosacral spine, decreasing lordosis and providing counter pressure for the abdominal wall when abdominal muscles are weak. Patients are instructed in Williams' exercises to strengthen the lumbar spine flexors, especially the abdominal muscles and the gluteus maximus.

Surgical Treatment. Operative removal of a herniated intervertebral disc is indicated if the attacks are severe, disabling, frequent, or persisting in spite of a well-planned conservative regimen of treatment. In a few cases, a sudden paraplegia or very severe nerve root compression with paralysis or paresis of muscle groups demands an emergency operation.

The operative procedure for removal of the herniated nucleus pulposus is one of laminectomy in which a small portion of the lamina and ligamentum flavum is removed at the site of the protrusion, the embarrassed nerve root retracted, and the prolapsed and herniating nucleus material removed. Concomitant spinal fusion is necessary only if there has been an extensive laminectomy, if there is associated degenerative disease of the intervertebral column or a congenital malformation, or when the patient is to return to very heavy manual labor.

DISORDERS OF THE LUMBOSACRAL JUNCTION

The lumbosacral junction is an unstable anatomic region because:

1. It is the junction of mobile and fixed portions of the vertebral column.
2. It is more suited to the quadriped position and is a disadvantage in the upright position of man.
3. It is the site of rotary movements which are often asymmetrical.
4. It is the site of great shearing strains.

Lumbosacral Strain

Lumbosacral strain occurs in both acute and chronic forms.

ACUTE. Acute lumbosacral strain may be precipitated by a sudden blow or fall which forces the joints of the lumbosacral region into positions beyond their normal range of movement. In such cases there may be severe pain in the back and occasionally root pressure, sciatic pain, and a sciatic scoliosis. Most patients, however, exhibit pain and tenderness at the lumbosacral junction with restriction of movement.

CHRONIC. Chronic lumbosacral strain is usually insidious in onset but may follow an acute strain which has been unrecognized or unsatisfactorily treated. The middle-aged woman with an obese abdomen and the tall, asthenic individual with poor musculature are both at risk. In the chronic cases symptoms vary from complaints of a "weak back," tiring easily, to others with very acute pain and real disability, although episodic in nature.

TREATMENT. Rest in bed for a period of 1 to 3 weeks is indicated, and as the symptoms subside, spinal and postural exercises are introduced. For those with chronic pain and particularly those with pendulous abdomens or poor musculature a lumbosacral support is advisable.

"Sprung Back"

"Sprung back" is a term devised by Newman to describe the syndrome of chronic low lumbar strain.

The patient is usually a female in the latter half of the second decade or in the third or fourth decade of life complaining of pain across the top of the sacrum often radiating to both buttocks and thighs as far as the knees. The pain is described as dull and nagging and becoming more severe toward the end of the day. There may be a history of a fall, a blow on the back, strain while lifting, difficulty with childbirth, or violent activity during adolescence.

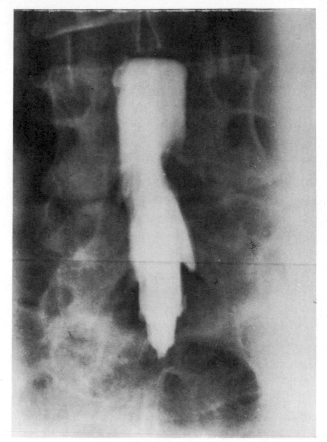

Fig. 43-11. Myelograph to show the deformed outline on the side due to a disc prolapse.

Characteristically, the pain is increased by lumbar flexion exaggerated by the slouch position, sleeping on a soft mattress, bending, stooping, lifting, or leaning forward over low objects as in washing, ironing, or cooking.

Clinical examination of these patients is mainly negative, although occasionally there may be restriction of active flexion with tenderness in the midline of the lower lumbar spine. There may be some widening of the spinous processes with deficiency of the supraspinous ligament. Indeed, it has been suggested that this condition is due to rupture or strain of the posterior ligaments, including perhaps the posterior longitudinal ligament and the annulus fibrosus.

Newman has advised against any temptation to label the condition as psychogenic. Treatment should consist of reassurance and the use of palliative measures such as heat, sedation, postural exercises, and lumbosacral support.

Sacralization of the Fifth Lumbar Vertebra

The lumbosacral region is liable to developmental disorders which diminish its strength and mobility. Small imperfections in this region may cause severe low back pain and sciatica following degenerative changes.

Sacralization of the last lumbar vertebra may vary in that the transverse processes, pedicles, and inferior facets may be transformed into the lateral masses of the sacral vertebra on one side or both. When both sides are sacralized and the vertebra is completely fused to the sacrum, the sacrum is lengthened by an extra vertebra at its upper end. This type of anomaly seldom produces symptoms.

Sacralization of the last lumbar vertebra gives rise to much more trouble when it is unilateral and incomplete (Fig. 43-12). The syndesmosis attaching the sacralized portion of the fifth lumbar vertebra to the sacrum allows some asymmetrical movement with wear and tear in the lateral articulation and the intervertebral disc. The symptoms tend to develop most frequently on the side which is not sacralized, where there is greater movement and a greater susceptibility to injury.

SPINAL OSTEOARTHRITIS AND SPONDYLOSIS

Osteoarthritis is a disease of synovial diarthrodial joints such as the posterior apophyseal joints of the vertebral column. It must be distinguished from spondylosis, which depends upon degeneration of the intervertebral discs, which are amphiarthrotic, and less movable joints possessing no synovial cavity of synovial membrane. Osteoarthritis of the facette joints can occur in the absence of disc disease or in association with it. The processes of osteoarthritis and degenerative disc disease are separate but frequently may coexist in the older patient.

Fig. 43-12. Radiograph of the left side of the fifth lumbar vertebra and the sacrum, showing unilateral sacralization with sclerosis around the abnormal syndesmosis.

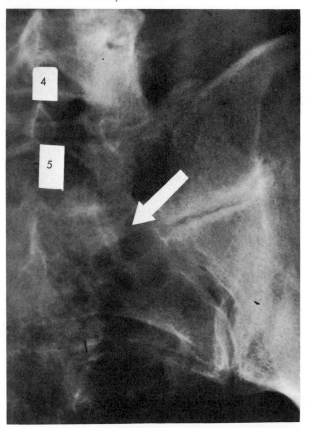

FIBROSITIS (LUMBAGO)

Fibrositis refers to cases of low backache in which there may be one or more tender nodules lying fairly superficially in the erector spinae or its attachments, or in the region of the muscular attachments to the crest of the ilium. Lumbago can be caused by some internal derangement of a low lumbar intervertebral joint. The pain comes on suddenly while the patient bends his back and is so severe that the lumbar region is at once immobilized by muscular spasm. After this acute phase, examination shows that lumbar extension is impossible. Treatment consists of rest in bed with heat and sedation.

TUMORS OF THE VERTEBRAL COLUMN

The vertebral column differs from other parts of the skeleton in reference to the relative incidence of various neoplastic lesions. Certain types of primary bone tumors including aneurysmal bone cysts and benign osteoblastomas predominate in the vertebral column, and one primary bone tumor, i.e., the chordoma, occurs exclusively in the axial skeleton. However, most types of primary bone tumors, including giant cell tumor, osteogenic sarcoma, chondrosarcoma, and fibrosarcoma occur less frequently in the spine than in other parts of the skeleton. Metastatic tumors commonly involve the spine and account for the majority of cases in any series of vertebral tumors in adults. Guri reported that the most common primary tumors affecting the vertebral column were multiple myeloma, fibrosarcoma, Hodgkin's disease, hemangioma, giant cell tumor, chondroma, and chondrosarcoma. In 50 cases of destruction of vertebrae by metastasis, 32 lesions were osteolytic lesions from carcinoma of the breast, 7 from carcinoma of the prostate, 3 from hypernephroma, and 1 from each of the following: Ewing's tumor, chondrosarcoma, bronchiogenic tumor, carcinoma of skin, rectum, and cervix, osteogenic sarcoma, and fibrosarcoma.

A classification of tumors of the vertebral column includes:

A. Primary tumors
   1. Malignant
      a. Myelomatosis
      b. Chordoma
      c. Giant cell tumor
      d. Ewing's tumor
      e. Chondrosarcoma
      f. Osteogenic sarcoma
      g. Fibrosarcoma
      h. Hodgkin's disease
   2. Benign
      a. Angioma
      b. Aneurysmal bone cyst
      c. Benign osteoblastoma
B. Secondary tumors
   1. Metastatic carcinoma

The symptoms produced by vertebral tumors depend upon their site, the speed of their growth, and the degree of involvement of cord and/or of nerve roots. In the early stages back pain is the most common symptom, and clinical signs may be restricted to tenderness over the area in which the disease process is present. Later, when the nerve roots or cord are involved, neurologic signs become manifest. It is important to look for signs of both upper and lower motor neuron involvement in any case in which vertebral tumor is suspected. Evidence of the *lower motor neuron* lesion is weakness or paralysis of individual muscles, decrease in muscle tone, reduction in tendon and cutaneous reflexes, which help to delineate the level of involvement, and wasting of muscle. *Upper motor neuron* disease of the pyramidal tract is characterized by loss of voluntary movement with spasticity, increased tendon reflexes, sensory changes, and an increased plantar reflex or a positive Babinski sign. The posterior columns of the posterior nerve roots or the peripheral nerve may also be involved.

Alteration of the spinal cord contents results from direct pressure on the tissues or, secondarily, because of a change in the blood supply to produce edema, hemorrhage, and degeneration. Autonomic system involvement may be evidenced by increased sweating with vasomotor and pilomotor reactions as well as a Horner syndrome when the inferior cervical ganglion is involved. The function of the sphincters must be carefully examined, since either incontinence or retention of urine or constipation or incontinence of feces may be present.

As with all bone tumors, radiologic examination and biopsy are important aids to diagnosis. Biochemical investigations are also important in recognizing myelomatosis, which has an abnormal electrophoretic pattern of the serum proteins, with a Bence Jones proteinuria. In metastatic prostatic carcinoma the serum acid phosphatase level may be elevated. Occasionally in osteoblastic lesions, such as a metastatic carcinoma of the prostate or of the lung, the serum alkaline phosphatase level may be elevated.

With circumscribed and presumably benign lesions, surgical excision is usually the treatment of choice, and this is a procedure which provides the histologic diagnosis. When, however, there is clinical uncertainty about the possibility of malignancy and when some other treatment such as radiotherapy is contemplated, elective biopsy must be undertaken in order to establish the nature of the lesion. Open surgical biopsy is the most desirable procedure, but this is not always possible, because of inaccessibility of the deep-seated vertebrae. In such cases, aspiration biopsy by the special techniques described by Ottolenghi and by Schajowicz may be used.

PYOGENIC OSTEOMYELITIS OF THE VERTEBRAL COLUMN

The most common organism responsible for this condition is *Staphylococcus aureus,* which spreads hematogenously from infective foci, such as boils, septic teeth, tonsillitis, or otitis media.

Pyogenic osteomyelitis in the vertebral column may occur at any age, but it is most common during adolescence and in young adulthood and considerably more common in males than females.

PATHOLOGY. Henson and Coventry and others have drawn attention to the urinary tract as a source of secondary spinal infection by hematogenous spread from the pelvic and abdominal viscera via the vertebral venous plexus described by Batson. However, vascular anatomy studies in relation to this condition by Wiley and Trueta indicate that although this venous plexus does exist, it is unlikely to be the route by which infection reaches the vertebrae.

The levels most commonly affected are the lumbar, thoracic, and cervical regions, in that order, and the actual site of infection is usually in the metaphyseal portion of the vertebra. It often rapidly spreads across the periphery of the disc to involve the metaphysis of the adjacent vertebra above or below, and sometimes two separate pairs of vertebrae are affected, or even three in succession. Wiley and Trueta maintain that this indicates arterial spread via ascending and descending nutrient branches of the posterior spinal arteries.

Marked collapse of the bodies with gibbus formation as in tuberculosis is quite uncommon in pyogenic vertebral osteomyelitis, as is large paravertebral abscess formation. Pus will spread along normal cleavage planes in the tissues to present in the retropharyngeal space in the cervical region, the mediastinum in the thoracic region, and the retroperitoneal space in the lumbar region with perirenal, psoas, and pelvic abscess formation. Occasionally the pus may track backward to form an epidural abscess with compression of the spinal cord.

CLINICAL MANIFESTATIONS. The acute fulminating type is most common in young patients and may be accompanied by very severe and intense toxemia. In the past the mortality rate in these cases was very high. The chronic type, which seems to be somewhat more common in the adult, usually presents as malaise, fever, and very severe spinal pain, which is aggravated by movement and not relieved by rest. Unrelieved or increasing back pain after posterior laminectomy should immediately raise the question of a disc space infection. Examination of these patients reveals marked tenderness over the spinous processes of the involved vertebrae and severe muscle spasm and rigidity of the vertebral column. If the symptoms are of long standing, an abscess may be detected, and if there has been involvement of the spinal cord, signs of partial or complete paraplegia may be evident.

It may be difficult to distinguish this condition, particularly in the subacute or chronic form, from tuberculosis. However, both in acute and chronic vertebral osteomyelitis there is a marked polymorphonuclear leukocytosis and a raised sedimentation rate. A positive blood culture is helpful both for obtaining the organism and determining its sensitivity. The staphylococcal antihemolysin titer may be elevated in osteomyelitis but is normal in tuberculosis.

RADIOLOGIC FEATURES. Radiologic evidence of the lesion may take from 10 days to 2 weeks to appear, although a small paravertebral abscess may be apparent before evidence of bony destruction. One of the earliest signs is slight haziness and loss of definition of bone structure in the end plates adjacent to the disc space. Later a more localized lesion becomes visible with destruction of adjacent vertebral bodies, new bone formation, and disc-space narrowing.

TREATMENT. This is based upon the three principles of treating bone infection, i.e., immobilization of the patient, both local and general, the use of the appropriate antibiotic, and surgical drainage of abscesses with debridement if at all possible.

Immobilization is best achieved by means of a plaster bed. Chemotherapy is selected from the results of culture of blood, urine, or pus aspirated from any localized abscess. The technique of surgical drainage varies, naturally, with the site of the abscess. In general, when surgical debridement is indicated, it is best carried out by an anterior approach to the spine with or without bone grafting.

Pain in the Chest Wall

Such pain may be referred or from local disease of the thoracic structures, i.e.,

1. In the spinal cord and its membranes from tumors or inflammation
2. In the posterior root ganglion from herpes zoster or tabes dorsalis
3. From disease of the vertebrae, such as tumor, tuberculosis, spondylolysis, osteophyte formation
4. From peripheral nerve lesions
5. From visceral disease of underlying lung, pleura, mediastinum, heart
6. Tietze's syndrome involving the costochondral junctions

DISORDERS OF MUSCLE

Anatomy

A single skeletal muscle consists of long cylindrical fibers collected together in many bundles, collections of which form the muscle as a whole. The muscle fibers are supported by fibrous connective tissue containing capillaries, nerve fibers, fibroblasts, histiocytes, and mast cells. A supporting fibrous connective tissue surrounds each individual muscle as the endomysium, from which it extends to enclose fiber bundles as the perimysium, and finally it extends to ensheathe the entire muscle to become the epimysium (Fig. 43-13).

The muscle fibers, which vary in length from 1 to 40 mm and in thickness from 50 to 100 μ, are enclosed in a structureless membrane known as the sarcolemma, which has four to eight nuclei arranged along its surface. Within

Fig. 43-13. The various parts of muscle mass, a muscle fiber, and a myofibril. (*Taken with permission from Mercer and Duthie [eds.], "Orthopaedic Surgery," Edward Arnold [Publishers] Ltd., London, 1972.*)

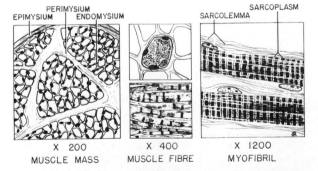

| EPIMYSIUM | PERIMYSIUM
ENDOMYSIUM | SARCOLEMMA | SARCOPLASM |

| X 200 | X 400 | X 1200 |
| MUSCLE MASS | MUSCLE FIBRE | MYOFIBRIL |

the sarcolemmic membrane lie many myofibrils, 1 to 2 μ in diameter, which form the basic internal unit of the muscle fiber and which are connected together by the sarcoplasm. The sarcoplasm contains numerous inclusion bodies such as glycogen and lipid granules. It also contains reticulum which provides the connecting link for the transmission of excitation impulses from the sarcolemmic membrane to the myofibrils as well as playing some part in the electrolytic exchanges across the sarcolemmic membrane. Chemical analysis of the sarcoplasm reveals that it is made up of a myogen fraction and several enzymes, i.e., zymohexase, phosphorylase, and dehydrogenase.

Biophysics of Muscular Contraction

Striated muscle is so named because of periodic cross striations lying perpendicular to the long axis of the fibers. When viewed under magnification with ordinary transmitted light, these striations are seen to be made up of alternate bands of A, or anisotropic (birefringent), and I, or isotropic, refringency. In the center of each A band is found a slightly less refractile region named the "H band," after Henson, and in the center of the I band is a narrow line of highly refractile material, which therefore looks dark on focusing, called the "Z line" from the German *Zwischenscheibe*, meaning "between disks." The basic unit of the muscle fiber has long been regarded as that area lying between two Z lines; this is called a "sarcomere."

Interference microscopy has been used to measure the relative amount of protein present in the A and I bands of the myofibrils, which consist of two basic protein filaments, myosin and actin. The myosin is confined to the A band, whereas the actin filaments stretch from the Z line through the I band into the A band, terminating at the H zone (Fig. 43-14).

Electron microscopy has shown that these structural proteins, actin and myosin, are arranged in longitudinal filaments spaced out a few hundred angstrom units apart. The myosin filaments, 100 to 110 Å thick and about 450 Å apart, extend from one end of the A band to the other. The actin filaments are thinner, 40 to 50 Å in diameter, and stretch from the Z line to the edge of the H zone. In the A band, each of the myosin filaments is arranged hexagonally and surrounded by six actin filaments, which it shares with its nearest neighboring myosin filament. This observation suggests that striated muscle is built up of two overlapping sets of filaments.

Muscle contraction and shortening occurs as the result of filaments interdigitating, i.e., according to the sliding filament theory of Huxley, who described two interdigitating sets of filaments. His electron microscope pictures of muscle fibers at resting length, contracted, or stretched confirm that the A band remains the same width but that the H zone changes in width according to alteration of the distance between the Z lines. Hence, both the I, or actin filaments, in the A, or myosin filaments, remain at constant length. The actual change in length of the sarcomere during contraction or during applied stretch is achieved by the two filaments sliding over each other. Cross bridges attached to the myosin with active groups at their ends are thought to physically attach to sites on the actin filaments and by some type of configurational change at the cross bridges mechanically translate one type of filament along adjacent filaments of the other type. This mechanical link is thought to accompany the enzymatic splitting of ATP (adenosine triphosphate).

Definitions of Function

The following are some of the definitions used when describing muscle function:

1. A *motor unit* consists of a single motor neuron, its axon, and a group of muscle fibers innervated by this single axon.
2. A *twitch response* is a brief phasic contraction of a muscle fiber or fibers of a muscle unit resulting from a single impulse. It is followed by depolarization of these muscle fibers.
3. *Tetanus* is maximal contraction in the fibers of a motor unit resulting from a series of stimuli or summation of responses from a single stimulus.
4. An *isotonic contraction* is one in which there is shortening of the fibers of the muscle under a constant tension and work is done.
5. An *isometric contraction* is one in which there is no shortening of the muscle fibers and in which no external work is done but tension is maintained.
6. The *equilibrium length* of a muscle is the length of the relaxed muscle at which the resting tension is zero.
7. The *resting, or optimal, length* of a muscle is that length at which maximal contraction tension develops.
8. *Latency relaxation* is the period between the stimulus and the contraction.
9. *Stress relaxation* is the slow loss of tension after a muscle is suddenly stressed and placed under a constant strain. The accompanying slow lengthening is called "creep."

MECHANICAL ASPECTS OF MUSCULAR CONTRACTION.
Tension is related to the length of the muscle fiber. Curve 1 in Fig. 43-15 shows the exponential development of tension in a resting muscle which is being passively stretched to increased percentages of its resting length. The resting tension develops almost immediately and is due to the sarcolemma, whereas later other components of the elastic series come into play. The peak tension which then develops is the same as the maximal isometric tetanic contraction.

For practical purposes, the equilibrium length and the optimal. or resting, length are considered the same. and in the resting state no tension is produced when the muscle is passively reduced to a shorter length. In curve 2 of Fig. 43-15 the developing tension is produced by contraction of the muscle after stretch, and the twitch response is maximal at 105 to 110 percent of equilibrium length, whereas tetany is maximal at 100 to 105 percent of optimal length. It is obvious. therefore, that the tetanic stimulation will allow better correlation with the maximum when nearest to the equilibrium length.

"Developed" tension represents the tension over and above the resting tension at a given length with one stimulus. It is dependent upon the number of sites available for cross-bridge formation and the status of elastic elements when the external load is imposed. The sum of these curves is the total tension, which is maximal at optimal length.

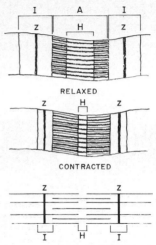

Fig. 43-14. Two primary protein filaments—myosin, in the A band, and actin, stretching from the Z line through the I band to terminate in the H zone. On contraction, the two filaments slide over each other. (*After Huxley. Taken with permission from Mercer and Duthie [eds.], "Orthopaedic Surgery," Edward Arnold [Publishers] Ltd., London, 1972.*)

There is a maximal length to which a muscle can be already stretched and then activated before the tension becomes zero. In maximally stretched fibers, the tension rises quite slowly, and a variant of this basic tension-length curve pattern can be demonstrated by adding the entity of an intact tendon, which introduces the phenomenon of stress relaxation and creep. As the tendon slowly lengthens, it allows a slight increase in the overlap of filaments and shows an earlier fall than that noted without tension.

Two further factors which correlate with tension and shortening are those of speed and load. Load can be compared to the tension of an isotonic contraction when the relation of force and speed of shortening is exponential. With a greater load, the muscles shorten much less and

Fig. 43-15. Relationship of tension of a muscle fiber during passive stretch (curve 1) and buildup of developing tension (curve 2) by contraction of muscle after stretch. (*Taken with permission from Mercer and Duthie [eds.], "Orthopaedic Surgery," Edward Arnold [Publishers] Ltd., London, 1972.*)

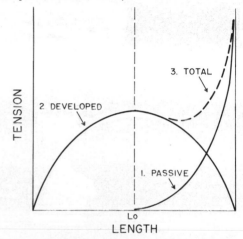

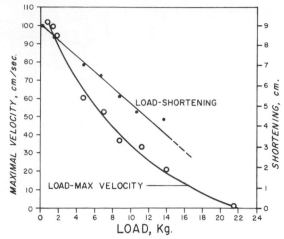

Fig. 43-16. Muscle length: comparing the speed or velocity of shortening against the load. (*Taken with permission from Mercer and Duthie [eds.], "Orthopaedic Surgery," Edward Arnold [Publishers] Ltd., London, 1972.*)

much more slowly. Of course, if a muscle were purely an elastic body, the velocity curve would be a straight line, but as seen in Fig. 43-16, the velocity is maximal with a zero load. With a load which a muscle just fails to lift and at zero velocity the maximal isometric tension is developed.

A. V. Hill has described isotonic contraction with increased load as follows:

1. There is an increased latent period equal to the time taken for the muscle to develop isometric tension equal to the isotonic load.
2. There is a decrease in maximal shortening.
3. There is a decrease in the initial velocity of shortening.

THE NEUROMUSCULAR JUNCTION (Fig. 43-17). A motor unit consists of a single anterior horn cell, its axon, and a variable number of muscle fibers which it supplies. The muscle fibers in the large motor units are supplied by thick fibers of 15 μ and the smaller by fine fibers of 4 μ. The

Fig. 43-17. Anatomy of the neuromuscular junction. (*Taken with permission from Mercer and Duthie [eds.], "Orthopaedic Surgery," Edward Arnold [Publishers] Ltd., London, 1972.*)

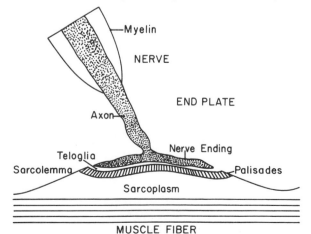

size of a motor unit varies inversely with the precision of the movements performed by the part; e.g., in the limb muscles, the unit may contain 150 muscle fibers, whereas in the eye it may contain fewer than five.

As the motor nerve fiber approaches a striated muscle fiber, it loses its medullary sheath, and the naked axis cylinder breaks up into terminal ramifications which make close and extensive contact with a specialized part of the muscle sarcoplasm known as the "motor end plate."

When an impulse arrives at the motor nerve terminal, there is released from the nerve terminal acetylcholine, which diffuses toward the motor end plate. The acetylcholine attaches to end plate receptors and produces a local end plate potential which alters the permeability of the membrane, allowing a free exchange of sodium and potassium. This process is known as "depolarization."

When the end plate potential reaches a certain critical magnitude, it depolarizes the surface membrane of the muscle fiber. When this local depolarization exceeds 30 to 40 mV, a spike potential in the muscle fiber is initiated which, when it attains an amplitude of 120 to 130 mV, results in muscular contraction.

After the acetylcholine is liberated at the end plate, it is rapidly hydrolized to choline and acetate by the enzyme cholinesterase. This enables the muscle fiber to become repolarized and to respond by contraction to further nervous stimuli. Certain extraneous factors may interfere with this chemical transmission of the nervous impulse, e.g., drugs, such as neostigmine or physostigmine, which are anticholinesterase compounds. These prevent the destruction of acetylcholine pooling, which results in the continued depolarization of the end plate and thus a failure to respond to further nervous stimuli. On the other hand substances such as curare will compete with receptor substances on the end plate for acetylcholine and counteract its effect, reducing the size of the end plate potential so that it can no longer excite the neighboring muscle membrane.

Muscle Paralysis and Spasticity

BASIC CONSIDERATIONS

Motor paralysis is the loss of voluntary muscle power either resulting from interruption of the motor or lower motor neuron pathways controlling it or due to some deficiency of the muscle itself, making it incapable of responding to nervous control. As a result of muscle paralysis, there will be changes in muscle tone, tendon reflexes, and the physical mass of the muscle or muscles involved.

MUSCLE TONE. The term "muscle tone" is used differently by the physiologist and the clinician. The physiologist defines it as a state of partial tetanus of the muscle which is maintained by an asynchronous discharge of impulses in motor neurons supplying it. It is reflexly produced from afferent nerve endings situated within the muscle itself and profoundly influenced by supraspinal mechanisms. Muscle tone provides the background of posture in which active movements occur and is an important element in the coordination of movement.

The clinician commonly estimates tone by the passive manipulation of limbs. This gives him a sense of the degree of tension, or elastic resistance, in the muscle. In lesions of the lower motor neuron muscle tone is abolished; this condition is called "flaccidity," or "flaccid paralysis." In lesions of the upper motor neuron muscle tone is increased, a condition of spasticity which occurs when the pyramidal tract is involved; when there is rigidity, the extrapyramidal tract is involved.

TENDON REFLEXES. The tendon reflexes are short-lived stretch reflexes elicited by tapping the tendon of the muscle, which evokes stimulation of the intrafusal muscle fibers of the muscle spindles. When muscle tone is increased, as in lesions of the upper motor neuron, the response to the tendon tap is increased, and the tendon jerk is thus increased in both amplitude and duration. Sometimes sudden stretching of the muscle will result in a repetitive jerk known as "clonus." The tendon reflex will be completely abolished by any interruption of the lower motor neuron reflex arc system on either the afferent or efferent loop.

PHYSICAL MASS OF MUSCLE. In upper motor neuron lesions the actual physical mass of the muscle remains unchanged, but in lower motor neuron lesions rapid wasting of the affected muscles will occur.

ATAXIA. "Ataxia" may be defined as imperfectly controlled or uncoordinated voluntary movements. It may be due to lesions of the cerebellum or the vestibular system. A sensory ataxia may arise from involvement of the pathways of proprioceptive and position sense, i.e., as seen in tabes dorsalis and in Friedreich's ataxia.

ELECTRICAL DIAGNOSIS AND ASSESSMENT OF MUSCLE DENERVATION. The method of obtaining the electrical "reaction" of muscle by faradic or galvanic stimulation applied to a muscle and its motor nerve has given place to more precise methods of greater complexity such as the intensity duration curve, electromyography, and nerve conduction velocity tests.

Intensity Duration Curve. Intensity duration curves (Fig. 43-18) are obtained by stimulating the muscle mass with pulses of known duration and intensity which produce characteristic patterns of contraction.

Electromyography. Electromyography (Fig. 43-19) is carried out with needle electrodes inserted into a muscle by means of which recordings are made of action potentials picked up within the muscles. The potential patterns reveal the presence or absence of denervation and of certain stages of regeneration of nerve.

Nerve Conduction Tests. Nerve conduction velocity tests are chiefly of value in defining peripheral nerve conduction interruption and together with electromyography form a useful basis in distinguishing among true motor neuron disease, peripheral nerve disease, and myopathy.

INTRINSIC DISEASES OF MUSCLE

Classification

A. Muscular dystrophies
  1. Progressive muscular dystrophy of Duchenne
  2. Fasciascapulohumeral dystrophy of Landouzy-Déjerine
  3. Dystrophia myotonica, or Steinert's disease

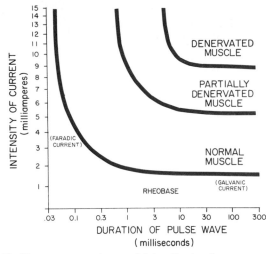

Fig. 43-18. Three common types of intensity duration curves. (*Taken with permission from Mercer and Duthie [eds.], "Orthopaedic Surgery," Edward Arnold [Publishers] Ltd., London, 1972.*)

B. Periodic diseases
  1. Myasthenia gravis
  2. Familial periodic paralysis
C. Other diseases of muscle
  1. Benign congenital hypotonia of Oppenheim-Walton
  2. Glycogen storage diseases of muscle
    a. Type 5, or McArdle-Schmid-Pearson disease
    b. Type 6, or Hers' disease
  3. Myotonia congenita, or Thomsen's disease
  4. Central core disease
D. Developmental defects of muscle
  1. Hypoplasia and aplasia
  2. Arthrogryposis
E. Constitutional disorders of muscle
  1. Neuromuscular atrophies
    a. Poliomyelitis
    b. Progressive muscular atrophy of Duchenne-Aran
    c. Infantile muscular atrophy of Hoffmann-Werdnig
    d. Peroneal muscular atrophy (Charcot-Marie-Tooth disease)

Fig. 43-19. Three electromyographic patterns of muscle fiber action potential showing normal potential curves (left), a myopathic lesion (middle), and lower motor neuron disease (right). (*Taken with permission from Mercer and Duthie [eds.], "Orthopaedic Surgery," Edward Arnold [Publishers] Ltd., London, 1972.*)

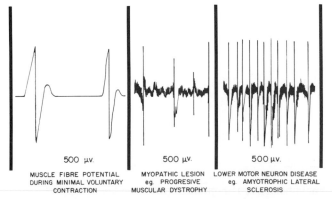

    e. Amyotrophic lateral sclerosis
    f. Syringomyelia
    g. Myelodysplasia
  2. Endocrine and metabolic disturbances
    a. Thyrotoxic myopathy
    b. Adrenal insufficiency
    c. Cushing's syndrome
    d. Hyperinsulinism
    e. Hyperkalemia and hypokalemia

In distinguishing the true myopathies from other causes of muscular paralysis, one must take into consideration the early age of onset, the familial history, and the progressive wasting of muscle groups without anatomic relation to any particular nerve supply. Other factors are the absence of fibrillation and the presence of normal tendon reflexes in the face of severe muscle wasting, and if necessary more specific data can be obtained by electromyography, muscle biopsy, and biochemical tests for serum aldolase and urine creatinine levels.

Muscular Dystrophies

PSEUDOHYPERTROPHIC MUSCULAR DYSTROPHY (DUCHENNE). The Duchenne type of muscular dystrophy is a progressive muscular disease which is usually manifested during the first three to six years, although it may be present in infancy or not recognized until adolescence. It affects boys primarily and is genetically determined by a sex-linked recessive gene. The presenting complaint is difficulty or instability in standing or walking. There may be an awkward waddling gait. The child gets up from the floor in a characteristic manner using his arms to get up on his legs to attain the upright posture. The child stands with increased lordosis, is weak, and usually has enlarged bulky muscles. The enlargement is conspicuous in the calves, the deltoids, and the quadriceps. The hands and the forearms usually are not involved. With progression, the pelvic musculature, erector spinae, and intercostals may be involved. Contractures occur early in the course of the disease and are first seen as equinovarus deformity of the foot. The cardiac muscle may be involved late in the course of the disease and may be responsible for death. Most patients are dead by the age of twenty years.

FASCIOSCAPULOHUMERAL TYPE OF MUSCULAR DYSTROPHY (LANDOUZY-DÉJERINE). This type of muscular dystrophy presents with facial and shoulder girdle involvement and is the most common form of muscular dystrophy in adults.

The facial muscles are involved early and may present in childhood or late adolescence. The cheeks droop, the lips pout, and the facies are immobile. Shoulder girdle involvement causes abnormal shoulder posture and difficulty in raising arms. Pelvic musculature is rarely involved. The heart may be affected, but life span is usually not shortened. It is transmitted by an autosomal dominant gene and may affect either sex.

LIMB GIRDLE TYPE OF MUSCULAR DYSTROPHY (ERB). This type of muscular dystrophy is much less common than Duchenne's and occurs later in life, usually in the second decade. Pseudohypertrophy is uncommon. The involvement begins first about the shoulder and pelvic girdles with involvement of the upper arm and thigh. The atrophy of the involved muscles produces striking contrast in the size of the arm, forearm, thigh, and leg in a typical case. The course is progressively downhill until there is involvement of all muscles and is more rapid, with earlier onset. Both sexes are involved. Inheritance is by an autosomal recessive gene.

OCULAR MUSCULAR DYSTROPHY. This is a dystrophic process involving first the levator palpebrae superioris and later the external ocular muscles. There may be weakness and wasting of other muscles about the face, head, and neck. Sexes are affected equally. Inheritance is by autosomal dominant gene.

PATHOLOGY OF MUSCULAR DYSTROPHY. The pathologic features of the various forms of muscular dystrophy are similar. The involved muscle is pink or gray and more whitish than normal. Microscopically there is greater variation of individual fiber size, from 10 to 200 mμ. On cross section fibers are rounded instead of polygonal, lose striation, and appear hyalinized in longitudinal section. There is no attempt at muscle regeneration. Fat and connective tissue replace degenerating muscle fibers. Sarcolemmic nuclei may be increased.

DIAGNOSIS. Early in the course of the disease, the diagnosis may be confused with polymyositis, since it may respond to medication. Serum enzymes, electromyography, and muscle biopsy are helpful in making the diagnosis of dystrophy, although the clinical features must be considered to distinguish the type of dystrophy.

In the Duchenne type of muscular dystrophy, the serum aldolase or creatine phosphokinase levels are invariably extremely high. Late in the disease, they may approach normal after muscle destruction has been complete. In the other dystrophies serum aldolase and creatine phosphokinase levels are raised according to the degree of muscle involvement, and the elevations are usually much lower than in the Duchenne type. Levels of creatine in the urine are increased above normal, while there is a reduction in the urinary excretion of creatinine which is probably related to a decrease in muscle mass. Urinary excretion of amino acid is also increased.

Electromyography of an involved muscle shows lower potentials and polyphasic pattern during voluntary contraction.

Muscle biopsy may be necessary in other dystrophies, but the diagnosis of Duchenne's dystrophy can be made on clinical grounds and on the basis of markedly elevated enzyme levels. The value of the muscle biopsy depends upon the selection of abnormal muscle, careful technique, and adequate tissue preparation. The selected muscle should be a muscle that is abnormal but not severely involved. The site of biopsy should be away from the insertion of the muscle where there is variation in the fiber size. A specimen at least $1\frac{1}{2}$ cm long and 1 cm wide is required for adequate study. The specimen should be gently stretched to the necessary length with ends fastened on a card or held in a special muscle clamp and placed in saline solution for 30 minutes and then fixed in formalin.

TREATMENT. There is no specific curative therapy for muscular dystrophy. Treatment is symptomatic. Vignos has shown that exercise is valuable in maintaining the patient's ability to ambulate and remain functional. The orthopedist should be aware that procedures which confine a patient to bed rest tend to accelerate the muscle weakness. Patients should not be confined to a wheelchair prematurely. Parents are instructed in stretching exercises of the lower extremities, hamstrings, spinal extensors, and gastrocnemius, and encouraged in a program of muscle strengthening exercises against active resistance.

Short and long leg braces for the lower extremities are used to keep the child standing and ambulating as long as possible. When equinus contractures are severe, heel cord lengthening may be carried out. The child should be fitted with a brace postoperatively and encouraged to ambulate within a few days. When spinal extensor and abdominal flexor weakness is severe and a wheelchair is required, the application of a torso body plaster may be of value in maintaining sitting posture.

Myotonias

MYOTONIC DYSTROPHY. This is a rare disorder in which there is a myopathy in combination with other abnormalities. The disorder is inherited as an autosomal dominant. The onset may be at any time during the first three decades of life. The onset commonly starts with dystrophy in the distal musculature and the muscles of the face and neck. Myopathic facies are common. Progress is slow, and proximal muscles may be involved much later. Percussion of a muscle or electric stimulation results in prolonged contraction of the muscle. Gonadal atrophy, cataracts, and frontal baldness occur in males with this disorder.

MYOTONIA CONGENITA, OR THOMSEN'S DISEASE. This is a rare hereditary disorder transmitted as an autosomal recessive or dominant gene. In all voluntary muscles there is difficulty in starting movement following rest. Symptoms may begin at infancy but usually appear between the ages of five and ten years. The patient gives the appearance of excessive muscle mass and muscular overdevelopment. Following repeated motion, the initial weakness improves to where muscle strength may be normal. Percussion of the muscle results in a myotonic sustained contraction. The disease is compatible with normal life expectancy.

PATHOLOGY AND DIAGNOSIS OF MYOTONIA. Histologic examination of a myotonic muscle reveals the presence of long chains of centrally placed nuclei in otherwise intact muscle fibers. Characteristically, some muscle fibers are enlarged. On cross section, the peripheral myofibrils have degenerated and surround a central group of normal fibrils. There is no regeneration, and connective tissue does not replace the muscle, thus accounting for the absence of contractures.

On electromyography, a characteristic shower of electrical activity occurs spontaneously after stimulation. Serum enzyme levels may be similar to those in the dystrophies other than Duchenne's, which has a marked elevation of creatine phosphokinase and serum aldolase levels.

TREATMENT. There is no effective treatment for myotonic dystrophy. However, patients with Thomsen's disease can be improved by the use of procaine amide, prednisone and quinine.

Inflammatory Disease

Myositis, or inflammation in muscles, may be due to specific etiologic agents such as a virus, parasite, bacterium, or spirochete. Myositis occurs in diseases of unknown cause such as the collagen vascular diseases, dermatomyositis, lupus, scleroderma, and rheumatoid arthritis. The term "polymyositis" is used to describe the changes in muscle associated with these conditions as well as those found in association with malignant tumors.

The clinical course of polymyositis is variable and may present as an insidious chronic muscle weakness, or it may begin with acute symptoms of high fever, marked muscle pain, spasm, and weakness. The heart muscle may be involved in any of these conditions. Skin changes associated with the primary diagnosis, i.e., lupus or scleroderma, will assist in making the diagnosis. The course of the disease is variable and may be rapidly progressive, resulting in death, or it may persist with episodes of remission and exacerbation. Spontaneous arrest may occur.

PATHOLOGY. Histologic examination of muscles reveals degeneration and necrosis of muscle fibers associated with infiltration by chronic inflammatory cells, both interstitially and about blood vessels. Serum enzyme studies are of little value in the diagnosis. Electromyography of the involved muscle reveals spontaneous fibrillation potential in the relaxed muscle, distinguishing polymyositis from muscular dystrophy.

TREATMENT. The treatment of polymyositis is directed at diagnosis of the primary condition. In elderly patients presenting with polymyositis, an unrecognized malignant tumor should be suspected. Most patients with polymyositis may be controlled dramatically with the use of cortisone preparations or ACTH. General treatment requires supportive care, physiotherapy in the form of exercise to maintain existing muscle power, appropriate bracing, and occasionally surgical treatment for contractures.

Orthopedic treatment is directed at control of deformities by appropriate bracing or surgical arthrodesis of neurotrophic joints.

POLIOMYELITIS

Poliomyelitis is an acute infectious disease caused by the poliomyelitis virus. The virus is present in the pharynx and feces of infected patients during the preparalytic and postparalytic stages. Invasion of the central nervous system is thought to take place by virus traveling proximally along the peripheral nerve to the spinal cord. Once established in the central nervous system, the virus causes anterior horn cell destruction, which results in a flaccid paralysis. With loss of innervation, the motor unit muscle fibers atrophy. Paralysis or deformity and leg-length discrepancies are the result.

CLINICAL COURSE OF THE DISEASE. In about one-third of patients with poliomyelitis infection an initial febrile illness develops consisting of headache, malaise, and low-grade fever, lasting 48 hours. Such a patient may recover completely or go on to a second, acute phase after 4 or 5 days of apparent good health. The acute phase may develop in the absence of the initial symptoms.

The acute phase lasts from a few days to a week and also may resolve without paralysis. The illness is characterized by meningeal symptoms including headache, fever, stiff neck, and muscle spasms in the spine or extremities. "Nonparalytic poliomyelitis" describes those patients who do not progress to the paralytic stage.

About the third or fourth day of the acute illness, paralysis may develop. There may be loss of deep reflexes, muscle spasm of the erector spinae, and even signs of bulbar paralysis. The lower limbs are involved twice as frequently as the upper extremities. Death may result from bulbar paralysis, due to respiratory insufficiency.

The convalescent stage begins after the acute illness and ends up to 2 years later at a point where there is no significant recovery in muscle power.

The residual stage occurs following changes in muscle recovery. Children will continue to improve in the residual stage because of their improved coordination.

TREATMENT. In the acute stage, treatment is directed at isolation of patients with the disease, general nursing care, and the treatment of respiratory difficulty by the use of mechanical respirators.

Treatment in the Recovery Stage. In the early stages of convalescence, treatment is directed at eliminating deforming tendencies, restoring joint motion, and training and protection of recovering muscles. Later on, the patient is fitted with suitable protective braces and taught resistance exercises to develop residual muscle power.

Muscle spasm is treated to prevent asymmetrical muscle tightness and soft tissue contractures. Trained therapists apply hot packs and give passive range-of-motion exercises. The patients must be nursed in the proper position, to prevent overstretching of paralyzed muscles and joint contractures. Appropriate splints are utilized, depending upon muscle weakness.

The patient is taught muscle reeducation to reestablish control of the extremities and joints as early as possible, when acute symptoms subside. When the patient is ambulatory, orthotic devices to protect and assist control of his paralyzed extremities are utilized.

Treatment in the Residual Stage. Treatment in the residual stage requires orthopedic surgical procedures to correct joint contractures, to improve joint power and function by appropriate muscle and tendon transfers, to stabilize joints by arthrodesis, and to correct leg-length inequality. The following surgical procedures are those most commonly used in poliomyelitis. The reader is referred to *Orthopaedic Surgery,* by Mercer and Duthie, and *Campbell's Operative Orthopedics,* edited by Crenshaw, for detailed discussion of these and other surgical procedures.

Principles of Reconstructive Surgery

TENDON TRANSFER. Tendon transfer is utilized to restore muscle balance to a joint, to restore lost function, and to increase active power of joint motions. Before undertaking tendon transfer, an expendable muscle of suitable strength and excursion must be available for transfer about a joint with a normal passive range of motion. Specific muscle power is graded on the Medical Research Council (MRC) scale, which is a clinical evaluation of muscle strength:

Grade	Muscle power
0	Complete paralysis
1	Flicker of contraction without joint excursion
2	Muscle power to effect partial range of motion
3	Muscle power to effect a full range of joint motion against gravity
4	Less than normal strength but full range of joint motion against resistance
5	Normal muscle strength

A muscle will lose one grade of strength following transfer, so that its power must be grade 4 or better. The muscle selected should have sufficient excursion to replace the lost function. Muscles from synergistic groups provide better results by making muscle reeducation more complete. Joint contractures should be corrected and a passive range of joint motion established prior to tendon transfer. Circulation to, and sensation in, the muscle should not be damaged during transfer. The tendon connecting the new origin and insertion should be as straight as possible to improve the efficiency of muscle action and should be placed in an area where gliding is possible.

BONY STABILIZATION. When muscle power is insufficient to protect or move the joint or when sufficiently expendable muscles are not available for transfer, arthrodesis of the joint will provide stability, prevent deformity, and even permit transfer of local muscles for other functions. A prerequisite of arthrodesis is the presence of adjacent mobile joints to compensate for the lost motion.

JOINT CONTRACTURES. Joint contractures are corrected by judicious stretching by a physiotherapist or by braces incorporating dynamic stretching. The joints may be gradually stretched into the corrected position by successive plaster-cast changes or plaster-cast wedging.

LEG-LENGTH EQUALIZATION. Leg-length discrepancy may be corrected by bone lengthening or shortening procedures. A 1-in. difference in leg length is usually of no practical significance. For patients with significant paralysis about the hip, moderate degrees of shortening facilitate bony stability by the motion of abduction. Before undertaking corrective surgical procedures of any type, the surgeon should be familiar with the patient's progress in reference to the rate of leg-length discrepancy and have an understanding of the degrees of shortening produced by such procedures as ankle arthrodesis and knee arthrodesis in flexion.

Treatment of Deformities

FOOT PARALYSIS. Paralysis from poliomyelitis may cause a wide variety of foot deformities (Fig. 43-20). Deformities are treated by proper bracing to maintain stability and prevent deformity until maximal recovery has occurred. When maximal recovery has occurred, tendon transfers or bony stabilization procedures are indicated. Bony stabilization other than the Grice extraarticular arthrodesis of the subtalar joint is not performed until bony maturity is achieved at age twelve to fifteen. Each foot deformity must be evaluated specifically, taking into consideration many factors including joint motion, other joints involved, and muscles available and their strength.

Valgus deformity is due to muscle imbalance from weakness or absence of functioning invertors which results in pronation of the forefoot and eversion of the calcaneus. The extraarticular arthrodesis of the subtalar joint (Grice) is an effective means of controlling this until bony maturity. A strut of tibial bone graft is wedged between the talus and the calcaneus, between the anterior and posterior components of the subtalar joint (Fig. 43-21*A*).

Varus deformity is due to muscle imbalance with paralysis of the peroneal muscles. Treatment is directed at restoring eversion power and strength. The anterior tibial may be transferred laterally to reduce its varus deforming force and improve eversion. The posterior tibial tendon may be released from its tendon sheath and allowed to ride in front of the medial malleolus. This effectively releases some inversion force. The posterior tibial tendon also may be transferred laterally through the interosseous membrane.

Calcaneus Deformity. Calcaneus deformity is the result of paralysis of the calf muscles. The unopposed dorsiflexors pull the foot into dorsiflexion, and the calcaneal foot results. This is a difficult deformity to control with bracing. The posterior or peroneal tendons may be transferred into the calcaneus, effecting partial improvement in plantar flexion power. Alternatives are tenodesis of the Achilles tendon, which will provide the fulcrum for push-off. At age twelve to fifteen years, triple arthrodesis may be required (Fig. 43-21*B*).

Equinus Deformity. Equinus deformity results from paralysis of the anterior tibial tendon, causing foot drop. This deformity may be controlled with a foot drop short leg brace. Forward transfer of the peroneals for dorsiflexion, combined with triple arthrodesis, may be accomplished at bony maturity. A Lambrinudi triple arthrodesis or Hoke triple arthrodesis may be effective in the absence of functioning peroneal muscles.

Claw Hallux Deformity. Extension of the metatarsophalangeal (MP) joint of the great toe with flexion of the interphalangeal (IP) joint commonly occurs with paralysis of the tibialis anterior. The overpull of the extensor hallucis longus results in dorsiflexion of the MP joint and clawing. Depression of the first metatarsal shaft is due to the unbalanced pull of the peroneus longus. This deformity can be effectively treated by the Jones procedure. This consists of transplantation of the extensor hallucis longus into the neck of the first metatarsal shaft, combined with stabilization of the IP joint by arthrodesis.

PARALYSIS ABOUT THE KNEE JOINT. Patients with isolated paralysis of the quadriceps get along satisfactorily if there is adequate power in the gastronemius and gluteus maximus to stabilize the knee in extension. Transplantation of the biceps combined with semitendinosis transfer to the patella may be indicated. However, the indications must be individualized and are based on the prerequisite of adequate posterior stability of the knee, including gastrocnemius power and gluteus maximus function.

PARALYSIS ABOUT THE HIP. Paralytic deformity of the hip results in severe disability through the disturbance of gait. The indications for treatment depend upon the avail-

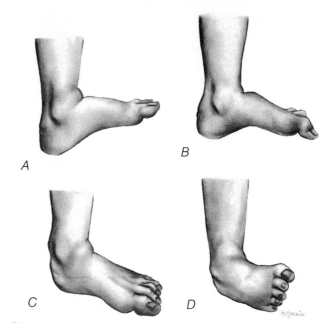

Fig. 43-20. Paralytic deformities of the foot. *A.* Calcaneal deformity. *B.* Cavus (claw) foot. *C.* Valgus deformity. *D.* Varus deformity.

Fig. 43-21. *A.* Grice procedure with a strut of tibial bone graft wedged between talus and calcaneus. *B.* Triple arthrodesis.

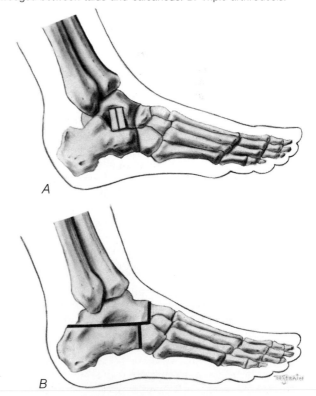

ability of function in adjacent muscles and the degree of disability. A posterior transfer of extensor fascia lata, lateral transfer of the iliopsoas (Mustard procedure), or erector spinae transfer for gluteus maximus paralysis give variable results. In the properly selected patients, a small gain in stability may result in great benefit by relieving fatigability of gait and pelvic stabilization. If a painful hip, subluxation, or frank dislocation due to muscle imbalance develops, arthrodesis may be necessary. Careful analysis of the paralysis in other joints, leg-length discrepancy, etc., in each patient must be considered before surgical treatment is undertaken.

PARALYSIS IN THE UPPER EXTREMITY. Shoulder. Paralysis of the deltoid and rotator cuff in the presence of remaining power in the scapular stabilizing muscles—trapezius, rhomboids, serratus anterior—may be treated by arthrodesis of the glenohumeral joint in the appropriate position. The resulting stabilization allows shoulder stability, adequate motion, and power from the function of scapulothoracic muscles.

Elbow. Surgical procedures to improve power across the elbow are directed primarily at restoring elbow flexion in paralysis of the biceps and brachialis. If normal power exists in the flexors of the wrist and fingers, Steindler's operation, which is the proximal transfer of the common flexor origin, will improve elbow flexion power. Alternative methods include transfer of the inferior portion of the pectoralis major or the sternocleidomastoideus attached to a free tendon graft.

Paralytic Hand. Paralysis of wrist extensors may be treated by dorsal transfer of the flexor carpi ulnaris or pronator teres into the extensor carpi radialis longus and brevis. Loss of thumb extension is treated by insertion of the flexor carpi radialis into the abductor pollicis longus and extensor pollicis brevis. The palmaris longus may be inserted into the extensor pollicis longus. Paralysis of the extensor digitorum communis may be treated by transfer of the flexor carpi ulnaris dorsally.

Loss of opposition of the thumb is a common finding in the paralytic hand due to poliomyelitis. Various procedures are available to restore opposition, including Bunnell's transfer of the flexor digitorum superficialis to the ring finger routed about a pulley on the flexor carpi ulnaris and inserted into the base of the thumb.

Wrist arthrodesis may provide stability of the hand and make available expendable tendons for transfer (see Chap. 50).

CEREBRAL PALSY

Cerebral palsy is a neurologic diagnosis of a condition in which there are nonprogressive but permanent upper motor neuron lesions occurring in children. The diagnosis excludes children with active or progressive disease. On examination, there may be disturbance of special senses, including sight, hearing, and peripheral sensation. Mental retardation alone is not cerebral palsy, but it may accompany upper motor neuron abnormalities.

INCIDENCE. Phelps estimated that cerebral palsy occurs in seven births for every 100,000 population. Of the seven patients, one will die within the first year, one will have subclinical involvement and pass unnoticed in the community, two will have such severe involvement as to require custodial care, and the remaining three will require orthopedic treatment.

ETIOLOGY. Cerebral palsy may be caused by a number of factors including head trauma at birth, head injury in childhood, anoxic brain damage, vascular accidents following treatment of brain tumor, involvement of the central nervous system from encephalitis, and other viral diseases, e.g., measles, cytomegalic inclusion body.

The pathologic lesions in the brain have not been well documented, and little information has been correlated between pathology and symptoms. Developmental defects, such as absence of the cerebellum or basal ganglia, may be responsible.

CLINICAL MANIFESTATIONS. Zuck estimates that 50 percent of all new patients are spastic, 25 percent are athetoid, 5 percent are ataxic, 5 percent are rigid, and the remainder have the mixed-type lesion.

Spasticity is due to an upper motor neuron lesion, involving the pyramidal tract. Clinical examination reveals hyperactive stretch reflexes. Sudden passive motion of a joint produced by spastic muscles activates this reflex, and clonus results. Weakness may be present in antagonistic muscle groups and contributes to the development of joint flexion contractures.

Cerebral spastic patients are of four types: sixty percent of all spastics are hemiplegic with paralysis of ipsilateral arm and leg; the patient with left-sided hemiplegia is more likely to have better preservation of intellectual function. The second most common type is the diplegic with symmetrical spastic involvement in the lower extremities and less severe involvement in the upper extremities. Paraplegic patients are uncommon, having involvement only of the lower extremities. The quadriplegic patient tends to have symmetrical involvement of all four extremities.

Athetosis is characterized by involuntary repetitive motion of a muscle group or extremity resulting in severe dysfunction. Athetotic motions may be worsened by sudden stress, tension, weight bearing, and even sudden changes of light. The defect is thought to be in the basal ganglia. Joint contractures are rare with this manifestation.

Ataxia is related to lesions of the cerebellum, causing deficient postural reflexes. There is commonly a voluntary tremor, hypotonia, and easy fatigability. The child walks with a staggering, broad-based gait. Reflexes are decreased and contractures uncommon.

Rigidity results from diffuse cerebral involvement, commonly from birth ataxia.

In *mixed types of cerebral palsy* spasticity commonly coexists with athetosis. Not infrequently, a child at age two to four with spasticity shows evidence of coexisting athetosis as he grows older.

Diagnosis can usually be made by an experienced physician during the first year of life. A history of difficult pregnancy, prolonged labor, delayed respiration, neonatal jaundice, postnatal irritability, or muscle twitching is suggestive.

Stiffness of extremities, weakness, or asymmetrical use of the limbs, retarded motor development, or athetoid movements may be evident in the history. Clinical examination should detect signs of spasticity, purposeless movements, delayed motor development, or incoordination. Any joint contractures should arouse the suspicion of spasticity.

TREATMENT. Adequate treatment of cerebral palsy requires a multidisciplined approach. The pediatrician, the orthopedic surgeon, the neurologist should collaborate with the social worker, psychologist, and teachers trained in the instruction of handicapped children. The total program of care requires understanding and participation by the parents.

Successful treatment is directly related to the intelligence of the child. About two-thirds of cerebral palsied children have IQs below 70, making education and treatment more difficult. There is a close correlation between motor ability and IQ. Motor ability is evaluated by the motor age test. The motor age test is a numerical expression of motor performance expressed as a percentage of age. The normal child would have a score of 100, the motor-handicapped child less than 100. By totaling the motor age and IQ a total is reached to which treatment results can be compared. When the total is below 130, intensive prolonged therapy is usually unrewarding. When the total of motor age and IQ is between 130 and 160, satisfactory results from a complete treatment program can be expected. Physiotherapy for muscle strengthening, gait training, and effective bracing are needed. Orthopedic surgical correction of deformities is important but is the least frequently required therapeutic approach.

Physiotherapy. Physiotherapy is directed at achieving controlled muscle function, which requires muscle relaxation and control of purposeless movements. Physiotherapy is applied under the guidance of the physiotherapist and carried out at home by the mother. Daily passive stretching is required to prevent flexion deformities. The child is taught through repetitive exercises and supervised play to obtain muscle relaxation and strengthen weakened muscles.

Bracing. Braces are necessary:

1. To prevent contractures from muscle imbalance and spasticity
2. To provide stability in the lower extremities, because of muscle weakness
3. To minimize purposeless motion
4. To provide evaluation prior to performing stabilization procedures

Braces have their greatest application to the lower extremities. A double upright, short leg caliper, with added T straps, will help to control varus or valgus deformities of the foot, provide stability in walking and standing, and assist in preventing contractures.

In the spastic child with the tendency to equinus contractures of the foot or flexion deformities of the knees, posterior plaster splints or bivalved plaster casts will assist in overcoming these deformities.

Long leg braces are applied to assist in preventing knee flexion contractures and valgus deformities and provide stability in the upright position. Bilateral long leg braces with a pelvic band provide additional stability at the hip joint.

Upper extremity bracing takes the form of plaster or metal splints to assist in holding the hand in the position of function and preventing flexion contractures at the wrists and fingers or adduction deformities of the thumb.

THERAPY FOR SPECIFIC AREAS. Hip. The effect of adductor spasticity with weakened abductors results in a valgus deformity of the femoral neck. With severe adduction, lateral displacement of the hips and increasing acetabular index develop. If these are not controlled with soft tissue procedure, tenotomy, and neurectomy, a subtrochanteric varus osteotomy with internal fixation is necessary (Fig. 43-22). Rotational deformity is corrected at the same time.

Knee. The knee develops flexion contractures because of isolated or combined problems of hip flexion deformity, spastic hamstrings, and equinus feet. Contractures can be

Fig. 43-22. Hip subluxation in spastic diplegia. *A.* AP of the pelvis showing lateral displacement of the right hip. *B.* AP of the pelvis showing maintenance of the head in the acetabulum following varus derotation osteotomy.

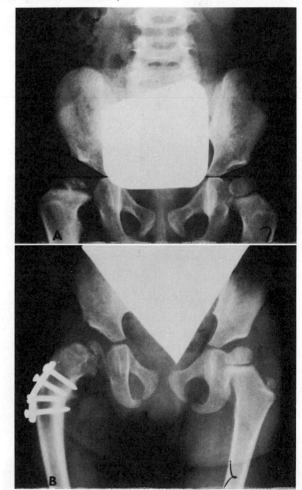

prevented by appropriate plaster night splints, bracing, and exercises. If a contracture has developed, it may be corrected by plaster-cast wedging. When this is unsuccessful, posterior capsulotomy or hamstring lengthening by Z-plasty may effectively relieve the contracture.

In the child walking in a crouched position with hips and knees flexed, surgical release of the hamstrings as described and modified by Eggers and Evans will assist in bringing both hip and knee to extension and improve the erect posture and gait. If there has been long-standing stretching of the anterior patellar retinacula and lengthening of the patellar ligament, effective quadriceps power can be improved by division of the posterior component of the patellar retinácula which allows any quadriceps power to be applied effectively to the stretched patellar ligaments.

Foot. Although any deformity may develop as the result of muscle weakness and spasticity in cerebral palsy, the equinovarus foot is most common. If an equinovarus contracture can be demonstrated with the knee extended but not with the knee flexed, contracture of the gastrocnemius is the cause, and its release is required. The Strayer procedure divides the gastrocnemius at its musculotendinous junction, effectively lengthening it, and does not disturb the underlying soleus.

Orthopedic Surgical Treatment

Orthopedic surgical treatment is used for:

1. Weakening spastic muscles by tendon lengthening
2. Improving joint motion by tendon transplantation
3. Stabilizing deformed or contracted joints by arthrodesis
4. Correcting deformity by osteotomy and correction of leg-length inequality

If children with cerebral palsy are put to bed for surgical procedures, their motor abilities deteriorate at least temporarily. For the athetoid child, surgical intervention is rarely indicated. As Phelps has shown, correction of the deformity at one level results in expression of the disorder at a more proximal level. Most surgical procedures are applied in the treatment of the spastic. Procedures which require stabilization are more likely to be successful, since muscle reeducation and patient cooperation are not required. When tendon transfers are indicated, a higher IQ and higher motor age are prerequisites.

UPPER EXTREMITY. Surgical treatment of the upper extremity is rarely indicated and is done to improve appearance and position of the hand, wrist, and forearm. The functional benefits are uncertain. The common deformity of the upper extremity spastic hemiplegic patient is an elbow in flexion with a forearm pronation contracture with wrist and fingers in flexion and the thumb closely opposed or adducted.

Arthrodesis of the wrist is done in extension and moderate ulnar deviation in order passively to improve thumb abduction. By eliminating wrist motion, finger power and control are improved.

An alternative method is transfer of the flexor carpi ulnaris tendon around the ulnar side of the forearm and insertion into radial wrist extensor tendons. This will improve wrist extension, though there is little effect on supination power.

Stabilization of the thumb by an iliac bone graft between the first two metacarpals may be necessary. Other procedures such as the flexor digitorum superficiallis tenodesis of Swanson and flexor carpi ulnaris transfers to the finger extensors following wrist fusion are rarely indicated.

LOWER EXTREMITY. The flexion adduction deformity of the hip is common in spasticity and requires treatment. The infant is splinted with an abduction splint, and daily passive stretching is carried out, to minimize deformity. When the child begins to walk, scissoring due to adductor spasticity may seriously interfere with gait.

Adductor tenotomy is done by surgical division of the major adductor origins from the pelvis. Postoperatively, abduction should be maintained by splints while abductor power is strengthened by exercise. When there is marked scissoring during attempts at walking, with little or no permanent contracture, obturator neurectomy is done, if tenotomy fails.

Internal rotation, which frequently accompanies adduction and flexion, may be treated by derotational osteotomy in the supracondylar or subtrochanteric areas. However, incision of the tendons of the gluteus medius and mimimus from the anterior portion of the greater trochanter followed by 6 months of immobilization in plaster is generally preferable.

Flexion deformity of the knee due to muscle spasm may be corrected by plaster wedging. When contracture is established and there is a weakened quadriceps or an overstretched patellar tendon with upward migration of the patella, the best procedure is posterior capsulotomy of the knee and Z-plasty lengthening of the hamstrings. The patellar tendon may be advanced, in addition, to aid the quadriceps to reach optimal length. Other procedures free the gastrocnemius from its femoral attachment or release the patellar retinaculum and transfer the hamstrings into the distal femur.

In the foot, the common equinus deformity may be treated by division of the nerve supply to the gastrocnemius or soleus muscles or by lengthening of the Achilles tendon or gastrocnemius. When the equinus deformity is present with knee flexed and extended, then lengthening of the Achilles tendon by Z-plasty with or without posterior ankle capsulotomy is necessary. Release of the posterior tibial tendon to allow it to ride forward of the medial malleolus will assist in overcoming the varus deformity. When bony maturity is reached, varus and valgus deformities may be treated by triple arthrodesis.

MYELODYSPLASIA (Spinal Dysraphism)

Myelodysplasia describes a developmental defect in the vertebral column with associated peripheral neurologic lesions. Lichtenstein used the term "spinal dysraphism" for congenital defects of the lumbosacral regions with failure of fusion of midline structures. The vertebral lesion may be present without involvement of the cord, i.e., as spina bifida occulta. However, spina bifida may be associated with meningocele, myelomeningocele, or myeloschisis, an open neural plate. Hydrocephalus is frequently associated with these lesions.

CLINICAL MANIFESTATIONS. Spina bifida occulta is frequently an incidental finding detected by x-ray and is not usually associated with neurologic abnormality. An occasional patient may have detectable muscle imbalance or sensory abnormalities of the foot which are quite localized.

Meningoceles (cystic enlargement of the lower meninges), myelomeningoceles (cystic enlargement of meninges and intradural contents), or myeloschisis (a frank open neural plate) may occur with spina bifida resulting in severe deformities of the lower extremity. Sharrard et al. have shown that when myelocele, myelomeningocele, or myeloschisis is present at birth, early surgical closure will prevent deterioration of the distal neurologic function. The neural sac is closed by mobilization of fascial flaps and full-thickness skin coverage. Associated hydrocephalus, which occurs in 80 percent of these patients, should be treated simultaneously. The prognosis for a child with these developmental abnormalities of the central nervous system will depend upon the degree of resultant lower extremity paralysis as well as neurologic abnormalities of the bladder and urinary tract.

ORTHOPEDIC MANAGEMENT. The deformities of the lower extremities are related to the level of spinal involvement, which may be complete or spotty in distribution. Neurologic evaluation should be repeated, as functional loss may increase with growth. If a complete lesion occurs at the first lumbar segment, flaccid paralysis is the result; treatment is directed at obtaining weight-bearing attitude in the lower extremities. When the level is between L_3 and L_4, hip adduction and flexion is present, whereas hip abduction and extension are absent, with resulting potential paralytic hip dislocation. The management of such paralytic deformities is similar to that of deformities which occur as a result of flaccid paralysis of poliomyelitis.

Foot and Ankle. Talipes equinovarus is the most common foot deformity resulting from muscle imbalance, although calcaneal valgus or varus also may occur. Management is directed at maintaining the weight-bearing position. If deformity is already present, plaster-cast correction of the foot is carried out and followed by short leg braces to control the muscle imbalance. Lack of sensation makes the possibility of pressure sores a chronic problem for these patients. For the valgus foot, the Grice procedure may be required. When bony maturity has been reached, triple arthrodesis is performed to stabilize the foot.

Knee Deformities. When a complete lesion occurs at the levels of L_3 and L_4, quadriceps function remains in the absence of the hamstring function, and hyperextension of the knee results. In such a patient, the deformity is managed by plaster casts, splints, and long leg braces to prevent recurvation of the knee. Osteotomy may be necessary to correct rotational deformities.

Hip. When a complete lesion occurs between L_3 and L_4 coxa valga and subluxation of the hip occur. It is important to recognize this deformity before actual dislocation results. Management is directed at restoring the muscle bal-

ance responsible for the deformity. Sharrard's lateral transfer of the iliopsoas through the wing of the ilium will improve hip abduction and extension and has given satisfactory results. Varus osteotomy and derotational osteotomy of the femur may also be necessary.

All the principles utilized in the treatment of paralytic poliomyelitis including correction of joint contractures by stretching, plaster-cast wedging, reinforcement of weak muscles by tendon transfers, arthrodesis of unstable joints, and correction of leg-length inequality are applicable in the treatment of deformities due to spinal dysraphism.

DEGENERATIVE DISEASES OF THE NERVOUS SYSTEM WITH SKELETAL DEFORMITY

Peroneal Muscle Atrophy (Charcot-Marie-Tooth Muscular Atrophy)

Peroneal muscular atrophy is a hereditary degenerative process beginning in the peroneal nerve and resulting in peroneal muscular weakness. As the disease progresses, nerve trunks supplying the distal parts of the extremities are involved. Degenerative changes may occur in the spinal nerve roots in pyramidal tracts.

CLINICAL MANIFESTATIONS. The disease usually manifests itself in the first or second decade and may occur as late as the third. The initial complaint is varus deformity of the feet, such that the child walks on the outer borders of his feet. With progressive involvement of the anterior tibial group and foot drop, the patient develops a slapping gait.

Neurologic examination reveals a decrease in reflexes of muscles supplied by involved nerve roots. Anesthesia may accompany the muscle atrophy. The disease is found in several generations and is transmitted as a dominant, recessive, or sex-linked recessive.

Treatment does not affect the slow progressive changes. Short leg braces may control the varus deformity.

Friedreich's Ataxia

Friedreich's cerebellar ataxia is a familial disease in which there is degeneration of spinocerebellar tracts, corticospinal tracts, and posterior columns of the cord.

CLINICAL MANIFESTATIONS. There is usually evidence of the disease in previous generations. It affects males more commonly than females. The onset is usually insidious in childhood, the first abnormality being one of gait or a tendency to fall easily. Later on, there is incoordination, followed by nystagmus, and speech disturbances. Thoracic scoliosis and pes cavus with claw toes are seen very commonly. The disease runs a steadily downhill course. Early in the course of this disease, orthopedic bracing procedures or even tendon transfers or bony stabilization may be indicated to maintain ambulation.

Syringomyelia

Syringomyelia is a degenerative condition of the spinal cord in which there is destruction of neurons in the central portion and proliferation of glial elements resulting in the formation of a cavity. It is usually related to defective development, but similar cavities may occur following vascular processes or trauma.

The sexes are affected with equal frequency. The onset usually is in the second or third decade. Rarely are symptoms severe before the age of twenty. The small muscles of the hands are frequently involved early in the course, with deformity and wasting of the hands as a result. Disturbances in sensibility with loss of pain sense result in trophic disturbances about the hands and upper extremities. There is progressive atrophy of the muscle supplied by the area of the cord, commonly the cervical area, less commonly the bulbar or lumbar area. Skeletal deformities such as kyphosis, scoliosis, and pes cavus may be evident. The diagnosis depends on finding the associated anesthesia with muscle wasting and skeletal deformity.

Fig. 43-23. Atrophy of the intrinsic muscles of the hand.

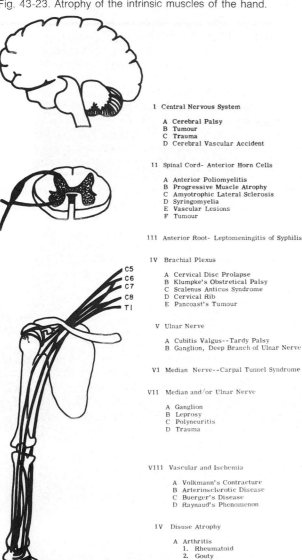

1   Central Nervous System

    A Cerebral Palsy
    B Tumour
    C Trauma
    D Cerebral Vascular Accident

11   Spinal Cord- Anterior Horn Cells

    A Anterior Poliomyelitis
    B Progressive Muscle Atrophy
    C Amyotrophic Lateral Sclerosis
    D Syringomyelia
    E Vascular Lesions
    F Tumour

111   Anterior Root- Leptomeningitis of Syphilis

1V   Brachial Plexus

    A Cervical Disc Prolapse
    B Klumpke's Obstetrical Palsy
    C Scalenus Anticus Syndrome
    D Cervical Rib
    E Pancoast's Tumour

V   Ulnar Nerve

    A Cubitis Valgus--Tardy Palsy
    B Ganglion, Deep Branch of Ulnar Nerve

V1   Median Nerve--Carpal Tunnel Syndrome

V11   Median and/or Ulnar Nerve

    A Ganglion
    B Leprosy
    C Polyneuritis
    D Trauma

V111   Vascular and Ischemia

    A Volkmann's Contracture
    B Arteriosclerotic Disease
    C Buerger's Disease
    D Raynaud's Phenomenon

1V   Disuse Atrophy

    A Arthritis
       1. Rheumatoid
       2. Gouty

    B Dupuytren's Contracture

If the disease occurs early in life, the prognosis is relatively serious. The disease may progress very slowly, and the patient may function for many years.

Orthopedic treatment is directed at control of deformities by appropriate bracing or surgical arthrodesis of neuropathic joints. Laminectomy may be required to relieve rapidly expanding cavities of the spinal cord.

See also Chap. 42.

ATROPHY AND WASTING OF INTRINSIC MUSCLES OF THE HAND

Atrophy and wasting of the intrinsic muscles of the hand may be due to involvement of the central nervous system, spinal cord, anterior horn cells, lesions of the brachial plexus or peripheral nerves, or vascular and ischemic disorders (Fig. 43-23).

ORTHOPEDIC MANAGEMENT OF STROKE

This field requires the same type of combined team approach as has been used with good effect in rehabilitation following poliomyelitis and following the more aggressive surgical treatment of meningomyelocele. However, the place of surgery in the management of the stroke patient is limited.

EARLY TREATMENT. The early general medical management of the stroke patient is well known, such as the maintenance of an adequate airway, the introduction of urinary catheter drainage with antibiotics if necessary, and attention to other general medical problems such as unrecognized coronary artery disease, pulmonary disease, or complications, etc. Rehabilitation of the stroke patient begins at the earliest possible time, usually on the third or fourth day after the stroke.

In the flaccid state the patient is in urgent need of external stimuli, to replace the proprioceptive impulses produced by movement of limbs. This deficiency of motion may be replaced by a trained physical therapist. Placing the patient in a wheelchair is far preferable to a horizontal view of the world.

Nursing care is of vital importance in preventing deformity. Correct positioning in bed by the use of a foot board may prevent equinus, and the use of a rolled blanket beneath the greater trochanters to roll the legs may prevent external rotation deformity and flexion of the knees. Correct support of the upper limbs by the use of a pillow in the axilla will maintain shoulder abduction and prevent "frozen shoulder."

Frequent change of position is also of vital importance to prevent hypostatic pneumonia and pressure sores. At each change of position the joints of the limbs are placed through a range of motion and positioned to maintain or increase their range of movement. The prone position should also be used to provide good drainage of secretions and to prevent hip flexion and knee flexion deformities.

ASSESSMENT. Pseudomotor changes are of value in assessing motor control deficits, and it may be possible to predict whether the involvement is bilateral or not.

The involvement of the extrapyramidal system is of importance, because of its potential reversibility. The classical signs of facial immobility, failure of accommodation, and flexor rigidity in the neck muscles are much later occurrences. In the early stages the most reliable sign of cog wheel rigidity is the test of internal/external rotation of the shoulder and, to a lesser extent, of the hip joint.

Difficulties in balance are often overlooked; it is essential to evaluate the patient in the upright position when attempting to assess his ability to walk. Only very occasionally does a stroke disturb the central control of balance. More frequently the inability to stand erect is related to a disturbance of the patient's body image, resulting from a lesion in the nondominant hemisphere of the brain.

The patient with a distorted body image will make no attempt to support or otherwise accommodate for the weight of that side and thus falls toward the involved side without making any effort to protect himself. Techniques to stimulate body awareness, walking aids, and braces are possible means of overcoming this inadequacy.

CONTROL OF SPASTICITY. The ideal method of controlling spasticity would decrease excessive muscle tone permanently without associated loss of motor control and without loss of sensation. Such a method is not yet available; the most useful clinical method is peripheral muscle release. However this has the disadvantage of causing associated muscle weakness, and the procedure cannot be undone. Because of this, a variety of techniques have evolved.

Peripheral nerve block to control spasticity by dilute phenol injections was reported by Khalili et al. Further results also have been reported by Mooney et al. With phenol, spasticity is reduced or abolished for a comparatively short period of time and begins to return at the second or third month.

A simpler technique for the reduction of spasticity has been described using intramuscular alcohol injection in the approximate locus of the motor point. This is an extremely simple technique involving the local infiltration of the affected muscle belly with 45 percent alcohol solution. The reduction of spasticity is comparable to that obtained using phenol. Its effect lasts about 3 months, but reinjection may be used with results similar to those obtained by the first injection.

SURGICAL CORRECTION OF DISABILITIES. Lower Limb Problems. The most common site of deformity in the stroke patient is the foot and ankle equinus. A reliable standing base is most important, and even a patient with very minimal motor control can achieve stability at the knee and hip provided a stable plantigrade position is obtainable at the foot. This deformity, whether due to actual contracture or to spasticity, is relieved by elongation of the tendon Achilles. The patient is encouraged to walk and stand 3 to 5 days following the surgery.

In order to control the varus deformity of the foot which is frequently associated with spasticity or contracture of the gastrocnemius and soleus, the tibialis anterior tendon transfer is a useful adjunct.

Knee flexion deformity is favored by a persistence of the primitive flexor pattern and lack of early stimulation of extensor patterns. Usually the flexed knee deformity is equally accountable to lack of quadriceps muscle tone as to excessive hamstring spasticity. Release of the hamstrings

by sectioning at the musculotendinous junction corrects this deformity.

Disability at the hip joint may arise from three causes:

1. Abductor and extensor weakness
2. Persistent hip flexion deformity
3. Excessive adductor motor tone

Abductor and extensor weakness often may be improved by the use of a walking stick carried in the opposite hand. Hip adduction contracture may be released by adductor division, or in the case of spasticity by obturator neurectomy.

Hip flexion deformity may be released. However it is important to demonstrate spasticity so severe and contractural deformity so marked that the subsequent weakness of hip flexion will be a less severe problem than the preexisting one.

Upper Limb. Surgical procedures in the upper limbs are usually carried out for problems of painful contracture, severe spasticity, or mechanical impairment of function.

The painful frozen shoulder is a major impairment to rehabilitation. Mild spasticity in the internal rotator adductor group at the shoulder is noted frequently in the third and fourth months following a stroke. Active assisted exercises combined with a positioning program may maintain or help regain a good range of shoulder movement.

The Flexed Spastic Elbow. Severe spasticity of the flexors of the elbow does not respond to exercising and positioning programs and may result in a flexion contracture. The deformity is unsightly and prevents the patient from positioning his hand. The contracture is frequently associated with a symptomatic adducted shoulder; both areas may be treated simultaneously during shoulder release surgery. Release procedures in the antecubital fossa are rarely called for, and the surgeon must be prepared to release or lengthen the biceps tendon, brachialis, brachioradialis, the forearm flexor muscles, and the elbow joint capsule.

The Spastic Forearm and Hand. Spasticity and poor motor control are common in the hemiplegic forearm and hand. Procedures to improve these may be considered when the general state of the patient is good and there is intact sensation associated with some selective motor control in the arm. If a patient with an apparent flexion deformity of the wrist and fingers is able to extend the wrist and fingers selectively following a nerve block, then a flexor slide procedure will be of value to weaken the spastic flexor pronators. However, when there is significant fixed flexion contracture in wrist and fingers, a simple muscle origin release procedure will not be sufficient.

POSTURE

Posture is the basis of all movement. All movements start from, and end in, posture. The regulation of normal posture in an intact animal depends upon the integrated activity of many reflex mechanisms. The anterior horn cell forms a convergent point for fibers from many dorsal nerve roots and for fibers from all levels of the brain and spinal cord. Only when the activity of all these converging pathways are properly coordinated does normal posture result.

In the spinal cord there are reflex mechanisms that subserve a variety of movements, but the maintenance of posture is thought to be exclusively a function of reflex arcs that have centers in the pons, medulla, and midbrain. The organization of movement is more complex. In the motor control involving posture and movement, the final common pathways from the anterior horn cells in the cord to the muscles have been found to contain both large alpha neurons, which directly innervate the muscle fibers, and small gamma fibers, which innervate only the intrafusal muscles of the sensory end organs in the muscle spindle. Excitation of these does not produce muscle contraction in the ordinary sense but, by producing contraction of the muscle within the spindles, sets up afferent impulses which return to the cord via the dorsal roots to produce a tonic facilitation of the large alpha neurons. This facilitation is essential to the development of the stretch reflex.

The gamma neurons may be stimulated to activity from the motor cortex, particularly from the tegmentum of the brain stem. There is also evidence that the gamma system of neurons may pass from higher levels of the central nervous system by many routes, one of which is probably the pyramidal or corticospinal system. Afferents which modify the discharge of centers giving rise to the long propriospinal or the reticulospinal tracts are responsible for the adjustments of posture produced by neck reflexes, labyrinthine reflexes, and righting reflexes.

Tonic neck reflexes appear in infants between the fourth and twelfth week, but it is not until the twenty-eighth week that an infant is able to raise his head and control it. By the fifth month the child can roll over, but is usually only creeping or moving forward in the prone position by the tenth month. By the thirty-sixth week he will be able to stand still for a short while without support but usually will not walk unaided before the age of twelve months.

The sensory end organs of ligaments play a significant role in maintaining the stability and position of joints. These act by limiting extreme ranges of movement as well as by indicating the actual position of the joint via proprioceptive pathways.

When assessing any disturbance of posture, one must inspect the child while he is standing, sitting, and lying and determine the presence or absence of any abnormal movements or response to movements. In addition, one should look for any laxity of joints or hypertonia of muscles. When the child stands erect, changes in the spinal column occur with the development of a cervical lordosis, a thoracic kyphosis, and a lumbar lordosis. In the standing position, the gravitational forces lie along lines passing through the mastoid processes, the greater trochanters, and the tibial tubercles, to reach the ground in line with the bases of the fifth metatarsals. A state of equilibrium between these forces occurs when a vertical line passes along the center of gravity but falls within the boundary of the supporting base of both feet.

Postural deformities resulting from habit, occupational attitudes, or body carriage in movement must be differentiated from static forces, which are concerned with bodies at rest, or the equilibrium of weights which are not moving. A postural deformity is dynamic in orgin, whereas a static deformity occurs because of weakened musculature.

Disturbances in Gait (Limping)

In normal gait there are three major phases through which the lower limbs alternate. These are the phases of stance, swing-through, and propulsion.

PHASE I—STANCE. When one leg is moving forward, the body is maintained in an upright position on the other supporting foot, and the center of gravity is balanced high at the level of the superior border of the sacrum. Under these conditions, the static forces passing through the lower extremity joints are immense. Denham has shown that the hip joint of the adult male may be subject to pressures of 350 ft-lb/in.[2]

Stability during this stance phase demands a locking mechanism in both the hip and knee. For the hip joint, Walmsley described this locking mechanism as internal rotation with some abduction in full extension so that the largest diameter of the femoral head will be accommodated within the acetabular socket, whereas Gilmour attributed the stability of the femoral head to a gripping mechanism served by the acetabular labrum, the capsule of the hip joint, and a cushion of synovial fluid.

Structural abnormalities can be aggravated by forces of gravity in all age groups. Postural abnormalities are usually correctible by changing the deforming force, whereas in static deformities the originating disease must be corrected as well.

The knee joint is stabilized and locked in full extension by the contraction of the vastus medialis and the popliteus muscle, which internally rotates the femoral condyle on the tibial plateau.

PHASE II—THE PENDULUM, OR SWING-THROUGH, PHASE. The swing-through phase of gait is characterized by dorsiflexion of the foot and toes and flexion of the knee and the hip. At the same time, a certain proportion of the total body weight is moved forward by means of hip abduction, external rotation of the leg, and rotation of the pelvis.

PHASE III—PROPULSION. The propulsion phase of gait is one of forward movement in which the body leans forward. At the same time the supporting limb is pushing off with plantar-flexed foot, extended toes, extended knee, and extended hip. These dynamic forces of propulsion are contributed to by those of body weight added to those of the muscular contraction.

REQUIREMENTS FOR EFFICIENT LOCOMOTION. These are:

1. Stability of joints, normal bone length, normal skeletal relationships
2. Normal joint range of movement and normal muscle power
3. Cortical control of voluntary muscle action
4. Normal muscle tone, including coordination as well as postural tone
5. Normal sensory modalities
6. Cerebellar control of muscle action, and intact ocular and auditory balance mechanism

Abnormal, or disturbed, gait of mechanical origin must be clearly distinguished from ataxic and other gait patterns of neurologic origin. This requires examination of the joints to determine normal range of motion and detect fixed flexion contractures. Abnormalities of the foot and ankle should be searched for and neurologic disorders evaluated.

NEUROLOGIC DISORDERS

Ataxic gait consists of an uncoordinated, awkward, unbalanced, wide-based gait with poor symmetry and repetition pattern. It may result from:

1. Disturbances of the cerebellum, such as thrombosis of the cerebellar artery, or tumors of the posterior cranial fossa
2. Lesions involving the posterior columns such as disseminated sclerosis, the Guillain-Barré syndrome, and Friedreich's ataxia
3. Lesions involving peripheral sensation and proprioceptive modalities, such as tabes dorsalis, or neuritis and subacute combined degeneration of the cord, which give a characteristic high-stepping gait

A spastic paraplegic gait is characterized by scissoring of the legs, which are held stiff in extension and adducted. If adduction deformity, which is common in cerebral palsy, is severe, the degree of pelvic rotation and elevation may be markedly exaggerated.

In hemiplegia the flail, or spastic, leg is used as a prop until the good leg can be brought forward for the propulsion phase.

MECHANICAL DISORDERS

JOINT DISORDERS. Among the numerous joint abnormalities which may produce gait disturbances are congenital dysplasia, congenital dislocation of the hip, slipped upper femoral epiphysis, Legg-Calvé-Perthes disease, and knee conditions such as juvenile arthritis, osteochondritis dissecans, discoid menisci, congenital genu valgum or varus, and congenital metatarsus varus, flatfoot, or congenital talipes equinovarus (clubfoot).

LEG-LENGTH DISCREPANCY. This may be the result of congenital or acquired shortening of the femur or tibia or soft tissue contractures of the hip or knee joint, secondary to joint or primary muscular disease.

MUSCULAR DISORDERS. Among the muscular disorders resulting in abnormal gait are those secondary to anterior poliomyelitis, cerebral palsy, nerve injury, spina bifida, myelodysplasia, primary motor neuron disease, and muscular dystrophy.

Spinal Deformities

The convexity of the thoracic and sacral curves, the primary curves of the vertebral column, result from the shape of the vertebral bodies, whereas the secondary, lordotic curves of the cervical and lumbar regions are due more to the shape of the intervertebral discs, which are wider anteriorly than posteriorly. In addition, the contour of the vertebral column is dependent upon the integrity of its supporting ligaments and the sacrospinalis and anterior abdominal musculatures.

The intervertebral discs, like arterial walls, reflect the age and tone of the body tissues. With increasing age, the nucleus pulposus loses its elasticity and fluid content, and the fibers of the annulus fibrosus lose their definition. These changes are very marked in those engaged in heavy work, but they are a feature of all aging spines.

Alterations in the normal anterorposterior curvature of the spine occur in both the young and the old and are the consequence of affections of bones, intervertebral discs, or spinal muscles.

KYPHOSIS

The term "kyphosis" refers to an increase in the normal posterior convexity of the thoracic spine, involving a number of vertebral bodies, if not the entire thoracic column. On the other hand, "gibbus" refers to an acute angular deformity resulting from a disease such as tuberculosis or a fractured vertebral body.

Kyphosis of Adolescence

MUSCULAR TYPE. The muscular type of adolescent kyphosis is seen in children of poor physical development and is characterized by a thoracic kyphosis, or "round shoulders." Such children are often slow and clumsy in their movements, i.e., uncoordinated. In the early stages, spinal movements are normal, but later the mobility of the spine decreases, and the kyphosis becomes fixed. Pain is not a common feature of the condition, but postural strain on ligaments may produce backache or pain in the feet or legs.

Early treatment aimed at improving musculature by exercise, swimming, deep breathing, and posture training produces dramatic improvement. External support by braces is not recommended.

OSSEOUS TYPE. This usually results from developmental disturbances such as arachnodactyly, osteochondral dystrophy, or acquired lesions such as tuberculosis. Tuberculosis as a result of bony destruction tends to produce an acute gibbus rather than a smooth kyphosis.

DISCOGENIC TYPE, OR TRUE ADOLESCENT KYPHOSIS (SCHEUERMANN'S DISEASE; VERTEBRAL EPIPHYSITIS). This condition occurs in both sexes between the ages of twelve and seventeen and is seen as marked thoracic kyphosis with round, drooping shoulders and a flat, narrow chest with prominent scapulae.

The cause of this condition, which is familial, is unknown, but possible factors are:

1. Circulatory disturbances affecting the nutrition of the vertebral epiphysis, with fragmentation and irregularities as seen on radiography (Fig. 43-24). Permanent wedging of the vertebral bodies may result.
2. Early disc degeneration consequent upon:
   a. A rapid increase in body weight.
   b. Multiple minor traumas.
   c. Shortening of the hamstrings, which produces hyperflexion strains at the thoracolumbar junction on stooping, or forward flexion.

Early active treatment in the form of spinal traction followed by hyperextension and spinal exercises can limit the progress of this deformity. Once spinal growth is complete at the age of sixteen to eighteen years, no further progression will occur.

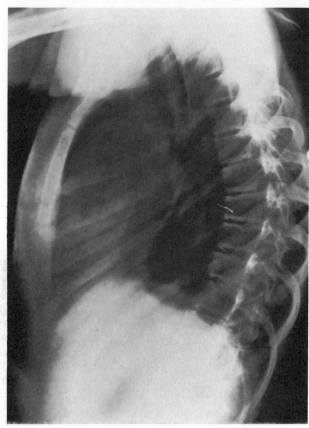

Fig. 43-24. Lateral radiograph showing fragmentation of the vertebral epiphysis in the thoracic spine in Scheuermann's disease.

Increasing spinal kyphosis is a common accompaniment of advancing years. It may result from a variety of pathologic changes affecting the different components of the spinal column.

"TRUE" SENILE KYPHOSIS. Especially in those engaged in heavy occupations, degeneration of the anterior portion of the annulus fibrosus leads to final disintegration of the intervertebral discs. This results in wedging of the anterior aspects of the vertebral bodies until they touch, by osteophyte formation as well as bony absorption.

SENILE OR POSTMENOPAUSAL OSTEOPOROSIS. In this condition, although the degree of osteoporosis of the vertebral bodies varies, it is evenly distributed throughout the vertebral column. There is absorption of the bony trabeculae, but the intervertebral discs remain normal or even tend to bulge into the atrophied spongy tissue of the vertebral body.

In the earliest phase the patient has great difficulty in carrying out extremes of movement, and there is often a history of attacks of "lumbago." Pain may never completely disappear. The individual loses his stature and carries himself stooping, the head and shoulders thrust forward. This loss in height must be differentiated from Paget's disease, Kümmel's disease, multiple myeloma, and secondary malignant deposits.

SCOLIOSIS

When viewed from the back any deviation from the normally straight spine to one side or the other, i.e., a lateral deviation, constitutes scoliosis.

CLASSIFICATION. There are many classifications, but the most simple and practicable is that suggested by Cobb and modified by Ponsetti and Freedman:

Classification of Scoliosis

I. Postural scoliosis
II. Structural scoliosis
   A. Idiopathic
     1. Cervicothoracic
     2. Thoracic
       a. Infantile—age of onset birth to three years
       b. Juvenile—age of onset four to nine years
       c. Adolescence—age of onset ten years to the end of growth
     3. Thoracolumbar
     4. Lumbar
     5. Combined thoracic and lumbar
   B. Osteopathic
     1. Congenital vertebral anomalies
     2. Thoracogenic following thoracoplasty or empyema
     3. Osteochondrodystrophy
   C. Neuropathic
     1. Congenital
     2. Postpoliomyelitis
     3. Neurofibromatosis
     4. Other neuropathies
       a. Syringomyelia
       b. Charcot-Marie-Tooth syndrome
       c. Friedreich's ataxia
       d. Cerebral palsy
   D. Myopathic
     1. Congenital scoliosis
     2. Muscular dystrophies

Postural Scoliosis

Postural scoliosis is seen most commonly in adolescent girls. The curve is usually slight, single, and characteristically a long left thoracolumbar scoliosis, without vertebral rotation, which disappears when the child hangs from a bar or bends forward. In recumbency, the spine appears straight, and when tested for lateral flexion it will bend equally well to both sides.

A short leg will cause a compensatory scoliosis convex to the side of the depressed pelvis, but correcting the shortening with a lift under the shoe, thus leveling the pelvis, will correct the scoliosis.

Treatment of postural scoliosis is the same as for poor posture in general, i.e., improvement in musculature by general spinal exercises.

Structural Scoliosis

CONGENITAL SCOLIOSIS. Congenital scoliosis is associated with demonstrable vertebral anomalies. There may be one hemivertebra or more involved with congenital absence of discs or fusions of vertebral bodies and ribs. In general, isolated vertebral anomalies have a good prognosis, but there are cases, particularly in the thoracic region, in which a long vertebral segment is involved and in which a gross scoliosis develops. Unfortunately, it is not easy initially to recognize which type is present.

It is preferable to determine and to treat surgically at a young age those with an anomalous vertebral development in association with undifferentiated posterolateral bony bars. Congenital scoliosis is more likely than other forms of scoliosis to lead to paraplegia, usually in the later years of growth, and for this reason must remain under observation until the end of the growth period.

PARALYTIC SCOLIOSIS. This most commonly results after anterior poliomyelitis and can be prevented or minimized by adequate initial management. In the young patient with paralytic poliomyelitis and asymmetrical involvement of trunk musculature, asymmetrical soft tissue contractures and subsequent disturbances of vertebral growth may develop.

The various curve patterns of paralytic scoliosis have been divided into high thoracic, thoracic, thoracolumbar, lumbar, and combined thoracic and lumbar scoliosis, and a telescoping spine.

The prognosis in paralytic scoliosis is less dependent on the localization of the primary curve than in idiopathic scoliosis. A more important prognostic factor is the age at which the disease first occurs, because the longer the imbalance of muscle affects vertebral growth, the more the distortion.

Idiopathic Scoliosis

PATHOLOGY. The true pathologic basis of idiopathic scoliosis is still unknown, but interesting animal experiments point the way toward the possible causes. Langerskiold and Michelsson produced a progressive scoliosis in rabbits by removing the posterior ends of five or six ribs as well as by hemilaminectomy of five of the thoracic vertebrae. The common factor was the loss of function of the posterior costotransverse ligaments, and cutting these ligaments alone produced similar deformities. Ponsetti and Shepard produced scoliosis by inducing lathyrism in rats. The skeletal deformities which resulted were due to lesions of the epiphyseal plates with loosening and detachments of the tendinous and ligamentous insertions.

NATURAL HISTORY. Idiopathic scoliosis will progress during growth in the majority of cases. Therefore the two important factors in deciding the prognosis of this condition are the *age of onset* and the *site of the curve.*

Risser and Ferguson first noticed the relationship between spinal growth and the increase of the deformity and also its cessation when the bony structure matured at the age of seventeen in boys and sixteen in girls. Later Risser observed that the completion of ossification of the iliac apophysis coincides with completion of spinal growth. Therefore any growth after this is minimal, as is deterioration in the curve. Thoracic curves beginning before the age of ten years carry a very poor prognosis and usually result in a severe deformity. Steindler, quoted by Crowe, noted that the maximal deterioration of scoliosis generally occurred between the ages of one and two years, between five and ten years, and at puberty when there was rapid growth of the spine. The author of the present chapter,

from a longitudinal growth study of 10 cases of infantile idiopathic scoliosis, found that there was deterioration during two main periods: first, shortly after diagnosis at the age of two to four years, when it was related to the midgrowth spurt, and, second, at the age of six to nine in boys and six to ten in girls. This latter deterioration followed the midgrowth spurt closely. The adolescent growth spurt had little influence on this particular form of scoliosis. Although the infantile idiopathic scoliosis makes up only 10 percent of all cases of scoliosis, it is exposed to the total effects of growth throughout its natural history and because of this has an extremely poor prognosis, producing the most progressive and severe of all curvatures.

In general, to prognosticate for any particular case of idiopathic scoliosis the following observations are required:

1. The site of the curve
2. The age of onset
3. The skeletal or physiologic age rather than the chronological age
4. The state of ossification of the iliac apophysis
5. The developmental age in relation to puberty

CLINICAL FEATURES OF IDIOPATHIC AND OTHER FORMS OF STRUCTURAL SCOLIOSIS. Medical attention is usually sought because of trunk asymmetry, a prominent hip, a prominent shoulder, or a hump on the back. There is occasionally a complaint of backache and fatigue, but severe pain is an unusual complaint. However, in adult life, particularly in lumbar scoliosis, pain due to secondary degenerative changes may produce symptoms.

Later complications of severe scoliosis include reductions in the vital capacity of the lungs and the development of cor pulmonale. Bergofsky et al. have described the correlation of cardiopulmonary pathologic changes in relation to the severity of the curvature.

The most common type of idiopathic scoliosis is a right thoracic curve, which occurs predominantly in girls (Fig. 43-25). The curvature of congenital scoliosis due to abnormal vertebral development is usually a short, sharp curve which is rigid and associated with much less rotational prominence of the posterior rib cage or lumbar area than the idiopathic and paralytic curves. An angular but short scoliosis in the presence of café au lait spots and subcutaneous nevi indicates neurofibromatosis.

Fig. 43-25. Features of an idiopathic scoliosis in a girl with a right thoracic curve.

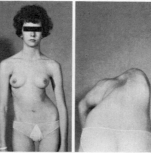
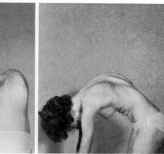

When a patient with scoliosis is examined, the shoulder girdles, the thoracic and lumbar areas of the trunk, and the iliac crests are assessed for asymmetry. The height of the iliac crest and the posterosuperior iliac spines is determined to note whether the pelvis is level. It is necessary to measure leg length in recumbency to exclude secondary scoliosis due to leg-length discrepancy. On forward flexion of the spine a rotational prominence of the transverse processes will be noted, particularly on the convex side of the curve.

The mobility of the spine is tested by traction applied to the head manually as well as by lateral bending in the erect position and lateral bending in the recumbent position. It will be noted that thoracic curves are usually more rigid than lumbar curves.

Finally a complete radiologic survey of the entire spine is essential including an anteroposterior view with the patient standing and recumbent views with the patient bending to the right and to the left. Lateral views of the spine are also required to assess any degree of congenital anomaly. From these it is possible to assess the site and degree of both the primary and secondary curves.

The primary curve is defined as:

1. The longest curve with the greatest degree of angulation
2. The least flexible curve as determined by clinical and radiologic examination
3. The curve toward which the trunk lists

The degree of angulation is measured on the radiograph in the manner described by Cobb. Perpendicular lines are erected to the superior surface of the proximal vertebra and the inferior surface of the distal vertebra involved. The angle formed by these two intersecting lines is the angle of the curve (Fig. 43-26).

Treatment of Scoliosis

CONSERVATIVE TREATMENT. The object of treatment is to obtain correction and to prevent any further increase in the deformity. In idiopathic scoliosis in particular, treatment requires regular clinical, radiographic, and photographic examination to observe and to record progress of the curvature during growth. General exercises are prescribed to obtain good posture and to maintain mobility of the spine.

With respect to external supports, the Moe brace (Fig. 43-27), which relieves pressure of the vertebral epiphyses on the concave side of the curve, is the most efficient appliance available. The efficient use of this brace permits the postponement of surgical treatment until final correction, and spinal fusion can be carried out at the age of ten years or more.

Paralytic scoliosis is treated more aggressively than idiopathic curvatures during development of the deformity. Initially in the very young child prolonged recumbency is advocated, and stretching exercises are instituted to maintain good spinal mobility and to prevent soft tissue contractures. Bent plaster shells such as the Murk-Jansen bed are used intermittently to counteract any deforming attitude in recumbency, and once correction is obtained, the vertebral column must be supported with a removable plaster jacket or a Milwaukee brace.

SURGICAL TREATMENT. Surgical treatment is required when the deformity cannot be controlled in the growing

Fig. 43-26. Idiopathic scoliosis treated by Harrington rod and massive bone graft. Goldstein technique. *A.* 85° right thoracic primary curve between T_5 and T_{12}. *B.* Lateral bend to the right corrects curve to 56°. *C.* Postoperative correction following Harrington rod instrumentation and bone grafting with massive autogenous cancellous bone. The curve is corrected to 37° and is fused to T_1.

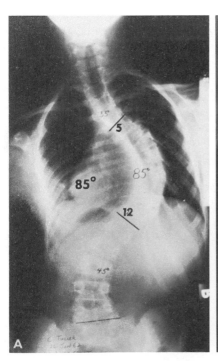
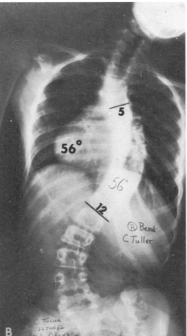
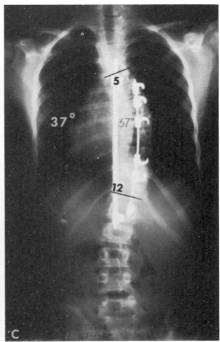

child by the use of the Milwaukee brace and in the case of any correctable deformity at or after maturity which is accompanied by pain. As a general rule, curves under 40° can be controlled by the Milwaukee brace, but when progression of the curve occurs, correction and spinal fusion is indicated. With progression of a paralytic scoliotic curve and instability of the trunk due to muscle imbalance, stabilization of the spine is indicated. In cases of congenital scoliosis where there is a definite undifferentiated bony bar in the concavity of the curve, early fusion over a short segment of the involved vertebrae is mandatory, since the curve will relentlessly progress without it. Congenital curves should be watched closely and fused early if there is progression. Specific indications for operation include curves over 60° and those involving the thoracic or thoracolumbar spine. A more conservative approach may be adopted for double major curves, which are usually balanced. Pain is rare in the adolescent scoliosis patient. Operative intervention is rarely required in adults unless there is severe pain.

The usual operative measures are those of posterior spinal fusion utilizing cancellous bone and some form of internal and external splintage after adequate correction has been obtained. The Harrington rod has added greatly to the ability to improve correction and, when utilized with sound spine fusion techniques, has lowered the rate of pseudarthrosis and loss of correction postoperatively. The Dwyer technique involves an anterior approach to the vertebral bodies, interbody fusion, and correction of the curve by the swadged cable fixed to screws attached to the vertebral bodies. For some types of rigid curves and severe thoracolumbar curves this technique is a definite advantage. When Harrington rod and posterior spine fusions are carried out, patients are immobilized postoperatively in a plaster cast extending from the chin and occiput to at least the groin and occasionally to include both thighs. Plaster cast immobilization is usually required for 4 to 6 months after surgery (Fig. 43-28).

Knee Deformities

GENU VALGUM

This deformity is characterized by an abnormal increase in the distance between the two medial malleoli when the extended knees are just touching each other. It may arise from disturbances of the epiphyseal plate, epiphysis, or ligamentous structures of the knee joint and after fractures of the lateral tibial or the lateral femoral condyle. A common cause used to be deficiency rickets with disturbance of the mineralization process in endochondral ossification. Rachitic deformities may still arise from congenital renal insufficiency such as Fanconi's syndrome or vitamin D–resistant rickets. Genu valgum is not an uncommon complication of rheumatoid arthritis, in which there is gradual attenuation of the medial ligament and collapse of the lateral tibial condyle. Similarly it may complicate postmenopausal osteoporosis.

However, the most common type of genu valgum, or knock-knee, is that seen in young children and is consid-

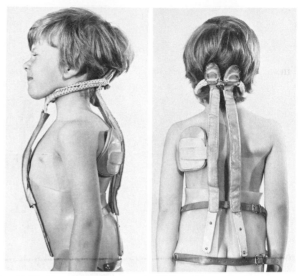

Fig. 43-27. Moe brace treatment of idiopathic scoliosis.

ered to be postural, or idiopathic, in type (Fig. 43-29). Indeed, it is so common during infancy that it might be considered a normal phase of development. Morley found that 22 percent of children of three to three and one-half years of age had genu valgum with an intermaleolar distance of 2 in. or more, whereas only 1 to 2 percent of children aged seven and over had an equivalent degree of genu valgum. The deformity arises because the line of weight transmission from the femur falls within the lateral side of the center of the knee joint, so that the lateral condyles of both the femur and the tibia bear more weight than their medial counterparts.

TREATMENT. Genu valgum in infants and children below the age of seven can be safely ignored if not excessive and in the absence of underlying causes. It may be advisable in certain cases to raise the inner edge of the heel by $\frac{1}{8}$ to $\frac{3}{16}$ in., especially as a measure of reassurance to the anxious parents.

Fig. 43-28. Localizer cast with windows cut allowing surgical exposure. A. Windows in place. B. Windows removed, showing access to the iliac crest and spine.

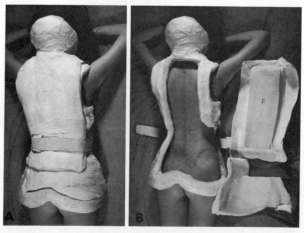

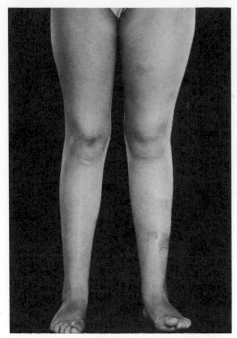

Fig. 43-29. Idiopathic genu valgum deformity.

Active treatment is occasionally necessary in the form of Jones walking genu valgum braces or mermaid night splints. In severe cases, some of which commence posturally and have been aggravated by obesity, operative correction in the form of supracondylar femoral osteotomy may be required.

Fig. 43-30. Genu varum deformity in an infant boy mainly arising from the tibiae.

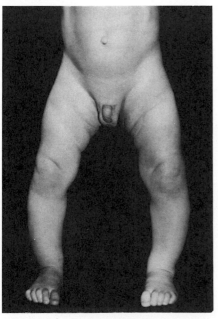

GENU VARUM

The pathogenesis of genu varum is similar to that outlined above for genu valgum. The idiopathic, or postural, variety in infancy is the most common clinical form of presentation.

A minor degree of the deformity is quite common in children up to three years of age, and the deformity is usually restricted to the tibia (Fig. 43-30). Occasionally, the deformity may be more apparent than real and is really a manifestation of an abnormal arc of rotation in the hips or persistent fetal alignment, in which there is excess of internal rotation over external rotation, due to marked anteversion of the femoral neck.

TREATMENT. As in genu valgum, most postural, idiopathic types without any evidence of underlying metabolic or congenital epiphyseal disorders regress spontaneously and require no treatment.

Foot and Ankle Deformities

In spite of its lightness and elasticity, the foot possesses tremendous strength. The architectural arrangement of its bones and joints into multiple elastic arches and levers provides two main functions: a stable support for the body's weight in standing and a resilient spring, or lever, for propulsion in walking.

The arch configuration of the foot is characteristic of man. Most textbooks describe three arches, two longitudinal and one transverse. The calcaneus forms the common posterior pillar for both the lateral and the medial longitudinal arches. The lateral longitudinal arch is completed by the cuboid and the lateral two metatarsals. The medial is completed by the talus, the cuneiform, and the inner three metatarsals. The third metatarsal, though a component of the medial arch, serves both longitudinal arches physiologically. Also, in forming the anterior pillar of the essential arch, it acts as a pivot to assist in shifting body weight from the lateral to the medial longitudinal arch during locomotion. The transverse arch usually refers to the anterior metatarsal arch, the existence of which as a functional element was denied by Morton, who demonstrated by means of special apparatus that all five metatarsal heads participate in weight bearing and that the foot does *not* distribute its weight like a tripod. Morton's experiment can be verified by standing barefoot on five slips of paper, one under each metatarsal head. If an assistant then attempts to pull out the strips, he soon discovers that the foot is no tripod.

The characteristically human, archlike structure of the foot is obvious in the cartilaginous skeleton at birth, but when the child begins to stand, the arch tends to flatten, and it is not for some years that it develops the ability to resist the forces of weight bearing. Postural tone of the leg muscles, which occurs somewhat late in human development, is essential in assisting the arch of the foot to resist these forces; should the development of this postural tone fail, the inherent bony arches of the foot become flattened, producing variable degrees and types of so-called "flatfoot."

MECHANICS OF THE FOOT. The function of muscles and ligaments in the control of the arch of the foot is much disputed, some emphasizing the ligaments and others favoring the muscles as the prime factor. Keith is largely responsible for the concept that muscles maintain the arch by their dynamic pull. However, many deny this, and Hicks, in an anatomic, electromyographic study of the foot, demonstrated that the leg muscles play no part in the configuration of the foot and are indeed inactive during standing. The arch of the foot should be considered as an inherent and characteristic structure based upon the architectural configuration of the skeletal elements aided by the numerous ligaments joining them and stabilized by the muscles acting upon them.

Hicks described the weight-bearing unit of the foot as a combination of beam action and arch action. An arch-shaped structure has its ends thrust apart when a weight is applied to it. Therefore the strength peculiar to a true arch is only acquired when the ends are prevented from coming farther apart. In the foot this function of the tie between the piers is produced by the plantar aponeurosis. However, when the ends of an archlike structure are not prevented from spreading farther apart, the structure cannot behave as an arch and behaves as a beam. A beam is subject to bending strain, and its strength depends upon the resistance of the material to being broken by bending. The concept of the foot, which is a structure composed of several pieces, as a beam is not acceptable unless there are tense intersegmental ties on the undersurface, the joints being at their limit of extension. In considering the weight-bearing unit of the foot, a distinction must be made between the beam action and the arch action. In the beam action there is bending strain in the bones which produces tension in the intersegmental ligaments, whereas in the arch action there is compression strain in the bones and a tension strain in the plantar aponeurosis.

In the flat standing position, the arch-flattening effect of body weight produces tension in the plantar aponeurosis, and the foot behaves as an arch, but when the line of weight moves forward through the foot as the heel begins to rise, the arch-flattening effect is resisted by both beam and arch mechanisms acting together. In the tiptoe standing position or the push-off phase of walking, the arch mechanism takes over from the beam action by virtue of the fact that the extension of the toes at the metatarso-phalangeal (MP) joints "winds up the windlass" of the plantar aponeurosis. The strain on the beam action therefore lessens, and in the extreme raised-heel position the arch mechanism assumes the whole load, and the arch rises.

FLATFOOT (Pes Planus; Pes Valgus)

Congenital Convex Pes Valgus (Congenital Vertical Talus)

See Chap. 44 on Congenital Orthopedic Deformities.

Peroneal Spastic Flatfoot

Although this condition may be produced by inflammatory and traumatic affections of the tarsal joints, Harris has shown that the most common cause is an abnormal

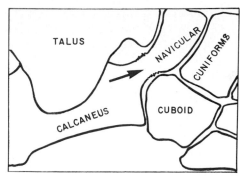

Fig. 43-31. Calcaneonavicular bar.

coalescence between two or more of the tarsal bones. This is in effect a congenital ankylosis which may be either complete or incomplete and may be osseous, cartilaginous, or fibrous.

In young children tarsal coalescence cannot be seen on x-ray, because it is cartilaginous and ossification does not occur until the age of nine or ten. Even in adulthood, special x-ray views and techniques such as tomograms are necessary to demonstrate the abnormal osseous anatomy. There are three common sites for such osseous coalescence between tarsal bones:

1. A calcaneonavicular bar (Fig. 43-31)
2. A talocalcaneal bar (Fig. 43-32)
3. A calcaneocuboid bar

Conservative treatment in the form of manipulation and the use of braces offer little chance of success. An operation is usually indicated. In young children if a bar can be demonstrated, simple resection may be successful, but usually the diagnosis is not made until adolescence or early adulthood when tarsal arthritis supervenes, necessitating triple arthrodesis.

Acquired Flatfoot

Acquired flatfoot may be divided into three pathologic types:

1. Osseous type, due to bony distortion produced by trauma or disease processes
2. Ligamentous type, which may follow rupture or avulsion of the ligamentous attachments of the foot, or sprain
3. Muscular imbalance, as in anterior poliomyelitis and cerebral palsy

Fig. 43-32. Talocalcaneal bar.

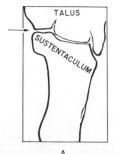

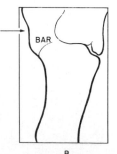

A.   B.

Flatfoot will arise whenever the muscles or ligaments fail to support the integral bony architecture of the arch. In the first efforts of walking a child usually walks with his feet flat and abducted. A good deal of this appears to be due to large deposits of fat over the medial aspect of the sole, but it is, in part, really due to inability of the leg muscles to support the arch. As postural tone develops, this deformity gradually disappears.

In an initially normal foot, there are certain predisposing extrinsic and intrinsic factors which may tend to transform it into a flat foot. All these factors will be considered under the following headings: Muscle Hypotonia, Excess of Muscular Fatigue, Footwear.

MUSCLE HYPOTONIA. The muscle hypotonia following recumbency accompanying long illness places the full strain of weight bearing and walking upon the bony and ligamentous structure of the arch. Stretching of these ligaments, which form the segmental ties of the archlike structure, will result in flattening of the foot.

EXCESS OF MUSCULAR FATIGUE. This is commonly an occupational hazard of nurses, policemen, and soldiers, and may also follow excessive exercises after a period of relative disuse. Relative muscular insufficiency as another factor in the development of acquired flatfoot is seen with sudden increases in body weight, a common occurrence in postmenopausal women accounting for much of the foot strain in this group.

FOOTWEAR. It has frequently been implied that unsuitable footwear is a basis of many of our foot troubles, but Hyman considered that this is unlikely, i.e., that ". . . most deformities of the foot and toes are developmental and it would be necessary to alter the genes rather than the children's footwear in order to prevent them."

Fig. 43-33. *A.* Line drawing of the lateral aspect of the foot to show the break occurring at the talonavicular and naviculocuneiform joints. *B.* Line drawing of the lateral aspect of the foot showing the correction of the talonavicular and naviculocuneiform joints, so that a straight line can be drawn through the axes of the talus, navicular, medial cuneiform, and metatarsals. (*After Jack, 1953.*)

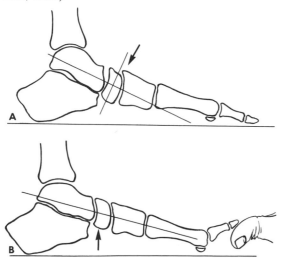

An extensive survey of school children's feet revealed that, between the ages of five and fifteen, hallux valgus was much more common in girls than in boys. In girls at the age of five the incidence of hallux valgus was 1.6 percent and by fifteen years had risen to 54 percent. In boys, on the other hand, at five years the incidence was 5.2 percent and at fifteen years had risen to only 14.8 percent. Therefore, the accelerated acquisition of this deformity must have begun before the age of nine, when there is virtually no difference in the footwear of the two sexes. However, Lam and Hodgson have shown significant increase in deformities in shoe-wearing populations in Hong Kong when compared with the unshod. Although there is no simple correlation between foot defects and unsatisfactory footwear, it is accepted that proper footwear is essential for the normal growth and development of the foot.

PATHOLOGY. If the calcaneonavicular ligament gives way, the talus deviates downward and mediad, and its body glides forward on the upper surface of the calcaneus. The calcaneus itself swings mediad, and its anterior end is depressed, with the result that the sustentaculum tali, the head of the talus, and the tuberosity of the navicular come to form prominences on the medial aspect of the foot.

Jack reviewed the anatomic types of flatfoot and pointed out that in lateral radiographs of the normal weight-bearing foot a straight line could be drawn through the axis of the talus, the middle of the navicular, the medial cuneiform, and the metatarsals. He described how a break would produce an unstable and everted foot of varying types depending upon the site of the break. A break may be at the talonavicular joint, producing the so-called "vertical talus deformity" or at the naviculocuneiform joint, or at both these joints combined (Fig. 43-33*A*). He demonstrated that dorsiflexion of the great toe restored the arch, particularly in cases of navicular cuneiform break, but not when the break occurred at other joints (Fig. 43-33*B*).

In time the displaced bones gradually alter in shape, and the navicular and cuneiform bones may become shaped like wedges with their apices situated dorsad. There is then permanent alteration in the architecture of the entire tarsus.

CLINICAL MANIFESTATIONS. The patient first notices that the feet become hot and uncomfortable after walking and standing. Later, they become stiff, especially after resting, and walking becomes increasingly painful. The gait becomes inelastic, clumsy, and "flatfooted," with no heel-and-toe rhythm, and severe pain and tenderness develop in the region of the navicular, the inferior calcaneonavicular ligament, the medial aspect of the sole, and the head of the first metatarsal. Finally, the awkward stiff, non-resilient gait results in abnormal weight distribution and the development of pressure points on the sole.

Four types of flatfoot may present themselves:

1. Foot Strain, or Incipient Flatfoot. This is the earliest stage, the period when pressure is first being exerted upon the ligaments. There is no evidence of deformity but simply symptoms of tenderness and pain.

2. Mobile Flatfoot.
   a. *Due to Faulty Postural Activity of Muscles.* This is seen in the very young child in whom there has been no development of postural tone.
   b. *Due to Short Calcaneus Tendon.* In these patients, the malalignment disappears on tiptoeing, but when the foot is correctly aligned, it is noted to be in planus.
3. Voluntary Flatfoot. This corresponds to the stage in which flattening of the arch has occurred but secondary adaptive changes have not yet ensued and the leg muscles, though they have lost their postural tone, can be used for volitional restoration of the arch.
4. Rigid Flatfoot. In these cases marked degenerative changes have occurred in the subtaloid and midtarsal joints, and the deformity has become fixed.

TREATMENT. The absolute indications for treatment are pain and impaired function. The existence of flatfoot per se does not necessarily mean that treatment is required. Many people with completely flat feet are able to go about their ordinary occupations without the slightest discomfort. Rigid flat feet are more likely to be symptomatic.

The ideal objectives of treatment, if indicated, are:

1. To correct the abnormal center of gravity in the foot so that the body weight is transferred to the outer side
2. To remove pressure symptoms

Treatment of Acute Foot Strain. Treatment of acute foot strain usually resolves itself into palliative measures, such as contrast footbaths, faradic footbaths, and foot exercises. Attention should also be directed toward the use of correct footwear, some features of which are outlined below.

The ideal shoe has a slightly concave inner border and a deep toe cap, and its width should be equal to, or a little greater than, that of the weight-bearing portion of the foot on standing. The sole should be firm over the heel and flexible over the forefoot, and the upper part must be made so as to form a well-fitting counter to support the heel and the high vamp over the instep.

For a short time following acute foot strain it is useful to thicken the medial portion of the sole of the shoe by about $\frac{1}{4}$ in., which deflects the body weight to the lateral side and spares the medial longitudinal arch. Special attention should be given to the fitting of correct footwear in children, but this is not always easy, as children rapidly outgrow rather than outwear their shoes. They should be fitted with Thomas heels, in which the medial border extends $\frac{1}{2}$ in. farther forward than the lateral, thus transferring the body weight to the lateral border of the foot.

Gait instruction and foot exercises are usual adjuncts in the management of foot strain from any cause. The patient should be taught to walk with the feet parallel, as the muscles supporting the arch are then activated and facilitate correction of the arch. Moreover, the heel-and-toe gait also brings into play the strong leg muscles which indirectly support the bony architecture of the foot.

Exercises, both active and against resistance, should be carried out twice daily. The rationale of these exercises is to stretch shortened structures such as the Achilles tendon and the soft parts of the lateral side of the foot and to strengthen relaxed muscles so that they are in a better condition to play their part in supporting the arch.

At the stage of voluntary flatfoot, in which there is still some possibility of volitional correction of the arch by muscle strength, exercises play a great part. While the muscles are being redeveloped, arch supports are often helpful in relieving symptoms. In the rigid and permanent types, however, the degenerative changes in the tarsal joints necessitate either triple arthrodesis or less extensive talonavicular fusions.

CONTRACTURE

The seventeenth-century term "contracture" means "a drawing together or becoming smaller." It implies, in pathologic terms, a permanent shortening and rigidity of muscles, joints, and fascial structures.

Contracture is a common sequel to joint immobility consequent upon disease, pain, etc. Experimental work in rats by Evans et al. has demonstrated that significant structural and progressive changes occur in muscle and intercapsular connective tissue planes after immobilization. Evans noted that these changes were partly reversible providing immobilization did not exceed 30 days, for beyond this time articular cartilage showed many irreversible changes such as matrix fibrillation, cleft separation, and subchondral bone destruction.

Contractures may be congenital or acquired.

CONGENITAL CONTRACTURES. Characteristic examples of congenital contractures are talipes equinovarus (clubfoot), sternocleidomastoid tumor (congenital torticollis), and the deformities associated with arthrogryposis multiplex congenita.

ACQUIRED CONTRACTURES. Acquired contractures of muscle, fascia, and ligaments involve disturbances of many tissue types, and it is therefore best to consider acquired contractures as primary or secondary with respect to their pathogenesis and tissue involvement.

Primary. *Muscle Contracture.* This includes primary muscular disorders such as progressive muscular dystrophy, the ischemia of Volkmann's contracture, and posttraumatic fibrosis.

Fascia. The classic primary, fascial type of contracture is that of Dupuytren's deformity affecting the palmar fascia and producing contractures of the fingers. It is occasionally seen in association with chronic barbiturism and may involve the plantar aponeurosis.

Joints. Many types of arthritic disorders such as rheumatoid arthritis, osteoarthritis, hemophilic arthropathy and infective and traumatic disorders of joints may result in contractures involving the intraarticular or periarticular structures, or both.

Secondary Contractures. These may be defined as contractures of muscles and joints as the result of primary disorders of nervous tissue such as anterior poliomyelitis, cerebral palsy, and many other types of neurologic disorders which produce paresis of muscle groups and unbalanced muscular activity. The skin may also develop severe contractures as a result of scarring, trauma, burns, and primary connective tissue disorders such as dermatomyositis and scleroderma.

Dupuytren's Contracture

This condition was first described in 1832 by Dupuytren, who demonstrated that it was caused by contracture of the palmar aponeurosis. Sir Astley Cooper had suggested the same cause some 10 years earlier.

INCIDENCE AND ETIOLOGY. Dupuytren's contracture chiefly affects people of European origin, and males are affected about twice as often as women. There is an increasing frequency with age. Inheritance of Dupuytren's contracture is well accepted, and family histories have been reported extending back for seven generations. It would appear that there is an autosomal inheritance with almost total penetrance in males, but to assume a single gene for Dupuytren's contracture is probably too simple an approach.

The ethnologic differences in incidence may simply indicate that the frequencies of certain autosomal characteristics are different in different racial groups.

The 40 percent incidence of Dupuytren's contracture demonstrated by Early and by Ling among Anglo-Saxon populations indicates that an autosomal system for Dupuytren's contractures among these populations is al-

Fig. 43-34. Pulling down of the ring finger by Dupuytren's contracture.

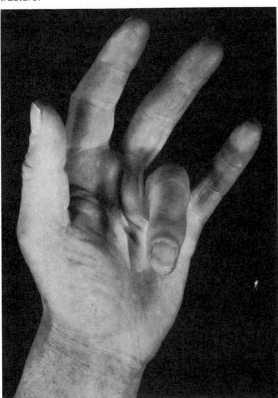

ways present but its expression is determined by other undetermined endogenous factors and less often exogenous factors such as injury, alcoholism, and pulmonary disease. It has been shown that there is a very strong association with epilepsy and a very high incidence among chronic invalids, particularly those with chronic pulmonary tuberculosis and alcoholism. On the other hand, no association can be demonstrated between Dupuytren's contracture and occupation, and indeed there is evidence suggesting that the condition might be aggravated by lack of, rather than excessive, manual activity.

PATHOLOGY. The earliest changes of palmar nodules, multifocal in distribution, arise within the palmar connective tissue on the anterior aspect of the palmar aponeurosis. Fibrosis of the nodule results in fixation of the skin and aponeurosis with contraction and thickening of the nodules and bands in the lines of maximal tension. Microscopically, there appears to be an increased vascularity of the palmar fibrofatty tissue. Perivascular cellular infiltration replaces the fat globules, and these hyperplastic foci finally mature into collagen bands. This process appears to commence on the palmar aspect of the aponeurosis and to extend along the formed fibrous elements of the palm including the aponeurosis and its intertendinous septums and the fine septums extending to the palmar skin and fingers. A similar process may occur in the plantar aponeurosis.

Factors such as epilepsy and alcoholism are often associated with severe local disease as well as with poor surgical results. Cases of fibrosis involving the dermal structures in the palm or overlying the proximal interphalangeal joint and "knuckle pads," or in the penis (Peyronie's disease), are examples of the extensive changes which can occur.

CLINICAL MANIFESTATIONS. Hueston described four clinical types:

1. Senile type. This consists of single discrete bands and a very slowly progressive deformity.
2. Middle-age type. This type often has multifocal proliferate nodules and slowly developing bands in one or both palms (Fig. 43-34).
3. Young fulminating type. This type has a tender palmar or digital thickening with pink, warm, and often sweaty skin and knuckle pads. Palmar lesions and sometimes deposits related to the palmaris longus and the insertion of the flexor carpi ulnaris may be found. The prognosis for this type is poor.
4. Feminine. This type demonstrates long-standing localized palmar plaques without deformity. There may be, however, slender bands in relation to these plaques, often very superficially placed and producing very minimal digital deformity. This "feminine" type is occasionally seen in men with delicate hand structure.

TREATMENT. Conservative Treatment. Good results have been claimed for many types of nonoperative treatment including the injection of fibrinolytic substances, cortisone, and radiotherapy, but apart from exercise aimed at hyperextension of the fingers, there is no real alternative to surgical treatment.

Surgical Treatment. The ultimate choice of procedure will depend upon the nature and the severity of the contracture and on the patient's general condition. Minor operations such as fasciotomy are useful where the main distribution of the contracture is limited to single fingers and especially where age or the circumstances of the patient prohibit more extensive procedures.

Radical excision of palmar fascia has the virtue of completely disposing of the affected tissue and must still be considered the method of choice in severe cases.

The ultimate result depends as much on postoperative treatment as on the actual operative procedure. The former involves protective splinting and physiotherapy.

Volkmann's Ischemic Contracture

In 1875 Volkmann described a contracture of the forearm muscles following the tight bandaging of an arm after fracturing the bones of the elbow. Such a contracture is due to ischemia of the muscles and is a common hazard in children following injuries about the elbow, particularly supracondylar fracture. Simultaneous damage to the brachial artery by inducing spasm or by thrombosis may produce segmental arterial spasm with severe ischemia of both muscle and nerves.

PATHOLOGY. The gross pathologic picture is one of muscle infarction in an elliptoid zone which has its axis near the anterior interosseous artery and its central point a little above the middle of the forearm. The greatest damage is usually to the flexor digitorum profundus and flexor pollicis longus, these being the deepest muscles lying in close relation to the anterior interosseous artery. The median nerve running near the anterior interosseous artery may also be involved in the ischemic process, and in very severe cases the ulnar nerve may be involved as well.

In the center of the ischemic mass the muscle fibers lose their nuclei and cross striations, and fuse into a homogeneous mass with little more than a defining membrane separating them. This picture is in contrast to muscle degeneration from other causes such as denervation and sepsis in which the appearance is one of diffuse interfibrillar fibrosis.

Seddon described some reversible changes following vascular ischemia in which dead muscle is removed and replaced by new. Hence, although it might appear initially that destruction is total, often after 2 or 3 months some of the muscles, particularly the extensor group, will recover. During this time, when recovery is occurring, treatment should be aimed at splinting to minimize contractures.

CLINICAL MANIFESTATIONS. The symptoms of pain, pallor, paralysis, and loss of radial pulse occur within a few hours of the injury, and usually intense pain is associated with either passive or active attempts to extend the fingers. Active and passive finger extension should be specifically checked in every patient with an elbow or forearm injury, since inability to extend in association with pain is the earliest sign of a Volkmann's ischemic contracture. Ultimately all voluntary motion is lost. Most of the damage occurs within the first few hours, so that initial treatment is urgent. After this period swelling gradually subsides, the muscles become hard and fibrotic, and as the fibrosis in-

creases, a characteristic deformity of the wrist and hand develops. When the wrist is flexed, extension occurs at the MP joints and flexion at the IP joints, while the forearm is often pronated and the elbow flexed.

PROPHYLAXIS. The circulatory and neurologic condition of the forearm and hand must be carefully watched in the early stage of treatment of all injuries or fractures about the elbow or forearm. It is inadvisable to treat fractures about the elbow, such as supracondylar fractures in children, with splints or bandages applied in a circular fashion.

TREATMENT. In the acute stage it is important to reestablish circulation before irreparable damage is done. The limb must be elevated, any circular bandages removed, and mild external warmth applied. Successful relief of spasm can sometimes be induced by ganglionic injection of the cervical sympathetic chain, but if this is unsuccessful, the artery should be exposed and papaverine applied to its surface. If this proves unsuccessful, complete interruption of the sympathetic reflex arc inducing spasm may be achieved by arteriectomy with resection of the artery and vein graft.

In established cases, prevention of contracture and maintenance of joint mobility can be obtained by splintage and physiotherapy of the fingers and thumb. Once maximal recovery is attained, operative procedures are necessary to remove the fibrotic muscular tissue. Such procedures have been described by Seddon and are preferable to indirect methods of correction such as shortening of forearm bones or carpal bone excision. Occasionally if the median nerve has been irreparably damaged and the ulnar nerve is intact, the latter has been used successfully as a pedicle nerve graft to restore maximal sensation to the hand.

EPIPHYSEAL DISORDERS (OSTEOCHONDRITIS)

General Considerations

The epiphysis is concerned with the growth in length of a bone. It also forms a part of joints and acts as an attachment for muscles and tendons. There are three types of epiphysis: (1) pressure epiphysis, which transmits weight from one bone to another, (2) traction epiphysis, or apophysis, which is situated at the point of attachment of muscles, and (3) atavistic epiphysis, which represents a part of the skeleton that has lost its function.

The epiphysis develops from a secondary center of ossification and is initially separated from the main bone by an area of unossified cartilage. Later, it joins the shaft to make the adult bone. The cartilage lying between the bony tissue and the diaphysis is known as the "epiphyseal cartilage." It does not ossify until bone growth has ceased, nor does the epiphysis become joined to the body of the bone until that time.

The term "osteochondritis," or "epiphysitis," is used to signify a derangement of growth at various ossification centers. The same pathologic process can underlie most epiphyses, though the particular location modifies its clinical manifestation. Unfortunately, in most instances, the lesions have come to be known by a series of eponyms (see the classification that follows).

Areas Involved with Epiphysitis

Primary centers of ossification:
    Vertebral body (Calvé, 1925)
    Carpal scaphoid (Preoser)
    Semilunar, adult (Kienböck, 1910)
    Patella (Köhler, 1908)
    Talus (Mouchet, 1928)
    Tarsal navicular (Köhler, 1908)
Secondary centers of ossification:
    Vertebral epiphysis (Scheuermann, 1921)
    Head of humerus (Hass, 1921)
    Capitellum of humerus (Panner, 1927)
    Head of radius (Brailsford, 1935)
    Pubic symphysis (Van Neck, 1924)
    Ischiopubic junction (Oldsberg, 1924)
    Head of femur (Legg, 1910)
    Patella (Sinding-Larsen, 1921)
    Tubercle of tibia (Osgood-Schlatter, 1903)
    Calcaneus (Sever, 1912)
    Metatarsals (Freiberg, 1914)

ETIOLOGY. The causes of epiphysitis have not been agreed upon; many causes, including genetic, infective, and hormonal, have been suggested. The theory presently favored is that a vascular disturbance, possibly following trauma, results in an avascular necrosis. Legg, in his early description, stated: "As a result of injury, there is an obliteration of a portion of the vascular supply of the epiphysis, which consequently undergoes the atrophy of anemia. A compensatory hyperemia of the adjacent portions of the diaphysis is the natural response, and is the starting-point of these hypertrophic changes which have been noted in the occurrence of broadening."

The traumatic factor is supported by a frequent history of injury, by the greater frequency of the condition in boys, and by the more usual location either in weight-bearing joints such as the hip or in epiphyses which are subjected to great strain, such as in the tibial tubercle. Legg-Calvé-Perthes disease has developed in a hip which was the site of congenital dislocation which had been reduced shortly prior to the manifestation of the disease. Minor degrees of Legg-Calvé-Perthes disease are common radiologic findings in old manipulated congenital hips.

A relationship between osteochondritis and skeletal growth has been described (see Table 43-3). It should be noted that the condition appears clinically (1) soon after the appearance of ossification, e.g., Legg-Calvé-Perthes disease at four years and Osgood-Schlatter disease at eleven years; (2) during or immediately after the midgrowth, or adolescent spurt, e.g., Scheuermann's disease, which is aggravated by adolescent growth spurt; and (3) earlier in girls than in boys, because the latter are slower in maturation.

PATHOLOGY. The pathologic changes in epiphyseal disorders are poorly described because of the paucity of operative material. Histologic sections have demonstrated avascular necrosis of the epiphyses with fibrosis in the metaphyseal region.

CLINICAL MANIFESTATIONS. The affection may be bilateral or unilateral. The onset is usually gradual in a patient with good general health who may offer a history of trauma. The local effects of the disease are similar to those of early tuberculosis and include slight pain, limp in a weight-bearing joint, limitation of the movement, and at times muscle spasm. The symptoms are usually mild. Many cases are asymptomatic and discovered only when deformities develop.

ROENTGENOGRAPHIC FINDINGS. The roentgenographic appearance is usually much more severe than the clinical picture would suggest. There is early osteoporosis with subsequent signs of repair. The epiphysis becomes fissured, fragmented, broadened, and irregular in outline. Areas of dense necrotic bone become evident. The process may involve both the epiphysis and metaphysis, and the former may be compressed and flattened. In the stage of regeneration, there is a gradual loss of osteoporosis with absorption of the dense necrotic bone in the epiphysis. This is fol-

Table 43-3. RELATIONSHIP BETWEEN EPIPHYSITIS DIAGNOSIS AND TIME
OF APPEARANCE OF EPIPHYSIS

Site of osteochondritis	Usual age at diagnosis	Range of age incidence	Sex incidence	Year of appearance of epiphysis	
				Male	Female
Upper femoral epiphysis (Legg-Calvé-Perthes disease)	5–9	$3\frac{1}{2}$–15	M > F	1	$\frac{1}{2}$
Tuberosity of tibia (Osgood-Schlatter disease)	12–15	10–23	M > F	11	11
Navicular bone (Köhler's disease)	3–8	$2\frac{1}{2}$–10	M > F	2–4	2–4
Calcanean apophysis (Haglund's disease)	$8\frac{1}{2}$–15	8–22	M > F	10	8
Head of second metatarsal bone (Freiberg's disease)	10–18	10–45	F > M	3	2
Upper and lower epiphyses of vertebrae (Scheuermann's disease)	10–21	. . .	M > F	10	10

SOURCE: From R. B. Duthie, 1959.

lowed by slowly advancing replacement of the necrotic bone by new bone until there is complete bony restitution. The amount of eventual deformity of restored bone depends on the stage at which the disease is first recognized and the nature of treatment applied.

Legg-Calvé-Perthes Disease

Osteochondritis of the hip, also known as "coxa plana," is essentially a disease of boys, occurring usually between the ages of five and nine, but may become manifest between two and eighteen years of age. It is bilateral in about 10 percent of the cases.

CLINICAL MANIFESTATIONS. There are three main stages: (1) the prodromal stage, (2) the active stage, and (3) the restoration stage. During the prodromal stage, the most constant early sign is a limp, which may or may not be accompanied by pain. Muscular spasm may be present in early stages of the disease. During the active stage, the spasm tends to disappear but leaves a residual limitation of mobility. The pain and tenderness also usually disappear. The limping may remit for short periods or may be marked with a completely fixed and painless hip in a position of slight flexion and adduction. The affected hip joint shows limitation of abduction, medial rotation, and flexion, initially because of spasm of adductive muscles and at a later stage because of true shortening of these muscles. Still later, the deformation of the femoral head results in a mechanical condition which prevents full degree of motion. The muscles on the affected side are usually atrophied, but, in spite of the considerable degree of deformity at the head of the femur, there is little if any shortening.

During the restoration stage, the subjective and objective signs gradually diminish, until the function of the hip is restored. Trochanteric thickening and limitation of range of abduction, however, persist through life.

It is usually not difficult to recognize the fully developed disease, particularly if roentgenograms are available. In the early stages, however, there are points of similarity with early tuberculosis involving bone. The distinguishing features between the two are that Legg-Calvé-Perthes disease usually affects boys from five to ten years of age, pain is an inconspicuous feature, extension and sometimes flexion are fairly free, and the patient is usually a healthy child. Tuberculosis may affect either sex at any age, though the subject is often young; all movements of the joints are usually limited, and the child is usually ill.

ROENTGENOGRAPHIC FINDINGS. Roentgenograms (Fig. 43-35) of the femoral head progressively demonstrate flattening, flattening plus fragmentation, flattening with fusion in the disorganized nucleus, and finally an expanded flattened head. The head is at first slightly reduced in its vertical diameter with no appreciable increase in its lateral extent. Later, there is a uniform increased radiodensity of the nucleus with irregular calcification. As fragmentation develops, there is some breaking up of the bony nucleus of the epiphysis with radiolucency apparent. At the same time, the head usually becomes more flattened and expands out of the acetabulum. The onset of the healing

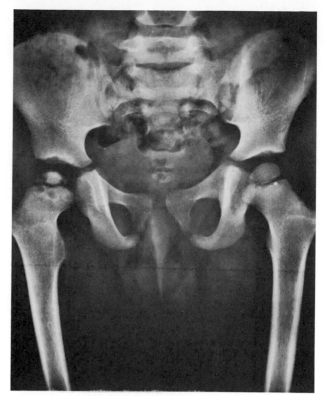

Fig. 43-35. Legg-Calvé-Perthes disease.

stage is marked with fusion changes. The bony fragments join, and the density of the epiphysis diminishes until the shadow becomes not only uniform but comparable to that of the other side. The head, however, remains flattened. Even after the lesion has healed, deformity of the head persists, usually throughout life. In rare cases in which there has been no weight bearing on the joint, the normal contour may be preserved.

In the neck of the femur, deformity can develop early in the disease, even before the head has demonstrated osteoporosis. The upper part of the neck is expanded, and its metaphyseal ends become rounded off. At the same time, the neck becomes progressively shorter. In the acetabular cavity, the distance between the medial pole of the head and the floor of the socket increases early in the disease. This may reach such a degree that the shadows of the head and the ischial bone no longer overlap but leave a gap. This sign may be caused by a grossly swollen ligamentum teres resulting in excavation of the acetabular roof by pressure.

An arthrogram may show whether the cartilaginous outline is nearly normal and can be used to determine the efficacy of treatment.

TREATMENT. It is generally agreed that no systemic measures are successful in modifying the pathologic process. The aim of treatment is to protect the weight-bearing area from pressure and preserve the normal contour of the femoral head. When first seen, if the patient has considerable spasm of hip musculature, a preliminary period of skin traction is indicated. After 5 to 10 days of bed rest and skin traction, the patient is usually comfortable. The patient may then be placed in bilateral, long-leg walking cast fixed with two transverse bars to maintain both hips in 45° of abduction and 5° to 10° of internal rotation as described by Petrie and Bitenc.

The child is allowed to walk with crutches, bearing full weight on the two casts. Plaster casts are changed at intervals of 3 to 4 months and continued until radiographs indicate that mature bone has replaced the avascular epiphysis. Total plaster time averages 19 months. A similar approach can be carried out using the Toronto brace described by Bobetchko et al. In order to reduce the long period of abduction immobilization to provide covering of the femoral head, a rotational-varus osteotomy of the upper femoral component may be performed.

COMPLICATIONS AND PROGNOSIS. Prognosis depends upon the degree of involvement of the femoral epiphysis, as well as the age and sex of the child. In general, with less involvement of the epiphysis, children under four and boys have a better prognosis. Catterall has called attention to specific radiographic signs, including (1) Gage's sign, (2) calcification lateral to the epiphysis, (3) lateral subluxation of the head, and (4) inclination of the growth plate to the horizontal as indicating a worse prognosis.

Ratliffe found that in patients followed into adult life, the overall results of treatment have been disappointing. Only 38 percent achieve good results, 38 percent fair results, and in 24 percent the results were poor. Although a high percentage of patients had no pain and good func-

tion, only 40 percent had a good hip roentgenographically, and there was evidence of arthritis in 51 percent. Failure of growth of the femoral neck with resultant shortening also may be a complication.

Osgood-Schlatter Disease (Tibial Tubercle Epiphysitis)

PATHOLOGY. The tibia is developed from four centers: one for the shaft, one for the lower epiphysis, and two for the upper epiphysis. The tuberosity usually arises as a tonguelike protrusion from the lower end of the upper epiphysis, but it may have two centers of ossification, one extending down from the epiphysis and the other reaching up from the shaft. While the center of ossification for the head appears first, it unites with the shaft last. Johnson has shown that the pathology of Osgood-Schlatter disease is comparable to a slipped epiphysis in which excessive traction on the growing epiphysis results in detachment of the epiphyseal plate and increased height of the tibial tubercle.

CLINICAL MANIFESTATIONS. Osgood-Schlatter disease occurs usually in patients from thirteen to fifteen years of age, and the history may suggest injury as a causative factor. The onset of pain and local tenderness is insidious. The patient first complains of some aching in the front of the knee after exercise. In many cases, the overexertion is the only history of trauma obtained. The pain is increased by full voluntary extension of the joint, since the affected epiphysis is pulled on by the contracted quadriceps muscle. There is also pain on passive complete flexion, because the epiphysis is dragged by the quadriceps stretch. The epiphysis itself is tender, and in many cases there is localized swelling and increased temperature.

The roentgenographic appearance is characteristic (Fig. 43-36). The tibial tubercle is irregular in contour and even fragmented. There may be localized haziness in the adjacent tibial metaphysis.

Osgood-Schlatter disease must be differentiated from osteomyelitis, sarcoma of the head of the tibia, bone cysts, and infrapatellar bursitis. It must also be differentiated from partial separation of the tuberosity associated with trauma, which is mainly caused by violent contraction of the quadriceps muscles in males between the age of sixteen and eighteen. In this instance, there is immediate pain over the affected site, and the pain is aggravated by attempts to straighten the knee. The tuberosity is tender and swollen, and the roentgenogram shows detachment of the tonguelike epiphysis.

TREATMENT. The condition is treated in a fashion similar to that used for an epiphyseal separation with severe symptoms. A cylinder plaster cast is applied initially for 6 weeks, during which time weight bearing is permitted. Following removal of the cast the knee is mobilized and the patient's activities modified, i.e., no contact sports or hard running are allowed for a number of months. When symptoms are mild, simple restriction of heavy athletic activity and running are usually sufficient to get the patient through the growth period without immobilization of the extremity.

PROGNOSIS. The end result of Osgood-Schlatter disease

Fig. 43-36. Osgood-Schlatter disease: tibial tubercle osteochondritis.

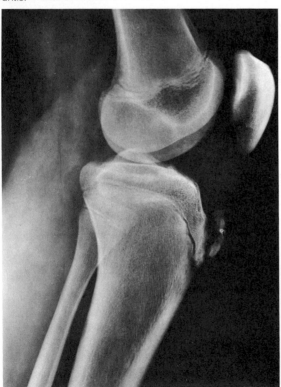

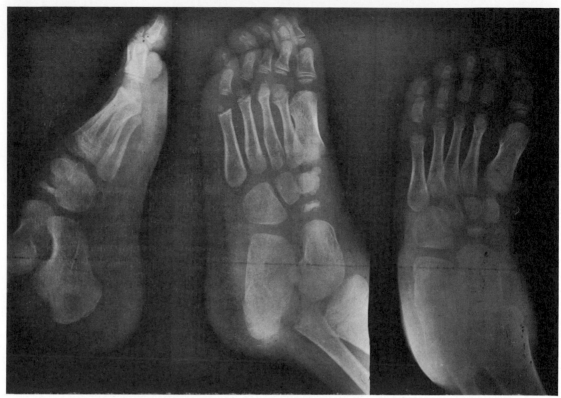

Fig. 43-37. Osteochondritis of the tarsal navicular: Köhler's disease.

is usually a prominent tibial tubercle which persists into adulthood. A rare complication is that of genu recurvatum. This results from early fusion of the anterior part of the upper tibial epiphysis such that, with continuing growth of the posterior part, recurvatum results.

Köhler's Disease of the Tarsal Navicular

As is true of the other forms of epiphysitis, Köhler's disease is probably an osteochondritis, but the cause has not been definitely established. It is analogous to Kienböck's disease, which affects the semilunar bone of adults. The navicular is the last bone of the foot to ossify, and since it forms the keystone of the long arch, it is subjected to considerable strain while in the cartilaginous state. Köhler's disease usually occurs in young children, especially between the ages of three and six.

CLINICAL MANIFESTATIONS. The symptoms and signs are often minimal, usually consisting of pain and swelling in the region of the tarsal navicular. The pain is exaggerated by weight bearing, and the affected region is sensitive to movement and may be tender. The condition is usually diagnosed by roentgenograms which reveal definite changes in the bone (Fig. 43-37). These consist of sclerotic narrowing in the anteroposterior diameter with no fragmentation of the bony nucleus. The joint spaces remain clear, and the neighboring tarsal and metatarsal bones are normal in appearance.

TREATMENT. The treatment is relatively simple, and symptomatic recovery usually occurs in a few months. A plaster cast should be applied to hold the foot in a slight varus position, and weight bearing is prevented by the use of crutches. After a few weeks the plaster is removed, and adhesive strapping is used to support the ankle and midtarsal region. The shoe is then fitted with a Thomas heel, i.e., with the medial half of the heel extended forward toward the sole, and sponge-rubber pads are inserted to relieve strain on the longitudinal arch, and, more particularly, on the navicular.

References

Pain

Adams, P., and Muir, H.: Qualitative Changes with Age of Proteoglycans of Human Lumbar Discs, *Ann Rheum Dis,* **35:**289, 1976.

Baker, D. R., and McHolick, W.: Spondyloschisis and Spondylosisthesis in Children (Demonstration), *J Bone Joint Surg* [*Am*], **38A:**933, 1956.

Batson, O. V.: The Role of the Vertebral Veins in Metastatic Processes, *Ann Intern Med,* **16:**38, 1942.

Campbell, A. M., and Phillips, D. G.: Cervical Disk Lesions with Neurological Disorder: Differential Diagnosis, Treatment, and Prognosis, *Br Med J,* **5197:**481, 1960.

Coomes, E. N.: Experimental Pain from the Hip Joint, *Ann Phys Med,* **7:**100, 1963.

Feinstein, B., Langton, J. W. K., Jamieson, R. M., and Schiller, F.: Experiments on Pain (Produced by Intervertebral Injection) Referred from Deep Somatic Tissue, *J Bone Joint Surg,* **36A:**981, 1954.

Frykholm, R.: Mechanism of Cervical Radicular Lesions Resulting from Friction or Forceful Traction, *Acta Chir Scand,* **102:**93, 1951.

Gaze, R. M., and Gordon, G.: Representation of Cutaneous Sense in Thalamus of Cat and Monkey, *Q J Exp Physiol,* **39:**279, 1954.

Guri, J. P.: Tumors of the Vertebral Column, *Surg Gynecol Obstet,* **87:**583, 1948.

Henson, S. W., Jr., and Coventry, M. B.: Osteomyelitis of Vertebrae as Result of Infection of Urinary Tract, *Surg Gynecol Obstet,* **102:**207, 1956.

Hueston, J. T., and Wilson, W. F.: Knuckle Pads, *Aust NZ J Surg,* **42:**274, 1973.

Killgren, J. H., and Samuel, E. P.: The Sensitivity and Innervation of the Articular Capsule, *J Bone Joint Surg [Br],* **32B:**84, 1950.

Livingston, W. K.: Phantom Limb Pain, *Arch Surg,* **37:**353, 1938.

McLeod, J. G.: The Representation of the Splanchnic Afferent Pathways in the Thalamus of the Cat, *J Physiol,* **140:**462, 1958.

Melzack, R.: The Perception of Pain, *Sci Am,* **204:**41, 1961.

Morgan, F. P., and King, T.: Primary Instability of Lumbar Vertebrae as a Common Cause of Low Back Pain, *J Bone Joint Surg [Br],* **39B:**6, 1957.

Newman, P. H.: Sprung Back, *J Bone Joint Surg [Br],* **30B:**30, 1952.

———: Spondylolisthesis: Its Cause and Effect, *Ann R Coll Surg Engl,* **16:**305, 1955.

O'Connell, J. E. A.: Discussion on Cervical Spondylosis, *Procr Soc Med,* **49:**202, 1956.

Ottolenghi, C. E.: Diagnosis of Orthopaedic Lesions by Aspiration Biopsy: Results of 1061 Punctures, *J Bone Joint Surg [Am],* **37A:**443, 1955.

Roche, M. B., and Rowe, G. G.: Incidence of Separate Neural Arch and Coincident Bone Variations: Survey of 4200 Skeletons, *Anat Rec,* **109:**233, 1951.

Rumbold, C.: Industrial Back Prevention, *J Occup Med,* **2:**132, 1960.

Rowe, M. L.: Newer Concepts of Low Back Pain, *J Occup Med,* **2:**219, 1960.

Schajowicz, F.: Aspiration Biopsy in Bone Lesions: Cytological and Histological Techniques, *J Bone Joint Surg [Am],* **37A:**465, 1955.

Smith, G. W., and Robinson, R. A.: The Treatment of Certain Cervical-spine Disorders by Anterior Removal of the Intervertebral Disc and Interbody Fusion, *J Bone Joint Surg [Am],* **40A:**3, 607, 1958.

Splithoff, C. A.: Lumbo-sacral Junction: Roentgenographic Comparison of Patients with and without Backaches, *JAMA,* **152:**1610, 1953.

Stewart, T. D.: Age Incidence of Neural-arch Defects in Alaskan Natives, Considered from Standpoint of Etiology, *J Bone Joint Surg [Am],* **35A:**937, 1953.

Weddell, A. G. M.: Observations on the Anatomy of Pain Sensibility, p. 47, in C. A. Keele and R. Smith (eds.), "The Assessment of Pain in Man and Animals," *Proc Intern Symp UFAW,* E. & S. Livingstone Ltd., Edinburgh, 1962.

———: Normal and Abnormal Sensory Patterns: Pain. II. "Activity Pattern" Hypothesis for Sensation of Pain in R. G.

Grenell (ed.), "Progress in Neurobiology," vol. 5, "Neural Physiology: Some Relationships of Normal to Altered Nervous System Activity," p. 134, Cassell & Co., Ltd., London, 1963.

Whitty, C. W. M., and Hockaday, J. M.: Patterns of Referred Pain in the Normal Subject, *Brain,* **90:**481, 1967.

Wiley, A. M., and Trueta, J.: The Vascular Anatomy of the Spine and Its Relationship to Pyogenic Vertebral Osteomyelitis, *J Bone Joint Surg [Br],* **41B:**796, 1959.

Wiltse, L. L.: The Etiology of Spondylolisthesis, *J Bone Joint Surg [Am],* **44A:**539, 1962.

Disorders of Muscle

Adams, R. D., Brown, D., and Pearson, C.: "Diseases of Muscles," Hansen and Broether, New York, 1962.

Baker, L. D., and Hill, L. M.: Foot Alignment in Cerebral Palsy Patient, *J Bone Joint Surg [Am],* **46A:**1, 1964.

Buchthal, F., Knappies, G. G., and Lindhard, J.: Bie Struktur der quergestreisten, legenden Muskelfaser des Frosches in Ruhe und wahrend der Kontraktion, *Scand Arch Physiol,* **73:**163, 1936.

Crenshaw, A. H. (ed.): "Campbell's Operative Orthopaedics," The C. V. Mosby Company, St. Louis, 1963.

Eggers, G. W. N., and Evans, E. B.: Surgery in Cerebral Palsy, instructional course lecture, American Academy of Orthopaedic Surgeons, *J Bone Joint Surg [Am],* **45A:**1275, 1963.

Elftman, H.: Biomechanics of Muscle with Particular Application to Studies of Gait, *J Bone Joint Surg [Am],* **48A:**363, 1966.

Goldner, J. L.: Reconstructive Surgery of the Hand in Cerebral Palsy and Spastic Paralysis Resulting from Injuries of the Spinal Cord, *J Bone Joint Surg [Am],* **37A:**1141, 1955.

Green, W. T., and Banks, H. H.: Flexor Carpi Ulnaris Transplant and Its Use in Cerebral Palsy, *J Bone Joint Surg [Am],* **44A:**1343, 1962.

Grice, D. S.: An Extra-articular Arthrodesis of the Subastragalar Joint for Correction of Paralytic Flat Feet in Children, *J Bone Joint Surg [Am],* **34A:**92, 1952.

———: Further experience with Extra-articular Arthrodesis of the Subtalar Joint, *J Bone Joint Surg [Am],* **37A:**246, 1955.

Hayes, J. T., Gross, H. P., and Dow, S.: Surgery for Paralytic Defects Secondary to Meningomyelocele and Myelodysplasia, instructional course lecture, American Academy of Orthopaedic Surgeons, *J Bone Joint Surg [Am],* **46A:**1577, 1964.

Hill, A. V.: Development of Active State of Muscle during Latent Period, *Proc R Soc Lond,* ser. B, **137:**320, 1950.

———: Does Heat Production Precede Mechanical Response in Muscular Contraction? *Proc R Soc Lond,* ser. B, **137:**268, 1950.

———: Is Muscular Relaxation Active Progress? *Nature,* **166:**646, 1950.

———: Mechanics of Contractile Element of Muscle, *Nature,* **166:**415, 1950.

———: Note on Heat of Activation in Muscle Twitch, *Proc R Soc Lond,* ser. B, **137:**330, 1950.

———: Series Elastic Component of Muscle, *Proc R Soc Lond,* ser. B, **137:**273, 1950.

Huxley, A. F.: Local Activation of Muscle, *NY Acad Sci,* **81:**446, 1959.

Lichtenstein, B. W.: Spinal Dysraphism and Spina Bifida and Myelodysplasia, *AMA Arch Neurol Psychiatr,* **44:**792, 1940.

Mercer, Sir W., and Duthie, R. B. (eds.): "Orthopaedic Surgery," Edward Arnold (Publishers) Ltd., London, 1972.

Phelps, W. M.: Prevention of Acquired Dislocation of the Hip in Cerebral Palsy, *J Bone Joint Surg* [*Am*], **41A:**440, 1959.

Sharrard, W. J. W.: Posterior Ilio-psoas Transplantation in Treatment of Paralytic Dislocation of the Hip, *J Bone Joint Surg* [*Br*], **46B:**426, 1965.

————, Zackary, R. B., Lorber, J., and Bruce, A. M.: A Controlled Trial of Immediate and Delayed Closure in Spina Bifida Cystica, *Arch Dis Child*, **38:**18, 1963.

Stamp, W. G.: Bracing in Cerebral Palsy, instructional course lecture, American Academy of Orthopaedic Surgeons, *J Bone Joint Surg* [*Am*], **44A:**1457, 1962.

Strayer, L. M.: Gastrocnemius Resection Five Year Report of Cases, *J Bone Joint Surg* [*Am*], **40A:**1019, 1959.

Thomasen, E.: "Myotonia: Thomsen's Disease, Paramyotonia, Dystrophia, Myotonia," Universities Forloget, Aarhus, Denmark, 1948.

Thompson, C. F.: Fusion of the Metacarpals to the Thumb and Index Finger to Maintain Functional Position of the Thumb, *J Bone Joint Surg*, **24:**907, 1942.

Vignos, P. J., and Watkins, M. P.: The Effect of Exercise in Muscular Dystrophy, *JAMA*, **197:**843, 1966.

Zuck, F. N.: *Proc U Cerebral Palsy Assoc*, Washington, 1957.

————: Cerebral Palsy, in Sir W. Mercer and R. B. Duthie (eds.), "Orthopaedic Surgery," chap. 10, Paralysis, Edward Arnold (Publishers) Ltd., London, 1964.

Orthopedic Management of Stroke

Khalili, A. A., and Betts, H. G.: Peripheral Nerve Block with Phenol in the Management of Spasticity, *JAMA*, **200:**1155, 1968.

Mooney, V., Frykman, G., and McLamb, J.: Present Status of Intra-neurol Phenol Injections, *Clin Orthop*, **63:**122, 1969.

Posture

Bergofsky, E. H., Turino, G. M., and Fishman, A. P.: Cardiorespiratory Failure in Kyphoscoliosis, *Medicine*, **38:**263, 1959.

Cobb, J. R.: Outline for the Study of Scoliosis, *Am Acad Orthop Surg Lect*, **5:**261, 1948.

Denham, R. A.: Hip Mechanics, *J Bone Joint Surg* [*Br*], **41B:**3, 550, 1959.

Duthie, R. B.: The Significance of Growth in Orthopaedic Surgery, *Clin Orthop*, **14:**7, 1959.

Gilmour, J.: The Relationship of Acetabular Deformity to Spontaneous Osteo-arthritis of the Hip Joint: An Investigation of the Intra-articular Factors Which Predispose to Osteoarthritic Degeneration, *Br J Surg*, **26:**700, 1938.

Harris, R. I., and Beath, T.: Etiology of Peroneal Spastic Flat Foot, *J Bone Joint Surg* [*Br*], **30B:**624, 1948.

Hicks, J. H.: Foot as Support, *Acta Anat* (*Basel*), **25:**34, 1955.

Hyman, G.: Children's Footwear, *Br Med J*, **1:**1189, 1959.

Jack, E. A.: Naviculo-cuneiform Fusion in the Treatment of Flat Foot, *J Bone Joint Surg* [*Br*], **35B:**75, 1953.

James, J. I. P.: Idiopathic Scoliosis: Prognosis, Diagnosis, and Operative Indications Related to Curve Patterns and Age at Onset, *J Bone Joint Surg* [*Br*], **36B:**36, 1954.

Keith, A.: Bone Growth and Bone Repair, *Br J Surg*, **5:**685, 1918.

Lam, S. F., and Hodgson, A. R.: A Comparison of Foot Form among the Non-shoe- and Shoe-wearing Chinese Population, *J Bone Joint Surg* (*Am*), **40A:**1058, 1958.

Langenskiöld, A., and Michelsson, J. E.: Experimental Progressive Scoliosis in the Rabbit, *J Bone Joint Surg*, **43B:**116, 1961.

Mair, W. G. P., and Druckman, R.: Aberrant Regenerating Nerve Fibres in Injury to Spinal Cord, *Brain*, **6:**448, 1953.

Morley, A. J. M.: Knock-knee in Children, *Br Med J*, **2:**976, 1957.

Outland, T., and Sherk, H. H.: Congenital Vertical Talus, *Clin Orthop*, **16:**214, 1960.

Ponsetti, I. V., and Friedman, B.: Prognosis in Idiopathic Scoliosis, *J Bone Joint Surg* [*Am*], **32A:**381, 1950.

———— and Shepard, R. S.: Lesions of the Skeleton and of Other Mesodermal Tissues in Rats Fed Sweet-pea (*Lathyrus odoratus*) Seeds, *J Bone Joint Surg* [*Am*], 36A:1031, 1954.

Risser, J. C., and Ferguson, A. B.: Scoliosis: Its Prognosis, *J Bone Joint Surg*, **18:**667, 1936.

Walmsley, T.: The Articular Mechanics of Diarthrosis, *J Bone Joint Surg.*, **10.**40, 1928.

Contracture

Early, P. F.: Population Studies in Dupuytren's Contracture, *J Bone Joint Surg* [*Br*], **44B:**602, 1962.

Evans, E. B., Eggers, G. W. N., Butler, J. K., and Blumel, J.: Experimental Immobilisation and Remobilisation of Rat Knee Joints, *J Bone Joint Surg* [*Am*], **42A:**737, 1960.

Hueston, J. T.: "Dupuytren's Contracture," E. & S. Livingstone Ltd., Edinburgh, 1963.

Ling, R. S. M.: Genetic Factors in Dupuytren's Disease, *J Bone Joint Surg* [*Br*], **44B:**219, 1962.

Seddon, H. J.: Volkmann's Contracture: Treatment by Excision of Infarct, *J Bone Joint Surg* [*Br*], **38B:**152, 1956.

Epiphyseal Disorders (Osteochondritis)

Bobetchko, W. P., McLaurin, C. A., and Motloch, W. M.: Toronto Orthosis for Legg-Perthes' Disease, *Artif Limbs*, **12:**36–41, 1968.

Cameron, J. M., and Izatt, M. M.: Legg-Calvé-Perthes Disease, *Scott Med J*, **5:**148, 1960.

Catterall, A.: The Natural History of Perthes' Disease, *J Bone Joint Surg* [*Br*], **53B:**37, 1971.

Duthie, R. B.: The Significance of Growth in Orthopaedic Surgery, *Clin Orthop*, **14:**7, 1959.

Haythorn, S. R.: Pathological Changes Found in Material Removed at Operation in Legg-Calvé-Perthes Disease, *J Bone Joint Surg* [*Am*], **31A:**599, 1949.

Johnson, L. C.: Histogenesis of Avascular Necrosis, Proceedings of the Conference on Aseptic Necrosis of the Femoral Head, St. Louis, Missouri, United States Public Health Service, p. 55.

King, E. S. L.: Localized Rarefying Conditions of Bone as Exemplified by Legg-Perthes Disease, Osgood-Schlatter Disease, Kümmell's Disease and Related Conditions, Edward Arnold (Publishers) Ltd., London, 1935.

Petrie, J. G., and Bitenc, I.: The Abduction Weight-Bearing Treatment in Legg-Perthes' Disease, *J Bone Joint Surg* [*Br*], **53B:**54, 1971.

Ratliff, A. H. C.: Pseudocoxalgia: A Study of Late Results in the Adult, *J Bone Joint Surg* [*Br*], **38B:**498, 1956.

Chapter 44

Congenital Orthopedic Deformities

by Robert B. Duthie and Franklin T. Hoaglund

A congenital malformation is present at or before birth, which implies that it is an inherited or genetically determined disorder. However, it may be difficult to determine whether it is truly of genetic or of environmental (intrauterine) origin. Carter described congenital conditions as resulting from (1) an abnormal genetic constitution, e.g., achondroplasia (a dominant mutant) and Morquio's disease (a recessive mutant); (2) environmental factors, e.g., cretinism; or (3) an interplay of both, such as is seen in congenital dislocation of the hip or talipes equinovarus deformity. Genes produce these effects by influencing either metabolic processes, e.g., in ochronosis, or the endocrine system, e.g., in the hypopituitary dwarf.

Stevenson has described three categories of congenital and/or hereditary disorders: (1) those malformations which are seen at birth but which have arisen during intrauterine life, i.e., true congenital malformations; (2) disorders or diseases determined by a single gene substitution or mutation; and (3) diseases in which the genetic contribution is made more complex by the presence of environmental factors or prenatal influences. Malformations due only to environmental causes are infrequent, e.g., viral infection of rubella or syphilis and the use of aminopyrine (amidopyrine) drugs and thalidomide. These produce teratogenic changes in the fetus, particularly during the first 4 weeks of pregnancy when the fetus is undergoing marked cellular differentiation and the mother's hormonal and nutritional milieu is also changing markedly. By considering embryonic development and its susceptibility to multiple factors it is possible to make a timetable (Fig. 44-1) of the appearance of various congenital malformations.

In a survey of 56,760 live births, McKeown and Record noted a total incidence of malformations 5 years after birth of 23.08 per 1,000. Talipes was found in 4.44 per 1,000, spina bifida and other spinal defects were noted in 3 per 1,000, and dislocation of the hip appeared in 0.67 per 1,000. Gentry et al. reported on congenital malformations found in 1,242,744 children born alive between 1948 and 1955. Malformations of the skeletal system and bones and joints were noted in 3,737 children.

DEFORMITIES RESULTING FROM IN UTERO POSITION

The in utero position has often been implicated as a deforming force, particularly of the lower extremities. Several moderately severe conditions are seen shortly after birth, but these can usually be treated by simple conservative measures:

1. Metatarsus adductus of one or both feet (Fig. 44-2).
2. Everted, or valgus, foot.
3. Talipes equinovarus deformity with one or more of four characteristics: forefoot adduction, inversion of the hind part of the foot, equinus of the whole foot at the ankle joint, and/or torsion of the tibia.
4. Unilateral externally rotated leg with an everted foot, the other leg being either in a neutral position or in internal rotation.
5. Bilateral internally rotated tibiae, which are aggravated by the prone position.
6. Adducted thigh and hip with some external rotation of the leg as a whole. This type of deformity has to be closely differentiated from congenital dysplasia or dislocation of the hip.

These conditions are often aggravated by the sleeping

COMPOSITE TIMETABLE FOR DEVELOPMENT OF
CONGENITAL LIMB ANOMALIES

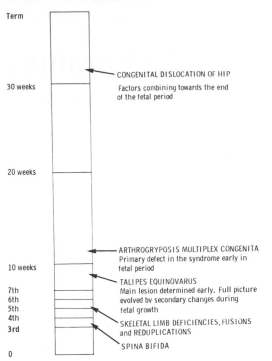

Fig. 44-1. Etiological timetable of some congential malformations.

or lying position of the child, e.g., the internally rotated leg and varus foot.

Resistance to achieving the full range of passive movements of the hip, knee, ankle, or midtarsal joints must be corrected by passive stretching exercises and by corrective appliances such as straight-last or reversed-last shoes, Denis-Browne splints with adjustable foot pieces, a pillow splint, or double diapers.

The postural deformity must be treated before the development of a static deformity with a structural disorder.

Fig. 44-2. Bilateral metatarsus adductus with medial displacement of the first rays.

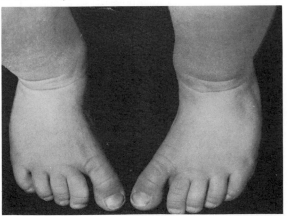

If soft tissue contractures develop and passive stretching cannot produce an anatomic position after about 6 weeks of treatment, corrective plaster of paris casting may be necessary, and the diagnosis of in utero position deformities may require revision.

On examining 5,000 newborn infants, Bick found 430 with some form of musculoskeletal malformation. Tibial torsion was seen in 30 children per 1,000 live births, subluxation of the hip in 17, metatarsus varus in 14, clubfeet in 8, deformity of the toes in 3, "bow legs" in 2, and other conditions such as polydactylism, birth fractures, birth palsy, and frank dislocation of the hip. The optimal time for a detailed musculoskeletal examination is between the third and fourth week.

CONGENITAL DYSPLASIA AND DISLOCATION OF THE HIP

Congenital dislocation of the hip consists of a partial or complete displacement of the femoral head from the acetabulum. It is very common, particularly in certain racial and ethnic groups such as the Northern Italian, the American Navaho Indian, and the Japanese. It is distinctly uncommon in the Hong Kong Chinese. Statistics vary depending upon criteria for detection but can be expected once in a thousand births in the Caucasian male, with a higher incidence in the Caucasian female. Its genetic and/or environmental causation has been reviewed by Carter and by Duthie and Townes.

PATHOGENESIS. The acetabulum appears as a condensation of mesoderm at the end of the fourth week of intrauterine life. It begins as a shallow socket, and later the socket is deepened by the progressive development of the posterosuperior rim, or buttress, in response to the head. A constant defect in congenital dislocation of the hip is an aplastic development of this osseous buttress and cartilage. Ossific hypoplasia of the capital femoral epiphysis may also be apparent at an early stage and is a constant feature of the later stage. Haas has classified this condition into a typical and an atypical group—the typical with its postnatal appearance, the atypical with its absence of prenatal development in association with other congenital anomalies such as arthrogryposis and intrauterine muscular dystrophy.

Complete dislocation of the hip in the typical group is seldom found in the immediate postnatal period. Haas found that the socket was only slightly reduced in circumference but corresponded in shape and depth to normal. The soft parts showed no abnormal change except for laxity of the capsule and iliofemoral ligament, permitting subluxation, which then became a frank dislocation.

Bone Changes. The acetabulum is shallower than normal; later its rounded shape disappears, and it becomes triangular with the base in front and below and the apex above and behind. X-ray examination shows that the outer surface of the ilium and the floor of the acetabulum lie in an almost straight line. Instead of containing the head of the femur, the acetabulum becomes occupied by an overgrowth of fibrocartilage, the remains of the ligamentum teres, and is covered over by adherent capsule. Above the acetabulum there is a depression on the ilium—a false acetabulum lined with periosteum—in which the head of the femur lies with a fold of the capsule intervening between the ilium and the head.

Ossification of the *head of the femur* is delayed, and there is marked discrepancy between the size of the cartilage head and the smaller acetabulum.

There is shortening of the *neck of the femur,* which is sometimes anteverted, so that the normal anteversion of 12° is increased until, in late cases, it may be almost 90°; i.e., the neck appears to project straight forward from the shaft.

When there is a bilateral dislocation, the *pelvis* is tilted forward and the normal lumbosacral lordosis increased.

Soft Part Changes. The *capsule* often becomes hourglass-shaped, one cavity containing the head, the other covering the acetabulum; the constriction is caused by the crossing iliopsoas tendon. The capsule becomes a hypertrophied suspensory ligament for the pelvis and supports most of the weight of the body. The ligamentum teres is usually attenuated and may be altogether absent, although in certain cases hypertrophy of the ligamentum teres occurs and blocks reduction.

There is considerable alteration in the *muscles.* There is shortening of the adductors, the hamstrings, and the gracilis, sartorius, tensor fasciae latae, pectineus, and the rectus femoris muscles. There is elongation of the obturators, the quadratus femoris, and the psoas tendon, with alteration in the function of the gluteal group.

In the development of congenital dislocation, subluxation is regarded as an intermediate stage from primary dysplasia to complete dislocation and is frequently associated with either predislocation or dislocation of the other hip.

The exact features responsible for migration of the femoral head from the predislocation stage to subluxation and dislocation are not known. The degree of primary hypoplasia affecting the cartilaginous roof of the acetabulum is probably the most important etiologic factor. Its ability to contain the head and to ossify in response to a correctly reduced head will determine the final result. Badgely considered that the primary dysplasia was produced by increased anteversion with an anterior primary position of the head and subsequent development of a flat socket.

In the early subluxated position the anteverted head can be palpated anteriorly when the legs are extended. The extension thrusts of the limb from the flexed position, which are a feature in the normal development of the growing infant, augment the pressure effect of the anteverted head. In the dysplastic hip, increased anteversion may stretch the capsule and fibrocartilaginous limbus and precipitate displacement.

In more advanced stages of subluxation, the head flattens the limbus and exerts a deforming pressure on the cartilaginous roof, causing further inhibition of ossification and actual flattening of the socket.

Dislocation occurs when the femoral head loses contact with the original acetabulum and rides up over the fibrocartilaginous rim. Arthrography demonstrates that in complete dislocation the fibrocartilaginous lip, or limbus, is inverted, as compared with the eversion which accompanies subluxation.

DIFFERENTIAL DIAGNOSIS. Coxa Vara. In this situation the limp is less severe, the head is not palpable in an abnormal position, nor is there any "telescoping." The x-ray appearance is characteristic.

Pathologic Dislocation. In these patients, there is usually a history of some previous hip joint trouble that developed after birth. There is general limitation of hip movements. The x-ray examination shows greater deformity and absorption of the head, while the acetabulum is usually well developed.

Paralytic Dislocation of Poliomyelitis. This condition simulates congenital dislocation in the waddling gait and shortness of the limb, but the hip joints are normal. There is obvious muscular paralysis.

Other Disorders. Cerebral palsy and septic arthritis must also be differentiated from congenital dysplasia and dislocation of the hip.

CONGENITAL HIP. Prognosis. Symptoms of congenital hip dysplasia depend upon the degree of acetabular dysplasia and whether the hip is subluxed or frankly dislocated. Patients with minor degrees of acetabular dysplasia might not be recognized at birth and only develop symptoms at age forty or fifty when a secondary osteoarthritis supervenes. Hirsch and Scheller have shown that when a positive Ortolani click sign is detected at birth, if the hips are appropriately splinted, clinical examination and x-ray findings on all hips are normal at age five. It is likely that these hips will be protected against osteoarthritis in later years as well.

At the other end of the scale, patients with untreated dislocated hips will carry the stigmata of the deformity throughout life. These patients walk with a short-leg–flexed-hip gait and are likely to have symptoms related to the hip in early adult life and certainly in the forties and fifties. They have diminished exercise tolerance and are more likely to complain of back symptoms as a result of their altered gait.

Symptoms attributable to hip joint with moderate dysplasia and a chronically subluxing hip resulting from inadequate diagnosis or treatment may appear in the early teens, depending upon the degree of anatomic distortion. The results of closed reduction depend upon the ability to restore a congruent stable hip joint relationship, and this depends upon age at which treatment is started. Muller and Sedden reported 50 percent excellent late results following closed reduction in children under three years of age. Platou, in a similar under-three age group, reported good short-term results in 80 percent and good anatomic results in 68 percent. Fourteen years later 68 percent of patients still had good functional results and 58 percent good anatomic results. Smith et al., analyzing patients up to 30 years after treatment of congenital hip dislocation, noted only 25 percent of patients normal in terms of symptoms, clinical examination, and x-ray evaluation. It is clear that maximal short-term and late results of congenital hip dysplasia depend upon early diagnosis and adequate treatment.

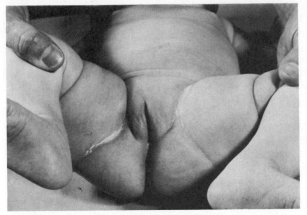

Fig. 44-3. Infant with congenital dislocation of the hips showing limitation of abduction on the right as compared with the normal left side. Examination is carried out with the hips in flexion and with an attempt to press the lateral aspect of the thigh on the examining table.

TREATMENT. The treatment of congenital dislocation of the hip depends on the degree of dislocation and the interpretation of the underlying pathology. The preliminary consideration in treatment is the accurate replacement of the femoral head in the acetabulum. Radiographic evidence of reduction, however, does not necessarily imply that development of the joint will proceed satisfactorily to form a normal articulation.

Fig. 44-4. *A.* Trendelenburg sign: left buttock rises slightly when the patient stands on her good right leg and the trunk is vertical. *B.* Same patient, standing on the side of the dislocated left hip. Right buttock drops, and the trunk now leans over the dislocated hip.

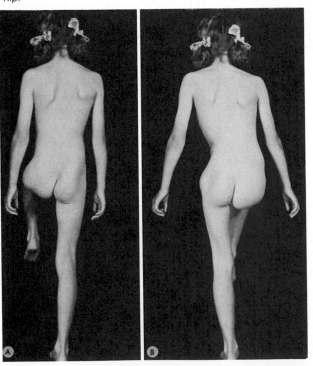

Reduction of a dislocation is complicated by secondary changes in the socket, the nature and significance of which remain the subject of much controversy. The secondary changes reported at operation will depend not only on individual interpretation but on the age of the patient, the duration of the dislocation stage, and the influence of preoperative attempts at closed reduction. Scaglietti and Calandriello found one or more of the following factors which prevented reduction of dislocated hips:

In 25 percent of cases—the iliopsoas muscle
In 31 percent of cases—an inverted limbus
In 33 percent of cases—a pericephalic insertion of the capsule
In 32 percent of cases—the ligamentum teres
In 16 percent of cases—capsular adhesions

CLINICAL MANIFESTATIONS. All babies must be examined at birth to determine the presence of congenital hip dysplasia, as successful treatment depends upon immediate diagnosis. If there is a family history of congenital hip dysplasia, difficult labor, or a breech presentation, the incidence of this defect is increased. In Sweden, where 99 percent of children are born in hospitals and examined by pediatricians, the rate of detection is extremely high. Over 600 new cases are diagnosed during the neonatal period, and only about 25 cases per year are detected after the newborn period. If the condition is not diagnosed until the head has dislocated from the acetabulum, the prognosis is much worse. Diagnosis at birth depends upon detection of the snap or click (Ortolani's sign) which is elicited when the head rides over the acetabular rim by abducting the flexed hip (Fig. 44-3). Hart has described the classic signs of dysplasia as being (1) Ortolani's sign, (2) limitation of hip abduction with the knees and hips flexed to 90° with the child on his back, and (3) apparent shortening of the thigh with the hip and knees flexed to 90°.

All children at follow-up examinations at six weeks and three months should be specifically examined for congenital hip dysplasia. If the click sign is no longer present, the only positive finding may be limitation of the symmetric abduction of both hips. If both hips are dysplastic, symmetric abduction may be present, in which case one should suspect dysplasia if adduction is limited to 75° or less. Minor degrees of acetabular dysplasia may go unnoticed throughout life until such time as a secondary osteoarthritis supervenes in the forties or fifties. If the hip progresses to a dislocation, the diagnosis will be apparent when the child begins to walk. The gait becomes abnormal, i.e., a ducklike waddle. The limb is particularly unstable, the trochanter ascending whenever the body weight is transmitted through the leg of the affected side. In a unilateral case, the child lurches toward the affected side. The gait results from inefficiency of the hip abductor muscles, which do not have the acetabular fulcrum. Leg shortening is evident, and lordosis often is noticeable, especially in bilateral cases. A Trendelenburg sign is seen when the child stands first on one foot and then on the other. In unilateral cases, when the child stands on the sound side, the buttock of the opposite side rises slightly, for the gluteus medius contracts in order to raise the pelvis and bring the trunk more directly above the limb which is sustaining the body

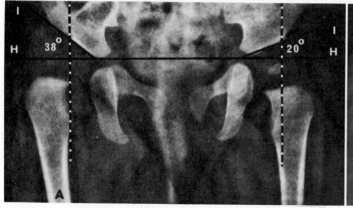
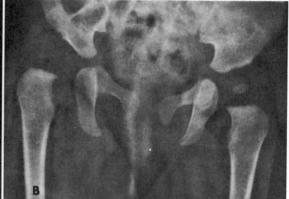

Fig. 44-5. Congenital dislocation of the hip. *A.* The right hip is held in the position of adduction compared with the left. The line parallel with the roof of the acetabulum intersecting Hilgenreiner's line indicates an acetabular index of 38° on the right and acetabular dysplasia. The dotted perpendicular line dropped from the outer margin of the acetabulum shows the proximal capital femoral epiphysis to be laterally displaced, indicating dislocation. The normal right side shows the dotted line at the outer margin of the proximal capital femoral epiphysis. *B.* Right proximal capital femoral epiphysis is much smaller than the left and is laterally displaced.

weight (Fig. 44-4*A*). When the child stands on the dislocated side, the opposite buttock drops, for the gluteus medius is relatively inefficient and the pelvis therefore cannot be raised or even be kept horizontal (Fig. 44-4*B*). In bilateral cases, the phenomenon is present on both sides.

The Trendelenburg test is not pathognomonic of congenital dislocation of the hip but occurs whenever the action of the gluteus medius is interfered with—e.g., in poliomyelitis and in coxa vara. Other signs are the position of the femoral artery, buttock creases, etc.

X-ray Appearance. X-ray examination is essential to establish the diagnosis, but in the young baby it must be realized that the cartilaginous structures involved are not visible on radiographs.

The relation of the head to the acetabulum can be established by Hilgenreiner's lines: the epiphyseal nucleus should be inside a vertical line drawn from the acetabular margin (Perkins line) and below the horizontal line drawn through the Y cartilages (Fig. 44-5*A*).

The slope of the osseous roof may be measured from the acetabular angle; the normal inclination is 22°, but in congenital dislocation it may be increased to 30 or 40°.

The outline of the femoral head should be noted, and it will be seen that the femur is displaced outward and upward. The epiphyseal shadow is usually smaller than normal and displaced outward in relation to the neck (Fig. 44-5*B*). The neck is foreshortened and may be anteverted. Anteversion is investigated by taking two plates, one with the patella pointing straight forward, the other with the leg in full medial rotation. Any anteversion is noted by the superimposition of the head on the trochanter in the first plate, while the second shows the outline of the head quite distant from the trochanter.

Arthrography of the hip gives further information of the underlying pathology in the different types of dislocation

and is of occasional value in deciding the appropriate treatment. The arthrogram reveals the extent of the cartilaginous roof in subluxation and in dislocations confirms the interposition of the limbus between the head and socket.

Predislocation. Infants with congenital hip dysplasia without subluxation or with initial subluxation stages diagnosed in the neonatal period of life are treated by simple abduction in a Freijka pillow splint or Von Rosen splint (Fig. 44-6). Hips recognized at birth usually need only 3 to 6 months of splinting until x-rays show normal acetabular and hip joint development.

Frame Reduction of Displacement. If the femoral head is

Fig. 44-6. Abduction splint maintaining the hip of a child with congenital hip dysplasia in the position of abduction.

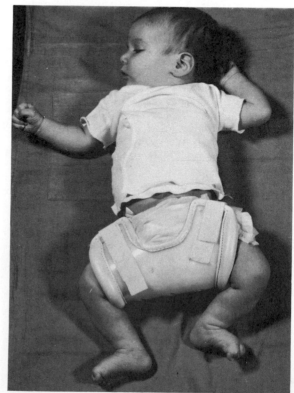

badly subluxated or dislocated, there is associated tightness of the adductor muscles which must be overcome before reduction is possible. Reduction by overhead traction or traction on a modified abduction frame followed by retention in a Batchelor-type plaster is preferred to manipulation under anesthesia and immobilization in the frog position in a plaster spica.

Osteochondritis or avascularity of the femoral head is more liable to follow manipulation than frame reduction. This may be due to the force necessary to overcome the tight adductors or to torsion of capsular vessels in the extreme frog position.

Frame reduction is a gradual process, but in the average case the head can be brought down and opposite the acetabulum in less than 3 weeks.

The child is placed on the frame and skin traction applied to the legs in slight abduction with the foot of the bed elevated. Fixed traction is sufficient in young children, but pulley traction may be necessary in the older child. After 1 week of preliminary traction, abduction is commenced by advancing each leg one opening of the abduction bar on alternate days. Abduction is increased, depending on relaxation of the adductors and the descent of the head as observed on x-ray. When the head arrives opposite the acetabulum, the leg traction is reduced to allow the head to sink into the socket (Fig. 44-7).

Failure of concentric reduction of the head in a correctly treated case usually indicates an obstruction to reduction which will not be affected by continued use of the frame.

Children under six years of age may be treated on the abduction frame, but reduction becomes increasingly difficult after the age of four. The indication for operative measures will depend on the degree of reduction achieved.

Abduction Plaster

Following successful reduction on the frame the hips must be protected until ossification of the acetabular roof provides a more stable socket. Plaster is applied under general anesthesia, and hips are flexed to more than 90°

Fig. 44-7. Abduction frame with a lateral pull on the dislocated right hip.

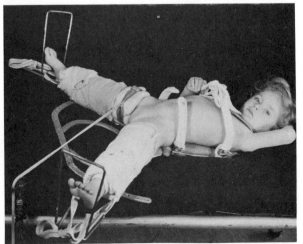

and in a position of about 45° abduction, the so-called "human position." Neutral rotation appears to be the safest position to maintain the hip, although some degree of external or internal rotation may be indicated depending upon stability. The duration of treatment depends upon the development of the acetabulum but is usually less than 1 year. Children are readmitted for plaster changes under anesthesia at 2 to 3 month intervals.

Subluxation. Subluxation presents no problem at initial reduction provided treatment is commenced before the development of irreversible secondary changes in the joint. In children who have borne weight for several years, the head may be enlarged and the cartilaginous roof of the acetabulum permanently deformed (Figs. 44-8A and B).

In younger children the subluxation is reduced on the frame and the reduction maintained by abduction plaster until ossification of the cartilaginous roof increases. Mobilization is then permitted, unless a marked degree of anteversion persists, in which case correction by derotation osteotomy of the femur should be carried out in order to maintain reduction and provide concentric stimulus to development of the osseous roof.

Dislocation. Dislocation implies complete displacement of the head and loss of contact with the articular surface of the original cartilaginous acetabulum.

Treatment even of the young child is difficult, because in complete dislocation, interposition of soft tissue may complicate reduction and subsequent joint development.

Differentiation between subluxation and dislocation may prove difficult in some cases without the aid of arthrography. Dislocation should be treated by conservative methods, provided the head appears accurately centered following frame reduction and application of abduction plasters. Any tendency for the head to stand out from the acetabulum after reduction or when freedom is permitted indicates the probable presence of an obstruction and requires open reduction.

OPERATIVE TREATMENT OF THE CONGENITAL HIP. Open Reductions. Open reduction of the dislocated hip is usually not required before the age of one year. As a separate operative procedure, it is contraindicated after the age of five or six, at which time other reconstructive operations are necessary.

In the series of 137 cases reported by MacKenzie et al., 58 percent of children under the age of three responded well to open reduction for failure of conservative treatment. Any soft tissue mass within the acetabulum such as an inverted limbus, hypertrophied ligamentum teres, or fibrofatty pad is looked for and, if found, turned outward and upward. The head is then rotated inward and the limb abducted to locate the head concentrically. The wound is closed and the leg placed in a plaster hip spica in a position in which maximal stability is attained. Open reduction is usually carried out in association with procedures to improve coverage of the head by some type of acetabuloplasty or redirection of the acetabulum.

Innominate Osteotomy. The acetabulum is not only deficient in size in congenital hip dysplasia but is maldirected, being open anteriorly and laterally. The procedure described by Salter of innominate osteotomy involves cutting the innominate bone immediately above the acetabulum with a Gigli saw and levering down (anteriorly and laterally) the acetabulum with its attached rami. The point of fulcrum for this rotation is at the symphysis pubis and not at the triradiate cartilage. A wedge of bone from the anterior crest of the ilium is wedged into the osteotomy defect between the upper ilium bone graft and acetabular portion of the innominate bone and fixed with two K wires. The procedure is usually carried out in conjunction with open reduction. Innominate osteotomy may be done without opening the hip joint when the hip is reduced but with significant degrees of persisting acetabular dysplasia. A similar procedure described by Pemberton involves levering down the roof of the acetabulum with an osteotomy and maintaining the position with an iliac bone graft. The Pemberton osteotomy obtains its correction at the triradiate cartilage.

Derotation Osteotomy of the Femur. In an attempt to restore a congruent relationship between the femoral head and the acetabulum in the presence of anteversion of the proximal femur, a derotation osteotomy of the femur is occasionally indicated. This may be carried out in association with an open reduction of the hip as an isolated procedure for severe anteversion and following acetabular surgery when severe anteversion has not been corrected.

The most suitable site for osteotomy is the subtrochanteric region. The lower fragment is externally rotated to the required angle as judged by rotational markers. The position is maintained by a four-hole Vitallium plate and screws. The femur is immobilized in hip spica for approximately 6 weeks.

The Chiari iliac osteotomy for the treatment of the irreducible hip subluxation in the child six years and older is an excellent alternative procedure.

Complications. Certain complications may follow the treatment of congenital dislocation of the hip. Some of these result from the operation itself, while others may be merely coincidental. As a direct result of the manipulative treatment, the femur sometimes is fractured, and occasionally the sciatic nerve may be traumatized.

Osteochondritis deformans juvenilis, which is due to avascular necrosis of the femoral head, may develop after reduction of a dislocated hip, but its occurrence in the normal hip in unilateral cases has also been recorded. Lima et al. studied 184 previously congenitally dislocated hips for vascularity and osteochondritis. He showed that the incidence was highest among patients treated by manipulation rather than frame reduction and also was related to the patient's age at start of treatment and completeness of reduction.

Pain and stiffness of the hip due to arthritis frequently follow manipulative reduction, particularly where the manipulation has been carried out with considerable force.

Palliative Operations. These are reserved for cases in which reduction is no longer possible either by closed or open methods. They are designed to improve stability, decrease lordosis, and control pain arising from the hip or lower back. The advisability of palliative procedures in the young patient with symptomless displacement of the hip is doubtful.

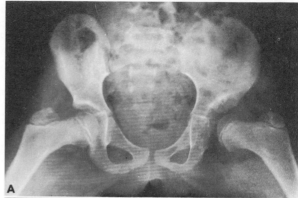

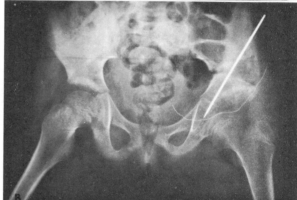

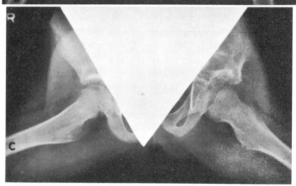

Fig. 44-8. Congenital hip dysplasia, diagnosed at age five. *A.* Position of abduction showing left acetabular dysplasia and subluxation of the femoral head. *B.* Ten weeks after innominate osteotomy with Steinmann's pin in place. *C.* One year following surgical treatment with maintenance of the head in the acetabulum and satisfactory acetabular coverage.

Palliative procedures fall into two categories: (1) arthrodesis and (2) osteotomy.

Arthrodesis. Hip fusion is a satisfactory procedure for relief of arthritic pain in the older patient with unilateral displacement. Arthritic pain occurs more commonly in subluxation than in dislocation unless there is a well-formed acetabulum.

Osteotomy. The primary object of osteotomy is deflection of weight bearing by angulation of the femur to bring the axis of the femoral shaft more in line with the direction of weight transmission.

Angulation osteotomy of the Schanz type is preferred to the bifurcation osteotomy of Lorenz, in which the upper end of the lower fragment is abducted and inserted into the acetabulum. The Lorenz procedure has the relative disadvantage of increased shortening, less mobility, and a greater likelihood of arthritic pain.

Total Hip Reconstruction. This procedure may be considered in middle-aged patients with pain as the main presenting feature. Special small acetabular cup and femoral prosthesis are usually required.

CONGENITAL DISLOCATION OF THE KNEE (CONGENITAL GENU RECURVATUM)

There are three types:

1. The developmental type, which is the most common and is considered to be due to malposition in utero. The legs may be caught by the chin or axilla with the knees extended.
2. A primary embryonic defect, accompanied by other defects, such as harelip, cardiac defects, spina bifida, and congenital dislocation of the hip. It is fortunate that this type is uncommon, since it is much more difficult to treat and usually requires operation.
3. Contracture of the quadriceps extensor muscle due to arthrogryposis.

CLINICAL MANIFESTATIONS. The knee is fixed in hyperextension with a varying degree of subluxation or dislocation of the tibia forward on the femoral condyles, and the skin over the anterior aspect of the joint shows several transverse creases. The patella is small or absent. On the posterior aspect of the joint, the hamstring muscles are palpable as tense cords, and the femoral condyles are felt projecting in the popliteal fossa.

TREATMENT. It may be possible to stretch the shortened quadriceps and replace the tibia in mild cases at birth. In more severe cases manipulation will be insufficient to overcome the contracture. Operative division or lengthening of the quadriceps and its lateral expansion—and occasionally of the iliotibial tract—will permit replacement.

Fig. 44-9. Characteristic deformities of talipes equinovarus, or clubfoot.

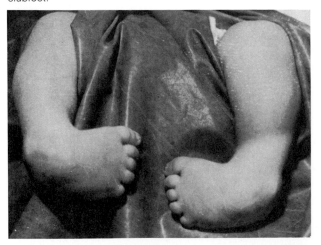

After operation, the corrected position is maintained by a splint or light plaster cast.

CONGENITAL PSEUDOARTHROSIS OF THE TIBIA

This is situated at the junction of the middle and lower thirds of the tibia, with sclerosis of bone ends and a gap between the fragments occupied by fibrous tissue. The leg is shorter. This lesion results from aplasia of a portion of the tibial shaft. A definite association with neurofibromatosis has been described.

TREATMENT. This is usually unsatisfactory, especially since the child may present after several attempts to obtain union and may never have walked on the limb. Leg discrepancy is marked, and the bones are markedly osteoporotic and underdeveloped, although the fibula is often intact.

Short of amputation, there are two possible methods of treatment: (1) by shortening the leg sufficiently to get good approximation and side-to-side apposition of the fragments and (2) by some method of bone grafting.

CONGENITAL TALIPES EQUINOVARUS (CLUBFOOT)

Congenital talipes equinovarus is a deformity involving four elements: flexion of the ankle, inversion of the foot, adduction of the forefoot, and medial rotation of the tibia (Fig. 44-9).

1. The "idiopathic" type may arise from such environmental factors as:
   a. Increased intrauterine compression because of change in the size of the uterus or reduction in the amount of amniotic fluid, e.g., oligohydramnios. Surprisingly little is known about intrauterine body mechanisms.
   b. Intrinsic anatomic disturbances in the talocalcaneal joint and in the innervation of the peroneal muscles with segmental changes in the spinal cord. Other factors have been described.
2. Genetic factors:
   a. Wynne-Davies has studied over 100 patients and their first-degree relatives. This deformity occurred in 2.9 percent of siblings, whereas in the general population there were 1.2 per 1,000 cases. No significant observations were possible concerning consanguinity, age of parents, birth order, etc.
   b. In the classic twin studies of Idelberger there was a 32.5 percent concordance in monozygous twins and only 2.9 percent in the dizygotic—the latter having the same incidence as that found in the nontwin sibling.

There is really no recognizable or acceptable inheritance pattern available as yet. However, there is a

1:800 chance of any individual having this deformity
1:35 chance of having it if any siblings have the deformity
1:3 chance if an identical twin is involved

There is real difficulty in defining this disease entity in detail, although from clinical experience two types can be recognized:

1. Those responding well to conservative management
2. A smaller percentage requiring operative therapy

PATHOLOGIC ANATOMY. The essential features are plantar flexion of the talus, inversion of the calcaneus (and with it the other tarsal bones), and adduction of the forefoot. At birth the bones of the foot are normal in shape but altered in position. Over the skin on the outer part of the foot there are usually dimples which may be so marked as to resemble scars. The lateral malleolus is prominent; the medial malleolus appears flattened and poorly developed.

Muscles and Tendons. The tendocalcaneus passes downward and inward to its insertion into the tilted calcaneus, while the plantar muscles, especially on the medial side, are contracted. The anterior muscles of the leg are elongated.

Ligaments. The ligaments on the medial and inferior surfaces of the talocalcaneonavicular joints are contracted, the plantar calcaneonavicular ligament being very small and short. The deltoid ligament of the ankle joint is similarly affected.

Bones. Bony changes appear as a result of the long-continued contraction of the soft parts. They are at first confined to the talus, but subsequently the calcaneus, the navicular, and the cuboid become appreciably altered.

At birth a small inverted heel and reduced calf muscles, suggesting a primary myodysplasia, may be seen. This type is difficult to correct and to maintain in correction.

In unilateral cases the deformity is never very severe, but the leg is obviously smaller and less well developed than on the healthy side.

DIAGNOSIS. The diagnosis is usually easy, but it is well to remember that an inverted position of the feet is frequently assumed by young infants. If this can be easily overcorrected by gentle manipulation and the foot can be dorsiflexed so that it touches the anterior shin without deviation, clubfoot can be excluded. In all cases search should be made for spina bifida and for evidence of poliomyelitis. Varying degrees of clubfoot should cause one to consider cerebral palsy or an arthrogryposis.

PROGNOSIS. Without treatment, the deformity increases, the gait becomes more unsightly, and the foot becomes more troublesome on account of calluses and ulceration. With early, effective, and continued treatment, all cases of clubfoot should be cured and a useful and properly shaped foot obtained. In older children the condition should be greatly improved.

TREATMENT. There are two objects of successful treatment: correction of the deformity and development of sufficient muscular power of the limb to maintain the correction. This implies constant supervision until the period of growth is over, since there is a distinct tendency to retrogression. The mode of treatment varies with the age and the extent of the deformity. The deformity of the hind part of the foot, which is the keystone to the function of such a deformed foot, must be brought into a vertical plane before the equinus deformity is corrected.

Treatment in an Early Case. Treatment of a clubfoot should begin while the child is still in the newborn nursery. The most effective treatment is application of serial corrective plaster casts to include the leg and foot, as described by Kite. It is extremely important to correct the forefoot adduction first, then the hindfoot varus, and not begin to dorsiflex the foot at the ankle until both forefoot adduction and hindfoot varus are completely corrected. Attempts at dorsiflexing the uncorrected hindfoot will result in the production of a rocker-bottom foot.

A single layer of sheet wadding or webril is applied to the leg and foot. On the very first cast, attention is directed at correcting the forefoot adduction, maintaining the foot in equinus, and correcting as much hindfoot varus as is possible. The cast is left on a few days to a week and then changed. At subsequent cast changes the forefoot adduction, hindfoot varus, and then equinus are further corrected. The duration of casting will depend upon the severity of the deformity. Most clubfeet can be corrected within a few weeks.

An alternative method is to manipulate the foot and then strap the foot in some type of L splint. A light lateral splint of aluminum covered with lint is applied to the outer side of the leg and foot, e.g., a Denis-Browne splint (Fig. 44-10). This allows full correction of the deformity and at the same time encourages the activity which is so important for muscular development. When the patient is capable of holding the feet naturally in the corrected position and the feet have full range of movement, the adhesive plaster and aluminum splint are discarded and replaced by a pair of boots riveted to the aluminum crosspiece to hold the feet in the same position as in the splint. These boots have open toes and unlace completely from one end to the other.

If it becomes apparent after some months that the equinus deformity has not been completely overcome, it is occasionally necessary to do a heel cord lengthening and a posterior capsulotomy of the ankle joint. After such operations the foot and leg are encased in plaster of paris with the foot in the slightly overcorrected position, the knee flexed, and plaster extended to the midthigh [Kite]. All children with clubfeet must be followed until bony maturation has taken place and usually require some type of corrective shoe or splint to maintain correction.

Treatment of Old and Relapsed Cases. However early and thoroughly congenital clubfoot is treated, in a certain percentage of cases, because of rigidity or a constant tendency to relapse, manipulative treatment will not suffice. Although a plantigrade foot may still be obtained by manipulation, the heel will remain inverted, and the navicular will still be in close contact with the medial malleolus. Any correction that takes place is between the cuneiform and the navicular, instead of between the navicular and the sustentaculum tali. To ensure a good result in this type of case, an operation is necessary to release the contracted ligaments between the tarsal bones, especially on the medial side of the foot. Goldner has recently called attention to the necessity of releasing the talus in the ankle joint in addition to extensive medial release of fascia and ligaments on the medial side of the foot.

Lateral transfer of the tibialis anterior tendon insertion has been recommended in addition to ligamentous and soft tissue release in order to remove a deforming force.

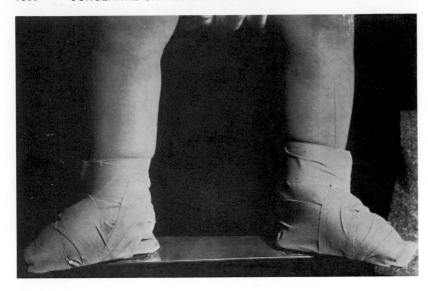

Fig. 44-10. Clubfeet immobilized in a Denis-Browne splint.

Heyman and colleagues have described a very satisfactory soft tissue release operation for the resistant forefoot adduction deformity. An incision is made across the dorsum of the foot, and the dorsal interosseous and intermetatarsal ligaments as well as the joint capsules are extensively dissected.

If the talipes equinovarus is due to arthrogryposis, the only consistently successful procedure to overcome this deformity is an astragalectomy, which allows positioning of a plantigrade foot.

Treatment in the Adult Patient. In the adult, no manipulation, tenotomy, or muscle operation is likely to be of benefit; operation on the bone is necessary in most cases. Cuneiform tarsectomy is the more certain and satisfactory operation.

In some cases, the best result will be obtained by stabilizing the foot as in the triple arthrodesis of Dunn. Here the midtarsal and subtaloid joints are arthrodesed as in some forms of flail foot.

CONGENITAL CONVEX PES VALGUS (VERTICAL TALUS)

This condition goes under a variety of names, including *congenital vertical talus* and *congenital rocker-bottom flatfoot*. It is thought to develop during pregnancy, but the cause is unknown. The pathology involves a primary dislocation of the talonavicular joint. The navicular articulates with the dorsal aspect of the talus, which is in a plantar-flexed or vertical position. The dorsal talonavicular ligament and the anterior aspect of the deltoid are both contracted, as is the calcaneal cuboid ligament. The muscles of the anterior compartment, peroneus brevis, and triceps surae are contracted.

CLINICAL FINDINGS. The deformity can be diagnosed at birth because of a rigid flatfoot. The sole of the foot has a rocker-bottom configuration. The head of the talus can be palpated on the medial plantar aspect of the foot.

The forefoot is abducted. The hindfoot is in equinovalgus, and the heel cord is tight. The child is able to walk on the foot without pain, although the gait may be awkward.

TREATMENT. Treatment is directed at early manipulative stretching and plaster correction of the forefoot into plantar flexion, inversion, and adduction. If manipulation and plaster cast immobilization can reduce the talonavicular dislocation, it is pinned with percutaneous K wires. If this is unsuccessful, open reduction is indicated at three months of age with a simultaneous tendoachilles lengthening. The calcaneal fibular ligament is also sectioned and posterior capsulotomy of the ankle and subtalar ligaments performed as necessary. Triple arthrodesis may be necessary in the older child.

ARTHROGRYPOSIS MULTIPLEX CONGENITA (MYODYSTROPHIA FETALIS)

There is marked muscular wasting with loss of mass, increased fibrous tissue around the joints, loss of mobility, and characteristic deformities. Bone changes are usually secondary to the overlying soft tissue changes. There may be unilateral or bilateral clubfoot and clubhand with marked rigidity of joints. In the lower limbs, there are also contractures of the knee and the hip, with occasional congenital dislocation.

PATHOGENESIS. Middleton first drew attention to the importance of muscular derangement in this disease. During the growth of the limb bud, before the bone skeleton is evolved, a bar of condensed mesenchyme becomes apparent at the situation where the skeleton subsequently appears. Gradually the mesodermal cells composing it are differentiated into cartilage and, later, into bone. At the same time, surrounding mesenchymal cells become differentiated to form muscle cells, the cells becoming oval and acquiring longitudinal striations, i.e., myoblasts. The transition from the myoblastic stage to the stage of fully developed muscle cell occurs at about the third month. After this there is progressive elongation to keep pace with the growth of the related skeletal tissues.

Middleton divided the pathology of the muscular derangement into three types:

1. There may be an arrest of development at the myoblastic stage.
2. The muscles may develop normally but fail to elongate.
3. The muscles, fully formed, may be the site of intrauterine degeneration, with progressive conversion into scar tissue (myodystrophia fetalis).

Many theories have been suggested, such as amyoplasia, abnormal intrauterine conditions, virus infection, developmental disturbance of the embryonic nervous system. Pathologically fibrous infiltration of the nerve bundles and peripheral nerves has been described. Microscopically the muscle is variable in appearance with greatly hypertrophied muscle fibers lying adjacent to hypoplastic fibers and infiltrated by fat. There is no systemic disturbance of biochemistry.

For the characteristics and treatment of the individual lesions which arise in myodystrophia fetalis see the discussions of congenital dislocation of the hip, congenital dislocation of the knee, and congenital talipes equinovarus earlier in the chapter.

CONGENITAL HIGH SCAPULA

Congenital high scapula (Sprengel's shoulder) was first described in 1863 by Eulenburg. It consists of an abnormally high and permanent elevation of the shoulder and is frequently associated with other deformities, such as congenital scoliosis, absence of vertebrae, fusion of ribs, or cervical rib, bony bridge to the spine, and errors in segmentation or position of the cervical spine.

PATHOGENESIS. This deformity is the result of deranged descent of the shoulder girdle, which first appears as a cervical appendage but normally descends by the end of the third month to the level of the upper part of the thorax.

The muscles suffer in their normal development, undergoing degeneration and necrosis at an early embryonic stage and becoming fibrous. This accounts for secondary contractures in the trapezius, levator scapulae, and rhomboidal group of muscles.

The scapula may be of normal shape or broadened. It lies at an unusually high level and may be attached to the vertebral column or the occipital bone by a band of imperfect muscle tissue or by fibrous tissue, or even by a bar of cartilage called the *omovertebral mass*. This mass is analogous to the suprascapular bone of the lower vertebrae, between the fourth cervical and the third dorsal vertebrae. The atlas may be in two halves, one or both of which may be fused to the occipital condyles.

CLINICAL MANIFESTATIONS. The scapula on one or both sides is 1 to 4 in. higher than usual. It is also tilted forward, so that the shoulder appears to be displaced upward and forward. When the arm is raised, the scapula does not move laterally, nor does its lower angle rotate when the arm is raised above the horizontal.

The deformity of the shoulders rather than any func-

tional disability of the arm attracts attention. There is only occasional weakness of the limb. All movements of the arm are complete except abduction and elevation to the vertical position. The neck frequently appears to be short, though the shortness is often more apparent than real, being caused or accentuated by the high position of the shoulder girdle. Torticollis is present in about 10 percent of cases. Cranium bifidum and spina bifida are often present. Congenital kyphosis affecting the thoracic region almost invariably accompanies the deformity, while scoliosis is quite frequently present as well. This deformity causes cosmetic disturbance or functional impairment, and it can cause pain.

The x-ray appearances are characteristic, the films showing the unduly high situation of the scapula. Other congenital defects in the neighborhood may also be apparent (Fig. 44-11).

PROGNOSIS. Prognosis depends upon the severity of the deformity. Mild cases need no surgery, although more severe cases can be improved at least cosmetically by surgery. Surgery is usually not done until the patient is three years old. Best results occur in the three-to-six age group, when associated deformities about the shoulder are fewer and there is a longer period of growth to adjust to the new position of the scapula.

TREATMENT. The omovertebral bone is removed and the band of fascia to the scapula tenotomized or excised. In severe deformities release of the multiple muscles attached to the scapula is necessary. The Woodward procedure

Fig. 44-11. Radiograph showing the abnormal high situation of the right scapula in Sprengel's deformity.

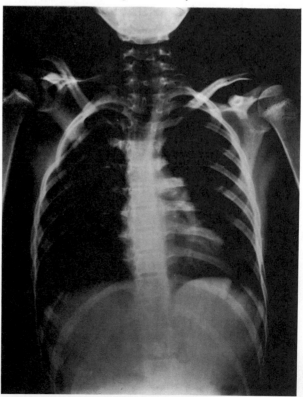

involves release of all the scapular stabilizing muscles, the trapezius, and the rhomboid major and minor from their origins on spinous processes. In addition to resection of the omovertebral bone, the levator scapula is released at its insertion. The aponeurosis of the trapezius and rhomboids are resutured to the spinous processes at a more distal level after the scapula has been displaced in a caudal direction.

CONGENITAL SHORT NECK (KLIPPEL-FEIL SYNDROME: BREVICOLLIS)

Klippel, in 1912, described the first such case with (1) short neck or absence of neck, (2) absence or limitation of movement of the head, (3) lowered hairline, and (4) often, an expressionless mongoloid type of face.

The neck is froglike and so short that the individual may appear to have no neck at all. Movement of the head is limited. The trapezius muscles are tense and produce a winglike appearance, which has given rise to the name *congenital webbed neck,* with a torticollis of muscular or bony origin. The posterior hairline of the scalp is so low that it reaches the upper part of the thoracic wall. Scoliosis, elevation of the scapula, and other congenital anomalies may be present.

Varying degrees of the deformity occur. In the slighter cases the cervical shortening is not marked. In the typical extreme case there is a fusion of the lower cervical vertebrae and usually the thoracic vertebrae into a solid mass. Less extreme cases vary from simple atlantooccipital fusion to all possible combinations of fusions of different vertebrae. Thus there is a considerable deformity of the cervical spine and usually numerical reduction of its component elements. Cervical spina bifida is usually present. As with other congenital defects, there are frequently associated defects in other parts of the body. Occasionally mental retardation is present. A few patients have shown functional impairment of the upper extremities suggestive of a common neurogenic origin.

This condition has to be differentiated from congenital torticollis, Pott's disease, and elevation of the scapula.

Treatment as a general rule is not indicated, but for patients with an extensive fold of skin a plastic operation may produce marked improvement.

CLEIDOCRANIAL DYSOSTOSIS SYNDROME

The syndrome was described by Marie and Fenton in 1897 and consists of (1) aplasia of the clavicles, (2) exaggerated development of the transverse diameter of the cranium, and (3) delayed closure of the fontanelles. Hereditary transmission is by a dominant expression affecting both sexes equally, although several cases have been reported with neither a familial nor a hereditary history.

Where the scapula is absent in addition, the deformity must be regarded as an aplasia of the whole shoulder girdle rather than a dysostosis. The deformities of the clavicles are always accompanied by variations in the muscles. Little or nothing is known of the cause of this condition.

CLINICAL MANIFESTATIONS. The patient usually presents with a coincidental pathologic condition or injury, but frequently no such history is obtained. Examination usually shows an apparently ununited fracture, defect in the midclavicle, or complete absence of the clavicle, and the patient can usually approximate the tips of his shoulders to each other below the chin. As a rule there is little or no disability or discomfort with abnormal mobility.

CONGENITAL WRYNECK (TORTICOLLIS)

This is a deformity characterized by lateral inclination of the head toward the shoulder, accompanied by torsion of the neck and dysplasia of the face. It is caused by unilateral contracture of the sternocleidomastoid, with secondary shortening of the fasciae and the other muscles of that side of the neck.

ETIOLOGY. Nové-Josserand and Vianny described how the middle part of the sternocleidomastoid muscle is supplied by an "end artery"—a branch of the superior thyroid—and they have noted how this sternocleidomastoid artery has been obliterated. It is generally believed that trauma is the primary cause of this deformity, producing a temporary acute obstruction of the veins followed by patchy intravascular clotting in the obstructed venous tree. In the early months of life this clotting is evidenced by the development of the sternocleidomastoid tumor of infancy, which eventually disappears, to be replaced by fibrous tissue which later contracts, very similarly to the so-called ischemic contracture of the flexor muscles of the forearm (Volkmann's contracture).

CLINICAL MANIFESTATIONS. The condition first becomes evident in the early months of life, when the mother notices an elongated swelling in the lower half of the sternocleidomastoid muscle. This swelling is at first tender, especially if the muscle is stretched. Gradually the swelling and the tenderness subside, but by the end of the first year of life the muscle becomes tense, pulling the head into the characteristic attitude, so that the ear on the affected side appears to be pulled down toward the sternoclavicular joint of the same side while the face is rotated toward the opposite side. If the deformity is not corrected, a gradual atrophy of the face on the affected side becomes increasingly evident with the growth of the child (Fig. 44-12).

PATHOLOGY. A sternocleidomastoid tumor appears about 2 or 3 weeks after birth as a spindle-shaped swelling affecting either the sternal head or frequently both heads. On microscopic examination it is found to consist of young cellular fibrous tissue, containing remnants of the original muscle fibers, which are seen to be undergoing degeneration.

The recognition of congenital wryneck should, theoretically, present no difficulty, but some cases are obscure. Every patient should be x-rayed to exclude any vertebral anomaly which may be the primary error. There is often a history of difficult birth. The early fusiform swelling may have escaped notice, but the later cordlike contraction of the sternocleidomastoid is characteristic. Hummer and MacEwen have pointed out that 20 percent of such patients have an associated congenital hip dysplasia, and this should be specifically looked for.

TREATMENT. The treatment should be begun at an early stage, as the development of the deformity can be arrested in mild cases. It is unwise to manipulate and stretch the sternocleidomastoid muscle when the tumor is tender; in these cases it may be better to excise the tumor as soon as the child will tolerate surgical treatment. The cause of the condition is thus removed, and further changes are prevented.

In later and mild cases, however, manipulation and exercises are sufficient. The head, having been grasped by the hand, is moved into a position in which the deformity is overcorrected, the object being to stretch the affected sternocleidomastoid. The manipulation must be performed gently. If this is carried out daily, there will probably be little or no evidence of contracture at the end of a few months.

When the child is not seen until the age of two or three years, operation is usually indicated. It can be performed through a comparatively short incision, so that the scar is insignificant. The muscular heads are defined and divided. When the muscle has retracted, the deep cervical fascia is divided and, if necessary, the carotid sheath and the scalenus anterior, as well. During the operation the head is gradually manipulated into the correct position, in order to bring any shortened structures into prominence.

The aftertreatment, which is of great importance, should be continued for about 6 months. It consists of active and passive movements to prevent any recurrence of the deformity.

CONGENITAL RADIOULNAR SYNOSTOSIS

One or both forearms are fixed at birth in a position midway between pronation and supination as a result of fusion of the proximal ends of the radius and ulna. In some cases the condition is inherited, and it is equally common in both sexes.

In the *true congenital radioulnar synostosis,* the upper end of the radius is imperfectly formed, being fused by bone to the ulna for a distance of several centimeters, and appears to grow from its upper end. The shaft of the radius angles forward more than usual and is longer and stouter than that of the ulna. The lower ends of the bones are almost invariably separate. Primary synostosis is usually bilateral; in over 80 percent of the recorded cases both forearms have been affected.

There may be congenital dislocation of an ill-formed head of the radius, the radius and ulna being anchored at some point a short way distal to their upper extremities, usually in the region of the coronoid process, by a short, thick interosseous ligament.

CLINICAL MANIFESTATIONS. The main feature is fixa-

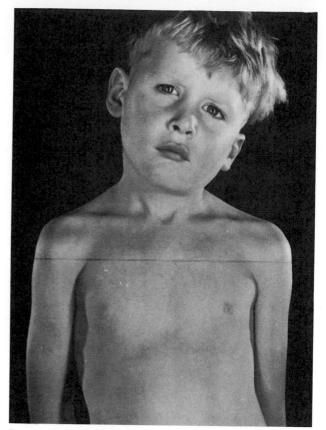

Fig. 44-12. Congenital wryneck on the left side with the head pulled down toward the shoulder, atrophy of the left face structure, and prominence of the shortened sternocleidomastoid muscle.

tion of the forearm in a position of midpronation. Extension of the elbow joint may be limited. Wrist movements are often unduly free.

TREATMENT. Although operation on the bony bridge would seem to be the obvious treatment, the soft tissues are not normally developed, and because of this the recorded results of operation are disappointing. In the type of condition associated with dislocation of the head of the radius, where the soft parts are more normal, the prospect of intervention is more hopeful. However, in any case prognosis should be guarded. If the pronation is extreme, it can be reduced by osteotomy.

MADELUNG'S DEFORMITY

Congenital subluxation of the wrist is due to defective development of the inner third of the growth cartilage at the lower end of the radius. This results in stunted growth of the epiphysis and diaphysis on the inner side. Growth of the outer two-thirds continues, and as a result the radial shaft is bowed backward, the interosseous space is increased, and the lower end of the ulna is subluxated backward.

The deformity is often bilateral, is most common in females, and appears frequently for the first time in adolescence. The hand and wrist are weak, and while flexion may be increased, other movements are restricted and may be painful.

The wrist appears enlarged, and dorsiflexion of the hand is impaired. In severe cases pronation and supination are limited.

TREATMENT. Operation is occasionally indicated and consists of an osteotomy of the lower end of the radius.

Darrach advocates the simpler operation of subperiosteal resection of the lower end of the ulna, since this gives as satisfactory a result as the more elaborate procedures.

CONGENITAL APLASIA AND/OR DYSPLASIA OF LONG BONES

These uncommon deformities, consisting of absence of an organ or part, are not recognized as inherited. Various maternal disturbances, e.g., thalidomide toxicity or rubella, can produce such changes. Also, Sanders, by extirpation procedures on the preaxial and postaxial parts of the early wing buds of chicks, has produced absence of the radius and radial half of the carpal and metacarpal bone and agenesis of the ulnar half, respectively.

Frantz and O'Rahilly have classified these various complex and poorly named abnormalities under the general heading of "congenital skeletal limb deficiencies," using a combination of the following terms:

melia, limb
podia, foot
dactylia, finger
preaxial, the thumb or big toe border of the limb
postaxial, the opposite border
terminal, either transverse or longitudinal

For example, an absence of the fibula and distal ray of the foot would be called *preaxial fibular hemimelia*, and the absence of the radius would be *radial preaxial hemimelia*.

Absence of the Radius

Absence of the radius is a rare developmental error but important because it is the commonest cause of clubhand, in which the hand is permanently deviated from the normal axis of the forearm. In less than half the cases the deformity is bilateral. The condition is sometimes hereditary and frequently coexists with other forms of congenital anomaly, notably harelip, cleft palate, and certain forms of congenital clubfoot. Riordin has also described an associated aplasia of the lung as well as Fanconi's syndrome with anemia.

PATHOLOGY. Usually the whole radius is absent, but occasionally, when the defect is only partial, a small portion of it remains generally at the upper end. When a small fragment of radius is present, the ulna may be fused to it, giving rise to a form of radioulnar synostosis. The ulna, which may attain a considerable size in many cases, is short, thick, and curved, and the concavity of its curvature is nearly always directed toward the radial side of the forearm.

The carpus often shows associated abnormalities, including absence of the scaphoid or fusion of that bone with neighboring carpal bones. More rarely the lunate is absent.

When the radius is totally absent, the biceps is usually inserted into the lacertus fibrosus, though in some cases the muscle is either completely absent or fused with the brachialis anterior or the coracobrachialis. Other disturbances in the brachialis, the extensor carpi radialis longus and brevis, the extensor digitorum communis, the extensor pollicis longus, the flexor pollicis longus, and the pronator quadratus are frequently seen. The radial nerve usually terminates at the elbow, and there is often no radial artery.

CLINICAL MANIFESTATIONS. Generally the affected arm shows some degree of atrophy, but this is most marked in the forearm, which is invariably short, stubby, and bowed with a posterior convexity. The hand is small and atrophic. It is also deviated to the radial side and slightly palmar-flexed—"radiopalmar clubhand." The thumb is occasionally absent. Despite these deformities the limb may retain a surprisingly good function, although grasping power is usually impaired.

TREATMENT. The treatment is aimed at relieving the deformity, weakness, inability to use the arm, and limitation of certain movements, such as dorsiflexion.

Riordin has pointed out that the aim should be to overcome the deformity as early as possible by splintage or by operative removal of the bony anlage which is producing the bowing defect as well as growth disturbance of the intact ulnar bone. Every attempt should be made to stabilize the carpus and hand to the ulnar bone in order to obtain stretching of muscle and any available growth.

Absence of the Ulna

This is a much more uncommon lesion than the absence of the radius and is most difficult to differentiate from the latter lesion.

Absence or Dysplasia of the Fibula

This is a relatively uncommon condition. The whole limb is seen to be shortened in length and reduced in girth. The tibia appears bowed in an anterior direction with the hind part of the foot in the equinovalgus position, and there may be absence of part of the lateral forefoot and toes. There is obvious soft tissue atrophy and development of contractures, e.g., tightness of the tendocalcaneous and peroneus muscles, as well as the lateral ligaments around the ankle. There may be bilateral involvement in about 30 percent of the cases. Radiography will show varying degrees of hypoplosia throughout the bones with delay in the appearance of their ossification centers.

TREATMENT. Because manipulation, casting, tendon lengthening, osteotomy of the tibia, etc., have not been very successful, early amputation, such as a Syme amputation of the foot, with fitting of a below-knee prosthesis, may be preferred.

Shortening of the Femur

Unlike the fibula, the dysplasia appears to affect mainly the proximal end of the femur rather than its center aspect. Steindler has described four types: (1) those with only rudimentary development of the upper third of femur and marked coxa vara, (2) coxa vara with a normal shaft, (3) overall shortening of shaft but a normal upper third component, and (4) dysplasia of the lower third with synostosis at the knee. As growth proceeds, the deformity becomes more severe with marked leg length discrepancy due to disturbance in all bones of the lower extremity. Often these children never put weight on the involved limb.

Treatment is directed toward providing some means of ambulation through an ischial-bearing, weight-relieving brace. Although bracing allows ambulation, it does not provide for the normal stimulation to growth or weight bearing, and, therefore, as well as the aplastic or dysplastic elements, the remaining "normal" components of bone fail to grow and develop. Thus, if the main disturbance is in the more distal components, early amputation with a prosthesis is indicated.

References

Congenital Disorders

Bick, E. M.: Congenital Deformities of the Musculo-skeletal System Noted in the Newborn, Am J Dis Child, 100:861, 1960.

Denis-Browne, R.: Congenital Postural Scoliosis, Proc R Soc Med, 49:395, 1956.

Fuller, D. J., and Duthie, R. B.: The Timed Appearance of Some Congenital Malformations and Orthopaedic Abnormalities, Am. Acad. Orthop. Surg., Instructional Course Lectures, The C. V. Mosby Company, St. Louis, 23:53, 1974.

Gentry, J. T., Parkhurst, E., and Bulin, G. V., Jr.: An Epidemiological Study of Congenital Malformations in New York State, Am J Public Health, 49:497, 1959.

McKeown, J., and Record, R. G.: Malformations in a Population Observed for Five Years after Birth, in G. E. W. Wolstenholme and C. M. O'Connor (eds.), Ciba Found Symp Congenital Malformations, p. 2, 1960.

Norton, P. L.: Pediatric Orthopedics, Med Clin North Am, 37:1427, 1953.

Stevenson, A. C.: Frequency of Congenital and Hereditary Disease: With Special Reference to Maturation, Br Med Bull, 17:3, 254, 1961.

Congenital Dislocation of the Hip

Badgely, C. E.: Etiology of Congenital Dislocation of the Hip, J Bone Joint Surg [Am], 31A:341, 1949.

Carter, C.: Genetics in Orthopaedics, J Bone Joint Surg [Br], 39B:4, 1957.

Duthie, R. B., and Townes, P. L.: The Genetics of Orthopaedic Conditions, J Bone Joint Surg [Br], 49B:2, 1967.

Gill, A. B.: End Results of Bloodless Reduction of Congenital Dislocation of the Hip, J Bone Joint Surg [Am], 25:1, 1943.

Haas, J.: "Congenital Dislocation of the Hip," Charles C Thomas, Publisher, Springfield, Ill., 1951.

Hirsch, C., and Scheller, S.: Result of Treatment from Birth of Unstable Hips: a Clinical and Radiographic Five-year Follow-up, Clin Orthop, 62:162, 1969.

Hummer, C.D., and MacEwen, G.D.: The Coexistence of Torticollis and Congenital Dysplasia of the Hip, J. Bone Joint Surg [Am], 54A:1255, 1972.

Lima, C., Esteve, R., and Trueta, J.: Osteochondritis in Congenital Dislocation of the Hip: A Clinical and Radiographic Study, Acta Orthop Scand, 29:218, 1960.

MacKenzie, I. G., Seddon, H. J., and Trevor, D.: Congenital Dislocation of the Hip, J Bone Joint Surg [Br], 42B:689, 1960.

Muller, G. M., and Seddon, H. J.: Late Results of Treatment of Congenital Dislocation of the Hip, J Bone Joint Surg [Am], 35B:342, 1953.

Pemberton, P. A.: Osteotomy of the Ilium with Rotation of the Acetabular Roof for Congenital Dislocation of the Hip, J Bone Joint Surg [Am], 40A:724, 1958.

Platou, E.: Luxatio Coxae Congenita: A Follow-up Study of Four Hundred and Six Cases of Closed Reduction, J Bone Joint Surg [Am], 35A:843, 1953.

Record, R. G., and Edwards, J. H.: Environmental Influences Related to the Aetiology of Congenital Dislocation of the Hip, Br J Prevent Social Med, 12:8, 1958.

Salter, R. B.: Innominate Osteotomy in the Treatment of Congenital Dislocation and Subluxation of the Hip, J Bone Joint Surg [Br], 34B:518, 1961.

Salvati, E. A., and Wilson, P. D., Jr.: Treatment of Irreducible Hip Subluxation by Chiari's Iliac Osteotomy, Rev Hosp Spec Surg, 1:49, 1971.

Scaglietti, C., and Calandriello, B.: Open Reduction of Congenital Dislocation of the Hip, J Bone Joint Surg [Br], 44B:257, 1962.

Scott, J. C.: Frame Reduction in Congenital Dislocation of the Hip, J Bone Joint Surg [Br], 35B:372, 1953.

Smith, W. S., Badgley, C. E., Orwig, J. B., and Harper, J. M.: Correlation of Post-reduction Roentgenograms and 31-Year Followup in Congenital Dislocation of the Hip, J Bone Joint Surg [Am], 50A:1081, 1968.

Symposium of the Swedish Orthopaedic Association; Prevention of Congenital Dislocation of the Hip Joint in Sweden: Efficiency of Early Diagnosis and Treatment, Acta Orthop Scand Suppl 130, 1970.

Wynne-Davies, R.: Acetabular Dysplasia and Familial Joint Laxity: Two Etiological Factors in Congenital Dislocation of the Hip, A Review of 589 Patients and Their Families, J Bone Joint Surg [Br], 52B:704, 1970.

Congenital Talipes Equinovarus (Clubfoot)

Crabbe, W. A.: Aetiology of Congenital Talipes, Br Med J, 2:1060, 1960.

Dunn, N.: Suggestions Based on Ten Years' Experience of Arthrodesis of the Tarsus in the Treatment of Deformities of the Foot, in "Robert Jones' Birthday Volume." Oxford University Press, London, 1928.

Goldner, J. L.: Congenital Talipes Equinovarus: Fifteen Years of Surgical Treatment, in J. P. Adams (ed.), "Current Practice in Orthopaedic Surgery," p. 61, vol. 4, The C. V. Mosby Company, St. Louis, 1969.

Heyman, C. H., Herndon, C. H., and Strong, J. M.: Mobilization of the Tarsometatarsal and Intermetatarsal Joints for the Correction of Resistant Adduction of the Fore Part of the

Foot in Congenital Club-foot or Congenital Metatarsus Varus, *J Bone Joint Surg [Am]*, **40A:**299, 1958.

Kite, J. H.: "The Clubfoot," Grune and Stratton, New York, 1964.

Steindler, A.: "Orthopaedic Operations, Indications, Techniques, and End Results," Charles C Thomas, Publisher, Springfield, Ill., 1940.

Wynne-Davies, R.: Family Studies and the Cause of Congenital Clubfoot: Talipes Equinovarus, Talipes Calcaneovalgus and Metatarsus Varus, *J Bone Joint Surg [Br]*, **46B:**445, 1964.

Congenital Convex Pes Valgus

Tachdjian, M. O.: Congenital Convex Pes Valgus, in "Symposium on Current Pediatric Problems," *Orthop Clin North Am,* **3:**131, 1972.

Congenital Limb Dysplasias

Darrach, W.: Colles Fracture, *N Engl J Med,* **226:**594, 1942.

Frantz, C. G., and O'Rahilly, R.: Congenital Skeletal Limb Deficiencies, *J Bone Joint Surg [Am]*, **43A:**1202, 1961.

Riordin, D. C.: Congenital Absence of the Radius, *J Bone Joint Surg [Am]*, **37A:**1129, 1955.

Sanders, J. W.: The Proximo-distal Sequence of Origin of the Parts of the Chick Wing and the Role of the Ectoderm, *J Exp Zool,* **108:**363, 1948.

Thompson, T. C., Straub, L. R., and Arnold, W. D.: Congenital Absence of the Fibula, *J Bone Joint Surg [Am]*, **39A:**1229, 1957.

Other Congenital Lesions

Green, W. T.: The Surgical Correction of Congenital Elevation of the Scapula (Sprengel's Deformity), *J Bone Joint Surg [Am]*, **39A:**1439, 1957.

———— and Rudo, N.: Pseudoarthrosis and Neurofibromatosis, *Arch Surg,* **46:**639, 1943.

McFarland, B. L.: Pseudarthrosis of the Tibia in Childhood, *J Bone Joint Surg [Br]*, **33B:**36, 1951.

Neibauer, J. J., and King, D. E.: Congenital Dislocation of the Knee, *J Bone Joint Surg [Am]*, **42A:**2, 1960.

Chapter 45

Generalized Bone Disorders

by Robert B. Duthie and Franklin T. Hoaglund

BONE

Composition

Bone is made up of organic and inorganic materials, and water.

ORGANIC PHASE. This is made up of osteogenic cells—i.e., the osteoblast, the osteocyte, and the osteoclast—the cartilage cell, or chondroblast, and the intercellular matrix, as well, which consists of approximately 89 percent collagen, 1 percent amorphous mucopolysaccharide complexes, and other proteins (Fig. 45-1). Collagen is a crystalline fibroprotein with a characteristic x-ray diffraction and electron microscopic pattern, having a periodicity of about 680 Å. Its length, diameter, and density vary with age; e.g., when old, its diameter may be over 1000 Å. Chemically it consists of a number of amino acids, such as alanine, leucine, glycine, arginine, glutamic acid, proline, and hydroxyproline with a total nitrogen content of 18.45 percent (glycine, proline, and hydroxyproline making up almost 60 percent of the total weight of collagen). Hydroxyproline is excreted in almost constant amounts in the urine of man at about 70 to 80 mg/24 hours and indicates collagen turnover.

Reticulin, present in small quantities, is a glycoprotein made up of polysaccharides such as glucose, mannose, and galactose combined with amino acids.

The intercellular matrix, or ground substance, which is sometimes called *osseomucoid*, is common to all connective tissues and contains protein, crystalloids, metabolites, and gases similar to plasma. Therefore, it forms the final diffusion or circulatory pathway for the exchange of nutritional substances from blood to the osteogenic cells through the various lacunae and canalicular systems. Osseous mucoid substance consists of (1) proteoglycans and (2) glycoproteins containing chondroitin sulfate, all having a great capacity for binding metal with various radionuclides and possibly calcium. In addition, plasma proteins, lipids, and peptides can be isolated from bone.

In certain inherited connective tissue diseases, these mucopolysaccharides are found in urine in increased amounts, e.g., Hurler's disease—chondroitin sulfate B and

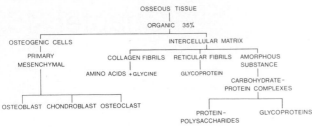

Fig. 45-1. Organic components of bone. (*Taken with permission from Mercer and Duthie, "Orthopaedic Surgery," London, 1974.*)

heparitin sulfate; Morquio's disease—keratosulfate; multiple exostoses—chondroitin sulfate A and C.

INORGANIC PHASE. In this phase, bone contains 99 percent of the total calcium and 90 percent of the phosphorus of the human body. It is made up of calcium, phosphate, hydroxyl, carbonates, and magnesium. The actual chemical composition of the bone crystal has not been fully determined but may be considered a hydroxyapatite crystal with the possible formulas of $Ca_{10}(PO_4)_6OH$ or $3Ca_3(PO_4)_2 \cdot Ca(OH)_2$. It is a single crystalline type with a molar calcium/phosphorus ratio of 1.3 : 2.1. The crystals are very small, and they are generally considered to be rod-shaped: $220\,\text{Å} \times 65\,\text{Å}$. However, Robinson has described them as being approximately $400\,\text{Å} \times 500\,\text{Å}$ in thickness with the shape of a hexagonal plate. The solution surrounding the crystal consists of many different ions and is in continuity with the body serum. The serum adjacent to a crystal is normally supersaturated with calcium and hypophosphate ions.

The chemical reactivity of the osteon is determined by the age of crystallization of its contents. Newly deposited crystals are highly hydrated and very imperfect in construction, with ion spaces in the crystal unfilled. Therefore, nearly all their ions are capable of rapid displacement. As aging proceeds, the crystals become larger, less hydrated, and more nearly perfect, with water displaced by mineral. This produces a reduction in the rate and extent of diffusion exchange and crystallization.

WATER OF BONE. Robinson has determined that 8 to 9 percent of the bone matrix, even in the fully mineralized state, is water in the form of either interstitial or extracellular fluid, or within the hydration shell of the apatite crystals. There is much water in the organic phase of mucopolysaccharide complexes, in collagen, in the inorganic component of bone, and in the marrow and osteocytic spaces of bone. Robinson has postulated that, as calcification of osteoid tissue takes place, water is displaced from the matrix, with reduction in the space between the crystals and other solids.

Also ions, such as calcium, sodium, phosphate, potassium, and chloride, require hydration for their movement or diffusion, and as the matrix calcifies, the rate of diffusion or exchange of calcium ions is reduced with slowing of crystallization. This calcification of matrix with reduction in diffusion is also seen in the zone of the mature chondroblasts in phase IV of the epiphyseal plate, where calcium is deposited with death of the chondroblasts and their disintegration into calcifying trabeculae.

CITRATE IN BONE. This represents 70 percent of the total body citrate in animals. It appears to be mainly on the surface of the apatite crystal but may be bound primarily to the calcium ion. As well as being concerned with the metabolic, oxidative processes of carbohydrate, fat, and protein in mammals, it forms soluble but complex compounds with calcium to facilitate absorption from the intestine, diffusion, and hence deposition of calcium into bone. It may also be concerned with making calcium in bone more soluble and, therefore, facilitating its removal without significant change in the local pH.

Not only does the citrate content of the serum parallel the calcium content but also there is a transport function performed by citrate in the cell membrane. Vitamin D in therapeutic doses causes a rise in serum citrate levels, which is also seen in hyperparathyroidism and hypercalcemic states. Normal serum citrate levels are decreased in conditions of hypoparathyroidism, rickets, and osteomalacia. Ordinarily excretion of citrate varies between 200 and 1,000 mg/day and reflects accurately the serum citrate levels.

In vitamin D deficiency rickets, the serum citrate level is low even when the calcium level remains normal; the administration of citrate as the sodium salt is followed by healing of the rachitic lesion of bone.

BONE ENZYMES. Bone cells contain the normal complement of enzymes similar, for example, to those found in liver cells. Bone cells have an active metabolism, the rate of oxygen consumption reaching 50 percent of that of liver cells. However, bone differs from other tissues in relying largely on glycolysis for energy production. Certain enzymes and enzyme systems have special importance in bone tissue:

Glycolytic Enzymes in Osteoclasts. These enzymes transform glucose into pyruvate with concomitant formation of adenosine triphosphate (ATP), which is used by the cell in various synthetic reactions. The pyruvate can then be metabolized further to lactate or to citrate. The production of lactic acid is an important factor in bone resorption, and the metabolism of osteoclasts is primarily glycolytic or anaerobic, which promotes lactate formation.

Acid Hydrolases. An example is cathepsin D, a protease with optimal activity at a pH of 3.6. The acid hydrolases are normally found within the lysosome. Thus, the extrusion or breakdown of the lysosomes in cells leads to the digestion of cells and their surrounding matrix when bone is resorbed by osteoblasts.

Collagenases. Bone contains enzymes that will specifically degrade collagen, a property that few proteases exhibit. Such enzymes are important in the breakdown of the organic matrix of bone during resorption, but little is known about them at present.

Alkaline Phosphatase. This is a phosphomonoesterase which is nonspecific and catalyzes orthophosphoric monoesters of phenol, alcohol, and sugars, and has an optimal activity at a pH of about 9. Its role is uncertain, but the serum level is altered in certain disorders of the skeletal and hepatobiliary systems (see Table 45-1). It is considered to be concerned with the preosseous cellular metabolism and with the subsequent elaboration of bone matrix before

Table 45-1. ALKALINE PHOSPHATASE LEVELS

Alkaline phosphatase levels	*Skeletal disease*	*Hepatobiliary disease*

Increased	Rickets and osteomalacia
	    In calcifying cartilage
	Paget's disease
	Osteosarcoma
	    At site of disease
	Carcinoma, osteoblastic
	    metastases
		Intra- and extra-hepatobiliary
		    obstructions
		Metastases
		Thorazine tox-
		    icity

Normal	Osteoporosis
	Osteopetrosis
	
	Healing fracture
	    Increase in phosphatase
	    locally
	Osteosclerosis
	Fibrous dysplasia
	    Variable level	

Decreased. . . .	Achondroplasia
	Deposition of radioactive
	    substances in bone
	Hypophosphatasia
	    Arrest of skeletal growth
	    with decreased osteo-
	    blastic activity
	Cretinism
	Scurvy	

the crystallization of calcium and phosphate ions. It is detectable in the serum of adults with normal levels of 35 to 80 I.U./liter and is also present in bone, calcifying cartilage, intestinal mucosa, liver, and kidneys.

Phosphorylase and Glycolytic Enzyme Systems. These are concerned with converting glycogen via the hexophospho-pyruvates into excess phosphate ions.

Acid Phosphatase. This is present in high levels in the osteoclasts and cells of the prostate. Serum levels in both sexes are very low under normal conditions. The enzyme is distinguished from alkaline phosphatase in that it has an optimal activity at a pH of 5.

Ossification

Much of the skeleton in the embryo is formed in the cartilage model by endochondral ossification, although some is formed in connective tissue by intramembranous ossification.

ENDOCHONDRAL OSSIFICATION. The long bones of the skeleton, with the exception of the clavicle, are all laid down primarily as hyaline cartilage in recognizable anatomic form. In the center of this cartilage model, at a certain stage depending upon cellular age and model mass, the cells undergo hypertrophy and accumulate glycogen. Phosphorylases and other enzymes with their glycolytic action appear in the cells and cartilage matrix to form the osseous centrum (Fig. 45-2).

Such changes in the cartilage are accompanied by ossification in the perichondrium and an ingrowth of vascular

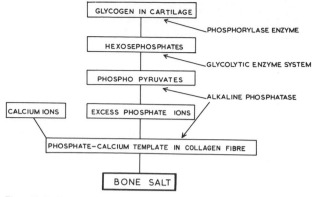

Fig. 45-2. Enzymes participating in endochondral ossification. (*Taken with permission from Mercer and Duthie, "Orthopaedic Surgery," London, 1974.*)

connective tissue which replaces the hypertrophied cartilage cells. Osteoblasts derived from this connective tissue then begin to lay down osteoid and fetal bone on the cartilage matrix. Hematopoietic cells appear from the invading tissues, and red marrow is soon identified.

The process extends up and down the shaft until the level of the future growth plates is reached at the epiphyseal-metaphyseal junction. Here the replacement of the cartilage model ceases, and the cartilage organizes into the proliferative epiphyseal growth plate.

During fetal and childhood osteogenesis, the endochondral growth of bone continues in the epiphyseal plate areas, as well as within the epiphysis. To maintain growth in length, further cartilage cells are added to the epiphysis from the juxtaepiphyseal apparatus or the perichondral ring of Lacroix. Streeter has described the classic five phases of the epiphyseal plate with the characteristic appearance of the cartilage cells (Fig. 45-3).

Accompanying such longitudinal and accretional growth there is remodeling to produce the tubular shape of bone as a result of cellular activity. Follis described how in the five normal processes of endochondral ossification there are three main phases which can undergo disturbance:

1. Disturbance in the actual growth and differentiation of cartilage, such as in achondroplasia
2. Disturbance in the osteogenic-osteolytic balance, such as in osteoporosis, osteosclerosis, and osteitis fibrosis
3. Disturbance in the deposition of the calcium phosphate crystals in the cartilage matrix and/or osteoid, such as in rickets or osteomalacia

INTRAMEMBRANOUS OSSIFICATION. This form of ossification occurs without any preformed cartilage model and is seen particularly in the development of the calvarium. The cells are developed from the germinal layers, and at a certain stage of differentiation the mesodermal cells condense and begin to proliferate in the area where bone will be formed. In this area the cells elaborate increased cytoplasm with an eosinophilic staining reaction and, at the same time, begin to secrete a metachromatic intercellular substance, as well as collagen fibrils. These cells soon become osteoblasts which continue to secrete much intracellular substance, or osteoid, which mineralizes to

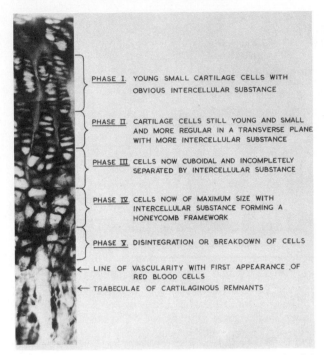

PHASE I.   YOUNG SMALL CARTILAGE CELLS WITH
           OBVIOUS INTERCELLULAR SUBSTANCE

PHASE II. CARTILAGE CELLS STILL YOUNG AND SMALL
           AND MORE REGULAR IN A TRANSVERSE PLANE
           WITH MORE INTERCELLULAR SUBSTANCE

PHASE III. CELLS NOW CUBOIDAL AND INCOMPLETELY
           SEPARATED BY INTERCELLULAR SUBSTANCE

PHASE IV. CELLS NOW OF MAXIMUM SIZE WITH
           INTERCELLULAR SUBSTANCE FORMING A
           HONEYCOMB FRAMEWORK

PHASE V.   DISINTEGRATION OR BREAKDOWN OF CELLS

←   LINE OF VASCULARITY WITH FIRST APPEARANCE OF
    RED BLOOD CELLS
←   TRABECULAE OF CARTILAGINOUS REMNANTS

Fig. 45-3. Photomicrograph of the epiphyseal plate and its division into Streeter's five phases. (*Taken with permission from Mercer and Duthie, "Orthopaedic Surgery," London, 1974.*)

form bone. From such centers of ossification the process spreads.

Remodeling

This consists of extensive but constructive resorption and deposition of new bone which, although most marked during growth and development, continues in the mature skeleton. With resorption there is the shift of both mineral and organic matrix into a fluid phase. During growth at the epiphyseal plate area the remodeling process is essential to change the shape and function of the bones, both in the longitudinal and in the circumferential planes and within the spongiosa of the medullary cavity (Fig. 45-4) in order to produce the normal tubular shape of the shaft. There is a morphologic remodeling process in the periosteal area, adjacent to the juxtaepiphyseal area or the perichondral ring of Lacroix, which contains large numbers of osteoclasts. However, there is a constant remodeling process taking place within the basic structure of bone, i.e., in the osteon itself. Vincent and Haumont have described how bone and its unit—the osteon—is one of two major reactive types, i.e., *metabolic,* undergoing continuous resorption because of its close relationship to the fluid phase or extracellular fluid with accretion, and *structural,* in which there is little exchange of state, because it is completely calcified and stable.

The marrow cavity is also widened during remodeling by osteoclastic activity on the endosteal surfaces of cortex and spongiosa.

RADIOLOGIC DIAGNOSIS OF BONE DISORDERS

The varying densities which may be seen on a radiograph are:

1. Background density of the film
2. Subcutaneous tissue
3. Fatty tissue
4. Fluids, edema, hemorrhage, joint effusion
5. Muscle (similar in consistency to that of water)
6. Cartilage
7. Bone—cancellous being less dense than cortical bone

The cortex encloses the cancellous bone and the medulla and may make interpretation within these structures difficult.

The following tissues are examined:

SOFT TISSUES. It is important to distinguish a soft tissue *swelling* from a soft tissue *mass.* A *soft tissue swelling* has a poorly defined expanded limit which is caused by extracellular fluid infiltrating the area and obscuring the normal soft tissue outlines. A *soft tissue mass* is clearly delineated, obscuring by its own density the normal anatomy of vessel and fat lines. A cyst or tumor would also produce such a finding. The shape of the mass may be significant, e.g., when gravity enlarges its inferior portion because of its fluid or purulent content.

Calcification or Ossification in Soft Tissues. Calcification is characterized by its uniform amorphous appearance, whereas ossification may be mature enough in formation and even remodeled to show cortex and trabecular pattern. Both may be seen in muscle (myositis ossificans), tendon (supraspinal calcification), joint capsule or ligament, or joint.

BONE. *"Apparent" expansion of bone* may be caused by destruction of the cortex followed by the deposition of new bone around the lesion. Thus, a simple bone cyst is never wider than the epiphyseal line. "Apparent" expansion is caused by remodeling above and below the lesion to such an extent that the lesion appears wider than normally remodeled bone.

Generalized decrease in bone radiodensity is seen as a diffuse decrease in bone density by narrowing the width of the diaphyseal cortices or by decreasing the width of the trabeculae or their number, as in osteoporosis, Sudeck's atrophy, and disuse atrophy of immobilization around a joint.

Increased radiodensity usually is seen in an area or segment of bone. It implies new bone formation on cortical bone or on trabecular bone, or an increase in the number of trabeculae in any unit area or compaction of trabecular bone, or a relative increase in density due to a surrounding area's losing its blood supply with decrease of its density, as in developmental osteopetrosis, fluorosis, and Paget's disease.

In *new bone formation,* trabecular bone can be laid down within the bone structure on preexisting trabeculae or filling between these structures. The amount of physical mass which is produced reflects the cause. For example, a staphylococcal infection will produce a much greater amount than a streptococcal infection. The disorganized deposition of new bone in a neuropathic joint, such as in Charcot's or Paget's diseases, will often completely obliterate the original trabecular pattern with a dense amorphous-appearing bone. The new bone pattern must be carefully examined for its degree of organization into trabeculae of normal shape, size, and amount, and the overlying cortex must be searched for evidence of osteon formation. It is important to differentiate *reactive new bone,* which is organized, and *tumor new bone,* which lacks this property. Periosteum will produce new bone in response to growth, infection, tumor, or vascular disturbances. Edeiken and Hodes have described two types of periosteal reactions. The first type is solid reaction of a single uniform layer more than 1 cm thick, which persists unchanged for weeks. It can be thin (eosinophilic granuloma), dense and undulating (vascular), dense and elliptical (malignant tumor or fracture), or Codman's triangle (malignant tumor or hemorrhage).

The second type is an interrupted reaction, either lamellated (onion skin) or perpendicular to the surface (sunburst). This occurs in active aggressive malignant tumors, infections, or subperiosteal hemorrhages or finally amorphous calcific densities lying between periosteal new bone and its adjacent bone cortex—and denoting malignant disease of bone. A localized bony protruberance arising from the surface of the cortex as an exostosis may be found in one or more bones.

Ossification must be distinguished from *calcification.* Ossification implies a cellular activity of depositing calcium phosphate complex crystals with an organized framework to form the structure of bone. Calcification is a chemical activity of laying down calcium phosphate crystals without structure or organization and usually is seen in soft tissue planes of tendons, bursae, etc.

Dysplasia is a disturbance of growth or metabolism without reaction of adjacent bone or periosteum to suggest an inflammatory or neoplastic process. Its location in the epiphyseal, metaphyseal, and diaphyseal areas of several bones suggests its multifocal origin. This may be an arrest of growth or a remodeling defect to produce alteration in shape and size of bones, as in developmental disorders.

JOINT TISSUES. Skin, subcutaneous tissues, and other soft tissue masses (ligaments, capsule) can be identified. Particular attention is given to the ballooning out of the normal layers by an effusion. Comparison should be made with the opposite joint for such soft tissue changes and for observing the normal width of the joint "space" which is formed by the adjacent articular cartilage surfaces or by the menisci of the knees, etc. The relationship of the bones making up the joint is studied, and rotational abnormalities around the hip joint, for example, can be noted by comparing how much of the lesser trochanter profile is visible or how far away the joint lines are displaced. The quality of these bones as regards their density, the presence of subchondral cyst formation in osteoarthritis, or subchondral erosion in rheumatoid arthritis should be noted. The symmetry or lack of it regarding the adjacent bone surfaces should be noted especially when destroyed

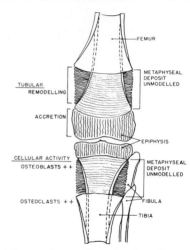

Fig. 45-4. Tubular remodeling and accretion of a long bone. (*After Keith. Taken with permission from Mercer and Duthie, "Orthopaedic Surgery," London, 1974.*)

by bone loss, resorption, or fragmentation of the growing epiphysis (Perthes' disease) or of the adult femoral head (avascular necrosis), or in the relationship of the upper femoral epiphysis to the femoral neck (Table 45-2).

CLASSIFICATION OF GENERALIZED BONE DISORDERS

I. *Developmental disorders* involving the organic phase of bone, i.e., collagen and cartilage matrix formation, calcification, and remodeling
   A. Achondroplasia
   B. Chondroosteodystrophy
   C. Dyschondroplasia
   D. Multiple enchondromas
   E. Metaphyseal aclasis
   F. Osteogenesis imperfecta
   G. Polyostotic fibrous dysplasia
   H. Osteopetrosis
II. *Metabolic disorders*
   A. Deficiency in inorganic constituents of bone
      1. Insufficient absorption of calcium or phosphates
         a. Low intake
            (1) Starvation
            (2) Rickets
            (3) Osteomalacia
         b. Defective absorption
            (1) Vitamin D deficiency
            (2) Defective fat absorption
               (*a*) Biliary deficiency
               (*b*) Pancreatic deficiency
               (*c*) Celiac disease
            (3) Chronic diarrhea
      2. Excessive secretion of calcium or phosphates
         a. Renal rickets, or osteodystrophy
            (1) Total renal insufficiency
            (2) Tubular insufficiency
               (*a*) Lignac-Fanconi syndrome
               (*b*) Hyperchloremic acidosis
               (*c*) Vitamin D-resistant rickets, or "phosphate rickets"

b. During pregnancy, via placenta and breast
   (1) Osteomalacia
c. Hyperparathyroidism
3. Decreased phosphate excretion
   a. Hypoparathyroidism
B. Deficiency in organic constituents of bone
  1. Decreased intake
    a. Starvation
    b. Chronic diarrhea
  2. Excessive utilization or loss
    a. Chronic infection
    b. Renal disease
    c. Liver disease
    d. Hormonal
      (1) Hyperthyroidism
      (2) Postmenopausal osteoporosis
      (3) Disuse atrophy
      (4) Stress
      (5) Cushing's disease
III. *Hormonal disorders*—normal, excessive, or deficient secretion, the effect being seen in a *child* as altered rate of epiphyseal growth and skeletal maturation and in an *adult* as alteration in the balance of osteolytic and osteoblastic activity
  A. Pituitary
  B. Sex glands
  C. Thyroid
  D. Adrenals
  E. Parathyroids
IV. *Reticulosis*—disease of bone marrow constituents such as
  A. Reticuloendothelial system
    1. Histiocytic granulomatosis
      a. Letterer-Siwe disease
      b. Eosinophilic granuloma
      c. Hand-Schüller-Christian disease
    2. Lipoid granulomatosis
      a. Gaucher's disease
      b. Niemann-Pick disease
      c. Xanthomatosis with hypercholesterolemia
  B. Lymphatic system
    1. Hodgkin's disease
    2. Lymphosarcoma
  C. Hematopoietic system
    1. Leukemia
      a. Lymphoblastic
      b. Myeloblastic
    2. Multiple myeloma
    3. Hemolytic anemia
      a. Mediterranean, or Cooley's, anemia
      b. Sickle cell anemia
      c. Erythroblastosis foetalis
V. *Vascular disorders*
  A. Paget's disease
  B. Osteodystrophy or Sudeck's atrophy
  C. Massive osteolysis, or "disappearing bones"

In the examination and diagnosis of these conditions Shearer said:

> If a bone lesion as seen radiographically does not show reactive change in the adjacent bone or periosteum, which suggests an inflammatory process or the invasive character of a neoplastic process, you should then have in mind the possibility of a dysplasia. Study then the localization; is it involving primarily metaphyseal bone or does it, in some conditions, involve only the epiphyses or only the small bones? Study then the nature of the abnormal process. Is it merely an arrest of growth; does the appearance suggest a cartilage dysplasia or a fibrous dysplasia? Then proceed to carry out a survey of the skeleton to show the distribu-

Table 45-2. RADIOGRAPHIC DIFFERENTIAL DIAGNOSIS OF GENERALIZED BONE DISORDERS

I. Reaction of adjacent bone and/or periosteum
  A. Tumor
  B. Inflammation
II. Normal adjacent bone and/or periosteum: dysplasia (disturbance of growth or metabolism) occurring in the
  A. Epiphysis
    1. Chondroosteodystrophy
    2. Gargoylism
    3. Epiphyseal dysplasia
    4. Achondroplasia
  B. Metaphysis
    1. Dyschondroplasia
    2. Multiple enchondromata
    3. Metaphyseal aclasia
    4. Polyostotic fibrous dysplasia
    5. Neurofibromatosis
  C. Diaphysis
    1. Engelmann's disease
    2. Dyschondroplasia
    3. Melorheostosis
  D. Marrow
    1. Leukemia
    2. Multiple myelomatosis
    3. Lymphadenoma—Hodgkin's disease
    4. Histiocytic granulomatosis
      a. Hand-Schüller-Christian disease
      b. Eosinophilic granuloma
      c. Letterer-Siwe disease
    5. Gaucher's disease
  E. Whole bone
    1. Porosis (decreased osteoblastic activity)
      a. Osteogenesis imperfecta
      b. Osteomalacia—rickets
      c. Sudeck's atrophy
      d. Osteoporosis
      e. Endocrine
        (1) Hyperparathyroidism
        (2) Hyperthyroidism
    2. Sclerosis (increased osteoblastic activity)
      a. Osteopetrosis
      b. Osteopathia striata
      c. Osteopoikilosis
      d. Melorheostosis
      e. Osteitis deformans
      f. Hypertrophic osteoarthropathy

tion of the abnormal bone. Do not forget to note whether the condition is associated with a generalized osteoporosis or whether bone, apart from the involved area, is normal. Then consider the findings in relation to the full history and clinical examination as well as biochemical blood analysis. Having done this I think you will at least make an intelligent approach to the correct diagnosis, and will usually reach a satisfactory conclusion.

DEVELOPMENTAL DISORDERS OF BONE

The common developmental diseases of bone apart from the obvious endocrine errors can all be arranged in two groups:

1. Errors in the proliferation and calcification of the cartilage model
   a. Achondroplasia
   b. Chondroosteodystrophy
   c. Dyschondroplasia
   d. Metaphyseal aclasis
   e. Multiple enchondromas
   f. Polyostotic fibrous dysplasia
2. Errors in the collagen and matrix formation
   a. Osteogenesis imperfecta
   b. Osteopetrosis

The epiphyseal cartilage proliferates normally in columnar fashion and in due course undergoes maturation, degeneration, and calcification. If the chondroblast is defective, multiple pathologic lesions may occur as a result of failure or irregularity in the maturation and calcification of the cartilage cells. If the failure of maturation and calcification is diffuse, the lack of the zone of preliminary calcification will result in delay of epiphyseal ossification and dwarfism.

A central chondroblast, if it continues to proliferate, will form an enchondroma which gives the bone a cystic appearance; if peripheral, this will result in an ecchondroma, or an exostosis may result instead of calcification to give a fibrous tissue mass. In general the following conditions are produced:

Achondroplasia—dwarfism
Metaphyseal aclasia—exostoses
Dyschondroplasia—cyst formation
Multiple chondromas—enchondromas
Chondroosteodystrophy—combination of all

Achondroplasia (Chondrodystrophia Fetalis)

The basic disturbance is in the calcification and remodeling of cartilage. Membranous bones, e.g., ribs and sternum, are formed, and all develop normally. The disease has been known since the earliest times, the Egyptian goddess Ptah having been pictured as achondroplastic. The severity can vary, and in very severe cases the fetus dies in utero. Achondroplasia is inherited as a dominant expression in the majority of those individuals who survive and reproduce.

The most evident histologic feature is the absence of cartilage proliferation and the columnar formation of cartilage. Ossification is irregular. Bone accretion at the periosteal surface is attached to the growth cartilage and may deposit a layer of compact bone over part of the metaphysis.

CLINICAL MANIFESTATIONS (Fig. 45-5). At birth, the typical infant with achondroplasia has a normal-sized body, very short, fat, flabby limbs, and a large head, with a characteristic depression at the root of the nose. Smallness in stature due to the absence of growth of the extremities becomes increasingly evident during childhood. A dwarf results. Walking occurs at the usual age, and dentition is normal.

When the patient stands erect, the tips of the fingers may only reach the great trochanter or the iliac crests, instead of normally reaching the lower part of the thigh. The achondroplastic hand is short and broad, with the fingers

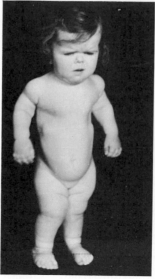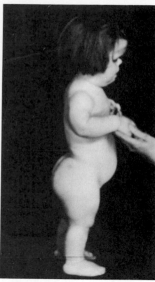

Fig. 45-5. Achondroplastic girl showing the decreased limb growth with foreshortening of the stature but normal trunk height.

of equal length, e.g., *main en trident*. The short limbs, especially the lower, are often curved, in contrast to the trunk, which is virtually normal. The sacrum is tilted, and, as a consequence, contracture of the pelvic inlet follows.

The head is enlarged, rounded, and markedly brachycephalic. The face is broad, and at the root of the short nose is a characteristic depression or indentation. The upper alveolar processes protrude, and prominence of the lower jaw results in prognathism.

Persons with achondroplasia usually have normal intelligence.

The *"long" bones of the limbs* are very short and curved with a "broadened" shaft. The epiphyses may be disproportionately large and roughly shaped.

The portion of the *skull* developed in cartilage—the base—is grossly abnormal and reduced, especially the presphenoid and postsphenoid and the basiocciput. The vault is more globular in form, and the fontanels are correspondingly enlarged.

Although the vertebral column is of normal length, the centers of ossification of the bodies may be smaller than normal. Often there is a long regular kyphosis at the lumbodorsal region. The most striking feature is the early synostosis between the body and the arch, which in some cases is so severe as to lead to marked diminution in the caliber of the vertebral canal.

Differential Diagnosis. This disorder has to be differentiated from rickets. Radiographically the epiphyseal outline is present with normal ossification in the abnormal epiphysis. In rickets, on the other hand, the epiphyseal outline is blurred and ossification delayed.

Achondroplasia may be confused with cretinism, but in the latter mental deficiency and retardation are evident. In cretinism the essential feature is delay in ossification. In some cases it is associated with stippling of the epiphyses and calcium deposits.

The achondroplastic person is a "dwarfed" individual

in whom the trunk length (crown to pubis) is normal, leg length (pubis to heel) is reduced, and the hand span (fingertip to fingertip) is reduced.

This form of dwarfism has to be differentiated from other forms of stunting in which there is a decrease in the trunk length while the leg length and hand span may or may not be normal, e.g., (1) osteogenesis imperfecta, (2) osteomalacia and rickets, (3) osteoporosis, (4) developmental diseases such as chondroosteodystrophy, metaphyseal aclasis, and (5) in adults, Paget's disease, spondylolisthesis, Charcot spine, neoplasia.

The prognosis varies with the degree of the affection, but an achondroplastic individual may live to a considerable age.

No known treatment is available.

Dyschondroplasia (Ollier's Disease)

In 1899, Ollier first described this condition of varying degrees of ossification of abnormal metaphyseal cartilage formation. The diagnosis can be made in early childhood.

Dyschondroplasia is more commonly diffusely unilateral or bilateral, but occasionally it may be confined to a single bone.

PATHOLOGY. The typical changes are in the ends of the diaphysis of long bones—humerus, femur, radius, etc.—or in the long bones of the hands and feet, where growth is most rapid. The metaphysis is usually broadened and cystic with trabeculae running in parallel lines in the long axis of the bone. Occasionally small exostoses project from the surface, and foreshortening is evident. In the short long bones, multiple enchondromas may form. The ilium, ischium, and pubis may appear stippled and varying in bone density because of the presence of small rounded areas of cartilage.

The differential diagnosis includes metaphyseal aclasis, multiple enchondromas, osteopathia striata, and osteopoikilosis. Dyschondroplasia may be associated with cavernous hemangiomas and phleboliths of the soft tissue, a syndrome described by Maffucci.

The prognosis for normal life expectancy appears to be good, but deformity and secondary arthritis are constant sequelae. Surgical intervention is indicated only when there is mechanical interference with joint function and after epiphyseal growth has ceased.

Multiple Enchondromas

This is a disturbance of growth in which multiple cartilaginous tumors are present in the shafts of the short long bones of the hands and feet. The lesion may be a variant of dyschondroplasia.

The bone may be grossly expanded, and the expansion may be regular, with faint bony striations along the periphery of the expanded area. As the chondromatous tissue grows, more and more of the bone is destroyed, until little of the affected bone may remain save a few scattered bony fragments embedded in irregular striped masses of exuberant chondromatous tissue. Pathologic fractures may occur and require bone grafting.

Metaphyseal Aclasis (Multiple Exostoses, Diaphyseal Aclasis, Hereditary Deforming Dyschondroplasia)

The disease affects only those bones arising from cartilage and from membrane. It is inherited in an autosomal dominant form.

The basic defect is in a failure of remodeling of the metaphysis with the formation of multiple outgrowths or exostoses from the surface of the shaft of long bones, leading to some stunting of skeletal growth (Fig. 45-6).

PATHOLOGY. The membranous bones of the skeleton, the tarsal and carpal bones, are not involved. The condition affects those parts of the long bones in which tubular remodeling is active, i.e., the distal end of the femur, the proximal ends of the tibia and fibula, the distal ends of the radius and ulna, and the proximal end of the humerus. It is also seen at the medial and lateral ends of the clavicle, the vertebral border of the scapula, and occasionally at the neurocentral synchondroses of the vertebrae.

The diaphysis is usually of normal cylindrical form and of normal caliber. The metaphysis is increased in diameter, with roughly parallel sides. Irregular projections—exostoses—appear on the surface.

Exostoses comprise the most singular feature. Normally most marked at the ends of the bone, they may be found at virtually any part of the shaft. Frequently an exostosis marks the junction of normal shaft and the expanded extremity. As the shaft increases in length, the exostoses which were initially near the epiphyseal cartilage are displaced farther up the shaft. In addition they may become obliquely disposed to the shaft, directed away from the extremity of the bone, and they are irregular in shape. The exostoses are composed of poorly trabeculated bone in direct continuity with the bone of the shaft. During the years of growth the exostosis is surmounted by a cap of cartilage, from which progressive growth in size of the exostosis may take place.

There is usually well-marked interference with growth in length of the affected bones with irregularity of the ossification at the epiphyseal plate. It is essentially a failure of maturation of the cartilage cells. In the leg, growth of the fibula lags behind that of the tibia. Adjacent exostoses may produce absorption of the adjacent surface of the neighboring bones.

Two occasional complications of metaphyseal aclasis occur:

1. Formation of a *chondroma* which projects from the surface of the bone near the epiphyseal cartilage and can become chondrosarcomatous
2. *Osteogenic sarcoma* or *chondrosarcoma*, which may arise in one of the exostoses

CLINICAL MANIFESTATIONS. In the diffuse type there may be extensive distortion. The stature is short or even dwarfed. In addition the limbs may show deformities of the nature of bowing or genu valgum. Fracture from slight trauma is common, but the fragments unite as readily as in normal individuals.

The most typical feature is the presence of numerous exostoses. These are most common at sites of active growth, such as the knee and shoulder. The projections are hard, the skin overlying them is normal, and the soft tissues move easily on them. They may be associated with pain if the tumor presses on a peripheral nerve or a nerve root or if the process is inadvertently fractured. They are also liable to interfere with the free play of associated tendons or may even act as a mechanical obstruction to joint movement, in which event they may give rise to considerable disability. A bursa may form over the projection and from time to time become inflamed.

Radiologic examination shows an irregularly expanded metaphyseal mass, with little or no compact cortical bone. The architecture of the interior is altered. The normal cancellous tissue is replaced by a mass of less dense tissue, in which islands of normal ossification may be observed. The exostoses appear as definite projections from the metaphyseal region. Their structure is similar to that of the metaphysis—a clear interior, with a thin shell of cortical bone.

PROGNOSIS AND TREATMENT. The disease has no effect on the general health, but there may be disability as a result of nerve pressure or interference with joint movement. The only treatment indicated is the removal of exostoses which are giving rise to symptoms or which have become malignant.

Polyostotic Fibrous Dysplasia (Osteodystrophy Fibrosa, Unilateral Recklinghausen's Disease, Albright's Syndrome)

The disease usually appears in childhood or puberty as cyst formation in the diaphysis or metaphysis, but rarely in the epiphysis, of long bones. The bones most frequently involved are the femur, tibia, humerus, and radius. Bending deformities of the weight-bearing bones and pathologic fractures with slow union or nonunion are frequent occurrences. On biopsy, there is usually a distinctive appearance of bony trabeculae formation in a stroma of fibrous tissue. Giant cells are not a usual feature except when the lesion has been traumatized. Blood calcium and phosphates are usually normal, and occasionally the alkaline phosphatase is raised, probably denoting compensatory osteogenesis.

The x-ray shows expansion of the bone and thinning of the cortex with numerous trabeculated cystic areas which contain giant cell collections, fibrous tissue, and collections of cartilaginous tissue. It is usually a unilateral disease affecting multiple long bones. When it affects only one bone, it is known as *monostotic fibrous dysplasia.*

This differential diagnosis includes hyperparathyroidism, which rarely occurs in the adolescent. The blood calcium and phosphate changes of hyperparathyroidism are absent, and on x-ray the unaffected parts of the bones have a normal appearance and do not present the diffuse osteomalacic appearance of hyperparathyroidism.

The treatment is of the deformities, and prognosis is good, as this is a self-limiting disease. However, certain lesions may require curettage and autogenous grafting.

Albright's syndrome is a variation of polyostotic fibrous dysplasia occurring in a female and accompanied by sexual precocity and flat pigmented areas of skin. This is thought by some to be due to excessive hormonal secretion.

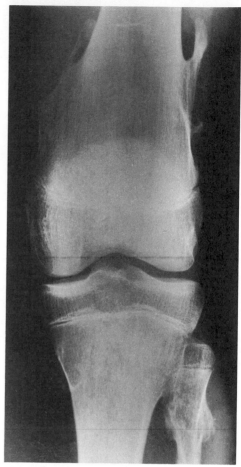

Fig. 45-6. AP radiograph of the knee joint showing bony spurring in the metaphyseal-diaphyseal area with minimal cap formation.

MONOSTOTIC FIBROUS DYSPLASIA

In this condition a single bone is the site of partial replacement of its substance by fibrous tissue, with or without the additional presence of osteoid. If present, osteoid is occasionally calcified, and cysts are occasionally formed. Any bone may be involved. The blood chemistry is within normal limits. The clinical findings are local swelling where the bone is superficial and pain if the lesion is near a joint. It has been suggested that the condition may represent a disturbance of the normal bone reparative process following trauma.

Osteogenesis Imperfecta

Osteogenesis imperfecta (fragilitas ossium, or Vrölich's disease), in which extreme fragility of bones is present, originates in fetal life. Dwarfism with micromelia occurs, and the patient's general condition is poor.

The classification of *brittle* bones includes:

A. Hereditary type—hereditary hypoplasia of the mesenchyme. Although this type is described as being congenital, it probably is inherited as a gene mutant, but this has been difficult to determine because of its lethal nature.

B. Nonhereditary congenital type—osteogenesis imperfecta (fragilitas ossium, osteopsathyrosis congenita of Vrölich): fetal, infantile, and adolescent (osteogenesis imperfecta tarda).
    1. Osteogenesis imperfecta with white sclera
    2. Osteogenesis imperfecta with blue sclera
C. Acquired type.
    1. Idiopathic
       a. Osteosclerosis fragilis generalisata (marble bone, or Albers-Schönberg disease)
    2. Osteoporosis
       a. Disuse
       b. Trophic
       c. Local disease
       d. Pressure
    3. Endocrine—hyperparathyroidism
    4. Vitamin deficiency
       a. Rickets
       b. Osteomalacia
       c. Scurvy

In the autosomal, dominant inherited form the stature is stunted, the joints are hypermobile, the sclera is blue, and deafness frequently appears after adolescence. Among adults with blue sclera 60 percent have associated fragile bones, and 60 percent have associated deafness.

PATHOLOGY. Knaggs has shown that in osteogenesis imperfecta the epiphyseal cartilage is normal, and the zone of calcified cartilage appears normal. However, in the zone of ossification the trabeculae are slender and delicate and widely separated by interstices filled with cellular connective tissue or fibrous marrow. No cross trabeculae are present as a general rule. The periosteum is thick, and

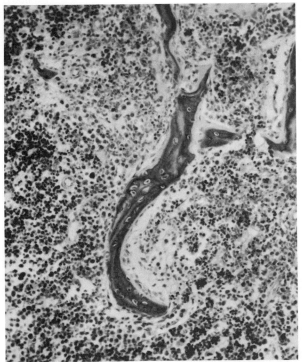

Fig. 45-7. Photomicrograph of tissue from osteogenesis imperfecta, in which there are numerous mesenchymal cells with poorly organized endochondral ossification, so that trabeculae are widely separated. (×150.)

there is no compact cortical layer of bone, but there are delicate and discrete subperiosteal trabeculae.

The bones are usually shorter and thinner than corresponding bones of normal individuals at a comparable age, so that the general skeletal development tends to be stunted.

In most cases there are many healed fractures, frequently in bad position. The consequent deformity, producing as it does shortening of the affected bones, adds to the dwarfing already present from the feeble osteogenesis.

The basic defect of osteogenesis imperfecta is a diffuse defect of the primitive mesenchymal cells, which fail to produce normal collagen. Studies have shown a deficiency or immaturity in the cross linkages. These abnormal cells enlarge to resemble cartilage cells in appearance. The endochondral arrangement and the Haversian systems are irregular (Fig. 45-7). A similar pathologic differentiation of the primitive mesenchymal cells occurs in the subperiosteal region, where there is no normal compact bone.

The bones are extremely fragile, because of the absence of a well-formed cortex, the sparse and widely separated trabeculae, and the nature of the osseous substance, which is less compact than the ordinary laminated bone. The bone is liable to undergo osteoclastic absorption and also, in late cases, appears to undergo spontaneous disintegration.

The raised serum alkaline phosphatase level, which is a frequent finding, is probably due to compensatory activity of bone repair.

CLINICAL MANIFESTATIONS. In the *fetal form,* the disease is severe, and the child is stillborn or survives only a very short time as a result of brain injury. There are multiple fractures, some healed at birth, while the cranium shows grossly imperfect ossification and consists merely of a membranous bag with a few plaques of poor bone embedded in it.

In the *infantile form,* the disease is less severe. At birth there may be some stunting and evidence of fractures, but the ossification of the skull is more advanced. The child survives for a year or two, but the bones are fragile and break at a touch. The skull may assume a globular shape and may appear large in proportion to the rest of the body. True hydrocephalus may develop and again may be related to intracranial damage at birth.

In the *adolescent type,* often called *osteogenesis imperfecta tarda,* the child may appear normal at birth and during childhood. The only disturbance observed may be a special liability to fractures from comparatively minor injuries. The ossification of the skull may be normal, but one or two soft areas may be found on examination. As time passes, the tendency to fracture decreases.

The disease may on rare occasions be encountered first in adult life, when a case which was slight at birth and during adolescence becomes active or when a case which has regressed spontaneously is reactivated.

Prominent features are:

1. Stunting of growth.
2. Fractures from trivial trauma. The fractures are often subperiosteal and unite readily, often more so than in normal bone,

and the callus is often more dense than in normal bone. The fractures are distinctive in that they cause little or no pain or tenderness—largely because they are subperiosteal. It is largely for this reason that so many are allowed to heal with deformity.

3. Blue sclera. This has been observed in the infantile and late types of fragility and is a result of increased visibility of the pigmented choroid through an abnormally translucent sclera due to alteration in the mucopolysaccharide content.

4. Characteristic skull, showing broadening of the forehead, angular projections above the zygoma, a downward tilting of the axis of the orbit, the ear, and the auditory canals, and an underhung jaw.

Radiologic Findings. In severe types the bones may show almost complete absence of cancellous texture, the cortex appearing as a faintly penciled line. The bones are shorter than normal and occasionally broader. In less severe types the long bones are stunted, are diffusely rarefied, and may have expanded club-shaped extremities. Fractures or old deformities following fractures are often apparent. In adult cases the shafts of the bones appear to shrink and have a dense, relatively thick cortex with no medulla. The ends of the bones are expanded and contain coarse cancellation with poor density. Ultimately the long bones may appear as two poorly calcified end bulbs joined by a slender rod of denser bone.

The ribs are usually bent sharply downward at their angles, and the thorax is therefore greatly deformed. This may be accentuated by scoliosis. The pelvis is asymmetric with irregular deformity. The skull has irregular ossification, with islands of denser bone in a poorly calcified matrix—the so-called Wormian bones.

Differential Diagnosis. The diagnosis is usually evident, but occasionally rickets may have to be excluded, especially since fractures are common. In rickets, however, the radiologic picture is characteristic: the epiphyseal cartilage is broad and fuzzy, the edge of the metaphysis to the zone of calcified cartilage is irregular and poorly defined, and the metaphysis itself is cup-shaped and expanded. On the other hand, the rarefaction of the rest of the bone is considerably less than in osteogenesis imperfecta.

PROGNOSIS AND TREATMENT. In the majority of cases early death is the outcome. Occasionally adult life is reached, but the constant occurrence of fractures and the repeated confinement to bed produce real disability.

No specific treatment is known. Dietetic and other measures to promote the general well-being are indicated. Care should be exercised in handling children, but when fractures occur, they are treated along the usual lines. When healing takes place with deformity, osteotomy may be carried out. Sofield and Millar have described how the limb bones when badly bowed and deformed can be re-aligned and reinforced by multiple osteotomies and intramedullary rod fixation.

Osteopetrosis (Albers-Schönberg Disease, Marble Bones, Osteosclerosis Fragilis Generalisata, Congenital Osteosclerosis)

Albers-Schönberg, in 1904, described this rare bone disease associated with increased density of the skeleton. Fewer than 40 cases have been described. The condition

Table 45-3. CLASSIFICATION OF OSTEOSCLEROSIS (INCREASE IN BONE DENSITY)

Generalized	Localized
Hypoparathyroidism	Infection—syphilis
Fluorosis	Chronic osteomyelitis
Osteopetrosis	Degenerative—arthritis
Osteopoikilosis	Mechanical—stress
Engelmann's disease	Ischemia
	Neoplasia—osteoblastic
	Metastasis—malignant tumor

has occasionally affected several members of a family as an autosomal recessive inheritance. A classification of osteosclerosis appears in Table 45-3.

PATHOLOGY. The characteristic change is the increased density and thickness with loss of trabeculation of the affected bone, in symmetric fashion, most commonly in the metaphysis. The increased thickness of the bone indicates that the condition affects not only the bone developed from the epiphyseal cartilage but that growing by accretion from the periosteum.

The most marked changes are found in the most rapidly growing extremities of the long bones—the lower end of the femur and radius, and the upper end of the tibia and humerus.

The ribs are similarly affected—thick, dense, and apparently structureless (Fig. 45-8). The vertebrae may be uniformly dense, or a dense zone at the upper and lower thirds of the body may be separated by a zone of normal density in the middle, indicating that the process is affecting the bone laid down from the cartilage end plates of the body. The skull may be so dense that no detail of its architecture can be made out. The bones of the carpus and tarsus are ringed by layers of dense bone, the result of peripheral accretions.

It is well known that so-called marble bones are liable to fractures, especially in the adolescent. It is said to be

Fig. 45-8. X-ray of a chest showing the thick, dense, structureless bones of the thorax characteristic of osteopetrosis, or marble bones.

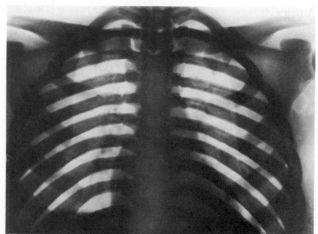

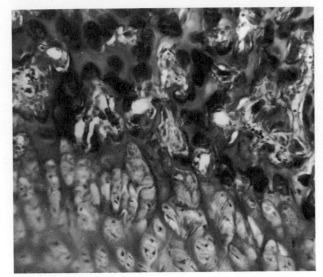

Fig. 45-9. Photomicrograph of tissue from osteopetrosis showing disorganized cartilage mass, abnormal bone, and fibrous tissue. (×200.)

possible to cut a so-called marble bone with a knife, the sensation experienced being similar to that on cutting chalk.

Microscopically the affected areas are seen to consist of a mixture of calcified cartilage masses, sclerotic bone, necrotic bone, and fibrous tissue (Fig. 45-9). It is noticeable that the tissues are avascular, the marrow spaces being filled with sclerotic tissue with very few capillaries. There, in the absence of true ossification or any lamellar system by osteoblastic activity, much of the sclerosis is due to excessive calcification of osteoid tissues.

The progressive sclerosis of the long bones gradually reduces the medullary cavity and the bone marrow to a degree incompatible with normal hematopoiesis, producing a true aplastic anemia, sometimes with enlargement of the liver and spleen.

In the skull the thickening is apt to restrict the size of the foramina, leading to pressure on, and paralysis of, the cranial nerves, to give blindness, nystagmus and ocular palsies, hydrocephalus, and occasionally signs of hypopituitarism.

MELORHEOSTOSIS

The condition was first reported by Léri in 1922. Its distinguishing features are (1) that the sclerotic changes are confined to one limb, (2) that the outline of an affected bone is definitely distorted, (3) the presence of pain, often severe, and (4) limitation of movement in the joints formed by the affected bone. The affection is usually limited to one limb and occasionally to one bone of a limb.

A portion of the cortex of one of the limb bones is irregularly enlarged, sufficiently to give rise to a swelling with an undulating surface. Between one undulation and another, a linear band of increased density may extend which has been likened to a "flow" of hyperostosis resembling "candle drippings."

OSTEOPATHIA STRIATA

In this condition, zones or striae of dense bone are found in the long axis of a long bone or in the ilium. The condition gives rise to a characteristic x-ray appearance. This is, perhaps, its main significance, for there is no clinical evidence, nor are there secondary pathologic changes.

Osteopoikilosis (Osteopathia Condensans Disseminata, or Spotted Bones)

This condition was described by Albers-Schönberg in 1915 and is characterized by the presence of dense spots in large numbers in the long and short bones but not in the skull, vertebrae, and ribs. The spots are usually uniformly dense but may have clear centers and are grouped toward the end of the bone in the epiphysis. They give rise to no symptoms and are usually discovered by chance. Schmorl found that they consisted of numerous closely packed trabeculae in the lamellae lying mostly in a longitudinal direction.

METABOLIC DISEASES

See "Metabolic disorders," in the Classification of Generalized Bone Disorders.

Metabolism of Calcium and Phosphorus

CALCIUM METABOLISM. Calcium is required in the processes of (1) blood coagulation, (2) transmission of neuromuscular impulses, (3) muscular excitability, (4) maintaining osmotic reactions in cellular permeabilities, (5) maintaining acid-base equilibrium, and (6) providing the mechanical strength of the skeleton.

Mitchell and his coworkers showed that a normal 70-kg adult male had over 1,000 Gm of calcium in his skeleton, over 10 Gm in the soft tissues, and less than 1 Gm in the blood and extracellular fluids. Calcium is readily absorbed from the intestine, particularly in the presence of vitamin D or a high-protein diet, or in any state of calcium demand, such as growth, pregnancy, or lactation (Fig. 45-10). For children, an adequate daily intake is approximately 1 Gm; adults require less, except during states of increased demand. Calcium is excreted in the urine, approximately 100 to 150 mg/day, and in feces, approximately 500 to 700 mg, during a balanced exchange reaction with normal bone accretion (i.e., positive balance) and bone resorption (i.e., negative balance). Neuman and Neuman have shown that over 99 percent of calcium going through the glomeruli is resorbed by the tubules. Serum calcium level is rigidly maintained at approximately 10 mg/100 ml, of which 70 percent is diffusible, the remainder being bound to protein.

Calcium metabolism is influenced by:

1. Thyroid extract. Thyrotoxicosis is characterized by increased urinary and fecal losses of calcium with the development of osteoporosis or a localized osteofibrosis. In myxedema there may be retention of calcium.
2. Growth hormone. Increase in total body mass is seen, and in

the active acromegalic individual serum inorganic phosphorus levels may be increased.

3. Adrenosteroids. In Addison's disease there may be an increased fecal and urinary loss of calcium with osteoporosis in the bone. This may be secondary to breakdown of the protein matrix.

Parathormone. Although Albright and Reifenstein suggested that the primary effect of this hormone was to increase the renal excretion of the phosphate with a resultant decrease in the serum phosphate level, this explanation can no longer be accepted.

The parathormone influences the levels of both serum calcium and serum phosphorus as well as the rate of bone absorption. In addition, it has some control over the urinary excretion of phosphate and through this controls the excretion of urinary calcium.

It should be emphasized that increased serum calcium levels can be obtained in animals after nephrectomy by giving parathyroid extracts. Parathyroid extracts may produce increased glomerular filtration, but decreased renal tubular resorption or increased renal tubular secretion is thought to be the primary mechanism.

Barnicot has demonstrated the direct local resorption of bone by crystals of parathyroid extract and grafts of parathyroid tissue placed in a rat's calvaria.

During hyperparathyroidism there is marked osteoclastic activity in bone, so that hypercalcemia and hypophosphatemia result, in spite of marked hypercalcinuria. Tetany or hypocalcemia will present as neuromuscular hyperirritability, convulsions, etc.

Talmage has emphasized the important role of the parathyroid gland in maintaining a constant level of ionic calcium in all tissue fluids of the body. A state of equilibrium between the calcium and phosphate concentrations is maintained between the liquid phase and the solid phase of bone, by removing ions from the fluid state and depositing them in bone. Talmage considers that the parathormone is acting in opposition to this equilibration gradient by removing calcium and phosphate from bone to return them to the fluid state and to maintain concentrations which are normal for the host.

McLean and Urist have proposed a feedback mechanism for the homeostatic regulation of serum calcium, in which the parathormone is particularly concerned with the regulation of calcium concentration in blood. Their mechanism consists of two parts: first, there is a compartment containing calcium in perfect chemical equilibrium with both the serum and labile fraction of bone minerals, i.e., approximately 70 percent of the total serum calcium content. Second, there is the feedback mechanism in which any fall in the serum calcium level results in an increased output of the parathormone. This in turn produces resorption in bone from the labile storage pool in the hydration shell of the surface of the crystal, the mobilization of additional calcium causing a rise in the calcium serum level back to the normal level of 10 mg/100 ml.

Parathyroidectomy produces a lowering of the calcium ion in the blood to about 7 mg/100 ml with the clinical evidence of tetany. Increase in parathormone causes increased bone calcium resorption with increased fibrous tissue formation and the condition of osteitis fibrosa.

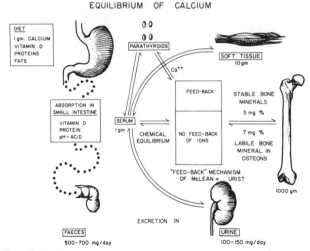

Fig. 45-10. Intake, homeostasis mechanism, and excretion of calcium. (*Taken with permission from Mercer and Duthie, "Orthopaedic Surgery," London, 1974.*)

Vitamin D deficiency is seen as hypocalcinemia and hypophosphatemia, with the development of rickets or osteomalacia, as well as retardation of growth. The action of vitamin D in rickets may be through suppressing the activity of the parathyroid gland.

Calcitonin. Calcitonin is a polypeptide secreted by the C cells of the human thyroid and other mammals and from the ultimobranchial glands of other vertebrates. It inhibits cell-mediated release of calcium from bone and directly inhibits resorption. It is thus important in controlling induced hypercalcemia, e.g., in Paget's disease and in bony metastases. This effect is of value in diagnosing osteolytic bone disease and controlling associated hypercalcemia of hyperparathyroidism, bone tumors, immobilization osteoporosis, and Paget's disease. Relief of bone pain in Paget's disease is an important therapeutic use of calcitonin.

PHOSPHORUS METABOLISM. Ninety percent of the body phosphorus is found in the skeleton, ten percent being found in the intracellular tissues and blood. An intake of less than 1 Gm/day is required by an adult, although more is required by growing children and pregnant women. Absorption is favored by the presence of calcium, and almost 60 percent of the intake is excreted in the urine. There does not appear to be any homeostatic control of the plasma levels, which in young children is 5 to 6 mg/100 ml and in adults is only 3 to 4 mg/100 ml. Almost all of the phosphorus is inorganic, in the form of orthophosphate with some pyrophosphate radicals, but some is found as phospholipid. Vitamin D may play a part in renal tubular reabsorption of phosphorus.

Serum inorganic phosphorus appears to be under the control of the parathyroids (which affect the resorption of phosphorus ions), the pituitary, and the thyroid. It is influenced by the level of circulating calcium and the excretion mechanism of the kidneys. The level is remarkably labile in a large number of pathologic and disease conditions.

Its serum level can be decreased by hyperparathyroidism, vitamin D deficiency, diabetes, and vitamin D–resistant rickets. They all tend to produce hyperphosphaturia and hypophosphatemia.

Vitamin D. Vitamin D is essential for the absorption of calcium and secondarily for the absorption of phosphorus from the intestine. Knowledge of the mechanism of action of vitamin D has expanded dramatically in the past few years as new metabolites of the vitamin have been identified. Vitamin D stimulates absorption of dietary calcium from the intestine and induces mobilization of bone mineral. Both effects supersaturate the plasma with calcium and phosphate, which allow normal mineralization.

Vitamin D produced from ultraviolet irradiation of 7-dehydrocholesterol in the skin is converted to 25-hydroxycholecalciferol in the liver and is secreted into the plasma. Current evidence suggests that the 25-hydroxycholecalciferol is converted to a polar metabolite in the kidney and passes into the systemic circulation and is involved in calcium transport by the mucosal cells of the small intestine. At physiologic levels, vitamin D is involved with mobilization of bone mineral and perhaps the uptake of calcium by the bone matrix. Current investigation suggests that various metabolites including 25-hydroxycholecalciferol; 21, 25-dihydrocholecalciferol; and other polar metabolites are present in bony extracts, although the active metabolite for mineral mobilization has not been delineated.

Calcification

This process consists of two phases, or systems: first, cellular differentiation to form a suitable medium of matrix osteoid, collagen fibrils, etc., and, second, the process of mineralization.

COLLAGEN AND MATRIX FORMATION. Osteoblasts secrete the organic matrix, or *osteoid,* which is made up of collagen fibers and an interfibrillar cement substance.

Jackson has demonstrated granules which pair within the osteoblast during the secretion of collagen and are thought to be an aminopolysaccharide and alkaline phosphatase, which is essential for developing calcifiable matrix. Sulfation first appears at the cell membrane along with prefibrillar collagen formation, and then the matrix contains the sulfated mucopolysaccharide chondroitin sulfate. This sulfation is defective in vitamin C scurvy, as noted by Reddi and Nörstrom. Any failure of alkaline phosphatase, of sulfation, or of vitamin C may alter the formation of osteoid and hence its calcification.

MINERALIZATION. Calcification involves the precipitation of mineral salts, i.e., calcium phosphate. The deposition of bone mineral requires two distinct steps: first, the grouping of a minimal number of ions capable of survival and growth (nucleation) and, second, the continued growth of these ions. Various theories are presented to explain this complicated process.

Bone cells, by increasing the local concentrations of calcium and phosphate ions, would precipitate the mineral. Robinson first proposed such a theory, suggesting that the local concentration of phosphate ions was elevated by the action of alkaline phosphatase on the phosphate esters. It is thought that these phosphate esters might arise from the phosphorolysis of glycogen. These theories are inadequate because bone is never the sole site of this reaction, and alkaline phosphatase is also abundant in tissues that do not calcify.

The components of matrix may contain specific mechanisms which create nucleating sites or remove barriers to these local calcification areas. It was shown by electron microscope that collagen fibrils are principally responsible for nucleation of bone mineral. The phosphorylation of collagen may be the important chemical reaction that enables nucleation to be initiated by the collagen. Histochemical and chemical analyses on the changes in the organic matrix on calcification indicate that the proteoglycan and phospholipid components may also be involved in mineralization.

Fleisch and his associates have suggested that the inorganic anion pyrophosphate present in bone and other tissues is an important controlling element in calcification. Pyrophosphate is the anhydride formed by condensation and removal of water from two molecules of orthophosphate. These investigations have suggested that calcification or mineral resorption is initiated by specific enzymes known as pyrophosphatases which remove inhibiting pyrophosphate by splitting it into two molecules of orthophosphate. Pyrophosphate in the concentrations found in bone and the body fluids will inhibit both the formation of hydroxyapatite and crystal growth from solutions containing calcium and phosphate ions at concentrations which otherwise spontaneously form hydroxyapatite. It will also prevent the transformation of amorphous calcium phosphate to crystalline hydroxyapatites.

The pyrophosphate theory could account for the absence of calcification, under normal circumstances, in tissues other than bone and cartilage. All these tissues contain concentrations of pyrophosphate sufficient to prevent spontaneous calcification. It is only bone and cartilage that contain the enzymes which remove these inhibiting concentrations of pyrophosphate.

It is suggested that, initially, there is a precipitate of calcium phosphate less basic than hydroxyapatite which is only subsequently converted to hydroxyapatite. There is evidence that this amorphous phase of calcium phosphate may be formed as packets within cells and be excreted into the matrix to form a nucleation center.

It is increasingly appreciated that proper calcification requires the coordinate activity in time and space of several distinct systems. Humoral factors are essential for the continuing supply of calcium and phosphate to the calcification sites. The activities of bone cells are involved both in the elaboration of the organic matrix and in its further transformations to a system that both permits and enhances calcification.

Scurvy

The antiscorbutic vitamin C is found in the majority of fresh foodstuffs—fruit juices, green vegetables, and to a lesser extent in potatoes, milk, and raw meat. Since it is destroyed by heating at 100°C, it is absent in dried, canned, and preserved foods, and in vegetables subjected to prolonged boiling. The absence of vitamin C from the diet gives rise to the clinical condition of scurvy.

The disease occurs most commonly in infants from six to eight months of age who have been fed exclusively on artificial food which has had its vitamin content destroyed. It also occurs in adults who are deprived of fresh food.

A diet deficient in vitamin C need not of necessity be deficient in the other vitamins. However, with a deficiency in vitamin D, a rachitic element may be added to the scorbutic in the case of the growing child, while in the adult there may be some evidence of osteomalacia.

PATHOLOGY. The cardinal feature of scurvy is a defect in the formation of intercellular substances which results in hemorrhage—from the gums, from the alimentary tract, from the subcutaneous tissues, and in bone. The hemorrhage is capillary in origin and occurs at sites at which new capillaries are sprouting, e.g., in bone, at the most actively growing metaphyses and beneath the periosteum (Fig. 45-11). Vitamin C controls the nutrition of capillary endothelium, or the amount of intercellular cement which binds the endothelial cells together.

From the capillary loops there occurs an irregular and patchy oozing of blood, so that small pools of blood collect and disrupt the newly forming bone, the calcified cartilaginous strata, and even the proliferating cartilaginous palisades. The blood clots and is replaced by fibrous tissue or by bone.

In very extreme cases, the hemorrhage may be sufficient to disrupt the growing area, with separation of the epiphyses. The subperiosteal hemorrhages are often extensive, the periosteum being stripped from the shaft for a considerable distance, with abnormal ossification.

CLINICAL MANIFESTATIONS. The child may or may not appear ill-nourished. The earliest features are restlessness and fretfulness, with one or more of the extremities not used. Handling of the parts produces extreme pain.

On examination there may be obvious swelling, fluid in character, in relation to the shaft of one or more of the long bones. The joints may appear swollen and are exquisitely sensitive to touch, appearing like an infective condition. On the other hand, the immobility of the parts may simulate paralysis, and this feature is often known as the *pseudoparalysis of scurvy.* Hemorrhages may also occur into and beneath the skin, and the gums may be swollen and spongy.

DIAGNOSIS. The conditions most liable to cause confusion in the early stages are anterior poliomyelitis, injury to joint, bone, and nerve, osteomyelitis, arthritis, and syphilitic osteochondritis—the latter being more common in the short long bones of hand and foot, the proximal end of the femur, and the distal end of the tibia.

The response to treatment in scurvy is dramatic, in sharp distinction to the other conditions enumerated.

The typical x-ray appearances are seen in Fig. 45-12.

TREATMENT. The administration of vitamin C in any of its forms leads to rapid cure. Within 24 hours pain and crying cease, and in a few days hemorrhages are beginning to heal. It is some months, however, before the bone remodeling occurs.

Rest in bed is indicated in the early stages, and, later,

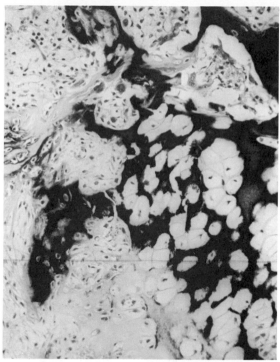

Fig. 45-11. Photomicrograph of tissue from the vicinity of an epiphysis in a seven-month-old child suffering from scurvy. It shows the irregular cartilage columns, abnormal new bone formation, and increased cellularity. (×200.)

exercises may be usefully employed to augment muscle tone. Unprotected weight bearing should be relieved by caliper until there is radiographic evidence of a return of bony structure, to prevent deformities.

Rickets

Rickets was formerly a disease of the lower classes and was common in industrial districts where poor housing, malnutrition, smoky atmosphere, and lack of sunlight were common. These factors favored a lack of vitamins, and it was generally assumed that rickets was a deficiency disease due to lack of vitamin D. However, Dent and Harris, in a classic description of inherited rickets and osteomalacia, have emphasized that rickets and osteomalacia in modern civilizations are usually due to primary metabolic abnormalities which are genetically determined. Most of the cases now appearing, although clinically similar to environmental or nutritional rickets, are vitamin D–resistant rickets, with or without an abnormality of renal tubular function but requiring massive dosages of vitamin D for cure. The primary defect of vitamin D deficiency intake or effect leads to a state of hypophosphatemia because of the decreased renal tubular resorption of phosphate.

The commonest type of the disease begins during the early years of infancy and is extremely rare after the age of four. It is known as *infantile rickets.* Comparable disturbances may arise at other age periods and are known as *late rickets and osteomalacia.*

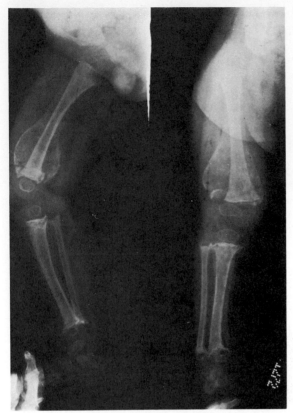

Fig. 45-12. X-ray of the lower limbs of a baby with scurvy showing the epiphyseal disturbance and calcifying periosteal hematoma formation.

PATHOLOGY. The normal epiphyseal line is a well-defined narrow strip of cartilage 2 mm deep, but in rickets it forms a wide irregular band, and the metaphysis is broad and irregular from excessive proliferation of the cells of the epiphyseal line. Mineralization is patchy in distribution and uniformly deficient.

The cartilage in the proliferating zone is hyperplastic, but instead of the normal palisade arrangement of the cells, the proliferated cells are arranged irregularly. Associated with this is a poor development of the bone marrow.

In the metaphysis the bony trabeculae are thinned with connective tissue hyperplasia, so that the extremity of the bone appears misshapen and unmodeled—particularly in the costochondral junctions, the lower end of the radius, etc. These changes are most marked in the most actively growing part of the bones. Bone formed before that is normal, while bone formed after the active phase of the disease is also normal.

When the child is able to crawl or to walk, the femur becomes bowed anteriorly and to the lateral side. The neck-shaft angle of the femur may be diminished (coxa vara), the tibia may be bowed, or the knee may assume a valgus attitude (Fig. 45-13). The whole pelvis may be flattened, or it may assume a trefoil shape as in osteomalacia causing obstetric difficulties. The skull is broad-

ened, the forehead square, and bosses of new bone may form in the parietal and frontal regions. The vertebral column may assume exaggerated curvatures.

CLINICAL MANIFESTATIONS. Cardinal manifestations include (1) restlessness associated with fear on moving limbs, (2) recurrent diarrhea and constipation, (3) evidences of irritability of the central nervous system, such as convulsions, laryngismus, or other types of spasmophilia, (4) large head, open fontanels, and craniotabes, (5) prominent abdomen, (6) narrow chest and rachitic rosary of costochondral junctions, (7) enlarged and tender epiphyses, (8) bowing of the long bones, (9) delayed dentition, with irregular, soft, decaying teeth, and (10) poorly developed muscles, with delay in walking.

Radiologic Findings. In the *acute stage,* the epiphysis is widened and lacks radiodensity, with delay in appearance of centers of ossification. The metaphysis is splayed out (Fig. 45-14). The periosteum is thickened, with fractures of the long bones frequently seen.

In the *chronic stage,* bowing occurs with the cortical part of the affected bone thickened on the side of the concavity (Fig. 45-15).

DIAGNOSIS. The disease is to be differentiated from congenital syphilis and infantile scurvy. The congenitally syphilitic child usually has other signs of syphilis, but occasionally the chief lesion may be a syphilitic osteochondritis. The epiphyseal region is tender, hot, and swollen; there is loosening and separation of the epiphysis, which can usually be moved on the shaft, with the production of muffled crepitus.

In infantile scurvy, swelling also occurs; it is not limited to the region of the epiphysis but encroaches on the shaft. There are usually hemorrhages in other situations, and the general signs of scurvy are present.

TREATMENT. Nutritional, or vitamin D deficiency, rickets may be cured by administration of one of the vitamin D–containing foods or by one of the standard preparations of the vitamin (e.g., calciferol, 3,000 I.U./day). The effect of this is enhanced by the addition of a calcium preparation (calcium carbonate or calcium phosphate).

Prevention of Deformity. When the bones are so soft, the child's movements should be so controlled that little or no pressure is exerted upon the limbs. He should not be allowed to stand or walk but should have physiotherapy in bed. For difficult children it is often advisable to fit rickets splints.

Treatment of the Established Deformity. Deformity is usually corrected by splints or by osteotomy.

Correction by Splinting. This method is used where the deformity is slight and the disease still active. It is employed particularly for young children, especially those below the age of four, and is most useful for deformities of the lower limb. The method is slow and requires continual supervision to ensure a good result and to prevent the formation of sores.

Correction by Osteotomy. Osteotomy should never be carried out until the radiograph shows eburnation, clearness, and regularity of outline. If corrective operations are attempted before this period, nonunion is likely to occur.

CELIAC RICKETS

Bone changes appear only in late and long-established cases, i.e., after the age of seven years, and are similar to those of rickets. The metaphysis is broad and irregular, the palisade arrangement of cartilage cells is lost, and instead there is an irregular hypertrophy of the cells. The zone of calcified cartilage is narrow, with poor calcification and ossification.

CLINICAL MANIFESTATIONS. In association with the characteristic appearances of celiac disease—pallor, cachexia, muscular hypotonicity, and abdominal swelling—there is lack of body development—stunting. In addition there may be skeletal deformity. Genu valgum is a common feature. Enlargement of the distal ends of the radius and ulna are also frequent signs, but occasionally still more extensive deformation may be present—enlarged costochondral junctions, Harrison's sulcus, kyphosis, coxa vara, bowleg, etc. Fractures may occur with mild trauma.

In celiac rickets there is invariably a lowered serum calcium content. Impaired fat digestion results in insoluble calcium soaps with decreased fat absorption.

The x-ray appearances are very variable, but the whole bone is usually fragile and porotic. The epiphyseal cartilage is broad and irregular with transverse striations of denser bone.

With celiac disease there is inadequate utilization of the fat of the diet and reduction in the source of vitamin D. The excess of free fatty acid leads to precipitation of the calcium in the diet as insoluble soaps, leading to a deficient absorption of these minerals from the alimentary tract. The absorption of calcium, though greatly diminished, appears to be sufficient to calcify the fragile bones of celiac disease so long as there is little or no growth, but when considerable growth appears, this defective absorption results in the development of rickets.

TREATMENT. Treatment is based upon high dosages of vitamin D and special diets.

RENAL OSTEODYSTROPHY

PATHOLOGY. The kidney lesions are mainly of two types:

1. Total renal insufficiency as found in chronic glomerulonephritis, focal nephritis, congenital cystic disease where there is a reduced glomerular function with failure to excrete phosphorus, as well as general uremia and acidosis. The main skeletal change accompanying this lesion is an osteitis fibrosis, with little osteoid formation, either as rickets or osteomalacia.
2. Tubular insufficiency. The resorption of phosphorus, amino acids, glucose, electrolytes, and water is impaired, particularly from the proximal convoluted tubules. If there is disease of the distal tubules, there is disturbance of potassium and creatinine secretion into the urine. As well as these defects of resorption or secretion, there is a marked disturbance in the general acid-base regulation of the body by alteration in the concentrations of bicarbonate, ammonium, and hydrogen ion, which are usually added to the urine to achieve the acid-base equilibrium.

CLINICAL MANIFESTATIONS. In a number of patients, symptoms are present from early days of life; in others, the child is normal for a few years before symptoms arise. *Features of the renal lesion* are polydipsia and polyuria,

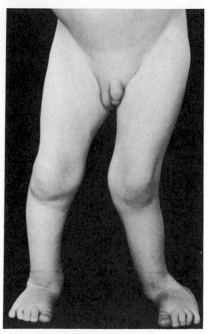

Fig. 45-13. Rachitic child showing the valgus deformity of the knees.

Fig. 45-14. X-ray of the hand and wrist of a three-year-old rachitic child showing the delay in the appearance of the carpal ossification center and the widening of the epiphysis with loss of bone density. (*Courtesy of Dr. R. C. Aicheson.*)

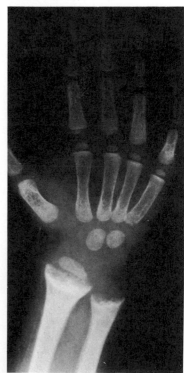

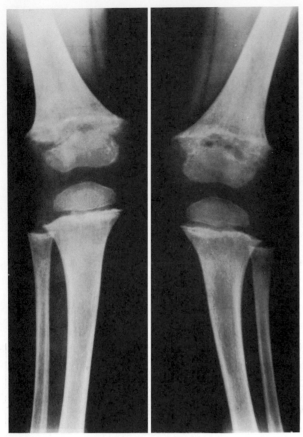

Fig. 45-15. X-ray of both knee areas during the healing phase of rickets showing the increasing ossification of the epiphyses but obvious valgus deformity of the knees and a tibia vara deformity.

with thirst. The urine is of low specific gravity, with an output of 1,200 to 3,700 ml daily. Albumin and casts are usually present at some stage of the disease, and cardiovascular symptoms of renal origin may appear. Ultimately, signs of kidney failure—headache, drowsiness, and gastrointestinal disturbance—arise, and death occurs from uremia. From the time of onset of the disease, tests of urinary function show a marked lowering of renal efficiency. The blood urea level is constantly raised, to 73 to 300 mg/100 ml.

Features of disturbance in growth include stunting in growth, often to a degree not equaled by any other form of infantilism. The body weight is correspondingly small, though malnutrition is not present, and the mental development is normal. The secondary sex characteristics do not develop.

Bone Changes. Genu valgum is common with enlargement of the epiphyses at the wrist and ankles, a costochondral rosary, Harrison's sulcus, or bowleg. The average age of recognition of deformity is between five and seven years.

Patients have been described with associated hyperplasia of the parathyroid glands, and these cases were interpreted as a composite picture of osteitis fibrosa and true rickets. The parathyroid hyperplasia may have resulted from the inability of the kidneys to secrete phosphorus and the parathyroid hyperplasia in turn responsible for the bone lesions.

Fanconi's Syndrome. Fanconi in 1931 described a case of renal diabetes in which there was retardation of growth. The features of Fanconi's syndrome are resistant and intractable rickets, hypophosphatemia, renal glycosuria, acidosis, and in some cases calcinosis. It is an affection of early life usually beginning within the first two years. Early signs are retarded development, loss of appetite, gastrointestinal disturbances, bouts of fever, and albumin and casts in the urine. The plasma phosphatase level is raised, and the excretion of calcium and phosphorus is excessive. Rachitic bowing of the legs and fractures may occur. Fanconi suggested that the condition is tubular renal rickets as opposed to glomerular renal rickets and results from hereditary inadequacy of the tubular epithelium, due to an autosomal recessive gene.

The Lignac-Fanconi Syndrome. This consists of a proximal tubular deficiency, with polydipsia, polyuria, anorexia, and vomiting. The children exhibit rickets as well as dwarfism and usually die before puberty. There is hyperphosphaturia with a low serum phosphate level but a normal calcium level, glycosuria which is sometimes accompanied by a mild ketonuria, and marked aminoaciduria, as well. The primary lesion appears to be an impaired resorption of glucose and phosphate because of some failure of phosphorylation in the tubules. Massive dosages of vitamin D may improve the skeletal disorder. Abnormal deposition of cystine crystals in the cornea, spleen, and lymph nodes gives the syndrome the name *cystinosis.*

Renal, or Hyperchloremic, Acidosis. In this condition, the primary defect is in the distal tubules, which fail to resorb water and to secrete ammonium. As well as excreting large amounts of water containing sodium, potassium, and calcium, there is a marked disturbance in the acid-base mechanism of the body with severe loss of bicarbonate and a corresponding retention of chlorides. The skeletal changes of either osteitis fibrosa or rickets are caused by the excessive mobilization of calcium from bone in response to the acidosis. This condition can be improved by administering excessive alkalizing salts, such as ammonium or calcium chlorides, and vitamin D.

Vitamin D–resistant Rickets, or "Phosphate Diabetes." As described by Fanconi and Girardet, this is characterized by a failure of phosphate resorption with a marked hyperphosphaturia and hypophosphatemia. Accompanying this, there is also excessive fecal loss of calcium leading to the typical changes of rickets in children or osteomalacia in adults. There appears to be some relationship between the resorption of bone as seen in von Recklinghausen's neurofibromatosis and that seen in this entity. Unlike vitamin D deficiency rickets, this form requires massive doses of vitamin D (i.e., 50,000 to 100,000 units) daily, which are thought to potentiate the diminished alkaline phosphatase required for transport of the phosphate ions within the tubules. These children tend to survive into adulthood, when they can present features of osteomalacia with reduction in the intestinal absorption of calcium and phosphates and, therefore, the possibility of a disturbed vitamin D metabolism.

Radiologic Findings. The diaphysis is osteoporotic, with the epiphysis broad and irregular. The metaphysis is broadened and its extremity uneven and ragged, like those seen in rickets.

In other forms the metaphysis is grossly enlarged, irregularly honeycombed or stippled or woolly, with subperiosteal resorption.

Calcification occurs in the kidneys with irregularities of the renal pelvis and ureters noted on pyelography. Calcium deposits in the kidney, with or without calculus formation, are usually more common in hyperparathyroidism than in chronic nephritis.

HYPOPHOSPHATASIA

This is an inherited rachitic disease which was first described by Rathbun in 1948 as a markedly impaired mineralization of the long bones and skull. The blood shows increased calcium, phosphorus, and nonprotein nitrogen levels, but a reduced alkaline phosphatase level. McCance et al. and Fraser et al. have shown that there is a large urinary excretion of phosphoethanoline without the other amino acids commonly seen in renal rickets.

Radiologically and pathologically, the lesion suggests severe rickets.

The metabolic defect lies in the osteoblast, which fails to secrete alkaline phosphatase. Severe metabolic disturbances are less marked after the age of sixteen or seventeen, with less liability to tetany, because the demand for calcium in ossification is much reduced. There may be remissions associated with improvement in kidney function and better excretion of phosphate. However, the ultimate prognosis for life depends on the renal pathologic condition, because of the liability of these patients to intercurrent infections. The occurrence of bone deformities is itself grave, and the average duration of life after their appearance is said to be less than 2 years. Therefore operative interference is directed toward restoring kidney function.

Where there is a congenital lesion of the renal tract, such as a posterior urethral valve, early surgical removal of the obstruction may be lifesaving. Surgical intervention, if it is to be successful, must be undertaken before puberty.

In hyperchloremic renal acidosis and nephrocalcinosis, an organic acid such as citric acid should be given in conjunction with sodium citrate to aid absorption of calcium from the intestines. Vitamin D should also be given in those cases to help calcification of the skeleton. In the active stage of the osteodystrophy, weight bearing should be prevented, and splints may be applied to limit deformity until spontaneous remission of the disease occurs.

Osteomalacia

Osteomalacia is a metabolic disease of adult bone in which there is a deficient mineralization of the bony matrix due to the lowered concentration of calcium or phosphorus or both in the body fluids. The diagnosis should be suspected in any patient with radiographic changes of osteoporosis or reduced skeletal mass. Reduced serum calcium or phosphorus may result from reduced dietary intake, impaired absorption from the gastrointestinal tract, increased renal excretion, or lack of vitamin D. Accompanying such change there is a generalized increase in the amount of osteoid, i.e., uncalcified, tissue.

PATHOLOGY. All the bones of the skeleton show decrease in bone density and strength. Frequently the bones are grossly deformed. The trabeculae are attenuated or absent, and the interstices of the spongy bone are filled with vascular or fibrofatty connective tissue, or osteoid tissue. Osteoclastic activity is marked and Howship's lacunae enlarged. The skeleton may become deformed, but bones subjected to muscular strains or to the influence of posture or gravity are the most grossly disturbed. The lower limb bones are therefore more affected than the arm bones, and curvatures of the femur and tibia, i.e., coxa vara, are common. Kyphosis is also frequent. Changes in the pelvis result from pressure of the femoral heads medially with displacement of the acetabula. The angle of the pubic symphysis therefore becomes more acute, and the pubis projects as a sharp beak. The sacral promontory rotates forward under the body weight to assume a trefoil shape. The rib deformities are similar to those of rickets. In some cases multiple almost symmetric radiotranslucent bands of diminished density resembling fractures appear in the cortex of the bone. A characteristic x-ray finding is that of Looser's zones or pseudofractures which are commonly seen in the tibia, in the ribs, or in the pelvic rami as translucent lines extending a short distance through the cortex.

The blood chemistry examination usually shows little deviation from normal values for calcium, but there may be reduced serum phosphorus as well as increased serum alkaline phosphatase.

OSTEOMALACIA OF PREGNANCY. In the late months of pregnancy large amounts of calcium are required for the fetal skeleton, and during lactation there is added excretion of calcium in the milk. However, the essential causative factors are a lack of sufficient calcium in the diet to supply the additional requirements or insufficient amount of vitamin D to permit the absorption of sufficient calcium.

STARVATION OSTEOMALACIA. This form is occasionally observed in circumstances of great food deprivation. It is due partly to an absolute lack of calcium in the diet and partly to avitaminosis.

OSTEOMALACIA OF IDIOPATHIC STEATORRHEA. In this disease there are fatty stools, dilatation of the colon, and anemia. Beginning in infancy, there is disturbance of skeletal development, i.e., celiac rickets with inability to absorb calcium as a result of the excess of free fatty acid in the bowel. At any time in the course of the disease, if the supply of calcium for absorption is insufficient for general requirements, the deficiency may be made good by withdrawing calcium from the bones, so that increased bone absorption occurs, resulting in osteomalacia.

The most common symptom is backache in association with a reduction in height from spinal collapse. There is also great muscular weakness, which may simulate paresis, especially where atrophy is present as well. The muscular hypotonicity may lead to an uncertain, feeble gait.

X-ray appearances of the vertebrae show wedge-shaped bodies or, more characteristically, fishtail-shaped bodies with marked biconcavity and enlarged disks. The vertebrae are most compressed in the lumbar region.

MILKMAN'S SYNDROME. Multiple spontaneous idiopathic symmetric fractures were described by Milkman in 1931. These are now considered not to be a disease entity but rather a clinical description of a condition revealed by x-ray examination and encountered in cases of demineralization of the skeleton. It occurs in association with osteomalacia, hunger osteopathies, celiac disease, idiopathic steatorrhea, and even severe rickets.

The syndrome is more common in females and occurs in adult life from ages twenty to sixty. The cause is usually osteomalacia. The onset is slow and insidious with periods of intermission. The patient suffers from back pain and tenderness before there is any x-ray evidence.

The bones are less dense than normal. The pseudofractures are inclined to be symmetric and have special and distinctive features. In addition to being seen in the long bones they are found at sites seldom if ever affected by fracture except from trauma, e.g., the rami of the pubis and ischium and the scapulae. In a typical Looser zone the clear band is not a mere line but one of considerable width, even as much as 1 cm. There is no callus and no sclerosis.

Parathyroid Osteodystrophy (Osteitis Fibrosa, or Von Recklinghausen's Disease)

The disease is caused by an increased secretion of parathormone, which stimulates the excretion of phosphate so that the serum phosphate level falls and the serum calcium level rises with mobilization of calcium phosphate from the bones. The excess of calcium is excreted along with the phosphate in the urine, and more calcium phosphate is resorbed from the bones. Parathormone also acts directly on the osteoclastic activity of bone. Many of the clinical features of hyperparathyroidism are discussed in Chap. 38, but certain aspects of the skeletal involvement will be discussed in this section.

PATHOLOGY. Skeletal changes consist of progressive absorption of the bones, and deformity, along with new bone formation. There are also collections of giant cells (osteoclastomas) and the formation of cysts containing a thin, brownish fluid.

Histologically, the significant change is the osteoclastic activity. The Haversian canals are enlarged into big irregular spaces lined by a zone of osteoclasts lying in lacunae in close apposition to the bone they are eroding. The spaces are filled with vascular tissue, with many capillaries, and endothelial cells, and as the bone is destroyed, spindle-shaped fibroblasts appear. Adjacent spaces eventually come to communicate with each other (Fig. 45-16).

New bone formation occurs in the mass of fibrous tissue, to form laminae of bone and osteoid.

Macroscopically, there are large reddish brown lesions which are made up of masses of giant cells, or osteoclasts, in a matrix of connective tissue. The distribution of the giant cell areas is of some significance. They are arranged in clusters around areas of hemorrhage or in relation to unabsorbed bony spicules, and their cytoplasm frequently contains red blood cells and hemosiderin.

It appears that in the stage of decalcification, the rapid removal of calcium is attended by marrow hemorrhages, probably as a result of damage to the capillary endothelium from the local concentration of calcium in the capillary vessels of the bone. It is only after the occurrence of the hemorrhage that the connective tissue proliferation and the giant cell accumulation are seen.

CLINICAL MANIFESTATIONS. The most common initial skeletal feature is increasing bone pain and tenderness felt especially in the lower limbs and back. Usually the pain is associated with general weakness and accompanied by pallor and debility. Hypotonia and muscular weakness are common. There may be a fracture from trivial injury, taking a long time to heal, often in a position of deformity. Occasionally, the development of a "brown tumor," in the maxilla or the mandible, may be the earliest evidence. Anorexia and nausea, vomiting, and abdominal cramps are common, and occasionally renal colic due to the development of a renal calculus may occur.

Radiologic Findings. The radiologic appearance consists chiefly of irregular diffuse osteoporosis with absorption of the compact bone and cystlike degeneration (Fig. 45-17). In the skull the bones show a well-marked stippling, but the opaque areas are pinhead in size, distinguishing them from the grosser mottling of Paget's disease. The vertebrae are less dense and show central collapse, the upper and lower surfaces being concave, and bulging of the intervertebral discs. The pelvis shows coarse striations among which large, clear cystlike spaces are usually visible. The earliest changes occur in the hand, the skull, and the outer end of the clavicle.

Fig. 45-16. Photomicrograph from a bone biopsy of a patient, showing the attenuated trabecular patterns with increased filling of the opened-up spaces by fibroblasts, capillaries, and endothelial cells. (×25.)

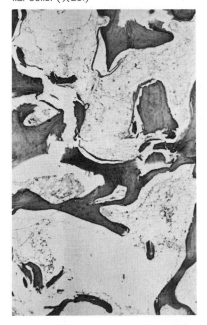

The femur shows loss of trabeculation. Deformity is common—coxa vara, bowing, and cystlike spaces may be present at the extremities and in the middle of the shaft. Over the cysts the bone may show a slight fusiform enlargement in the long as well as the short bones of the hand and foot.

Loss of the lamina dura around the teeth and severe demineralization of the distal ends of the clavicles, and tufts of the fingers are characteristic though not irreversible changes.

DIFFERENTIAL DIAGNOSIS OF BONE LESIONS (Table 45-4). **Senile Osteoporosis.** In this condition, the blood calcium level is normal, and the age of onset is late, in contradistinction to fibrocystic disease. Nevertheless, the tendency to fracture, deformity, and bone pain may lead to some confusion, and the radiographic bone changes are

not dissimilar to the changes of the milder forms of hyperparathyroidism.

Osteitis Deformans. The occasional occurrence of cysts and of hypercalcemia may render it difficult to distinguish from parathyroid osteodystrophy. The radiologic appearances, the age of onset, and the absence of blood changes will lead to a correct diagnosis.

Osteomalacia. In this disease there is deformity of the bones rather than fracture, the serum calcium level is low, and there is rapid response to vitamin D therapy.

Multiple Myeloma. The radiologic appearance of multiple myeloma may simulate closely the appearance of parathyroid osteodystrophy, especially in the collapse of the vertebrae, the occurrence of punctate areas of diminished density in the skull and long bones, and fine mottling of the pelvic bones. The blood calcium/phosphorus ratio is

Table 45-4. POINTS IN DIFFERENTIAL DIAGNOSIS BETWEEN HYPERPARATHYROIDISM AND OTHER BONE DISEASES

| Disease | Differential points | | | Serum | | Alkaline phosphatase‡ | Miscellaneous |
	Symptoms	X-ray appearance	Biopsy	Calcium*	Phosphorus†		
Hyperparathyroidism with bone involvement	Bone pain, deformity, fracture, tumor; polyuria; symptoms related to stones	Increased radiability; generalized deformity; cysts; tumors; fractures; stones	Rarified bone; fibrosis of marrow; osteoclasts + + +; osteoid tissue only slightly increased; osteoblasts + + +	High	Low	High	All age groups
"Senile" osteoporosis	No bone tumor, polyuria, or stones	No cysts, tumors, or stones	No fibrosis of marrow; osteoclasts normal; osteoid tissue normal or decreased; osteoblasts decreased	Normal	Normal or low	Normal	Old age
Paget's disease	Bones enlarged; no polyuria; stones infrequent	Polyostotic but not generalized; bones hypertrophied, e.g., thickened skull	May occasionally be difficult or impossible to differentiate	Normal or slightly high	Normal or slightly high	Very high	Runs in families; predilection for weight-bearing bones; seldom seen in patients under 40; arteriosclerosis + + +
Osteomalacia	No bone tumor, polyuria, or stones	No tumors or stones; bending deformities + + +	Osteoid tissue + + +; osteoblasts + +; osteoclasts decreased	Normal or low	Low	High	Virtually absent in this country except with fatty diarrhea
"Solitary" cysts	Confined to cysts	No generalized changes; cysts may be multiple	Cannot differentiate if taken from lesion	Normal	Normal	Normal	
Solitary benign giant cell tumor	Confined to tumor	No generalized changes	Cannot differentiate if taken from lesion	Normal	Normal	Normal	
Osteogenesis imperfecta	Fractures + + +; no bone tumor, polyuria, or stones	Cysts rare; no tumors or stones	No fibrosis of marrow; osteoclasts normal	Normal	Normal	Normal or very slightly elevated	Hereditary, often coupled with blue sclera and deafness; improves after cessation of growth
Multiple myeloma	Can cause some bone symptoms and renal symptoms	Can be almost indistinguishable	Tumor tissue	Normal or high	Normal or high	Normal	Bence Jones proteinuria

*Normal values for calcium 9–11 mg/100 ml.
†Normal values for phosphorus 2.5–5 mg/100 ml.
‡Normal values for alkaline phosphates 35–80 I.U./liter.
SOURCE: After Albright. Taken with permission from W. Mercer and R. B. Duthie, "Orthopaedic Surgery," 7th ed., Edward Arnold (Publishers) Ltd., London, 1974.

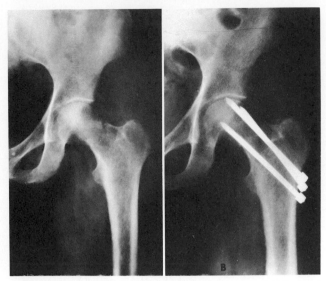

Fig. 45-17. *A*. X-ray of pelvis and upper femur of a middle-aged woman who presented with a stress fracture of the femoral neck and a serum calcium level of 12 mg/100 ml. *B*. X-ray of the same patient after internal fixation of pathologic fracture with three Knowles pins.

as a rule normal, while an abnormal protein—the Bence Jones proteose—may appear in the urine. A raised blood protein level frequently results in a raised total blood calcium level, but the diffusible fraction is usually normal. A biopsy may be required.

Diagnosis of parathyroid osteodystrophy depends upon the demonstration of hypercalcemia and hypophosphatemia in association with characteristic bone changes. In late hyperparathyroidism, renal damage may result in a rise in the renal phosphate threshold and a consequent rise in the blood phosphate level with a lowering of the blood calcium level. Hypercalcinuria also frequently accompanies parathyroid osteodystrophy but may also be seen in osteolysis of bone in malignant conditions, multiple myeloma, and sarcoidosis, in immobilization for chronic diseases, in hypervitaminosis D, and in renal rickets.

TREATMENT. Parathyroidectomy is the treatment of the basic disorder. Following this procedure the prognosis is generally good with immediate relief of bone pain and gain in weight and in strength of the bones. Orthopedic treatment is directed toward adequate protection of the softened bones with reduction in all deforming stresses and strains. After the disease has been arrested and recalcification of bone has taken place, any established deformity can be corrected by osteotomy or other measures.

Osteoporosis

This condition has been defined by Sissons as a structural change in bone whereby the supporting tissue is reduced in amount but remains highly mineralized. Albright and Reifenstein have pointed out that it is a disorder of protein metabolism which is reflected in abnormal trabeculae formation, but the metabolism of calcium is normal, and the trabeculae present are normally calcified.

Because of this definition Cooke, in a complete review of this subject, has emphasized how osteoporosis must be clearly differentiated from such terms as "decalcification," in which the radiologic or postmortem appearance of the bones is deficient in minerals, or "halisteresis," in which the bone mineral is removed to leave only a proteinlike structure in osteoid tissue, or "uncalcified matrix," an artificial state which does not occur naturally.

ETIOLOGY. Osteoporosis is a response of the bony skeleton to a variety of factors.

Mechanical Factors. Mechanical factors are those of immobilization of the whole body or a part of it for the treatment of fractures, prolonged postoperative bed rest, tuberculosis, etc. Osteoporosis can result from conditions such as anterior poliomyelitis, rheumatoid arthritis, and traumatic paraplegia. The condition is general or local. Accompanying muscle loss and osteoporosis is a negative nitrogen balance, resulting from an increased urinary excretion of nitrogen.

Nutritional Factors. Severe protein deficiency resulting from malnutrition or failure in absorption or abnormal protein excretion can result in osteoporosis. With such a deficiency, the calcium and phosphorus intake is reduced and forms part of the circumstances leading to senile osteoporosis. Scurvy due to deficiency in vitamin C can also produce osteoporosis.

Endocrine Factors. Osteoporosis is a common complication in Cushing's syndrome, of a basophil adenoma of the pituitary, or in disease of the adrenal cortex. These give rise to an excess of the antianabolic S hormone, or glucocorticoid hormone, which also acts on sugar metabolism. The adrenal corticoids are considered to withdraw amino acids from protein synthesis, during glyconeogenesis, with disturbance in *matrix formation*. Accompanying the generalized osteoporosis are other endocrine changes such as sexual characteristics, obesity, and diabetes mellitus.

In von Recklinghausen's disease, with hyperparathyroidism resulting from an adenoma, as an early manifestation there may be osteoporosis of the skull and spine, before the appearance of the fibrocystic lesions, osteoclastomas, and stone formation.

Postmenopausal osteoporosis may result from ovarian insufficiency with diminution in estrogen secretion. That there is some sex hormonal factor in this condition may be inferred from the much higher incidence for women.

In other endocrine diseases, such as acromegaly and gigantism, or in the hypothyroidism of cretinism or myxedema in which there is excessive utilization of nitrogen-containing substances for caloric needs, reduction in matrix formation and osteoporosis occur.

Thyrotoxic Osteoporosis. In thyrotoxicosis there is a marked increase in the general metabolism with an associated nitrogen loss to produce osteoporosis. Krane et al., by radioactive calcium studies, have shown both increased bone resorption and increased bone formation in this state. Biochemically, there is hypercalcinuria with a negative calcium balance and increased serum phosphorus and alkaline phosphatase concentrations. In hyperthyroidism, the serum calcium and phosphorus levels are normal, but there is exaggerated excretion, sometimes to as much as eight times the normal. In association with this, the bones undergo marked rarefaction, through increased osteoclastic activity, and eventually become so weak that spontaneous fractures occur. Apart from definite fractures, deformities may arise from weight bearing or from muscular action. Thus kyphosis or scoliosis and pelvic asymmetry may be present. Deformity is less common in the long bones.

Other Factors. Other pathologic conditions in which the normal bone architecture is replaced, e.g., myelomatosis and tumor invasion, are etiologic factors in osteoporosis.

PATHOLOGY. There is reduction in the thickness of the cortex, especially of the endosteal surfaces, the intermedullary contents being made up of a yellow and fatty cancellous bone tissue. On microradiography of undecalcified bone specimens, a reduction is seen in the number and size of the trabeculae and in the number of osteoblasts present. This results in a marked reduction in the mechanical strength of the involved bone, which therefore is fractured or crushed by minor trauma.

Fundamentally, there appears to be a disturbance of the normal balance between *bone formation* (osteoblastic activity) and bone resorption (osteoclastic activity). Osteoblastic activity is greatest during growth and repair of bone but is also stimulated by physical activity. However, in osteoporosis there appears to be a decrease in osteoblastic activity with the usual bone resorption of the osteons, leading to a state of imbalance. Nordin describes how there is a mineral loss as well as resorption of matrix to give a negative calcium balance but no real evidence of impaired osteoblastic activity. This negative calcium balance is seen in calcium intake deficiency, faulty resorption, faulty mobilization and transport of calcium, or excessive loss of phosphorus. It also may be accompanied by a negative nitrogen balance.

CLINICAL MANIFESTATIONS. Most patients are in the senile and postmenopausal groups. The other forms of osteoporosis are usually discovered incidentally to the main disease process, by radiology. Pathologic fractures, especially of the femoral neck, commonly arise because of this condition.

Pain is in the nature of a lumbar backache which radiates around the trunk or down the lower limbs. It is aggravated by movement or jarring, and although suggestive of a nerve root compression, this is rarely seen. Acute sudden onset of pain with localized tenderness in the chest or back is most suggestive of a pathologic fracture of a rib or vertebral body.

Loss of height may have been noted by the patient, with the appearance of a thoracic kyphosis and an approximation of the rib margin to the iliac crests.

Radiologic Findings. The involved bone has a "ground glass" appearance (a late manifestation) because of loss of definition of the trabeculae. In the spine, the vertebral bodies become flattened but biconcave with increase in the intervertebral spaces. Varying degrees of collapse and wedging may be seen (Fig. 45-18). Healing of the pathologic fracture is usually accompanied by little callus formation.

Biochemistry. The serum calcium, phosphorus, and alkaline phosphatase levels are within normal limits. The total

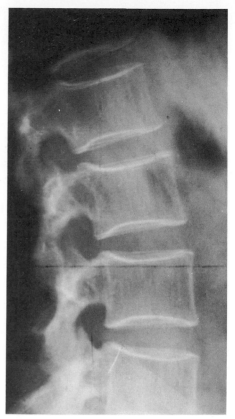

Fig. 45-18. X-ray of the spine of a patient with osteoporosis. Note the "ground glass" appearance, biconcavity of vertebral bodies, and increase in the intervertebral spaces.

plasma protein and plasma albumin levels may be low, but this is of little value from the diagnostic aspect. A measurement of urinary calcium excretion over a 24-hour period may be of some help, particularly if the daily intake can be estimated.

Biopsy. Specimens can be obtained by trephining from the iliac crest or the spinous processes of the lumbar vertebrae and are of value.

DIFFERENTIAL DIAGNOSIS. *Osteomalacia* is a condition of hypocalcification which radiologically may resemble osteoporosis but results from a failure in calcification of the bone matrix due to a calcium and vitamin D deficiency. The plasma phosphorus level is lowered with an increase in the serum alkaline phosphatase.

As a general rule, osteoporosis is seen in the spine and pelvis with frequent pathologic fracturing, whereas osteomalacia is more commonly seen in the extremities, with more deformity than fractures and osteofibritis. Osteitis fibrosa is particularly common in the skull.

Secondary osteoporosis of other diseases such as hyperparathyroidism, either primary or secondary, Cushing's syndrome, and acromegaly can be identified by the features of the primary disease. Metastatic carcinoma, multiple myeloma, and rheumatoid arthritis with excessive corticoid therapy are also included in the differential diagnosis.

TREATMENT. *Ambulation* must be encouraged and support given to the diseased spine in the form of a light plaster jacket or a brace, or to the pathologic fracture of the femur by a walking non-weight-bearing caliper. Internal fixation is sound in principle because of the loss in mechanical strength of the surrounding bone. A high-protein-high-calcium diet should be prescribed.

Hormonal Therapy. Estrogen therapy has been shown to produce hyperossification in animals. It can be given as 1 mg/day orally or by injection as estrogen dipropionate, 2 mg/day, for a period of 4 weeks with a following rest of 2 weeks before recommencing the drug. This may produce uterine bleeding, which is an indication to stop treatment.

Androgen therapy has been shown to produce an increase in the bone matrix, body weight, and musculature. Because of this Cooke recommends administering testosterone propionate, 10 to 20 mg/day, by injection or methyltestosterone, 30 mg/day, by mouth in combination with the estrogens. The latter combination may prevent the masculinizing effects of the androgen.

Hormonal administration can induce both a positive nitrogen and calcium balance and improvement in matrix and bone formation, but the side effects have proved to be difficult and disturbing. A more recent anabolic hormone—methandrostenolane, or Dianabol, appears to have greater potency in doses as low as 2.5 to 5 mg/day. A weekly measurement of the body weight is recommended to check for edema. Therapy is still very controversial but is required to decrease bone resorption and/or increase bone formation. Calcitonin and the diphosphonates have not proved useful. The estrogens, synthetic anabolic hormones, calcium, and any such combinations are believed only to slow the progression of bone loss. Combinations of fluorides, calcium, and vitamin D may enhance bone formation.

Pituitary Disturbances

The anterior lobe of the pituitary gland, by its secretion of the thyrotropic, adrenocorticotropic, and gonadotropic hormones, "controls" the activity of the thyroid, adrenal cortex, and sex glands. However, there is the reciprocal relationship of feedback, or control by the amount of circulating hormone, as well as indirect relationships of the hormones to each other. In addition to this endocrine control there is the integration of the endocrines with the nervous system by the hypothalamus.

The *anterior lobe* of the pituitary is made up of:

Clear chromophobe cells ⟶   Acidophil cells   Basophil cells
              ↓   ╱   ╲ |
Hypopituitarism (by pressure)   Hypersecretion   Hyposecretion   Hypersecretion
                                      | | |
                                 Gigantism or   Infantilism   Cushing's syndrome
                                 acromegaly   ╱   ╲
                                         Lorain's or Froehlich's syndrome
                                                    |
                                            Simmonds' disease

The *posterior lobe* is made up of neurologic cells and fibers which are connected to the supraoptic nuclei of the hypothalamus. Secretion of oxytocin or vasopressin from

the posterior lobe of the pituitary does not appear to have any direct effect upon osseous tissues.

PITUITARY DWARFISM

The term *dwarf* is applied to an individual whose physical dimensions are less than those peculiar to his race.

There are two main types:

1. *Froehlich's adiposogenital type,* in which skeletal stunting is associated with general obesity, genital hypoplasia, and often stupidity or idiocy.
2. The *Lorain type,* in which there is no mental change and no physical change except lack of skeletal growth; i.e., children with Lorain's syndrome are "attractive and graceful children."

The usual cause of hypopituitarism is a tumor or cyst (suprasellar cyst) compressing and destroying the gland. In some cases where the dwarfing is already present at birth, there is said to be aplasia of the gland, or a failure of differentiation of the eosinophil cells.

PATHOLOGY. The growth of all parts of the skeleton is delayed or arrested. The epiphyses remain ununited for a prolonged period, and the metaphysis terminates in a line of dense bone. The histologic change is an absence of division of the cartilage cells in endochondral bone and absence of division of the primitive connective tissue cells in the membrane bones.

DIAGNOSIS. The differential diagnosis of dwarfism, or reduction in all structural diameters, which can be made before the age of five years includes (1) achondroplasia (usually inherited and present at birth), (2) osteogenesis imperfecta, (3) chondroosteodystrophy, (4) pituitary dwarfism, (5) renal dwarfism, (6) nutritional dwarfism—steatorrhea, rickets, and (7) cretinism.

HYPERPITUITARY SYNDROMES

Gigantism

This condition begins before the epiphyses have closed, and there is an increase both in the rate of epiphyseal growth and in the maturation of the skeleton. The mental development is subnormal and the body strength often surprisingly slight. In the majority of cases some of the features of acromegaly develop later.

Pathology. The bones of the skeleton show increased thickness and length; the membrane bones are also hypertrophied.

At the epiphyseal cartilage growth of the cartilage cells is active, but the orderly palisade arrangement is lost, the cells being arranged in irregular groups. The amount of matrix is increased. The number of vascular buds and of advancing osteogenic cells is increased.

Acromegaly

The manifestations of acromegaly appear after skeletal growth has ceased, and the disease is characterized by an unevenly distributed exaggeration of ossification, due to the effects of local pressure and traction.

Acromegaly results from abnormal secretion of the eosinophil cells of the anterior lobe of the pituitary, with either hyperplasia or a tumor—an eosinophil adenoma.

Pathology. Abnormal bone formation occurs in the alveolar margins of the jaws, leading to great elongation of the face and projection of the chin, but the ramus of the jaw is narrow and elongated. The malar bones and the vault of the skull may be thickened. The skull change begins or is most marked in the frontal bone, and the deposits or osteomas grow from the inner table of the skull. The foramen magnum is usually displaced forward and the pituitary fossa enlarged from the presence of the adenoma.

The thorax is massive, because of the increased length of the ribs, which is partly the result of the exaggerated bone growth and partly the result of the hypertrophy of the lungs.

In the long bones the most obvious changes are found toward the extremities, which are more massive than normal and less well modeled. Muscular insertions and tuberosities and ridges are usually accentuated.

The short long bones are thick and usually elongated. Muscular and tendinous insertions are again prominent, and at the articular ends lipping may be pronounced.

In the vertebral column there is new subperiosteal bone, which is thickest on the anterior surface of the body and gradually diminishes as the body is traced around to the vertebral canal. This phenomenon is occasionally referred to as *acromegalic spondylitis.*

Acromegalic arthritis may affect any of the limb or spinal joints. In osteoarthrosis the earliest change consists of attenuation and ultimate disappearance of the articular cartilage at the points of greatest pressure. In acromegaly, articular cartilage thickens under the stimulus of growth hormone and subsequently degenerates.

Congenital Hypothyroidism (Cretinism)

When the thyroid gland is completely absent (athyrosis) or is destroyed in early infancy by disease, cretinism with decrease in cartilage proliferation and osteoblastic activity is produced.

The prominent features of cretinism are signs of mental deficiency, anomalies in genital growth, and generalized growth disturbances.

The cretin is a dwarf because of delayed ossification and retardation in growth and skeletal maturation. The long bones are short, while the ossification of the skull is delayed, and the fontanel closes late—as late, sometimes, as at twenty years. The root of the nose is depressed, from defective growth of the base of the skull. The vault of the skull may appear large in comparison with the body.

The principal skeletal changes are the late appearance of the epiphyses and of bones whose ossific nuclei develop after birth, e.g., the carpal and the tarsal bones, and delayed union of the epiphyses.

The shafts of the long bones appear short, with a thick cortex, but their caliber is diminished. Toward the extremities of the bones the size more nearly approximates the normal. The epiphyses are not only late in appearing but are small and often irregular in ossification, appear fragmented, and show a superficial resemblance to those of a patient with osteochondritis.

There may be delay or arrest in fusion between the two halves of the neural arch or the neurocentral synchondrosis, with disturbance of normal ossification of the vertebral bodies.

The administration of thyroid extract is curative if treatment is begun in infancy. It is interesting to note that since epiphyseal fusion is delayed, the administration of thyroid may produce growth in stature even of the adult.

Mucopolysaccharidoses

Abnormalities of mucopolysaccharide metabolism result in skeletal deformities in addition to involvement of other systems including the central nervous, cardiovascular, and reticuloendothelial systems. McKusick has reviewed the inheritance of the various disorders and correlated the clinical findings with the biochemical abnormalities (Table 45-5).

DIAGNOSIS. Chondroitin sulfate A accounts for 80 percent of normally excreted urinary mucopolysaccharide; chondroitin sulfate B, 10 percent; and heparitin sulfate, 10 percent. Approximately 3 to 15 mg is excreted each 24 hours. Excessive excretion of any of the above or the presence of keratosulfaturia is abnormal.

Metachromatic granules may be present in circulating leukocytes, lymphocytes, and bone marrow cells and should be investigated.

Mucopolysaccharidosis I (Hurler Syndrome). This rare condition, inherited as an autosomal recessive trait, is recognizable in infancy or early childhood. There is severe mental deterioration, dwarfism, and clouding of the corneas. Hepatosplenomegaly is present. The skull is large with a saddle-like nose. The tongue is large and lips are patulous with mouth open (gargoyle facies). The neck is short, and the dorsal spine has a kyphosis with a gibbus at the dorsal lumbar area. The abdomen is protuberant and the lower thorax flared as a result of the hepatosplenomegaly. X-ray examination of the spine shows wedge-shaped bodies with anterior beaking. Varus or valgus knees and foot deformities are frequently present, and joints are stiff. Radiographic changes in the extremities include expansion of the medullary cavity, cortical thinning, and shortened phalanges. The fundamental defect is an abnormality of metabolism of heparitin sulfate and chondroitin sulfate B.

Mucopolysaccharidosis II (Hunter Syndrome). The Hunter syndrome is inherited as a sex-linked recessive trait with abnormality of mucopolysaccharide metabolism similar to that of the Hurler syndrome. The disease is clinically similar although less severe in all aspects including dwarfing, hepatosplenomegaly, and the gargoyle facies.

Table 45-5. THE GENETIC MUCOPOLYSACCHARIDOSES (as classified in 1972)

Designation	Clinical features	Genetics	Excessive urinary MPS	Substance deficient
MPS I H Hurler syndrome	Early clouding of cornea, grave manifestations, death usually before age 10	Homozygous for MPS I H gene	Dermatan sulfate Heparan sulfate	α-L-iduronidase (formerly called Hurler corrective factor)
MPS I S Scheie syndrome	Stiff joints, cloudy cornea, aortic regurgitation, normal intelligence, normal life span	Homozygous for MPS I S gene	Dermatan sulfate Heparan sulfate	α-L-iduronidase
MPS I H/S Hurler-Scheie compound	Phenotype intermediate between Hurler and Scheie	Genetic compound of MPS I H and I S genes	Dermatan sulfate Heparan sulfate	α-L-iduronidase
MPS II A Hunter syndrome, severe	No clouding of cornea, milder course than in MPS I H but death usually before age 15	Hemizygous for X-linked gene	Dermatan sulfate Heparan sulfate	Hunter corrective factor
MPS II B Hunter syndrome, mild	Survival to 30's to 50's, fair intelligence	Hemizygous for X-linked allele for mild form	Dermatan sulfate Heparan sulfate	Hunter corrective factor
MPS III A Sanfilippo syndrome A	Identical phenotype: Mild somatic, severe nervous system effects	Homozygous for Sanfilippo A gene	Heparan sulfate	Heparan sulfate sulfatase
MPS III B Sanfilippo syndrome B		Homozygous for Sanfilippo B (at different locus)	Heparan sulfate	N-acetyl-α-D-glucosaminidase
MPS IV Morquio syndrome (probably more than one allelic form)	Severe bone changes of distinctive type, cloudy cornea, aortic regurgitation	Homozygous for Morquio gene	Keratan sulfate	Unknown
MPS V Vacant				
MPS VI A Maroteaux-Lamy syndrome, classic form	Severe osseous and corneal change, normal intellect	Homozygous for M-L gene	Dermatan sulfate	Maroteaux-Lamy corrective factor
MPS VI B Maroteaux-Lamy syndrome, mild form	Severe osseous and corneal change, normal intellect	Homozygous for allele at M-L locus	Dermatan sulfate	Maroteaux-Lamy corrective factor
MPS VII β-glucoronidase deficiency (more than one allelic form?)	Hepatosplenomegaly, dysostosis multiplex, white cell inclusions, mental retardation	Homozygous for mutant gene at β-glucoronidase locus	Dermatan sulfate	β-glucoronidase

SOURCE: Taken with permission from V. A. McKusick, "Heritable Disorders of Connective Tissue," 4th ed., The C. V. Mosby Company, St. Louis, 1972.

Mental deterioration is slower, and there is neither the lumbar gibbus nor the clouding of the cornea. Patients may survive well into the thirties.

Mucopolysaccharidosis III (Sanfilippo Syndrome). This syndrome is rare, inherited as an autosomal recessive trait, and associated with excessive production of urinary heparitin sulfate. Severe mental retardation is the predominant finding, although skeletal changes may be present. Stiffness in the joints occurs, but dwarfing may be mild. Corneal clouding has not been reported.

Mucopolysaccharidosis IV (Morquio-Brailsford Syndrome, Chondroosteodystrophy). This syndrome, inherited as an autosomal recessive trait, was described independently in 1929 by both Morquio and Brailsford. The defect is an abnormality in keratosulfate metabolism.

The patient appears normal at birth, but dwarfism becomes apparent within the first two years of life. Lumbar spinal changes are similar to those of the Hurler syndrome, are recognizable within the first year of life, and progress to flat or platyspondylitic vertebrae. Wrists are enlarged, and a pigeon-breasted thorax develops. Clouding of the cornea is progressive.

Radiographs of the long bones reveal shortening and wide metaphyses with increase in the thickness of epiphyseal and articular cartilages. Epiphyseal centers of ossification begin as multiple foci and become distorted, resulting in joint incongruity. Genu valgum and flatfoot with a posture of hip and knee flexion are common.

Mucopolysaccharidosis V (Scheie Syndrome). This is a rare variant of the Hurler syndrome, transmitted as an autosomal recessive and related to a defect in mucopolysaccharide metabolism of chondroitin sulfate B. Height is usually low-normal to normal, joints are stiff, and corneal clouding is the most striking finding. Intellect is normal or above normal.

Mucopolysaccharidosis VI (Maroteaux-Lamy Syndrome, Polydystrophic Dwarfism). In this syndrome the dominant findings are severe osseous abnormalities in the presence of normal intellect. Metaphyses are irregular and epiphyses deformed. Vertebral bodies are flattened and may be wedge-shaped. Hepatosplenomegaly, deafness, and corneal clouding are common.

It is apparent that there are other abnormalities of mucopolysaccharide metabolism, and as the biochemistry is clarified, other syndromes will be recognized and correlated. Current treatment for these conditions is based on empiric treatment of orthopedic deformities, although progress rests upon an exact understanding of the biochemical defect.

OSTEITIS DEFORMANS

Osteitis deformans was described in detail by Sir James Paget in 1876 and is often known as *Paget's disease*. The disease has a universal distribution in the human race but has also been identified in horses and monkeys.

ETIOLOGY. The origin of Paget's disease is not known. Paget believed it to be inflammatory in origin.

Brailsford regarded the disease as a primary localized vascular disturbance with a secondary adverse effect on the bone. Mercer and Duthie consider that the vascular disturbance is produced by some form of an arteriovenous malformation not yet demonstrated. They found an increase in the bone blood flow sufficient to produce circulatory disturbances compatible with those resulting from an arteriovenous shunt and high blood pressure. In such cases death from congestive heart failure is not an unusual occurrence. The basic lesion appears to be an acceleration of bone turnover with an associated increase in urinary hydroxyproline.

PATHOLOGY. The *bone changes* are characterized by thickening, softening, and deformity, and later by ossification. Knaggs described three stages in the pathology of the skull changes: In the first, or *vascular,* stage, there is a deposit of finely porous bone beneath the pericranium with permeation of a very vascular connective tissue. In the second stage, that of *advancing sclerosis,* the thickness of the skull is increased and the calvarial sutures obliterated. In the stage of *diffuse complete sclerosis* the condensed type of bone is present for the most part throughout the whole thickness of the calvaria.

In the *spine* there is thickening, with osteoporosis of the various parts, and as a consequence of the weight-bearing function some of the bodies may collapse. Secondary changes—synostosis of adjacent bodies, even ankylosis of a segment of the spine—are common. These changes may lead to marked reduction in stature. The thickening of the neural arch leads to a reduction in the caliber of the vertebral canal, which may reach a sufficient degree to give rise to evidence of spinal cord compression.

In the *long bones* there are marked resorption of bone and ingrowth of vascular connective tissue, which subsequently ossifies. The periosteum is normal. The thickening of the bone leads to irregularity on the surface, with marked reduction in the medullary cavity. In the stage of softening and enlargement the bone is apt to become deformed, partly because the soft bone yields to normal gravitational weight bearing or muscular stresses and partly, in the forearm and leg, because one bone may be more involved than its neighbor.

In the early stages of the disease there is a diffuse infiltration by young granulation tissue, and the trabeculae of the bone are attenuated. Howship's lacunae are enlarged and occupied by granulation tissue cells or osteoclasts. In the stage of osteogenic activity the sections show numerous trabeculae of new bone containing an irregular lamellar system which appears typically as a mosaic pattern (Fig. 45-19). These are elaborated from the connective tissue and are irregular in their distribution. They are so numerous that adjacent struts may fuse to enclose an irregular space, or lacuna, containing connective tissue.

CLINICAL MANIFESTATIONS. The disease usually begins between the ages of thirty-six and fifty years. Incidence in the sexes is equal. Pain in the lower limbs, thighs, or hips is often the initial feature and present in 30 percent of patients with this disease. It may be aggravated by exercise or be more pronounced at night. Gradual bowing of the legs and/or the development of a spinal curvature are common, with gait abnormality.

The circumference of the head may gradually increase. Headache and vertigo may result from the cranial thickening. Compression of the cranial nerves in the foramina appears when the lumen of the foramen is encroached upon with resulting auditory and visual disturbances. Spi-

Fig. 45-19. Microscopic section in Paget's disease (see text).

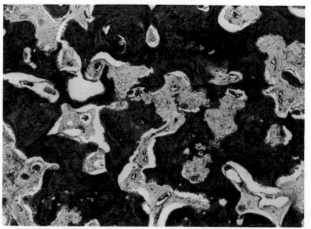

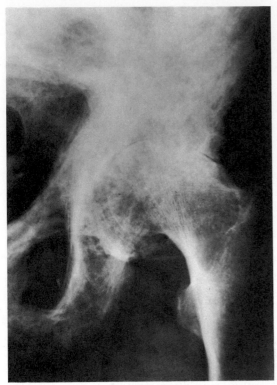

Fig. 45-20. X-ray of the pelvis and femur of a patient with Paget's disease.

nal cord compressions producing paraplegia have also been reported in a number of instances.

Trivial violence can result in spontaneous fractures, especially in the femur and the tibia. Development of osteogenic sarcoma in one of the affected bones may present as increased pain or pathologic fracturing.

Osteitis deformans usually begins in the monostotic form, most commonly in the tibia, but in 75 percent of cases this will progress to give the generalized, or polyostotic, form.

Radiologic Findings. The bones most commonly involved, in order of frequency, are the skull, tibia, femur, pelvis, radius, bones of the hand, bones of the foot, humerus, and ulna.

The earliest change in the *skull* is blurring of its surface outline, together with some flattening. New bone formation is irregular and appears as irregular islands of dense bone, giving the calvaria a mottled or coarsely piebald appearance. The base of the skull may show comparable changes.

Changes in the spine consist of a woolly appearance of the bodies, with coarse striae at the periphery and horizontal striae near the upper and lower surfaces. The bodies may be fatter and squatter than normal, and abnormal curvatures may be present.

The *pelvis* tends to assume a trefoil shape, as a result of the pressure of the femoral heads. The bone appears thick and massive, but the texture of the bone is altered; it now appears mottled and blurred, while occasionally

coarse striae are apparent throughout the cortex (Fig. 45-20).

The *long bones* are thickened from enlargement of the cortex. The natural curves of the bone are accentuated, but sometimes the deformities are more bizarre.

Fairbank has described four typical radiologic appearances which can be seen in most bones: (1) a honeycomb, or spongy, appearance, which is the commonest and most widespread manifestation; (2) a striated appearance, as seen in the pelvis, sacrum, and calcaneum; (3) a uniform and increased density, which is most frequently seen in the vertebrae; and (4) true cystic areas, as seen in the pelvis or long bones.

Laboratory Findings. The serum calcium and the serum phosphorus levels are usually normal, but there is a very high serum alkaline phosphatase content. The urinary excretion of calcium and phosphorus is on occasion increased, and pathologic calcification may occur in arterial walls and in the interventricular septum of the heart.

TREATMENT. No curative treatment of Paget's disease is known, and the most that can be done in the usual case is to relieve the pain. Radiotherapy is of benefit in alleviating the bone pain. Recently three drugs have been used for the relief of bone pain: (1) fluorides, which are effective only in doses producing other severe skeletal changes; (2) diphosphonates, which have been shown to produce rickets by blocking vitamin D metabolism; and (3) the calcitonins (porcine, salmon or human), which markedly reduce bone turnover, with minimal side effects.

Internal fixation by some form of intramedullary nailing for all fractures is worthwhile to relieve pain. Resection of sarcomas should be attempted and the area replaced by some form of prosthesis.

RETICULOSES

The cells forming the lining of the minute blood vascular channels of the bone marrow are part of the reticuloendothelial system. The other cellular elements of the system are certain adult connective tissue cells (fibrocytes), the endothelium lining blood and lymph vessels, the reticulum cells of the spleen, and certain of the large mononuclear cells of the blood.

The cells of the reticuloendothelial system are believed to be the scavengers of the body, and their activity is concerned mainly with the removal from the circulating fluid of dead and damaged cells, bacteria, and other foreign or noxious material. They are also energetic in the disposal of such metabolic substances as hemoglobin and cholesterol.

Red bone marrow consists of blood-forming cells as well as reticuloendothelial cells. Affections of any of these resulting in increased volume or vascularity will result in absorption of the adjacent bony trabeculae. In response to continued strain new bone is laid down to buttress the weak site. Hodgkin's disease usually affects the spine, skull, and pelvis; leukemia, the long bones; and chloroma, usually bones of the orbit.

In the adult the red marrow is confined to irregular or

flat bones or to the ends of long bones. It is here that malignant involvement and bony changes first occur.

The reticuloendothelial tissue of bone is found mainly at the ends of the long bones and in the spongy bone of the flat and short bones, and it is here that any affections occur most markedly.

RETICULOSES—DISEASES OF BONE MARROW CONSTITUENTS

A. Reticuloendothelial system
  1. Histiocytic granulomatosis
    a. Letterer-Siwe disease
    b. Eosinophilic granuloma
    c. Hand-Schüller-Christian disease
  2. Lipoid granulomatosis
    a. Gaucher's disease
    b. Niemann-Pick disease
    c. Xanthomatosis with hypercholesterolemia
B. Lymphatic system
  1. Hodgkin's disease
  2. Lymphosarcoma
C. Hematopoietic system
  1. Leukemia
    a. Lymphoblastic
    b. Myeloblastic
  2. Multiple myeloma
  3. Hemolytic anemia
    a. Mediterranean, or Cooley's, anemia
    b. Sickle cell anemia
    c. Erythroblastosis foetalis

Hodgkin's Disease

Autopsy records show that involvement of the bone marrow in Hodgkin's disease is more frequent than clinical studies would lead one to suspect.

PATHOLOGY. The bodies of the vertebral column and pelvis are the bones most often involved. The cancellous tissue of the upper end of the femur is also a common site. Of the other bones, the diploë of the skull, the ends of the tibia, the lower end of the femur, and the ends of the humerus are less commonly affected.

In the cancellous tissue and red marrow of the affected bone, an infiltrating mass of tissue with destruction of bone develops. In the vertebrae the destruction is usually so extreme that collapse of one or more of the bodies occurs. In the pelvis, areas of rarefaction are surrounded by areas of sclerosis, while in the skull the infiltration is predominantly osteolytic. In the ribs, complete destruction of the affected segment is the rule and is pathognomic. In the long bones there is often subperiosteal new bone formation which may be so marked that the lesion resembles chronic osteomyelitis. In other cases the lesion resembles a lymphosarcoma in which the lesions are purely osteolytic with invasion throughout bone.

CLINICAL MANIFESTATIONS. The sexes are equally liable, and age bears no relationship to the severity or the frequency of the bone changes. In most cases pain is the first indication of the osseous spread with delay in radiologic evidence. The pain is of a dull aching or lancinating character and may be so severe as to interfere with the function of the neighboring joints. In the spine there may be girdle pains, and in some cases evidences of cord compression have subsequently arisen. The bone changes have little or no effect on the constitutional course of the disease. Differential diagnosis includes lymphogranuloma of bone.

TREATMENT. In common with the other lesions of Hodgkin's disease the bone changes appear to respond to x-ray therapy. The pain is relieved, and in some cases reparative changes appear in the affected bones.

HISTIOCYTIC GRANULOMATOSIS

A combined syndrome is a more appropriate consideration, because the permanent and constant pathologic feature is the presence of numerous histiocytes and granulomatous tissue (Table 45-6). Anatomically the underlying lesion in eosinophilic granuloma is related to the lesion of Hand-Schüller-Christian disease and that of Letterer-Siwe disease. These three conditions have been described as different clinicoanatomic expressions of the same disorder.

LIPOID GRANULOMATOSIS

Disturbances in lipoid metabolism may give rise to a specific pathologic change in the reticuloendothelial system involving the spongy skeleton. In Gaucher's disease a lipoprotein of the cerebroside type is at fault; in Niemann-Pick disease, a phosphatid lipoid; in Tay-Sachs syndrome, a cerebroside protein; and in Hand-Schüller-Christian disease, cholesterol. In all these, bone changes have been reported or observed, though the main effects of the disease are found in the extraosseous portions of the reticuloendothelium. Hand-Schüller-Christian disease has particular orthopedic importance.

PATHOLOGY. There is an increased lipoid content of the circulating body fluids with the reticuloendothelial cells absorbing and depositing the substance. It is suggested that a congenital or acquired deficiency of liver and lungs increases the reticuloendothelium elsewhere—especially in bone. In the skeleton, the diploë of the skull, cancellous tissue of the mandible, clavicle, ribs, pelvis, and vertebrae are affected. In addition, the pleura, the lungs, the liver, and the cerebellum have been the sites of typical deposits. In this situation, the deposits appear as multiple circumscribed, rounded tumors, golden yellow or brownish yellow.

These "tumors" are composed of large, often multinucleated reticuloendothelial cells, with small nuclei and a finely reticulated cytoplasm. The cytoplasm contains for the most part innumerable globules of lipoid which give the cell a "foamy" appearance. The largest foam cells are found away from the vessels; around the vessels are arranged smaller reticuloendothelial cells. The presence of the deposits of lipoid produces granulation tissue around the deposits. This causes destruction of the bone without new bone reaction, to give rise to large defects with irregular margins (Fig. 45-21).

The condition in a typical case is marked on the skull base in the vicinity of the sella turcica. The pituitary gland may be compressed or obliterated, and the lipogranulomatous tissue may extend through the superior orbital fissure to collect behind the globe of the eye and push it forward.

Table 45-6. DIFFERENTIAL DIAGNOSIS BETWEEN HAND-SCHÜLLER-CHRISTIAN DISEASE, EOSINOPHILIC GRANULOMA, AND LETTERER-SIWE DISEASE

	Hand-Schüller-Christian disease	*Eosinophilic granuloma*	*Letterer-Siwe disease*
Age	Early childhood but occasionally in adults	Older children, adolescents, and young adults	Infants
Clinical features	Triad of exophthalmos, polyuria, polydipsia, swelling; N.B.: other pituitary dysfunction	Pain, swelling, and local tenderness; systemic manifestations of fever, loss in weight	Low fever, pain and swelling; low-grade anemia; short and rapidly fatal course in most cases
Localization	Base of skull, spine, ilium, mandible—most common in "membranous bones"; liver and spleen sometimes	72%—solitary lesion involving all bones but mainly ribs, skull, femur, pelvis, humerus; soft tissues rare	Multiple lesions of liver, spleen, glands, skin, lungs, and mainly skull
Pathology	Secondary deposition of cholesterol in "foam cells" following formation of granuloma; (?) unknown infection	Granuloma formation with histiocytes, eosinophils in large numbers, multinucleated cells and areas of necrosis	Eosinophils + +; foam cells sometimes present; true reticuloendotheliosis
Radiology		Cannot be differentiated	
Blood picture and biochemistry	Normal; hypercholesteremia in most cases	"Circulating" eosinophilia; normal	Anemia; normal
Prognosis	Slow and benign except in 25% of cases	Good but guarded in multiple lesions	Fatal

SOURCE: Taken with permission from W. Mercer and R. B. Duthie, "Orthopaedic Surgery," 7th ed., Edward Arnold (Publishers) Ltd., London, 1974.

CLINICAL MANIFESTATIONS. The disease as originally described consisted of a distinctive syndrome—defects in the membranous bones, exophthalmos, with thirst and polyuria (diabetes insipidus). It is to this triad of effects that the term Hand-Schüller-Christian syndrome is given. The exophthalmos is the result of the retrobulbar accumulation of lipoid-laden reticuloendothelial cells, while the diabetes insipidus is the sequel to the distortion of the hypothalamus.

Thus interference with the pituitary may lead to retardation of growth, and the irritation or tension on the dura mater to irritability and restlessness. Should the extraosseous reticuloendothelium be affected, splenomegaly or hepatic enlargement may be present, and in the latter case jaundice may be observed. The blood shows a cholesterol content which may be increased to 280 mg/100 ml. Biopsy with histologic examination will give an accurate diagnosis.

TREATMENT. The disease tends to be progressive, and in many published cases death has resulted. An attempt is made to reduce the hypercholesteremia by dietetic means. Deep radiotherapy is employed to control the deposits, while in the event of polyuria and thirst from dia-

Fig. 45-21. Lipoid granulomatosis demonstrating destruction of bone with large defects, irregular margins, and absence of new bone reaction.

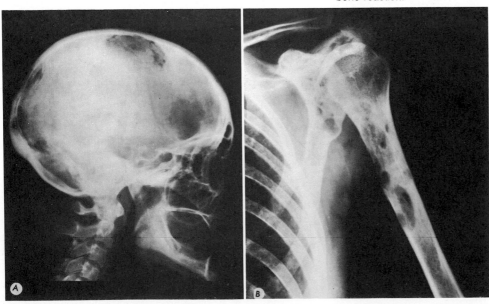

betes insipidus pituitary extract may be given. Any pathologic fractures should be immobilized by internal fixation devices.

EOSINOPHILIC GRANULOMATOSIS

This is an affection of the young, 64 percent of patients being under twenty years of age. The cause is unknown, though it is believed to be an infection or toxin of some sort. The lesions, usually multiple, affect the skeleton almost exclusively, although in some cases lymph glands and the lungs may also be involved. The local lesion, though frequently silent, may give rise to local pain and tenderness and even swelling. The illness may be initiated by fever. Where the skull is affected, headache is often a complaint. Blood examination is not characteristic, although eosinophilia may be present.

The radiologic appearance varies and may simulate other types of disease. Most commonly the lesion is oval or circular, translucent, and cystlike. It may be accompanied by some periostitis adjacent to the osteolytic area. The confluences of the translucent areas, particularly in the skull, sometimes gives the appearance of the "geographic" skull. In the long bones the lesions are endosteal and usually affect the shafts; only occasionally is a lesion seen in the epiphysis. Vertebra plana due to eosinophilic granuloma has been described by Compere et al. Biopsy was carried out in their four cases and demonstrated the typical eosinophilic granulomatosis lesion. However, an inflammatory lesion must be excluded, in which case rest and splinting will cause the symptoms to disappear, and even the deformed and flattened vertebral body may reossify.

The lesion may resolve spontaneously; it may heal after curettage without the aid of radiotherapy or after radiotherapy alone.

The contents of a relatively early lesion consist of soft brownish granulation tissue which may be streaked with yellow necrotic material. Patches of hemorrhage may be present. Histologically it shows histiocytes, eosinophils in large numbers, and leukocytes, and large multinuclear giant cells, especially near hemorrhage or necrosis.

Diagnosis must differentiate this condition from Hand-Schüller-Christian disease (Table 45-6), in which there is often exophthalmos, diabetes insipidus, and a characteristic histologic appearance, and from myelomatosis by the lesions in the skull, which are larger and less numerous, and by the absence of Bence Jones protein in the urine. Polyostotic fibrous dysplasia also has to be excluded.

LETTERER-SIWE DISEASE

This very rare condition, a reticuloendotheliosis, occurs in infants up to the age of three or four and is regarded as an acute form of Hand-Schüller-Christian disease. It usually runs a short and rapidly fatal course without the secondary deposits of cholesterol esters in the cells of the granulomas. The soft tissues, particularly of the viscera, are chiefly affected, although in most cases destructive lesions are found in the skeleton. There is a low and progressive anemia, and lesions are found in the liver and spleen (which are usually enlarged) as well as in glands, lungs, skin, and the bones of the skull. The x-ray picture

closely resembles that of the Hand-Schüller-Christian disease. If the base of the skull is involved, the characteristic symptoms of Hand-Schüller-Christian disease—exophthalmos and diabetes insipidus—may develop, although the lesions are without foam cells. Histologically there is difficulty in distinguishing the condition from the other two forms of histiocytic granulomatosis. (See Table 45-6.)

In most cases death ensues within a few weeks.

HEMATOPOIETIC SYSTEM

Leukemia

Lymphoblastic leukemia most commonly produces bony changes. Myeloblastic leukemia has a lower incidence of bony changes because of its shorter acute course. In aleukemic leukemia bony changes do occur in spite of its very rapid course.

These lesions can be found in any part of the skeleton, although they most commonly occur in the knee and shoulder regions around the metaphysis. The skull is rarely involved.

On x-rays, the characteristic lesion is a translucent zone adjacent to the metaphysis, but there may be a diffuse spotty osteolysis with vertebral collapse and deformity as well as abnormal periosteal ossification. The metaphyseal translucent zone is not specific for these diseases but is seen in numerous unrelated conditions such as prolonged immobilization of the limb or scurvy.

The main differentiation is from juvenile rheumatism; both may present as a polyarticular "arthritis" with pain, swelling, and loss of movement.

Treatment with ACTH and folic acid antagonists has been successful in some of these diseases.

Multiple Myeloma

Marrow develops from the primitive undifferentiated mesenchyme cell, and in the process of differentiation progeny of distinctive characteristics are produced. There are the reticulum cell with its fibrils, the plasma cell with its typical cartwheel nucleus eccentrically placed and showing in the basophilic cytoplasm a characteristic clear area, the cells of the lymphocyte series, and the forerunners of the polymorphonuclear cells and erythrocytes of the blood. Tumors arising in the marrow can therefore exhibit a wide variation in cell type, resembling in greater or lesser detail the cells normally found and affording ample opportunity for complex classification. Such discussion, however, is of little clinical significance.

PATHOLOGY. The affected bones show replacement of their marrow and the bone trabeculae without reactive new bone formation, so that the tumors bear a close resemblance—on inspection as well as on radiologic examination—to diffuse carcinomatosis. Hemorrhage with cyst formation is common, and pathologic fracture is frequent. When the disease is extensive, there may be gross restriction of the absolute amount of red marrow, with anemia.

Myelogenous tumors are most commonly encountered

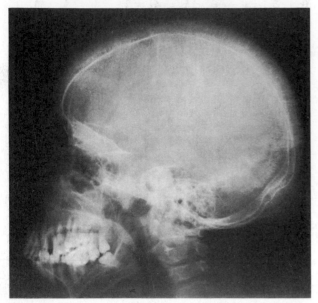

Fig. 45-22. Skull x-ray of a patient with hemolytic anemia, demonstrating the "brush" appearance.

in the skull and vertebrae, ribs, pelvis, femur, and humerus, but the bones of the peripheral parts of the limbs are only occasionally the site of disease. The sternum frequently contains tumors, and sternal puncture in consequence may be a valuable diagnostic procedure. The disease is closely related to the leukemias except that in myelomatosis the plasma cell is the predominant cell type.

In myelomatosis metabolic disturbance is common, the blood calcium level is raised, and there is hyperproteinemia, the globulin being raised. In 50 percent of patients, globulin (Bence Jones protein) is present in the urine, a fact which, however, can also occur in leukemia, skeletal carcinomatosis, and rarely in nephritis.

Amyloid deposits in muscles and joints have been described in 10 percent of cases of myelomatosis and are particularly common when large amounts of globulin are present in the urine. Renal insufficiency is another frequent complication. This is believed to be due to plugging of the renal tubules by globulin casts, and the cortex may be eroded from the marrow surface.

In certain myelomas, when the tumor is sectioned, the cut surface is bright green, which is due to a pigment the character of which is not fully understood. The color rapidly fades. To this group of tumors the name *chloroma* has been given.

CLINICAL MANIFESTATIONS. The disease is one of adult life and chiefly affects men between the ages of forty and sixty years. A history of trauma preceding the development of individual local lesions is often obtained. Pain is a common initial symptom, but pathologic fracture or paraplegia have frequently been the presenting symptoms. Multiple myeloma, Paget's disease, and metastasis constitute the commonest causes of pathologic fracture. Backache as an initial symptom is noteworthy, and the condition should be borne in mind as the cause of such symptoms in the elderly, especially in the presence of

osteoporosis and where the pain is not relieved by rest. Fever may be observed in the course of the disease, and pathologic fracture is not infrequent; eggshell crackling may be noted on examining the individual lesion.

The tumors appear as multiple circumscribed areas of destruction in which all parts of the bone are involved.

DIFFERENTIAL DIAGNOSIS. Radiologic examination of the skull, ribs, and vertebrae, estimation of the total serum proteins and serum albumin and globulin, examination of the urine for Bence Jones protein, and sternal marrow puncture are necessary.

The multiple nature of the lesions, the absence of pulmonary metastases, the late age period, and the osteolytic character of the radiologic picture are the significant features. The most likely error is a diagnosis of diffuse secondary carcinomatosis, and a thorough investigation for a demonstrable focus in breast, thyroid, prostate, or uterus must be undertaken.

TREATMENT. When the disease is generalized, with pyrexia, loss of weight, and pain, the administration of such alkylating agents as phenylalanine, nitrogen mustard, and cyclophosphamides may produce bone marrow depression with regression of the disease. When there is thrombocytopenia, hypercalcemia, or renal failure, prednisolone will improve the blood counts.

Solitary Myeloma

Rarely, cases have been described of solitary lesions of bone in which on careful examination the histologic picture has been that of a myeloma typical of the plasmacyte type and in which other lesions have not been demonstrated. Patients with a condition of this character in which the local lesion has been resected or treated by radiation have survived without evidence of recurrence or of other foci developing elsewhere in the skeleton. Accordingly it is now accepted that solitary myeloma constitutes a definite disease entity. Curettage is contraindicated, since it may disseminate disease.

Hemolytic Anemia

Both Mediterranean, or Cooley's, anemia and sickle cell anemia produce bone marrow changes in the vertebral bodies and, most prominently, in the bones of the skull and face. The skull shows a striking picture similar to periosteal "sun ray" formation and is called the "brush skull" (Fig. 45-22); avascular necrosis of the femoral head is also common.

References

Anatomy and Physiology of Bone

Albright, F., and Reifenstein, E. C.: "The Parathyroid Glands and Metabolic Bone Disease," The Williams & Wilkins Company, Baltimore, 1948.

Barnicot, N. A.: Local Action of Parathyroid and Other Tissues on Bone in Intracerebral Grafts, *J Anat,* **82:**233, 1948.

Bourne, G. H.: "The Biochemistry and Physiology of Bone," vol. 1, "Structure," 2d ed., Academic Press, Inc., New York, 1972.

————: "The Biochemistry and Physiology of Bone" vol. 2, "Physiology and Pathology," 2d ed., Academic Press, Inc., New York, 1972.

————: "The Biochemistry and Physiology of Bone," vol. 3, "Development and Growth," 2d ed., Academic Press, Inc., New York, 1972.

Brailsford, J. F.: "The Radiology of Bones and Joints," J. & A. Churchill Ltd., London, 1944.

Dixon, T. F., and Perkins, H. R.: The Chemistry of Calcification, chap. 10 in G. H. Bourne (ed.), "Biochemistry and Physiology of Bone," Academic Press, Inc., New York, 1956.

Duthie, R. B., and Barker, A. N.: Autoradiographic Study of Mucopolysaccharide and Phosphate Complexes in Bone Growth and Repair, J Bone Joint Surg [Br], 38B:304, 1955.

Edeiken, J., and Hodes, P. J.: "Roentgen Diagnosis of Diseases of Bone," The Williams and Wilkins Company, Baltimore, 1967.

Fleisch, H.: Mechanism of Calcification: Inhibitory Role of Pyrophosphate, Nature, 195:911, 1962.

Follis, R. H.: A Survey of Bone Disease, Am J Med, 22:469, 1957.

Freeman, S., and Chang, T. S.: Role of Kidney and of Citric Acid in Production of Transient Hypercalcemia following Nephrectomy, Am J Physiol, 160:335, 1950.

Glimcher, M. J.: Calcification in Biological Systems, Symp Am Assoc Adv Sci Washington 1958, vol. 64, p. 421, 1960.

Gutman, A. B., and Yü, T. F.: A Concept of the Role of Enzymes in Endochondral Calcification, Metab Interrelations Trans Conf 2d, vol. 2, p. 167, 1950.

Harrison, H. E.: The Interrelation of Citrate and Calcium Metabolism, Am J Med, 20:1, 1956.

Hass, G. M.: Studies of Cartilage: Morphologic and Chemical Analysis of Aging Human Costal Cartilage, Arch Pathol, 35:275, 1943.

Heinz, E., Müller, E., and Rominger, E.: Citronensäure und Rachitis, Z Kinderheilkd, 65:101, 1947.

Jackson, S. F.: The Fine Structure of Developing Bone in the Embryonic Owl, Proc R Soc Lond [Biol], 146:270, 1957.

Keith, A.: Bone Growth and Bone Repair, Br J Surg, 5:685, 1918.

Knaggs, R. L.: "Inflammatory and Toxic Diseases of Bone," Wright, Bristol, England, 1926.

Lacroix, P.: "Radiocalcium and Radiosulphur in the Study of Bone Metabolism at the Histological Level," Proc Radioisotope Conf 2d, Oxford Engl, 1:134, 1954.

McLean, F. C., and Urist, M. R.: "Bone: An Introduction to the Physiology of the Skeletal Tissue," The University of Chicago Press, 1972.

Neuman, W. F., and Neuman, M. W.: The Nature of the Mineral Phase of Bone, Chem Rev, 53:1, 1953.

Reddi, K. K., and Nörstrom, A.: Influence of Vitamin C on Utilization of Sulphate Labelled with Sulphur-35 in Synthesis of Chondroitin Sulphate of Costal Cartilage of Guinea Pig, Nature (Lond), 173:1232, 1954.

Robinson, R. A.: Crystal-Collagen-Water Relationships in Bone Matrix, Clin Orthop, 17:69, 1960.

Shearer, W. S.: Review of Radiographic Features of Some General Affections of Skeleton, Edinburgh Med J, 61:101, 1954.

Sheldon, H., and Robinson, R. A.: Electron Microscope Studies of Crystal Collagen Relationships in Bone. IV. The Occurrence of Crystals within Collagen Fibres, J Biophys Biochem Cytol, 3:1011, 1957.

Siffert, R. S.: Role of Alkaline Phosphatase in Osteogenesis, J Exp Med, 93:415, 1951.

Talmage, R. V.: "Action of Parathyroids on Bone Studied with Radio-isotopes," Blackwell Scientific Publications, Ltd., Oxford, 1962.

Vincent, Y. J., and Haumont, S.: Autoradiographic Identification of Metabolic Osteones after the Administration of Ca 45, Rev Fr Etud Clin Biol, 5:348, 1960.

Metabolic Bone Disorders

Bauer, C. C. H., Carlsson, A., and Lindquist, B.: Bone Salt Metabolism in Human Rickets Studied with Radioactive Phosphorus, Metabolism, 5:573, 1956.

Dent, C. E.: Some Problems of Hyperparathyroidism, Br Med J, 2:1495, 1962.

———— and Harris, H.: Hereditary Forms of Rickets and Osteomalacia, J Bone Joint Surg [Br], 38B:204, 1956.

Fanconi, G., and Girardet, P.: Familiärer persistierender Phosphatdiabetes mit D-Vitamin-resistenter Rachitis, Helv Paediatr Acta, 7:14, 1952.

Fleisch, H., Russell, R. G. G., Bisaz, S., Termine, J. D., and Posner, A. S.: Influence of Pyrophosphate on the Transformation of Amorphous to Crystalline Calcium Phosphate, Calcif Tissue Res, 2:49, 1968.

Fraser, D., Leeming, J. M., Cerwerka, E. A., and Kenyers, K.: Studies of the Pathogenesis of the High Renal Clearance of Phosphate in Hypophosphatemic Vitamin-D Refractory Rickets of the Simple Type, Am J Dis Child, 98:586, 1959.

Gutman, A. B., and Yü, T. F.: Metab Int 2d Conf, 1950, 1967.

McCance, R. A., Morrison, A. B., and Dent, C. E.: Excretion of Phosphoethanolomine and Hypophosphatasia: Preliminary Communication, Lancet, 1:131, 1955.

McKusick, V. A.: "Heritable Disorders of Connective Tissue," 3d ed., The C. V. Mosby Company, St. Louis, 1966.

Rathbun, J. C.: "Hypophosphatasia": New Developmental Anomaly, Am J Dis Child, 75:822, 1948.

Snapper, I., and Nathan, D. J.: Rickets and Osteomalacia, Am J Med, 22:939, 1957.

Osteoporosis

Cooke, A. M.: Osteoporosis, Lancet, 1:877, 1955.

Krane, S. M., Brownell, G. L., Stanbury, J. B., and Corrigan, H.: Effect of Thyroid Disease on Calcium Metabolism in Man, J Clin Invest, 35:874, 1956.

Nordin, B. E. C.: Osteomalacia, Osteoporosis and Calcium Deficiency, Clin Orthop, 17:235, 1960.

Sissons, H. A.: Osteoporosis and Epiphyseal Arrest in Joint Tuberculosis, J Bone Joint Surg [Br], 34B:275, 1952.

Reticuloendothelial Disturbances in Bone

Compere, E. L., Johnson, W. E., and Coventry, M. B.: Vertebra Plana (Calvé's Disease) Due to Eosinophilic Granuloma, J Bone Joint Surg [Am], 36A:969, 1954.

Griffith, D. L.: "Modern Trends in Blood Diseases," Butterworth & Co. (Publishers), Ltd., London, 1955.

Mercer, W., and Duthie, R. B.: Histiocytic Granulomatosis, J Bone Joint Surg [Br], 38B:279, 1956.

Meyer, K., Grumbach, M. M., Linker, A., and Hoffman, P.: Excretion of Sulfated Mucopolysaccharides in Gargoylism (Hurler's Syndrome), Proc Soc Exp Biol Med, 97:275, 1958.

Generalized Bone Disorders

Albers-Schönberg, W.: Roentgenbildung einer seltenen Knochen-
erkrakung, *Munch Med Wochenschr,* **51:**365, 1904.

———: Einer seltener bisher nicht Bekannter Structuranomalie des
Skellets, *Fortschr Geb Roentgenstr Nuklearmed,* **23:**174, 1915.

Bailey, J. A.: Orthopedic Aspects of Achondroplasia, *J Bone Joint
Surg* [*Am*], **52A:**1285, 1970.

Brailsford, J. F.: "The Radiology of Bones and Joints," J. & A.
Churchill Ltd., London, 1944.

Knaggs, R. L.: "Inflammatory and Toxic Diseases of Bone,"
Wright, Bristol, England, 1926.

Milkman, L. A.: Pseudofractures (Hunger Osteopathy, Late Rickets, Osteomalacia): Report of Case, *Am J Roentgenol,* **24:**29,
1930.

Sofield, H. A., and Millar, E. A.: Fragmentation, Realignment and
Intramedullary Rod Fixation of Deformities of the Long
Bones in Children, *J Bone Joint Surg* [*Am*], **41A:**8, 1371,
1959.

Chapter 46

Tumors of the Musculoskeletal System

by **Robert B. Duthie and Franklin T. Hoaglund**

Biologic Properties

Classification of Bone Tumors

True Bone Tumors

Osteoma
Osteoid Osteoma
Osteosarcoma (Osteogenic Sarcoma)
Chondroma
Benign Chondroblastoma (Codman's Tumor)
Chondrosarcoma
Fibroma
Fibrosarcoma
Osteoclastoma (Giant Cell Tumor)

Nonosteogenic Tumors of Bone

Unicameral (Solitary) or Juvenile Bone Cyst
Periosteal Fibrosarcoma
Ewing's Tumor
Reticulum Cell Sarcoma

Blood Vessel Tumors

Aneurysmal Bone Cyst
Hemangioma
Angiosarcoma (Angioendothelioma)

Tumors Arising from Included Tissues

Adamantinoma
Neurilemmoma
Chordoma

Malignant Tumors of Soft Tissues

Metastatic Tumor of Bone

In response to injury, infection, or hormonal disturbance, localized overgrowth of bone, cartilage, or fibrous tissue may occur to give rise to a bony swelling, or "tumor," but these are not neoplasms. In bone there are not only "osteogenic" tissues but many other tissues, i.e., hematopoietic tissue, fat, nerves, blood vessels, which give rise to tumors within bone.

New bone formation may result during *malignant* ossification, i.e., bone formed by malignant osteoblasts, and *benign* ossification, i.e., bone formed by normal osteoblastic activity in malignantly formed cartilage, osteoid, or collagenous tissues or as reactive bone by normal tissue response to the adjacent malignant process.

Destruction or resorption of bone may result from increased vascularity, by pressure of the tumor or by mechanical compression of the blood vessels with consequent ischemic necrosis and sequestrum formation.

BIOLOGIC PROPERTIES

In relating the site of origin of musculoskeletal tumors to the cellular activity in that area (Fig. 46-1), Johnson has shown that the giant cell tumor commonly arises in the juxtametaphyseal area, where there is much osteoclastic activity, required for remodeling; the osteogenic-osteolytic sarcoma is seen just below this area, whereas the fibrosarcoma is in relation to the endosteum and the round cell sarcoma occurs within the medullary cavity.

The terms "benign" and "malignant" are relative terms; Foulds emphasized that it is the tumor's response to its environment, or any change in this environment, which should be used as a guide to the subsequent behavior of the tumor and, hence, prognosis.

The relative age incidence shows the first peak of mortality between the ages of fifteen and twenty years and a secondary peak from the age of thirty years up to about seventy-five years. The first peak is due mainly to the primary malignant tumors of bone, e.g., osteogenic sarcoma, whereas the second peak is due to malignant neoplasia in such preexisting conditions as Paget's disease.

In the development of a malignant condition there may be either (1) chromosomal or genetic factors or (2) extrachromosomal factors. At the present time, no one single etiologic agent has yet been determined, and probably there are a number of etiologic factors taking part. In studying skeletal neoplasia there are only four known examples of premalignant change:

1. Diaphyseal aclasis (rare) $\longrightarrow$ chondrosarcoma
2. Fibrous dysplasia (few) $\longrightarrow$ fibrosarcoma
3. Irradiated tissues $\longrightarrow$ osteogenic sarcoma
4. Paget's disease (10–20%) $\longrightarrow$ multiple sarcomas (both osteogenic sarcomas and chondrosarcomas)

In diaphyseal aclasis, which is inherited from a dominant mutant gene, lesions rarely undergo chondrosarcomatous changes. In Paget's disease, which is present in about 3 to 4 percent of the European population over the age of forty years, 10 to 20 percent of the patients have been observed postmortem to have developed sarcomas.

Growth patterns and their hormonal backgrounds may have some significance in the development of osteogenic

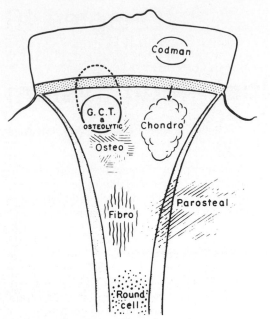

Fig. 46-1. Common sites of origin of bone tumors. (*Used with permission of L. C. Johnson, 1953.*)

sarcoma in males and females. Price has shown that the greatest incidence in females occurs between the ages of five and fourteen years, whereas in males it is between the ages of fifteen and twenty-four years, because males grow longer and larger and, therefore, there are more cells available to undergo malignant change. Extraneous carcinogenic agents are now well recognized; e.g., hydrocarbons, aromatic and azo dyes which can produce fibrosarcoma, and radiation both from internal sources—e.g., plutonium, radium, yttrium, strontium—and from external sources of x-radiation are also well known etiologic factors in osteosarcoma.

CLASSIFICATION OF BONE TUMORS

A. *True bone tumors*—neoplasms arising from cells of mesenchymal origin, whose function is primarily skeletal bone formation. These tumors fall into four main groups according to the predominant cell type present:

B. *Tumors arising from tissues normally found in bone but not participating in bone formation:*
  1. Tumors arising from fibrous tissue
     a. Periosteal fibroma
     b. Periosteal fibrosarcoma
  2. Tumors arising from bone marrow
     a. Myeloma
     b. Reticulum cell sarcoma
     c. Hodgkin's disease of bone
     d. Lymphosarcoma
     e. Ewing's tumor
  3. Tumors from blood vessels
     a. Hemangioma
     b. Hemangioblastoma
     c. Aneurysmal bone cyst
     d. Angiosarcoma
  4. Tumors arising from adipose tissue
     a. Lipoma
     b. Liposarcoma
  5. Tumors arising from nerves
     a. Neurilemmoma
     b. Neurofibroma
C. *Tumors arising from included tissue:*
     a. Chordoma
     b. Adamantinoma
D. *Metastatic tumors*

TRUE BONE TUMORS

Osteoma

This small, sessile, rare tumor is found in the orbit, nasal sinuses, external auditory meatus, and oral side of the mandible. The tumor is dense and hard and is termed *ivory exostosis.*

Bone may form from abnormal growth or imperfect remodeling, and a variety of names have been given depending on the site and etiology.

Irritative exostosis results from lesions causing a proliferation of fibroblasts or granulation tissue with ossification.

Traumatic osteomas are most frequently seen on the femur in relation to the adductor magnus (the so-called "rider's bone") or in relation to the medial collateral ligament of the knee joint (Pellegrini-Stieda disease).

Osteoid Osteoma

This lesion occurs in young males between the ages of ten and thirty years, particularly in the bones of the lower

Cell type predominating	Simple tumor types	Malignant
1. Osteoblast: tumor cells show active ossification.	Osteoma 　Osteoid osteoma 　Benign osteoblastoma	Osteosarcoma 　Primary 　Parosteal
2. Chondroblast: tumor cells show active cartilage formation.	Chondroma 　Benign chondroblastoma 　Chondromyxoid fibroma	Chondrosarcoma 　Primary 　Secondary
3. Fibroblast: tumor cells show active collagen formation.	Fibroma 　(?) Solitary bone cyst 　Nonosteogenic fibroma	Fibrosarcoma Rhabdomyosarcoma
4. Osteoclast: tumor cells show active bone destruction by giant cells.	Osteoclastoma	Malignant 　osteoclastoma

extremities. There is doubt as to whether this is a true tumor.

The patient presents with pain, frequently felt during the night and not aggravated by exercise or position but often relieved specifically, although empirically, by salicylates.

On radiography, a zone of bony sclerosis is seen surrounding a radiolucent nidus (Fig. 46-2).

This condition has to be distinguished from (1) the sclerosing nonsuppurative osteomyelitis of Garre, (2) Brodie's abscess, (3) osteogenic sarcoma, (4) Ewing's tumor, (5) nonossifying fibroma.

Three characteristic regions have been described by Jaffe: (1) an inner region of vascular granulation tissue containing osteoblasts and (2) a zone of calcification and osteoid formation which is surrounded by (3) a zone of trabecular formation of bone in various stages of reorganization (Fig. 46-3).

Complete resection, if possible, will provide cure, but partial removal of the sclerotic bone and the nidus is often sufficient for symptomatic improvement.

Ossifying fibroma is almost exclusively seen in the jawbones of adolescents. It is often asymptomatic, being discovered during dental examinations. Histologically it consists of dense fibroblastic proliferation within compact bone.

Osteosarcoma (Osteogenic Sarcoma)

These tumors arise from cells concerned with bone formation. There are various forms, or types, including myxosarcoma, pseudomyxoma, and osteochondrosarcoma.

Osteosarcoma is rare, about 1 in 75,000 of the population, with a predilection for the second decade.

The tumor occurs in the metaphysis of the femur (52 percent), in the upper end of the tibia (20 percent), and in the humerus (9 percent). Less usual sites are the radius, the ulna, the ilium, and the scapula. The short long bones are rarely affected.

The tumor may originate beneath the periosteum or more centrally in the shaft of the bone and extend in two directions: (1) toward the medulla and (2) to the subperiosteal area, with destruction of bone trabeculae. Initially the periosteum is a barrier and is raised off the bone with new bone formation to produce a fusiform swelling. The intramedullary part of the tumor rarely transgresses the cartilage of the epiphysis.

The tumor may be soft, fleshy, vascular, and destructive, or it may be grayish white, containing cartilage or bone. The new bone may be arranged as scattered islands throughout the tumor which impart a gritty sensation on cutting, and in the form of spicules radiating from the periosteum, giving the "sun ray" appearance on radiography. On the diaphyseal side of the tumor the periosteum is often raised for a short distance, with new bone formation, triangular in shape, and is called Codman's triangle. Pathologic fractures may occur.

Histologically, cells are small and spindle-shaped, with hyperchromatic nuclei with great variation in cell form and shape. The degree of pleomorphism is most marked in the

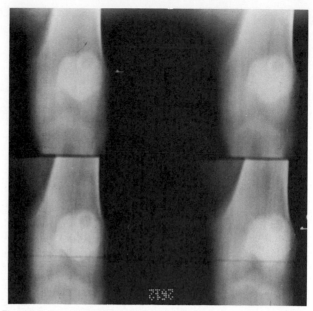

Fig. 46-2. Tomographs of a patella showing an osteoid osteoma in the right upper quadrant. (*Used with permission from Mercer and Duthie, "Orthopaedic Surgery," 1974.*)

extremely anaplastic tumors in which there are often giant multinucleated cells of bizarre shapes. Mitosis is evident. The intercellular substance may be scanty in amount and in character, being myxomatous, cartilaginous, osteoid, or osseous, according to the degree of differentiation and metaplasia taking place (Fig. 46-4). Blood vessels are thin-walled and numerous.

Pain, especially at night, is usually the first symptom and is caused by periosteal irritation. Such pain in the long bone of a young adult should arouse suspicion of sarcoma. The clinical history of trauma is unreliable. The general

Fig. 46-3. Photomicrograph to show zone 3 of an osteoid osteoma with trabecular bone formation and numerous osteoblasts. (×300.)

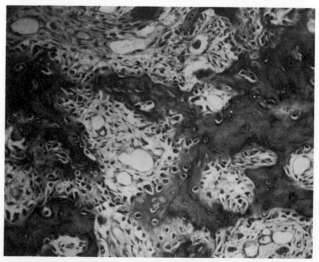

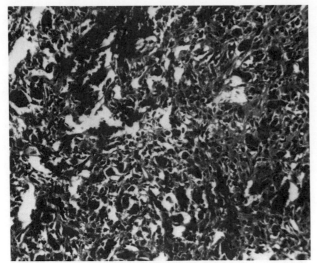

Fig. 46-4. Photomicrograph showing numerous "malignant" osteoblasts and pleomorphic cells of an osteogenic sarcoma with new bone formation. (×300.)

condition is good until a late stage with spread when rapid deterioration occurs.

Later, general dissemination of the tumor takes place. While the lymphatic stream occasionally plays a definite role, spread by the blood vessels is predominant. Pulmonary metastases are the most frequent. The first clinical signs of these lesions are usually those of a diffuse bronchitis, but occasionally the cough, dullness, fever, and leukocytosis suggest a diagnosis of pneumonia. Dilated veins may be evident at an early stage.

Pathologic fracture is not typical of osteogenic sarcoma, since the swelling and pain usually keep the patient off his feet. There may be some initial pain and effusion into the nearest joint, but movement is free and painless.

The x-ray appearances (Fig. 46-5) have been categorized:

1. The sclerotic type, usually found at puberty, where dense new irregular bone occurs in the metaphysis and there may be a few spicules projecting from its surface.

Fig. 46-5. Osteogenic sarcoma of the femur. The films show characteristic bone destruction, soft tissue mass, new bone formation, and sclerosis limited to the metaphysis of the lower femur.

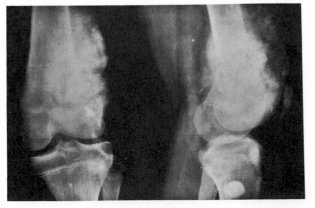

2. The osteolytic type, usually metaphyseal. An eccentric translucent gap is found and at its edges a gradual increase of density compared to that of the normal bone.
3. The radiating spicule type, the least common, usually found at puberty in the metaphyseal region.

The radiologic diagnosis may be obvious in the early lesion, but histologic evidence is required and biopsy is indicated. The added risk of any biopsy in view of the already grave prognosis appears justified when compared with the chance that amputation may be carried out unnecessarily on equivocal clinical and radiologic findings.

Until recently the standard treatment has been intensive irradiation with delayed amputation, giving a 5-year survival of about 20 percent. However, with the discovery of Doxorubicin (adriamycin) in 1970, Cortez et al. demonstrated a marked regression in patients with pulmonary metastases. In 1972 Jaffe reported similar results with the use of high-dose methotrexate and citrovorum, hemopoietic tissue-rescue factor. Following these successes, primary amputation with chemotherapy is now producing over 50 percent survivals.

Osteogenic sarcoma has been shown to possess specific tumor-associated antigens. Therefore, attempts are now being made to enhance the host's immune mechanisms either by specific antibodies to the tumor-specific antigen or by sensitized lymphocytes.

Recently Morton et al. reported management of extremity, skeletal, and soft tissue sarcomas with preoperative intraarterial adriamycin and radiation therapy, radical surgical resection, and postoperative chemotherapy or immunotherapy. Some patients in whom bone was resected and replaced with cadaver allografts remained free of disease with functional extremity for as long as 34 months.

OSTEOSARCOMA IN PAGET'S DISEASE. In 10 percent of cases of Paget's disease sarcomatous changes occur. The histologic appearance is similar to that arising de novo in younger patients but appears at a much later age—usually over fifty years. The tumor is more diffuse in character and can arise simultaneously at multiple sites; i.e., it can be polyostotic. Osteosarcoma in Paget's disease has the lowest rate of survival of any of the tumors of the sarcoma series.

PAROSTEAL SARCOMA. This occurs in older age groups and presents as a painful tumor mass, near the knee joint. It is juxtacortical and usually is densely ossified with areas of less ossified or calcified cartilage. There are usually no periosteal reactions, or "sun rays." Growth is slow, but eventual destruction of the cortex with invasion of the medullary cavity by malignant bone and osteoid tissue with malignant connective tissue stroma occurs. Parosteal sarcoma has a better progress than osteosarcoma, particularly when treated with a primary amputation.

Chondroma

Chondroma is a benign tumor arising from the cartilaginous elements of developing bone with slow growth. Calcification frequently occurs in the fibrous septums dividing the lobules. Microscopically there is a chondroid matrix containing cartilage cells; encapsulation and lobulation are present. When ossification does occur, the lesion is known as *osteochondroma*.

If malignancy develops, it does so after the age of thirty-five and occurs most commonly in tumors of the large long bones. If this type of tumor presents as a centrally placed mass of such a bone or of a flat bone, e.g., the ilium or scapula, one must seriously consider a low-grade chondrosarcoma.

When a chondroma occurs in the small bones of the hand or foot, it is known as a *solitary cystic chondroma*, and when it occurs elsewhere within a bone, as a *single enchondroma*. Radiologic features are characteristic. There is a dense shadow, with a feathery outline composed of calcified spicules.

SOLITARY CYSTIC ENCHONDROMA. This occurs in the short long bones of the hand and foot in the metaphyseal region of a proximal phalanx or metacarpal. The tumor arises asymptomatically and is brought to attention by trauma or even a pathologic fracture. If cortical expansion or pathologic fracture occurs, the cyst should be curetted with bone grafting. When the cyst wall is thick and asymptomatic, it should be left alone.

CARTILAGINOUS HYPERTROPHY. This always arises from existing cartilage; when it occurs mainly in the confines of bone, it is known as *enchondroma* and when on the surface, *ecchondroma*.

The common sites are the epiphyseal plates, the cartilaginous parts of ribs (Fig. 46-6), and the symphysis pubis. Such lesions may be part of a generalized chondroosteodystrophy. They rarely, if ever, become malignant and may be multiple, especially in the short long bones of the hand and foot. The well-formed fibrous capsule enables the tumor in most cases to be cleanly excised.

MULTIPLE ENCHONDROMAS. Multiple enchondromas occur in childhood and affect the short long bones of the hand and foot, so that the part may be distorted and appear to be of excessive size. They arise in the center of the shaft as a collection of cartilage cells which, in the process of growth, gradually expand the surrounding cortex (Fig. 46-7).

Operative treatment is indicated when the tumors are rapidly growing and have become unsightly or a source of inconvenience. Complete excision, with curettage and autogenous bone grafting, is the treatment of choice.

Benign Chondroblastoma (Codman's Tumor)

The lesion occurs in an earlier age group, i.e., in the first and second decades, in which the epiphyseal line has not yet closed, and its origin may be from a primitive cartilage cell type.

There is often a long history of a painful swelling with loss of joint function. On x-rays (Fig. 46-8) the typical lesion in the epiphysis is an osteolytic one which contains calcium deposits. Extension into the metaphysis and articular cartilage may occur, but the margin is always discrete and demarcated by a zone of sclerotic or condensed bone. This tumor is most commonly confused with a sarcoma or an inflammatory process such as tuberculosis.

On biopsy, the lesion is found to be very vascular and

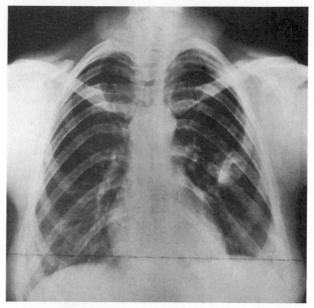

Fig. 46-6. Chondroma of the rib.

gritty. Histology shows much chondroid material with "chondroblastic"-appearing cells, which exhibit strong metachromasia and a positive periodic acid–Schiff reaction. Osteoid tissue and calcified areas are seen.

Treatment consisting of adequate curettage and cancellous bone grafting gives excellent results.

Fig. 46-7. Multiple enchondromas of the hand.

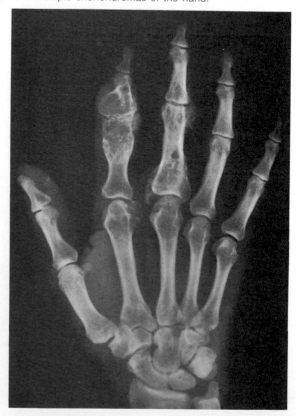

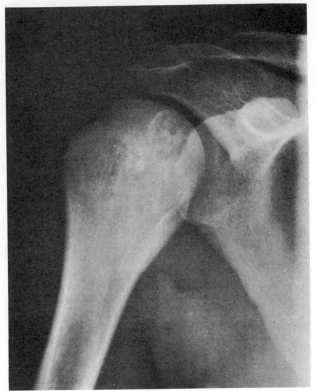

Fig. 46-8. Benign chondroblastoma (Codman's tumor) of the humerus.

Chondrosarcoma

This tumor occurs mainly between the ages of twenty and sixty years. It occurs as a primary malignant tumor in the earlier age groups but as secondary malignant change in such conditions as an osteochondroma, in Paget's disease, or diaphyseal aclasia.

The bones most commonly involved are the pelvis, the

Fig. 46-9. Chondrosarcoma of the upper femur showing an expanding lesion with irregular mottling of calcified tissue. No definite periosteal reaction or spiculation is seen.

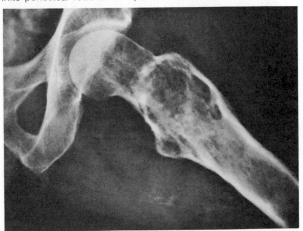

ribs and sternum, and the femur. Dahlin and Henderson have stated that the nearer a cartilaginous tumor is to the axial skeleton and the larger it is, the more likely it is to be malignant.

On x-ray (Fig. 46-9), there is often frank destruction of trabecular bone and cortex with an expanding lesion which contains irregular flecking or mottling of calcified tissue. With this tumor periosteal new bone formation may be present, in which case it often extends outward.

On biopsy, the sarcomatous mass appears as grayish, translucent, fairly vascular tissue. Histologically, varying degrees of pleomorphism, hyperchromatism, mitotic figures of cartilage cells, and chondroid formation with calcification and ossification are seen (Fig. 46-10).

Thomson and Turner-Warwick have divided this tumor into three types of malignancy:

1. *Low-grade,* a well-differentiated tumor, in which the cells are cartilaginous in type although increased in number, with the matrix well formed. Nearly three-quarters of these patients were alive 10 years after treatment.
2. *Average-grade,* in which there is a reduction in the amount of matrix and an increase in the cellularity, the cells varying in size and shape with nuclear irregularities. Less than half the patients were alive at 5 years, and only one-third were alive at 10 years.
3. *High-grade,* a poorly differentiated cartilaginous pattern with anaplastic cells common, frequent mitoses, and only occasional islands of cartilage seen. This type of tumor behaves similarly to osteosarcoma; i.e., only 1 of 10 patients survived 3 years. Treatment should be excision, using a wide margin, or amputation, especially if recurrence takes place after resection.

Secondary chondrosarcoma arises in a preexisting chondroma, osteochondroma, multiple exostoses, and Ollier's disease, occurring mainly in the pelvis, the vertebrae, the femora, and the humeri.

Fibroma

Benign fibrous tumors of bone are rare lesions and closely allied to the fibrous dysplasias.

The cellular and collagenous fibrous content varies but is usually arranged in whorls. Growth is slow and unlimited with mucoid or necrotic degeneration. Ossification is also common but differs in that the bone is laid down in an irregular manner without the organized compact bone of a true osteoma (Fig. 46-11).

Included in this group is the *nonosteogenic fibroma* (nonossifying fibroma) (Fig. 46-12).

These lesions are usually discovered incidentally by x-rays in children. Roentgenographically, they present as small cortical areas of translucency in the metaphysis. During growth some will disappear. However, a few are displaced toward the center of the bone, where they may grow large, with thinning of the sclerotic cortex.

On biopsy, the tissue is fibrous, containing both fibroblasts and "small" giant cells in a relatively large amount of collagenous fibrous tissue in which rarely there are delicate trabeculae of bone which help to differentiate these lesions from fibrous dysplasia.

Curettage or local resection is indicated.

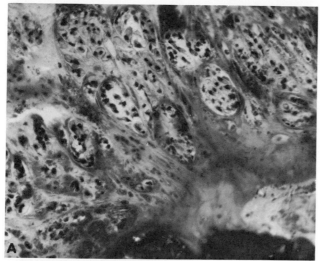

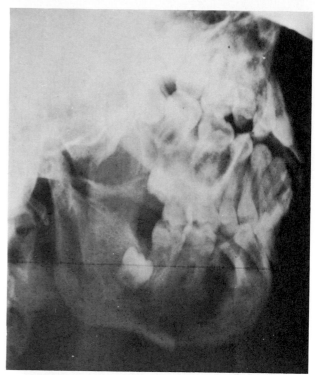

Fig. 46-11. Ossifying fibroma of the mandible in a fourteen-year-old boy with a 1-year history of gradual, painless swelling.

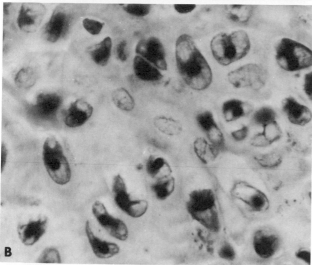

Fig. 46-10. *A*. Photomicrograph of a chondrosarcoma showing the pleomorphism of the "cartilage" cells with chondroid formation. (×250.) *B*. Photomicrograph of the same tissue showing the characteristics of the malignant cartilage cells. (×500.)

Fig. 46-12. Nonossifying fibroma of the left fourth rib. The patient was asymptomatic, the lesion having been detected on routine chest x-ray.

Fibrosarcoma

Medullary fibrosarcomas are characterized by definite collagen formation as the predominant feature, and early destruction of bone. These tumors appear to have a much more favorable prognosis than osteosarcoma, with a 25 percent 5-year survival rate by radical surgical treatment or x-radiation and local excision. Among the patients of Thomson and Turner-Warwick, over 50 percent of those who died had pulmonary metastasis, and a few had malignant deposits in lymph nodes. Thomson and Turner-Warwick differentiate fibrosarcoma from a spindle cell sarcoma, which is distinguished by the complete lack of intercellular substance, by its occurrence in a younger age group, and by its greater radiosensitivity.

Fibrosarcomas have been reported at all ages and as a secondary malignant degeneration in Paget's disease of the

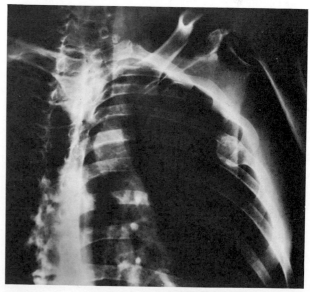

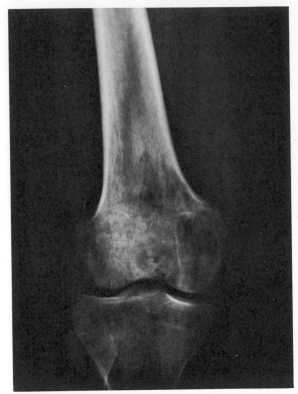

Fig. 46-13. Fibrosarcoma of the lower femur. The films show a lytic lesion apparently of medullary origin on the distal end of the femur. The lesion is destroying cortex. There is no evidence of sclerosis and new bone formation or any definite soft tissue mass.

skull, etc. They usually occur in long bones around the knee joint, as a central lesion which expands and partially destroys the cortex (Fig. 46-13).

Osteoclastoma (Giant Cell Tumor)

The typical osteoclast is a large cell containing a variable number of centrally placed but distinct nuclei, which are identical in vesicular appearance, ovoid, and basophilic on staining with hematoxylin and eosin. Its cell of origin is unknown, since it is found in many states and conditions of bone. For example, these cells are commonly found in areas where bone is being remodeled, in recesses named *Howship's lacunae*. They also follow hemorrhage into the marrow or during cyst formation and are particularly prominent in hyperparathyroidism or osteitis fibrosa cystica during the formation of the "brown tumor." They are also found in such bone lesions as nonosteogenic fibroma, unicameral bone cysts, aneurysmal bone cyst, fibrous dysplasia, chondroblastoma, osteosarcoma, and histocytic granulomatosis, but these must be clearly differentiated from a giant cell tumor.

The critical feature of this tumor is the vascular and cellular stroma, which is made up of oval-shaped cells containing a small, elongated, darkly stained nucleus with little eosinophilic cytoplasm on staining with hematoxylin and eosin. The stroma cells show a varying degree of

malignancy with the typical features of mitotic activity, pleomorphism, and hyperchromatism (Fig. 46-14). In the more frankly malignant giant cell tumors, the giant cells become anaplastic, with areas of necrotic material and hemorrhage. These true neoplasms occur primarily in the second and third decades with an equal sex distribution. They are seen mainly in the ends of long bones, particularly in the vicinity of the knee and at the lower end of the radius. They commonly arise in the metaphyseoepiphyseal area and are related to the usual osteoclastic activity of remodeling in this area.

On x-rays, the metaphyseoepiphyseal areas are seen to be enlarged and occupied by a clear cystic tumor (Fig. 46-15). The cortex is thin and may sharply limit the tumor from the surrounding soft tissues, with a sharp line of demarcation between the tumor and the unaffected shaft in contradistinction to sarcomas and bone cysts. The expanding osteolytic lesion can continue to destroy the

Fig. 46-14. *A.* Photomicrograph of tissue from a giant cell tumor containing numerous giant cells and scanty stroma. (×300.) *B.* Photomicrograph of the same tissue showing that the nuclei of the stroma appear similar to those of the giant cells. (×500.)

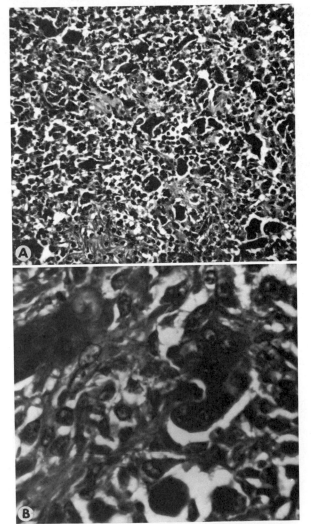

cortex, although usually it leaves some external rim. The tumor grows eccentrically to destroy the epiphyseal cartilage, and it may penetrate the articular cartilage, but rarely does it extend into a joint. Pathologic fractures occur.

Clinically these patients present because of pain and loss of function around the joint, which may even suggest a possible inflammatory lesion or a swelling of an asymmetric nature.

Although in the past these tumors have been regarded as relatively benign, up to 30 percent behave with malignant characteristics despite a benign histologic appearance. There are varying degrees of malignancy of this tumor; because of this, excision is indicated. With curettage there is up to a 50 percent local recurrence rate. Treatment is therefore directed to a complete and total local resection if at all possible. Amputation is occasionally indicated. Radiotherapy has not been shown by Dahlin's group to decrease the recurrence rate, and 10 percent of tumors given such treatment underwent sarcomatous degeneration.

Malignant giant cells are found in osteosarcomas. These are found especially in the more anaplastic lesions and contain a variable number of nuclei but seldom so many as in the osteoclast. The cells and nuclei are irregular in form and size. These features serve to differentiate such malignant giant cells from the osteoclast.

NONOSTEOGENIC TUMORS OF BONE

Unicameral (Solitary) or Juvenile Bone Cyst

This lesion occurs during the years of active bone growth, particularly in the metaphyseal area of long bones, such as the upper end of the humerus and femur. It usually presents because of a pathologic fracture without previous symptoms except for a minor injury.

On x-ray (Fig. 46-16) a characteristic expanding lesion is seen in the metaphysis with thinning of the cortex as a shell, but it rarely, if ever, penetrates or passes through the still open epiphysis like a giant cell tumor. It is loculated with relatively large cystlike areas.

On biopsy, these cysts are seen to contain a clear, glary fluid with a fine fibrous framework which is relatively avascular. Histologically, the thin fibrous framework is in continuity with the fibrous wall, but there is little cellular activity unless a pathologic fracture has occurred (Fig. 46-17).

This lesion must be differentiated from:

1. *Osteitis fibrosa cystica,* either the generalized form of von Recklinghausen's disease or the localized form. The latter usually occurs during adolescence in the metaphysis, but it tends to spread down the shaft more often. On biopsy, the obvious feature of vascular connective tissue invading cortex and cancellous bone, with degeneration and cyst formation, is observed.
2. *Hydatid disease.* This usually occurs in the long bones of adults, in which there are localized "solid" masses of hydatid material replacing the marrow, cancellous, and cortical components of bone to extend into the soft tissues.
3. *Tumors.* Giant cell tumors occur in older age groups, and al-

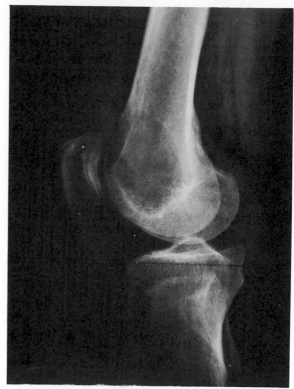

Fig. 46-15. Benign giant cell tumor of the lower femur. The films show a sharply demarcated area of decreased density in the lateral condyle of the femur, extending through the cortex. Some soft tissue swelling around the lesion is visible.

Fig. 46-16. Simple bone cyst of the humerus.

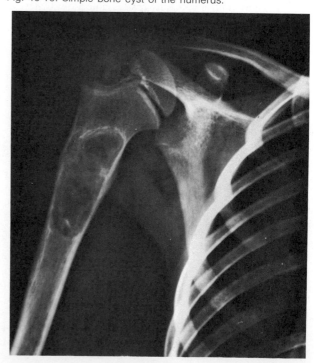

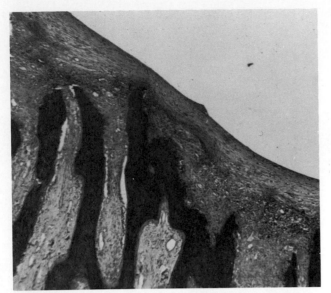

Fig. 46-17. Photomicrograph of the wall of a unicameral bone cyst which is lined with relatively acellular fibrous tissue above the trabeculae of the bone. (×200.)

though the x-ray appearance may be similar, the histologic character is obviously different. Chondromas, myelomas, sarcomas, neurofibromatosis, and secondary metastases must also be differentiated. In sarcoidosis, also to be considered, the tumors are usually multiple, involving the short, miniature bones, such as the metacarpals or phalanges.

Treatment is surgical and directed toward total obliteration of the cavity by a guttering and curetting procedure or collapsing down of the surrounding and thinned cortex by compression. Bone grafting, to restore continuity, is then carried out both with autogenous cancellous bone and overlying cortical matchstick grafts.

Periosteal Fibrosarcoma

This tumor originates in the outer nonosteogenic fibrous layer of the periosteum. It is a fascial sarcoma and similar in character to those arising in other sites in the soft tissues. It is extracortical and neither invades nor infiltrates the bone. The tumor remains encapsulated for a long time; as it grows, it pushes aside the soft tissues but rarely infiltrates them.

Secondary changes eventually appear in the underlying bone, but they result from the pressure and the contact of the tumor. Saucer-shaped erosions may occur where the cortex is in contact with the tumor and areas of new periosteal bone formation at the periphery.

The tumor may appear to be encapsulated, but the capsule merely consists of the condensed surrounding tissues. It remains localized for a considerable time, but ultimately, as the vascularity and cellularity increase, it becomes more malignant. At this stage secondary metastases usually occur in the lungs.

Histologically the tumor is a spindle cell fibrosarcoma with a variable degree of collagen formation. There is no true ossification, but calcification can occur.

Radical removal of the tumor is the operation of choice, with a favorable prognosis when the tumor is encapsulated. If the operation is incomplete, it may be followed by local recurrence and general metastases. The operation should be supplemented by a prolonged course of deep x-ray therapy, although its beneficial effects are questionable.

Ewing's Tumor

In 1921 Ewing described a rare lesion of bone characterized by the development of a tumor from the endothelial marrow of the diaphysis of the long bones, occurring in childhood and associated with febrile attacks. The tumor rapidly involved other parts of the skeleton and was radiosensitive. Willis demonstrated that many of the cases diagnosed clinically and radiologically as "Ewing's tumor," because the histologic pattern demonstrated a rosette formation, were really neuroblastomas, and a primary tumor could be found in the adrenal. Ewing's tumor must also be differentiated from reticulum cell sarcoma (Table 46-1) and from chronic osteomyelitis.

Ewing's tumor usually appears between the ages of five and fifteen. The bones most commonly affected are the tibia, the fibula, the humerus, and the femur. Regional lymph glands may be involved, and polyostotic lesions may be present.

The tumor begins in the diaphyseal marrow; it is grayish white with areas of necrosis and hemorrhage causing destruction of trabeculae and suggesting osteomyelitis. From the medulla the tumor extends to the periosteum, where new bone formation occurs. This has been aptly described as "onion layers."

The tumor is very cellular; the cells are small, round or polyhedral, and arranged in solid cords or sheets with little intercellular substance. The nuclei are always prominent, and mitosis is frequent (Fig. 46-18).

Many tumors show a rosette arrangement, and within the center of the rosette, by special staining methods, fibrils can sometimes be demonstrated, similar to those of a

Table 46-1. DIFFERENTIAL DIAGNOSIS OF EWING'S TUMOR AND RETICULUM CELL SARCOMA

Ewing's tumor	Reticulum cell sarcoma
1. Under 20 years	1. 35–40 years
2. Much periosteal reaction with some bone destruction	2. Little periosteal reaction, but destructive and expanding lesion
3. Small cells with compact chromatin and less well-defined cytoplasm	3. Larger, round, or oval cells with indented, or kidney-shaped, nucleus but poorly defined and stained cytoplasm; delicate framework of interlacing fibers with pattern
4. Radiosensitive	4. Radiosensitive
5. No 5-year survivors	5. 50% 5-year survivors

SOURCE: From W. Mercer and R. B. Duthie, "Orthopaedic Surgery," 7th ed., Edward Arnold (Publishers) Ltd., London, 1974.

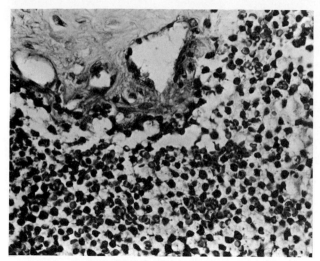

Fig. 46-18. Photomicrograph of tissue from the Ewing's tumor of the scapula, to show the marked cellularity with small round cells and little intercellular substance. (× 250.)

neuroblastoma. The vessels of both the tumor and the lymphatics may contain obvious emboli, for the tumor spreads by the blood and lymphatic systems.

CLINICAL MANIFESTATIONS. A history of trauma may be elicited, and chronic pain may occur. There may be febrile attacks and leukocytosis. X-rays demonstrate a circumscribed osteoporotic area in the center of the shaft, extending for a considerable distance. Later, the periosteum shows onion-skin layers parallel to the shaft and rather like osteomyelitis, or more commonly small spicules appear (Fig. 46-19). Pathologic fracture seldom occurs. When the vertebrae are involved, there is severe root pain or paralysis. Death usually results from metastatic involvement of the lungs.

TREATMENT. Deep x-ray therapy may cause the local lesion to disappear, but subsequent local recurrence is the rule. Accordingly it has been the practice to follow primary radiation with amputation. Such treatment will not affect the ultimate prognosis in those cases where the tumor has metastasized. Survival is usually about 2 years, and it is commonly stated that the lesions of the so-called 5-year survivors have been misdiagnosed and have really been reticulum cell sarcoma. Dahlin et al. reviewed their experience of Ewing's sarcoma treated at the Mayo Clinic and emphasized that the 5-year survival rate of 133 patients was only 15 percent, 95 patients having died within 2 years of the time of diagnosis.

Reticulum Cell Sarcoma

This tumor occurs in patients between twenty and forty years of age and particularly affects the femur, tibia, and humerus. Pain is often the first complaint, preceding the formation of a tumor which may invade a large part of the shaft.

Radiologically there is an osteolytic lesion in the end of the diaphysis which later extends throughout the length, and pathologic fracture may occur.

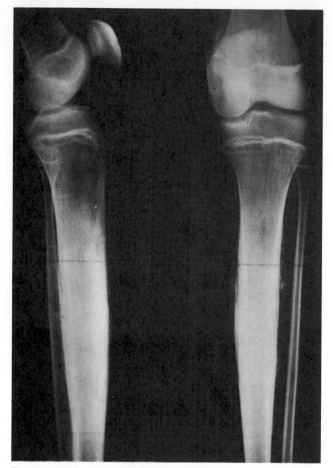

Fig. 46-19. Ewing's tumor of the tibia. The films show diffuse bone reaction with periosteal lifting and onion-skin thickening of the cortex plus some spiculation.

The tumor is made up of a pinkish gray granulation tissue, and the cells are larger than a lymphocyte and have round, oval, indented, or lobulated nuclei with considerable cytoplasm. Delicate reticulum fibers pass between the cells, which often show a large number of mitotic figures (Fig. 46-20).

Although the initial response to radiation is good, local recurrence may take place, and therefore radiation should be followed by amputation or radical resection.

BLOOD VESSEL TUMORS

Aneurysmal Bone Cyst

This lesion occurs in the metaphyses of long bones in young people. X-rays show a characteristic lesion of an eccentrically placed osteolytic expansion of the cortex, with some extension into the surrounding soft tissues, and periosteal new bone formation. On biopsy, there is a mass of blood spaces filled with frank blood. Histologically, the characteristic feature consists of cavernous spaces built by fibrous tissue containing some osteoid tissue, but rarely an

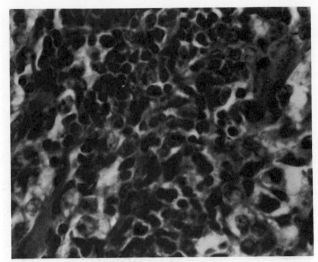

Fig. 46-20. Photomicrograph of tissue from a reticulum cell sarcoma showing the rounded or indented cells with large numbers of mitotic figures. (×300.)

endothelial lining. Giant cells may be present, particularly in the more cellular areas of the tumor. Stroma cells are usually fibroblastic and have to be differentiated from those of a giant cell tumor. Local curettage, with or without bone grafting, will give an adequate result.

Hemangioma

Vascular tumors of bone are rare, but the most common sites for these lesions are in the skull and vertebral column. In the vertebral column when the body is affected, the appearance may suggest tuberculosis, secondary neoplasm, or Paget's disease. Collapse of the vertebral body occurs with pressure on the cord.

These tumors are benign in a majority of instances. Treatment is difficult on account of the location of the tumor, but should the lesion be peripheral, radical excision has been advised.

Angiosarcoma (Angioendothelioma)

This is *extremely* rare and must be differentiated from the reticulosarcoma, which may mimic it closely because of the potential endothelial function of reticular cells.

TUMORS ARISING FROM INCLUDED TISSUES

Adamantinoma

Adamantinoma, or adamantine epithelioma, occurs in the jaw and more rarely in the tibia. The long-bone tumors may not be related to adamantinomas of the jaw, since no enamel has been found in them. Pain accompanied by tenderness is commonly the first symptom.

It is a slow-growing tumor the origin of which is unknown. This epithelial tumor may be a basal cell or squamous cell carcinoma. Microscopically it consists of solid strands, sheets, or whorls of dark-staining polygonal or spindle-shaped cells, often with a tendency toward a syncytial character. It shows a tendency to form clefts and cysts, and in most cases there are collections of cuboidal cells arranged in irregular acini. The treatment of choice is amputation, preferably through the more proximal bone. Metastasis has been proved by biopsy in several cases, further emphasizing the need for radical surgical treatment, especially with local bone destruction.

Neurilemmoma

This is a type of nerve sheath tumor which may grow in bone. Clinically the tumor may present as a cystic swelling, and the x-rays show a destruction of the bone. The common and often only symptom is the physical presence of a tumor. This is always single and circumscribed. The clinical course appears to be benign, and local removal appears to be adequate.

Chordoma

Chordoma is a rare malignant neoplasm found at either end of the spinal axis. It is generally accepted as originating from embryonic remnants of the notochord. Although in the adult remnants of the notochord persist in the intervertebral disks in the form of the nucleus pulposus, the majority of chordomas arise in either the spheno-occipital or sacrococcygeal region. Sixty percent occur in the latter area. The physical presence of a tumor is usually the first symptom, though there is often pain in the back with sacral tumors. The tumors are locally invasive and tend to recur after removal.

The radiogram usually shows destruction of bone with an expanding soft tissue shadow (Fig. 46-21). There is nothing characteristic in the bony erosion, and the diagnosis, though it may be guessed at from the site, is usually made by biopsy. The tumor is slow-growing but malignant and kills by invasion of vital structures.

Microscopically chordomas are distinguished with difficulty from atypical chondromas and mucoid, or signet-ring cell, carcinomas arising in the gastrointestinal tract. Myeloblastomas originating in the sacrococcygeal region are usually interpreted as chordomas. The chordoma cells are more epithelial in appearance than cartilage and more variable in size. There is a great tendency for vacuolization and variability in the size of the nuclei.

An attempt at complete surgical extirpation must be made, since these growths are radioresistant.

MALIGNANT TUMORS OF SOFT TISSUES

FIBROSARCOMA OF MUSCLE. These are of two types: differentiated fibrosarcoma with malignant fibroblasts and malignant fibrosarcoma with anaplastic cells. Both usually infiltrate widely, and the patient presents with a painful and large tumor mass, particularly in the thigh.

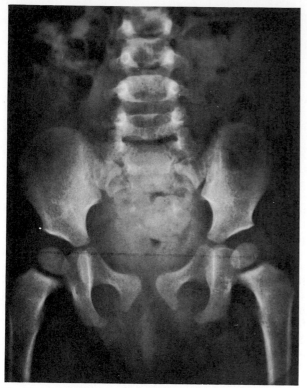

Fig. 46-21. Chordoma destroying the coccyx of an infant.

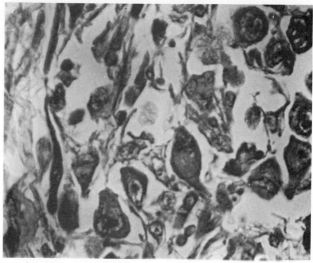

Fig. 46-22. Photomicrograph of tissue from a rhabdomyosarcoma to show the giant rhabdomyoblasts with multiple nuclei. (× 350.)

LIPOSARCOMA. This occurs in the soft tissues of the extremities and is one of the more common malignant soft tissue tumors. It presents in the middle age groups with little difference between the sexes. It occurs commonly in the thigh, in the popliteal area as well as in the inguinal and gluteal regions. It does not appear to arise in simple lipomas. Like the fibrosarcoma, these tumors are of two types, well-differentiated and anaplastic. Curative treatment is directed toward wide surgical excision, because their radiosensitivity varies.

RHABDOMYOSARCOMA. This is a malignant tumor involving the striated muscle cells. It occurs commonly in infants and young adults. It has a high incidence of blood metastasis with rapid growth and fungation. Histologically it is characterized by giant rhabdomyoblasts with multiple nuclei which attempt to form myofibrils (Fig. 46-22). It is rarely radiosensitive.

SYNOVIAL SARCOMAS. These occur in subcutaneous tissue as well as in deeply placed muscle layers and have no obvious continuity with joint tissue, although it is supposed that they arise from embryologically sequestered "synovioblastic cells" (Fig. 46-23). They infiltrate and spread locally. Total radical local excision should be carried out and should include the main muscle mass involved.

RETICULUM CELL SARCOMA. This also arises in subcutaneous as well as in muscle layers and develops at any age, growing rapidly and infiltrating widely with metastasis via the bloodstream to the lungs. These tumors have to be differentiated from Ewing's sarcoma.

MALIGNANT GIANT CELL TUMORS. These tumors can arise in subcutaneous tissues as well as joint structures, tendons, and tendon sheaths. Their malignancy is variable and can be evaluated by their histologic pattern.

DESMOID TUMOR. This appears to be a very low-grade fibrosarcoma which is locally invasive but does not tend to metastasize by blood. It occurs in the deep muscle masses as a painful tumor or swelling. It has a much better prognosis than a fibrosarcoma, even though it occurs in young people, but it can recur following inadequate resection. Therefore, it is advisable to remove the involved muscle mass in its entirety.

GENERAL PRINCIPLES OF TREATMENT OF SOFT TISSUE MALIGNANT TUMORS. Bowden and Booher have pointed out that usually no capsule surrounds the malignant cells but by rapid growth the surrounding soft tissues may be

Fig. 46-23. Photomicrograph of tissue from a synovial sarcoma to show the large synovioblastic cells forming a villuslike structure. (×350.)

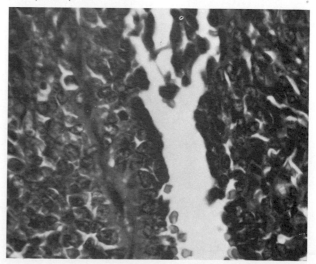

compressed to form a pseudocapsule. More often this capsule is made up of the peripherally situated neoplastic cells. Therefore, if the malignant tumor is only enucleated, a shell of neoplastic cells will be left behind. The entire muscle bundle surrounding the sarcoma must be removed from its point of origin to its insertion, by sharp dissection as well as ligation of all major tributaries. Amputation is indicated when the anatomic location requires it.

Although in recent decades heroic attempts have been made to reduce the mortality and morbidity of malignant tumors in the upper aspect of both extremities, by such operations as the forequarter and hindquarter amputations, for such tumors as osteosarcoma, Ewing's tumor, etc., these procedures have proved of little value in prolonging life. Their main indication appears to be the need to prevent fungation or ulceration and to relieve local symptoms, except in malignant tumors of soft tissues arising high in the buttock or thigh, such as liposarcoma, fibrosarcoma, or secondary chondrosarcoma. Modification of the classic hemipelvectomy has been described by Sherman and Duthie in which there is less deformity and dysfunction but still an adequate tumor excision. With operation it is possible to obtain a 30 to 40 percent 5-year survival rate.

METASTATIC TUMORS OF BONE

The skeleton is one of the most common sites for metastases, accounting for more than half the cases of malignant bone tumors. Their actual incidence is probably higher than that recorded, since the skeleton is inadequately examined at necropsy. Abrams and his colleagues, in 1,000 consecutive autopsies on patients with carcinoma, described metastases in 27 to 84 percent from prostatic carcinomas, 73 percent from breast, 50 percent from thyroid, and 32 percent from bronchogenic carcinomas. The carcinomas which commonly metastasize to bone arise in the

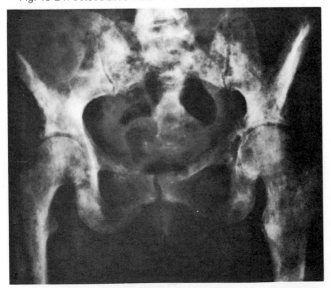

Fig. 46-24. Osteoblastic metastases from carcinoma of the breast.

breast (about 30 percent; Fig. 46-24), prostate, thyroid, kidney, and lung, as well as from adrenal neuroblastoma. However, skeletal metastases have been found in virtually all types of malignant tumors including melanomas, carcinoids, and testicular, ovarian, and intestinal tumors.

METHOD OF SPREAD. Bone may be involved as a result of direct spread from an overlying tumor such as from squamous carcinoma of the skin in the facial bones and in the calvarium and in the ribs from bronchogenic and mammary carcinoma. However, the usual route is via the bloodstream. This may be by the systemic circulation with the cells entering veins in the tumor, passing through the pulmonary circulation to the arterial bloodstream, and then to the capillary beds. This does not explain the selective distribution of skeletal metastases in the dorsal and lumbar spine, pelvis, rib cage, skull, and proximal end of the femur.

In an attempt to explain the high incidence of metastases in the axial skeleton, Batson has described an alternative route for the dissemination of malignant cells. He has shown that the vertebral venous system, which contains no valves, communicates freely with venous channels of the chest wall and the intrathoracic and abdominal viscera. When the intrathoracic or intraabdominal pressure rises as in coughing or sneezing, the flow of blood in the venous vertebral system can be reversed. By this method malignant cells may be carried into the bodies of the vertebrae or reach the central nervous system.

DIAGNOSIS. Conventional methods of diagnosing skeletal metastases are inaccurate. Of 86 patients with advanced mammary carcinoma, all of whom had skeletal metastases evident on x-ray, only 65.1 percent complained of pain at any stage of the disease, tenderness was elicited in only 16 percent, and the alkaline phosphatase level was raised in only 66 percent. Pain may be localized to a few sites and is not associated with every metastasis.

The serum phosphorus level is raised only when there is associated renal failure with phosphate retention. The serum acid phosphatase concentration is usually elevated in patients with skeletal metastases from prostatic carcinoma.

X-rays also are unreliable. Metastases start growing in the medulla and from there involve the cortex. It has been shown that at least 50 percent of the medulla must be destroyed before a lesion will be seen radiologically. Tomograms are more sensitive.

There is now evidence which indicates that radioisotopes may be more sensitive than x-rays for the early detection of skeletal metastases. Of the bone-seeking isotopes available, the most sensitive would appear to be fluorine 18, although good results have been obtained with ^{47}Ca ^{85}Sr, and ^{87}Sr.

The vast majority of skeletal metastases evoke an osteoid reaction by the invaded bone. The degree of osteoid and new bone formation varies from tumor to tumor. It is most marked in prostatic carcinoma. Because this osteoid has an increased avidity for the bone-seeking isotopes, they can be used for the early detection of skeletal metastases.

The separation of skeletal metastases into lytic or sclerotic, depending on their radiologic appearance, is reinforced by histologic examination. In all metastases there is a combination of destruction due to the tumor and new bone formation caused by the reaction of the bone to the lesion.

Hypercalcemia is found particularly in association with bronchogenic and mammary carcinoma. It is usually produced as a result of the destruction of the skeleton by metastases. As the bone is destroyed, the calcium is released into the circulation. If the kidneys are functioning, the calcium is excreted in the urine as a hypercalcinuria. However, if the kidneys are unable to excrete the increased load, the serum calcium level rises to produce hypercalcemia. Hypercalcemia may also be caused by the secretion of a parathormone-like or parathyrotropic principle by the tumor, which is sometimes found in a bronchogenic carcinoma, by the excretion of a vitamin D–like principle, or by the excretion of specific osteolytic sterols which have been isolated from mammary carcinoma.

TREATMENT. Treatment of skeletal metastases is essentially palliative, although there have been cases described where a solitary metastasis from a hypernephroma has been removed, after the primary tumor was treated, with apparent cure (Fig. 46-25). As many patients may live for months or years with skeletal metastases, it is important to relieve their symptoms.

Pain may occur only in association with hypercalcemia. Once the hypercalcemia has been treated, the pain will be relieved. It may be associated with a pathologic fracture; again, the pathologic fracture must be treated. Large lytic metastases with impending fracture may also produce pain and require treatment. If the patient has a hormonally dependent tumor such as carcinoma of the breast or prostate, the pain is often relieved by hormonal therapy. In carcinoma of the prostate, therapy with diethylstilbestrol diphosphate (stilbestrol), orchidectomy, or a combination of both frequently relieves pain. In mammary carcinoma approximately 27 percent of patients respond objectively to hormonal therapy. In the premenopausal woman this usually consists of an oophorectomy. In the postmenopausal woman diethylstilbestrol is usually given. In both groups when the primary treatment fails to produce a remission, androgens, progestogens, or corticosteroids have been tried; if these fail, endocrine ablative surgery is usually indicated. This includes procedures such as adrenalectomy, hypophysectomy, or pituitary ablation using rods of [90]yttrium.

Where hormonal therapy is not indicated or not effective, radiotherapy to a localized area of pain will frequently produce relief. Where the pain is not controlled by radiotherapy or hormonal therapy, analgesics must be given without concern over drug addiction. Interruption of the nerve supply to the painful area is sometimes indicated. This may take the form of phenol blocks, rhizotomies, and even a spinothalamic tactotomy.

Large lytic lesions with impending fracture should be internally fixed. They usually occur in the shafts of the femur or humerus or in the neck of the femur. Lesions in the shafts should be fixed with a closed nailing using a Küntschner nail. For lesions in the neck of the femur a Massie nail pin and plate are required. Following inter-

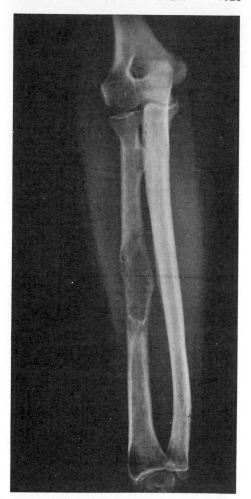

Fig. 46-25. Solitary metastasis in the radius from hypernephroma. The lesion characteristically involves the more proximal bones such as the humerus and femur.

nal fixation the area is irradiated. Where radiotherapy is given prior to internal fixation, a pathologic fracture may occur, making treatment more difficult.

More than 50 percent of patients in whom a pathologic fracture occurs die of the disease within 3 months, although survivals of 6 years or more after pathologic fracture have been known. Without treatment the fracture will not heal. Since the most common site is the femur, the patient will become bedridden.

When several vertebrae have collapsed, some form of brace may be required. Occasionally compression fractures may be associated with involvement of the spinal cord or cauda equina with sensory, motor, or bladder disturbances. Laminectomy and decompression is urgently indicated, since once paraplegia is established, it is very rarely relieved by surgery. Radiotherapy is very useful for treating pain but usually does not improve an established paraplegia. However, a laminectomy can be carried out only if there is sufficient bone in the vertebral body to prevent complete collapse and instability of the spinal column.

References

Abrams, H. L.: Skeletal Metastases in Carcinoma, *Radiology,* **55:**534, 1950.

———, Spiro, R., and Goldstein, N.: Metastases in Carcinoma: Analysis of 1000 Autopsied Cases, *Cancer,* **3:**74, 1950.

Batson, O. V.: The Role of the Vertebral Veins in Metastatic Processes, *Ann Intern Med,* **16:**38, 1942.

Bowden, L., and Booher, R. J.: The Principles and Technique of Resection of Soft Parts for Sarcoma, *Surgery,* **44:**6, 1958.

Collins, D.: Paget's Disease of Bone: Incidence and Subclinical Forms, *Lancet,* **2:**51, 1956.

Cortez, E. P., Holland, J. F., and Wang, J. J.: Doxorubicin in Disseminated Osteogenic Sarcoma, *JAMA,* **221:**1132, 1972.

Dahlin, D. C.: "Bone Tumours," Charles C Thomas, Publisher, Springfield, Ill., 1957.

———, Coventry, M. B., and Scanlon, P. W.: Ewing's Sarcoma: A Critical Analysis of 165 Cases, *J Bone Joint Surg [Am],* **43A:**185, 1961.

——— and Henderson, E. D.: Chondrosarcoma, A Surgical and Pathological Problem: Review of 212 Cases, *J Bone Joint Surg [Am]* **38A:**5, 1956.

Edelstyn, G. A., Gillespie, P. J., and Grebbell, F. S.: The Radiological Demonstration of Osseous Metastases: Experimental Observations, *Clin Radiol,* **18:**158, 1967.

Foulds, L.: Experimental Study of Tumour Progression: Review, *Cancer Res,* **14:**327, 1954.

Gordan, G. S.: Medical Staff Conference: Hypercalcemia of Malignant Disease, *Calif Med,* **107:**54, 1967.

Grimes, B. J., Fisher, B., Finn, F., and Danowski, T. S.: Steroid-resistant Hypercalcemia and Parathyroid Hyperplasia in Non-osseous Cancer, *Acta Endocrinol (Kbb),* **56:**510, 1967.

Guri, J. P.: Tumors of the Vertebral Column, *J Surg Gynecol Obstet,* **87:**583, 1948.

Jaffe, H. L.: "Osteoid-osteoma": Benign Osteoblastic Tumour Composed of Osteoid and Atypical Bone, *Arch Surg,* **31:**709, 1935.

———: "Tumors and Tumorous Conditions of the Bones and Joints," Lea & Febiger, Philadelphia, 1958.

Jaffe, N.: Recent Advances in the Chemotherapy of Metastatic Osteosarcoma, *Cancer,* **30:**1627, 1972.

Johnson, L. C.: A General Theory of Bone Tumours, *Bull NY Acad Med,* **29:**2, 1953.

Lichtenstein, L.: "Bone Tumors," 3d ed., The C. V. Mosby Company, St. Louis, 1965.

McKenna, R. J, Schwinn, C. P., Soong, K. Y., and Higinbotham, N. L.: Sarcomata of the Osteogenic Series (Osteosarcoma, Fibrosarcoma, Chondrosarcoma, Parosteal Osteogenic Sarcoma, and Sarcomata Arising in Abnormal Bone): An Analysis of 552 Cases, *J Bone Joint Surg [Am],* **48A:**1, 1966.

Marcove, R. C., Miké, V., Hajek, J. V., Levin, A. G., and Hutter, R. V. P.: Osteogenic Sarcoma under the Age of 21: A Review of 145 Operative Cases, *J Bone Joint Surg [Am],* **52A:**411, 1970.

Marsh, B., Flynn, L., and Enneking, W.: Immunological Aspects of Osteosarcoma and Their Relationship to Therapy, *J Bone Joint Surg [Am],* **54A,** 1367, 1972.

Milch, R. A., and Changus, G. W.: Response of Bone to Tumor Invasion, *Cancer,* **9:**340, 1956.

Morton, D. L., Eilber, F. R., Townsend, C. M., Jr., Grant, T. T., Mirra, J., and Weisenburger, T. H.: Limb Salvage from a Multidisciplinary Treatment Approach for Skeletal and Soft Tissue Sarcomas of the Extremity, *Ann Surg,* **184:**268, 1976.

Plimpton, C. H., and Gelhorn, A.: Hypercalcemia in Malignant Disease without Evidence of Bone Destruction, *Am J Med,* **21:**5, 1956.

Price, C. H. G.: Primary Bone-forming Tumours and Their Relationship to Skeletal Growth, *J Bone Joint Surg [Br],* **40B:**574, 1958.

Sherman, C. D., and Duthie, R. B.: Modified Hemipelvectomy, *Cancer,* **13:**1, 1960.

Sissons, H. A., and Duthie, R. B.: "British Surgical Practice: Surgical Progress," Butterworth & Co. (Publishers), Ltd., London, 1959.

Spjut, H. J., Dorfman, H., Feckner, R., and Ackerman, L.: "Tumors of Bone and Cartilage," ser. 2, Armed Forces Institute of Pathology, Washington, 1971.

Thomson, A. D., and Turner-Warwick, R. T.: Skeletal Sarcomata and Giant-cell Tumour, *J Bone Joint Surg [Br],* **37B:**266, 1955.

Willis, R. A.: "Pathology of Tumours," 2d ed., Butterworth & Co. (Publishers), Ltd., London, 1953.

Chapter 47

Fractures and Joint Injuries

by Franklin T. Hoaglund and Robert B. Duthie

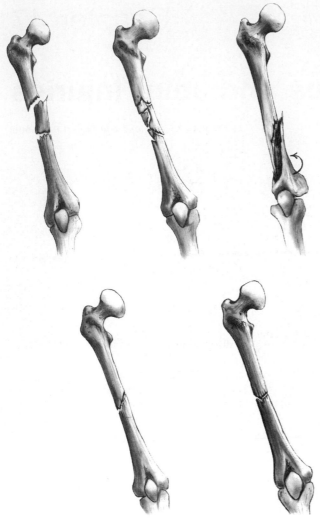

Fig. 47-1. Types of fractures. Top row, segmental, comminuted, and spiral; bottom row, oblique and transverse.

GENERAL CONSIDERATIONS

Definitions

A fracture is a linear deformation or discontinuity of bone produced by forces exceeding the modulus of elasticity of the bone. The strength of bone may be below normal because of pathologic conditions such as tumor, infection, or metabolic bone disease, which impair its normal viscoelastic properties. If bone is normal, excessive force will cause a fracture. The force applied to the bone may be direct, as when a car bumper strikes a tibia causing a fracture at the site of impact. The force may be applied indirectly by torsional stress, resulting in fracture occurring at a distance from the area of force application.

Fractures are classified anatomically as to location in the bone, e.g., epiphyseal, metaphyseal, or diaphyseal. Fractures are also characterized according to the plane of the fracture surface (Fig. 47-1). In a transverse fracture the plane of the fracture surface is perpendicular to the long axis of the bone. A spiral fracture is one in which the fracture surface is spiral and is produced by torsional stress which fractures the bone along the line of maximal sheer. In an oblique fracture the fracture surface forms an angle with the axis of the shaft. Comminution indicates more than two fragments or potential fragments are present.

A fracture is undisplaced when a plane of cleavage exists in the bone, without angulation or displacement. If separation of bone fragments exists, the fracture is said to be displaced. The direction of displacement is described by the relationship of the distal fragment with respect to the proximal fragments as medial, lateral, posterior, etc. Displacement is measured in terms of the thickness of the shaft; e.g., the distal fragment is displaced laterally one-half the diameter of the shaft. Angulation indicates angular deformity between the axes of the major fragments. It is also described by the position of the distal fragment with respect to the proximal one. Rotational deformity is expressed in similar fashion.

A *closed*, or simple, fracture is one in which the fracture surface does not communicate with the skin or mucous membranes. An *open*, or compound, fracture is one with communication between the fracture surface and the skin or mucous membrane. A *pathologic* fracture is a discontinuity occurring in the bone at an area of weakness caused by pathologic processes including tumor, infection, or metabolic bone disease. A *stress*, or fatigue, fracture is the response of bone to repeated stress, none of which by itself is sufficient to cause a fracture. The earliest pathologic process in stress fracture is osteoclastic resorption, followed by periosteal callus, in an attempt to repair and strengthen the bone. If the repeated stress is halted in time, actual discontinuity of the bone does not occur. A *compression* fracture results when a compression force causes compaction of bone trabeculae, resulting in decreased length or width of a portion of the bone, e.g., compression wedging in thoracic spine fractures. A *greenstick* fracture is an incomplete fracture with the opposite cortex intact. A *torus* fracture is one in which one cortex is intact with buckling or compaction of the opposite cortex (Fig. 47-2).

Diagnosis

The clinical manifestations of fracture are (1) pain, (2) swelling, (3) deformity, (4) ecchymosis, (5) instability, (6) crepitus. The most reliable diagnostic signs are instability and crepitus. Crepitus should not be tested for specifically, since it increases the local soft tissue injury. A specific diagnosis requires two plane film x-rays at right angles to each other, taken at the level of the fracture site. When the patient is examined a few minutes after injury, swelling and ecchymosis may not be present. In such situations, reexamination and/or x-ray diagnosis is necessary. The surgeon should not place absolute faith in the x-rays in ruling out undisplaced or chip fractures. When the patient has significant symptoms and the x-rays are negative, the patient should be treated with splints and re-x-rayed at 14 to 21 days, when sufficient resorption or periosteal new bone formation is present about the fracture site.

Evaluation of the Injured Patient

The immediate threat to a patient's life from an injured extremity is rare but does occur. Associated injuries to the thoracic, peritoneal, and cranial cavities are potentially more serious and should be immediately evaluated and receive priority for treatment. Shock is not usually caused by one injured extremity, although multiple fractures including pelvic fractures may be responsible. Shock is treated by replacement therapy, while splinting of the fractures continues. It is imperative to determine the presence of a fractured spine and prevent subsequent spinal cord injury by proper handling of the patient. At the scene of the accident and/or when the patient arrives in the emergency room, the spine is carefully palpated for tenderness. Before allowing the patient to sit, stand, or be turned, appropriate spine x-rays should be obtained to determine its stability.

Evaluation of the Injured Extremity

The injured extremity is examined immediately for neurovascular, soft tissue, and bone injury. The presence of peripheral pulsations, capillary flow, and peripheral muscle and nerve function are evaluated to determine vascular competence. Neurologic function is determined by evaluating motor power, as well as skin sensation of touch and pinprick. It may be difficult to get the patient to contract muscles which are injured at a fracture site, but with proper splinting a determination of function, based on an accurate knowledge of peripheral nerves, can usually be made.

The presence of intact skin indicates a closed fracture. However, if the skin is severely damaged or abraded and is nonviable, subsequent skin loss may convert a closed fracture to an open wound. Proximity of sharp bone spicules in relation to the skin should be observed and attempts made to prevent further skin damage from the underlying bone. If there is sufficient skin damage and open-fracture surgical treatment cannot be given within the first 6 hours, it may have to be delayed until the skin is healed.

Emergency Splinting of Fractures

After close scrutiny and evaluation of neurovascular injuries and local skin trauma, splinting of the fracture is carried out to minimize further soft tissue or neurovascular injury. If the wound is compound, exposed bone which has been contaminated is not replaced into the depths of the wound until debridement is complete. Splinting of fractures of the knee or distal to the knee or elbow is done with an air splint if available (Fig. 47-3). A pillow splint may be used to bind an injured ankle, or folded magazines bound with loose mesh gauze may be used on forearm fractures. Fractures involving the humerus or shoulder girdle can be splinted by the use of a sling and a swath bandage. Fractures involving the femur require the application of traction over a Thomas splint.

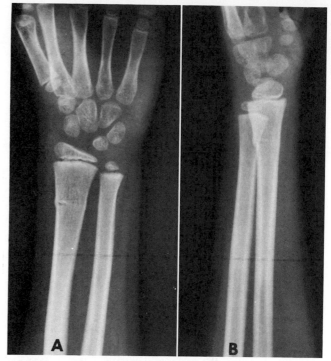

Fig. 47-2. Torus, or buckle, fracture. *A.* AP x-ray, on which the radiolucent line is visible proximal to the distal radial epiphysis. *B.* Lateral x-ray, showing a buckling of the distal cortex of the radius.

Anesthesia for Fracture Reductions

When reduction of fractures is indicated, anesthesia is usually required. An exception to this is the dorsally angulated distal radius in a child, which may be reduced with deft manipulation.

The use of local infiltration anesthesia to the fracture site hematoma can be effective, safe, and minimally hazardous to the patient.

TECHNIQUE. The area overlying the fracture site is cleansed with 2% aqueous iodine and alcohol. An area of undamaged skin is infiltrated with local 2% Xylocaine; a sensitivity to Xylocaine must be determined by the history. The fracture site is entered and infiltrated with a few milliliters of 2% Xylocaine. The hematoma is partially evacuated to accommodate the increased volume of local anesthetic solution. In the case of fractures of both bones of the forearm or bimalleolar fractures both fracture sites

Fig. 47-3. Long leg air splint about the lower extremity.

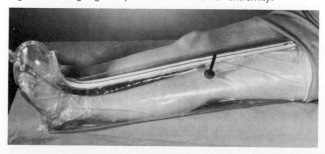

must be anesthetized. Manipulation of the fracture is not carried out until at least 10 to 30 minutes following fracture site injection.

Peripheral nerve block, spinal anesthesia, general anesthesia, or intravenously administered procaine plus a tourniquet may be required in some closed fractures and is invariably necessary for open wounds.

Open Fractures

An open, or compound, fracture has a direct pathway of communication through the skin or mucous membrane. Regardless of how the injury is sustained, there is resultant contamination of the fracture site and potential infection, i.e., osteomyelitis. Less than adequate treatment by the initial surgeon may result in delayed union, skin loss, loss of joint motion, chronic osteomyelitis, and even amputation. The degree of initial injury to the bone and surrounding soft tissue with its attendant circulation to the bone determines the end result. The union of fractures requires adequate circulation to the bone fragments. When the periosteum, muscle, and skin have been severely traumatized by injury or further devitalized by ill-advised and ill-applied surgical technique, complications, from nonunion to infection, are the end result. Once infection complicates a fracture, adjacent bone may be rendered avascular, which interferes with or prevents union. When circulation to an area of infected bone is still present, the normal response of the bone is to lay osteoid seams about the contaminating bacteria. In so doing, the bacteria are contained, but normal mechanisms of bacterial destruction by phagocytosis are prevented, and chronic osteomyelitis may result.

The major aim in the treatment of open fractures is to prevent infection and provide an environment for bone union. This is accomplished by excising sources of contamination and devitalized tissue without further compromise to local, viable, uninjured tissue. Since all open wounds are contaminated from the instant the bone comes in contact with skin, antibiotic therapy is always indicated. This should in no way be construed as prophylactic antibiotic treatment. However, the umbrella of antibiotic coverage is not a substitute for meticulous, complete, surgical debridement of the wound. Both antibiotic treatment and debridement are basic necessities in the proper management of open fractures. Immobilization of the fragments is needed to prevent further soft tissue devitalization and promote union.

Debridement of open wounds is optimally done within the first 6 hours after injury. In some wounds it may be possible to cover these structures with muscle or skin and to institute appropriate drainage at a distance from tendons, nerves, and blood vessels. Primary closure of open wounds is hazardous and rarely indicated. Secondary closure at 5 to 7 days is preferable.

TECHNIQUE. The following technique is outlined for the treatment of an open tibial shaft fracture with a 6-in. wound over the medial subcutaneous surface of the tibia. Steps in treatment of this wound apply generally to most open fractures.

1. The wound is covered with a sterile bandage and placed in a long leg air splint, as soon as evaluation of the injury is complete.
2. Intravenously administered penicillin, 2 million units, and 1,000 ml of glucose and water are started as soon as the patient arrives in the emergency room (after questioning as to penicillin sensitivity). One gram of streptomycin is given intramuscularly. A booster dose of tetanus toxoid is given, or appropriate human tetanus antitoxin. If the patient does not have an adequate blood level at the time of surgical intervention, 1 Gm of crystalline local penicillin is instilled into the wound prior to closure.
3. In the operating room, under regional or general anesthesia, a sterile sponge is placed over the wound and skin, which has been shaved and prepared with antiseptic, taking care not to contaminate the wound further.
4. Skin edges of the wound are excised, taking only those amounts of tissue necessary to remove avascular and contaminated skin. Relatively clean areas require only a 1- to 2-mm excision. The first set of instruments is then discarded. The leg is then carefully redraped and all devitalized tissue debrided from the depths of the wound. Avascular muscle is recognized by noncontractility, blue or black color, and soft fish-flesh consistency.
5. If necessary, the skin incision is enlarged to expose the fracture site properly. Careful evaluation of damaged skin and a basic knowledge of circulation to skin flaps are required to prevent further devitalization of skin adjacent to the wound.
6. The ends of the bone are exposed with a bone hook, and the fracture surface is gently curetted to remove all sources of debris. Small, detached fragments are removed. Larger fragments are curetted and left in place as judgment indicates.
7. The fracture is aligned and the skin approximated over exposed bone if possible. As a rule, some area of the wound is left open; if there is any question about adequate debridement, the entire wound is left open. Only under optimal conditions should the wound be closed tightly.
8. The leg is immobilized in a well-molded plaster cast over two thicknesses of sheet wadding. If there is a question of viability of the foot or difficulties with position of fracture fragments, skeletal traction through the os calcis, with the leg on a Böhler-Braun frame, may be used.
9. Intravenous Keflin or another appropriate antibiotic is administered prior to and during debridement in order to have therapeutic levels at the fracture site hematoma. Antibiotics are continued for a minimum of 10 to 14 days postinjury. The cast is split to relieve swelling of the leg, as necessary. The wound is inspected at 5 to 7 days, and secondary closure carried out. If the wound is not sufficiently clean at that time, the wound may be left open and early weight bearing started.

In an occasional fractured tibia with a 1-mm puncture wound caused by penetrating bone from the inside with good evidence that it did not penetrate the pants leg of the patient, surgical exposure of the bone may not be necessary. In the rare case where these conditions prevail, antibiotics are indicated and continued for a minimum of 2 weeks.

Vascular Injury

Major arterial injury should be suspected with any fracture-dislocation or trauma to an extremity. The first diagnostic consideration must be the determination of vascular competence. A maximal time limit for irreversible change from complete muscle ischemia is 6 to 8 hours, and delay in diagnosis may result in ultimate amputation. Arterial injury may accompany any fracture or dislocation, although certain fractures or dislocations, such as supracondylar fractures of the humerus or femur, femoral shaft fractures, and knee dislocations, carry a higher incidence. Gunshot wounds and open fractures have the highest incidence.

The diagnosis of vascular compromise may be difficult. One should never hesitate to seek experienced consultation when the diagnosis is in doubt. Diagnosis depends on evaluation of skin color, warmth, capillary return, ischemic pain, motor and sensory nerve function, and the presence of arterial pulsations. In the upper extremity, the ability of the patient to extend the fingers actively or passively in the absence of pain and in the presence of good capillary return is good evidence for adequate circulation. The absence of a radial pulse in the presence of these findings is not in itself an indication for vessel exploration. However, the hand must be normal in all aspects. If the radial pulse is absent and hand circulation is in doubt, because of associated local injury, exploration of the proximal arterial supply is indicated.

In the lower extremity, the determinations of pedal pulsations may be difficult. Oscillometric or Doppler determinations will aid in the diagnosis and assist in localization of pulsatile arterial flow. Capillary flow, skin color, warmth, and sensation are difficult to evaluate. Pain due to ischemia is characteristically severe and unrelenting, and continues after the fracture is splinted, reduced, or immobilized. Most patients show marked improvement in comfort when a fracture is immobilized. This is not true of the patient with a fracture and associated arterial insufficiency. Glovelike anesthesia is an important early sign of ischemia.

Griffiths has categorized the signs of vascular compromise by the four P's: pain, pallor, pulselessness, and paralysis, either sensory or motor. When two of these signs are present and vascular insufficiency cannot be ruled out, exploration is indicated. It must be emphasized that the injured limb must be evaluated and reexamined at intervals. Initial injury may produce only intimal trauma, resulting in delayed thrombosis with delayed onset of signs of vascular compromise.

Hypoxemia and the Fat Embolism Syndrome

Tachakra and Sevitt have shown that 50 to 60 percent of patients with femoral shaft fractures will have reduced arterial blood oxygen concentrations either immediately or within 2 to 3 days post injury. Fat macroglobules from the marrow or other sources occluding the pulmonary circulation are the most likely cause. About 10 to 20 percent of patients with femoral shaft fractures will also develop skin petechiae and/or central nervous system depression in addition to hypoxemia within 3 days post injury. This combination of signs is referred to as the fat embolism syndrome. The incidence is greatest in patients with femoral shaft involvement, occurs not infrequently with tibial fractures, and may occur with any fracture or other conditions such as sepsis where bone has not been injured. The diagnosis is a clinical one. Tests for urinary and sputum fat or serum lipase have not proved specific.

All patients with femoral shaft fractures should have

their arterial blood gas tested on admission to hospital; if it is low, the patient should be given oxygen and his or her condition should be carefully monitored both for clinical signs of fat embolism and for subsequent changes in arterial blood oxygen concentration. In patients not responding to oxygen administration, corticosteroids may be of some benefit. Other therapeutic agents include the use of dextran to improve microcirculatory flow and decrease platelet adhesiveness, low-dose heparin for its plasma-clearing effect, and Lasix, especially if there is any question of fluid overload.

Peripheral Nerve Injuries

Soft tissue injuries and fractures of the extremities are not infrequently accompanied by injuries to the peripheral nerves (see Chap. 42). The clinical manifestations and course depend on the degree of injury. With the least severe of nerve injuries, which has been referred to as "neurapraxia," there is a physiologic interruption of nerve conduction manifested by a transient incomplete or complete paralysis and associated with recovery within a 10-week period postinjury. This type of lesion occurs with minor stretch injuries and contusions, and as a result of local continuous pressure on the nerve. With severe stretch injuries, as in brachial plexus stress, or trauma associated with fractures Wallerian degeneration of the axon may occur while the Schwann sheath remains intact, i.e., axonotmesis takes place. In this circumstance, there may be axonal regeneration, and the prognosis is good. The most severe lesion is complete division of the nerve, neurotmesis, which can accompany violent stretch in open or closed fractures.

The axiom that closed soft tissue wounds and fractures cause nerve injuries in continuity, i.e., neurapraxia or axonotmesis, is generally reliable. Peripheral nerve injuries associated with open wounds are more likely to result in actual division of the nerve. Peripheral nerve injuries in continuity should be allowed to heal spontaneously, while transected nerves require nerve suture at a time when surgical repair is feasible. The conservative treatment of a closed fracture should not be altered because of associated peripheral nerve injury. However, attention should be given to splinting the limb in order to maintain the function of unopposed paralyzed muscles and avoid contractures. If treatment of the fracture requires open reduction, this affords an opportunity to inspect the nerve. It is not always possible to recognize the extent of local nerve injury at the initial surgical procedure, since local inflammation, which persists for about 10 days, interferes with determination of the junction between injured and normal nerve.

Neurotmesis, or division of the nerve, requires exact approximation of the nerve ends, so that regeneration of the axon can proceed into the distal portion of the severed tube. Peripheral nerve injuries which should be repaired primarily are sharp lacerations without adjacent stretch, a situation which does not commonly pertain when there are associated soft tissue injuries or fractures. Divided digital nerves are difficult to repair secondarily if length is a problem and do well with primary repair because of their pure sensory character.

At the time of debridement for open fractures, the nerve should be inspected and, if in continuity, should be left undisturbed. If transected, the nerve ends may be loosely approximated and this procedure followed by early delayed repair when the extent of the lesion can be accurately defined. The operative microscope can facilitate examination of the extent of injury and allow primary repair in some situations. It may be necessary to delay repair until the fracture is healed. In general, nerve suture is technically easier after 10 days, at which time the sheath has thickened. Following nerve injury and/or nerve repair, continued critical evaluation by physical examination and a variety of specific tests is necessary to determine the progress of healing.

Injury to Bone

After injury to bone there are three main morphologic sequences that overlap in time and space. These are concerned with actual injury to cells and tissues, with defense and demolition, and with healing and regeneration.

IMMEDIATE INJURY. The immediate injury results in structural and chemical changes in cells and tissues, which may or may not die; vascular changes (hemorrhage, clotting, and exudation); and neurogenic changes. Miles has described two early phases: an early phase, mediated by the local release of histamine from mast cells, platelets, and other blood cells, and a delayed phase, in which there is activation of peptide systems to form plasma kinins, as well as the globulin permeability factor of Spector and Willoughby. The vasoconstrictor amine epinephrine may also be inactivated locally.

Wilhelm has characterized permeability factors as belonging to three main groups: (1) the proteases, e.g., plasmin (fibrolytic), kallikrein (vasodepressor), and the globulin permeability factor; (2) the polypeptides, e.g., leukotaxine, bradykinin, and kallidin; and (3) the amines, e.g., histamine, 5-hydroxytryptamine, epinephrine, and norepinephrine. These substances are believed to produce increased permeability, cellular migration, small vessel dilation (similar to the triple response of Lewis), and alteration in the diffusion mechanisms of the intercellular matrix or ground substance.

From damaged capillaries or from increased capillary permeability, protein-rich plasma and numerous cells—lymphocytes, neutrophils, and eosinophils—leak out. Plasmacytes are thought to be derived from these lymphocytes and are believed to hold or synthesize within their cytoplasm nucleoproteins liberated by the autolysis of cells, the necrosis of tissues, and protein leak.

Following this, a clot of insoluble fibrin forms. This protein is derived from the circulating soluble fibrinogen by the addition of two amino acids—phenylalanine and lysine—in the presence of thrombin, calcium, platelets, and other clotting factors. The amino acids are derived from serum albumin, γ-globulin, and the globulin of red blood cells from the extravasated blood. Fibrinogenesis provides a screen, or framework, of fibrin fibers to collect plasma proteins and extravasated cells. This framework is invaded by reticuloendothelial cells, e.g., macrophages, round cells, and histocytes; by endothelial cells, which undergo mitosis to form capillaries; and finally by fibroblasts. The fibrin filaments are oriented to provide a framework for the fibroblasts and capillaries to follow along definite patterns. The fibroblasts arise from undifferentiated mesenchymal cells and synthesize acid mucopolysaccharides, which are used later in collagen formation. Although mast cells contain acid mucopolysaccharides in their cytoplasmic granules, they are not the direct source of this material for collagen synthesis.

DEFENSE AND DEMOLITION. In the defense-and-demolition stage there are significant vascular reactions that affect inflow of tissue fluids and cellular infiltration. The arterioles and efferent veins particularly are involved. There is redistribution of blood flow through capillary channels by shunt mechanisms under poorly understood neurogenic reflexes.

Wray and Lynch have shown a quantitative increase in vascular volume of fractures by enlargement of existing vessels, as well as formation of new ones. Rhinelander and Baragry, in bone microangiographic studies, saw a marked opening of the existing medullary arterial tree within the first day, but it was not until the fourth day that periosteal vessels were seen entering the fracture site. Accompanying these changes was a marked infiltration of polymorphonuclear leukocytes, lymphocytes, and monocytes. This infiltration alters the physical state of the ground substance from a solution to a gel and produces autolysis, phagocytosis, and digestion of debris. Plasmin, with its fibrinolytic and permeability effects, is formed from the circulating but inactive serum protein plasminogen. Plasmin is considered to be able to digest necrotic mesodermal tissues and to release further active substances. Lack has demonstrated its autolytic digestion of articular cartilage. Mast cells may influence white cell migration because of their heparin content and stimulate phagocytic activity because of their 5-hydroxytryptamine content, but these actions have not yet been clearly demonstrated.

HEALING AND REGENERATION. Blastema formation results from hyperplasia and proliferation of undifferentiated mesenchymal cells, from monocytes, from lymphocytes, and from pseudolymphocytes, which form fibroblasts. The phylogenic characterization, or specific naming of cells, is much more certain in this stage, because their functions and environments are more clearly understood; e.g., fibroblasts form collagen, myxoblasts form ground substance, chondroblasts form cartilage, and osteoblasts form bone. Such changes are very rapid. Tonna and Cronkite have demonstrated marked proliferation of local mesenchymal cells making up the periosteum within 16 hours of wounding. Within 3 days the proliferative reaction spreads some distance along the shaft away from the fracture site.

There have been many attempts to determine the stimulus for such proliferation. Abercrombie reviewed various "wound hormones" and suggested that increased mitosis and increased migration of cells are produced by one chemical stimulus. A possible factor which accelerated the healing of skin wounds has been demonstrated in cell-free extract of human granulation tissue. A wound factor in amphibian tissues produced by damaged tissue at the time and site of wounding has been proposed. It also has been demonstrated that injured cells liberate a growth-promoting factor in the inflammatory exudate. The stimulation factor also had been thought to be present in the organized blood clot of the fracture hematoma, and to promote new bone formation by the "chronic irritation of the necrosis and hemorrhage."

During a study of fracture repair in rats, Duthie and Barker noted the accumulation of mast cells in greater numbers than those seen in the opposite (control) leg within 48 hours of the fracture, which persisted for the next 7 days. Because of this, it was suggested that mast cell appearance was related to the trauma, and that these cells might function in the ensuing regeneration processes, especially because of their cytoplasmic content of histamine, heparin, and 5-hydroxytryptamine. Mast cells subsequently were observed during the response of standard fractures to various systemic and hormonal change, as well as to locally applied drugs.

The result of the hyperplasia and proliferation of mesenchymal cells is the callus which obliterates the medullary cavity and connects the two ends of bone by irregularly surrounding the fracture defect. With sufficient organization of this callus the fracture site becomes clinically stable. The early bone of the callus is fiber bone which has spicules perpendicular to the cortical surface. This is gradually replaced and remodeled with osteonal bone. Conversion and remodeling continue up to 3 years following an acute fracture. Motion plays a role in the amount of cartilaginous tissue formed. Anderson has shown that when fractures are initially fixed with compression, eliminating motion, there is little callus from the endosteum and none from the periosteum. There is direct bridging of the fracture site by endosteal callus and bone formation.

The use of weight-bearing treatment for fractures of long bones has raised questions about the need for strict immobilization to achieve union. When patients bear weight on a healing fracture, motion at the fracture site results. Despite this, the stability of the callus formation is greater sooner, resulting in more rapid union. It is possible that rapidity of union is explained by better approximation of bone ends and compression forces across the fractured surfaces, but it seems likely that altered circulation either from rhythmic contraction of muscles or from changes in medullary blood flow as a result of this are responsible. Further experimental work in this area is needed.

All processes involved in fracture healing occur much more rapidly in children, accounting for the rate of fracture union and the almost unheard of nonunion in this age group.

Delayed Union and Nonunion

Delayed union is an ill-defined term arbitrarily applied to fractures taking longer than average to heal. It should be defined in relation to the specific fracture for which it is used.

Nonunion refers to a fracture in which healing cannot be expected even with prolonged immobilization. X-ray examination of a nonunion will reveal sclerosis of bone ends, plugging off of the medullary canal with sclerotic bone, rounding of the adjacent fracture surfaces, and a definite defect between the fragments, consisting of fibrous tissue, cartilage, etc.

Wray has pointed out that the normal contribution of fracture callus is primarily from the surrounding soft tissues and vascularization of the callus occurs from the same soft tissues. Most nonunions are of local origin and are the result of inadequate callus or vascularization of this fracture callus. They frequently occur in young adults in whom there has been excessive soft tissue destruction or infection.

Inadequate reduction of a fracture may result in, or be caused by, interposition of soft tissue between the bone ends, interfering with callus formation. Inadequate immobilization predisposes to the formation of fibrous or cartilaginous tissue instead of osteoid or bone. The most common cause of nonunion is local damage to the soft tissues surrounding the fracture. A frequent cause is ill-advised operative reduction of fractures. When open reduction of fractures is done, every attempt should be made to minimize periosteal stripping and devitalization of the fracture area. Local infection, destroying adjacent soft tissue, may contribute to delay or nonunion, but the possibility exists for healing in the presence of infection.

Pathologic Fractures

Fractures occurring through abnormal bone which has been weakened by a preexisting pathologic condition is considered a pathologic fracture (Fig. 47-4). Whenever fractures occur with minor trauma, consideration should be given to generalized or local bone disease.

In children, developmental diseases such as osteogenesis imperfecta, osteopetrosis, or nutritional deficiencies such as rickets or scurvy may result in pathologic fractures. Unicameral bone cysts, aneurysmal bone cysts, eosinophilic granulomas, fibrous dysplasia, and any of the primary or secondary malignant processes also may weaken a bone sufficiently to cause pathologic fracture.

Idiopathic osteoporosis in the adult is a common cause of pathologic fractures, as is osteoporosis associated with prolonged cortisone therapy. Hyperparathyroidism should always be considered, since it is a correctable lesion.

Patients with slow-growing metastatic bone tumors, for example, from breast or kidney, should be carefully followed in an attempt to prevent pathologic fractures. Sizable bone lesions occurring in the femoral or humeral shafts should be prophylactically nailed, since this may save the patient considerable morbidity.

Stress Fractures

Stress fractures occur in characteristic locations in specific age groups and certain occupational situations. Stress or fatigue fractures are the end result of repeated stress to a bone which would not be injured by isolated forces

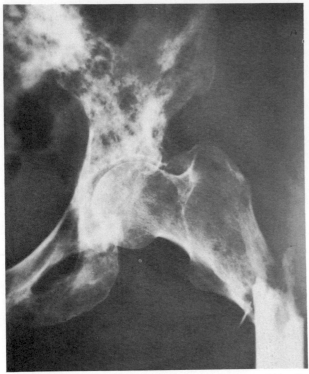

Fig. 47-4. Pathologic fracture. Metastatic carcinoma with pathologic subtrochanteric fracture of the femur. There is diffuse involvement of the adjacent pelvis.

of the same magnitude. Johnson et al. have shown that repeated stress causes accelerated osteoclastic remodeling in areas of bone which have not yet been converted to osteonal bone. Following osteoclastic resorption, with a loss of normal structural mass, there is new periosteal bone

formation in an attempt to strengthen the weakened area. If the repeated stress is discontinued, the bone may not go on to fracture. Patients complain of aching pain following unusual activity during the early phases of this process and go on to complete fracture if the stress activity is not discontinued.

Stress fractures commonly occur in young soldiers required to force-march. The second and third distal metatarsal shafts, proximal tibia, distal fibula, and calcaneus are common sites (Fig. 47-5). Early in the course of the symptomatology, x-ray findings may reveal only subtle osteoporosis at the stressed area, but later new periosteal bone formation occurs with incomplete or complete fracture.

Treatment of stress fracture is immobilization and discontinuance of the fatiguing activity.

Epiphyseal Plate Injuries

Longitudinal growth of bone occurs by cartilaginous growth at the epiphyseal plate and conversion to bone by endochondral ossification. Interference with normal epiphyseal growth will result in abnormalities of length of the affected bone or deformity. Epiphyseal separations occur consistently between the uncalcified hypertrophying cells and the zone of provisional calcification, which is the weakest area through the plate. In such an injury, normal growth will continue, since the proliferating cells are still attached to their blood supply in the bony epiphysis. Any injury which damages the proliferating cells or interferes with circulation may cause growth disturbance.

Salter and Harris have devised a classification of epiphyseal plate injuries, with a rationale for treatment. Type I is a complete separation of the epiphysis from the me-

Fig. 47-5. Stress fracture of the distal second metatarsal shaft. Note periosteal new bone formation about the transverse defect proximal to the second metatarsal head.

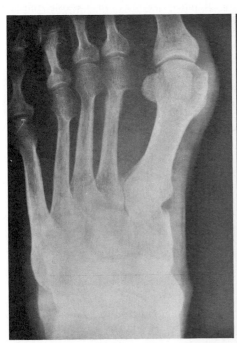
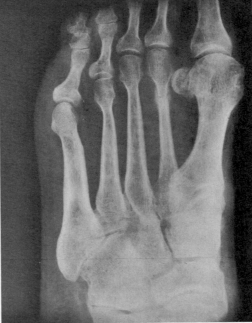

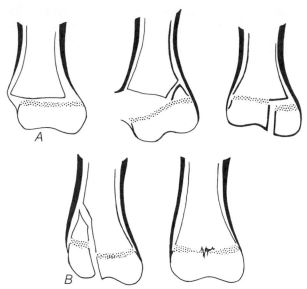

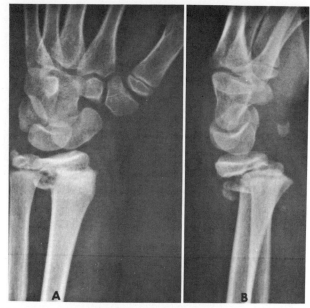

Fig. 47-6. Salter and Harris classification of epiphyseal injury Type I. See text for description. *A*. Types I to III. *B*. Types IV to V.

Fig. 47-7. Type II epiphyseal separation at the distal radius. Distal radial epiphysis is displaced dorsad and ulnarward with a fragment of the metaphysis.

taphysis without bone fracture (Fig. 47-6). Such injuries occur at birth or in early childhood in scorbutic bones. Treatment is by closed reduction, and the prognosis is excellent, since the proliferating cells and blood supply have not been damaged.

Type II is a separation along part of the epiphyseal plate with a fracture through the metaphysis (Fig. 47-7). It commonly occurs at the distal radial epiphysis or distal tibial epiphysis. Treatment is closed reduction, and the prognosis is excellent, even though reduction is not anatomic (Fig. 47-8).

Type III, epiphyseal plate injury, is an intraarticular

fracture, extending from the joint surface through the bony epiphysis to the plate and then along the plate to the periphery.

Accurate reduction is necessary to minimize articular deformity. The prognosis is good if the blood supply to the fractured portion has not been compromised.

Type IV is also an intraarticular epiphyseal injury. The fracture line extends through the joint surface across the bony epiphyseal plate and through a portion of the metaphysis. The commonest Type IV injury is a fracture of the lateral condyle of the humerus. Anatomic reduction and usually open reduction are required to prevent union across the epiphyseal plate at the fracture site and growth abnormality.

Fig. 47-8. *A* and *B*. AP and lateral x-rays showing lateral displacement of the distal tibial epiphysis with the fracture line extending into the distal metaphysis and also through the medial malleolus with fracture of the distal fibular shaft. *C* and *D*. Oblique and lateral x-rays in plaster following successful closed manipulation.

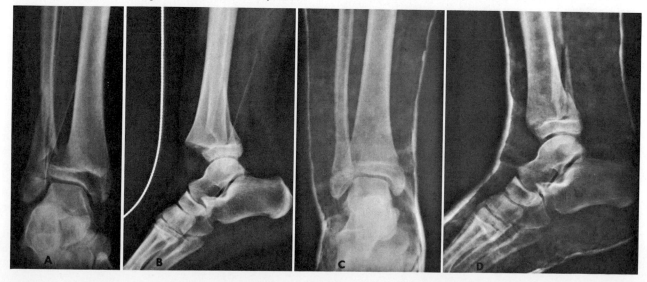

Type V epiphyseal plate injuries are those in which severe crushing damages the epiphyseal plate. Displacement is not common, and the initial severity may go unrecognized. Because of crushing injury to the proliferating cartilage cells, growth disturbances may occur.

With any injury or suspected injury to an epiphyseal plate, the parent of the child should be cautioned that growth abnormalities are possible. Type IV and Type V injuries are more likely to cause growth disturbances. Injuries which interfere with the blood supply to the epiphysis or damage proliferating cells will result in greater deformity in the young child. However, if neither of these occurs, the younger child has greater remodeling potential where accurate reduction cannot be obtained.

Fractures in Children

A fracture in a child presents different problems from those of a similar fracture in the adult. Compound fractures are much less common than in the adult. Nonunion is almost unheard of in children. Fracture healing is more rapid with the younger patient.

The challenge in handling children's fractures is in recognizing and understanding what degree of fracture site angulation, displacement, and shortening will be corrected, in relation to remaining growth potential. The presence of healing fracture callus in the neighborhood of an epiphysis causes epiphyseal stimulation. If a displaced femoral shaft fracture is reduced anatomically, overgrowth and leg length inequality will ensue. If rotational deformity at a fracture site involving a long bone is not corrected, permanent deformity results. However, certain degrees of angulation, displacement, and shortening will be corrected and remodeled depending upon the age of the child. Shaft fractures in the long bones must not be opened because of the hazard of infection or epiphyseal growth disturbance and deformity. However, certain articular and epiphyseal fractures must be recognized and anatomically reduced.

Closed Reduction versus Open Reduction

The optimal method for handling a specific fracture should (1) permit rapid union, (2) reestablish length and alignment of the injured extremity, (3) restore complete painless range of motion of adjacent joints, and (4) return the patient to gainful functional activity, with as little morbidity and hazard to the patient as possible.

The closed treatment of fractures has the advantages of little or no risk of infection or subsequent interference with local blood supply to the fracture site. However, closed treatment requires prolonged traction or immobilization which may cause restriction of joint motion, and accurate anatomic restoration of length and alignment may not be possible.

In order to obviate the difficulties of prolonged immobilization and overcome the problems of inaccurate reduction, open reduction and internal fixation have been proposed. However, open reduction carries the risks of local infection and delayed union resulting from compromise of local blood supply to fracture fragments. Also, internal fixation may not provide sufficient immobilization of fracture fragments to permit early motion of adjacent joints.

Despite the disadvantages of each technique, closed treatment is frequently indicated for some situations, while open reduction is mandatory for others. The system of internal fixation devices has been developed by Muller and colleagues; it provides stainless steel plates fixed to bone with a modified bone screw and employs the principle of compression across fracture surfaces. This technique has allowed early joint motion when sufficient stabilization of the fracture site has been accomplished, which may allow earlier and more complete return of joint function. Surgeons using this technique should bear in mind the hazards of open reduction outlined above.

Application of Plaster Casts

External immobilization for fractures and dislocations is obtained by the application of plaster casts. Plaster consists of anhydrous calcium sulfate, which solidifies with hydration. Plaster, to which water is added, sets up in minutes but does not completely dry for 36 to 48 hours. It comes in rolls or strips of crinoline bandage to which anhydrous calcium sulfate has been added.

Plaster in rolls is applied circumferentially to make a cast but never wrapped directly on the skin. Strips are used to construct splints by applying a strip of plaster to one surface of an extremity without intervening padding. When plaster is applied for an acute injury, sufficient padding should be employed to accommodate the anticipated swelling. As a general rule, one layer of stockinet and one layer of sheet wadding or webril is sufficient with extra padding for bony prominences. The cast is applied smoothly and molded over bony prominences and articulations. In order to permit evaluation of peripheral circulation, the toes or digits are never completely enclosed with plaster.

Postinjury patients in plaster casts should be placed in bed with the extremity elevated. The nursing staff and house staff should be completely familiar with cast complications and signs of impending vascular insufficiency. The patient should never be sent home when the possibility of circulatory compromise exists.

COMPLICATIONS OF PLASTER CAST TREATMENT. The most serious complication associated with plaster casts is the development of vascular insufficiency due to unrelieved swelling. The cast will not shrink, but it may restrict soft tissue swelling to the point of gangrenous necrosis. Unrelieved pain, pulselessness, pallor, and sensory or motor paralysis are signs of this complication. Unrelenting pain should be investigated immediately and not allowed to progress to the point where other signs are present. Narcotics are administered with great caution to patients in plaster. Unrelieved pain beneath the cast should be treated by splitting the cast with parallel cuts on the opposite sides of the extremity, to allow anteroposterior swelling. The cast is split down to include the underlying padding, since blood-soaked padding may be as resistant as plaster and not allow sufficient expansion. Leg casts are split medially and laterally in their entirety, and forearm

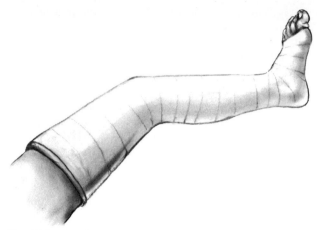

Fig. 47-9. Long leg cast.

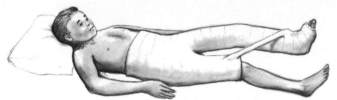

Fig. 47-11. A 1½ hip spica.

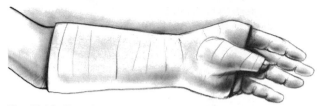

Fig. 47-12. Short arm cast.

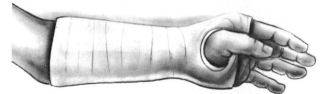

Fig. 47-13. Gauntlet cast.

casts split along the radial and ulnar borders of the arm.

Patients who complain of burning pain at a localized site in the cast should be suspected of a pressure point from the plaster. This commonly occurs over the site of a bony prominence. This is investigated by cutting an appropriate window and inspecting the underlying skin. Skin necrosis may result and be associated with pain relief due to damage of sensory receptors. When a point of pressure is detected, the cast window should be hollowed out and sufficient padding applied to relieve the pressure. Windows in the cast should always be replaced, or local swelling will occur through the window and cause pressure on the skin at the window margins.

TYPES OF PLASTER CASTS. Casts for fractures should immobilize the joint above and the joint below the fracture. Plasters which include the ankle are extended to the bases of the toes to prevent swelling, edema, and irritation of the forefoot. A long leg cast extends from the bases of the toes to include the knee and thigh as high as possible (Fig. 47-9). A boot cast extends to the level of the tibial tubercle (Fig. 47-10). A cylinder cast is a circular cast which extends from just above the ankle to include leg, knee, and thigh. It is used for immobilization of the knee.

A hip spica is a plaster designed to immobilize the hip. A single hip spica extends from the nipple line or upper abdomen to include the pelvis and one thigh and lower leg. A double hip spica immobilizes the pelvis and extends to include both thighs and lower legs. A 1½ hip spica extends only as far as the knee on one side (Fig. 47-11).

A short arm cast extends from below the elbow to the proximal palmar crease, leaving the entire thumb free (Fig. 47-12). A gauntlet cast is similar but includes the thumb (Fig. 47-13). A long arm cast extends from the proximal palmar crease, leaving the thumb free to include the elbow and arm as far as the axilla (Fig. 47-14). A shoulder spica is a body jacket with the plaster immobilizing the shoulder and elbow.

Body casts are applied for immobilization of the spine

Fig. 47-10. Boot cast.

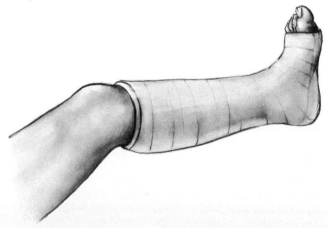

Fig. 47-14. Long arm cast.

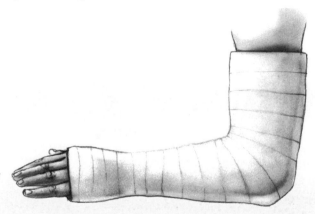

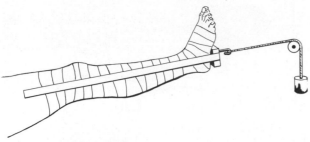

Fig. 47-15. Buck's traction.

and extend to the groin and as high as the sternum, anteriorly. They may be applied with plaster straps across the shoulders. A scoliosis plaster, or localizer plaster for scoliosis correction, extends to the groin anteriorly, to the sacrum posteriorly, and as far proximally as to provide a distracting force on the chin and occiput. Distally, the distracting force is applied by well-molded pressure areas across the crest of the ilia.

Traction

Traction is used in orthopedics:

1. To overcome muscle spasm and apply reducing force in fractures of the long bones
2. To provide immobilization of long bone fractures
3. To provide immobilization and distracting force for painful and diseased joints
4. To correct joint deformities or contractures

Skin traction is applied by tapes attached to the skin and skeletal traction by pins or screws affixed to bone. The maximal weight tolerated by adhesive tapes to the skin is about 10 lb. In children, skin traction is usually sufficient to overcome muscle pull in the reduction and treatment of fractures. The most common form of skin traction is Buck's traction, in which tapes with attached weights are applied to the leg and thigh (Fig. 47-15). This is commonly used prior to surgical treatment in the immobilization of intertrochanteric hip fractures. Skin traction is used with Russell's traction (Fig. 47-16), which is designed to apply traction to the femoral shaft with the knee flexed. A fem-

Fig. 47-16. Russell's traction.

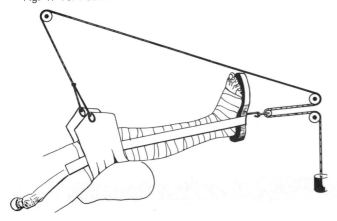

oral shaft fracture in a small child may be treated with Bryant's traction. In this technique, skin traction is attached to both legs, which are suspended from the bed.

Skeletal traction (Fig. 47-17) is usually applied to a Steinmann pin or Kirschner wire driven percutaneously across the distal femoral shaft or proximal tibia. A traction bow is affixed to the metal wire and weight applied. Kirschner wires drilled across the olecranon may be used for supracondylar or humeral shaft fractures. Crutchfield tongs affixed to the outer table of the skull and the halo device, which has a similar purchase on the skull, are other forms of skeletal traction.

FRACTURES AND JOINT INJURIES IN THE UPPER EXTREMITY

SHOULDER MOTION. The act of moving the hand from the anatomic position to a position of full abduction requires normal function in the glenohumeral joint, the acromioclavicular joint, the sternoclavicular joint, and the scapulothoracic joint. Interference with any of these joints will limit full shoulder motion.

Inman and colleagues have worked out the ranges of motion occurring at these joints during normal shoulder function. During the first 30° of abduction or 60° of forward flexion, the scapula seeks a position of stability with the humerus. This occurs by lateral or medial motion of the scapula on the chest wall or by motion at the glenohumeral joint, with the scapula remaining fixed. When the position of 30° of abduction or 60° of forward flexion has occurred, there is a simultaneous 10° of glenohumeral joint motion for each 5° of scapula rotation on the thorax during the continued elevation of the arm.

The rotation of the scapula involves motion of the sternoclavicular and the acromioclavicular joints. As the arm is elevated, elevation of the clavicle occurs at the sternoclavicular joint. It is almost complete during the first 90° of arm elevation. For every 10° of elevation of the arm, there are 4° of elevation of the clavicle. Motion at the acromioclavicular joint is approximately 20° and occurs during the first 30° of abduction and after 135° of elevation. On the long axis of the acromioclavicular joint during the position of 60 to 180° of elevation of the arm, 40° of clavicular rotation occurs. It is apparent, from this anatomic description, that fusion or disruption of any one joint will interfere with the elevation of the arm.

Sternoclavicular Joint Injuries

Injuries to the sternoclavicular joint occur from direct lateral force to the shoulder applied in an axial direction to the clavicle. Dislocations are commonly anterior, but in some cases, when posterior and lateral forces are applied, retrosternal dislocation of the sternoclavicular joint occurs.

Reduction is necessary in retrosternal dislocations, because of compression of neurovascular structures. When closed manipulation and lateral traction are not sufficient, open reduction is indicated. With interior dislocation, reduction is not critical. However, for best results, closed reduction and maintenance of position are required. Old, unreduced dislocations, if symptomatic, require excision of the proximal end of the clavicle.

Fractures of the Clavicle

Fractures of the clavicle occur at any age from direct downward force to the shoulder or from forces applied indirectly as in falling on the extended arm. Fractures may occur at any level but are most common at the junction of the middle and distal thirds (Fig. 47-18). In older age groups, fractures of the distal tip of the clavicle are more common.

CLINICAL MANIFESTATIONS. The patient presents supporting the affected extremity by his opposite hand, with his head tilted to the affected side, and chin rotated away. There is local swelling and direct tenderness at the site of the fracture. Any motion of the extremity causes pain. The diagnosis is confirmed by x-ray.

TREATMENT. The clavicle is difficult to immobilize, because of its anatomic location and muscle attachments. In spite of this, nonunion is rare (about $\frac{1}{2}$ percent) with conservative treatment. The weight of the shoulder causes the distal fragment to be inferiorly angulated or depressed, while the proximal fragment is superiorly angulated by the pull of the sternocleidomastoid and upper fibers of the trapezius.

Treatment in Children. Both shoulders are drawn back and elevated by a figure-of-eight apparatus, which may be constructed of felt padding covered with stockinet (Fig. 47-19). The axillae are padded with large gauze pads to prevent irritation of the skin and compression of the neurovascular bundle. The figure-of-eight should be maintained in a taut position by frequent adjustment by the parents. Warning is given about swelling in the hands from venostasis. This is relieved by having the patient lie supine while elevating the arms overhead. Fracture reduction in children is not important. Bayonet overriding is accepted and will remodel with age. The figure-of-eight is left in place for 2 weeks in infants and until the fracture is clinically solid in older children, 4 to 6 weeks if necessary.

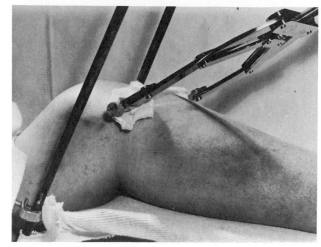

Fig. 47-17. Skeletal traction. Traction bow is attached to a transverse Steinmann pin through the tibial tubercle for a supracondylar or femoral shaft fracture.

Treatment in Adults. When growth of the clavicle has been completed, accurate reduction and maintenance of position is required to prevent cosmetic deformity. It is difficult to maintain a displaced fractured clavicle in the reduced position with any ambulatory apparatus. However, in men and older women, a figure-of-eight apparatus for 6 weeks would provide sufficient immobilization for union but may leave a cosmetic deformity. In women who desire a cosmetic result, supine bed rest with a small sandbag placed in the interscapular area and lateral traction on the abducted arm are required for 4 to 6 weeks. Open surgical reduction with intramedullary fixation will minimize angular deformity at the fracture site but leaves a scar and may result in nonunion.

Acromioclavicular Injuries

The acromioclavicular joint is injured by forces applied downward from the point of the shoulder. Such injuries occur frequently during blocking and tackling in football (Fig. 47-20) and in all contact sports. The age incidence coincides with that of people participating in sports, usually the latter part of the second decade or the third or fourth decades. Acromioclavicular joint injuries may occur

Fig. 47-18. *A.* Fracture of the middle third of the clavicle with complete displacement and overriding. *B.* Healing of a clavicle fracture in 6 weeks with internal callus formation.

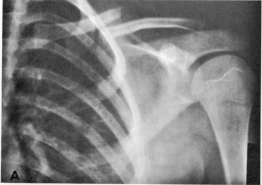

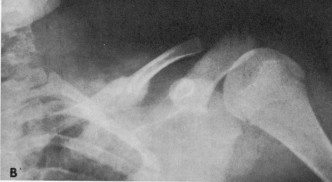

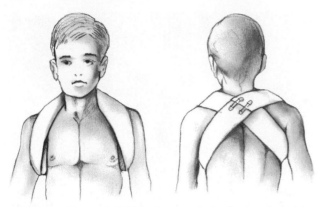

Fig. 47-19. Figure-of-eight for treatment of a fractured clavicle. The axillae are padded with gauze pads over which a figure-of-eight of felt and stockinet is applied.

in the elderly, but fractures of the distal third of the clavicle are more common in this age group, with the same type of trauma. The integrity of the acromioclavicular joint is primarily dependent upon the coracoclavicular ligaments, the conoid and trapezoid, which run upward, backward, and laterally from the base of the coracoid process to the inferior surface of the clavicle. Superior and inferior acromioclavicular ligaments contribute little to the stability of the joint.

CLINICAL MANIFESTATIONS. Signs of acromioclavicular joint injury include local swelling and tenderness over the acromioclavicular joint and palpable deformity. The patient cocks his head to the affected side to relax the sterno-

Fig. 47-20. Acromioclavicular dislocation incurred from a direct fall on the shoulder while playing football.

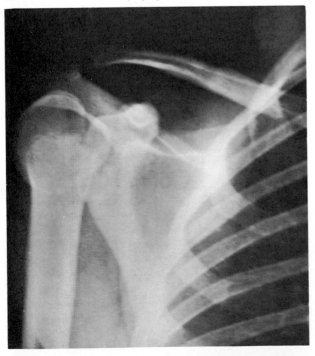

cleidomastoid and supports his arm with the opposite hand to relieve the weight of the shoulder distracting the joint.

When the patient is examined lying supine, a subluxation may reduce spontaneously, making diagnosis difficult. In the upright position or in the obese patient, or with sufficient local swelling, the diagnosis may not be readily apparent. The diagnosis is made by obtaining comparable AP x-rays of both acromioclavicular joints with the patient standing. With a subluxation, it may be necessary to have the patient suspend a 10-lb weight in the affected hand to distract a partially disrupted acromioclavicular articulation.

TREATMENT. The treatment of minor sprains or subluxations is symptomatic. It is accomplished by a sling on the affected side, supporting the weight of the arm. Complete dislocation of the acromioclavicular joint will not be held with less than open reduction or the suspension cast of Stubbins and McGaw, which applies relocation pressure to the clavicle.

In treating complete dislocations of the acromioclavicular joint, consideration should be given to the patient's age and occupation. Jacobs and Wade have shown that there is no significant improvement in results whether conservative treatment (sling) or open surgical reduction is used. For young men with the desire to continue sports activities and reacquire maximal strength, surgical treatment of the type described by Neviaser or Weaver and Dunn may be indicated. Open reduction is also indicated for young women who will accept the surgical scar in the place of a permanent high-riding clavicle. However, for older patients symptomatic treatment for the initial dislocation is all that is necessary. In any patient with persistent symptoms from a subluxed or painful acromioclavicular joint, excision of the distal end of the clavicle generally provides good results.

Technique of Open Reduction. A curved incision is made over the outer half of the clavicle at its anterior border and extends to the outer border of the acromion. The deltoid fibers attaching to the clavicle are stripped subperiosteally. The coracoacromial ligament and the acromioclavicular joint are exposed. No attempt is made to repair the coracoclavicular or acromioclavicular ligaments. The dislocation is reduced and maintained with a Kirschner wire, transfixing the acromion and the clavicle but placed behind the acromioclavicular joint. The tip of the wire extending lateral to the acromion is bent to prevent inward migration.

The coracoacromial ligament is detached from its coracoid attachment by reflecting a small piece of bone from the coracoid process. With the normal attachment of ligament distad to the undersurface of the acromion, the proximal end is then reflected over the acromion, where it is sutured with catgut sutures and turned back across the acromioclavicular joint and affixed to the clavicle by catgut sutures passing through the drill holes in the clavicle.

The patient's shoulder is immobilized in a sling and swath for 4 to 6 weeks. The pin is then removed and motion begun.

Fractures of the Scapula

Fractures of the body of the scapula and glenoid are invariably the result of severe trauma, either to pedestrians or automobile occupants. Such injuries are usually associated with injuries to the brachial plexus, fractured ribs, and cardiopulmonary trauma. Treatment of such patients is aimed primarily at the associated injuries. Symptomatic immobilization of the shoulder is preferable to open reduction.

Dislocations of the Shoulder

ACUTE ANTERIOR DISLOCATIONS

The humeral head may be dislocated from the glenoid in any direction. For superior dislocation to occur, fracture of the overlying acromion must be present. Anterior dislocations include subglenoid and subcoracoid dislocations. The humeral head is dislocated anteriorly when an extension force is applied to the abducted arm. The initial injury is typically one involving a fall with the arm in the abducted position or direct trauma to the abducted arm as may occur with football injuries. Less force is required to dislocate the shoulder when there is a congenital defect in the labrum or with paralysis of shoulder musculature. The humeral head is driven anteriorly, tearing the anterior shoulder joint capsule and detaching the labrum from the glenoid, producing a compression fracture in the posterior lateral aspect of the humeral head, as it is wedged between the anterior-lying subscapularis tendon and the anterior rim of the glenoid.

CLINICAL MANIFESTATIONS. The patient holds his arm in slight abduction and is unable to bring his elbow to the side. There is flattening of the normal deltoid prominence with a depression laterally beneath the acromion. The humeral head creates a prominence anteriorly, although in the obese person these findings may be difficult to define. Any attempt at arm motion causes severe pain. In a small percentage of cases, injury to the axillary nerve is incurred, as it is stretched around the neck of the humerus. This diagnosis may be made before reduction by localizing an area of sensory loss overlying the deltoid muscles and supplied by the superficial branch of the axillary nerve. Postreduction, weakness, or loss of power in the deltoid may be demonstrable.

Anteroposterior x-rays of the shoulder will reveal the head displaced medially into the subcoracoid or subglenoid position (Fig. 47-21).

TREATMENT. The dislocation should be reduced immediately. Closed reduction can be accomplished within the first 2 to 3 weeks, but open reduction may be required when dislocations are neglected for longer periods.

Over 90 percent of acute anterior dislocations may be reduced by a modification of the Milch maneuver (Fig. 47-22). Under mild analgesia, the patient is placed supine on a stretcher with his elbow extended and the arm in the position of 90° forward flexion, hanging off the side of the stretcher. A pail of water is attached to the arm

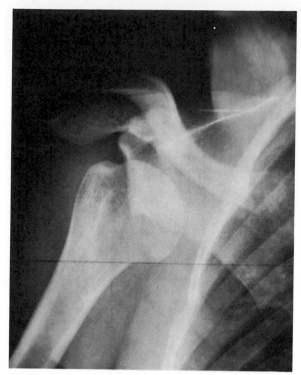

Fig. 47-21. Anterior subcoracoid dislocation of the shoulder. The articular surface of the humeral head can be seen medial to the glenoid fossa and inferior to the coracoid process.

Fig. 47-22. Reduction technique for anterior dislocation of the shoulder. With the patient in the prone position and the arm in the position of forward flexion, water is added to the bucket, and traction is gradually increased.

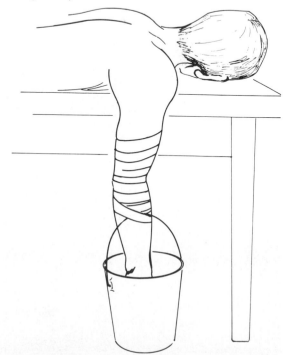

with an Ace bandage. Water can gradually be added to the bucket and traction increased. A few minutes of this traction is sufficient for the shoulder to reduce gradually, but in more muscular individuals 30 minutes may be required. In some instances, it is necessary to rotate the humeral head internally while maintaining traction. In the few instances where this treatment is insufficient, general anesthesia and a Hippocratic maneuver is accomplished by applying manual traction with countertraction applied by the stockinged foot of the operator to the axilla.

Postoperative management is as important as the closed reduction. The arm is bound to the side with the elbow flexed at 90° across the abdomen. A sling and swath are applied and are not disturbed for 6 weeks in young individuals. In patients over fifty, 4 weeks is sufficient, and in elderly patients mobilization of the shoulder is begun after 2 or 3 weeks.

RECURRENT ANTERIOR DISLOCATIONS

With adequate initial treatment and postreduction immobilization, the majority of patients will not redislocate unless subjected to significant trauma. However, redislocations occur when the initial dislocation is not immobilized in sufficient time and may do so with minor trauma. Some patients abducting the arm in getting dressed or reaching out to open a door may incur a recurrent dislocation.

TREATMENT. A number of surgical repairs are used in the treatment of recurrent dislocations, including the methods of Magnuson and Stack, Eden, Hybbinette,

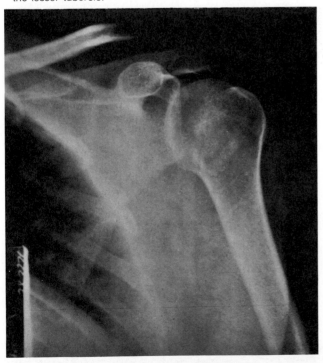

Fig. 47-23. Posterior dislocation of the shoulder. AP x-ray shows an indistinct border of the humeral head, superimposed upon the glenoid rim. There is also compression fracture in the region of the lesser tubercle.

Bankhart, and Bristow. Before instituting any of these, it is mandatory to document the direction of the dislocation. Excellent results have been obtained using the Putti-Platt procedure.

Technique. The shoulder is exposed through a standard deltopectoral incision. The clavicular origin of the deltoid is incised, leaving a $\frac{1}{2}$-cm attachment to the clavicle, in order to make resuture easier. The coracoid process is osteotomized at its tip and muscle origins of the pectoralis minor, and coracobrachialis retracted, medially. The axillary approach, as proposed by Leslie and Ryan, dividing the pectoralis major insertion is also used and has the advantage of leaving a less disfiguring scar.

The veins delineating the lower borders of the subscapularis tendon are located and ligated. The subscapularis tendon is divided 1 in. medial to its insertion on the lesser tuberosity. The capsule is divided vertically at the same level of the incision in the subscapularis tendon. The lateral capsule and subscapularis tendon are sutured to the inferior surface of the medial capsule and glenoid rim with interrupted heavy silk sutures. The medial capsule is then sutured anterior to this. The distal end of the proximal stump of the scapularis is then reattached to the lesser tuberosity to limit external rotation beyond neutral. A reefed shoulder capsule with a shortened subscapularis tendon limits external rotation and assists retention of the humeral head. The patient is immobilized with sling and swath, or Velpeau bandage, for 6 weeks, and then mobilization is begun. The results of this treatment are excellent in preventing repeated dislocation.

CHRONIC DISLOCATIONS. In patients with chronic complete anterior dislocation, arthrodesis of the shoulder at 45° of abduction, 15° of internal rotation, and 20° of forward flexion will eliminate pain and restore shoulder function.

POSTERIOR DISLOCATIONS

The shoulder dislocates posteriorly during epileptiform convulsions, during electroshock therapy, and in automobile accidents in which the arm is axially loaded in the position of forward flexion. Any patient complaining of shoulder pain following a convulsion should be considered to have a dislocated shoulder until proved otherwise.

Clinical findings on examination reveal prominence of the humeral head posteriorly, loss of the anterior shoulder contour, limitation of full abduction, and complete loss of external rotation.

Routine AP x-rays may reveal the diagnosis, but an axillary x-ray will confirm the location of the humeral head posterior to the glenoid fossa. On the AP x-ray, the humeral head will appear smaller than the opposite side, since it is closer to the x-ray film (Fig. 47-23). In the normal shoulder, there is an overlap of the shadow of the humeral head on the posterior lip of the glenoid, which gives a *sharp* half-moon shadow. When the head is dislocated posteriorly, this half-moon shadow will be blurred or absent. Proof of posterior dislocation is by an axillary x-ray. Frequently, the lesser tuberosity is fractured at the time of the dislocation. The presence of this finding should

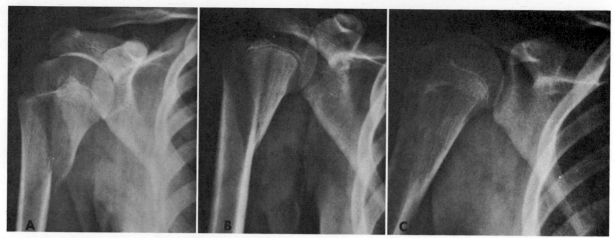

Fig. 47-24. Fracture of the proximal humerus in a twelve-year-old girl. The fracture is an epiphyseal separation with a large metaphyseal fragment attached to the epiphysis. *A.* Initial fracture position. *B.* Slight improvement after closed reduction. *C.* Healed fracture with remodeling changes at 1 year postinjury. The patient has a normal range of shoulder motion.

suggest a posterior dislocation or a reduced posterior dislocation.

TREATMENT. Reduction is accomplished by the modified Milch maneuver under analgesia or general anesthesia or by direct traction. Following reduction, the shoulder is immobilized in 30° of abduction, in external rotation, with a modified shoulder spica. This permits adequate healing of the posterior capsule in the shortened position.

A few posterior dislocations are recurrent. Treatment of posterior recurrent dislocations is accomplished by a bone block applied to the posterior glenoid or reefing of the infraspinatus tendon, which is the posterior analog of a Putti-Platt procedure.

FRACTURE DISLOCATIONS OF THE SHOULDER

A fracture of the neck of the humerus may occur in combination with an anterior dislocation. The initial treatment is the same but generally requires closed reduction and manipulation under general anesthesia. Traction is applied in the long axis of the shaft of the humerus in the position in which it lies. Direct counterpressure is applied in a posterior direction over the head of the humerus. If the dislocation can be reduced, subsequent treatment is the same as for fractures of the humeral neck. In the young, when it is not possible to reduce such fracture dislocations, open reduction and internal fixation of the fracture are indicated.

Fractures of the Proximal Humerus

The most common fracture of the proximal humerus is a fracture of the surgical neck. It is prevalent in older individuals but may occur at any age. In children, a similar injury results in a fracture of the anatomic neck, with epiphyseal displacement, usually of Type II of the Salter and Harris classification (Fig. 47-24). The treatment of

such an injury in a child is by closed reduction with manual traction, followed by hanging cast immobilization. Moderate degrees of displacement may be accepted if there is sufficient growth potential remaining in the epiphysis. It may be necessary to place the arm at full abduction in a shoulder spica, to hold position.

Fractures of the surgical neck of the humerus have a varus deformity at the fracture site. A hanging cast or sling and swath are sufficient to hold reduction of most fractures of the surgical neck. When manual reduction and sling and swath are unsuccessful in maintaining reduction, skin traction applied to the adducted arm will maintain position. However, in some patients, open reduction with blade plate fixation, staples or screws, or Rush pinning may be necessary. Neer has described an excellent system for classification and treatment of proximal humeral fractures.

Fractures of the greater tuberosity should be reduced anatomically to maintain normal function. If this cannot be obtained by closed means, open reduction and screw fixation of the fragment are necessary. In all fractures of the humerus, it is necessary to begin early shoulder motion as soon as stability at the fracture site can be ascertained. With fractures of the surgical neck in elderly patients, shoulder motion and gentle pendulum exercises may be started as early as 7 to 10 days to minimize shoulder stiffness. In younger individuals with displaced fractures, motion is not started before 3 to 4 weeks.

Fractures of the Humeral Shaft

Fractures of the humeral shaft (Fig. 47-25) occur from direct blows to the humerus, which cause transverse or comminuted fractures, or by indirect force, i.e., torsional stress, as in falling on the elbow. On physical examination, there is swelling, ecchymosis, and deformity, with inability to elevate the arm because of painful instability. It is necessary to determine the presence or absence of associated neurovascular injuries, which are common, especially with serious traumatic forces. The radial nerve is the most commonly injured nerve, but any of or all the major nerves may be stretched or interrupted with either closed or open

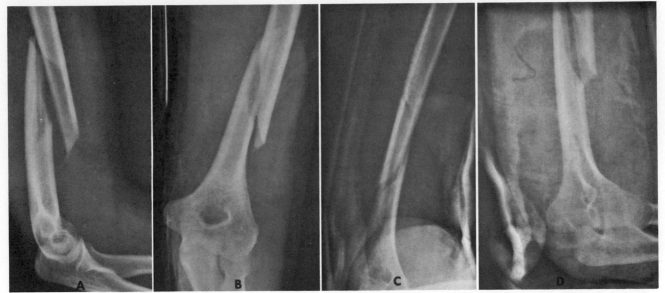

Fig. 47-25. Spiral fracture at the junction of the middle and distal thirds of the humeral shaft. *A.* Lateral x-ray showing displacement with angulation. *B.* AP x-ray. *C* and *D.* AP and lateral x-rays showing postreduction positions after closed reduction and the application of coaptation splints. The patient had a complete radial nerve palsy (axonotmesis) from which there was complete recovery in 8 months.

fractures. Holstein and Lewis have described an oblique fracture at the junction of the middle and distal thirds of the humerus, in which radial nerve injury is commonly encountered.

TREATMENT. Various methods of treatment have been devised for this injury, but the most successful has been to reduce the fracture with gentle longitudinal traction, injecting 2% Xylocaine at the fracture site as necessary. With the patient in a sitting position, a coaptation plaster splint is applied to the medial surface of the arm, as high in the axilla as possible, encompassing the elbow and continuing over the lateral surface of the arm with a small extension of the plaster over the superior surface of the shoulder. While the plaster is hardening, it is circumferentially wrapped to the arm with a soft bandage roll. The elbow is flexed 90° across the abdomen, and the entire arm is bound to the side with a Velpeau, or sling and swath, dressing. The weight of the arm in this situation acts like a hanging cast to apply gentle traction for the fracture. This method of coaptation is superior to the hanging cast, because it provides more immobilization and comfort with less hazard of distraction from overweighted plaster.

In individuals with multiple injuries who require bed rest, the reduction may be maintained with skin traction applied to the arm. Two or three pounds is sufficient for lateral traction; when greater weight is added, the hazard of distraction is likely. With either method, when the fracture is clinically stable, the arm is placed in a sling and active elbow and shoulder motion started.

Spontaneous recovery ensues in over 95 percent of the patients with associated traction injuries to the radial nerve. The presence of such a lesion is not an indication for open reduction or primary exploration of the nerve.

When primary repair of a brachial artery is required, internal fixation of the humeral shaft is necessary. This is accomplished by plate and screw fixation of the AOI type but may also be effected by intramedullary fixation.

Primary open reduction of the closed humeral shaft fracture is indicated when it is not possible to get bony apposition because of marked displacement or interposition of soft tissue.

In all humeral shaft fractures, it is necessary to get biplanar check x-rays at intervals during the first 3 weeks and make traction or plaster adjustments as necessary.

Fractures and Dislocations about the Elbow

The motions at the elbow joint are flexion and extension from the hinge joint between the distal end of the humerus and the proximal radius and ulna, and pronation and supination of the forearm, which requires motion of the proximal radioulnar joint and radiohumeral joint. Significant injury to any area of these articulations may interfere with both forearm motion and elbow flexion and extension. Because of this complex articulation, the elbow is less able to withstand minor degrees of anatomic distortion. Injuries involving this articulation have a propensity for stiffness if immobilized too long and for production of new periosteal bone or myositis ossificans if irritated during the immediate postinjury period. Because rather minor injuries can produce subtle fractures, it is imperative not only to have standard AP and lateral x-ray views of the elbow joint but also oblique x-rays; in difficult diagnostic situations comparable views of the opposite normal side should be obtained. With children, in the presence of incompletely or unossified bony epiphyses, interpretation of x-rays following trauma is difficult, making it mandatory to have comparably positioned x-rays of the normal side.

Fractures of the Radial Head and Neck

Fractures of the head of the radius usually occur from falls on the outstretched hand. This force drives the head of the radius against the capitellum, which causes various degrees of cartilage contusion on the capitellum or head of the radius or fractures of the radial head.

CLINICAL MANIFESTATIONS. Patients with isolated fractures of the radial head may notice immediate stiffness of the elbow. As the hematoma and effusion increase, further limitation is noted, and pain becomes constant and severe. On examination, there is localized tenderness over the radial head, with painful limitation of motion.

TREATMENT. Successful treatment of radial head fractures is dependent upon the establishment of early joint motion. The initial treatment consists of aspiration of the joint hematoma and instillation of 2 to 3 ml of 2% Xylocaine. Following this, the patient should have improved motion and comfort. The patient is treated with a sling, and active motion within the range of pain tolerance is encouraged. After 3 weeks, the sling is discarded, but the patient is instructed to refrain from lifting heavy objects for 6 weeks. If the patient is still unable to pronate and supinate in the midrange of joint motion, excision of the radial head is indicated, because of mechanical block. Immediate range of motion is started following excision of all fragments of the radial head.

FRACTURES OF THE RADIAL NECK IN CHILDREN

The mechanism of injury causing a fracture of the radial head in adults produces a fracture of the radial neck (Fig. 47-26) in young children. This fracture is reduced by manipulation. The elbow is angulated into varus, while direct digital pressure is applied to the valgus-angulated radial head.

Fig. 47-26. AP and lateral x-rays of a fracture of the radial neck in a child.

Blount states that if less than 45° of angulation is present, the end result will be excellent. However, if residual angulation is more than 45°, open reduction during the first week is indicated. After 3 weeks open reduction is not justified. The radial head should never be excised in a child, because of the resultant shortening which will develop from loss of the proximal radial epiphysis.

Fractures of the Proximal Ulna

Isolated fractures of the olecranon occur most commonly in adults and are very infrequent in children. They are caused by forced flexion of the elbow against the actively contracting triceps, as when a patient falls on an outstretched hand. The olecranon is avulsed by the triceps.

In children, the fractures are, as a rule, undisplaced and can be treated with immobilization in extension.

When the fracture is displaced in adults, operation is invariably indicated if local skin condition is satisfactory. For noncomminuted fractures, open reduction and internal fixation of the fracture with a rigid olecranon screw is the treatment of choice. For very comminuted fractures, it may be necessary to excise the olecranon fragments and resuture the triceps aponeurosis to restore active extension.

Supracondylar Fractures of the Humerus

The supracondylar fracture (Fig. 47-27) accounts for the majority of fractures sustained about the elbow in children. The same injury occurs in adults but is rare in comparison with its incidence in children. It is usually caused by a fall upon the extended elbow; a small percentage of these fractures occur with the elbow flexed and should be recognized, so that the treatment and immobilization can be applied in extension.

A supracondylar fracture is the most hazardous fracture treated by the orthopedist, because of the vascular com-

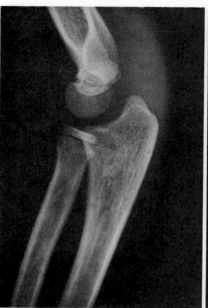
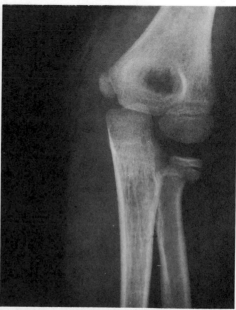

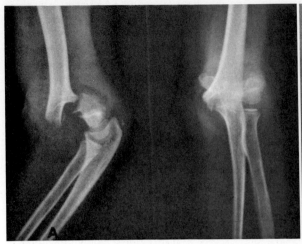
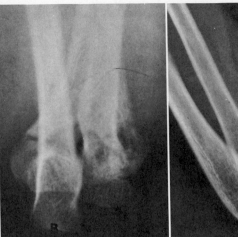
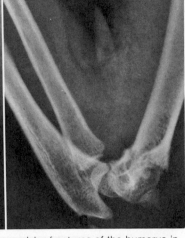

Fig. 47-27. Displaced supracondylar fractures of the humerus in a child. *A.* AP and lateral x-rays on initial examination. *B* and *C.* AP and lateral x-rays obtained following closed manipulation after the local instillation of 2% Xylocaine.

plication of Volkmann's ischemic contracture. As the humeral condyles are driven back into extension, the brachial artery may be stretched, contused, or lacerated over the distal end of the proximal fragment during the initial injury. An injury to the brachial artery may cause collateral vasospasm, producing ischemia to the flexor forearm muscles and resulting Volkmann's contractures.

Fig. 47-28. Position of skeletal traction (Smith) for supracondylar fracture of the humerus.

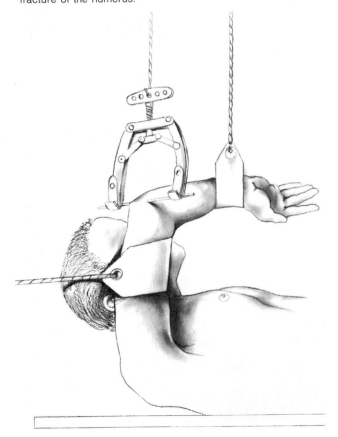

CLINICAL MANIFESTATIONS. Children with displaced supracondylar fractures present with marked swelling about the elbow, deformity, and ecchymosis when initially seen. Undisplaced fractures may have considerable swelling and symptoms of pain, but without deformity. Before instituting treatment, it is necessary to determine the presence of circulation to the hand and the presence or absence of a radial pulse. A small percentage have injuries to the radial or median nerves in the presence of normal circulation. If the radial pulse is absent, it is imperative to reduce the fracture immediately.

TREATMENT. Manipulation reduction can be accomplished after local anesthetic infiltration of the fracture site with 2% Xylocaine or using general anesthesia. With countertraction applied to the axilla, one hand of the operator grasps the biceps, placing the thumb over the distal fragment. Traction is applied to the forearm with the opposite hand, and when the fracture fragments have been disengaged by slight hyperextension, the elbow is brought into the position of maximal flexion. While holding the elbow in maximal flexion, x-rays are obtained to determine the accuracy of reduction. If reduction is satisfactory and the radial pulse is present or has returned, the arm is immobilized at 90° with the forearm in neutral or slight pronation, in a collar and cuff, with plaster splints. All patients with supracondylar fractures should be hospitalized so that possible changes in circulation can be monitored.

If the radial pulse disappears with maximal flexion, the elbow is brought toward a right angle into a position in which the pulse is present but with as much flexion as possible. If the pulse does not return and there is good capillary circulation to the hand, the patient has no pain, and he can fully extend the fingers without discomfort, it is sufficient to temporize and evaluate these findings each 1 or 2 hours. If at any time circulation to the hand is in doubt in the presence of pain or if inability to extend the fingers painlessly develops, exploration of the brachial artery where it crosses the fracture site is indicated, along with release of the antebrachial fascia.

If fracture reduction and its maintenance are not possible, the patient should be placed in a traction device described by Smith (Fig. 47-28). A $\frac{3}{32}$-in. Kirschner wire is driven across the crest of the ulna, 1 in. distal to the tip of the olecranon process, and a traction bow is attached. With the patient lying supine in bed and the arm in forward flexion of 90°, enough weight is suspended overhead to reduce the fracture with the elbow at 90° of flexion and the forearm suspended in an overhead sling. The accuracy of reduction is determined by aligning the bony prominences with the distal humerus and comparing it with the opposite side. X-ray check is made to determine the degree of apposition and rotation of fracture sites, but alignment is best determined by the visual method of Smith. Traction is removed at 14 days, and the arm is placed in a long arm cast.

Reversal of the carrying angle, or so-called gunstock deformity, results when medial angulation of the distal fragment is not corrected. It also may be due to stimulation of the lateral condylar epiphyses from the fracture itself, since deformities have been noted following undisplaced fractures.

FRACTURES OF THE LATERAL EPICONDYLE IN CHILDREN

These injuries occur from hyperextension of the elbow with a valgus force. The child complains of pain with minimal swelling. If adequate x-rays are not taken and compared with the opposite side, this fracture may be overlooked. The fracture is either undisplaced or pulled from its normal location (Fig. 47-29) and rotated into the joint by the extensor muscles of the forearm attached to the fragment.

TREATMENT. This is a Type IV epiphyseal injury of the Salter and Harris classification, and requires anatomic reduction. Even if reduction is successful and the elbow is placed in acute flexion, when muscle tone is recovered following anesthesia, the fragment will be displaced again. As a rule, only undisplaced fractures do not require surgical treatment.

The elbow is exposed through a Kocher incision. The fracture fragment is anatomically reduced and fixed with two small Kirschner wires or by periosteal suture. The elbow is immobilized in neutral position at 90° flexion for 3 weeks, after which the pins are removed. Unreduced fractures may be opened up to 3 or 4 months postinjury. Beyond this time it is best to accept the nonunion, limitation of motion, and cubitus valgus which occurs.

FRACTURES OF THE MEDIAL EPICONDYLE IN CHILDREN

A sudden valgus strain of the elbow in a child may avulse the medial epicondylar apophysis. Minor degrees of displacement need not be anatomically reduced. If there has been a temporary dislocation of the joint with avulsion and incarceration of fragments in the joint or if ulnar nerve symptoms are present, open reduction and pinning of the fragments are required.

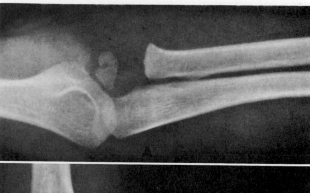
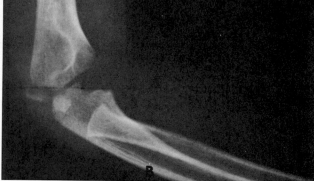
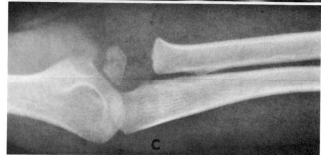

Fig. 47-29. AP, lateral, and oblique x-rays showing Type IV epiphyseal fracture of the lateral epicondyle with displacement and rotation.

COMMINUTED FRACTURES OF THE DISTAL HUMERUS

Comminuted fractures of the distal end of the humerus are uncommon and usually result from a direct fall on the elbow or automobile collisions. Open reduction and internal fixation carried out through a posterior approach is the treatment of choice. If sound fixation can be obtained, early elbow motion at 7 to 10 days is started. If secure internal fixation cannot be anticipated, traction through an olecranon pin is used, followed with motion as soon as callus can be demonstrated. Residual disability from such an injury is painless loss of motion.

Dislocations of the Elbow

A posterior dislocation of the elbow without associated fracture is more likely to occur in a child than an adult but is not a common injury. The injury is caused by falling on an outstretched arm with extension confined by adduction or abduction forces applied across the joint. The entire

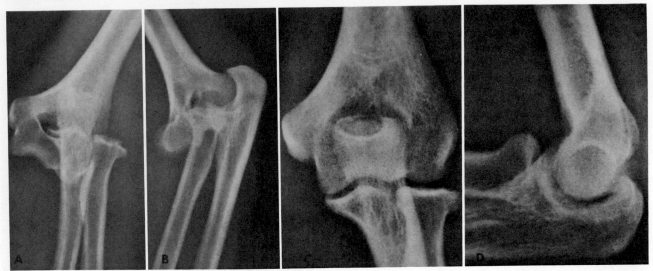

Fig. 47-30. Posterolateral dislocation of the elbow with a fracture of the radial head. *A* and *B*. AP and lateral x-rays prior to reduction. *C* and *D*. Postreduction x-rays showing satisfactory reduction with a minimally displaced small fracture of the radial head.

anterior capsule is torn with damage to medial and lateral ligaments of the elbow.

These patients have severe pain and marked swelling. In contrast to fractures of the supracondylar region, the dislocation is quite stable.

TREATMENT. The treatment is immediate reduction. The reduction may be carried out under local anesthesia into the joint or by use of analgesics. In large muscular individuals, general anesthesia may be necessary. Traction is applied to the axis of the forearm in the position in which it lies, maintaining countertraction on the humerus. When reduction has been accomplished, the elbow is brought to

a 90° flexion, and check x-rays are obtained. The arm is then immobilized in a collar and cuff in maximal flexion; active exercises are started in 3 weeks in children.

Adults are put in a posterior splint at 90° in neutral rotation. The splint is discarded at 10 days, and the arm is placed in a sling. Active motion is begun within the tolerance of pain. The treatment of lateral dislocations is the same.

FRACTURE-DISLOCATIONS OF THE ELBOW

In addition to a posterior dislocation of the elbow, there may be a fracture of the coronoid process, the head of the radius (Fig. 47-30), or the lateral condyle. In the coronoid process it is usually a small chip fracture and is caused by the insertion of the brachialis, avulsing this portion of the bone during the dislocation. Its significance is that postreduction position of the elbow is more unstable, and immobilization is continued for a longer interval (3 weeks). If the radial head is fractured, the elbow is treated in the same manner as a posterior dislocation (reduction and immobilization). If motion does not return, radial head excision is indicated.

Monteggia's Deformity

Monteggia described deformity in which there was a dislocation of the radial head with a fracture of the proximal third of the ulna (Fig. 47-31). In 85 percent of the cases the radial head is dislocated anteriorly, and in 15 percent, posteriorly. The deformity may be caused by a direct blow on the ulna, fracturing it and driving the radial head anteriorly. Evans has shown that the injury is usually caused by a forced pronation and that reduction can be accomplished by closed methods.

Whenever an x-ray reveals a fracture of one bone of the arm or dislocation of one end, the concomitant injury

Fig. 47-31. Monteggia's deformity. *A*. Midshaft ulna fracture with anterior bowing and anterior dislocation of the radial head. *B*. Midshaft ulna fracture with posterior bowing and posterior dislocation of the radial head (most common).

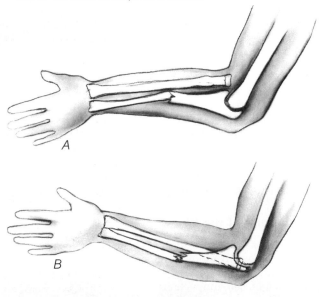

to the adjacent bone should be ruled out by x-rays of the entire forearm.

If reduction of the ulna can be maintained, closed reduction of the radial head is usually possible by maintaining the arm in supination. If the ulnar fracture is displaced, intramedullary fixation (except in children) is required. After stabilization of the ulna, supination of the forearm and direct pressure over the radial head will accomplish its reduction. If the radial head is still not reduced, open reduction and suture of the annular ligament are carried out. If the radial head is anterior, the elbow is reduced and maintained in flexion. If the radial head is posterior, reduction and immobilization are carried out in full extension with the forearm in supination. Following reduction, immobilization is maintained with a circular plaster cast.

SUBLUXATION OF THE RADIAL HEAD IN CHILDREN

One of the most common injuries of children under the age of five is the "nursemaid's elbow," or "pulled elbow." The usual history is that the child's hand is suddenly pulled, forcing the elbow into extension and causing the sudden onset of pain in the elbow. The child avoids motion of the arm. Passive, painless elbow flexion is possible from 30 to 120°. X-rays of the elbow are negative.

Salter has demonstrated that the thin distal attachment of the annular ligament to the periosteum of the radial neck is torn when traction is applied to the pronated radius. The radial head escapes beneath the anterior part of the annular ligament, which is caught between the joint surfaces.

Treatment is effected by the deft maneuver of firm supination with the elbow held at 90° flexion. The arm may be in a sling 1 week, and the parents should be cautioned against repeated traction injury to the elbow.

Fractures of the Capitellum

Fractures of the capitellum may occur in the same manner as fractures of the radial head. The patient complains of pain with any attempt at motion, and flexion is limited, depending upon the degree of displacement of the fracture.

TREATMENT. In some cases, closed reduction is sufficient. This is accomplished by extending the elbow while applying adduction force to the elbow joint. While traction is maintained, local digital pressure is applied to the fragment. The elbow is then maintained in marked flexion for 3 to 4 weeks, at the end of which time active motion is begun.

If closed manipulation fails, the elbow is exposed through a lateral Kocher approach. If the fragment is small, it is excised; if large, it is reattached with a Kirschner wire or screw fixation. When the capitellar fracture is recognized after 4 weeks, excision and early motion are necessary.

Fractures of the Forearm

Fractures of the forearm are most common in children, but occur at any age from falls on the outstretched arm or direct trauma. Clinical findings include deformity, local swelling, tenderness and instability. Anteroposterior and lateral x-rays are obtained of both bones and should include views of the elbow and wrist. If only one bone is fractured, dislocation of the proximal or distal joint should be suspected.

ANATOMIC CONSIDERATIONS. The radius has both a slight lateral bow and a posterior bow. The ulna has less medial bow but also has a slight dorsal curve. Any loss of this anatomic feature or compression of the interosseous space will interfere with rotation.

The pronator quadratus attached to the distal radius tends to pull it ulnaward and encroach upon the interosseous space. Both supinators act upon the proximal radial fragment. In fractures of the proximal third, the proximal radius will usually be in supination. The attachments of the pronator teres and the brachioradialis act to shorten the deformity and increase the lateral bow of the radius. Interference with the interosseous membrane from scarring will interfere with rotation.

In other diaphyseal fractures, alignment is the only consideration. However, in fractures of both bones of the forearm, because of the interrelationship required for rotation, anatomic restoration is required for normal function. If this can be accomplished by the closed method, there will be less scarring from surgical trauma, and the patient is more likely to have normal function. However, if the anatomic features cannot be restored by closed means, open reduction is indicated.

METHODS OF CLOSED REDUCTION. General anesthesia or axillary block anesthesia is required for reduction of forearm fractures. With the elbow flexed 90°, traction is applied to the long axis of the forearm by grasping the thumb and index finger of the patient and applying countertraction to the humerus. This may be done with the help of an assistant or by suspending the thumb and index finger with traction and adding weight over the humerus proximal to the flexed elbow as countertraction. When length has been regained, the fracture fragments are grasped by the operator, angulation increased, displacement corrected, and the fracture reduced.

If there is more than one fracture, reduction of the transverse fracture is accomplished first. Using the length gained from this reduction, reduction of the adjacent bone is then effected. The arm is immobilized in a position in which stability is greatest. For proximal-third fractures, this is supination, and for distal-third fractures, pronation, although there are exceptions to this rule. A well-molded, minimally padded plaster from the proximal palmar crease to the axilla, with the elbow at 90° flexion, is used. X-rays are obtained to determine accuracy of reduction. Interpretation may require comparison with the normal side. It is necessary to take check x-rays at intervals during the first 3 weeks to be certain that position is maintained. When position is lost, open reduction may be necessary.

The fractures most often requiring open reduction are displaced fractures of the proximal third and oblique fractures of the radius. Segmental fractures also require open reduction and internal fixation.

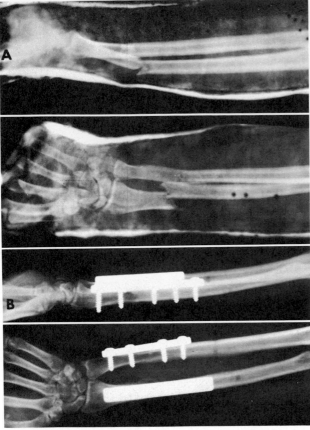

Fig. 47-32. Fracture of both bones of the forearm with open reduction and internal fixation. *A.* AP and lateral x-rays following closed reduction, showing displacement of distal radial fragment. *B.* AP and lateral x-rays showing anatomic position following open reduction and fixation with compression plates.

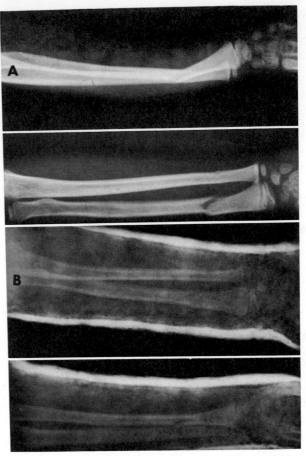

Fig. 47-33. *A.* Greenstick fracture of the radius with torus fracture of the ulna. *B.* Satisfactory position following manipulation and application of plaster.

Open reduction of the radius is carried out through the approach of Henry. The ulna is exposed through a separate incision, along its subcutaneous border. A compression plate is an ideal means of internal fixation for open reduction, although both bones may be fixed with intramedullary nails (Fig. 47-32).

Postoperative immobilization is continued until union has occurred. The approximate time is 10 to 12 weeks, but a considerably longer period may be required. Open fractures, if clean and treated immediately after injury, may be fixed with internal fixation, although we prefer debridement, closure, and skeletal pin fixation. Skeletal fixation is accomplished with a Kirschner wire through the bases of the second and third metacarpals, incorporated in plaster.

FOREARM SHAFT FRACTURES IN CHILDREN

Operative reduction of shafts of both bones is almost never indicated in the young child. Treatment of these injuries is by closed reduction and immobilization in plaster. However, in children twelve years of age and older (i.e., close to epiphyseal maturity), there will be minimal remodeling, and operative reduction may be required.

TREATMENT. Greenstick fractures with angulation (Fig. 47-33) should be manipulated to correct the deformity and at the same time break the unbroken cortex. Otherwise, deformity will occur in the cast. The apex of the deformity is deftly snapped over the operator's knee, a maneuver which will usually correct the deformity.

The principles of reduction of displaced fractures in children are the same as for displaced fractures in adults. If both bones are displaced, one bone is reduced, and using this as a lever the adjacent bone is reduced. The forearm is then immobilized with the elbow at 90° and in the position of greatest stability: supination for proximal-third, pronation for distal-third, and neutral position for midshaft fractures. Check x-rays are obtained immediately post-reduction and at 7 to 10 days to be certain that reduction is maintained. If it is not possible to hold both bones reduced, fixed traction as outlined by Blount, in which skin traction is applied to the fingers and attached to an outrigger splint from the cast, is necessary. Experience is required in judging what degrees of angulation will be corrected with remodeling. The closer the fracture to the growing epiphysis, the greater remodeling possible. In general, 30° of shaft angulation in an infant will correct itself. However, this should not be accepted in the older child.

Fractures of the Distal Radius

COLLES FRACTURE

A fracture of the distal radius with dorsal angulation produces a typical silver fork deformity, as was described by Abraham Colles in 1814. Since Colles was describing a clinical deformity before the use of x-ray, the use of the term *Colles fracture* has come to mean dorsally angulated fractures of the distal radial metaphysis with an associated fracture of the ulnar styloid (Fig. 47-34) and not fracture of the distal ulnar shaft, which occurs in children.

CLINICAL MANIFESTATIONS. Distal radial fractures usually occur in patients over the age of fifty, more commonly in women, and are produced by a fall on the outstretched hand. The term "silver fork" offers an appropriate clinical description. Depending upon the degree of comminution, there may be considerable instability, tenderness, and swelling about the wrist. Palpation of the wrist will reveal a more proximal position of the tip of the radial styloid. On examination, it is important to rule out the presence or absence of a concomitant median nerve injury. X-ray examination should include AP, lateral, and both oblique views. A carpal dislocation can clinically simulate this deformity.

TREATMENT. The aim of treatment of this injury is to obtain a functional hand and wrist and, secondly, to minimize cosmetic deformity. In the past, many operative skeletal traction methods have been used in an attempt to improve the cosmetic deformity. Unfortunately, immobilization of the hand required of these methods compromises hand function. The best results in this fracture have been obtained by closed reduction and plaster immobilization.

Manipulation Technique. With an assistant applying countertraction to the humerus and with the elbow flexed, traction is applied to the radial side of the hand for disimpaction of the distal radial fragment, which is displaced and angulated in a radial and dorsal direction.

Fig. 47-34. Colles fracture in a twenty-five-year-old woman. *A.* AP and lateral x-rays postinjury. *B.* AP and lateral x-rays after closed reduction under local anesthesia and cast immobilization.

While traction is maintained, the operator grasps the distal radial fragment between thumb and index finger and displaces it anteriorly to correct the displacement. At the same time, counterpressure is applied in a dorsal direction, with the opposite hand applied to the anterior surface of the forearm. Simultaneously, the wrist is brought into maximal flexion and ulnar deviation while pronating the forearm.

If reduction has been accomplished, there will be palpable dorsal step, and the tip of the radial styloid will be at least 1 cm distal to the ulnar styloid. It may be necessary to repeat the manipulation.

Over two layers of sheet wadding a well-molded plaster cast is applied which includes the elbow, with the wrist in maximal ulnar deviation, 30° of palmar flexion. Check x-rays are obtained immediately and at 7 to 10 days to be certain that reduction has been maintained.

The patient should be encouraged to keep the hand elevated for 2 or 3 days or until swelling has subsided. The patient is instructed in exercises to maintain a full range of motion of all interphalangeal (IP) and metaphalangeal (MP) joints. The patient should maximally flex the IP joints with the MP joints in extension and flex the MP joints with the IP joints in extension. Patients who are able to do this have little difficulty in mobilizing the wrist following 6 weeks of plaster immobilization. Patients should do range-of-motion shoulder exercises daily. This prevents the occasional episodes of shoulder stiffness that accompany Colles fractures. Shoulder stiffness may be due to traction on the shoulder joint from the weight of the cast or from a primary capsular injury at the time of initial injury. If the wrist is placed in maximal palmar flexion, median nerve compression in the carpal tunnel may ensue. If median nerve paresthesias occur, decrease in the amount of wrist flexion is necessary. If unrelieved, the flexor retinaculum is incised surgically.

SMITH FRACTURE

A fall on the dorsum of the wrist may cause a reverse Colles or Smith fracture. In such fractures position is difficult to maintain (Fig. 47-35) because of comminution.

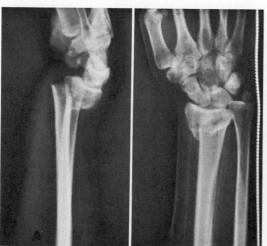
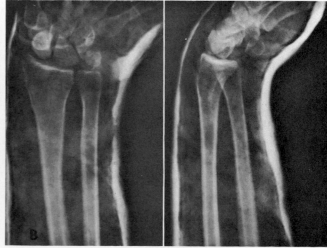

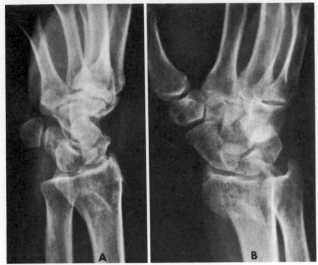

Fig. 47-35. Smith fracture. *A*. Lateral x-ray. *B*. Oblique x-rays showing minimal anterior angulation and displacement of the distal fragments.

Plaster immobilization in the position of dorsiflexion of the wrist is required. If this will not maintain position, continuous skeletal traction to the thumb metacarpal or open reduction and screw fixation are necessary.

Injuries to the Wrist

A person falling on the outstretched wrist may sprain the anterior radial carpal ligament, with resulting synovial effusion and wrist pain, and limitation of motion. It is important to distinguish this from a fractured navicular or dislocation of the lunate, which have similar signs.

FRACTURES OF THE NAVICULAR

Young adults who fall on the outstretched hand frequently fracture the navicular (Fig. 47-36) against the unyielding anterior radial carpal ligament. In elderly patients, a Colles fracture occurs, because the distal radius is the point of least resistance. There is tenderness to direct pressure over the tuberosity of the navicular, with limitation of wrist flexion and extension. With any wrist injury, it is imperative to rule out a fractured navicular by x-ray examination.

In addition to AP, lateral, and oblique x-rays of the carpal bones, with the wrist in neutral position, a special 17° angled AP x-ray view of the wrist is needed. If the patient has tenderness over the tuberosity of the navicular and x-ray examination is negative, the patient is presumed to have a fractured navicular, treated as such, and then re-x-rayed when there has been some resorption at the fracture site (3 weeks). At 3 weeks, if clinical and x-ray examination are still negative, the wrist is mobilized.

There is little or no displacement with fractures of the navicular. Arterial supply enters the distal third of the bone constantly. The proximal-third blood supply may be only by communication in the bone from the vessels entering distad. Fractures transecting the waist or proximal third may interrupt the entire circulation to the proximal third. Because of this, nonunion or avascular necrosis of the proximal fragments is not uncommon.

TREATMENT. When there is little or no displacement and the injury is diagnosed accurately, the optimal treatment is by plaster cast immobilization. Plaster is applied from the tip of the thumb to include the elbow. By immobilizing the elbow, pronation-supination, which causes motion at the fracture site, is prevented.

Most navicular fractures require 16 weeks of adequate plaster immobilization. The patient is seen at monthly intervals and the cast replaced, if loose, without disturbing the position of the wrist. X-rays out of plaster are obtained at 8 weeks and at subsequent 4-week intervals. When all tenderness from direct pressure over the tuberosity of the navicular has disappeared and x-rays show obliteration of the fracture site, plaster immobilization is discontinued. In some situations, 6 months or longer is necessary.

When a patient has an acute fracture in which displacement cannot be corrected, the best treatment is open reduction and the insertion of a McLaughlin lag screw. This is preferable to accepting a possible nonunion or the long delay necessary for union of the displaced fracture. Displaced fractures usually occur as the result of, and in combination with, perilunar dislocation of the carpus.

When the interval between trauma and diagnosis is less than 6 months, prolonged plaster immobilization (6 to 9 months) will usually result in union.

NONUNION OF NAVICULAR FRACTURES. With a simple nonunion of navicular fractures, without avascular necrosis and without degenerative arthritis at the wrist, an autogenous bone graft is indicated. In patients with significant degenerative changes adjacent to the nonunion, excision of the radial styloid gives satisfactory pain relief and maintenance of wrist power. When the proximal fragment is small and avascular, excision will give satisfactory results. However, if large, bone grafting is the procedure of choice.

DISLOCATIONS OF THE LUNATE

Dislocations of the lunate are uncommon but occur from trauma causing hyperextension of the wrist. Patients complain of pain, swelling, and limitation of motion. Median nerve symptoms are frequent. The diagnosis is made by AP and lateral x-rays. On the lateral x-ray of the wrist, the semilunar shape of the lunate is displaced anterior to the distal radial articular surface. On the AP x-ray, the normal quadrilateral shape of the lunate appears triangular and larger than on the opposite side.

TREATMENT. Treatment is by closed reduction and plaster immobilization. Reduction is accomplished by hyperextending the wrist and applying direct pressure of the operator's thumb over the dislocated lunate. After it is reduced, the wrist is brought into the flexed position. There is a high incidence of avascular necrosis following this injury, for which lunate excision is indicated. Kienböck's disease, which is avascular necrosis of the lunate, may occur without known trauma. The onset of symptoms, which include wrist pain, stiffness, and local swelling, is insidious. Treatment is excision of the avascular lunate.

A similar mechanism of injury may produce a perilunar

dislocation of the carpus with or without fracture of the scaphoid or rotatory subluxation of the scaphoid—so-called traumatic instability of the wrist. The diagnosis of the former is obvious radiographically, but attention should always be directed at the scaphoid-lunate relationship to detect subtle signs of scaphoid subluxation. The reader is referred to the work of Linscheid et al. for discussion of therapy.

Fractures and Dislocations in the Hand

METACARPAL FRACTURES

Metacarpal fractures occur from direct violence to the hand, as in crushing injuries, although the most common mechanism is by striking the hand against an opponent (Fig. 47-37). Fractures of the necks of fourth and fifth metacarpals invariably occur in young men as a result of altercations. There is local swelling involving the fracture site which minimizes the actual degree of anterior angulation of the head of the metacarpal. Therefore, the degree of angulation can be determined only by x-ray. Rotational deformity of such a fracture must be determined clinically. Each finger, when flexed individually into the palm, points to the navicular, and any deviation from this is an indication of rotational deformity of the finger or its metacarpal shaft.

TREATMENT. Treatment of the acute metacarpal neck fractures is by closed manipulation, making certain that rotational deformity is corrected. The finger is then splinted with the MP and the IP joints in 45° of flexion and with the tip pointing toward the navicular. It is not always possible to hold the fracture by this method, and some cosmetic deformity of the knuckle may persist. However, since there is mobility at the carpometacarpal joints of the fourth and fifth fingers, the grip will not be compromised. It is preferable to accept some degree of anterior angulation without rotation rather than immobilize the MP joint at 90° with pressure on a fully flexed IP joint, as has been described.

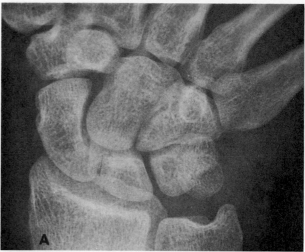

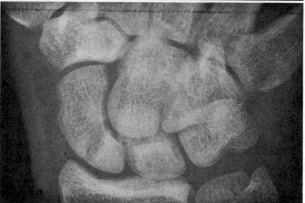

Fig. 47-36. Fracture of the carpal navicular. *A.* AP x-ray 1 day postinjury is negative for fracture. *B.* Patient was persistently tender over the navicular tuberosity. X-ray at 3 weeks reveals fracture at the junction of the proximal and middle thirds. Fracture subsequently healed without avascular necrosis.

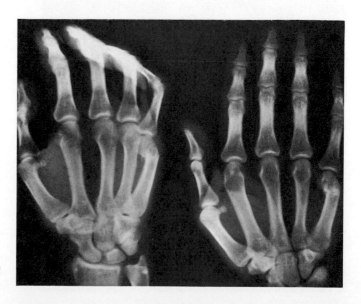

Fig. 47-37. AP and oblique x-rays of a fracture of the neck of the fifth metacarpal which occurred during an altercation.

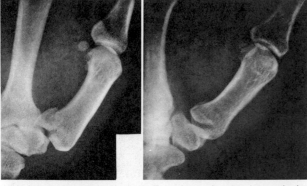

Fig. 47-38. Bennett's fracture. Two views showing intraarticular fracture of the base of the proximal first phalanx with displacement. Such an injury requires reduction and maintenance of position by plaster or open reduction.

Metacarpal shaft fractures which are oblique or spiral usually require nothing more than anterior splinting for 2 to 3 weeks. Anterior angulated fractures of the second and third metacarpals which do not have carpometacarpal mobility must be protected against anterior angulation, or interference with grasp will result. Multiple fractures of metacarpal shafts may require intramedullary fixation. This is done by inserting a single intramedullary wire percutaneously from distal to proximal direction, starting on the lip of the metacarpal head and avoiding the articular surface. Comminuted fractures of the metacarpal heads involving the articular surface are difficult to treat because

Fig. 47-39. A. Lateral x-ray of the dorsal dislocation of the proximal interphalangeal joint of an index finger. B. After closed reduction under local anesthesia, postreduction position was maintained on a metal splint in the position of function.

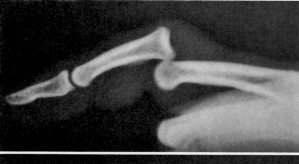

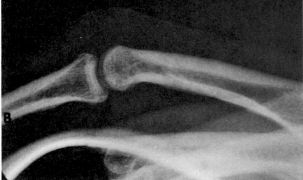

of the extensive damage to the articular surface. Such fractures should be immobilized in a position of function over a metal splint and motion started at 2 to 3 weeks.

Fracture dislocations of the carpometacarpal joint occur very rarely. A typical mechanism of injury is severe force applied to a hyperextended wrist. If possible, it is preferable to maintain closed reduction of a carpometacarpal fracture dislocation. However, there may be interposition of tendons and soft tissue, necessitating open reduction. Kirschner wire fixation across the carpometacarpal junction is used to maintain the reduction.

BENNETT'S FRACTURE

Bennett's fracture is an intraarticular fracture involving the base of the carpometacarpal joint of the thumb (Fig. 47-38). Such an injury is the result of forcible abduction on the thumb. There is an oblique fracture which involves the base of the metacarpal and which transects the proximal articular surface. The resulting instability causes subluxation of the shaft and the remaining articular surface. If such a fracture is unreduced, the normal range of abduction and carpometacarpal joint motion will be compromised.

Closed methods may hold reduction of minimally displaced and undisplaced fractures. Traction is applied to the axis of the shaft of the metacarpal, which is then brought into abduction, while direct adduction pressure is applied over the base of the carpometacarpal joint. If displacement persists, closed reduction and percutaneous wire fixation of the first carpometacarpal joint will hold the fracture. If this is not sufficient, open reduction and Kirschner wire fixation across the fracture is indicated.

PHALANGEAL FRACTURES

Undisplaced fractures of phalangeal shafts require splinting with the MP joints in 70° flexion and IP joints in slight flexion. The finger is placed on a metal splint and taped in this position without traction. If the fracture is displaced, it is manipulated into position and placed on a metal splint as for undisplaced fractures.

A small chip fracture involving an IP joint is treated symptomatically by the use of a splint for 2 weeks followed by early motion. Interphalangeal dislocations (Fig. 47-39) require closed reduction and splinting in a position of function. Open reduction is rarely necessary.

Distal Phalanx

A crushed fingertip with resultant fracture of the distal phalanx is one of the most common injuries seen in an emergency room. Initial treatment is aimed at cleansing the skin and relieving the pain by splinting the finger. There is usually no intraarticular involvement, and position of fragments is rarely a consideration.

Mallet Finger

When the distal phalanx is forcibly flexed against the taut extensor tendon, avulsion of the extensor tendon may occur with or without a fragment of bone from its insertion on the distal phalanx. This causes a characteristic dropped finger; the last 15 to 20° of active extension is lost, although full passive extension is possible. There is local tenderness and swelling over the dorsal aspect of the distal interphalangeal (DIP) joint.

Many types of treatment have been tried for this lesion. If the tendon has been avulsed without a bone fragment, the finger is splinted over a metal splint with the DIP joint in maximal extension or hyperextension and with the proximal interphalangeal (PIP) joint in 60° of flexion. The splint needs to be repeatedly inspected and adjusted. Care should be taken not to cause excessive pressure over the DIP joint. If active extension is not gained in 6 weeks, splinting should be continued for another 2 or 3 weeks. Incomplete extension is not always associated with disability. However, if the patient shows symptoms, surgical reefing of the lengthened extensor tendon is indicated.

When avulsion occurs with a fragment of bone (Fig. 47-40) involving one-third of the distal articular surface, open reduction and Bunnell pullout wire fixation are required. If the bone chip is small or does not involve the articular surface, the treatment may be the same as with a pure tendon avulsion.

In crush injuries of any IP joint with severe comminution of articular surface the phalanges should be splinted in a position of function at 45° of flexion and consideration given to early arthrodesis, if symptoms are evident.

Compound fractures involving the hand invoke the same principles as those applied to other compound fractures.

FRACTURES AND JOINT INJURIES IN THE LOWER EXTREMITY

Fractures of the Proximal Femur

Fractures of the proximal femur are a challenge to everyone responsible for the care of patients with such injuries. The hospital mortality of 25 percent encountered with this injury, as reported by Horowitz, is an indication of the severity of the problem. Prior to the introduction of internal fixation, such fractures were treated by bed rest and traction, with a much higher mortality rate. The age of most patients with fractures of the proximal femur is in the sixties or seventies. Complications of immobility imposed by this fracture in this elderly age group are responsible for the high mortality. Operative fixation will allow early mobility and relief of pain and is the treatment of choice. Only in the occasional younger individual with this injury can bed rest and traction be tolerated.

FEMORAL NECK FRACTURES

Femoral neck fractures usually occur in the elderly but may occur in young adults or children when severe trauma is involved. Fractures are commonly produced by a fall, although the history may suggest that the fracture occurred from a twist or indirect type of force and the patient fell as the fractured femoral neck gave way.

CLINICAL MANIFESTATIONS. The patient is usually unable to stand on the side of the affected hip and has increasing pain as a tense hemarthrosis develops. On clinical examination, the affected leg may be slightly shorter

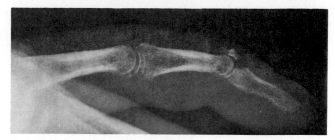

Fig. 47-40. Mallet finger. Lateral x-ray of a finger with avulsion of the extensor tendon at its bony insertion. There is minimal subluxation, and open reduction and direct suture of the fragment are indicated.

and held in a position of external rotation of 30 to 40°. Attempts at motion cause excruciating pain. There may be ecchymosis over the trochanter, but local swelling is not prominent.

Anteroposterior and tube lateral x-rays demonstrate interruption between the trabeculae of the head and neck. The head is rotated into varus with posterior angulation. There are varying degrees of comminution of the posterior neck at the fracture site.

CLASSIFICATION. Garden has classified femoral neck fractures according to displacement and comminution (Fig. 47-41): Type I fractures are incomplete fractures; Type II, complete fractures without displacement; Type III, partially displaced fractures; and Type IV, complete displacement. This classification is useful in evaluating therapy, since displaced fractures have a higher rate of nonunion and avascular necrosis.

Fig. 47-41. Types of subcapital fracture (Garden; see text).

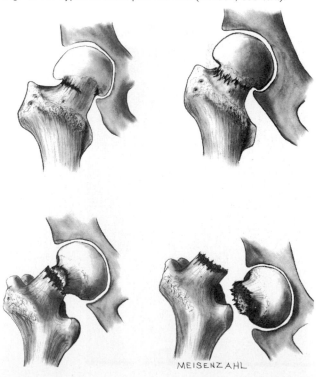

MEISENZAHL

TREATMENT. The prognosis of this fracture depends upon the attainment of union, without development of avascular necrosis. In adults, the blood supply to the femoral head is via the metaphyseal vessels (which are interrupted by the fracture), the artery of the ligamentum teres, and the lateral epiphyseal vessels. The location of a fracture site high on the neck with associated displacement may damage the lateral epiphyseal vessels. If the artery of the ligamentum teres provides insufficient circulation, avascular necrosis may ensue.

The periosteum on the neck has no cambium layer, so that external callus does not develop. The absence of external callus and the precarious circulation contribute to the high incidence of nonunion.

Massie and Deyerle have shown that early reduction and adequate immobilization of the fracture site can overcome these difficulties. Despite the apparent medical contraindication for surgical treatment in these patients, internal fixation will relieve pain, allow mobilization, and at the same time facilitate union and minimize the incidence of avascular necrosis.

Impacted Femoral Neck Fractures

Type I (Garden) subcapital fractures or Type II fractures which are impacted may be treated conservatively. Some patients have walked with the fracture by the time of examination. If the fracture is impacted in slight valgus with less than 15 to 20° of anterior angulation at the fracture site, it is worthwhile to attempt nonoperative management, as outlined by Crawford. The patient is instructed not to bear weight or use leverage with the leg. The patient is kept in bed until he can actively control the leg without discomfort. This usually takes from a few days to a week. In Crawford's series, the few impacted

Fig. 47-42. Subcapital fracture fixed with Deyerle plate and pins.

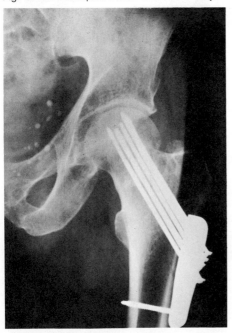

fractures, which subsequently were displaced, all occurred within the first 10 days. If displacement occurs, closed reduction and internal fixation are indicated.

Displaced Fractures of the Femoral Neck

Treatment. Pain, associated with such fractures, causes rapid deterioration in the patient's condition, making the treatment of this fracture a surgical emergency. If a patient is in congestive heart failure, diabetic acidosis, or a state of dehydration, i.e., in a condition which can be alleviated within 24 hours, this time should be invested for correction of the condition. Mortality rates are lower when such fractures are fixed immediately. It is not sufficient to place the patient in traction, expecting his condition to improve for surgical treatment, because this does not relieve the pain, and the complications of pneumonia, pulmonary emboli, decubitus ulcer, urinary tract infection, or paralytic ileus will occur.

Technique of Reduction and Fixation. *Reduction.* Under spinal or general anesthesia, the patient is placed on a standard fracture table equipped for AP and lateral x-rays to be taken during surgical procedures.

Closed reduction is done by manipulation. The affected leg is grasped in both hands, and with the knee flexed traction is applied in the long axis of the thigh with the hip in 20 to 30° of abduction and 30 to 40° of external rotation. As part of the same motion, the hip is flexed about 45°, internally rotated 15°, and then slowly brought toward extension to a position of 15° of flexion. While traction is maintained manually, the foot is taped to the foot plate of the fracture table in 30 to 45° of internal rotation, in 10° of abduction, and with sufficient tension to hold the reduction.

Check x-rays are obtained to determine the adequacy of reduction. If reduction is not satisfactory, repeat manipulation is carried out. A satisfactory reduction is one in which the head is in a position of a few degrees of valgus, with the medial point of the proximal fracture surface displaced a millimeter or two lateral to the calcar on the distal fragment. On the lateral x-ray, the head should be anatomically aligned with the neck.

Internal Fixation (Deyerle Method.) A lateral incision is used to expose the lateral aspect of the proximal femur. The skin, subcutaneous tissue, and fascia lata are divided in line with the incision. The vastus lateralis is separated by muscle-splitting incisions close to the linea aspera. The intermedius and periosteum are separated from the proximal femoral shaft, exposing the base of the greater trochanter. A guide pin is inserted in a $\frac{1}{4}$-in. drill hole placed $1\frac{1}{4}$ in. below the flare of the greater trochanter and at a point midway between the anterior and posterior cortices. The guide pin is inserted through the bone across the fracture site into the head. A Deyerle guide plate (Fig. 47-42) is then passed over the guide pin and affixed to the shaft. The appropriate nine holes using the guide plate are predrilled with a $\frac{9}{64}$ drill. The guide plate is then removed and the regular plate affixed to the shaft with the screw. Nine Deyerle pins of appropriate length to give secure fixation of the femoral head are inserted. Selection of pins is monitored by biplane check x-rays. After all pins have been inserted, traction is removed from the extremity, and the fracture site is impacted using the impactor applied to the plate.

Although superior results have been reported with the Deyerle procedure, the Massie nail technique is also suitable. The Smith-Petersen nail is no longer recommended, because it does not control rotation satisfactorily.

When closed reduction is not satisfactory for routine fractures, open reduction, through either a Watson-Jones or Smith-Petersen incision, is required prior to internal fixation. Primary insertion of a femoral head prosthesis may also be used.

Postoperative Management. Postoperatively, patients are mobilized as rapidly as possible. They are allowed out of bed the following day and mobilized to use crutches without weight bearing as soon as possible. Check x-rays are obtained at monthly intervals to follow the progress of healing. Approximately 4 to 6 months is required for sufficient healing across the fracture site. Unprotected weight bearing is not allowed until union is solid.

If nonunion exists in the presence of a viable head, reconstructive surgical treatment, with bone grafts, or osteotomy may be required. In elderly patients, excision of the femoral head and insertion of a prosthesis is a satisfactory solution when this complication occurs.

Insertion of Femoral Head Prosthesis

Because nonunion and avascular necrosis are problems, attempts have been made to obviate these difficulties by the insertion of a primary femoral head prosthesis (Fig. 47-43). Such measures taken on a routine basis do not give as good results as hip nailing. Hinchey and Day list spastic hemiplegia, severe arthritis of the fractured hip, pathologic fracture, the need for ambulatory care because of blindness, extreme age, or poor general health contraindicating a second operation as indications for a primary prosthesis. If the complications of avascular necrosis or nonunion develop in the aged patient, a femoral head replacement prosthesis is indicated.

Technique. The prosthesis may be inserted from anterior or posterior approaches, although we have found the posteroinferior exposure of Austin Moore to be satisfactory.

The patient is placed in a lateral or semiprone position, lying on the normal side. An incision is started 2 to 3 in. lateral to the posteroinferior spine of the ilium and is extended across, and parallel with, the fibers of the gluteus maximus to the tip of the great trochanter and then approximately 4 in. distad along the lateral aspect of the trochanter. Fibers of the gluteus maximus are separated at the junction of the superior three-quarters and inferior one-quarter of the muscle. Sharp dissection is used to split the fascia lata where the inferior fibers of the gluteus maximus are inserted. If necessary, the gluteus maximus insertion on the gluteal tubercle may be partially divided. The sciatic nerve is next located, identified, and retracted medially. The short external rotators, piriformis, gemellus inferior and superior, and obturator internus are divided just proximal to the insertion on the femur. If necessary, the upper fibers of the quadratus femoris are divided also.

The hip capsule is exposed and incised. The detached

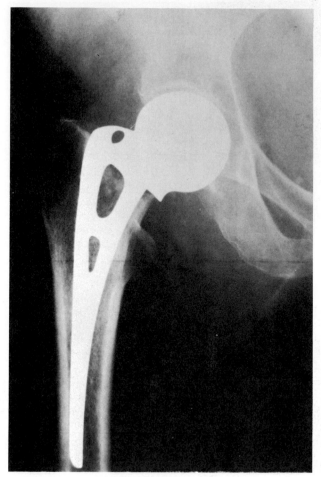

Fig. 47-43. Austin Moore's appliance inserted for displaced fracture of the femoral neck.

femoral head is then gently levered from the joint. The neck is fashioned to accept the Austin Moore prosthesis, and the medullary cavity is reamed with an Austin Moore rasp. Care should be taken to insert the reamer accurately in the proper position of 20° of anteversion and also to seat the prosthesis sufficiently laterally. Excessive reaming may result in a loose prosthesis with pain.

An Austin Moore or Thompson prosthesis which matches the size of the excised femoral head is driven into the proximal femur. If it is not possible to match it exactly, a slightly smaller prosthesis is accepted, in order to reduce the hazard of postoperative dislocation. If the femoral canal is large and osteoporotic, the prosthesis may be fixed with methyl methacrylate to minimize subsequent loosening.

The head of the Austin Moore prosthesis, which is securely driven into the femoral shaft, is then relocated in the acetabulum. The capsule is closed, if possible, and the short external rotators reapproximated.

Postoperative care is extremely important. Nursing care should prevent adduction, flexion, and internal rotation, which is the position in which dislocation occurs. The patient is allowed out of bed in 2 or 3 days. Protected

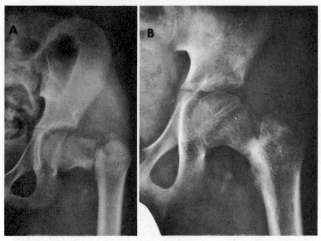

Fig. 47-44. *A.* Fracture of the femoral neck in a nine-year-old boy with varus deformity. *B.* AP x-ray showing united fracture 1 year postinjury in satisfactory position. Russell's traction was the method of treatment.

weight bearing (50 percent) is started early using crutches or a walker. Patients may progress to a cane held in the opposite hand at 3 months if able to walk painlessly and without a limp.

Femoral Neck Fractures in Children

Fractures of the femoral neck occur in children (Fig. 47-44) only after severe trauma, such as in pedestrian injuries or in falls from a great height. Since there are usually associated injuries, operative treatment is not always possible. If satisfactory reduction can be obtained by Russell's traction, it is continued until union is sound, usually for 10 to 16 weeks, depending upon the age of the child. If union is not sound, a hip spica will not protect against loss of position into varus. If closed reduction is not satisfactory, operative internal fixation treatment, as

in adults, is indicated. The fracture should be pinned with three parallel Knowles pins. There is a high incidence of avascular necrosis of both the head and neck in children.

INTERTROCHANTERIC AND SUBTROCHANTERIC FRACTURES

Intertrochanteric and subtrochanteric fractures occur very commonly in the elderly from a direct fall onto the hip. They also occur from severe traumatic forces in younger individuals as in automobile accidents or crush injury.

There is considerably more instability to this type of fracture than intracapsular fractures of the femoral neck. On clinical examination there is shortening and external rotation, which may be 90°, and swelling about the anterior and proximal thigh.

In treatment of this type of fracture in the elderly patient indications for open reduction are the same as in intracapsular fractures. The main aim of treatment is to relieve pain and mobilize the elderly patient to prevent the complications of immobility. In younger individuals who can tolerate bed rest, the conservative treatment, such as Russell's traction or skeletal traction and balanced suspension, will maintain reduction if there are contraindications to surgical treatment. If traction is decided upon, it must continue until union is solid, which may require 16 weeks or longer with bed rest. Surgical treatment involves closed or open reduction on a fracture table, combined with internal fixation (Fig. 47-45). A Jewett blade plate appliance or Richards compression screw will provide satisfactory internal fixation.

Subtrochanteric fractures should have a sufficiently longer fixation on the shaft than intertrochanteric fractures. There should be at least 3 to 4 screw holes below the lowest point of the subtrochanteric fracture (Fig. 47-46). An ex-

Fig. 47-45. Intertrochanteric hip fracture. *A.* AP x-ray postinjury. *B* and *C.* AP and lateral x-rays showing postoperative fracture position with a Jewett plate in satisfactory position.

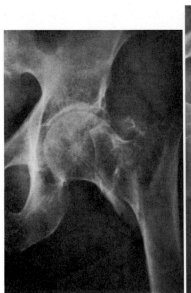
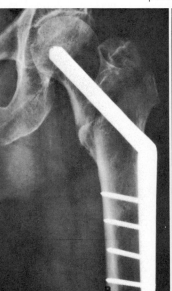
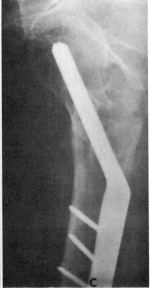

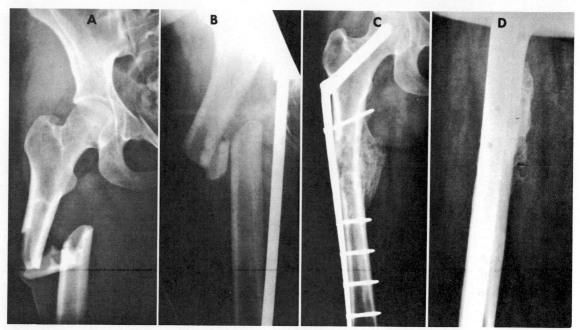

Fig. 47-46. Comminuted fracture of the femoral shaft incurred in automobile accident. *A* and *B*. AP and lateral x-ray before treatment. *C* and *D*. AP and lateral x-rays at 9 months showing union with a Jewett appliance in place.

cellent device for subtrochanteric fractures, especially in younger patients, is the Zickel nail.

The patient is placed in bed for 2 or 3 days and then mobilized from chair to non-weight-bearing crutch walking. Four months is the average time for union. Weight bearing should not be allowed until union has occurred.

Postoperative care should include attention to proper hydration and pulmonary hygiene. Prophylactic anticoagulation or dextran (which have been shown to prevent embolic complication) is indicated. The medical aspects of the patient's condition are a challenge to the surgeon and are at least as important as the technique and insertion of internal fixation devices.

Fractures of the Femoral Shaft

Femoral shaft fractures occur at any age, from severe violence, but injuries in children may occur from less severe indirect torsional stress applied to the leg. When major trauma is involved, associated injuries of the chest, head, and abdomen are common and should be the first consideration. When a patient with a fractured femur is in shock, other injuries requiring immediate attention should be suspected, although hemorrhage into a thigh may produce severe hypotension.

CLINICAL MANIFESTATIONS. Patients with a fractured femoral shaft have severe pain with any attempt at motion of the extremity. There is usually rotational deformity, shortening of the affected leg, with prominent swelling of the thigh.

The most important immediate local consideration with fractures of the femoral shaft is whether there has been damage to the femoral or popliteal vessels. If the patient has good pedal pulses, with normal sensation and motor power in the foot, major arterial injury is unlikely. However, when signs of ischemia are present or cannot be ruled out, arteriography and/or exploration of the vessels are indicated. This may be a difficult judgment, and consultation with the most experienced surgeon should be obtained.

TREATMENT. Emergency treatment at the scene of the accident should include splinting the leg to the adjacent extremity or, optimally, traction applied to the foot over a Thomas splint. If the wound is compound and the bones are protruding, they should not be repositioned until proper debridement has been carried out.

Femoral shaft fractures in children are treated exclusively by closed methods. Internal fixation is contraindicated because of potential damage to the epiphyseal plate and growth disturbances of the femur. Anatomic reduction is not required (Fig. 47-47). With a displaced femoral shaft fracture in a child, 1 cm of overriding is acceptable as long as there are no more than a few degrees of angulation and rotational deformity has been completely corrected. The epiphyseal stimulation provided by the presence of healing callus will make up 1 cm of shortening. In the very young child, where a maximum of 2 lb can be used to reduce the fracture, Bryant's traction provides an effective means for reduction. However, the child's ability to dorsiflex his great toe should be repeatedly inspected to be certain that an anterior compartment syndrome or vascular compromise is not developing in either lower extremity. Russell's traction is used for older children. Repeat check x-rays are obtained at intervals to be certain that position and reduction are maintained. It is imperative that reduction be accomplished in a few days, because by 10 days most fractures in children are clinically firm. When the fracture is clinically stable and nontender and callus

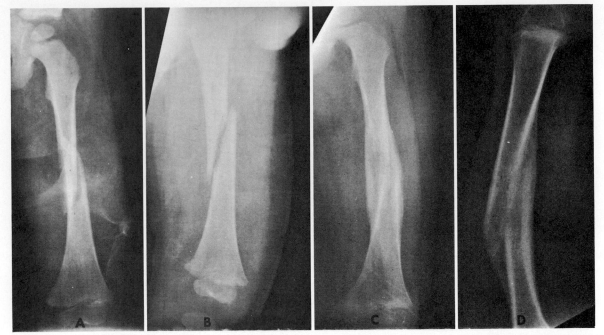

Fig. 47-47. Femoral shaft fracture in a child treated by traction. *A* and *B*. AP and lateral x-rays in satisfactory position in skin traction. *C* and *D*. AP and lateral x-rays of healed fracture showing satisfactory position. The anterior angulation at the fracture site will remodel itself.

is present by x-ray, the child is placed in a 1½ hip spica. Progressive weight bearing between crutches is started when bony union is solid.

Treatment of shaft fractures in adults may be accomplished by either closed methods or open reduction. Methods employing intramedullary fixation or plate reduction have been used, at times with disastrous results. If a shaft fracture is transverse or of a short oblique type without comminution and occurs at the narrowest portion of the medullary cavity, intramedullary fixation may be indicated provided the skin is normal and the patient is in optimal condition for operative intervention. Intramedullary fixation requiring an open reduction of the fracture site has a high incidence of wound sepsis (6 percent) and an increased incidence of delayed union. An infection at the site of an intramedullary nail means 3 to 4 years of treatment, stiff joints, and the possibility of chronic osteomyelitis.

Closed intramedullary nailing using the technique of Küntscher is superior to that in which the fracture site must be opened. Küntscher's technique relies upon reaming of the medullary cavity, allowing good fixation of both fracture fragments when the fracture site is not at the narrowest portion of the medullary canal. The incidence of infection with blind nailing is much less than with exposure of the fracture site. This may be nearly as safe as the treatment with skeletal traction. It is imperative that the operator be familiar with the technique and be equipped with a fracture table as well as an image intensifier for accomplishing the closed reduction and blind nailing.

Femoral shaft fractures, by virtue of the surrounding muscle mass, require skeletal traction to maintain length and alignment. Traction is applied to a threaded Steinmann pin placed across the supracondylar area or proximal tibia. When there is associated knee injury, it is best to insert the Steinmann pin through the supracondylar area and not to apply skeletal traction across the injured knee.

Technique of Insertion of the Steinmann Pin. The supracondylar region is prepared and draped under aseptic conditions. Local anesthesia is infiltrated to the skin and periosteum both medially and laterally, at a point just proximal to the femoral condyles. A threaded Steinmann pin is then drilled across the supracondylar region from medial to lateral, making certain that the pin is placed as far posterior as possible, to prevent crossing the suprapatellar pouch.

If the fracture is in the distal femoral shaft, the Steinmann pin is inserted from lateral to medial at the level of the tibial tubercle in order to prevent damage to the lateral popliteal nerve. The leg is placed in a balanced suspension apparatus with weight applied to the skeletal traction bow on the Steinmann pin. If conditions permit, the fracture is manipulated into position and held there with skeletal traction.

Repeat AP and lateral x-rays are obtained in traction, and skeletal traction is adjusted accordingly. When the fracture is stable and firm, i.e., with no tenderness at the fracture site, and shortening does not occur when traction is removed, the patient is ready for immobilization in a 1½ hip spica if the fracture is high at the junction of the upper and middle thirds. A cast brace is applied and weight-bearing treatment instituted if the fracture is in the middle or distal third of the femur.

Cast Brace Treatment (Fig. 47-48). Cast brace treatment for fractures of the midshaft and distal one-third of the femur treated initially with skeletal traction allows more rapid mobilization of the patient and results in more rapid union and better functional return of knee motion than with spica cast immobilization. It may be possible to mobilize some fractures in a cast brace as early as the first or second week postinjury.

Technique of Cast Brace Application. A well-molded total contact plaster cast is applied to the thigh. An elastic Spandex sock is placed over the thigh, over which one layer of webril is wrapped snugly about the thigh. Elastic plaster of paris is wrapped over these layers, following which standard plaster, which has greater strength, is applied. The proximal rim is fashioned with an adjustable plastic quadrilateral rim or constructed in standard fashion. An elastic bandage is applied about the knee, following which a well-molded short leg cast is applied with the ankle at 90° and the foot in neutral position. When both plasters have dried, a single axis or polycentric knee joint hinges are applied medially and laterally connecting the two plasters with the knee hinge.

The patient is instructed in quadriceps exercises and knee range-of-motion exercises in the cast brace. He is allowed to bear increasing weight on the fractured extremity between crutches as tolerated. The brace is changed if it loosens and is discontinued when the patient can bear full weight painlessly without crutches, usually an additional 6 to 8 weeks from the time of its application. Mooney et al. have reported the mean healing time of $14\frac{1}{2}$ weeks for fractures in the distal femur treated with skeletal traction and the cast brace technique.

Delayed union when the cast brace technique is used is uncommon. However, if it occurs, it requires a reinforcing bone graft of circumferential iliac autogenous cancellous bone strips tied in place with catgut as indicated. In some instances it may be necessary to use internal plate fixation or intramedullary rod fixation in addition to autogenous iliac bone graft. Restriction of knee motion with the method of cast brace mobilization is uncommon but may occur when a $1\frac{1}{2}$ hip spica is applied.

Supracondylar Fractures

Supracondylar fractures of the femur and Y or T intracondylar fractures occur in all age groups from trauma occurring in automobile accidents, pedestrian injuries, falls, and various other accidents. Patients with this injury present with the usual signs of fracture, i.e., local swelling, instability, deformity. In some cases, the patient will appear to have only a knee effusion. Supracondylar fractures are intraarticular fractures, since they communicate with the suprapatellar pouch of the knee. Scarring in this region may obliterate the suprapatellar pouch and interfere with knee motion.

The supracondylar fragment is angulated posteriorly from the pull on the gastrocnemius muscle, attached to the posterior aspect of the femoral condyles. The pull of the quadriceps and hamstrings acts to increase shortening and the posterior angulation. The supracondylar fragment may have a valgus deformity produced by the strong pull of the adductors on the proximal femoral fragment. In T

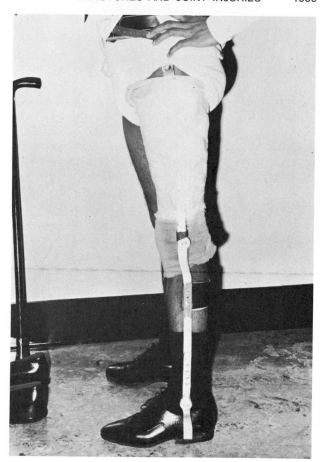

Fig. 47-48. Ischial weight-bearing brace, quadrilateral plaster thigh socket for fractured femur.

or Y condylar fractures, the proximal fragment tends to be wedged between the condylar fragments by the existing muscle pull.

TREATMENT. Results of treatment of fractures in this region have been discouraging. With optimal treatment, a third of patients have significant restriction of knee motion. In attempting to overcome the poor results, open reduction and internal fixation have been tried, but the results are still inferior to conservative traction treatment.

A Steinmann pin is inserted through the tibial tubercle, and through this skeletal traction is applied. If persistent posterior angulation at the fracture site occurs, a trans-supracondylar Steinmann pin is inserted and 3 to 5 lb of additional traction applied at right angles to the shaft of the femur. Reduction is monitored by check x-rays.

Quadriceps exercises are begun at 10 days and are continued in the traction apparatus until clinical stability is attained, at approximately 6 weeks. The cast brace technique of Mooney may be used when the fracture is stable.

TRAUMATIC EPIPHYSEAL SEPARATION OF THE DISTAL FEMUR

This injury occurs from forced hyperextension of the knee, in the adolescent child. Treatment should be immediate closed reduction and plaster immobilization. Open reduction of this injury is indicated only when the fracture is causing circulatory embarrassment.

Ligamentous Injuries of the Knee Joint

Injuries to the ligamentous supporting structures of the knee occur in all types of athletic endeavors but are especially common in sports utilizing cleats where the foot becomes fixed to the ground and direct or indirect force is applied to the knee joint. A similar mechanism occurs in skiing, where the long lever arm of the ski applies torque or stress to the knee joint, resulting in ligamentous damage. It must be emphasized that determination of ligamentous damage is dependent upon clinical examination and that routine x-rays add little information.

MEDIAL COLLATERAL LIGAMENT

The medial collateral ligament consists of a superficial portion which originates from the medial femoral epicondyle proximally and is attached distally a handbreadth below the knee joint on the medial aspect of the tibia beneath the pes anserinus. In addition to the medial collateral ligament are capsular ligaments which form a half-sleeve medially extending from the popliteal space behind to the patellar tendon in front. The anterior portion is represented by the anterior knee capsule with a contri-

Fig. 47-49. Knee ligament injuries from valgus force. Anterior cruciate is interrupted near its femoral origin. Medial collateral may avulse at the upper and lower ends of rupture in the middle as well as be disrupted from its meniscal attachment. (*After O'Donoghue.*)

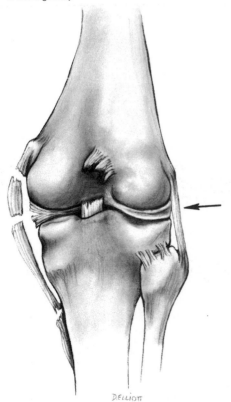

DElliott

bution from the vastus medialis retinaculum. The anterior capsular ligament is tight when the knee is flexed and relaxes as the knee is extended. The middle portion of the capsular ligament is also referred to as the deep layer of the medial ligament or the short internal lateral ligament. The upper part of the middle portion of the capsular ligament is attached to the medial femoral condyle slightly forward of the superficial tibial collateral ligament and is fixed to the middle third of the medial meniscus (the meniscal femoral ligament). The lower portion continues distally from the meniscus and is attached to the tibia just below the articular margin (the meniscal tibial ligament). The middle one-third is taut in all positions of flexion. The posterior part of the medial capsular ligament is a portion of the posterior capsule. When the knee is extended, the posterior ligament tightens; it slackens as the knee is flexed.

With increasing valgus stress to the knee and usually with simultaneous external rotation of the tibia upon the femur, medial capsular ligaments rupture, followed by rupture of the tibial collateral ligament. If the force continues, rupture of the anterior cruciate may occur (Fig. 47-49).

CLINICAL MANIFESTATIONS. With an acute injury to the medial ligamentous structures, symptoms and findings will vary according to the degree of damage. With a mild sprain without complete disruption of any of the components, the patient may only complain of pain and have a mild hemarthrosis. Occasionally, there is no hemarthrosis as the bleeding is external to the capsule. If clinical examination of the knee does not reveal instability or increased motion as compared with the opposite knee, the injury can be treated as a sprain with temporary immobilization and restriction of activity. When the force results in complete disruption of the ligaments, the findings are usually obvious, and there is no difficulty in deciding upon the need for surgical repair.

The real difficulty lies in moderate degrees of instability on clinical examination. If there is any doubt as to the integrity of the ligaments on clinical examination, the examination should be repeated under anesthesia and surgical exploration carried out as necessary. The uninjured knee is examined first and all examinations repeated on the injured side and compared with the normal.

The knee joint is flexed 20° to relax the posterior capsule, and valgus stress is applied to the knee. Opening up of the medial joint space is abnormal and indicates ligamentous discontinuity. The knee is then flexed to 90° and AP stability tested by pulling the tibia forward on the femur. This is carried out with the tibia in internal rotation, external rotation, and neutral rotation. Motion of the medial tibial condyle greater than 5 mm is abnormal and is a sign of rotational instability with damage to the medial capsular ligament. Forward motion of both condyles is an indication of anterior cruciate damage. When varus stress applied to the knee in 20° of flexion causes greater opening up of the lateral joint than the normal, it indicates lateral collateral and iliotibial band disruption. Valgus and varus testing is carried out on the extended knee to determine the integrity of the posterior capsule. Instability in this position indicates posterior capsule damage in addition to medial or lateral collateral ligament injury.

ANTERIOR CRUCIATE LIGAMENT RUPTURE

The anterior cruciate ligament may be ruptured in association with complete tears of the medial collateral ligaments. Isolated tears occur as the result of hyperextension or internal rotation of the tibia on the femur but may be due to a direct blow on a flexed knee. Determination of anterior cruciate rupture depends upon demonstrating forward displacement of both tibial condyles on the femur usually of more than 5 mm when compared with the opposite uninjured knee. This test is best carried out with the knee in near-extension. Interpretation of the findings is subjective, and great experience is necessary in this examination.

TREATMENT OF MEDIAL COLLATERAL AND CRUCIATE LIGAMENT INJURIES. Mild sprains of the medial collateral ligament when there is no evidence of instability are treated symptomatically. A tense hemarthrosis may be aspirated with considerable relief. The limb is splinted in a position of extension with a compression bandage or a posterior plaster splint. The patient is started on immediate isometric quadriceps exercises performed hourly. He may bear partial weight between crutches with the quadriceps set and the knee in full extension. It is helpful to reevaluate the knee in a few days in order to confirm the findings of stability.

Complete tears of the medial collateral ligaments, medial capsular ligaments, or anterior cruciate require surgical repair. This should be carried out as soon as possible but certainly within 2 weeks. A detached ligament may be retracted from its attachment with resultant healing in a lengthened or lax position. At the present time, there is no way to determine this without surgical exploration.

Operative Technique. The knee is exposed through an incision overlying the medial collateral ligament. When the subcutaneous tissue is entered, the site of ligamentous rupture will be marked by localized ecchymosis if surgical treatment is carried out within 24 hours of the time of injury. After ligamentous damage has been assessed, the knee joint is entered through a separate peripatellar incision in the capsule, and the anterior cruciate and menisci are evaluated. If the meniscus is torn, it is excised. Ruptures of the anterior cruciate ligament occurring in its substance are irreparable, and its remaining portion should be excised with attention then directed to an accurate repair of the medial ligamentous structures. If the anterior cruciate is pulled from its bony attachment, it is reattached with silk sutures passing through the substance of the femoral condyle or tibial condyle.

The medial collateral ligament is reattached to bone with silk sutures passed through drill holes in bone, and ruptures in the substance are repaired with silk approximating the torn ends. Postoperatively, the leg is immobilized in a long leg plaster cast from toes to groin with the ankle at neutral position and the knee in 40° flexion and maximal internal rotation. The cast is changed if there is sufficient loosening. Plaster immobilization is continued 6 to 8 weeks. The knee is mobilized gradually, with active motion strengthening both quadriceps and hamstrings. Protection against weight bearing is continued until full extension is possible and power of the quadriceps is near normal.

INJURIES TO THE LATERAL COLLATERAL LIGAMENT

The lateral collateral ligament is interrupted when a varus force is applied to the knee. The lateral popliteal nerve, by virtue of its location and fixation as it winds around the neck of the fibula, is commonly stretched by the same injury. The treatment of this acute injury requires open exploration repair of the avulsed ligament from the femoral condyle or head of the fibula. The iliotibial band crossing the knee joint is commonly ruptured and requires repair. The nerve should be examined at the time of surgical treatment, but since this is usually a stretch injury, delayed repair depending upon follow-up evaluation is necessary. Injuries to the posterior cruciate ligament occur rarely as isolated injury but may accompany medial lateral collateral ligamentous injuries. Repair of the posterior cruciate is similar to the repair of the anterior cruciate, i.e., by utilizing drill holes through the femur or tibia.

CHRONIC LIGAMENTOUS INJURIES TO THE KNEE

Persistent laxity of the collateral ligamentous structures or cruciate ligaments results in knee joint instability. Such injuries, if severe, are disabling and may require the competitive athlete to discontinue competition. With minor degrees of instability, symptoms may be apparent only with vigorous athletics. When severe, the knee may be chronically effused, painful, and unstable with normal activity. Patients give a history of pain, locking, sudden giving way, or feeling of instability.

Reconstruction of the chronically unstable knee is difficult and is not always successful in returning a patient to athletics. Reefing the posterior medial capsule, shortening the medial collateral structures, and pes anserinus transfer are of value for medial collateral instability. Similar procedures are available for the lateral side. It is occasionally difficult to separate medial from lateral instability in the chronically unstable knee, in which case stress x-rays should be obtained.

INJURIES OF KNEE MENISCI

The tibia rotates laterally upon the femur as the knee joint goes from flexion to extension, and medial with the opposite motion. If this simultaneous rotation is interfered with or forcibly reversed, the semilunar cartilage may be injured. A common injury occurs when the football player catches his cleated shoe while weight is applied to the flexed knee. Similarly, a person squatting with the knees fully flexed and suddenly twisting his knee without simultaneous movement into extension will suffer an acute meniscus tear. Helfet believes that only the fibrotic medial meniscus of the elderly is actually torn by pressure grinding between the femoral and tibial surfaces.

In the young adult, rotation without flexion or extension causes the cartilage to straighten out. If the force is excessive, the cartilage is unable to accommodate, and a tear occurs at its inner free border, usually about the midpoint.

The cartilage may be detached from its attachment to the anterior cruciate or be split longitudinally to produce a bucket-handle tear, or it may be injured in its posterior portion by detachment from its posterior capsular attachments (Fig. 47-50). The medial meniscus is injured at least nine times as commonly as the lateral in the Caucasian, although lateral meniscal tears are more common in the Oriental. The medial meniscus is fixed to the capsule and is relatively immobile, whereas the lateral meniscus is not fixed to the capsule and has the popliteus muscle to assist in controlling its position.

CLINICAL MANIFESTATIONS. Meniscal injuries are commonly found in the young male individual who is using his knee vigorously, either for athletics or vocationally. Such injuries are less common in women.

The injury causes acute pain, which may subside rapidly. If the cartilage is undisplaced, there may be no immediate interference with motion. A joint effusion, with associated discomfort and stiffness, gradually develops in response to the injury. This will occur sooner and more severely if the meniscal damage is at its peripheral attachment, where blood vessels may be interrupted.

The diagnosis of a torn meniscus will depend on an accurate history, which should include the position of the knee and the direction of the rotational force at the time of the injury. The patient should be questioned about locking, instability, episodes of giving way or buckling, and previous injuries to the knee.

Examination of the knee after an acute injury may reveal varying degrees of joint effusion. There is local tenderness over the meniscus, which is greatest at the site of injury. Stability of the knee ligaments should be examined by valgus, varus, and anteroposterior stress.

The knee motion is examined with special emphasis on testing for synchronous rotation as the knee goes into full extension. By grasping both heels, both knees are passively brought to full extension and any limitation determined. Normally, the tibial tubercle in full extension aligns with

Fig. 47-50. Types of meniscal injuries. Top left, complete bucket-handle tear; top right, complete detachment of the meniscus from its peripheral margin; lower left, posterior tab tear; lower right, anterior tab tear of the medial meniscus.

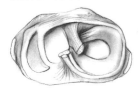
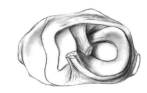
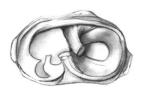
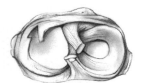

the lateral border of the patella. If rotation has been compromised, the tibial tubercle will align with the central axis of the patella. In carrying out extension motions, there is localization of pain to medial or lateral aspects of the joint, at the site of the injury to the meniscus. Palpation of the joint line may indicate displacement of the meniscus. The test described by McMurray to delineate meniscal tears is occasionally helpful. The maneuver is elicited by passively flexing hip and knee of the supine patient. The foot is gradually externally rotated, while abduction stress is applied to the knee as it is gradually brought into extension. A displaced portion of the medial meniscus, catching between the femur and tibia, will cause a definite click and pain.

The diagnosis of acute meniscus injury may be difficult. Unless there is definite evidence of locking or displacement of the meniscus, the patient should be treated conservatively and reevaluated when the acute symptoms subside. Knee effusion, if severe, is aspirated, and the knee is brought to maximal extension and immobilized in a splint or compression bandage. The patient is allowed to bear weight between crutches with his quadriceps taut. The patient is reevaluated at weekly intervals and meniscectomy carried out only when the diagnosis is certain.

Arthrography is extremely helpful when the diagnosis is not absolutely certain. It is also of value in ruling out damage to the opposite meniscus. The technique of arthrography is demanding and requires exact positioning of the knee at the time of x-ray and experience in interpreting the arthrograms. The technique of Fryberger involves injection of air and absorbable contrast media into the joint. The x-ray beam is centered on the meniscus, and x-rays are taken in various positions of rotation for both medial and lateral menisci. The technique of arthroscopy increases the accuracy of the diagnosis when it is questionable. Even in patients with locked knees, when arthrotomy cannot be avoided, arthroscopy will delineate pathologic change in the other meniscus.

TREATMENT. When the diagnosis is established, meniscectomy is indicated to prevent the further cartilage and ligamentous damage associated with displaced menisci.

Technique. If injury to the patella is suspected, meniscectomy should be carried out through a median parapatellar incision, so that better exposure of the patella can be obtained. If the diagnosis can be localized to the meniscus, a transverse incision is used. A transverse incision is made parallel to, and immediately above, the medial meniscus between the patellar ligament and the anterior border of the medial collateral ligament. The anterior capsule is split vertically above the meniscus, and the joint is inspected through this incision.

The anterior horn of the meniscus is detached from its attachment to the cruciate and upper tibial plateau and the peripheral edge incised by sharp dissection as far posteriorly as possible. The interval of dissection is in the most peripheral portion of the meniscus and not between the capsule and meniscus, which would cause hemorrhage. By externally rotating the tibia on the femur, it is possible to view the posterior attachment of the meniscus. However, in some instances, it may be necessary to make a second vertical incision posterior to the medial collateral ligament in order to define the posterior third attachment. When the meniscus has been detached peripherally, it is displaced into the intracondylar notch, and the posterior attachment to the tibial surface is divided under direct vision. The wound is closed in routine fashion.

Postoperatively, the leg is immobilized in a position of full extension and the patient started on hourly quadriceps exercises. He is allowed out of bed when he can control his leg without pain and can bear partial weight between crutches with his quadriceps taut. Gradual knee flexion is started between 2 and 3 weeks, and the patient should be back to full activity in 6 weeks.

Injuries to the lateral meniscus are much less common and are handled in similar fashion. Discoid meniscus and cysts of the lateral meniscus also require meniscectomy.

Fractures of the Patella

Patellar fractures are usually due to direct trauma to the patella but also occur with sudden forced flexion of an actively contracting quadriceps. Fractures are more commonly transverse or comminuted but may take any direction. As the patella is an integral part of the extensor mechanism, separation at the fracture site is an indication that the adjacent patellar retinacula have been interrupted and active extension will not be possible (Fig. 47-51). Treatment is aimed at restoring a smoothly gliding extensor mechanism.

TREATMENT. Undisplaced fractures require a plaster cylinder cast for 6 to 8 weeks to prevent separation of the fragments. Check x-rays in plaster should be obtained at 7 to 10 days to be certain that displacement has not occurred. The patient is instructed in quadriceps exercises and may bear partial weight between crutches.

Transverse fractures with separation of the fragments require operative intervention to restore continuity of the extensor mechanism. Although some surgeons advocate circumferential wire suture to hold the fragments together, there is usually enough comminution in the region of the subchondral surface of the patella that an irregular articular surface of the patella will remain. For this reason, excision of the smaller fragments, usually the lower half, is indicated, combined with reattachment of the patellar ligament through drill holes on the raw fracture surface of the proximal fragment. At the same time, the patellar retinaculum is surgically repaired.

For grossly comminuted fractures of the patella, immediate excision of all fragments is carried out and the quadriceps mechanism repaired. Postoperatively, the limb is maintained in extension, and quadriceps exercises are immediately instituted. At 4 weeks, the cast is removed and beginning range-of-motion exercises started. At 6 weeks, active flexion is begun.

The same principles apply to open fractures of the patella.

The quadriceps may be ruptured or the patellar ligament avulsed from its insertion on the patella when acute flexion

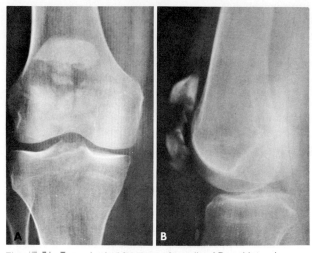

Fig. 47-51. Comminuted fracture of patella. AP and lateral x-rays showing comminuted patella with separation of the upper and lower major fragments indicating interruption of the extensor mechanism.

forces are applied to the contracting extensor mechanism. Immediate diagnosis and surgical repair are required.

Recurrent Dislocation of the Patella

The patella may be dislocated in any direction. Upward dislocation is the result of rupture of the patellar ligament. Medial dislocation is uncommon but may occur from severe injury or, rarely, after poliomyelitis. Lateral dislocation is the most common type. This may occur with severe injury or poliomyelitis but is most commonly seen in young women or girls after minor trauma. It is related to the increased valgus angle of the female knee but may also be the result of hypoplastic development of the external condyle of the femur, congenital abnormalities of the patella, or congenital contractures of the vastus intermedius.

The patient complains of the knee's giving way as the patella momentarily slips laterally over the lateral femoral condyle and spontaneously reduces. In more severe cases the patella may become lodged lateral to the femoral condyle, requiring manipulative reduction. Following spontaneous relocation of the patella, the patient has symptoms of mild synovitis and effusion.

Treatment for the acutely dislocated patella is manual reduction followed by immobilization of the knee in full extension in plaster and rehabilitation of quadriceps muscle power. It is necessary to treat the initial dislocation by plaster immobilization of the knee, or the medial patellar retinaculum will heal with capsular laxity, allowing subsequent dislocation. By maintaining the tone of the vastus medialis, there may be sufficient muscle power to prevent subsequent dislocation. With recurrent dislocations, surgical treatment is usually necessary. Before epiphyseal closure, the Roux-Goldthwait operation may be done. This consists of transposing the lateral half of the patellar ligament at its insertion medially beneath the undisturbed medial insertion. At the same time, an ellipse of capsule and medial patella retinaculum is excised and the capsule reefed to hold the patella medially. After the age of fourteen, the Hauser procedure, a medial transposition of a block of bone encompassing the attachment of the patellar ligament, is utilized. With recurrent dislocation the progression of chondromalacia to severe damage to the undersurface of the patella may necessitate patellectomy and quadricepsplasty.

Fractures of the Tibial Plateau

Fractures of the tibial plateau occur at any age but are more common in the middle-aged or elderly. Fractures of the lateral tibial plateau occur when there is a sudden valgus stress to the knee joint, when there is an axial load applied to the femoral shaft. Common causes involve an automobile bumper striking the knee joint of a pedestrian or a worker falling from a scaffolding. The medial collateral ligament may be ruptured, concomitantly.

Types of fractures are (1) a simple split fracture of the lateral tibial plateau, (2) severe comminution of the lateral tibial plateau, and (3) fractures of both condyles with a vertical fracture line into the region of the tibial spines.

TREATMENT. If the medial collateral ligament is ruptured, surgical repair is indicated. If there is severe displacement of the lateral tibial plateau, open reduction in an attempt at elevation of the depression may be required.

However, most fractures can be handled with best results by the method of Weissman and Harold. Large hemarthroses are aspirated. The knee is splinted in extension for 1 week during which time hourly quadriceps and straight-leg-raising exercises are instituted. When normal quadriceps muscle power has been regained, flexion exercises are

started; a posterior splint is reapplied between exercises. The splint is gradually discontinued as power and motion improve. Partial weight bearing is permitted between 4 and 6 weeks, and full weight bearing at about 8 to 10 weeks. Despite the apparent severity of these fractures as seen by x-ray, good results usually can be obtained.

Tibial Shaft Fractures

Fractures of the tibial shaft occur from direct trauma and may occur when an automobile passenger strikes his leg against the dashboard or when the leg of a pedestrian is struck by a car bumper (Fig. 47-52). Fractures also may occur by indirect torsional forces as with sports injuries, such as in skiing. In falling, the skier applies torsional force to the shaft of the tibia, via the long lever of the attached ski. Some fractures of the tibia occur from simple falls.

Tibial shaft fractures occur at any age. About 70 percent of such fractures are closed and 30 percent open. Indirect torsional forces cause oblique or spiral fractures, whereas direct trauma may result in transverse, segmental, or comminuted fractures of the tibial shaft. There is no difference in the rate of healing of tibial shaft fractures according to the location of the fracture or the plane of the fracture surface. Rate of healing is correlated with the severity of trauma. Fractures caused by high-energy trauma from automobile accidents with or without open wounds have the longest rate of healing. The presence of an intact fibula results in a more rapid rate of union.

CLINICAL MANIFESTATIONS. Undisplaced fractures may

Fig. 47-52. Fracture of the proximal tibia shaft with fracture of the neck of the fibula incurred by an automobile bumper's striking a pedestrian. *A* and *B*. AP and lateral x-rays postinjury. *C* and *D*. AP and lateral x-rays showing postreduction position in a long leg cast.

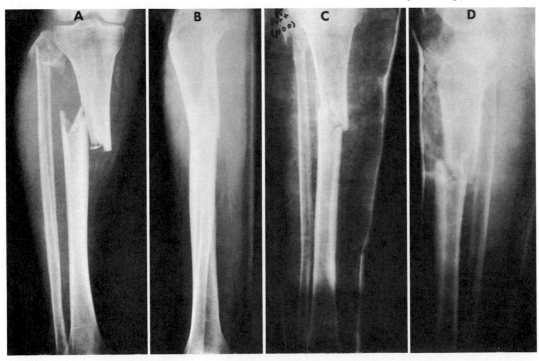

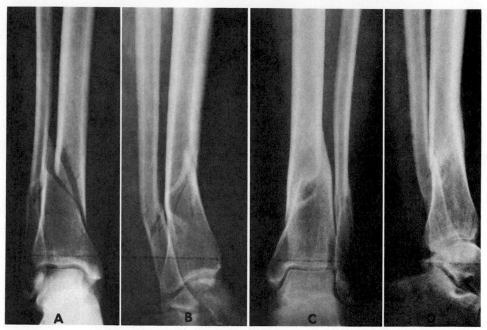

Fig. 47-53. Fracture of the distal tibia and fibula shafts. *A* and *B*. AP and lateral x-rays postinjury. *C* and *D*. AP and lateral x-rays showing healed fracture in satisfactory position.

have only tenderness and swelling at the site of fracture, but patients are unable to put weight on the affected extremity. Undisplaced spiral fractures occur in the very young. Such fractures may be quite stable, and diagnosis is suggested by the fact that the child will not use the affected leg.

Displaced fractures result in deformity with swelling and ecchymosis. Anteroposterior and lateral x-rays will characterize the fracture.

TREATMENT. Closed tibial shaft fractures are best handled by closed conservative measures (Fig. 47-53). Dehne et al. and Sarmiento, using plaster methods and allowing early weight bearing, have achieved rapid union with no infection and a low incidence of delayed union.

Technique of Closed Reduction

With the patient under analgesia or local anesthesia to the fracture site and lying supine with both legs flexed at the knees, hanging over the end of the table, most tibial shaft fractures can be realigned and deformity corrected by gentle manipulation. The opposite leg is used as a guide to determine correction of rotation and deformity.

Over one layer of stockinet and one layer of sheet wadding, a well-molded plaster cast is applied to the knee with the foot in 10 to 15° of plantar flexion or, if possible, at a right angle. When the plaster has hardened, the knee is brought to full extension and the plaster extended to include the thigh. The reduction is checked by AP and lateral x-rays. The patient is hospitalized with the leg elevated and ice applied over the region of the fracture site. Circulation to the foot and the patient's ability to dorsiflex and plantar flex toes comfortably is checked every 2 hours to be certain that vascular insufficiency or com-

partment syndromes are not occurring. If necessary, the cast is split to relieve swelling.

When the patient is comfortable and can actively control the affected extremity, he is allowed up on crutches to bear as much weight as pain tolerates. The patient may continue in the long leg cast until union is complete, or at 3 weeks the plaster may be changed to a below-knee cast appropriately molded about the tibial condyles and patellar ligament to control rotation, as described by Sarmiento.

Any type of fracture including transverse, comminuted, or oblique spiral fractures may be treated in this fashion. Approximately a ½-cm shortening can be anticipated from the weight-bearing treatment in addition to whatever shortening is present at the time of the closed reduction. If this seems unacceptable, pins may be placed above and below the fracture site to control length and weight bearing not allowed. The weight-bearing method of treating tibial shaft fractures is clearly the best method available with the lowest incidence of complication. The average time until plaster removal is about 13 weeks.

Management of Compound Fractures. Compound fractures must be immediately debrided and fractures immobilized. Depending upon the kind of wound and adequacy of debridement, the skin may be closed, but the indications for this are extremely rare. Secondary closure of the wound may be carried out or the wound left open to granulate beneath a weight-bearing plaster cast as described by Brown and Urban. The use of internal fixation in open fractures is not justified because of the hazard of infection, skin loss, and nonunion.

Administration of antibiotics is continued until the wound is healed and followed with appropriate check x-rays during the first month to make certain that position is being maintained. Cast wedging or remanipulation may be required to restore alignment.

Compartment Syndromes

After fractures, soft tissue injury, prolonged limb compression (as in drug-overdosed patients), and arterial operations, progressive muscle ischemia may occur in any of the fascial compartments of the limbs. In the upper extremity this includes the anterior compartments of the forearm, and in the lower extremity the four anterior and posterior compartments. The mechanism involved is unrelieved swelling in the tight osseofascial compartments. The arteries may continue to pulsate while the ischemia is developing, since the latter occurs when the capillary filling pressure is exceeded. Hence the clinical signs depend upon detection of change in muscle function, i.e., loss of motor power or extreme pain with passive stretch. Patients should also be observed for ischemic pain (severe pain at rest) or pain not responding to analgesics. Distal pulses of the extremity are usually present early in the course and may persist until complete and irreversible necrosis has occurred.

Prevention of sequelae depends upon early recognition and surgical decompression of the individual compartments. Compartment pressures can be determined by direct measurement, as with the Wick catheter, but when in doubt surgical exploration (and decompression) is indicated. It is important to consider the possibility that compartment syndromes may develop after open fractures or during elective tibial osteotomies. In those instances compartments should be decompressed prophylactically.

Ankle Injuries

ANATOMY. Motion of the tibiotalar joint is pure flexion and extension. Inversion and eversion of the foot is accomplished at the subtalar and midtarsal joints. The upper surface of the talus is dome-shaped in the anteroposterior plane, with a narrower articular surface, posteriorly. The talus is without muscular origin or insertion and is attached to its related articulations by capsule and ligaments. The ankle mortise is formed by the downward medial and lateral projections of malleoli grasping the dome of the talus. Maintenance of the normal mortise is a prerequisite for painless ankle motion. Stability of the talus in the mortise is dependent on the distal tibiofibular ligaments and interosseous membrane, as well as the anterior and posterior talofibular ligaments, calcaneofibular ligaments laterally, and a strong deltoid ligament medially.

MECHANISMS OF INJURY. Ankle injuries are caused by a sudden application of force which exceeds the strength of the ligaments or malleoli. Applied across the ankle joint, the force rotates the foot into inversion-eversion, or adduction-abduction in relation to the tibia, or rotates the tibia similarly in relation to the fixed foot. Athletic injuries account for a large proportion of ankle injuries, although a simple fall or sudden misstep may be sufficient to cause a severe fracture-dislocation. All combinations of ligamentous injuries and fractures are possible, depending upon the severity and direction of force.

The injured ankle should be carefully examined for the location of tenderness, swelling, and deformity. If the patient was able to walk on the ankle immediately after the injury, this indicates stability but does not rule out undisplaced fracture. Caution should be applied in diagnosing injuries on the football field before all signs have had time to develop.

The ankle should be splinted with an air splint or with a pillow splint until x-ray examination is complete. Three x-ray views are necessary for x-ray evaluation of the ankle joint. Standard AP and lateral x-rays are required and, in addition, a 30° medial oblique view to determine the competence of the mortise.

LIGAMENTOUS INJURIES

The most common ankle injury which involves portions of the lateral collateral ligaments is caused by a sudden inversion force applied to the foot. The anterior talofibular ligament is usually involved. On examination, there is local tenderness and ecchymosis at the midpoint or attachments of the anterior talofibular ligament or calcaneofibular or posterior talofibular ligaments.

If the patient has minimal swelling and tenderness on examination, can walk with minimal discomfort, and x-rays are normal, it is sufficient to treat the injury as a sprain by adhesive strapping for 2 to 4 weeks. Tenderness on the medial side of the joint immediately after the injury is an indication of sufficient lateral damage to allow subluxation to produce stretch or injury to the deltoid ligament. If there has been complete division of any component of the lateral collateral ligament, stress films are indicated, for which the ankle is anesthetized under local or general anesthesia and the foot brought into maximal inversion. X-rays taken with the foot in this position will reveal tilting of the talus in the mortise, if there is discontinuity of any portion of the lateral collateral ligaments. If a talar tilt is present, immobilization in a short leg plaster with the foot in neutral position and the ankle at a 90° angle is required for 6 weeks. Plaster immobilization may be elected in the absence of stress films. With any ankle injury requiring plaster, it is necessary to obtain check films immediately after reduction and also at 10 to 14 days to ensure maintenance of position. If patients continue to have instability after conservative treatment, secondary open repair of the involved lateral ligaments can be performed.

Distal Tibiofibular Diastasis

With eversion injuries to the ankle, there may be interruption of the ligamentous continuity of the distal tibiofibular joint, resulting in a diastasis of the ankle mortise. The patient's ankle is unable to bear weight, and marked swelling occurs in the region of the tibiofibular joint.

It is rarely possible to maintain reduction without operative intervention. A 1½-in. vertical incision is made over the distal fibula and the periosteum elevated from the fibula, proximal to the level of the tibiotalar articulation. A lag screw is inserted across an overdrilled hole in the fibula to close the diastasis. This is accomplished with the ankle at 90° and not with the foot in plantar flexion. When the foot is in plantar flexion, the narrowest portion of the talus is in contact with the tibia, and permanent limitation

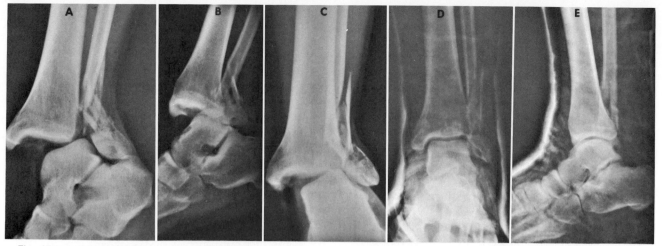

Fig. 47-54. Compound fracture-dislocation of the ankle. *A, B,* and *C.* AP, lateral, and oblique x-rays postinjury showing comminuted fracture of the distal fibula and posterior dislocation of the ankle. The deltoid ligament was avulsed from the medial malleolus, which protruded through the skin. *D* and *E.* AP and lateral x-rays following debridement and closed reduction.

of dorsiflexion will result. At 8 weeks, the cast is removed and the screw excised at a second operation.

FRACTURES AND DISLOCATIONS (Fig. 47-54)

Undisplaced fractures of malleoli require immobilization in plaster for 8 weeks. The most common isolated malleolar fracture is an oblique fracture of the lateral malleolus caused by an external rotation injury. If the ankle mortise is not involved, a well-molded plaster cast is applied with the foot in neutral varus-valgus position and maintained for 6 weeks. Check x-rays are obtained to be certain that reduction has not been lost. If there is a fracture of the lateral malleolus with lateral displacement of the talus, this is corrected by manipulation under local or general anesthesia and the hind part of the foot placed in maximal inversion with the ankle at 90° of dorsiflexion.

Medial Malleolar Fractures

Undisplaced fractures of the medial malleolus with an intact mortise are treated by plaster immobilization. Bimalleolar ankle fractures with dislocation require accurate reduction until union is solid. The usual mechanism of injury of a bimalleolar fracture is by external rotation and eversion. If the talus is displaced laterally, reduction is necessary. Most fractures can be handled by closed reduction.

Technique of Closed Reduction. With local or general anesthesia and the leg hanging over the end of the table, traction is applied to the hind part of the foot in the long axis of the leg. With traction maintained, the hind part of the foot is gradually brought into inversion, to correct the lateral displacement, while lateral countertraction is applied to the medial subcutaneous surface of the tibia. Simultaneously, the foot, which is resting on the knee of the operator, is brought into 90° of dorsiflexion. The reduction should be stable when the foot is held at 90° of

dorsiflexion at maximal inversion. A well-molded cast is applied over one thickness of stockinet and one thickness of sheet wadding. The cast is then extended to include the knee. Check x-rays are obtained and the patient admitted to the hospital for evaluation of circulation. If the medial malleolus fracture extends to the point where the vertical and horizontal articular cartilage meet at the distal end of the tibia, sufficient medial buttress will not be present to hold a closed reduction, and open reduction will be required.

Technique of Open Reduction. A 2-in. vertical incision is centered over the medial malleolus. The fracture site is exposed, and the medial malleolar fragment retracted distad by hinging it upon its deltoid attachment, thus exposing the joint. Intraarticular fragments are removed. Soft tissue dissection, for inspection of the joint, is minimized. The fragment is reduced anatomically, held with a towel clip, and fixed with a 2-in. standard bone screw. Using a reconstituted medial malleolar buttress, closed reduction is carried out and the foot held in maximal inversion. X-rays are obtained to determine reduction, and a well-molded long leg cast is applied with the knee at 20° of flexion, the ankle at 90° of dorsiflexion, and the foot in maximal inversion. Plaster immobilization is continued for 8 weeks, and weight bearing is not allowed before 12 weeks.

Posterior Malleolar Fractures

The posterior malleolus is usually fractured in combination with medial or lateral malleolar fractures. The importance of the posterior malleolus is to maintain anteroposterior stability of the ankle joint. When 30 percent of the tibial articular surface is involved in the posterior malleolar fracture, instability will ensue if anatomic reduction is not obtained.

Anatomic reduction of a large posterior malleolar fragment can be maintained only with internal fixation. The posterior malleolar fragment is exposed through a posteromedial or posterolateral incision and fixed with a screw to the major tibial fragment. Trimalleolar fractures with small posterior fragments and good anteroposterior stabil-

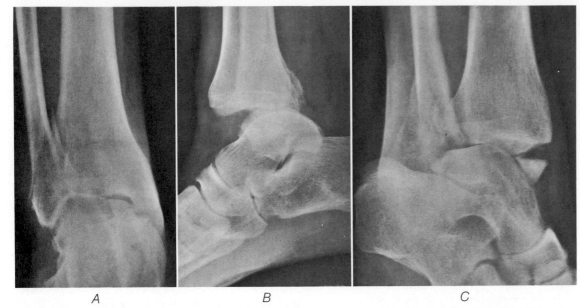

A	*B*	*C*

Fig. 47-55. Trimalleolar ankle fracture-dislocation. AP, lateral, and oblique x-rays showing posterior dislocation of the talus and fractures of the medial malleolus, the lateral malleolus, and a small fragment from the posterior malleolus.

ity require maintenance of reduction of the mortise, and the posterior fragment can be disregarded (Fig. 47-55).

Fractures involving the anterior articular surface occur from severe trauma, as in falls from heights and in automobile injuries. The anterior portion of the distal tibial articular surface may be fractured or crushed, but usually this is in association with adjacent malleolar fractures. Such injuries are serious, because there is an associated crush injury to the articular cartilage which may cause difficulty, regardless of the reduction.

Attempts should be made to realign the articular surface by closed manipulation. In some cases, it may be possible to perform open reduction, although when comminution is severe, subsequent ankle arthrodesis may be necessary.

Fractures and Dislocations of the Foot

FRACTURES AND DISLOCATIONS OF THE TALUS

The talus is fractured in its distal portion, through the neck or body. Neck fractures account for the majority of talus injuries. Fractures of the neck occur from forcible dorsiflexion of the foot, such that the neck is driven against the anterior margin of the distal tibia.

If the vertical force continues, a subtalar dislocation may complicate the fracture. Still greater force is associated with fractures of the neck of the talus, subtalar dislocation, and posterior displacement of the body from the ankle joint. Such fracture-dislocations are commonly compound. In some cases, the patient presents with the posterior body of the talus having been driven out through the wound and left at the scene of the accident.

The subtalar joint may be dislocated by maximal inversion stress in the position of plantar flexion. In such a case, the foot is dislocated medially, beneath the body of the talus. Greater force results in dislocation of the talus from the ankle joint, resulting in total dislocation of the talus.

If there is sufficient damage across the neck of the talus, avascular necrosis of the body may ensue. In the series by Dunne et al., avascular necrosis developed in 69 percent of neck fracture-dislocations and 50 percent of body fractures.

TREATMENT. Fractures of the neck are treated by closed reduction and plaster cast immobilization until bony union is complete. Displaced fractures with dislocation are reduced by closed manipulation carried out with the foot in the talipes equinus position. If accurate closed reduction cannot be accomplished, open reduction through a lateral approach is indicated. Care is taken not to devitalize soft tissue attachments. Kirschner wires are used for internal fixation. Postoperative plaster immobilization is continued until union is evident (3 months or longer).

Undisplaced fractures of the body of the talus may be treated by immobilization in neutral position. For severe compression fractures, primary tibial-talar fusion using the method of Blair may be indicated. Avascular necrosis, which develops in the majority of cases, is not a deterrent to a good result if immobilization is continued until union is solid and weight bearing is prevented until revascularization occurs.

Complete talar dislocations or subtalar dislocations are reduced by placing the foot in maximal inversion and, with direct pressure over the talus, bringing the calcaneus and forefoot into eversion. Considerable force and general anesthesia may be necessary to accomplish reduction of the completely dislocated talus. The foot is then immobilized until soft tissue healing is complete.

FRACTURES OF THE CALCANEUS

Fractures of the calcaneus commonly occur from falls in which the maximal force is applied to the calcaneus.

It has been shown experimentally by Thoren that the type of fracture is related to the position of the subtalar joint at the time of impact. Involvement of the posterior articular facet is least likely to occur when the foot is in maximal pronation. The main fracture line is oblique, creating two major fragments, an anteromedial fragment and a posterolateral fragment. Fractures of the anterior portion of the calcaneus or the tuberosity also may occur.

A suitable classification of fractures of the calcaneus has been described by Dart and Graham (Fig. 47-56). Type I isolated fractures include beak fractures of the tuberosity or fractures of the anterior part of the calcaneus with minimal calcaneocuboid joint involvement. Type II includes fractures of the body without joint surface involvement. Type IIIa consists of depressed fractures of the posterior facet with minimal depression of Böhler's angle. Böhler's angle (tuberosity joint angle) is the angle formed by the axis of the subtalar joint and the superior surface of the tuberosity. Type IIIb is severe depression of Böhler's angle. Type IV fractures are grossly comminuted fractures (Fig. 47-57), involving subtalar and calcaneocuboid joints. Type V consists of avulsions of the tendocalcaneus with a portion of bone from the posterior portion of the calcaneus.

Approximately 25 percent of patients presenting with fractures of the calcaneus have associated injuries, including compression fractures of the spine, pelvic fractures, or fractures in the lower extremities.

TREATMENT. Treatment of severely comminuted calcaneus fractures is difficult because of the associated soft tissue injury, which contributes to chronic swelling as well as to interference of subtalar joint motion. Compression of the cancellous calcaneus makes stable reduction difficult. The patient should be hospitalized; regardless of what course of treatment is decided upon, the limb must be immediately elevated to prevent swelling and minimize hematoma formation. Types I and II are treated by bed rest, elevation, and early range-of-motion exercises. Patients are allowed to ambulate with crutches after 2 to 3 weeks, and weight bearing is prevented for 3 months. In Type III fractures, Böhler's angle should be corrected by the method of Essex-Lopresti. This involves the insertion of a Steinmann pin through the tendocalcaneus and posterior fragment, which is then forcibly depressed, correcting the tuberosity-joint angle. The pin is then driven across the anterior fragment and/or calcaneocuboid joint. Any significant widening of the calcaneus is corrected by manual compression. The foot and protruding Steinmann pin are immobilized in plaster for 6 weeks. At 6 weeks, range-of-motion exercises are started, and weight bearing is allowed at 3 months.

One may elect the same type of treatment for Type IV fractures, although triple arthrodesis may be indicated when the acute swelling has subsided, approximately 6 weeks after injury.

For Type V fractures, the fragment should have open reduction and screw fixation of the tendocalcaneus insertion.

Many patients, in spite of early active motion and physiotherapy, will have stiffness, chronic swelling of the foot,

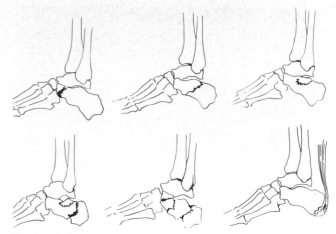

Fig. 47-56. Types of fracture of the calcaneus (after Dart and Graham).

and broadening of the heel. If the early active motion can be instituted, there will be less difficulty due to swelling and less restriction of motion.

METATARSAL FRACTURES

Fractures of the Fifth Metatarsal

The base of the fifth metatarsal may be fractured during inversion injuries of the foot (Fig. 47-58). The attachment of the peroneus brevis to the base of the fifth metatarsal avulses this portion of the bone during sudden, forceful inversion. The patient may sustain an associated sprain of the anterior talofibular ligament at the same time. On examination, there is local tenderness over the base of the fifth metatarsal. The patient may be unable to bear weight because of discomfort.

Fig. 47-57. Comminuted (Type IV) fracture of the calcaneus incurred from a fall from a two-story window. A. Lateral x-ray. B. Axial view of calcaneus and subtalar joint.

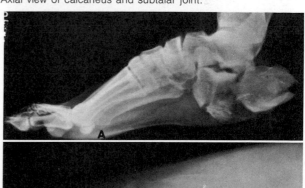

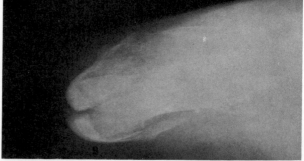

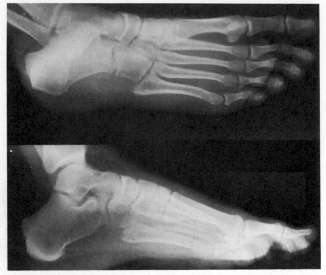

Fig. 47-58. Avulsion fracture of the base of the fifth metatarsal. Lateral and oblique x-rays showing undisplaced fracture. Treatment was by boot walking cast for 6 weeks.

Treatment of this injury is symptomatic. For some individuals, taping of the foot and ankle to provide immobilization in the position of eversion is all that is necessary. Most patients, however, are best managed with a short leg walking plaster which will provide stability and comfort for a 4- to 6-week period.

Multiple Metatarsal Fractures

Fractures of the metatarsal shafts may occur with severe traumatic or crush injuries to the foot. Isolated fractures of the necks of fourth and fifth metatarsals may also occur. Stress fractures of the shafts of the second and third metatarsals should be suspected when the patient complains of insidious pain, without acute injury.

Fracture-dislocations occur at the tarsometatarsal junction, with associated fractures of the bases of metatarsals. Such injuries occur from severe trauma, such as cycling injuries or crush injuries to the feet. There is commonly associated severe soft tissue damage with or without compounding. In closed fractures, reduction should be accomplished by closed efforts, but in some instances Kirschner wire fixation is required. The handling of multiple fractures of the metatarsal shafts should include an attempt at alignment to restore painless weight bearing.

PHALANGEAL FRACTURES

Fractures of the phalanges of the toes may occur at any age from direct trauma to the forefoot, as in the dropping of heavy objects upon the toes or striking the toes against a door or foot of the bed. Such an injury may dislocate MP or IP joints as well.

Treatment of phalangeal fractures is directed at alignment and relief of pain. Reduction should be accomplished and the toes splinted to adjacent toes with adhesive tape. The patient may be allowed to walk if symptoms are tolerated.

PELVIC AND SPINE INJURIES

Acetabular Fractures and Hip Dislocations

Dislocation of the hip with or without associated fracture of the acetabulum is caused by force applied to the proximal femur. Such injuries may result from automobile collisions, pedestrian injuries, or falls from a great height. The type of fracture and dislocation is dependent upon the position of the hip and the direction of the force at the moment of impact. Force applied to an abducted femur may result in an anterior hip dislocation without fracture. Striking the knee on a dashboard of a car with the hip in a position of adduction and flexed at 90° may result in a posterior dislocation (Fig. 47-59) with or without a fracture of the posterior acetabular rim. Direct trauma to the trochanter with the hip in various positions will result in inner wall or bursting fractures of the acetabulum, including central dislocation.

Patients with fracture-dislocations about the hip may have other, more serious injuries, as with any fractures of the pelvis. Regardless of the type of dislocation, reduction should be accomplished as soon as possible, to minimize the change of avascular necrosis of the femoral head.

ANTERIOR HIP DISLOCATIONS

Such injuries occur from extreme abduction or trauma applied anteroposteriorly to an abducted thigh. Patients with this dislocation have the thigh held in abduction, flexion, and external rotation. Reduction is accomplished by applying force to the anesthetized patient in the direction of the deformity. When muscle resistance has been overcome and the femoral head has been pulled laterally to the rim of the acetabulum, the leg is adducted in flexion and internally rotated. Check x-rays are obtained to be certain that bone fragments are not displaced into the acetabulum. If bone fragments are obstructing reduction, open excision of the fragments must be accomplished.

The patient is maintained in traction, with the hip in extension for 10 to 14 days, following which active range of motion is carried out. Crutch walking with partial weight bearing is continued for 6 weeks, and then full weight bearing is allowed.

POSTERIOR HIP DISLOCATIONS

Posterior hip dislocations occur when axial force is applied to the flexed, adducted femur. The hip may be dislocated through a rent in the posterior capsule or with the posterior rim of the acetabulum driven off by the femoral head (Fig. 47-60). The diagnosis is usually apparent on clinical examination. The clinical deformity reveals the hip in a position of flexion, adduction, and internal rotation. Attempts to lower the limb to the table are met with severe resistance and anguish from the patient. Reduction of a dislocation should be accomplished immediately, but not before x-rays define the lesion. A standard AP x-ray of the pelvis is required, but a lateral x-ray of the hip joint may be necessary to demonstrate the dislocation accurately.

TREATMENT. Before moving the patient from the x-ray

table, reduction should be accomplished by the method of Bigelow. Most patients can be reduced under mild analgesia or with local anesthesia to the hip joint, but a few require general anesthesia. The basic principle is to pull the dislocated femoral head back through the rent in the capsule. If a large fragment has been fractured from the acetabulum, reduction may not be difficult.

Technique of Reduction. With the patient lying supine and with countertraction exerted across the pelvis, traction is applied to the long axis of the femoral shaft, with the knee flexed, and with the hip in a position of flexion, adduction, and internal rotation. When the femoral head has been brought to the level of the posterior acetabular rim, the femur is then gradually abducted, externally rotated, and placed in extension. If this cannot be accomplished gently or if the hip does not reduce with a sudden click, it should not be forced, or fracture of the femoral neck may occur. The stability or tendency to redislocation should be estimated after reduction, to decide whether screw fixation of this fragment is indicated. Anteroposterior, oblique, and lateral check x-rays are obtained to delineate the position of the posterior rim of the acetabulum to be certain that fragments are not displaced intraarticularly and that the posterior acetabular rim has been satisfactorily reduced. As a general rule, the acetabular rim requires open reduction. It is important to reduce the dislocation promptly and carry out open reduction of the acetabular rim when the patient's condition warrants, usually within the first week.

The uncomplicated dislocation is reduced, and the patient is placed in skin traction of 10 lb for 10 to 14 days, and weight bearing is prevented for an additional 4 weeks. Aspirin is administered to minimize progression of the cartilage injury sustained at the time of dislocation. All patients with hip dislocations should be followed indefinitely after this injury, because of the incidence of avascular necrosis and degenerative arthritis. Avascular necrosis,

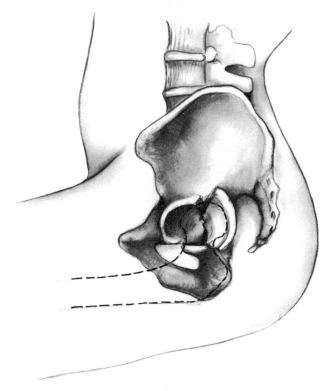

Fig. 47-59. Posterior dislocation of the hip with fracture of the posterior acetabular rim. Axial force applied to the femur drives the femoral head from the acetabulum and the posterior rim of the acetabulum along with it. Such injuries are common to automobile passengers.

the incidence of which is directly related to the delay of reduction, develops in about 20 percent of patients and is usually clinically apparent by the 2-year interval. Traumatic arthritis occurs in about 50 percent of patients and may occur as late as 5 years postreduction.

Technique of Open Reduction of Acetabular Rim Fractures. The patient is placed in a semiprone position with the affected hip close to the edge of the table. The posterior approach of Osborne or Austin Moore will expose the hip joint. The short external rotators of the hip are divided just proximal to their insertion and reflected medially, pro-

Fig. 47-60. Posterior dislocation of the hip with fracture of the acetabular rim. *A.* AP x-ray postinjury showing the femoral head, which appears smaller than that of the opposite side and is superiorly displaced. *B.* AP x-ray showing the relocation of the femoral head with persistent displacement of the acetabular fragment. *C.* AP x-ray following open reduction and screw fixation of the acetabular fragment.

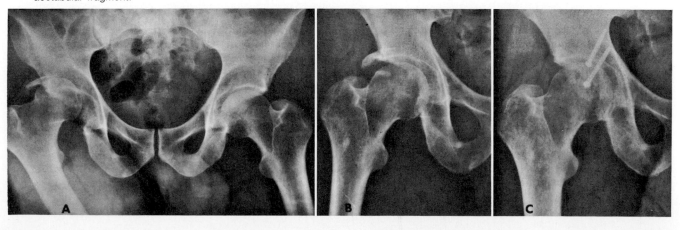

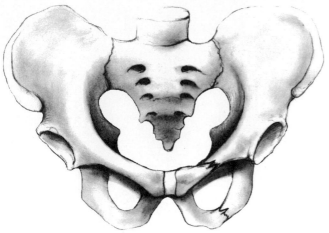

Fig. 47-61. Undisplaced fracture of both pubic rami.

tecting the sciatic nerve. The hip joint may be inspected through the fracture defect, which commonly consists of a large fragment of the posterosuperior rim of the acetabulum. The joint is inspected and any small, loose fragments removed. Compression of articular cartilage and underlying cancellous bone in the acetabulum are gently elevated with a periosteal elevator. Large fragments are accurately reduced and fixed with screws inserted at an angle and directed toward the midcrest of the ilium. The wound is closed, and skeletal traction of 10 lb is maintained for about 6 to 8 weeks, followed by plaster spica immobilization for another 6 weeks. Weight bearing is not allowed before 4 months or until union of the fragment has occurred.

FRACTURES OF THE INNER WALL
OF THE ACETABULUM

Fractures of the inner wall of the acetabulum represent the most common type. If there is a central dislocation of the femoral head and the superior dome of the acetabulum is intact, reduction of the dislocation should be ac-

Fig. 47-62. Displaced fracture of all pubic rami, suggesting injury to the pelvic viscera.

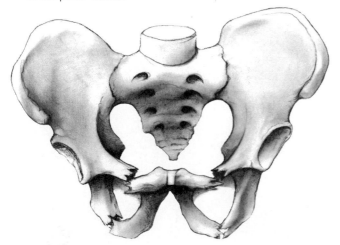

complished by manipulation and maintained with skeletal traction for 8 weeks. It is important to reduce the femoral head into a normal relationship with the intact superior weight-bearing portion of the acetabulum. Active motion of the hip is then begun. Protected weight bearing between crutches is not allowed until the fractures are consolidated, about 4 months after injury.

Fractures of the Superior Acetabulum

Bursting or superior wall fractures have the worst prognosis of acetabular fractures. The ultimate result will depend upon the severity of comminution of the superior dome, as well as the restoration of the superior dome relationship to the femoral head. Attempts should be made to restore this relationship by closed or conservative methods. However, in some instances, open reduction through an anterior approach or even a combined anterior and posterior approach is necessary.

Pelvic Fractures

The pelvic ring, composed of the coxae and sacrum, provides protection for the pelvic viscera, attachments of muscles, and the transmission of weight-bearing forces from the lower extremities. Only the posterolateral wings, which connect the acetabula with the sacrum, function in the transmission of weight.

Injuries to the pelvic ring may occur at any age and from various types of violence. Elderly patients with osteoporosis who fall may sustain isolated fractures of the pubic rami (Fig. 47-61) or undisplaced fractures of the acetabula, the coccyx, or even the sacrum but usually do not have disruptions of the weight-bearing segments. The most common cause of the pelvic fracture is automobile collision. Passengers, drivers, pedestrians, and cyclists sustain pelvic injuries by direct crushing of the pelvis and combinations of rotational stress on the iliac wings.

CLINICAL MANIFESTATIONS. Patients with an acute fracture of the pelvis are unable to bear weight without discomfort. If this is an isolated fracture of the pubic ramus, weight bearing on the affected side causes pain in the groin. There may be local tenderness and swelling at the site of the fractured pubic ramus.

The examiner should test the stability of the pelvis by anterior compression with direct pressure over the symphysis and should determine lateral stability by compressing the pelvis in a frontal plane and applying direct pressure over both iliac wings. Both hips should be put through a range of motion. Any pain associated with these maneuvers requires AP, lateral, and oblique x-ray views of the pelvis to delineate fractures and displacement.

TREATMENT. The treatment of the acute pelvic fracture is first directed at the detection and treatment of associated injuries to the pelvic viscera or abdominal viscera, as well as treatment for shock. One-third of patients with pelvic fractures die as a result of local hemorrhage. Patients with severe retroperitoneal or pelvic hemorrhage complain of abdominal or back pain. There may be signs of hemorrhage into the scrotum or buttocks. If there is any doubt of intraabdominal hemorrhage, laparotomy is indicated.

The risk of laparotomy is far outweighed by the hazard associated with missing an intraabdominal lesion. Ten to twelve percent of patients with pelvic fractures, especially bilateral pubic rami fractures, have an associated injury to the bladder or urethra. Therefore a large indwelling catheter should be inserted immediately and retrograde cystograms obtained. Lesions of the lumbosacral plexus also should be suspected.

Isolated fractures occurring in elderly patients from a single fall are treated by bed rest for a few days, until acute symptoms subside. The patient is then gradually mobilized, and weight bearing is allowed as it is tolerated. Since the anterior arch is not contributing to weight bearing, there is no problem of pelvic stability. Thrombophlebitis and ileus with urinary retention are common complications.

Bilateral fractures of the pubic rami (Fig. 47-62) have the highest incidence of associated injuries and mortality of any pelvic fractures. Some degree of immobilization of bilateral pubic rami fractures can be obtained by bed rest and a pelvic sling.

Symphysis pubis separations account for a small percentage of all pelvic fractures. The main complication is damage to the urethra and bladder. There may be an associated subluxation or dislocation of one sacroiliac joint (Fig. 47-63). Reduction is accomplished by placing the patient in the lateral position on the sound side and, with direct downward and forward pressure, rotating the displaced hemipelvis into position. The patient may then be nursed in a pelvic sling, or if there is an isolated injury, a double hip pantaloon spica may be applied, with the patient lying on his side. If there is an upward displacement of the hemipelvis, skeletal traction to the femur may be required to hold the reduction. All combinations of fracture, including unilateral pubic rami fracture with separation of the sacroiliac joint or separation of the symphysis with a fracture through the wing of the ilium, are handled in similar fashion.

It is not always possible to reduce these fractures anatomically. Every attempt should be made to restore the pelvic outlet in young women of childbearing age. Open reduction is rarely indicated.

Isolated fractures of the iliac wing are usually the result of a direct blow to the crest of the ilium. If the major portion of the iliac wing is intact, weight bearing will not be affected. Fractures of the sacrum (Fig. 47-64) may occur from direct trauma or in association with fractures of the hemipelvis. Fractures of the coccyx occur from a direct blow to the coccyx as in a fall to a sitting position. The patient is treated by having him sit on a support beneath his thighs to take the direct pressure from the coccyx. In refractory situations, the coccyx may be excised.

Fractures and Dislocations of the Spine

Fractures and dislocations involving the cervical, thoracic, or lumbar spine are most commonly the result of injuries sustained by pedestrians, motorcyclists, or automobile occupants but may occur with any severe trauma. The prognosis in these injuries is dependent on whether

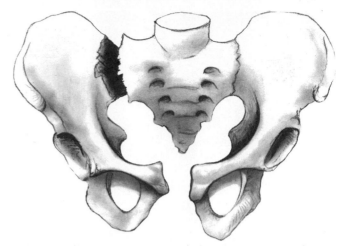

Fig. 47-63. Disruption of the hemipelvis by separation of symphysis pubis and sacroiliac joint.

there is associated cord injury. Fractures or dislocations without cord damage can result in normal function.

MANAGEMENT OF THE ACUTE INJURY. Everyone responsible for the first-aid care of patients at the scene of an accident should be well versed in the hazards of spine injuries and well informed in the transportation of these patients, to prevent or minimize neurologic damage.

Any patient complaining of neck or back pain from an automobile collision or serious fall should be presumed to have an unstable spine until completely examined both clinically and radiologically by a competent physician. Patients sustaining a neck injury with or without acute cord damage should be placed supine on a stretcher with sandbags beside the head to hold it in neutral position. Since half of the cervical spine fractures occur from hyperextension, the neck should be positioned midway between flexion and extension.

Patients with thoracic or lumbar spine injuries should be transported in a position to minimize motion of the spine. The patient is placed supine or prone on a board

Fig. 47-64. Vertical fracture through the sacrum at the neural foramina.

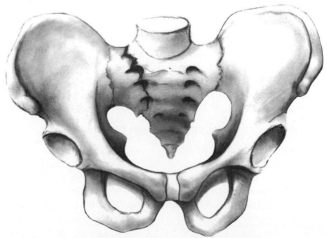

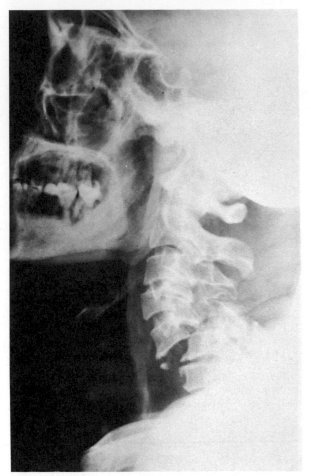

Fig. 47-65. Fracture-dislocation of C_5 upon C_6. Lateral x-rays show complete displacement of C_5 with fracture of the neural arch. The patient was paraplegic immediately following his injury.

or rigid stretcher, which can be moved to the x-ray table so that repositioning is not necessary. If the patient has other injuries, including chest, head, or abdominal hemorrhage, these should be treated first with the establishment of airway, resuscitation, and blood replacement.

A neurologic examination is accomplished as soon as possible. Appropriate AP and lateral x-rays of the cervical, thoracic, or lumbar spine are obtained before moving the patient from the stretcher. If x-rays indicate stability of the spine, oblique x-rays of the cervical spine may be obtained to supplement the AP and lateral x-rays. Immediate and continued immobilization is indicated if there is any question of instability.

CERVICAL FRACTURES AND DISLOCATIONS

Flexion injuries of the cervical spine occur when there is acute forcible flexion of the head upon the neck. With this type of injury, the first lesion to occur is compression of the vertebral body, resulting in an anterior wedge compression fracture of the vertebral body. The common areas are the lower three cervical vertebrae. For this reason, it is imperative to be sure that x-ray diagnosis includes the

entire cervical spine and the relationship between C_7 and T_1.

As the flexion force continues, the posterior longitudinal ligament may be ruptured, and one or both facets may be subluxated or dislocated. Beatson has shown that a unilateral facet dislocation results in only forward displacement of less than one-fifth the anteroposterior diameter of the vertebra. With bilateral facet dislocations, forward displacement may be greater than one-half the anteroposterior diameter. Cord injuries occur when the neural canal is compromised by forward dislocation and are more common with bilateral dislocations of the facets.

When a compression force (vertical load) is applied to the cervical spine, a bursting fracture of a vertebral body may occur. This may result in backward displacement of the posterior portion of the vertebral body, resulting in impingement upon, and damage to, the spinal cord. Combinations of flexion, compression, and rotation may occur, resulting in pedicle or lamina fractures, causing dislocation with or without cord damage (Fig. 47-65).

Forsythe has called attention to the hyperextension injury of the cervical spine. Patients from automobile accidents may present with a contusion of the forehead, and x-rays may reveal forward displacement of an upper vertebra upon the one below it. As the upper cervical spine is driven into extension, the anterior longitudinal ligament is ruptured, causing a compression force at the facet joints. As the force continues and the head is driven back, secondary flexion and forward displacement of an upper vertebra occurs upon the adjacent lower vertebra. Lateral x-rays reveal horizontal facet fracture or fracture of the anteroinferior border of the cervical spine body. Care must be taken in these injuries not to hyperextend the neck, or subsequent cord damage may result. Hyperextension injuries may result without a facet or body fracture and spontaneously be reduced. The cord is driven back against the sharp edge of the lamina, resulting in cord damage. With the head brought into neutral position, the dislocation may be spontaneously reduced, and the x-rays may appear normal, although the patient is paraplegic.

Injuries of the transverse process in the cervical spine are rare and represent avulsion fractures. Fractures of the spinous processes may also occur and have been characterized as the clay shoveler's fracture. A sudden stress on the supraspinous ligament pulls off the tip of the spinous process. Also, a direct blow to the spinous process may cause fracture.

Fractures of the atlas occur when compression force is applied to a thin posterior ring by downward force on the head (Jefferson's fracture).

Fractures of C_2, involving the odontoid or posterior elements, may occur from flexion and extension or rotational forces. In children under the age of six, injuries to the odontoid result in an epiphyseal displacement and associated subluxation or dislocation of atlas upon the axis.

MANAGEMENT OF CERVICAL SPINE FRACTURES AND DISLOCATIONS WITHOUT NEUROLOGIC INJURY. Unstable fractures must be immobilized and dislocations or subluxations reduced. Patients arriving at the emergency room are placed in a cervical halter traction, which will provide immediate stability, while appropriate x-rays or associated conditions are managed. For the long-term immobilization of these injuries, skeletal traction is required. This is accomplished by the use of a halo apparatus. The halo purchases with four pins inserted under local anesthesia onto the outer table of the skull. To this skeletal traction device 5 lb is added for upper cervical lesions and as much as 30 lb for lower cervical lesions.

Dislocations and fractures are reduced with skeletal traction. When the dislocation or fracture is reduced, the halo device is connected to a body plaster jacket molded over the iliac crests and the patient is allowed to walk until stability has ensued, a period of approximately 12 weeks. The patient is then immobilized in a four-poster cervical brace for an additional period. Before immobilization is discontinued, flexion and extension films are obtained to determine stability. When stability cannot be anticipated with immobilization alone, spine fusion is carried out after a 6-week interval.

In some undisplaced fractures, such as a pedicle or lamina fracture, where stability is certain, an initial Minerva plaster jacket may be elected. However, if there is uncertainty about stability, skeletal traction, followed by Minerva plaster, is the safest procedure.

Rogers reported an incidence of 12 percent recurrent instability following the conservative management of unstable fractures and dislocations. For this reason, he and Forsythe have recommended early posterior spine fusion with wiring of spinous processes. Their procedure is to resolve the acute general injuries, during which time skeletal traction is maintained and is then continued during posterior spine fusion. Spine fusion in the face of instability is not recommended before 6 weeks, until ligamentous healing has added some stability. Anesthesia will relieve the protective muscle spasm of the unstable spine, and the very act of positioning such a patient at surgery is not without hazard. The technique is to wire together the spinous process of the affected adjacent vertebrae.

Autogenous iliac bone is applied to the roughened posterior lamina and spinous processes. If satisfactory stability is obtained by wiring, the patient is kept in a four-poster cervical spine brace until bone union is solid (12 to 16 weeks).

CERVICAL FRACTURES AND DISLOCATIONS WITH ASSOCIATED NEUROLOGIC INJURY. There is disagreement about the indications for open laminectomy and decompression of acute fracture-dislocations of the cervical spine with associated cord injury. There is little disagreement that patients who present with minimal neurologic findings and have progressive neurologic deficits require immediate laminectomy and exploration. Another indication is unsuccessful reduction and persistence of bone fragments in the spinal canal. Proponents of the nonexploration attitude argue that irreparable damage has been done from the time of the initial injury and will not be influenced by decompression and subsequent exploration, which in themselves are life-threatening procedures. Also, if the lesion is partial, surgical procedures may further endanger the cord. The operative school base their indications on the fact that occasionally a displaced disc or fragment of bone will compress the cord and unrelieved swelling may further damage a cord capable of recovery.

THORACOLUMBAR FRACTURES AND DISLOCATIONS

Fractures and dislocations involving the upper thoracic and midthoracic regions are uncommon because of the stability afforded by the adjacent rib cage. The principles involved in treatment of such injuries are the same as in thoracolumbar spine fractures.

Holdsworth has clearly shown that flexion force applied to the thoracolumbar spine results in anterior wedge compression fractures which are stable by virtue of intact posterior structures and longitudinal ligaments (Fig. 47-66). Wedge compression fractures may occur in any osteoporotic spine from relatively minor trauma. Wedge compression fractures also occur in normal spines from severe flexion forces common in mine cave-ins, automobile collisions, and falls from a height.

When rotation is combined with flexion, the posterior

Fig. 47-66. Wedge compression fracture L₂. *A.* Lateral x-ray shows compression wedging of the upper portion of L₂. *B.* AP x-rays do not demonstrate the fracture.

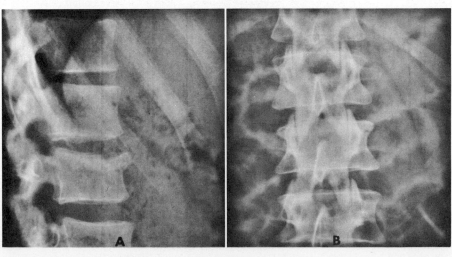

ligaments rupture or the articular processes fracture, and a wedge-shaped fracture may occur through the upper border of the lower vertebral body, resulting in a fracture-dislocation (Fig. 47-67). Extension injuries may cause dislocation with rupture of the anterior longitudinal ligaments and may cause posterior dislocation. This is rare in the lumbar region. When compression force (vertical load) is applied to the line of vertebral bodies, especially at the thoracolumbar area and upper lumbar spine, the result is a bursting fracture with the posterior fragments displaced into the spinal canal.

MANAGEMENT OF ACUTE INJURIES OF THE THORACO-LUMBAR SPINE. Patients with acute traumatic injury to the spine should be presumed to have an unstable situation and potential paraplegia until proved otherwise. They should be placed prone or supine on a stretcher and not moved until AP and lateral x-rays delineate the lesion.

Clinical examination will give some indication of the extent of the lesion. The patient should be inspected for signs of impact, abrasion over one shoulder causing flexion and rotation, etc. If the supraspinous ligaments are ruptured, a defect between the spinous processes will be evident. With any compression fracture, there is tenderness over the affected vertebrae.

Interpretation of the AP and lateral x-rays is important. Flexion injury causing compression wedging will be evident on the lateral x-ray but not on the AP x-ray.

When the "slice wedge" fracture of the upper part of the lower vertebrae is seen on both AP and lateral x-rays without dislocation, instability should be suspected. Such

Fig. 47-67. Posterior fracture-dislocation of the thoracic spine. Lateral x-rays show backward displacement of T_7 upon T_8 with fracture involvement of the neural arch. Patient was paraplegic upon arrival.

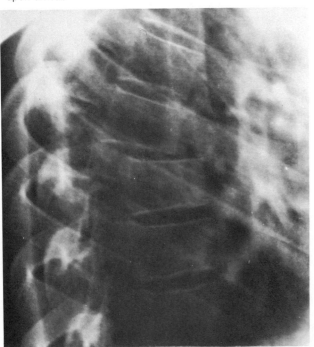

fractures are so unstable that they are reduced just by placing the patient supine. Any displacement in the lumbar spine is an indication of instability.

Treatment of fractures of the thoracolumbar spine will depend on the degree of instability caused by the trauma. Wedge compression fractures are usually stable. Patients are confined to bed rest until symptoms allow mobilization. The patient should be watched for paralytic ileus. Prescribing a liquid diet for a few days to minimize these problems is worthwhile. When patients are comfortable, they are taught hyperextension exercises, which are continued for 6 to 12 weeks. No reduction for a stable wedge compression fracture is necessary, since the deformity rarely causes disability. Bursting fractures are usually stable but may not be. Stable fractures are immobilized in plaster, and spontaneous fusion across the involved disc will usually result. If instability is present or questionable, the patient should be treated on a Foster frame and spine fusion performed at 6 weeks.

Pure dislocations in the thoracolumbar region are rare; when they occur, they require spine fusion.

Fracture-dislocations without injury to the cord may be handled by immobilization on a Foster frame for 6 to 8 weeks and then plaster cast immobilization for another 6 to 8 weeks. Union across adjacent involved vertebrae usually occurs.

A different situation exists when injury to the cauda equina is associated with this rotational fracture-dislocation. The fracture must be adequately reduced to free the nerve roots from pressure. Immobilization must be maintained to prevent recurrent injury during the early post-fracture period. For this reason, Holdsworth employs early stabilization above and below the site of injury. The best method for stabilization is the use of Harrington rods. Others feel that exploration is not indicated and Foster frame reduction and immobilization are sufficient.

MANAGEMENT OF SPINAL CORD INJURY. See Chaps. 42 and 52.

References

Evaluation

Griffiths, L. L.: The Management of Acute Circulatory Failure in an Injured Limb, *J Bone Joint Surg [Br]*, **30B:**280, 1948.

Mercer, W., and Duthie, R. B.: "Orthopaedic Surgery," 6th ed., Edward Arnold (Publishers) Ltd., London, 1964.

Seddon, H. J.: Three Types of Nerve Injury, *Brain,* **66:**237, 1943.

Tachakra, S. S., and Sevitt, S.: Hypoaxemia after Fractures, *J Bone Joint Surg,* **57B:**197, 1975.

Healing and General Treatment

Abercrombie, M.: "Advances in Biology of Skin: V. Wound Healing," Pergamon Press, New York, 1964.

Aegerter, E., and Kirkpatrick, J. A.: "Orthopaedic Diseases," W. B. Saunders Company, Philadelphia, 1964.

Anderson, L. D.: Compression Plate Fixation and the Effect of Different Types of Internal Fixation on Fracture Healing, instructional course lecture, American Academy of Orthopaedic Surgeons, *J Bone Joint Surg [Am]*, **47A:**191, 1965.

Bier, A.: Beabactungen über Regeneration beim Menschen, *Dtsch Med Wochenschr,* **43:**705, 1917.

Duthie, R. B., and Barker, A. N.: An Autoradiographic Study of Mucopolysaccharide and Phosphate Complexes in Bone Growth and Repair, *J Bone Joint Surg [Br],* **37B:**304, 1955.

Johnson, L. C., Stradford, H. T., Geis, R. W., Dineen, H. R., and Kerley, E. R.: Histogenesis of Stress Fractures, *Armed Forces Inst Pathol Annu Lec,* 1963.

Lack, C. H.: Increased Vascular Permeability, Chondrolysis and Cortisone, *Proc R Soc Med,* **55:**113, 1962.

Miles, A. A.: Local and Systemic Factors in Shock, *Fed Proc,* **20**(*Suppl* 9):141, 1961.

Muller, M. E., Allgower, M., and Willenegger, H.: "Technique of Internal Fixation of Fractures," Springer-Verlag, Inc., New York, 1965.

Ray, R. D., Sankaran, B., and Fetro, K. O.: Delayed Union in Non-union Fractures, instructional course lecture, American Academy of Orthopaedic Surgeons, *J Bone Joint Surg [Am],* **46A:**627, 1964.

Rhinelander, F. W., and Baragry, R. A.: Microangiography in Bone Healing, *J Bone Joint Surg [Am],* **44A:**1273, 1962.

Salter, R. B., and Harris, R. W.: Injuries Involving the Epiphyseal Plate, instructional course lecture, American Academy of Orthopaedic Surgeons, *J Bone Joint Surg [Am],* **45A:**587, 1963.

Tonna, E. A., and Cronkite, E. P.: Cellular Response to Fracture Studied with Tritiated Thymidine, *J Bone Joint Surg [Am],* **43A:**352, 1961.

Wilhelm, D. L.: "The Inflammatory Process," Academic Press, Inc., New York, 1965.

Wray, J. B.: Factors in the Pathogenesis of Non-union, instructional course lecture, American Academy of Orthopedic Surgeons, *J Bone Joint Surg [Am],* **47A:**168, 1965.

—— and Lynch, C. J.: The Vascular Response to Fracture of the Tibia in the Rat, *J Bone Joint Surg [Am],* **41A:**1143, 1959.

Fractures and Joint Injuries to the Shoulder and Girdle

Bankart, A. S. B.: Recurrence of Habitual Dislocation of the Shoulder Joint, *Br Med J,* **2:**1132, 1923.

"Campbell's Operative Orthopaedics," chap. 5, p. 366, The C. V. Mosby Company, St. Louis, 1963.

Inman, V. T., Saunders, J. B., and Abbott, L. C.: Observations on the Function of the Shoulder Joint, *J Bone Joint Surg [Am],* **26A:**1, 1944.

Jacobs, B., and Wade, P. A.: Acromioclavicular Joint Injury and End Result Study, *J Bone Joint Surg [Am],* **48A:**475, 1966.

Lacey, T., III, and Crawford, H. B.: Reduction of Anterior Dislocation of the Shoulder by Means of Milch Abduction Techniques, *J Bone Joint Surg [Am],* **34A:**108, 1952.

Leslie, J. T., and Ryan, T. J.: The Axillary Incision to Approach the Shoulder Joint, *J Bone Joint Surg [Am],* **44A:**1193, 1962.

Neviaser, J. S.: Acromioclavicular Dislocations Treated by Transference of the Coraco-acromio Ligaments, *Arch Surg,* **64:**292, 1952.

Nobel, W.: Post-traumatic Dislocation of the Shoulder, *J Bone Joint Surg [Am],* **44A:**523, 1962.

Osmond-Clark, H.: Habitual Dislocation of the Shoulder: The Putti-Platt Operation, *J Bone Joint Surg [Br],* **30B:**19, 1948.

Rowe, C. R.: Symposium on Dislocation of the Shoulder, instruc-tional course lecture, American Academy of Orthopaedic Surgeons, *J Bone Joint Surg [Am],* **44A:**998, 1962.

Stubbins, S. G., and McGaw, W. H.: Suspension Casts for Acromio-clavicular Separation and Clavicle Traction, *JAMA,* **169:**672, 1959.

Weaver, J. K., and Dunn, H. K.: Treatment of Acromioclavicular Injuries, Especially Complete Acromioclavicular Separation, *J Bone Joint Surg,* **54A:**1187, 1972.

Fractures and Joint Injuries to the Humerus, Elbow, and Forearm

Adler, J. B., and Shaftan, G. W.: Radial Head Fractures: Is Excision Necessary? *J Trauma,* **4:**115, 1964.

Blount, W. P.: "Fractures in Children," The C. V. Mosby Company, St. Louis, 1955.

Cave, E. F.: "Fractures and Other Injuries," Year Book Medical Publishers, Inc., Chicago, 1961.

Darrach, W.: Colle's Fracture, *N Engl J Med,* **226:**594, 1942.

Evans, E. M.: Pronation Injuries of the Forearm with Special Reference to the Anterior Monteggia Fracture, *J Bone Joint Surg [Br],* **31B:**578, 1949.

Gould, N.: Early Mobilization of the Joint in Intra-articular Fractures with Special Attention to the Elbow Joint, *Surg Gynecol Obstet,* **115:**575, 1962.

Holstein, A., and Lewis, G. B.: Fractures of Humerus with Radial Nerve Paralysis, *J Bone Joint Surg [Am],* **45A:**1382, 1963.

Hughston, J. C.: Fracture of the Forearm in Children, instructional course lecture, American Academy of Orthopaedic Surgeons, *J Bone Joint Surg [Am],* **44A:**1678, 1962.

Miller, W. E.: Comminuted Fractures of the Humerus in the Adult, instructional course lecture, American Academy of Orthopaedic Surgeons, *J Bone Joint Surg [Am],* **46A:**644, 1964.

Neer, C. S.: Displaced Proximal Humeral Fractures: Part 1. Classification and Evaluation, *J Bone Joint Surg,* **52A:**1077, 1970.

——: Displaced Proximal Humeral Fractures: Part II. Treatment of Three Part and Four Part Displacements, *J Bone Joint Surg,* **52A:**1090, 1970.

Neviaser, J. S.: Complicated Fractures and Dislocations about the Shoulder Joint, instructional course lecture, American Academy of Orthopaedic Surgeons, *J Bone Joint Surg [Am],* **44A:**984, 1962.

Salter, R. B., and Harris, R. W.: Injuries Involving the Shoulder Joint, instructional course lecture, American Academy of Orthopaedic Surgeons, *J Bone Joint Surg [Am],* **45A:**587, 1963.

—— and Zaltz, C.: Anatomic Investigations of the Mechanism of Injury and Pathologic Anatomy of "Pulled Elbow" in Young Children, *Clin Orthop,* **77:**134, 1971.

Scuderi, C. S.: Operative Indications in Fractures of Both Bones of the Forearm, instructional course lecture, American Academy of Orthopaedic Surgeons, *J Bone Joint Surg [Am],* **44A:**1671, 1962.

Smith, L.: Deformity following Supracondylar Fractures of the Humerus, *J Bone Joint Surg [Am],* **42A:**235, 1960.

Fractures and Joint Injuries to the Wrist and Hand

Barnard, L., and Stubbins, S. G.: Styloidectomy of the Radius in the Surgical Treatment of Non-union of the Carpal Navicular: A Preliminary Report, *J Bone Joint Surg [Am],* **30A:**98, 1948.

Boyes, J. H.: "Bunnel's Surgery of the Hand," J. B. Lippincott Company, Philadelphia, 1964.

Linscheid, R. L., Dobyns, J. H., Beabout, J. W., and Bryan, R. S.: Traumatic Instability of the Wrist. Diagnosis, Classification and Pathomechanics, *J Bone Joint Surg,* **54A:**1612, 1972.

Fractures of the Hip and Femur

Banks, H. H.: Healing of Femoral Neck Fractures, *Proc Conf Aseptic Necrosis Femoral Head, St. Louis,* 1964.

"Campbell's Operative Orthopaedics," The C. V. Mosby Company, St. Louis, 1963.

Clawson, D. K.: Trochanteric Fractures Treated by the Sliding Screw Plate Fixation Method, *J Trauma,* **4:**737, 1964.

———, Smith, R. F., and Hausen, S. T.: Closed Intramedullary Nailing of the Femur, *J Bone Joint Surg [Am],* **53A:**681, 1971.

Crawford, H. B.: Conservative Treatment of Impacted Fractures of the Femoral Neck: A Report of 50 Cases, *J Bone Joint Surg [Am],* **42A:**471, 1960.

Deyerle, W. M.: Multiple Pin Peripheral Fixation in Fractures of the Neck of the Femur: Immediate Weight Bearing, *Clin Orthop,* **39:**135, 1965.

Dimon, J. H., and Hughston, J. C.: Unstable Intertrochanteric Fractures of the Hip, *J Bone Joint Surg [Am],* **49A:**440, 1967.

Furuya, M., Harrison-Stubbs, M. O., and Freiberger, R. H.: Arthrography of the Knee: Analysis of 2101 Arthrograms and 623 Surgical Findings, *Rev Hosp Spec Surg,* **2:**11, 1972.

Garden, R. S.: Stability and Union in Subcapital Fractures of the Femur, *J Bone Joint Surg [Br],* **46B:**630, 1964.

Harris, W. H., Salzman, E. W., and Desanctis, R. W.: The Prevention of Thromboembolic Disease by Prophylactic Anticoagulation: A Controlled Study in Elective Hip Surgery, *J Bone Joint Surg [Am],* **49A:**81, 1967.

Hinchey, J. J., and Day, P. L.: Primary Prosthetic Replacement in Fresh Femoral Neck Fractures, *J Bone Joint Surg [Am],* **46A:**223, 1964.

Horowitz, B. G.: Retrospective Analysis of Hip Fractures, *Surg Gynecol Obstet,* **123:**565, 1966.

Lowell, J. D.: Fractures of the Hip, *N Engl J Med,* **275:**1418, 1966.

Massie, W. K.: Avascular Sequelae of Femoral Neck, Studied by a Radioisotope Technique, *Proc Conf Aseptic Necrosis Femoral Head, St. Louis,* 1964.

———: Fractures of the Hip, instructional course lecture, American Academy of Orthopaedic Surgeons, *J Bone Joint Surg [Am],* **46A:**658, 1964.

Stewart, M. J., Sisk, D., and Wallace, S. L.: Fractures of the Distal Third of the Femur, instructional course lecture, American Academy of Orthopaedic Surgeons, *J Bone Joint Surg [Am],* **48A:**784, 1966.

Trueta, J., and Harrison, M. H.: The Normal Vascular Anatomy of the Femoral Head in Adult Man, *J Bone Joint Surg [Br],* **35B:**442, 1953.

Zickel, R. E.: A New Fixation Device for Subtrochanteric Fractures of the Femur. A Preliminary Report, *Clin Orthop,* **54:**115, 1957.

Fractures and Injuries of the Knee Joint, Patella, Tibia, and Fibula

Brown, P. W., and Urban, J. G.: Early Weight-Bearing Treatment of Open Fractures of the Tibia: An End-Result Study of 63 Cases, *J Bone Joint Surg [Am],* **51A:**59, 1969.

Dehne, E., Metz, C. W., Deffer, P. A., and Hale, R. M.: Nonoperative Treatment of the Fractured Tibia by Immediate Weightbearing, *J Trauma,* **1:**514, 1961.

Goldthwait, J. E.: Slipping or Recurrent Dislocation of the Patella with Report of Eleven Cases, *Boston Med Surg J,* **150:**169, 1904.

Hauser, E. D. W.: Total Tendon Transplant for Slipping Patella: New Operation for Recurrent Dislocation of the Patella, *Surg Gynecol Obstet,* **66:**199, 1938.

Helfet, A. J.: "The Management of Internal Derangements of the Knee," J. B. Lippincott Company, Philadelphia, 1963.

Hoagland, F. T., and States, J. D.: Factors Influencing Rate of Healing in Tibial Shaft Fractures, *Surg Gynecol Obstet,* **124:**71, 1967.

Karlen, A.: Congenital Fibrosis of the Vastus Intermedius Muscle, *J Bone Joint Surg [Br],* **46B:**488, 1964.

Kennedy, J. C., and Fowler, P. J.: Medial and Anterior Instability of the Knee: An Anatomical and Clinical Study Using Stress Machines, *J Bone Joint Surg [Am],* **53A:**1257, 1971.

Mooney, V., Nickel, V. L., Harvey, J. P., Jr., and Snelson, R.: Cast-Brace Treatment for Fractures of the Distal Part of the Femur, *J Bone Joint Surg [Am],* **52A:**1563, 1970.

Nicoll, E. H.: Fractures of the Tibial Shaft: A Survey of 705 Cases, *J Bone Joint Surg [Am],* **46B:**373, 1964.

O'Donoghue, D. H.: Surgical Treatment of Fresh Injuries to the Major Ligaments of the Knee, *J Bone Joint Surg [Am],* **32A:**721, 1950.

Sarmiento, A.: A Functional Below-the-Knee Cast for Tibial Fractures, *J Bone Joint Surg [Am],* **49A:**885, 1967.

Slocum, D. B., and Larson, R. L.: Rotatory Instability of the Knee: Its Pathogenesis and a Clinical Test to Demonstrate Its Presence, *J Bone Joint Surg [Am],* **50A:**211, 1968.

Weissman, S. L., and Harold, Z. H.: Fractures of the Tibial Plateau, *Clin Orthop,* **33:**194, 1964.

Ankle Injuries, Fractures, and Dislocations of the Foot

Dart, D. E., and Graham, W. D.: Treatment of the Fractured Calcaneum, *J Trauma,* **6:**362, 1966.

Dunne, L. R., Jacobs, B., and Campbell, R. D.: Fractures of the Talus, *J Trauma,* **6:**443, 1966.

Morris, H. D., Hand, W. L., and Dunn, A. W.: The Modified Blair Fusion for Fractures of the Talus, *J Bone Joint Surg [Am],* **53A:**1289, 1971.

Thoren, O.: Os Calcis Fractures, *Acta Orthop Scand Suppl,* 70, 1964.

Watson-Jones, Sir Reginald: "Fractures and Joint Injuries," vol. II, chap. 28, p. 813, and chap. 29, p. 862, 4th ed., The Williams & Wilkins Company, Baltimore, 1956.

Pelvic and Spine Injuries

Beatson, T. R.: Fractures and Dislocations of the Cervical Spine, *J Bone Joint Surg [Br],* **45B:**21, 1963.

Flesch, J. R., Leider, L. L., Erickson, D. L., Chou, S. N., and Bradford, D. S.: Harrington Instrumentation and Spine Fusion for Unstable Fractures and Fracture-Dislocation of the Thoracic and Lumbar Spine, *J Bone Joint Surg,* **59A:**143, 1977.

Forsythe, H. F.: Extension Injuries of the Cervical Spine, instructional course lecture, American Academy of Orthopaedic Surgeons, *J Bone Joint Surg [Am],* **46A:**1792, 1964.

Holdsworth, F. W.: Fractures, Dislocations, and Fracture-Dislocations of the Spine, *J Bone Joint Surg [Br]*, **45B:**6, 1963.

McCarroll, J. R., Braunstein, T. W., Cooper, W., Helpren, M., Seremetis, M., Wade, P. A., and Weinberg, S. B.: Fatal Pedestrian Automobile Accidents, *JAMA,* **180:**127, 1962.

Peltier, L. F.: Fractures of the Pelvis, instructional course lecture, American Academy of Orthopaedic Surgeons, *J Bone Joint Surg [Am]*, **47A:**1060, 1965.

Rogers, W. A.: Treatment of Fracture Dislocation of the Cervical Spine, *J Bone Joint Surg [Am]*, **24:**245, 1942.

Rowe, C. R., and Lowell, J. D.: Prognosis of Fractures of the Acetabulum, *J Bone Joint Surg [Am]*, **43A:**30, 1961.

Stewart, M. J., and Milford, L. W.: Prevention of Disability after Traumatic Dislocation of the Hip, and End Result Study, *J Bone Joint Surg [Am]*, **36A:**315, 1964.

Watson-Jones, Sir Reginald: "Fractures and Joint Injuries," vol. II, chap. 32, p. 934, and chap. 33, p. 946, 4th ed., The Williams & Wilkins Company, Baltimore, 1956.

Chapter 48

Diseases of Joints

by Franklin T. Hoaglund and Robert B. Duthie

The problem of joint injury or disease is common. An estimated 2 to 8 percent of the population have rheumatic complaints at some time in their lives. Virtually everyone over the age of fifty years has sufficient degenerative changes in joints to have some restriction of some joint motion, although only a small percentage show symptoms. Injuries frequently involve joints; the immobilization imposed by every fracture or injured extremity results in restriction of joint motion either temporarily or in some cases permanently.

ANATOMY

Joints are either fibrous or cartilaginous. A fibrous joint, or synarthrosis, consists of two bones united by fibrous tissue, such as the syndesmoses or sutures of the skull.

Cartilaginous joints consist of bones united by either hyaline cartilage or fibrocartilage. An example of a primary cartilaginous joint is an epiphyseal plate. Examples of fibrocartilaginous joints are the pubic symphysis and the intervertebral discs.

Diarthrodial joints are movable joints in which the cartilage-covered bone ends are united by a capsule lined with synovium (Fig. 48-1).

The plane or planes of motion occurring in the synovial joint characterize the joints as uniaxial, i.e., ginglymus (hinge), trochoid (pivot), biaxial, or multiaxial. The motion permitted in a diarthrosis depends upon the configuration of the articular surface, adjacent capsule, and supporting musculature, and upon the unique properties of articular cartilage.

ARTICULAR CARTILAGE. Normal articular cartilage is blue-white, has a smooth surface, and is slightly compressible. The thickness of articular cartilage varies in different locations of specific joints.

Articular cartilage is composed of chondrocytes, which

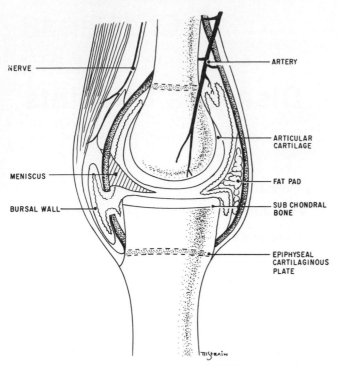

NERVE

ARTERY

ARTICULAR
CARTILAGE

MENISCUS

FAT PAD

BURSAL WALL

SUB CHONDRAL
BONE

EPIPHYSEAL
CARTILAGINOUS
PLATE

Fig. 48-1. Schematic drawing of synovial joint structures.

are embedded in a network of collagen fibers, surrounded by a matrix of proteoglycans. It is separated from the underlying supporting subchondral bone by a thin layer of calcified cartilage. Histologically, there are four distinct layers of normal cartilage: in the superficial, or surface, layer the cells are numerous, flattened, and smaller than in the deeper layers; the intermediate zone blends imperceptibly with the surface layer, but the cells are larger; the deep zone contains larger cells and lies upon the calcified cartilage. In the immature animal in the deeper layers of the articular cartilage, there are two zones which show evidence of cell reproduction and growth. The deepest layer is responsible for circumferential epiphyseal enlargement, and the more superficial zone is responsible for growth of the articular surface. Cell reproduction does not occur in normal healthy adult articular cartilage. After injury and in degenerative disease of articular cartilage, the rate of deoxyribonucleic acid (DNA) synthesis is increased, indicating cell replication.

CARTILAGE MATRIX. The cartilage cells produce the intercellular substances composed of matrix, or ground substance, and collagen fibers. The matrix, proteoglycan, is a complex substance and contributes to the maintenance of the water content and resiliency of the cartilage. Proteoglycan is composed of a linear protein to which aggregates of chondroitin 6-sulfate, chondroitin 4-sulfate, or keratan sulfate are attached. The amounts of each vary with age; keratan sulfate is present in trace amounts in the young and may reach 50 percent in the elderly.

COLLAGEN. The collagen of articular cartilage is different from that of bone and contains three a_1 (II) chains with more hydroxyline residues and increased glycolosylation of

hydroxylysine. The network of collagen fibrils in normal hyaline cartilage ranges from the normal characteristic banding of 645 to 700 Å down to widths of 50 to 250 Å. The collagen fibers have a definite arrangement. In the depths of the cartilage, the fibers are at right angles to the surface of the subchondral bone. At the articular surface, the fibers curve to run parallel with the surface. The resulting network is called Benninghoff's arcades.

In the adult, cartilage is nourished by diffusion of substances from the synovial fluid on the surface and in the immature animal before the basal layer calcifies, also by diffusion from the underlying capillaries on the subchondral bone.

SYNOVIAL MEMBRANE. The synovial membrane is composed of secretory and phagocytic cells, which are arranged in depths of one to three cells over subsynovial connective tissue. The latter consists of a vascular network surrounded by fibroblasts, macrophages, fat cells, and mast cells. Over ligaments, the synovium is quite thin, while in regions of the fat pads and loose capsule there is considerable areolar tissue beneath the synovium. Circulation to the synovium comes from the main blood vessels about the joint which first supply the fibrous capsule. The synovium is much more vascular, with a large plexus immediately beneath the synovial surface. At the synovial membrane junction with the articular cartilage, the vessels are continued as the circulus articuli vasculosus. The blood vessels in the synovia are continuous and communicate with metaphyseal and epiphyseal blood vessels.

The secretory cells produce the hyaluronate of the synovial fluid. In addition, electrolytes and certain plasma proteins diffuse from the synovial capillaries into the joint space. Normal synovial fluid is a weakly alkaline, viscous, clear, pale yellow nonclottable fluid. The viscosity is dependent upon the presence of hyaluronate, a sulfate-free mucopolysaccharide, containing glucuronic acid and N-acetylglucosamine. When hyaluronate is depolymerized, the viscosity is reduced.

The concentration of α- and β-globulins in synovial fluid is the same as in serum, but α_2- and γ-globulin levels are lower. Albumin accounts for about three-fourths of the total protein in the synovial fluid. The protein molecules with molecular weight greater than 160,000 such as fibrinogen, α- and β-macroglobulin, and β-lipoprotein are absent in normal joint fluid. However, when capillary permeability is increased during inflammation, the clotting proteins will enter the joint space.

Normal synovial fluid contains up to 200 nucleated cells consisting of polymorphonuclear leukocytes, lymphocytes, and monocytes. Electrolytes and glucose are present. Nonprotein nitrogen and uric acid concentrations are approximately the same as in serum.

Joint fluid nourishes cartilage and has the added function of joint lubrication. The coefficient of friction of cartilage on cartilage with synovial fluid as a lubricant is extremely low. There is disagreement as to whether this is an example of hydrodynamic or boundary lubrication. Another theory incorporates the hydrodynamic theory with a "weeping" lubrication in which the synovial fluid oozes from the articular cartilage.

The nerve supply of each synovial joint is by articular twigs from nerves supplying muscles responsible for the control of motion of that joint. The distribution and location of these branches is quite variable, making complete denervation of a joint difficult. The capsule and ligaments are the most pain-sensitive structures in a joint. Synovium also contains free nerve endings, but the areas of pain sensation are variable and ill defined.

Nerve fibers accompany arteries into bone, and this may be the basis for bone pain in certain inflammatory conditions about joints. The pain from the joint is difficult to localize and is often referred distally. There are proprioceptive endings in the capsule and joint ligaments which are sensitive to stretch and are indicators of joint position. Articular cartilage is without sensation.

EXAMINATION

The diagnosis of joint disease is dependent upon:

1. Clinical history of joint symptomatology
2. Clinical examination of all joints
3. X-ray examination
4. Synovial fluid analysis
5. Serologic tests

The patient is questioned about the specific onset of the joint complaint and any relation to trauma. Information about aggravation and relief of pain, and history of previous joint complaints, morning stiffness, locking, giving way, swelling, erythema, and symptoms related to other joints are necessary. Complete clinical history regarding other systems is always required.

CLINICAL EXAMINATION. The involved joint or joints should be inspected for signs of swelling and effusion, and evidence of erythema and local skin temperature increase. In unilateral involvement, the opposite side is used for comparison. The ligaments responsible for stability are examined and ranges of joint motion recorded. Active motion is examined by asking the patient to put the joint through a range of motion. Passive motion is measured by putting the joint through the maximal range of motion with muscles relaxed. The proximal and distal joints are always examined to be certain that the complaint is not due to referred pain. Muscle girth is determined by measurement, and muscle power is graded. Clinical examination is incomplete without evaluation of all joints in both upper and lower extremities, as well as a complete physical examination.

X-RAY EXAMINATION. Standard biplanar x-rays of the involved joints are necessary. The x-rays should clearly show the margins of the joint, as well as the adjacent bone metaphysis. In some situations, oblique x-rays and laminograms are necessary to delineate the adjacent bone and specific lesion. X-rays may be required in positions of flexion and extension to test for subluxation and dislocation. In certain traumatic situations, i.e., ankle and knee injuries, x-rays may be required with stress applied to the joint to determine the continuity of ligaments. Arthrography with the injection of radiopaque dyes is useful in

delineating the shoulder capsule and rotator cuff, as well as soft tissue structures involved in congenital dislocation of the hip.

SYNOVIAL FLUID EXAMINATION. The examination of synovial fluid may give a specific diagnosis in pyogenic arthritis, tuberculous arthritis, gout, and pseudogout, and may add valuable diagnostic information in most other types of arthritis, including degenerative and rheumatoid arthritis, and in traumatic injuries. The technique of aspiration of a joint will depend on an accurate knowledge of anatomy of the specific joint to be aspirated. The following technique is suggested for the knee joint in which there are moderate degrees of fluid evident in the suprapatellar pouch (Fig. 48-2):

With the patient lying supine and the knee flexed 20° over a small pillow, the entire knee region is prepared with Betadine. With scrupulous aseptic technique, the skin immediately proximal and lateral to the upper pole of the patella, as well as the underlying capsule, is anesthetized with a few milliliters of 2% lidocaine. Using a #18 needle or larger and with the patella pointing toward the ceiling, the insertion is made with the needle parallel with the floor and just anterior to the anterior surface of the femur at the upper pole of the patella.

A large-bore needle is used, since thick, purulent secretion may not be withdrawn through a smaller needle. The joint is completely evacuated of all fluid by displacing fluid from other areas of the joint to the region of the site of entry of the needle. The fluid is collected in (1) a culture tube, (2) a tube with a few crystals of EDTA, and (3) an empty tube.

The synovial fluid is examined for color, appearance, and viscosity. Bacterial culture, Gram stain examination, mucin clot test, white blood cell count, crystal examination, and glucose concentration determination are made (Fig. 48-3).

Color, Turbidity, and Viscosity. Normal synovial fluid is slightly straw-colored. In gout, the fluid may be white or yellow, depending upon the concentration of urate crystals. Septic joint fluid may be gray, thin, and watery or white, purulent, and thick.

A tube of normal joint fluid is completely clear, and

Fig. 48-2. Site of needle penetration for aspiration of the knee joint effusion.

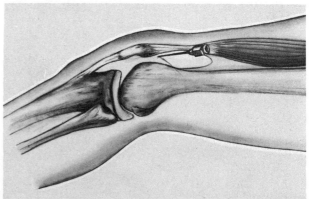

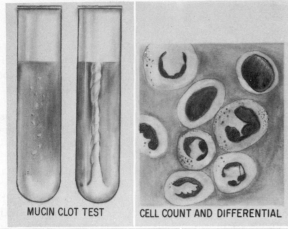

MUCIN CLOT TEST   CELL COUNT AND DIFFERENTIAL

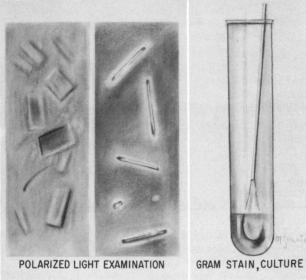

POLARIZED LIGHT EXAMINATION   GRAM STAIN, CULTURE

Fig. 48-3. Synovial fluid analysis.

newsprint can be read through it. When the white cell count is increased or crystals present, turbidity is increased. Viscosity is tested by spreading a drop of fluid between the thumb and index finger. It is usually possible to spread the stringy viscous fluid for 2 in. before it separates. Viscosity is due to the property of the hyaluronic acid polymerization; in conditions of inflammation, it is depolymerized, and thus viscosity is reduced.

Mucin Clot Test. The mucin clot test is an indication of the character of the protein polysaccharide complex of the synovial fluid. The simplest test is the Ropes test, which is performed by adding a few drops of synovial fluid to a small test tube containing 10 ml of 5% acetic acid. A good clot is a firm, ropey clot which on agitation will not separate or fragment. These characteristics are dependent upon normal polymerization and normal concentration of mucin. A good clot is present in normal joints and with degenerative arthritis. A poor clot is one which is small and fragments immediately with agitation. When the

mucin is very poor, only a turbid suspension of fragments may occur. Poor clots occur in the presence of inflammation such as rheumatoid arthritis, gout, or septic arthritis.

Fluid removed at the bedside should be cultured aerobically and also plated on anaerobic media such as chocolate agar if gonoccocal arthritis is suspected. Aspirates should be cultured in hypertonic growth media in order to detect the presence of atypical bacterial forms. Routine cultures for tuberculosis as well as guinea pig inoculation may be carried out if tuberculous arthritis is suspected.

Cell Count and Other Determinations. A total cell count is carried out on the fluid, to which EDTA has been added. If normal white cell counting solution is used, the acidity will precipitate the mucin and make the count inaccurate. The joint fluid is diluted with saline solution to which a drop of methylene blue is added, and a routine count is done in a white cell counting chamber. A differential white blood cell count is done on smears of this fluid stained with Wright's stain.

Joint fluid is examined for the presence of urate or calcium pyrophosphate crystals. It is important not to perform this on fluid to which oxylate or EDTA has been added. The fluid is first centrifuged to concentrate the white blood cells. Supernatant is removed and the sediment examined under polarized light. Urate crystals will be rod-shaped with rounded ends and exhibit strongly negative birefringence under polarized light. Calcium pyrophosphate crystals are rodlike or rhomboid with sharp ends. Under polarized light, they show weakly positive birefringence. If there is doubt about the type present, uricase is added to dissolve the urate crystals.

Glucose determination is performed on the synovial fluid. At the same time, a fasting blood glucose is determined. In conditions with a high white cell count, such as rheumatoid arthritis or infection, the gradient between blood and joint fluid may be 50 mg/100 ml or greater. In the normal, there is 10 mg/100 ml less glucose in joint fluid than in blood.

PYOGENIC ARTHRITIS

If the diagnosis of septic arthritis can be made very early, the chances of restoring a normal joint are excellent. If the diagnosis is missed and the purulent destructive process goes unchecked, disability due to chronic arthritis is the end result.

PATHOGENESIS. Joints may become infected by:

1. Hematogenous spread from septicemia
2. Direct infection by traumatic wounds or at surgical treatment
3. Extension of an adjacent osteomyelitis

In hematogenous infection, a nidus of bacteria is lodged in the synovium and if not destroyed erupts into the joint space. Inflammatory response results in passage of plasma proteins, fibrinogen and plasminogen, into the joint space because of the increased capillary permeability. Leukocytes are attracted into the joint fluid by chemotaxis. The end result of this inflammation is an abscess in the joint space. This abscess is no different from an abscess in other areas of the body, with the exception that the lining or synovial wall may be more permeable to systemic antibiotics.

Proteolytic enzymes from the lysozymes of disintegrating white blood cells and activated plasminogen degrade the proteoglycan of the articular cartilage, exposing collagen fibers. Phemister has pointed out that the white blood cell is necessary for cartilage destruction. The first microscopic change in the articular cartilage is in the central pressure or weight-bearing area where cartilage is in contact with adjacent cartilage. It has been postulated by Curtiss and Klein that the matrix is first lost, exposing the collagen fibers to pressure denaturation. The collagen fibers are then subject to degradation by white blood cell enzymes. The chondrocytes may be killed by bacterial toxins, and, because of poor or absent regenerative capacity, chronic arthritis supervenes.

Staphylococcus aureus and hemolytic streptococci are the two most common organisms producing a pyogenic arthritis. The actual incidence is not important, since the bacterial type in each infection must be determined. Coliform organisms, *Hemophilus influenzae,* pneumococci, meningococci, and *Brucella,* may be the etiologic agents.

CLINICAL MANIFESTATIONS. Septic arthritis may occur at any age but has a higher incidence in patients with debilitating disease and/or on cortisone therapy, or in those with rheumatoid arthritis. Premature infants have a high incidence of septic arthritis of the hip joint.

Patients with hematogenous spread may have more than one joint involved, although localization is commonly confined to one large joint, e.g., knee, hip, shoulder, or elbow; however, any joint may be involved. The patients complain of malaise, chills, fever, and general lassitude. An increase in the white blood cell count with increased polymorphonuclear leukocytes is usually noted. However, in some patients, an elevated sedimentation rate may be the only abnormality.

Examination of the involved joint will reveal the classic signs of inflammation, local tenderness, erythema, swelling, and extreme pain with attempts at motion. The joint will assume a position which is influenced by muscle spasm and pressure/volume relationship. For the knee joint, this is about 20° of flexion. Usually, the patient will not allow complete examination of the joint because of the excruciating pain. In some low-grade infections the range of joint motion may be close to normal early in the course of the disease.

X-rays of a septic joint will show only soft tissue swelling and joint effusion. Bone changes will not be present on the initial x-ray examination (Fig. 48-4). In a child with lax joint capsule and ligaments, the shoulder or hip joint may be subluxed or dislocated as a result of the pressure from the synovial abscess.

DIAGNOSIS. The diagnosis of pyogenic arthritis is made by joint aspiration and synovial fluid analysis. The physician should be cautioned to be reasonably certain that the joint is infected and that the symptoms are not coming

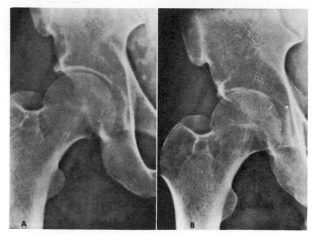

Fig. 48-4. Pyogenic hip joint. *A.* AP x-ray of hip joint taken 48 hours after onset of acute hip pain associated with minor hip injury. Joint space is normal. No bone changes are seen. *B.* Three and one-half weeks later there is complete loss of joint space with no bone changes. Cartilage destruction was due to *Hemophilus influenzae* septic arthritis.

from an overlying cellulitis. This problem occurs in children in whom an infected prepatellar bursitis develops with secondary effusion of the knee joint. If ill-advised aspiration is done through an overlying infection, the joint may be directly inoculated with bacteria. If there is doubt, however, the joint should be aspirated away from the area of superficial infection.

At the time of aspiration, every attempt is made to evacuate the joint completely by compressing fluid into the suprapatellar pouch, from which it is aspirated. The fluid is immediately sent for anaerobic and aerobic cultures, as well as examination for fungus and tuberculosis. A mucin clot test, white blood cell count, and differential and joint fluid glucose determination are carried out on the remainder of the fluid. Blood sugar is drawn simultaneously and the blood sugar synovial fluid gradient determined. An immediate Gram stain examination is carried out on the synovial fluid as well. If organisms are seen in the fluid and the culture is positive, this is diagnostic of sepsis. A poor mucin clot, a white blood cell count between 23,000 and 250,000 with 90 percent polymorphonuclear leukocytes, and a blood/synovial fluid glucose gradient of more than 40 mg/100 ml are consistent with the diagnosis of septic arthritis.

TREATMENT. The treatment of septic arthritis begins with complete aspiration of the joint, which is done for diagnostic purposes. If the Gram stain is positive, immediate antibiotic treatment is instituted. If the Gram stain is negative and the diagnosis is still strongly suspected, antibiotic therapy should be started. Choice of antibiotics will depend upon the suspected organism and the age of the patient. For children, antibiotic coverage for *H. influenzae* should be included; ampicillin is appropriate. For an adult patient with suspected resistant staphylococci, methicillin should be included in the antibiotic regimen.

Surgical Drainage. As soon as the culture report is available, surgical drainage of the involved joint is considered. Surgical drainage is the treatment of choice, but daily aspiration and systemic antibiotic treatment are occasionally indicated. With joints previously damaged by rheumatoid arthritis and where it is possible to evacuate the joint completely by aspiration, or with streptococcal infections where complete daily aspiration is possible, omission of surgical drainage may be appropriate. However, when it is not possible to evacuate the joint completely because of loculated collections of fluid or when biopsy is necessary, surgical drainage should be undertaken as soon as the diagnosis is certain. All infections of the hip must be drained, since the surrounding musculature makes it difficult to monitor the adequacy of needle aspiration drainage. For the knee joint, two parapatellar incisions are necessary, while the hip joint usually requires one well-placed posterior incision. Septic hips of children should always be drained surgically in order to minimize the chance of dislocation from pressure of the intraarticular abscess.

Technique of Posterior Drainage of the Hip Joint. An incision is made parallel with the femoral neck, beginning at the base of the greater trochanter and directed toward the posterior superior iliac spine. The gluteus maximus is split in line with its fibers and the short external rotators divided after retracting the sciatic nerve. The distended capsule is then incised longitudinally and the joint evacuated. Drains are inserted down to the capsule but not into the joint.

Postoperatively, antibiotics are continued, and the patient is nursed supine with the leg in 8 to 10 lb. of Buck's traction.

Adjunctive Measures to Treatment. In addition to surgical drainage and treatment with systemic antibiotics, the patient and joint should be placed at rest. In the case of the knee or hip joint, skin traction is applied to the leg for purposes of immobilization, and an attempt is made to minimize cartilage compression at the point of contact. Where traction is not possible, i.e., for the elbow or wrist, a posterior plaster splint is applied to the joint for immobilization in a position of function.

Antibiotic therapy is continued for a minimum of 4 weeks or until the sedimentation rate returns to normal. If the septic arthritis is an extension of adjacent osteomyelitis, antibiotic treatment is indicated until osteomyelitis has been successfully controlled, i.e., 6 weeks or longer.

Restoration of Joint Motion. If the joint has been treated by closed methods, i.e., aspiration and antibiotics, when the joint remains dry and asymptomatic, early active range-of-motion exercises are started. If treated by surgical drainage, joint motion is not begun until the wounds are granulating or completely closed. Early motion is important in giving a good result.

If damage to the articular cartilage occurs, patients may have residual stiffness, deformity, and a painful joint. Depending upon the severity of symptoms, reconstructive procedures including arthrodesis, arthroplasty, or osteotomy may be necessary.

BONE AND JOINT TUBERCULOSIS

General Considerations

Skeletal tuberculosis is now an uncommon infection in the United States, although it is still a major problem in parts of Asia and Africa. The incidence in the United States has dropped remarkably because of the control of bovine sources, protective measures for infected patients, and the effective use of antituberculous chemotherapy.

Tuberculosis involving the spine or peripheral joints is always secondary to infection elsewhere in the body. The primary infection is usually pulmonary.

PATHOLOGY. The most common site of skeletal involvement with tuberculosis is the spine. The highest incidence occurs in the vertebral bodies opposite the kidney. Hodgson et al. believe that infection is spread via the veins or lymphatics from the kidneys. Once infection starts in a vertebral body, it may spread across the disc space margin to involve the adjacent vertebrae. By tracking beneath the anterior longitudinal ligament, it may spread through Batson's plexus of veins. Infection in the dorsal spine usually is contained beneath the anterior longitudinal ligament, but in the lumbar spine the intimate origin of fibers of the psoas muscle results in spread into the psoas and formation of a psoas abscess.

Peripheral joint tuberculosis involves synovial membrane, bone, and cartilage. It is not certain whether the bone or synovium is infected first, but the result is involvement of both structures. Tuberculous synovitis with tubercle formation and synovial pannus develops, which gradually covers the cartilage and invades the underlying subchondral bone. The cartilage is the last structure to be involved. In contrast to pyogenic joints which have increased leukocytic protease activity, the cartilage in tuberculous joints is destroyed by interference with its underlying circulation. The end result of this process is complete destruction of the joint. Fibrous ankylosis of adjacent surfaces is a common sequel, but spontaneous bony ankylosis is rare.

CLINICAL MANIFESTATIONS. Any chronic monarthritis should be suspected of being tuberculous. There is frequently a history of pulmonary disease, although tuberculous monarthritis may be the first presentation of the systemic illness. Any of the large joints may be infected. Tuberculous arthritis may occur at any age but is more common in children.

The clinical course is insidious, and patients have symptoms for weeks or months prior to seeking consultation. Low-grade pain occurring at night is common. Limitation of joint motion with local synovial swelling is present. Examination of the joint reveals local synovitis out of proportion to the content of synovial fluid. There may be limitation of joint motion and signs of higher local temperature over the joint, but erythema is uncommon. Frequently, in children, the onset of tuberculosis of the hip is suggested by a limp and a history of pain and night crying.

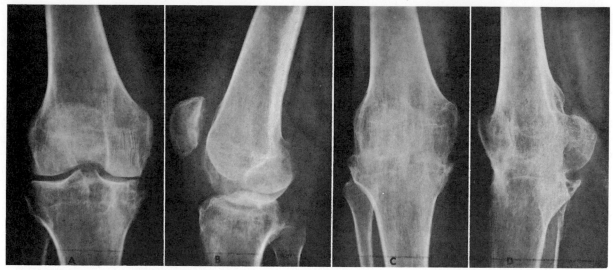

Fig. 48-5. Tuberculosis of the knee joint. *A* and *B*. AP and lateral x-rays of the knee showing erosion of the margins of the medial tibial plateau and medial femoral condyle. There is only minimal joint space narrowing. *C* and *D*. Postsurgical arthrodesis of the knee.

ROENTGENOGRAPHIC FINDINGS. Early in the course of the infection, there may be roentgenographic evidence of soft tissue swelling and adjacent osteoporosis. As the disease progresses, marginal erosion occurring at the cartilage synovial junction may be seen on both sides of the joint (Fig. 48-5). The joint space commonly maintains its integrity because cartilage destruction occurs late in the course of the disease.

In children with long-standing tuberculous synovitis, there may be enlargement of the adjacent growing epiphyses due to chronic inflammation. In long-standing disease in adults, the joint may be completely destroyed with areas of necrosis secondary to undermining, and "kissing" sequestra develop.

DIAGNOSIS. The specific diagnosis of tuberculous arthritis is dependent upon the recovery of organisms from the joint or demonstration of organisms in granulomas on pathologic section. The demonstration of pulmonary lesions or other joint infections as well as positive Mantoux test results are helpful but are not pathognomonic. Joint aspiration, smear, and culture or guinea pig inoculation with the synovial fluid should be carried out in all suspected cases. Synovial fluid analysis will reveal a leukocytic response of less than 20,000 and a poor mucin clot. If the diagnosis cannot be made by joint fluid aspiration, open biopsy should be done without hesitation, since early treatment is mandatory.

TREATMENT. Treatment of skeletal tuberculosis includes (1) general supportive measures, (2) chemotherapy, (3) local treatment of the involved joint or joints, (4) surgical treatment.

General supportive measures include adequate protein and caloric intake, hydration, and proper rest. Patients are started on antituberculous chemotherapy. If the chemotherapy is started before significant necrosis and caseation or walling off has occurred, treatment is associated with a high success rate.

Patients are started on triple-drug therapy until culture reports of the specific organisms are available. Streptomycin is administered in 1-Gm doses daily for 2 or 3 months and then twice weekly for an additional 3 months. Para-aminosalicylic acid (PAS) is administered in doses of 12 Gm/day in three or four divided doses. Isoniazid (INH) is administered at the rate of 3 to 5 mg/kg of body weight, which is about 300 mg for an adult. When the cultures are available and if resistance to one or all of these is present, other agents such as viomycin, Pyrazinamide, oxytetracycline, or cycloserine may be indicated. Tuberculous chemotherapy is continued for at least 18 months.

The treatment of the specific joint involves immobilization by traction, plaster splinting, or casts, combined with bed rest. If the infection is diagnosed early, local immobilization combined with chemotherapy may be sufficient. However, if the joint does not respond to these measures or if the disease has already progressed to involve subchondral bone, surgical joint clearance including synovectomy and excision of tuberculous foci is necessary. Joint debridement with the excision of involved tissues may be quite successful in controlling the local infection and still allow a partially mobile joint. If the joint is totally destroyed, arthrodesis of the involved joint is the treatment of choice.

Tuberculosis of the Spine

Tuberculous spondylitis (Pott's disease) is the most common form of skeletal tuberculosis (Fig. 48-6). The infection is located in the anterior border of the vertebral body, commonly in the thoracic region. Multiple areas may be involved. The infection spreads across the disc space to

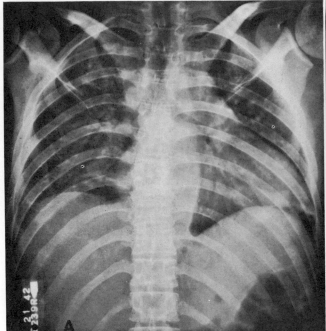
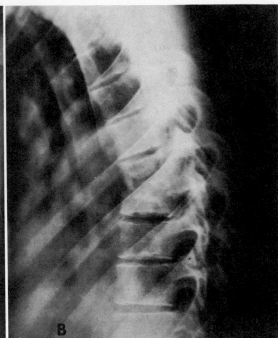

Fig. 48-6. Spinal tuberculosis (Pott's disease). *A.* AP x-ray of thoracic spine showing large paravertebral abscess. *B.* Lateral x-ray of thoracic spine showing disruption of the T_7–T_8 interspace with kyphotic deformity.

involve the adjacent upper or lower vertebrae. The disc space is lost because of loss of fluid from the disc. Actual destruction of the disc does not occur early, because of lack of proteolytic enzymes. The disc may be sequestrated into the paraspinal abscess which develops if treatment is delayed.

If there is sufficient destruction of the involved vertebrae, damage to the posterior-lying spinal cord may occur from the pressure of abscess formation or from angular deformity at the site of infection.

Symptoms of Pott's disease include back pain, limitation of spinal motion, paraspinal muscle spasm, and the systemic signs of infection, as well. With cord involvement, the patient will have neurologic signs and symptoms involving the lower extremities.

Treatment requires specific diagnosis. The x-ray findings of tuberculous spondylitis and staphylococcal disc space infection are the same. The diagnosis rests on the recovery of organisms or characteristic histologic evidence from the site of infection. The direct anterior approach to the spine, as described by Hodgson and Stock, provides an effective means for early diagnosis and stabilization of the spine at the same time.

Patients suspected of having spinal tuberculosis are started on triple-drug chemotherapy and bed rest in anterior and posterior plaster shells. After adequate chemotherapy has been established, the spine is exposed by the anterior approach and biopsy material obtained. All infected disc and bone are excised and the adjacent vertebral bodies stabilized with autogenous rib or iliac bone grafts.

Postoperatively patients are nursed in plaster shells or Bradford frames until consolidation has occurred at the site of bone grafting. If paraplegia is present, immediate decompression of the spinal cord is mandatory via the same anterior approach or, occasionally, costotransversectomy. Laminectomy is contraindicated, because it decreases posterior spine stability and allows the anterior-lying abscess, which is not drained, to increase pressure on the dural contents.

Tuberculosis of the Hip

When the diagnosis of tuberculosis of the hip is made early, bed rest with skin traction to the hip, combined with antituberculous chemotherapy, may suffice. If the infection cannot be controlled, open arthrotomy through the Smith-Petersen approach and joint debridement should be carried out to remove the necrotic material. Postoperatively, the patient is kept in traction until the wound is healed. Chemotherapy is continued, and early active motion of the joint is instituted. With severe destruction of the hip joint, surgical arthrodesis by the method of Trumbell or Brittain may be required.

GONOCOCCAL ARTHRITIS

Gonococcal arthritis occurs in females secondary to gonococcal cervicitis or vaginitis. Since the clinical manifestations of the primary cervical infection are relatively occult, treatment may not be effected, and the patient is subject to gonococcal septicemia and gonococcal arthritis. In contrast, the male with gonococcal urethritis has symptoms, seeks early medical treatment, and rarely presents with a gonococcal joint infection.

CLINICAL MANIFESTATIONS. Symptoms usually begin with migratory polyarthralgia, followed by localization in one or two joints. The knee, elbow, and wrist are common sites of infection. A variable febrile course may occur concomitantly with the joint infection.

DIAGNOSIS. The diagnosis is dependent upon the recovery of gonococcal organisms from the septic joint. Cultures of joint fluid are performed on chocolate agar and incubated in 10% carbon dioxide. Aspirates should be cultured in hypertonic broth media to detect the presence of bacterial L forms. It is important to inoculate the culture medium at the bedside and to withhold antibiotics until the culture has been taken.

Synovial fluid analysis will reveal white cell counts in the region of 20,000, with poor mucin and depressed glucose content, which are not in themselves diagnostic of gonococcal infection.

X-rays early in the course of the disease will show only soft tissue swelling.

Cervical smears and cultures should be obtained to prove the primary focus of the infection.

TREATMENT. Intramuscular penicillin G, 1 to 2 million units/day for 2 weeks, is sufficient to eradicate the primary focus and the intraarticular infections completely. With a patient failing to respond to penicillin therapy, other organisms, Reiter's syndrome, or early rheumatoid arthritis should be considered. Local treatment of the joint by immobilization is required and provides additional symptomatic relief. With early adequate penicillin treatment, recovery of a normal joint is the rule.

RHEUMATOID ARTHRITIS

General Considerations

Rheumatoid arthritis is a systemic disease affecting any organ of the body including those of the cardiovascular, respiratory, nervous, and musculoskeletal systems.

PATHOLOGY. The pathologic features of rheumatoid arthritis are found in the diarthrodial joints as well as in adjacent tissues, tendons, tendon sheaths, and bursa.

Articular Changes. The synovitis associated with rheumatoid arthritis is variable and depends on the duration and location of the inflammation. The synovium is congested and edematous with fibrin exudates on the surface or diffusely dispersed throughout the synovium itself. There may be diffuse infiltration of polymorphonuclear leukocytes with localized and nodular collections of small lymphocytes. Plasma cells are commonly arranged about small blood vessels. The end result is thickened hypertrophied villous synovial tissue, covered with fibrin and infiltrated with both acute and chronic inflammatory cells. These changes are not specific for rheumatoid arthritis.

The articular cartilage may be covered by the synovial granulation tissue called pannus (Fig. 48-7). At the cartilage synovial junction, the synovial granulation tissue in-

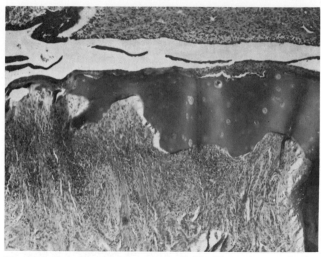

Fig. 48-7. Pathology of rheumatoid arthritis. Photomicrograph of articular cartilage of the metacarpal head showing synovial pannus on the surface of articular cartilage with pannus invading, destroying, and undermining the articular cartilage in the region of the subchondral bone.

vades the subchondral bone, causing erosive changes, which are visible by x-ray. New periosteal bone formation develops in the region of the capsular attachments, and subchondral bone becomes osteoporotic.

As the granulation tissue and pannus increase, the articular cartilage is eroded. The area of calcified cartilage increases in thickness, effectively diminishing the thickness of the uncalcified cartilage. Roentgenographically, the joint space is narrower, because of the advancement of calcified cartilage as well as the loss of surface contour. The end result of the cartilage destruction and synovial inflammation may be complete disintegration of the joint and instability, with or without superimposed degenerative changes. The joint may undergo fibrous or bony ankylosis.

Subcutaneous Nodules and Other Lesions. In about 25 percent of patients subcutaneous nodules develop commonly over the subcutaneous border of the ulna, olecranon process, dorsal aspects of the fingers, or any area receiving recurrent trauma. There are characteristic histologic findings in the usual subcutaneous nodule consisting of a central area of fibrinoid necrosis surrounded by a second layer of palisading fibroblasts, enveloped by a third layer of diffuse chronic inflammatory cell infiltration. Similar nodules occur in the tenosynovial lining of tendons. Ruptures, due to attrition or invasion by the rheumatoid process, may result.

Skeletal muscle commonly has scattered foci of chronic inflammatory cells. Aggregations of lymphocytes and chronic inflammatory cells may be present in the endoneurium and perineurium of peripheral nerves. The granuloma-like lesions resembling the subcutaneous nodules may occur in valve leaflets or any of the layers of the heart. Pericarditis is present in about 40 percent of cases of rheumatoid arthritis. Granulomatous lesions also occur in the lungs. Anthracite-coal miners develop silicotic nodule formation coupled with rheumatoid arthritis. Rheumatoid arthritis patients may demonstrate uveitis or episcleritis. There may be involvement of lacrimal and salivary glands with lymphoid infiltration.

CLINICAL MANIFESTATIONS. Rheumatoid arthritis affects two or three females to one male and occurs at any age with the peak incidence in the thirties and forties. Involvement of joints may be sudden but is usually insidious without antecedent cause. Patients commonly have stiffness of the hands or affected joints in the morning or after inactivity. Muscular weakness and atrophy occur and may be related to the joint pain but are also due to lymphocytic infiltration of the muscles.

DIAGNOSIS. The diagnosis of a patient with long-standing classic rheumatoid arthritis and deformity is not difficult, but in the early stages and with unusual presentations the diagnosis may be quite difficult. There is no specific histopathologic character, since the pathologic findings in the arthritis associated with lupus, dermatomyositis, or periarthritis may be indistinguishable from classic rheumatoid arthritis. Laboratory tests such as the sheep cell agglutination test and latex fixation test are not specific and are positive in other diseases. Because of the difficulty and confusion associated with this diagnosis, the committee on diagnosis of the American Rheumatism Association, under Marion Ropes, set up criteria to aid in this diagnosis. The following features of the disease should be considered:

1. Morning stiffness present for longer than 15 minutes
2. Pain with motion or direct tenderness in at least one joint
3. Swelling unrelated to bony overgrowth of at least one joint for at least 6 weeks
4. Swelling observed in a second joint within a 3-month interval
5. Symmetric joint swelling excluding distal interphalangeal (DIP) joints
6. Presence of subcutaneous nodules over bony prominences
7. X-ray changes consistent with rheumatoid arthritis
8. Positive sheep cell agglutination test or latex fixation test

Fig. 48-8. X-ray findings in rheumatoid arthritis: soft tissue swelling about MP joints and IP joints; erosive changes in the third metacarpal head, right; marked joint space narrowing of the right PIP joint of the index finger; marked destruction and loss of joint space of the carpal bones; erosion of the styloid bilaterally.

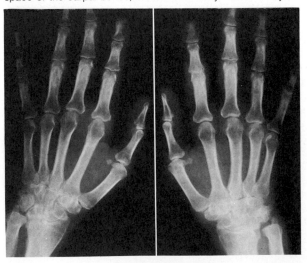

9. Poor mucin clot on synovial fluid analysis
10. Characteristic histopathologic changes in the synovial membrane on biopsy
11. Characteristic histopathologic changes in nodules

Classic rheumatoid arthritis would have seven of the above criteria with continuous joint swelling for 6 weeks. A definite diagnosis requires five criteria with continuous joint swelling for at least 6 weeks. A "probable rheumatoid" has three of the above criteria and joint symptoms for at least 4 weeks.

A possible diagnosis of rheumatoid arthritis is suggested if two or more of the following symptoms are present for at least 3 weeks:

1. Morning stiffness
2. Recurrent pain on motion
3. Observed joint swelling
4. Subcutaneous nodules
5. Elevated sedimentation rate
6. Iritis

Rheumatoid arthritis is excluded if a diagnosis of lupus, polyarteritis nodosa, or erythema nodosum can be made. Similarly, rheumatic fever, gout, tuberculous arthritis, Reiter's syndrome, hypertrophic pulmonary osteoarthropathy, ochranosis, multiple myeloma, or lymphomas may simulate the joint findings.

LABORATORY FINDINGS. A normochromic or hyperchromic, normocytic anemia of moderate severity occurs with rheumatoid arthritis. The sedimentation rate is elevated and is a good index of the activity of the disease.

In the serum of 90% of adult patients with rheumatoid arthritis the anti-γ-globulin factor called *rheumatoid factor* is present. Only 20 percent of juvenile patients with rheumatoid arthritis have positive results of tests for rheumatoid factor. Rheumatoid factor is measured by the sheep cell agglutination test or latex fixation test.

Positive lupus erythematosus (LE) cell preparation may be present in less than one-fourth of patients. Serum complement level may be normal or elevated.

Synovial Fluid Analysis. Analysis of synovial fluid from a rheumatoid joint will reveal a poor mucin clot, decrease in synovial fluid glucose, joint fluid leukocytosis reaching 50,000 or more, and decreased viscosity.

ROENTGENOGRAPHIC FINDINGS. The roentgenographic findings (Figs. 48-8, 48-9) in the extremities of early rheumatoid arthritis are related to the presence of destructive influences of the hyperplastic synovia. As the disease progresses, degenerative or responsive changes in the joint may be superimposed upon the rheumatoid process. The earliest x-ray changes are best identified in the involved hands. Similar processes and changes may occur in any joint.

The earliest finding is soft tissue swelling. This fusiform swelling may be about the proximal interphalangeal (PIP) joint, metatarsophalangeal (MP) joints, or radiocarpal joint. The presence of persistent synovial swelling causes osteoporosis in the ends of the bones adjacent to the inflammation. With long-standing arthritis, osteoporosis is a common finding and is in part related to disuse atrophy of the bone.

The presence of synovial and capsular inflammation produces new periosteal bone in the region of capsular attachment. This is noted particularly in the region of capsular attachments about the PIP and MP joints. Proximal to the capsular attachment, there may be cortical involvement with irregularity produced by osteoclastic resorption. The presence of rheumatoid synovium causes erosion at the cartilage synovial junction and on the so-called bare area of bone. Erosions occur commonly on the metacarpal heads, PIP joints, radial margin of the navicular, ulnar styloid, and ulnar aspect of the triquetrum. The damage caused by the synovium when seen in profile appears to be a pseudocyst. The presence of vascular tenosynovium in the region of the radial styloid or on the dorsal aspect of the first metacarpal may cause resorption of bone resulting in irregularity of the bone cortex.

Joint space narrowing may occur quite early in the disease or late. The presence of joint space narrowing in the absence of sclerosis or degenerative changes is indicative of an inflammatory process of the rheumatoid type. With progression of the rheumatoid process, joint subluxations, ulnar deviation at the MP joints (Fig. 48-10), and dislocation may occur. If the patient is actively using this hand, superimposed degenerative changes may occur.

In the juvenile, the presence of rheumatoid synovitis causes soft tissue swelling and osteoporosis. Increased local vascularity results in circumferential enlargement and change in shape of the epiphyses. Leg length inequality may occur as a result of unilateral epiphyseal stimulation. Juvenile rheumatoid arthritis is more likely to go on to ankylosis in comparison with the erosion and instability which predominates in adults.

Management

Treatment of patients with rheumatoid arthritis should be a multidisciplined approach. Ideally, a team should consist of a rheumatologist, orthopedist, physiotherapist, occupational therapist, and social worker. Only by combining the efforts and interests of these individuals can maximal therapy be rendered to the arthritic. The team should strive for early diagnosis and, therefore, early treatment.

By nature of the systemic manifestations of rheumatoid arthritis, it is, at present, a surgical disease only by default. In previous years, many patients with rheumatoid arthritis were treated surgically for established deformity with no attempt at prevention of deformity. The orthopedic surgeon should be involved in the care of every rheumatoid patient. The basic aim of treatment is to halt the progressive destruction caused by this disease, to relieve the patient's pain, and to allow him to continue functioning without the hazard of progressive deformity. This is not possible for all patients, but the progress of the disease usually can be minimized with adequate medical and physical therapy and well-timed surgical intervention.

MEDICAL MANAGEMENT

Medical management includes administration of antiinflammatory drugs and analgesics, as well as physical and

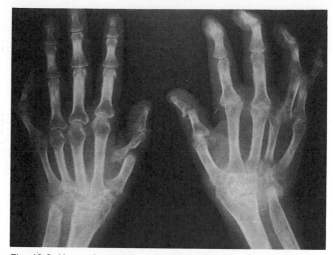

Fig. 48-9. X-ray changes in rheumatoid arthritis: severe destruction of radiocarpal articulation with subluxation and ulna deviation at the wrist; loss of ulna styloid bilaterally due to the rheumatoid process; dislocation of the PIP joint of the left thumb and dislocation of the right fourth and fifth finger MP joints and left MP joint; diffuse joint space narrowing of many IP joints.

Fig. 48-10. Dorsal and ventral photographs of a rheumatoid arthritic hand showing a mild degree of ulnar deviation with MP joint swelling.

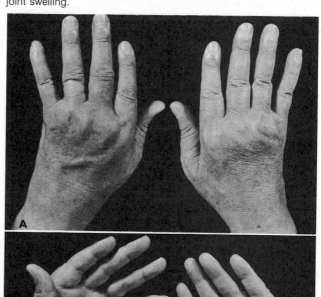

emotional supportive treatment. The drugs now available for treating this form of arthritis are numerous, but Huskisson has suggested a simple classification:

1. Simple analgesics, e.g., aspirin in small doses (2 mg daily), paracetamol, codeine.
2. Analgesics with minor anti-inflammatory properties, e.g., ibuprofen, naproxen, nefenamid acid.
3. Analgesics with major anti-inflammatory properties, e.g., indomethacin, phenylbutazone, aspirin (at least 3.6 Gm daily).
4. Pure anti-inflammatory drugs, e.g., corticosteroids, corticotropin.
5. "Slow-acting" drugs, e.g., gold, penicillamine, the antimalarials, and immunosuppressives.

Corticosteroids have a place in the management of rheumatoid arthritis, especially in life-threatening situations of vasculitis or severe exacerbations of the disease, but are contraindicated as routine treatment.

ORTHOPEDIC MANAGEMENT

PHYSICAL THERAPY. The patient should be informed about deforming forces on inflamed joints. For example, patients with MP joint involvement should understand that grasping heavy objects between thumb and forefingers or grasping objects over long periods which requires excessive force will put undue strain on the inflamed capsule, contributing to subluxation and ulnar drift. Patients with acutely swollen knees should be cautioned about putting excessive stress on the knees when arising from a chair, walking, or standing for long periods. Patients with hip disease should be cautioned to use crutches during acute flare-up of the joint disease.

Inflamed joints should be protected against mechanical trauma that aggravates and complicates the inflammatory destruction. An inflamed joint assumes the position in which the greatest volume of fluid can be accommodated in the joint with the least capsular pressure. In the knee, this is about 20° of flexion. If a contracture in the position of 20° flexion occurs, the patient will have difficulty walking and will superimpose mechanical trauma on the joint inflammation. Wrists go into flexion, which weakens grip. Metatarsophalangeal joints drift into flexion and ulnar deviation, weakening grasp and function.

Anterior plaster shells should be constructed to hold the

Fig. 48-11. Night wrist splint for rheumatoid hand. Wrist is in slight radial deviation, in dorsiflexion with MP joints in extension and IP joints in slight flexion.

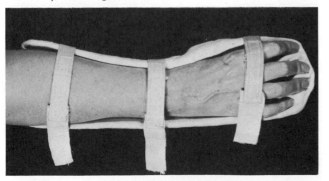

wrists in 30° of dorsiflexion, MP joints in extension, and interphalangeal (IP) joints in slight flexion (Fig. 48-11). Posterior plaster shells are constructed to maintain the knees in full extension and the ankles at 90°. Splints are always worn at night and may be worn continuously during the acute episode.

It is extremely important for patients with joint disease to maintain active muscle power. Patients are instructed to carry out daily range-of-motion exercises. This should be done without putting undue force on the capsule of the joint. Knee joints should be exercised while the patient is sitting or lying without body weight applied. Patients should do isometric exercises in a position of function, i.e., full extension for the knees. Patients with cervical spine involvement are urged to maintain a range of full extension. Inflamed hips will develop flexion deformities which can be minimized by passive stretching daily. The patient accomplishes this by lying in a prone position for 15 to 20 minutes twice a day.

The deformities and disabilities from rheumatoid arthritis are insidious. The surgeon should be prepared to fit patients with lower extremity braces as well as wrist splints. The patient who must continue to work and walk with severely involved knees can be helped by the use of a long leg brace with the knee locked in full extension. Valgus and varus deformities involving ankle and subtalar joints can be stabilized by the use of double upright short leg braces.

SURGICAL TREATMENT OF RHEUMATOID ARTHRITIS. The presence of inflamed rheumatoid synovium is intimately associated with joint destruction, but the mechanism has not been defined. When the biochemical processes are understood, it is hoped that systemic or local pharmacologic agents will be developed to interrupt the destructive processes. At the present time, when proper joint rest, modification of activity, and systemic anti-inflammatory medications are unable to control the rheumatoid process, early synovectomy is indicated. If this is carried out before there is significant joint space narrowing and bony collapse, it can protect against joint destruction and effectively relieve pain. As reported in multicenter trials, after 3 years, knees treated by early synovectomy were less painful and tender than those treated by conservative measures and had less effusion. This procedure did not halt the irreversible changes in all treated joints but significantly slowed the development of further pathological changes in some knee joints. However, the results from metacarpophalangeal joints when treated by synovectomy showed no advantage over control joints at 3 years, either clinically or radiographically.

Synovectomy is particularly applicable when synovitis is concentrated in a few joints. However, when the synovitis is generalized, early synovectomy is indicated, especially in the hands and knees.

TECHNIQUE OF KNEE SYNOVECTOMY

Under tourniquet control, a long, curved, median parapatellar incision is made, starting 2 in. proximal to the patella, curving medially over the medial condyle of the femur, and extending distally to end in the region of the tibial tubercle. The capsule and medial patellar retinaculum are divided in line with the incision. The incision is carried across the insertion of the vastus medialis and extends proximally into the quadriceps tendon.

The synovium is excised with meticulous dissection from the suprapatellar pouch en bloc by finding the avascular plane between synovium and capsule or femur. Pannus encroaching upon margins of articular cartilage is wiped off with a sponge or dissected free by sharp dissection. Care is taken to excise all synovium from both lateral and medial recesses. Menisci usually are excised. Synovium invading and surrounding cruciate ligaments is excised. Fibrillated cartilage from the undersurface of the patella is excised with a scalpel. The tourniquet is removed prior to closure, and all bleeders are cauterized. The quadriceps tendon and patellar retinaculum are repaired with interrupted chromic catgut sutures, and the skin is closed in a routine fashion. The knee is splinted in extension for 5 days, during which time the patient does hourly isometric quadriceps exercises. In 5 days the posterior splint is removed and active knee flexion started. The patient is allowed to continue active knee motion within pain tolerance and is allowed out of bed for non-weight-bearing crutch walking. The patient should have 90° of knee flexion by 3 weeks. If not, the knee is manipulated into flexion under general anesthesia.

This technique excises the anterior two-thirds of the synovium. In some instances, it may be necessary at the second operation to excise the posterior one-third through a lateral or posterior incision.

KNEE SURGERY FOR INSTABILITY

If the rheumatoid process has progressed to the point where cartilage substance has been lost, there is concomitant relative lengthening of the collateral ligaments and, therefore, instability. There may be a varus or valgus deformity associated with the cartilage destruction. Synovectomy alone at this stage of the disease is not sufficient to relieve pain and provide knee stability. Such patients require total knee arthroplasty (Fig. 48-12), in which the femoral surface is replaced with metal and the tibial surface with high-density polyethylene. If collateral ligament damage or bone destruction is severe or marked flexion contractures are present, total knee prosthesis with built-in stability (constrained or semiconstrained) is necessary. In rare situations the problem will require the use of a hinge prosthesis.

As a salvage procedure, arthrodesis of the knee is an effective means for controlling pain and relieving instability. However, the patient should have a good ipsilateral hip joint and a mobile functioning contralateral knee joint.

Total knee arthroplasty presently is being used for patients with severe damage to the knee joint as an alternative to arthrodesis. The principle is similar to that used in total hip arthroplasty in which the components are fixed to the bone with acrylic cement. This procedure is in an early period of development but promises to be a significant advance for the unstable knee.

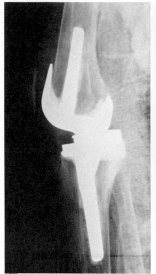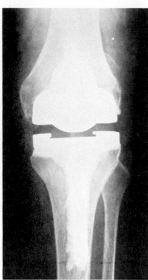

Fig. 48-12. *A*. Internal x-ray of Murray-Shaw total knee prosthesis. *B*. Anteroposterior x-ray of Murray-Shaw total knee prosthesis.

HIP SURGERY

At the present time, there has been insufficient experience with prophylactic synovectomy in the rheumatoid hip with early involvement. However, for the patient with moderate or severe hip disease with disabling pain, total hip replacement is the treatment of choice. (See Total Hip Replacement, under Osteoarthritis.) When there is failure of total hip replacement or infection, the Girdlestone pseudarthrosis will provide pain relief and good hip mobility.

TECHNIQUE FOR GIRDLESTONE PSEUDARTHROSIS

The femoral head is excised at the base of the neck. The lateral portion of the acetabulum is osteotomized and excised to construct a parallel surface to articulate with the osteotomized base of the neck. In selected cases, the iliopsoas tendon may be reinserted distad on the anterior aspect of the femoral shaft to assist in stability. Postoperatively, the patient is maintained in 6 to 8 lb of Buck's traction in a balanced suspension apparatus for 4 weeks. After soft tissue and capsular healing, active exercises including adduction, flexion, and extension are initiated. The patient is allowed on crutches and at 6 to 8 weeks bears weight using an ischial weight-bearing brace. Crutches are converted to a cane as pain is tolerated. Most patients develop sufficient stability about the hip to discard the ischial weight-bearing brace. Most patients achieve improved motion and marked relief in comfort and continue to improve to as long as 3 years postoperation.

ANKLE AND FOOT

Most rheumatoid deformities about the ankle and hind part of the foot can be controlled by adequate bracing techniques. An occasional patient will require bony stabili-

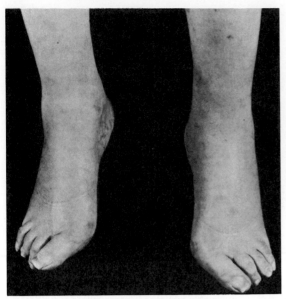

Fig. 48-13. Rheumatoid synovitis involving the hind part of the foot and the forefoot. Note claw toes with lateral deviation of all toes.

zation with correction of deformity at the ankle or subtalar joints. The insertion of a total ankle in which the damaged joint surfaces are replaced with metal and polyethylene may eliminate the need for arthrodesis.

FOREFOOT

The rheumatoid process occurs almost as frequently in the MP joints of the toes (Fig. 48-13) as in the hands. Claw toes with dislocation of the MP joints and flexion of the IP joints is the resultant deformity. The patient is unable to displace forefoot weight between the toes and the metatarsal heads. With the loss of fat pad beneath metatarsal heads and increased weight over this area, painful calluses develop, and difficulty in ambulation occurs. The Hoffman operation, which consists of proximal partial

Fig. 48-14. Hoffman operation used in rheumatoid deformities of the forefoot to relieve metatarsal head pressure and improve toe function and alignment. Metatarsal head and proximal portions of phalanges are excised through transverse dorsal incision.

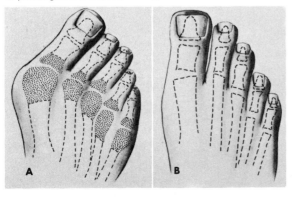

phalangectomy of all MP joints and excision of the metatarsal heads, will give great relief to the patient and improve gait (Fig. 48-14).

SURGICAL REHABILITATION OF THE RHEUMATOID HAND. The rheumatoid process commonly involves the PIP joints, MP joints, carpal joints, and the tenosynovium of the flexor and extensor tendons about the wrist.

The rheumatoid synovitis of the MP joints causes capsular distension and laxity of collateral ligaments (Fig. 48-10). As the disease progresses, the MP joints sublux anteriorly and ulnarward, causing ulnar drift of the fingers. The extensor tendons are dislocated into the gutters between the metacarpal heads, accentuating the deformity.

Joint involvement of the MP joints as well as rheumatoid disease involvement of the intrinsic muscle mass may produce flexion contracture of the MP joints, hyperextension of the PIP joints, and flexion of the DIP joints. This is the so-called "swan-neck deformity of the intrinsic-plus hand."

Involvement of the PIP joint may result in rupture of the central slip of the extensor tendon crossing the PIP joint, which allows the lateral bands to sublux anteriorly, and a typical boutonnière flexion deformity of the PIP joint develops.

With synovial distension of the MP joint of the thumb, lateral instability occurs, usually with a flexion deformity due to damage or attrition of the extensor pollicis brevis as it inserts into the proximal phalanx. Synovitis may similarly injure the interphalangeal joint of the thumb. Destruction of the carpometacarpal joint may interfere with opposition.

Synovial inflammation of the carpal joints will result in limitation of wrist dorsiflexion and cause anterior subluxation of the wrist. Involvement of the distal radioulnar joint may cause dorsal dislocation of the ulna, interference with wrist rotation, flexion, and extension.

Tenosynovitis occurs about the extensor tendons, and rheumatoid nodules may develop in the tendons themselves. The tendon may stretch or rupture because of the tenosynovial inflammation process or because of mechanical erosion from the involved distal radioulnar joint. The common tendon ruptures occur in those tendons crossing the distal radioulnar joint, the extensor tendons to ring and small finger, and the extensor digiti minimi proprius (Fig. 48-15). The extensor pollicis longus may be involved along its path across the dorsum of the wrist.

Flexor tenosynovitis is commonly overlooked because of the deep position of these structures. With sufficient tenosynovitis, there may be compression of the median nerve in the carpal tunnel. Tenosynovitis of the flexor tendons will cause limitation of active motion of the fingers in the absence of MP or IP joint involvement.

METATARSOPHALANGEAL JOINT SYNOVECTOMY

Metatarsophalangeal joint synovectomy is indicated when the synovitis cannot be controlled by conservative measures. Minimal subluxation can be corrected at the same time, but if severe ulnar drift is present, arthroplasty is required.

TECHNIQUE. Under tourniquet control, a transverse incision is made across the dorsal midpoint of the finger metacarpal heads (Fig. 48-16). Care is taken not to interrupt the veins draining the fingers. A vertical incision is made on the radial side of the MP joint extensor hood, radial to the extensor tendon. A plane is developed between the extensor hood and the underlying capsule and synovium, which are excised en bloc. Pannus is excised from the cartilage as well. The synovial recesses between collateral ligaments and metacarpal heads are also excised.

Ulnar subluxation of the extensor tendons is corrected by reefing the capsule at the time of closure. Involvement of the MP joint of the thumb requires synovectomy through a dorsal curved incision.

Postoperatively, the hand is immobilized in a bulky compression dressing, keeping the MP joints in full extension and neutral position with all IP joints in a position of 45° of flexion. The compression dressing is continued for 3 to 4 weeks and active motion instituted.

If an intrinsic-plus deformity is present, Littler releases in addition to MP joint synovectomy are carried out. Individual dorsal incisions are made over each MP joint, and the lateral triangular bands which represent intrinsic insertions, responsible for extension of the PIP joint, are divided and excised. Postoperatively, the MP joints are kept in extension and the PIPs in 45° flexion.

ARTHROPLASTY

When there is subluxation or dislocation of the MP joint which cannot be corrected by crossed intrinsic muscle transfer, MP arthroplasties are indicated. The technique of arthroplasty using an implant described by Swanson or Niebauer is recommended.

FLEXIBLE IMPLANT ARTHROPLASTY (SWANSON). A transverse incision is made across the necks of the metacarpals. Dorsal veins are retracted but not divided. A longitudinal incision is made on the ulnar aspect of each extensor hood. The neck of the metacarpal is divided, and the metacarpal head, lateral ligaments, synovium, and capsule removed. Appropriate soft tissue releases are carried out in order to reduce and displace the proximal phalanx dorsal to the metacarpal. Osteophytes are removed from the base of the proximal phalanx. The intramedullary canal of the metacarpal and phalanx are curetted out to accept the stems of a Swanson silastic prosthesis. After insertion of silastic prostheses, the radial aspects of the extensor hoods are reefed so that the extensor tendon is displaced slightly to the radial side of the center of the joint. After closing the skin, a bulky hand dressing is applied to splint the MP joints in extension and the IP joints in flexion. A dynamic brace is applied on the fourth or fifth postoperative day, and active motion is started. A similar procedure may be carried out on the proximal interphalangeal joints, appropriately modified if the deformity is of the boutonniere or swan-neck type.

TENOSYNOVIAL INVOLVEMENT OF EXTENSOR TENDONS

Unrelieved tenosynovitis of the dorsum of the wrist will result in attrition or destruction of tendons. Early dorsal

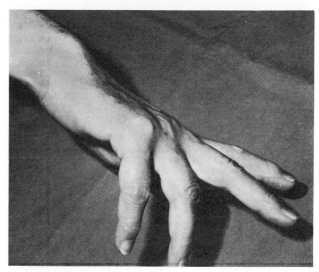

Fig. 48-15. Rupture of extensor tendon on the ring finger and small finger from direct invasion of rheumatoid synovium about the distal radial ulnar joint. Note inability to extend ring and small finger at the MP joint and a prominent ulna styloid which is dorsally subluxed.

tenosynovectomy should be carried out when possible. At the same time, the distal $\frac{3}{4}$ in. of the ulnar shaft and styloid should be excised with adjacent diseased synovium of the distal radioulnar joint.

TREATMENT OF TENDON RUPTURES

The extensor tendons of the ring and small fingers are commonly ruptured with any long-standing process in the

Fig. 48-16. Synovectomy of MP joints for rheumatoid arthritis. *A.* Transverse incision is made over the dorsal aspect of the MP joints. *B.* Incision is made on the radial side of the ulnar deviated extensor tendon, and the synovium is excised. *C* and *D.* Extensor hood is reefed in a radial direction to improve tendon alignment over metacarpal heads.

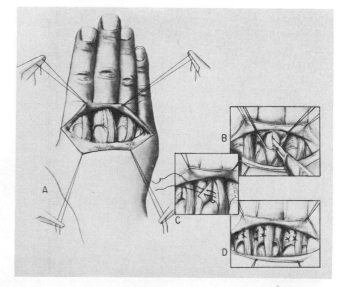

dorsum of the wrist. The extensor pollicis longus may also rupture. When rupture has occurred, tenosynovectomy is indicated, during the repair of the tendons. The tendons are repaired by attaching the distal stumps to the intact extensors of the index and long fingers. In the case of the extensor pollicis longus, a new motor tendon is attached to the distal stump. This is best supplied by the extensor indicis proprius, if available.

FLEXOR TENOSYNOVITIS
AND THE CARPAL TUNNEL SYNDROME

In rheumatoid arthritic patients, flexor tenosynovitis may encroach on the available space for the median nerve as it passes through the carpal tunnel. The patient complains of pain in the thumb, index finger, or long finger with weakness of grasp due to thenar muscle weakness. The patient is commonly awakened at night and shakes his hand in an attempt to relieve the discomfort. On examination, there may only be minimal swelling due to the flexor tenosynovitis. A positive Tinel sign, thenar weakness, and atrophy and numbness in the median nerve distribution may be present in varying degrees. Frequently there is only a history of night pain with paresthesias in the median distribution.

Flexor tenosynovitis may limit active flexion of the fingers with or without median nerve compression. The patient should always be examined for his ability to flex fingers actively to the same degree as that achieved in passive motion. When passive motion is significantly increased over active, flexor tenosynovitis is the diagnosis.

THUMB DEFORMITIES

With sufficient destruction of the MP or IP joint, the functioning of the hand may be severely limited. Instability is corrected by MP arthrodesis (Fig. 48-17) in the position of 15 to 20° of flexion. The pulp of the thumb should be rotated into the position of opposition. In some instances, it may be necessary to fuse the IP joint. Painful involve-

ment of the carpometacarpal joint with subluxation or limitation of motion will require an arthroplasty by excision of the trapezium.

OTHER RHEUMATOID DEFORMITIES
IN THE UPPER EXTREMITY

The rheumatoid process may cause severe painful instability of the elbow. Pain is controlled by proper splinting of the elbow, which is usually sufficient. If ankylosis of the elbow occurs bilaterally or flexion is limited bilaterally, so that the patient cannot feed himself, an arthroplasty may be necessary. This is carried out by excision of the distal humerus and proximal ulna and radius with interposition of fascia lata.

Acromioclavicular involvement which is painful may require excision of the distal clavicle. Rheumatoid disease of the glenohumeral joints is quite difficult to manage. Local injection of cortisone may be helpful in managing the acute stage. These problems are best handled by physical therapy to maintain shoulder motion.

OSTEOARTHRITIS

Osteoarthritis is a term used to describe degenerative changes in diarthrodial joints. The primary change is in the articular cartilage, which is characterized by softening, fibrillation, and abrasion of the articular surface. Since inflammation is not a primary mechanism, *osteoarthrosis* or *degenerative joint diseases* are, perhaps, more accurate terms. Degenerative joint changes occur secondarily in joints previously damaged by inflammation or trauma.

Fig. 48-17. Flexion deformity of the thumb in a patient with long-standing juvenile rheumatoid arthritis, treated by arthrodesis of the MP joint. *A.* Joint space narrowing of the MP joint with inability to extend the thumb beyond 45° flexion. *B.* Crossed Kirschner wire fixation following excision of articular surfaces. *C.* Eight months postfusion with solid arthrodesis in functional position.

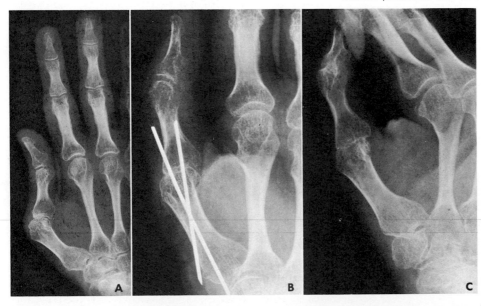

PATHOLOGY. The first recognizable changes in osteoarthritic joints occur in the articular cartilage. There is a loss of metachromasia followed by fissuring in the surface of the cartilage. On gross examination, the cartilage appears softer and yellower than its normal blue-gray color.

As the process progresses, flaking of the articular cartilage and fibrillation of its surface occur. Chondroitin sulfate is decreased in osteoarthritic cartilage, although turnover of matrix is actually increased, as indicated by sulfate utilization. Thymidine uptake indicates increased synthesis of DNA and thus an attempt at cell replication. The earliest changes, since they are present only in the articular cartilage, are not demonstrable by x-ray until there has been some joint space narrowing.

With loss of cartilage, the underlying subchondral bone may be exposed and eburnated. Osteophytes occur at the margins of the articular surfaces or in the capsule and ligamentous attachments at the joint margins. The osteophytes on the joint margins are usually covered with a layer of hyalin or fibrocartilage. The earliest roentgenographic change may be sharpening of the normally smooth, rounded marginal contours of the subchondral bone. Bone proliferates in the area below cartilage fibrillation and accounts for sclerosis, which is manifested roentgenographically by increased density in the subchondral region.

Cysts may develop in the subchondral bone. In this situation, the marrow has undergone mucoid degeneration; trabeculae are lost, and sclerotic new bone encircles the cystic rarefied area. The zone of calcification of the base of the articular cartilage advances into the uncalcified cartilage, which accounts for further loss of joint space seen by x-ray.

Concomitant with changes in the underlying bone, the subsynovial layers develop increasing amounts of fibrous tissue with capsular scarring. There may be moderate degrees of villous synovitis if the joint has been repeatedly injured.

PRIMARY AND SECONDARY OSTEOARTHRITIS. Joints deranged by any process will develop secondary osteoarthritic changes. Secondary osteoarthritis is particularly common in the hip following congenital dysplasia, Legg-Calvé-Perthes disease, slipped capital femoral epiphysis, aseptic necrosis of the femoral head, or fractures involving the acetabulum. In joints damaged by crystal deposition, such as in gout or pseudogout, by ochronosis, or by hemophilia and neurogenic lesions, secondary osteoarthritis develops.

When there is no predisposing cause for the articular cartilage change, the osteoarthritis is considered primary. There is no known cause of primary osteoarthritis and no known reason for the basic change in the cartilage. The majority of persons over forty have some changes compatible with the diagnosis of primary osteoarthritis. Whether these changes are attritional and associated with age or represent a primary disease entity is still under discussion. In a postmortem study of hip joints, Byers et al. were able to separate aging changes from the progressive changes of osteoarthritis.

Kellgren and Moore have described an entity called *primary generalized osteoarthritis.* It occurs mainly in females, with onset during menopause, and involves multiple joints to include the DIP, in which Heberden's nodes develop. Heberden's nodes are osteophytic growths on the proximal aspects of the distal finger phalanges. The symptoms in this type of arthritis tend to be more acute, with clinical evidence of local inflammation at the articular sites.

Certain factors predispose to specific joint osteoarthritis. Trauma or repetitive stress to a joint may be a contributing factor, but hereditary factors as yet unknown are also implicated. Patients with obesity have a significantly higher incidence of osteoarthritis of the knees. The carpometacarpal joints of seamstresses and manual workers are involved with greater frequency than those of other workers. Elbows of pneumatic drill operators are frequently involved. Population and genetic studies indicate a higher incidence of affected relatives with osteoarthritis in patients who have Heberden's nodes.

CLINICAL MANIFESTATIONS. Although radiologic and pathologic studies indicate that the incidence of osteoarthritic joints increases with age, only a small percentage have symptoms related to the joint pathology. It is estimated that only 5 percent of all individuals past fifty have clinical symptoms, and the percentage increases to 20 to 30 percent after the age of sixty. Clinical manifestations are more common in women, although pathologic changes are found with equal incidence in both sexes.

Secondary osteoarthritis may affect any joint in which there is an underlying pathologic condition; i.e., a previously injured hip joint or knee joint may be the only symptomatic joint. Primary osteoarthritis tends to affect the large weight-bearing joints—hips or knees (Fig. 48-18). Osteoarthritis without underlying trauma or other inflammatory joint disease only rarely involves elbows, wrists, or MP joints.

The onset of osteoarthritis symptoms is commonly in-

Fig. 48-18. Primary osteoarthritis of the knee. AP and lateral x-rays showing varus deformity of the knee with joint space narrowing, osteophyte production on medial, lateral, and posterior aspects of the tibia, on anterior aspects of femoral condyles, and on both upper and lower poles of the patella. There is minimal cyst formation and sclerosis of subchondral bone of the medial joint space.

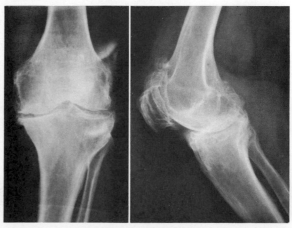

sidious; at the time of presentation the x-ray changes indicate that bone and joint abnormality has long been present. Except in the primary generalized osteoarthritis of Kellgren and Moore, there are no systemic manifestations. Local symptoms include pain with motion, relieved by rest. Stiffness occurs after rest and resolves after the joint has been repetitively exercised. Muscle atrophy is not common. On examination, there is restriction of joint motion.

There are no specific laboratory examinations to prove the diagnosis. All blood tests including latex fixation are normal. Occasionally, the sedimentation rate may be slightly elevated. The synovial fluid contains a white blood cell count below 2,000, a good mucin clot, and a normal synovial fluid/blood glucose gradient.

X-ray findings may be quite normal in the very early stages of cartilage change. As the disease progresses, joint space narrowing, subchondral bone sclerosis, osteophyte formation, and subchondral bone cysts are present in varying degrees (Fig. 48-19). The presence of such x-ray signs should not be interpreted as the cause of the patient's symptoms, since these x-ray findings may exist without symptoms. The patient may have underlying rheumatoid disease, gout, or even septic arthritis, superimposed on a degenerative joint.

Conservative Treatment

Most patients with osteoarthritis can be treated by conservative measures. The pain in an osteoarthritic joint is probably due to irritation of the capsular and ligamentous structures of the joint. The abnormal articular surface and incongruous articulation predisposes to minor sprains of the joint capsule and ligaments. In later stages, underlying vascular change in the bone may account for the local and referred pain which persists following rest of the affected joint.

Conservative measures should be attempted and can be successful for the relief of pain.

Fig. 48-19. Bilateral osteoarthritis of the hips showing marked osteophyte formation, sclerosis, acetabular cysts, obliteration of joint space, and partial subluxation.

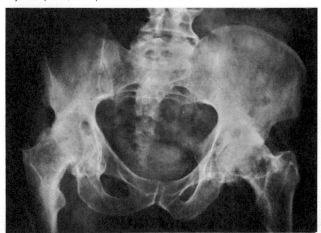

Immobilization of a painful osteoarthritic joint is dramatic in its relief of pain. Frequently, protection of a painful joint for a few days or weeks is sufficient to alleviate symptoms, and the patient can return to his previous activity. Since most symptoms are due to minor strains on the mechanically abnormal joint, the patient should be instructed in ways to minimize further injury. The patient should understand the differences between osteoarthritis and rheumatoid arthritis, etc., and be given reassurance of his good prognosis.

All factors adding to stress across the symptomatic joint or joints should be minimized or eliminated. Obese patients should be put on a reducing diet. Muscle power which will stabilize the damaged joint should be strengthened. The patient should be instructed to rest the joint when minor symptoms return so as to prevent the pain–muscle-spasm–limitation-of-motion cycle. In some situations, weight-relieving calipers or braces or splints will effectively protect the joint. Daily and occupational activities should be evaluated and activities modified, if possible. Range-of-motion and muscle-strengthening exercises may be helpful because of the protective stabilizing effect to a deranged joint.

Analgesic drugs are helpful in controlling symptoms, but under no circumstances should the patient be started on narcotic or habit-forming drugs. Aspirin, in addition to its analgesic action, has a direct anti-inflammatory effect on cartilage, as well as on periarticular structures. Phenylbutazone and indomethacin are also helpful. The local instillation of hydrocortisone into a painful joint may afford relief if conservative splinting and local rest measures fail. Although there have been reports of neurotropic joints developing following excessive injections, Hollander has had good results and minimal complications with local cortisone.

Orthopedic Management

Surgical treatment of osteoarthritis is indicated when conservative measures fail to control pain or when joint motion is significantly limited and symptomatic. Procedures available for relief of pain of an osteoarthritic joint include arthrodesis, arthroplasty, osteotomy, pseudarthrosis, and neurectomy.

Arthrodesis eliminates motion and relieves the irritation of pain-producing structures. Arthroplasty and pseudarthrosis provide increased mobility of a joint but may be less effective in relieving the discomfort. Osteotomy is effective in correcting deformity and realigning joints and has the added benefit of pain relief by mechanisms incompletely understood at the present time. Neurectomy is indicated in rare situations, but because of the gross overlap of articular innervation, complete denervation of a joint is difficult.

SPECIFIC JOINT INVOLVEMENT

THUMB CARPOMETACARPAL JOINT OSTEOARTHRITIS.
In clothing workers, seamstresses, and surgeons osteoarthritis of the carpometacarpal joint of the thumb may develop. The patients have pain with any motion of the

thumb and marked interference with grasp, due to pain.

Painful DIP joints afflicted with osteoarthritis are rarely unstable. Conservative treatment will usually suffice, and rarely arthrodesis or flexible implant arthroplasty of one of these joints may be indicated.

WRIST, ELBOW, AND SHOULDER. Surgical treatment is infrequently required for wrist, elbow, and shoulder osteoarthritis, which usually result from injuries. Wrist pain due to posttraumatic arthritis not responding to conservative measures may be treated by arthrodesis of the radiocarpal and intercarpal joints. Management of the painful posttraumatic elbow may require excision of the radial head, because of radiohumeral joint subluxation. In sedentary individuals and office workers, a fascia lata arthroplasty will allow motion, although it will increase instability. For laborers who are unable to change occupations, arthrodesis of the elbow in the correct position will provide pain relief and stability. Posttraumatic symptomatic acromioclavicular and sternoclavicular joints may be treated by arthroplasty. In the case of the acromioclavicular joint, the distal 1 in. of the clavicle is removed, and for the sternoclavicular joint, the proximal 1 in. of the clavicle is excised.

OSTEOARTHRITIS OF THE HIP. Osteoarthritis of the hip may be primary or secondary as a result of abnormalities of the acetabulum or shape and alignment of femoral head and neck. Patients with significant acetabular dysplasia, post-Legg-Calvé-Perthes disease with femoral head enlargement, and slipped epiphyses tend to become symptomatic a decade sooner, in their forties and fifties, than patients with primary osteoarthritis of the hip.

In primary osteoarthritis of the hip, two patterns develop: In the *adduction–external-rotation type* the only remaining mobility is usually that of flexion. The most severe bony changes of cyst formation and sclerosis occur in the superior part of the joint with marked osteophyte formation and a valgus position of the neck. In the *non-adducted type,* although the only mobility may be flexion with external rotation, the femur is in a neutral or abducted position. The most severe bony changes occur in the deepest part of the joint.

Clinical Manifestations

The presenting complaint with osteoarthritis of the hip is invariably pain. In the early symptomatic stages, pain is intermittent with episodes occurring after excessive activity and followed by asymptomatic remissions. Pain is aching in character, referred to the groin, the lateral aspect of the thigh, and frequently as far distally as the medial aspect of the knee. Pain is more severe with activity following joint rest, either in the morning or after sitting. With increased activity, the symptoms are less severe. Later in the course of the disease, pain may be severely aggravated by activity, followed by rest pain lasting a few hours.

The origin of pain in an osteoarthritic hip is still conjectural, but it can arise from (1) disease in the subchondral bone, which contains blood vessels and their nerve fibers; (2) muscle spasm and contractures of the muscles around the diseased joint, i.e., the adductors, iliopsoas, and rectus femoris; (3) disease within the sensitive capsule, which is particularly sensitive to the stimulus of tension and trac-

tion; (4) disease in the synovium, although it is unknown whether this tissue is sensitive to painful stimuli or whether transmission is from adjacent joint capsule; or (5) disease in the periosteum.

Patients with osteoarthritis of the hip are usually unaware of restriction of motion early in the disease. As the disease progresses, restriction may be severe. The earliest loss of motion is that of internal rotation but also with associated loss of abduction and extension. Patients may present with an adduction–external-rotation flexion contracture.

The loss of mobility results from (1) articular cartilage destruction with marked loss of joint space and incongruity of the joint surfaces, (2) muscle spasm and contractures with fibrosis of overlying fascia and their musculotendonous junctions, (3) capsular contracture, or (4) mechanical blocking by loose bodies or from large osteophytes. Patients walk with a characteristic hip limp of the Trendelenburg type or an abductor lurch, because they spend less time on the involved hip during the stance phase of gait.

Treatment

Conservative treatment should be attempted. It may be sufficient to allow the patient to continue activities with modification, and while conservative treatment is in progress, the physician can evaluate the patient's cooperation and motivation prior to undertaking reconstructive surgical procedures.

Rest in bed with skin traction to the leg or non-weight-bearing crutch walking during acute episodes are helpful when the pain is severe. The simple maneuver of having the patient carry a cane in the opposite hand to relieve weight load across the contralateral hip may dramatically relieve symptoms. Salicylates are administered. Often, modification of the patient's activities and job requirements will allow him to continue working. If conservative measures fail, surgical procedures are available, each with advantages and disadvantages but all requiring a patient who is a good operative risk (Fig. 48-20).

Arthrodesis. For the young individual who experiences repetitive stress to a hip and who must stand for long periods, hip arthrodesis (Fig. 48-20A) may be the procedure of choice. The most frequent indications are sepsis (pyogenic or tuberculous) and cases in which implant arthroplasty is contraindicated. Surgical arthrodesis requires a patient who is physiologically young enough to undergo this treatment, and who will tolerate the plaster cast immobilization and bedrest for 3 to 6 months. Patients with previous back injuries or disease are not suitable candidates for this procedure because of the added stress to the lumbar spine. Patients with bilateral hip disease or involvement of other joints in the lower extremities should be considered for other surgical procedures.

Femoral Osteotomy. The displacement osteotomy (Fig. 48-20B) described by McMurray may provide dramatic pain relief and allow hip joint mobility. In young patients with early osteoarthritis, before bone collapse, and with 90° of hip flexion, displacement osteotomy is a good procedure with a high rate of pain relief and minimal risk to

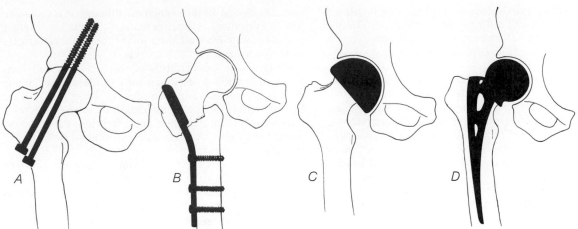

Fig. 48-20. Surgical treatment of hip disease. *A.* Arthrodesis. *B.* Displacement osteotomy. *C.* Cup arthroplasty. *D.* Femoral head replacement arthroplasty.

the patient. In the early stages of osteoarthritis, this procedure can provide complete pain relief and a mobile hip, which can be expected to last for many years. Compared with hip arthrodesis or cup arthroplasty, there is less risk to the patient in this procedure, and if unsuccessful (10 to 20 percent of patients) anatomy is not distorted, and other procedures may be undertaken. The femoral shaft is divided immediately above the lesser trochanter and displaced mediad about one-half the width of the shaft. It is then affixed to the proximal fragment in abduction or adduction, depending upon preoperative joint motion and x-ray studies which show the best seating of the head in the acetabulum. The reason for pain relief, improvement in joint motion, and reestablishment of the joint space is not understood. Possible explanations have to do with changing the vascular bed of the underlying subchondral bone and decreasing the force of tight muscles about the hip. The indications for displacement osteotomy require an osteoarthritic joint in its early stages, before joint motion is severely restricted and before bone collapse.

Cup Arthroplasty. Cup arthroplasty employs the interposition of a well-fitting metal cup between the femoral head and acetabulum (Fig. 48-20C), which are shaped to accommodate the cup. The healing process covers the raw bone surfaces with a regenerated arthroplasty surface resembling articular cartilage. Insertion of the cup requires precision, and patients must be willing to have the cup modified by a second surgical procedure if satisfactory results are not obtained. The postoperative management is complicated and requires experienced physiotherapists and a well-motivated patient to continue the exercises. This operation can be done in severely involved hips or even ankylosed joints. The best results are obtained in patients with good preoperative ranges of motion. One can expect relief of disabling pain in about 85 percent of patients including 25 percent with complete relief, unlimited walking in 25 percent, walking without support in 30 percent, and walking with a cane or stick in 55 percent. Since the advent of total hip replacement, the need for cup arthroplasty is rare.

Femoral Head Replacement Arthroplasty. This operation (Fig. 48-20D) is used when there is severe damage to the

femoral head in the presence of a normal acetabulum. The indications include nonunion of the femoral neck or avascular necrosis of the femoral head secondary to fracture or other causes. The operation should not be considered in primary or even secondary degenerative arthritis where there are abnormalities on both sides of the articulation.

Total Hip Replacement. All reconstructive procedures on the adult hip must be evaluated in the light of the superior results being obtained with total hip replacement arthroplasty. The total hip arthroplasty replaces both sides of the joint with a prosthetic femoral head and prosthetic acetabular component (Fig. 48-21). The concept for this is not new, dating to 1938 when Wiles designed a stainless steel femoral head with a matching acetabulum, both of which were fixed mechanically to bone. Charnley, and McKee and Watson-Farrar, who began work in the early 1950s, must receive the credit for the current state of total hip replacement arthroplasty.

Indications for Total Hip Arthroplasty. Total hip replacement surgery has been utilized for various types of disabling hip diseases such as osteoarthritis, primary or secondary, and rheumatoid arthritis. It is also used for reconstruction of previously unsuccessful hip surgery such as osteotomy or cup arthroplasty and in any type of joint disorder where infection is not present. Since component-part wear can be expected and loosening may occur in patients who put high demands and excessive forces on their hips, the operation is currently limited to older patients or younger patients with shortened life expectancy or diminished physical capacity. The operation has the best short- or medium-term results of any type of hip reconstructive operation. The uncertainties, of course, are whether the fixation of the component parts to bone can be maintained, how long the bearing surfaces will wear, and whether there is any long-term toxicity to the cement or wear debris. If a patient develops an infection following total hip arthroplasty, either acutely or as a delayed phenomenon, removal of the prosthesis will likely be necessary. The loss of stock results in a Girdlestone pseudarthrosis. In essence, the patient is gambling on an operation

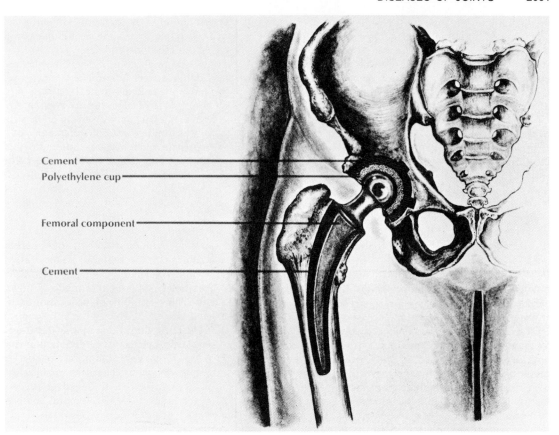

Cement
Polyethylene cup
Femoral component
Cement

Fig. 48-21. Schema of total hip replacement (Charnley-Muller prosthesis). (*From S. Graves et al., RN Magazine, 34:35, 1971.*)

which has a high rate of success but severe disability if complications due to infection develop. The operation has the advantage that severely damaged joints can be reconstructed; there is no urgency in early timing of the procedure as there is, for example, with displacement osteotomy.

Bioengineering Considerations. Total hip replacement requires (1) an understanding of forces across the prosthesis or hip joint, as well as of friction, wear, and lubrication of the component parts of the prosthesis; (2) fixation of the prosthesis to bone; and (3) biologic acceptance of the prosthetic materials.

Forces across the Hip. In the normal walking cycle it has been shown that loads across the hip joint vary between zero and four times the body weight. With the patient standing on one foot, the weight of the body is balanced by the simultaneous contraction of the abductor muscles of the hip in the stance phase. Since the body weight is working on a lever arm, about three times the length of the lever arm across which abductor muscles have their force application, the multiplication of forces about the hip can be accounted for. Recognition of these lever arm forces demands attention to prosthetic materials capable of withstanding the loads. Because of the leverage applied to the hip joint, the acetabular component of the total hip must be placed as mediad as possible, with a corresponding lateral displacement of the greater trochanter. This requires reaming of the acetabulum and osteo-

phytes on the medial acetabulum in order to displace the center of the total hip device mediad. Increasing the length of the prosthetic neck will necessarily displace the greater trochanter laterally, thereby increasing the leverage of the abductor muscles and reducing the force across the joint.

Friction, Wear, and Lubrication of the Total Hip Appliance. The introduction of an appliance system into the body in which there is motion between two components involves considerations of friction, wear, and lubrication between the parts. Bearing material utilized in total hip replacement is of two types, metal on metal and metal on plastic. To prevent corrosion arising in the biologic system, similar metals are necessary. Alloys of cobalt, chromium, and molybdenum as are used in the McKee-Farrar prosthesis have been shown to be suitable for this. Motion between similar metals in either the dry or lubricated state has a higher coefficient of friction than in the metal-plastic type of prosthesis used in the Charnley or T-28 types. In the Charnley prosthesis, a stainless steel femoral head is in contact with a high-density polyethylene acetabular component. Reducing the size of the femoral head component reduces the frictional resistance between the surfaces and minimizes the tendency of the components to separate from bone. The optimal femoral head size should be one which is small enough to minimize the volume of wear debris and at the same time maintain sufficient mechanical strength. Characteristics of the fluid lubricating the surfaces of a total hip replacement in vivo are not known but may correspond closely to normal synovial fluid. Wear of the metallic surfaces in a metal-to-metal prosthesis is of the adhesive wear type in which separation of welded asperities results in metal transfer and loose wear particles. Abrasive wear, in which a harder surface such as the metal erodes through the softer surface of the plastic, occurs in the metal-plastic type. Information on the tribiologic characteristics of total hip replacement is incomplete. The reader is referred to the work of Dowson and Wright and Scales and Lowe.

Fixation of the Prostheses to Bone. The marked long-term relief of pain with a total hip replacement is attributed to the optimal mechanical relationship and stability between prosthesis and the bone. This is accomplished by the use of cold curing acrylic cement, methyl methacrylate, which acts as a force diffuser between the stem of the prosthesis and the bone or between the acetabular prosthesis and the pelvis. The methacrylate does not adhere to the bone but acts only by mechanical interdigitation. Force across the prosthesis is transmitted to a much greater surface area of bone by the interposition of the acrylic. Thus, the force on any given area of bone is insufficient to cause resorption, and stability is maintained.

The acrylic cement is prepared by mixing liquid methyl methacrylate monomer and dimethyl-*p*-toluidine stabilized with hydroquinone and a fine powder of polymethyl methacrylate and 2% benzoyl peroxide. After a few minutes of mixing, a doughlike substance is obtained which increases its viscosity over the next few minutes. When the doughy consistency is reached, the material is pushed into the roughened medullary canal or acetabulum. When the cavity has been filled, the stem of the prosthesis, or acetabular prosthesis, is inserted and excess cement removed. Total curing time is about 8 minutes for Surgical Simplex. Depending upon the mass of acrylic used, temperatures of 90°C may be attained. There is concern for the amount of tissue damage resulting from the exothermic reaction. Just prior to the acute rise in temperature, expansion of the Simplex occurs by $1\frac{1}{2}$ percent, and during the cooling period contraction of 1 percent occurs.

Biologic Acceptance of the Prosthetic Materials. Within the time frame of methacrylate use, there has been no evidence of carcinogenic or toxic reactions of the acrylic. Absorption of methacrylate constituents at the time of surgery may result in hypotension. At the bone cement interface, both experimentally and in prostheses removed at postmortem, there is a fibrous layer of tissue between cement and bone. Wear debris from a metal-to-metal prosthesis can be seen as particulate material in macrophages in the regenerated capsule. There is little information about the fate of wear debris from high-density polyethylene.

Types of Total Hip Joint Replacement. *McKee-Farrar Prosthesis.* The McKee-Farrar prosthesis is a metal-to-metal prosthetic design in which both femoral head and acetabular components are made of a cobalt chrome alloy and designed so that the components are fixed with methyl methacrylate. Two head sizes are in standard use, $1\frac{3}{8}$ and $1\frac{5}{8}$. The acetabular cup has a rim with multiple studs for fixation with acrylic cement. The large size adds stability to the articulation, making the technique of insertion less

demanding. The rate of loosening with this device is greater than when the acetabular component is made of high-density polyethylene.

Charnley Prosthesis. The Charnley prosthesis consists of a stainless steel femoral component with a head of 22.25 mm fabricated of surgical stainless steel. The acetabular cup is made of high-density polyethylene with an external diameter of 42 mm. Varying stem sizes are available as well as smaller external diameters of the cup. The cup contains a reference wire for radiographic determination of wear. This device generates less frictional torque due to the smaller head size and the improved frictional characteristics of metal on plastic. The smaller head size and the wide cup thickness demand exacting surgical technique to minimize dislocation.

Charnley-Muller Prosthesis. The Charnley-Muller prosthesis is a modification of the Charnley and consists of a cobalt chrome femoral component with a head size of 28 mm with standard long and short necks available. The acetabular component is made of high-density polyethylene. The possibility of dislocation is less with the larger head size.

Other modifications of the metal-on-metal and metal-on-plastic designs are available and include the Amstutz, T-28, Harris, and Stanmore types.

Ring Prosthesis. The Ring prosthesis is a metal-on-metal prosthesis which is designed to be used without cement or acrylic fixation. The femoral component is a modification of Austin Moore's prosthesis. The acetabular component consists of a cup with a long threaded stem for fixation into the weight-bearing line of the ilium. The design has eliminated cement. It is anticipated that loosening of the components will be increased with this design.

Technique of Insertion of a T-28 Prosthesis. With the patient lying in the lateral position, a standard Harris approach to the hip is carried out. A gently curved incision is centered at the posterior border of the trochanter and extending to $1\frac{1}{2}$ in. posterior and distal to the anterior spine of the ilium, the distal limb being symmetric with the proximal. The greater trochanter is osteotomized and retracted proximally with its attached abductors. The short external rotators are divided from the greater trochanter and retracted posteriorly. The exposed capsule of the hip joint is excised and the femoral head dislocated by flexing, adducting, and externally rotating the hip. Using an oscillating saw, the femoral head and neck are removed at a point just above the lesser trochanter. The iliopsoas is divided for better mobility of the proximal femur as necessary. The acetabulum is then reamed, taking care to remove acetabular debris and osteophytes from the medial acetabulum in order to attain medial cup displacement. Two $\frac{1}{2}$-in.-diameter holes are drilled into the iliac portion of the acetabulum. Two additional holes are drilled through the acetabulum into the superior ramus of the pubis as it joins the acetabulum and also the ischial ramus. The holes are undercut with a curet. Hemostasis is maintained by gel foam packs into the holes.

Methyl methacrylate cement is mixed; when it becomes of doughy consistency, it is inserted as a mass into the acetabulum and drill holes. A T-28 acetubular component is then inserted as far medially as possible and held in a position of 45° abduction and 10° anteversion. Excess cement is removed. Acrylic cement projecting around the rim of the cup after hardening is trimmed with an osteotome. The proximal femur is then reamed using an appropriate rasp. The femoral component with the correct neck length is then inserted into the femur without cement and a trial reduction carried out. If this is satisfactory, the prosthesis is cemented into the proximal femur in a position of 10 to 15° anteversion using acrylic cement. The greater trochanter is reattached with steel wire through two drill holes across the lateral cortex of the proximal femur. Closed suction drainage is applied to the wound. Postoperative management includes bed rest in balanced suspension followed by early partial weight bearing between crutches. Protected weight bearing is continued until union of the trochanter has occurred.

Complications of Total Hip Replacement. The dread complication of total hip replacement is a wound infection. This may occur as an acute postoperative complication or as a delayed phenomenon months or years after primary wound healing. Prevention of wound infection from total hip replacement requires scrupulous operative technique on the part of operating personnel. Surgery is often carried out in operating theaters equipped with positive-pressure rapid air changes with high-efficiency particle filters. Penicillinase-resistant antibiotics are administered preoperatively, intraoperatively, and postoperatively. Infection rates in total hip replacement series vary from as low as less than 1 percent to as high as 10 percent.

Thrombophlebitis and pulmonary embolism are complications of any type of hip surgery, and total hip replacement is no exception. Prophylactic measures against thrombophlebitis are indicated, such as administration of Coumadin or low-molecular-weight dextran. Both lower extremities should be elevated postoperatively. Patients should be cautioned against sitting for even short periods until hip motion and activity have been restored.

The prosthesis can be dislocated. The incidence of this is low and can be minimized by accurate positioning of the prosthetic components and positioning of the operative extremity until soft tissue healing has occurred.

Loosening of the prosthetic components is a late complication and may be evident if the patient begins to experience pain in the characteristic hip distribution. Loosening can be determined by unusual resorption of bone at the bone-cement interphase. It may be necessary to do an arthrogram or bone scan for diagnosis.

Charnley has reported follow-up results on 379 hips followed between 4 and 7 years postoperatively. Ninety percent of the patients maintained excellent results. Late mechanical failure occurred in 1.3 percent of patients. The overall infection rate was 3.8 percent, 2.2 percent being late infections. The average degree of acetabular prosthesis wear varied from 1 mm in 5 years to absence of wear at 7 years postsurgery. Preoperative range of motion was improved in all patients, and there was no tendency to decrease motion with increasing time of follow-up.

CHONDROMALACIA OF THE PATELLA. Chondromalacia of the patella represents degeneration, or the first stage of osteoarthritis, involving the cartilage surface of the patella. Changes in this cartilage are common by the age of thirty, although symptomatology is infrequent in terms of incidence of the pathologic change. The earliest changes occur on the medial facet of the patella. The cause of chondromalacia is unknown, but trauma, such as striking the knee on the dashboard of a car, and mechanical factors of an incongruent relationship of the patella with the femoral condyle may play a role. In teen-agers, especially girls, mild degrees of recurvatum and valgus knees are associated with subluxing patella with attendant chondromalacia. Chondromalacia is not uncommon with clinical symptoms after immobilization of a fractured femur for prolonged periods.

Clinical Manifestations. The onset may be insidious; the patient is aware only of minor discomfort in the knee with acute flexion or in descending stairs or kneeling. Often the onset is acute following a direct blow to the knee. Chondromalacia frequently presents with symptoms of subluxation or even frank dislocation of the patella. The patient may be aware of crepitus. Synovial effusion, although uncommon, does occur. Physical examination will demonstrate tenderness if the patella is pressed distad in its groove while the quadriceps is actively contracted. By displacing the patella, mediad, the undersurface can be palpated and also may reveal tenderness. Atrophy of the vastus medialis is uncommon.

Radiographs are negative early in the course of the disease but are taken to rule out other causes for discomfort. With progressive change, osteophytes may be present on the proximal and distal pole of the patella, progressing to frank osteoarthritis of the entire knee joint. Other causes of knee pain must be excluded, i.e., rheumatoid arthritis, loose bodies, and meniscal injuries, some of which have patellar symptoms in addition to the primary condition.

Treatment. The majority of patients with symptoms are managed by conservative treatment. The patient is taught quadriceps-strengthening exercises. He is cautioned to sit with his knee extended and to avoid flexion until symptoms subside (1 to 3 weeks). In some cases, crutches or posterior plaster splints are necessary.

Surgical Treatment of Chondromalacia. Patients not responding to conservative treatment or having persistent recurrent episodes may require excision of the diseased cartilage, realignment of the quadriceps patellar mechanism by tibial tubercle transfer or similar procedures, or even patellectomy when the condition has progressed to severe osteoarthritis of the patellofemoral joint.

The knee is explored through a median parapatellar transverse incision, and the undersurface of the patella is examined. If the cartilage destruction is not severe or less than one-third of the undersurface is involved, the diseased cartilage is excised. If there are clinical findings of patellar subluxation, a tibial tubercle transfer may be carried out. If involvement is greater or large osteophytes are present, patellectomy may be necessary (Fig. 48-22).

Postoperative treatment requires an initial period of immobilization and quadriceps-strengthening exercises. The knee is placed in a posterior splint or circular plaster cylinder, and hourly quadriceps exercises are instituted. In

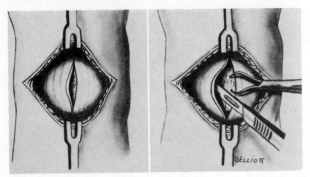

Fig. 48-22. Patellectomy. Patella exposed through transverse skin incision and excised through vertical incision in its tendinous envelope.

the case of cartilage excision, active knee flexion and range-of-motion exercises are started at 2 to 3 weeks. The patient is allowed to bear full weight when range of motion and quadriceps power are normal.

For postpatellectomy management, a cylinder is applied for 3 to 4 weeks, and then gradual active flexion within pain tolerance is begun within 4 to 6 weeks. Weight bearing is allowed when there is 90° of knee flexion and quadriceps power is normal.

OSTEOARTHRITIS OF THE KNEE. Osteoarthritis of the knee does not commonly require surgical intervention. Patients are reassured and activity is modified. Salicylates and quadriceps-strengthening exercises are usually sufficient to overcome discomfort.

If symptoms can be localized to the patellofemoral joint, patellectomy is indicated. If symptoms do not respond to conservative treatment and there is a mild varus or valgus

Fig. 48-23. Charnley compression arthrodesis of the knee.

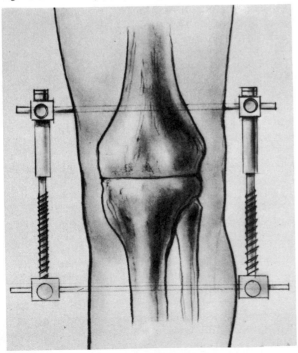

deformity of the knee, realignment by proximal tibial osteotomy may afford dramatic relief. The mechanism by which osteotomy is beneficial is not understood. Part of the value lies in realignment of the knee joint, although the change in vascularity to the subchondral bone may be of importance. In severe osteoarthritis of the knee of posttraumatic causation, arthrodesis may be indicated when other joints are normal (Fig. 48-23). Total knee joint replacement appears to be a significant advance in osteoarthritis of the knee in older patients and should be considered when osteotomy is contraindicated. An alternative procedure is the insertion of MacIntosh prostheses.

OSTEOARTHRITIS OF THE ANKLE AND FOOT. Osteoarthritis of the ankle is usually the result of injury. Attempts at modifying discomfort or deformity should be made with a short leg brace, the ankle fixed in appropriate position to minimize medial-lateral and flexion-extension forces. Arthrodesis may be required. Similarly, subtalar joint problems requiring treatment are more likely the result of posttraumatic osteoarthritis. Again, arthrodesis may be indicated.

Hallux Valgus (Bunion)

Hallux valgus, or lateral deviation of the great toe, is a disease of the shoe-wearing population. Hodgson has shown that foot deformities have a much greater incidence in the shoe-wearing population in Hong Kong than in those without shoes. The incidence of hallux valgus is much greater in the female than in the male and is certainly precipitated by improper shoe wear. A short first metatarsal or metatarsus primus varus may contribute to or initiate deformity. Once the great toe starts to deviate laterally, there is little conservative treatment can do to overcome deformity. With lateral deviation of the great toe, the long flexor and extensor tendons are bow-stringed laterally across the joint and maintain and increase the deformity.

Traction on the capsule of the MP joint at its attachment to the metatarsal head, as well as local shoe pressure over the medial aspect of the metatarsal head, contribute to the development of a large exostosis with an overlying soft tissue bursa, a bunion. Contracture in the adductor hallucis contributes to hallux valgus with further displacement of the first metatarsal mediad. The lateral sesamoid may become displaced in the direction of the lateral side of the foot. Changes occur in the articular cartilage which resemble the early stages of osteoarthritis. The end result is an osteoarthritic MP joint. Hallux rigidus is a stiff MP joint and is associated with pain during attempts to bear weight and during the push-off phase of walking.

Clinical Manifestations. Hallux valgus is a common deformity, although few are symptomatic. The most common complaint is the inability to wear the modern shoe with its narrow forefoot. Patients may complain intermittently of pain over the bunion due to acute bursitis from local shoe pressure. Such patients wear old shoes and commonly take their shoes off after a day's work.

With sufficient deformity and lateral deviation and rotation of the great toe, there is less distribution of weight between metatarsal heads and toes. The result is increased pressure on metatarsal heads during the push-off phase of gait. Callosities develop over the second and third metatarsal heads because of this increased pressure.

Treatment. If hallux valgus has already developed, symptoms from the bursa and osteophyte over the metatarsal head can be minimized with appropriate modification of shoes. Symptoms due to metatarsalgia from abnormal weight distribution from the malaligned great toe may be handled with insoles and metatarsal arches to distribute the weight proximally away from the metatarsal head pressure area. A metatarsal bar on the external surface of the sole may assist in accomplishing the same changes in weight distribution. There are over 100 different operations for bunions and hallux valgus which attest to the inefficiency of the various procedures. The most common surgical procedure for bunions is the Keller arthroplasty (Fig. 48-24). This consists of excision of the proximal one-half of the proximal phalanx of the great toe and excision of the osteophyte on the medial dorsal surface of the metatarsal head. Following this surgical procedure, the great toe is shorter, but long tendons take up the slack, restoring function to the great toe. This procedure is applicable to any degree of hallux valgus and has a high rate of success.

In the young female with minimal osteoarthritic changes and essentially normal joint flexion and extension, the McBride procedure or a modification of it will give a satisfactory result. The procedure involves a dorsal incision between the first and second metatarsal heads in which the fibular sesamoid is excised. This interrupts the adductor insertion on the great toe. Through a second incision over the dorsal medial aspect of the MP joint, the osteophyte is excised, and the abductor tendon and capsule insertion are reefed to hold the toe in neutral, but not varus, position. McBride reattaches the adductor to the first metatarsal neck to assist in controlling the varus of the first metatarsal shaft. The capsules of the first and second metatarsal heads are sutured together to assist in controlling the metatarsus primus varus.

The end result of this procedure is realignment of the toe with function and normal length maintained. Another approach is to osteotomize the adducted, or varus, first metatarsal. This should be done before significant MP joint changes have occurred. The procedures which excise only the bursa overlying the metatarsal head or its exostosis do not usually result in relief of symptoms.

GOUT

Gout is a metabolic disease in which crystals of sodium urate monohydrate are deposited in and about joints. Patients with gout have an increase in serum uric acid concentration. Patients may have complicating renal diseases due to urate deposition.

Gout is said to be primary when it is due to an inborn error of metabolism. Secondary gout may be due to other diseases such as myeloproliferative disorders, leukemia, hemolytic anemias, or glycogen storage disease. It is generally accepted that the hyperuricemia of primary gout has a hereditary transmission. However, the hyperuricemic rela-

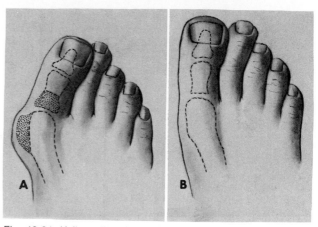

Fig. 48-24. Keller arthroplasty. *A.* Exostosis and proximal phalangectomy carried out through dorsal medial incision. *B.* Postoperative position.

tives of patients with gout have an incidence of gout symptoms of only 20 percent, suggesting that there are other factors than hyperuricemia determining the clinical condition.

Hyperuricemia must be defined for each laboratory. With colorometric methods, the upper limit of normal in the male is about 6.4 mg/100 ml and 5.8 in females. Population studies indicate that hyperuricemia may be transmitted by an autosomal dominant or sex-linked dominants. Other information suggests that polygenic transmission is also operative. Hyperuricemic patients of primary gout both overproduce and underexcrete uric acid. Both processes may operate in varying degree in patients with clinical gout.

The incidence of gout is less than 1 percent in Europe and the United States. It is much higher in Filipinos and reaches the incidence of 8.2 percent in the Chamorros of the Mariana Islands and Carolinians of the Caroline Islands. In most series only 3 to 7 percent of cases of primary gout occur in the female. The clinical onset is rare before the third decade. The mechanism by which an acute attack is precipitated is still unknown. When crystals of sodium urate are injected experimentally into animals or human beings, acute arthritis will ensue whether the patient has hyperuricemia or is normal. Following injection of urate crystals, joint pressure increases, and the pH of synovial fluid drops. The change in pH is related to lactic acid produced by leukocytes. Leukocytes ingest the urate crystals, a mechanism which is blocked by treatment with colchicine.

Seegmiller and Howell propose a cycle of crystallization of sodium urate from supersaturated body fluids. Once crystals enter the joint, leukocytosis increases lactate production, causing a fall in local pH and a tendency for further crystal deposition. The mechanism of initiation of deposit of the crystals in the joint is not known. Certain clinical situations such as trauma, stress, and ACTH withdrawal are associated with a high incidence of acute gout in the hyperuricemic.

PATHOLOGY. Urate crystals are deposited in cartilage, subchondral bone, and the periarticular structures and kidneys, as well. The tophaceous deposit consists of urate crystals surrounded by an inflammatory granuloma. The crystalline deposit may calcify and be detectable on roentgenograms.

Tophi may occur anywhere in the body but are common in the external ear, in the olecranon, and about tendons and bursae. Secondary degenerative joint changes occur in response to urate deposits. Urate crystals may be deposited in the kidney and be surrounded by giant cell granulomas.

CLINICAL MANIFESTATIONS. The classic presentation of an acute attack is in a male over the age of thirty who experiences sudden onset of a monarticular arthritis, usually involving the MP joint of the great toe (Fig. 48-25). The onset is dramatically acute with swelling, erythema, and tenderness about the affected joint. Untreated, an attack lasts from a few days to 2 weeks. The initial attack is most common in the big toe but may involve any of the weight-bearing joints of the foot, ankle, or knee. Occasionally, an olecranon bursa is the location for the first attack.

Following an acute attack, the patient may be completely asymptomatic for many months or years. However, subsequent attacks may involve other joints and follow a longer and febrile course. In less than half the patients

Fig. 48-25. Severe gouty arthritis involving the MP joint of right toe with destruction of the metatarsal head. Proximal phalanx with joint space narrowing. Note large soft tissue gouty tophus.

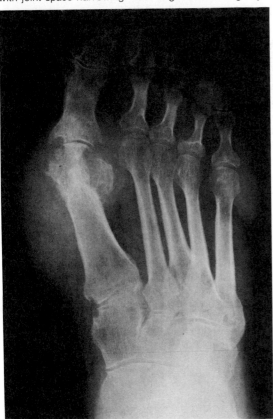

with recurrent attacks chronic gouty arthritis develops. Chronic gouty arthritis may develop gradually without preceding acute symptoms in a specific joint. Tophi may ulcerate and drain urate material intermittently. Acute gonococcal arthritis, acute rheumatoid arthritis, or acute rheumatic fever may simulate an acute gouty arthritis. In less typical situations, gout may resemble any of the chronic arthritides.

The diagnosis is confirmed when urate crystals can be detected by polarized light microscopy of fluid aspirated from an acutely affected joint. The serum uric acid level is commonly elevated during an acute attack but during the interval stage may be within normal limits. Patients with an acute attack may have leukocytosis and an increased sedimentation rate. The presence of tophi aids in the diagnosis, and aspiration will reveal urate crystals. In chronic tophaceous gout, characteristic punched-out lesions in the regions of the subchondral bone and at capsular attachments of involved joints are found. Such findings, however, may be seen in rheumatoid arthritis, sarcoid, hyperparathyroidism, and other conditions, making x-ray interpretation nonspecific.

TREATMENT. Management of the Acute Attack. Colchicine has been known to be effective since the days of Hippocrates. Recently, it has been shown that colchicine interferes with the metabolic activity of leukocytes. Colchicine in a dose of 0.65 mg is given each hour or 2 hours, until acute symptoms subside or until diarrhea or vomiting results. The response to colchicine is quite often dramatic and diagnostic of acute gout. Phenylbutazone, 200 mg, two or three times daily during the acute stage, is an alternative. Indomethacin will also result in rapid resolution of symptoms.

The acutely inflamed joint should be immobilized and the patient put at bed rest.

Subsequent Management. Since not all uric acid is derived from exogenous sources but much of it is synthesized in the body, a strict dietary limitation of purines will not prevent subsequent attacks. However, the diet should be limited in this respect, although even with complete abstinence from purines attacks will recur.

Patients should be maintained on continued colchicine dosage in attempts to reduce the frequency of recurrences of acute symptoms. Most patients are managed with one or two colchicine tablets per day, increasing the dosage at the first signs of recurrence.

The formation of new tophi and recurrent attacks can be reduced by uricosuric agents: probenecid and salicylates. Allopurinol, a xanthine oxidase blocking agent, will reduce serum uric acid concentration and is effective in reducing chronic tophaceous deposits.

Chronic Gouty Arthritis. Treatment of chronic gouty arthritis is almost exclusively by medical measures. When severe joint destruction has occurred, surgical reconstruction including arthrodesis and arthroplasty may be required. Large tophaceous deposits causing irritation of overlying skin about joints may be excised with considerable benefit to the patient. Tophaceous deposits requiring excision have also been responsible for median nerve compression in the carpal tunnel.

Pseudogout (Chondrocalcinosis, or Crystal Deposition Disease)

McCarty has called our attention to the condition of calcium pyrophosphate crystal deposition disease. Prior to the characterization of articular chondrocalcinosis and the discovery that calcium pyrophosphate crystals could induce an acute arthritis, these patients were thought to have a type of gout. The incidence of pseudogout may be more common than gout, but it is not as well recognized. It occurs in males $1\frac{1}{2}$ times as commonly as females. The age of onset is commonly in the middle or the late decades but may be in the twenties.

CLINICAL MANIFESTATIONS. An acute attack may be similar to gout and occurs frequently after joint trauma or in postoperative patients. The onset may be acute, with symptoms increasing in a joint over 1 to 2 days in contrast to the more abrupt onset of gout. The joint most commonly involved is the knee joint. It is quite uncommon in the MP joint of the great toe. Patients with acute attacks have asymptomatic intervals. One-third of such patients have an elevation of the serum uric acid level.

A small percentage of patients will have continuous acute attacks, but the most frequent pattern is that of progressive chronic arthritis of large joints. Hypertension and diabetes are associated with one-fourth to one-half of patients with pseudogout.

The patients complain of acute pain in the involved joint with stiffness, local swelling, tenderness, and erythema overlying the joint. In the chronic presentation, the joint may resemble a degenerative arthritis.

The diagnosis is dependent upon finding calcium pyrophosphate crystals in the synovial fluid or in leukocytes of synovial fluid. Polarized light microscopy reveals the crystals to show weakly positive birefringence. X-rays reveal crystalline deposits in the articular cartilage (Fig. 48-26) as well as in fibrocartilaginous structures as menisci (Fig. 48-27) and ligaments in joint capsules. The distal radioulnar nerve and symphysis pubis, as well as glenoid and acetabular labra, may show calcification. The calcification of the articular cartilage is in the midzonal layer and appears as a radiopaque line, paralleling the subchondral bone.

Treatment of an acute attack is by aspiration of the synovial effusion and the local injection of cortisone. Systemic phenylbutazone and salicylates may be helpful, but colchicine is not. At present, there is no means of halting the progressive deposition in joints.

HEMOPHILIC ARTHRITIS

The major problem confronting the hemophiliac between episodes of acute bleeding is his disability due to hemophilic arthropathy. Duthie et al. have shown spontaneous bleeding occurs only with 0 percent circulating Factor VIII; severe bleeding after minor injury occurs when Factor VIII is between 1 to 5 percent, and excessive bleeding after minor injury or operation at 5 to 25 percent of normal (Fig. 48-28). Classic hemophilia is due to Factor

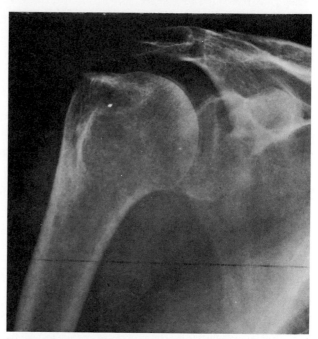

Fig. 48-26. Pseudogout chondrocalcinosis. Note calcification of the articular cartilage of the humeral head.

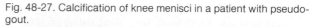

Fig. 48-27. Calcification of knee menisci in a patient with pseudogout.

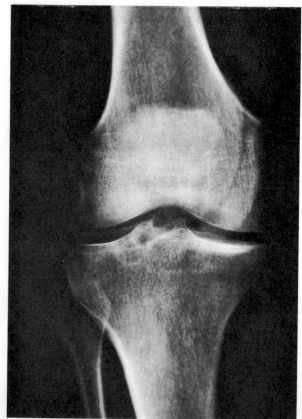

Factor VIII level (% average normal)	Haemorrhagic manifestations
50 – 100	None
25 – 50	Excessive bleeding occasionally after serious injury or major operation
5 – 25	Excessive bleeding after minor injury or surgery
1 – 5	Severe bleeding after minor injury. Occasional haemarthrosis and spontaneous bleeding
0	Severe haemophilia with spontaneous bleeding into muscles and joints.

Fig. 48-28. Relationships of blood Factor VIII levels to hemorrhagic manifestations.

VIII deficiency, while Christmas disease is due to a deficiency of Factor IX.

Synovia and capsule have no tissue thromboplastin. In the hemophiliac with inability to generate circulating thromboplastin, the absence of tissue thromboplastin allows hemorrhage due to injury or spontaneous hemorrhage to occur and go unchecked in joint cavities. Repeated hemorrhage into growing joints results in progressive deterioration and chronic arthritis.

PATHOLOGY. The synovium is thickened with hyperplasia of the synovial lining cells. There are diffuse areas of chronic and acute inflammatory cells with hemosiderin deposition in the surface and the depths of the synovial

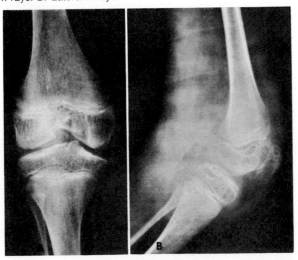

Fig. 48-29. Hemophilic arthritis. AP and lateral x-rays of the knee joint showing enlargement of epiphyses of the knee, joint space narrowing, with irregularity and squaring of the lower end of the patella. Note also the soft tissue swelling about the knee. A. AP x-rays. B. Lateral x-rays.

tissue. New blood vessels and fibrous tissue increase in the subintimal synovial tissue.

The adjacent growing epiphyses enlarge and change shape, findings which are demonstrated by x-ray. There is osteoporosis of the adjacent epiphyses and metaphyses. Cartilage destruction occurs in varying degrees and increases with severity and chronicity of the joint hemorrhage. Cysts may occur in the subchondral bone in long-standing cases. Degenerative changes are superimposed if the patient survives.

CLINICAL MANIFESTATIONS. In the severe hemophiliac, bleeding into one of the large joints occurs spontaneously or with mild trauma. The most common joint of involvement is the knee, followed by elbow, ankle, and shoulder, with joint hemorrhage in any joint a possibility. If unchecked by coagulation therapy, hemarthrosis becomes acute, and the joint assumes that position which accommodates the greatest volume of fluid and comfort, i.e., 20° of flexion for the knee or adduction and external rotation for the hip joint. The patient will not move the joint because of pain and associated muscle spasm.

The hemorrhage tends to run in cycles, one or two joints being repeatedly affected, followed by other joints with recurrent episodes. In the chronic stage, with sufficient joint destruction and arthritis, there is limitation of motion, fixed contracture, and deformity.

In the acutely involved joint, x-ray findings may show only soft tissue swelling and the presence of effusion. With repeated hemorrhage, adjacent epiphyses enlarge and change the configuration. The characteristic findings in the knee joint (Fig. 48-29) are a squared-off lower pole of the patella, enlargement of femoral condyles, and increase in size of the intercondylar notch. Osteoporosis may be marked, and joint space is narrow. In the chronic state, the residual changes in epiphyseal configuration are superimposed with sclerosis and osteophytes of degenerative change.

TREATMENT. If joint hemorrhage can be minimized, the chronic arthritis will not ensue. Patients with the first sign of hemorrhage into the joint should be treated with appropriate coagulation factors, i.e., Factor VIII. The joint is splinted with a compression bandage until effective blood clotting ensues. Weight-bearing joints are protected with crutches until the range of motion of the joint returns and the joint effusion resolves. Joints subjected to repeated hemorrhage must be protected with bracing to limit motion and prevent recurrence. The short leg brace preventing ankle motion is used for the ankle, and a light plastic splint is used for repeated hemorrhage into the knee.

If contractures have developed, these are corrected by reversal dynamic traction. When the contracture has been corrected, an immobilizing brace is applied. A Quingle-type cast may be used for severe degrees of subluxation of the knee. Ischial weight-bearing braces may be required for serious involvement of the hip joints. With adequate prophylaxis and early treatment, severe deformity can be prevented. Reconstructive surgery for joint deformities is now being carried out in specialized centers where the clotting factor deficiency can be reversed for the healing and rehabilitation phases.

SYNOVIAL LESIONS

Pigmented Villonodular Synovitis

Pigmented villonodular synovitis is an inflammatory process of unknown cause which occurs in monarticular form in young adults. The peak incidence of this condition is in the thirties, with men more frequently involved than women.

Patients present with symptoms of pain and swelling which may be intermittent and are frequently of long duration. The most commonly involved joint is the knee, but any single large joint may be involved. On examination there is usually evidence of synovial thickening with effusion. Joint aspiration characteristically reveals bloody or dark brown sanguineous fluid. X-ray evaluation may reveal soft tissue swelling and occasionally cystic erosion of joint margins.

The pathologic finding is a villous, thickened, brownish proliferation of synovial tissue which has nodules and pedicles of synovium projecting into the joint. Microscopic examination reveals proliferated synovial cells with large, round, stromal connective cells beneath the surface. Hemosiderin and cholesterol are diffused throughout the synovium in the intercellular space and in multinucleated giant cells.

Treatment of this condition depends upon its early recognition and removal by synovectomy. If there is recurrence after synovectomy, repeat surgical treatment is required and is usually successful. The same process may occur as a localized nodular form, and a similar pathologic condition may occur in a bursa or as a localized nodular tenosynovitis.

Synovial Chondromatosis

Synovial chondromatosis is a condition occurring in synovium, bursa, or tendon sheaths in which metaplastic cartilage growth occurs. Such growths may ossify and persist in the synovium or become detached and displaced into the joint cavity as a loose body. The condition occurs as a monarticular arthritis in middle-aged adults. The knee is most commonly involved, but any large joint may be affected. Clinical examination reveals signs of inflammation with effusion. X-rays show evidence of calcified bodies in the synovium or joint space. The remainder of the joint may be normal or secondarily degenerative because of mechanical trauma from the loose body. Synovectomy is the treatment of choice.

Acute Synovitis of the Hip in Childhood

Children in the Legg-Calvé-Perthes age group, age three to ten years, may present with an acutely painful hip. The mother may note a hip limp of several days' duration in the child. In other situations, the discomfort is acute enough so that the child will not bear weight. X-rays of the hip may reveal soft tissue swelling of the hip in the absence of bone changes of the capital femoral epiphyses.

Immediate evaluation should attempt to rule out acute septic arthritis by hip joint aspiration. Acute synovitis of the hip is a diagnosis of exclusion. If an initial sepsis can be ruled out, the child is placed at bed rest with the leg in Buck's traction. When the acute symptoms resolve, he is allowed to ambulate with non-weight-bearing crutch walking. Repeat x-rays are obtained in 6 weeks to be certain that Legg-Calvé-Perthes disease is not developing. In the absence of signs of Legg-Calvé-Perthes disease, the child is allowed weight-bearing ambulation.

HYPERTROPHIC PULMONARY OSTEOARTHROPATHY

Hypertrophic pulmonary osteoarthropathy is a syndrome affecting bone and joints of the extremities and occurring in association with intrathoracic pathologic conditions. Patients develop insidious asymptomatic clubbing of the fingers, which is an increased nail bed convexity with loss of the normal angle between the proximal nail beds and the distal covering of the dorsal surface of the phalanx. The nail may be brittle and striated with an underlying vascular engorgement. Associated with the clubbing may be a synovitis of a peripheral joint. X-ray examination of the extremities may reveal new periosteal bone along the shafts, including distal phalanges. This is responsible for the clubbing effect.

When clubbing is noted, a thoracic pathologic condition should be immediately suspected. Bronchiectasis, chronic emphysema, tuberculosis, valvular disease of the heart, and, especially, pulmonary malignant tumors are possible causes.

The exact cause is unknown, but is thought to be associated with changes in tissue oxygenation or arteriolar blood flow as a consequence of lung disease. Treatment depends upon diagnosis and treatment of the underlying lung condition. It is not uncommon to excise a pulmonary neoplasm and have peripheral joint symptoms completely resolve.

NEUROPATHIC, OR CHARCOT, JOINTS

A neuropathic joint, or Charcot joint, is a condition which occurs as a consequence of various neurologic diseases. Tabes dorsalis, syringomyelia, leprosy, or diabetes may be associated with the development of neuropathic joints. Neuropathic joints have also been described in association with insensitivity due to peripheral nerve lesions and in rare situations where no neurologic lesion is evident.

The prevailing opinion as to the mechanism of destruction in such joints has been repeated trauma on structures rendered insensitive by sensory interruption. However, some patients do have pain associated with these lesions, suggesting that other factors may be responsible.

CLINICAL MANIFESTATIONS. The onset is commonly insidious with the patient unaware of the degree of joint disability developing. There may be minor discomfort in a weight-bearing joint—hip, knee, ankle, or tarsus—with diffuse swelling about the joint, but medical aid may not be sought until gross instability and deformity are present. The knee joint may have a massive effusion with gross instability of all ligamentous supporting structures. Associated with this may be varying degrees of edema and swelling involving the leg. In the case of the tarsal joints, swelling with erythema and valgus or varus deformity are common presentations.

Radiographic findings (Fig. 48-30) include extreme dissolution of bone ends with frank dislocation, enlarged joint space, and large collections of bone fragments deposited

Fig. 48-30. Neuropathic knee due to tabes dorsalis showing marked destruction of medial femoral condyle. Clinically there was marked synovial swelling and effusion with marked instability due to the loss of bone substances.

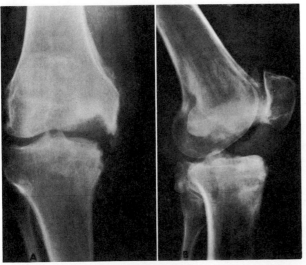

in the enlarged synovial cavity. A rapid rate of change by x-ray, with bone loss and destruction, is suggestive of a neuropathic joint. Infection frequently complicates the diagnosis of neuropathic joints, due to diabetes.

TREATMENT. The rate and degree of destruction of bone ends with marked ligamentous instability make conservative treatment difficult. A well-fitting ischial weight-bearing brace may benefit a patient with a Charcot knee or hip joint. If this is not tolerated, surgical arthrodesis of the knee, using the principles of Charnley or hip arthrodesis, is indicated.

In the insensitive foot of the diabetic, plaster cast immobilization has resulted in spontaneous fusion. Molded orthopedic shoes with contoured arch supports and metatarsal bars have been used for diabetics and lepers with severe neurotropic destruction of the tarsal joints. The end result in the diabetic is usually below-knee amputation.

PAINFUL SHOULDER

Spontaneous pain or pain after minor strains of the shoulder are extremely common after the age of thirty-five. The most common lesion responsible for shoulder pain in this age group is that of lesions of the rotator cuff, bicipital tendonitis, or subacromial bursitis. Before ascribing the diagnosis to a local lesion, it is mandatory to rule out disease of the cervical spine and central nervous system, as well as lesions of the brachial plexus, caused by Pancost's tumor, and referred pain from the heart, lungs, or gastrointestinal tract.

Lesions of the Rotator Cuff

The rotator cuff consists of the common tendinous insertion of supraspinatus, infraspinatus, and teres minor muscles as well as the subscapularis tendon. These tendons form a continuous fibrous sheath, which is intimately adherent to the underlying shoulder capsule. When the shoulder is moved from the anatomic position to the position of full elevation or abduction, the rotator cuff comes in contact with the undersurface of the coracoacromial ligament and is subject to mechanical irritation, and degenerative change occurs. With sufficient degeneration, bursitis may develop in the intervening subacromial bursa, which separates the undersurface of the acromion and coracoacromial ligament from the rotator cuff. With changes in the tendon, deposition of calcium occurs in the worn and degenerative tendon, as well as in the subacromial bursa.

CLINICAL MANIFESTATIONS. In the absence of preexisting symptomatology, a patient may note the spontaneous acute onset of severe unrelenting pain in the shoulder and in the region of the glenohumeral joint, occasionally referred into the arm and elbow. The onset may occur after unusual vigorous exercise or sports activities in the patient over thirty-five years. The patient may awaken with minor discomfort in the shoulder, which gradually increases in severity. The pain is unimproved by position and may require narcotics for relief.

On examination, there is local tenderness over the greater tuberosity of the humerus. Any motion of the shoulder causes pain. Routine x-rays of the shoulder may be negative or show a calcium deposit in the subacromial bursa or supraspinatus tendon.

TREATMENT. Untreated, the lesion will take about 5 to 10 days for relief of symptoms. If the patient is seen when symptoms are resolving, sling immobilization combined with analgesia may be sufficient. In the acutely painful situation, the bursa should be needled, 2% Xylocaine injected, and an aspiration of the bursa contents attempted. One milliliter of cortisone is then introduced. The results of this treatment are often dramatic. After injection, the shoulder is immobilized until pain relief is complete; then gradual shoulder-motion exercises of the pendulum type are instituted.

If the shoulder symptoms do not completely resolve, repeat cortisone injection is considered.

CHRONIC SUPRASPINATUS TENDONITIS

The presentation of degenerative lesions of the rotator cuff are often insidious. The patient complains of low-grade discomfort in the shoulder with sudden motion and with certain positions, such as full internal rotation and the extremes of abduction. These may be aggravated by increase in shoulder activity.

X-ray examination in such instances is more likely to show evidence of calcification in the supraspinatus tendon (Fig. 48-31). The treatment of this lesion should start with conservative therapy. The shoulder is immobilized in a sling and swathe for 10 days to 2 weeks until relief from pain is complete. Then gradual range-of-motion exercises are started. If this does not produce a response, cortisone is injected into the shoulder, or the shoulder is treated with diathermy or ultrasound.

RUPTURES OF THE ROTATOR CUFF

A rupture of the rotator cuff occurs commonly in middle age but may also occur in late adolescence and in the elderly. Occupation has no relationship to incidence. Minor strain or injury will cause a rupture in a previously degenerative tendon. The patient may have had preexisting chronic low-grade shoulder symptoms. The patient has difficulty in achieving full active shoulder motion, although there is no contracture on examination.

If radiopaque solution is injected into the shoulder, the solution will enter the subdeltoid bursa if there is discontinuity in the rotator cuff. X-ray evidence of fracture of the greater tuberosity indicates that the tendon has been avulsed. If the rupture has been present for a few weeks, the muscles involved, such as the supraspinatus, may show evidence of atrophy. If a calcium deposit is present, it is unlikely that rupture has occurred.

TREATMENT OF ROTATOR CUFF RUPTURES. Since 25 percent of shoulders at postmortem, in the absence of previous symptoms, have had evidence of torn or degenerated cuffs, immediate surgical treatment is not indicated. Most patients will recover with conservative treatment. The acute symptoms are treated by immobilization in a sling. When pain is resolved, gradual range-of-motion

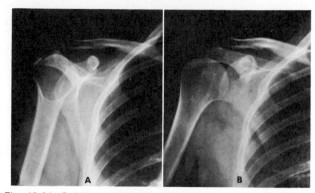

Fig. 48-31. Calcific supraspinatus tendonitis. *A.* AP x-ray of the shoulder with internal rotation shows calcium deposit in the region of the supraspinatus tendon. *B.* External rotation shows calcific shadow superimposed over the greater tuberosity.

exercises are instituted. If symptoms do not resolve within a few months with this type of treatment, open surgical repair, as described by McLaughlin, is done.

BICIPITAL TENDONITIS

Shoulder symptoms resembling supraspinatus tendonitis may be due to a bicipital tendon which has become irritated and inflamed in its groove and long passage through the shoulder joint. The symptoms are quite similar, but differentiation may be made on the basis of pain and tenderness extending farther distad over the bicipital groove. Treatment is by conservative means—cortisone, short-wave diathermy, immobilization—followed by return of motion. An occasional patient will require surgical exploration.

References

Anatomy

Barnett, C. H., Davies, D. V., and MacConaill, M. A.: "Synovial Joints: Their Structure and Mechanics," Charles C Thomas, Publisher, Springfield, Ill., 1961.

Curtiss, R. H.: Changes Produced in the Synovial Membrane and Synovial Fluid by Disease, instructional course lecture, American Academy of Orthopaedic Surgeons, *J Bone Joint Surg [Am]*, **46A:**873, 1964.

Examination

Hollander, J. L.: "Arthritis and Allied Conditions," Lea & Febiger, Philadelphia, 1966.

Pyogenic Arthritis

Clawson, B. K., and Dunn, A. W.: Management of Common Bacterial Infections of Bones and Joints, instructional course lecture, American Academy of Orthopaedic Surgeons, *J Bone Joint Surg [Am]*, **49A:**164, 1967.

Curtiss, P. H., and Klein, L.: Destruction of Articular Surfaces in Septic Arthritis. I. In Vitro Studies, *J Bone Joint Surg [Am]*, **45A:**797, 1963.

Hollander, J. L. (ed.): "Arthritis and Allied Conditions," Lea & Febiger, Philadelphia, 1966.

Phemister, D. B.: The Effect of Pressure on Articular Surfaces in Pyogenic and Tuberculosis Arthritides and Its Bearing on Treatment, *Ann Surg,* **80:**481, 1924.

Bone and Joint Tuberculosis

Henderson, M. S.: Tuberculosis of Joints with Special Reference to Knee, *Aust NZ J Surg,* **6:**27, 1936.

Hodgson, A. R., and Stuck, F. E.: Anterior Spine Fusion for the Treatment of Tuberculosis of the Spine, *J Bone Joint Surg [Am],* **42A:**295, 1960.

————, Wong, W., and Yau, A.: "X-ray Appearances of Tuberculosis of the Spine," Charles C Thomas, Publisher, Springfield, Ill., 1969.

Somerville, E. W., and Wilkinson, M. C.: "Girdlestone's Tuberculosis of Bone and Joint," Oxford University Press, London, 1965.

Gonococcal Arthritis

Ford, D. K.: Gonorrheal Arthritis, in J. L. Hollander (ed.), "Arthritis and Allied Conditions," Lea & Febiger, Philadelphia, 1966.

Rheumatoid Arthritis

Arthritis and Rheumatism Council and British Orthopaedic Association: Controlled Trial of Synovectomy of Knee and Metacarpophalangeal Joints in Rheumatoid Arthritis, *Ann Rheum Dis,* **35:**437, 1976.

Casagrande, P.: Surgical Rehabilitation of the Upper Extremities in Rheumatoid Arthritis, in Dixon, A. S. (ed.), "Progress in Clinical Rheumatology," chap. 6, Little, Brown and Company, Boston, 1965.

Clayton, M. L.: Surgery of the Thumb in Rheumatoid Arthritis, *J Bone Joint Surg [Am],* **44A:**1376, 1962.

————: Surgery of the Lower Extremity in Rheumatoid Arthritis, instructional course lecture, American Academy of Orthopaedic Surgeons, *J Bone Joint Surg [Am],* **45A:**1517, 1963.

Flatt, A. E.: "Care of the Rheumatoid Hand," The C. V. Mosby Company, St. Louis, 1963.

Hoffman, P.: An Operation for Severe Grades of Contracted or Claw Toes, *J Orthop Surg,* **9:**441, 1916.

Huskisson, E. C.: Report on Rheumatic Diseases, No. 54, Arthritis and Rheumatism Council, London, 1974.

Littler, J. W.: Basic Principles of Reconstructive Surgery of the Hand, *Surg Clin North Am,* **40:**383, 1960.

MacIntosh, D. L., and Hunter, J. B.: The Use of Hemiarthroplasty Prosthesis for Advanced Osteoarthritis and Rheumatoid Arthritis of the Knee, *J Bone Joint Surg [Br],* **54B:**244, 1972.

Mercer, S. W., and Duthie, R. B.: "Orthopaedic Surgery," Edward Arnold (Publishers) Ltd., London, 1972.

Murray, W. R., Lucas, D. B., and Inman, V. T.: Femoral Head and Neck Resection, *J Bone Joint Surg [Am],* **46A:**1184, 1964.

Niebauer, J. J., Shaw, J. L., and Doren, W. W.: Silicone-Dacron Hinge Prosthesis. Design, Evaluation, and Application, in J. S. Calnan and P. J. L. Holt (eds.): "Workshop on Artificial Finger Joints," vol. 28, pp. 56–58, British Medical Association, London, 1969.

Sokoloff, L.: Pathology of Rheumatoid Arthritis and Allied Diseases, in J. L. Hollander, "Arthritis and Allied Conditions," Lea & Febiger, Philadelphia, 1966.

Swanson, A. B.: Flexible Implant Arthroplasty for Arthritic Finger

Joints: Rationale, Technique, and Results of Treatment, *J Bone Joint Surg [Am],* **54A:**435, 1972.

Osteoarthritis

Aufranc, O. E.: "Constructive Surgery of the Hip," The C. V. Mosby Company, St. Louis, 1962.

————: Mould Arthroplasty of the Hip, in W. D. Graham (ed.), "Modern Trends in Orthopaedics," vol. 5, p. 23, Appleton Century Crofts, New York, 1967.

Byers, P. D., Contepomi, C. A., and Farkas, T. A.: A Post Mortem Study of the Hip Joint, Including the Prevalence of the Features of the Right Side, *Ann Rheum Dis,* **29:**15, 1970.

Charnley, J.: The Long-Term Results of Low Friction Arthroplasty of the Hip Performed as a Primary Intervention, *J Bone Joint Surg [Br],* **54B:**61, 1972.

Copeman, W. S. C.: Osteoarthrosis, in W. S. C. Copeman (ed.), "Textbook of the Rheumatic Diseases," E. & S. Livingstone Ltd., Edinburgh, 1964.

Denham, R. A.: Hip Mechanics, *J Bone Joint Surg [Br],* **41B:**550, 1959.

Dowson, D., and Wright, V.: Lubrication, Friction and Wear of Total Hip Replacements, in M. Jayson (ed.), "Total Hip Replacement," J. B. Lippincott Company, Philadelphia, 1971.

Girdlestone, G. R.: Acute Pyogenic Arthritis of the Hip, *Lancet,* **1:**419, 1943.

Harris, N. H., and Kirwan, E.: The Results of Osteotomy for Early Primary Osteoarthritis of the Hip, *J Bone Joint Surg [Br],* **46B:**477, 1964.

Hoaglund, F. T.: Osteoarthritis, *Orthop Clin North Am,* **2:**3, 1970.

Jackson, P., and Waugh, W.: Tibial Osteotomy for Osteoarthritis of the Knee, *J Bone Joint Surg [Br],* **45B:**618, 1963.

Jayson, M.: "Total Hip Replacement," J. B. Lippincott Company, Philadelphia, 1971.

Keller, W. L.: Surgical Treatment of Bunions and Hallux Valgus, *NY Med J,* **80:**741, 1904.

Kellgren, J. H., and Moore, R.: Generalized Osteoarthritis and Heberden's Nodes, *Br Med J,* **1:**181, 1952.

Kettelkamp, D. B., Wenger, D. R., Chao, E. Y. S., and Thompson, C.: Results of Proximal Tibial Osteotomy: The Effects of Tibiofemoral Angle, Stance-Phase Flexion-Extension and Medial Plateau Force, *J Bone Joint Surg,* **58A:**952, 1976.

McBride, E. D.: Hallux Valgus, Bunion Deformity: Its Treatment in Mild, Moderate, and Severe Stages, *J Int Coll Surg,* **21:**99, 1954.

McKee, G. K., and Watson-Farrar, J.: Replacement of Arthritic Hips by the McKee-Farrar Prosthesis, *J Bone Joint Surg [Br],* **48B:**245, 1966.

Mankin, H. J.: Biochemical and Metabolic Aspects of Osteoarthritis, *Orthop Clin North Am,* **2:**19, 1971.

Pearson, J. R., and Riddell, D. M.: Idiopathic Osteoarthritis of the Hip, *Ann Rheum Dis,* **21:**31, 1962.

Scales, J. T., and Lowe, S. A.: Some Factors Influencing Bone and Joint Replacement: With Special Reference to the Stanmore Total Hip Replacement, in M. Jayson (ed.), "Total Hip Replacement," J. B. Lippincott Company, Philadelphia, 1971.

Sokoloff, L.: The Pathology and Pathogenesis of Orthoarthritis, chap. 51, in J. L. Hollander (ed.), "Arthritis and Allied Conditions," Lea & Febiger, Philadelphia, 1966.

Walker, P. S., and Bienenstock, M.: Fixation Properties of Acrylic Cement, *Rev Hosp Spec Surg,* **1:**27, 1971.

West, F. E., and Soto-Hall, R.: Recurrent Dislocation of the Patella in the Adult: End Results of Patellectomy and Quadriceps Plasty, *J Bone Joint Surg [Am]*, **40A:**386, 1958.

Wiles, P., Andrews, T. S., and Bevas, M. B.: Chondromalacia of the Patella, *J Bone Joint Surg [Br]*, **38B:**95, 1956.

Gout

Burch, T. A., O'Brian, W. M., Kurland, L. T., Need, R., and Bunim, J. J.: Hyperuricemia and Gout in the Marianas Islands, *Arthritis Rheum*, **7:**296, 1964.

McCarty, D. J.: Pseudogout: Articular Chondrocalcinosis Calcium Pyrophosphate Crystal Deposition Disease, chap. 56, in J. L. Hollander (ed.), "Arthritis and Allied Conditions," Lea & Febiger, Philadelphia, 1966.

————, and Hollander, J. L.: Identification of Urate Crystals in Gouty Synovial Fluid, *Ann Intern Med*, **54:**452, 1961.

Seegmiller, J. E., and Howell, R. R.: The Old and New Concepts of Acute Gouty Arthritis, *Arthritis Rheum*, **5:**616, 1962.

————, ————, and Malowista, S. E.: The Inflammatory Reaction to Sodium Urate: Its Possible Relationship to the Genesis of Acute Gouty Arthritis, *JAMA*, **180:**469, 1962.

Smyth, C. J.: Hereditary Factors in Gout: A Review of Recent Literature, *Metabolism*, **6:**218, 1957.

Stecher, R. M., Hersh, A. H., and Solomon, W. M.: The Heredity of Gout and Its Relationship to Familial Hyperuricemia, *Ann Intern Med*, **31:**595, 1949.

Wyngaarden, J. B.: Etiology and Pathogenesis of Gout, chap. 54, in J. L. Hollander (ed.), "Arthritis and Allied Conditions," Lea & Febiger, Philadelphia, 1966.

————, Rundles, R. W., Silberman, H. R., and Hunter, S.: Control of Hyperuricemia and Hydroxypyrazolopyrimidine, a Purine Analogue Which Inhibits Uric Acid Synthesis, *Arthritis Rheum*, **6:**306, 1963.

Hemophilic Arthritis

Atprup, T., and Sjolini, K. E.: Thromboplastic and Fibrinolytic Activity of Human Synovial Membrane in Fibrous Capsular Tissue, *Proc Soc Exp Biol*, **92:**852, 1958.

Duthie, R. B., Matthews, J. M., Rizza, C. R., and Steel, W. M.: "The Musculoskeletal Problems in the Haemophilics," Blackwell Scientific Publications, Oxford, England, 1972.

Synovial Lesions

Chung, S. M. K., and James, J. M.: Diffuse Pigmented Villonodular Synovitis of the Hip Joint, *J Bone Joint Surg [Am]*, **47A:**239, 1965.

Jaffe, H. L., Lichtenstein, L., and Seutro, C. J.: Pigmented Villonodular Synovitis, Bursitis, and Tenosynovitis, *Arch Pathol*, **31:**731, 1941.

McIvor, R. R., and King, D.: Osteochondromatosis of the Hip Joint, *J Bone Joint Surg [Am]*, **44A:**87, 1962.

Murphy, A. F., and Wilson, J. N.: Tenosynovial Osteochondroma in the Hand, *J Bone Joint Surg [Am]*, **40A:**1236, 1958.

Hypertrophic Pulmonary Osteoarthropathy

Smyth, C. J.: Rheumatism and Arthritis: Sixteenth Rheumatism Review, *Ann Intern Med*, **61**(*Suppl* 6):3, 1964.

Neuropathic or Charcot Joints

Charnley, J., and Baker, S. L.: Compression Arthrodesis of the Knee: A Clinical and Histological Study, *J Bone Joint Surg [Am]*, **34A:**187, 1952.

Johnson, J. T. H.: Neuropathic Fractures and Joint Injuries: Pathogenesis and Rationale of Prevention and Treatment, *J Bone Joint Surg [Am]*, **49A:**1, 1967.

King, E. J. S.: On Some Aspects of the Pathology of Hypertrophic Charcot's Joints, *Br J Surg*, **18:**113, 1930.

Mooney, V., and Mankin, H. J.: A Case of Congenital Insensitivity to Pain with Neurotrophic Arthropathy, *Arthritis Rheum*, **9:**821, 1966.

Painful Shoulder

McLaughlin, H.: Rupture of the Rotator Cuff, instructional course lecture, American Academy of Orthopaedic Surgeons, *J Bone Joint Surg [Am]*, **44A:**979, 1962.

Milone, F. P., and Copeland, M. M.: Calcific Tendonitis of the Shoulder Joint: Presentation of 136 Cases Treated by Irradiation, *Am J Roentgenol Radium Ther Nucl Med*, **85:**901, 1961.

Chapter 49

Amputations

by Seymour I. Schwartz

GENERAL CONSIDERATIONS

Indications

The indications for amputation of part or all of an extremity include (1) trauma which is sufficiently extensive to preclude repair; (2) tumor of the bone, soft tissue, muscles, blood vessels, or nerves; (3) extensive infection which does not respond to conservative measures or contributes to septicemia; and (4) a variety of peripheral vascular diseases. Refinement in surgical technique as applied to blood vessels and peripheral nerves has markedly reduced the indications for amputation following trauma and has permitted reimplantation of totally amputated extremities.

Amputations accounted for 2 percent of all operations performed in Veterans Administration hospitals in 1964. Presently, more than two-thirds of the amputations on civilians in Western society are performed for peripheral vascular disease in patients over the age of fifty.

AMPUTATION OF ISCHEMIC LIMBS

Amputations are performed for four main categories of vascular disease: (1) arteriosclerosis obliterans, (2) arteriosclerosis obliterans with diabetes, (3) thromboangiitis obliterans, and (4) miscellaneous conditions such as embolic occlusion, peripheral aneurysm, vascular trauma, and venous obstruction. The specific indications for amputation in these patients are severe arterial insufficiency with necrosis of all or part of an extremity, intractable and severe pain which disables the patient, and infection which is spreading or unresponsive to therapy. In a few patients, extrarenal azotemia and hyperkalemia secondary to tissue necrosis constitute specific indications for amputation.

Amputation performed on a patient with compromised circulation requires special consideration. The patients are generally more brittle and require more intensive preoperative preparation. The compromised vascular supply within the limb necessitates meticulous and somewhat refined techniques, as described below. It is more difficult to achieve healing of the stump, and even after it has healed, breakdown related to the trauma of a prosthesis may occur. Finally, the patients are generally less vigorous and less adept at handling prostheses.

Selection of Site

Several factors contribute to the decision concerning level of amputation. When amputation is performed for malignant disease, the principal factor is wide excision of grossly apparent tumor. In the case of amputation subsequent to trauma or for peripheral vascular disease, the major factor determining the optimal level is usually the extent of healthy tissue. Other factors include the length of the stump sufficient for function of a prosthesis, the cosmetic effect of a prosthesis, and the placement of the scar so that it will neither break down nor compromise the fitting of the prosthesis.

In general, the longer the amputation stump, the more functional the limb and the better control the patient has of his prosthesis. For traumatic amputations with irregular damage to the skin, grafting procedures and mobilization of flaps are indicated to maintain as much of the bony length as possible. Regarding the upper extremity, as much length as possible should always be saved, even if there is only a very short below-elbow or humeral stump. There are exceptions to the general rule of "the longer, the better." For the lower extremity, proximal to the Syme amputation, the best level below the knee as far as prosthetic fitting is concerned is at the gastrocnemius musculotendinous junction. Proximal to knee disarticulation, an amputation which removes at least 4 in. of the distal femur is indicated, so that a prosthetic knee joint can be fitted with less difficulty. For children, disarticulation is frequently the procedure of choice in order to save the growing epiphysis and minimize the problem of distal bone overgrowth.

Other factors which contribute to selection of amputation site are the patient's general condition and, particularly, the feasibility of rehabilitation. More proximal amputations are indicated for bedridden patients who require nursing care, since these procedures are associated with a higher incidence of primary healing. If there is established contracture, it is usually preferable to plan to amputate above the level of contracture, to permit rehabilitation.

Factors which influence selection of the level of amputation in patients with peripheral vascular disease vary with the region. At all levels, healing ability is a function of nutritional skin blood flow. The status of the skin circulation may be evidenced by the extent of skin circulation. More recently, the clearance of radioxenon, measured at the anterior incision line, has been shown to correlate well with the healing of amputations. In one series no patient with a flow exceeding 0.6 ml/100 Gm tissue per minute failed to heal because of ischemia, and no patient with a lower flow was able to heal a BK amputation.

A correlation has been reported between the healing of both digital and transmetatarsal amputations and the presence of peripheral pulses. In patients with a palpable popliteal pulse, healing at this level occurred twice as effectively as in those in whom only femoral pulse was demonstrated. Potential for healing minor forefoot amputations has been predicted by determining ankle pressures using Doppler Ultrasound. No amputations in this region healed with a pressure of less than 60 mmHg. Although the presence of a palpable popliteal pulse generally ensures adequate circulation below the knee, several series have reported that the presence or absence of the pulse did not affect the healing of a BK amputation. Oscillometry may be applied to determine the level of pulsatile circulation, and arteriography is helpful in determining the patency of major vessels in significant collateral circulation around the knee.

The recent advances in rehabilitation and the application of the immediate prosthetic fitting have increased the indications for BK amputations and reduced the incidence of AK amputations. In selecting between these two sites, there are two additional factors which have to be assessed, viz., the patient's general condition and the prospect for rehabilitation.

Preoperative Management

Amputations for massive trauma should be performed early to reduce the extent of contamination and the potential for infection. When an amputation is being considered for ischemia, care of the patient and the involved and uninvolved extremities is critical. Atelectasis, pneumonia, and decubiti must be prevented in elderly bedridden patients. This can be accomplished by frequently turning the patients and providing them with a trapeze which can also be used to condition muscles to be used postoperatively. If the patient is diabetic, it is generally preferable to revert to a regimen of crystalline insulin rather than long-acting medications, since this is easier to regulate on the day of the operation and postoperatively.

Care of the ischemic extremity and also the contralateral extremity, which is frequently compromised, involves strict avoidance of injuries to areas of deficient circulation. The strength of wasted muscles and the motion of the critical joints must be preserved or, frequently, restored. Efforts should be made to heal necrotic or infected lesions, and only after direct arterial reconstruction and occasionally sympathectomy have failed to evidence improvement of the lesion is amputation indicated. The leg is usually kept in a slightly dependent position, and Buerger's exercises may be applied to improve the circulation. In the face of infection, drainage and local wet dressings of warm saline solution coupled with the appropriate antibiotic are employed. Intense heat and soaks are contraindicated, and if no infection is apparent and there is dry gangrene, wet dressings should not be used. Injury to ischemic areas is avoided by moving the patient frequently and preventing pressure to the heel by placing the foot on a pillow or lambskin mat. Foot care is administered to all areas without open lesions and to the uninvolved extremity. In some instances of digital gangrene, spontaneous amputation will occur, and this is frequently preferable to an operative procedure.

Refrigeration may be used preliminary to amputation to improve the condition of the patient by decreasing the metabolic by-products of the necrotic limb and also decreasing the absorption of these products and infectious material. Refrigeration also relieves pain, but the technique should not be employed if there is any hope of salvaging the extremity. The technique involves the placement of ice bags below the proposed level of amputation and may require use of mild narcotics.

Wrapping of the extremity in towels impregnated with antiseptic materials such as hexachlorophene for 12 hours prior to operation has been advised as a method of reducing the incidence of wound infection. Either spinal or inhalation anesthesia may be used for lower extremity amputations, while regional block may be applicable for distal upper extremity amputations.

Principles of Technique

The three general classes of amputations are (1) the standard or conventional amputation, (2) the osteomyoplastic or myodesis amputation, and (3) the provisional, or open (guillotine), amputation.

The conventional amputation is performed by constructing curved skin and fascial flaps which have their base at the level of amputation. The muscles, major blood vessels, and bone are divided at the level of amputation, while the major nerves are put on slight stretch and transected so that they retract approximately 1 in. proximal to the level of amputation. The muscles may be tapered so that not too much soft tissue remains over the bone end, and the distal inch of periosteum may be removed to avoid leaving a detached segment which can cause bone spur formation. After the amputation has been completed, the deep and superficial fascia are approximated over the bone, and the skin is loosely closed. The wound may be closed without drainage, or drainage may be established by soft rubber tubes or preferably a catheter connected to a closed section suction apparatus.

The osteomyoplastic amputations and myodesis provide for improved function and have been employed with increasing frequency when immediate postsurgical prosthetics (IPOP) are applied. Skin and fascial flaps are prepared in a manner similar to that used during conventional amputation, and the nerves and blood vessels are also divided in a routine fashion. In the osteomyoplastic technique, the muscles are divided 2 in. distal to the level of bone transection, and, prior to amputation of the bone, an osteoperiosteal flap is developed so that it may be sutured to the opposing periosteum in order to cover the bone and plug the marrow cavity. Then, with the remaining extremity in neutral position, i.e., extension for BK amputation and hip extension for AK amputation, the antagonistic muscles are sutured across the bone ends. Closure and drainage is similar to that employed in conventional amputations. In the case of myodesis, the distal ends of the transected muscle are attached to the bone by suturing through drill holes through the distal end. The muscles should be attached at a point that will put them under moderate tension so that they will become fixed along their normal pathway in a position slightly beyond rest length and therefore capable of providing maximal function.

Open, or provisional (guillotine), amputations should be regarded as drainage procedures and are rarely indicated. They are of historical interest in that they represent the most commonly employed procedures prior to the age of modern surgery. The procedure is still employed to release a person whose extremity is caught under an immovable object and is used for severely ill and toxic patients who are considered unable to tolerate a definitive amputation. All tissues are cut circularly, but the bone is transected higher than the fascia, which, in turn, is cut higher than the skin, in the hope that the soft tissue will ultimately cover the bone end with the help of traction. The results are generally poor, and a large scar, which adheres to bone, often results. The operation is frequently followed by a long healing period, exuberant granulation tissue, fibrosis, muscle retraction, prolonged drainage, reinfection, and exposure of the bone; definitive reamputation is frequently required.

AMPUTATIONS FOR PERIPHERAL VASCULAR DISEASE

Under no circumstance should a tourniquet or constricting bandage be applied, and throughout the procedure undue trauma should be avoided. Short skin and fascial flaps with minimal undermining are employed.

For patients who are to be fitted with an IPOP, the technique is modified. The anterior incision is made at the level of the anticipated bone division, and no anterior flap is constructed. Skin coverage is achieved with a thick posterior flap which includes subcutaneous tissue and fascia. Extreme gentleness is used throughout the procedure. Careful hemostasis is necessary to prevent hematoma formation and subsequent infection. If there is any question of compromised blood supply at the level of amputation, that site of amputation is abandoned and a higher site immediately used. In the case of midthigh amputation for peripheral vascular disease, some surgeons have advised routine ligation of the ipsilateral common femoral vein to obviate embolism.

Postoperative Management

The conventional postoperative care has been directed toward providing an adequate period of rest for tissues by splinting, firm compression over the injured tissue to prevent postoperative edema, exercises and positioning to prevent contracture, and rehabilitation (see Chap. 52) to provide the patient ultimately with a prosthesis compatible with both his vocational demands and ability.

A lightly compressive dressing is applied to the stump immediately after the operation and until the sutures are removed. Following this, elastic bandages are repeatedly applied to minimize the postoperative edema. Contractures are prevented by stump exercises and stretching the proximal joint in the hope of achieving full motion of the remaining joints of the amputated extremity. Rehabilitation requires the services of an experienced physiotherapist, occupational therapist, and prosthetist. In the case of lower extremity amputees, the sequence progresses from balance to crutch walking to use of temporary prosthesis with eventual application of permanent prosthesis. The upper extremity amputee frequently requires intensive training in the activities of daily living and of his specific vocation.

IPOP have recently achieved popularity in the management of extremity amputees. In this situation, a rigid dressing is applied at the operating table. This is accomplished by covering the stump with a sterilized sock and elastic plaster of paris bandages. Relief is provided for areas sensitive to pressure, and a prosthetic unit which includes socket attachment flaps may be applied immediately after the rigid dressing has dried. The patient is then encouraged to walk between parallel bars 24 hours after the operation, and weight bearing is increased daily. At 48 hours, a window may be cut in the plaster of paris to permit removal of the drain, and the material removed to provide the window is immediately replaced with plaster bandage. The rigid dressing is kept in place for approximately 2 weeks, at which time the sutures are removed and a new socket is applied without delay. Ten days later the second socket is removed, and at that time stump measurements and a cast are made for permanent prosthesis. Another temporary socket is provided until the permanent prosthesis is available. With both IPOP and the conventional management, shrinkage of the stump occurs in time and may necessitate a new socket for use with a permanent prosthesis.

Prognosis, Morbidity, and Mortality

Mortality and morbidity statistics and the incidence of rehabilitation are frequently difficult to evaluate, since many amputations have been performed by general surgeons with minimal training in postoperative rehabilitation, by orthopedic surgeons who are not experienced in the principles of operating on ischemic tissue, or all too often the most junior resident with the least training. The operative mortality for amputations performed for isolated tumor, trauma, or infection is less than 3 percent. By contrast, the mortality for amputations performed for peripheral vascular disease has been reported to be 22 and 29 percent in two large series. The mortality rate was doubled in patients who exhibited signs of arteriosclerotic disease of other systems and was increased twofold by postoperative complications. Diabetes did not apparently influence the mortality rate. The mortality rates were generally higher for more proximal amputations in the lower extremity; e.g., the mortality rate for AK amputations was 28 percent as compared with 10 percent for BK amputations. This could be related to the greater frailty of patients subjected to more proximal procedures. The results of recent series are more encouraging, with mortality rates of 3 percent and failure rates of 4 percent reported.

In a recent series reported by Couch and associates the operative mortality rate was 13 percent, with the most frequent causes being cardiac (52 percent) and pulmonary (26 percent) complications. Dale and Capps noted that pulmonary embolism caused 39 percent of deaths in their series. The high incidence of pulmonary embolism and other embolic phenomena has been stressed by Thompson and associates, who reported that in 4 percent of amputees pulmonary infarcts developed, 3 percent had myocardial infarctions, and 3 percent experienced cerebrovascular accidents in the postoperative period.

Phantom limb pain occurred relatively infrequently in most series, and the incidence has been reduced by avoiding the incorporation of nerve in scar tissue of the stump and by IPOP.

The median hospital stay for upper extremity amputees is between 2 and 3 weeks, whereas the average stay for lower extremity amputees was 11 weeks.

In a recent series of 130 patients with unilateral amputation, 70 received prostheses and 84 percent of these had successful rehabilitation. However, of the total group of those receiving unilateral amputations, only 30 percent of the AK group were successfully rehabilitated, while 66 percent of the BK group walked on prosthesis. In those patients with bilateral amputations, 30 percent have had successful rehabilitation, and this required that at least one of the amputation sites be at the BK level. Moore and associates compared the results of amputation and IPOP with the standard procedure. The IPOP group had a lower mortality, a higher primary healing rate, a reduction of time from amputation to fitting of a permanent prosthetic, and an increased rate of rehabilitation.

AMPUTATIONS OF THE LOWER EXTREMITY

The overwhelming majority of amputations in the lower extremity (Fig. 49-1) are performed for ischemia. A variety of eponyms have been applied to specific levels of amputations and refinements of technique, but the most commonly employed procedures are AK and BK amputations. Transmetatarsal and digital amputations are less frequently applicable in patients with peripheral vascular disease. The Syme amputation, knee disarticulation, hip disarticulation, and hemipelvectomy are usually reserved for malignant and traumatic lesions. At each level, the operative procedure and postoperative management are directed at achieving primary healing, a painless stump which will withstand the pressures of a prosthesis, and relatively unrestricted ambulation.

Toe Amputations

Amputations of one or more toes may be performed for gangrene or osteomyelitis. The procedure is rarely indicated for deformity, because excision of a toe results in deviation of adjacent toes. A transphalangeal level may be used if necrosis is distal to the proximal interphalangeal (PIP) joint and if there is absence of cellulitis, necrosis, and edema in the skin to be used for the flaps. If a more proximal amputation is required, transmetatarsal resection with removal of the head is preferable to disarticulation. The latter is associated with an increased incidence of breakdown, since the stump is bulky, and in the face of infection or poor vascular supply the exposed cartilage resists infection less effectively than bone. The incidence of healing at both the transphalangeal and transmetatarsal level has been relatively poor, with reports ranging from 40 to 60 percent. A direct relationship has been demonstrated between healing at these levels and the presence of popliteal and pedal pulses, suggesting that the poor results have been related to poor selection of amputation sites. Holden reported that digital amputations led to major amputations in 37 percent of cases and reported a mortality rate of 23 percent for these patients.

Transphalangeal Amputation

Either lateral or anteroposterior flaps may be used, and in either instance they should be sufficiently long to cover anticipated bone length. If an anteroposterior flap is employed, the plantar flap should be longer, so that the scar is placed dorsad. After the flaps have been established, the tendons and nerves are placed under slight tension and transected to permit retraction. The bone is transected and the skin and subcutaneous tissue closed loosely.

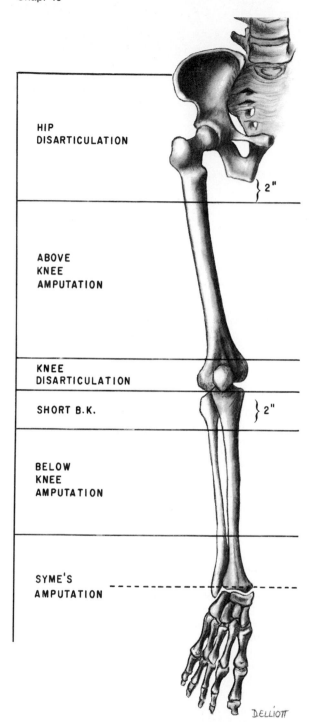

HIP
DISARTICULATION

} 2"

ABOVE
KNEE
AMPUTATION

KNEE
DISARTICULATION

SHORT B.K.

} 2"

BELOW
KNEE
AMPUTATION

SYME'S
AMPUTATION

D.ELLIOTT

Fig. 49-1. Levels of amputations in the lower extremity.

Transmetatarsal Amputation (Fig. 49-2)

A racquet incision is usually employed. In the case of a second, third, and fourth toe, the long limb is positioned on the dorsum of the foot, whereas it is placed on the medial and lateral surface for the great and small toes, respectively. Skin and subcutaneous tissue flaps are devel-

oped, and the head and neck of the metatarsal is amputated. Excessive skin is removed, and a closure without tension is accomplished.

The foot should be elevated in the immediate postoperative period, and ambulation may begin as soon as the incision is healed. There is no need for a special shoe.

Transmetatarsal Foot Amputations

The indications for this procedure include necrosis proximal to the PIP joint but distal to the level of the transmetatarsal incision. Necrosis in the interdigital creases constitutes a relatively frequent indication. Although Bradham and Smoak reported a failure rate of 66 percent in patients with atherosclerosis, the combined statistics reported by Warren et al. indicated that between two-thirds and three-fourths of the patients achieved healing, which in 10 to 50 percent of the instances was delayed. In one series, primary healing was achieved in 54 percent of patients with absent pedal pulses. Prior lumbar sympathectomy apparently did not alter the rate of healing.

TECHNIQUE (Fig. 49-3). Skin incisions and subcutaneous flaps are established so that the plantar flap is longer than the dorsal flap in order to maintain the thicker skin and permit placement of the scar on the distal surface. The plantar incision extends to within a centimeter of the crease between the base of the toes and the ball of the foot, and this flap is left as thick as possible, while the dorsal incision is developed directly to the bone and not established as a flap. Metatarsals are divided just proximal to the level of the dorsal incision, the specimen is removed, and the skin and fascia are closed in layers.

POSTOPERATIVE MANAGEMENT. The amputation provides a good stump, and preservation of the tibialis anterior tendon and intrinsic flexors and the fat pad help to maintain the short arch. The patients generally walk within 3 weeks after the operation, using a shoe with a pad of cotton in the toe.

Syme Amputations

This procedure is usually performed when most of the foot has been destroyed by trauma. Terminal arterial disease involving the distal part of the foot constitutes one of the few peripheral vascular disorders for which the Syme amputation is indicated. Functionally, it represents an excellent level for amputation since it maintains the length of the extremity, and preservation of the heel skin provides an excellent weight-bearing stump. However, the prosthesis is more difficult to fit, and because it is bulky, a BK amputation is preferable for females.

TECHNIQUE (Fig. 49-4). The incision extends from the anteroinferior border of the medial malleolus around the sole to the lateral maleolus and thence around the anterior aspect of the ankle to complete the circumference. The soft tissue is incised in a line down to the bone, avoiding trauma to the posterior tibial artery and its branches. The calcaneus is dissected from the skin and shelled from its attachments to permit removal of the foot. The tibia and fibula are then cleared and transected proximal to the flare

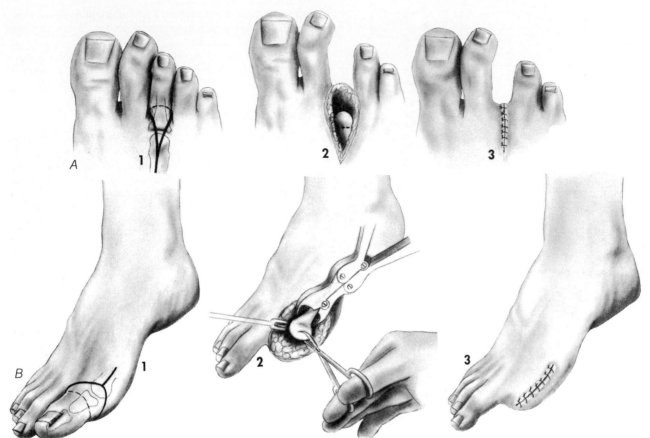

of the tibial malleolus. The long plantar flap is sutured to the anterior portion of the incision, with care to center the heel flap.

POSTOPERATIVE MANAGEMENT. In the conventional approach, the position of the heel pad is supported by tape. Since weight bearing occurs at the end of the stump, healing should be advanced and the heel flap firmly fixed to the end of the stump before the patient is permitted to walk either on the stump or on the prosthesis. The Canadian Syme prosthesis, which incorporates a SACH (solid ankle cushion heel) foot and ankle and an end-bearing socket on foam rubber, is one which is frequently employed. Excellent results have been obtained with immediate fitting of a prosthesis following the Syme procedure. Some of the weight-bearing load is transferred to the patellar tendon and the flares of the tibial condyles, and it is not necessary to immobilize the knee joint. Weight bearing is then begun within 24 hours when the stump is mature and stable, measurements for a permanent prosthesis are made, and the stump is replaced in a plaster bandage until the prosthesis is available. The permanent prosthesis is usually applied earlier with this approach than with the conventional management.

Below-the-Knee Amputations (BK)

This level is being employed with increasing frequency since the advent of IPOP. Major functional advantages of

Fig. 49-2. Transmetatarsal toe amputation. *A.* Technique for amputation of any of the middle three toes. 1. Racquet incision made. 2. Toe disarticulated and line of transection of the head of the metatarsal indicated. 3. Skin closure. *B.* Transmetatarsal amputation of the great or little toe. 1. Racquet incision with long limb on the side of the foot. 2. Toe disarticulated and the head of the metatarsal resected. 3. Lateral skin closure.

the BK amputation over the AK level are the ability to provide a more functional prosthesis for complete rehabilitation, the ability of the patient to move more easily in and out of bed, and a reduction in the incidence of phantom limb pain. Even a BK stump which is too short to accept a BK prosthesis is superior to an AK stump and can be fitted with a bent-knee prosthesis. BK amputations constitute the level of choice for ischemic lesions of the foot which do not extend above the malleoli but are generally not applicable if the gangrene extends in continuity above the ankle. Ischemic rigor of the calf muscles is another contraindication. Contracture of the knee or hip represents a relative contraindication, since it negates the functional advantages of this level.

The choice between the BK and AK amputation is determined by the patient's general health and potential for rehabilitation and an evaluation of the vascular status at the proposed level of amputation. No essential difference in healing rate was noted when patients with or without palpable popliteal pulses were evaluated, and, similarly, healing was not influenced by the presence or

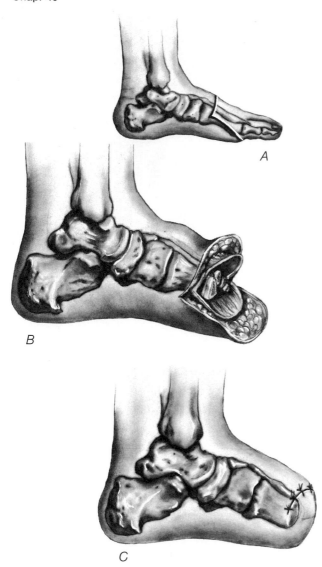

Fig. 49-3. Transmetatarsal foot amputation. *A*. Skin incision is outlined. Note the short dorsal flap and longer plantar flap. *B*. Distal part of the foot has been removed, and the head of the metatarsals have all been amputated. *C*. Fascia and skin have been closed so that the scar is located dorsad.

stump. Equally short anterior and posterior flaps may be made, or a longer posterior flap may be combined with a short anterior flap or only a longer posterior flap made with no anterior flap. When possible, the skin flaps are fashioned so that they are longer to permit an even closure, but if there is compromised circulation, short skin and subcutaneous flaps are reflected together. The posterior incision is beveled to reduce the bulk of muscle in order to provide a better stump. The tibia is usually transected 2 in. above the distal level of the skin flap, and the fibula is transected approximately 1 in. above the tibial level. The tibia may be beveled approximately 45° both anteriorly and mediad to provide a better stump. The nerves are pulled down gently and transected so that they are allowed to retract, and the vessels are ligated above the level of the end of the tibia. If a myodesis is performed (see Fig. 49-5*B*), the muscles are sutured to the tibia by drilling small holes through the bone into the marrow and suturing the muscles so that they are attached under moderate tension along their normal pathways, in a position slightly beyond rest length. The fascia and skin are loosely closed, and either a through-and-through drain or a catheter which will be connected to suction apparatus may be used for 2 days.

Fig. 49-4. Syme amputation. *A*. Incision is outlined. *B*. Foot has been amputated by disarticulating the calcaneus. Tibia and fibula are transected proximal to the flare of the tibial malleolus. *C*. The long plantar flap is sutured to the anterior part of the incision, with care to center the heel flap.

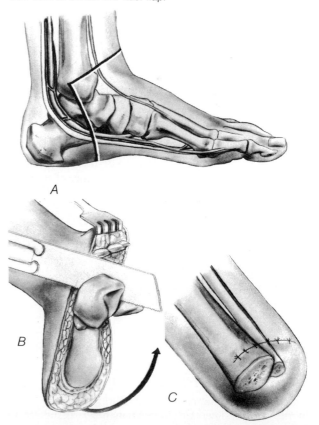

absence of diabetes. Healing of BK amputations has been reported in 68 to 90 percent of cases in large series as compared with healing rates of 82 and 98 percent, respectively, for AK amputations. By contrast, considering the relative general status of the patients, a higher percentage of BK amputees walk on prosthetics. Precise figures are difficult to evaluate since they reflect the efforts and aggressiveness of the rehabilitation team. The range of reported figures for rehabilitation of BK amputations in patients with ischemia is from 50 to 90 percent.

TECHNIQUE (Fig. 49-5). The amputation should be performed proximal to the lower third of the tibia, since the preponderance of tendinous structures distal to this area predisposes to poor circulation and an unstable, painful

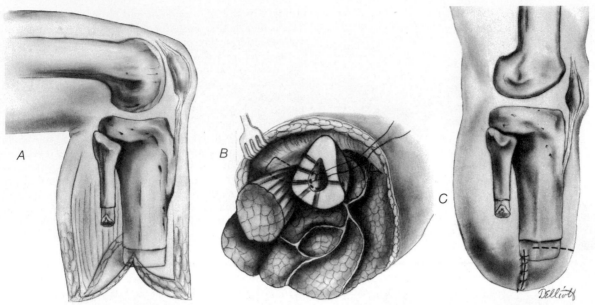

Fig. 49-5. BK amputation. *A.* Equally short anterior and posterior flaps have been made (a long posterior flap may be combined with a very short anterior flap). The muscles have been beveled, and the fibula is transected approximately 1 in. above the tibia. The periosteum has been removed from the distal portion of the bones. *B.* Myodesis: individual muscle fibers are sutured to the tibia through small drill holes. *C.* Fascia and skin are closed (dotted lines indicate skin closure when a long posterior flap is used).

POSTOPERATIVE MANAGEMENT (Fig. 49-6). With the conventional management, a small splint is applied in the operating room to prevent flexion of the knee joint. The splint is usually removed on the second day, and joint motion is then begun. Measurements for a temporary prosthesis may be made on the second day, and walking on this temporary prosthesis, with which the weight is borne on the ischium, may be performed within 3 days. When the patient is physically capable and the stump is well healed, a permanent prosthesis with which the weight is borne on the patellar tendon and tibial flares is provided. Walking on this permanent prosthesis should be possible about the fourth postoperative week.

IPOP may be applied, in which case the patient is encouraged to stand and bear weight on the first postoperative day and activity is rapidly increased. A permanent prosthesis can usually be applied at the time of the second cast change, i.e., at 3 weeks when the stump is sufficiently mature. In a series of cases, the use of IPOP at this level has not been associated with a single incidence of sustained phantom limb pain.

Knee Disarticulation

This is most commonly employed in children in whom there is a reason for maintaining the epiphysis for bone growth. Other advantages of the disarticulation are that it provides maximal length and good weight bearing and lends itself to a good fit between stump and socket. The disadvantages are that the end of the stump is bulky and has bony prominences which may result in skin breakdown. The procedure is rarely indicated when there is impaired circulation.

TECHNIQUE. The skin incision is placed about 1 in. above the stump end posteriorly, and the anterior flap is fashioned approximately 4 in. distal to the inferior border of the patella. The skin and subcutaneous tissue are re-

flected together. The femoral condyles and patella are usually not disturbed. If the patella is displaced or damaged by disease, it should be excised, leaving the quadriceps tendon or patellar ligament intact. Myodesis is easy to perform at this level. If the patella has been left in place, the patellar tendon is then sutured to the cruciate ligaments posteriorly. If the patella has been removed, the remaining tendon and quadriceps tendon are brought down through the intercondylar notch and sutured to the cruciate ligaments posteriorly. The hamstring tendons may also be brought down through this notch and sewn to the cruciate ligaments.

POSTOPERATIVE MANAGEMENT. The postoperative care and the application of a prosthesis is similar to that which is described below for the AK amputations.

Above-the-Knee Amputations (AK)

This level has generally been selected when gangrene extends above the level of the malleoli. Absolute indications for the procedure include extension of skin gangrene above a level which would permit BK amputation and rigor of the calf muscles. Peripheral gangrene coupled with contracture of the knee or hip constitutes a relative indication, since there is no advantage to a BK amputation.

The AK amputation is associated with the highest healing rate in patients with peripheral vascular disease; in series reviewed by Warren and Kihn this ranged between 84 and 100 percent. The rate of reamputation is lower, which is an important consideration in elderly and debilitated patients. These characteristics contribute to the fact that the mortality rate is higher than that reported for other levels of amputation of the lower extremity. The procedure has been associated with a relatively high incidence of pulmonary embolism, and some have advised routine anticoagulation or ligation of the ipsilateral femoral vein.

TECHNIQUE (Fig. 49-7). Anterior and posterior skin flaps are fashioned of equal length, and if there is any question of compromised vascular supply, as is frequently the case, short skin flaps are used. The skin and subcutaneous tissue are reflected together, taking care not to compromise the circulatory status. When possible, the adductor and hamstring muscles are beveled to provide a cylindrical stump rather than a bulbous one, but if there is a severe vascular problem, beveling is contraindicated. The vascular bundles are divided individually at the level of proposed transection of the femur, and gentle traction is applied to the sciatic nerve. Ligature of the nerve may be required if there is a significant vessel within, and the nerve is transected so that it retracts proximal to the stump of the femur. The periosteum of the femur is incised circularly and scraped to avoid leaving detached periosteum in the stump and consequent bone formation. The femur is transected at a level proximal to the condyles at a distance approximately equal to one-half the anteroposterior diameter of the thigh proximal to the most distal point of the skin flap. The edge of the bone is beveled to provide a smooth radius.

If myodesis is performed (see Fig. 49-5B), the muscles are attached through several small holes extending through the bone to the marrow, approximately 1 in. proximal to the distal end of the bone. Slight tension is applied to the anterior, medial, and posterior muscle groups, and these are sutured individually to the bone. The muscle should be able to effect maximal contraction and provide good function for the use of a prosthesis. Subcutaneous tissue and skin flaps are loosely approximated.

POSTOPERATIVE MANAGEMENT. With conventional management, a small dressing and stockinet are employed. The patient is positioned in bed so that there is no hip flexion and is turned frequently to the prone position. He is not allowed to sit in a chair or bed until he is able to hyperextend the stump. Measurements may be performed for a temporary prosthesis as early as the second day, since the weight is borne on the ischium, gluteal region, and thigh. The weight of the permanent prosthesis is borne either on the end of the stump, if it is end-bearing, but more usually on the ischial tuberosity, gluteal, and thigh regions. Fitting of the permanent prosthesis may take several months because of stump shrinkage but may occur as early as 4 to 6 weeks after amputation. A suction contact may be used for young patients with long stumps, but a suspension apparatus (Fig. 49-8) with a purchase across the iliac crest is more frequently employed. The incorporation of a single-action friction knee or a hydraulic mechanism which incorporates swing phase control depends upon the degree of rehabilitation required. A SACH foot and ankle are usually incorporated.

If an IPOP is used, a rigid dressing is applied in the

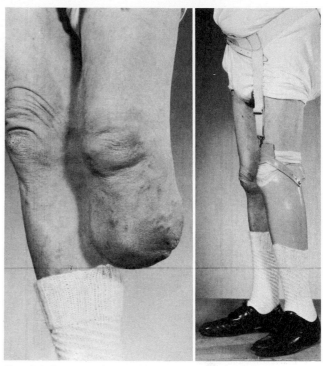

Fig. 49-6. Postoperative rehabilitation for BK amputation. Left. BK stump. Right. Prosthesis fitted.

operating room in such a fashion that the ischial tuberosity is resting on the posterior brim incorporating a waist belt and harness for suspension. The patient is encouraged to stand as soon as possible after the first postoperative day and to progress rapidly toward ambulation. Rehabilitation toward ambulation usually requires more time than with BK amputations.

Hip Disarticulation

The indications usually include bone tumors, soft tissue tumors, and extensive traumatic injuries. Flaps are fashioned so that they will come together anteriorly, and the posterior flap is constructed so that it forms a unit of skin, fascia, and muscle to swing forward in order that the patient may sit comfortably in the socket of his prosthesis. The femoral vessels are ligated anteriorly, and after the posterior dissection is completed, the femur is disarticulated. The sciatic nerve is cut high and tied in order to prevent bleeding from vasa nervorum. The undersurface of the gluteal muscle is tapered to facilitate approximation of the structures to the lower abdominal wall. Prostheses are available to permit ambulation, and have been applied to this level. A specially constructed Canadian prosthesis is used for these patients (Fig. 49-9).

Hemipelvectomy

This procedure has been used in the treatment of malignant tumors of the upper thigh, particularly those of soft tissue and bone, when it is felt that hip disarticulation

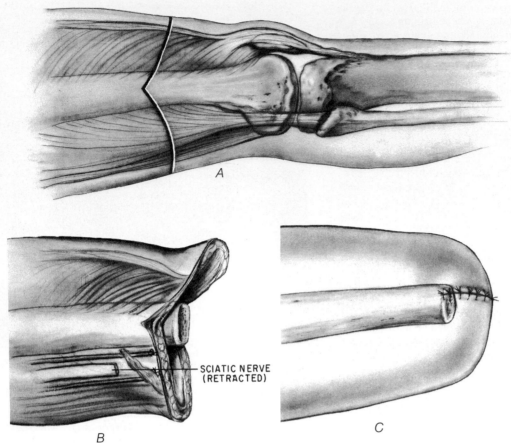

SCIATIC NERVE
(RETRACTED)

B

C

Fig. 49-7. AK amputation. *A*. Outline of short anterior and posterior flaps. *B*. Amputation completed with muscles beveled. Note that the sciatic nerve has been cut after tension had been applied in order that it retract proximal to the bone end. *C*. Skin closure which does not interfere with fitting of prosthesis.

would give a questionable margin of clearance around tumor. Soft tissue sarcomas have a predilection for extension along tissue planes between the muscles, and they continue to the muscular attachment in the pelvis. Hemipelvectomy or a modification thereof avoids local recurrence to a greater extent in these cases. Modification of the classic procedure by dividing the ileum through the greater sciatic notch requires less surgical manipulation and results in less shock. The adjustment to a prosthesis is better when a leaf of the ileum and pubic rami are left as supporting points for the socket. Following this procedure, patients have also been permitted to ambulate with a special Canadian prosthesis.

AMPUTATIONS OF THE UPPER EXTREMITY

In most instances, upper extremity amputations (Fig. 49-10) are performed for trauma. Malignant disease represents the second most common indication. Peripheral vascular disease, particularly thromboangiitis obliterans, constitutes a rare indication.

In all circumstances, the treatment is directed at conserving as much viable tissue as possible and, with more distal amputations, maintaining the function of the hand

as a grasping organ. The latter requires preservation of intrinsic muscle-tendon systems of the hand and the longer and more powerful flexors and extensors originating in the arm. The technique employed for amputations in the upper extremity is directed at producing minimal scar tissue, and the procedure is planned so that the scar is in an area as far removed as possible from bones, tendons, nerves, and points of external contact. Above the level of the metacarpals, opposing tendons should be fixed in order to preserve muscle length and tone.

In view of the precise nature of surgical technique, tourniquets are frequently employed to provide a bloodless field and facilitate identification of critical structures. They are best tolerated high in the upper arm with the cuff inflated to 280 mm Hg. Digital tourniquets, such as rubber bands, should not be used, because of the danger of thrombosis. Anesthesia is frequently best accomplished by the use of regional block, particularly since many of the patients present with multiple injuries and a full stomach and cannot tolerate general anesthesia at the preferred time for operation.

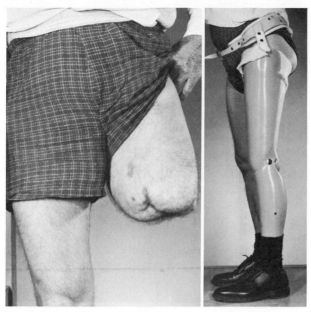

Fig. 49-8. Rehabilitation for AK amputation. *A.* Healed AK stump. *B.* Prosthesis for AK amputation. Note that the weight is not borne on the end of the stump.

Amputations in the Hand (See Chap. 50)

AMPUTATION OF DIGITS

When part or all of the distal phalanx requires amputation, an attempt should be made to create a longer volar flap and a shorter dorsal flap, so that the scar may be positioned dorsad away from pressure. Neither bone nor

Fig. 49-9. Rehabilitation following hip disarticulation. *A.* Healed amputation site. *B.* Patient fitted with special Canadian prosthesis.

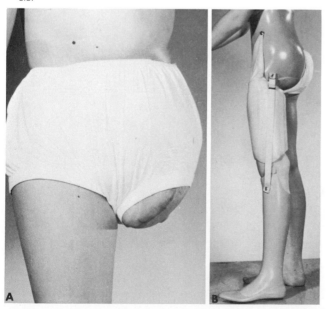

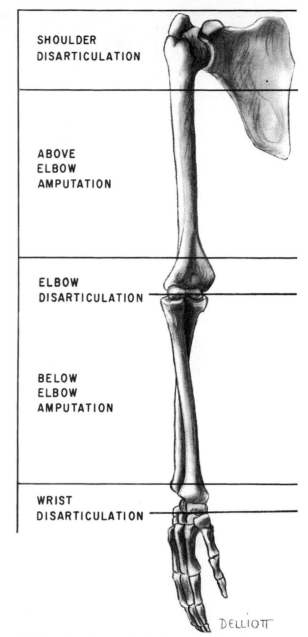

Fig. 49-10. Levels of amputation in the upper extremity.

viable soft tissue should be sacrificed to produce an ideal flap. If the amputation removes less than one-half the nail, it is preferable to retain the nail bed, but if more than half the nail is removed, the entire root should be excised. When it is necessary to disarticulate at the distal interphalangeal joint, the cartilage should be removed from the head of the middle phalanx, and the flexor digitorum profundus tendon should be withdrawn, transected, and allowed to retract.

Amputations of fingers distal to the PIP joint leave function which is useful for pinching and finer movements.

Amputations through the middle phalanx result in little alteration of extension when only the more distal portion of the dorsal expansion of the extensor digitorum communis tendon is cut. By contrast, the flexor digitorum superficialis tendon has a long insertion on either side of the phalanx, and if a significant portion of this insertion cannot be left intact, disarticulation may be necessary. Whenever possible, amputation through the proximal phalanx is preferable to disarticulation at the metacarpophalangeal joint, since the stump, however short, has function.

When one or more fingers must be removed in entirety, attention should be directed at the hand as a working unit. When the long and ring fingers are both removed, the adjoining fingers may continue to function perfectly, or they may deviate toward each other, and deviation weakens flexion. If only the long or ring finger is removed, it is best also to remove the head of its metacarpal to allow the adjoining metacarpals to approximate each other. This tends to prevent adjoining fingers from rotating and crossing toward each other. As a secondary procedure, the index (in the case of amputation of the long finger) or the little finger (in the case of amputation of the ring finger) may be moved over by resecting the metacarpal of the missing finger through the proximal third of its shaft and shifting the adjoining finger on to the stump (Fig. 49-11).

When the middle finger plus either the index or little finger are removed together, the heads of the metacarpals should be obliqued to produce a smooth contour. When the index finger has been disarticulated, the metacarpal should be partially excised to improve the final appearance of the hand and to avoid interference with function. In the case of the little finger, it is preferable to resect the whole metacarpal.

The thumb is the most important of the digits, and every bit should be saved, since even the smallest stump is preferable to a prosthesis. When only the thumb and small finger remain, a rotation osteotomy of the metacarpal of the thumb may be performed to permit approximation and grasping.

A variety of prostheses are available for more major amputations of the digits. These include functional terminal devices, such as hooks and cosmetically acceptable plastic hands. The selection of the prosthesis is dependent upon the patient's individual needs.

AMPUTATION THROUGH THE CARPOMETACARPAL LEVEL

After dorsal and volar skin and subcutaneous tissue flaps have been established, the digital extensor tendons are pulled down, transected, and allowed to retract, while the tendons of the carpal extensors are separated from their attachments to the metacarpal bases and left long so that they may be inserted into the carpal bone. The thenar and hypothenar muscles are tapered to make a smoothly rounded stump. The long flexor tendons are transected after applying gentle traction so that they will retract. After the metacarpals have been disarticulated from the carpals and the synovial cartilage has been removed from the distal carpals, the flexor carpi radialis and the tendons of carpal extension are sutured to the carpal bones. The skin and subcutaneous tissue then must be closed.

Fig. 49-11. Shifting of finger. *A.* Middle finger has been amputated at a transmetacarpal level. *B.* The remaining portion of the shaft of the middle finger metacarpal has been resected, and the metacarpal of the index finger has been transected and the distal portion secured to the base of the metacarpal of the middle finger by means of a Kirschner wire.

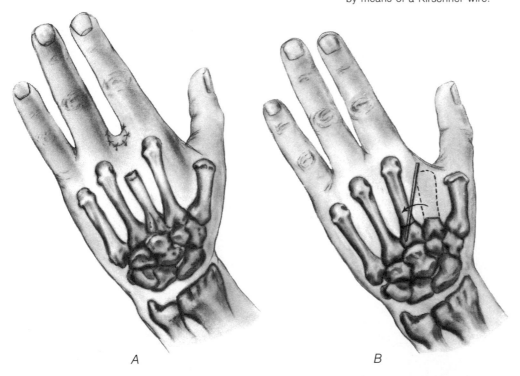

A   *B*

The stump is capable of more motion than a forearm stump, since there is more pronation and supination and good flexion and extension at the wrist. It accepts prostheses to provide a cosmetic hand and also more versatile and functional hooks.

Wrist Disarticulation

This level preserves greater length and provides better prosthetic control than amputations proximal to the wrist joint. The tendons of the hand should be transected with the muscles at rest length, so that they may be sutured to the ligaments and periosteum in order to prevent retraction and atrophy. The brachioradialis should not be disturbed. The styloid processes should be removed to permit a smoother fit for the prosthesis. The articular cartilage should also be removed and covered with a fascial flap to prevent limitation of pronation and supination by scar formation.

Although the stump is less strong and less versatile than when the carpal bones are left in, a less conspicuous prosthesis can be used. In women, amputations are generally carried a little higher in order to reduce the size of the prosthetic wrist by removal of the bulbous mass of bone at the end.

Forearm Amputations

In order to avoid excessive scarring and immobility of skin, skin flaps should not be dissected extensively from the fascia. The long flexor and extensor muscles and tendons are dissected and tapered so that they adhere to underlying tissue. After the bones have been transected, about $\frac{1}{2}$ in. of periosteum should be removed to prevent spur formation, and the fascia should be closed over the end so that muscle length is maintained.

With longer stumps, the actions of pronation and supination should be preserved, and the tendinous muscles and bones are therefore treated atraumatically to prevent fibrosis. Even if only a short stump can be achieved, this is superior to an above-elbow amputation. The formation of a functioning stump through the upper forearm can be successful if there is only a short segment of either radius or ulna which may be preserved distal to the tuberosity. This can be lengthened secondarily with a bone graft or flap.

The biceps and pectoralis muscles have been used in cineplastic operations as prime movers of artificial limbs in this situation. The plastic procedure is usually performed secondarily after the stump has healed. An inverted skin flap is formed and sutured into a tube and drawn through a tunnel of muscle in the biceps. The biceps tendon is divided at the midpoint and skin graft applied to cover the defect from the inverted flap (Fig. 49-12). The biceps can then transmit its force externally, while the brachialis muscle remains as a flexor of the forearm. The transmission of force is accomplished by attaching the rod through a muscle to a cable which exercises power over a hook.

The Krukenberg operation may be used in the forearm

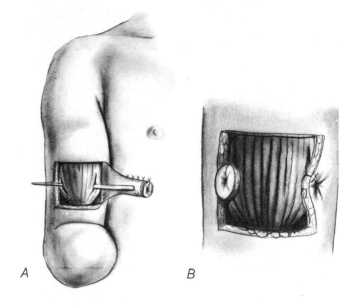

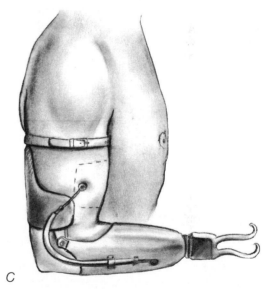

Fig. 49-12. Cineplastic procedure for forearm amputation. *A.* Amputation has healed, and an inverted skin flap has been fashioned into a tube. *B.* Dermal tube has been brought through a tunnel of biceps muscle, and the biceps tendon is divided at the midpoint. A skin graft is then applied to cover the defect on the inverted flap. *C.* Prosthesis fitted. The transmission of force is accomplished from the biceps muscle to the cable which powers the hook.

when amputation is performed on a blind patient. With this procedure, a cleft is constructed between the radius and ulna to provide a grasping terminus which possesses tactile sensation.

Elbow Disarticulation

Flaps are created as in the case of forearm amputations so that the closure of skin and fat will not lie directly over the fascial incision. In order to obviate a bulky stump, the epicondyles are removed, and the cartilage is excised from the end of the bone. The tendons of the biceps, brachialis, and triceps muscles are sutured over the end at rest length. A cineplastic procedure to develop power for a functional terminal device may be performed secondarily.

Amputation through the Humerus

Every attempt should be made to preserve as long a stump as possible, since the longer the stump, the greater the applicability of subsequent cineplastic procedures for functional prosthesis. If a high amputation is necessary, it is preferable to preserve the head of the humerus, since this maintains the width of the shoulder and acts as a support for a prosthesis.

After anterior and posterior flaps are developed, the muscles are transected so that there is sufficient length of biceps and brachialis tendons and triceps muscle so that these muscles can be joined over the end of the bone to avoid retraction. In the case of shorter stumps, the biceps and triceps may be fixed to the humerus in a fashion similar to that described for myodesis procedures in the lower extremity. The skin and muscles are then closed loosely.

As soon as the stump is mature, it can be fitted with a prosthesis with a terminal device operated by a shoulder cable and with an elbow which can be fixed at varying degrees of flexion. The type of elbow joint utilized depends upon the type of function required by the patient. The most functional terminal devices are hooks which may be voluntarily opened. In the case of the adult unilateral amputee, the prosthesis usually functions only as an aid for the contralateral hand.

Disarticulation of the Humerus and Forequarter Amputation

The former procedure is usually performed for extensive trauma, whereas the latter operation may be indicated for malignant disease of the proximal upper extremity.

In most instances, care must be taken in individually ligating the vessels and nerves. In the case of disarticulation of the humerus, the flaps are fashioned to provide covering of the glenoid fossa, and the deltoid muscle is retained to be incorporated in this closure. Forequarter amputation includes excision of the scapula and clavicle followed by closure of the chest and back muscles over the chest wall and coverage with previously established skin flaps. A prosthetic device operated by the opposite shoulder may be applied.

LIMB REPLACEMENT

A 1970 review limited to replacement of the arm transected at or above the wrist revealed sufficiently detailed data on 51 patients, including 15 with complete amputa-

tions, 24 with near-complete amputations, and 12 failures in replacement. Only 23 of the 39 successful replacements were evaluated as to long-term result. Full functional recovery was not achieved.

References

General Considerations

Aitken, G. T.: Surgical Amputations in Children, *J Bone Joint Surg [Am]*, **45A:**1735, 1963.
Burgess, E. M., and Romano, R. L.: Immediate Postsurgical Prosthesis Fitting, *Bull Prosthetic Res,* vol. 10, no. 4, 1965.
Jansen, K.: Amputation: Principles and Methods, *Bull Prosthetic Res,* vol. 10, no. 4, 1965.
Warren, R., and Record, E. E.: "Lower Extremity Amputations for Arterial Insufficiency," Little, Brown and Company, Boston, 1967.

Amputations of the Lower Extremity

Baker, W. H., and Barnes, R. W.: Minor Forefoot Amputation in Patients with Low Ankle Pressure, *Am J Surg,* **133:**331, 1977.
Couch, N. P., David, J. K., Tilney, N. L., and Crane, C.: Natural History of the Leg Amputee, *Am J Surg,* **133:**469, 1977.
Dale, W. A., and Capps, W., Jr.: Major Leg and Thigh Amputations, *Surgery,* **46:**333, 1959.
Hansson, J.: The Leg Amputee: A Clinical Follow-up Study, *Acta Orthop Scand Suppl* 69,1964.
Harris, P. D., Schwartz, S. I., and DeWeese, J. A.: Midcalf Amputation for Peripheral Vascular Disease, *Arch Surg,* **82:**381, 1961.
Holden, W. D.: Arteriosclerotic Ischemic Necrosis of the Lower Extremities, *Surgery,* **22:**125, 1947.
Moore, W. S.: Determination of Amputation Level: Measurement of Skin Blood Flow with Xenon-133, *Arch Surg,* **107:**798, 1973.
———, Hall, A. D., and Lim, R. C., Jr.: Below the Knee Amputation for Ischemic Gangrene, *Am J Surg,* **124:**127, 1972.
Nagendran, T., Johnson, G., Jr., McDaniel, W. J., Mandel, S. R., and Proctor, H. J.: Amputation of the Leg: An Improved Outlook, *Ann Surg,* **175:**994, 1972.
Sherman, C. D., and Duthie, R. B.: Modified Hemipelvectomy, *Cancer,* **13:**51, 1960.
Stahlgren, L. H., and Otteman, M. G.: Review of Criteria for the Selection of the Level for Lower Extremity Amputation of Arteriosclerosis, *Ann Surg,* **162:**886, 1965.
Warren, R., Crawford, E. S., Hardy, I. B., and McKittrick, J. B.: The Transmetatarsal Amputation in Arterial Deficiency of the Lower Extremity, *Surgery,* **31:**132, 1952.
——— and Kihn, R. B.: A Survey of Lower Extremity Amputations for Ischemia, *Surgery,* **63:**107, 1968.
——— and Record, E. E.: "Lower Extremity Amputations for Arterial Insufficiency," Little, Brown and Company, Boston, 1967.

Amputations of the Upper Extremity

Burnham, P. J.: Regional Block of the Great Nerves of the Upper Arm, *Anesthesiology,* **19:**281, 1958.

———: Amputation of the Upper Extremity, *Clin Symp,* **11:**107, 1959.

———: Regional Block at the Wrist of the Great Nerves of the Hand, *JAMA,* **167:**847, 1958.

Chase, R. A., and Laub, D. R.: The Hand: Therapeutic Strategy for Acute Problems, *Curr Probl Surg,* 1966.

Limb Replacement

McNeill, R. E., and Wilson, J. S. P.: Problems of Limb Replacement, *Br J Surg,* **57:**365, 1970.

Malt, R. A., Remensnyder, J. P., and Harris, W. H.: Long-Term Utility of Replanted Arms, *Ann Surg,* **176:**334, 1972.

Chapter 50

Hand

by **Robert A. Chase and Lester M. Cramer**

Congenital Abnormalities

Syndactyly
Polydactyly
Circumferential Grooves and Amputations
Missing Parts
Macrodactyly

Hand Infection

Subcutaneous Abscess
Paronychia
Felon
Bacterial Tenosynovitis
Palmar Space Infections
Acute Suppurative Arthritis
Unusual Infections

Hand Injuries

Hand Amputation
Replantation of Amputated Digits

Elective Incisions

Postoperative Care

Unusual Pain Syndromes

The philosophic exaltation of the hand by scholars of antiquity is equaled by the profound regard for its complexity and versatility held by functional anatomists and surgeons. Its capabilities depend on the intricate relationships between its architectural, motor, and sensory elements with the brain and its peripheral linkages. Therefore, an understanding of the anatomy and unique healing capacities of nerves, tendons, bone, skin, and blood vessels is not the only prerequisite essential for the hand surgeon. He also must understand the functional contribution of each part of the hand in order to be able to judge what the expectations for function may be if parts in various combinations are rendered functionless.

Diseases and injuries of the hand covered in other chapters are burns of the hand (Chap. 7), diseases of muscle and Dupuytren's contracture (Chap. 43), tumors (Chap. 46), fractures and joint injuries (Chap. 47), and diseases of joints (Chap. 48).

CONGENITAL ABNORMALITIES

The genetic and environmental factors cited as etiologic agents in other congenital anomalies also apply in upper limb abnormalities. Anomalies fall into no fixed pattern, but generally they consist of specific deficits, supernumerary parts, fusions, clefts, or hypertrophy or atrophy.

Syndactyly

Webbing of the fingers is the most common of all congenital hand abnormalities. The condition varies from a thin web between otherwise normal digits to fusion of skeletal elements as well as soft tissues. It is characterized by phenotypic variability and genetic heterogeneity. However, in many of the families reported, there has been dominant autosomal inheritance. A dominant gene may give various expressions of syndactyly in association with preaxial and/or postaxial polydactyly. Syndactyly is also an integral part of many different syndromes such as anhidrotic ectodermal dysplasia, Laurence-Moon-Bardet-Biedl syndrome, Poland syndactyly, oculodentodigital dysplasia, and acrocephalosyndactyly (Apert's Syndrome). Very frequently, both the hands and the feet are involved at the same time.

Digits are not separated in fetal life until about the sixth week. The arrest of digital separation at this stage creates this abnormality. The incidence is variously reported as 1 in 1,000 to 1 in 3,000 births. Males are affected more frequently than females in a ratio of about 2:1. Roentgenographic examination is helpful in assessing the nature of skeletal involvement.

TREATMENT. The timing of surgical intervention has been a subject of debate. When digits of different growth rates are involved, separation of the bony junctures is recommended prior to age one year, to prevent growth retardation of the larger digit and progressive deviation of the connected ones. After this has been attended to or if there has been no concern with the growth problem, it is advisable to wait until the end of the second year of life for surgical intervention. Surgical correction must be planned to avoid compounding the problem by creating scar contractures. Because there is inadequate local skin to achieve complete closure and a functioning web space, a combination of local flap tissue supplemented by free skin grafting is essential.

The operation (Fig. 50-1) involves creation of geometric interdigitating skin flaps on the adjacent sides of the two involved digits. If more than two digits are involved, the procedures should be staged; working on both sides of any single digit would endanger its vascular supply. The interdigitating flaps with the grafts will avoid linear closure

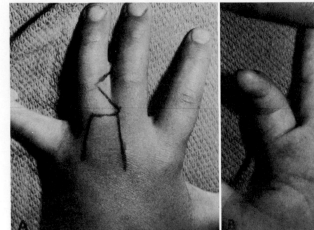
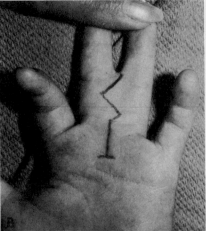
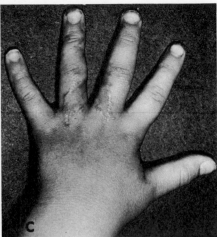

Fig. 50-1. Congenital syndactyly. *A.* Incisions outlined to create interdigitating flap and web space pedicle. *B.* Palmar incision. *C.* Result after syndactyly correction.

which would result in scar contracture. The web requires special attention to avoid scar fixation of the digits in a position of adduction toward one another. The flaps of skin and subcutaneous tissue of both dorsal and palmar skin are designed to interdigitate within the web cleft for this purpose. The areas of skin deficit at the time of exposure are covered with free full-thickness skin grafts obtained either from the inguinal crease or from the arch of the plantar surface of the foot.

Polydactyly

Extra digits are a manifestation of embryologic duplication. They may appear as supernumerary phalanges, duplications of whole extremities, or any degree of variation between these extremes. The most common form of polydactyly consists of a rudimentary digit without its own tendons. It may be associated with an extra metacarpal, or it may extend from another metacarpal which is Y-shaped. Fortunately, the supernumerary digit is usually on the radial or ulnar margin of the hand, where it may be removed without difficulty. Duplications of the thumb are most common. When duplication involves the whole thumb, it is occasionally difficult to tell which is the prime digit and which is vestigial. Supernumerary digits must be amputated precisely, with care to preserve tendons and sensory nerves to the digit left in situ.

Circumferential Grooves and Amputations

Shallow or deep circumferential grooves in the extremities are not uncommon congenital anomalies. There is controversy as to whether the defect is a result of intrauterine environmental factors such as amniotic bands or of influences transmitted genetically. It seems most reasonable (although admittedly on incomplete evidence) that circumferential grooves and congenital amputations are influenced by growth and developmental changes determined genetically.

If the grooves do not threaten survival of the part, they may be ignored or treated by Z-plasty for cosmetic im-

provement. Rarely, the constriction is so severe that the survival of the extremity or part is threatened. Surgical release and Z-plasty then become more urgent.

Missing Parts

Children born with specific parts of the hand and arm totally absent or represented by a small vestige may have numerous combinations of deformities. There are, however, a few common combinations of absences. Parts of digits or whole rays (phalangeal and metacarpal) may be absent. Absence of the thumb or a vestigial first ray preventing good prehensile grasp is very disabling. Missing central rays result in a cleft or lobster-claw-like hand. Congenital absence of the whole hand is an obvious disaster. Absence of segments of the forearm, much more commonly the radius than the ulna, are found in combination with hand losses or as an independent anomaly. Total absence of the extremity or an extremity nub with vestigial hand is recognizable as the phocomelia deformity, such as was seen in the thalidomide cases.

Surgical reconstruction is individualized for each specific deformity. For example, the child born with absence of the first ray may have four normal digits, or there may be five fingers with no opposable thumb unit. Surgical reconstruction is planned after careful study of the deformity, including level of function of each of the digits, and roentgenograms. When four normal fingers exist but the thumb ray is totally absent, pollicization of the index digit is a reasonable procedure (Fig. 50-2). This is best and most safely performed at the age of four to five years, before the child enters school. Some surgeons prefer to carry out the procedure in the first year of life.

Macrodactyly

Digital gigantism, localized symmetric enlargement of one or more digits, is most common in the index finger, most often unilateral, more common in the male, and

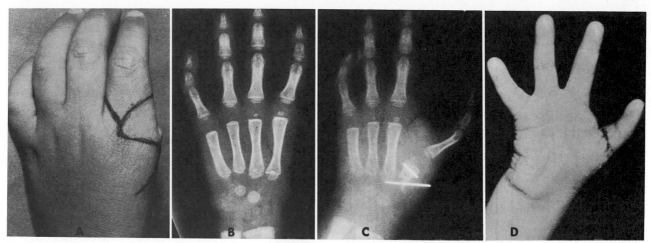

Fig. 50-2. Congenital absence of thumb. *A.* Incision outlined for transfer of index digit to thumb position. *B.* Preoperative x-ray. *C.* Postoperative x-ray. *D.* Index digit pollicized.

frequently accompanied by such other congenital anomalies as syndactyly, café au lait spots, neurofibromas arteriovenous fistulae, nevi, polydactyly, and hemangiomas. Commonly this is a form of neurofibromatosis. Treatment is difficult. Obviously, if there is a single, functionless, grotesque digit, amputation of the finger or the ray would be the treatment of choice. If it is a functional single digit, particularly in children, multiple operations of bone remodeling, epiphyseal arrest, and excision of the excessive soft tissues including longitudinal excision of hypertrophic nerves constitute a reasonable approach.

HAND INFECTION

The vulnerability of the hand to frequent wounding makes the hand a common portal of entry for bacterial invasion. This, coupled with the concentration of tendons (with their poor blood supply), as well as the difficulty in sustaining natural immobilization, sets the stage for grave local infections. The hand is so important in every form of activity that one is not likely to protect or immobilize it when early infection occurs. The potential spaces and moist synovial sheaths are a fine environment for bacterial growth, particularly because of constant massaging motion and lack of luxuriant blood supply so important in mobilizing local resistance to infection.

A succinct but specific history and general physical examination must precede the examination of the hand. In addition to noting influencing diseases, such as diabetes, arthritis, cardiopulmonary or renal disorders, and drug addiction, the infection symptomatology of fever, tachycardia, nausea, vomiting, malaise, and polycytosis should be sought. The amount and quality of pain is important. Severe pain is ominous, but the absence of pain can be misleading. Local signs of spread along the lymphatic system, ascending lymphangitis or lymphadenopathy, must be examined for. The three primary lymph node drainage sites are the epitrochlear nodes for the ring and little fingers, the axillary nodes for the thumb and index finger, and the deltopectoral nodes for the middle finger. Inspection of the suspected infection will reveal erythema, edema, tenderness, and perhaps purulent drainage; gentle palpation can reveal fluctuance.

Injuries that are particularly susceptible to subsequent infection are those where crushing is a factor, those occurring in a filthy environment (some meatcutting plants, farmyards, some types of manual labor, city streets), puncture wounds involving a contaminated or irritating foreign body (plant thorns, fish hooks) or the injection of human or animal saliva (bites, fights), and the drug addict's self-inflictions (needles, glass droppers). There is an ever-increasing incidence of severe and exotic hand infections in the drug culture. As the proximal veins become obstructed or thrombosed, brawny edema of the hand develops, causing addicts to use digital veins as a portal of entry. At this site extravasation of contaminated materials will lead to disastrous infections and sloughing of chemically injured, contaminated tissues.

Many of the common and less serious infections can be treated on an ambulatory basis. A position-of-function splint and a brachial sling are used for rest and elevation, appropriate antibiotics and pain medications are given, and multiple soakings are advised. If pus is localized, many subcutaneous abscesses and most paronychiae can be drained in the emergency department or office. Narcotics, sedatives, and/or tranquilizers may be needed. The patient should always be lying down, his arm on a side table, sterility assured, and a brachial tourniquet in place. In the office or emergency room, a blood pressure cuff can be used to record the blood pressure and then left on the arm to act as the tourniquet, subsequently being inflated just prior to incision. During the cleansing of the skin and the application of the sterile drape, the arm is kept elevated so that when the cuff is inflated to 280 mm Hg, there will be a minimum of congestion in the hand. The need for a bloodless field to assure accuracy is critical, even for the most seemingly insignificant drainage procedure. The brachial cuff for a tourniquet is preferred in all situations, but there are some surgeons and emergency physicians who feel that a digital tourniquet suffices for fingertip procedures. A rubber band should never be used as a digital tourniquet, as pressure is difficult to control, it may injure the digital nerves, and it might easily be left in place accidentally. Soft rubber tubing held in place by an artery clamp is preferred. Inducing hand ischemia by distal-to-proximal wrapping as is done in elective, clean surgery is contraindicated, since this can encourage proximal spread via synovial sheaths or lymphatics, enhancing the spread of infection.

Postoperative care consists of rest, constant elevation of the hand higher than the heart, an absorptive and non-constricting dressing with a position-of-function splint incorporated, pain control with narcotics, and sedatives for sleep.

For the more seriously ill, immediate hospitalization may be needed, and antibacterial therapy should be instituted immediately by the intravenous route. All incision and drainage operations should be done in the operating room, except for the few exceptions noted above.

The judicious use of antibiotics is important, and urgency may justify initiating the appropriate agent on the basis of a smear or characteristics of the clinical picture prior to receipt of culture and sensitivity reports. Empiric selection of a proper antibiotic is guided by the following considerations:

1. Familiarity with the usual pattern of infection, since the pathophysiology of the lesion makes diagnosis more definitive (Fig. 50-3)
2. The local and systemic response to the lesion
3. Knowledge of the local bacterial ecology
4. Gram stain, if material is available
5. Total health picture of the patient
6. The properties of the antibiotic agent

Staphylococci are present in nearly 80 percent of hand infections. Over one-half are penicillinase-producing. Beta-hemolytic streptococci, *Escherichia coli*, *Proteus* species, and *Pseudomonas* species account for the remaining. Over one-third of all infections have a mixed flora; the most frequent combination is *Staphyloccus aureus*, beta-hemolytic streptococci, and *E. coli*. Fungal superinfection may develop after several days of high doses of antibiotics, especially if used in combinations.

When an area shows the signs of early inflammation and possible infection, the differential diagnosis must include chemical or metabolic synovitis, gout, rheumatoid arthritis, Reiter's syndrome, and nonspecific tenosynovitis. If these are not prime suspects, the inflammatory lesion should be treated promptly, although the antibiotic is difficult to select as usually there is no area to culture. Systemic antibiotics often can be supplemented by local instillation or topical applications of antibiotic solutions or ointments. If the process subsequently progresses to one requiring incision

Fig. 50-3. *A*. Diagram of the locations of common infections showing spreading and pointing. 1. Dorsal subcutaneous abscess. 2. Paronychia. 3. A vesicle or pustule indicative of felon beneath. 4. Felon. 5. Abscess in volar fat pad; this can point in a palmar direction or track to the dorsum before pointing; the flexion creases frequently act as barriers to spread. 6. Abscess in palmar fat pad may spread by perforating dorsad, by passing the flexion crease barrier through bacterial action and going proximally to the subcutaneous tissue in the palm, or by spreading via the lumbrical canal to a palmar space. *B*. The collar-button abscess. This advanced lesion, with abscess cavities on both the palmar and dorsal aspects, is common in the area of the metacarpophalangeal joint. It has the potential for spreading beneath the palmar fascia or into the dorsal compartment opposite the web space, or it may fill the web space and extend along the tendons into the midpalmar space or to the thenar space.

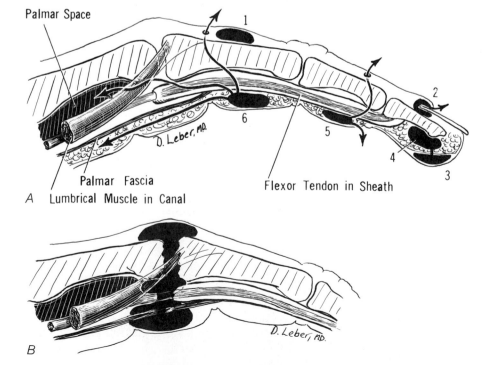

Palmar Space

Palmar Fascia

A Lumbrical Muscle in Canal

Flexor Tendon in Sheath

D. Leber, MD.

B

D. Leber, MD.

and drainage or if purulence is already apparent at the initial examination, prompt surgery is recommended.

When an infection is not hospital-acquired, a penicillin is the best choice of antibiotic at the outset. For ambulatory outpatients or for lesions of apparent staphylococcus infections to which there is good body response, oral dicloxacicin may be used. If the lesion is not localizing well and lymphangitis is prominent, penicillin should be added, since it is so much more effective against the nonpenicillinase-producing staphylococci and against beta-hemolytic streptococci. If the patient is allergic to penicillin and needs antistaphylococcal treatment, either gentamicin or lincomycin is recommended. Daily evaluation at 24 and 48 hours is essential to assess the response and the patient's compatibility with the antibiotic. The specific cultural sensitivities will determine subsequent continuation or change of drug. If more than one antibiotic is being used, only the best one needs to be continued.

When severe infection has supervened, intravenous administration of antibiotics must be begun immediately and a hospital surgical procedure performed when there is adequate antibiotic within the patient's system.

For the gram-positive cocci, methicillin or nafcillin are recommended as intravenous therapy; if the infection appears to be less well localized or mixed, cephalothin is added.

If there is an impending tenosynovitis in a critically ill patient, the treatment is cephalothin or carbenicillin to which are added methicillin or nafcillin. In a compromised host, e.g., a diabetic or drug addict, and especially if the infection is mixed, either gentamicin or ampicillin may be added. Ampicillin is not commonly recommended for treating hand infections unless there is specific positive cultural information. Despite the possibility of encouraging a superinfection, it is best to slightly "overtreat" a severe infection initially and be able to withdraw a *possibly* unnecessary antibiotic when the culture information is available rather than have the infection progress rapidly because of a delay. Special note should be made of infections from human bites or those caused when the fist strikes the tooth of an opponent. In the latter situation there is often some crush of tissue plus the injection of organisms into tendon sheaths or joints. Early aggressive antibiotic therapy with penicillin and tetracycline is indicated.

Subcutaneous Abscess

These abscesses are quite common, accounting for about 15 percent of all infections of the hand. Most of them are situated on the palmar aspects of the middle and proximal segments of the fingers or in the palm; only a few will occur on the dorsal surfaces of the fingers or hand. They frequently follow a needle or thorn prick and thus are very common in gardeners. Other cases may follow blistering from hard manual work. They usually present in the stage of cellulitis with diffuse redness and swelling of the fingers, which must be differentiated from some of the deeper and more dangerous infections. The tenderness generally is confined to the small area at the site of the abscess, although all have the potential for spreading out laterally or

deeply to become the initiating sites for deeper infections. Treatment with rest, elevation, and antibiotics sometimes will abort the process, but most abscesses will localize and require drainage. Abscesses may point in a palmar direction or at the side of the finger, but even a palmar lesion may point to the dorsum. This situation, if not treated promptly by antibiotics and drainage, can lead to acute suppurative tenosynovitis, acute suppurative arthritis, osteomyelitis, and occasionally gangrene.

Paronychia

Infection around the nail bed occurs because the area is frequently subject to injury which creates a portal of entry for bacteria, and also because the nail juncture with soft tissues is a weak area of defense against local invasive infection. The initiating cause may be hangnails, ingrowing nails, manicure trauma, unclean subungual areas, steel wool slivers, or other foreign bodies. Once the paronychia is established, the cornified nail acts as an intrinsic foreign body, perpetuating the infection. Staphylococcus is usually the offending organism. Combined infection with staphylococcus and streptococcus is resistant to treatment and requires not only incision and drainage but appropriate antibiotics and intensive soaking. Frequently a portion of the nail must be removed (Fig. 50-4), since the pathologic process has progressed. Occasionally a chronic paronychia may need long-term treatment with frequent applications of antifungal agents.

Felon

Infection of the digit pulp has certain important characteristics. The fibrous septa to the skin limit swelling of the part, and pressure builds up in the pulp space. This gives rise to deep ischemic necrosis. Thus more culture medium is created, and severe deep infection with osteomyelitis of the distal phalanx may result. All this occurs before pointing and spontaneous external drainage. Erythema, pain, and tenderness characterize the felon. The pulp space should be incised and drained before deep necrosis occurs (Fig. 50-5).

Bacterial Tenosynovitis

As bacteria invade the more proximal areas in the digit, they find a receptive site for growth in the slippery synovial sheaths around the flexor tendons. The area is characterized by poor natural resistance to infection and the presence of nearly avascular tendon. It takes little disruption to convert living tendon into a collagenous foreign body with its tendency to augment the infectious process.

The anatomy of the tendon sheaths varies significantly, but the general pattern should be known in order to predict routes of natural extension of the infection (Fig. 50-6). For example, a single felon in the pulp of the little finger may extend to the flexor tendon sheath, then along a natural anatomic route to the ulnar bursa. From this site in the hand it may readily extend to the radial bursa and into the thumb flexor tendon sheath. Where the anatomy is of

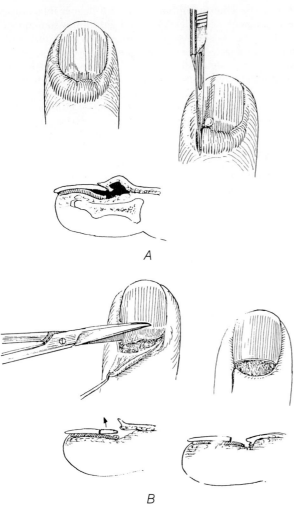

Fig. 50-4. *A.* Surgical drainage of the paronychial abscess is best performed through an incision proximal to the corner of the involved nail. *B.* If the abscess extends around the nail base or lateral margin, the base or margin should be excised to assure adequate drainage and removal of nonviable nail which serves as a foreign body. The fingernail will regenerate from the nail bed.

the classic pattern, the little finger infection would be more likely to extend to the thumb than to the adjacent ring finger or the middle or index fingers.

When the flexor tendon sheath is infected, the posture assumed by the involved digit is one of mild flexion at all points. Active or passive attempts to extend the finger elicits local pain. Swelling, inflammation, and local temperature elevation may not be striking but are observed on close examination. The differential diagnosis between true bacterial tenosynovitis and acute rheumatoid or nonspecific tenosynovitis can be difficult. Roentgenograms for calcium deposits may be helpful in diagnosing a reactive chemical (nonbacterial) local inflammation. A history of previous episodes of tenosynovitis, rheumatoid disease, gout, recent local or systemic infection, injury, or excessive use of the part may provide the clue for the correct diagnosis. Aspiration of the tendon sheath for smears and culture may be helpful.

Proper therapy (Fig. 50-7) for established bacterial tenosynovitis is surgical drainage and administration of appropriate antibiotics. The tendon sheath must be adequately opened with a midaxial (ulnar or radial side of digit along joint axes) incision. Once drainage is performed, vigorous treatment is required to achieve early wound closure to preserve the flexor tendons.

Palmar Space Infections

The deep spaces in the hand between the deep flexor tendons and the metacarpals with their interposed interosseous muscles are potential receptive pockets (Fig. 50-6). The subtendinous palmar area is divided into a thenar space and midpalmar space by a thick vertical septum from the palmar fascia to the third metacarpal. Frequently one of these deep spaces becomes the seat of grave infection without involvement of the other. The localized swelling, redness, and tenderness make diagnosis quite straightforward. These spaces may be surgically drained through any of a variety of incisions, with care to avoid violating the general principle of not crossing areas of flexion (Fig. 50-8).

Fig. 50-5. *A.* Incision and drainage of felon with preservation of sensory digit pulp. (*From R. A. Chase and D. R. Laub, The Hand: Therapeutic Strategy for Acute Problems, in "Current Problems in Surgery," Year Book Medical Publishers, Inc., Chicago, 1966. By permission of Year Book Medical Publishers, Inc.*) *B.* A centrally located incision permits excellent drainage and decompression. This alternate incision lies between innervation areas but does leave a scar in the finger pad.

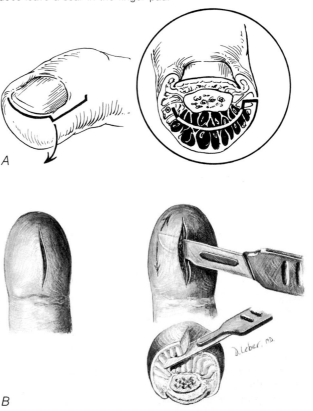

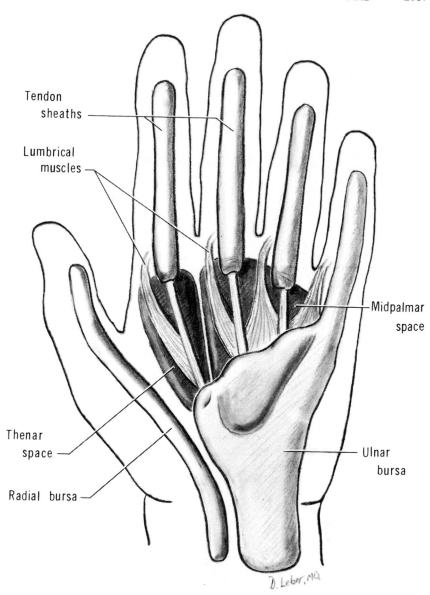

Fig. 50-6. The anatomy of the synovial sheaths and deep spaces in the hand.

Acute Suppurative Arthritis

When the joints are involved with a purulent disease, they are most commonly secondarily affected from a penetrating wound or from the direct spread from a neighboring abscess. Also, with the increasing incidence of venereal disease, monarticular gonococcal arthritis is becoming more common. Early surgery supplemented by both systemic and articular infusion antibiotics (Fig. 50-9) may preserve function, but prognosis for a normal joint is always guarded.

Unusual Infections

A group of severe infections which must be watched for carefully includes acute streptococcal hemolytic gangrene, necrotizing fasciitis, streptococcal myositis, clostridial cellulitis, gram-negative anaerobic cutaneous gangrene, and progressive bacterial synergistic gangrene. Although these severe soft tissue infections occur infrequently, early recognition is important to prevent progressive destruction secondary either to continuing bacterial action or to ischemic necrosis from pressure produced by swelling. The diagnosis should be entertained for a hand or forearm that has had recent trauma or surgery and presents with extensive swelling and systemic toxicity without the usual signs of local acute inflammatory process. Figure 50-10 presents a brief summary of the differential diagnostic characteristics of common hand infections.

HAND INJURIES

A large proportion of accidental injuries in industry, at home, or in automobile accidents involve the forearm and

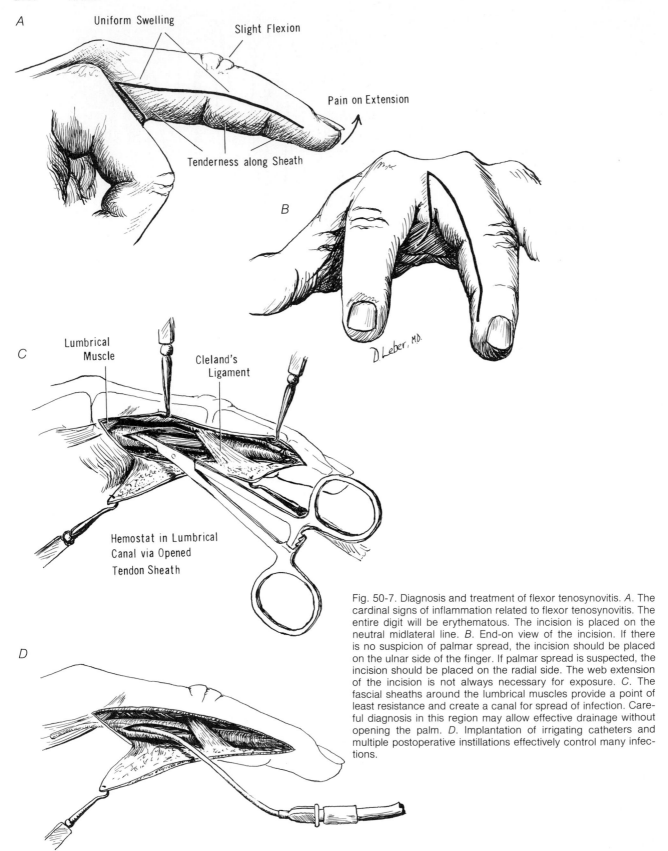

A. Uniform Swelling

Slight Flexion

Pain on Extension

Tenderness along Sheath

B

D. Leber, M.D.

C Lumbrical Muscle

Cleland's Ligament

Hemostat in Lumbrical Canal via Opened Tendon Sheath

D

Fig. 50-7. Diagnosis and treatment of flexor tenosynovitis. *A.* The cardinal signs of inflammation related to flexor tenosynovitis. The entire digit will be erythematous. The incision is placed on the neutral midlateral line. *B.* End-on view of the incision. If there is no suspicion of palmar spread, the incision should be placed on the ulnar side of the finger. If palmar spread is suspected, the incision should be placed on the radial side. The web extension of the incision is not always necessary for exposure. *C.* The fascial sheaths around the lumbrical muscles provide a point of least resistance and create a canal for spread of infection. Careful diagnosis in this region may allow effective drainage without opening the palm. *D.* Implantation of irrigating catheters and multiple postoperative instillations effectively control many infections.

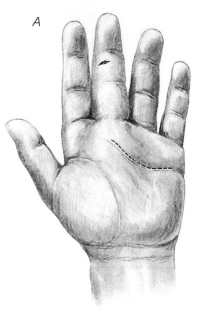

A

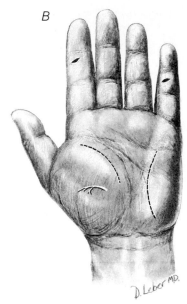

B

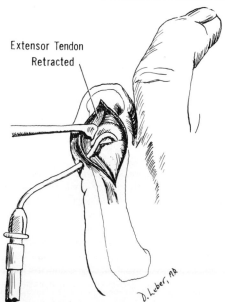

Fig. 50-8. Spread of digital infection into the palm. *A.* Incision for drainage of the midpalmar space. *B.* Incisions for drainage of the radial bursa and the ulnar bursa. *C.* Palmar digital infections frequently create extremely swollen regions on the dorsum of the hand, because the lymphatic drainage runs from the palmar to dorsal aspects. A common error is to expect to drain such a lesion at this lymphadenitis point. When there are dorsal infections, incision and drainage will be performed dorsally. *D.* The incision for drainage of the thenar space.

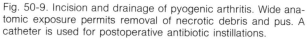

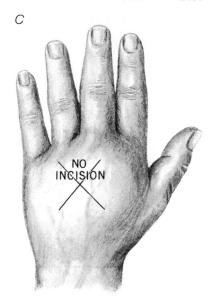

C

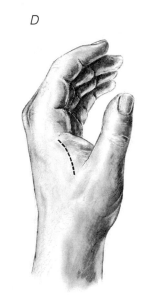

D

Fig. 50-9. Incision and drainage of pyogenic arthritis. Wide anatomic exposure permits removal of necrotic debris and pus. A catheter is used for postoperative antibiotic instillations.

Extensor Tendon
Retracted

	Paronychia	Terminal pulp infection	Acute cellulitis
Time of presentation from onset	2–5 days	4–5 days	12–24 hours
Cause	Nail biting. Manicuring.	Puncture wound	Prick or not known
Organism	Mixed	Staphylococcus	Streptococcus
Symptoms	Tender swelling round nail fold.	Throbbing pain confined to the end of the finger increasing daily and preventing sleep.	Hot red finger. Malaise shivering and tenderness up arm to axilla.
Physical Signs	Fluctuant swelling of nail fold. Often subcuticular pus.	Hot red tense and tender pulp. Often subcuticular pus. Rest of the finger normal.	Hot red finger. Not very swollen.
Movements	Full. Painless.	Full. Painless.	Practically full. Painless.
Temperature	Normal	Normal	Raised
Lymphagitis	No	No	Yes
Differential diagnosis	1 Early acute cellulitis 2 Lateral pulp infection 3 Late subungual haematoma	1 Acute cellulitis 2 Early paronychia 3 Haematoma of pulp following trauma	Early pulp infection especially apical infection

Fig. 50-10. Differential diagnosis of hand infection. (*From J. Sneddon, The Care of Hand Infections, The Williams & Wilkins Company, Baltimore, 1970.*)

hand. The hand is frequently used as a protective shield, it is generally unclothed, and it is the probe with which man explores his environment. It is no surprise that it is frequently subject to trauma. The complexity of its anatomy and the compact proximity of all its elements set the stage for every injury to be a threat to subsequent normal function, and the surgeon must be alert to subtle functional losses when specific nerves, tendons, or architectural elements are compromised. Systematic, precise examination of the hand is necessary even when the injury appears to be minor.

CLINICAL MANIFESTATIONS. History. One must know the circumstances leading to the injury in order to outline and execute an optimal program of treatment. Knowledge of the time elapsed since the injury, the character of the wounding agent, the nature of first-aid care, and the patient's general health are important; an elderly patient on steroid therapy for an unrelated disease who sustained a laceration while working with a garden tool several hours before being seen presents an entirely different problem from a healthy teen-ager brought directly to an emergency suite with a cut from broken glass.

Sensibility. The distribution of sensory nerves in the hand is such that they are subject to frequent injury. In adults it is simple to assess areas of anesthesia by simple touch and pinprick testing. If there is doubt about the patient's response or if one is dealing with a small child, peripheral nerve injury may be assessed by a more objective test: Using Ninhydrin as a reagent, one may demonstrate presence or absence of sudomotor (sweating) function in the digits. Fingerprints are made on test paper and processed with the reagent. When sensory nerves are transected, there is loss not only of sensibility but also of sympathetic sweating function. The patterns of anesthesia clearly document which of the sensory nerves has been injured. Testing for sensibility must be done before local anesthetic agents are used and before any wound exploration is done.

Tendon sheath infection	Boil or carbuncle	Palmar and web infection	Infective arthritis
6–36 hours	2–3 days	2–3 days	1–3 days from onset infection Up to 3 wks from time of original injury
Midline injury with sharp instrument	Often not known	Puncture wound—often splinter	Cut or puncture over dorsum of the joint
Streptococcus	Staphylococcus	Staphylococcus	Mixed
Hot red swollen finger. Extremely painful especially on movement. Malaise. Tenderness up arm to axilla.	Painful swelling on the back of the hand or fingers. History of previous boils.	Throbbing pain in the palm and gross swelling of the back of the hand.	Painful swelling all round the infected joint and discharging wound on the dorsum
Whole finger hot, red and swollen. Maximal on dorsum. Tenderness along course of the sheath maximal in proximal compartment in the palm.	Cellulitis and oedema of dorsum, with triangular spread to the wrist. Later, discharging lesion.	Infected puncture wound in palm brawny, red and tender. Swelling and pitting oedema of dorsum. In web infections fingers separated. Best seen from the dorsum.	Cellulitis of whole finger. Swelling tenderness maximal all round the infected joint. Discharging wound on dorsum.
Extremely painful, especially extension.	Full	Slight limitation by pain in fingers.	Flexion and extension limited and painful. Lateral movement increased and crepitus present.
Raised	Slightly raised	Slightly raised	Normal
Yes	Sometimes	Sometimes	No
1 Acute cellulitis 2 Middle or proximal space infection 3 Fascial infection	Palmar or web infection	1 Early carbuncle 2 Tendon sheath infection involving proximal compartment	1 Infected laceration not involving the joint 2 Neglected acute paronychia 3 Mallet finger

Extrinsic Muscular Function. *Distal Interphalangeal (DIP) Joint Flexors.* The tendons of the profundus muscles and the flexor pollicis longus insert on the distal phalanges of the fingers and thumb, respectively. Inability actively to flex the distal phalanx means loss of functional integrity of the tendon, the muscle, or its innervation (Fig. 50-11A).

Superficialis Muscles. The superficialis flexors primarily flex the proximal interphalangeal (PIP) joints. They operate independently of one another and thus are responsible for independent interphalangeal flexion of a single finger. If one checkreins the profundus tendon by holding other fingers in extension, the ability to flex the finger at the interphalangeal level is dependent upon the integrity of the superficialis mechanism (Fig. 50-11B).

Long Extensors. The extensor digitorum, the extensor digiti minimi, and the extensor indicis are prime extensors of the metacarpophalangeal joints of the fingers. Transection of the extensors to a single digit results in a flexion drop of the finger at the metacarpophalangeal joint and inability actively to extend it. The presence of intertendinous bridges leads to diagnostic errors by masking a proximal injury of a solitary extensor, since some extension will be retained. Independent extension exists only in the index and little fingers. Loss of this independence is diagnostic of transection or paralysis of the extensor indicis or extensor digiti minimi.

Intrinsic Muscular Function. Although there is considerable minor variation in the patterns of innervations of the intrinsic muscles of the hand, the classic pattern is generally reliable for proper diagnosis of nerve injuries.

The thenar muscles on the radial side of the flexor pollicis longus (abductor pollicis brevis, opponens pollicis, and superficial head of the flexor pollicis brevis), and the first two lumbrical muscles are innervated by the median nerve. The test for function of the thenar muscles is palmar abduction of the thumb into position for pulp-to-pulp opposition with the fingers (Fig. 50-12). One may readily observe tensing of the abductor pollicis brevis, the most superficial muscle in the thenar group.

The ulnar nerve innervates all the hypothenar and inter-

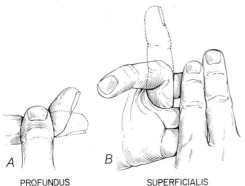

PROFUNDUS   SUPERFICIALIS

Fig. 50-11. Test for long digital flexors. *A.* Flexion of distal interphalangeal joint dependent upon profundus tendon. *B.* Flexion of proximal interphalangeal joint with remaining fingers checkreined is dependent upon an intact superficialis tendon. (*From R. A. Chase and D. R. Laub, The Hand: Therapeutic Strategy for Acute Problems, in "Current Problems in Surgery," Year Book Medical Publishers, Inc., Chicago, 1966. By permission of Year Book Medical Publishers, Inc.*)

osseous muscles and the third and fourth lumbricals. If innervation is lost to these muscles, the patient cannot abduct or adduct his fingers (Fig. 50-13*A*). This is particularly obvious when he attempts to abduct (radially) the index finger. One may readily observe tensing of the prominent first dorsal interosseous muscle in the first web space when ulnar nerve function is intact. The ulnar-innervated intrinsic muscles are responsible also for primary flexion of the metacarpophalangeal joints. If these joints can be held in flexion while the interphalangeal joints are in extension, ulnar-innervated intrinsic muscles are intact (Fig. 50-13*B*).

Retaining Ligaments. In recent years excellent descriptions of the structure and function of the retaining ligaments of the hand have been presented by Landsmeer, Kaplan, and Milford. These ligaments are dense, fibrous

Fig. 50-12. Test for median nerve–innervated intrinsic muscles in the thenar eminence. Palmar abduction of the thumb for pulp-to-pulp opposition of thumb with other digits is possible only with these muscles. (*From R. A. Chase and D. R. Laub, The Hand: Therapeutic Strategy for Acute Problems, in "Current Problems in Surgery," Year Book Medical Publishers, Inc., Chicago, 1966. By permission of Year Book Medical Publishers, Inc.*)

MEDIAN INTRINSIC

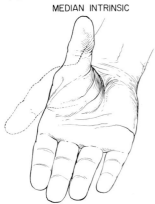

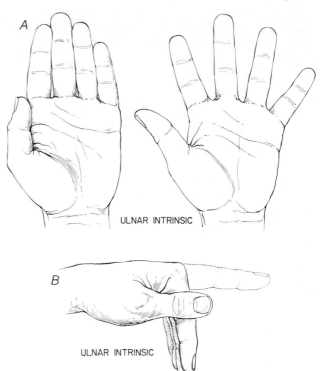

ULNAR INTRINSIC

ULNAR INTRINSIC

Fig. 50-13. Testing for ulnar nerve–innervated intrinsic muscles of the hand. *A.* Abduction and adduction of the fingers. *B.* Flexion of the metacarpophalangeal joints with the interphalangeal joints in extension. (*From R. A. Chase and D. R. Laub, The Hand: Therapeutic Strategy for Acute Problems, in "Current Problems in Surgery," Year Book Medical Publishers, Inc., Chicago, 1966. By permission of Year Book Medical Publishers, Inc.*)

bundles that retain either the skin (Cleland's ligaments, Grayson's ligament, peritendinous ligaments) or the extensor mechanism (oblique retinacular ligament, transverse retinacular ligament, and the sagittal bands).

Cleland's cutaneous ligaments radiate in two planes on either side of the interphalangeal joints of each digit, connecting the joints to the skin. They lie dorsal to the digital neurovascular bundle; palmar to the bundle are similar fibers. Together, these fibers form a protective tunnel for the neurovascular structures. They are excellent surgical landmarks in finger exploration and are used in some reconstructions. The peritendinous fibers hold the skin creases in position over the respective interphalangeal joint.

The retaining ligaments of the extensor mechanism have more functional significance. The transverse retinacular ligament originates from the palmar aspect of the PIP joint capsule and flexor tendon sheath, passes superficial to the fibers of Cleland's ligament (acting as a sling for them), and inserts mainly on the lateral margin of the lateral tendon of the extensor mechanism. Its major function is to act as a stabilizer for the lateral tendon of the extensor mechanism. The oblique retinacular ligament is more tenuous in character. Its fibers arise from the bone of the distal fourth of the proximal phalanx and pass lateral to the lateral extensor tendon palmar to the axis of rotation of the

PIP joint when the joint is flexed. The fibers traverse distad along the palmar portion of the lateral bands and insert dorsal to the axis of rotation of the DIP joint. Because of its relation to these axes, this ligament does not allow easy flexion, either active or passive, of the DIP joint when the PIP joint is in extension. Contraction of this ligament, either in cases of arthritis or secondary to trauma, can cause constant hyperextension of the DIP joint when the PIP joint is partially extended; if the PIP joint becomes fully extended, it may prevent flexion of the DIP joint.

The sagittal bands originate from the deep transverse intermetacarpal ligament, project perpendicular to the long axis of the finger, and insert on the lateral margin of the extensor tendons. They actually continue over the dorsum of the tendon on the dorsum of the hand to become continuous with the sagittal bands of the opposite side of the digit. As pointed out by Tubiana, these structures are important in helping to balance the extensor and flexor mechanisms.

X-rays. X-rays should be considered for every major hand injury, not only to assess bone and joint injury but also to reveal radiopaque foreign bodies.

Vascular Integrity. The simple notation of color, capillary emptying and filling, peripheral pulses, bleeding, and temperature of the hand may require refinement by Allen's test for determining the integrity of vascular arches, and tourniquet blushing for evaluating blood supply to flaps of soft tissue or whole composite units of the hand. If the arm is emptied of blood by elevation and a pneumatic tourniquet is inflated to a level above systolic blood pressure, reactive hyperemia results when the tourniquet is released after 5 minutes of ischemia. This hyperemia may help demarcate the vascularized from the nonvascularized parts. Ultrasonic probes are also useful.

TREATMENT. The Wound. Initial wound care has been discussed in Chap. 8. Cleansing and debridement are particularly important, since the achievement of a closed wound at the earliest possible date is crucial to salvaging functional parts of the hand.

Exploration of Acute Wounds. When there is suspicion that deeper structures are injured, probing is contraindicated, because it may cause further injury and inoculate the wound with organisms which produce infection; functional testing can accurately determine the extent of injury. The wound is immediately and thoroughly cleansed and covered with a sterile protective dressing. Figure 50-14 shows the most common approaches for enlarging hand wounds to provide maximal exposure with minimal secondary scar or contracture.

Control of Hemorrhage. Vigorous bleeding rarely calls for clamping, since indiscriminate and/or successful efforts to clamp arteries can lead to median nerve (radial artery) or ulnar nerve (ulnar artery) injury. Furthermore, the artery itself should not be injured until decision for or against arterial repair is made. With the patient supine and the hand and extremity maximally elevated, external pressure should be applied. This will control bleeding in almost all situations. If not, a brachial tourniquet is applied after the limb is rendered ischemic, and under sterile conditions the bleeding vessel is clamped and ligated or the artery is

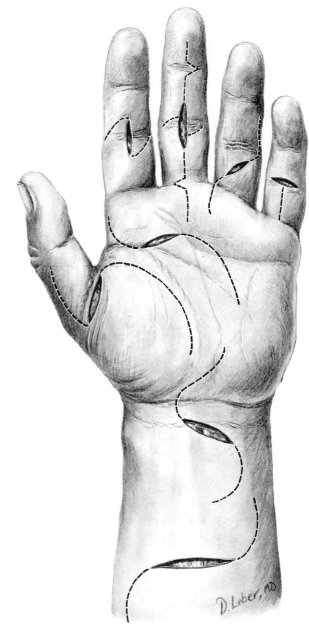

Fig. 50-14. Incisions for exploration of laceration following acute trauma. Flexion creases should not be traversed; if the laceration has traversed the crease, a Z-plasty should be created. Following the natural creases of the hand will give the best final scar. Incisions should be long enough to provide adequate exposure. When curved, the curve should be gradual to prevent long flaps. In the forearm, incisions should be transverse when possible; to provide exposure, a gently curved vertical component is required.

repaired; ×2 magnification is recommended to ensure nerve protection.

Principle of Delayed Closure. Most civilian injuries will qualify as "tidy" wounds for which primary closure of the skin with maximal repair of the tendons, nerves, and bones is indicated. Experiences with military injuries as well as with crushing injuries caused by farm instruments and industrial machines have shown that not all hand wounds should be closed immediately after injury. Staged closure is indicated for explosive injuries of the hand, considerable foreign body contamination, delay of initial treatment, or significant crush injury. In these situations, an initial debridement is accomplished and the hand reevaluated for closure 72 to 96 hours later. It is well to reemphasize that most civilian hand injuries should be closed primarily; only the unusual, difficult, and/or contaminated wounds should be considered for staged management.

Wringer Injuries. A very common injury, particularly of the very young or very old, is crushing of a hand and upper limb by the wringer of a washing machine. This must be differentiated from the severe crushes seen from industrial or farm machinery in which there is frequently complicating deep tissue destruction, impending ischemia, and severe burns. Most victims of home wringer injuries will require only the wound care and/or suturing needed at the initial examination. Even though 25 percent of the patients will need surgery later, this is commonly a small skin graft to replace the skin lost by the friction burns; the need for subsequent grafting can almost always be determined reliably at the time of the initial examination. Less frequently will there be nerve injury, hematoma or edema leading to vascular occlusion or nerve pressure. This may require fasciotomy of the hand or forearm. Dislocation of joints and fractures may result during more severe wringer injuries. The possibility of a developing Volkmann's ischemic contracture must not be overlooked, but the occurrence after a home wringer injury is not common.

Recommended treatment involves evaluation of the history and experienced examination of the skin, nerves, and pulse; x-rays only if there are signs of fractures; suture of lacerations; and application of an absorptive noncompressive dressing with an incorporated splint to keep the elbow straight and the wrist extended. Hospitalization is recommended for those patients in whom there is doubt raised by the physical findings or by the judgment that the parents cannot assume the responsibility for reliable outpatient care.

Patients with complex wringer injuries obviously will need to be hospitalized and will probably require early debridement and either prompt or staged skin coverage by grafting or by flaps. Fasciotomies may be necessary. Definitive nerve, tendon, or bone surgery is delayed except for stabilization of obviously unstable bone fragments. If blood vessels are damaged, they must be repaired initially, either by suture or by graft, or be ligated.

Crush Syndrome after Limb Compression. An increasing and easily overlooked problem produced by the growing number of drug addicts is the appearance of the crush syndrome in a comatose patient. The weight of the patient's body upon an extremity compromises the vascularity, resulting in erythema, induration, ulceration, vesiculation, and paralysis. Swelling of the limb may not be seen early but always develops subsequently. An early reliable sign of impending muscle damage is increased turgor involving a muscle compartment, with pain on passive muscle stretch. Myoglobinemia and myoglobinuria should be tested for as evidence of muscle necrosis. Nerve involve-

ment will be indicated by both sensory and motor loss. The peripheral pulse will frequently be normal upon palpation. Recognition of the crush syndrome is critical because prompt replacement of fluid deficits and careful renal management will diminish the threat of renal shutdown and early fasciotomy may preserve the function of the involved limb by decreasing the severity of damage to nerves and muscles.

The Injured Fingertip. Lacerations should be meticulously debrided and closed as soon as possible. If the nail bed is injured, it should be approximated carefully. When crush injury is involved, conservative amputation may be indicated. In some people, a crush injury will produce a secondarily painful fingertip; however, a secondary amputation in a few months is preferable to an immediate amputation unless there is loss of viability immediately after the injury. Distal transverse amputations are best treated with a thin split-thickness skin graft on the end of the tip. If the absent tissue contained the pulp and the bone or a tendon is exposed, a cross finger flap should be considered. If the pulp injury preserves the pad, a free full-thickness skin graft is satisfactory. Fractures of the tuft of the distal phalanx rarely require internal fixation. If they are badly comminuted and lack sufficient tissue cover, shortening them and covering them with available local tissues or covering the stump with a free skin graft are the procedures of choice. If the bone is not fractured but is uncovered by loss of soft tissues at the fingertip, flap tissue either from an adjoining finger or from the palm will preserve the length of the finger and give it a protective covering with reasonable sensibility.

Nerve Injury. Injury to peripheral nerves results in a specific pattern of sensory and motor loss. Ultimate recovery may depend upon proper surgical management of the injured nerve.

Nerve Transection. There has been much debate over whether peripheral nerves should be repaired at the time of initial wound therapy or secondarily after a short delay. In sharp transections a precise repair should be done primarily in any wound clean enough to close primarily. Careful realignment of funiculi is aided by realigning the tiny blood vessels found on the nerve surface. Fine nonabsorbable sutures placed only in the nerve sheath should be used (Fig. 50-15).

Nerves may be successfully repaired as far distally as the proximal third of the distal phalanges. Arborization of digital nerves beyond this point makes nerve repair difficult. Adequate regeneration for protective sensibility occurs with precise wound closure alone. Microsurgery, using extremely small nylon suture material, improves the repair significantly by allowing accurate separate suture of major funiculi in a large mixed peripheral nerve.

Purposeful or unintentional delay in repairing a peripheral nerve does not measurably alter the ultimate result unless the delay interval is extensive; delayed repair in the first 3 months after nerve transection may achieve a result indistinguishable from that following primary repair. The axons at the proximal cut end of the nerve sprout and attempt to regrow distally. In a receptive distal nerve sheath where wallerian axonal degeneration occurs, the

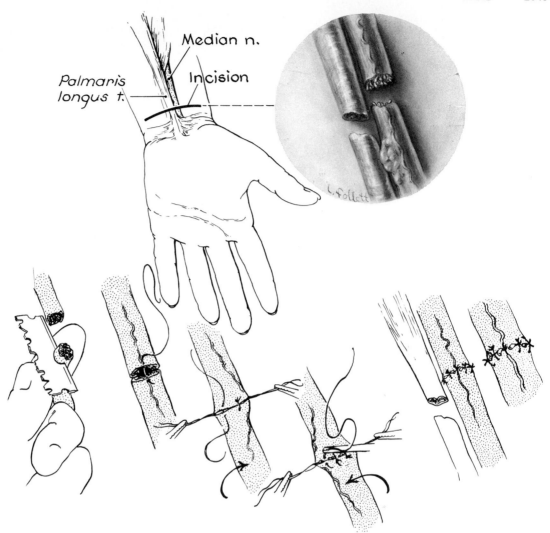

Fig. 50-15. Technique of nerve repair, showing sharp retransection, sutures in the sheath only, and careful axial alignment using surface blood vessel as a guide. *(From R. A. Chase and D. R. Laub, The Hand: Therapeutic Strategy for Acute Problems, in "Current Problems in Surgery," Year Book Medical Publishers, Inc., Chicago, 1966. By permission of Year Book Medical Publishers, Inc.)*

regrowing axons are directed to peripheral sensory end organs and motor end plates. As time passes, the peripheral sheath becomes less receptive, and denervation atrophy in peripheral muscles makes them nonreceptive to reinnervation. The time scale is variable, but generally nerve repair is progressively less effective after 6 months after injury. After 2 years results are generally poor, but there are enough exceptions to make late repair worthwhile.

Recovery after nerve repair progresses in a predictable manner. Sensibility return starts at the proximal area of anesthesia and moves distally as the axons regenerate and grow down the sheath. Nerve regeneration proceeds, on the average, at the rate of 1 mm/day, but this varies depending on the site (proximal regeneration is faster than peripheral) and the age of the patient (regeneration is faster and more complete in young children than in adults). Regeneration may be followed clinically by observation of the distal progress of Tinel's sign, an electric-shock-like sensation on percussion over the regenerating nerve; specific sensibility testing; motor return observation; electromyography; and sudomotor testing (Fig. 50-16).

Nerve Stretching or Compression. Injuries which do not transect the nerve have a better prognosis and faster recovery than those involving nerve transection. Electromyography may be very helpful in assessing the nature of a closed injury to a peripheral nerve. If compression can be released and stretching relaxed by appropriate surgical treatment and splinting, no direct nerve operation is necessary.

Nerve Gaps. Millesi et al. have made a major recent contribution by demonstrating that when injury results in a loss of nerve substance, the best results are achieved if the nerve gap is overcome by accurate interposition of fascicular nerve autografts. The key to his successes, corroborated by the authors and others, is the absence of any tension

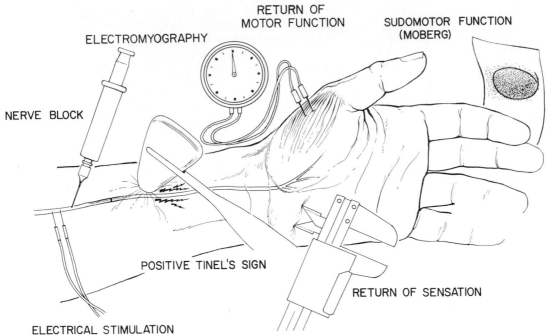

RETURN OF
MOTOR FUNCTION

SUDOMOTOR FUNCTION
(MOBERG)

ELECTROMYOGRAPHY

NERVE BLOCK

POSITIVE TINEL'S SIGN

RETURN OF SENSATION

ELECTRICAL STIMULATION

Fig. 50-16. Methods of assessment of recovery following nerve injury. (*From R. A. Chase and D. R. Laub, The Hand: Therapeutic Strategy for Acute Problems, in "Current Problems in Surgery," Year Book Medical Publishers, Inc., Chicago, 1966. By permission of Year Book Medical Publishers, Inc.*)

upon the proximal or distal suture lines. The results are much superior to those previously achieved by rerouting the peripheral nerve and positioning joints to gain enough length in the nerve to overcome the nerve gap. Unfortunately, nerve homografts (allografts) are not successful. Thus, the patient exchanges one deficit for another, since a donor nerve must be used with resulting loss of its prime function. The best donor for nerve is the sural. Allografts of nerve, notoriously unsuccessful in the past, remain so despite efforts to decrease their antigenicity by immunosuppressive agents.

Neuroma. When a peripheral nerve is left unrepaired, the sprouting axons at the proximal cut end form a tumor mass with local fibroblasts. This neuroma is tender to palpation and percussion, and electric-shock-like sensations interpreted as coming from the area previously innervated are bothersome. The best treatment is nerve repair, directing the axons peripherally. When this cannot be done, the cut nerve end should be placed deep in soft tissue away from the superficial scar. Protection from repeated trauma may serve to relieve the symptoms.

Substitution after Nerve Injury. Where peripheral nerve function is permanently lost, sensibility reorientation peripherally, appropriate tendon transfers, and selected arthrodeses may be substituted.

Restoration of Sensibility. When peripheral nerve repair or grafting is impossible, alternative measures for restoring sensibility may be considered. Nerve crossing by transfer of a digital nerve from a secondary digit to a prime digit has been used. The restored sensibility is not as normal or exact as that resulting from transfer of the nerve together with a patch of its innervated soft tissue on a vascular pedicle. The versatility of such innervated and vascularized islands of skin and subcutaneous tissue is great. The radial arrangement of the digital vessels and nerves

lends itself to this method. A prime digit such as the thumb may be restored by simultaneous correction of skin and sensory deficit, using an island pedicle flap from the protected sides of the long or ring fingers. The transferred sensibility is precise and immediate, although the switch does result in misidentification of the source of a stimulus; i.e., a touch stimulus on the thumb resurfaced by an island pedicle from the long finger will be interpreted as a touch on the long finger in the early period after transfer and sometimes permanently.

Substitution for Irreversible Motor Paralysis. When there is irreversible paralysis of muscles innervated by a peripheral nerve, muscles innervated by intact motor nerves may be transferred to overcome lost function. For example, when the median nerve is irreversibly damaged, usable muscles innervated by the radial and ulnar nerves are transferred to substitute for the paralyzed muscles. There are several standard patterns of tendon transfers and many additional individually tailored transfers.

Median Nerve Palsy. Low median nerve loss (wrist level) results in paralysis of the thenar thumb-positioning muscles (abductor pollicis brevis, opponens pollicis, and superficial head of the flexor pollicis brevis) and the radial two lumbricals. The important functional deficit is inability to position the thumb for proper pulp-to-pulp opposition with the fingers. Transfer of the tendon of an unparalyzed muscle (e.g., ring finger superficialis) to the insertion of the abductor pollicis brevis will substitute its pull for that of the median-innervated thenar muscles.

High median nerve palsy produces the same pattern of

peripheral intrinsic muscular paralysis plus paralysis of the flexor carpi radialis, all superficialis muscles, the flexor pollicis longus, the profundus muscles to the index finger, and the pronators (teres and quadratus). The serious functional deficit is loss of phalangeal flexion in the thumb and index finger and diminished strength and independence of flexion in all fingers. The ulnar-innervated abductor digiti minimi may be swung across the palm as an opponens substitute. The index finger profundus tendon and even the flexor pollicis longus may be sutured side-to-side to the intact ulnar-innervated profundus tendons above the wrist.

Ulnar Nerve Palsy. All the intrinsic muscles of the hand except the thenar thumb-positioning muscles and the radial two lumbricals are paralyzed by interruption of the ulnar nerve at the wrist. If the ulnar nerve is interrupted before it enters the forearm, the flexor carpi ulnaris and the ulnar two or three profundus muscles are also paralyzed. Functionally, the important loss is in the hand, with paralysis of the intrinsic muscles as evidenced by loss of isolated flexion of the metacarpophalangeal joints of the fingers and strong side pinch between the thumb and fingers. Claw deformity results, because the metacarpophalangeal extensors are unopposed. As the metacarpophalangeal joints are pulled into extension and hyperextension, the effect of the long flexors on the interphalangeal joints is accentuated, and clawing (intrinsic minus) position is assumed. This is less marked with high ulnar nerve paralysis, since the profundus flexors are also paralyzed.

Any procedure which restricts hyperextension of the metacarpophalangeal joints is helpful (volar plate advancement, or tenodesis). One of several specific muscle substitutions is the Brand operation, which substitutes a major wrist extensor (extensor carpi radialis longus) for the interossei. In this operation a tendon graft divided into four separate tails routed below the intermetacarpal ligaments and inserted into the lateral bands of the fingers creates a dynamic substitute for the digital intrinsic function. An abductor pollicis substitution using a superficialis tendon from a finger with an intact profundus is commonly done in combination with the Brand operation.

Radial Nerve Palsy. Radial nerve interruption at the axilla or interruption of its motor branches in the proximal half of the arm results in paralysis of the triceps muscle. The radial nerve passes through the spiral groove of the humerus and enters the forearm adjacent to the brachioradialis, which it innervates. It then passes through the supinator muscle to innervate it as well as the wrist and digital extensors. Thus if the radial nerve itself is interrupted, the extensor-supinator group of muscles in the forearm is paralyzed.

The most serious disability results from paralysis of the major wrist extensors (extensor carpi radialis longus and brevis). This may be overcome by releasing the pronator teres from its insertion on the radius and transferring it to the wrist extensors. These are immediately superficial to the pronator insertion and need not be interrupted for the surgical insertion of the tendinous portion of the pronator teres.

Other muscles available for transfer as substitutes for muscles paralyzed by radial nerve interruption are the median- and ulnar-innervated superficial palmar forearm muscles. A variety of transfers of the flexor carpi radialis, flexor carpi ulnaris, palmaris longus, and superficialis tendons can supply motor power to the finger and thumb extensors.

Tendon Injuries. The healing of a tendon is a dynamic event dependent upon local cellular activity. In this respect there is no basic difference initially from the healing of any other injured structure. Because of the relative avascular nature of tendons, the slow metabolism of the very few cells within the tendon substance, and the great reactivity of the vascular pedicle (mesotendon) and the layering covering structures, later phases of tendon healing are somewhat different. Later healing is further influenced by the physicochemical nature of the milieu, remodeling of the tendon callus, and differential development of tendon healing and gliding capability (see Chap. 8). Atraumatic repair must bring cut tendon ends into precise coaptation without interfering seriously with the physiologic elements important for healing and callus differentiation (Fig. 50-17). Technical finesse will contribute to the final result by minimizing scar formation. However, there remain many situations where unavoidable adhesions negate good results. Many efforts are being aimed at systemic control of scar tissue (see Chap. 8). In addition, the local use of silicone rods to create channels for tendon sliding has proved useful in special circumstances. Specific treatment for individual tendon injuries varies greatly because of differences in anatomy and functional demands on each tendon or group of tendons in the hand.

Extensor Tendon Injuries. The relatively short excursion of the long extensors of the digits and their location in loose areolar tissue favors a good prognosis after injury and repair. Adhesions between the tendon at its site of injury and the overlying skin wound rarely restrict function significantly, because the mobility of the dorsal hand and

Fig. 50-17. Technique of end-to-end tendon repair using double-armed, single nonabsorbable suture with final knot away from repair site. (*From R. A. Chase and D. R. Laub, The Hand: Therapeutic Strategy for Acute Problems, in "Current Problems in Surgery," Year Book Medical Publishers, Inc., Chicago, 1966. By permission of Year Book Medical Publishers, Inc.*)

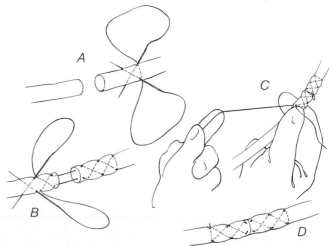

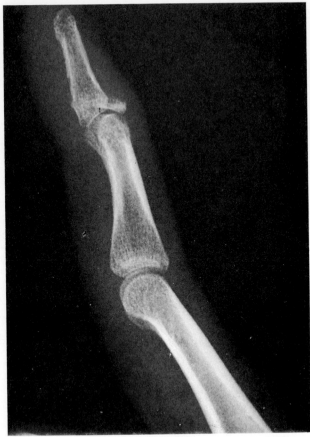

Fig. 50-18. X-ray of mallet finger deformity. Because a significant surface of the DIP joint is fractured, open reduction of this closed fracture is indicated. Most situations are handled by closed reduction and internal fixation.

finger skin is as great as the physiologic excursion of the extensor tendons.

Injuries to the Extensor Mechanism on the Hand. The technique of repair can be that shown in Figure 50-17 or the figure-of-eight pullout technique using wire or other nonabsorbable suture material (Fig. 50-18). The latter uses the skin as a backing, thus avoiding the pulling of sutures through the longitudinally aligned extensor tendon fibers. Postoperative splinting is for 5 weeks with the wrist and metacarpophalangeal joints in extension the entire time. The PIP joint should be held in extension for 2 weeks and then placed in 15° of flexion.

Fig. 50-19. Closed reduction and internal fixation of mallet finger deformity. The PIP joint is kept in mild flexion by a dorsal splint.

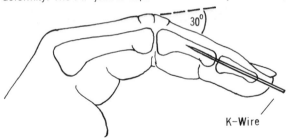

K-Wire

Injuries to the Extensor Mechanism in the Finger

Boutonniere Deformity. Transection of the central extensor tendon near its insertion into the middle phalanx is frequently accompanied by a tear in its lateral extension into the lateral bands. This results in displacement of the lateral bands palmar to the axis of rotation of the PIP joint, causing the bands to lose their extensor function at this joint and to actually become PIP joint flexors. The joint loses both its extrinsic and its intrinsic extensors and assumes an attitude of flexion. Attempts to extend the joint actively accentuate its flexion and are transmitted to the DIP joint through the lateral bands and the oblique retinacular ligament, causing hyperextension of the DIP joint. The defect in the digital extensor apparatus assumes the shape of a buttonhole, through which the PIP joint protrudes.

The injury creating this acute boutonniere deformity is usually a laceration but may be a closed injury. In the closed injuries, immobilization of the PIP joint in extension and usually the whole finger and wrist as well for a 5-week period will avoid the chronic progressive deformity. If the injury is a laceration, the extensor mechanism should be repaired and the same immobilization schedule followed.

Dropped Tip, or Mallet, Finger. Injuries of the extensor insertion into the distal phalanx are common and challenging. The closed injury, such as a baseball finger or the pressure of a football or other object on the end of the finger, causes an avulsion of the insertion of the extensor mechanism. X-rays must be taken to determine the presence or absence of an associated avulsion fracture of the distal phalanx. The configuration of the associated fracture may determine proper management. If a minimal amount of the joint surface is involved, closed reduction and correct joint positioning is the treatment of choice. The PIP joint should be kept flexed for 2 weeks, using an external splint (Fig. 50-19). The DIP joint should be kept at 0°, not in hyperextension; a temporary internal fixation using a Kirschner wire across this joint for 6 weeks is the most secure means of immobilization. After 2 weeks DIP joint fixation by the wire is supplemented with a volar splint, and splinting of the PIP joint is discontinued and mild active and passive flexion begun. After 6 weeks the wire is removed and graded exercise begun for the DIP joint.

Flexor Tendon Injuries. The management of lacerations of flexor tendons of the forearm, wrist, hand, and fingers has been the subject of debate for many years. There are no absolute rules for correct treatment, but several facts should be considered. An injury which involves several tendons, nerves, vessels, surrounding fascia, joints, and soft tissues heals as a single wound. Tendons with repairs in contact with one another are very likely to become adherent to one another as healing progresses. Wherever a tendon repair is adjacent to a fixed fibrous structure, it may become fixed to it by scar tissue. The flexor tendon anatomy is such that there are certain sites where the functional success following primary repair is poor. Better understanding of anatomy and physiology and technical advances during the past several years have improved the prognosis for these situations.

The long flexor tendons (superficialis and profundus) in each digit pass through a rigid tunnel of fascia which extends from the distal palmar crease to the middle phalanx, providing the necessary mechanical action to prevent ventral bowstringing during flexion. In addition there is a major pulley mechanism at the wrist, where the thick, resistant, fibrous flexor retinaculum constitutes the roof of the carpal tunnel.

Forearm lacerations involving multiple tendons will commonly lacerate the median or ulnar nerves, or both. All the involved structures should be repaired primarily. In the wrist portion, because of the unyielding nature of the fibrous retinaculum, rarely are all the tendons within the carpal tunnel actually sectioned. If all these tendons are lacerated, only the profundus tendons and flexor pollicis longus should be repaired. Elimination of repair of the superficialis tendons gives more space within the tight tunnel and better functional results.

Verdan (Fig. 50-20) has designated six zones of the hand correlated with prognosis. Zone 1, distal to the digital tunnel, is an area where prognosis is good. Repair of the profundus tendon should be performed primarily at this level. In zone 6, the wrist area, only the profundus tendon should be repaired. In zone 5, in the palm, both the superficial and profundus tendons should be repaired. Tendon lacerations in zone 2, "no-man's-land," the region of the fibrous digital tunnel, remain controversial in terms of treatment. For children, all surgeons agree on primary repair of the profundus tendon or the flexor pollicis longus. In adults, the trend appears to be toward immediate repair of the profundus tendon in the digit provided the laceration is clean, there is minimal associated injury (at least one digital nerve intact), and treatment is prompt. Proper attention to technique, good wound care, and early and intensive physiotherapy seem to produce adequate results in the hands of some surgeons following primary repair at this level. An alternative procedure, thorough wound toilet and only primary skin closure and digital nerve repair as necessary initially, may be performed when there has been a jagged laceration, if treatment is delayed, or by the surgeon's preference. After the digit has been mobilized passively and after a suitable delay for wound healing, a free or attached tendon graft is performed. One anastomosis then is placed in the palm, where there is no fixed fibrous sheath, and the other is at the site of insertion on the distal phalanx. In this circumstance, anastomosis is usually made by end-to-end suturing (Fig. 50-17). The distal anastomosis is made at the site of tendon insertion in the distal phalanx, where there is no need for sliding (Fig. 50-21, 50-22).

Hand Amputation

Hand amputations should follow careful assessment of critical levels of function and appearance for each digit (Fig. 50-23). Preservation of bony architecture to encourage stronger grasp is preferable for manual laborers (Fig. 50-24*A*), while people who require finer movements and/or are predominantly concerned with appearance have different functional and aesthetic needs (Fig. 50-24*B*).

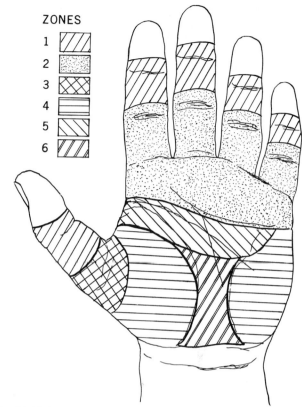

Fig. 50-20. Verdan's zones of flexor injury.

With injuries to many digits, normally unimportant digits or partial digit lengths attain prime importance after partial or complete amputation of the damaged digits.

The thumb is the most important digit by virtue of being the opposable unit for all the fingers. Any length which can be salvaged by conservative surgical treatment should be preserved. When an injury results in loss of soft tissue in excess of bone, the protruding bone should be preserved by immediate coverage with vascularized soft tissue, using a local or distant pedicle flap or even a primary vascularized island pedicle flap.

The peripheral fingers (index and little fingers), if foreshortened seriously, may be best treated by ray amputation (amputation through the proximal metacarpal), particularly if there is associated metacarpophalangeal joint injury. The index finger is very important and versatile. It functions primarily by pinching and manipulating with its pulp opposing the pulp of the thumb. Any amputation of the index finger proximal to the PIP joint leaves insufficient length for useful pinching. It then becomes an impinging nub in the new web space between the thumb and the middle finger, which assumes the role of primary pinching finger. Therefore, all length possible should be saved in amputations distal to the PIP joint, but when amputation is proximal to this joint, immediate closure by further shortening may be done. Within the first few months after injury, an index finger may become stiff and painful or may lack sensation, deterring rehabilitation of the rest of the hand. Early amputation of an index finger, including

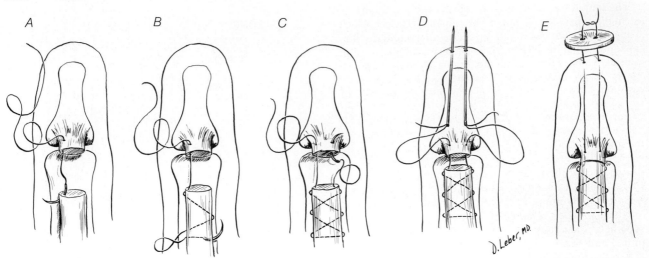

Fig. 50-21. Atraumatic, removable suture technique for distal attachment of profundus tendon or a tendon graft. A flexible, strong, and slippery material has replaced wire; this simplifies the placement of the suture and allows distal removal in a more efficient and painless manner.

the second metacarpal, may well result in the best final cosmetic and functional result.

Even when the central fingers (the middle and ring) are amputated, they can contribute to efficient handling of small objects as long as some of the proximal phalanx remains. Thus any salvage of length beyond the metacarpophalangeal joint is helpful. If the injury is confined to a central finger, there is no reason to use complicated procedures to preserve length. The traumatic amputation may be immediately revised and closed. Amputation at the metacarpophalangeal joint leaves a space between digits with the hand cupped or in a fist. If this creates palmar incontinence, allowing small objects to fall through the resulting space, transfer of the adjacent peripheral finger and its metacarpal should be considered.

Amputation of all fingers and the thumb at the metacarpophalangeal joint level leaves an endpiece for a hand which has little function. Later reconstruction to increase

function should include deepening of the space between the thumb metacarpal and the rest of the hand.

Replantation of Amputated Digits

With the advent of blood vessel repair and more recently with refinement of microsurgical repair of vessels, many reports have appeared of replantation of amputated portions of the upper limb. Initially, replantation of whole arms or of arms amputated through the forearm was reported. This has been followed in the last several years by reports of replantation of digits or parts of digits. These technical triumphs have opened up new opportunities to salvage hand elements that heretofore were irreversibly lost.

Whenever new technology develops, there follows a period during which sensible indications for use of that technology settle in place. In the case of replantation it is particularly important that sound reasoning be applied to indications and more significantly to contraindications for its application. To achieve survival of a part which is useless or even detrimental can represent a serious breach of the doctrine, "first, do no harm."

Some principles in replantation surgery are well established.

1. The replantable part must be important enough to balance the risk of the procedure.
2. The prospect of subsequent useful function after replantation must be adequate to make the part worthy of replantation.
3. The risks of the procedure must be assessed by carefully noting the patient's general health and associated injuries or disorders requiring simultaneous treatment.
4. All the technical requisites must be met including (a) the condition of the amputated part, (b) nature of the wound, (c) time elapsed since amputation, (d) status of the amputation site, (e) facilities and professional team.

Fig. 50-22. A variation of distal profundus tendon or graft insertion.

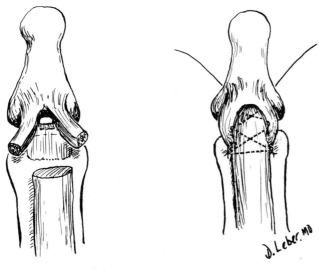

In general the farther distal the amputation occurs with a replantable part, the better the final return of sensibility and function will be. Except under unusual circumstances, replantation of single fingers in the absence of other digital losses is not indicated. Amputation of the thumb is an indication for surgical replantation when it is technically possible. Amputation through the hand and wrist or low forearm is an ideal level in terms of indication for replantation, all other things being equal. Amputations above the elbow may be an indication for replantation, particularly in children. Even if hand function fails to return and distal sensibility is lost to the point that elective amputation and prosthesis replacement are decided upon, salvage of a functional elbow by replantation makes rehabilitation by prosthesis far better than amputation at the original level.

With replantation at its present level of reliability, it behooves the surgeon who first sees the patient suffering an amputation to know how to handle the wound and amputated part prior to transfer of the patient to the replantation team for decision and definitive treatment. The wound should be treated with as little manipulation as possible to avoid further injury to the cut vessels and nerves. A tourniquet or pressure dressing is preferable to instrumentation of the wound for hemostasis. The amputated part should be kept clean in sterile dressings and when possible it should be placed in a plastic bag and kept in a cool atmosphere (4°C) but not a freezing one. Placing the watertight, wrapped part on ice is appropriate, but the part should not be immersed in fluid unprotected.

If decision of the replantation team is to attempt replantation, veins, arteries, nerves, and selected tendons will be repaired after skeletal fixation is achieved. Sometimes repeated procedures must be done in the first several days if vessel occlusion occurs.

ELECTIVE INCISIONS

Elective incisions in the hand must be planned to avoid contractures and to avoid scars in an area of importance for sensory perception.

Scars lack elasticity and have a tendency to heal by contraction. Any scar which ends up where stretching of its length is important for full function will cause disability. Thus scars on the palmar surface of the hand where the skin is tethered to the underlying palmar fascia should not cross the hand creases without changing direction. When the fingers are fully flexed there are areas where palm skin from one phalanx contacts that of another like the pages of a book. The diamond-shaped area of contact is like similar areas at all major palmar creases (see Fig. 50-25). Any incision crossing from one-half of the diamond to the other across the crease may result in contracture as the wound heals. One may elect freely to make incisions which do not violate this principle.

POSTOPERATIVE CARE

Success following surgery or trauma to the hand is facilitated by the control of pain, principally by appropriate

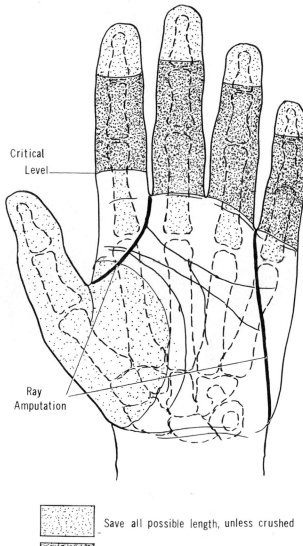

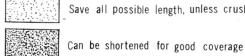

Save all possible length, unless crushed

Can be shortened for good coverage

Fig. 50-23. The recommended levels for elective amputations or for completion of traumatic amputations.

rest and elevation. Comfortable elevation of the traumatized hand by a compressive nonconstricting immobilization dressing is a cardinal principle. Supportive drugs (analgesics, narcotics, tranquilizers, and sedatives) should be administered to ensure rest, relieve anxiety, and control pain. Activity of adjacent parts that do not need rest is extremely important in reducing sensitivity to pain; exercise of the shoulder and elbow can be most helpful for early rehabilitation. Patient motivation, including preoperative, operative, and postoperative encouragement and reassurance, is another key to rapid and successful rehabilitation.

Early hand motion is important. The earliest day to start active motion, guarded passive motion, energetic passive motion, dynamic splinting, or whirlpool manipulations is determined by the injury received and the procedure per-

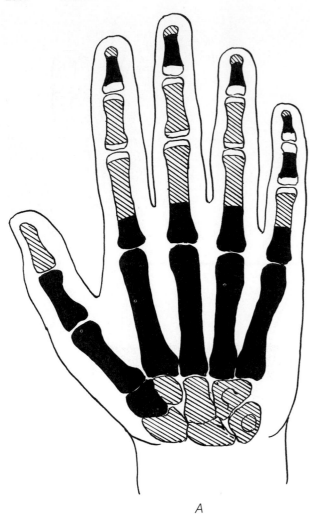

A

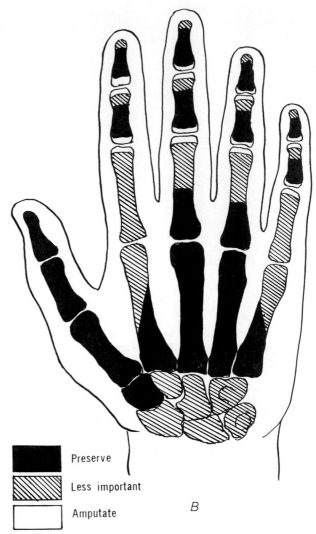

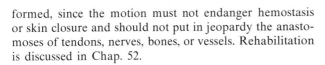

Preserve

Less important

Amputate

B

Fig. 50-24. Recommended levels for amputation in the hand, showing the bony architecture. *A.* For those requiring heavy-labor strength. *B.* This variation may be more critical for patients who need fine motion or for whom appearance is of paramount importance. Efforts to maintain extra digital length must be correlated to the sensation possible in the covering skin.

formed, since the motion must not endanger hemostasis or skin closure and should not put in jeopardy the anastomoses of tendons, nerves, bones, or vessels. Rehabilitation is discussed in Chap. 52.

Unusual Pain Syndromes

Some discomfort is to be expected after operations on the hand. Since it is used to perceive and evaluate the environment, the hand has a concentration of sensory nerves and end organs. It is sensitive to ischemia resulting from swelling or compression; thus when pain occurs postoperatively, the surgeon must examine the hand sufficiently to assure himself that there is no impending or existing complication.

When pain persists or appears after healing is complete, thorough diagnostic evaluation is mandatory. Pain may be a result of continuing ischemia, as when marginal blood supply remains after a severe injury. Nerve injuries with resulting neuroma at the injury site may give rise to pain from repeated trauma to the neuroma site.

Very trying for the patient and the surgeon are the

sympathetic dystrophies which occur after hand injuries or operations. True causalgia (burning pain) generally follows partial nerve injuries in the limb. This is a disabling syndrome consisting of severe burning pain set off by motion of the part, touching the part, and even emotional trials. Sympathetic outflow touches off the pain, and it is commonly relieved by sympathetic stellate ganglion block. Such treatment and even sympathectomy should be instituted early.

Other forms of reflex sympathetic dystrophy may occur after hand and arm injuries. Vascular syndromes with coldness, cyanosis, and atrophic changes in the skin and nails may predominate, or osseous atrophy (Sudeck's atrophy) may be prominent in sympathetic dystrophies. Elements within the healing wound which might trigger such reflex dystrophies should be corrected as the first therapeu-

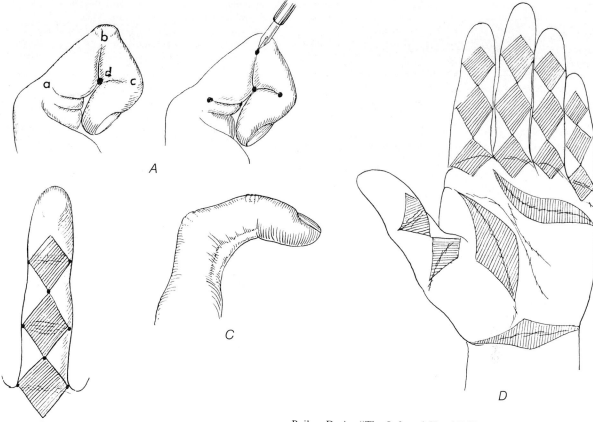

A

B

C

D

Fig. 50-25. In maximum flexion, skin folding results in skin-to-skin contact in diamond-shaped areas. Any incision which crosses from one-half of the diamond to its contact area in the other half may result in flexion contracture as the wound heals. *A.* In each of the fingers the contact areas may be seen by flexing the finger, marking the dorsal extent of each skin crease (*a, b,* and *c*), and marking the point of contact in the palmar midline where skin from all three finger segments meets. *B.* Extension of the finger and connection of these marks by lines makes visible the contact triangles. *C.* Any longitudinal incision crossing from proximal to distal triangle across flexion creases may result in flexion contracture. *D.* The same incision principles must be adhered to in contact areas at flexion creases in the hand and wrist if contracture and concomitant scar hypertrophy are to be avoided. Free choice of incision may then be made as long as none of the diamonds resulting are crossed from contact surface to contact surface.

tic approach. For example, neuromas should be excised, unhealed areas should be covered with skin, crushed useless finger parts should be amputated, and irreversible ischemic elements should be removed.

Some of the persistent pain syndromes may be amenable to psychotherapy, transcutaneous sensory counterstimulation, or physiotherapy; some are relieved simply by time.

References

Babcock, W. W.: Standard Techniques for Operations of Peripheral Nerves with Special Reference to Closure of Large Gaps, *Surg Gynecol Obstet,* **45:**364, 1927.

Bailey, D. A.: "The Infected Hand," Harper & Row, Publishers, Incorporated, New York, 1963.

Barsky, A. J.: "Congenital Anomalies of the Hand and Their Surgical Treatment," Charles C Thomas, Publisher, Springfield, Ill., 1958.

Baxter, C. R.: Surgical Management of Soft Tissue Infections, *Surg Clin North Am,* **52:**1483, 1972.

Bonica, J.: Regional Anesthesia for Surgery, *Clin Anesth,* **2:**123, 1969.

Boyes, J. H.: "Bunnell's Surgery of the Hand," 5th ed., J. B. Lippincott Company, Philadelphia, 1970.

———— and Stark, H. H.: Flexor-Tendon Grafts in the Fingers and Thumb: A Study of Factors Influencing Results in 1000 Cases, *J Bone Joint Surg* [*Am*], **53A:**1332, 1971.

Chase, R. A.: "Atlas of Hand Surgery," W. B. Saunders Company, Philadelphia, 1973.

———— and Laub, D. R.: The Hand: Therapeutic Strategy for Acute Problems, June, *Curr Probl Surg,* 1966.

Chong, J. K., Cramer, L. M., and Culf, N. K.: Combined Two-Stage Tenoplasty with Silicone Rods for Multiple Flexor-Tendon Injuries in "No-Man's-Land," *J Trauma,* **12:**104, 1972.

Cramer, L. M., and Chase, R. A.: "Symposium on the Hand," The C. V. Mosby Company, St. Louis, 1971.

Edshage, S.: Peripheral Nerve Suture, *Acta Chir Scand* [*Suppl*], **3:**31, 1964.

El Shami, I. N.: Congenital Partial Gigantism, *J Surg,* **65:**683, 1969.

Guth, L.: Degeneration in Mammalian Peripheral Nervous System, *Physiol Rev,* **36:**441, 1956.

Hunter, J. M., and Salisbury, R. E.: Flexor-Tendon Reconstruction in Severely Damaged Hands, *J Bone Joint Surg [Am]*, **53A:**829, 1971.

Kanavel, A. B.: "Infections of the Hand," Lea & Febiger, Philadelphia, 1912.

Kaplan, E. B.: "Functional and Surgical Anatomy of the Hand," 2d ed., J. B. Lippincott Company, Philadelphia, 1965.

Landsmeer, J.: The Anatomy of the Dorsal Aponeurosis of the Human Finger and Its Functional Significance, *Anat Rec,* **104:**31, 1949.

Lendvay, P., and Owen, E.: Microvascular Repair of Completely Severed Digits, *Med J Aust,* **2:**818, 1970.

Lucas, G. L.: "Examination of the Hand," Charles C Thomas, Publisher, Springfield, Ill., 1972.

Milford, L. W.: "Retaining Ligaments of the Digits of the Hand," W. B. Saunders Company, Philadelphia, 1968.

————: "The Hand," The C. V. Mosby Company, St. Louis, 1971.

Millesi, H., Meissl, G., and Berger, A.: The Interfascicular Nerve-Grafting of the Median and Ulnar Nerves, *J Bone Joint Surg [Am]*, **54A:**727, 1972.

Minkowitz, S., and Minkowitz, F.: A Morphological Study of Macrodactylism, *J Pathol,* **90:**323, 1965.

Moberg, E.: Objective Methods for Determining the Functional Value of Sensibility in the Skin, *J Bone Joint Surg [Am]*, **37A:**2, 1955.

Peacock, E. E.: Treatment of Finger Tip Injuries, *Ann Surg,* **173:**812, 1971.

Schreiber, S. N., Leibowitz, R., and Bernstein, L.: Limb Compression and Renal Impairment (Crust Syndrome) following Narcotic and Sedative Overdose, *J Bone Joint Surg [Am]*, **54A:**1683, 1972.

Seddon, H. J.: Practical Value of Peripheral Nerve Repair, *Proc R Soc Med,* **42:**427, 1949.

Simeone, F. A. (ed.): Symposium on Operative Nerve Injuries and Their Repair, *Surg Clin North Am,* vol. 52, no. 5, October 1972.

Smith, J. W.: Microsurgery of Peripheral Nerves, *Plast Reconstr Surg,* **33:**317, 1964.

Sneddon, J.: "The Care of Hand Infections," The Williams & Wilkins Company, Baltimore, 1970.

Stenstrom, S. J.: Functional Determination of the Flexor-Tendon Graft Length, *Plast Reconstr Surg,* **43:**633, 1969.

Stone, N. H., Hursch, H., Humphrey, C. R., and Boswick, J. A., Jr.: Empirical Selection of Antibiotics for Hand Infections, *J Bone Joint Surg [Am]*, **51A:**899, 1969.

Symonds, F. C.: Pitfalls in Management of Penetrating Wounds of the Forearm, *J Trauma,* **11:**47, 1971.

Temtamy, S., and McKusick, V. A.: Synopsis of Hand Malformations with Particular Emphasis on Genetic Factors in "The First Conference on the Clinical Delineation of Birth Defects," pt. III, "Limb Malformations: Birth Defects," Original Article Ser, vol 5, no. 3, pp. 125–184, The National Foundation—March of Dimes, New York, 1969.

Tsuge, K.: Treatment of Megalodactyly, *Plast Reconstr Surg,* **39:**590, 1967.

Tubiana, R.: Surgical Repair of the Extensor Apparatus of the Fingers, *Surg Clin North Am,* **48:**1015, 1968.

———— and Valentin, P.: The Anatomy of the Extensor Apparatus of the Fingers, *Surg Clin North Am,* **44:**897, 1964.

Verdan, C.: Basic Principles of Surgery of the Hand, *Surg Clin North Am,* **47:**355, 1967.

White, W. L.: Secondary Restoration of Finger Flexion by Digital Tendon Grafts: An Evaluation of 76 Cases, *Am J Surg,* **91:**662, 1956.

————: Restoration of Function and Balance of the Wrist and Hand by Tendon Transfers, *Surg Clin North Am,* **41:**427, 1960.

Williams, S. B.: New Dynamic Concepts in the Grafting of Flexor-Tendons, *Plast Reconstr Surg,* **36:**377, 1965.

Woodhall, B., and Beebe, G. W.: "Peripheral Nerve Regeneration: A Follow-up Study of 3,656 World War II Injuries," Veterans Administration Medical Monograph, 1956.

Woolf, C. M., and Woolf, R. M.: A Genetic Study of Polydactyly in Utah, *Am J Hum Genet,* **22:**75, 1970.

Zancolli, E.: "Structural and Dynamic Bases of Hand Surgery," J. B. Lippincott Company, Philadelphia, 1968.

Chapter 51

Plastic and Reconstructive Surgery

by Lester M. Cramer and Thomas J. Brobyn

HISTORICAL BACKGROUND

Surgery had its origin in procedures which are traditionally considered in the field of plastic surgery today. Many of the initial thrusts were attempts by man to correct deformity, since, in the centuries before anesthesia and asepsis, surgical procedures were limited to the body surface.

Among the earliest operations performed were those by Hindu surgeons for restoration of missing parts. Our present-day approach to total and subtotal nose reconstruction does not differ in principle from that of at least 4,000 years ago. An account of Hindu manners and customs written in 1800 mentions punishment of highway robbers by amputation of the right hand and nose, and amputation of the noses of conquered warriors as well as those of women who incurred their husbands' jealousy. Susruta, about 600 B.C., repaired the injured nose with a patch of "living flesh slided off the region of the cheek." This popular procedure employed by the Hindus now bears the name "Indian method." This technique for nose construction migrated from East to West. The Brancas, a family of Sicilian laymen, became prominent around 1430, when it was learned that they could repair noses, ears, and lips with flaps from the cheek or forehead. Antonius, the youngest of the Brancas, perfected the method now referred to as the "Italian method" for nose reconstruction by using a skin flap taken from the arm.

In the fifteenth century, the renowned Gasparo Tagliacozzi produced his classic volume on reconstruction of the nose and other parts by pedicle flap surgical methods. Having the advantage of the printing press, Tagliacozzi disseminated knowledge of the details of the techniques of reconstruction. However, following this era, operations for reconstruction of missing parts fell into disrepute for about 200 years. The procedures once again appeared in the eighteenth century in England. Carpue of London gave a detailed account of the restoration of lost noses. In the nineteenth century, von Graefe and Dieffenbach recorded several techniques for reconstruction of missing parts.

In the twentieth century, Gillies in England, Davis, Ivy, and Kazanjian in the United States, and Filatov in Russia were stimulated by World War I tragedies to pioneer newer methods of wound closure and tissue transfer. The next generation of pioneers, McIndoe, Mowlem, and Kilner in England, Wallace in Scotland, and Blair, Brown, Cannon, Bunnell, Webster, and Pierce in the United States received impetus for further development from problems raised by World War II injuries.

WOUND HEALING

The principles and the specifics discussed in Chap. 8 are especially important for plastic and reconstructive surgery.

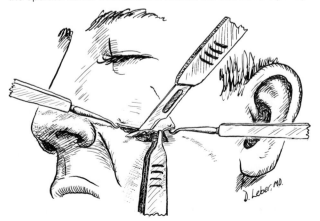

Fig. 51-1. The final result of suturing lacerations is greatly improved if careful wound toilet and debridement is supplemented by fastidious skin management. Technically, three-point fixation of the skin facilitates accurate excision, permitting straight-line execution and cutting of tissues at right angles to the surface. The assistant holds the skin hooks under moderate tension, and the operator varies the amount of tension needed with the pickup.

Metabolic and genetic characteristics greatly influence the final outcome of surgical wounds, and the knowledge and ability of the surgeon are even more critical in determining most results. Attention to detail and meticulous wound closures have become identified with plastic and reconstructive surgery. Halsted's principles and those outlined by Esmarch in 1877 have become self-evident requirements in proper wound care. Techniques are critical in avoiding excessive scar formation but are not the only factors.

Abnormalities of wound healing leading to hypertrophic scars, mismatched scars, and large secondary iatrogenic markings (crosshatches from large suture material tied too tightly) are mainly avoidable by the critical attention to known facts. Scar tissue can be further controlled either by the systemic use of biochemical antagonists or by the local injection of steroids. Keloid scar, as differentiated from hypertrophic scar, is a true metabolic anarchy of scar tissue. It is much more difficult to control but can be judiciously handled by working totally within the keloid lesion and by the intralesional injection of steroids at the time of surgery.

The implantation of prosthetic materials is increasingly applied. There are two types, according to the surface presented. The first is totally inert, a smooth *macro* surface such as that presented by silicone or Teflon. The body reacts minimally, but walling-off by a lining membrane does occur. This membrane, a mesothelia-like surface, allows these implanted substances to remain in situ for long periods of time, perhaps indefinitely, but infection is a hazard. Smooth-surfaced prostheses also can be used to create tissue channels, the prosthesis later being electively removed in order to insert moving surfaces, such as tendons, through these channels (see Chap. 50). The second type of tissue implant works on the principle of capture. These implants are purposely felted or veloured, in the case of materials such as Dacron or polypropylene, or sintered, in the case of ceramics. By presenting *micro* surfaces to the body, membrane formation is avoided, and a true tissue-prosthetic interface without walling off is created. This type of implant has a better opportunity for long life, since it is less liable to become infected.

TECHNICAL CONSIDERATIONS

Wound Closure

The principles outlined in this section pertain to all wounds, but their importance in achieving a cosmetically acceptable result is magnified in the face and neck regions and usually the extremities. The wound should be thoroughly cleaned; if the edges are ragged, they should be revised (Fig. 51-1). Subcutaneous undermining to achieve closure without tension is essential. The dermal and subcutaneous tissue trimming should be fashioned so that subcuticular sutures will hold the skin edges in approximation. Fine absorbable subcutaneous sutures positioned so that the knots are tied in the depth of the wound lend strength to the wound closure during the critical first weeks

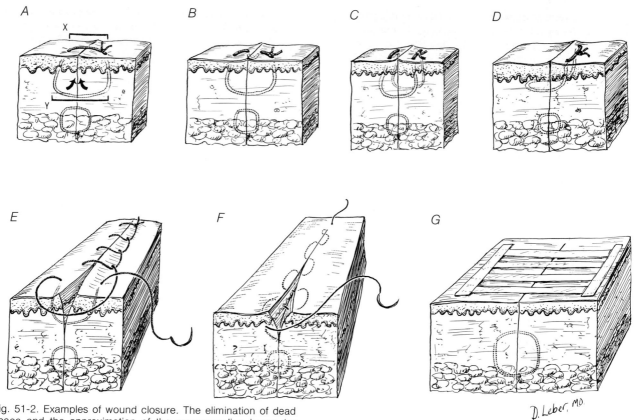

D. Leber, MD.

Fig. 51-2. Examples of wound closure. The elimination of dead space and the approximation of the corresponding layers (or levels) of tissue are desirable. The transcutaneous suture is best placed by ensuring that the deeper portion of the suture (y) is wider than the superficial portion (x). This causes the wound pressures to encourage slight edge eversion (curved arrow), an excellent way of preventing edge inversion. Inversion would delay wound healing and result in a wider cutaneous scar. With all these closure methods, the cutaneous perforation should never exceed 3 mm from the wound edge, and it should be appropriately closer on the face. A suture should never be tied tightly. *A.* Simple conventional suture. *B.* Vertical mattress suture. *C.* Horizontal mattress suture. *D.* Half-buried mattress suture, the preferred method on most flaps. This is especially useful on the corners of lacerations or on Z-plasties because of its slight interference with the blood supply. *E.* Running lockstitch, infrequently indicated. *F.* Running subcuticular stitch of Halsted, the recommended method of wound closure and the one most commonly employed by the authors. *G.* Nonsuture closure of wounds with nonallergic, porous tape.

of healing. Fine-caliber skin sutures have been employed to achieve accurate epidermal and dermal coaption and to diminish the skin wound interface. The use of subcuticular running pullout sutures accomplishes the same tissue coaption without having extra external markings across the wound. In many instances accurate placement of the subcuticular and subcutaneous closure requires approximation only with porous, nonallergic tape, completely obviating skin sutures (Fig. 51-2). Early removal of sutures is not necessary, particularly if they have been placed carefully and have been loosely tied for the wound approximation. Since suture support of the scar can improve

the final result and since a subcuticular pullout suture causes less tissue reaction both at the surface and in the depth because it does not cross the dermal-subcutaneous juncture, the use of subcuticular pullout sutures takes on added importance.

Skin Grafting

Skin which is completely removed from its donor site and transplanted into a recipient area is a *graft*. A graft is composed of epidermal and dermal tissue whose survival in the recipient bed is via a plasmatic circulation until capillary juncture occurs. A graft differs from a *skin flap*, which is composed of epidermal, dermal, and subcutaneous tissue whose survival in the recipient bed is via a well-maintained or surgically reestablished vasculature. A skin flap is never devoid of its blood supply. Transplantation by graft or flap has become a commonplace and practical surgical procedure for covering open wounds or for replacing the skin after surgical excision of scars or tumors.

HISTORICAL BACKGROUND. Aulus Cornelius Celsus in 30 A.D. wrote of eyelid surgery and mentioned the possibility of free skin grafts in his *De re medica,* Book VII. During the Middle Ages, there were few references to free transplantation of tissue, although isolated instances were recorded. Sancassani described a female street vendor, who, in order to prove the efficacy of a certain salve, removed a piece of skin from her leg, passed it around the audience on a plate, replaced it in its original position, and covered it with the salve. The subsequent reunion was such that the site of operation was described as "scarcely discernible." In the nineteenth century, Baronio carried out a series of successful experiments on animals, mainly sheep, in which he transplanted pieces of skin. Reverdin and Guyon independently reported the use of pinch grafts to achieve healing on human granulating wound surfaces, although Frank Hamilton of New York initially suggested the implantation of a piece of skin 20 years prior to Reverdin's report. Hamilton's presentation concerned a patient on whom Reverdin had successfully carried out skin grafting with "two small bits of epidermis raised with the point of a lancet from the patient's right arm." The work was ridiculed by many, including David Page, then president of the Royal Medical Society of Edinburgh, who remarked, "It is not likely to occupy a permanent position in minor surgery." In 1870, in a paper entitled "On the Transplantation of Portions of Skin for the Closure of Large Granulating Surfaces," Lawson laid down the following dicta, which are still applicable: (1) that the new skin should be applied to a healthy granulating surface, (2) that only skin which is devoid of fat should be taken, (3) that the portion of skin should be accurately and firmly applied to the granulating surface, and (4) that the new skin should be kept in its new position without interruption.

In 1872, Ollier announced his new method of skin grafting in which he transplanted large squares of epidermis,

up to 8 cm long, as free grafts. Shortly thereafter, Thiersch suggested using a razor to cut thin skin grafts, which were actually very thin split-thickness grafts devoid of dermal elements.

In 1875, Wolfe, an oculist in Glasgow, suggested grafting full-thickness segments of skin for correction of ectropion deformity. He also pointed out the importance of removing fat beneath the skin to be transferred and emphasized that "after a lapse of a fortnight, massage should be started with lanolin or cold cream," exactly the orders one would give today. Although skin grafting was rarely employed in World War I, with the development of the Padgett dermatome the technique became established in the 1930s. With the use of electric dermatomes developed by Brown and McDowell, and facilitated by the techniques developed in World War II, grafting become a routinely used operative procedure.

SKIN STRUCTURE (Fig. 51-3). The skin is a complex organ, varying in thickness, elasticity, color, and texture.

Fig. 51-3. Diagrammatic representation of the skin with correlation for use as graft donor sites. Split-thickness skin grafting is possible because the epithelial appendages in the donor dermis allow healing by proliferation and migration of the epithelial cells left behind. Healing is faster when there are more of these cells, as when the site is hairy or the donor graft is thin, and when the cells are metabolically active, as in young and healthy patients. When the graft contains more of the donor dermis, it probably is more serviceable and cosmetically superior. But the thicker the graft removed, the more epithelial cells removed; the fewer cells remaining at the donor site will determine slower healing. When the full thickness of the skin is removed, the wound is usually closed by undermining the skin and approximating it by sutures. If the wound is extremely large, a split-thickness skin graft would be needed.

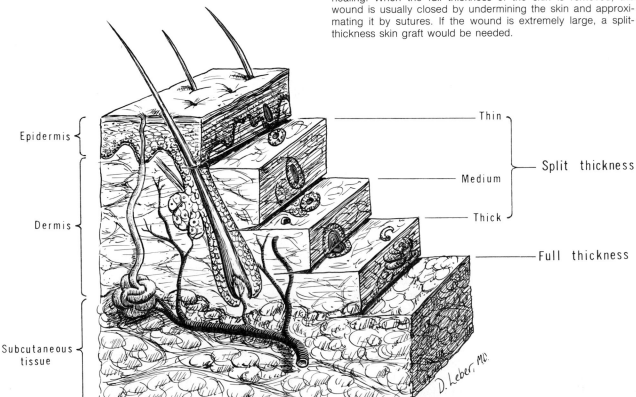

These traits are influenced by age, sex, and state of nutrition. Use of a portion of skin as a donor to be transplanted elsewhere involves donor site selection based on the function and appearance of the skin in its recipient site and the proclivity of the donor site to heal. The latter is determined by the character of the remaining dermis, its thickness, and the number of epithelial appendages remaining. Because donor site healing may leave some scarring, it is advisable to remove the skin from an area that will be socially inconspicuous. The donor sites should also be selected to match the recipient area in texture and color when possible, e.g., grafting to the face mandates a donor site from the blush area (skin above the level of the nipples, on the ventral aspect of the body).

SPLIT-THICKNESS GRAFTS

A skin graft in which the epidermis and a partial thickness of the dermis is employed is referred to as a *split-thickness graft*. There are several advantages in this procedure. The donor site will heal spontaneously by reepithelialization through retained epidermal appendages such as sweat glands and hair follicles. Also the likelihood of graft survival, or "take," is high, because the thin skin can survive on the plasmatic nutrition while the blood supply is being restored by capillary juncture.

Indications for split-thickness skin graft are many and varied: Whenever there is a large wound with a well-vascularized bed which cannot be readily closed by suture or local flaps, a split-thickness skin graft is appropriate, although a local flap is superior to free skin grafts. The skin deficit may exist as a result of trauma, surgical excision, a burn wound healing by secondary intention, or skin loss from infection now under control. The recipient site must be cleaned and well vascularized to be receptive to split-thickness skin grafting. The selection of the donor site and thickness of split-thickness skin graft to be used is dependent upon the need at the recipient site. For example, if a skin graft is to be used as permanent skin coverage in an area of wear where contraction of the wound is undesirable, a thick (0.018- to 0.025-in.) split-thickness graft should be used. In an area where circumstances are not perfect for skin graft application, a slightly thinner, or moderate-thickness, split-thickness skin graft 0.012 to 0.018 in. thick may take more reliably and yet be thick enough to prevent contraction of the wound at the graft site. Skin grafts thinner than 0.01 in. are thin split-thickness skin grafts. These provide excellent early coverage for large granulating burn wounds, and the donor site can be used two or three times because the healing is more rapid. It is important to achieve the proper color match between the skin graft and its recipient site, particularly on the face and hands. When color match is not important, skin grafts are taken from the inconspicuous places, usually from the high thigh, buttock, or abdominal areas.

Split-thickness skin grafts are commonly taken with mechanical dermatomes which precisely control thickness. There are many varieties of drum dermatomes which pick up skin with a mechanically attached blade, controlling thickness by adjustment of the blade. Electrified or air-driven mechanical dermatomes are useful in rapidly procuring large lengths of split-thickness skin for coverage of burned areas requiring grafting. Special knives are also used, either with or without mechanical guards to determine thickness, to take freehand grafts. Large sheets can be obtained with all these techniques.

The split-thickness skin graft is carefully fitted to the recipient site and under most circumstances is best sutured in place with nonabsorbable suture. Usually the peripheral stitches are left long so that they can be tied over a dressing to immobilize it upon the graft site to apply pressure and prevent motion. In some wounds, particularly granulating ones, the split-thickness skin graft is best left unsutured and exposed during the early phases of healing. It must be protected in place by proper splinting. Exposure will allow meticulous postoperative wound care, such as removal of fluid accumulated beneath the graft, to facilitate the graft take.

FULL-THICKNESS GRAFTS

A full-thickness skin graft, as the name implies, consists of the full thickness of both epidermis and dermis (Fig. 51-4). There are several advantages in using the full thickness of skin. The donor site may be closed; when small grafts are required, a sutured donor site is less bothersome than a raw healing split-graft donor area. There is no limitation on the area which may be used for the donor site, a situation which does not pertain to grafts taken with a freehand knife or a dermatome. The postauricular area, upper eyelid, flank, groin, arm, and wrist are examples of the areas which are excellent sources of full-thickness grafts (Fig. 51-5). No special instrument is required to procure the graft, and skin appendages remain intact. Although the take is somewhat less reliable, once the survival is secure, the full-thickness graft is much more

Fig. 51-4. Full-thickness free skin grafts. Removal from donor site free of subcutaneous fat and areolar tissue.

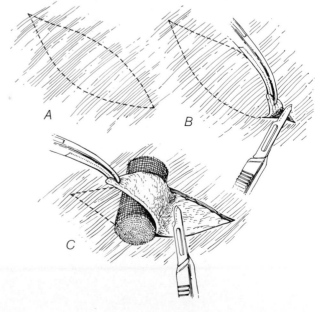

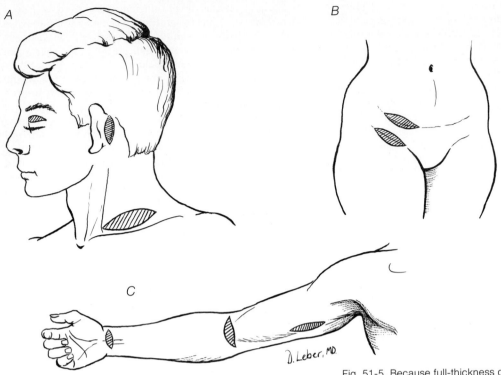

durable and more acceptable in consistency and color. Because of these attributes, full-thickness grafts may be employed for cosmetic reasons in some areas and are particularly applicable in areas in which the skin must withstand pressure or repeated trauma such as the fingers and palm.

COMPOSITE GRAFTS

A composite graft consists of skin, in combination with other tissue, which is transferred without its blood supply

Fig. 51-6. Composite graft from ear to furnish both lining and alar skin.

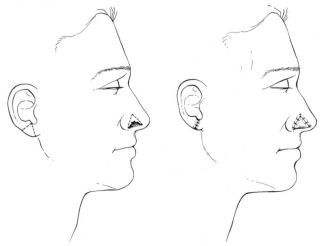

Fig. 51-5. Because full-thickness grafts are cosmetically superior on the face, the appropriate donor sites must be determined according to availability, color match, and texture. *A.* Correct design on the upper eyelid, retroauricular area, and supraclavicular region allow closure with a linear scar and minimal noticeable defect. *B* and *C.* Nonfacial full-thickness-graft donor sites, primarily for use on the hands and occasionally on the feet. These allow maximal availability and a linear closure with minimal discomfort and an inconspicuous scar.

as a free graft from the donor to the recipient area. As rapid vascularization is needed for survival of the composite graft, its use is restricted to recipient areas of good blood supply. Under optimal circumstances and for relatively small defects, it is a reliable graft.

The classic composite graft is a free graft of skin, subcutaneous tissue, and cartilage from the ear to the nose (Fig. 51-6). This is applicable for through-and-through defects in the nose, especially those involving the alar edge. The composite graft which matches the defect is procured from the edge of the ear incorporating both anterior and posterior ear skin and interposed cartilage.

Free composite grafts from the hair-bearing scalp have been employed for eyebrow reconstruction for many years (Fig. 51-7). In recent years, the treatment of male pattern baldness has become popularized. Multiple circular grafts of hair follicles, each graft containing approximately six hairs, are transferred from the posterior region to the anterior bald portion. These are interspersed with short linear segments of 8 to 10 hairs apiece. Eventual luxuriant growth of these hairs can camouflage the bald region effectively. Transfer of total-thickness segments of lip, usually from the lower lip to the upper lip without a pedicle, also illustrates the use of composite grafts.

PEDICLE TISSUE TRANSFERS

The salient feature in the technique of pedicle transfer of tissue is that the tissue being transferred is never devoid of blood supply; the pedicle is the handle by which the tissue maintains its attachment and blood supply during the first stage of the transfer. Once the transferred tissue heals to the recipient site, its nourishment is supplied by the recipient site, and the pedicle may be severed. A better final result can be achieved if the pedicle is a permanent one, maintaining its original blood and nerve supply for better trophism. Thus, local pedicle flaps are the best tissue, and if they can be geometrically devised, they become the best replacement.

Knowledge of the blood supply of the skin allows correct design. Tracing this blood supply from the aorta out to the dermal capillaries categorizes the vessels into the following groups: (1) segmental, (2) perforator, and (3) cutaneous.

Segmental branches are direct branches of the aorta, such as the internal mammary or the inferior epigastric systems, which lie deep to the muscles.

Perforators are the branches from the segmental vessels, connecting to the cutaneous vessels and supplying muscles as they pass through them. Examples are the thoracoacromial or the anterior and posterior humeral circumflex.

Cutaneous branches represent the third level and are most important to understand for flap design. They supply the skin directly and are the principal determinants of flap survival. They are the musculocutaneous arteries and the direct cutaneous arteries. The musculocutaneous arteries individually supply a small area, but collectively are the predominant blood supply to the skin. The direct cutaneous arteries run parallel to the skin surface, each perfusing a much greater area, but are quite limited in number and location throughout the body. A summation of the characteristics of cutaneous arteries is presented in Table 51-1.

Excellent examples of named direct cutaneous arteries upon which well-conceived flaps have been designed are the following: (1) superficial temporal, (2) superficial inferior epigastric, (3) superior thoracic, (4) superficial external pudendal, (5) lateral thoracic, (6) intercostal–internal mammary (Bakamjian et al.), (7) superficial circumflex iliac artery (McGregor), (8) dorsal artery of the penis.

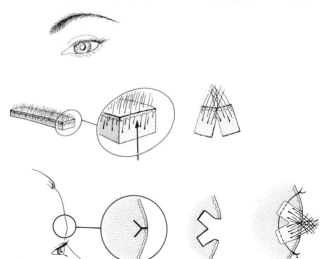

Fig. 51-7. Composite free graft from hair-bearing scalp for eyebrow reconstruction. Note that the graft is split and interposed in the recipient area so that the hairs interdigitate and give an eyebrow effect.

Flap Design. Flap design based on specific length/width ratios have clinical application, on a statistical basis, for the different parts of the body. They are positively influenced when there are major named direct cutaneous arterial systems. In the head and neck region, length/width ratios as high as 3:1 or even 4:1 can be safely used; in other regions such as the deltopectoral or the ilioinguinal, such high ratios or higher have been accomplished on the named systems, giving long lengths of tissues on relatively narrow bases. However, in most parts of the body it is difficult to make a flap of a higher ratio than 2:1, and below the knee rarely is the safe limit for a primary transfer any higher than 1:1. It is important to understand that the viable lengths of such skin flaps are really only indirectly related to their widths. Flaps of varying widths all survive to the same length provided they have similar conditions of blood supply; decreasing the width will decrease the chance of the pedicle's containing large vessels.

Delay. The principle of delay allows safer transfer when a larger amount of tissue is needed than can be supplied by designing a flap from the local region. When this would exceed the safety factor of the vasculature, the dimensions of the flap needed can be augmented by one or more preliminary operations which consist of incising portions of the flap periphery or depth in stages. This old concept is based on the observation that the blood supply of a part is better after it has been previously partially separated from its blood supply.

Reinisch has done much to help explain the incompletely understood pathophysiology of the delay phenomenon. His experimental model shows substantial blood supply in the distal ends of flaps which are designed to be longer than their predicted surviving length. This circulation is contained in thick, nonnutritive arteriovenous channels, controlled by the sympathetic nervous system. Elevation of a flap denervates it, allowing the arteriovenous

Table 51-1. CHARACTERISTICS OF CUTANEOUS ARTERIES

Musculocutaneous	Direct
Dominant	Supplementary
Ubiquitous	Fixed
Regional variations	Anatomic variations
Perpendicular	Parallel: deep subcutaneous
Single vein	Paired venae comitantes + associated subdermal veins

SOURCE: Classification of Williams and Daniel.

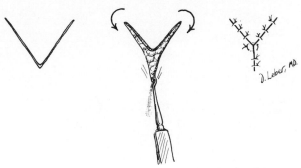

Fig. 51-8. The V-Y advancement principle, allowing the apex of the V to advance along the axis of a scar to facilitate lengthening.

shunts to open, thus causing lethal bypassing of nutrient capillaries in areas of decreased circulation. Delay of the flap causes denervation and retains enough residual blood supply to provide adequate flow through both capillaries and dilated shunts. Because the difference between an ischemic flap (leading to a successful delay) and a necrotic flap is frequently very small, judgment and experience in delay design and execution are critical.

LOCAL PEDICLE FLAPS. A local pedicle, as differentiated from a distal pedicle, involves tissue with its blood supply intact reaching the recipient area without moving the recipient area or without intervening stages of donor area movement. These most useful reconstructive procedures include the following:

V-Y advancement
Z-plasty
Rotation
Advancement
Transposition
Interpolation
Bilobed
Bipedicle
Island
Microvascular

Fig. 51-9. The clinical application of a V-Y advancement.

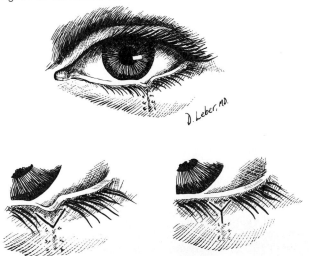

Potentially bewildering, this array of local tissue shifts is easily understood and should receive primary consideration for all wounds that cannot be closed by direct suture. When they can be used, they are superior to free graft, because of more reliable healing, easier wound management, and better cosmetic and functional results. In addition an avascular recipient site, e.g., the cortical bone devoid of its periosteum, cartilage devoid of its perichondrium, or a previously heavily irradiated area, will be unable to support a free graft.

The V-Y advancement (Fig. 51-8) obtains small amounts of length along a correct axis when the apex of the V-flap is placed on that axis. It is useful in a few highly selected instances of scar revision, particularly at free borders (Fig. 51-9).

Much more useful, perhaps the most commonly employed reconstructive procedure, is the Z-plasty (Fig. 51-10). By changing the direction of a laceration or a scar, using the geometric principles of a parallelogram, great advantage is gained in added length.

Transposition (Fig. 51-11), rotation (Fig. 51-12), and interpolation flaps (Figs. 51-13, 51-14) all use the attached local tissues, widely undermined, to close the wound.

The bipetal, or bilobed, flap, popularized by Zimany, has been a useful modification, because it eliminates the need for grafting the donor site defect when it might otherwise have been necessary to employ such a skin graft to close the donor site (Fig. 51-15).

The bipedicle flap is still a very useful maneuver, despite notoriety gained from lack of understanding of its design. It is commonly employed in the pretibial region to cover compound fractures on the night of injury. The donor site of this flap must always be grafted, and the correct proportions of the flap accurately maintained by a curved incision allowing two wide bases (Fig. 51-16).

The island pedicle flap diminishes the size of the pedicle which carries nourishment so that it incorporates only the major blood vessels and allows movement of composite tissue blocks without a skin bridge, the bridge being these blood vessels and some surrounding subcutaneous and dermal tissue. Since the introduction of this technique by Gersuny, Monks, and Esser, its versatility has encouraged increasing use, particularly as knowledge of direct cutaneous arteries and microsurgical technique improve, so that the principle of vascularized island pedicle transfer is now widely applied. Loops of bowel are shifted to areas well away from their normal residence on a pedicle of mesenteric vessels alone. Esophageal substitution and bladder substitution with bowel are classic examples. Composite tissue carried on the temporal vessels has great value in facial reconstruction (Fig. 51-17). Total eyebrow reconstruction may be carried out using composite hair-bearing scalp shifted on a pedicle of the temporal vessels. Vascular pedicle grafts which incorporate digital nerves have been useful in hand surgery to transfer tissue to the critical area of denervation of the thumb and index finger.

DISTANT PEDICLE FLAPS. These include *jump flaps,* either direct or via a carrier, and *tubed flaps.*

Direct jump flaps are those which are elevated and left attached to their nourishing pedicle while the recipient site

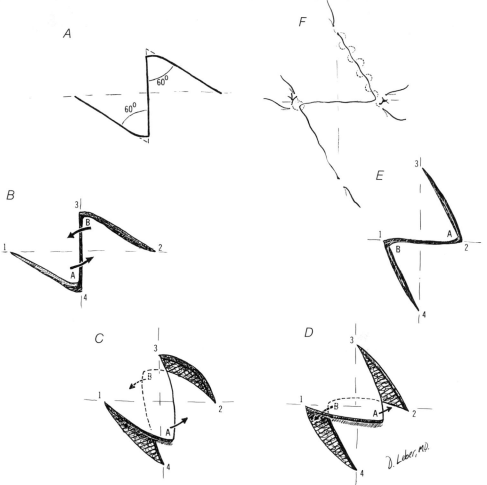

Fig. 51-10. Principles of the Z-plasty. Construction of two identical equilateral triangles based on any scar line makes two triangular flaps which together constitute a parallelogram. Interchanging these two flaps will lengthen the original line by 50 percent. This is easy to understand by noting that the short leg of a parallelogram is exchanged for the long leg.

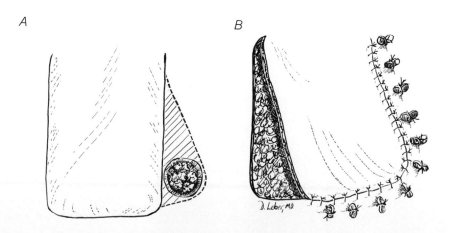

Fig. 51-11. A transposition flap.

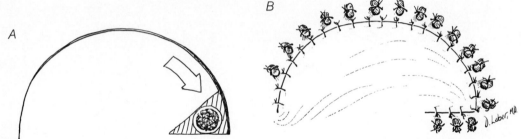

Fig. 51-12. A rotation flap.

is moved to an adjacent position. These may be of many sizes and shapes. Some involve only small amounts of tissue being brought to a critical area, such as a cross finger flap (Fig. 51-18). They may involve massive tissue shifts, such as truncal flaps to the hand from the abdominal wall (Fig. 51-19), or the shoulder region (Fig. 51-20).

When the tissue cannot be made to reach the place for which it is intended, a carrier can be devised, such as attachment to the wrist, as an intermediate phase. A series of operations then will be performed to eventually transfer the tissue to the recipient site.

Tubed flaps are used less frequently as better designs of local or jump flaps become available, because tubed flaps involve more inherent complications and many more operations in sequence. However, when tissue must be transferred over a considerable distance, the tubed flap,

despite the possible complications, must be considered because of the provision for constant tissue nourishment and the reliability of a completely closed wound. Gillies has been generally credited with popularizing this technique, but it was probably initially reported by Filatov in 1917.

The tubed pedicle is created by fashioning two parallel incisions and closing the pedicle edge to edge, resulting in a handle effect (Fig. 51-21). This creates the closed wound, which incorporates the blood supply and the soft tissue in addition to the skin. Later the pedicle is transferred to a new site (Fig. 51-22). One end of the pedicle is initially transected and positioned over the recipient site about 3 or 4 weeks later. After another 3 or 4 weeks, the opposite end also may be transected, so that the entire tube pedicle now has been moved to the distant site. During

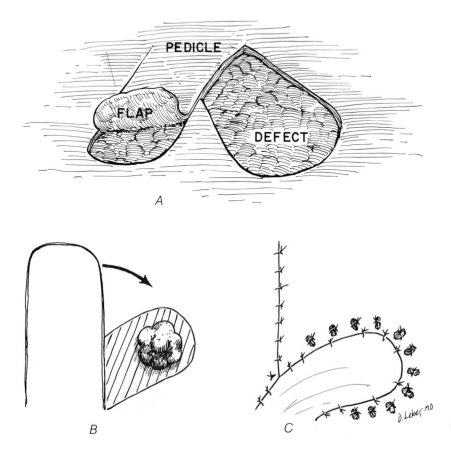

Fig. 51-13. Interpolation pedicle flap.

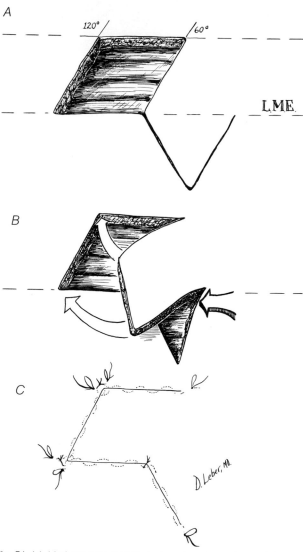

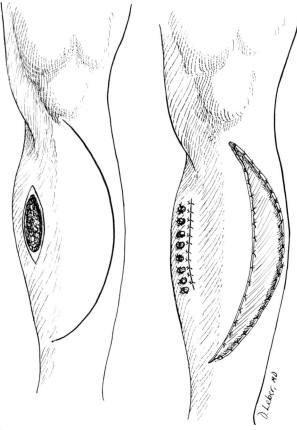

Fig. 51-16. A bipedicle flap.

Fig. 51-14. Limberg flap. This is designed as shown by excision of a 60° rhomboid, oriented correctly in relation to the lines of maximum extensibility (LME) of the skin. *A.* Excision of the 60° rhomboid, showing correct orientation with regard to the LME. The flap is constructed by extending the short diagonal (short axis) by its own length and constructing a third side arranged at a 60° angle to the extended short diagonal and equal in length to any side. *B.* Elevation and transposition of the Limberg flap. The heavy arrow emphasizes the closure of the donor defect parallel to the LME, a critical consideration in the design and execution of this flap. *C.* Completed closure.

Fig. 51-17. Island pedicle graft. Vascularized islands of composite tissues may be transferred over a wide area of the face when carried solely on temporal vessels. This allows the surgeon to pass the tissue and its pedicle to the recipient area through a subcutaneous tunnel. The blood supply is permanently retained, and there is no need for a second stage to cut the carrying pedicle and set the composite graft in place.

Fig. 51-15. A bipetal (bilobed) flap.

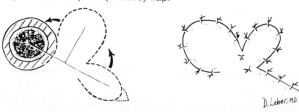

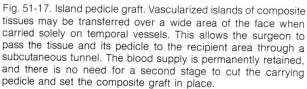

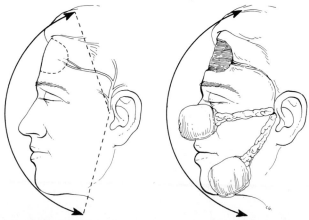

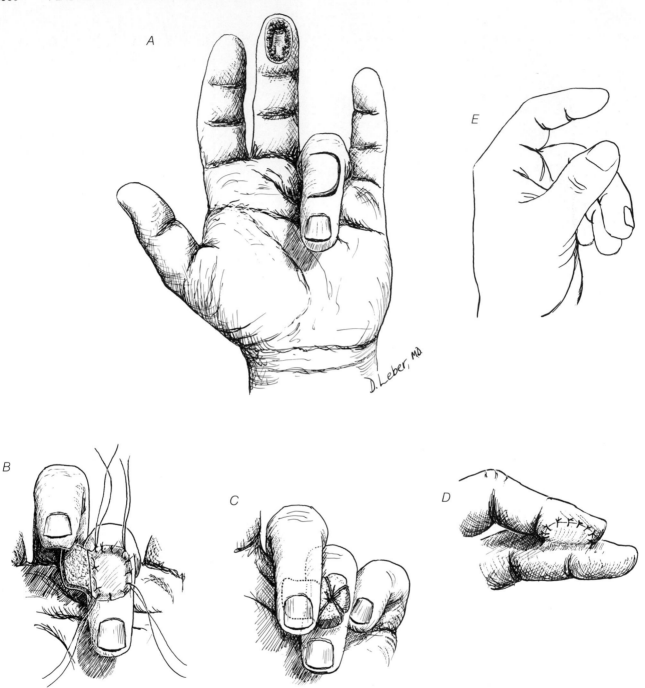

Fig. 51-18. The cross finger flap. *A.* The dorsum of the next digit in the ulnar direction is the usual donor site. *B.* The donor site and some of the carrier are grafted with a medium split-thickness skin graft so that there will be a closed wound system. *C.* An example of the tie-over dressing to maintain pressure and immobilization on a split-thickness skin graft. The material best suited is sponge rubber. *D.* The flap replacing the defect. *E.* When the replacement area is the touch strip on the volar aspect of the thumb, the best donor site is not on the index finger but on the middle finger, because the position of the thumb in relation to the index finger creates acute angles in the joints, leading to pain and potential stiffness.

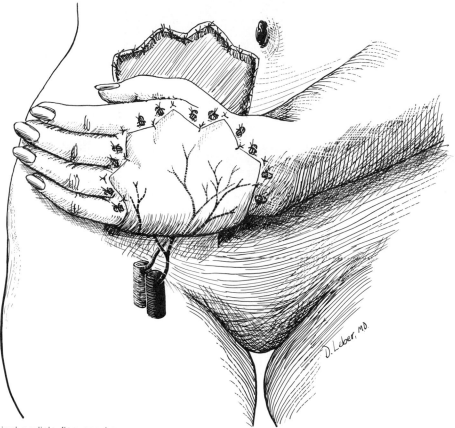

Fig. 51-19. An extremely large abdominal pedicle flap can be constructed without delay because of the inferior epigastric system. The major disadvantage of using this flap to resurface the hand is that the dependent position of the hand increases edema. The donor site and flap carrier portion are skin-grafted. The deltopectoral flap popularized by Bakamjian for reconstruction in the head and neck area is also excellent for hand coverage, because it makes available a large amount of tissue without delay while allowing the hand to be in a position for dependent drainage. This flap is based on the internal mammary vasculature. Its only disadvantage is that the donor site is left with a more visible scar.

these intervals, the transferred tissue becomes nourished by the recipient site and no longer requires its original vascular supply.

Myocutaneous Flaps. The use of multiple large, compound muscle-skin flaps has recently been described in detail by McCraw et al. Utilization of these flaps provides new avenues of approach to reconstruction problems, with definite advantages. They provide a blood supply to an avascular area and bulk for filling defects or covering bone grafts, and they make possible the creation of longer viable flaps. Delay procedures may be decreased or avoided.

Myocutaneous flaps consist of a "carrier" muscle segment and the overlying skin and subcutaneous tissues. Vascularity is provided to the carrier muscle by a dominant pedicle and its segmental blood supply. This pedicle will support a large muscle segment even when the remaining pedicles are ligated. Complete detachment of the myo-

cutaneous flap except for its blood supply is possible, providing an increase in its effectiveness for reconstruction.

Independent myocutaneous vascular territories which have been described include the sternomastoid, upper trapezius, latissimus, lower sacrospinalis, upper and lower rectus abdominus, thoracoepigastric, upper and lower sartorius, rectus femoris, gracilis, biceps femoris, and gastrocnemius.

The viable muscle length, location of the dominant vascular pedicle, and functional expendability of the muscle are among the essential considerations.

Muscle Flaps. The reconstructive problems of the lower extremities, such as nonunion of the tibia, soft tissue loss with exposed bone, chronic tibial osteomyelitis, or venous stasis ulcers, have long been appreciated. Correction has required prolonged hospitalization and carries significant morbidity. The use of available lower extremity muscle flaps, popularized by Ger, has greatly facilitated the treatment of these conditions.

The principle is transposition of an available muscle with its intact neurovascular bundle to provide soft tissue coverage and an immediately suitable bed for split-thickness skin grafting. This bed is not dependent on surrounding pathologic tissue for vascularity.

Muscles suitable for transposition must be of adequate length and must have a vascular pedicle located near the muscle origin to provide satisfactory rotation. If there are

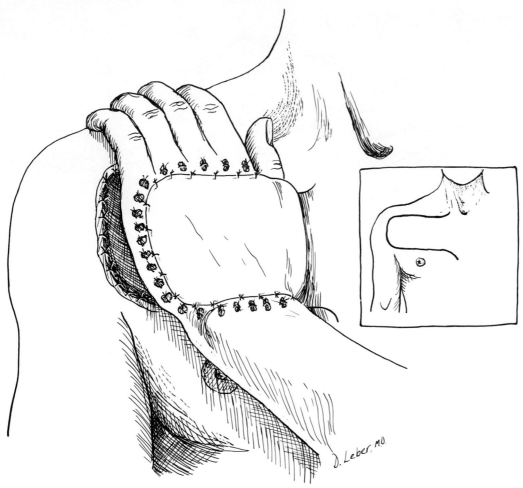

Fig. 51-20. The deltopectoral flap (Bakamjian). A direct cutaneous internal system provides a large amount of tissue in one stage.

multiple vascular pedicles, delay may be necessary. Also, synergistic muscles must be present to replace the lost function of the transposed muscle.

The muscles most suitable for transposition have been cataloged into areas: (1) tibia (upper third)—medial head gastrocnemius; (2) tibia (middle third)—soleus and flexor digitorum longus; (3) tibia (lower third)—peroneus and flexor digitorum longus; (4) tibia (upper two-thirds)—gastrocnemius, soleus, peroneus, flexor digitorum longus; (5) medial malleolus—abductor hallucis; (6) lateral malleolus—abductor digiti minimi; (7) calcaneus—flexor digitorum brevis.

In addition to the lower extremity flaps, muscles flaps for tissue defects in other areas have been used. Vasconez et al. described use of the deltoid for scapular coverage, abductor digiti quinti for the wrist, sartorius for the pubis, and paravertebral muscles for the ilium.

Bone Flaps. Osteocutaneous flaps consisting of all or part of the clavicle in a tubed flap have been described for mandibular reconstruction. The flap is transferred in stages, and there is evidence to show that the bone remains viable in the tube. Preservation of the periosteal circulation maintains bone viability.

Omental Flaps. Large defects in the chest wall can be corrected by combined use of the greater omentum and split-thickness skin grafting. The omentum can be freed from the stomach and, utilizing either the right or the left gastroepiploic vessels, transposed to the chest wall. Choice of the pedicle depends on whether the right or left chest wall is to be reconstructed. Segments of omentum have been transferred to repair skull defects and hemifacial atrophy.

Free Flaps. Successful one-stage distant transfer of an island flap using microvascular anastomosis was first reported a few years ago. This *free flap* has since become well established as a feasible alternative to multistaged flap transfer. A high level of microvascular expertise is required to successfully perform this procedure, since anastomosis of vessels less than 1 mm in diameter may be necessary. Also, there must be a predictable vascular supply in the donor flap and suitable recipient vessels. Use of the free flap technique carries a higher risk of failure than other methods of tissue transfer. The technique is not limited to flaps of skin and subcutaneous tissue but has been described for direct transfer of lower extremity muscle to

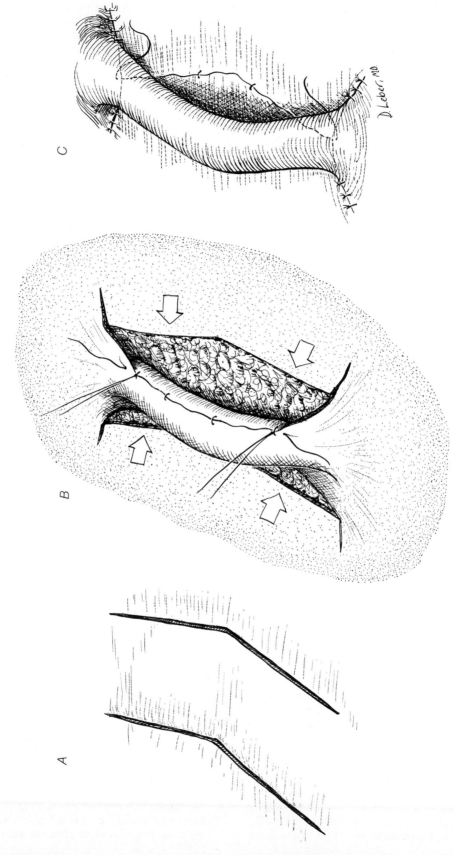

Fig. 51-21. Tubed pedicles are used much less frequently than in the past because of better understanding of direct tissue transfer possibilities. Their construction necessitates careful adherence to length/width ratio (A) and meticulous, atraumatic technique. Proper undermining and advancement (B) allow direct closure of nearly every tube pedicle donor site.

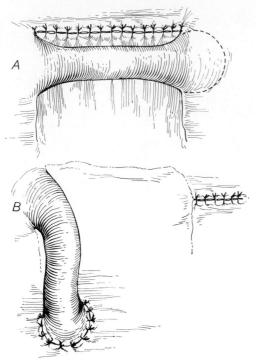

Fig. 51-22. Transfer of tubed pedicle flap. *A.* Tubed pedicle constructed. *B.* After healing, the tissue at one end of the tube may be transferred, retaining its blood supply through the tube.

reanimate the face in selected cases of facial nerve paralysis.

Although several donor sites have been described for free skin flaps, the best is one based on the superficial circumflex iliac and superficial inferior epigastric systems—the "regional" iliofemoral flap. Flaps as large as 15 by 24 cm may be transferred in one stage. This flap has the disadvantage of a short pedicle and excess bulk in obese patients. A satisfactory alternative is a free deltopectoral flap based on the second and third perforators of the internal mammary vessels. Skin flaps based on the dorsalis pedis vessel can also be taken from the dorsum of the foot.

Microsurgery

Magnification techniques have made possible the abundant transfer of composite units by vascular restoration. Microsurgery has extended the use of tissue transfer to whole organs and composite units whose vascular supply is from small vessels, allowing successful anastomosis of blood vessels less than 1 mm in diameter with rather predictable reliability. The reconstructive surgery that has developed with these improved techniques has been exciting and imaginative. Previously unmanageable problems can now be solved by the use of microsurgical anastomoses of arteries, veins, and nerves. Approximately seven to nine interrupted sutures of monofilament nylon are required for an artery 1 mm in external diameter, while six to seven

sutures are needed for a 1 mm vein. The flap vasculature is not irrigated, but the vascular stumps are washed out with diluted heparin solution. Postoperative systemic heparinization is not used, but dextran, aspirin, and Persantin may be employed. In the first 12 to 24 hours postoperatively, it is mandatory to monitor the patient closely by Doppler radar, for an embarrassed flap may be saved by early thrombectomy.

Large units of skin can be transferred by using donor sites from the groin (superficial circumflex iliac artery and vein or superficial epigastric artery and vein), the scalp (superficial temporal artery and vein), the deltopectoral region (second perforating branch of internal mammary artery and vein), the dorsum of the foot (dorsalis pedis artery and vein), and the skin of the lateral chest wall (the thoracodorsal artery and vein).

Large segments of omentum utilizing vascular stalks of the gastroepiploic vessels have been transferred to repair skull defects, chest wall defects, and hemifacial atrophy.

Reconstruction of the thumb by free total toe transplantation is now a reality, utilizing neurovascular anastomosis. Replantations of digits and extremities have been reported with increasing frequency. Successful replantation after total scalp or penile avulsion also is now possible with these techniques.

Free transplantation of muscle by microneurovascular techniques has been successful in treatment of Volkmann's contracture, using the pectoralis major, and in facial palsy, using the gracilis. Free bone transplantation has also been done by making pedicles of the ribs and the intercostal vessels.

It is now possible to determine units of the body from which the muscle and the overlying skin can be transplanted as a unit. The most reliable unit is the rectus femoris muscle and its skin; others that have been employed are the gracilis and skin and the latissimus and skin.

Skin Banking

At the time of the creation of a surgical defect (e.g., the large donor site of a deltopectoral flap being used for a pharyngoesophageal reconstruction) or the grafting of an already existing wound (e.g., debridement of a granulating wound or a burn), one may wish to postpone the grafting procedure for a few days. Such postponements are occasioned by such specific factors as inadequate hemostasis, unhealthy wound bacteriology, or poor patient condition necessitating termination of the operation. The split-thickness skin graft preserved for usage within the next week, by either in vitro or in vivo banking, is an *autograft.* In the past in vitro preservation has been best accomplished by maintaining the tissue in a balanced salt solution containing antibiotics at 4°C. More recently, it has become apparent that skin replaced upon its donor site is better preserved, as there is less chance for infection and improved opportunity for a more satisfactory take when the skin is eventually used. Skin banked in this way can be easily removed at the bedside without anesthesia, using narcotic sedation, in the first few days. It is still readily removed up to 10 days, although after 6 days it is much more firmly attached and causes more pain and increased bleeding on removal.

Allograft skin is being used much less frequently at present. However, as tissue typing procedures become more sophisticated and are more extensively applied by national and international computer systems, the uses for allografts will resurge.

Currently, the most commonly used nonautograft of skin is the pig *xenograft*. It has become readily commercially available and has assumed a very important place in wound management. As these xenografts do not take in the classic sense, they do not evoke classic immunologic responses and their sequential re-use is possible. They effectively combat fluid loss and wound organisms, and successfully prepare granulating wounds for early subsequent autografting. They may be used fresh, lyophilized, or freeze-dried with nearly equal success, although the fresh product appears to have some slight advantage.

Scar Placement and Correction

Every area in the body has lines of least skin tension (Fig. 51-23). The placement of incisions or the redirection of lacerations or scars should be guided by these anti-tension lines. In the face (Fig. 51-24) these natural lines created by animation should never be electively crossed by incisions. When incorrectly oriented wounds are created by trauma, it may be wise to revise and alter the wounds by Z-plasty or other geometrically conceived techniques (Fig. 51-10). The wound in the new direction can be predicted by placing points along the desired line in the face and dropping parallel lines to the scar or laceration, creating a Z for interchange of flaps. If a scar or laceration crosses the nasolabial fold, the segment which crosses the fold can be altered to fall in the fold itself (Fig. 51-25*A*). Notches in borders are likewise easily corrected by Z-plasty technique (Fig. 51-25*B*).

In order to correctly orient scars or to aid in planning for flap rotation, knowledge of the lines of skin extensibility is essential. It is possible to determine a line of maximum extensibility (LME) and a line of minimum extensibility perpendicular to it. In the face, skin crease lines and the lines of minimum extensibility are the same. If elliptical facial excisions are oriented with the long axis of the ellipse parallel to the skin crease lines, excision of the maximum amount of tissue that allows direct wound closure is possible.

When an elliptical incision is employed to remove a lesion, "dog ears" may be obviated by planning adjustment excisions at the ends of the wound. These adjustments can be avoided if the ellipse is made four times as long as its greatest central width. When this is not feasible, the adjustments can be made at the ends of the wound by geometric excisions (Fig. 51-26*A*).

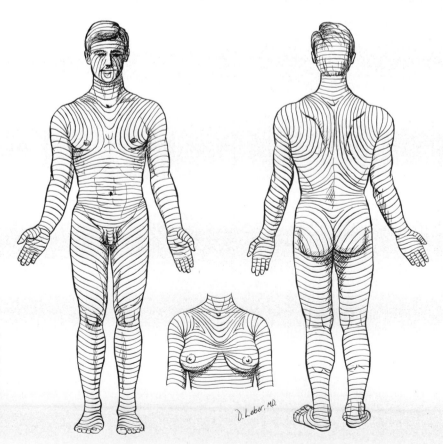

Fig. 51-23. In nearly every area of the body the line of least tension is readily discernible. It is generally related to the direction of the muscle fibers beneath and to the orientation of the collagen in the dermis, appearing to be at right angles to these determining factors. The correct lines for the presternal, deltoid, and interscapular regions are difficult to determine. Except for these areas, placing incisions in the direction of the line will enhance the chance of an excellent scar.

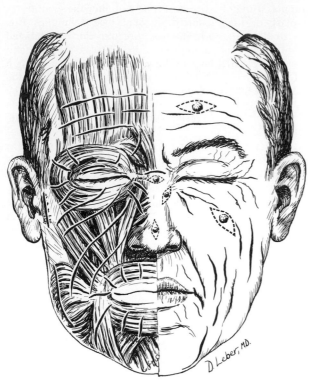

Fig. 51-24. The relation of the elective lines of tension in the face to the underlying mimetic musculature. Only in the lower eyelid are these lines not perpendicular to the muscles. The left side of the drawing shows the use of this principle when excising common facial lesions.

Other methods of scar control are either mechanical or biochemical. Early and continuous pressure can prevent scar contracture as demonstrated by Cronin and by Larson et al.; this has important application in the treatment of the scars following burns. The biologic control of scars by chemical or metabolic means is a promising frontier. The experimental uses of beta-aminoproprionitrile, D-penicillamine, and *cis*-hydroxyproline all may lead to effective scar control in the clinical situation.

Dermabrasion

The casual observation that lacerated wounds accompanied by traumatic abrasions over their surfaces seemed to heal with less perceptible scars stimulated the elective use of dermabrasion. Purposeful abrasion of the skin using air-driven carborundum wheels planes the skin to remove pitted scars, deep wrinkles, and superficially embedded dirt. Perhaps the most frequent use of dermabrasion is in the treatment of the face pitted by previous acne. The sharp edges of the acne pit are abraded down to diminish the shadow cast in the pits, making them less perceptible. The technique is particularly useful when the acne pits do not have acutely angled borders.

Dermabrasion is also important in treating traumatic wounds containing particulate matter, efficiently removing

this matter to prevent permanent tattooing. It can also remove some embedded pieces secondarily.

Dermabrasion is useful in abrading a scar revision to help camouflage.

Tattooing

Skin tattooing has been used to establish proper color match between facial skin and that transferred to the face from an alien donor site. It can also provide stippling over a non-hair-bearing skin graft implanted on the bearded area in the male to make the repair less conspicuous. Camouflage in the area of an eyebrow graft with poor hair growth can be provided, and the lip vermilion can be evened by the use of tattooing pigment.

Perhaps its most widespread use has been to cover a facial capillary hemangioma (port wine stain), although it is still very difficult to mix the pigments to obtain the correct color match.

Cartilage Grafts

Reconstruction of the ear, the nasal tip, and the eyelid will frequently require the use of cartilage to ensure proper

Fig. 51-25. Common clinical applications of Z-plasty.

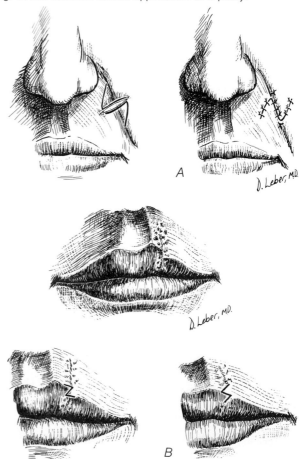

size and consistency. Free cartilage grafting is most successful when autografting is performed, although irradiated homografts have been successful in many instances. The best donor sites are the ribs and the concha of the nonaffected ear.

Bone Grafts

The ribs and the iliac crest are the best sources for bone when large amounts are needed for stability. Cancellous bone has a higher survival rate but may need cortical struts for the necessary strength. Alternate methods include using small bone chips or mechanically pulverized bone dust which will act as a nidus for new bone formation. Urothelium can also form bone in ectopic placement but has not been useful clinically as a graft. The newest pedicle methods include placement of the bone at the end of a muscle pedicle and transfer of a segment of rib as a free graft, utilizing microvascular anastomosis of the intercostal vessels.

Muscle Grafts

Muscle can be transplanted by free grafting (without vessel and nerve anastomosis). To function successfully, the muscle must be small in volume, the recipient bed must be very vascular, and the environment must be favorable to motor neurotization by ingrowth. Preliminary denervation of the donor muscle a few weeks prior to transplantation is recommended. Grafting of muscle as a free flap, utilizing microneurovascular anastomoses, is now feasible, its major applications being the treatment of Volkmann's contracture and the correction of facial palsy.

FACIAL TRAUMA

General Considerations

In the management of injuries to the head and neck, top priority is assigned to the control of the life-threatening problems of airway obstruction and hemorrhage. Tracheotomy is frequently necessary in severe facial injuries,

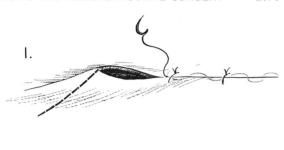

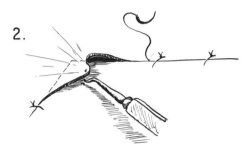

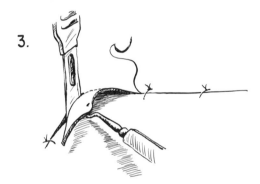

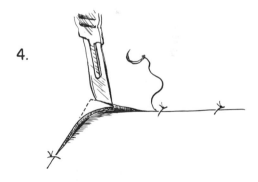

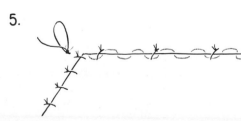

B

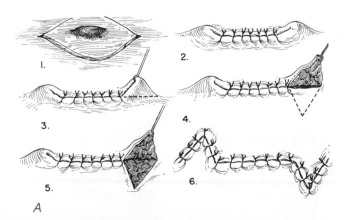

A

Fig. 51-26. Adjustment for wound dog ears by appropriate geometric excision.

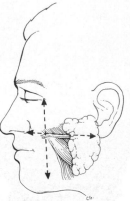

Fig. 51-27. Surface projection of the parotid duct on a line between the earlobe and nasal alar origin. The oral entry is found at the bisection of this line by a vertical line from the lateral canthus of the eye.

particularly when both the maxilla and mandible are fractured or when there is an associated injury to the trachea, larynx, or chest. Even though a fractured, and thus flail, mandible removes support from the tongue and the floor of the mouth tracheotomy for the airway obstruction resulting from a fracture of the mandible alone may be obviated by clearing the air passages of mucus, blood, dirt, and dentition and providing judicious support of the mandible. Tracheal intubation via the nose or mouth for sev-

Fig. 51-28. Facial nerve laceration. *A.* Small superficial laceration. Note marginal (mandibular) branch paralysis of facial nerve. *B.* Stab wound below mastoid. Note total facial paralysis.

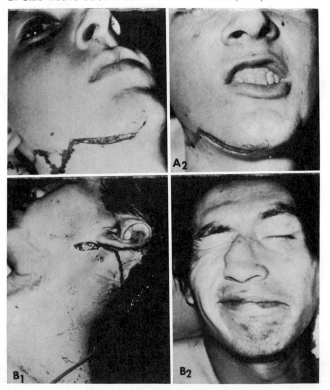

eral hours may also make tracheotomy unnecessary. In general, hemorrhage is best managed initially by pressure until the injured structures are carefully assessed.

Meticulous closure and primary revision of traumatic wounds should be performed only if there are no life-threatening injuries of higher priority. The liberal use of free skin grafts and tissue shifts to achieve the objective of early wound closure is very important at the time of primary care. However, before any specific efforts at skin closure are undertaken, a careful examination must assess injury to anatomic structures which cross the site of the wound. Injuries to the facial nerve, parotid duct, salivary glands, and facial bones represent some of the situations which must be evaluated. The parotid duct may be probed transorally to determine its integrity if the wound falls across a line from earlobe to alar cartilage posterior to a vertical line dropped from the lateral canthus of the eye (Fig. 51-27). Before any local anesthesia is administered, the function of the facial nerve should be evaluated for the integrity of its multiple branches, and sensation should also be assessed (Fig. 51-28).

When the face is abraded on a roadway or dirty surface, the dark particles are frequently ground deeply into the skin; retention will result in permanent tattooing. Treatment consists of thorough irrigation and cleansing with a stiff brush, followed by abrading with fine carborundum. This procedure must be carried out at the time of primary wound care, since secondary removal is much more difficult and not as successful.

Facial Fractures

Facial fractures, themselves, do not constitute life-threatening injuries and therefore are not assigned top priority in the patient with multiple wounds. However, facial fractures are frequently associated with serious head trauma and central nervous system injury. Under these circumstances, treatment of the fracture is deferred until the patient is stable, in order to avoid the additional hazard of anesthesia, but temporary wound approximation frequently can be accomplished with a few well-placed sutures and microporous tape.

DIAGNOSIS. The clinical diagnosis of facial fractures incorporates careful examination for a variety of specific physical findings (Fig. 51-29).

Deformity or Depression. Shortly after injury, there may be obvious evidence of architectural abnormality when one looks down on the face from above. Depression of the zygoma or zygomatic arch with asymmetry is frequently apparent.

Anesthesia or Paresthesia. An area of numbness over a major branch of the trigeminal nerve suggests fracture involving specific bones through which branches of this nerve pass. Anesthesia or hypesthesia over the distribution of the mental nerve suggests mandibular fracture, whereas the same finding over the distribution of the infraorbital nerve should arouse suspicion of a fracture of the zygoma or of the orbitomaxillary complex.

Ocular Disparity. Enophthalmos, depression of the globe, incomplete extraocular movement, double vision, and oc-

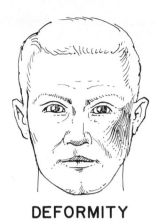

DEFORMITY

FACIAL FRACTURE DIAGNOSIS

(CLINICAL)

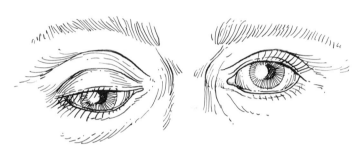

OCULAR DISPARITY

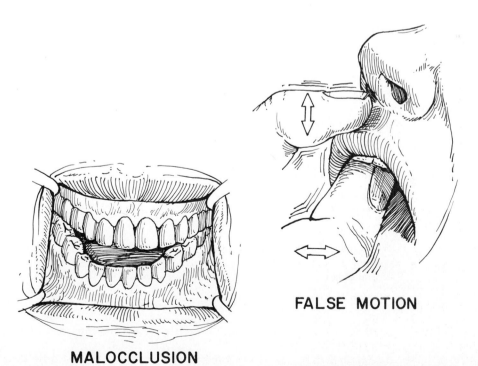

MALOCCLUSION

FALSE MOTION

Fig. 51-29. Common physical findings in facial fractures.

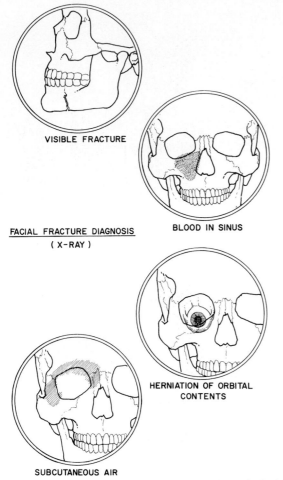

VISIBLE FRACTURE

FACIAL FRACTURE DIAGNOSIS
(X-RAY)

BLOOD IN SINUS

HERNIATION OF ORBITAL
CONTENTS

SUBCUTANEOUS AIR

Fig. 51-30. Common roentgenographic findings in facial fractures.

casionally exophthalmos all suggest facial fracture involving the orbit.

False Motion. Palpable crepitation and demonstrable false motion are diagnostic of facial fracture. These signs should be very gently elicited.

Malocclusion. This finding is characteristic of fractures of the mandible or maxilla or both with displacement. It is a reliable sign of architectural disruption in the normal maxilla-to-mandible relationship and also provides later evaluation of the reduction of major maxillary and mandibular fractures.

RADIOLOGIC FINDINGS (Fig. 51-30). Although careful clinical examination, even of an uncooperative patient, usually allows quite accurate diagnosis, very specific roentgenograms taken at very specific angles supplement the clinical diagnosis by defining the exact location, direction, and nature of the facial fracture (Fig. 51-31). The gymnastic positions needed to take roentgenograms that are capable of interpretation contraindicate these studies until the patient is stable and cooperative. Because of the intricate picture produced by multiple superimposed facial bones, stereo views or laminography may be necessary for final specific diagnosis in some instances. In addition to direct visual evidence of interruption of osseous continuity, other features which may be demonstrated on roentgenogram include hemorrhage into sinuses, herniation of orbital contents or teeth into the sinuses, foreign bodies, and subcutaneous air indicative of fracture into the nose or sinus.

TREATMENT. If an open wound exposes the fracture sites and the patient's condition is satisfactory, immediate fracture reduction and fixation are recommended. In all other cases, *early* reduction and fixation are the procedures of choice, usually a few days following the injury when the patient's status has been completely evaluated. If an extremely serious accompanying injury necessitates a long

Fig. 51-31. Chart for x-ray for facial bone fractures.

Bone	X-Ray
Mandible	
Condylar and coronoid processes Ascending ramus and body	Right and left lateral obliques of mandible
Symphysis, parasymphyseal Body and ascending rami	Posterior–anterior of mandible
Condyle and condylar neck	Towne's (modified) Anterior–posterior of base of skull
Anterior arch	Occlusal of anterior mandible
Maxilla & Zygoma	Water's (posterior–anterior oblique) Anterior–posterior of face Lateral of face
Zygomatic arch	Submental–vertex
Orbital Floor	Water's Stereo Water's Laminography
Nasal Bone	Superior–inferior of nose Lateral of nose

waiting period, this should be no longer than 2 weeks. After this, successful reduction is difficult to achieve, and severe cosmetic and functional deformity, nonunion, or osteomyelitis may ensue.

Attaining preinjury occlusion is the prime goal if either the maxilla or mandible is fractured, and restoration of vision, airway, and cosmesis are the aims of treatment of the other fractures. Cerebrospinal fluid rhinorrhea, diagnosed by testing for glucose in the nasal secretions, is usually successfully managed by exact reduction. Occasionally a delayed dural repair or graft may be needed.

Fixation is accomplished by applying wires, bars, or splints to the teeth, reestablishing occlusion, and fixing one jaw to the other by attaching the appliances to each other. Open reduction and internal fixation by wires, bars, or clamps across the fracture site frequently is necessary, particularly if muscle or fat interposed between the fracture fragments prevents their reduction by external means or if the direction of the fracture and the muscle pull will make a closed reduction unstable. External splints with wires or pins inserted transcutaneously may also be helpful in securing final fixation.

ZYGOMA

The prominence of the cheek, formed by the zygoma, may be depressed by a blow to the side of the face fracturing the zygoma. This usually manifests itself in one of three ways: (1) fracture of the arch of the zygoma (Fig. 51-32), (2) crushing of the bone of the cheek, or (3) fracture-dislocation with rotation of the zygoma in a downward and outward or downward and inward direction (Fig. 51-33).

Frequently the result of a fight or a fall, the isolated zygoma fracture is very common, or it may be accompanied only by associated nasal bone injury. When it is the result of high-speed trauma, an increasing occurrence, it is one of a group of facial and skull fractures and is accompanied by fracture of the maxilla, frontal bone, temporal bone, nasoethmoidal complex, and mandible. Common findings are disparities of the eye level, palpable notches in the inferior orbital rim (zygomaticomaxillary suture) and at the lateral rim (zygomaticofrontal suture), anesthesia in the distribution of the infraorbital nerve, and a characteristic lateral subscleral hemorrhage (Fig. 51-34). The diplopia present is predominantly horizontal, with images side by side, because of the direction of the displacement and the injury to the lateral rectus muscle. If the eye level drops because of injury to Lockwood's ligament, there will be a concomitant vertical aspect accompanying this horizontal diplopia. However, when vertical diplopia is the predominant or only finding, it usually indicates injury to the inferior rectus muscle, perhaps injury to the inferior oblique muscle, and trapping of these muscles by an injured orbital floor. Trismus may occur as a fragment of the zygomatic arch impinges on the temporalis muscle and coronoid process of the mandible. Techniques for treatment include completely closed reduction, a closed reduction through small incisions, and open reductions with internal fixation. For reduction employing an elevator inserted from small incisions, temporal, oral,

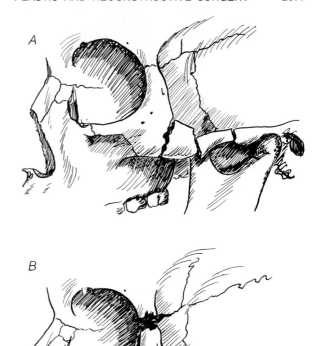

Fig. 51-32. *A.* A depressed fracture of the zygomatic arch, which may impinge upon the mandible and prevent opening or closing (trismus). *B.* The "tripod," or "tripartite," fracture of the zygoma which will dislocate when separated at its three suture lines where the fractures manifest: the zygomaticofrontal, zygomaticotemporal, and zygomaticomaxillary. The orbital floor and wall are always injured with this fracture, sometimes in a linear fashion and at other times by being comminuted or disrupted.

or antral insertion approaches will be employed, each with specific indications. If the zygomatic fracture is displaced and/or rotated, open reduction and fixation using interosseous wiring are usually necessary. If, in addition, the orbital floor is so crushed and sagging that it can be supported only from below, packing the sinus may aid in its reduction, but this is not usually necessary. A portion of the orbital floor may be missing; this allows herniation of the orbital contents into the maxillary antrum and may result in trapping of the inferior rectus and inferior oblique muscles within the defect. These injuries may also occur in the absence of other fractures of the zygomatic maxillary complex, such as following a direct blow to the globe. When occurring in this pure form, these classic "blowout" fractures may be inapparent unless the clinician is alert. They are manifested by *vertical* diplopia (one image above the other image), particularly on upward gaze; enophthal-

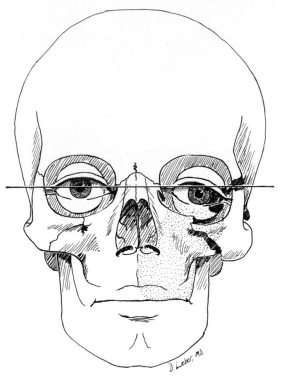

Fig. 51-33. Fracture-dislocation of the zygoma with rotation, disparity of eye level, lateral subscleral hematoma, and a surface representation of anesthesia of the infraorbital nerve.

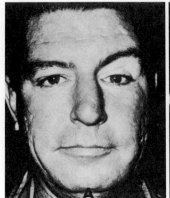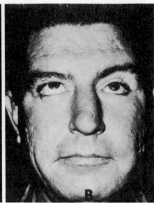

Fig. 51-35. Blowout fracture. *A.* Blowout fracture of orbital floor. Note depression of globe. *B.* Upward gaze shows incarceration of inferior rectus.

mos; and depression of the globe (Figs. 51-35 and 51-36). Such fractures require open reduction, deliverance of the orbital contents back into the orbit, and primary orbital floor reconstitution with the fracture fragments, prosthetic implants, or a bone or cartilage graft. Only occasionally must this treatment be supplemented by packing of maxillary antrum.

MAXILLA

Maxillary fractures frequently result from a direct anteroposterior blow to the middle third of the face, de-

Fig. 51-34. *A.* A lateral, subscleral hematoma confined anteriorly, due to direct trauma. White sclera is visible behind the hematoma when the patient moves the globe in the opposite direction. *B.* The lateral subscleral hematoma secondary to zygomatic fracture or frontal bone trauma does not allow visualization of white sclera behind it, because the blood has dissected forward subperiosteally and subconjunctivally.

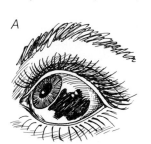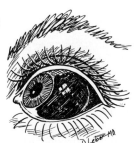

pending upon the magnitude, direction, and site of the blow (Fig. 51-37). The upper dentition, the maxillary sinus, the orbital floor, and the maxillary division of the fifth cranial nerve are important anatomic structures to be considered in the diagnosis and therapy of maxillary fractures.

A displaced maxillary fracture is characteristically manifested by gross malocclusion. Anesthesia over the cheek and upper lip, which are areas innervated by the infraorbital nerve, may be demonstrable. Enophthalmos with

Fig. 51-36. A blowout fracture of the orbital floor with characteristic hanging drop sign.

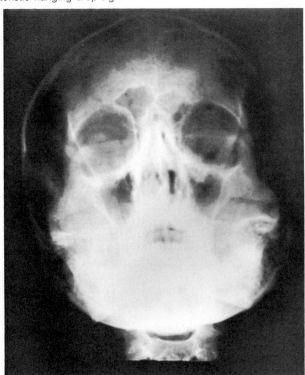

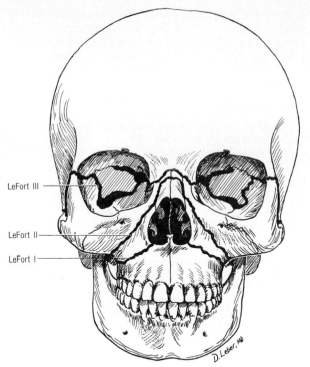

Fig. 51-37. The common levels of fracture of the middle and upper face, based on the work of LeFort. (*After R. LeFort, Experimental Study of Fractures of the Upper Jaw, Rev Chir [Paris], 23:208, 23:360, 1901.*)

depression of the globe is an important diagnostic finding. Subcutaneous emphysema with palpable crepitus over the cheek suggests communication between the antrum and subcutaneous space through the fracture site. False motion may be demonstrated by palpation or grasping of the upper teeth and noting movements separate from the cranium. With marked displacement and true craniofacial disjunction, the patient may present a "long-faced" appearance. Roentgenograms are indicated to confirm the presence of maxillary fractures and may demonstrate

fluid or herniation of orbital contents into the maxillary sinus.

Fixation may be accomplished by wiring the maxillary and mandibular teeth in occlusion or by open reduction, intraosseous wiring, and packing the maxillary antrum. In true craniofacial dysjunction, the entire maxillary complex must be wired to the frontal bone, since this represents the only adjacent fixed skeletal unit.

MANDIBLE

The mandible is the most frequently fractured bone within the facial complex. Knowledge of the sites and frequencies aids the diagnosis immensely (Fig. 51-38). About 60 percent of mandibular fractures are bilateral. The powerful muscles of mastication inserting on the mandible may account for continuing displacement of the fractures unless fixation is achieved by treatment. The complex temporomandibular joint, lower teeth, and mandibular division of the fifth cranial nerve are important anatomic structures related to fractures of the mandible. Examination may reveal deformity or malocclusion, with crepitation and swelling as characteristic signs. Anesthesia over the chin and lower lip suggests injury to the inferior alveolar nerve.

Accuracy of reduction and immobilization are important to avoid nonunion and also the late development of temporomandibular joint symptoms resulting from malocclusion. The majority of mandibular fractures may be successfully treated by wired fixation of the teeth in occlusion. Some fractures must be treated by the addition of open reduction to remove interposed muscle and fat and replace the bones in anatomic position; this reduction is maintained by interosseous wires, plates, or compression devices. When there are not enough teeth present, the occlusal fixation can be supplemented by imaginative dental prostheses which are attached either to the teeth or to the bones themselves. When the mandible is completely edentulous and the patient is elderly, a direct approach to the mandible under local anesthesia is indicated, fixing the parts securely with internal, interosseous wires or compression.

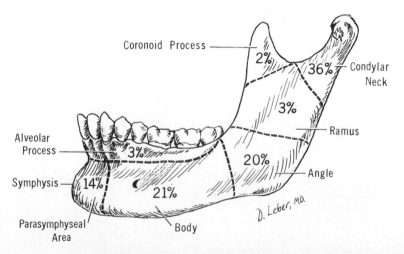

Fig. 51-38. The common mandibular fracture sites. (*After R. O. Dingman, and P. Natvig, "Surgery of Facial Fractures," W. B. Saunders Company, Philadelphia, 1964.*)

NOSE (Fig. 51-39)

Nasal fractures are very common but assume clinical significance only if they are displaced. Immediate reduction of the nasal bones and septum is generally achieved without difficulty under local anesthesia. The crushed and depressed nasal bridge may be elevated with intranasal manipulation at the same time that the bones are manipulated from the external nasal surface.

It must be emphasized that straightforward nasal fractures may be accompanied by major injuries to the septum or contiguous structures. The septum may be grossly displaced laterally, or it may be telescoped up under the dorsum. With any injury to the nose, the septum must be carefully inspected for a submucosal hematoma. If not evacuated, this may lead to pressure necrosis and secondary infection causing septal perforation. Associated injuries to adjacent structures will include disruption of the medial canthal ligament or injury to the base of the skull resulting in cerebrospinal fluid leak. These need to be treated in the operating room under general anesthesia.

The nose can be properly splinted by using individually fashioned splints made from dental compounds, plaster of paris, or plastic-impregnated gauze. Intranasal packing can help maintain the parts in proper reduction.

Soft Tissue Facial Injuries

Soft tissue injuries of the face may be associated with considerable deficits in function in addition to disturbance in a normal appearance. A simple laceration is "simple" only if it does not involve important ingredients of normal facial, ocular, aerodigestive, and aesthetic function. Therefore, a careful assessment of function of structures in anatomic proximity to a facial injury is essential prior to any instrumentation or injection of an anesthetic agent.

FACIAL NERVE

The wide distribution and relatively superficial position of the branches of the facial nerve in the face and upper neck make these structures vulnerable to injury with even small lacerations (Fig. 51-28). To administer anesthetic agents prior to careful assessment of function of this purely motor nerve is to eliminate the only possibility of assuring that the injury and not the treatment is responsible for partial facial motor deficit. A sterile pressure dressing should be used to control hemorrhage during assessment of facial nerve function, since the indiscriminate application of hemostats may in itself result in nerve injury (Fig. 51-40).

Fig. 51-39. The severity of fractures of the nose varies from simple (A, B) to the more complex (C, D, E). A will need no treatment, and B can be successfully reduced under local anesthesia in the office or emergency department. C, D, and E require adequate sedation and anesthesia to allow the manipulations necessary to prevent secondary cosmetic defects or obstructed breathing. In addition, the more severe fractures may need additional treatment to the ethmoid region or the medial canthal ligament.

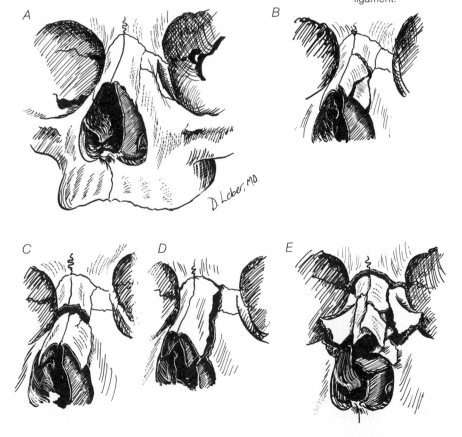

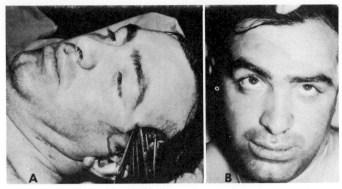

Fig. 51-40. Facial nerve trauma. *A.* Laceration of temple with arterial hemorrhage. Note multiple hemostats. *B.* Forehead branch facial palsy secondary to injury (?) or instrumentation (?).

Branches of the facial nerve should be repaired if significant motor deficits exist. Microsurgical techniques have increased the successes of such repairs. If facial nerve injury results in paralysis of the orbicularis oculi muscle, the eye must be protected during the postoperative period. Temporary tarsorrhaphy, i.e., surgical attachment of the upper lid to the lower lid, in the region of the lateral canthus may be necessary if ointments, external support by tape, and glasses cannot protect the eye from exposure keratitis.

TRIGEMINAL NERVE

Trauma to the trigeminal nerve interferes with sensation in the face, and, as in the case of facial nerve injuries, evaluation of the areas of sensory loss must be carried out prior to any manipulation or treatment. The losses of sensation are of diagnostic significance in localizing fractures and soft tissue injuries. Anesthesia of the chin and lower lip on one side suggests injury of the mandibular division. If the loss of sensation is localized to this area, the injury is peripheral at the mental foramen. However, if the lower teeth are also anesthetic, this indicates that the inferior alveolar nerve has been injured more proximally or by a mandibular fracture. Anesthesia in the ear region and detectable weakness in mastication or tongue anesthesia are suggestive of even more proximal injury of the mandibular division.

PAROTID

The parotid duct lies caudad to a line drawn from earlobe to the nasal ala and enters the mouth at a point where this line is bisected by an imaginary vertical line from the lateral canthus of the eye (Fig. 51-27). Transection of the parotid duct usually occurs in its superficial portion where it lies over the masseter; this is frequently associated with injury of the buccal branches of the facial nerve. Repair of the duct over a polyethylene tube represents optimal therapy, but ligation may be indicated in the case of severe injury. Lacerations through the parotid gland substance per se are best treated by careful repair of the gland capsule and simple drainage of the wound. Postoperatively, parotitis and temporary salivary drainage are the rule, but spontaneous remission and closure generally occur. The postoperative management should include the avoidance of gustatory stimulation by diet and the use of anticholinergic drugs to reduce secretion.

LACRIMAL DUCTS

Lacerations in the region of the medial canthus of the eye must be carefully evaluated for lacrimal duct injury. The ducts should be probed to assure their integrity. Lacerations are best repaired over a small polyethylene stent carried from the punctum to the nasal cavity.

AREAS OF AESTHETIC IMPORTANCE

HAIRLINE. Injuries and surgical procedures which involve the forehead hairline require careful consideration. Local flaps of hair-bearing skin may be used to construct the hairline in its proper position. Conversely, if hair-bearing scalp is initially used to cover a traumatically or surgically created defect in a non-hair-bearing area close to the scalp hairline, it should be removed later and restored with non-hair-bearing skin to avoid grossly noticeable deformity.

EYEBROW. Precise realignment of the eyebrow which has been divided is important, since a 1- or 2-mm stepwise offset is noticeable at conversational distance. Sharp lacerations which are closed simply may leave an area of alopecia in the eyebrow. This occurs because of the obliquity of the hair roots which are transected by the laceration. Retrimming wound edges parallel to hair follicles prior to closure will avoid this problem (Fig. 51-41). When lacerations cross the eyebrow, the eyebrow should be repaired first, and the remaining portion of the laceration

Fig. 51-41. Avoidance of alopecia during repair of eyebrow laceration. *A.* Oblique projection of eyebrow hairs creates eyebrow alopecia at the laceration site unless the wound is revised parallel to hair follicles. *B.* Laceration crossing the eyebrow. *C.* Precise realignment of eyebrow elements is important.

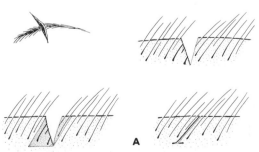

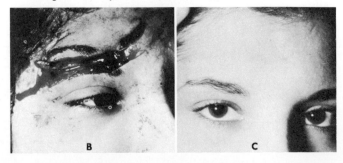

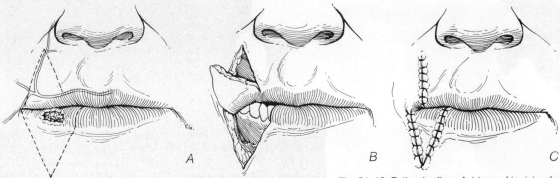

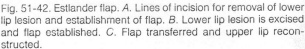

Fig. 51-42. Estlander flap. *A.* Lines of incision for removal of lower lip lesion and establishment of flap. *B.* Lower lip lesion is excised and flap established. *C.* Flap transferred and upper lip reconstructed.

may then be shifted or revised to conform with the eyebrow repair.

EYELID. The healing and normal wound contraction associated with vertical lacerations of the eyelid result in a predictable contracture. The incisional direction may be altered by performing a primary Z-plasty to avoid this contracture and ugly, uncontrolled exposure of the eye. When soft tissue has been lost by avulsion, primary skin grafting may be essential. Potential donor sites for eyelid skin include the contralateral eyelid, the posterior auricular area, low cervical supraclavicular areas, and the prepuce. These sites furnish skin which is pliable and of appropriate color.

NASOLABIAL FOLD. Hypertrophic bridging scars occur when a laceration crosses this fold. Such lacerations should be altered to place part of the scar within the nasolabial fold per se, employing the technique of Z-plasty (Fig. 51-25).

VERMILION BORDER OF LIP. An offset in this area produces an abnormal step which is apparent at conversational distance. Therefore, precise coaptation of this important landmark deserves primary attention at the time of initial repair. During the repair, the first suture should be placed at this ridge; adjustments of the rest of the wound then can be made accordingly.

HEAD AND NECK TUMORS

Since head and neck tumor therapy (see Chap. 16) may result in functional and/or cosmetic deformity, principles of reconstructive surgery are particularly applicable in this area.

Lip

A small lesion up to 1 cm can generally be readily excised by a shield-shaped resection, and the wound closed with minimal deformity. However, larger tumors which require removal of half or more of the lower lip should have restorative surgical treatment using local soft tissue in various geometric shifts. Such an example is the Estlander flap (Fig. 51-42), which makes use of a segment of the upper lip rotated around at the commissure, with the marginal vessels (coronary vessels) preserved for blood supply. The Abbe modification of the Estlander flap also takes tissue from the upper lip to fill the lower lip deficit (Fig. 51-43). In this instance, the upper lip wedge is connected to the upper lip by a vascular pedicle which crosses the opening of the mouth, preserving the commissure. This results in a double oral stoma which is reconverted to the single stoma about 2 weeks later. Preserving the commissure is a major advantage, because commissure reconstruction is so difficult.

The Bernard procedure (Fig. 51-44) has been applied to allow movement of cheek skin mediad in order to reconstruct larger defects of the lower lip. A similar procedure devised by Webster can be used to reconstruct the upper lip. Nasolabial triangles are the key to the tissue

Fig. 51-43. Abbe modification of Estlander flap. *A.* Incisions outlined. *B.* Tumor excised from lower lip, and upper lip flap established. *C.* Upper lip flap turned down to fill defect in lower lip. Note double oral stoma. *D.* Upper-to-lower lip pedicle transected, with single stoma as a result.

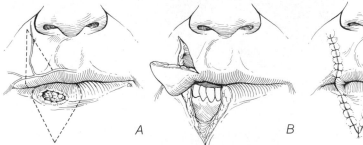

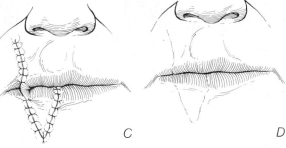

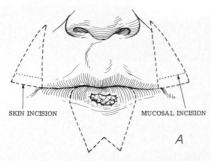

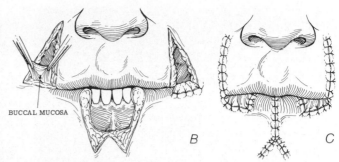

Fig. 51-44. Bernard procedure. *A.* Outline of skin incisions for removal of tumor and skin plus mucosal incision for removal of nasolabial triangles. *B.* Tumors and nasolabial triangles excised and buccal mucosa turned down to enlarge lower lip. *C.* Incisions closed.

movement; their removal allows the advancement of full thicknesses of the cheek into the medial position to make a lip. For the lower lip, cheek rotations of the mucosa are used for the vermilion reconstruction.

Tongue

If the lesion is small, adequate excision may be accomplished by a wedge resection, if this is located in the free margin of the tongue. This is applicable to very few malignant tumors (Fig. 51-45). Most tumors of the anterior portion of the tongue are best treated by a combination of supervoltage radiation followed by hemiglossectomy, partial mandibulectomy, and cervical node dissection. Selecting the proper combinations of radiation, surgery, and adjunctive chemotherapy, for each situation is critical. Proper dental splinting to control mandibular fragments and the imaginative use of flaps of the forehead, neck, or chest will help control the cosmetic and functional deformity.

Fig. 51-46. *A.* Carcinoma of the nose. *B.* Wide through-and-through resection of tumor. *C.* Forehead flap reconstruction. *D.* Result after healing.

Nose

Reconstructive surgical treatment is frequently indicated for the cosmetic deformity which results from removal of a tumor. The procedures generally employ a forehead, a cheek, or occasionally a distant pedicle flap to replace the resected tissue (Fig. 51-46).

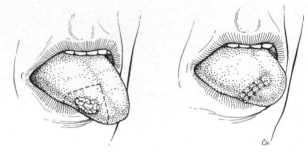

Fig. 51-45. Wedge excision of small anterior tongue lesion and primary closure.

Eyelid

The functional and cosmetic deficit created by excision of eyelid tumors must usually be reconstructed immediately. Loss of function, if not corrected, may result in

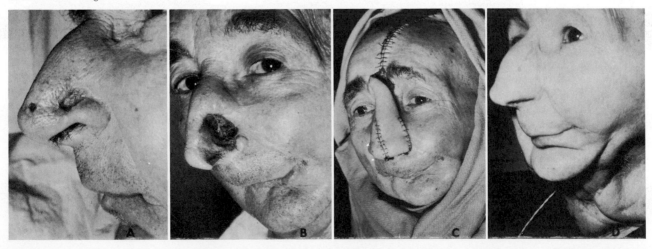

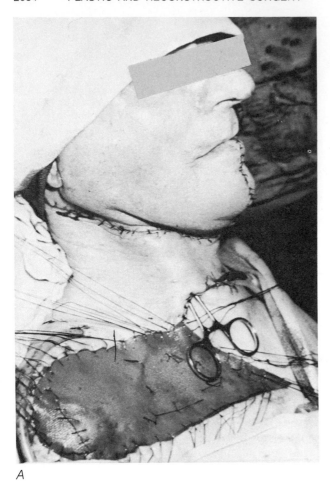

A

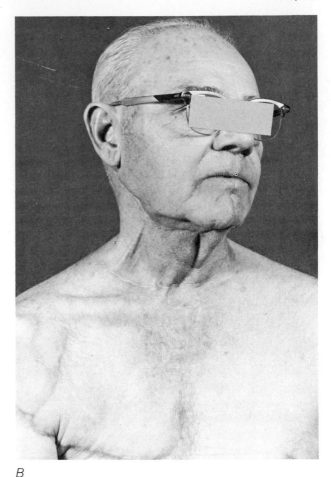

B

Fig. 51-47. Five months after composite resection including a large portion of the tongue and pharynx, rehabilitation is accomplished by only two operations: (1) the original extirpation and reconstruction with deltopectoral flap, and (2) insetting of the flap and return of its base to the chest wall. *A.* A deltopectoral flap has been raised from the right shoulder and chest, rotated upward, tubed upon itself, and used to reconstruct the pharynx and esophagus. The large clamp is in this skin-lined tube; the end of the clamp is in the mouth. This has accomplished the reconstruction at the time of the resection. Only one further procedure will be needed approximately 10 weeks later to transect the flap, close the fistula, and return the base of the flap to its original position. *B.* Note that there are no vertical scars on the neck (use of the MacFee incisions) or the shoulder donor site of the pharyngeal wall. *C.* The lip-splitting incision leaves a permanent but not objectionable scar. Forty percent of the mandible has been removed from the right side. *D.* Deviation is controlled by the special dental metal outrigger on the right, attached to an acrylic splint. The lighter area on the left is the upper end of the shoulder tissue forming the lateral pharyngeal wall. (*Source: R. Goldwyn (ed.), "The Unfavorable Result in Plastic Surgery: Avoidance and Treatment," Little, Brown and Company, Boston, 1972.*)

permanent damage to vision. Local flaps, utilizing available skin, and full-thickness skin grafts are the most common methods of repair. Large cheek rotation flaps or eyelid flaps may be required in some cases.

Soft Tissue Losses

Excision of large tumors of the head and neck frequently results in major losses of soft tissue and consequent contour defects. The lining of the mouth and pharynx, as well as the cutaneous surfaces, are generally best replaced by pedicle flap reconstruction, although split-thickness skin grafts are serviceable in certain regions. When flaps are used, they are preferably obtained locally from the head, neck, or chest, unless all the donor sites have been subjected to irradiation or are otherwise compromised. When this occurs, pedicle flaps from distant sites may be carried on the upper extremity or may be moved end over end in stages, as popularized by Gillies. These multiple transfer flaps have been mainly replaced by the newer flap techniques (Fig. 51-47), which usually close defects by primary reconstruction. If the reconstruction cannot be accomplished early, a defect may present secondarily. Before any secondary defect is closed, all necrotic bone and cartilage must be removed from the depths of the wound, since they

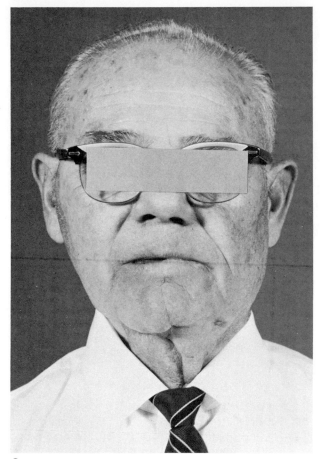

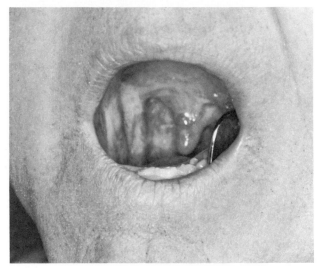

D

C

Fig. 51-47. *(continued).*

represent nonviable active foreign bodies which will perpetuate draining and interfere with healing. Orocutaneous, pharyngocutaneous, or esophagocutaneous fistulas may be covered and closed with flaps such as a forehead tissue flap transferred to the area on a pedicle of temporal vessels (island pedicle flap) (Fig. 51-48). This same type of technique is particularly applicable to the covering of defects in heavily irradiated areas, because the flap provides its own permanent blood supply. Free skin grafts (Fig. 51-49) are also frequently used for closing defects left after excision of cancer of the head and neck. Care must be taken to match color, consistency, and hair-bearing characteristics.

Bone Losses

The major areas of loss of bone are from the calvarium, maxilla, mandible, or nose. Each of these areas has its own particular specifications for replacement. The calvarium is best replaced by rib grafts, split longitudinally, or by plates made of metal or plastic. The maxilla is best replaced by soft prosthesis, preferably sponges made from silicone. The mandible may be replaced either with bone grafts or by an implanted synthetic prosthesis. The best donor site for a mandible graft is the ilium, since autogenous cancellous

Fig. 51-48. (See Fig. 51-17.) Repair of orocutaneous fistula in irradiated area. *A.* Note osteoradionecrosis of mandible. *B.* Some time after mandibular resection. Fistula closure started. *C.* Island pedicle flap taken from the forehead carried solely on the temporal vessels prepared to be passed subcutaneously to the fistula site where vascularized soft tissue is needed. *D.* Healing with the island pedicle flap furnishing skin and subcutaneous tissue with blood supply from the temporal vessels, which now course subcutaneously from the temporal area to the large composite skin patch.

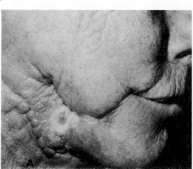

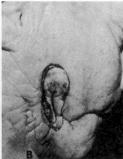

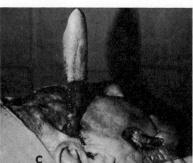

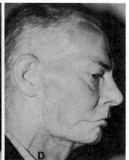

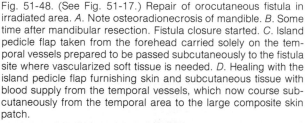

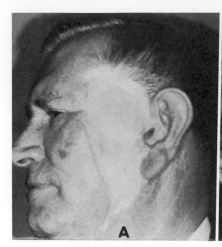
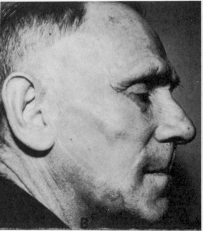
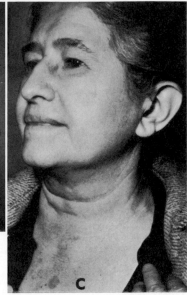

bone appears to have the best chance for survival. Problems of immobilization of the jaws are challenging and require the ingenious use of dental wiring or splints, external fixation appliances, and bone carpentry with internal fixation by means of wires, plates, or compression devices. Defects of nasal losses can be replaced by cancellous bone, cartilage, or a solid silicone prothesis. In all these situations it is critical that adequate soft tissue coverage and lining is provided to prevent secondary extrusion.

CONGENITAL ANOMALIES OF THE HEAD AND NECK

Cleft Lip and Palate

One in eight hundred living neonates has cleft deformity of the lip and/or palate. Today, children with this defect may be completely rehabilitated through combined surgical, orthodontic, otologic, psychologic, and speech therapy. Although the treatment is very individualized, each patient benefits greatly if the specialists in these many disciplines are closely allied as a diagnostic and therapeutic team.

CLASSIFICATION. Clefts of the palate and lip are classified by various criteria according to whether the primary palate (lip and alveolar ridge) or the secondary palate (hard and soft palate), or both, are involved in the fusion failure. Clefts of the primary palate may be incomplete (Fig. 51-50A and B), involving only part of the vertical lip dimension, or they may extend into the nostril (Fig. 51-50C). The clefts may be bilateral or unilateral, and they may or may not involve the alveolar bone (tooth-bearing alveolus). Clefts of the lip and alveolar ridge may extend to involve the hard and soft palate (secondary palate); these are classified as complete unilateral clefts of the lip and palate (Fig. 51-50C and F) and complete bilateral clefts of the lip and palate (Fig. 51-50D and G). The fusion defect may be limited to the secondary palate, in which case it is termed an incomplete cleft of the palate (Fig. 51-50E).

Fig. 51-49. Free skin grafts to cover soft tissue losses. A. Face skin graft with poor color match. Donor site, abdomen. B. Skin graft of face with good color match. Donor site chosen for proper match. C. Full-thickness graft to face from supraclavicular area. Note good color match and texture.

TREATMENT. Prior to any surgery, the dental specialist and the surgeon evaluate the patient. This applies to the neonate, since appropriate neonatal dental obturators may be important in preventing subsequent arch deformity. The newborn patient with a cleft lip and palate is a true emergency for both the plastic surgeon and the dentist. The plastic surgeon's therapy begins as soon after birth as is feasible, even though no surgery may be planned for several weeks. Counseling of parents can be best accomplished by the plastic surgeon who has the longitudinal depth of knowledge of this problem.

Timing of Surgery. There is little disagreement that our knowledge to date supports the notion that cleft lip should be repaired early (i.e., during the first three months of life,) and that the cleft palate should be repaired a little later (i.e., when the patient is 1 to 1½ years of age). Whether the lip should be repaired at birth or at age three months depends on the individual preference of the surgeon, since the results are equivalent. The authors prefer to carry out the definitive repair when the baby is approximately ten to twelve weeks of age; when general anesthesia may be used with greater safety, the repair can be technically more precise, since the lip elements are larger, and conversion to cup or dropper feeding in the postoperative period is somewhat easier. When the lip has been repaired at birth prior to the baby's exposure to the parents, they may not adequately appreciate the severity and problems of this deformity and thus may not be as gratified by the surgical repair. This is important because the parents' satisfaction or dissatisfaction may be transmitted to the child.

It is customary to repair the palate when the child is between 1 and 1½ years of age, and the younger the better,

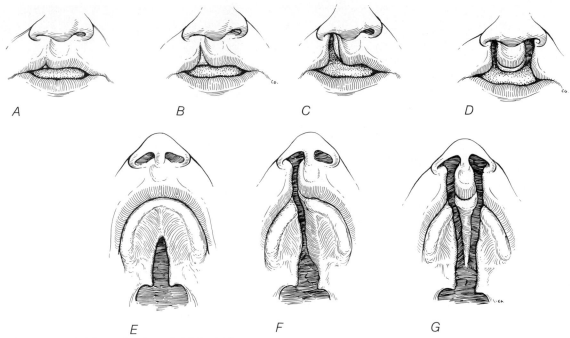

Fig. 51-50. Classification of cleft lip and palate. *A.* Minimal incomplete cleft of the lip (primary palate). Note nostril asymmetry. *B.* Moderately severe incomplete cleft of the lip (primary palate). Note nostril asymmetry. *C.* Complete unilateral cleft lip and palate (primary and secondary palate). *D.* Complete bilateral cleft lip and palate (primary and secondary palate). *E.* Incomplete cleft of the palate (secondary palate). *F.* Unilateral complete cleft of lip and palate (primary and secondary palate). *G.* Bilateral complete cleft of lip and palate (primary and secondary palate).

so that there will be a repaired palate during a major initial speech effort. However, repair earlier than at one year is hazardous, because blood loss may represent a significant percentage of the child's blood volume. Blood transfusions are rarely indicated or necessary in these operations. It also has been noted that repairs of the cleft palate prior to the age of eighteen months result in a much higher percentage of children with normal speech, greater than 70 percent. If the procedure is delayed to three or more years after

Fig. 51-51. Millard infranasal Z-plasty. *A.* Lines of incision outlined. *B.* Closure demonstrated. *C.* Preoperative photograph. *D.* Postoperative photograph.

birth, the speech is not as good.

Techniques. The unilateral incomplete cleft of the primary palate (lip) may be repaired so that the defect is barely perceptible. The goal is to achieve adequate length from the nostril floor to the vermilion ridge, to match precisely the contralateral side of the lip. The usual techniques for closure of the cleft lip are variations of a Z-plasty. The various methods proposed by Skoog, Tennison, LeMesurier, Millard and Pigott, Randall, and Wynn differ in the vertical level at which the Z-plasty is performed, but all represent the application of surgical geometry with an interdigitation of flaps. The type of Z-plasty repair selected (occasionally a straight-line, i.e., Rose-Thompson repair) is determined by the anatomy of the defect. The authors of this chapter generally employ the Millard infranasal Z-plasty (Fig. 51-51), since it places the primary scar along the normal philtrum line. The Millard technique is applicable to all types of clefts, but is most suitable when there is a large infraalar portion of white lip on the cleft side. When the lip cleft is a complete one and is

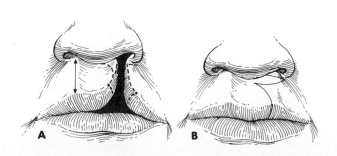

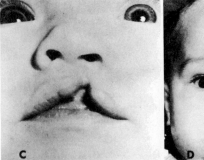

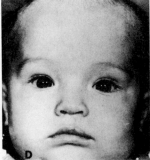

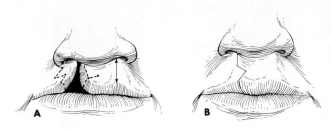

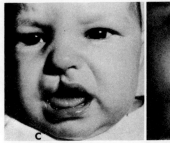
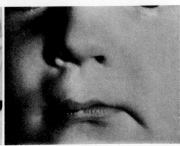

Fig. 51-52. Tennison Z-plasty. *A.* Lines of incision outlined. *B.* Closure demonstrated. *C.* Preoperative photograph. *D.* Postoperative photograph.

particularly wide, even though primary closure can be accomplished, it may be desirable to perform a preliminary operation, or "lip adhesions." This procedure is performed 8 weeks prior to definitive cheiloplasty, best at age four to six weeks. The cleft is bridged by two matching quadrangular flaps designed from the tissues on the borders of the cleft that eventually would have been discarded. This operation achieves four important goals: (1) it molds anterior alveolus, (2) it directs nasal ala to correct direction, (3) it stimulates local growth processes, and (4) it increases the amount of tissues available for subsequent repair.

When the local pathologic anatomy is such that the rotation-advancement technique of Millard will encounter a difficulty in adding vertical length, the authors favor the supravermilion triangular flap Z-plasty, described by Tennison and modified by Randall (Fig. 51-52).

Occasionally, the nostril deformity common to all clefts is minor and can be corrected completely at the primary operation. The distortions of the nostril can be corrected considerably during these early operations, to lessen the deformity during the growing years. However, most nostril distortions will require corrective procedures at secondary operations when the child is older, at age five, age eight, and finally a definitive rhinoplasty just prior to the teens.

Bilateral clefts of the lip and palate are an even greater challenge. Repair of the lip may be performed in one or two stages, care being taken to preserve the prolabium (central portion of the lip between the clefts), because it

becomes the central segment of the reconstructed lip and will grow in an amazing fashion when it has been connected to the lateral segments. This creates an intact muscular lip arch which will help mold the alveolar ridge into the correct position, with adjunctive orthodontic devices guiding the ridge. The repaired lip itself is acting as an orthodontic traction to bring elements of the alveolar dental arch into the proper relation (Fig. 51-53).

Additional orthodontic methods are required for complete clefts of the palate in order to mold the alveolar arch and prevent its collapse. Although early orthodontic treatment remains popular, the early grafting of bone across the cleft is decreasing in applicability, since the long-term benefits have not been forthcoming, and there is perhaps less growth in the area where bone grafting has been done. However, after the age of five there are many instances when only bone grafting can obtain the proper arch and facial configuration. The clefts of the soft and hard palate are closed by a modification of the Kilner operation (Fig. 51-54) or by the Langenbeck technique.

All patients with cleft palate have drainage problems

Fig. 51-53. Effects of lip closure on alveolar dental arch. *A.* Complete cleft of lip and palate. *B.* Closure of defect of lip brings alveolar segment in anatomic position. *C.* Note correction of alveolar arch. Guidance of the parts by intraoral appliances may be necessary to enhance correct positioning.

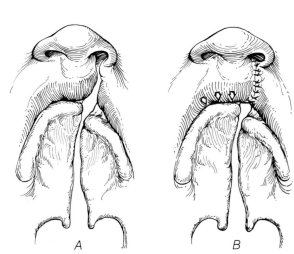
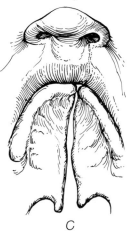

A   *B*   *C*

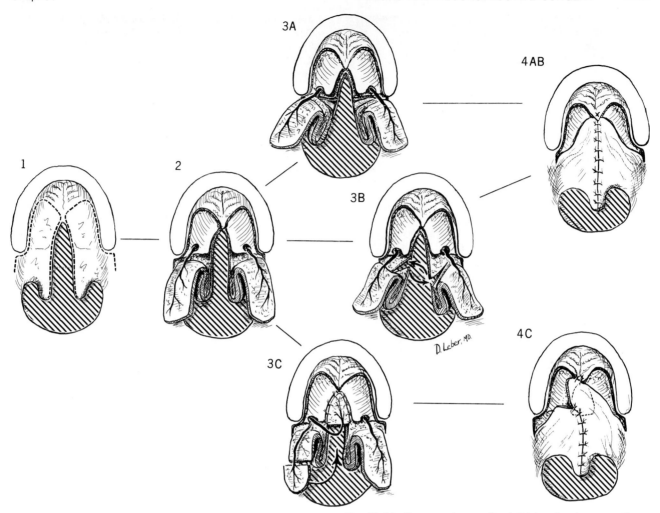

Fig. 51-54. Common types of palatal lengthening operations. Retropositioning during the repair of a cleft is a logical means of improving speech. 1. Long flaps are designed; note the anterior shape and the incisions along the cleft and laterally. 2. The mucoperiosteal flaps are elevated, with isolation and preservation of the greater palatine vessels and nerves. The nasal mucosa is widely undermined from the hard palate on the nasal side. 3. The handling of the nasal mucosa (a) in a palate that is long; the mucosa does not need to be transected, only widely mobilized; the soft palate aponeurosis is separated from the posterior edge of the hard palate, and the levator palati muscles are repositioned posteriorly. (b) When the palate is short, the nasal mucosa is sectioned obliquely; these angled incisions form a Z-plasty which lengthens the palate and prevents linear contracture from tension. (c) If the palate is short and the cleft wide, a turned-over island flap to bridge the gap is useful, although necessary only occasionally. 4. (a and b) The second and third layers of the closure are now completed using a row of buried sutures to approximate the muscles, in addition to the row of mucosal sutures already present. The only raw surfaces left are overlying the bony palate. (c) The method of closure when an anterior island has been used for closing the nasal surface superiorly.

of the middle ear. These frequently require drainage at an early age, usually supplemented with insertion of tubes for more permanent drainage. Upper respiratory tract infections must be even more closely monitored and promptly treated with decongestants, anti-inflammatory agents, and antibiotics guided by appropriate cultures.

The appearance of the patients and their dental occlusion is important, but of equal or more significance is their communication, as the speech results are intimately intertwined with hearing and motivation. Speech therapy is helpful for all patients. Careful assessment clinically, aerodynamically, and radiographically is imperative. Both static roentgenograms (Fig. 51-55) and cineradiography in lateral, frontal, and superoinferior planes are helpful. Secondary procedures include methods of adding length to the palate itself, reinforcing the elevation properties of the palate, occlusion of the space by attachment of a flap of the posterior pharyngeal wall to the palate, or techniques to make the pharyngeal port smaller either by retropharyngeal implantation or by procedures to decrease the size of the opening by protrusion of the pharyngeal muscle and mucosa.

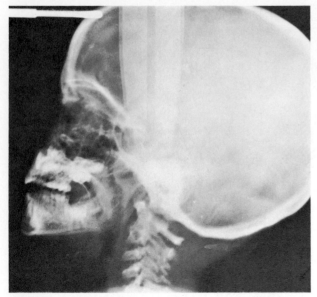

A

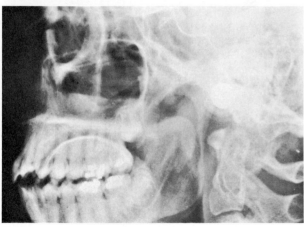

B

Fig. 51-55. Cephalometric speech studies. *A.* The head-holding cephalostat which is used so that the film can have its exact parameters duplicated at any subsequent time. Note that during a maximal effort at stimulating the palate it hangs loosely so that there is a wide gap in the pharynx communicating to the nose. This patient will have excessive escape of air and unintelligible speech, and will need a surgical procedure of the pharyngeal flap type. *B.* In marked contrast is this soft palate which has elevated excellently, although a gap between it and the posterior pharyngeal wall can still be noticed. For a palate such as this a lengthening procedure or a pharyngeoplasty procedure would be effective, and a pharyngeal flap is not needed.

Congenital Microtia

Severe hypoplastic malformations of the ear, which occur in 1 of 15,000 births, represent branchial arch deformities. There may be partial or complete absence of the external, middle, and/or inner parts of the ear. Frequently, the external auditory meatus and canal are totally absent, and there may be associated anomalies of the facial

nerve, the temporomandibular joint, and the mandible. The unilateral situation is about six times as frequent as bilateral.

TREATMENT. When radiologic and audiologic examination reveals a functioning hearing apparatus and the patient has bilateral atresia of the canals, surgery on one side should be attempted to alleviate the total deafness. In unilateral situations, no surgery is recommended to improve the hearing on the affected side.

Reconstruction of the absent or nearly absent external ear is usually recommended, because of the great improvement in the surgical techniques of cartilage reconstruction. As prosthetic techniques improve, both in the materials to design the prostheses and the glues used to attach them, there is a growing feeling that surgery can be replaced by an excellent prosthesis. However, at this date the authors still recommend surgical reconstruction. Cartilage is still preferred. The initial successes with prosthetic implanted ears described by Cronin and others have had to be modified, as long-term results indicate that the implants become extruded, although autogenous fascia lata coverage has improved the retention rate. Even though a perfect ear is not reproduced, the results of cartilage reconstructions seem to be more reliable and satisfactory.

Any of these ear reconstructions require multiple operations. They are best performed when ear growth is nearly complete, so that further contralateral growth will not cause a size disparity, and when the child is old enough to have well-developed costal cartilages. This usually means that the first stage should be deferred until the child is approximately six or seven years old. The first-stage operation is designed to place the remaining visible ear elements in their proper relationship, so that they will accept the supporting material at a later date in the correct position. This initial operation is also the time when unsightly, nonusable tags of skin and fragments of cartilage may be discarded. At the second stage the supporting material is obtained from the ribs and carved. It is inserted beneath the mastoid skin as the architectural framework. At a third stage, the posterior surface of a reconstructed ear is grafted with skin after it has been elevated from its mastoid bed (Fig. 51-56).

Thyroglossal Anomalies

About 6 percent of the masses found in the neck are of congenital origin. The most common lesions, which represent two-thirds of the total, are cysts or sinuses of the thyroglossal duct. The thyroid gland has its embryonic origin in the middle of the anterior pharynx in an area which later becomes the tongue. The thyroid anlage migrates into the neck but remains attached at the foramen cecum by the thyroglossal duct. Normally, this connection becomes obliterated early in embryonic life, but occasionally it may persist as a sinus tract, which becomes enclosed by the fused elements of the hyoid bone, or as a cyst (Fig. 51-57).

The lesions appear in the midline or just off the midline of the neck at some point between the isthmus of the thyroid gland and the hyoid bone. The cystic lesions may

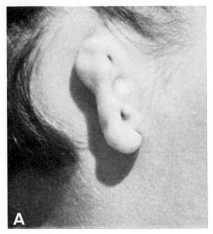 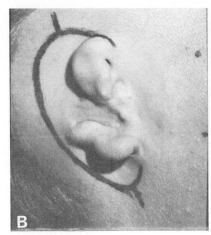 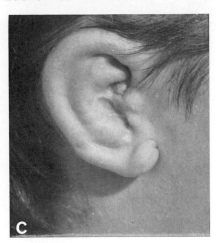

Fig. 51-56. A multistaged ear reconstruction in microtia. *A.* The original defect—congenital absence of normal ear cartilage and malposition of the lobule. *B.* The first stage. Repositioning of the lobule has been accomplished by the use of a Z-plasty. The marks indicate the correct size and angle for reconstruction. Measurement of the opposite normal ear, acrylic models, and photography are essential to correct placement. *C.* The completed ear. Costochondral cartilage is used to form the structure.

be identified by their position and rubbery characteristics. These may become infected and rupture spontaneously or require surgical incision. Once the cyst has become infected, it will persist with repeated episodes of abscess formation and drainage until the entire cyst and its tract are removed. A midline sinus, which is diagnostic of a persistent thyroglossal duct, should also be surgically excised.

Incomplete removal represents the most common error in treatment of thyroglossal anomalies. Removal of either cyst or sinus requires excision of the central hyoid segment if recurrence is to be avoided (Sistrunk procedure). If the mass is of significant size, the presence of thyroid tissue in its normal position should be demonstrated in order to avoid the possibility of removing the patient's only functioning thyroid from the base of the tongue.

Branchial Anomalies

Abnormalities in the cervicofacial complex result from arrest and alteration of the developing branchial arches and clefts. Congenital cysts, sinuses, fistulas, and growth alterations in the head and neck fall into a pattern which is specific for each branchial cleft and arch. As a group, these represent the second most common congenital lesion of the neck.

EMBRYOLOGY. Each of the five branchial arches seen in early embryonic life (Fig. 51-58) is separated from the adjacent arch by a cleft. Normally, the clefts close and disappear, and the arches coalesce to create a smooth continuity of the face and neck tissues. The first arch provides the building blocks for the maxillomandibular complex and part of the auricle. The second arch gives rise to the cervical structures and part of the auricle. Between these two arches is the first branchial cleft, which

is the embryonic origin of the eustachian apparatus and auditory canal. The third branchial arch derivatives are neck structures in the hyoid region. The second cleft anatomically runs from the tonsillar fossa anteriorly to the lower neck. It normally closes prior to birth. Parts of the larynx and cervical vascular structure have their origin in the fourth and fifth arches. Anomalies in the fourth and fifth arches rarely cause abnormalities and will not be considered in this section.

FIRST BRANCHIAL ARCH ANOMALIES. These become manifest as abnormal development confined to the mouth, mandible, and anterior parts of the ear, referred to as the *oromandibuloauricular syndrome.* More frequently, the anomalies are not confined, and parts derived from the second arch are also abnormal.

FIRST BRANCHIAL CLEFT ANOMALIES. A cyst, sinus, or fistula which lies between the external auditory canal and

Fig. 51-57. Sagittal section indicating tract of thyroglossal duct. Originating at the foramen cecum, it passes through the hyoid bone in the midline and continues to the skin at the suprasternal notch.

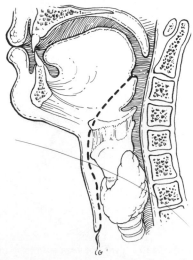

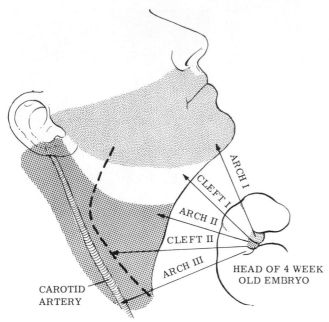

Fig. 51-58. Contribution of the embryonic branchial arches to the parts of the adult face. (*Modified from Knute Berger.*)

the submandibular area originates from the first branchial cleft. Proximity of such sinuses to the facial nerve may make removal difficult (Fig. 51-59).

SECOND BRANCHIAL CLEFT ANOMALIES. The vast majority of branchial anomalies represent remnants of the second branchial cleft. These commonly present as a cyst

Fig. 51-59. Pathologic consequences of incomplete embryonic dissolution of the first and second branchial grooves and clefts. (*Modified from Knute Berger.*)

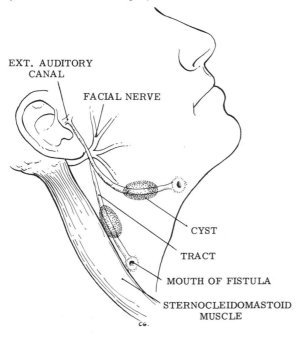

which is located anterior to the sternocleidomastoid muscle in the middle third of the anterior triangle of the neck (Fig. 51-59). The cyst is lined with squamous or columnar epithelial tissue and contains a greenish mucuslike detritus, which accumulates in the lumen and gradually causes the cyst to increase in size. It may become secondarily infected or may cause pressure symptoms by sudden increase in size. The original internal opening of the branchial cleft is in the tonsillar fossa, and sinuses can connect to the tonsillar fossa from the cyst or extend all the way to the skin. Treatment is by excision of the cyst and its tract. Since the tract descends between the internal and external branches of the carotid artery, care must be taken during the surgical procedure.

COSMETIC SURGERY

Scar Revision

Facial scars resulting from trauma, infection, previous surgical treatment, chemical and radiation therapy, or dermatologic disorders frequently are dramatically improved by surgical renovation. Not all scars can be eliminated completely, but improvement is accomplished by excision and precise closure to achieve the best per primam healing. The lines of the scar may be altered by geometric reorientation to avoid crossing normal facial lines of tension. Scar characteristics such as pigmentation, depigmentation, depression, hypertrophy, improper alignment, tattooing, and ragged edges are correctible by excision, reclosure with or without Z-plasty, or other geometric reorientation techniques.

Distorting contractures and unsightly hypertrophy may necessitate excision and replacement with skin graft. If no contour defect exists, free skin grafts are employed. These should be obtained from areas with the same characteristics, i.e., color, texture, hairlessness, and thickness, as the area of skin to be grafted (Fig. 51-49). Small defects on the face may be successfully and inconspicuously covered with free full-thickness grafts from the postauricular area or the supraclavicular region. The thin eyelid skin is best replaced by contralateral lid skin or from the prepuce in the uncircumcised male.

If the facial scar is accompanied by an abnormality in contour, pedicle flap reconstruction is essential. A graft fashioned from local tissue is superior, because it creates the least conspicuous correction as far as color and texture are concerned. The copious blood supply in the head and neck assures the success of local pedicle flaps even when the pedicle is reduced to a vascular bundle. If local tissue is not available, pedicles may be carried from a distant site, in which case multiple stages of advancement may be required.

Eyebrow Reconstruction

An eyebrow which has been destroyed by trauma, leprosy, radiation, or another cause creates a noticeable defect. The hair-bearing eyebrow may be replaced by a free

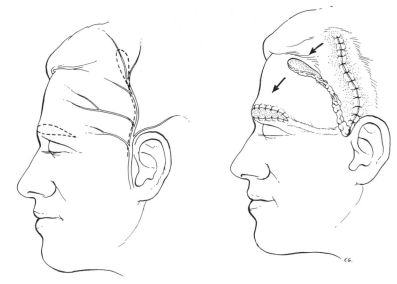

Fig. 51-60. Eyebrow restoration using a vascularized hair-bearing scalp island carried on the temporal vessels.

composite graft from the scalp (Fig. 51-7) or contralateral eyebrow or, even more reliably, by using a temporal vascular island pedicle flap from the scalp (Fig. 51-60). Since the replaced eyebrow hair maintains the characteristics of the donor site, it must be clipped regularly, just as one cuts the hair on his head.

Prominent Ears

Prominent ears with no antihelix fold and, frequently, overdevelopment of the concha occur in both sexes. Corrective surgical procedures consist of weakening the cartilage on its anterior surface, resecting a portion of the hypertrophic conchal wall, suture fixating the antihelix fold, and removing excesses of helix tail and retroauricular skin excisions. This can result in near-perfect restoration. The optimal age for correction is not determined, but it is best done the summer before entering school, either under local or general anesthesia (Fig. 51-61).

Rhinoplasty

Nasal size and contour are largely dependent upon the bony and cartilaginous framework. Occasionally the skin and soft tissue over this underlying architecture may be the cause of the deformity, as in rhinophyma. Deformities may result from trauma to the nasal skeleton, previous surgical treatment, infection, or simple inherited characteristics.

Rhinoplasty represents the most frequently considered cosmetic surgical procedure. With today's reliable, safe, and simple procedures to overcome nasal deformity, whether congenital or traumatic, it seems unduly conservative to consider rhinoplasty as unnecessary surgical treatment. In some individuals, these deformities, even though purely cosmetic, are psychically disturbing. The psychosocial readjustment that frequently follows the op-

eration is most rewarding in patients who have been carefully selected and assessed prior to operation (Fig. 51-62).

The usual cosmetic nasal deformities are correctible by revision of the bony and cartilaginous architecture, allowing the soft tissues to readjust naturally. The nasal bones, like the roof of a house, support one another at the midline of the nose. They are joined at this point by the nasal septum. When a permanent nasal hump is removed, the nasal bones and septum remain as three separate elements creating a broad nasal bridge. During rhinoplasty, the hump is removed and the nasal bones are fractured through lateral osteotomies in the nasal processes of the maxilla, so that the bridge of the nose may be made narrow at the same time.

The nasal tip and septal support are entirely cartilaginous, and they may be reshaped by trimming the alar, upper lateral, and septal cartilages appropriately.

Very frequently deformity of the septum causes obstruction to breathing. The majority of septal resections may

Fig. 51-61. *A.* Congenital prominence of ears. *B.* After otoplasty.

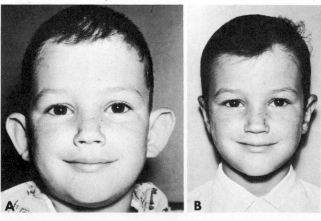

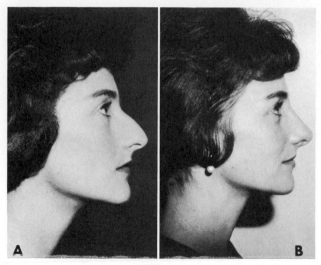

Fig. 51-62. Cosmetic rhinoplasty. *A.* Preoperative photograph. *B.* Postoperative photograph.

accompany the rhinoplasty. However, if the septal removal will compromise support of the dorsum of the nose, the combined septal resection and rhinoplasty should not be done and either one or the other electively deferred for a few months.

Rhytidectomy (Face-lifting) and Blepharoplasty

The aging face may create significant problems among people whose occupations depend upon their appearance. Premature looseness of facial tissues or wrinkling of facial skin and eyelid skin can be a psychologic barrier impossible to overcome; surgical correction may be urgently indicated. Although this type of aesthetic surgery occupies an extremely important place in American medical practice, it is poorly understood by many physicians who must be supportive toward their patients and recognize their need when making the difficult preoperative decisions. The gratifying results to such a high percentage of patients are eloquent testimony to the fulfillment of *realistic* needs.

The fine wrinkles and grooves in the skin are best treated by chemical peeling or dermabrasion. Looseness and ptosis of the skin are corrected by excising excessive skin at a site where the residual scar is not readily visible. From these incisions in the hairline and around the ear, there is wide undermining of the facial and cervical skin, allowing it to be rotated upward and backward to permit the excess to be removed in order to accomplish tightening by this overlapping at the incision site. In the eyelids, age expresses itself by sagging and wrinkling of the eyelid skin and also weakening of the lids' orbital septums, allowing protrusion of the intraorbital fat into the lids. This will give the appearance of constant tiredness, or even a deceptive look of debauchery. Resections of the excessive eyelid skin and removal of the fat herniations, a procedure known

as blepharoplasty, may precede, accompany, or follow a face-lifting procedure.

FACIAL CONTOUR DEFECTS

Loss of soft tissue substances or skeletal support results in facial contour defects which are cosmetically unattractive and occasionally grotesque. A number of useful techniques are available to restore facial contour and symmetry. Free autogenous grafts of bone, cartilage, dermis, and fat have been employed in the standard techniques for many years. Nonreactive plastic materials recently have been refined to the extent that they are now being used with increasing frequency as contour-restoring tissue substitutes.

FREE GRAFTS. Autogenous bone grafts are useful in correcting defects in the orbital margins, over a depressed zygoma, and over the mandible where the support beneath the skin and subcutaneous tissue is normally firm. In the cheek areas, defects are better corrected with soft tissue grafts of dermis and fat, or with prostheses. During vascularization of free autogenous grafts, some atrophy and loss of fat occurs; for this reason the graft should overcorrect the deformity initially. Spontaneous readjustment generally takes place 6 months to 1 year after operation.

PEDICLE GRAFTS. Subcutaneous tissue and dermis may be transferred from a local area or a distant site using a tubed pedicle in order to fill contour defects. Since the transfer tissue is never devoid of blood supply, atrophy does not occur to the same extent as noted in free grafts. Therefore, overcorrection is not essential with this technique.

PLASTIC MATERIALS. Of the various plastic materials available for implantation, silicones have proved to be the most useful. Dacron, Teflon, polyethylene, and acrylics each have many specific indications. Medical-grade silicone is chemically inert, readily fabricated, easily sterilized, and noncarcinogenic. It can be manufactured in a wide variety of consistencies from semiliquid to sponge to rigid. Studies of the tissue reactions both to silicone and to the other materials mentioned suggest that there is minimal foreign body response, although a bursal separation is common around the smoother types. The smaller the fiber presented to the patient's tissues, the less the total reaction. Studies are still in progress to determine the total longevity of these materials. Injectable liquid silicone is still experimental.

Distorted Maxillomandibular Relationship

Distortion of the anatomic relationship of the maxillary and mandibular units may be associated with minimal abnormality of aesthetic significance or severe disproportion of a disfiguring nature. Disproportion may be due to congenital malformation, growth abnormality, infection, trauma, or surgical procedures. Skeletal aberration may or may not be associated with dental occlusion. Conversely, malocclusion in itself may be responsible for distorted facial patterns. In the latter case, orthodontic therapy alone is sufficient.

MANDIBULAR RETRUSION

Inadequate mandibular substance with foreshortening of the mandible is called *micrognathia*. This may be congenital or may result from injury to the condylar epiphysis. With unilateral mandibular growth disturbance, there are asymmetry and problems with lateral occlusion. With temporomandibular joint disease, ankylosis of this joint is the problem.

Surgical relief of ankylosis is achieved by osteotomy and removal of sufficient bone of the condyle to allow free motion of the mandible. Interposition of soft tissue or silicone aids in preventing recurrent ankylosis. To achieve appropriate correction of the mandibular retrusion, precise measurements must be made roentgenographically, photographically, and with dental models. Correction is accomplished by osteotomy with or without bone grafting, which may produce dramatic results. Both the abnormal occlusal relationship and the cosmetic aberration can be corrected. When the deformity is severe and there is no major occlusion problem, a bone graft or sponge silicone implant over the point of the chin is corrective.

MANDIBULAR PROTRUSION

Prognathism, or protrusion of the mandible, represents another disproportion between the mandible and maxilla. Malocclusion usually occurs, and osteotomy and recession of the mandible are the preferable approach. Vertical, sagittal, and horizontal osteotomies applied in many geometric variations are used. Once the bilateral osteotomy has been performed, the teeth are brought into proper occlusal relation, maintained there by an interdental acrylic occlusal wafer, and then immobilized by intermaxillary fixation for 10 to 12 weeks so that proper healing will ensue.

MAXILLARY RETRUSION

Flattening and depression of the middle third of the face, referred to as the "dish-face deformity," may represent a familial trait and is commonly associated with congenital cleft palate. Trauma may also result in maxillary retrusion. Correction of maxillary retrusion by osteotomy and adjustment of occlusion is more difficult than correction of the distortions of the mandible. Substitution for the cosmetically important flattened area can be achieved by onlay grafts or silicone implantation. Prosthetic devices as part of an upper denture also may be helpful.

Craniofacial Anomalies

Severe craniofacial anomalies such as those seen in Apert's syndrome, Crouzon's disease, and hypertelorism are now amenable to correction. Pioneer surgery by Tessier et al., Converse et al., Dingman and Natvig, Edgerton et al., and Murray and Swanson has proved the worth of the combined intracranial-transfacial approach to correct the abnormal facies by complicated osteotomies and bone grafts. These are extremely complex and exacting procedures, requiring a well-trained team of plastic surgeons, neurosurgeons, anesthesiologists, and dental specialists.

FACIAL PARALYSIS

The causes of facial nerve palsy vary from the incompletely understood Bell's palsy to complete or partial transection of the nerve by trauma or surgical procedure. The proximal intratemporal portion of the nerve is characterized by a lengthy and circuitous passage through the temporal bone. The nerve emerges via the stylomastoid foramen, enters the parotid gland, and arborizes with considerable variability as it passes anteriorly through the gland. The peripheral motor branches, i.e., temporal, zygomatic, buccal, mandibular, and cervical, lie just deep to the very superficial facial musculature. The diffuse spread of these branches coupled with their superficial position makes them subject to injury in face lacerations. Operations in the parotid region, middle ear, or intracranially in the auditofacial area may all result in facial nerve injury.

Localization of the lesion requires a knowledge of nerve anatomy and an appreciation of the function of individual branches. Central (supranuclear) palsy characteristically presents with paralysis of the facial muscles with the exception of the forehead and eyelid musculature. The paralysis is contralateral to the site of the lesion. The intratemporal portion of the nerve gives rise to the chorda tympani nerve and therefore may be assessed by testing taste from the anterior two-thirds of the tongue. The nerve to the stapedius is difficult to test, but the greater superficial petrosal nerve supplies taste to the soft palate. All muscles of facial expression, the platysma, and the buccinator are supplied by the intraparotid portion of the nerve. Except for a few sensory fibers to the ear carried in the posterior auricular branch, the extratemporal facial nerve is purely motor.

Facial Nerve Repair

Paralysis of the facial nerve may pose two separate problems for reconstruction: one involves a direct approach to the nerve itself, while the other consists of methods to overcome the functional and cosmetic disability which results from irreversible paralysis.

Intratemporal nerve decompression and repair of the nerve with grafting techniques are procedures which are now performed regularly with acceptable success. The extratemporal nerve should be repaired as soon as the diagnosis is established, and studies of nerve conduction, chronaxie, and electromyography are all helpful in this regard. The application of an operating microscope has facilitated precise repair of small facial nerve branches.

When gaps exist as a result of loss of nerve substance, nerve grafts may be used. For many years surgeons have experimented with nerve crossings using proximal ends of the spinal accessory, hypoglossal, phrenic, glossopharyngeal, and descendens hypoglossi nerves sutured to the distal end of the transected facial nerve. These techniques have resulted in diminished atrophy and improved tone of the facial muscles. The most satisfactory results have been achieved with the hypoglossal nerve (Fig. 51-63). In this case, the anticipated paralysis of one-half of the tongue

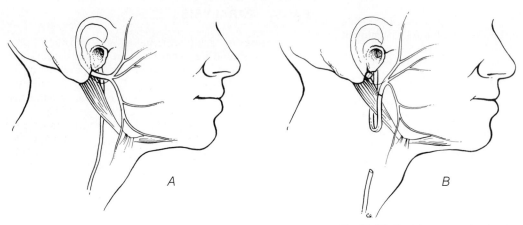

Fig. 51-63. Facial nerve graft using hypoglossal nerve. *A.* Normal relationship between descendens hypoglossi and facial nerves. *B.* Nerve graft from proximal descendens hypoglossi to distal facial nerves.

and occasional difficulty in swallowing, unless the descendens hypoglossi is preserved, should be explained to the patient prior to the operation. Substitution via the trigeminal nerve has been less effective. Spontaneous return of some function has been noted after complete transection of the facial nerve without subsequent repair.

Reconstructive Procedures

EYE. The loss of the protective function of the eyelid musculature is the most pressing problem associated with total irreversible facial paralysis. Exposure keratitis and epiphora not only are troublesome but may result in severe corneal damage and ultimate blindness (Fig. 51-64). If nerve recovery is anticipated, the patient must be taught to protect the eye from exposure by wearing glasses, using ophthalmic ointments, and, at times, applying a patch to the eye. The best surgical procedure for ocular protection is lateral tarsorrhaphy, i.e., attaching the upper lid to the lower lid by tissue overlapping. A medial canthoplasty is

Fig. 51-64. Exposure keratitis and leukoma formation as a result of facial nerve paralysis.

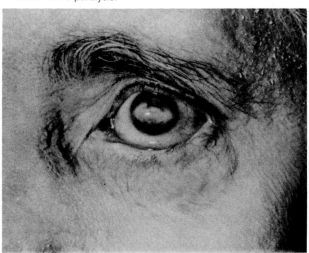

the procedure used to tighten the loose lower lid and turn the punctum in against the globe to diminish epiphora.

Transfer of intact motor power to the eyelids may be achieved by the Gillies operation (Fig. 51-65). This procedure consists of turning down the central portion of the temporalis muscle, which is innervated by the fifth nerve, from the temporal fossa and extending temporalis fascial strips from the lateral canthus through the upper and lower lids. The strips are attached at the medial canthal ligament. The procedure allows dynamic function of the eyelids and supplies enough tone to keep the lower lid against the globe.

Another useful palliative procedure for the paralyzed eyelid is the insertion of a palpebral spring as advocated by Morel-Fatio and Lalardrie. This can be done through small incisions with minimal scarring under local anesthesia in the outpatient clinic.

FACE. The contorted appearance of the face creates a great deal of anxiety for the patient with total unilateral facial palsy. The marked asymmetry is contributed to by excessive activity of facial muscles on the contralateral unparalyzed side. Surgical measures to overcome asymmetry consist of operations to substitute for paralyzed muscles, to diminish the pull of antagonistic muscles, or to excise skin in order to overcome redundancy.

Muscle substitution may be static, using slings of fascia or tendon extending from the temporalis fascia down into the lips and eyelids (Fig. 51-66). Dynamic substitution may be achieved by attaching these slings to muscles of mastication, such as the temporalis or masseter, which have been diverted from their primary function. Segments of muscles may be redistributed into the facial muscles directly as in the Gillies procedure. For example, the anterior one-half of the masseter may be reflected forward into the orbicularis oris as a dynamic support (Fig. 51-67).

Thompson has reported on the successful free graft of skeletal muscle in man. Using the muscle bellies of the extensor digitorum brevis muscles applied directly to the temporalis muscle, the tendons are passed subcutaneously

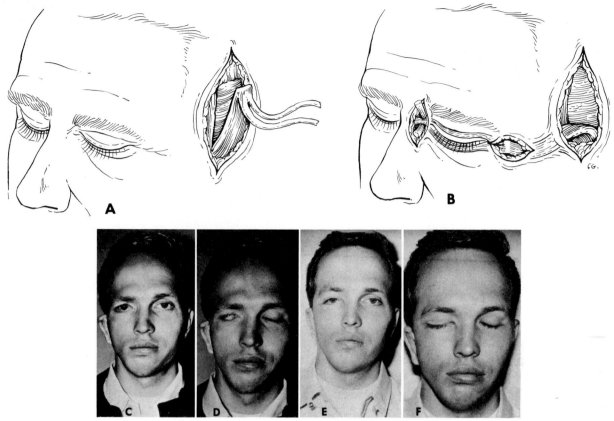

Fig. 51-65. Gillies' procedure to establish motor power for eyelids. *A* and *B*. Temporalis muscle reflected forward with strips of its own fascia passed through the upper and lower lids to the medial canthal ligament. *C* and *D*. Preoperative eyelid paralysis. *E* and *F*. After Gillies' operation.

along the eyelid margins and are anchored to the medial palpebral ligament. Neurotization of the free graft occurred, as proved by clinical motion and electromyography. In dogs, this has been corroborated by cholinesterase staining of motor end plates.

Fig. 51-66. Facial palsy treated with slings of fascia lata.

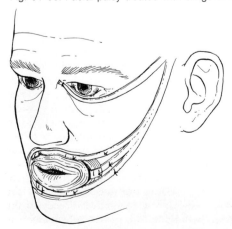

Facial Nerve Surgery. The two newest methods of re-innervating the face both show great promise. One of these is the previously mentioned transplantation of the gracilis muscle by microneurovascular anastomosis. The other, also a microsurgical technique, has been popularized by J. W. Smith. It incorporates the use of extremely long sural nerve grafts, anastomosed to fascicles on the normal side and passed subcutaneously to the paralyzed side, where they

Fig. 51-67. Facial palsy treated with transfers of portions of muscles of mastication and a static sling to the zygomatic arch.

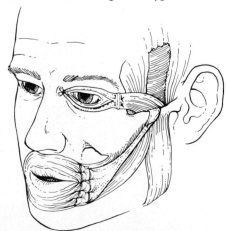

are tagged to be identified 6 months later, when they are anastomosed to their respective facial nerve branches.

The antagonistic, unparalyzed muscles on the contralateral side of the face may be surgically paralyzed or excised to diminish asymmetry. Selective neurectomy after preoperative trial with nerve blocks is useful in creating proper facial balance. The mandibular and the temporal branches of the facial nerve are most frequently transected surgically to overcome specific asymmetry in the face with unilateral facial palsy. Excision of segments of muscle on the unparalyzed side of the face selectively weakens these muscles without creating paralysis and an expressionless appearance.

Removal of redundant skin by "face-lifting" techniques is helpful in overcoming gross asymmetry. In general, a combination of slings, muscle transfers, myectomy, neurectomy, and removal of redundant skin produces the best results in patients with this difficult problem.

MISCELLANEOUS PROCEDURES

Surgery for Decubitus Ulcer

Skin and soft tissue defects in the trunk and extremities are frequently the result of pressure necrosis from prolonged pressure because of lack of sensation or because of inability to move secondary to unconsciousness or debility. Any disease or trauma which destroys sensation removes the protective barrier against destruction by pressure. The ulceration and ultimate loss of fingers and toes in leprosy, diabetic neuropathy, familial sensory neuropathy, and peripheral nerve injuries are all attributable to loss of pain sensitivity. It is also this pathway which is implicated in the formation of decubiti in patients with spinal cord injury. The majority of decubitus ulcers occur in elderly patients who are confined to bed for long periods of time.

Restoration of soft tissue and skin losses usually requires pedicle flaps. In the paraplegic, particularly, these operations are difficult to plan and tedious to execute, and necessitate meticulous and time-consuming wound care both pre- and postoperatively. The flap donor sites invariably need a skin graft for closure, creating even another wound, the skin donor site, which also may need very special attention for healing. The skeletal prominences in the base of the pressure ulcers, most frequently the greater trochanter, the ischial tuberosity, or the posterior surface of the sacrum, must be resected along with the infected bursae overlying them. In addition to the skin flaps that will cover them they frequently can best be protected by the local rotation of muscle flaps. Well-conceived plans can often secure healing and diminish the likelihood of reulceration, but constant vigilance by the patient, the families, attendants, and paramedical as well as medical personnel may be unable to ward off recurrences.

Surgery of the Breast

MALIGNANT AND PREMALIGNANT DISEASE

Cooperation between general and oncologic surgeons and the reconstructive surgeon can benefit the patient with breast disease. Too few women are given the opportunity to benefit from reconstruction after they have been cured of this malignant breast disease. Reconstruction of the

Fig. 51-68. Breast reconstruction after mastectomy. *A.* The patient had had a modified radical mastectomy through a transverse incision; good skin flaps and pectoralis bulk were present. *B.* Postoperative appearance, showing the breast mound recreated.

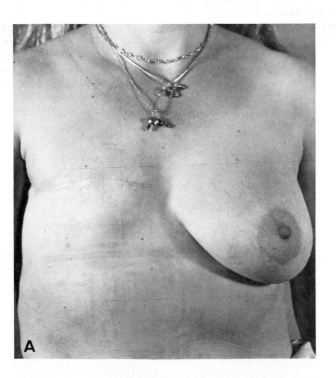
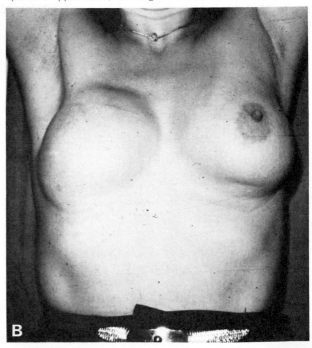

missing breast can be accomplished readily in most instances, particularly if a transverse incision has been used for the extirpation. If a modified radical mastectomy has been performed, the reconstruction is done in one stage. The result is cosmetically superior, and the pectoralis muscle may provide excellent protective covering for the prosthesis that is implanted (Fig. 51-68). If the surgical cure necessitated a more extensive procedure so that there is less skin, more scar, and perhaps an irradiated field, the reconstruction may be more complicated, entailing preliminary flap rotation procedures. These results are still gratifying, even though they are not as cosmetically good as the reconstruction after the modified extirpation.

Patients who do not have breast cancer but are at high risk should be considered for breast removal. This may be performed by a subcutaneous mastectomy with immediate or delayed prosthesis implantation. If a total mastectomy is done, the nipple is left attached to the specimen and the areola is removed to be grafted to the skin covering the prosthetic implants.

Of special note is the patient who has had a breast involved and is at high risk for contralateral breast involvement. If this patient is young and the breast texture or the radiograph is difficult to interpret, or if the patient is excessively bothered by the situation, prophylactic total mastectomy with implantation of a prosthesis and free areola graft is recommended.

REDUCTION MAMMOPLASTY

FEMALE. Enlargement of the female breasts is a much misunderstood clinical problem. It can occur in adolescence and become quite massive, or it can occur gradually through the developmental years and then with loss of support and the addition of ptosis become even more of a problem. The psychologic strains associated with this deformity are great. In addition the physical symptoms of postural deformity, backache, shoulder pain and ulceration from brassiere straps, inframammary skin eruptions, and mastodynia are all most bothersome and frequently incapacitating. Surgical correction will handle both the physical and psychologic problems, and the functional result is also aesthetically pleasing. Many varieties of procedure have been proposed. Rarely is it necessary to resort to an amputation of the breast with subsequent free transplantation of the nipple and areola. This must be reserved only for the most massive of breasts. Usually the technique can retain the nipple-areolar complex on a dermal pedicle to preserve its sensation and function. The geometric design is not complex but does take understanding and planning (Fig. 51-69).

MALE. In approximately 10 percent of the normal male population adolescent gynecomastia will occur. The great majority recede spontaneously. For those which do not, a subcutaneous mastectomy performed through a circumareolar incision is recommended to remove the breast with a minimal scar.

AUGMENTATION MAMMOPLASTY

The augmentation of breast size for cosmetic purposes has become an acceptable procedure in carefully selected patients. A multiplicity of prosthetic breasts are available. The silicone breasts devised by Cronin and Greenberg have been used most and have the greatest longevity of clinical experience. Recently other materials such as polyurethanes have been recommended. In addition inflatable prostheses are now being investigated.

The operation consists of implanting the prosthesis in a plane beneath the breast tissue if any is present. Most surgeons prefer to place the prosthesis upon the superficial surface of the fascia overlying the pectoralis muscles, although there are some who prefer placing it behind the pectoralis muscle.

When patients have extensive cystic disease of the breast which has been painful and recurrent and for which a simple mastectomy is indicated, a subcutaneous mastectomy is a good alternative. Either at the same procedure or several weeks later, a breast prosthesis is implanted so the woman does not feel neutered. The aesthetic result is good, but the complication rate is 10 to 15 percent.

Hypospadias

The congenital hypospadias deformity, incomplete masculinization of the external genitalia, occurs once in every 300 to 400 boys born in the United States. Chromosomal studies have shown no consistent abnormalities associated with hypospadias. Failure of the embryonic fusion during the second month of development gives rise to this deformity, which is often minimal. A useful clinical classification is the following: glans, distal penile, midpenile, penoscrotal junction, scrotal, and perineal. The more distal lesions, i.e., glans, distal penile, and midpenile, usually do not have any associated anomalies. Those situated more proximally need more extensive work-up, since they are more likely to be associated with abnormalities of the upper urinary tract.

All varieties of hypospadias are frequently accompanied by chordee, a ventral curvature of the penis caused by the replacement of the dartos fascia, Buck's fascia, and corpus spongiosum by a band of tough fibrous tissue in a triangular area extending from the urethral meatus to the edge of the hooded prepuce.

When a newborn infant is seen with a hypospadias, two important steps must be taken at once: The first is to evaluate the urethral opening to determine whether it is constricted, necessitating a meatotomy. The second is to prevent circumcision, even that required by ritual. All patients should eventually have cystoscopy, intravenous pyelography, and sex chromatin studies. Surgery is best performed during the latter portion of the second year, with the ultimate goals of providing (1) a straight penis, (2) the urethral opening at the tip of the penis, (3) normal voiding, (4) normal appearance, and (5) normal erection.

Reconstruction of the urethra and release of the chordee can be accomplished in simultaneous operations, although most surgeons will precede the urethroplasty by the chordee release (Fig. 51-70A to D). During the stage of the urethral reconstruction, urinary diversion is accomplished, usually through a perineal urethrostomy although occasionally by a suprapubic drainage procedure. Of the many procedures that have been advocated, the authors favor either the buried-strip method proposed by Denis-Browne (Fig. 51-70*E* and *F*) or the free skin graft (Fig. 51-71). Success is usually possible without fistula formation (Fig. 51-72).

Body Contouring

Abdominoplasty, thigh lift, and reduction of upper arm skin redundancy are most frequently considered in patients who have undergone massive weight loss after years of obesity. Frequent pregnancies with resulting flaccid abdominal skin and diastasis recti, surgically denervated abdominal wall musculature, or lipodystrophy are also indications. Surgical correction requires extensive mobilization of tissues and will cause scars of great length. The surgeon must carefully plan scar placement to provide the best aesthetic result.

Vaginal Reconstruction

Successful construction of a vagina for agenesis is best accomplished by creation of a perineal pocket lined with a skin graft. After vaginectomy or pelvic exenteration for malignant disease, however, lack of sufficient bony coverage makes skin grafting less satisfactory. Local flaps, distant flaps, and colonic interposition have been utilized with only limited success. Use of myocutaneous flaps based on the gracilis muscle, as described by McGraw et al., provides an excellent reconstructive modality. The procedure can be performed in one stage, resulting in primary wound healing and decreased morbidity. Good sensibility and successful intercourse are reported.

Transsexual Surgery

Transsexual surgery has received increasing publicity since its popularization in 1952. Increasing numbers of patients are requesting sexual reassignment, and several medical centers have formed interdisciplinary medical teams for the evaluation, diagnosis, and treatment of this difficult problem. Although the primary modality of diagnosis is psychiatric, an adequate medical team should include plastic surgery, gynecology, urology, endocrinology, genetics, neuropsychiatry, and psychology.

TECHNIQUES: MALE TO FEMALE. After exhaustive psychiatric evaluation and cross-gender role adaptation with hormonal therapy, selected patients are started on a course of operative procedures. In addition to removal of testes and penis and construction of a vagina, this may also include adjunctive procedures such as breast augmentation, rhinoplasty, and reduction of thyroid cartilage. The most satisfactory method of vaginal construction utilizes the skin and subcutaneous tissue of the penis as an inverted pedicle for a surgically created perineal pocket. The glans is used as a clitoral substitute, and labia are constructed from scrotal skin. "Normal" sexual intercourse has been reported in many patients.

TECHNIQUES: FEMALE TO MALE. This conversion is more difficult but far less common. Most often, a phallus is

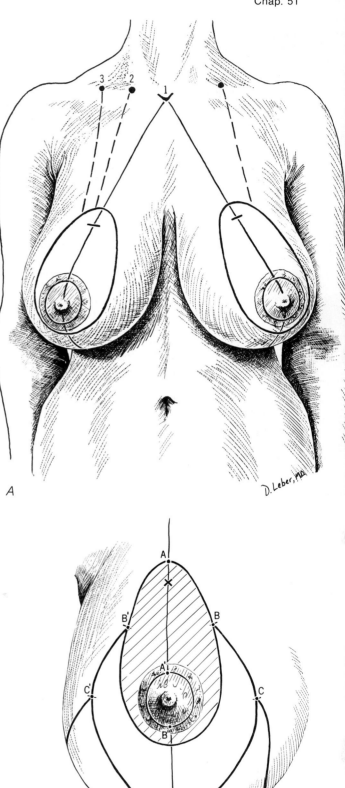

A

B

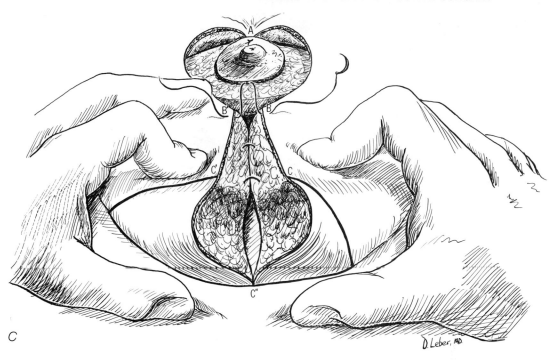

C

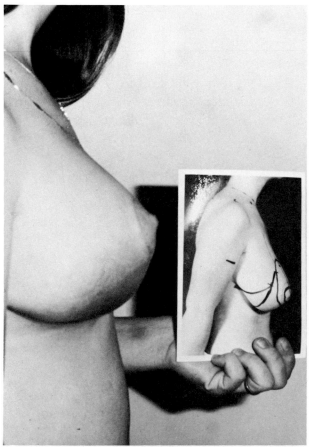

D

Fig. 51-69. Reduction mammaplasty. *A.* Correct location of the new nipple site is determined by measuring from the midclavicular line and the sternal notch. An equilateral triangle is recommended, extending from the sternal notch to both nipples, each side measuring between 20 and 23 cm according to height and torso. *B.* The crosshatched area is deepithelialized to preserve the vasculature just beneath the dermis; this dermal pedicle ensures survival of the nipple and areola. The circumference of the area demarcated by a line from *A* to *B* to *B'* to *A* must be approximately 13 cm to accommodate the areolar area, which has a diameter (*A'B''*) of 4 cm. The line *B'C'* must equal the *BC* and measure 4.5 to 6.5 cm; these lines are joined to form the new vertical dimension of the inferior breast. The wedge resected beneath the areola and between lines *C'C''* and *CC''* frequently may weigh as much as 1,500 Gm. *C.* Repositioning the breast tissues: The suspending suture at *A* for the top of the areola and the reconstructions beneath the areola at *BB'*, *CC'*, and *C''* give the new breast its size and shape. Additional breast tissue, the two triangles on either side of the sagittal closure, is resected just above the inframammary fold. *D.* Before and after breast reduction and reconstruction.

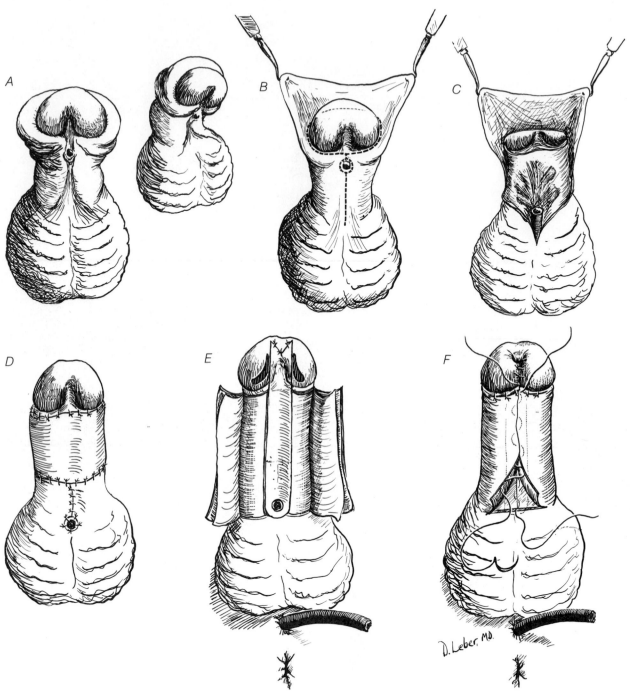

Fig. 51-70. *A.* Hypospadias of the midpenile area with chordee. *B.* Release of the chordee in a preliminary operation always drops the urethral opening back to a more proximal position. Circumcision now can be accomplished but without discarding any skin. *C.* The dorsal hooded prepuce is rearranged by moving it to the ventral surface to cover the defect left by the straightening. *D.* The Denis-Browne technique: The perineal urethrostomy has been accomplished. The parallel lines are made from the tip of the glans and extend proximally around the urethral orifice. This buried strip of skin accomplishes tubing without suturing. It is necessary to have good skin closure over this strip. *E* and *F.* Reliable closure is accomplished with running pullout sutures in three layers, the dartos fascia, Buck's fascia, and the skin.

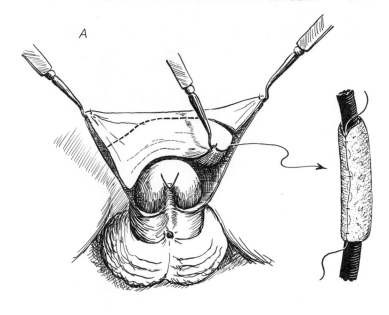

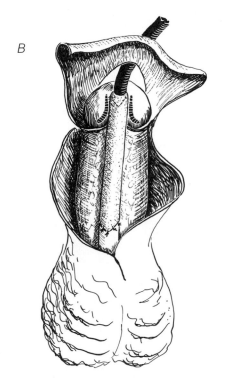

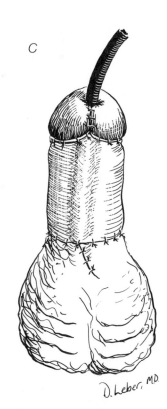

Fig. 51-71. Urethroplasty by the free skin graft method. *A.* The inner surface of the prepuce is removed and made into a tube around a catheter, the skin side against the catheter. If the patient has been previously circumcised, hairless skin from the inner arm is substituted. *B.* The catheter is placed within the urethra and the skin graft sutured to the distal portion of the urethra. Coverage is accomplished by using the hooded prepuce, moving it to the ventral surface. *C.* The completed procedure. In this case the diversion is accomplished by the catheter, obviating a perineal urethrostomy.

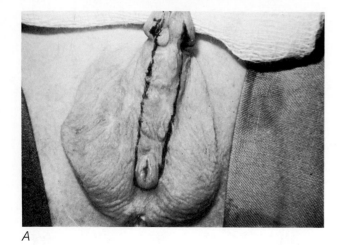

A

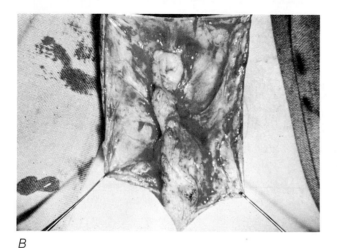

B

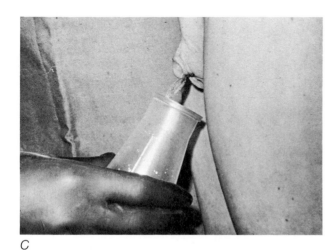

C

Fig. 51-72. Urethroplasty by the Denis-Browne method. *A.* The chordee has been released 3 months previously; the design of the buried strip is shown. *B.* Wide undermining is necessary to accomplish good closure to prevent fistula formation. *C.* The functional result.

constructed from a midline abdominal tube flap, with a urethra formed from a section of ilium. A silicone rod may be implanted to increase rigidity, and testes may be simulated with inflatable prostheses. Adjunctive procedures may include subcutaneous mastectomy to improve body contour. Liquid silicone has been injected into the vocal cords to deepen the voice.

References

Historical Background

Esser, J. F. S.: Island Flaps, *NY Med J,* **106:**264, 1917.

Gersuny, R.: Platischer ersatz der Wangenschleimhaut, *Zentrlbl Chir,* **14:**706, 1887.

Gillies, H. D.: The Tubed Pedicle in Plastic Surgery, *NY Med J,* **111:**1, 1920.

Lawson, G.: On the Successful Transplantation of Portions of Skin for the Closure of Large Granulating Surfaces, *Lancet,* **2:**708, 1870.

Maltz, M.: "Evolution of Plastic Surgery," Froben Press, New York, 1946.

Ollier, Leopold Louis Xavier Edouard: Sur les greffes cutanées ou autoplastiques, *Bull Acad Med Paris,* **1:**243, 1872.

Rogers, P. O.: Historical Development of Free Skin Grafting, *Surg Clin North Am,* **39:**289, 1959.

Tagliacozzi, Gasparo: "De curtorum chirugia per insitionem," libri duo, Gaspari Bindonus, Jr., Venice, 1597.

Thiersch, C.: Über Hautverpflanzung, *Verh Dtsh Ges Chir,* **15:**17, 1886.

Von Graefe, C. F.: "Rhinoplastik, oder die Kunst den Verlust der Nase organisch zu ersetzen in ihren früheren Verhaltnissen erforscht und durch neue Verfahrungsweisen zur hoheren Vollkommenheit gefordert," Berlin, 1818.

Wolfe, J. R.: A New Method of Performing Plastic Operations, *Br Med J,* **2:**360, 1875.

Technical Considerations

Bakamjian, V. Y., Culf, N. K., and Bales, H. W.: The Versatility of the Medially Based Delto-pectoral Skin Flap in Primary Reconstruction in Head and Neck Surgery, *Trans 4th Int Cong Plast Surg (1967) Amsterdam,* Excerpta Medica Foundation, New York, 1969, p. 808.

Barron, J. H., and Emmett, J. J.: "Subcutaneous Pedicle Flaps," *Br J Plast Surg,* **18:**51, 1965.

Brobyn, T. J., Cramer, L. M., Hulnick, S. J., and Kodsi, M. S.: Facial Resurfacing with the Limberg Flap, *Clin Plast Surg,* **3:**481, 1976.

Brown, J. B., and McDowell, F.: "Skin Grafting," 3d ed., J. B. Lippincott Company, Philadelphia, 1958.

Cronin, T. D.: The Use of a Molded Splint to Prevent Contracture after Split Skin Grafting on the Neck, *Plast Reconstr Surg,* **27:**7, 1961.

Daniel, R. K., and Taylor, G. I.: Distant Transfer of an Island Flap by Microvascular Anastomoses, *Plast Reconstr Surg,* **52:**111, 1973.

———, and Williams, H. B.: The Free Transfer of Skin Flaps by Microvascular Anastomoses, *Plast Reconstr Surg,* **52:**16, 1973.

Ger, R.: Surgical Management of Ulcerative Lesions of the Leg, *Curr Probl Surg,* p. 1, March, 1972.

Grabb, W. C., and Myers, M. B.: "Skin Flaps," Little, Brown and Company, Boston, 1975.

————, and Smith, J.: Plastic Surgery: A Concise Guide to Clinical Practice, Little, Brown and Company, Boston, 1968.

————, Ohmori, K., and Ohmori, S.: Successful Clinical Transfer of Ten Free Flaps by Microvascular Anastomosis, *Plast Reconstr Surg,* **53:**259, 1974.

————, ————, and Shuhei, T.: Free Gracilis Muscle Transplantation, with Microneurovascular Anastomosis for the Treatment of Facial Paralysis, *Plast Reconstr Surg,* **57:**133, 1976.

Ikuta, Y., et al.: Free Muscle Transplantation by Microsurgical Technique to Treat Severe Volkmann's Contracture, *Plast Reconstr Surg,* **58:**407, 1976.

Kubacek, V.: Transposition of Flaps on the Face on a Subcutaneous Pedicle, *Acta Chir Plast (Praha),* **2:**108, 1960.

Larson, D. L., Abston, S., Evans, E. B., Dobrkovsky, M., and Linares, H. A.: Techniques for Decreasing Scar Formation and Contractures in the Burned Patient, *J Trauma,* **11:**807, 1971.

Lewis, J. R., Jr.: "The Surgery of Scars," McGraw-Hill Book Company, New York, 1963.

Longacre, J. J.: "Scar Tissue: Its Use and Abuse," Charles C Thomas, Springfield, Ill., 1972.

McCraw, J. B., et al.: Vaginal Reconstruction with Gracilis Myocutaneous Flaps, *Plast Reconstr Surg,* **58:**176, 1976.

————, Dibbel, D. G., and Carroway, J. H.: Clinical Definition of Independent Myocutaneous Vascular Territories, *Plast Reconstr Surg,* **60:**341, 1977.

McFarlane, R. M., Heagy, R. M. R., Aust, J. C., and Wermuth, R. E.: A Study of the Delay Phenomenon in Experimental Flaps, *Plast Reconstr Surg,* **35:**245, 1965.

McGregor, I. A.: Fundamental Techniques of Plastic Surgery, 4th ed., The Williams & Wilkins Company, Baltimore, 1968.

Mathes, S. T., McCraw, J. B., and Vasconez, L. O.: Muscle Transposition Flaps for Coverage of Lower Extremity Defects: Anatomic Considerations, *Surg Clin North Am,* **54:**1337, December, 1974.

Milton, S. H.: Pedicled Skin-Flaps: The Fallacy of the Length: Width Ratio, *Br J Surg,* **57:**502, 1970.

Myers, M. B., and Cherry, G.: Augmentation of Tissue Survival by Delay, *Plast Reconstr Surg,* **39:**397, 1967.

———— and ————: Mechanism of the Delay Phenomenon, *Plast Reconstr Surg,* **44:**52, 1969.

Ohmori, S. (ed.): Microsurgery, in *Trans 6th Int Cong Plast Reconstr Surg,* Sec. 2, p. 33, Masson et Cie, Paris, 1976.

Peacock, E., and Van Winkle, W: Surgery and Biology of Wound Repair, W. B. Saunders Company, Philadelphia, 1970.

Peet, E. W., and Patterson, T. J. S.: The Essentials of Plastic Surgery, F. A. Davis Company, Philadelphia, 1963.

Reinisch, J. F.: The Role of Arteriovenous Anastomosis in Skin Flaps, in W. C. Grabb and M. B. Myers (eds.), "Skin Flaps," p. 81, Little, Brown and Company, Boston, 1975.

Smith, P. J., Foley, B., McGregor, I. A., and Jackson, I. T.: The Anatomical Basis of the Groin Flap, *Plast Reconstr Surg,* **49:**41, 1972.

Taylor, G. I., and Daniel, R. K.: The Anatomy of Several Free Flaps Donor Sites, *Plast Reconstr Surg,* **56:**243, 1975.

Thompson, N.: A Review of Autogenous Muscle Grafts and Their Clinical Applications, *Clin Plast Surg,* **1:**349, 1974.

Vasconez, L. C., Bostwick, J., and McCraw, J. B.: Coverage of Exposed Bone by Muscle Transposition and Skin Grafting, *Plast Reconstr Surg,* **53:**526, 1974.

Facial Trauma

Dingman, R. O., and Natvig, P.: Surgery of Facial Fractures, W. B. Saunders Company, Philadelphia, 1964.

Georgiade, N. G., (ed.): "Plastic and Maxillofacial Trauma Symposium," vol. 1, The C. V. Mosby Company, St. Louis, 1969.

Grabb, W. C.: Emergency Department Facial Injuries, in "Techniques in Surgery." Ethicon, Inc., New Jersey, 1972.

LeFort, R.: Experimental Study of Fractures of the Upper Jaw, *Rev Chir Paris,* **23:**208, 1901; reprinted in *Plast Reconstr Surg,* **50:**497, 1972.

Rowe, N. L., and Killey, H. C.: Fractures of the Facial Skeleton, 2d ed., The Williams & Wilkins Company, Baltimore, 1968.

Mustarde, J. C.: Repair and Reconstruction in the Orbital Region, The Williams & Wilkins Company, Baltimore, 1966.

Head and Neck

Bakamjian, V. Y.: A Two-Stage Method for Pharyngoesophageal Reconstruction with a Primary Pectoral Skin Flap, *Plast Reconstr Surg,* **36:**173, 1965.

————, Culf, N. K., and Bales, H. W.: The Versatility of the Medially Based Delto-pectoral Skin Flap in Primary Reconstruction in Head and Neck Surgery, *Trans 4th Cong Plast Surg (1967) Amsterdam,* Excerpta Medica Foundation, New York, 1969, p. 808.

Bromberg, B. E., Song, I. C., and Craig, G. T.: Split-Rib Mandibular Reconstruction, *Plast Reconstr Surg,* **50:**357, 1972.

Cramer, L. M., and Culf, N. K.: Complications of Radical Neck Dissection, in R. Goldwyn, "The Unfavorable Result in Plastic Surgery: Avoidance and Treatment," Little, Brown and Company, Boston, 1972.

Elliott, R. A.: Rotation Flaps of the Nose, *Plast Reconstr Surg,* **44:**147, 1969.

Gaisford, J. C.: Symposium on Cancer of the Head and Neck, The C. V. Mosby Company, St. Louis, 1969.

MacComb, W. S., and Fletcher, G.: Cancer of the Head and Neck, The Williams & Wilkins Company, Baltimore, 1967.

Rappaport, I., Boyne, P. V., and Nethery, J.: The Particulate Graft in Tumor Surgery, *Am J Surg,* **122:**748, 1971.

Webster, J. P.: Crescentic Peri-alar Cheek Excision for Upper Lip Flap Advancement, *Plast Reconstr Surg,* **16:**434, 1955.

Congenital Anomalies

Bill, A. H.: Branchiogenic Cysts and Sinuses, in C. D. Benson, W. T. Mustard, M. M.: Ravitch, W. H. Snyder, Jr., and K. J. Welch (eds.), "Pediatric Surgery," vol. 1, Year Book Medical Publishers, Inc., Chicago, 1962.

Converse, J. M., Horowitz, S. L., Valauri, A. J., and Montardon, D.: The Treatment of Nasal Maxillary Hypoplasia: A New Pyramidal Naso-orbital Maxillary Osteotomy, *Plast Reconstr Surg,* **45:**527, 1970.

Cronin, T. D., Greenberg, R. L., and Brauer, R. O.: Follow-up Study of Silastic Frame for Reconstruction of External Ear, **42:**522, 1968.

LeMesurier, A. B.: A Method of Cutting and Suturing the Lip

in the Treatment of Complete Unilateral Clefts, *Plast Reconstr Surg,* **4:**1, 1949.

Millard, D. R., Jr., and Pigott, R. W.: Rotation-Advancement in Wide Unilateral Lip Clefts, *Trans 4th Int Cong Plast Surg Rome 1967,* Excerpta Medica Foundation, Amsterdam, 1969, pp. 349–355.

Murray, J. E., and Swanson, L. T.: Mid-Face Osteotomy and Advancement for Cranio-synostosis, *Plast Reconstr Surg,* **41:**299, 1968.

Obwegeser, H. L.: Surgical Correction of Small or Retrodisplaced Maxillae, *Plast Reconstr Surg,* **43:**351, 1969.

Randall, P.: A Triangular Flap Operation for the Primary Repair of Unilateral Clefts of the Lip, *Plast Reconstr Surg,* **23:**331, 1959.

———: A Lip Adhesion Operation in Cleft Lip Surgery, *Plast Reconstr Surg,* **35:**371, 1965.

Skoog, T.: Repair of Unilateral Cleft Lip Deformity: Maxilla, Nose and Lip, *Scand J Plast Reconstr Surg,* **3:**109, 1969.

Tanzer, R., and Converse, J. M.: Deformities of the Auricle, in J. M. Converse (ed.), "Reconstructive Plastic Surgery," vol. II, W. B. Saunders Company, Philadelphia, 1964.

Tennison, C. W.: The Repair of the Unilateral Cleft Lip by Stencil Method, *Plast Reconstr Surg,* **9:**115, 1952.

Tessier, P., Guiot, G., Rogerie, J., et al.: Ostéotomies cranio-naso-orbito-faciales: Hypertélorisme, *Ann Chir Plast,* **12:**103, 1967.

———: Ostéotomies totales de la face. *Ann Chir Plast,* **12:**273, 1967.

Wynn, S. K.: Lateral Flap Cleft Lip Surgery Technique, *Plast Reconstr Surg,* **26:**509, 1960.

Cosmetic Surgery

Brown, J. B., and McDowell, F.: "Plastic Surgery of the Nose," Charles C Thomas Company, Springfield, Ill., 1965.

Denecke, H. J., and Meyer, R.: "Plastic Surgery of Head and Neck," vol. 1, "Corrective and Reconstructive Rhinoplasty," Springer-Verlag New York Inc., New York, 1967.

Edgerton, M. T., Knorr, N., and Hoopes, J.: Psychiatric-Surgical Approach to Adolescent Disturbance in Self Image, **41:**248, 1968.

Webb, W. L., Slaughter, R., Meyer, E., and Edgerton, M. T.: Psychosomatic Medicine: Mechanism of Psychosocial Adjustment in Patients Seeking "Face-Lift" Operation, **27:**183, 1965.

Facial Paralysis

Babcock, W. W.: Standard Techniques for Operations of Peripheral Nerves in Special References to Closure of Large Gaps, **45:**364, 1927.

Beahrs, O. H.: Use of Nerve Grafts for Repair of Defects in the Facial Nerve, *Ann Surg,* **153:**433, 1944.

Conley, J. J.: Treatment of Facial Paralysis, *Surg Clin North Am,* **51:**403, 1971.

Edgerton, M. T.: Surgical Correction of Facial Paralysis, *Am J Surg,* **120:**82, 1970.

Freeman, B. S.: Facial Palsy, in J. M. Converse (ed.), "Reconstructive Plastic Surgery," vol. III, W. B. Saunders Company, Philadelphia, 1964.

Hanna, D. C., and Gaisford, J. C.: Facial Nerve Management in Tumors, *Plast Reconstr Surg,* **35:**445, 1965.

Kessler, L.: Twelfth Nerve to Seventh Nerve Anastomosis for Treatment of Facial Paralysis, *Neurology,* **9:**118, 1959.

Morel-Fatio, D. (ed.): Facial Palsy, in *Trans 6th Int Cong Plast Reconstr Surg,* Sec. 6, p. 330, Masson et Cie, Paris, 1976.

———, and Lalardrie, J. P.: Palliative Surgical Treatment of Facial Paralysis: The Palpebral Spring. *Plast Reconstr Surg,* **33:**446, 1964.

Niklison, J.: Contribution to the Subject of Facial Paralysis, *Plast Reconstr Surg,* **16:**276, 1956.

Rees, T. D., Rhodes, R. D., and Converse, J. M.: The Palliation of Facial Paresis, *Am J Surg,* **120:**82, 1970.

Smith, J. W.: Advances in Facial Nerve Repair, *Surg Clin North Am,* **52:**1287, 1972.

Sunderland, S., and Cossar, D. F.: The Structure of the Facial Nerve, *Anat Rec,* **116:**147, 1953.

Thompson, N.: Autogenous Free Grafts of Skeletal Muscle, *Plast Reconstr Surg,* **48:**11, 1971.

———: Investigation of Autogenous Skeletal Muscle Free Grafts in the Dog: With a Report on a Successful Free Graft of Skeletal Muscle in Man, *Transplantation,* **12:**353, 1971.

———: Treatment of Facial Paralysis by Free Skeletal Muscle Grafts, *Trans 5th Int Cong Plast Reconstr Surg Aust 1971,* Butterworth Scientific Publications, London, p. 660.

Miscellaneous Procedures

Broadbent, T. R., and Woolf, R. M.: Augmentation Mammoplasty, *Plast Reconstr Surg,* **40:**517, 1967.

———, ———, and Toksu, E.: Hypospadias: One-Stage Repair, *Plast Reconstr Surg,* **27:**154, 1961.

Browne, D.: An Operation for Hypospadias, *Proc R Soc Med,* **42:**466, 1949.

Conway, H., and Smith, J. W.: Breast Plastic Surgery: Reduction Mammoplasty, Mastopexy, Augmentation Mammoplasty and Mammary Construction, *Plast Reconstr Surg,* **21:**8, 1958.

Cronin, T. D., and Greenberg, R. L.: Our Experiences with Silastic Gel Breast Prosthesis, *Plast Reconstr Surg,* **46:**1, 1970.

Edgerton, M. T., and Meyer, J. K.: Surgical and Psychiatric Aspects of Transexualism, in C. Horton (ed.), "Plastic and Reconstructive Surgery of the Genital Area," p. 117, Little, Brown and Company, Boston, 1973.

Griffith, B. H., and Schultz, R. C.: Prevention and Surgical Treatment of Recurrent Decubitus Ulcers in Patients with Paraplegia, *Plast Reconstr Surg,* **27:**248, 1964.

Hoopes, J. E., Edgerton, M. T., and Shelley, W.: Organic Synthetics for Augmentation Mammoplasty: Their Relation to Breast Cancer, *Plast Reconstr Surg,* **39:**263, 1967.

Horton, C. E., and Devine, C. J.: Hypospadias and Epispadias, *Ciba Found Symp,* **24:**2, 1972.

Maliniac, J. W.: "Breast Deformities and Their Repair," Grune & Stratton, Inc., New York, 1950.

McCormack, R. M.: Simultaneous Chordee Repair and Urethral Reconstruction for Hypospadias, *Plast Reconstr Surg,* **13:**257, 1954.

Strombeck, J. O.: Breast Reconstruction: I. Reduction Mammoplasty, *Mod Trends Plast Surg,* **1:**237, 1964.

Webster, J. P.: Mastectomy for Gynecomastia through a Semicircular Intra-areolar Incision, *J Surg,* **124:**557, 1946.

Chapter 52

Rehabilitation

by J. Herbert Dietz, Jr., and Howard A. Rusk

PRINCIPLES OF REHABILITATION

The principles of rehabilitation are those of readaptation of each disabled individual to the situation and the setting in which he or she must survive, with maximum independent function, comfort, and emotional support, for whatever time of life is allowed. This entails the setting of an appropriate goal—whether preventive, restorative, supportive, or palliative—for each person. All patients are candidates for appropriate effort directed toward adaptation to disability or distress. Rehabilitation is a dynamic concept and active program.

Following severe trauma or surgical treatment, there is an increased nitrogen loss in peripheral skeletal muscles, the principal nitrogen donor, resulting in a decrease in muscle mass. Since much of physical therapy is directed toward use or reeducation of muscle, nitrogen intake during this phase is important. Planning and regulation of oral or parenteral nutrition may become an essential part of the rehabilitation process.

Disabilities result from the interference by disease with bodily functioning and control, or they may follow trauma or result from surgical procedures, radiation therapy, chemotherapy, or immunotherapy.

Disabilities may be primary or secondary. Primary disability is a direct result, while secondary disability arises from restrictions and conditions which evolve in the course of treatment and convalescence. Primary disabilities include loss of limb, sensory perception, motor function, or communication; restriction in cardiopulmonary reserve; impaired vision; or alterations in organ function. Secondary disabilities include muscle atrophy, joint contraction, osteoporosis, urinary calculi, phlebothrombosis, pneumonia, decubitus ulcers, and psychologic deterioration.

Inactivity in bed results in 3 percent loss of strength and endurance daily. The value of early postoperative mobilization was demonstrated in 1893 by Emil Ries and reconfirmed by John H. Powers in the light of modern science. Nutritional intake during inactivity is converted primarily to fat, while under the influence of programmed exercising, muscle-mass improvement results.

TECHNIQUES OF REHABILITATION

Rehabilitation should begin at the earliest possible opportunity, at times in the preoperative period, and should continue throughout the entire course of care until maximal benefit is achieved. Treatment measures should be directed toward appropriate care for any disability, as soon as recognized, and toward the reduction or prevention of predictable disability, whenever possible. Prompt assessment of the entire clinical picture of the disabled patient will permit the setting of an appropriate rehabilitation goal of prevention, restoration, support, or palliation. Rehabilitation of the patient is best conducted by a team which may include physicians, surgeons, physiatrists, psychiatrists, nurses, physical therapists, social workers, orthotists or prosthetists, and volunteers. The family should be involved, whenever appropriate, in the acceptance of and assistance to the patient with emotional, cosmetic, or physical disability.

Basic techniques include (1) physical therapy; (2) occupational therapy; (3) training in activities of daily living (A.D.L.); (4) application of mechanical devices including splints, braces, prostheses, and ortheses; (5) educational, vocational, and psychosocial services.

Physical Therapy

EXERCISES AND MUSCLE REEDUCATION

1. Objectives of exercise:
    a. Power. Exercises for power are based on maximal active effort with few repetitions and are especially helpful where atrophy is the result of disease.
    b. Endurance. Exercises for endurance are designed to increase tolerance. They are based on submaximal effort with many repetitions and are especially useful following a period of convalescence.
    c. Coordination. Exercises for coordination are designed to develop an efficient pattern of function. They are based on the principle that practice and repetition lead to precision in performance.
    d. Range of motion. Exercises designed for maintaining or increasing range of motion are of value whenever there is limitation or potential limitation of normal range from any cause.
    e. Speed. Exercises for speed are designed to shorten activity time. Speed is attained by frequent repetition of functional activities during the final phase of the rehabilitation program.
2. Types of exercise:
    a. Passive. Exercise accomplished by the therapist or apparatus with no active participation by the patient. The main purpose is to prevent contractures by maintaining the normal range of joint motion.
    b. Active assistive. Exercise accomplished by active voluntary movement by the patient with the assistance of the therapist or mechanical device. This is the first step in a program of muscle reeducation. The use of mechanical or hydrotherapeutic modalities is often prescribed during this phase of treatment.
    c. Active. Free exercise accomplished by the patient without either assistance or resistance.
    d. Resistive active. Exercise accomplished by the patient against added resistance, either manual on the part of the therapist or by the use of mechanical resistance. Resistive exercises are usually given when a muscle is rated "good" to "normal." The major effect of any resistive exercise program is the development of strength, and the exercises must be graduated to the patient's tolerance.
    e. Stretching. Exercises accomplished by applied force, either vigorous and of short duration or moderate and prolonged. The therapeutic use of stretching is designed to restore the normal range of motion where limitation of this range is due to loss of elasticity of the soft tissue.
    f. Functional. Exercises that are the foundation for a training program in functional performance. They may be done in the patient's bed, on an exercise mat, on a training apparatus unit, on parallel bars, or on crutches and include techniques of ambulation.
    g. Special exercises. Included are breathing exercises and coughing, which are useful to correct or minimize respiratory function deficit, eliminate secretions, improve alveolar ventilation, and maintain a clear airway. The patient is taught to put forth repeated slow and gentle maximal effort during inspiration and to utilize the diaphragm to full extent. Strengthening exercises for the abdominal muscles are of help in the presence of restrictive or obstructive lung disease. Proper voluntary coughing, with appropriate splinting, and regional costal expansion are taught, with consideration given to the patient's functional needs and restrictions and to whether it is before or after the operation. When the patient requires the assistance of a respirator, he can be taught to perform glossopharyngeal breathing for use during periods when he must be off the respirator. The patient who has been given a tracheostomy should be instructed in adequate "huffing" to clear secretions.

AMBULATION

Training in adequate ambulation with or without supportive devices such as crutches, walker, or canes and with or without bracing is part of physical therapy. Ambulation training is necessary for patients with neuromuscular dysfunction, including ataxia, and for those who have lost the use of a leg, either temporarily due to injury or local surgery or permanently due to amputation. If there is leg-length discrepancy following trauma or surgery, or if the patient cannot clear a cast or splint, a lift under the shoe on the uninvolved side will facilitate walking.

HEAT

Heat may be used to relieve pain, increase circulation, or increase the local metabolic activity. The physiologic effects of heat are most applicable in lesions affecting the musculoskeletal system such as bursitis, arthritis, myositis, tenosynovitis, tendinitis, fractures, dislocations, contusions, sprains, and strains. Externally applied heat causes vasodilatation and an increase in circulation. Sedation, relief of pain, and reduction in muscular tension may also result.

Heat is not used in acute inflammation or acute trauma until the initial reaction has subsided. Obstructed venous or arterial circulation present definite contraindications, and heat must be cautiously applied when the circulation is even partially impaired. The increase in circulation and capillary engorgement associated with heat therapy creates a tendency toward the formation of edema. Heat alone is not used over areas involved by neoplastic disease, except in conjunction with radiation therapy. The use of thermotherapy in cancer treatment is still under investigation. Heat is contraindicated in the presence of noninflammatory edema. Special precautions should be taken when sensation is absent or impaired and when an infant or psychotic patient is unable to report the onset of unpleasant sensation of heat. The therapeutic application of heat usually involves radiant, conductive, or conversive mechanisms.

SUPERFICIAL HEAT. The increase in temperature is maximal in the skin, with no significant rise in temperature occurring beyond 1 to 2 cm depth of tissue. Most sources of superficial heat require from 20 to 30 minutes to produce the desired effect. Commonly used means of therapeutic application include luminous or nonluminous radiation and various forms of dry or moist heat. Effects are superficial and topical or reflex.

Infrared Radiation. A simple and safe device for applying infrared radiation to fairly large areas, such as the back or both thighs, is the luminous heat "baker." The baker consists of several luminous bulbs mounted in the center of a semicircular metal reflector on adjustable legs. The intensity can be varied by changing the distance from the lamp to the skin. The patient should feel comfortably warm, and at the end of the treatment period, the skin should be warm, pink, and moist.

Hydrotherapy. Heat given by immersion in warmed water has some advantages over radiant heat. The buoyancy of the water provides gentle support without hindering movement.

Whirlpool Bath. The usual temperature ranges from 102 to 104°F except where there is an impairment of circulation, in which case the water temperature should not exceed 100°F. It is indicated principally for the treatment of extremities and can be used where there are open wounds and denervated areas. One disadvantage is that the immersed extremity is dependent and edema may develop.

Whirlpool provides heat, gentle massage, relief of pain, muscular relaxation, and assists in debridement. When used with a large tub, it is useful in the treatment of burns and decubitus and other ulcers, and in facilitating performance of range of joint motion exercises.

Hubbard Tank. All of the body except the head and neck is immersed in heated water at a temperature of 98 to 104°F. The water is usually agitated gently like the whirlpool. It provides a means of giving heat and gentle exercise and is especially useful where disease or disability affects many joints of the body or where burns, ulcerations, or denervated areas exist.

Hot Packs. These are effective in the relief of tenderness and muscle spasm, for localized areas, and for reflex vasodilation in the lower extremities from lumbar region application. Moist rather than dry heat is used.

Paraffin. Application is especially useful in localized or chronic joint diseases such as arthritis.

DEEP HEAT. Deep heat sources include ultrasound, microwave, and ultra-short-wave diathermy. The most effective agent for heating of periarticular tissues is ultrasound, and because of its characteristics it is safe to use in the presence of implanted metallic pins, plates, or prostheses. Muscle heating is obtained through use of microwave or short-wave diathermy.

Deep heat is contraindicated when there is a bleeding tendency, over a pregnant uterus, and over a fracture site before callus has formed. Microwave therapy should not be used over superficial accumulations of fluid and should be applied cautiously over growing or superficial bones, over eyes and testes, and when metal is present in the area. Ultrasound is contraindicated in or about the brain, eyes, ears, nasal sinuses, heart, reproductive organs, and epiphyses of growing bones. It should be used with caution over large nerves.

COLD THERAPY. Ice bags, cold-water bags, and cold compresses are used to minimize the initial reaction of tissues to local traumatic injuries such as contusions and sprains. It has been suggested that the beneficial effects of ethyl chloride spray for painful joints and muscles are due to direct and reflex effects of the change in tissue temperature produced by the spray. Induced hypothermia and refrigeration anesthesia for surgical purposes are widely used, but these phases of cold therapy are not within the scope of this chapter.

ULTRAVIOLET. Decubitus ulcers and some indolent ulcers respond favorably to ultraviolet, especially with the use of cold quartz mercury lamps. Ulcers resulting from Raynaud's disease, thromboangiitis obliterans, and chronic varicosities do not respond. Specific contraindications to this therapy are photogenic diseases of the skin, such as pellagra, lupus erythematosus, hydroa aestivale, and xeroderma pigmentosum. Certain antibiotics and other medications result in a photosensitivity which also contraindicates ultraviolet therapy. It has been suggested that ultraviolet should not be used in patients with hyperthyroidism, diabetes, advanced cachexia or inanition, nephritis, or myocarditis.

ELECTROTHERAPY

A variety of currents can be used to stimulate motor and sensory nerves. The interrupted direct and the faradic currents are used mainly for electrodiagnosis. Interrupted direct current may also be used for stimulation of denervated muscles. The therapeutic objective of stimulation for temporarily denervated muscles is to maintain the muscle in as normal a state as possible during the period of nerve recovery. Conduction deficit without denervation (neurapraxia) is usually a temporary condition but may last for several weeks, and stimulation during this period may be of definite benefit. The best results have been obtained with frequent brief periods of stimulation; 25 to 50 contractions a session, four times a day, can be performed by the patient with his own portable battery unit, when he is properly instructed.

MASSAGE

Manual massage exerts the effect of direct displacement of fluid in vascular and lymphatic channels. There is also direct and reflex dilation of the smaller vessels leading to an increase in rate of flow and interchange of substances between bloodstream and tissue cells. Lymphatic flow is assisted and edema is reduced. Mechanical stretching and disruption of connective tissue fibers can be effectively accomplished by the friction type of massage where undesirable fibrosis has occurred in subcutaneous and superficial muscle layers. Light stroking massage results in relaxation of involuntary muscular contraction.

Pain threshold can be increased by slowly increasing stimuli to the central nervous system beginning with light stroking movement and slowly increasing the intensity of the massage. Massage may be used to assist in the accommodation of tissue to pressure, for example, the preparation of an amputation stump prior to the use of a prosthesis. The effect is obtained by progressing from gentle kneading and tapping to firm pounding and weight bearing. Massage will not prevent atrophy or loss of strength

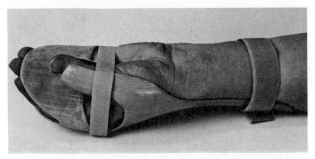

Fig. 52-1. Plastic splint, molded directly or to a positive cast of the patient's hand, maintains the spastic hand in a functional position, preventing flexion contractures of the fingers or thumb.

due to inactivity or denervation, nor will it increase muscular strength. Only active exercise will strengthen muscles. Even the most vigorous massage will not reduce local deposition of fat.

Massage is indicated where the following effects are sought: (1) relief of pain, (2) relaxation of muscle tension, (3) improvement of circulation, (4) reduction of induration or edema, and (5) stretching of adhesions. Local application of heat is commonly used prior to massage, because it enhances the desired effects. Both heat and massage are frequently used prior to active or passive exercise, because the combined effects enable a patient to get maximal benefit from the exercise.

Contraindications for massage include (1) acute inflammation, since massage may result in systemic spread; (2) skin lesions; (3) malignant tumors; (4) acute circulatory disturbances such as phlebitis, thrombosis, or lymphangitis.

Occupational Therapy

Occupational therapy has been described as functional (physical or kinetic), vocational (prevocational therapy or work adjustment), and supportive (psychiatric or diversional). The goals of therapy are (1) to assist in the increase of range of motion of affected joints; (2) to assist in the increase of muscle strength; and (3) to develop motor coordination, skills, and work tolerance.

Fig. 52-2. Molded plastic cuff with a spring-steel pencil clip compensates for loss of opposition in writing. A small extension on the ulnar side permits dialing a telephone or operating a keypunch.

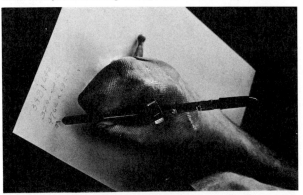

Functions of the upper extremities are concentrated upon. Training is given also to patients with upper extremity prostheses or orthoses in the proper use of the particular device and its application to the activities of daily living and of work.

The purposes of vocationally oriented occupational therapy are (1) prevocational evaluation for the patient who has never had a vocation or vocational objective; (2) a vocational exploration utilizing present physical capacities for the patient who may need to consider changing vocations because of his disability; (3) work adjustment for the patient needing to regain lost work skills, habits, or tolerance; and (4) development of skills for the patient who is considering a further academic career.

ACTIVITIES OF DAILY LIVING

The purpose of an A.D.L. program is to train the patient to perform his maximum in the daily activities inherent in his life. The degree to which a patient can carry out these activities determines his level of independence. There are three functional abilities required: (1) self-care, (2) mobility, and (3) communication. Activities in daily living are divided into the following groups: (1) bed activities, (2) wheelchair activities, (3) self-care activities, (4) miscellaneous hand activities, (5) ambulation and elevation activities, (6) traveling activities, and (7) kitchen and household activities.

ORTHOTICS AND PROSTHETICS

This is a field of knowledge relating to orthopedic devices which are either static or dynamic in character. Static units provide support and correction and dynamic units actively aid or provide elements of function. These devices can be helpful in promoting self-sufficiency for the patient with permanent, severe disability. They may be directed toward providing positioning and support for extremities, increasing the function of permanently weakened muscles, replacing the function of muscles, and assisting in the control of incoordination (Figs. 52-1 to 52-5).

SPLINTS AND BRACES. These control the action of specific joints to prevent or decrease motion, provide support, maintain position, and prevent contracture. Splints and braces may be used for flaccidity, spasticity, incoordination, contracture, or protection from pain and trauma. Splints may be classified as (1) static, those designed to support the involved segment, to prevent contracture, and to protect a painful, weakened, or injured part; and (2) dynamic, those designed to add active mechanical assistance to therapeutic exercise and functional use.

MANAGEMENT OF PSYCHIATRIC PROBLEMS AND PAIN

Emotional and motivational attitudes can have a decisive effect on the outcome of the rehabilitation process. In about 50 percent of adults with physical disability such factors are of major importance. In children the figures run considerably higher, approximately 75 percent. Important problems which frequently need psychiatric assistance are management of persistent pain and drug addiction, and sexual problems.

Physical disability may be accompanied by pain. Since

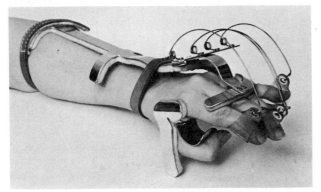

Fig. 52-3. Dorsal cockup splint keeps the wrist in extended position, and the C-bar positions the thumb for better opposition. The lumbrical bar prevents hyperextension of the metacarpophalangeal joints, while the spring-steel outriggers and plastic finger rings encourage finger extension and permit active flexion.

pain can inhibit activities and lead to interpersonal difficulties, its proper management may determine the success or failure of rehabilitation. Pain produces emotional changes even in well-adjusted individuals. It is not a static condition but changes with circumstances. It tends to be exaggerated at night because of fear, aloneness, and absence of diverting interests. Patients vary in their threshold to painful stimuli, and certain disabilities present special problems. In the paraplegic patients, pain *below* the level of the cord lesion is common and can be quite severe, despite total sensory loss below the test level.

Successful management of pain requires accurate medical diagnosis, as well as analysis of psychologic, emotional, and socioeconomic factors. Measures for relief include adequate counseling, the use of nonnarcotic drugs, physical therapy, radiation therapy, anesthetic block, and surgical procedures. The use of acupuncture and transcutaneous neural electrostimulation has been extensively investigated, but dependable, reproducible response has not been documented. Selected patients, especially those with suitable psychological characteristics, may respond to these modalities. Inquiry into the presence of possible sources of painful reaction to life situations should be considered. If methods are properly employed, narcotics can be avoided, and the disabling problem of addiction can be obviated.

In physically disabled persons, sexual function may be interfered with in two ways: (1) local anatomic injury or neurologic deficit, which may make normal sexual functioning impossible, and (2) psychologic changes resulting from the disability, such as doubts about adequacy and attractiveness. A serious problem for both male and female patients is loss of control of bladder and bowel function. When assistance in care is needed from husband or wife, additional sexual problems may result. The presence of a colostomy or the absence of a uterus or breast may cause anxiety and distaste. Maturity and understanding increase adjustive capacity.

SOCIAL SERVICE

The social worker should meet with the patient and his family as soon as feasible following his admission. The

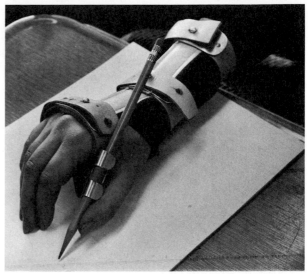

Fig. 52-4. Simple leather and spring-steel dorsal wrist cockup splint has a double dorsal leather strip into which spring-steel bands are inserted. The number required depends on the weight of the hand and the degree of residual wrist extension. A palmar pocket holds standard eating and grooming utensils, typing sticks, or an adapted pencil holder.

Fig. 52-5. Wrist-driven flexor hinge splint utilizes residual wrist power to obtain pincer or three-point grasp between the thumb, index, and middle fingers or gross grasp employing the thumb web space. A rachet on the metal bar locks for static holding and releases with slight pressure.

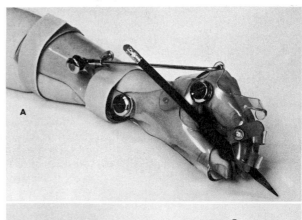

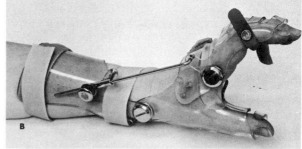

interview has many purposes: (1) to give the patient and his family information and understanding regarding the services that are available to him; (2) to evaluate from the patient's social history his environmental resources and his abilities to utilize the services; (3) to refer the patient and his family to the appropriate resource, outside the hospital, for alleviating environmental problems.

In permitting the patient to adjust to interpersonal relations and relative independence, vocational evaluation and counseling may be employed. Returning the patient to his home environment as a fully functioning member may necessitate preparation of special home programs.

VOCATIONAL REHABILITATION

Vocational rehabilitation assistance should be sought for any patient whose residual disability limits his capacity to return to his previous occupational activity or potential.

Directly or through the medical social worker, the patient can be referred to the State Vocational Rehabilitation Service counselor for evaluation, guidance, and eligible financial support for definitive treatment, rehabilitation therapy, and any indicated training or retraining for work. This includes driver training for the handicapped driver and provision of needed controls for the car.

REHABILITATION OF PATIENTS WITH SPECIFIC PROBLEMS

Musculoskeletal Problems

Programs are directed at the goals of efficient function with painless and free motion, good alignment and posture, and adequate coordinated muscular control. Deformities are prevented by immobilizing affected parts in optimal position, supervising bed posture, and avoiding unnecessary fixation of the joints. The function of uninvolved parts should be maintained, and this may involve electrical stimulation of the muscles which patients cannot move. Mobilization is carried out as early as possible without jeopardizing healing. This program will retard atrophy, prevent permanent scar formation, preserve joint range of motion, stimulate reciprocal muscle function, and reduce the extent of the disability. Pain should be relieved before performing any therapeutic exercises. The patient's weaknesses should be protected by avoiding activities for which he does not have the required strength and by using splints and braces when needed.

Involved muscles are treated specifically with selective exercise, while involved joints are treated extremely gently, avoiding forced motions and combining complete rest with short periods of motion of the painful joints. The plan is carried out as early as possible. Limited weight bearing may be achieved in deep water in a therapeutic pool or using parallel bars, a walker, or crutches.

FRACTURES

During the period of required fracture immobilization, the major goal of rehabilitation is directed toward the prevention of osteoporosis, atrophy of muscles, contracture of ligaments, and edema of soft tissue. Immobilization should be limited to include only the joints proximal and distal to the fracture site. All other joints in the involved extremity should be permitted free motion and carried through their full range at least once daily. With time, this activity should increase.

As soon as possible after cast application, active exercises should be carried out at levels proximal and distal to the immobilized area. Pain should be minimal, and severe pain represents an indication for investigation of the cast or fracture position. At all times, the use of narcotics should be minimized.

Control of swelling and edema is particularly important during the first 5 to 7 days of treatment. Elevation of the involved areas should be started immediately postoperatively and maintained for prolonged periods of time. Application of intermittent massage may relieve the discomfort, aid circulation, and reduce edema.

Isometric muscle-setting exercises are effective, especially when extremities cannot be actively moved. They are of great potential value because of their widespread applicability, but their effective use requires careful planning and explanation to the patient. The precaution of instructing each patient in strict avoidance of breath holding (creating a Valsalva maneuver) during muscle-setting exercises must be observed. Such precaution is to prevent impairment of coronary circulation and possible occlusion. Isometric exercises should be followed, after termination of immobilization, by active exercise through full range of motion. In the lower extremity, isometric quadriceps exercises are directed at preventing loss of stability of the knee. In the upper extremities, attention is particularly directed toward hand function and prevention of contracture of the fingers. In all these situations rehabilitation should be initiated within 24 hours after treatment of the injury, sequentially employing passive motion, isometric exercises, and active exercises.

Immediately following cast removal, active exercises should be started with direction toward return of full joint range of motion.

Current concepts of care for patients with metastatic bone cancer with impending or actual pathological fracture have introduced procedures of hip replacement and intramedullary nailing and use of methylmethacrylate which allow the patients to regain activity on a schedule similar to that offered patients after procedures for trauma, arthritis, or aseptic necrosis.

JOINT DISABILITIES

TRAUMATIC ARTHRITIS. Joint damage may result from a single major trauma, such as a fracture extending into the joint space, but more commonly it follows from repeated small traumas. The latter may be related to occupational stresses, joint instability, postural derangement, or torn ligaments. The arthritic joint has a decrease in functional efficiency and range of motion, and movement may be associated with pain and swelling.

Treatment of the traumatic arthritic joint should be directed toward (1) elimination of any residual etiologic factor, (2) relief of pain, (3) therapeutic exercise, and (4) protection of the joint against further wearing. The latter is attained only by reducing the amount of physical work or weight imposed on the damaged joint structure. Definitive therapy includes physical activity, therapeutic exercises to build periarticular muscle power and the dependent joint stability to a maximum, and transfer of stress to other uninvolved joints through the use of such measures as shoe lifts, stabilizing supports, crutches, canes, braces, and energy-saving devices.

INFECTIOUS ARTHRITIS. In the acute active phase of the infection, the objectives of physical medicine are analgesia and the maintenance of motion of the involved joint to prevent deformity. Heat applied locally is usually indicated, and warm, moist heat in the forms of compresses or packs is generally best tolerated. In the less acute phase, hydrotherapy in the form of whirlpool baths or the Hubbard tank may be used more effectively to permit early active exercising. Even in the active phase of a specific infectious arthritis, the involved joint should be carried passively through normal range of motion at least once a day to prevent capsular and tendinous tightening and the development of deformity. Pain sedation with non-narcotic medications and intermittent rest periods should spell the exercise or movement efforts. As the process subsides, an active exercise program should be initiated to maintain normal range of motion and to prevent muscle atrophy.

Following the eradication of the infection, the problem of physical rehabilitation is contingent upon the degree of muscle weakness which has resulted, the range of motion which may have been lost, and the extent of structural intraarticular damage produced by the infection. The first two conditions should be actively treated with stretching and range-of-motion exercises and progressive resistive exercises. Active range-of-motion exercises or use may prevent intraarticular damage from causing increasing range restriction.

AMPUTATIONS

In the United States, more than 75 percent of lower extremity amputations are performed in treatment for peripheral vascular disease problems on individuals over the age of sixty. Since many people in this age group fail to achieve even the minimal standards of success with the use of prostheses, it is necessary to be selective in the planning of rehabilitation programs. Most of the failures can be directly attributed to medical factors such as (1) coexisting cardiovascular disease or advanced peripheral vascular disease in the unamputated extremity; (2) personal factors such as lack of insight, motivation, or opportunity in the use of a prosthesis; or (3) the prosthesis itself, which may be ill-conceived or improperly prescribed for the patient's individual needs. Diagnoses of cancer and trauma account for about 10 percent each of the remaining amputations performed.

Successful physical and vocational rehabilitation is dependent upon (1) the reason for the amputation, (2) general health and the presence or absence of other disabilities, (3) the level and characteristics of the amputation stump, (4) personal characteristics of the individual,

(5) preparation for function, (6) prescription for the prosthesis, (7) the quality of training with the prosthesis and the nature of rehabilitation facilities available to the patient. Rehabilitation of the amputee is achieved through the following progressive procedures:

PRELIMINARY ORIENTATION. The patient and his family should be informed in general terms regarding the future procedures and estimated timetable.

SURGERY.* The amputation stump in most cases is the key to determining whether or not the patient will be successful in developing skill with a prosthesis. The surgeon is responsible for creating a stump which tapers from above downward and in which all the tissues have been treated in such a manner that the patient can be fitted with conventional prosthetic equipment, leading to a high degree of function.

Each of the tissues encountered in the amputation can be responsible for creating a problem formidable enough to interfere with good function. Flexion contractures are often created by closing amputation stumps with the proximal joint in acute flexion. No tension should exist in the skin closure. Skin flaps which are tightly stretched across the end of the stump remain painful and often break down under conditions of function. The fascia should be used as a barrier between the deep tissues and the skin flaps, so that the skin flaps remain freely movable over the end of the stump. The muscles must be anchored down to, and in some instances in the form of myofascial flaps across, the end of the bone, so that they provide good control and do not retract upon movement of the stump. Such myodesis or myoplasty is particularly mandatory when immediate postoperative application of a prosthesis is planned for the above- or below-knee amputee. The bone requires accurate cutting without piling up the periosteum at the end, since this inevitably will result in the development of exostosis, which may create pain with the use of the prosthesis.

Hemostasis during and after surgical procedures is an extremely important factor. The accumulation of hematoma under the skin flaps not only may jeopardize healing of the wound but may eventually result in a hard, painful scar which can interfere with comfort. Nerves should be pulled down and cut as high as possible, so that they are not incorporated in the scar at the end of the stump. All severed nerves form neuromas, but when a neuroma is in the scar or low in the stump where it may be compressed against the solid wall of a prosthesis, it can become extremely painful and may preclude the possibility of the amputee's developing tolerance for weight bearing. The postoperative dressing is related to hemostasis, and if an efficient compressive dressing or the cast for an immediate prosthesis cannot be applied, drainage should be employed.

The degree of function achieved with a prosthesis is directly proportional to the amount of the functioning limb

---

* Adapted from Allen R. Russek, management of Lower Extremity Amputees, *Arch Phys Med Rehabil,* vol. 42, September, 1961; and E. M. Burgess, R. L. Romano, and J. H. Zettle, "Management of Lower Extremity Amputations," U.S. Government Printing Office, Publication TR10-6, August, 1969.

remaining. In the upper extremity, the general principle holds of saving as much bone length as possible. Myoelectric control units are still experimental, and claims vary, but usefulness is limited to below-elbow-level amputees.

Standard sites of amputations are recognized. In the upper extremity, the most proximal amputation is the interscapulothoracic or forequarter amputation. Below that level there are standard amputations of disarticulation at the shoulder, above-elbow or below-elbow amputations, disarticulation at the wrist, and partial-hand amputations. Amputations of individual digits, especially through the thumb and index finger, may require special surgical reconstructive procedures following the initial surgical procedure. Finger and thumb stumps may be built out and webbed spaces deepened to improve ultimate hand function.

In the lower extremity, the standard amputations are the hemipelvectomy, hip disarticulation, above-knee and below-knee amputations, Syme amputation, and partial foot amputations. Amputations within 2 in. immediately above or below the knee are undesirable. When amputating above the knee it is preferable to sever the bone not closer than 4 in. from the knee joint. This makes it possible to use conventional prosthetic equipment, whereas if the amputation is performed closer to the knee joint, there may be asymmetry of the position and function of the normal and prosthetic knee joints. Very short stumps of less than 2 in. below the knee create frequent interference with anatomic knee function and satisfactory prosthetic fit and function.

Because of the appearance of the prosthesis, the Syme amputation is frequently unacceptable to women. However, it is a good amputation for men. Partial foot amputations result in a complicated weight-bearing stump and have the tendency to break down, particularly following trauma. They are seldom selected, and amputation is more often performed at a Syme level.

Successful translumbar amputation (hemicorporectomy) has been performed by disarticulation at the L_4-L_5 or L_5-S_1 levels, with prosthetic replacement and rehabilitation to complete independence including ability to drive a car.

STUMP AND PREPROSTHETIC STAGE. The muscles of the amputation stump and the remaining limb should be strengthened. It is necessary to make sure that all the joints can be carried through their full range of motion with control. The patient's ability to balance independently on the remaining leg should also be noted. Training should be given with crutches for standing and balance and eventual ambulation on the remaining limb. It is necessary that the patient achieve a safe, stable, and secure crutch-walking gait without pain in the calf of the remaining leg and without the development of dyspnea from effort. The patient's posture on the remaining leg and the stability of his pelvis are very important to develop and control. Excessive weight is a serious problem and requires a positive approach.

Immediate postoperative or early postoperative (within 14 days) application of a lower extremity prosthesis provides excellent concomitant stump conditioning and shaping. The snug cast and early partial weight bearing are positive forces and increase control, utilize proprioception, and limit phantom sensations.

When techniques for the early application of the prosthesis are not used, the stump requires conditioning, shaping, shrinkage, and a full range of motion in the proximal joints. Conditioning of the stump is achieved by a graded program of exercise: at first gentle active, later assistive, and finally resistive exercises. For midthigh amputations it is important to make sure that there is no flexion or abduction contracture at the hip and that all the muscles controlling the amputation stump and the leverage of the stump are strong and reliable. Shrinkage of the tissues and shaping of the stump are accomplished by means of proper wrapping with elastic bandages and/or use of elastic stump-shrinking socks.

Wrapping of the proximal mass of tissues is as important as wrapping the distal tissues, since the anatomic points of fitting are proximal rather than distal and these will shrink rapidly with the use of prosthesis and should be prepared prior to the application of the prosthesis. Most patients are unable to apply the bandage properly by themselves. The repeated encircling of the limb with turns of elastic bandage can actually constitute a tourniquet. Bandaging should be tight, with exertion of pressure only distad. The proximal turns should be relatively loosely applied, as they are used only to hold the wrapping in place. Elastic stump-shrinking socks are preferred. These have a predetermined degree of compression necessary for shaping and shrinkage of the stump and are far superior to bandaging by an inexperienced patient or attendant. Wrapping or shrinker socks must be carried high on the stump to eliminate formation of bulging flesh at the top.

PERSONAL CHARACTERISTICS OF THE AMPUTEE. Throughout the management of the patient, his personal characteristics require understanding. His type of employment should be considered. The age of the patient is an important factor, and his insight, understanding, ability to cooperate, and motivation require detailed attention and a positive approach. When personality problems present themselves, investigation of the psychologic factors associated with this difficulty is essential, if the patient does not emerge from this state voluntarily by gaining confidence.

PRESCRIPTION FOR A PROSTHESIS. The prescription is based upon individual needs. Components prescribed should provide the degree of function and stability needed. Patients with good potentials are given prescriptions which allow unobstructed use of all joints in conventional alignment. Others will need limited function components and added assistive devices. Prescription is best made with the advice of a physiatrist or prosthetist.

TRAINING. Training is a graded procedure and should begin by making the patient familiar with the prosthesis. He then learns to care for the prosthesis and keep it clean, to utilize and wash stump socks, to maintain good hygienic care of the skin, and to avoid stresses on the remaining limb. The achievement of skill requires practice and effort, and the patient should be informed of the need for his participation in the training program. When the prescription for the prosthesis is made, some estimate of the expected achievements of the patient should be established. It is obvious that not all patients reach a safe, acceptable level of function. The classifications of function are important to recognize, and each patient should be informed as to his potential and his individual goal.

Class 1—full restoration. This indicates that the individual has been functionally restored and trained with his prosthesis. Despite his physical handicap, he is able to function maximally. Few people attain such an objective.

Class 2—partial restoration. The patient who achieves this level of function, when trained with a proper artificial limb, will be able to work. He may possibly have to make changes in his job. He lives a normal life, may dance or even play golf, but he has very definite limitations in nonessential areas.

Class 3—self-care plus. While people in this class are disabled and have physical limitations, they are capable of doing everything for themselves in terms of their personal needs. Many are able to work at jobs that do not require much standing and walking. They give up competitive sports and long walking, but they are still able to maintain a satisfactory degree of function, which permits them to live without modification of their normal standards. They may require fairly frequent services of the prosthetist to keep the prosthesis in a satisfactory serviceable condition.

Class 4—self-care minus. People in this category are better off with a prosthesis than they are without one. Their best achievement, however, falls somewhat short of taking care of all their needs. They require the help of another person. They have frequent difficulty in maintaining comfort in the artificial limb. People in this class may be quite functional for short periods and may have a tolerance of several hours of the use of the prosthesis but cannot wear it all day. Others may be quite functional all day but are uncomfortable and need to remove the prosthesis from time to time.

Class 5—cosmetic plus. Amputees in this group are better off with a prosthesis than without one, but the difference is quite small. They do little more than they would without the prosthesis, but for personal reasons and appearance the prosthesis serves a definite function. Also in this class are people for whom the prosthesis serves one single function of personal import, such as getting in and out of a car, or standing when changing from one chair to another, or possibly going to the bathroom unassisted.

Class 6—not feasible. There are some patients for whom no clear objective, not even a cosmetic one, justifies the prescription of a prosthesis. In these instances, the patient should be trained to do as much as he can for himself from a wheelchair.

When prescribing a prosthesis for an amputee, it must be understood that the various medical and psychologic problems which affect amputees may detract from their potential function. The amputee suffers from a summation of problems which affect him. If several factors unrelated to each other each interfere with function, he will not achieve a great degree of skill. For example, a patient without motivation and short, above-knee stump with a flexion contracture has three unrelated problems, each of which, on its own, will interfere with function. Awareness of problems which interfere with function will help establish the class in which each patient falls when the prosthesis is prescribed. Establishment of the goal is important, since this determines the extent of training. In addition, it is possible to tell the patient in advance how far he may expect to go, so that he does not hope to achieve more than is possible.

IMMEDIATE AND EARLY PROSTHETIC FITTING. Efforts can frequently be directed toward fitting patients with temporary prostheses in the operating room. This is preceded by myoplasty or myodesis in the closure of the amputation stump so that all opposing muscle groups are firmly anchored to opposing fascia or to the end of the bone and the amputation stump is shaped in the operating room to accommodate a total contact socket for weight bearing, quadrilateral for the above-knee and patellar tendon–bearing for the below-knee procedure. This has been highly satisfactory for early weight bearing. It does not jeopardize the healing of the wound and is considered by many to enhance healing. Fitting with temporary prostheses in the operating room has resulted in readiness of the patient to wear a permanent prosthesis at between 4 and 6 weeks following major amputation above or below the knee, and a return to work within 2 months.

Another concept is that of early fitting, when only the elastic plaster of paris dressing cover is applied postoperatively. In the normal uncomplicated case, the dressing and sutures are removed after about 2 weeks, and the patient is measured then for a temporary prosthesis. Conditioning, shaping, and shrinking of the amputation stump are accomplished in the ensuing 3 or 4 weeks with the use of the temporary prosthesis. Thereafter, the patient can be fitted with a permanent prosthesis.

UPPER EXTREMITY AMPUTATIONS. Excellent prostheses are now available for patients with upper extremity amputations at any level. These prostheses consist of plastic laminated sockets made from corrected plaster casts of the amputation stumps. They are harnessed by means of a split figure-of-eight strap, one end of which suspends the prosthesis while the other end operates a cable within a housing. The cable in turn activates the functional terminal device, which may consist of one of the available split hooks or a functional hand. Cosmetic hands are also obtainable and are interchangeable with the other terminal devices. Myoelectric control units are still in the experimental stage and are limited principally to below-elbow amputations. It is more difficult to fit patients with certain partial hand amputations where only part of the palm remains, since there is no satisfactory functional equipment for such an amputation. Whenever such a part of a hand is left, if no practical function is achieved below the wrist, it may then be better to disarticulate at the wrist, making it possible to use commercially available prosthetic equipment.

Application of immediate postoperative prosthesis to the upper extremity is limited. Experience has been gained in both below-elbow and above-elbow techniques, however, and the plaster dressing can be fitted with a terminal device with shoulder harness. Rehabilitation is speeded, especially in the case of the double amputee.

AMPUTATIONS IN CHILDREN. Some children are ready to use upper extremity prostheses before three years of age.

Most children learn rapidly and well. The objective for the young child is the achievement of complete physical rehabilitation by the time he enters school. In the management of children who have had an extremity removed because of a malignant tumor, it is generally agreed that the restored function and cosmesis afforded by prosthetic fitting are of practical and psychologic value to both the child and his parents. Data from recent studies indicate that a significant percentage of amputees with malignant tumors survive for 1 to 5 years postoperatively and wear prostheses successfully for 1 year and longer. The majority of these patients are full-time users of their prostheses. If there is no evidence of metastasis and the stump is suitable for fitting, a limb should be provided at the earliest possible date.

HIP-REPLACEMENT SURGERY

Hip-replacement surgery allows postoperative weight-bearing activity earlier than pinning procedures for fractures. Austin-Moore-type prosthetic hips, without an artificial acetabular socket, will allow start of weight bearing by 2 to 3 weeks postsurgery. Acetabular replacement requires an additional 2 to 3 weeks of limited weight bearing. The patient's age, condition of tissues at time of surgery, absence of other diseases, and the basic diagnosis (trauma, osteoarthritis, cancer) need assessment in setting time for progression in activity.

WIDE RESECTION OF EXTREMITY SOFT TISSUE

Wide resection of soft tissue, including muscle groups, fascia, and nerves, creates functional loss directly related to the structures involved. Postoperative rehabilitation, particularly for lower extremity disability, may require prescription of appropriate bracing to stabilize against quadriceps, gastroc-soleus, or anterior tibial muscle deficit. Loss of sensation precludes application of heat and requires attention to foot protection and cover. Forearm soft tissue resections may benefit from supportive static splinting or from a dynamic, functional tenodesis splint to provide grasp through wrist extension, when finger flexors have been lost or resected.

Grafts placed over surgical defects require protection from trauma, particularly during healing in the early postoperative period.

LONG-BONE RESECTION

Long-bone resection, such as total or *en bloc* bone resection for cancer, requires special programming for rehabilitation of the patient. Such a procedure as the Tikhov-Linberg resection of scapula, clavicle, and upper humerus for malignant tumors of the scapular and shoulder region preserves the neurovascular bundle and leaves the patient with a functional forearm, wrist, and hand, limited only by lack of stabilization to the body. Sling and swathe support of the arm and forearm assists the patient in hand use.

The problems which follow long-bone excision and replacement include deficient muscle attachment to the internal prosthetic replacement for movement control and power, minimal cover over the internal prosthesis potenti-

ating infection after skin break, potential fracture of the internal prosthesis, hip joint instability, and prolonged interval prior to allowance of joint activity or weight bearing. These patients can be permitted ambulation, initially without weight bearing and with the support of combined ischial seat and double-bar long leg bracing over a Jordan splint. Subsequent gradual increase in weight bearing in the brace has been successful after 4 to 8 months. Unhandicapped, free use of the limb cannot be expected. Consistent care must be paid toward protection of the skin from injury where it covers the artificial knee joint and the prosthesis.

THE HAND

Rehabilitation of the patient with a poorly functioning hand requires the closest collaboration between the disciplines of surgery and rehabilitation. The benefits of active and passive exercise, heat, massage, and related techniques may not be optimal unless superficial scars, densely adherent tendons, and nerve injuries are repaired. Maximal surgical benefit to the patient will not accrue, in many instances, unless rehabilitation measures are also supplied.

TENDONS AND TENDON TRANSFERS. Freshly lacerated tendons are frequently repaired within the early hours after injury. Should the fear of infection or the loss of superficial tissues dictate delay in repair, such repair may well be postponed for several months. During this time, physiotherapeutic efforts designed to maintain the mobility of the joints and the integrity of the muscles are instituted. Whenever the repair of the involved tendons is carried out, whether early or late, immobilization for about 3 weeks is usually mandatory for the development of firm union at the suture lines. The position of the hand during immobilization will depend in great part upon the nature of the surgical repair, but in general the principle to be followed is to avoid tension at the suture line while keeping the joints, as nearly as possible, in the neutral position of function. Optimal position for immobilization of the hand is in slight dorsiflexion at the wrist, flexion at the metacarpophalangeal joints, minimal flexion of the fingers, and moderate abduction and slight flexion of the thumb. After termination of immobilization, progressive and intensive efforts must be directed toward the reestablishment of function.

In general, the period of rehabilitation following tendon transfer is longer than that following tendon repair or tendon grafting. This is because of (1) the problem of reeducation of the muscles to perform unaccustomed tasks, (2) the usual loss of one grade of power in the muscle of the transferred tendon, and (3) the generally more extensive disability in the patient requiring the tendon transfer.

POSTTRAUMATIC BACK PAIN

Pain in the back may result from single or multiple incidents of external violence, from a pathologic condition of an intervertebral disc, from neoplasm, from excessive effort, and from cumulative prolonged stress and strain. It may develop without apparent cause, perhaps from emotional stress or instability. It is necessary to determine the cause before appropriate treatment can be given.

In the majority of cases of acute strain or sprain of a ligament, the pathologic condition will spontaneously resolve when the local tissue damage has healed. Acute injuries of the back, without damage to the bony structures, usually heal spontaneously under protected conditions of rest and support. When a patient fails to respond to therapy and pain becomes prolonged, detailed reexamination should be performed.

When a positive diagnosis of herniated intervertebral disc has been made, the treatment should be conservative at first, since a significant percentage of cases can be brought under satisfactory control without surgical intervention. If recurrences of pain are frequent or insufficient relief follows conservative treatment, then surgical measures should be considered. Most authorities agree that the best results following surgical treatment are obtained in the patients operated on fairly early. Because of the secondary changes in muscles, posture, habits, and emotional reactions with passage of time, it may be too late for surgical procedures to relieve more than a small part of the complex problem after a case has become chronic.

In general, a patient who has suffered recent back trauma should be placed at rest, muscular spasm released, range of motion of the trunk restored, weight bearing gradually introduced, tolerance to activities developed according to individual needs, and continuous reassurance given to prevent excessive concern. The relief of pain during the treatment period must be achieved in order to permit the patient to cooperate.

The patient should be kept at rest on a firm mattress, preferably on one under which a bed board has been placed. Sedative and analgesic drugs should be used to control pain. Active setting exercises for the gluteal, abdominal, and back muscles should be begun as soon as they can be tolerated. Non-weight-bearing stretching exercises in the bed are sometimes effective in relieving tension from spasm. The use of muscle-relaxant drugs during the acute or chronic stage has not proved effective. When symptoms begin to subside, the use of local heat by means of moist hot packs, tub bath, or Hubbard tank should follow. Focal pain may be relieved by ultrasound application to joint or muscle but not to nerve structures. As the symptoms permit, passive stretching of tight muscles should be attempted. Exercises for 20 minutes in a Hubbard therapeutic tank with the water at 100°F are frequently followed by rapid improvement in range of motion. Occasionally, walking in the deep end of a therapeutic pool restores coordination and elasticity of muscles.

When the patient is capable of resuming activities on a progressive basis, it may be useful to protect the back from the stresses of movement and to support body weight by the use of reinforced belts or braces. The "chair back" and Knight-Taylor types of braces provide best limitation of motion of the thoracic and upper lumbar spine, and a lumbar corset or belt is best for midlumbar and lower lumbar regions (where motion is actually aggravated by the application of a long back brace). The patient should be kept on a sustained program of exercises of increasing intensity, designed to rebalance the supporting musculature of the trunk and pelvis, while he is wearing these

supports. The brace or belt may be removed later, when the patient has a muscular corset of his own sufficient to handle the stresses. If symptoms have been severe and the patient's usual work is strenuous, it may be advisable to discuss a change in occupation in order to avoid recurrence under working conditions. If the patient fails to respond to these methods and chronic back pain persists, he may develop numerous psychogenic superimposed symptoms which complicate the picture. Such patients should obtain the supportive therapy of professional personnel such as psychologists, social workers, vocational counselors, and psychiatrists, when necessary. Chronic or recurrent backache is one of the most frequent symptoms of psychologic and emotional disturbances.

Diseases of the Nervous System

FACIAL PARALYSIS

Although facial paralysis is usually due to idiopathic Bell's palsy, it may be the result of tumor, abscess, or cyst, or a consequence of head and parotid trauma or surgical treatment. The majority of patients with a benign process exhibit spontaneous improvement within 6 weeks after the onset of the paralysis.

Initial treatment is primarily symptomatic and includes local application of warmth to the involved muscles, attention to eye hygiene, and protective glasses or a patch. Gentle perioral and periorbital massage several times daily in front of a mirror is prescribed. The massage should be begun at the medial and inferior margins of mouth or eye, gradually stroking upward with a circular motion in the direction of the muscle fibers. Attempts at volitional movement should be made or practiced regularly with the aid of a mirror. The therapeutic use of electrical stimulation is controversial and is usually not recommended beyond the acute stage. It is considered to be of little value when volitional movement has returned. Facial splints and supports of many types have been designed to prevent stretching and asymmetry. A simple one extends over the ear on the affected side and hooks into the angle of the mouth.

There frequently will be transient synkinetic movement of the platysma or other facial musculature, which may distress the patient. Mild sedation and reassurance are commonly all that is required in managing the patient. If there is no improvement within 2 weeks after the onset of the paralysis, electrodiagnostic studies may prove invaluable in prognosticating recovery or permanence of denervation. If no recovery is seen in 6 weeks, surgical intervention should be considered.

PERIPHERAL NEUROPATHY

Peripheral neuropathy may be caused by nerve trauma including complete division, crushing, stretching, and pressure. Although the disability is primarily due to the resultant muscle paralysis, superimposed contractures and atrophic changes complicate the situation. Proper rehabilitation procedures instituted early can do much to prevent or to correct problems.

Following traumatic interruption of a nerve, suture is essential. Proper subsequent treatment requires an accurate diagnosis of the involved nerve and the extent of the pathologic condition, and knowledge of the motor ramifications. Electrodiagnostic testing techniques are invaluable for this purpose, but the examination is best deferred for 2 or 3 weeks, to allow for possible wallerian degeneration and permit detection of denervation potentials and measure nerve conduction velocity change. In occasional instances, nerve blocks are of diagnostic value, and, in specific instances, surgical exploration may be necessary.

Periodic retesting is necessary in many cases to determine the prognosis. Serial changes in the electrical studies frequently presage obvious clinical improvement. Return of function may be measured clinically by the development and progression of Tinel's sign, alteration in the extent and character of the sensory deficit, retrogression of the vasomotor signs, and gradual return of motor function.

The rehabilitation program for the patient with peripheral nerve involvement must frequently be of long duration, in view of the fact that regeneration occurs from the proximal portion of the nerve and is considered to occur at an average of 1.5 mm/day. The initial approaches are preventive. Passive motions are utilized to prevent joint contractures and the development of adhesions between tendons and their sheaths. These exercises and massage may frequently retard but cannot prevent reduction in muscle volume and tone. Electrical stimulation is also useful for this purpose but in no way appears to influence the rate of neuron regeneration. Special splints, slings, casts, or braces may be needed to prevent overstretching of the muscle by the intact antagonist or by gravity. If these are used, they should be so designed as to allow daily passive movements of the involved joints. Attempts to stimulate the circulation of the involved part consist of gentle massage, the cautious administration of heat with padded hot packs or warm baths, with or without whirlpool.

When voluntary motion begins to return, the program is supplemented by intensive muscle reeducation procedures. At first these are performed with gravity eliminated, but they are gradually increased until progressive resistive exercises are employed.

Causalgia is a distressing symptom which is frequently very difficult to treat. The limb may have to be carefully protected from inclement weather and minor trauma by adequate padding and support. Moist heat and gentle massage may be applied. Despite the discomfort, the importance of passive motion must be emphasized in instructions to the patient, and it should be carried out regularly if at all possible. Nerve block to determine the presence of a neuroma may be considered. Psychotherapy may be indicated. Sympathetic block, followed, if successful, by preganglionic sympathectomy, may be needed to relieve causalgic pain.

SPECIFIC PERIPHERAL NEUROPATHIES. The *long thoracic nerve* may be involved by direct injury, surgical procedure, or sudden stretching; the result is paralysis of the serratus anterior muscle. With the lack of scapular fixation

it is difficult or impossible for the patient to raise his arm above the horizontal level. In selected patients, it has been possible to stabilize the scapula and restore a great deal of arm function by the use of a special brace, designed with firm scapular plates and a firmly affixed breast plate. The *axillary nerve* may be involved by injuries or lesions in the region of the neck of the humerus. During treatment the arm is splinted in a shoulder-abducted position while the usual program for peripheral nerve lesions is instituted. The *musculocutaneous nerve* is seldom involved alone, but it may be injured by direct trauma or dislocation of the head of the humerus. The forearm should be supported by a sling during treatment.

The *radial nerve* is commonly damaged by injuries to the humerus, dislocations in the axilla, or a crutch or other pressures (abduction and pressure on the operating table, malpositioning). A splint providing for extension of the wrist and of the fingers with moderate metacarpophalangeal flexion is essential. Spring and elastic extensions for the fingers, extending over the dorsum of the hand and fixed to a rigid wrist support, or a spring-assisted bar to extend the proximal phalanges of the fingers are used to provide active motion at the metacarpophalangeal joints.

The *median nerve* is most commonly injured in civilian life by lacerations of the wrist. In some cases the ulnar nerve may also be damaged. A splint to keep the thumb in a position of abduction and opposition is recommended. Causalgia may be a serious problem and hamper rehabilitation. The *ulnar nerve* may be involved as the result of injuries in the region of the elbow. A splint designed to posture the hand in a position of flexion at the metacarpophalangeal joints with extension of the interphalangeal (IP) joints is of value.

The *femoral nerve,* although vulnerable to many pathologic processes, is most commonly involved with fractures of the pelvis. The resulting weakness of the quadriceps can be compensated for in many individuals by the use of elastic devices running from the waist or upper thigh to the anterior margin of the lower leg, by special knee braces with spring action to retard knee flexion, or by a long leg brace, depending on the degree of weakness.

The *sciatic nerve* terminates as the common peroneal and tibial nerves. It and its many branches are very susceptible to injury, and one of the complicating features is associated causalgia. The *common peroneal nerve* is frequently injured by trauma involving the upper end of the fibula. Compression bandages also represent common causes. Usually the peroneal muscles are more involved than the anterior tibial group. In addition to providing range of motion, it is necessary to prevent and compensate for foot drop and equinovarus deformity. If the patient is bedridden, the foot may be supported by the use of a posterior molded splint or a footboard. In ambulatory patients, the use of a high-topped shoe is frequently all that is necessary to correct a slight foot drop. In others, a posterior spring brace, made of molded, fitted plastic or of metal, inserted into the shoe heel or attached to a foot plate, is needed to provide support. Occasionally, it is necessary to use a short leg brace with either a spring or a 90° plantar flexion stop at the ankle. The *tibial nerve* is less commonly involved. Care must be taken to prevent the common tendency toward the formation of trophic ulcers. Paralysis of the triceps surae muscles creates gait difficulties and calcaneus deformity of the foot. Short leg braces with stirrup attachment and 90° dorsiflexion stop are needed.

PARAPLEGIA OR QUADRIPLEGIA

The patient with paraplegia or quadriplegia needs a coordinated program designed (1) to prevent decubitus ulcers, (2) to maintain range of motion, (3) to prevent contractures, (4) to improve the power of those muscles which are intact, (5) to strengthen weakened muscles to their maximal capacity, (6) to establish a satisfactory bowel and bladder program, and (7) to reestablish independence in activities of daily living.

Any paralyzed patient, either operative or nonoperative, should, at the onset, be kept in an extended neutral position. Special nursing care, with particular attention to nutrition, skin care, and posture, is mandatory.

SKIN CARE. The patient must be turned at least every 2 hours, day and night, in order to prevent decubitus ulcers. Nurses should inspect the skin carefully over the following pressure points: sacrum, trochanters, iliac crests, ischial tuberosities, knees, and heels. As the patient is turned, these areas should be cleansed very carefully with soap and water, dried gently, and massaged lightly, and a bland oil or neutral ointment should be applied.

CONTROL OF DECUBITUS ULCERS. This requires adequate relief of local pressure by application of surrounding polyurethane foam pads or use of alternating pressure mattresses or pads, multiple bolsters, flotation pads or beds, Stryker frames, or Circle beds. Adequate debridement of slough and frequent changes of dry, soft, sterile dressings aid control or healing. Various dressings from sugar to dried plasma or red cells have been used with success. Hyperbaric oxygen may be beneficial to healing, and application of mild electric currents to ulcer surfaces has aided infection control and granulation.

MAINTENANCE OF RANGE OF MOTION. All joints of the affected extremities should be taken through a complete range of motion twice daily. Patients who have residual muscle power but with some weakness should be encouraged to carry through their range of motion actively, as far as possible, and the therapist should then assist the patient or complete the range of motion with passive movement. These patients are prone to develop short heel cords with subsequent equinus deformity. To prevent this, bedclothes should *not* be pulled down tightly over the foot of the bed. The patient's feet must be kept at right angles to the legs at all times, either by means of a footboard and pillow or sandbag support, or by a carefully padded posterior splint.

THERAPEUTIC EXERCISE. Muscle-strengthening exercises should emphasize conditioning the shoulder depressor, including the latissimus dorsi, and the triceps brachii. These are the muscles which the patient with paraplegia must utilize in order to walk with braces and crutches. Exercises for these muscle groups should be started early and increased in intensity as rapidly as possible.

CONTRACTURES. Prevention of contractures is fundamental. To neglect this preventive procedure may delay rehabilitation by weeks or even months. Special care must be given to the hip and knee joints, where flexion contractures are most prone to occur. These can be prevented by full range-of-motion exercises performed passively twice daily and periods of lying on the abdomen. Prolonged sitting should be avoided. A tilt table can be used to elevate the patient with hips and knees kept in extension. Severe spasticity may be relieved by intramuscular or perineural injection of dilute phenol solution.

DRUGS. Habit-forming narcotics should be avoided, except when absolutely necessary during postoperative periods. Most paraplegic pain can be controlled with a mild analgesic. Persistent pain which is not relieved by these drugs may require neurosurgical or orthopedic intervention. It is virtually impossible to rehabilitate the paralyzed patient who has become addicted to drugs.

EARLY STANDING. Quadriplegic or paraplegic patients should be put in a standing position by means of a tiltboard as soon as possible. Usually this can be accomplished 10 days to 2 weeks following surgical treatment, depending on the clinical condition of the patient. Patients without cord transection, with a hope of return of muscle function but with spine injury that remains unstable, must be carefully protected to avoid further cord damage. Here, it is best to be conservative and withhold tilting.

In the absence of abdominal muscle function, the use of a Scultetus binder or canvas corset with stays is recommended during tilting. At the onset the angle of inclination is usually 20 to 30°. The angle of inclination and length of time that the patient can stand are increased rapidly, so that at the end of 2 to 3 weeks the patient should have reestablished circulatory equilibrium and be able to stand in a vertical position for a minimum of 1 hour daily.

It has been pointed out that an hour of standing each day will help retard osteoporosis in the lower extremities and decrease the incidence of urinary calculi and genitourinary infection, which are frequent causes of death in patients with paraplegia and quadriplegia. Circulation and nutrition, as well as morale, are also aided by keeping the patient in an upright position for several hours each day. When maximal physiologic response has been obtained, plastic repair of decubitus ulcers should be performed.

Bladder and bowel care and training for all paraplegic and quadriplegic patients involves careful initial urologic evaluation, appropriate handling of catheter drainage and irrigation, and training in autonomous or automatic reflex emptying. Adequate fluid intake and control of infection are necessary. Bowel training is less complex and usually requires added glycerine suppositories, occasional enemas, stimulant medications by mouth or rectally, and regular digital stimulation as well as removal of scybala or impaction. Neurogenic uropathy is discussed in detail below.

Upon completion of definitive medical and surgical treatment, the rehabilitation program becomes the primary therapeutic regimen. A full day's program, usually extending from 4 to 6 hours, is indicated. General conditioning exercises performed on the mat should be stressed for 2 to 3 hours daily if the physical condition of the patient is satisfactory. Exercises should be designed to strengthen the muscle groups of the upper extremities, particularly the shoulder depressors and triceps brachii, and the abdominal and trunk muscle groups. The patient is also taught sitting balance. Short sawed-off crutches or wooden blocks may be used to practice push-ups on the mat while sitting. These exercises are designed to prepare the patient for training in transfers, in activities of daily living, and for ambulation with braces and crutches where feasible.

BRACES. Patients with lesions at the T_{10} level and above are usually given double-bar long leg braces with a pelvic band and a Knight spinal attachment for back support. These braces are fitted with sliding box-type locks at the hip and knee joints. The ankle joints should have stirrup attachments to the shoes with a 90° plantar-flexion stop. Patients with lesions from T_{10} to L_1 are given double-bar long leg braces with a pelvic band, and those with lesions below L_1, depending upon the specific functioning muscle groups around the hips, are given ordinary long leg braces. It is better, at first, to prescribe too much bracing than too little.

ACTIVITIES OF DAILY LIVING. The program in activities of daily living includes training in bed, toilet, eating, dressing and undressing, hand, wheelchair, elevation, walking, climbing, and traveling activities.

All quadriplegic and paraplegic patients have emotional and social problems as well as physical disability. Each patient should be seen as early as possible by the social service worker and, when indicated, by the psychologist. As the patient becomes more proficient in his activities of daily living, more and more emphasis should be placed on vocational testing, counseling, and training.

QUADRIPLEGIA. Most of these patients have lesions at the C_6 or C_7 level or above. The patient with traumatic quadriplegia resulting from a cervical fracture or dislocation requires immediate skeletal traction, which is continued for approximately 8 weeks. It may be necessary to provide some type of neck support for 2 to 4 months following removal of traction, particularly if cervical laminectomy has been required.

Extremities should be carried through a complete range of motion of all joints twice daily. Extreme care must be taken by the therapist to protect the vertebral traction. Little can be done at this time toward strengthening the remaining muscles. Modified isometric exercises may be started with care. After the patient is released from traction, gradually placing him in a standing position by means of a tiltboard is initiated. Again, as with the patient with paraplegia, standing an hour or more a day with the use of the tiltboard helps prevent urinary infection and calculi. The majority of patients with quadriplegia are not braced for ambulation.

These patients usually need the care of an attendant. Electric devices are available which can be controlled with the pressure of a shoulder, by one functional muscle in the forearm or elbow, by the touch of the chin or the teeth, by breath impulse, and also by reflected light from the corneas of the eyes to the control units. These devices will operate electric wheelchairs, feeder arm supports, special telephones, and other mechanisms.

NEUROGENIC UROPATHY

Urinary tract complications and infections (see Chap. 40) are the most frequent causes of death in quadriplegic and paraplegic patients. In the beginning, there is stasis which is readily followed by infection. Subsequent to infection, calculus formation, renal obstruction, and gradual loss of renal function ensue as part of the vicious cycle.

Following traumatic lesions of the spinal cord with the stage of spinal shock and also with lower motor neuron lesions involving the posterior sacral roots, the bladder immediately becomes atonic. The detrusor reflex is abolished, and the sensation of fullness is absent. As mechanical pressure overcomes the forces of external urethral resistance, small amounts of urine are emptied periodically. In contrast, lesions affecting both afferent and efferent limbs of the reflex arc leave the bladder completely autonomous and capable of exerting expulsive force by myoneural activity of the vesical ganglionic plexuses within the wall. Emptying is by overflow dribbling only.

In quadriplegic and paraplegic patients with upper motor neuron lesions, spastic reflex bladder occurs following the stage of spinal shock. Bladder capacity in these patients is small, and variable amounts of urine are passed without warning. Occasionally, erection, fullness in the head, and autonomic reactions such as transient hypertension, flushing, or sweating may precede involuntary evacuation of the bladder. In addition, spasticity of the external sphincter may cause interruption of the stream at any point.

The uninhibited neurogenic bladder rarely follows traumatic lesions of the cord and is more commonly associated with acquired lesions of the cerebral cortex as an accompaniment of hemiplegia from tumor or following craniotomy. In this situation, sensation is intact, and there is usually great urgency coupled with an inability to control sphincter contraction with resultant incontinence.

MANAGEMENT. Treatment of the flaccid bladder is by catheterization adhering strictly to the principles of catheter management outlined in Chap. 40. In these patients, a low-grade infection is almost always present, and chemotherapy is directed at preventing acute episodes of urinary tract infections rather than eliminating the low-grade infection. The atonic stage may last for a period of several weeks depending on the level of spinal lesion. Cystometric examination helps define the status of detrusor activity.

Urinary tract complications which are encountered in quadriplegics and paraplegics include cystitis, acute pyelonephritis, formation of calculi, hydronephrosis, and epididymitis. Complications require immediate treatment and control, as urinary tract problems are generally the most serious and dangerous which the patient has to face.

BLADDER TRAINING PROGRAM. In the urologic rehabilitation of the patient with quadriplegia or paraplegia, efforts are directed toward achieving complete or nearly complete evacuation of the bladder. This goal is rarely attained in the paraplegic patient, particularly in those individuals with spastic reflex activity of upper motor neuron lesions. The surgical conversion of upper into lower motor neuron lesions usually results in more predictable bladder function. Even though sensation of bladder fullness is seldom present, the patient may aid emptying by straining and Credé maneuvers performed at regular intervals. The functionally adequate spastic reflex bladder has an unpredictable action, and a majority of patients require some type of external collection apparatus. A variety of surgical procedures have been employed and are directed at the elimination of obstruction and consequent residual urine. These include transurethral resection of bladder neck or prostate, pudendal neurectomy, sacral rhizotomy, spinal cordectomy, and intrathecal alcohol injection.

Transurethral resection is best applied in patients with lower motor neuron lesions in whom voiding is accomplished by straining and Credé maneuvers but where an obstructive outlet pathologic condition is found. Pudendal neurectomy is used in patients with upper motor neuron lesions, particularly at the cervical and upper thoracic levels, to effect relaxation of muscles of the pelvic floor and the external urinary sphincter. The potential efficacy of this procedure can be tested by local anesthetic block of the pudendal nerves.

Anterior and posterior sacral rhizotomy converts an upper motor neuron lesion into a lower motor neuron lesion and may be indicated in paraplegic and quadriplegic patients with severe peripheral spasticity and a spastic reflex bladder. Preliminary sacral nerve blocks can be used to determine the potential value of this procedure. Spinal cordectomy or the intraspinal injection of alcohol represent relatively radical procedures to create a more completely autonomous bladder and are indicated only where no motor function return in the lower extremities can be expected.

Pulmonary and Cardiovascular Procedures

The goals of therapy include (1) improvement in ventilation by techniques of proper breathing and coughing; (2) prevention of postural deformity with maintenance of the strength of neck, shoulder girdle, and upper extremity musculature and range of joint motion; (3) facilitation of bronchopulmonary drainage by postural exercises and coughing. Humidification, bronchodilators, mucolytic agents, and incentive spirometers are frequently employed and directed at these aims. The intermittent positive-pressure breathing (IPPB) machine has been found less useful, except for assistance in administration of nebulized medications and as an adjunct when assistance in respiratory function is needed.

During surgical procedures, muscles may be divided or stretched causing resultant dysfunction, progressive structural scoliosis, and alteration in shoulder girdle mobility. The position of the patient during the operative procedure may be attended by unintentional trauma to the subclavicular portion of the brachial plexus, resulting in palsy of one of its branches or of the radial, median, or ulnar nerves.

Rehabilitation of patients undergoing thoracic surgical procedures is initiated preoperatively and continued during the postoperative period. The object of preoperative therapy is to educate the patient with a program of breathing exercises and instruction in coughing which are pertinent to adequate ventilation and maintenance of a clear airway. Preoperative training includes deep breathing with pursed-lip expiratory phase, diaphragmatic breathing, regional costal breathing, and instruction in adequate voluntary productive coughing. Postoperatively the instructions are continued as appropriate, and assistance is given by splinting the chest with hand support. Range-of-motion activity of the shoulder arm and hand on the side operated on are encouraged, as well as frequent change of position while in bed, both to prevent limitation and to promote stimuli to cough.

Radical Mastectomy

Rehabilitation is directed toward aiding psychologic adjustment, restoring external appearance, and maintaining good function of the ipsilateral arm and shoulder. The patient frequently experiences disappointment and depression from the loss of a symbol of femininity and anxiety regarding her future. She is therefore in need of support and encouragement from members of the family, her physicians, and the members of the hospital team. Early return to normal activity affords a significant psychologic boost. Shortly after the wound is healed, a suitable prosthesis should be provided for the patient. A variety of uncomplicated prostheses are available and can usually be obtained in the larger department stores. The nurse, the physical therapist, and the medical social worker can act with teamwork to counsel and instruct the patient. The surgeon's office nurse can afford prime help to the patient both pre- and postoperatively. The American Cancer Society's "Reach to Recovery" program is widely available to provide trained volunteers, who are mastectomy patients themselves, to help and instruct patients in the hospital and at home.

Current concepts of reconstruction potential following mastectomy allow for the consideration for selected patients of silicon prosthetic implants as replacement, as well as cosmetic reconstructive procedures. Implants or procedures may be performed as immediate operations or may follow the mastectomy by a year, depending on the choice of the surgeon. The use of such approaches depends on the attitude and desires of the patient, the type of mastectomy performed, and the status of the chest wall, including the opposite breast. Plastic surgeons are increasingly aware of the potential of reconstruction or prosthetic implant replacement after mastectomy.

In order to prevent adhesions about the shoulder joint, a routine exercise schedule should be instituted in the immediate postoperative period, with emphasis on elevation and abduction of the arm coupled with active exercises of the arm, forearm, and hand.

Postmastectomy lymphedema in the ipsilateral extremity frequently causes concern. It varies markedly among patients and the areas involved. Slight swelling may occur in the immediate postoperative period and then subside. Swelling which occurs weeks or months postoperatively is more likely to be persistent or progressive and may cause disability in addition to disfigurement. Prevention is more effective than treatment. Each patient should be instructed carefully in prevention of injury, burns, and infection, during her work or recreation. Injections or venipuncture should be avoided in the arm on the side operated on. Advice should be given covering proper rest positioning by frequent elevation of arm, forearm, and hand, so as to promote gravity-assisted outflow of tissue fluids. The patient should also avoid exposure to sunburn, to heat, or to hot water, and to the stress of prolonged vigorous work with the arm on the mastectomized side. The patient should be made aware of the need for immediate attention to the slightest sign of infection in a local site.

Once edema occurs and persists, treatment can be less than satisfactory. Use of elastic sleeves and daily, repeated 20- to 30-minute applications of intermittent compression by air sleeve, salt-free diets, diuretics, and mechanical massaging have all been used with varying effect. For severe intractable edema, the transposition of the partially detached omentum as a pedicle graft (Goldsmith procedure) to the axilla and upper arm has afforded relief in selected patients. Also, the insertion of a series of parallel nylon threads down the arm and forearm in the subcutaneous fat has been reported occasionally helpful. Lymphedema which has progressed to cause paralysis, weeping and chronic infection may require high amputation or shoulder disarticulation of the arm.

The patient may be the victim of recurrent attacks of cellulitis of the arm and will require antibiotics as both preventive and definitive treatment. After several years of lymphedema a lymphangiosarcoma may develop, and this possible change must be kept in mind.

Colostomy and Ileostomy

The formation of a colostomy is associated with a variety of problems requiring adjustment. Concern over leakage, noisy expulsion of gas, and the presence of odor results in anxiety. Care of the colostomy usually requires the establishment of a routine. Dietary changes may be required. Impotence occurs in 50 percent of male patients following abdominal perineal resection of the rectum.

Rehabilitation should begin in the preoperative period when the surgical procedure and the immediate and long-term function of the colostomy is described. Initial post-operative care of the colostomy is directed at avoiding massive evacuation or soiling. It is frequently preferable immediately to employ and maintain cover of the stoma with a disposable plastic collecting bag. During the patient's postoperative hospitalization, he should be instructed in self-care, using either the irrigation or nonirrigation technique. Instruction and assistance in irrigation need to be consistent and should be regularly given by the same nurse or the enterostomal therapist. Most patients are more readily managed by irrigation, using a regular enema administered via catheter and bulb syringe. Commercial kits are available. A daily routine enema at any time which is preferable for the given patient should be established and adhered to. In many patients, a small gauze pad is all that is required to cover the colostomy, but some patients gain a sense of security by wearing a disposable plastic bag. The nonirrigation technique is not widely used but may have merit where toilet facilities are not satisfactory or when regulation has not been accomplished with the irrigation method. Assistance may be obtained from "stomal care" clinics and colostomy clubs, which are widespread. The colostomy may require occasional or regular digital dilation. In general, the patient with a well-regulated colostomy may carry out all activities without concern.

In contrast to the colostomy, the ileostomy requires a collecting appliance. The location of the stoma should be determined with consideration for the appliance to be used and prior to performing the abdominal incision, which distorts the abdominal wall. A variety of satisfactory appliances are available. These are secured to the anterior abdominal wall so that there is no leakage. Ileostomy clubs offer help or counseling to the patient. A well-fitted ileostomy appliance should permit the patient normal and unimpeded activities.

Maxillofacial Surgery

Surgical treatment for tumors of the face and mouth may be attended by severe cosmetic problems. Impairment of mastication may result in nutritional deficiency. Resection of the tongue may be followed by difficulties with speech and swallowing. Enucleation of the eye creates a reduction in the total field of vision, changes in accuracy of depth perception, and cosmetic needs for prosthetic replacement, as well. Care should begin in the preoperative period and should include counseling of the patient and family. Careful oral hygiene and dental preparatory care should precede all orofacial surgery and radiation therapy. The anticipated ultimate cosmetic and functional results should be defined, and if staged procedures are to be carried out, a description and timing should be outlined.

Temporary and permanent maxillofacial prostheses may play a significant role in rehabilitation by lessening the disfigurement and restoring function. Reconstructive surgical procedures may be needed to improve appearance and function. Speech therapy can assist most patients in overcoming the major portion of this disability. Frequently, the most difficult problem is the disfigurement itself. Efforts with the patient, his family, and associates are directed toward preventing the patient from assuming an attitude of social withdrawal. Prostheses, prosthodontic procedures, and plastic reconstructive surgery help according to individual indications.

Laryngectomy

While hemilaryngectomy and radiation therapy may permit effective phonation, total laryngectomy is followed by total loss of speech. There is also frequently a temporary loss of the sense of taste, which returns reasonably well as the patient recovers. Speech instruction should be initiated by trained therapists shortly after discharge from the hospital. Esophageal voice training, which is successful in up to 80 percent of cases, is more satisfactory than a prosthetic appliance as far as articulation, intelligibility, and phonation are concerned. Patient "clubs," such as "Lost Chord" and "New Voice" societies, are very helpful in promoting confidence and motivation. When esophageal speech is unsuccessful, the patient may resort to electronic devices such as a hand-held artificial larynx. There also are surgical procedures, such as devised by Asai, with construction of a skin tube from tracheostomy to pharynx, which will vibrate to produce sound when the tracheostomy is covered, and by Taub, to utilize a pharyngostomy to carry the sound created by a reed apparatus applied to the tracheostomy. These have worked well, but in contrast to esophageal speech, they immobilize one of the patient's hands during speech. In care of the permanent tracheostomy, tubes, gauze pads, tape for covering, plastic stoma protectors for showering, disposable bibs, and portable suction apparatus with catheters are employed. The patient should avoid exposure to fumes and dust, and small boating is usually contraindicated because of the tracheostomy-associated danger of drowning.

Radical Neck Dissection

Extensive radical neck dissection may result in shoulder disability in addition to cosmetic defect. Disability is related to section of the spinal accessory nerve, which may result in paralysis of the trapezius muscle and a dropped, painful shoulder with rotation of the scapula. Support of the arm and shoulder in a sling or on a padded roll or bar hand rest may be helpful. Exercises are used to promote fixation of the scapula by the rhomboid and serratus anterior muscles, so that the scapula is stabilized during shoulder activities. The results of these maneuvers are frequently discouraging. A nerve graft may be used to replace the excised segment of the accessory nerve, and electromyographic testing of the trapezius will determine return of innervation. In the interim, supportive passive motion and electrical stimulation of the trapezius are useful. Occasional patients have partial or full direct innervation of the trapezius muscle from C_1, C_2, and C_3 motor roots and sustain less or little disability.

Radiation Therapy

Radiation therapy causes changes in normal tissues. Fibrosis occurs in the lungs and in joint tissues. Patients with respiratory problems need support and understanding. There is little specific therapy other than establishment of good voluntary respiratory patterns and controlled and paced breathing to limit dyspnea on exertion. Joints which are affected need gentle active and assisted range-of-motion exercises. Any forceful stretching is contraindicated.

Radiation necrosis of soft tissue is rare, but interference with wound healing in previously radiated tissue may be encountered, as well as decrease in the resistance of such areas to stress or trauma. Exposure of bone may be followed by aseptic radiation necrosis. All these factors involve limitations when activities involving stress may be ordered or contemplated for the patient. Patients who have had their full tolerance dose of radiation therapy should be protected from any further exposure to diagnostic or therapeutic radiation, except when under the advice and guidance of a radiation therapist.

Exposure of the hospital staff to patients treated with radioactive implants should be monitored by the wearing of radiation monitor badges, regularly checked. Staff exposure to patients treated by after-loading techniques must be kept at a maximum of 2 to 3 minutes, and distance from the patient maintained as appropriate and possible.

Bone Marrow Replacement

The current research in the treatment of myelogenous neoplasia by the use of bone marrow replacement introduces periods of immunodeficient susceptibility for the patients. Protection from exposure to infection by laminar flow and reverse isolation requires that recommended activity programs be provided in limited space areas and by properly trained personnel.

Advanced Disease

To this point our consideration has been for patients whose goals could be set for restoration or long-term support. Care for many other patients requires planning for a course of advanced or terminal disease. This is particularly a need for cancer patients with extended disease and widespread metastases. Such patients must be evaluated for and helped in the maintenance of maximum comfort, independence in physical function, reduction of complications such as pain, lymphedema, or decubiti, and provision of emotional support. Palliation can be accomplished by an active program of adjustment and instruction in activity, recreation therapy, and positive involvement within the capacity of the individual patient. The stabilizing effects of a regular schedule of modified physical and emotional support therapy prevent these patients from feeling isolated and abandoned during the remainder of the life they must live.

References

Brompton Hospital Physiotherapy Department, "Physiotherapy for Medical and Surgical Thoracic Conditions," 3d rev. ed., Brompton Hospital, London, 1967.

Burgess, E. M., Romano, R. L., and Zettle, J. H.: "The Management of Lower Extremity Amputation," TR 10-6, Superintendent of Documents, Government Printing Office, Washington, 1969.

Cicenia, E. F., and Hoberman, M.: Braces and Brace Management, *Am J Phys Med*, **36**:136, 1957.

Dietz, J. H., Jr.: Rehabilitation of the Cancer Patient, *Med Clin North Am*, **53**:607, 1969.

———: Rehabilitation of the Surgical Patient, *Contemp Surg*, **4**(5):22, 1974.

———: Rehabilitation of the Cancer Patient: Its Role in the Scheme of Comprehensive Care, *Clin Bull, Memorial Sloan-Kettering Cancer Center*, **4**(3):104, 1974.

———: Rehabilitation of the Mastectomy Patient, *Breast*, **2**(3):7, 1976.

Druss, R. G., O'Connor, J. P., and Stern, L. O.: Psychologic Response to Colectomy, *Arch Gen Psychiat,* **20:**419, 1969.

Friedmann, L. W.: Rehabilitation of Amputees, in S. Licht (ed.), "Rehabilitation and Medicine," Elizabeth Licht, New Haven, Conn., 1968.

Katona, E. A.: Learning Colostomy Control, *Am J Nurs,* **67:**534, 1967.

Krusen, F. H., Kottke, F. J., and Ellwood, P. M., Jr.: "Handbook of Physical Medicine and Rehabilitation," 2d ed., W. B. Saunders Company, Philadelphia, 1972.

Lauder, E.: "Self Help for the Laryngectomee," 2d ed., Lauder, San Antonio, Texas, 1969.

Moskowitz, E.: "Rehabilitation in Extremity Fractures," Charles C Thomas, Publisher, Springfield, Ill., 1968.

Myers, S. J. (ed.): "An Orientation to Chronic Disease and Disability," The Macmillan Company, New York, 1965.

Rusk, H. A.: "Rehabilitation Medicine," 3d ed., The C. V. Mosby Company, St. Louis, 1977.

Schottstaedt, E. R., and Robinson, G. B.: Functional Bracing of the Arm, *J Bone Joint Surg* [*Am*], **38A:**477, 1956.

Snyderman, R. K. (ed.): "Symposium on Neoplastic and Reconstructive Problems of the Female Breast," vol. 7, Educational Foundation of the American Society of Plastic and Reconstructive Surgeons, The C. V. Mosby Company, St. Louis, 1973.

Turnbull, R. P.: Instructions to the Colostomy Patient, *Cleve Clin Q,* **28:**134, 1961.

————: Construction and Care of the Ileostomy, *Hosp Med,* **2:**145, 1966.

Weiss, A. A.: The Phantom Limb, *Ann Intern Med,* **44:**668, 1956.

Wilson, A. B.: Limb Prosthetics—1970, *Artif Limbs,* **11:**1, 1970.

Name Index

Subject Index